Differential Diagnosis
in Surgical Pathology

THIRD EDITION

Differential Diagnosis in Surgical Pathology

PAOLO GATTUSO, MD
The Otho S.A. Sprague Professor of
Pathology
Director of Anatomic Pathology
Rush Medical College of Rush University
Chicago, Illinois

VIJAYA B. REDDY, MD, MBA
Professor and Associate Chair
Department of Pathology
Rush Medical College of Rush University
Chicago, Illinois

ODILE DAVID, MD
Associate Professor and Director of
Cytopathology
University of Illinois at Chicago
Chicago, Illinois

DANIEL J. SPITZ, MD
Chief Medical Examiner
Macomb and St. Clair Counties, Michigan
Clinical Assistant Professor of Pathology
Wayne State University School of
Medicine
Detroit, Michigan

MERYL H. HABER, MD
Borland Professor and Chairman of
Pathology, Emeritus
Rush Medical College of Rush University
Chicago, Illinois

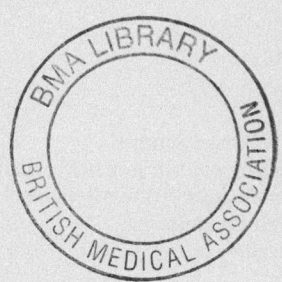

ELSEVIER
SAUNDERS

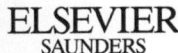

1600 John F. Kennedy Blvd.
Ste 1800
Philadelphia, PA 19103-2899

DIFFERENTIAL DIAGNOSIS IN SURGICAL PATHOLOGY, THIRD EDITION   ISBN: 978-1-4557-7013-7

Notices

Knowledge and best practice in this field are constantly changing. As new research and experience broaden our understanding, changes in research methods, professional practices, or medical treatment may become necessary.

Practitioners and researchers must always rely on their own experience and knowledge in evaluating and using any information, methods, compounds, or experiments described herein. In using such information or methods they should be mindful of their own safety and the safety of others, including parties for whom they have a professional responsibility.

With respect to any drug or pharmaceutical products identified, readers are advised to check the most current information provided (i) on procedures featured or (ii) by the manufacturer of each product to be administered, to verify the recommended dose or formula, the method and duration of administration, and contraindications. It is the responsibility of practitioners, relying on their own experience and knowledge of their patients, to make diagnoses, to determine dosages and the best treatment for each individual patient, and to take all appropriate safety precautions.

To the fullest extent of the law, neither the Publisher nor the authors, contributors, or editors assume any liability for any injury and/or damage to persons or property as a matter of products liability, negligence or otherwise, or from any use or operation of any methods, products, instructions, or ideas contained in the material herein.

Library of Congress Cataloging-in-Publication Data
Differential diagnosis in surgical pathology. – Third edition / [edited by] Paolo Gattuso, Vijaya B. Reddy, Odile David, Daniel J. Spitz, Meryl H. Haber.
    p. ; cm.
  Includes bibliographical references and index.
  ISBN 978-1-4557-7013-7 (hardcover : alk. paper)
  I. Gattuso, Paolo, editor of compilation. II. Reddy, Vijaya B., editor of compilation. III. David, Odile, editor of compilation. IV. Spitz, Daniel J., editor of compilation. V. Haber, Meryl H., 1934- editor of compilation.
  [DNLM: 1. Neoplasms–pathology. 2. Neoplasms–surgery. 3. Diagnosis, Differential. 4. Pathology, Surgical. QZ 268]
  RD57
  617'.075–dc23
                                                                                            2013046614

Content Strategist: William Schmitt
Content Development Specialist: Janice M. Gaillard
Publishing Services Manager: Anne Altepeter
Project Manager: Ted Rodgers
Designer: Ellen Zanolle

Printed in the United States of America

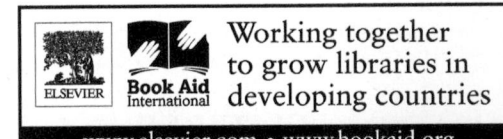

Last digit is the print number: 9 8 7 6 5 4 3

Contributors

SYLVIA L. ASA, MD, PhD
Pathologist-in-Chief
Laboratory Medicine Program
University Health Network
Professor
Department of Laboratory Medicine and Pathobiology
University of Toronto
Toronto, Ontario, Canada

LAURA BARISONI, MD
Professor of Pathology
University of Miami Miller School of Medicine
Miami, Florida

PINCAS BITTERMAN, MD
Professor of Pathology
Rush University Medical Center
Chicago, Illinois

ELIZABETH J. COCHRAN, MD
Professor of Pathology
Medical College of Wisconsin
Milwaukee, Wisconsin

KUMARASEN COOPER, MBChB, FRCPath, DPhil
Professor of Pathology and Laboratory Medicine
Director of Anatomic Pathology
Department of Pathology and Laboratory Medicine
Perelman School of Medicine at the University of
   Pennsylvania
Philadelphia, Pennsylvania

BYRON E. CRAWFORD, MD
Professor of Pathology
Director of Anatomic Pathology
Tulane University School of Medicine
New Orleans, Louisiana

MICHAEL CRUISE, MD, PhD
Assistant Professor of Pathology
Johns Hopkins Hospital
Baltimore, Maryland

KOSSIVI DANTEY, MD
Clinical Instructor of Pathology
University of Vermont College of Medicine and Fletcher
   Allen Health Care
Burlington, Vermont

ADEL K. EL-NAGGAR, MD, PhD
Professor of Pathology and Head and Neck Surgery
Program Director, Head and Neck Pathology Fellowship
The University of Texas MD Anderson Cancer Center
Houston, Texas

MARK F. EVANS, PhD
Research Assistant Professor
Department of Pathology
University of Vermont College of Medicine
Burlington, Vermont

SANDRA E. FISCHER, MD
Consultant Pathologist
Laboratory Medicine Program
University Health Network
Assistant Professor
University of Toronto
Toronto, Ontario, Canada

JULIA TURBINER GEYER, MD
Assistant Professor of Pathology and Laboratory
   Medicine
Weill Cornell Medical College
New York, New York

RICHARD J. GROSTERN, MD
Assistant Professor of Pathology and Ophthalmology
Rush University Medical Center
Chicago, Illinois

RALPH H. HRUBAN, MD
Professor of Pathology
Johns Hopkins Hospital
Baltimore, Maryland

ALIYA N. HUSAIN, MD
Professor of Pathology
University of Chicago
Chicago, Illinois

ALEXANDRA N. KALOF, MD
Associate Professor of Pathology
University of Vermont College of Medicine
Attending Physician, Department of Pathology
Fletcher Allen Health Care
Burlington, Vermont

ROBIN D. LEGALLO, MD
Assistant Professor of Pathology
University of Virginia School of Medicine
Charlottesville, Virginia

CRISTINA MAGI-GALLUZZI, MD, PhD
Professor of Pathology
Lerner College of Medicine of Case Western
    Reserve University
Director of Genitourinary Pathology
The Cleveland Clinic
Cleveland, Ohio

MARIA J. MERINO-NEUMANN, MD
Chief of Translational Surgical Pathology
National Institutes of Health
National Cancer Institute
Bethesda, Maryland

CESAR A. MORAN, MD
Professor and Deputy Chair
Department of Pathology
The University of Texas MD Anderson Cancer Center
Houston, Texas

ATTILIO ORAZI, MD
Director of Hematopathology Division
Department of Pathology and Laboratory Medicine
Weill Cornell Medical College
New York, New York

HREEM N. PATEL, MD
Resident Physician
Ophthalmology
Rush University Medical Center
Chicago, Illinois

ROBERT E. PETRAS, MD
Associate Clinical Professor of Pathology
Northeastern Ohio Medical University
Rootstown, Ohio
AmeriPath Institute of Gastrointestinal Pathology and
    Digestive Disease
Oakwood Village, Ohio

MICHAEL R. PINS, MD
Chairman and Professor
Department of Pathology
Chicago Medical School of Rosalind Franklin University
    of Medicine and Science
Chairman, Department of Pathology
Advocate Lutheran General Hospital
Park Ridge, Illinois

SONAM PRAKASH, MD
Health Sciences Associate Clinical Professor
UCSF School of Medicine
University of California, San Francisco
San Francisco, California

VIJAYA B. REDDY, MD, MBA
Professor and Associate Chair
Department of Pathology
Rush Medical College of Rush University
Chicago, Illinois

E RENE RODRIGUEZ, MD
Section of Cardiovascular Pathology
Department of Anatomic Pathology
The Cleveland Clinic
Cleveland, Ohio

JOHN J. SCHMIEG, MD, PhD
Assistant Professor of Pathology
Department of Pathology and Laboratory Medicine
Tulane University School of Medicine
New Orleans, Louisiana

SAUL SUSTER, MD
Chairman and Professor
Department of Pathology and Laboratory Medicine
Medical College of Wisconsin
Milwaukee, Wisconsin

PAUL E. SWANSON, MD
Professor of Pathology
University of Washington School of Medicine
Seattle, Washington

CARMELA D. TAN, MD
Section of Cardiovascular Pathology
Department of Anatomic Pathology
The Cleveland Clinic
Cleveland, Ohio

MARK R. WICK, MD
Associate Director of Surgical Pathology
University of Virginia Health System
Charlottesville, Virginia

MICHELLE D. WILLIAMS, MD
Associate Professor of Pathology
Director, Surgical Pathology Fellowship Program, Head
    and Neck Section
The University of Texas MD Anderson Cancer Center
Houston, Texas

MATTHEW M. YEH, MD, PhD
Associate Professor
Director of Gastrointestinal and Hepatic Pathology
University of Washington School of Medicine
Seattle, Washington

MING ZHOU, MD, PhD
Professor of Pathology and Urology
Director of Surgical Pathology and Urological Pathology
NYU Medical Center Tisch Hospital
New York, New York

Preface

I find it hard to believe that more than a decade has passed since the initial concept of writing a "new" textbook of pathology was proposed by a few residents and an attending pathologist in the Department of Pathology at Rush Medical College. The concept was for a different type of pathology textbook—simple in design, not encyclopedic, and one that would be useful for students, residents, and pathologists. To achieve these ends, the text would have to be limited, with a relatively simple format—a succinct outline-type style with a focus on more frequently seen conditions. Additionally, to be really useful, hundreds of photographs and photomicrographs inserted in parallel along with text descriptions would be required. To achieve these ends, considerable time, effort, and expertise would be demanded. After three years of development and the finding of a publisher, the first edition of *Differential Diagnosis in Surgical Pathology* was published in 2002. Its success immediately became evident. Now, some 14 years after the original concept for this textbook was approved, *Differential Diagnosis in Surgical Pathology* has been translated into other languages and is widely accepted as a useful addition to the pathologist's library—both for teaching pathology to students and residents, and for assisting in the diagnosis of a variety of pathologic conditions.

Dr. Vijaya Reddy spearheaded the writing and production of the third edition. In this edition, new authors have been added; some former authors no longer appear. New photographs and photomicrographs facilitate the text, and references for each section have been updated. Biomarkers, which are assuming an evermore significant importance in pathologic diagnosis, have taken a prominent place in sections of the text. Medical diseases of the kidney have been added. But, as in previous editions, the book is organized by systems, and within each disease category specific entities are discussed using an outline approach that begins with clinical features and then goes on to explore the pathologic hallmarks, criteria for diagnosis, including pertinent laboratory findings, and differential diagnosis. Selected references are appended. The photographs continue to be reproduced in the highest quality of color. We believe that this is the best and most complete edition of this textbook yet, but, more important, it continues to achieve our most important goal—to be a useful diagnostic aid for practicing pathologists and a valuable teaching adjunct for resident pathologists and students of medicine and the health sciences.

MERYL H. HABER, MD
March 26, 2014

Acknowledgments

We thank all our contributors for their expertise, knowledge, and invaluable role in the continued success of this book.

The editors also gratefully acknowledge the work of authors who have contributed to this book in its previous editions.

We thank Irma Parker and Mira Davis for their secretarial assistance. We are thankful to our publisher, Elsevier, and William R. Schmitt, executive editor, for his support and encouragement in the production of a third edition. A special thanks to Janice M. Gaillard, senior content development specialist at Elsevier, for her patience and competence in keeping the book on course over the past year, and to Ted Rodgers, production editor at Elsevier, for overseeing the final stages of the publication process.

VIJAYA B. REDDY, MD

Table of Contents

Chapter 1

Special Diagnostic Techniques in Surgical Pathology

ALEXANDRA N. KALOF • MARK F. EVANS • KOSSIVI DANTEY • KUMARASEN COOPER

CHAPTER CONTENTS

LIGHT MICROSCOPY

TISSUE PROCESSING OVERVIEW

- Fixation
  - Preserves tissues in situ as close to the lifelike state as possible
  - Ideally, fixation will be carried out as soon as possible after removal of the tissues, and the fixative will kill the tissue quickly, thus preventing autolysis
- Dehydration
  - Fixed tissue is too fragile to be sectioned and must be embedded first in a nonaqueous supporting medium (e.g., paraffin)
  - The tissue must first be dehydrated through a series of ethanol solutions
- Clearing
  - Ethanol is not miscible with paraffin, so nonpolar solvents (e.g., xylene, toluene) are used as clearing agents; this also makes the tissue more translucent
- Embedding
  - Paraffin is the usual embedding medium; however, tissues are sometimes embedded in a plastic resin, allowing for thinner sections (required for electron microscopy [EM])
  - This embedding process is important because the tissues must be aligned, or oriented, properly in the block of paraffin
- Sectioning
  - Embedded in paraffin, which is similar in density to tissue, tissue can be sectioned at anywhere from 3 to 10 μm (routine sections are usually cut at 6 to 8 μm)
- Staining
  - Allows for differentiation of the nuclear and cytoplasmic components of cells as well as the intercellular structure of the tissue
- Cover-slipping
  - The stained section on the slide is covered with a thin piece of plastic or glass to protect the tissue from being scratched, to provide better optical quality for viewing under the microscope, and to preserve the tissue section for years

FIXATION

- There are five major groups of fixatives, classified according to mechanism of action
  - Aldehydes
    - Formalin

- Aqueous solution of formaldehyde gas that penetrates tissue well but relatively slowly; the standard solution is 10% neutral buffered formalin
- A buffer prevents acidity that would promote autolysis and cause precipitation of formol-heme pigment in the tissues
- Tissue is fixed by cross-linkages formed in the proteins, particularly between lysine residues
- This cross-linkage *does not harm the structure of proteins greatly, preserving antigenicity*, and is therefore good for immunoperoxidase techniques
  - Glutaraldehyde
    - The standard solution is a 2% buffered glutaraldehyde and must be cold, buffered, and not more than 3 months old
    - Fixes tissue quickly and therefore is ideal for EM
    - Causes deformation of α-helix structure in proteins and therefore *is not good for immunoperoxidase staining*
    - Penetrates poorly but gives best overall cytoplasmic and nuclear detail
    - Tissue must be as fresh as possible and preferably sectioned within the glutaraldehyde at a thickness of no more than 1 mm to enhance fixation
- Mercurials
  - B-5 and Zenker
    - Contain mercuric chloride and must be disposed of carefully
    - Penetrate poorly and cause tissue hardness but are fast and give excellent nuclear detail
    - Best application is for *fixation of hematopoietic and reticuloendothelial tissues*
- Alcohols
  - Methyl alcohol (methanol) and ethyl alcohol (ethanol)
    - Protein denaturants
    - Not used routinely for tissue because they dehydrate, resulting in the tissues becoming brittle and hard
    - *Good for cytologic smears because they act quickly and give good nuclear detail*
- Oxidizing agents
  - Permanganate fixatives (potassium permanganate), dichromate fixatives (potassium dichromate), and osmium tetroxide cross-link proteins
  - Cause extensive denaturation
  - Some of these have specialized applications but are used infrequently
- Picrates
  - Bouin solution has an unknown mechanism of action
  - It does almost as well as mercurials with nuclear detail but does not cause as much hardness
  - Picric acid is an explosion hazard in dry form
  - Recommended for fixation of tissues from testis, gastrointestinal tract, and endocrine organs
- Factors affecting fixation
  - Buffering
    - Fixation is optimal at a neutral pH, in the range of 6 to 8

- Hypoxia of tissues lowers the pH, so there must be buffering capacity in the fixative to prevent excessive acidity; acidity causes formation of formalin-heme pigment that appears as black, polarizable deposits in tissue
  - Common buffers include phosphate, bicarbonate, cacodylate, and veronal
- Penetration
  - Fixative solutions penetrate at different rates, depending on the diffusibility of each individual fixative
  - In order of decreasing speed of penetration: formaldehyde, acetic acid, mercuric chloride, methyl alcohol osmium tetroxide, and picric acid
  - Because fixation begins at the periphery, thick sections sometimes remain unfixed in the center, compromising both histology and antigenicity of the cells (important for immunohistochemistry [IHC])
  - It is important to section the tissues thinly (2 to 3 mm)
- Volume
  - Should be at least a 10:1 ratio of fixative to tissue
- Temperature
  - Increasing the temperature, as with all chemical reactions, increases the speed of fixation
  - Hot formalin fixes tissues faster, and this is often the first step on an automated tissue processor
- Concentration
  - Formalin is best at 10%; glutaraldehyde is generally made up at 0.25% to 4%
- Time interval
  - Formalin should have 6 to 8 hours to act before the remainder of the processing is begun
- Decalcification
  - Tissue calcium deposits are extremely firm and do not section properly with paraffin embedding because of the difference in densities between calcium and paraffin
  - Strong mineral acids such as nitric and hydrochloric acids are used with dense cortical bone because they remove large quantities of calcium at a rapid rate
  - These strong acids also damage cellular morphology and thus are not recommended for delicate tissues such as bone marrow
    - Organic acids such as acetic and formic acid are better suited to bone marrow because they are not as harsh; however, they act more slowly on dense cortical bone
    - Formic acid in a 10% concentration is the best all-around decalcifier

PEARLS

- *Prolonged fixation can affect immunohistochemical results owing to alcohol precipitation of antigen at the cell surface; to optimize antigenicity of the tissue for IHC, the American Society of Clinical Oncology/College of American Pathologists (ASCO/CAP) guidelines recommend fixation of tissue destined for IHC in neutral buffered formalin for a minimum of 6 hours and a maximum of 48 hours (see Wolff et al., 2007)*
- *Urate crystals are water soluble and require a nonaqueous fixative such as absolute alcohol*

- *If tissue is needed for immunofluorescence (e.g., kidney or skin biopsies) or enzyme profiles (e.g., muscle biopsies), the specimen must be frozen without fixative; enzymes are rapidly inactivated by even brief exposure to fixation*
- *For rapid intraoperative analysis of tissue specimens, tissue can be frozen, and frozen sections can be cut with a special freezing microtome ("cryostat"); the pieces of tissue to be studied are snap-frozen in a cold liquid or cold environment (–20° to –70° C); freezing makes the tissue solid enough to section with a microtome*

HISTOLOGIC STAINS

- The staining process makes use of a variety of dyes that have been chosen for their ability to stain various cellular components of tissue
- Hematoxylin and eosin (H&E) stain
  - The most common histologic stain used for routine surgical pathology
  - Hematoxylin, because it is a basic dye, has an affinity for the nucleic acids of the cell nucleus
  - Hematoxylin does not directly stain tissues but needs a "mordant" or link to the tissues; this is provided by a metal cation such as iron, aluminum, or tungsten
  - The hematoxylin-metal complex acts as a basic dye, and any component that is stained is considered to be *basophilic* (i.e., contains the acid groups that bind the positively charged basic dye), appearing blue in tissue section
  - The variety of hematoxylin stains available for use is based partially on choice of metal ion used, which can vary the intensity or hue
  - Conversely, eosin is an acid aniline dye with an affinity for cytoplasmic components of the cell
  - Eosin stains the more basic proteins within cells (cytoplasm) and in extracellular spaces (collagen) pink to red *(acidophilic)*

Connective Tissue

- Elastin stain
  - Elastin van Gieson (EVG) stain highlights elastic fibers in connective tissue
  - EVG stain is useful in demonstrating pathologic changes in elastic fibers, such as reduplication, breaks or splitting that may result from episodes of vasculitis, or connective tissue disorders such as Marfan syndrome (Figure 1-1)
  - Elastic fibers are blue to black; collagen appears red; and the remaining connective tissue is yellow
- Masson trichrome stain
  - Helpful in differentiating between collagen fibers (blue staining) and smooth muscle (bright red staining) (Figure 1-2)
- Reticulin stain
  - A silver impregnation technique stains reticulin fibers in tissue section black
  - Particularly helpful in assessing for alteration in the normal reticular fiber pattern, such as can be seen in some liver diseases or marrow fibrosis
- Jones silver stain

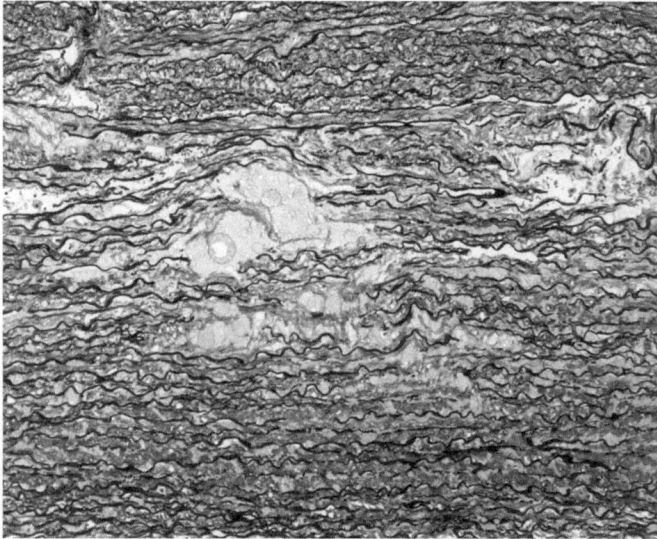

Figure 1-1. Elastin/Alcian blue stain. Aortic cystic medial degeneration in Marfan syndrome. Elastin stain highlights fragmentation of elastic fibers (*brown-black*) and pooling of mucopolysaccharides (*blue*) within the media.

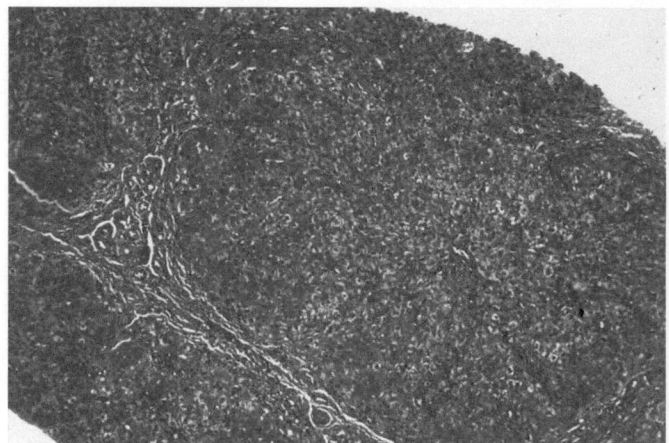

Figure 1-2. Masson trichrome stain. Cirrhosis of the liver characterized by bridging fibrosis (*blue*) and regenerative nodule formation (*red*).

  - A silver impregnation procedure that highlights basement membrane material; used mainly in kidney biopsies (Figure 1-3A)

Fats and Lipids

- Oil red O stain
  - Demonstrates neutral lipids in frozen tissue
- Sudan black stain
  - Demonstrates neutral lipids in tissue sections
  - Mainly used in hematologic preparations such as peripheral blood or bone marrow aspirations for demonstration of primary granules of myeloid lineage

Carbohydrates and Mucoproteins

- Congo red stain
  - Amyloid is a fibrillar protein with a β-pleated sheath structure

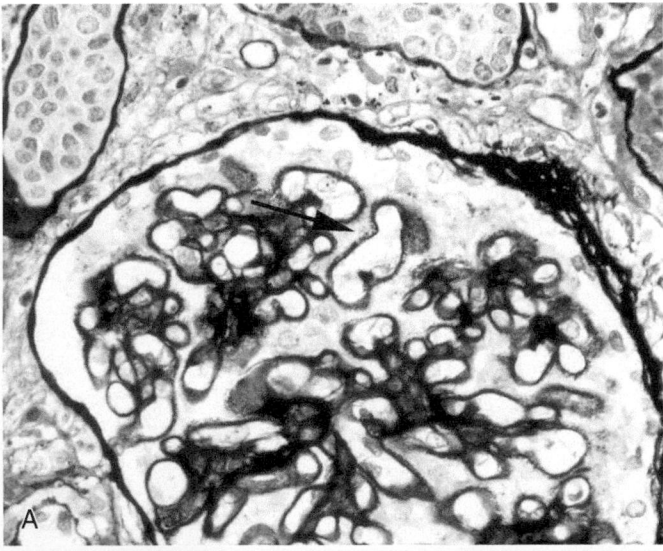

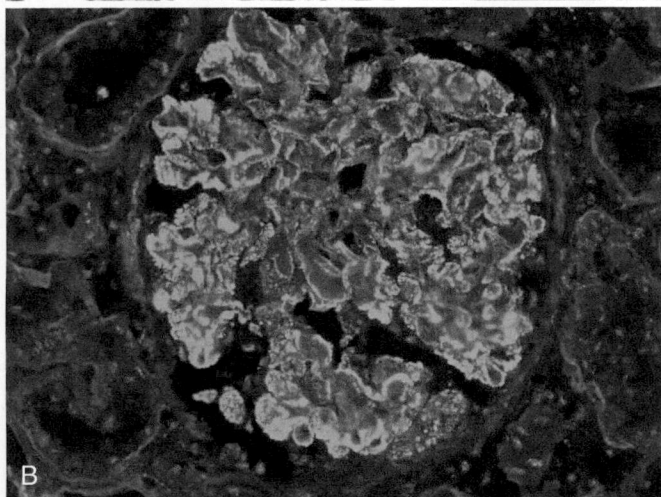

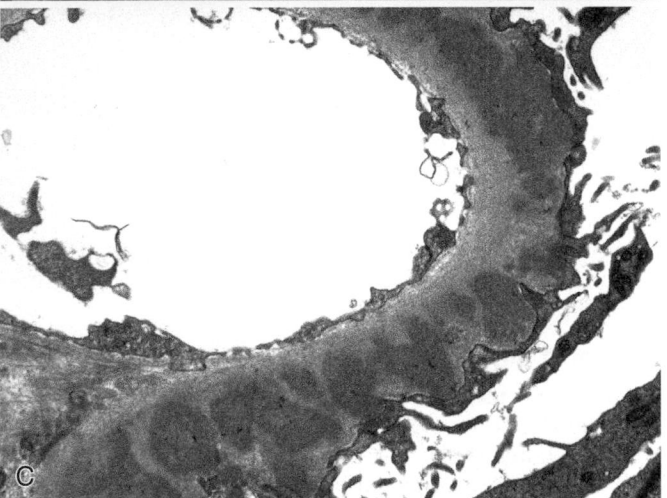

Figure 1-3. Membranous glomerulopathy. A, Jones silver stain highlighting basement membrane "spikes" (*arrow*) along glomerular capillary loops corresponding to basement membrane material surrounding intramembranous immune complexes. **B,** Direct immunofluorescence showing diffuse, granular staining of the glomerular capillary basement membranes with goat antihuman immunoglobulin G. This technique requires fresh-frozen tissue sections. **C,** Electron microscopy showing intramembranous electron-dense immune complexes within the glomerular capillary basement membranes. *(Courtesy of Pamela Gibson, MD, University of Vermont/Fletcher Allen Health Care, Department of Pathology, Burlington, VT.)*

- Amyloid deposits in tissue exhibit a deep red or salmon color, whereas elastic tissue remains pale pink (Figure 1-4A)
- When viewed under polarized light, amyloid deposits exhibit apple-green birefringence (Figure 1-4B)
- The amyloid fibril-Congo red complex demonstrates green birefringence owing to the parallel alignment of dye molecules along the β-pleated sheath
- The thickness of the section is critical (8 to 10 μm)
- Mucicarmine stain
  - Demonstrates epithelial mucin in tissue sections
  - Also highlights mucin-rich capsule of *Cryptococcus* species
- Periodic acid–Schiff (PAS) stain
  - Glycogen, neutral mucosubstances, basement membranes, and fungal walls exhibit a positive PAS (bright rose)
  - *PAS with diastase digestion*: diastase and amylase act on glycogen to depolymerize it into smaller sugar units that are then washed out of the section
  - Digestion removes glycogen but retains staining of other substances attached to sugars (i.e., mucopolysaccharides)
- Alcian blue stain
  - May be used to distinguish various glandular epithelia of the gastrointestinal tract and in the diagnosis of Barrett epithelium
    - pH 1.0: acid sulfated mucin positive (colonic-like)
    - pH 2.5: acid sulfated mucin (colonic-like) and acid nonsulfated mucin (small intestine–like) positive
    - Neutral mucins (gastric-like) negative at pH 1.0 and 2.5

Pigments and Minerals

- Ferric iron (Prussian blue), bilirubin (bile stain), calcium (von Kossa), copper (rhodanine), and melanin (Fontana-Masson) are the most common pigments and minerals demonstrated in surgical pathology specimens

Nerves and Fibers

- Bielschowsky stain
  - A silver impregnation procedure that demonstrates the presence of neurofibrillary tangles and senile plaques in Alzheimer disease (Figure 1-4C)
  - Axons stain black
- Luxol fast blue stain
  - Demonstrates myelin in tissue sections
  - Loss of staining indicates myelin breakdown secondary to axonal degeneration
  - Gray matter and demyelinated white matter should be almost colorless and contrast with the blue-stained myelinated white matter (Figure 1-5)

Hematopoietic and Nuclear Elements

- Toluidine blue stain
  - Demonstrates mast cells in tissue
- Giemsa, Wright, and May-Grünwald stains
  - For cellular details, including hematopoietic (peripheral blood or bone marrow) and cytology preparations
- Leder stain (chloracetate esterase)
  - Identification of cytoplasmic granules of granulocytes and myeloid precursors

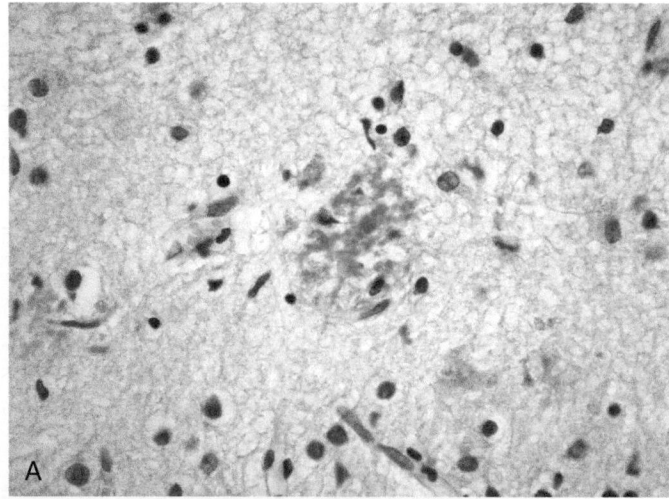

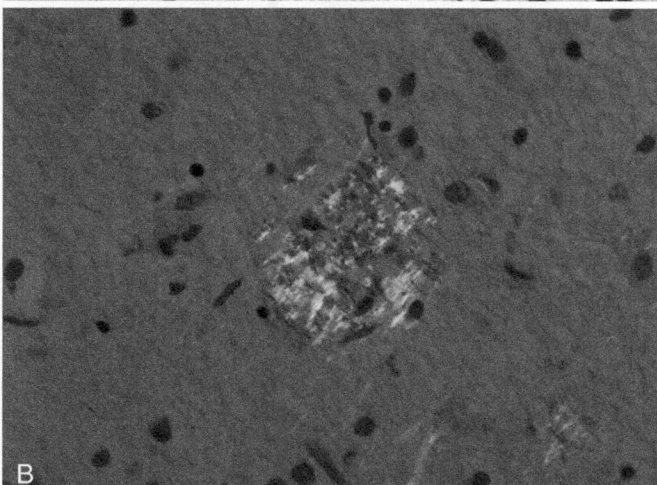

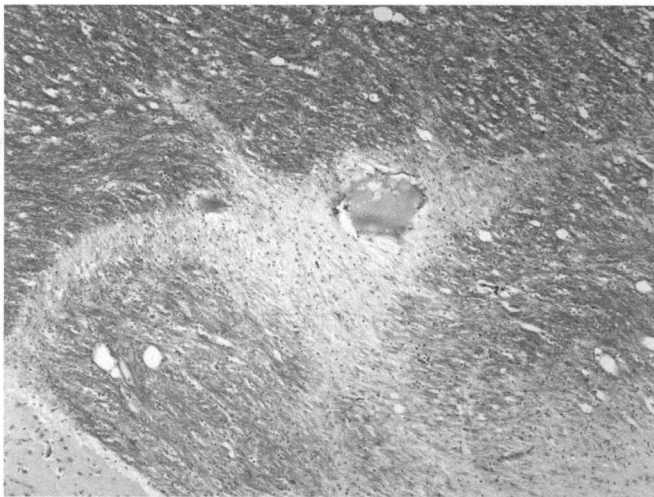

Figure 1-5. Luxol fast blue stain. Demyelination in multiple sclerosis (*colorless regions*).

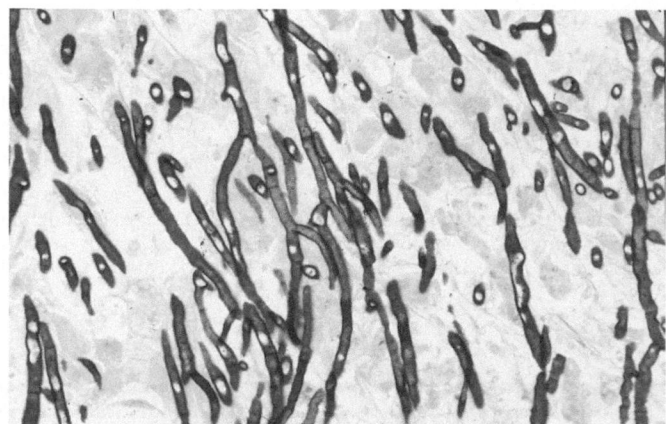

Figure 1-6. *Aspergillus* organisms in the lung stained by Grocott methenamine silver stain.

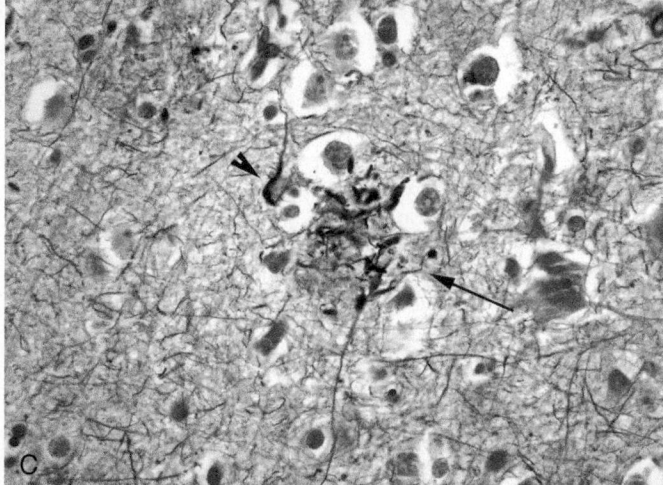

Figure 1-4. Alzheimer disease. A, Congo red–positive core of Alzheimer disease plaque. **B,** Apple-green birefringence of amyloid core under polarized light. **C,** Bielschowsky stain highlighting Alzheimer disease plaque (*arrow*) and neurofibrillary tangle within neuronal cell bodies (*arrowhead*).

Microorganisms: Bacteria, Fungi, Parasites

- Brown and Brenn Gram stain
  - Demonstration of gram-negative (red) and gram-positive (blue) bacteria in tissue
- Giemsa stain

  - Demonstration of bacteria, rickettsia, and *Toxoplasma gondii* in tissue sections
- Grocott methenamine silver (GMS) stain
  - Demonstration of fungi or *Pneumocystis* organisms (fungi may also be demonstrated by PAS-amylase stain) (Figure 1-6)
- Warthin-Starry and Steiner stains
  - Silver impregnation technique for spirochetes (e.g., *Borrelia burgdorferi*, *Treponema pallidum*) in tissue sections
  - *Note:* all bacteria are nonselectively blackened by silver impregnation methods such as the Warthin-Starry and Steiner stains
  - These methods are more sensitive for small gram-negative bacteria (e.g., *Legionella* species, *Helicobacter pylori*, and *Bartonella* species) than tissue Gram stain
- Ziehl-Neelsen method for acid-fast bacteria (AFB)
  - Detect the presence of acid-fast mycobacteria (bright red) in tissue sections (background light blue) (Figure 1-7)
  - Fite method should be used to demonstrate *Mycobacterium leprae* or *Nocardia* species, both of which are weakly acid fast

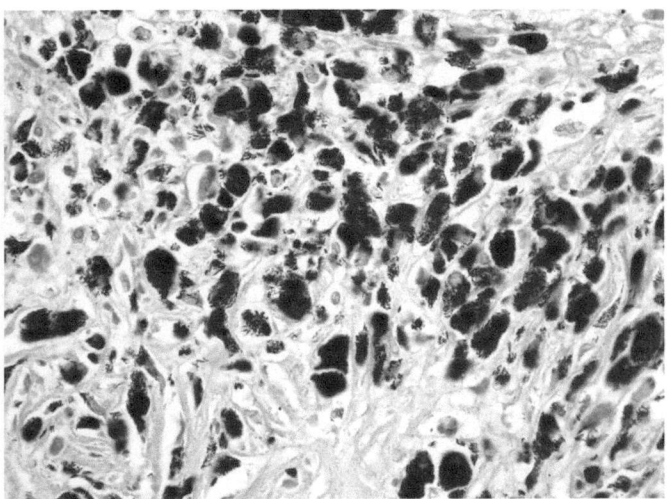

Figure 1-7. Ziehl-Neelsen stain for acid-fast bacilli. Abundant *Mycobacterium avian intracellulare* organisms (*red*) within macrophages in the lung.

SELECTED REFERENCES

Bancroft JD, Gamble M: Theory and Practice of Histochemical Techniques, 5th ed. Philadelphia, Elsevier, 2001.
Carson FL: Histotechnology: A Self-Instructional Text, 2nd ed. Chicago, American Society for Clinical Pathology (ASCP) Press, 1997.
Wolff AC, Hammond ME, Schwartz JN, et al: American Society of Clinical Oncology/College of American Pathologists Guideline Recommendations for Human Epidermal Growth Factor Receptor 2 Testing in Breast Cancer. Arch Pathol Lab Med 131:18-43, 2007.

FLUORESCENCE MICROSCOPY

- Tissue is exposed to short-wavelength ultraviolet (UV) light (2500 to 4000 angstroms) through a mercury or halogen lamp; the energy is absorbed by molecules that then release the energy as visible light (4000 to 8000 angstroms)
- In immunofluorescence techniques, antibodies are labeled with a fluorescent dye such as fluorescein isothiocyanate (FITC)
- Direct immunofluorescence
  - Fluorescein-labeled antihuman globulin primary antibodies are applied to frozen, unfixed tissue sections to locate and combine with antibodies, complement, or antigens deposited in tissue
- Indirect immunofluorescence
  - Unlabeled primary antibody is applied to the tissue section, followed by application of an FITC-labeled antibody that is directed against a portion of the unlabeled primary antibody
  - More sensitive and more expensive
  - Primary application in surgical pathology is detection of autoimmune diseases involving the skin and kidney (Table 1-1)

SELECTED REFERENCES

D'Agati VD, Jennette JC, Silva FG: Non-neoplastic Kidney Diseases. AFIP Atlas of Nontumor Pathology, vol 4. Washington, DC, Armed Forces Institute of Pathology, 2005.
Kalaaji AN, Nicolas MEO: Mayo Clinic Atlas of Immunofluorescence in Dermatology: Patterns and Target Antigens. New York, Informa Healthcare, 2006.

TABLE 1-1 IMMUNOFLUORESCENCE PATTERNS AND DISEASE ASSOCIATIONS			
Disease	**Antibodies**	**Pattern**	**Histologic Manifestation**
Skin			
Pemphigus vulgaris	Antidesmosomal	Intercellular chicken-wire IgG in epidermis	Suprabasal vesiculation
Bullous pemphigoid	Antiepithelial BM; anti-hemidesmosome (collagen XVII [BP180])	Linear IgG along BM; in salt-split skin, reactivity along roof	Subepithelial vesiculation
Epidermolysis bullosa acquisita (EBA)	EBA Ag	Linear IgG along BM; in salt-split skin, reactivity along floor	Subepithelial vesiculation
Dermatitis herpetiformis	Anti-gluten	Granular IgA, especially in tips of dermal papillae	Subepithelial vesiculation
Kidney			
Anti–glomerular basement membrane (anti-GBM) disease	Anti-GBM COL4-A3 antigen	Linear GBM staining for IgG, corresponding granular staining for C3	Crescentic GN
Membranous glomerulopathy	Subepithelial deposits secondary to in situ immune complex formation (antigen unknown; associated with lupus nephritis, hepatitis B, penicillamine, gold, malignancy)	Diffuse, granular GBM staining for IgG and C3	Diffusely thickened glomerular capillary loops with lacelike splitting and "spikes" identified on Jones silver stain
IgA nephropathy	Deposited IgA polyclonal: possible increased production in response to exposure to environmental agents (e.g., viruses, bacteria, food proteins such as gluten)	IgA ± IgG, IgM, and C3 in mesangium	Focal proliferative GN; mesangial widening
Membranoproliferative glomerulonephritis	Type I: immune complex Type II: autoantibody to alternative complement pathway	Type I: IgG + C3; C1q + C4 Type II: C3 ± IgG; no C1q or C4	Mesangial proliferation; GBM thickening; splitting

BM, basement membrane; GBM, glomerular basement membrane; GN, glomerulonephritis; Ig, immunoglobulin.

ELECTRON MICROSCOPY

- The electron microscope has a magnification range of 1000 to 500,000 diameters (×) (the upper limit of light microscopy is about 1000 diameters), thereby allowing for analyzing the ultrastructure of a cell
- There are two types of EM:
  - Transmission EM
    - Two-dimensional (2D) black-and-white image is produced
    - Tissue either transmits electrons (producing "lucent" or clear areas in the image) or deflects electrons (producing electron "dense" or dark areas in the image)
    - Useful in the diagnosis of non-neoplastic diseases of the kidney
  - Scanning EM
    - Three-dimensional (3D) black-and-white image results as an electron beam sweeps the surface of the specimen and releases secondary electrons
    - Lower resolution than transmission EM and used primarily in the research setting to study cell surface membrane changes
- Application in surgical pathology: EM is a useful diagnostic technique to supplement morphologic, immunohistochemical, cytogenetic, and molecular analysis of tissues
- Immunoperoxidase techniques have largely replaced EM for tumor diagnosis in surgical pathology
- EM is useful in
  - Renal, skin, myocardial, nerve, and muscle biopsies
  - Undifferentiated or poorly differentiated neoplasms
  - Diagnosis of lysosomal storage disorders
  - Ciliary dysmorphology
  - Visualization of infectious agents

TECHNICAL OVERVIEW

- The main fixative used for EM is glutaraldehyde, which penetrates tissues more slowly than formalin; cubes of tissue 1 mm or smaller are needed
- Processing postfixation with osmium tetroxide, which binds to lipids in membranes for better visualization; dehydration with graded alcohols; infiltration with propylene oxide and epoxy resin; embedding in epoxy resin
- 1-μm sections (semithin) are cut and stained with toluidine blue to verify that the area of interest has been selected for EM
- 100-nm sections (ultrathin) are cut and collected on copper grids
- Tissues are stained with heavy metals (uranyl acetate and lead citrate)
- *Electron dense*: darker in color as a result of heavy impregnation with heavy metal
- *Electron lucent*: lighter in color

ULTRASTRUCTURE OF A CELL

Nucleus

- Nuclear membrane
- Nuclear pore
- Nucleolus

- Dense, rounded basophilic structure that consists of 80% to 90% protein
- Produces most of the ribosomal RNA
- Mitotically or metabolically active cells have multiple nucleoli
- Chromatin
  - Heterochromatin: stainable, condensed regions of chromosomes seen as intensely basophilic nuclear material in light microscopy
  - Euchromatin: nonstainable, extended portions of the chromosomes that consist of genetically active DNA

Cytoplasm

- Plasma membrane
  - Appears as two electron-dense (dark) layers with an intervening electron-lucent (light) layer
- Basement membrane = basal lamina (lamina densa + lamina lucida) + lamina reticularis + anchoring fibrils + microfibrils
  - Lamina densa
    - Electron-dense membrane made up of type IV collagen fibers coated by a heparan sulfate proteoglycan
    - About 30 to 70 nm thick with an underlying network of reticular collagen (type III) fibrils, which average 30 nm in diameter and 0.1 to 2 μm in thickness
- Mitochondria
  - The energy-producing component of the cell; these membrane-bound organelles undergo oxidative reactions to produce energy
  - Energy generation occurs on the cristae, which are composed of the inner mitochondrial membrane
  - Most cells contain shelflike mitochondrial cristae
  - Steroid-producing cells (i.e., adrenal cortex) contain tubular cristae
  - Mitochondrial crystals are always pathologic
  - Hürthle cell change occurs when the cytoplasm of a cell becomes packed with mitochondria
- Ribosomes
  - Sites of protein synthesis
  - Usually responsible for the basophilic staining of the cytoplasm on H&E-stained sections
- Endoplasmic reticulum
  - Membrane-bound channels responsible for the transport and processing of secretory products of the cell
  - Granular or rough endoplasmic reticulum is abundant in cells that actively produce secretory products (e.g., plasma cells producing immunoglobulin and pancreatic acinar cells producing digestive enzymes); the granular appearance is due to attached ribosomes
  - Smooth endoplasmic reticulum is abundant in cells that synthesize steroids (i.e., adrenal cortex, Sertoli-Leydig cells) and in tumors derived from these types of cells
- Golgi apparatus
  - Concentrates and packages proteins into secretory vesicles for transport to the cell surface
  - Prominent in cells that secrete proteins

Single Membrane–Bound Structures

- Cytoplasmic granules are classified based on size and morphology (Table 1-2)

TABLE 1-2	**CYTOPLASMIC GRANULES**				
Type	**Size**	**Morphology**	**Product**	**Cell Type/Tumor**
Mucigen	0.7-1.8 μm	Electron lucent	Glycoprotein	Mucin secreting
Serous, zymogen	0.5-1.5 μm	Electron dense	Proenzyme/enzyme	Example: acinar cells of pancreas
Neuroendocrine	100-300 nm	Dense core	Example: biogenic amines	Neuroendocrine cells

- Lysosomes
  - Contain enzymes that assist in digesting material to be disposed of in the cell
  - Endogenous and exogenous pigments can be collected in lysosomes; can be large and filled with undigested cellular components in lysosomal storage disorders
- Dense core granules: seen in cells and tumors with neuroendocrine differentiation (Figure 1-8)
- Melanosomes and premelanosomes are specific single membrane–bound structures
- Weibel-Palade bodies are specific for endothelial cells
- Birbeck granules are seen in Langerhans cell histiocytosis (Figure 1-9)

Filaments and Tubules

- Filaments are classified based on size (Table 1-3)
- Microtubules are seen in association with the mitotic spindle and in cells or tumors of neural origin (e.g., neuroblastoma)

Cell Surface

- Cell processes are seen in cells that are capable of movement; some tumors, such as schwannomas and meningiomas, demonstrate interdigitating processes
- Villi are prominent and regular in cells or tumors of glandular origin (Figure 1-10)
- Terminal web and rootlets in villi are seen in foregut derivatives (e.g., colon)
- Junctions are seen in virtually all cells except those of hematopoietic origin

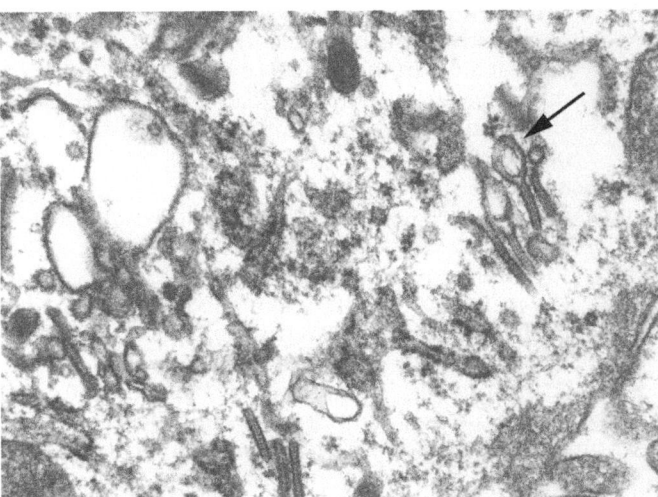

Figure 1-9. Electron microscopy. Birbeck granules *(arrow)* in Langerhans cell histiocytosis. *(Photo courtesy of Janet Schwarz, Senior Research Technician, Microscopy Imaging Center, University of Vermont, Burlington, VT.)*

TABLE 1-3	**FILAMENTS AND TUBULES**	
Component	**Diameter**	**Location**
Microfilaments (actin, nonmuscle myosin)	6-8 nm	Cytoskeleton of all cells
Intermediate filaments	10 nm	
Cytokeratin	> 19 proteins 40-68 kd	Epithelial cells
Glial fibrillary acid protein	55 kd	Astrocytes
Neurofilament	68, 160, 200 kd	Neural tissue
Vimentin	57 kD	Mesenchymal tissues
Desmin	53 kD	Muscle
Microtubules	25 nm	Neural derivatives (e.g., neuroblastoma)

kD, kilodaltons; nm, nanometers; 50 kD = ~4 nm.

- Basal lamina is seen surrounding all endodermal and ectodermal derivatives; cells with muscle differentiation also may have a basal lamina, which may be incomplete

Extracellular Matrix

- Collagen shows a regular structure amyloid
  - Fibrils measuring approximately 10 nm in diameter, with an electron-lucent core
  - Fibrils are straight, nonbranching, and arranged randomly

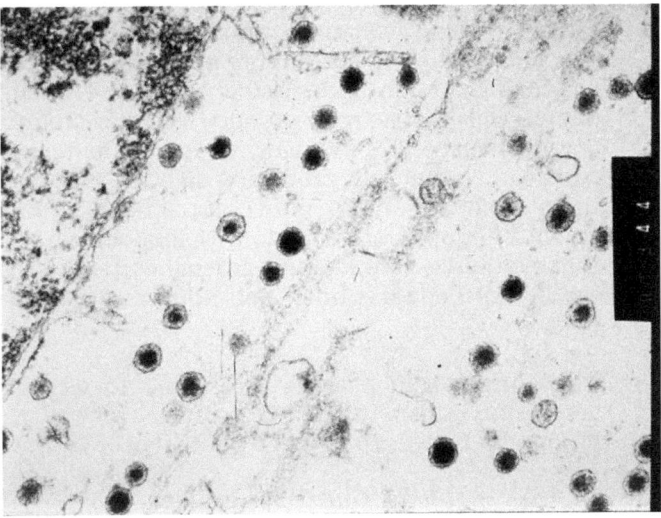

Figure 1-8. Electron microscopy. Neuroendocrine granules in small cell carcinoma of the lung.

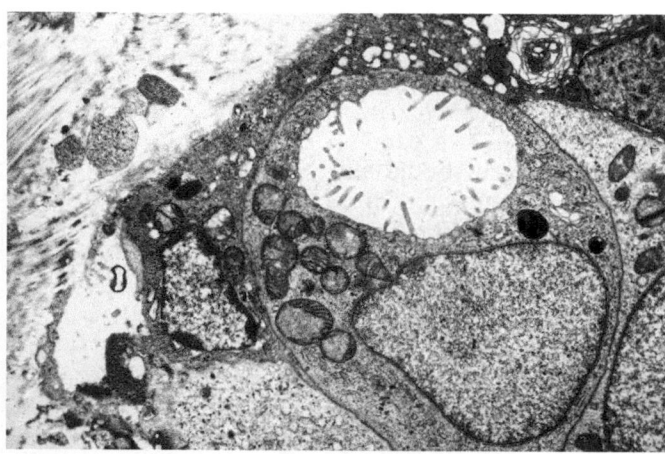

Figure 1-10. Electron microscopy. Short villi lining an intracytoplasmic lumen in adenocarcinoma of the breast.

SELECTED REFERENCES

Ghadially FN: Diagnostic Electron Microscopy of Tumors. Boston, Butterworth-Heinemann, 1986.

Ghadially FN: Diagnostic Ultrastructural Pathology, 2nd ed. Boston, Butterworth-Heinemann, 1998.

Ghadially FN: Ultrastructure of the Cell and Matrix, 4th ed. Boston, Butterworth-Heinemann, 1997.

IMMUNOHISTOCHEMISTRY

INTRODUCTION

Immunohistochemistry (IHC) combines anatomic, immunologic, and biochemical techniques to identify specific tissue components using a specific antigen-antibody reaction labeled with a visible reporter molecule. This binding is then visualized through the use of various enzymes that are coupled to the antibodies being used. The enzyme acts on a chromogenic substrate to cause deposition of a colored material at the site of antibody-antigen bindings. Hence, IHC permits the visualization and localization of specific cellular components within a cell or tissue while importantly preserving the overall morphology and structure of the tissue section. Key improvements in protein conjugation, antigen preservation and antigen retrieval methods, and enhanced immunodetection systems have enshrined IHC as a major adjunctive investigative tool for both surgical and cytopathology. IHC is not only critical for the accurate diagnosis of malignancies but also plays a pivotal role in prognostic evaluation (e.g., estrogen and progesterone receptors in breast cancer) and treatment strategies (e.g., c-kit protein for gastrointestinal stromal tumors and *HER-2-neu* in certain breast cancers).

TECHNICAL OVERVIEW

- Formalin cross-links proteins in tissues; success of immunohistochemical staining depends on the availability of an antigen after fixation
  - Various techniques may unmask antigens, such as digestion by enzymes (e.g., trypsin) or antigen retrieval using heat, metallic mordants, or alkaline buffers
  - Commonly used enzymes include peroxidase, alkaline phosphatase, and glucose oxidase

- Most commonly used chromogen substrates produce brown (DAB) or red (AEC) reaction products
- Definition of terms
  - *Polyclonal antibody:* conventional antiserum produced by multiple plasma cells of an animal that had been injected with an antigen; a polyclonal antibody may have multiple determinants (binding sites)
  - *Monoclonal antibody:* produced by fusion of a malignant cell with a plasma cell producing antibody to a specific epitope; antibodies may be grown in tissue culture
- Antibodies for the detection of cellular components
  - Intermediate filaments (see Table 1-3)
  - Other cellular and tissue components: (e.g., α_1-antitrypsin, myeloperoxidase, synaptophysin and chromogranin, myoglobin)
- Leukocyte antigens and immunoglobulin components commonly used in paraffin-embedded tissues
  - T-cell
    - CD1a: thymocyte; also marks Langerhans cells
    - CD3: Pan–T-cell marker that shows cytoplasmic and membrane staining
    - CD5: Pan–T-cell marker also expressed by some B-cell lymphomas
    - CD43: Pan–T-cell marker also expressed by some B-cell lymphomas
    - CD45RO (UCHL-1), CD4, CD8: T-cell markers
  - B-cell
    - CD20: Pan–B-cell marker
    - Immunoglobulin heavy and light chains: used for demonstration of clonality in B-cell neoplasms
  - Myeloid
    - CD15 (Leu-M1): pan-myeloid antigen that also marks Reed-Sternberg cells of Hodgkin lymphoma
  - Monocyte and histiocyte
    - CD163, CD68
  - Natural killer cell
    - CD57 (Leu-7)
    - CD56 (neural cell adhesion molecules, NCAM, Leu-19)
  - Megakaryocyte
    - CD41
    - Factor VIII–von Willebrand factor (vWF)
    - *Ulex europaeus* agglutinin-1 (UEA-1)
- Hormones and hormone receptors
  - Presence may have prognostic significance
  - Estrogen and progesterone receptors in breast carcinomas
  - Androgen receptors
- Infectious agents
- Oncogenes and oncogene products
  - May correlate with prognosis
  - *bcl-1, bcl-2, bcl-6* in lymphoid neoplasms
  - *HER-2-neu* and *C-erbB2* in breast carcinomas (Figure 1-11)
- *p53* tumor suppressor gene: mutations are seen in a variety of malignant tumors

GROUND RULES FOR QUALITY APPLICATION OF IMMUNOHISTOCHEMISTRY IN SURGICAL PATHOLOGY

- Technique
  - It is imperative that the pathologist work closely with the immunohistotechnologist to optimize, validate,

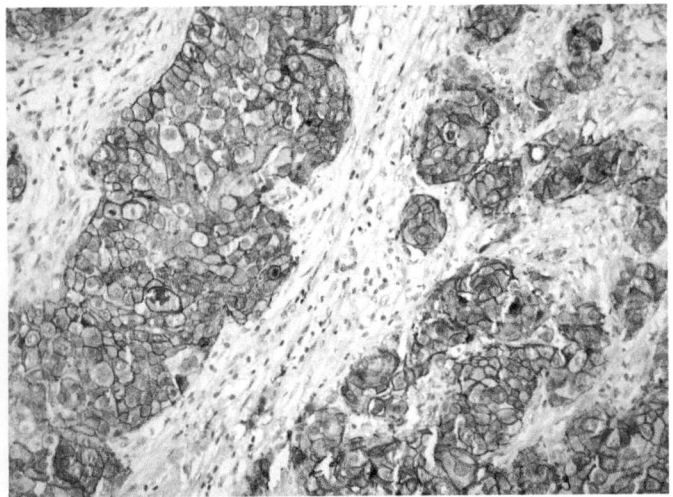

Figure 1-11. Immunohistochemistry for *HER-2-neu* in a breast adenocarcinoma showing (3+) membranous staining.

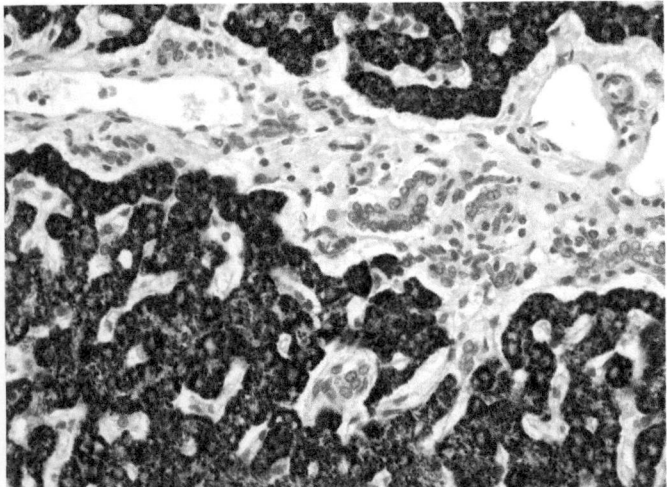

Figure 1-12. Immunohistochemistry for HepPar-1 highlighting strong cytoplasmic staining of normal hepatic parenchyma.

- Avoid using a single antibody in isolation (because this may result in a potentially erroneous diagnosis), and always use more than one antibody to target a specific antigen
- The choice of a panel of antibodies to target a specific antigen should always be made in the context of the morphology and clinical presentation of any neoplasm; avoid use of the "buckshot" approach in hope that an IHC assay returns a positive reaction
- Avoid preordering an IHC panel of antibodies before previewing the morphology; remember that IHC is an ancillary or adjunctive technique to the quality practice of surgical pathology and not vice versa
- Interpretation
  - Interpretation of IHC should always be made in the context of the known subcellular localization or distribution of the targeted antigen (e.g., membranous, cytoplasmic, nuclear, or perinuclear "Golgi pattern" of immunoreactivity) (Figures 1-12 and 13)
- Controls
  - Finally, the importance of adequate incorporation of appropriate tissue and reagent (both positive and negative) controls in every run of IHC cannot be

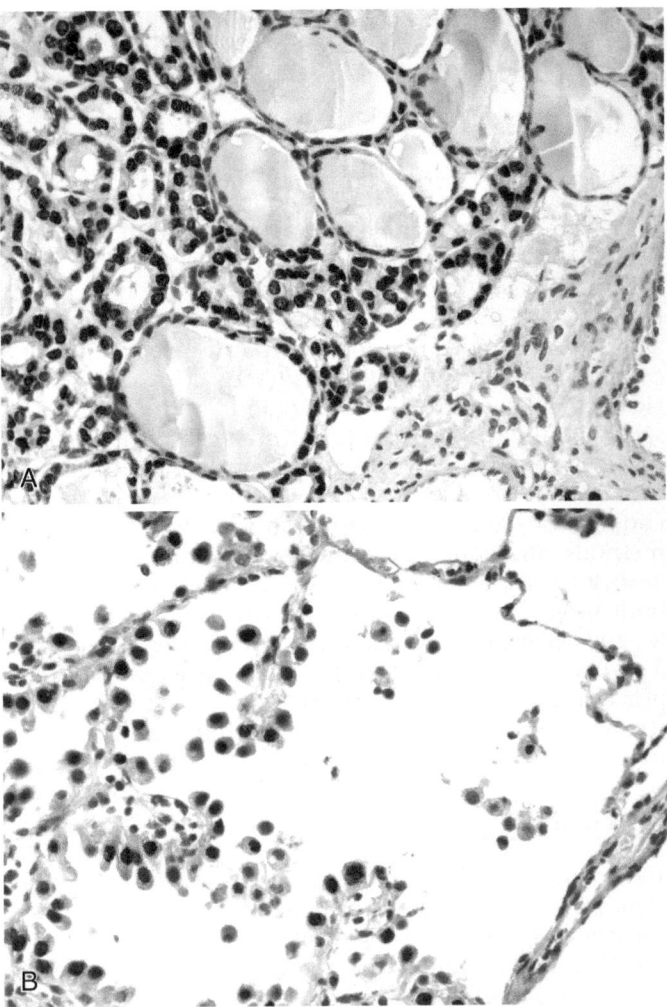

Figure 1-13. Immunohistochemistry for TTF-1. **A,** Nuclear immunoreactivity in normal thyroid parenchyma. **B,** Nuclear immunoreactivity in pulmonary adenocarcinoma.

and interpret the IHC assay for any particular antibody reagent
- Adequate fixation of tissue or specimen in 10% buffered formalin is essential to high-quality IHC; it is probably better to overfix (because modern antigen retrieval systems can unmask epitopes) rather than underfix (because inadvertent alcohol fixation during tissue processing precipitates and masks epitopes)
- It is best to use a polymer-based detection system, which has the advantage of being avidin-biotin free, thereby avoiding false immunoreactivity with endogenous biotin
- Appropriate antigen retrieval systems should be optimized for each antibody (noting that different antibodies require unique systems, and some require none)
- Antibody choice
  - A generic screening panel of antibodies should be chosen initially, followed algorithmically by a specific panel to further characterize a neoplasm

overemphasized; this is ultimately the highest form of quality control of the IHC assay and should be reviewed daily to avoid false-positive and false-negative interpretation

A PRACTICAL TABULAR APPROACH TO USING IMMUNOHISTOCHEMISTRY FOR COMMON DIAGNOSTIC PROBLEMS

- Because a complete technical overview of IHC and comprehensive listing of available antibodies is beyond the scope of this chapter, our goal is to provide a practical approach to IHC application in surgical pathology; the following tables are presented as guidelines to assist with the choice of an antibody panel when confronted with certain differential diagnoses (Tables 1-4 through 1-36)

PEARLS

- *Tumors are not 100% specific or sensitive to a particular immunoreagent; interpretation of these tables should be used in this context to avoid diagnostic pitfalls*
- *Always target the IHC panel in the context of the morphologic differential diagnosis*

SELECTED REFERENCES

Dabbs D: Diagnostic Immunohistochemistry, 2nd ed. Philadelphia, Churchill Livingstone, 2006.
Leong AS-Y, Leong TY-M: Newer developments in immunohistology. J Clin Pathol 59:1117-1126, 2006.
Jagirder J: Immunohistochemistry: Then and now. Arch Pathol Lab Med 132:323-509, 2008.
Yaziji H, Barry T: Diagnostic immunohistochemistry: what can go wrong? Adv Anat Pathol 13:238-246, 2006.

FLOW CYTOMETRY

INTRODUCTION

- Flow cytometry is widely used to immunophenotypically detect clonal hematopoietic populations (e.g., leukemia and lymphoma)
- When performed on peripheral blood, bone marrow, and lymph nodal tissue, single-cell suspensions are required
- Manipulation of solid tissue samples into single-cell suspensions can sometimes compromise the integrity of the cell surface

TECHNICAL OVERVIEW

- Single-cell suspension is split into multiple tubes
- Various fluorescent-labeled antibodies against different cell surface antigens (each with a different attached fluorochrome) are added to each tube
- One by one, the cells are run through the flow cytometer; as the cells pass through the counting chamber, multiple data points are collected
  - Degree of forward light scatter (FSC): indicator of cell size
  - Degree of 90-degree light scatter or side scatter (SSC): indicator of nuclear complexity and cytoplasmic granularity
  - Intensity of fluorochrome on the cell surface: detects expression of cell surface antigens (e.g., CD45, leukocyte common antigen)
- Gating: the cells of interest are digitally selected for interpretation; for example, if lymphocytes are to be examined, one would "gate" around the cells that exhibit low side scatter (little cytoplasmic granularity) and strong CD45 (leukocyte common antigen) expression (Figure 1-15)
- Typical findings in mantle cell lymphoma would include a CD20-positive population (B cells) exhibiting coexpression of CD19 and CD5 (narrowing the differential to small lymphocytic lymphoma and mantle cell lymphoma), with light chain restriction supporting

TABLE 1-5 **IMMUNOPHENOTYPIC DISTRIBUTION OF CYTOKERATINS 7 AND 20**		
Carcinoma Type*	**CK7**	**CK20**
Colorectal and Merkel cell	–	+
Hepatocellular	–	–
Salivary gland	+	–
Lung, non–small cell carcinoma	+	–
Lung, neuroendocrine carcinoma	–	–
Breast, ductal	+	–
Ovarian, serous, and endometrioid	+	–
Endometrial and endocervical	+	–
Renal cell	–	–
Prostatic	–	–
Urothelial	+	+
Pancreas	+/–	+/–
Mesothelioma	+	–

*Only about 70% to 90% of these tumors follow the given CK7/20 immunoprofile; therefore, reliance solely on this profile to determine the primary site of carcinomas is not recommended.
CK, cytokeratin; +, positive; –, negative; +/–, variably positive.

TABLE 1-4 **IMMUNOHISTOCHEMISTRY APPROACH TO UNDIFFERENTIATED TUMORS**						
	Pan-CK	**EMA**	**S-100**	**SALL4**	**LCA**	**CD138**
Carcinoma	+	+	–	–/v	–	–
Melanoma	–/v	–	+	–	–	–
Germ cell	v	–	–	+	–	–
Lymphoma	–	–	–	–	+	–
Anaplastic plasmacytoma/myeloma	–	+	–	–	–/+	+

EMA, epithelial membrane antigen; LCA, leukocyte common antigen; Pan-CK, pan-cytokeratin; SALL4, sal-like4; v, variable; +, positive; –, negative; –/+, rarely positive.

TABLE 1-6   SPECIFIC ANTIBODY REAGENTS TO IDENTIFY PRIMARY SITE OF METASTATIC CARCINOMA

Carcinoma Type	Antibody	Signal Localization	Other Tumors Identified
Breast	GCDFP-15	Cytoplasmic	Salivary, sweat gland
Breast	Mammaglobin	Cytoplasmic	Salivary, sweat gland
Colon	CDX2	Nuclear	Subset of pancreas, gastric
Hepatocellular	HepPar-1 Ag	Cytoplasmic	Hepatoid carcinomas of stomach, ovary
Hepatocellular	pCEA or CD10	Bile canaliculi	Hepatoid carcinomas
Hepatocellular	GPC-3	Membranous and cytoplasmic	Melanoma, a subset of chronic active hepatitis
Lung and thyroid except mucinous adenocarcinoma in situ (formerly mucinous BAC)	TTF-1	Nuclear	Neuroendocrine carcinoma extrapulmonary
Lung squamous cell carcinoma	p40	Nuclear	—
Ovarian serous	WT-1, p16	Nuclear	Mesothelioma (WT-1)
Prostate	PSA, PAP	Cytoplasmic	
Squamous, urothelial, thymic	p63	Nuclear	Salivary gland, neuroendocrine, subset prostate
Thyroid	Thyroglobulin	Cytoplasmic	—
Urothelial	Uroplakin III	Membranous	—
Renal, clear	RCC	Membranous	

BAC, bronchoalveolar carcinoma; GCDFP-15, gross cystic disease fluid protein-15; GPC-3, glypican 3; PAP, prostatic acid phosphatase; pCEA, polyclonal carcinoembryonic antigen; PSA, prostate-specific antigen; RCC, renal cell carcinoma; TTF-1, thyroid transcription factor-1; WT-1, Wilms tumor gene protein 1.

Modified from Kakar S, Gown AM, Goodman ZD, Ferrell LD: Best practices in diagnostic immunohistochemistry: hepatocellular carcinoma versus metastatic neoplasms. Best practices in diagnostic immunohistochemistry: hepatocellular carcinoma versus metastatic neoplasms. Arch Pathol Lab Med 131:1648-1654, 2007; Bishop JA, Teruya-Feldstein J, Westra WH, et al: p40 (ΔNp63) is superior to p63 for the diagnosis of pulmonary squamous cell carcinoma: Mod Pathol 25:405-415, 2012.

TABLE 1-7   IMMUNOHISTOCHEMISTRY PANEL FOR INTERPRETATION OF LUNG MESOTHELIOMA AND ADENOCARCINOMA

Antibody	Epithelioid Mesothelioma (Percentage Positive)	Sarcomatoid Mesothelioma (Percentage Positive)	Adenocarcinoma (Percentage Positive)
Epithelial Marker			
Naspin A	Negative	Negative	83 (lung)
mCEA	3	—	81
Ber-Ep4	10	0	80
B72.3	7	0	80
CD15 (Leu-M1)	7	0	72
MOC-31	7	0	93
TTF-1	Negative	0	72 (lung)
Mesothelial Marker			
Cytokeratin 5/6	83	13	15
Calretinin	82	88	15
WT-1	77	13	4
D2-40	86-100	0	36 (weak)
Mesothelin	100	0	—

mCEA, monoclonal carcinoembryonic antigen; TTF-1, thyroid transcription factor-1; WT-1, Wilms tumor gene protein 1.

Modified from Marchevsky AM: Application of immunohistochemistry to the diagnosis of malignant mesothelioma. Arch Pathol Lab Med 132:397-401, 2008; Bishop JA, Sharma R, Illei PB: Naspin A: and thyroid transcription factor-1 expression in carcinomas of the lung, breast, pancreas, colon, kidney, thyroid, and malignant mesothelioma. Hum Pathol 41:20-25, 2010.

clonality. Lack of CD23 expression helps to exclude small lymphocytic lymphoma, which would have an immunophenotype similar to that of mantle cell lymphoma, except for CD23 expression and dimmer light chain expression. Follicular lymphoma would also consist of a population of CD20-positive B cells that express CD10 and lack CD5

SELECTED REFERENCE

Carey JL, McCoy P, Keren DF: Flow Cytometry in Clinical Diagnosis, 4th ed. Chicago, ASCP Press, 2007.

CYTOGENETIC ANALYSIS

- Technical overview
  - Fresh tissue is incubated in short-term culture, and metaphase chromosomes are spread on glass slides
  - After staining of the chromosomes, specific chromosomal abnormalities can be detected
- In surgical pathology practice at University of Vermont/Fletcher Allen Health Care, we routinely submit fresh tissue in Hanks solution for cytogenetics in the following cases

TABLE 1-8   IMMUNOHISTOCHEMISTRY PANEL FOR LUNG ADENOCARCINOMA AND BREAST ADENOCARCINOMA

Immunostain	Lung Adenocarcinoma (Percentage Positive)	Breast Adenocarcinoma (Percentage Positive)
TTF-1	77	0
Napsin A	83	0
Mammaglobin	17	85
GCDFP-15	2	53
ER	4	72

ER, estrogen receptor; GCDFP-15, gross cystic disease fluid protein-15; TTF-1, thyroid transcription factor-1.
Data from Takeda Y, Tsuta K, Shibuki Y, et al: Analysis of expression patterns of breast cancer-specific markers (mammaglobin and gross cystic disease fluid protein 15) in lung and pleural tumors. Arch Pathol Lab Med 132:239, 2008; Striebel JM, Dacic S, Yousem SA: Gross cystic disease fluid protein (GCDFP-15): Expression in primary lung adenocarcinoma. Am J Surg Pathol 32:426, 2008; Bishop JA, Sharma R, Illei PB: Naspin A and thyroid transcription factor-1 expression in carcinomas of the lung, breast, pancreas, colon, kidney, thyroid, and malignant mesothelioma. Hum Pathol 41:20-25, 2010.

TABLE 1-9   IMMUNOHISTOCHEMISTRY COMPARISON OF SPINDLE CELL AREAS IN METAPLASTIC CARCINOMA, PHYLLODES TUMOR, AND FIBROMATOSIS OF THE BREAST

	CD34	SMA	34βe12	Pan-CK	β-catenin	Desmin	p63
Metaplastic carcinoma	–	+/–	+/–	–/+	–	–/+	+
Phyllodes	+/–	+/–	–	–	–	–/+	–
Fibromatosis	–	+/–	–	–	+	–	–
Myofibroblastoma	+	+/–	–	–	–	+	–
Myoepithelial tumor	–	+/–	+/–	+	–	–/+	+/–

Pan-CK, pan-cytokeratin; SMA, smooth muscle actin; +, positive; –, negative; +/–, often positive; –/+, rarely positive.
Modified from Dunne B, Lee AH, Pinder SE, et al: An immunohistochemical study of metaplastic spindle cell carcinoma, phyllodes tumor and fibromatosis of the breast. Hum Pathol 34:1009-1015, 2003.

TABLE 1-10   USEFUL ANTIBODY PANEL TO DEMONSTRATE MYOEPITHELIAL AND BASAL CELLS IN BREAST LESIONS TO DISTINGUISH BENIGN (+) FROM INVASIVE (–) CARCINOMA

	Myoepithelial/Basal Cells	Stromal Myofibroblasts
Smooth muscle heavy-chain myosin	+ (Cytoplasmic)	–/+
p63	+ (Nuclear)	–
α-SMA	+ (Cytoplasmic)	+/–
S-100	+ (Nuclear and cytoplasmic)	v
Calponin	+ (Cytoplasmic)	–/+
D2-40*	–/+	–

*D2-40 is a useful marker to highlight lymphatic endothelium in lymphovascular invasion (LVI) by carcinoma but may in addition occasionally stain myoepithelial and basal cells—hence the use of D2-40 to demonstrate that LVI should always be accompanied by p63/SMHCM immunohistochemistry.
SMA, smooth muscle actin; v, variable; +, positive; –, negative; –/+, rarely positive.
Modified from Rabban JT, Chen YY: D2-40 expression by breast myoepithelium: potential pitfalls in distinguishing intralymphatic carcinoma from in situ carcinoma. Hum Pathol 39:175-183, 2008.

- All renal tumors (except for urothelial carcinomas of the renal pelvis)
- Any soft tissue tumor larger than 5 cm (including adipocytic neoplasms) (Figure 1-16)
- In addition, a portion of fresh tissue (1 cm³, if available) is snap-frozen for potential molecular analyses for tumor-specific translocations or for potential treatment protocols
- Oncogenes (Table 1-37) and tumor suppressor genes (Table 1-38) of importance in surgical pathology
- Cytogenetic abnormalities of importance in surgical pathology (Table 1-39)

SELECTED REFERENCES

Gersen SL, Keagle MB: The Principles of Clinical Cytogenetics, 2nd ed. Totowa, Humana Press, 2004.
Korf B: Molecular medicine: Molecular diagnosis (part I). N Engl J Med 332:1218-1220, 1995.
Korf B: Molecular medicine: Molecular diagnosis (part II). N Engl J Med 332:1499-1502, 1995.
Richmond JA, Tang M, Cooper K: Cytogenetic and clinicopathologic analysis of benign lipomatous tumors. Arch Pathol Lab Med 129:553, 2005.

MOLECULAR PATHOLOGY METHODS

INTRODUCTION

Molecular tests are now widely relied upon as standard of care assays in the diagnosis of a variety of pathologic conditions. Ongoing advances in molecular pathology, genomics, epigenetics, proteomics, and infectious diseases research, as well as technological developments continue to expand the potential of molecular assays to improve

TABLE 1-11   IMMUNOHISTOCHEMICAL PANEL APPROACH TO DIFFERENTIAL DIAGNOSIS OF HEPATOCELLULAR CARCINOMA

	Arginase1	HepPar-1	CK19	MOC-31	GPC-3	pCEA	CDX-2	TTF-1	RCC	Inhibin/Melan-A/D2-40
Hepatocellular carcinoma	+	+	–	–/+	+	+	–	–*	–	–
Cholangiocarcinoma	–/+	–	+/–	+/–	–	–	–	–	–	–
Metastatic adenocarcinoma										
Colon	–	–	–	–	–	–	+	–	–	–
Thyroid, lung	–	–	–	–	–	–	–	+	–	–
Tumors with polygonal cells										
RCC	–	–	–	+	–	–	–	–	+	–
Adrenocortical carcinoma	–	–	–	–	–	–	–	–	–	+
Neuroendocrine tumors†	–	–	–	+	–	–	–	v		
Hepatoid carcinoma (e.g., gastric, ovary)	–	+								

*Certain TTF-1 antibody reagents may highlight the cytoplasm of liver cells (only nuclear immunoreactivity should be interpreted as being of thyroid or lung origin in the correct clinical setting).
†Strong synaptophysin and chromogranin support neuroendocrine tumor; TTF-1 may notoriously highlight extrapulmonary neuroendocrine tumors.
CK, cytokeratin; p-CEA, canalicular pattern of staining; RCC, renal cell carcinoma; TTF-1, thyroid transcription factor-1; v, variable; +, positive; –, negative; +/–, often positive; –/+, rarely positive.
Modified from Kakar S, Gown AM, Goodman ZD, Ferrell LD: Best practices in diagnostic immunohistochemistry: hepatocellular carcinoma versus metastatic neoplasms. Arch Pathol Lab Med 131:1648-1654, 2007; Yan BC, Gong C, Song J, et al: Arginase-1: a new immunohistochemical marker of hepatocytes and hepatocellular neoplasms. Am J Surg Pathol 34:1147-1154, 2010.

TABLE 1-12   IMMUNOHISTOCHEMISTRY PANEL INTERPRETATION FOR GASTROINTESTINAL AND ABDOMINAL SPINDLE CELL TUMORS

	WT-1	DOG1	CD117	CD34	SMA	Desmin	S-100 Protein	β-Catenin
Leiomyoma	–/+	–	–	+	+	–		
Leiomyosarcoma (LMS)*	+/–	–	–/+*	+	+	–		
Inflammatory myofibroblastic tumor	–	–	–	+/–	–	–		
Inflammatory fibroid polyp	–	–	+	+/–	–	–		
Solitary fibrous tumor	–	–	+	–	–	–		
Desmoid fibromatosis	–	–	–	+	–/+	–		+ (Nuclear)
Gastrointestinal schwannoma	–	–	–	–	–	+		
Metastatic melanoma	–	+/–	–	–	–	+		
Desmoplastic small round cell tumor	+	–	–	–	–	+	–	
GIST	+	+	+	+/–	–/+	–/+		

*Retroperitoneal LMS may be positive.
GIST, gastrointestinal stromal tumor; SMA, smooth muscle actin; +, positive; –, negative; +/–, often positive; –/+, rarely positive.
Modified from Miettinen M, Sobin LH, Sarlomo-Rikala M: Immunohistochemical spectrum of GISTs at different sites and their differential diagnosis with a reference to CD117 (KIT). Mod Pathol 13:1134-1142, 2000; Sah SP, McCluggage WG: DOG1 immunoreactivity in uterine leiomyosarcomas. J Clin Pathol 66:40-43, 2013; Hill DA, Pfeifer JD, Marley EF, et al: WT1 staining reliably differentiates desmoplastic small round cell tumor from Ewing sarcoma/primitive neuroectodermal tumor: an immunohistochemical and molecular diagnostic study. Am J Clin Pathol 114:345-354, 2000.

TABLE 1-13   IMMUNOPHENOTYPE OF PRIMARY OVARIAN AND METASTATIC COLORECTAL ADENOCARCINOMA

	Mucinous Ovarian Tumors		Endometrioid Adenocarcinoma	Metastatic Colorectal Adenocarcinoma
	Intestinal Type	Endocervical Type		
CK7	+++/+	+++	+++	–
CK20	–/+/+++	–	–	+++
mCEA	+	–	–	++
CDX2	+	–	–/+	++
ER	–	+	+	–

ER, estrogen receptor; mCEA, monoclonal carcinoembryonic antigen; +++, diffusely positive; +, focally positive; –, negative.
Modified from McCluggage WG: My approach to and thoughts on the typing of ovarian carcinomas. J Clin Pathol 61:152-163, 2008.

TABLE 1-14 IMMUNOHISTOCHEMISTRY PANEL FOR PRIMARY AND METASTATIC ADENOCARCINOMA OF THE OVARY

	PAX2	PAX8	CK7	CK20	CDX2	DPC4
Primary mucinous, intestinal type	−	−	+	+	+/−	+
Primary endometrioid	+	+	+	−	−	+
Metastatic colorectal	−	−	−	+	+	+
Metastatic pancreas	−	−	+/−	+/−	−	−
Metastatic thyroid		+				
Metastatic renal		+				
Metastatic thymic		+				

CK, cytokeratin; DPC, deleted in pancreatic carcinoma; +, positive; −, negative; +/−, often positive.

Modified from Ji H, Isacson C, Seidman JD, et al: Cytokeratins 7 and 20, Dpc4, and MUC5AC in the distinction of metastatic mucinous carcinomas in the ovary from primary ovarian mucinous tumors: Dpc4 assists in identifying metastatic pancreatic carcinomas. Int J Gynecol Pathol 21:391-400, 2002; Ozcan A, Liles N, Coffey D: PAX2 and PAX8: Am J Surg Pathol 35:1837-1847, 2011.

TABLE 1-15 IMMUNOHISTOCHEMISTRY: HIGH-GRADE SEROUS CARCINOMA AND POORLY DIFFERENTIATED ENDOMETRIOID ADENOCARCINOMA OF THE OVARY AND ENDOMETRIUM

	Serous	Endometrioid
WT-1	+++	−/+
p53	+++	−/+/+++*
p16	+++	−/+
β-Catenin	Membranous	Membranous/nuclear

*The +++ expression corresponds to some high-grade carcinomas.

WT-1, Wilms tumor gene protein 1; +++, diffusely positive; +, focally positive; −, negative.

Modified from McCluggage WG: My approach to and thoughts on the typing of ovarian carcinomas. J Clin Pathol 61:152-163, 2008.

TABLE 1-16 IMMUNOHISTOCHEMISTRY APPROACH TO OVARIAN SEX CORD–STROMAL TUMORS AND ENDOMETRIOID ADENOCARCINOMA

	FOXL2	Inhibin	Calretinin	CD99	EMA	Pan-cytokeratin
Granulosa cell tumor	+	+	+	+	−	−/+
Sertoli-Leydig cell tumor	+/−	+	+	+	−	+/−
Endometrioid adenocarcinoma	−	−	−	−	+	+

EMA, epithelial membrane antigen; +, positive; −, negative; +/−, often positive; −/+, rarely positive.

Modified from Mount SL, Cooper K: Tumours with divergent müllerian differentiation of the uterine corpus. Curr Diagn Pathol 11:349-355, 2005; Al-Agha OM, Huwait HF, Chow C, et al: FOXL2 is a sensitive and specific marker for sex cord-stromal tumors of the ovary. Am J Surg Pathol 35:484-494, 2011.

TABLE 1-17 IMMUNOHISTOCHEMISTRY APPROACH TO ENDOCERVICAL ADENOCARCINOMA AND ENDOMETRIOID ENDOMETRIAL ADENOCARCINOMA

	mCEA	Vimentin	ER/PR	p16	HPV DNA
Endocervical	+	−	−	+	+
Endometrial	−	+	+	−/+	−

ER/PR, estrogen/progesterone receptor; HPV, human papillomavirus; mCEA, monoclonal carcinoembryonic antigen; +, positive; −, negative; −/+, rarely positive.

Modified from Staebler A, Sherman ME, Zaino RJ, Ronnett BM: Hormone receptor immunohistochemistry and human papillomavirus in situ hybridization are useful for distinguishing endocervical and endometrial adenocarcinomas. Am J Surg Pathol 26:998-1006, 2002.

TABLE 1-18 IMMUNOHISTOCHEMISTRY IN THE DIFFERENTIAL DIAGNOSIS OF SQUAMOUS AND GLANDULAR LESIONS OF THE UTERINE CERVIX

	p16*	MIB-1 (Ki-67)
LSIL (CIN I)	+/–	Increased
HSIL (CIN II-III)	+	Increased (full thickness)
Adenocarcinoma in situ	+	+
Atypical immature metaplasia	–	–/+
Reactive squamous or glandular atypia	–	+
Tubal metaplasia	+/–	–

*Expression of p16 (nuclear and cytoplasmic) is a surrogate marker for high-risk human papillomavirus (HPV), for example, HPV-16 and HPV-18. In LSIL, the p16 expression may be confined to the lower one third or one half of the squamous epithelium or show focal immunoreactivity (the latter being a pattern of expression, albeit cytoplasmic only, that may be seen in reactive squamous epithelia). HSIL p16 immunoexpression usually involves two thirds or full thickness of the squamous epithelium.

CIN, cervical intraepithelial neoplasia; HSIL, high-grade squamous intraepithelial neoplasia; LSIL, low-grade squamous intraepithelial neoplasia; +, positive; –, negative; +/–, often positive; –/+, rarely positive. MIB-1, monoclonal antibody directed against the Ki-67 antigen, a nuclear antigen expressed by all human proliferating cells.

Modified from Kalof AN, Cooper K: p16INK4a immunoexpression: surrogate marker of high-risk HPV and high-grade cervical intraepithelial neoplasia. Adv Anat Pathol 13:190-194, 2006.

TABLE 1-19 P57^KIP2 IMMUNOREACTION AND _HER-2_ FLUORESCENCE IN SITU HYBRIDIZATION (FISH) ANALYSIS IN MOLAR PREGNANCY

	Villous Cytotrophoblasts	Villous Stroma	Syncytiotrophoblasts	_HER-2_ FISH Analysis
Complete hydatidiform molar pregnancy	–	–	+	Diploid
Partial hydatidiform molar pregnancy	+	+	+	Triploid
Hydropic abortion	+	+	+	Diploid

Note: p57^KIP2 is a paternally imprinted, maternally expressed gene protein. Hence, complete moles comprising only paternal genes will not express this protein.

Modified from Hoffner L, Dunn J, Esposito N, et al: p57^KIP2 Immunostaining and molecular cytogenetics: combined approach aids in diagnosis of morphologically challenging cases with molar phenotype and in detecting androgenetic cell lines in mosaic/chimeric conceptions. Hum Pathol 39:63, 2008; and LeGallo RD, Stelow EB, Ramirez NC, et al: Diagnosis of hydatidiform moles using p57 immunohistochemistry and her2 fluorescent in situ hybridization. Am J Clin Pathol 129:749, 2008.

TABLE 1-20 IMMUNOHISTOCHEMICAL APPROACH FOR TROPHOBLASTIC LESIONS

Trophoblastic Lesion	CK18	p63	hPL	MIB-1 LI (%)
Exaggerated placental site	+++	–	+++	<1
Placental site trophoblastic tumor	+++	–	+++	>1
Placental site nodule	+++	+++	–/+	<10
Epithelioid trophoblastic tumor	+++	+++	–/+	>10
Choriocarcinoma	+++	–/+	++	

Note: Expression of p63 highlights mononucleated trophoblasts corresponding to cytotrophoblasts, and human chorionic gonadotropin selectively stains syncytiotrophoblasts; this combination is indicative of choriocarcinoma.

CK, cytokeratin; hPL, human placental lactogen; LI, labeling index; MIB-1, Ki-67 proliferation marker; +++, diffusely positive; ++, focally positive; –, negative; –/+, rarely positive.

Modified from Shih IM, Kurman RJ: p63 Expression is useful in the distinction of epithelioid trophoblastic and placental site trophoblastic tumors by profiling trophoblastic subpopulations. Am J Surg Pathol 28:1177-1183, 2004.

disease characterization and patient care. This section provides an overview of the molecular techniques applicable to pathology practice.

NUCLEIC ACID EXTRACTION METHODS

Background

- The extraction of nucleic acids from pathology samples involves cell lysis followed by selective DNA or RNA isolation, and a quantity and quality assessment relative to the requirements of the end-diagnostic test
- Pathology samples that can be used include biopsy or surgical material (fresh or formalin-fixed, paraffin-embedded [FFPE] tissue), body fluids (amniotic, saliva, stools, urine), buccal cell scrapes, cervical scrapes, fine-needle aspiration, hair root, peripheral blood, primary cell culture

TABLE 1-21   IMMUNOHISTOCHEMISTRY FOR SELECTED GERM CELL TUMORS

	SOX2	SALL4	c-kit	OCT3/4	CD30	AFP	GPC-3	D2-40	β-hCG
Germinoma	−	+	+	+	−	−	−	+	−*
Embryonal carcinoma	+	+	−	+	+	−	−	−	v
Yolk sac tumor	−	+	−	−	−	v	+	−	−
Choriocarcinoma	−	+/−	−	−	−	−	−	−	+

*Except for syncytiotrophoblastic giant cells in seminoma.
AFP, α-fetoprotein; β-hCG, β-human chorionic gonadotropin; GPC-3, glypican-3; SALL4, sal-like4; SOX2 (also known as SRY [sex determining region Y]-box2); v, variable; +, positive; −, negative; +/−, often positive.
Modified from Ulbright TM: The most common, clinically significant misdiagnoses in testicular tumor pathology, and how to avoid them. Adv Anat Pathol 15:18-27, 2008; and Young RH: Testicular tumors: Some new and a few perennial problems. Arch Pathol Lab Med 132:548-564, 2008.
Cao D, Li J, Guo CC: SALL4 SALL4 is a novel diagnostic marker for testicular germ cell tumors. Am J Surg Pathol 33:1065-1077, 2009; Gopalan A, Dhall D, Olgac S, et al: Testicular mixed germ cell tumors: a morphological and immunohistochemical study using stem cell markers, OCT3/4, SOX2 and GDF3, with emphasis on morphologically difficult-to-classify areas. Mod Pathol 22:1066-1074, 2009.

TABLE 1-22   IMMUNOHISTOCHEMISTRY PANEL TO DISTINGUISH RENAL CELL NEOPLASMS

	RCC	CD10	CK7	AMACR	CA IX	Melan A or HMB45	TFEB	TFE3	CD117	PAX2	PAX8
Clear cell carcinoma	+/−	+	−	−	+		−	−		+	+
Chromophobe carcinoma	−	−	+/−	−	−		−	−	+	−	+
Papillary carcinoma	+/−	−/+	+/−	+	−		−	−	−	−/+	+
Oncocytoma	−	−	−/+	−	−		−	−	+/−	−	+
Xp11/TFE3 translocation renal carcinoma		+	−	+				+	−		
RCC with t(6,11)						+	+				

AMACR, α-methylacyl coenzyme A racemase (P504S); CA IX, carbonic anhydrase 9; CK, cytokeratin; PAX2, paired box gene-2; PAX8, paired box gene-8; RCC, renal cell carcinoma; TFE3, transcription factor E3; +, positive; −, negative; +/−, often positive; −/+, rarely positive.
Modified from Truong LD, Shen SS: Immunohistochemical diagnosis of renal neoplasms. Arch Pathol Lab Med 135:92-109, 2011; Ozcan A, de la Roza G, Ro JY, et al: PAX2 and PAX8 expression in primary and metastatic renal tumors: a comprehensive comparison. Arch Pathol Lab Med 136:151-154, 2012; Suárez-Vilela D, Izquierdo-García F, Méndez-Álvarez JR, et al: Renal translocation carcinoma with expression of TFEB: presentation of a case with distinctive histological and immunohistochemical features. Int J Surg Pathol 19:506-509, 2011.

TABLE 1-23   SELECTED IHC TO DISTINGUISH VASCULAR NEOPLASM

Neoplasm	IHC
Angiosarcoma*	CD31, CD34, ERG
Hemangioendothelioma	CD31, CD34, ERG
Kaposi sarcoma	HHV8, CD31, CD34, ERG

*Angiosarcoma is also cytokeratin and EMA positive (+). Al-Abbadi MA, Almasri NM, Al-Quran S, Wilkinson EJ: Cytokeratin and epithelial membrane antigen expression in angiosarcomas: an immunohistochemical study of 33 cases. Arch Pathol Lab Med 131:288-292, 2007.
ERG, v-ets erythroblastosis virus E26 oncogene homologue; ETS family transcription factor present at 22q12.
From Miettinen M, Wang ZF, Paetau A, et al: ERG transcription factor as an immunohistochemical marker for vascular endothelial tumors and prostatic carcinoma. Am J Surg Pathol 35:432-441, 2011.

TABLE 1-24   IMMUNOHISTOCHEMISTRY APPROACH TO ATYPICAL GLANDULAR PROLIFERATIVE LESION IN THE PROSTATE*

Lesion	Basal Cell Markers (HMWCK 34βE12, CK5/6, p63)	AMACR (p504S)
Atrophic glands	+	−
Post–atrophic hyperplasia	+	−
Basal cell hyperplasia	+	−
Atypical adenomatous hyperplasia (adenosis)	+/− (patchy)	−/+
Prostatic intraepithelial neoplasia	+	+
Prostate carcinoma	−†	+

*See Figure 1-14.
†Rarely, p63 may demonstrate immunoreactivity in prostate carcinoma (see Ali TZ, Epstein JI: False positive labeling of prostate cancer with high molecular weight cytokeratin: p63 a more specific immunomarker for basal cells. Am J Surg Pathol 32:1890-1895, 2008).
AMACR, α-methylacyl coenzyme A racemase; CK, cytokeratin; HMWCK, high-molecular-weight cytokeratin; +, positive; −, negative; +/−, often positive; −/+, rarely positive.
Modified from Paner GP, Luthringer DJ, Amin MB: Best practices in diagnostic immunohistochemistry: prostate carcinoma and its mimics in needle core biopsies. Arch Pathol Lab Med 132:1388-1396, 2008.

DNA Extraction Methods

- Classical methods were time consuming (~3 days) and required relatively large quantities of tissues (100 mg to > 1 g)
- Numerous extraction kits are now available that utilize glass-fiber filters that selectively bind DNA following tissue treatments with a protease and chaotropic buffers

TABLE 1-25 IMMUNOHISTOCHEMISTRY PANEL TO DISTINGUISH PROSTATE AND UROTHELIAL CARCINOMAS

	GATA3	CK7	CK20	PSA	Uroplakin	p63
Prostate carcinoma	–	–/+	–/+	+	–	–/+
Urothelial carcinoma	+	+/–	+/–	–	+/–	+

CK, cytokeratin; PSA, prostate-specific antigen; +, positive; –, negative; +/–, often positive; –/+, rarely positive. GATA3, GATA binding protein3
Notes:
- Only CK7/20 negativity (prostate carcinoma) and CK7/20 positivity (urothelial carcinoma) reliably distinguish between these two carcinomas. Any other permutation is unreliable.
- Uroplakin is highly specific for urothelial carcinoma but has a low sensitivity, being focally present in about 50% to 60% of tumors.
- Expression of p63 is used more often to highlight basal cells in benign prostate glands but may rarely be positive in the prostate carcinoma itself (see Ali TZ, Epstein JI: False positive labeling of prostate cancer with high molecular weight cytokeratin: p63 a more specific immunomarker for basal cells. Am J Surg Pathol 32:1890-1895, 2008).
Modified from Hammerich AH, Ayala GE, Wheeler TM: Application of immunohistochemistry to the genitourinary system (prostate, urinary bladder, testis, and kidney). Arch Pathol Lab Med 132:432-440, 2008; Chang A, Amin A, Gabrielson E, et al: Utility of GATA3 immunohistochemistry in differentiating urothelial carcinoma from prostate adenocarcinoma and squamous cell carcinomas of the uterine cervix, anus, and lung. Am J Surg Pathol 36:1472-1476, 2012.

TABLE 1-26 RECOMMENDED ANTIBODY PANEL FOR COMMON PLEOMORPHIC CUTANEOUS SPINDLE CELL TUMORS

	CD10	p63	Cytokeratins (Pan, HMW, CK5/6)	S-100 Protein	Melanocytic (HMB-45, Melan-A)	Smooth Muscle Actin	Desmin	Endothelial (CD31, CD34)
Sarcomatoid squamous cell carcinoma	–	+	+	–	–	–	–	–
Melanoma	–	–	–/+	+	+/–	–	–/+	–
Atypical fibroxanthoma	+	–/+	–	–	–	–/+	–	–
Leiomyosarcoma	–	–	–	–/+	–	+	+/–	–/+
Angiosarcoma	–	–	–/+	–	–	–	–	+

+, positive; –, negative; +/–, often positive; –/+, rarely positive.
Modified from Folpe AL, Cooper K: Best practices in diagnostic immunohistochemistry: pleomorphic cutaneous spindle cell tumors. Arch Pathol Lab Med 131:1517, 2007; Hultgren TL, DiMaio DJ: Immunohistochemical staining of CD10 in atypical fibroxanthomas. J Cutan Pathol 34:415-419, 2007; Dotto JE, Glusac EJ: p63 is a useful marker for cutaneous spindle cell squamous cell carcinoma. J Cutan Pathol 33:413-417, 2006.

TABLE1-27 MIB-1(KI-67) MEMBRANOUS AND CYTOPLASMIC STAINING

	MIB-1 (Ki-67); Clone MIB-1, 1:700; Dako, Glostrup, Denmark Staining Pattern
Hyalinizing trabecular tumor of the thyroid	Cytoplasmic staining*
Pulmonary sclerosing hemangiomas	Membrane and cytoplasmic staining[†]

From Hirokawa M, Carney JA: Cell membrane and cytoplasmic staining for MIB-1 in hyalinizing trabecular adenoma of the thyroid gland. Am J Surg Pathol 24:575-578, 2000.
[†]*From Kim BH, Bae YS, Kim SH, et al: Usefulness of Ki-67 (MIB-1) immunostaining in the diagnosis of pulmonary sclerosing hemangiomas. APMIS 121:105-110, 2013.*

TABLE 1-28A IMMUNOHISTOCHEMISTRY PANEL FOR THE INTERPRETATION OF LOW-GRADE (SMALL) B-CELL LYMPHOMA

	CD23 (%)	CD5 (%)	Cyclin D1 (%)	CD10 (%)	bcl-1 (%)
SLL/chronic lymphocytic leukemia	85	80	0	0	2
Mantle	2	80	75-100	2	85
Marginal zone	8	0	0	2	0
Lymphoplasmacytic	0-30	5	0	3	0
Follicular	0-25	0	0	85	0
Extranodal marginal	0	0	0	0	0

SLL, small lymphocytic lymphoma.
Modified from http://surgpathcriteria.stanford.edu.

TABLE 1-28B BASIC IMMUNOPHENOTYPIC APPROCH TO LYMPHOMAS OF SMALL B CELL TYPE (CD20+ AND LOW KI-67)

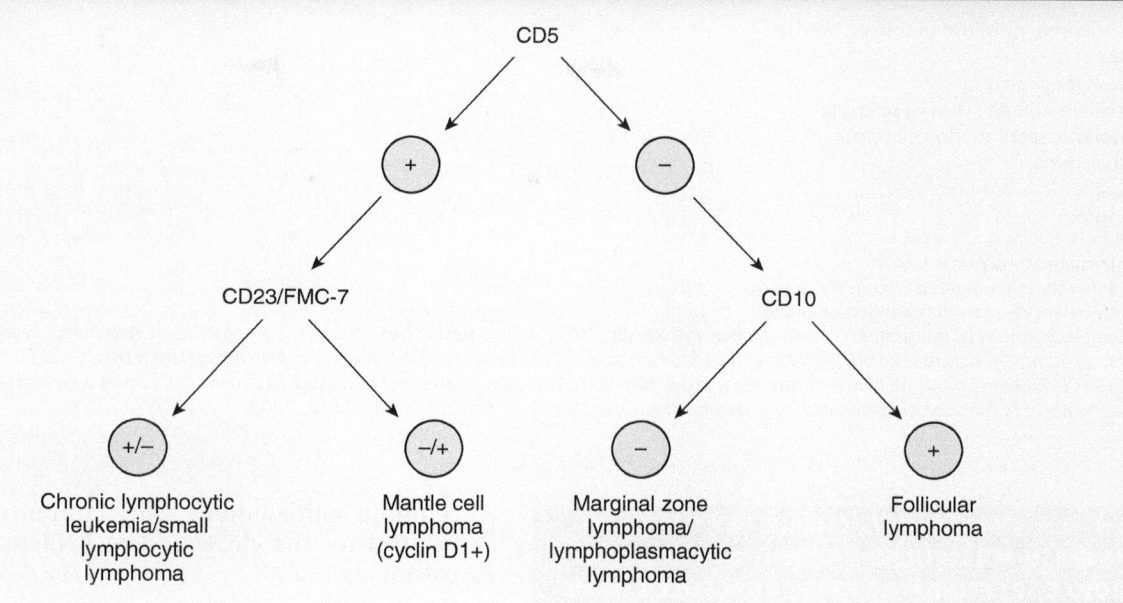

TABLE 1-29 ANTIBODY PANEL FOR DIFFERENTIAL DIAGNOSIS OF HODGKIN LYMPHOMA

	CD30	CD15	CD20	CD45 (LCA)	ALK
Hodgkin lymphoma	+	+	–/+	–	–
ALCL	+	–	–	–/+	+
DLBCL	–/+	–	+	+	–

ALCL, anaplastic large cell lymphoma; ALK, alkaline kinase; DLBCL, diffuse large B-cell lymphoma; EMA, epithelial membrane antigen; LCA, leukocyte common antigen; +, positive; –, negative; –/+, rarely positive.

TABLE 1-30 IHC CLASSIFICATION OF DIFFUSE LARGE B CELL LYMPHOMA INTO GERMINAL CENTER B-LIKE CELL (GCB) AND NON-GCB

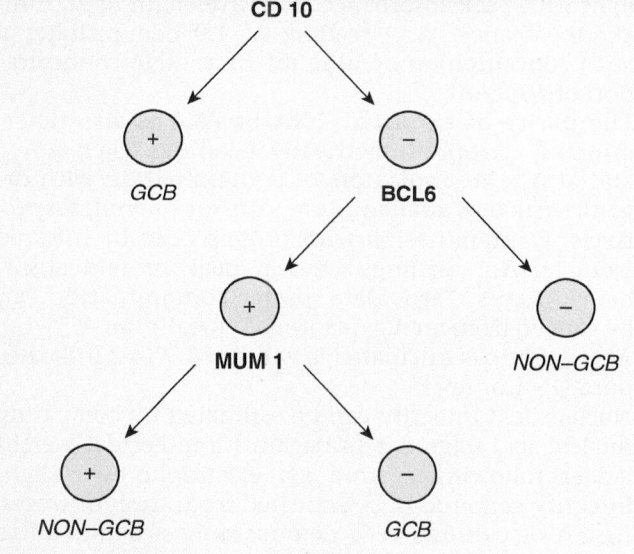

From Hans CP, Weisenburger DD, Greiner TC: Confirmation of the molecular classification of diffuse large B-cell lymphoma by immunohistochemistry using a tissue microarray. Blood 103:275-282, 2004.

(which disrupt protein and DNA secondary structures); the glass fibers, typically loaded in mini-columns, are washed to rinse away cellular debris, extraction solution reagents, and pathology tissue processing chemicals; the DNA is then recovered from the resin/glass-fiber by low-salt buffer rinses; pure DNA recovery from diverse pathology samples is possible within several hours by these procedures

• Automated DNA extraction platforms are available for the processing of multiple patient samples

RNA Extraction Methods

• Classical methods required the rapid homogenization of large quantities of fresh tissues in protease/guanidinium thiocyanate solution to denature ubiquitous endogenous RNases that otherwise degrade cellular RNA

• Current methods allow the relatively rapid (1-day) recovery of RNA again following tissue homogenization in a chaotropic guanidinium salt solution that leaves RNA contained in an aqueous phase and protein and DNA in an organic phase. Admixture of the aqueous phase with nucleic acid binding glass filters allows the recovery of pure total RNA by elution from the glass filters with a low-salt buffer. mRNA can be purified from total RNA by passage through oligo(dT)

TABLE 1-31   IMMUNOPROFILE OF SMALL ROUND CELL TUMORS

	FLI-1	Pan-CK	CD99	Desmin	Myogenin	WT-1	CD56
Ewing sarcoma, primitive neuroectodermal tumor	+	v	+	−	−	−	v
Rhabdomyosarcoma	−	−	v	+	+	−	+
Poorly differentiated synovial sarcoma[†]	−	+	+	−	−	−	+
Desmoplastic small round cell tumor	+	+	v	+	−	+	v
Neuroblastoma	−	−	−	−	−	−	+
Lymphoblastic lymphoma[‡]	+	−	+	−	−	−	−
Wilms tumor	+	v	v	+	v*	+	+

*In rhabdomyomatous Wilms tumor.
[†]Epithelial membrane antigen is frequently positive.
[‡]Frequently leukocyte common antigen negative.
FLI-1, Friend leukemia virus integration-1; Pan-CK, pan-cytokeratin; WT-1, Wilms tumor gene protein 1; +, positive; −, negative; v, variable.
Modified from Barami A, Truong LD, Ro JY: Undifferentiated tumor: true identity by immunohistochemistry. Arch Pathol Lab Med 132:326-348, 2008.
Folpe AL, Hill CE, Parham DM, et al: Immunohistochemical detection of FLI-1 protein expression: a study of 132 round cell tumors with emphasis on CD99-positive mimics of Ewing's sarcoma/primitive neuroectodermal tumor. Am J Surg Pathol 24:1657-1662, 2000.

TABLE 1-32   IMMUNOHISTOCHEMISTRY PANEL TO DISTINGUISH FOLLICULAR VARIANT OF PAPILLARY THYROID CARCINOMA (FVPTC) FROM FOLLICULAR ADENOMA (FA)

	HBME1 (%)	CK19 (%)	Galectin-3 (%)
FVPTC	96	91-100	98
FA	7-11	44-68	30

Note: The combination of HBME1 and CK19 has the greatest utility in differentiating FVPTC from benign follicular lesions.
From Erickson LA, Lloyd RV: Utility of a panel of immunohistochemical markers in the diagnosis of follicular variant of papillary thyroid carcinoma. Adv Anat Pathol 15:59-60, 2008.

TABLE 1-33   IHC TO DETECT THE GAIN OR LOSS OF PROTEIN EXPRESSION

	Loss of SMARCB1 (INI-1) Expression (%)
Medullary carcinoma of kidney	100
Malignant rhabdoid tumor (Glypican 3 +)*	98
Epithelioid sarcoma (classic and proximal type)	90
Epithelioid MPNST	50

	Loss of Succinate Dehydrogenase B (SDHB) Expression[†]
Succinate dehydrogenase-deficient wildtype GISTs, paragangliomas, and pheochromocytomas	− (no expression)
Sporadic GISTs (association with KIT or PDGFRA mutations)	+ (expression)

*Glypican 3 positive in malignant rhabdoid tumor and negative in epithelioid sarcoma. Kohashi K, Nakatsura T, Kinoshita Y, et al: Glypican 3 expression in tumors with loss of SMARCB1/INI1 protein expression. Hum Pathol 44:526-533, 2013.
[†]Barletta JA, Hornick JL: Succinate dehydrogenase-deficient tumors: diagnostic advances and clinical implications. Adv Anat Pathol 4:193-203, 2012.
From Am J Surg Pathol Oct; 35(10), 2011.

cellulose spin columns. Mini-columns have been developed for the extraction of RNA from all types of pathology sample

DNA and RNA Quantification, Purity, and Integrity Assay

- High-integrity nucleic acids are best extracted from fresh tissue specimens. Extraction from tissues preserved in liquid nitrogen is the next best option. Commercially available storage reagents (e.g., RNA*later*, Ambion, Inc., Foster City, CA) preserve tissue morphology and nucleic acids integrity. Disaggregated cells/cell cultures can be stored at −20°C in 70% ethanol with efficient nucleic acid preservation. DNA and RNA extracts from FFPE tissues tend to be degraded. In general, the quality of nucleic acids extractable from FFPE blocks decreases with block age
- The concentration of extracted nucleic acids is assessed spectrophotometrically. Both DNA and RNA absorb UV light with peak absorbance at a wavelength of 260 nm; an Absorbance (A_{260}) reading of 1.0 demonstrates a DNA concentration of 50 µg/mL or an RNA concentration of 40 µg/mL
- The purity of extracted DNA or RNA is also determined spectrophotometrically. Readings taken at A_{230} and at A_{270} are indicators of contamination with organics (such as guanadinium salts) or phenol, respectively. Contamination with proteins can be inferred from an A_{280} reading, whereat peak protein absorbance occurs. Particulate matter contamination can be gauged from an A_{320} reading. Typically, an $A_{(260-320)}$: $A_{(280-320)}$ ratio is calculated; a value of 1.7 to 2 indicates pure DNA or RNA
- Nucleic acid integrity can be estimated by comparing nucleic acid fragment size against a molecular weight ladder following agarose gel electrophoresis. High-integrity genomic DNA extracted from fresh or frozen tissues or cultured cells demonstrates a band > 30 to 40 kilobase pairs (kb) in size. The presence of a smear extending to smaller sized fragments indicates degraded DNA. DNA extracted from FFPE tissues typically appears as a smear extending from ~1 kb to < 100 base

TABLE 1-34 IHC TO DETECT THE GAIN OR LOSS OF PROTEIN EXPRESSION

	MSH2	MSH6	MLH1	PMS2
Tumor positive for microsatellite instability (highly suspicious for Lynch syndrome); germline mutation of MSH6	Present	Loss	Present	Present
Tumor positive for microsatellite instability (highly suspicious for Lynch syndrome); germline mutation of MSH2	Loss	Loss	Present	Present
Tumor positive for microsatellite instability (highly suspicious for Lynch syndrome); germline mutation of PMS2	Present	Present	Present	Loss
Tumor positive for microsatellite instability; majority of colon cancers with this pattern of protein loss are associated with somatic changes (not inherited mutation); follow-up testing should include a BRAF mutational analysis or methylation of MLH-1 testing	Present	Present	Loss	Loss
—Presence of the BRAF V600E mutation and MLH1 promoter hypermethylation provide confirmation of a sporadic MSI tumor (loss of MLH1 secondary to promoter hypermethylation, not due to inherited mutation)				
—Absence of BRAF V600E and negative MLH1 promoter hypermethylation is highly suggestive of a germline mutation of MLH1				
Tumor negative for microsatellite instability; germline mutation unlikely (however, up to 10% of Lynch syndrome patients may have retained expression of these 4 MMR proteins)	Present	Present	Present	Present

Loss, negative nuclear staining; Present, positive nuclear staining.
Courtesy of Rebecca Wilcox, MD, University of Vermont/Fletcher Allen Health Care.

TABLE 1-35 IHC FOR GENE PRODUCTS DETECTION FROM SPECIFIC MUTATIONS

Antibodies Against Gene Products from Specific Mutations

Gene	Malignancy
BRAF V600E	Melanoma (37/38)[*]
	Hairy cell leukemia (32/32)[†]
	Papillary thyroid carcinoma (72/144)[‡]
EGFR	Non-small cell lung cancer[§]

[*]From Long GV, Wilmott JS, Capper D, et al: Immunohistochemistry is highly sensitive and specific for the detection of V600E BRAF mutation in melanoma. Am J Surg Pathol 37:61-65, 2013.
[†]From Andrulis M, Penzel R, Weichert W, et al: Application of a BRAF V600E mutation-specific antibody for the diagnosis of hairy cell leukemia. Am J Surg Pathol 36:1796-1800, 2012.
[‡]From Koperek O, Kornauth C, Capper D, et al: Immunohistochemical detection of the BRAF V600E-mutated protein in papillary thyroid carcinoma. Am J Surg Pathol 36:844-850, 2012.
[§]From Hasanovic A, Ang D, Moreira AL, Zakowski MF: Use of mutation specific antibodies to detect EGFR status in small biopsy and cytology specimens of lung adenocarcinoma. Lung Cancer 77:299-305, 2012.

pairs (bp). Total RNA integrity is gauged in terms of the presence of 28S (~5 kb) and 18S (~2 kb) ribosomal RNA (rRNA). Discrete 28S and 18S bands, with minimal smearing, indicate intact RNA species, whereas partial or absent bands and smeared rRNA indicate a degraded sample
- Instruments such as the NanoDrop spectrophotometer (Thermo Fisher Scientific, Wilmington, DE), and the Agilent 2100 Bioanalyzer (Agilent Technologies, Inc., Santa Clara, CA) have facilitated rapid DNA and RNA quantitation and purity analyses, and RNA integrity assay, respectively

Nucleic Acids Storage
- DNA is generally stored at 4°C for assays performed within 1 week to 1 month of extraction, and in aliquots at −20°C or −80°C for longer-term storage; repeated freeze-thawing may lead to DNA degradation
- RNA is more labile than DNA and is susceptible to degradation by RNases that are a pervasive laboratory hazard. For short-term use, RNA is stored at −20°C, and at −80°C or under liquid nitrogen for longer-term storage

TISSUE MICRODISSECTION METHODS

Background
- Microdissection enables the targeted collection of cells or tissues from slide mounted cytologic specimens, or frozen or FFPE tissue sections. Sample tissues may be treated for nucleic acids or protein extraction

Methods
- In the simplest approach, lightly stained tissue sections are viewed by dissecting microscope and after dampening the tissues with 70% ethanol, tissues are selectively scraped off the slides using a syringe needle. DNA is extracted from the collected tissues after digestion with proteinase K. A glass-fiber mini-column method allows further purification
- Laser capture microdissection (LCM) (Figure 1-17) requires specialized microscopy apparatus such as the ArcturusXT system (MDS Analytical Technologies, Sunnyvale, CA)
- The procedure involves overlaying the tissue of interest with a thermoplastic film contained in a cap. LCM can be applied to frozen or FFPE tissues, or to

TABLE 1-36 SELECTED SOFT TISSUE TUMORS WITH CORRESPONDING IHC	
CD 34+ Spindle Cell Tumors	
Cellular angiofibroma (ER/PR +)	
Angiomyofibroblastoma (ER/PR +)	
Superficial myofibroblastoma (ER/PR +)	
Solitary fibrous tumor (CD99 +)	
Spindle cell lipoma	
Dermatofibrosarcoma protuberans	
Kaposi sarcoma	
IHC for Liposarcomas (LPS)	
Myxoid LPS	S100 protein + (mature fat cells and lipoblasts)
Well-differentiated/atypical lipomatous tumor	MDM2 +
	CDK4 +
	p16 +
	MDM2 +
Dedifferentiated liposarcoma	CDK4 +
IHC for Myxoid Spindle Cell Tumors	
Myxofibrosarcoma	Vimentin +
Low-grade fibromyxoid sarcoma	MUC4 +
	Vimentin +
Myxoid LPS	S100 protein + (mature fat cells and lipoblasts)
Extraskeletal myxoid chondrosarcoma	S100 protein + (17%)*
	Vimentin +
Chordoma	Brachyury +
	CK +
	EMA +
	S100 protein +
Myxoid leiomyosarcoma	Desmin +
	h-Caldesmon +
	DOG1 −/+
Myxoid malignant peripheral nerve sheath tumor (MPNST)	SMA + (50%)
	S100 + (50%) focal
	CD34 +/−
Myxoid dermatofibrosarcoma protuberans (DFSP)	CD34 +
	Apolipoprotein D +
Myxoid solitary fibrous tumor (SFT)	CD99 +
	CD34 +
	BCL2 +
Myxoid monophasic synovial sarcoma	Keratin +
	CD99 +
	TLE1 +

+, positive; −, negative; +/−, often positive; −/+, rarely positive.
*Oliveira AM, Sebo TJ, McGrory JE, et al: Extraskeletal myxoid chondrosarcoma: a clinicopathologic, immunohistochemical, and ploidy analysis of 23 cases. Extraskeletal myxoid chondrosarcoma: a clinicopathologic, immunohistochemical, and ploidy analysis of 23 cases. Mod Pathol 13:900-908, 2000.
MUC4 (mucin 4 gene): Doyle LA, Möller E, Dal Cin P, et al: MUC4 is a highly sensitive and specific marker for low-grade fibromyxoid sarcoma. Am J Surg Pathol 35:733-741, 2011.
MDM2, CDK4, and p16: Thway K, Flora R, Shah C, et al: Diagnostic utility of p16, CDK4, and MDM2 as an immunohistochemical panel in distinguishing well-differentiated and dedifferentiated liposarcomas from other adipocytic tumors. Am J Surg Pathol 36:462-469, 2012.
Apolipoprotein D: West RB, Harvell J, Linn SC, et al: Apo D in soft tissue tumors: a novel marker for dermatofibrosarcoma protuberans. Am J Surg Pathol 28:1063-1069, 2004.
TLE1 (transducer-like enhancer of split 1): Foo WC, Cruise MW, Wick MR, Hornick JL: Immunohistochemical staining for TLE1 distinguishes synovial sarcoma from histologic mimics. Am J Clin Pathol 135:839-844, 2011.
From Jambhekar NA, Rekhi B, Thorat K, et al: Revisiting chordoma with brachyury, a "new age" marker: analysis of a validation study on 51 cases. Arch Pathol Lab Med 134:1181-1187, 2010.

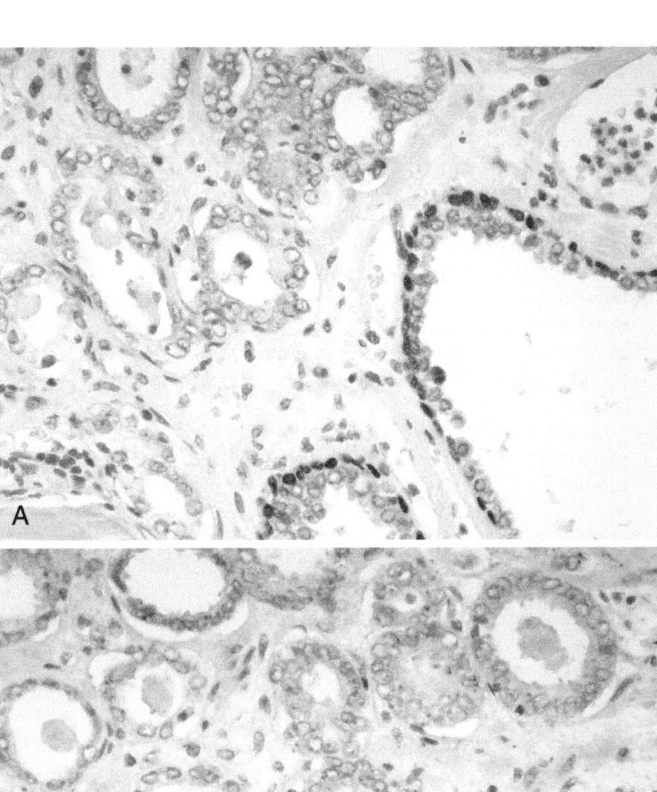

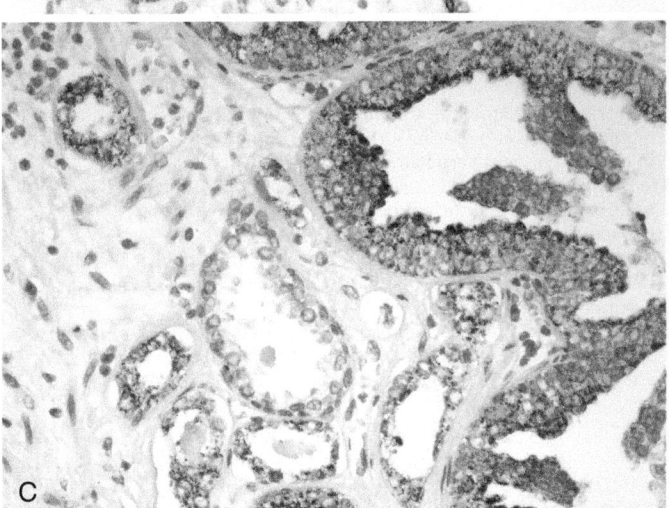

Figure 1-14. Immunohistochemistry in prostate adenocarcinoma. Both p63 **(A)** and 34βE12 **(B)** highlight an intact basal cell layer surrounding benign glands and loss around small acini of invasive adenocarcinoma. **C,** P504S immunohistochemistry shows strong, granular luminal staining in invasive adenocarcinoma and prostatic intraepithelial neoplasia. Normal glands are negative.

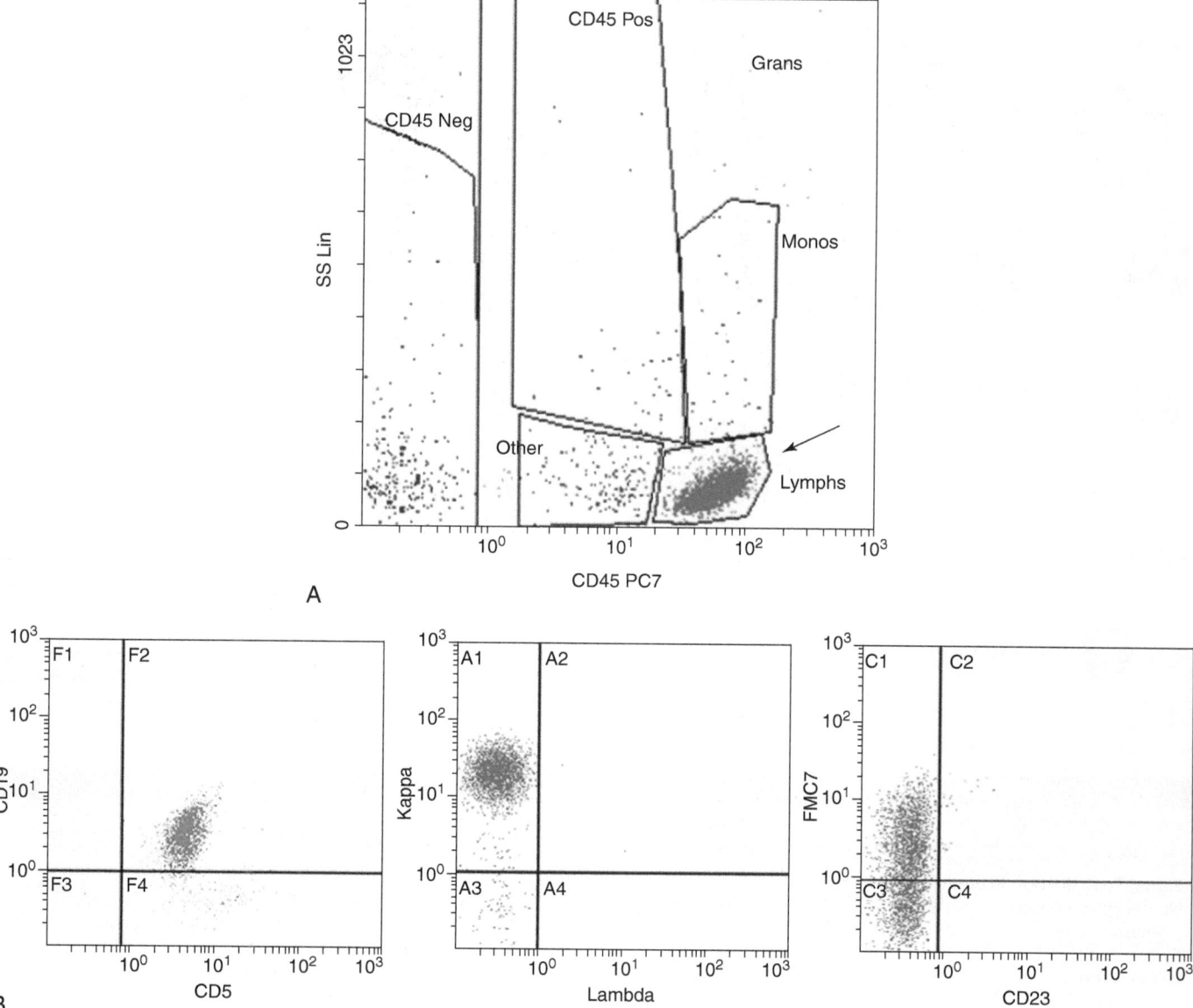

Figure 1-15. Flow cytometry. A, Gating for lymphocytes (CD45 versus side scatter, linear scale [SS Lin]) shows the relative locations of granulocytes (Grans), monocytes (Monos), and lymphocytes (Lymphs) (*arrow*). **B,** Mantle cell lymphoma. Flow cytometric analysis of a lymph node specimen shows that nearly all of the lymphocytes express CD19, CD5, and kappa immunoglobulin light chains. A subset coexpresses FMC7, whereas the cells are negative for CD23. Expression of CD20 is not dim (data not shown). This immunophenotypic profile fits with involvement by mantle cell lymphoma. *(Courtesy of Michael R. Lewis, MD, MBA, Department of Pathology, University of Vermont/Fletcher Allen Health Care, Burlington, VT.)*

blood smears, or cytologic or cell culture samples. Tissues can be unstained or histochemically or immunohistochemically stained (chromogenic or fluorescence). A pulsed laser beam is targeted against the selected cells, which fuses them to the thermoplastic film. The cap is then removed from the tissue section surface and nucleic acids are recoverable from the cells adhered thereto after cell lysis treatments applied directly to the cap film

Applications

- Microdissection is primarily a research application, but it is useful in surgical pathology practice when there is a suspicion of patient sample cross-contamination.

Polymerase chain reaction (PCR)–based identity testing comparing the known patient sample with the queried tissue supports verification of a patient diagnosis

GEL ELECTROPHORESIS METHODS

Background

- Gel electrophoresis, as a method for separating, identifying, or purifying nucleic acids, was conceived in the mid-1960s by Vin Thorne at the Institute of Virology, Glasgow, UK, who was interested in analyzing different forms of the polyomavirus
- Nucleic acids are negatively charged at neutral pH due to the phosphate in the sugar-phosphate backbone of

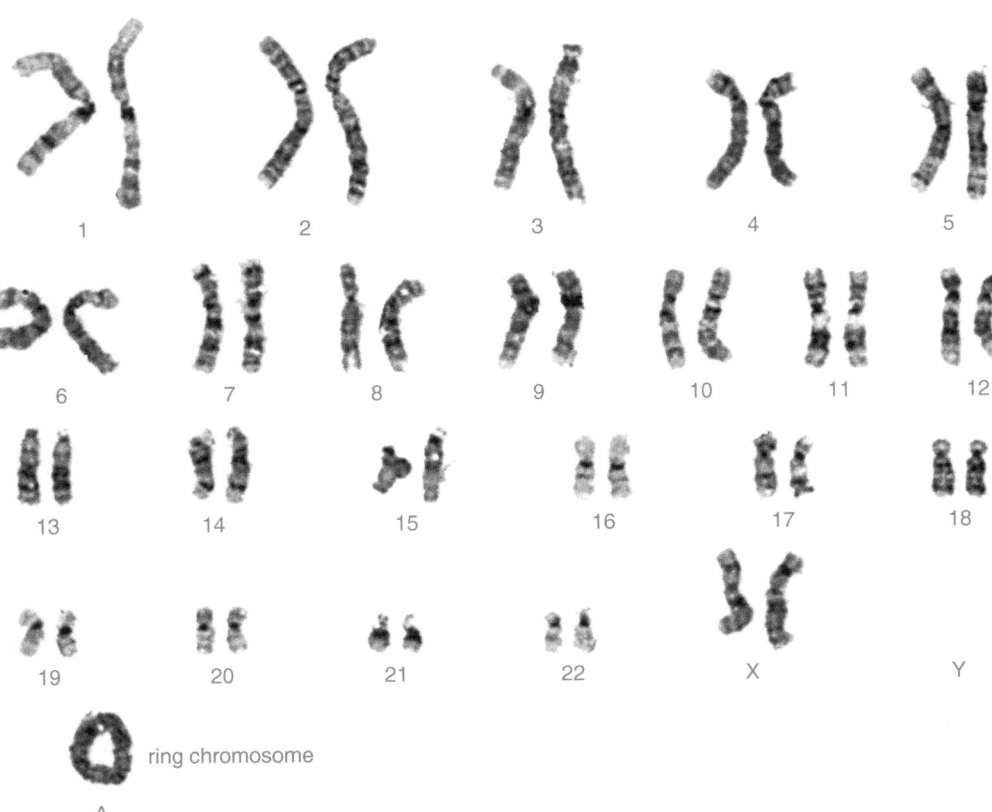

Figure 1-16. Well-differentiated liposarcoma. Karyotype analysis of a deep retroperitoneal lesion revealed a giant ring chromosome. *(Courtesy of Mary Tang, MD, Cytogenetic Laboratory, University of Vermont/Fletcher Allen Heath Care, Burlington, VT.)*

TABLE 1-37	ONCOGENES OF IMPORTANCE IN SURGICAL PATHOLOGY		
Category	**Proto-Oncogene**	**Mode of Activation/Location (Chromosome)**	**Association**
Signal Transduction Proteins			
Nonreceptor tyrosine kinase	*ABL*	Translocation/9q34	Chronic myeloid leukemia/acute lymphoblastic leukemia. t(9;22)(q34;q11) (Philadelphia chromosome) forming bcr-abl fusion protein
GTP-binding	*KRAS*	Point mutation/12p12	Colon, lung, pancreatic carcinomas
	NRAS	Point mutation/1p22	Melanomas, hematologic malignancies
	HRAS	Point mutation/11p15	Bladder and kidney tumors
RAS signal transduction	*BRAF*	Point mutation/7q34	Melanoma
WNT signal transduction	*Beta-catenin*	Point mutation	Hepatoblastomas, hepatocellular carcinoma
	bcl-1 (PRAD-1)	11q13	Parathyroid adenomatosis; mantle zone lymphomas with translocation to 14q32
	bcl-2	18q21	Block of apoptosis; translocation to 14q in follicular lymphomas
	bcl-6	3q27	Diffuse large cell lymphoma
Growth Factor Receptors			
	erbA	17	Erythroleukemia
	erbB1 (EGFR)	Overexpression/7p11-12	Squamous cell carcinoma of lung, gliomas
	neu (erbB2, HER-2)	Overexpression/17q11-12	Breast carcinoma, gastric and esophageal carcinoma
	KIT	Point mutation	Gastrointestinal stromal tumors, seminomas, leukemias
	PDGFRB	Overexpression, translocation	Gliomas, leukemias
	Ret	10q11.2	Medullary and papillary thyroid carcinomas
	FLT3	Amplification	Breast and ovarian carcinomas
Nuclear-Regulatory Proteins			
Transcriptional activators	*L-MYC*	Amplification/1p32	Small cell carcinoma of lung
	N-MYC	Amplification/2p23-24	Neuroblastoma, small cell carcinoma of lung
	C-MYC	Translocation/8q24	Burkitt lymphoma
Cell Cycle Regulators			
Cyclins	Cyclin D	Translocation	Mantle cell lymphoma
		Amplification	Breast and esophageal carcinomas
	Cyclin E	Overexpression	Breast carcinoma
Cyclin-dependent kinase	*CDK4*	Amplification or point mutation	Glioblastoma, melanoma, sarcoma

TABLE 1-38 TUMOR SUPPRESSOR GENES OF IMPORTANCE IN SURGICAL PATHOLOGY

Gene	Location (Chromosome)	Association
RB (retinoblastoma)	13q14	Retinoblastoma, childhood osteosarcoma
p53	17p13.1	Mutations in cancers of colon, breast, lung, leukemia, sarcoma; progression to diffuse large cell lymphoma (germline mutation of p53 forms the basis for Li-Fraumeni syndrome)
WT-1	11p13	Wilms tumor; desmoplastic small round cell tumor
EWS	22q12	Ewing/primitive neuroectodermal tumor, soft tissue clear cell sarcoma, desmoplastic small round cell tumor, myxoid liposarcoma, acute myelogenous leukemia
BRCA1 and BRCA2	17q21	Breast and ovarian carcinomas
APC/B-Catenin	5q21	Familial adenomatous polyposis coli; carcinomas of colon, stomach, pancreas
PTEN	10q23	Endometrial and prostate cancers/Cowden syndrome
NF1	17q11	Schwannomas, neuroblastomas, neurogenic sarcomas
NF2	22q12	Central schwannomas, meningiomas

TABLE 1-39 CYTOGENETIC ABNORMALITIES OF IMPORTANCE IN SURGICAL PATHOLOGY

Tumor	Chromosomal Abnormality	Fusion Transcript, Involved Genes
Hematopoietic Neoplasms		
Acute myelogenous leukemia (AML)		
—AML-M1	t(9;22)	*BCR-ABL*
—AML-M2	t(8;21) (favorable)	*CBFα-ETO*
—AML-M3	t(15;17)	*RARα/PML*
—AML-M4eo	inv(16) (favorable)	*CBFβ/MYH11*
Chronic myelogenous leukemia	t(9;22)(q34;q11)	*BCR-ABL*
B-cell acute lymphoblastic leukemia	t(12;21)	*CBFα-ETV6*
Chronic lymphocytic leukemia	Trisomy 12, deletions of 11q, 13q and 17p	
Burkitt lymphoma	t(8;14), t(8;22), t(4;8)	Involving *c-myc* and Ig loci
Follicular lymphoma	t(14;18)	*BCL2* gene
Mantle zone lymphoma	t(11;14)	*BCL1* (cyclin D1) and immunoglobulin H
Primitive Precursor Cell Neoplasms		
Ewing sarcoma/primitive neuroectodermal tumor	t(11;22)(q24;q12)	*EWS-FLI1* fusion
Medulloblastoma	del 17q	
Neuroblastoma	del 1p (poor prognosis); double minute chromosomes	*N-myc* amplification
Retinoblastoma	del 13q (band q14)	
Wilms tumor	del 11p (band p13)	
Epithelial Neoplasms		
Colorectal carcinoma	del 17p	
Mesothelioma	del of 1p, 3p, 22p	
Renal cell carcinoma (RCC)		
Clear cell carcinoma	del 3p	
Papillary RCC	Trisomy 7 and 17	
Chromophobe RCC	Loss of chromosome 1, 2, 6, or 10	
Oncocytoma	Loss of chromosome 1; translocation involving 11q13	
Small cell carcinoma	del 3p	
Soft Tissue Neoplasms		
Alveolar soft part sarcoma	t(X;17)(p11;q25)	*TFE3-ASPL* fusion
Chondrosarcoma, extraskeletal myxoid	t(9;22)(q22;q12)	*EWS-NR4A3* fusion
Clear cell sarcoma	t(12;22)(q13;q12)	*EWSR1-ATF1* fusion
Desmoplastic small round cell tumor	t(11;22)(q24;q12)	*EWSR1-WT-1* fusion
Dermatofibrosarcoma protuberans	Ring form of chromosomes 17 and 22	*COL1A1-PDGFB* fusion
Fibrosarcoma, infantile	t(12;15)(p13;q26)	*ETV6-NTRK3* fusion
Hibernoma	Translocation at 11q13	
Inflammatory myofibroblastic tumor	t(1;2)(q22;p23)	*TPM3-ALK* fusion
Leiomyoma	t(12;14), del 7q	
Leiomyosarcoma	del 1p	
Lipoma	Rearrangement of 12q15	*HMGIC* fusion
Liposarcoma (myxoid)	t(12;16)(q13;p11)	*TLS/CHOP*
Liposarcoma (well differentiated)	Ring chromosome 12	
Rhabdoid tumor	Deletion of 22q	*INI1* inactivation
Rhabdomyosarcoma (alveolar)	t(2;13)(q35;q14)	*PAX3-FKHR*
Rhabdomyosarcoma (embryonal)	Trisomies 2q, 8, and 20	
Synovial sarcoma	t(X;18)(p11;q11)	*SYT-SSX1/SYT-SSX2*
Central Nervous System Neoplasms		
Atypical teratoid rhabdoid tumor	Deletion of 22q	*INI1* inactivation
Oligodendroglioma	del 1p, 19q (improved response to chemotherapy)	
Schwannoma	Deletion of 22q	*NF-2* inactivation

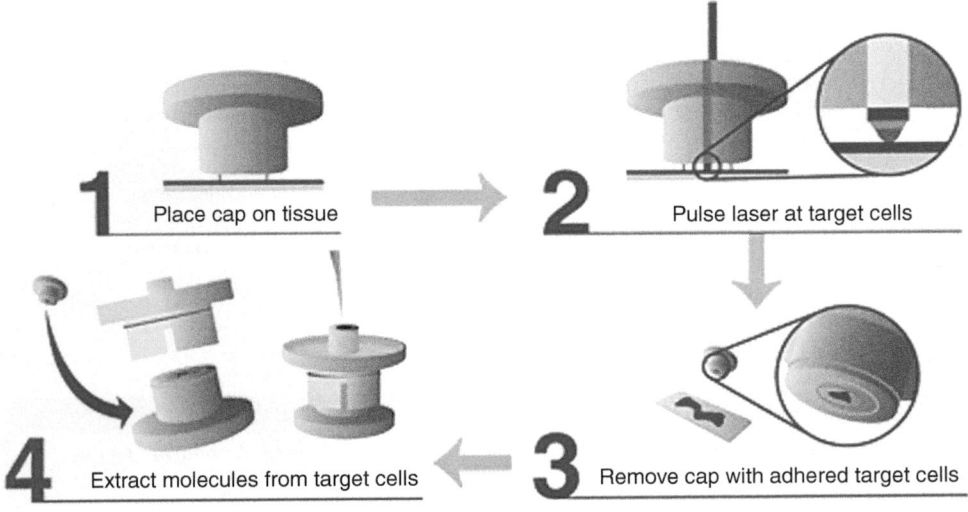

1 Place cap on tissue

2 Pulse laser at target cells

4 Extract molecules from target cells

3 Remove cap with adhered target cells

Figure 1-17. Laser capture technology. Target tissues are overlaid with a cap using microscope guidance. Cells are adhered to the thermoplastic film of the cap by laser pulsing. Lifting the cap removes the target cells for nucleic acids or protein extraction. *(Courtesy of Molecular Devices, Sunnyvale, CA.)*

DNA or RNA. Accordingly, in the presence of an electric field, nucleic acids will migrate from the cathode to the anode; migration through a sieving matrix (gel) depends on the size of the nucleic acid molecule, its conformation (secondary folding), net charge (dependent on the pH of the gel buffer), and pore size of the gel

- Agarose gel and polyacrylamide gel are the basic forms of electrophoresis. Variations on these methods include pulsed-field gel electrophoresis (PFGE), capillary gel electrophoresis (CGE), denaturing gradient gel electrophoresis (DGGE), and temperature gradient gel electrophoresis (TGGE)

Agarose Gel Electrophoresis

- Agarose is manufactured from seaweed such as Rhodophyta. It consists of multiple linked repeat units of the disaccharide agarobiose (D-galactose and 3,6-anhydro-L-galactose)
- Agarose gel is prepared by heating agarose powder to near boiling in electrophoresis buffer. The concentration of the agarose determines the gel pore size, which in turn determines the size range of DNA fragments that can be resolved. The higher the agarose concentration, the smaller the pore size. At low agarose concentrations, small DNA fragments pass rapidly through the gel and cannot be resolved, whereas large DNA molecules are size sorted; at high agarose concentrations, the mobility of large DNA molecules through the gel is limiting and large fragment sizes cannot be resolved, whereas the resistance to the passage of smaller fragments is sufficient for their resolution
  - A 0.5% agarose gel resolves DNA fragment sizes in the range ~0.7 to 25 kb
  - A 0.8% agarose gel resolves DNA fragment sizes in the range ~0.5 to 15 kb
  - A 1% agarose gel resolves DNA fragment sizes in the range ~0.4 to 10 kb
  - A 1.5% agarose gel resolves DNA fragment sizes in the range ~0.2 to 4 kb
  - A 2% agarose gel resolves DNA fragment sizes in the range ~0.05 to 2 kb
- The gel is poured into a horizontal casting tray and a comb is inserted at one end to mould wells

- When set, the "slab" gel is placed in an electrophoresis tank and immersed under electrophoresis buffer
- DNA sample is combined with a gel-loading dye. The loading dye (typically bromophenol blue containing sucrose and/or glycerol) ensures the DNA sample sinks into the well and indicates how far the samples have migrated during electrophoresis. Electrophoresis is generally conducted at 5 V/cm measured as the distance between the negative and positive electrodes
- A DNA ladder is also run so that sample DNA fragment sizes can be estimated
- DNA is most commonly visualized in agarose gels by staining with ethidium bromide, which intercalates double-stranded DNA and fluoresces under UV illumination. Less toxic (noncarcinogenic) alternatives to ethidium bromide, such as SYBR, EvaGreen, or GelStar dyes, stain DNA and with higher sensitivity
- Applications
  - Agarose gel electrophoresis is commonly used for the analysis of end-point PCR/reverse transcription (RT)–PCR assays where the presence or absence of amplicons defines the interpretation of the test; for example, the detection of a fusion transcript or a pathogen
  - The analysis of restriction fragment length polymorphism (RFLP) assays (see RFLP section) generally requires agarose gel electrophoresis
  - The technique is used routinely in molecular biology for the analysis of recombinant DNA experiments and can be used for the purification of probes for ISH and blot hybridization by excision of DNA fragments from a gel followed by minicolumn purification

Pulsed-Field Gel Electrophoresis (PFGE)

- PFGE is an electrophoretic method for the improved resolution of high molecular weight DNA. Standard agarose gel electrophoresis separates DNA under a constant and uniform electric field. Under these conditions, DNA >50 kb is poorly distinguished from DNA in the size range of 30 to 50 kb
- The improved resolution of PFGE is accomplished by alternating the direction of the electrical field. In the simplest approach, the direction of field is constantly

reversed so that the DNA spends some time moving backward. More refined techniques alternate the field so that the DNA moves through the gel in a zigzag pattern

- Applications
  - PFGE can be used for the identification of microorganismal strains such as *Escherichia coli* O157:H7, *Salmonella*, *Shigella*, *Listeria*, or *Campylobacter*. High-molecular-weight DNA extracts (from culture) are digested with a restriction enzyme (see the Southern blotting section). The PFGE electrophoretic DNA "fingerprint" helps identify the infective strain. The Centers for Disease Control and Prevention (CDC) maintain databases of PFGE standardized molecular subtypes for the identification of microorganisms
  - In combination with Southern blot analysis, PFGE can be used in the evaluation of autosomal dominant ataxia

Polyacrylamide Gel Electrophoresis

- Polyacrylamide is produced from monomers of acrylamide in a reaction initiated by free radicals generated by reduction of ammonium persulfate by TEMED (*N,N,N',N'*-tetramethylene diamine). These linear strands of polyacrylamide form into a gel after cross-linkage by *N,N'*-methylenebisacrylamide. The higher the concentration of acrylamide the finer the resolution of DNA fragments. The advantage of polyacrylamide over agarose is that size differences at the base pair bases can be distinguished
  - A 5% polyacrylamide gel resolves DNA fragment sizes in the range ~80 – 500 bp
  - An 8% polyacrylamide gel resolves DNA fragment sizes in the range ~60 – 400 bp
  - A 12% polyacrylamide gel resolves DNA fragment sizes in the range ~40 – 200 bp
  - A 15% polyacrylamide gel resolves DNA fragment sizes in the range ~25 – 150 bp
- Polyacrylamide "slab" gels are set between glass plates and run under a buffer in a vertical gel apparatus. Samples and DNA ladder plus loading dye, are loaded into wells and DNA fragment progression is estimated from the dye migration
- Polyacrylamide gels may be stained for DNA with ethidium bromide, SYBR dyes and the like, or silver nitrate. PCR amplicons can be detected by autoradiography when one primer is labeled with a radioisotope; the gel is dried then fastened with an x-ray film in a cassette. Gel/image analysis apparatuses fitted with a laser-induced fluorescence (LIF) detector can be used to analyze PCR amplicons that include a fluorophore-labeled primer
- Applications
  - End-point PCR fragment analysis where fragment size differences are slight
  - The discrimination of PCR fragments of identical size (bp) but containing different sequences (mutations or variants) can be performed by several polyacrylamide gel–based techniques, including single-stranded conformational polymorphism (SSCP) analysis, and denaturing gradient gel electrophoresis (DGGE)
    - The SSCP assay combines PCR with polyacrylamide gel electrophoresis. PCR is performed on a known normal/wild-type sample and on a test sample. The amplicons are rendered single-stranded and are then subjected to polyacrylamide gel electrophoresis under native (nondenaturing) conditions; the single-strand amplicons fold into conformations dependent on sequence-specific intramolecular base-pairing. Migration of DNA through the gel is dependent on size, charge, and conformation. The presence of a mutant sequence may significantly alter single strand-folding resulting in an altered migration relative to the normal control. The assay can be used for any mutant screening test (e.g., for *BRCA1* mutations in breast cancer)
    - The DGGE technique requires the formation of a gel containing a "denaturing" gradient. The gradient is created by combining two solutions (polyacrylamide reagents plus denaturants [formamide and urea]) during the pouring of the gel. The result is a gel with an increasing concentration of denaturants from the cathode to anode. In TGGE, a heat gradient is established using a specialized gel apparatus. As DNA migrates to the anode it encounters the denaturing gradient. The first regions of the PCR amplicons to denature will be those with a high A+T (adenine and thymine) base content as the A:T base pair are bound by two hydrogen bonds. The last to denature will be those high in G+C (guanine and cytosine) content due to G:C sharing three hydrogen bonds (this effect is sometimes referred to as the GC clamp). The formation of melted "domains" retards the migration of DNA fragments through the gel; normal and variant/mutated sequences may then be distinguished after gel staining on the basis of altered patterns of migration through the gel when the altered base affects domain melting. The power of the technique to detect altered sequences can be improved by comparing band gel migration of a "normal" control, the "abnormal" sample, and a "normal/abnormal" (heteroduplex) hybrid. This technique has the potential for application in mutation screening application (e.g., cystic fibrosis *CTFR* mutation screening)
  - Polyacrylamide slab gels are used for sequencing assays and for microsatellite marker-based assays using autoradiography or fluorescently labeled fragments

Capillary Gel Electrophoresis

- Capillary gel electrophoresis supports automated DNA sequencing and fragment analyses
- The technique involves the electrophoresis of DNA molecules through a solution phase polyacrylamide-based gel matrix contained within a 20- to 50-inch silica capillary with a 25- to 100-μm bore
- Proximal to the anode end of the capillary is a LIF detector. The light emissions from fluorescence labeled DNA fragments (e.g., by way of PCR using a fluorescence-labeled primer) are registered by the LIF detector, which can detect up to four different emission wavelengths
- Given the LIF detector location, all DNA fragments are sieved through the complete length of gel prior to detection. This supports the accumulation of data having high resolution; single base differences can be distinguished. Emission data are recorded using dedicated computer software that integrates the data collected

during the time course of the electrophoresis. The final data are presented in terms of peak heights and areas (relative to a fluorescence emissions scale [representing DNA amplicons/fragments]) and with reference to a DNA size marker

- Applications
  - Capillary gel electrophoresis is widely used for sequencing and microsatellite assay data analyses

BLOT HYBRIDIZATION METHODS

Southern Blotting

- Background
  - Dr. E.M. Southern developed the Southern blot technique in 1975 as a method for transferring DNA out of an agarose slab gel onto a solid support (a nitrocellulose or nylon membrane)
  - The method involves the use of restriction endonucleases to cut (restrict) genomic DNA into differently sized fragments that are size-fractionated by gel electrophoresis. After transfer, the membrane is hybridized with a labeled probe specific to the target sequence of interest
  - Can be used to detect chromosomal rearrangements, DNA amplifications, deletions, loss of heterozygosity, and to assess clonal status
  - The technique (Figure 1-20, presented later in the chapter) generally requires relatively large quantities of high-molecular-weight DNA (5 to $10\,\mu g$ per restriction endonuclease treated sample)
- Applications
  - The Southern blot method is widely used in restriction fragment length polymorphism (RFLP) applications. The number of restriction sites for a given restriction endonuclease in the site of a gene may vary because of normal (polymorphic) variation between individuals or due to sequence mutations. These differences can result in altered restriction fragment patterns. Altered fragment sizes between individuals may also result when the restriction fragment contains a variable number of tandem repeat (VNTR) sequences. VNTR regions contain microsatellite or minisatellite repeats comprising $\sim < 6\,bp$ or ~ 10 to $100\,bp$ repeat sequences, respectively. Differences in the number of these repeat units may be detectable as altered fragment sizes (see Figure 1-8). The size differences may be simple polymorphisms or can reflect a disease condition. For example, the $(CGG)_n$ microsatellite trinucleotide in the *FMR1* gene is repeated ~ 5 to 44 times among normal individuals, whereas in patients with Fragile X syndrome the number of repeats is expanded > 230 up to 1000s of times. The detection of this expansion by Southern blot analysis also involves the use of a methylation-sensitive restriction endonuclease that fails to cut a restriction site that is unmethylated in normal individuals but methylated in Fragile X syndrome patients
  - Despite the requirement for relatively large quantities of DNA and time-consuming procedures, Southern blotting may have advantages over PCR in certain applications. For example, when available sequence data are insufficient to design PCR primers specific to the site of a chromosomal rearrangement or where competition from normal cells in a sample will mask the detection of an anomaly by PCR
  - The detection of clonality by Ig gene rearrangements in B-cell lymphoproliferative disorders can aid the diagnosis of minimal residual disease. PCR tests for B-cell clonality may have a false-negative rate of up to 30%, and the gold standard test for the detection of Ig clonal rearrangements may be Southern blot analysis. Clonality can be inferred from a comparison of normal and B cell tumor tissue restriction fragment sizes following hybridization with a region of the Ig gene. The normal sample will demonstrate a single band representing the germline Ig gene, whereas a B-cell tumor also demonstrates a unique band size as a consequence of gene rearrangement and altered restriction site position(s)
  - Southern blotting can also have an advantage over PCR in the detection of Fragile X syndrome. PCR can be used in this diagnosis by designing primers that include the $(CGG)_n$ repeat unit within the amplicon. However, especially when the expansion involves hundreds to thousands of (CGG) repeats, PCR amplification can be problematic and may fail
  - Southern blotting can be combined with PCR. Hybridization with a target-specific probe can be used to confirm PCR amplicons represent the target and are not anomalous products resulting from incidental primer annealing events. PCR amplicon RFLP analyses may also be performed by Southern blotting
  - Examples of Southern blot clinical applications include the following:
    - Autosomal dominant ataxia evaluation (in combination with PFGE)
    - Beckwith-Wiedemann syndrome
    - Myotonic dystrophy evaluation
    - EBV clonality assay
    - Fragile X syndrome
    - Hemophilia A analysis for inversion, deletion and carrier
    - Immunoglobulin gene rearrangement
    - *MLH1* deletion/duplication screen
    - *MSH2* deletion/duplication screen
    - *MSH6* deletion/duplication screen
    - Partial DMD deletion/duplication assay (females only)
    - T-cell receptor gene rearrangement
    - Alpha-globin gene analysis (PCR/Southern blot deletion assay as part of a thalassemia and hemoglobinopathy evaluation test panel)

Northern Blotting

- Northern blotting is used in the analysis of mRNA expression. mRNA constitutes up to 5% of the total cellular RNA. Extracted mRNA is denatured with formaldehyde or glyoxal to prevent the formation of secondary RNA structures. Digestion of the RNA into smaller fragments is not required as native mRNA fragment sizes range from ~ 300 to $\sim 12,000$ nucleotides; the average size is 1000 to 3000 nucleotides. Following agarose gel electrophoresis, RNA is transferred to a membrane by a capillary, vacuum, or electrotransfer process and the membrane is hybridized with a labeled probe to the gene target. The resulting data indicate whether the gene is over- or underexpressed, or if an abnormally sized transcript is expressed. The method requires relatively large amounts of high integrity RNA, is time consuming, and requires a high level of laboratory skill, all of which limits the clinical utility of northern blotting

Dot Blotting

• Dot blot hybridization involves spotting denatured DNA or RNA onto a membrane for hybridization with a labeled probe. The method allows confirmation that a genomic DNA or RNA sample or a PCR product is positive for the probe target. The method can also be used semiquantitatively to assess or compare target sequence load within a sample
• Reverse-line dot blot hybridization
  • An alternative approach to the standard dot-blot is to fix an array of unlabeled probes onto the membrane and hybridize this with labeled nucleic acids/ PCR products
  • Applications
    • A variety of "line probe assays" (LiPA) have been developed. These include screening tests for ApoE mutations, cystic fibrosis mutations, HBV and HPV genotyping, HLA typing, and mycobacteria detection
    • Outside the United States, Conformité Européenne (CE) marked LiPA tests are available for PCR-based HPV clinical screening
      • The SPF$_{10}$-INNO LiPA Human Papillomavirus (HPV) Genotyping Test (Innogenetics, Ghent, Belgium) allows the specific genotyping of 25 different HPV types
      • The Roche Linear Array (LA) HPV genotyping test (Roche Molecular Systems, Inc., Branchburg, NJ) detects 37 different HPV types
      • With both systems, biotinylated PCR product is hybridized with a membrane strip affixed with a line of HPV genotype-specific probes. Detection of the PCR product label indicates the HPV genotype(s) for which the patient is positive

AMPLIFICATION METHODS

The Polymerase Chain Reaction (PCR)

• Background
  • PCR (Figure 1-18) is a method for the in vitro amplification of DNA involving automated cycles of denaturation, annealing, and extension/synthesis performed in a thermocycler
  • End-point PCR (first-generation PCR) consists of performing 30 to 50 cycles of amplification followed by analysis of the PCR product
  • In real-time quantitative PCR (second-generation PCR) continuous cycle-by-cycle monitoring of product accumulation is performed by measuring fluorescent signal generated from the amplicons

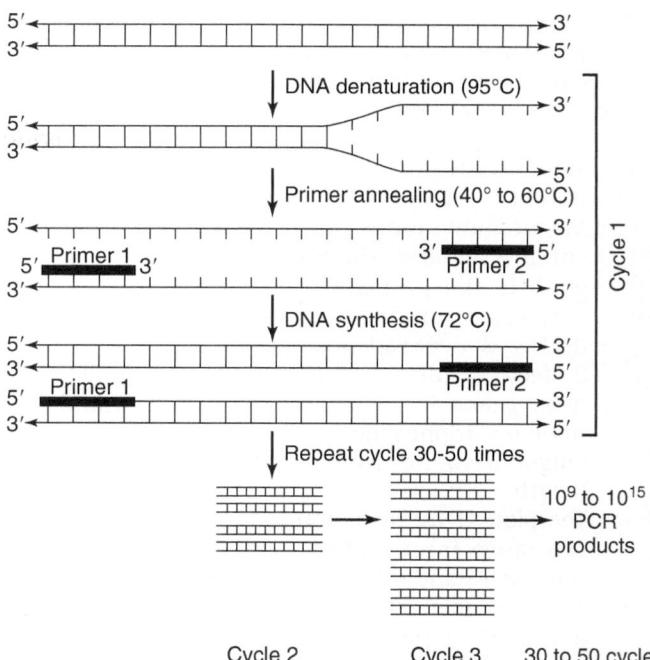

Figure 1-18. Polymerase chain reaction (PCR). A PCR cycle consists of denaturation, primer annealing, and DNA synthesis or extension steps. Following the first PCR cycle, there is (theoretically) a per-cycle doubling in the number of copies of the PCR product. *(Modified from Leonard DGB [ed]: Diagnostic Molecular Pathology. Philadelphia, WB Saunders, 2003.)*

  • In digital PCR (third-generation PCR) ~40 cycles of PCR are performed on a reaction tube containing 20,000 droplet partitioned reactions; each droplet is then assessed individually for fluorescent signal generated from PCR amplicons
• Basic PCR method
  • During the denaturation stage, sample specimen DNA is rendered to a single-stranded form by heating to 94° to 98°C
  • In the annealing step, oligonucleotide primers hybridize with the target sequences they have been designed to complement. The annealing temperature depends on the deoxyribonucleoside triphosphate (dNTP) composition of the primers and is typically in the 40° to 60°C range
  • During the extension step (72°C), the annealed primer/target DNA seeds the (5′→3′) synthesis by thermostable DNA polymerase of a new DNA strand
  • DNA amplification is accomplished by repetition of the denaturation, annealing, and extension cycle, 30 to 50 more times
  • The time period for each of the denaturation, annealing, and extension steps can vary from 10 seconds to > 1 minute and depends on reaction volume size, amplicon base composition and length, thermostable DNA polymerase activity (~1000 bp are extended per minute), and thermal cycler hardware specifications
  • The essential ingredients in a PCR include the following:
    • DNase/RNase free pure water: final PCR reaction volumes typically vary from 10 μl to 50 μl

- Buffer: pH is typically maintained using a Tris-HCl based buffer. Other ingredients include KCl, which can aid primer template annealing (K$^+$ ions offset the repulsive force between negatively DNA strands), non-ionic detergents, and bovine serum albumin (BSA) to aid Taq DNA polymerase enzyme stability
- Magnesium cations: Mg^{2+} is an essential ingredient and stabilizes the interaction between the oligonucleotide primer, template DNA, and Taq DNA polymerase enzyme
- dNTPs: 2'-deoxyadenosine 5'-triphophate (dATP), 2'-deoxycytidine 5'-triphosphate (dCTP), 2'-deoxyguanosine 5'-triphosphate (dGTP), and thymidine 5'-triphosphate (TTP also referred to as dTTP)
- Oligonucleotide primers: typically 18 to 25 bases in length
- Template DNA: the amount of sample in a reaction can range from 1 ng to 1 µg, with ~100 ng representing a standard quantity for many applications
- Thermostable DNA polymerase enzymes such as *Taq* DNA polymerase extracted from *Thermus aquaticus* isolated from a hot-springs dwelling bacterium of the Deinococcus-Thermus phylum
- PCR efficiency
  - Optimization experiments are required to ensure PCR test efficiency approaches ideal efficiency and to avoid false-negative data. Potentially, each component of the PCR setup can be manipulated for improved PCR sensitivity and specificity

PCR Contamination Control

- The sensitivity of PCR incurs the potential defect of false-positive data due to the amplification of cross-contaminating DNA from an exogenous source. Strict measures are required from patient sample collection through to PCR assay to ensure authentic data and to avoid false-positive data
- Ideally, laboratory space should be arranged such that DNA sample extraction, PCR setup, and post PCR manipulations all occur in physically distinct areas, and utilizing PCR-grade reagent aliquots, dedicated equipment, and laboratory coats specific for each area. PCR products from previous rounds of PCR represent the major potential source for contamination

PCR Method Variations

- PCR technique is a highly adaptable technique, enabling its applicability in a wide range of research and clinical niches
- Modifications centered on primer design/usage:
  - *Multiplex PCR* supports the simultaneous detection of more than one target by the use of multiple primer pair sets
  - *Consensus PCR* can be used to amplify a single target that has variable sequences or multiple targets that have similar (common) sequences
  - *Degenerate PCR* is also used in the amplification of a variable sequence target and involves a primer design that incorporates alternative sequences at a particular primer base sequence

- *Nested PCR* is a method for improved PCR sensitivity and specificity. Standard PCR is performed; the PCR product obtained is then used as DNA template for a second round of PCR with nested primers
- Amplification refractory mutation system (ARMS)/Allele-specific PCR (AS-PCR)/PCR amplification of specific alleles (PASA) supports sequence-specific PCR by designing the 3'-base at the end of a primer to match critical target
- LA PCR stands for long and accurate PCR and allows the amplification of sequences 5 to >20 kb in length

Reverse Transcription (RT) PCR

- RT-PCR (Figure 1-19) allows the investigation of RNA expression via PCR. Thermostable DNA polymerases require DNA as a substrate; the first step in RT PCR is thus the conversion of (DNA-free) total RNA or mRNA into single-stranded complementary DNA (cDNA). The two most commonly used reverse transcriptase enzymes are the avian myeloblastoma virus (AMV) or Moloney murine leukemia virus (M-MuLV) reverse transcriptases
- In addition to the general determinants of standard PCR success, RT-PCR efficiency depends on RNA sample quality and the effectiveness of the reverse transcriptase step

Real-Time Quantitative (q) PCR

- In end-point PCR, the final product obtained after 30 to 50 PCR cycles is the object of data interpretation. Although end-point PCR can be semiquantitative, it is essentially a qualitative assay. QPCR is used for the accurate quantification of a DNA or RNA (via cDNA) target in a sample. Fluorescent dyes or amplicon-specific probes are used to monitor amplicon accumulation at each cycle of PCR

Digital PCR

- Digital PCR (dPCR) or droplet digital PCR (ddPCR) is the latest development in PCR technology. The technique allows absolute quantification of a target sequence. This is in contrast to QPCR, where the quantification is relative to standard curve data derived from assays preformed using known amounts of target copies
- The procedure involves setting up a 20 µL PCR, which is then partitioned into 20,000 droplets (i.e., 20,000 self-contained individual PCRs in one tube). Target and nontarget sequences are randomly distributed among the droplets. After 40 cycles of PCR, droplets are analyzed one by one for the detection of fluorescence released by an amplicon. The fraction of fluorescence positive droplets supports quantification calculation based on Poisson distribution analyses
- The technique enables the highest analytic sensitivity of any molecular method allowing the detection of rare targets in a complex background with sensitivity down to one target copy in 10^{15} bases. DPCR has been used to confirm rare cases of HIV clearance in individuals previously diagnosed as HIV positive. The method can also be used to investigate copy number variation, mutation detection, and gene expression

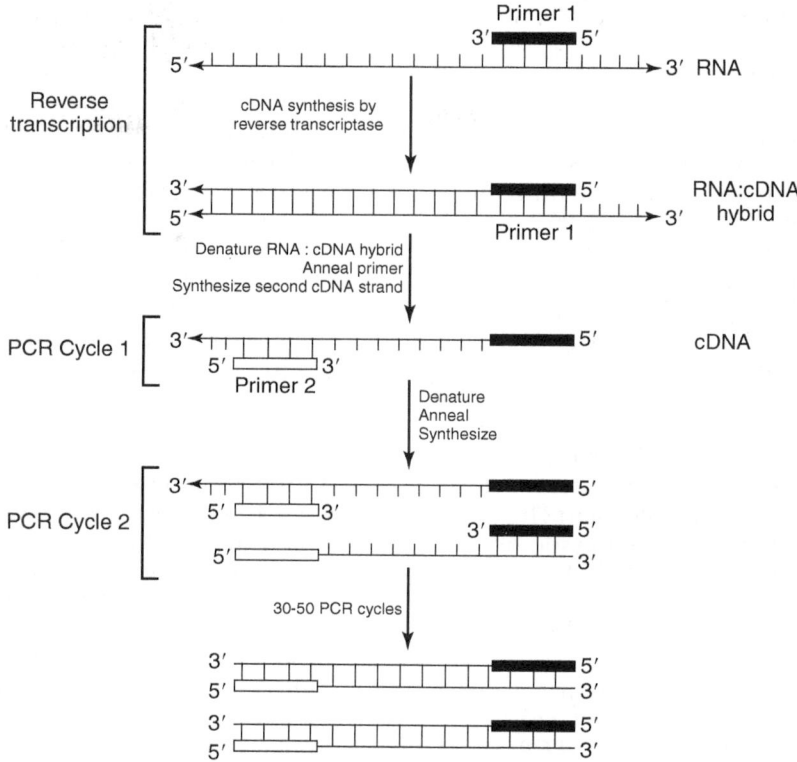

Figure 1-19. Reverse transcription polymerase chain reaction (RT-PCR). Complementary DNA (cDNA) is synthesized from an RNA sample by a reverse transcriptase enzyme; thereafter, the cDNA is available for PCR amplification. *(Modified from Leonard DGB [ed]: Diagnostic Molecular Pathology. Philadelphia, WB Saunders, 2003.)*

PCR Tests in Pathology Practice

- PCR is highly adaptable for use in a wide variety of clinical applications including the following:
  - Infectious pathogens detection
  - Genetic diseases diagnosis
  - Hematologic diseases diagnosis (e.g., chimeric RNA transcripts detection such as the bcr-abl translocation product characteristic of chronic myelogenous leukemia)
  - Sarcoma diagnosis by signature gene fusion detection (e.g., *EWS/FLI1* in Ewing sarcoma/peripheral neuroectodermal tumor)
  - Solid tumor characterization (e.g., HNPCC/Lynch syndrome mutation analyses)
  - Identity testing
  - Detection of circulating tumor or pathogen nucleic acid signatures
- PCR-based tests that have been approved and cleared by the U.S. Food and Drug Administration (FDA) include assays for avian flu (qRT-PCR), *Bacillus anthracis* (qPCR), *Chlamydia trachomatis*, warfarin sensitivity (qPCR), enteroviral meningitis (qRT-PCR), *Francisella tularensis* (qPCR), HBV, HCV, HLA typing, MRSA screening (qPCR), West Nile virus (qPCR), and *Yersinia pestis* (qPCR)
- There are also many non-FDA approved tests in widespread clinical diagnostics usage including the following:
  - Infectious pathogen detection
    - Adenovirus (qPCR), *Bartonella henselae*, BK virus, cytomegalovirus, enterovirus, hepatitis B virus, HHV-6, human metapneumovirus (hMPV), JC

virus, *Legionella* RNA, Lyme disease, malaria, parvovirus B19, varicella-zoster virus
  - Genetic diseases diagnosis
    - Bloom syndrome mutation analysis, Fabry disease known mutation factor IX gene known mutation familial amyloidosis DNA sequence, familial dysautonomia, Fragile X syndrome, Gaucher disease, mutation Fanconi anemia, mutation analysis, galactosemia gene analysis, hemochromatosis, Prader Willi/Angelman, spinobulbar muscular atrophy, Tay-Sachs disease
  - Tumor characterization/diagnosis
    - BCR/ABL (qRT-PCR), DSRCT (RT-PCR), Ewing sarcoma (RT-PCR), HNPCC, JAK2 V617F mutation detection, microsatellite instability, PML/RARA (qPCR), RET/PTC rearrangements (RT-PCR), synovial sarcoma (RT-PCR)
    - The Oncotype DX breast cancer assay is a qRT-PCR array test that screens 21 genes (16 tumor-related genes, 5 reference genes). The test is applicable to patients with stage I, II, or IIIa invasive breast cancer that is estrogen-receptor positive (ER+) and human epidermal growth factor receptor negative (HER2-). Based on the gene expression profile, a recurrence score (RS) is calculated indicating prognosis and treatment path. The Oncotype DX DCIS test screens for 7 cancer-related and 5 reference genes. Oncotype DX prognostic tests are also available for colon and prostate cancer.

- Several automated platforms incorporate PCR amplification steps
  - Roche COBAS 4800 system performs automated DNA extraction and is capable of multiplex PCR (using TaqMan fluorescent probes); for example, the FDA-approved COBAS HPV test performs a threefold screening assay: HPV-16, HPV-18, and 12 other high-risk HPV types; additionally, a β-globin PCR assay is performed to confirm amplifiable quality DNA was extracted from a patient sample. COBAS platforms are also available for HBV, HCV, and HIV detection
  - Luminex xTAG technology combines multiplex PCR, followed by multiplexed primer extension assays that incorporates labeled dNTPs. The extended products are captured on fluorescent microspheres. Coincident dual detection of the microsphere and extension product fluorescent signatures confirms detection of a given target in a specimen. The methodology is FDA cleared for screening cystic fibrosis, respiratory viruses, gastrointestinal pathogens and for polymorphisms associated with CYP2D6 drug metabolism and has also been developed for numerous other applications
  - AutoGenomics' BioFilmChip microarray assay multiplexes ARMS-type PCR of target sequences. Fluorescent dCTP is incorporated into PCR amplicons. A successfully amplified target is immobilized by sequence-specific capture probes embedded in a fluorescent-labeled hydrogel matrix. Coincident dual detection of the hydrogel and amplicon fluorescent signatures confirms detection of a given target in a specimen. The assay is FDA-cleared for CYP2C19 and warfarin metabolism sensitivity as well as for coagulation factor (Factor II, Factor V Leiden) assessments
  - The GenMark Dx eSensor XT-8 assay involves multiplex PCR of target sequences followed by incubation with exonuclease III, which results in single-stranded amplicon DNA. A hybridization reaction is then preformed with a ferrocene labeled probe; hybridization occurs if the target sequence has been amplified from the patient specimen. Next, the hybrid solution is pumped through a microfluidics cartridge containing a series of gold disk electrodes. Each electrode is tagged with a unique capture probe. Voltage is applied to the cartridge; a current will be detected at the electrode at which probe-hybridized-amplicon has been immobilized by the capture probe. The assay is FDA cleared for investigation of cystic fibrosis, respiratory viruses, thrombophilia, and warfarin sensitivity
- Several assays combine PCR with other molecular manipulations
  - Multiple Ligation-dependent Probe Amplification (MLPA) is a proprietary technology of MRC-Holland, Amsterdam, The Netherlands, that allows multiplex assaying of disease biomarkers
  - The technique involves two steps: ligation followed by PCR. First, denatured specimen DNA is hybridized overnight with multiple target-specific primer pairs; for example, primers could be specific for a variety of alternative mutations. If two oligonucleotides hybridize directly adjacent to each other, they can be ligated to form one continuous DNA molecule by the enzyme DNA ligase. At the 5'-end of the forward oligonucleotide is a universal PCR primer sequence "X" that does not hybridize to specimen DNA sequences. At the 3'-end of the reverse oligonucleotide is a second universal primer sequence "Y." This second primer also contains a nonhybridizing "stuffer sequence" of variable length intermediate between "Y" and the 5'-sequence that binds to target. The length of the "stuffer sequence" is linked to the specific target that the oligonucleotide can hybridize with. The total length of the first oligonucleotide is 50 to 60 bp and the second oligonucleotide is 60 to 450 bp in length; PCR amplified products range from 130 to 450 bp in length
  - PCR is then performed on the ligation product using two primers complementary to X and Y. The length of the PCR product will depend on which (if any) oligonucleotide pairs initially hybridized and were ligated; that is, the length of the "stuffer sequence" indicates which biomarket target was present in the sample
  - Applications
    - MLPA is applicable for the detection of mutations/SNPs, deletions, and amplifications. Nonamplification with a particular probe indicates the presence of a mutation, SNP, or deletion; "excess" amplification demonstrates an amplification event
    - MLPA tests (none are currently FDA cleared/approved) are available for the diagnosis of a large variety of pathologic conditions including these:
      - Familial cancers: ataxia telangiectasia, BRCA1 and BRCA2 testing, colon polyposis (APC), MLH1/MSH1/MSH2/MSH6/PMS2 testing, Li-Fraumeni syndrome, multiple endocrine neoplasia, neurofibromatosis types 1 and 2, Peutz-Jeghers syndrome, retinoblastoma, Von Hippel-Lindau syndrome, Wilms tumor
      - Tumor analyses: melanoma (Uveal), mismatch repair genes, neuroblastoma, oligodendroma, PTEN, rhabdoid tumors, tumor suppressor genes
      - Prenatal and postnatal screening: aneuploidy (Down, Edwards, Patau), mental retardation syndromes, microdeletion syndromes (Prader-Willi/Angelman; RETT/Xq28 duplication and others)
      - Pharmacogenetics: DPYD deficiency
      - Specific syndromes: cystic fibrosis, Turner/Klinefelter, typical uremic, Wilson disease
- PCR/oligonucleotide ligation assay (OLA)
  - Whereas MLPA involves an oligonucleotide ligation step followed by rounds of PCR, PCR/OLA involves multiplex PCR (up to 40 cycles) followed by cycles (up to 10) of multiplex ligation amplification of oligonucleotides to PCR product
  - PCR/OLA is FDA cleared for cystic fibrosis gene mutation panel screening (CELERA, Alameda, CA)

OTHER NUCLEIC ACID AMPLIFICATION METHODS

Transcription-Mediated Amplification (TMA)

- TMA supports the amplification of RNA targets, including species-specific ribosomal RNA (rRNA) sequences. The method involves an isothermal reaction containing the following ingredients:
  - RNA sample
  - A target specific "forward" primer with an RNA polymerase promoter sequence at the 5'-end
  - Reverse transcriptase (RT) with active RNase H activity (e.g., avian myeloblastosis virus reverse transcriptase [AMV-RT])
  - A target-specific "reverse" primer
  - RNA polymerase (e.g., SP6, T3, or T7 RNA polymerase)
- Applications
  - TMA is a proprietary technique of Gen-Probe, Inc. (San Diego, CA). FDA-cleared TMA tests are available for the detection of *Chlamydia trachomatis, Neisseria gonorrhoeae, Mycobacterium tuberculosis,* and *Streptococcus* infections. FDA-approved TMA assays for high-risk type HPV *E6/E7* RNA, for HCV, and for gastrointestinal infectious agents have also been developed. There is also an FDA-approved test for prostate cancer gene 3 (PROGENSA PCA3) mRNA detected from urine samples

Nucleic Acid Sequence-Based Amplification (NASBA)

- NASBA is an isothermal amplification technique and can be used for the amplification of a DNA or RNA target. The technique requires an initial heat denaturation step when DNA is the sample to render the target as single-stranded sequences
- The technique is essentially identical to TMA but uses a separate RNase H enzyme and FRET-based detection technology. NASBA amplifies its target by a factor of 10^9 in a 90-minute reaction at 41°C
  - Applications: FDA-rated NASBA assays have been developed by bioMérieux, Inc. (Durham, NC) for the detection of cytomegalovirus (CMV), enterovirus, and human immunodeficiency virus (HIV) RNA

Displacement Amplification

- Several amplification strategies have been developed for use with DNA polymerases that have "strand displacement" activity, e.g., Bst DNA polymerase, (derived from *Bacillus stearothermophilus*) or Phi29 DNA polymerase (derived from the *Bacillus subtilis* phage phi29 [Φ29])
  - As with other DNA polymerases, DNA is synthesized in the 5'→3' direction; unlike other polymerases having initiated DNA polymerization from an upstream primer binding site, these enzymes will displace a double-stranded DNA region resulting from synthesis initiated at a downstream region. This displacement property supports isothermal DNA amplification as it is not necessary to (cyclically) heat-denature DNA to produce a single-stranded template
  - Applications: Two of these approaches have FDA-cleared proprietary tests

- Strand displacement amplification (SDA) tests have been developed for the detection of *Chlamydia trachomatis, Neisseria gonorrhoeae,* and *Legionella pneumophila* (BD ProbeTec ET systems for each microorganism; Becton, Dickinson and Company, Sparks, MD)
  - The method involves generating a target-specific sequence using microorganism primers that also incorporate a restriction enzyme (RE) site into the polymerized product; exponential amplification of these targets follows triggered by nicks to the amplified DNA at the RE sites
  - In excess of 10^9 copies of the target may be produced within 15 minutes
- Loop mediated isothermal amplification (LAMP) tests are available for a wide range of targets including *Clostridium difficile,* groups A and B *Streptococcus,* and mycoplasma (Meridian Bioscience, Inc., Cincinnati, Ohio)
  - This self-contained complex isothermal reaction involves the judicious use of multiple primers resulting in the continuous generation of target-specific DNA structures. The pyrophosphate ions released during DNA synthesis bind to magnesium ions forming a white precipitate of magnesium pyrophosphate. The resultant turbidity is measured by assay instrumentation; the presence or absence of threshold turbidity indicates the infectious status of the patient sample

Helicase Dependent Amplification (HDA)

- HDA is an in vitro isothermal amplification technique that uses DNA helicase to unwind and separate double-stranded helix into single-stranded DNA (ssDNA). SsDNA-binding proteins (SSBs) included in the HDA reaction inhibit ssDNA reannealing and degradation. Sequence-specific primers (one labeled) hybridize with the target (if present), and DNA polymerase synthesizes a complementary strand. This dsDNA product is rendered single-stranded by the DNA helicase and so on, resulting in an exponential amplification cascade
- An FDA-approved test for HSV is available from BioHelix (Beverly, MA)

SIGNAL AMPLIFICATION TECHNIQUES

- The assays described earlier are based on the amplification of target nucleic acid sequences to a threshold of detection. Alternatively, an amplification signal can be generated from a DNA probe(s) hybridized to target sequences
- Signal amplification techniques may be less susceptible to false-positive data resulting from patient sample cross-contamination than methods generating multiple copies or target sequences

Branch DNA (bDNA)

- This method involves the capture of specimen RNA or DNA in a microtiter plate well, followed by a sequential four-step detection procedure
- Multiple "capture" probes specific to the sequence(s) of interest and lining the microwell hybridize and

bind the specimen RNA or denatured DNA. A set of "target" probes is then applied; part of each target probe hybridizes with the captured sequence. "Preamplifier" sequences are then added; these in turn partly hybridize with the target probe and an extended region is available to hybridize with multiple "amplifier" constructs applied following the preamplifier. Finally, alkaline phosphatase-labeled probes bind to the amplifier constructs. Alkaline phosphatase activity is demonstrated by chemiluminescence using a dioxetane substrate

- bDNA technology allows highly specific and quantitative nucleic acid assays
- Applications
  - FDA-approved bDNA tests are available for HCV and for HIV quantification (VERSANT HCV RNA 3.0 Assay and VERSANT HIV-1 RNA 3.0 Assay, respectively [Siemens Healthcare Diagnostics, Deerfield, IL]). bDNA research applications are available from Panomics, Inc. (Fremont, CA)

Invader Chemistry

- Invader chemistry (HOLOGIC, Bedford, MA) is a proprietary technique for the specific and accurate detection of single-base changes, insertions, deletions, and changes in gene and chromosome number
- The method involves two simultaneous isothermal reactions; a primary reaction detects the DNA target of interest and a second reaction generates detectable signal
- Invader chemistry can be adapted for combined use with PCR for even greater detection sensitivity
- Applications
  - An FDA–cleared Invader chemistry assay screens for 46 cystic fibrosis mutations (InPlex Molecular Test). An FDA-cleared assay is also available to identify patients homozygous for abnormal UDP glucuronosyltransferase 1A1 (UGT1A1) genes (Invader UGT1A1 Molecular Assay). Patients with seven instead of six TA repeats in the TATA box region of the gene metabolize the chemotherapeutic agent irinotecan (CAMPTOSAR, Pfizer Corporation) poorly and require lowered dosages to avoid a toxic response
  - An Invader assay for high-risk HPV genotype screening is awaiting FDA clearance/approval
- Mutation/variant screening Invader tests have been developed for Factor V Leiden, Factor II, methylenetetrahydrofolate reductase 677 (MTHRFR 677), MTHRFR 1298, cytochrome P450, and vitamin K genes. A kit to detect the six major hepatitis C virus genotypes is also available

Hybrid Capture

- The Hybrid Capture assay (QIAGEN, Germantown, MD) involves an in vitro solution hybridization of a target DNA sequence with an RNA probe, followed by a signal amplification step
- Applications
  - The *digene* HPV Test utilizes Hybrid Capture 2 (hc2) technology and is currently the only FDA-approved HPV screening assay

- The test screens for 13 high-risk HPV genotypes (16, 18, 31, 33, 35, 39, 45, 51, 52, 56, 58, 59, and 68)
  - The test requires the majority of cell samples remaining after routine cytology testing and has a detection sensitivity of 1000 to 5000 copies of HPV target per sample
- FDA-cleared hybrid capture assays are also available for the detection/quantitation of cytomegalovirus (CMV), *Chlamydia trachomatis,* and *Neisseria gonorrhoeae.* Assays are also available for hepatitis B virus (HBV) and herpes simplex virus (HSV)

Verigene Nanosphere

- The Verigene Nanosphere (Nanosphere, Inc., Northbrook, IL) proprietary instrumentation supports a range of FDA-cleared tests, including ones for respiratory viruses, gram-positive and gram-negative blood culture, *C. difficile*, *F5/F2/MTHFR*, warfarin metabolism, and *CYP2C19*
- Automated DNA extraction from patient samples is followed by sonication to fragment the DNA, which is then flowed through a cartridge containing target-specific capture probes. Gold "nanospheres" coated with sequence-specific probes are then flowed through the cartridge for hybridization to patient DNA immobilized by the capture sequences. Silver ions, hydroxyquinone, and an electric current are then passed through the cartridge. Silver ions are reduced to silver atoms on the surface of nanospheres localized to target sequences. The increase in nanosphere diameter due to silver deposition is detected by automated imaging of the cartridge, allowing inference of target detection
- The main advantages of this technique are its rapidity, minimal pipetting steps, and complete absence of any nucleic acid amplification

DNA MICROARRAY TECHNOLOGY

- DNA microarrays make up a solid support (a silicon chip) imprinted with sequence-specific oligonucleotide probes. Fluorescence-labeled sample DNA or cDNA is hybridized with the microarray, and the detected emissions demonstrate qualitatively or quantitatively the nucleic acid species present in the sample
- DNA microarrays can be used to examine gene expression by simultaneously hybridizing the array with cDNA from normal and diseased tissues; each cDNA preparation is labeled with a different fluorophore. Analysis of the intensities of the different labels demonstrates genes that are or under, over, or unchanged in expression
- A similar assay using labeled DNAs and chromosome-specific probes can be performed to infer chromosome losses or gains. DNA microarrays can also be used to screen for SNPs
- Potentially, thousands of sequences can be screened using a single microarray. Limited target (< 100) set arrays designed toward cell pathways (e.g., apoptosis, angiogenesis, cell cycle, cytokines, signal transduction), or tumor nucleic acid signatures, have also been developed
- Microarray assay affordability, standardization, and clinical interpretability are issues limiting clinical array applications

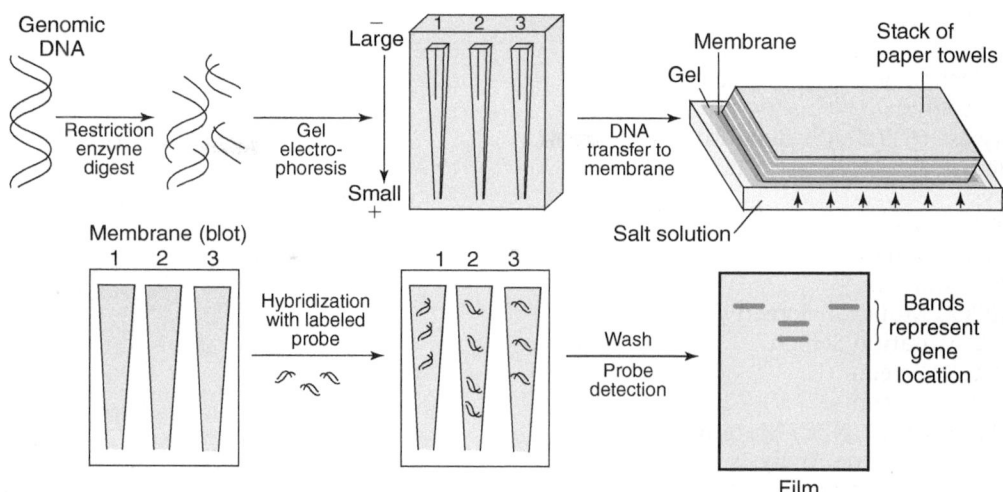

Figure 1-20. Southern blot analysis. Following agarose gel electrophoresis of restriction endonuclease-treated genomic DNA, alkali-denatured DNA is transferred onto a nylon membrane by capillary action. The recovered membrane is screened for target sequences by hybridization with a labeled probe. *(Modified from Leonard DGB [ed]: Diagnostic Molecular Pathology. Philadelphia, WB Saunders, 2003.)*

- Applications
  - There are two FDA-cleared microarray tests; each requires fresh tumor tissue samples
  - The MammPrint test (Agendia, Inc., Irvine, CA) screens 70 genes to assess the likelihood of recurrence in patients who have undergone breast cancer surgery. The expressed gene data indicate patients who are at high- or low-risk of disease recurrence. The test is applicable to lymph node negative patients under 61 years of age with stage 1 or 2 tumors ≤ 5 cm.
- The Pathwork Tissue of Origin Test (Pathwork Diagnostics, Sunnyvale, CA) aids identification of the origin of a tumor. The test measures the expression pattern of more than 1500 genes in the "uncertain" tumor. This pattern is compared to expression patterns of a panel of 15 known tumor types, representing 60 morphologies overall. An objective, probability-based score is generated relative to each of the 15 potential tumor types supporting assignment or exclusion of the uncertain tumor to each panel type

NUCLEIC ACID SEQUENCING

- The most widely used nucleic acid sequencing technique has been the chain termination method originated by Frederic Sanger in the mid-1970s. This technique has since been adapted to include PCR technology and fluorescently labeled nucleotides leading to the development of dye terminator sequencing that allows routine automated sequence analyses

- Dye terminator sequencing involves a reaction that includes the DNA sample, one PCR primer specific to the target area, DNA polymerase, the four regular dNTPs, and four dideoxynucleotides (ddNTPs [ddATP, ddGTP, ddCTP, and ddTTP]). Each ddNTPs is labeled with a different fluorophore. ddNPTs are like regular DNA but lack a 3'-hydroxyl group. This means that once a ddNTP has been incorporated into a nascent DNA strand, no further extension is possible because the hydroxyl group is missing to form a 3'-5' phosphodiester linkage with a distal nucleotide. The proportion of dNTPs and ddNTPs in the reaction mix ensures that DNA fragments are generated representing all possible lengths of the target and typically yielding sequence order data for up to ~700 nucleotides. The generated fragments are sieved by capillary gel electrophoresis. ddNTP fluorophore emissions are detected as the fragments pass through the gel revealing the base sequence order (Figure 1-21)
- Applications
  - DNA sequencing represents the gold standard confirmation of a mutation. However, the detection of a mutation may be compromised in heterogeneous samples (e.g., tumor cells in a high background of normal cells). Pyrosequencing techniques (Pyrosequencing, Inc., Westborough, MA) may overcome this potential defect by allowing the simultaneous detection of mixed genotypes within a sample
  - Clinical applications generally involve PCR amplification of a defined target region followed by sequencing; available tests include the following:

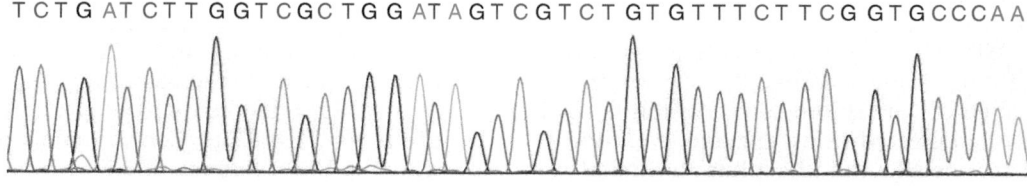

TCTG AT CTT GGT CGC TGG ATA GT CGT CT GT GTTTCT TCG GTGCCCAA

Figure 1-21. Electropherogram showing DNA sequencing data output.

- Autosomal Recessive Polycystic Kidney Disease (*ARPKD*) Mutation Screen
- Biotinidase Deficiency (*BTD*) Gene Analysis
- *CFTR* Gene Analysis
- 21-Hydroxylase (*CYP21A2*) Gene Analysis
- Dentatorubral-Pallidoluysian Atrophy (*DRPLA*) Gene Analysis
- Fabry Disease Gene Analysis
- Galactose-1-phosphate uridyltransferase gene (*GALT*) Gene Analysis
- *MLH1* HNPPCC Mutation Screen
- *MLH1/MLH2* Mutation Screen
- *MSH2* Mutation Screen
- *MSH6* Mutation Screen
- Niemann-Pick type C (NPC) Mutation Screen
- Progranulin (*GRN*) Gene Analysis
- Von Hippel-Lindau (*VHL*) Gene Analysis
- FDA-cleared sequencing assays are available for HIV drug resistance testing (ViroSeq HIV-1 Genotyping System, Celera Diagnostics, CA, and, TruGene HIV-1 Genotyping and Open Gene DNA Sequencing System, Siemens Healthcare Diagnostics, Deerfield, IL)
- Next-generation sequencing (NGS) platforms allow millions up to billions of sequences to be decoded in relatively short time periods (hours/days). The method involves shearing extracted genomic DNA or cDNA (size range ~500 ± bp) followed by primer ligation to the fragment ends. This fragment library is then amplified (e.g., by PCR) followed by massively parallel sequencing and alignment of the sequence reads
  - NGS was originally developed to facilitate whole genome sequencing. For pathology diagnostics, targeted sequencing assays are more appropriate and involve directing the assay to a subset of genes or defined regions in a genome. The main advantage over Sanger sequencing may be for the multiplex detection of minority aberrant sequences in high background of wild-type ones. Standard of care diagnostic applications for NGS are at the developmental stage
- NGS platforms include MiSeq/HiSeq (Illumina, San Diego, CA), SOLiD (Life Technologies, Carlsbad, CA), and 454 pyrosequencing (454 Life Sciences, a Roche company, Branford, CT)

IN SITU HYBRIDIZATION

- ISH enables the direct visualization of nucleic acid targets in relation to cytologic, histologic, or karyotypic features (Figure 1-22)
- ISH was first described in 1969 using radiolabeled probes and slide autoradiography to assess hybridization data. ISH methods employing ³H, ¹²⁵I, ³²P, ³³P, or ³⁵S labeled probes are still used in a research setting but are hazardous and may require long exposures
- Chromogenic ISH (CISH) techniques were developed during the 1980s using biotin, 2,4-dinitrophenyl (DNP), digoxigenin, or fluorescein hapten-labeled probes. Labels are detected using enzyme (e.g., horseradish peroxidase or alkaline phosphatase) linked reagents followed by a chromogenic substrate. Two label

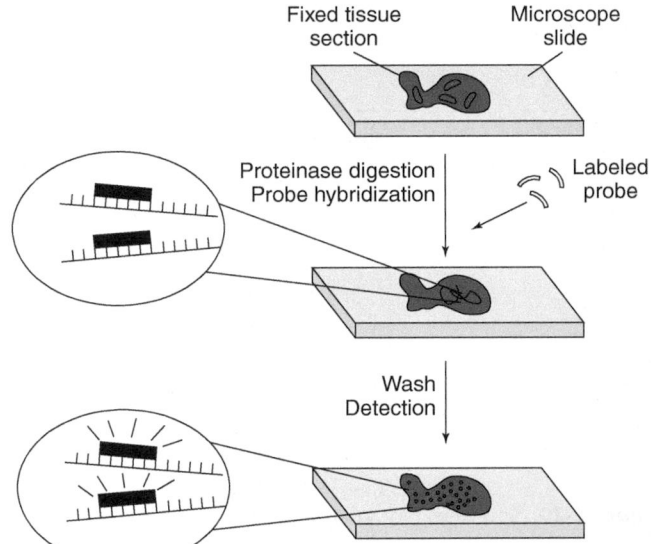

Figure 1-22. In situ hybridization (ISH). Slide-mounted tissues are pretreated/protease digested to facilitate labeled probe access to nucleic acid targets for hybridization. Chromogenic ISH involves the detection of a hapten-labeled probe with enzyme-labeled secondary reagents and a chromogenic substrate. Fluorescence ISH involves the use of fluorophore-labeled probes or fluorescence-labeled secondary detection reagents. *(Modified from Leonard DGB [ed]: Diagnostic Molecular Pathology. Philadelphia, WB Saunders, 2003.)*

CISH assays can be performed by combing two different labels with two different enzyme detection steps
- Metallographic ISH (MISH) methods include silver-enhanced in situ hybridization (SISH) and gold-facilitated in situ hybridization (GOLDFISH). MISH and CISH assays can be combined using two different hapten labels
  - SISH clinical assays are available as a proprietary formulation for Ventana Medical Systems, Inc. (Tucson, AZ). After hybridization and stringency washes, DNP-labeled probe is detected with rabbit antibody against DNP. A goat antirabbit antibody conjugated with horseradish peroxidase (HRP) is then applied followed by incubation with silver acetate, hydroquinone, and hydrogen peroxide: silver ions are reduced by hydroquinone to silver atoms by chemical interaction with HRP and hydrogen peroxide. Silver atoms are deposited at the site of probe hybridization and appear as black signals under microscopy
  - Combined SISH/CISH. The FDA-approved INFORM HER2 Dual ISH DNA Probe Cocktail (Ventana Medical Systems, Inc.) combines SISH with CISH for the dual color assessment of HER2 amplification. After hybridization with the dual probe (HER2 locus and centromeric region of chromosome 17 [Cen 17]), SISH is performed as above followed by detection of the digoxigenin-labeled Cen 17 probe by serial incubation with mouse antidig antibody, goat antimouse antibody conjugated with alkaline phosphatase followed by naphthol fast red chromogen. The assay allows the ratio of HER2 to Cen17 signals to be estimated allowing the inference of HER2 amplification status (Figure 1-23)

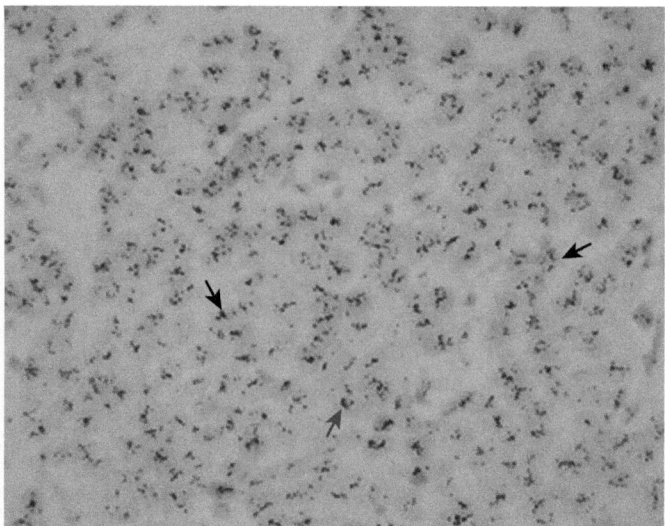

Figure 1-23. HER2 amplification in a breast carcinoma demonstrated using the INFORM HER2 Dual ISH DNA Probe Cocktail (Ventana Medical Systems, Inc.). The test combines a SISH assay to demonstrate HER2 amplification status (black signals) with CISH to demonstrate chromosome 17 centromeric signals *(red signals)*. *(Image courtesy of Dr Abiy Ambaye, MD, Pathology and Laboratory Medicine, Fletcher Allen Health Care, Burlington, VT.)*

- Fluorescence ISH (FISH)
  - FISH techniques can be practiced using fluorophore labeled nucleic acid probes or using fluorophore-labeled secondary reagents against hapten-labeled probes
  - FISH can be performed using multiple probes each labeled with a different fluorescent dye (Figure 1-24), which is the main advantage of FISH. Its main

disadvantage is that tissue morphology has to be interpreted on the basis of fluorescent counterstains, whereas CISH or MISH signals can be assessed in conjunction with hematoxylin counterstaining and bright field microscopy

- RNA in situ hybridization
  - RNA in situ hybridization (sometimes referred to as RISH) can be performed using isotopic or hapten-labeled oligonucleotide, plasmid probes, PCR generated probes, or riboprobes
  - The detection of low-copy RNA sequences has been facilitated by the development of a branched DNA (bDNA) type amplification adapted for use in ISH. The proprietary technology is independently marketed as RNAscope (Advanced Cell Diagnostics, Hayward, CA) and as QuantiGene ViewRNA (Affymetrix Panomics, Santa Clara, CA). Multiple oligoprobes are hybridized to target sequences. Preamplifier sequences are hybridized to the probes followed by amplifiers to the preamplifiers and the labeled probes to the amplifiers. The assay can be performed as a CISH or FISH test. RNAscope CISH for human papillomavirus (HPV) in cervical lesions is shown in Figure 1-25
- ISH is applicable to all pathology sample preparations including cytologic samples, primary cell cultures, chromosome spreads, FNAs, ThinPrep smears, frozen tissue sections, and FFPE specimens
- Applications
  - ISH techniques are amenable to a wide range of applications including investigation of genetic instability, gene amplification, gene expression, and chromosomal rearrangements. The extensive list of pathogens that can be detected by FISH includes cytomegalovirus, Epstein-Barr virus

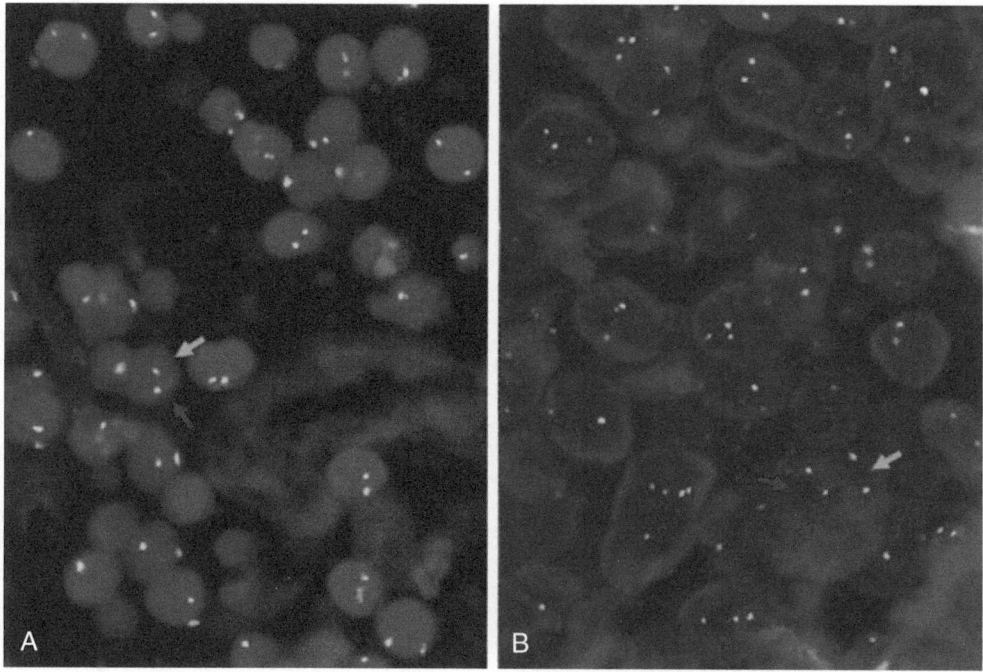

Figure 1-24. Fluorescence in situ hybridization (FISH). FISH assay (PathVysion, Abbott Molecular, Inc., Des Plaines, IL) of breast carcinoma tissues for *HER-2* gene amplification. Nonamplification **(A)** is indicated by a balanced ratio of green signals (chromosome 17 centromere) (*green arrows*) to orange signals (*HER-2* locus-specific probe [17q11.2-q12]; *red arrows*). Amplification **(B)** is indicated by a relative excess of *HER-2* signals.

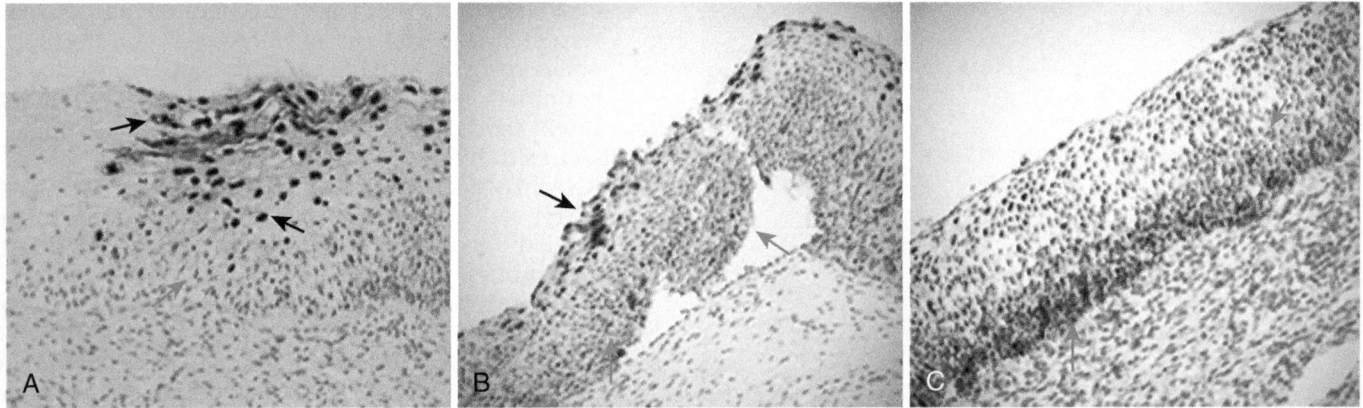

Figure 1-25. HPV *E6/E7* RNA demonstrated in CIN I **(A)**, CIN II **(B)**, and CIN III **(C)** by RNAscope CISH (Advanced Cell Diagnostics, Hayward, CA). Diffusely stained nuclei *(black arrows)* indicative of productive phase HPV infections are present in the superficial layers of CIN I and II lesions but are relatively absent in CIN III, which is characterized by the detection of fine dotlike nuclear and cytoplasmic signals throughout the epithelial layer *(blue arrows)*.

(DNA or mRNA), hepatitis C viral RNA, herpes simplex virus, human papillomavirus (Figure 1-25 and Figure 1-26), hantavirus, influenza virus, parvovirus B19, and varicella zoster. FISH is used in the diagnosis of diverse hematologic and sarcomatoid disorders, in the diagnosis of breast (Figure 1-23 and Figure 1-26), and bladder cancer, for prenatal screening, and for assessing sex mismatched bone-marrow transplantation success

- FDA-cleared/approved FISH-based tests are available for use in the diagnosis of acute myeloid leukemia diagnosis, B-cell chronic lymphocytic leukemia, bladder cancer, breast cancer (*TOP2A* gene amplification, *HER2* amplification, prenatal abnormalities, sex-mismatched bone marrow transplantation, *Candida albicans*, *Enterococcus faecalis*, *Staphylococcus aureus*, *Escherichia coli*, and *Pseudomonas aeruginosa*); CISH assays include *HER2* amplification detection; a combined CISH/SISH test is also available for dual *HER2* and centromere 17 enumeration
- Many non-FDA-listed tests are in widespread clinical diagnostics usage, for example:
  - ALL (B-cell, T-cell), AML, BCR/ABL, biliary tract malignancy, Cri-du-chat, 5p del, EWS, 22q12 rearrangement, FKHR 13q14 rearrangement, IMT 2p23 rearrangements, Kallmann, Xp22.3, MDS, Miller-Dieker, 17p13.3 del, *N-myc* amplification, NF1, 17q11.2 del, SRY Yp11.3, STS Xp22.3, SYT 18q11.2, T-cell lymphoma, Williams syndrome, Wolf-Hirschhorn, 4p del

PROTEIN ANALYTIC METHODS

- Aberrant protein expression consequent to disrupted nucleic acids or infective pathogens is detectable by protein analytic techniques
- Immunohistochemistry (see the Immunohistochemistry section of this chapter) demonstrates protein expression at the morphologic level. "Genogenic" IHC supports the detection of chimeric proteins, such as the EWS-FLI1 protein (Ewing sarcoma) that can arise following translocation events

- Western blotting consists of polyacrylamide gel electrophoresis of proteins followed by electroblotting onto a nitrocellulose membrane. The membrane is incubated with labeled antibodies directed against the protein of interest and expression is measured by the detection of the label
- The enzyme immunoassay (EIA) technique involves the capture of a specimen antigen (or antibody) in an antibody (or antigen) coated microtiter plate well. Secondary enzyme-labeled (e.g., HRP) antibodies are applied and the label is detected by a colorimetric substrate reaction that can be qualitative or quantitative
- Line immunoassays (LIA, Innogenetics, Ghent, Belgium) involve incubation of patient serum/plasma with a membrane strip prefixed with a range of purified, recombinant, or synthetic antigens. CE-approved INNO-LIA assays are available for the detection of HCV, HIV, HTLV, and syphilis
- Membrane immunochromatographic (ICT) tests for infectious agents have been developed (NOW-Technologies) by Binax, Inc. (Scarborough, ME). FDA-cleared tests are available for *Legionella pneumophila* serogroup 1 antigen in urine specimens, malaria—Plasmodium falciparum (P.f.) antigen, and the antigen common to all Pan malarial species: Plasmodium vivax (P.v.), Plasmodium ovale (P.o.), and Plasmodium malariae (P.m.) in whole blood—reparatory syncytial virus (RSV) fusion protein antigen in nasal wash and nasopharyngeal swab, *Streptococcus pyogenes* group A antigen from throat swab specimens, the *Streptococcus pneumoniae* antigen test for urine of patients with pneumonia, and in the cerebral spinal fluid (CSF) of patients with meningitis
- Matrix-assisted laser desorption/ionization-time of flight (MALDI-TOF) mass spectrometry is used for the rapid identification of pathogenic bacteria and fungi. Patient specimen is mixed with a "matrix" compound and irradiated by a laser, which vaporizes and ionizes the matrix-specimen combination into charged particles. The mass-to-charge (m/z) ratio of the particles is detected by MALDI-TOF instrumentation. The charge mass profile generated is compared to known pathogen profiles allowing microorganism identification.

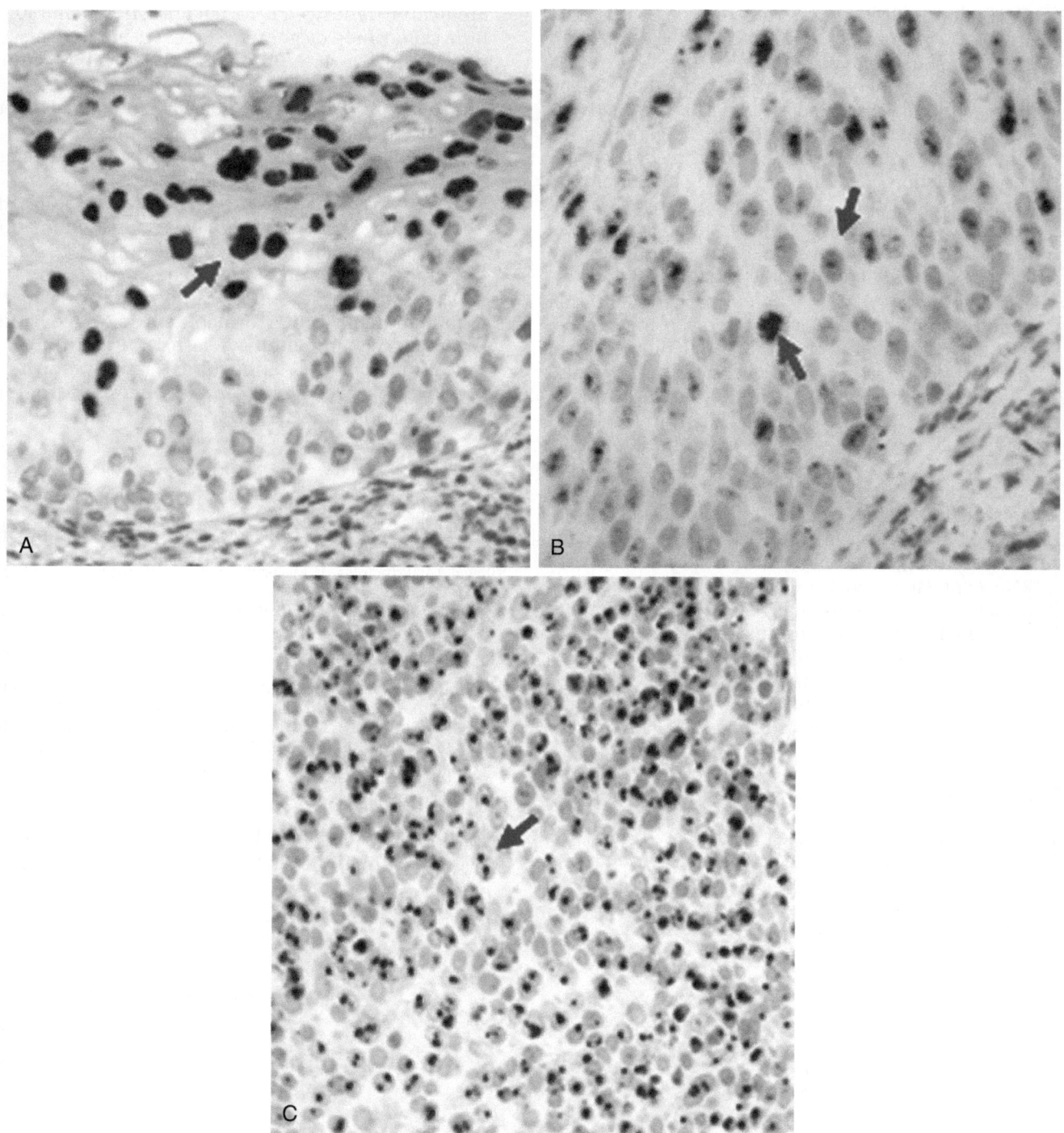

Figure 1-26. Chromogenic in situ hybridization (CISH). Human papillomavirus (HPV) DNA detected by CISH in cervical tissue; low-grade lesion **(A)**, high-grade lesion **(B)**, and squamous cell carcinoma **(C)**. "Diffuse" signals (*blue arrows*) are indicative of episomal HPV, and "punctate" signals (*red arrows*) are indicative of HPV integrated into the cell genome.

The two main platforms for this assay are the Vitek MS (bioMérieux, Inc., Durham, NC) and the MALDI Biotyper (Buker Corporation, Inc., Billerica, MA)

EMERGING METHODOLOGIES

- DNA methylation assays are likely to increase in significance as more is discovered about the importance of epigenetic factors in disease etiology. Abnormal methylation, which can result in gene silencing, is a recognized diagnostic factor for Angelman, Prader-Willi, and Beckwith-Wiedemann syndromes and is implicated as a general tumor characteristic. Methylation can be detected by Southern blot RFLP analysis using methylation-sensitive restriction endonucleases (as in the current assays for Beckwith-Wiedemann syndrome, etc.) or by PCR in combination with sample DNA treatment with bisulfite. Bisulfite converts dCTP residues to dUTP; during PCR, the dUTP is replaced with dTTP. Methylated cytosine is unaffected by bisulfite treatment. A comparison of bisulfite-treated and -untreated PCR amplicon sequences (by direct sequencing or restriction endonuclease analysis) reveals the methylation status of investigated sequences. Epigenomic AG (Berlin, Germany) has developed PCR-based assays for the early detection of colon cancer using blood samples and has a test for confirming malignant lung disease in patients with inconclusive cytology that uses bronchial fluid specimens. Next-Gen sequencing techniques also support DNA methylation characterization

- MicroRNA (miRNA), short single-stranded RNA that can bind complementary mRNA, preventing protein translation, is emerging as a potential biomarker of pathologic conditions. Array technology may also prove useful in screening for pathology defining miRNA species expression. For example, Rosetta Genomics (Philadelphia, PA) has developed several miRNA-based clinical assays. These include microarray tests for the tissue-of-origin of metastatic tumors; a test to classify tumors of the kidney as clear cell, papillary, chromophobes or as oncocytomas; a test for mesothelioma from other lung carcinomas; and a qRT-PCR test for miRNA expression signatures for the identification of nonsmall cell lung carcinoma (NSCLC), non-squamous NSCLC, small cell lung carcinoma, or carcinoid tumors. ISH assays for miRNA detection have been developed by Exiqon A/S (Vedbaek, Denmark), using locked nucleic acids (LNA) technology, and by Affymetrix Panomics (Santa Clara, CA), using QuantiGene ViewRNA assay

RESOURCES

- FDA cleared/approved nucleic acid based tests are listed at www.fda.gov/MedicalDevices/Productsand MedicalProcedures/InVitroDiagnostics/ucm330711. htm. Companion diagnostic devices are listed at www.fda. gov/MedicalDevices/ProductsandMedicalProcedures/ InVitroDiagnostics/ucm301431.htm
- The following websites include educational aids for understanding molecular pathology techniques:
  - The Dolan DNA Learning Center's Gene Almanac (www.dnalc.org/home.html) is a comprehensive biology educational resource. The Biology Animation Library (www.dnalc.org/ddnalc/resources/animations. html) includes animations of DNA restriction, gel electrophoresis, PCR, and Sanger sequencing
  - Davidson College, North Carolina, has prepared an animation of RT-PCR, available at www.bio.davidson. edu/courses/Immunology/Flash/RT_PCR.html
  - Real-time PCR animations are shown at www.biosearchtech.com/products/fluorogenic-probes-and-primers.aspx

SELECTED REFERENCES

Cheng L, Zhang DY (eds): Molecular Genetic Pathology. Totowa, NJ, Humana Press, 2008.

Coleman BC, Tsongalis GJ (eds): Molecular Diagnostics for the Clinical Laboratorian, 2nd ed. Totowa, NJ, Humana Press, 2006.

Killeen AA. Principles of Molecular Pathology. Totowa, NJ, Humana Press, 2004.

Leonard DGB (ed): Molecular Pathology in Clinical Practice. New York, Springer, 2007.

McPerson M, Møller S: PCR, 2nd ed. New York, Taylor & Francis Group, 2006.

Roulston JE, Bartlett JMS (eds): Molecular Diagnosis of Cancer: Methods and Protocols, 2nd ed. Totowa, NJ, Humana Press, 2004.

Tubbs RR, Stoler MH: Cell and Tissue Based Molecular Pathology: A Volume in the Foundations in Diagnostic Pathology Series. Philadelphia, Churchill Livingstone, 2008.

Acknowledgments

The authors would like to thank Lisa Kapoor for her assistance and support during the preparation of the chapter.

Chapter 2
Skin and Adnexal Structures

VIJAYA B. REDDY

CHAPTER OUTLINE

INFLAMMATORY CONDITIONS

SUPERFICIAL PERIVASCULAR DERMATITIS

Dermatitis with Minimal Epidermal Changes

SUPERFICIAL DERMATOPHYTOSIS (TINEA)

Clinical Features

- Caused by three genera of imperfect fungi—*Epidermophyton, Trichophyton,* and *Microsporum*—that cause superficial infections involving keratinized tissues such as the cornified layer of epidermis, the hair, and the nails
- Dermatophytosis involving different anatomic sites are named with site-specific terms such as tinea capitis (scalp), tinea barbae (beard area), tinea faciei (face), tinea corporis (trunk), tinea cruris (intertriginous areas), tinea pedis et manus (feet and hands), and tinea unguium (nails)
- Typical lesions of superficial dermatophytosis present as sharply demarcated patches and plaques with an arcuate border
- Tinea capitis and tinea barbae present as folliculitis; tinea unguium is characterized by yellow-gray discoloration of nails

Histopathology

- Focal parakeratosis with neutrophils and mild epidermal spongiosis (Figure 2-1A)
- Mild, superficial perivascular lymphocytic infiltrate

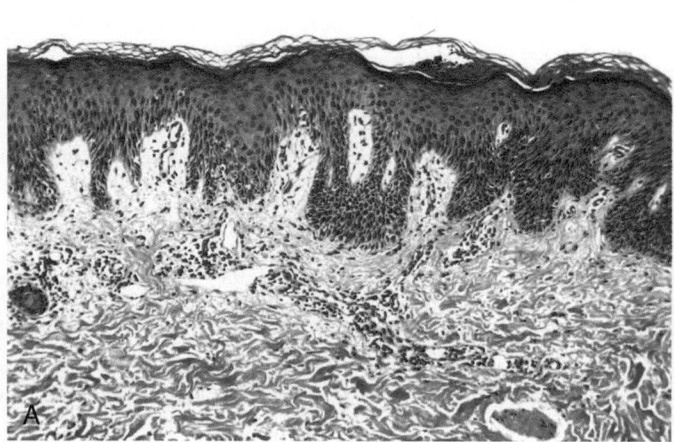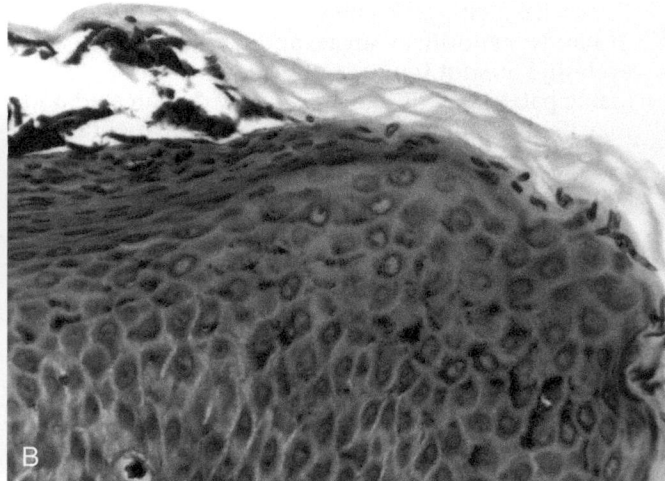

Figure 2-1. Dermatophytosis. A, Hematoxylin and eosin-stained section shows focal parakeratosis with neutrophils and mild superficial perivascular inflammation. **B,** Periodic acid-Schiff (PAS) stain shows the fungal hyphae within the cornified layer.

- Fungi are present as filamentous hyphae, spores, or yeast forms in the cornified layer and in the hair shafts in cases of tinea capitis and tinea barbae

Special Stains and Immunohistochemistry
- Periodic acid–Schiff (PAS) reaction stains fungi deep red to pink, and Gomori methenamine silver (GMS) stains fungi black (Figure 2-1B)

Other Techniques for Diagnosis
- Microbiologic cultures are useful in identifying the genera and species of the fungal organisms
- Polymerase chain reaction (PCR) techniques are particularly helpful for detecting dermatophyte infections of the nail (onychomycosis)

Differential Diagnosis
- Vitiligo and Urticaria
  - Should be considered in cases with minimal histologic changes
  - Demonstration of the fungal organisms with special stains confirms the diagnosis of dermatophytosis
- Candidiasis
  - Seen in patients with impaired host response, especially patients with hematologic malignancies and diabetes
  - Can present as cutaneous, mucocutaneous or systemic infection
  - Histologic sections show spongiotic or subcorneal pustules in which yeast forms and pseudohyphae can be demonstrated with PAS or GMS stain
- Pityriasis (Tinea) Versicolor Caused by Genus *Malassezia*
  - Affects upper trunk with brownish discoloration that may become hypopigmented
  - Histologic sections show slight hyperkeratosis, round spores, and thick, short hyphae ("spaghetti and meatballs") recognizable as faintly basophilic, refractive structures in routine hematoxylin and eosin (H&E)–stained sections
  - Folliculitis pattern of dermatophytosis may be similar to *Malassezia (Pityrosporum)* folliculitis

PEARLS

- *Identification of fungal organisms on routine H&E-stained sections may be aided by lowering the microscope condenser, which enhances the refractile nature of the fungi*
- *Fungi in the cornified layer are sandwiched between a lower zone of parakeratosis and an upper zone of orthokeratosis ("sandwich sign"); diagnosis can be confirmed by demonstration of fungi with special stains*
- *The presence of neutrophils in a slightly parakeratotic cornified layer and mild superficial perivascular dermatitis should always prompt a PAS stain in search of fungal elements*
- *Deep folliculitis with intense acute and granulomatous inflammation due to dermatophyte infection is known as "Majocchi granuloma"*

SELECTED REFERENCES

Gottlieb GJ, Ackerman AB: The "sandwich sign" of dermatophytosis. Am J Dermatopathol 8:347, 1996.
Havlickova B, Czaika VA, Frieddrich M: Epidemiologic trends in skin mycosis worldwide. Mycoses 51(suppl 4):2-15, 2008.
Ilkit M, Durdu M, Karakaş M: Majocchi's granuloma: a symptom complex caused by fungal pathogens. Med Mycol 50:449-457, 2012.
Kondori N, Tehrani PA, Strömbeck L, Faergemann J: Comparison of dermatophyte PCR kit with conventional methods for detection of dermatophytes in skin specimens. Mycopathologia 176:237-241, 2013.
Vermout S, Tabart J, Baldo A, et al: Pathogenesis of dermatophytosis. Mycopathologia 166:267-275, 2008.

VITILIGO

Clinical Features
- Acquired, possibly autoimmune disease with strong familial association
- Characterized by patches of pigment loss in skin
- Localized disease may show linear, segmental pattern

- Generalized vitiligo involves face, upper trunk, dorsa of hands, periorificial areas, and genitalia; scalp and eyelashes are not typically affected
- Stable patches of vitiligo are sharply demarcated and may be surrounded by a zone of hyperpigmentation; in active lesions, areas of total depigmentation may be surrounded by a zone of partial depigmentation and have a slight rim of erythema at the border

Histopathology

- Low-power examination shows mostly unremarkable skin or mild superficial perivascular inflammation with scattered melanophages
- Total absence of melanocytes is seen in well-established lesions and in the depigmented center of expanding lesions of vitiligo
- A few melanocytes may be seen in the hypopigmented areas; in the outer border of the patches, prominent melanocytes with long dendritic processes filled with melanin granules and a mild superficial perivascular inflammation are present
- Mild superficial perivascular and patchy lichenoid lymphocytic infiltrate and vacuolar alteration of the basal cell layer can be seen in normal-appearing skin adjacent to the vitiliginous patches

Special Stains and Immunohistochemistry

- Silver stains or the dopa reaction (Fontana-Masson) highlight loss of melanin pigment (Figures 2-2A and 2B)
- Immunohistochemical stains for S-100 protein or Melan-A can be useful in confirming the absence of melanocytes

Other Techniques for Diagnosis

- Noncontributory

Differential Diagnosis

- On routine H&E-stained sections, other diseases manifesting with minimal histologic alterations (normal-appearing skin), such as tinea versicolor, urticaria, and macular variant of urticaria pigmentosa, should be considered

PEARLS

- *Studies show that autoimmune mechanisms and genetic predisposition are the most likely causative factors*

- *Vitiligo can be seen in association with other autoimmune disorders such as thyroid disorders, pernicious anemia, and alopecia areata*

SELECTED REFERENCES

Attili VR, Attili SK: Lichenoid inflammation in vitiligo: a clinical and histopathologic review of 210 cases. Int J Dermatol 47:663-669, 2008.

Le Poole IC, Das PK: Microscopic changes in vitiligo. Clin Dermatol 15:863-873, 1997.

Le Poole IC, Luiten RM: Autoimmune etiology of generalized vitiligo. Curr Dir Autoimmun 10:227-243, 2008.

Malhotra N, Dytoc M: The pathogenesis of vitiligo. J Cutan Med Surg 17:153-172, 2013.

Silverberg JI, Silverberg NB: Clinical features of vitiligo associated with comorbid autoimmune disease: a prospective survey. J Am Acad Dermatol 69:824-826, 2013.

URTICARIA

Clinical Features

- Presents with pruritic, raised, erythematous, and edematous areas known as *wheals* or *hives*
- Acute urticaria lasts less than 6 weeks and is more common in the pediatric age group
- Chronic urticaria lasts more than 6 weeks and is more common in adults
- An underlying predisposing condition can be identified in up to 25% of patients; certain foods, drugs, contact allergens, and physical stimuli such as pressure, cold temperature, and occult infections may be factors
- Urticarial vasculitis is a syndrome consisting of recurrent urticaria, arthralgia, and abdominal pain; individual cutaneous lesions persist for more than 24 hours
- In angioedema, dermal edema extends into subcutaneous fat and presents with large wheals

Histopathology

- Interstitial edema, dilated vessels, and a sparse perivascular mixed inflammatory cell infiltrate composed of lymphocytes, eosinophils, and neutrophils (Figure 2-3)
- Urticarial vasculitis shows features of early leukocytoclastic vasculitis characterized by mild perivascular infiltrate of neutrophils, neutrophilic nuclear dust, and extravasated red blood cells; minimal or absent fibrin deposits in the vessel walls

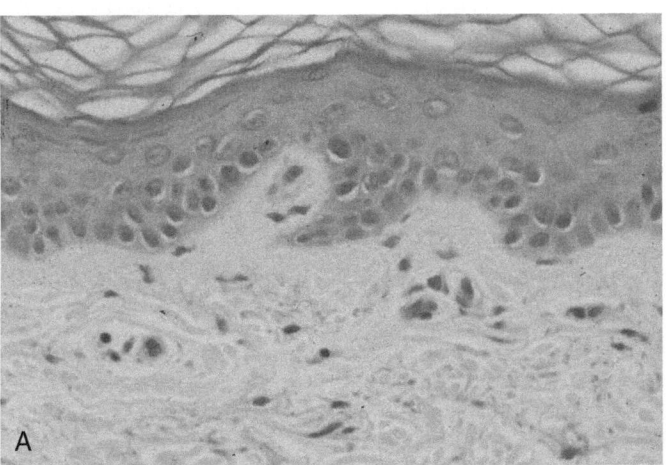
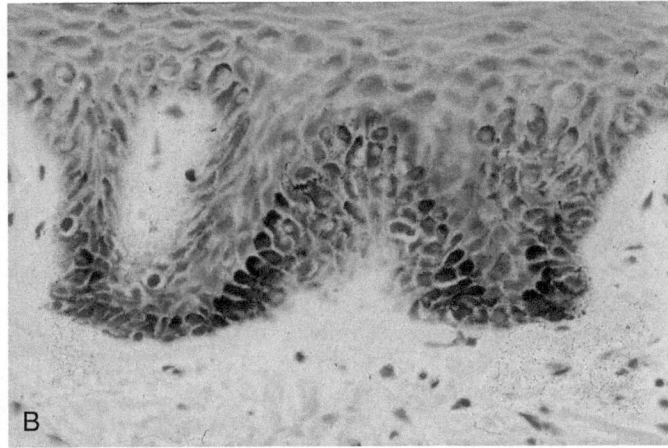

Figure 2-2. A, Vitiligo. Fontana-Masson stain shows loss of pigmentation at the basal cell layer. **B,** Normal skin. Fontana-Masson stain shows normal pigmentation at the basal cell layer.

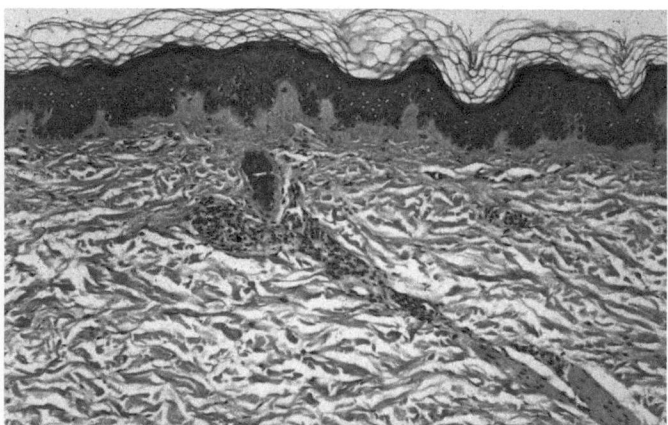

Figure 2-3. Urticaria. Histologic section shows mild superficial perivascular mixed inflammatory cell infiltrate and interstitial edema.

Special Stains and Immunohistochemistry
* Noncontributory

Other Techniques for Diagnosis
* Hypocomplementemia is seen in 32% of patients with urticarial vasculitis; measurements of CH50 and C1q binding assays are helpful
* Patients with hereditary angioedema have a low serum level of esterase inhibitor of first component of complement
* Direct immunofluorescence studies: vascular deposits of immunoglobulins, complement, or fibrin are seen in one third of patients with urticarial vasculitis

Differential Diagnosis
* Macular Variant of Urticaria Pigmentosa (Telangiectasia Macularis Eruptiva Perstans)
  * Generally occurs as an extensive eruption of brownish red macules
  * Histologic sections show dilated blood vessels in the upper dermis and a mild superficial perivascular mononuclear cell infiltrate composed mostly of mast cells; eosinophils are generally absent; dermal edema is not prominent (Figure 2-4A)
  * Giemsa, toluidine blue, Leder, or immunohistochemical stain for mast cell tryptase can help demonstrate the increased number of mast cells (Figure 2-4B)

* Other Causes of Leukocytoclastic Vasculitis
  * Should be considered in the differential diagnosis of urticarial vasculitis

PEARLS

* *In hereditary angioedema, a form of dominantly inherited angioedema, recurrent attacks of edema involve skin and oral, laryngeal, and gastrointestinal mucosa; death due to laryngeal edema can occur if not treated*
* *Urticarial vasculitis may be associated with infectious mononucleosis, infectious hepatitis, and autoimmune diseases such as systemic lupus erythematosus*

SELECTED REFERENCES

Beltrani VS: Urticaria and angioedema. Dermatol Clin 14:171-198, 1996.

Cugno M, Castelli R, Cicardi M: Angioedema due to acquired C1-inhibitor deficiency: a bridging condition between autoimmunity and lymphoproliferation. Autoimmun Rev 8:156-159, 2008.

Gibbs NF, Friedlander SF, Harpster EF: Telangiectasia macularis eruptiva perstans. Pediatr Dermatol 17:194-197, 2000.

Młynek A, Maurer M, Zalewska A: Update on chronic urticaria: focusing on mechanisms. Curr Opin Allergy Clin Immunol 8:433-437, 2008.

Stitt JM, Dreskin SC: Urticaria and autoimmunity: where are we now? Curr Allergy Asthma Rep 13:555-562, 2013.

Wisnieski JJ: Urticarial vasculitis. Curr Opin Rheumatol 12:24-31, 2000.

Interface Dermatitis
LICHEN PLANUS
Clinical Features
* Disorder of unknown etiology involving skin, mucous membranes, hair follicles, and nails
* Typically presents as pruritic, flat-topped violaceous papules with a fine scale
* Predilection for flexor surfaces of extremities, lower back, and glans penis
* Surface of lesions may show a network of white lines known as *Wickham striae*
* Oral lesions may be seen as sole manifestation or in association with skin involvement and consist of lacy, reticular network of papules involving buccal mucosa or tongue
* Association with hepatitis C

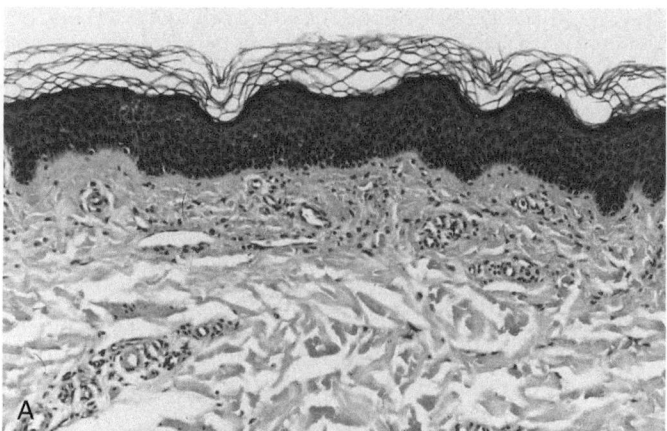
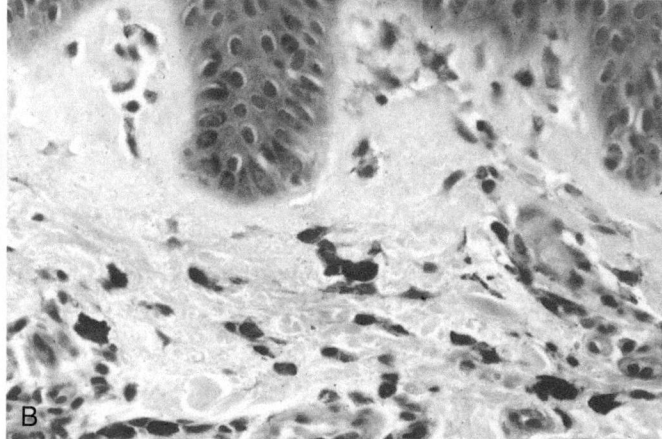

Figure 2-4. Urticaria pigmentosa, macular type. A, Hematoxylin and eosin–stained section shows dilated blood vessels in the superficial dermis surrounded by a mild perivascular infiltrate of cells. Without a high degree of suspicion and special stains, it might be difficult to notice that the cells are predominantly mast cells. **B,** Giemsa stain highlights the mast cells in the infiltrate.

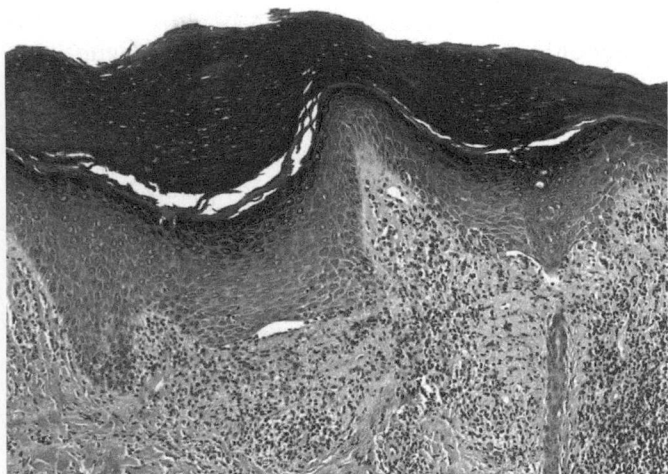

Figure 2-5. Lichen planus. There is hyperkeratosis, hypergranulosis, irregular epidermal hyperplasia, and a bandlike, predominantly lymphocytic infiltrate that obscures the dermoepidermal junction. Melanophages are present in the dermal infiltrate.

Histopathology

- Compact hyperkeratosis and wedge-shaped hypergranulosis that corresponds to the openings of follicles and acrosyringia (Figure 2-5)
- Irregular epidermal hyperplasia with a sawtooth appearance and a bandlike, predominantly lymphocytic infiltrate in the superficial dermis that obscures the dermoepidermal junction
- Eosinophilic colloid bodies or Civatte bodies are present at the dermoepidermal junction and usually represent damage to the basal cell layer
- Small clefts known as *Max-Joseph spaces* may be seen between the epidermis and dermis
- Chronic lesions show hyperkeratosis and papillomatous epidermal hyperplasia (hypertrophic lichen planus)
- Oral lesions show parakeratosis, less epithelial hyperplasia, and frequent ulceration
- Lichen planus of hair follicles (lichen planopilaris) shows a dense lymphocytic infiltrate surrounding the follicular epithelium; in later stages, there is perifollicular fibrosis with advanced stages resulting in scarring alopecia

Special Stains and Immunohistochemistry

- Lymphoid infiltrate is composed predominantly of T cells

Other Techniques for Diagnosis

- Noncontributory

Differential Diagnosis

- Lichenoid Drug Eruption
  - Focal parakeratosis and necrotic keratinocytes particularly at and above the dermoepidermal junction
  - Presence of eosinophils in the inflammatory cell infiltrate favors a diagnosis of lichenoid drug eruption
- Lichen Planus–Like Keratosis (Benign Lichenoid Keratosis)
  - Solitary lesion that shows parakeratosis in addition to lichenoid pattern of inflammation
  - Adjacent areas may show changes of solar lentigo
  - Lichenoid Graft-versus-Host Disease (GVHD)
  - Generally the inflammatory cell infiltrate is sparse

- Foci of parakeratosis and thinning of epidermis may be present
- Lichen Striatus
  - More common in children than adults and presents as a unilateral eruption along Blaschko lines on extremities, trunk, or neck
  - Lichenoid inflammatory cell infiltrate similar as in lichen planus
  - Distinguishing features include the presence of inflammatory cell infiltrate deep in the reticular dermis around hair follicles and sweat glands
  - Epidermal spongiosis and an admixture of histiocytes in the inflammatory cell infiltrate can be present
- Lichen Nitidus
  - Asymptomatic dermatosis of childhood, characterized by round, flat-topped papules that measure only a few millimeters
  - Histologically, the inflammatory cell infiltrate is bandlike but the lesion is small and discrete; infiltrate is confined to widened dermal papillae and enclosed by elongated rete, which gives an appearance of a claw clutching a ball
  - Frequent histiocytes in the infiltrate, epidermal atrophy, and focal parakeratosis are helpful in differentiating lichen nitidus from lichen planus
- Lichen Planopilaris Versus Alopecia Areata
  - Presence of lymphocytes mostly at the base of the follicular bulb rather than along the infundibulum favors alopecia areata
  - Scarring is generally not a feature of alopecia areata

PEARLS

- *Parakeratosis is not a feature of cutaneous lichen planus, and its presence should prompt consideration of other causes of lichenoid inflammation*
- *Koebner phenomenon (formation of a linear configuration of lesions due to scratching) can be seen in lichen planus*

SELECTED REFERENCES

Birkenfeld S, Dreiher J, Weitzman D, Cohen AD: A study on the association with hepatitis B and hepatitis C in 1557 patients with lichen planus. J Eur Acad Dermatol Venereol 25:436-440, 2011.

Boyd AS, Neldner KH: Lichen planus. J Am Acad Dermatol 25:593-619, 1991.

Johnson H, Soldano AC, Kovich O, Long W: Oral lichen planus. Dermatol Online J 14:20, 2008.

Kang H, Alzolibani AA, Otberg N, Shapiro J: Lichen planopilaris. Dermatol Ther 21:249-256, 2008.

Shai A, Halevy S: Lichen planus and lichen planus-like eruptions: pathogenesis and associated diseases. Int J Dermatol 31:379-384, 1992.

Shiohara T: The lichenoid tissue reaction: an immunological perspective. Am J Dermatopathol 10:252-256, 1988.

ERYTHEMA MULTIFORME

Clinical Features

- Erythema multiforme is an acute cytotoxic cell-mediated hypersensitivity reaction to infections, most commonly herpes simplex virus infection, and drugs, in particular sulfonamides
- The eruption is multiform and consists of macules, papules, vesicles, and occasionally large flaccid bullae; often associated with fever

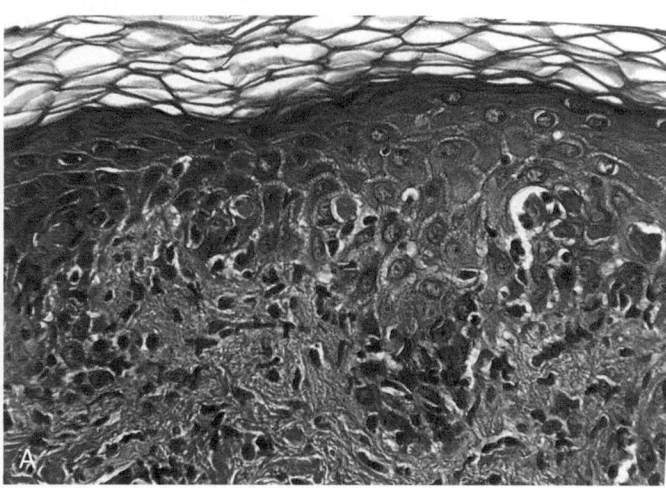 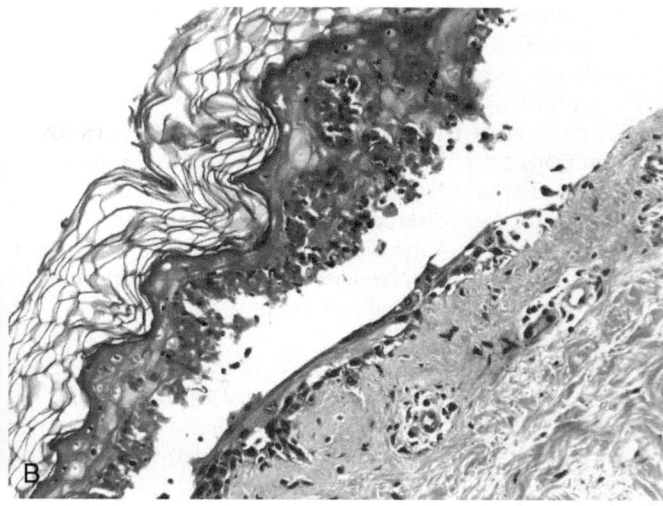

Figure 2-6. A, Erythema multiforme. Vacuolar alteration of the basal cell layer above which there are necrotic keratinocytes. **B,** Toxic epidermal necrolysis. Full-thickness epidermal necrosis with separation at the dermoepidermal junction is seen. The cornified layer is unaltered, attesting to the acute nature of the process, and there is only a minimal inflammatory cell infiltrate.

- Herpesvirus-associated erythema multiforme involves the extremities and presents with typical target-like lesions, whereas that associated with drugs shows truncal involvement and a purpuric type of macular eruption; mucosal involvement (Stevens-Johnson syndrome) is characteristic
- In the most severe form, toxic epidermal necrolysis (a widespread blotchy erythema) is soon followed by large flaccid bullae with detachment of epidermis; this is most often caused by drugs, including sulfonamides, β-lactam antibiotics, and nonsteroidal anti-inflammatory drugs; associated with a high mortality rate

Histopathology

- Cornified layer is unaltered, attesting to the acute nature of the disease
- Vacuolar alteration of the basal cell layer and a sparse superficial perivascular lymphocytic infiltrate may focally obscure the dermoepidermal junction (Figure 2-6A)
- The hallmark of erythema multiforme is the presence of necrotic keratinocytes, initially as single cells and later as small clusters; the necrosis is more widespread in drug-induced erythema multiforme; in bullous lesions and toxic epidermal necrolysis, there is full-thickness epidermal necrosis resulting in subepidermal bullae (Figure 2-6B)
- In late lesions, the papillary dermis may contain melanophages (a sign of damage to the basal cell layer)

Special Stains and Immunohistochemistry

- Noncontributory

Other Techniques for Diagnosis

- Immunofluorescence studies show immunoglobulin M (IgM) and C3 in the walls of superficial dermal vessels
- Herpes simplex virus DNA has been detected within lesions of erythema multiforme using polymerase chain reaction (PCR) and in situ hybridization (ISH)

Differential Diagnosis

- Staphylococcal Scaled-Skin Syndrome
  - Clinical appearance may be similar to toxic epidermal necrolysis
  - Microscopically, staphylococcal scaled-skin syndrome shows a split in the granular layer, whereas in

toxic epidermal necrolysis, there is separation at the dermoepidermal junction, a feature most helpful in distinguishing the two entities
- Acute GVHD Disease
  - May be histologically indistinguishable from early erythema multiforme
- Drug Eruptions, Including Fixed Drug Eruptions
  - Characterized by the presence of necrotic keratinocytes
  - Presence of eosinophils and deeper infiltrate in fixed drug eruption

PEARLS

- *Erythema multiforme, Stevens-Johnson syndrome, and toxic epidermal necrolysis are best regarded as a spectrum of the same disease process*
- *Presence or absence of mucosal lesions in bullous forms of erythema multiforme does not appear to correlate with severity or prognosis*

Selected References

Ackerman AB, Ragaz A: Erythema multiforme. Am J Dermatopathol 7:133, 1985.
Borchers AT, Lee JL, Naguwa SM, et al: Stevens-Johnson syndrome and toxic epidermal necrolysis. Autoimmun Rev 7:598-605, 2008.
Gerull R, Nelle M, Schaible T: Toxic epidermal necrolysis and Stevens-Johnson syndrome: a review. Crit Care Med 39:1521-1532, 2011.
Mockenhaupt M: The current understanding of Stevens-Johnson syndrome and toxic epidermal necrolysis. Expert Rev Clin Immunol 7:803-813, 2011.
Roujeau JC: Stevens-Johnson syndrome and toxic epidermal necrolysis are severity variants of the same disease which differs from erythema multiforme. J Dermatol 24:726-729, 1997.
Sokumbi O, Wetter DA: Clinical features, diagnosis, and treatment of erythema multiforme: a review for the practicing dermatologist. Int J Dermatol 51:889-902, 2012.

GRAFT-VERSUS-HOST DISEASE (GVHD)

Clinical Features

- Occurs most frequently in bone marrow transplant recipients and less commonly in recipients of blood products and solid organ transplants

- Incidence is 30% to 40% in related donor-recipient versus 60% to 80% when unrelated; risk increases with age
- Acute phase
  - Presents with the triad of skin lesions, hepatic dysfunction, and diarrhea; develops within 3 months after transplant
  - Skin lesions are characterized by extensive erythematous macules, purpuric to violaceous papules and plaques, and, in severe cases, toxic epidermal necrolysis–like eruption; oral lesions may be present
- Chronic phase
  - Occurs > 3 months to a year after transplantation
  - In the early lichenoid stage, the eruption is similar to lichen planus
  - Late sclerotic stage is characterized by skin induration and tightening

Histopathology

- Acute phase
  - Grade I: vacuolar alteration of the basal cell layer, which may be focal or diffuse
  - Grade II: necrotic keratinocytes occasionally surrounded by lymphocytes (satellite necrosis) are seen in the epidermis (Figure 2-7)
  - Grade III: more widespread necrosis of keratinocytes with separation at the dermoepidermal junction
  - Grade IV: full-thickness necrosis and loss of epidermis
  - Sparse superficial perivascular lymphocytic infiltrate is usually present in acute GVHD
  - Occasionally follicular papules are seen clinically, and histologic changes similar to those of epidermis can be seen in the follicular epithelium
- Chronic phase
  - Early lichenoid phase shows histologic features of lichen planus; satellite necrosis may still be seen in GVHD
  - Late sclerotic phase shows changes similar to scleroderma with dermal sclerosis extending into subcutaneous fat and loss of adnexal structures; however, epidermal atrophy is present in GVHD

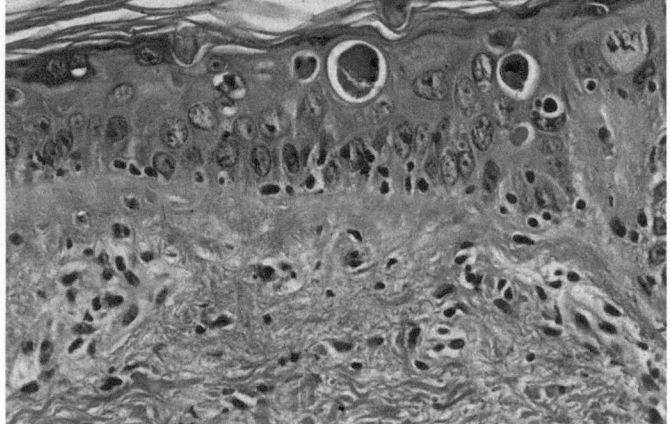

Figure 2-7. Acute graft-versus-host disease. Vacuolar alteration of the basal cell layer is seen with scattered necrotic keratinocytes within the epidermis. Lymphocytes are present at the basal cell layer and extending into the epidermis, where they may surround the necrotic keratinocytes (satellite necrosis).

Special Stains and Immunohistochemistry
- Noncontributory

Other Techniques for Diagnosis
- Noncontributory

Differential Diagnosis
- Erythema Multiforme
  - Acute GVHD shows histologic changes and a spectrum of severity indistinguishable from that of erythema multiforme
- Lichen Planus
  - Lichenoid phase of GVHD may be indistinguishable from lichen planus
- Scleroderma
  - Epidermal atrophy, if present, helps in differentiating sclerotic phase of GVHD from scleroderma

PEARLS

- *Acute phase of GVHD is caused by the attack of donor immunocompetent T lymphocytes against histocompatibility antigens exposed on recipient cells*
- *Chronic phase of GVHD is caused by immunocompetent lymphocytes that differentiate in the recipient*
- *Target cells in GVHD are the stem cells in the regenerating compartment—that is, the basal keratinocytes in skin and the epithelial cells at the base of the crypts in the gastrointestinal tract*

Selected References

Aractingi S, Chosidow O: Cutaneous graft-versus-host disease. Arch Dermatol 134:602-612, 1998.
Häusermann P, Walter RB, Halter J, et al: Cutaneous graft-versus-host disease: a guide for the dermatologist. Dermatology 216:287-304, 2008.
Martí N, Martin JM, Monteagudo C, et al: Follicular graft-versus-host disease: a rare manifestation of chronic cutaneous graft versus host disease. Am J Dermatopathol 30:620-621, 2008.
Paun O, Phillips T, Fu P, Novoa RA, et al: Cutaneous complications in hematopoietic cell transplant recipients: impact of biopsy on patient management. Biol Blood Marrow Transplant 19:1204-1209, 2013.
Wu PA, Cowen EW: Cutaneous graft-versus-host disease-clinical considerations and management. Curr Probl Dermatol 43:101-115, 2012.
Zhou Y, Barnett MJ, Rivers JK: Clinical significance of skin biopsies in the diagnosis and management of graft-vs-host disease in early post-allogeneic bone marrow transplantation. Arch Dermatol 136:717-721, 2000.

CUTANEOUS LUPUS ERYTHEMATOSUS

Clinical Features
- Lupus erythematosus is a chronic multisystem autoimmune disease that affects the connective tissue and vasculature of various organs
- Cutaneous changes are seen in the three classic forms of lupus: chronic discoid, subacute, and systemic lupus
- Discoid lesions of cutaneous lupus erythematosus appear as mildly scaling, erythematous, edematous, sharply demarcated plaques measuring up to 15 cm, involving scalp, face, upper trunk, and upper extremities (photosensitive distribution); follicular plugging may be seen
- Older lesions appear atrophic with variable pigmentation
- Tumid form of lupus presents as indurated plaques and nodules without overlying erythema or atrophy

- Verrucous lesions due to epidermal proliferation are seen in 2% of patients with chronic cutaneous lupus erythematosus
- Panniculitis may be seen in some patients with chronic cutaneous or systemic forms of lupus erythematosus
- Subacute lupus erythematosus may present as symmetric eruption of psoriasiform or annular plaques in photodistribution

Histopathology

- Histologic features of discoid lupus erythematosus are characteristic and include hyperkeratosis with follicular plugging, atrophy of epidermis, vacuolar alteration of the basal cell layer, and marked thickening of the basement membrane (Figure 2-8A)
- Variable amount of lymphocytic infiltrate obscures the dermoepidermal junction and surrounds the adnexal structures and dermal blood vessels
- Interstitial deposits of mucin are noted in many cases
- Epidermal hyperplasia with papillomatosis is seen in the verrucous form of lupus
- In the tumid form of lupus erythematosus, there is superficial and deep perivascular and periadnexal lymphocytic infiltrate with interstitial mucin but no epidermal changes
- In lupus panniculitis, there is a lobular lymphocytic panniculitis with hyaline fat necrosis and interstitial mucin, with or without epidermal changes (Figure 2-8B)
- Subacute cutaneous lupus erythematosus and neonatal lupus erythematosus show prominent changes

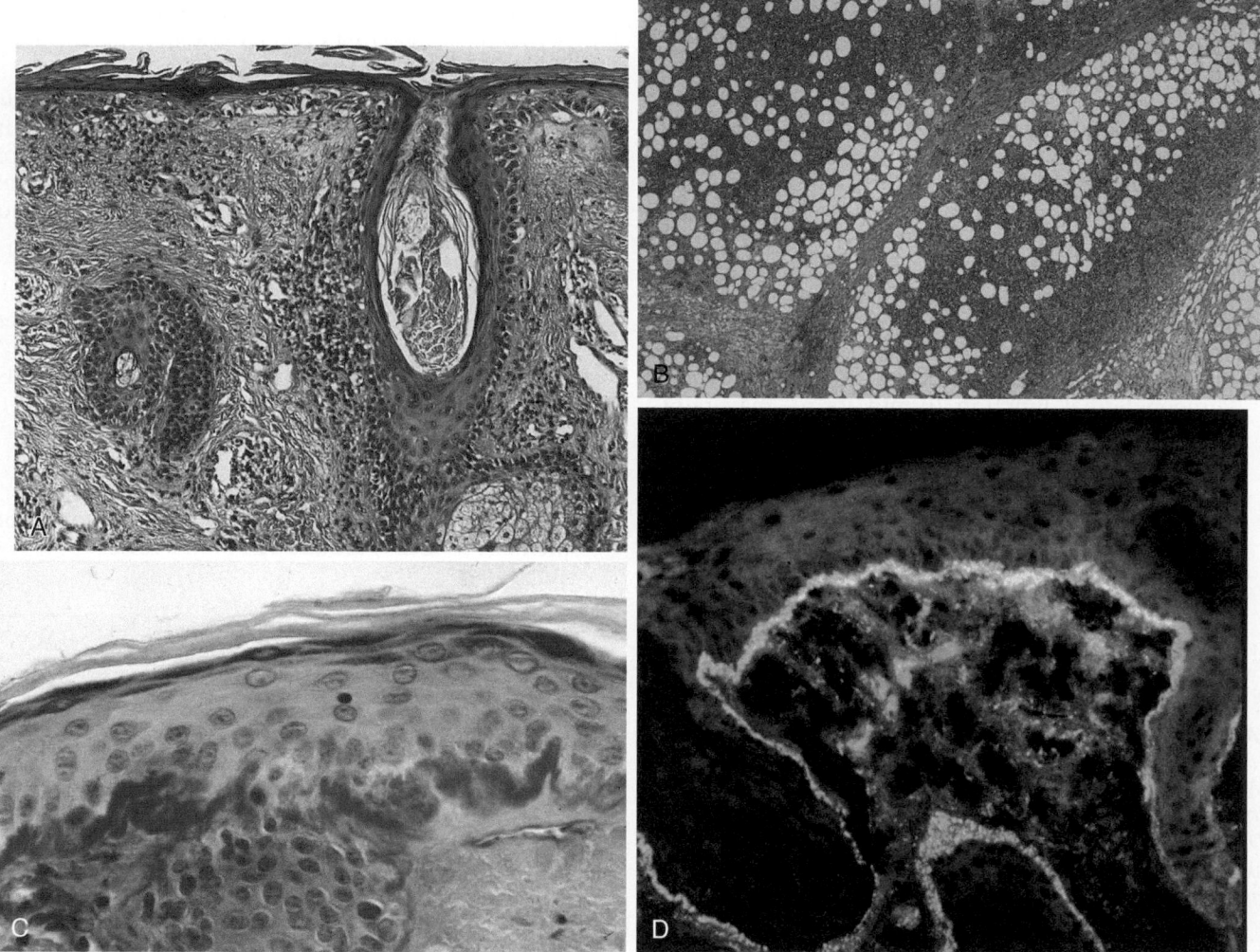

Figure 2-8. **Cutaneous lupus erythematosus.** **A,** Hematoxylin and eosin–stained section demonstrates hyperkeratosis with follicular plugging, atrophy of the epidermis, marked vacuolar alteration of the basal cell layer, and a thickened and smudged basement membrane. Perifollicular lymphocytic infiltrate is present. **B,** Lupus profundus. Section shows a predominantly lobular pattern of lymphocytic panniculitis with associated hyaline fat necrosis. **C,** PAS stain demonstrates the thickening of the basement membrane. **D,** Direct immunofluorescence studies show bandlike granular positivity along the basement membrane of the epidermis and the adnexal epithelium. Positive fluorescence may be seen with immunoglobulin G (IgG) or IgM and C3.

at the dermoepidermal junction but less prominent hyperkeratosis and inflammatory cell infiltrate than discoid lupus erythematosus
- Cutaneous lesions of systemic lupus may show changes of discoid lupus or subacute lupus, but more often the histologic changes are subtle

Special Stains and Immunohistochemistry
- PAS stain is helpful in demonstrating the thickened basement membrane (Figure 2-8C)
- Colloidal iron stain can highlight interstitial mucin deposits

Other Techniques for Diagnosis
- Direct immunofluorescence shows a continuous granular deposition of immunoglobulin G (IgG), IgM, and C3 in a band along the dermoepidermal junction (Figure 2-8D)

Differential Diagnosis
- Dermatomyositis
  - May show histologic changes similar to those of subacute lesions of cutaneous lupus erythematosus
  - Lupus band test is generally negative
- Lichen Planus
  - The epidermal changes of discoid lupus erythematosus may resemble lichen planus
  - Presence of hypergranulosis, irregular epidermal hyperplasia with sawtooth appearance, and absence of interstitial mucin deposits favors a diagnosis of lichen planus
- Polymorphous Light Eruption
  - Superficial and deep perivascular lymphocytic infiltrates of lupus (especially tumid form) must be differentiated from polymorphous light eruption, which usually shows marked edema of papillary dermis
- Lymphoma
  - Superficial and deep dense lymphocytic infiltrate of lupus, when seen in the absence of changes at the dermoepidermal junction (tumid form), may raise the possibility of lymphoma or leukemia; interstitial deposits of mucin are present in lupus, and the lymphoid cells are small and mature
  - In the differential diagnosis of lupus profundus panniculitis, subcutaneous panniculitis-like T-cell lymphoma may be considered; however, the lymphoid cells in T-cell lymphoma panniculitis are atypical, lymphocyte nuclei are present within the cytoplasm of histiocytes (emperipolesis), and there is rimming of the subcutaneous fat cells by the neoplastic T cells (Figure 2-8D)

PEARLS

- *Well-defined lesions of discoid lupus erythematosus occur in 15% of patients with subacute lupus erythematosus*
- *Direct immunofluorescence studies are positive in lesional skin only in discoid lupus and positive in both lesional and nonlesional skin in systemic lupus (lupus band test)*

SELECTED REFERENCES

Arps DP, Patel RM: Lupus profundus (panniculitis): a potential mimic of subcutaneous panniculitis-like T-cell lymphoma. Arch Pathol Lab Med 137:1211-1215, 2013.
Biazar C, Sigges J, Patsinakidis N, Ruland V, et al: Cutaneous lupus erythematosus: first multicenter database analysis of 1002 patients from the European Society of Cutaneous Lupus Erythematosus (EUSCLE). Autoimmun Rev 12:444-454, 2013.
Jerdan MS, Hood AF, Moore GW, et al: Histopathologic comparison of the subsets of lupus erythematosus. Arch Dermatol 126:52, 1990.
Lee LA, Weston WL: Cutaneous lupus erythematosus during the neonatal and childhood periods. Lupus 6:132-138, 1997.
Patel P, Werth V: Cutaneous lupus erythematosus: a review. Dermatol Clin 20:373-385, 2002.
Yu C, Chang C, Zhang J: Immunologic and genetic considerations of cutaneous lupus erythematosus: a comprehensive review. J Autoimmun 41:34-45, 2013.

DERMATOMYOSITIS

Clinical Features
- Dermatomyositis is a connective tissue disease characterized by inflammatory myositis involving the proximal muscles and cutaneous lesions consisting of heliotrope rash, Gottron papules, and erythematous-edematous lesions over the upper chest and back in a photodistribution
  - *Heliotrope rash* refers to violaceous, slightly edematous periorbital patches involving the eyelids
  - *Gottron papules* are discrete red-purple papules over bony prominences of knuckles, knees, and elbows
- The disease has two peaks, one in childhood and one between the ages of 45 and 65 years

Histopathology
- Histologic changes of the erythematous-edematous lesions of the skin may be similar to those seen in subacute lupus erythematosus and consist of epidermal atrophy, vacuolar alteration of the basal cell layer, and a sparse superficial perivascular lymphocytic infiltrate (Figure 2-9)
- Interstitial mucin deposits may be present
- Subepidermal fibrin deposits can be seen
- Sections of Gottron papules show epidermal hyperplasia in addition to mild interface changes
- Panniculitis and calcification of the subcutaneous tissue may be seen at a later stage

Special Stains and Immunohistochemistry
- Noncontributory

Other Techniques for Diagnosis
- Direct immunofluorescence studies may show complement (C5b-C9) around the blood vessels

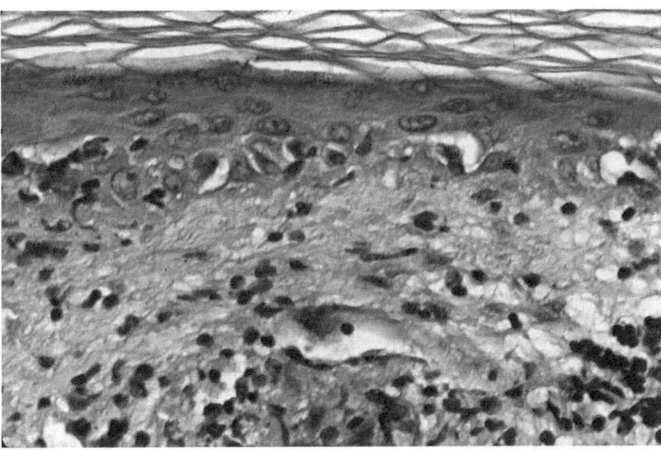

Figure 2-9. Dermatomyositis. Vacuolar alteration of the basal cell layer, epidermal atrophy, and a mild perivascular inflammatory cell infiltrate are seen.

Differential Diagnosis

- Subacute Cutaneous or Systemic Lupus Erythematosus
  - Histologic changes of dermatomyositis can be indistinguishable from those of lupus, and clinical correlation including evaluation for myositis is critical
  - A negative lupus band test is generally helpful, especially in early stages of dermatomyositis when the muscular weakness is not apparent

PEARLS

- *Dermatomyositis has been shown to be associated with malignancy, particularly ovarian carcinoma; exact incidence, however, is controversial*

SELECTED REFERENCES

Callen JP: Dermatomyositis. Lancet 355:53-57, 2000.

Femia AN, Vleugels RA, Callen JP: Cutaneous dermatomyositis: an updated review of treatment options and internal associations. Am J Clin Dermatol 14:291-313, 2013.

Hill CL, Zhang Y, Sigurgeirsson B, et al: Frequency of specific cancer types in dermatomyositis and polymyositis: a population-based study. Lancet 357:96-100, 2001.

Sontheimer RD: Cutaneous features of classic dermatomyositis and amyopathic dermatomyositis. Curr Opin Rheumatol 11:475-482, 1999.

Epidermal Spongiosis
SPONGIOTIC DERMATITIS
Clinical Features

- *Spongiotic dermatitis* refers to a heterogeneous group of disorders characterized histologically by the presence of intercellular edema (spongiosis) in the epidermis
- This group includes allergic contact dermatitis, photoallergic dermatitis, nummular dermatitis, atopic dermatitis, dyshidrotic dermatitis, and Id reaction
- Allergic Contact Dermatitis
  - Most commonly caused by poison ivy, nickel, and rubber compounds
  - Presents with pruritic, edematous, erythematous papules and occasional vesicles usually within 1 to 3 days after exposure
- Photoallergic Dermatitis
  - Due to topical application (photocontact) or ingestion of an allergen
  - Shows pruritic and erythematous papulovesicular lesions on sun-exposed skin; usually on face, arms, and neck
- Nummular Dermatitis
  - Disease of unknown etiology characterized by coin-shaped, pruritic, erythematous, scaly, crusted plaques on exterior aspects of extremities
- Atopic Dermatitis
  - Inherited chronic, pruritic, scaly eruption affecting face and extensor aspects of extremities in children
- Dyshidrotic Dermatitis
  - Characterized by numerous pruritic vesicles along sides of fingers and toes and palms and soles
- Autoeczematization or Id Reaction
  - Refers to a sudden localized or generalized eruption of pinhead-sized vesicles developing in association with a defined local dermatitis or with infection
  - Most common cause is a remote dermatophyte infection

Histopathology

- Spongiotic dermatitis, irrespective of the specific type, may be acute, subacute, or chronic
- Acute Spongiotic Dermatitis
  - Shows variable degree of epidermal spongiosis with vesiculation in extreme cases (Figure 2-10A)
  - Mild papillary dermal edema and a superficial perivascular lymphohistiocytic inflammation are present
  - In allergic contact dermatitis, eosinophils may be present in the dermis and spongiotic foci (Figure 2-10B)
- Subacute Spongiotic Dermatitis
  - Shows parakeratosis with plasma, mild to moderate spongiosis, epidermal hyperplasia, and superficial perivascular lymphohistiocytic infiltrate
- Chronic Spongiotic Dermatitis
  - Spongiosis is mild or absent, but changes of chronicity include a hyperkeratotic cornified layer, marked epidermal hyperplasia, and fibrosis of papillary dermis
  - Dermal inflammatory cell infiltrate is mild

Special Stains and Immunohistochemistry

- PAS stain may be useful in excluding dermatophytosis with spongiosis

Other Techniques for Diagnosis

- Noncontributory

Differential Diagnosis

- Includes many causes of dermatitis that show foci of spongiosis such as seborrheic dermatitis, pityriasis rosea, insect bite reactions, and dermatophyte infections
- Seborrheic Dermatitis
  - Spongiosis is mild and associated with a parakeratotic scale at the openings of the follicular infundibula
- Pityriasis Rosea
  - Spongiosis is focal and associated with mounds of parakeratosis and extravasated red cells
  - Identical changes are also seen in superficial form of erythema annulare centrifugum
- Spongiotic Drug Eruptions and Insect Bite Reactions
  - Show deeper infiltrate of inflammatory cells that also include eosinophils
- Psoriasis
  - Chronic spongiotic dermatitis (lichen simplex chronicus) may resemble psoriasis but generally lacks confluent parakeratosis with neutrophils and thinning of suprapapillary plates

PEARLS

- *Eczema is a nonspecific term used clinically to describe erythematous vesicular lesions with scaly crust that show spongiotic dermatitis on histologic examination*

SELECTED REFERENCES

Ackerman AB, Chongchitnant N, Sanchez J, et al: Histologic Diagnosis of Inflammatory Skin Diseases. Baltimore, Williams & Wilkins, 1997.

Ackerman AB, Ragaz A: A plea to expunge the word "eczema" from the lexicon of dermatology and dermatopathology. Am J Dermatopathol 4:315, 1982.

Weedon D: Skin Pathology, 2nd ed. New York, Churchill Livingstone, 2002, p 112.

INCONTINENTIA PIGMENTI
Clinical Features

- Incontinentia pigmenti is an X-linked–dominant dermatosis that affects mostly females

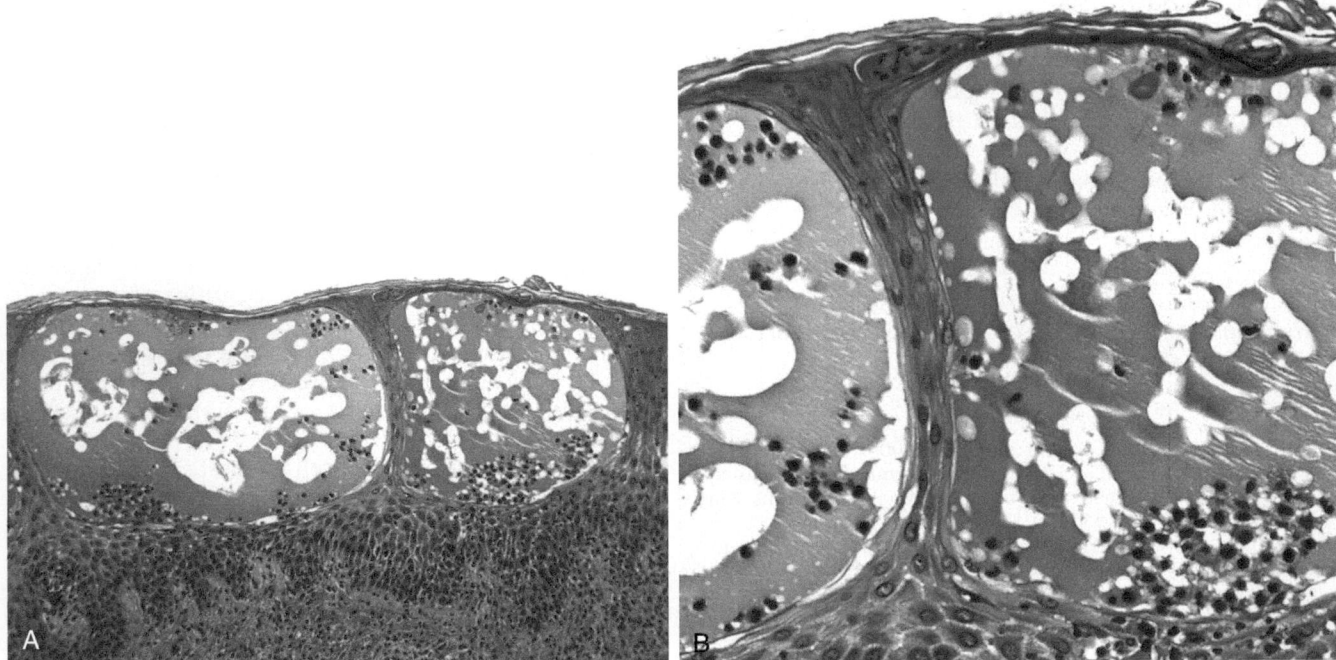

Figure 2-10. Spongiotic dermatitis. A, Marked epidermal spongiosis with formation of spongiotic vesicles and a superficial perivascular mixed inflammatory cell infiltrate are seen. **B,** Higher-power view shows abundant eosinophils within the spongiotic vesicle, which favors a diagnosis of contact dermatitis.

- Characteristic cutaneous manifestations seen at birth include crops of vesicles and bullae on extremities arranged in a linear or whorled pattern
- Lesions heal with hyperkeratosis and verrucous epidermal hyperplasia; the verrucous lesions heal with streaks and whorls of hyperpigmentation that are later replaced by faint hypochromic patches

Histopathology
- Vesicular stage is characterized by marked epidermal spongiosis with eosinophils, single dyskeratotic keratinocytes, and whorls of squamous cells with central keratinization (Figure 2-11)
- Verrucous stage is characterized by hyperkeratosis and papillomatous epidermal hyperplasia with dyskeratotic cells and occasional eosinophils
- Hyperpigmented stage is characterized by numerous melanophages in the upper dermis
- Hypopigmented stage shows epidermal atrophy, decreased melanin in the basal cell layer, and absence of adnexal structures

Special Stains and Immunohistochemistry
- Noncontributory

Other Techniques for Diagnosis
- Noncontributory

Differential Diagnosis
- Spongiosis with eosinophils can be seen in allergic contact dermatitis and in the early stages of pemphigus and bullous pemphigoid; clinical history is essential
- Verrucous stage resembles epidermal nevus
- Changes in the hyper- and hypopigmented stages are those of postinflammatory pigmentary alteration

Toxic Erythema of Newborn
- Eosinophils are typically abundant, but spongiosis is much less prominent

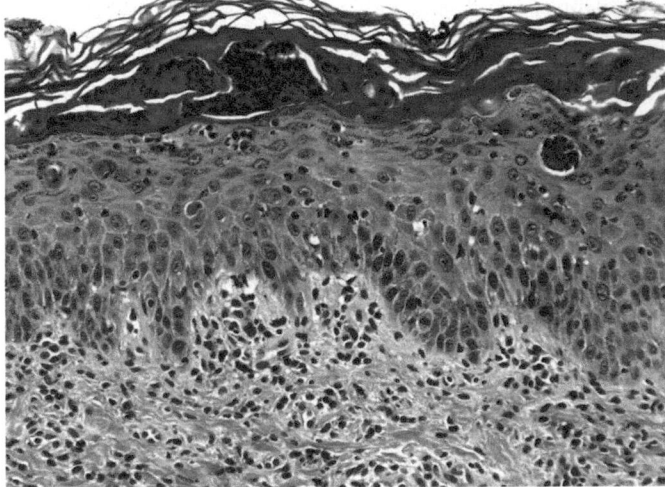

Figure 2-11. Incontinentia pigmenti. Intraepidermal spongiosis, dyskeratosis, and collections of eosinophils both within the epidermis and in the dermal inflammatory cell infiltrate are seen.

PEARLS

- *Eosinophilic chemotactic activity has been shown in the blister fluid of patients with incontinentia pigmenti*
- *In up to 80% of patients, systemic findings with involvement of the central nervous system and eye may be seen; teeth abnormalities may be present*
- *Extent of systemic involvement determines the clinical course*
- *The genetic defect in the familial form has been traced to a mutation in the IKBKG- gene (called NEMO) localized to Xq28 region*

SELECTED REFERENCES

Ackerman AB, Chongchitnant N, Sanchez J, et al: Histologic Diagnosis of Inflammatory Skin Diseases. Baltimore, Williams & Wilkins, 1997.

Ehrenreich M, Tarlow MM, Godlewska-Janusz E, Schwartz RA: Incontinentia pigmenti (Bloch-Sulzberger syndrome): a systemic disorder. Cutis 79:355-362, 2007.

Nelson DL: NEMO, NFkappaB signaling and incontinentia pigmenti. Curr Opin Genet Dev 16:282-288, 2006.

Sulzberger MB: Incontinentia pigmenti (Bloch-Sulzberger). Arch Dermatol Syph 38:57, 1938.

Psoriasiform Dermatitis

PSORIASIS

Clinical Features

- Chronic dermatosis of unknown etiology affecting up to 2% of the population
- Males and females affected equally
- Predilection for areas with trauma, including scalp, lumbosacral skin, and extensor surfaces of elbows and knees
- Variably sized well-demarcated plaques covered by thick, silvery white scale
- Localized or generalized pustular psoriasis, eruptive or guttate psoriasis, and erythrodermic psoriasis are other manifestations of the disease
- Involvement of nails, oral mucosa, and tongue can occur

Histopathology

- Parakeratosis that is often confluent and contains neutrophilic collections (Munro microabscesses)
- Hypogranulosis corresponding to zones of parakeratosis
- Regular epidermal hyperplasia with elongation of rete ridges and thinning of suprapapillary plates (Figure 2-12)
- Dilated tortuous blood vessels in the dermal papillae
- Mild superficial perivascular lymphocytic infiltrate
- In pustular psoriasis, there are prominent spongiform pustules (pustules of Kogoj)
- In guttate psoriasis, the changes are those of early lesion of psoriasis with less pronounced epidermal hyperplasia
- In erythrodermic psoriasis, the histologic changes may be nonspecific

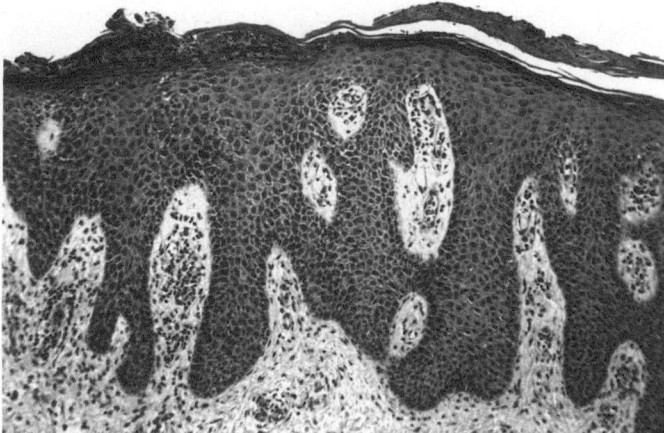

Figure 2-12. Psoriasis. Confluent parakeratosis with collections of neutrophils, diminished granular layer, regular (psoriasiform) epidermal hyperplasia with thinning of suprapapillary plates, dilated blood vessels in the papillary dermis, and mild superficial perivascular inflammation are seen.

Special Stains and Immunohistochemistry

- PAS stain is helpful in excluding dermatophytic infections

Other Techniques for Diagnosis

- Noncontributory

Differential Diagnosis

- Chronic spongiotic dermatitis such as contact or nummular dermatitis should be considered in the differential diagnosis of psoriasiform dermatitis
  - Presence of spongiosis and eosinophils in spongiotic dermatitis may be helpful in differentiation
- Dermatophytes and Bacterial Impetigo
  - Parakeratosis with neutrophils and spongiform pustules should prompt PAS and Gram stains to rule out dermatophytes and bacterial impetigo
- Pityriasis Rubra Pilaris
  - Shows epidermal hyperplasia and parakeratosis and may resemble psoriasis
  - However, in pityriasis rubra pilaris, the suprapapillary plates are thick, the granular layer is prominent, and neutrophils are absent in the parakeratotic cornified layer

PEARLS

- *Removal of the scale on a psoriatic plaque results in a tiny bleeding point (Auspitz sign)*
- *Psoriatic arthritis is seen in about 15% of patients with psoriasis and characteristically involves terminal interphalangeal joints*
- *Severe expression of psoriasis is seen in patients with AIDS who may present with extensive erythroderma, inverse psoriasis, and palmoplantar psoriasis*

SELECTED REFERENCES

Barker JN: Pathogenesis of psoriasis. J Dermatol 25:778-781, 1998.

De Mozzi P, Johnston GA, Alexandroff AB: Psoriasis: an evidence-based update. Report of the 9th evidence-based update meeting, 12 May 2011, Loughborough, UK. Br J Dermatol 166:252-260, 2012.

Nestle FO: Psoriasis. Curr Dir Autoimmun 10:65-75, 2008.

Nickoloff BJ: The immunologic and genetic basis of psoriasis. Arch Dermatol 135:1104-1110, 1999.

Ragaz A, Ackerman AB: Evolution, maturation, and regression of lesions of psoriasis. Am J Dermatopathol 1:199, 1979.

Stern RS: Psoriasis. Lancet 350:349-353, 1997.

PITYRIASIS RUBRA PILARIS

Clinical Features

- Pityriasis rubra pilaris is a chronic follicular-based erythematous papular eruption of unknown etiology that progresses to form orange-red scaly plaques that contain islands of normal-appearing skin
- With progression, a generalized erythroderma may occur
- Palmoplantar keratoderma and scales on face and scalp may be seen

Histopathology

- Sections of fully developed erythematous lesions show alternating orthokeratosis and parakeratosis in horizontal and vertical directions (Figure 2-13A and B)
- Epidermal hyperplasia with broad and short rete, thick suprapapillary plates
- Mild superficial perivascular lymphocytic infiltrate

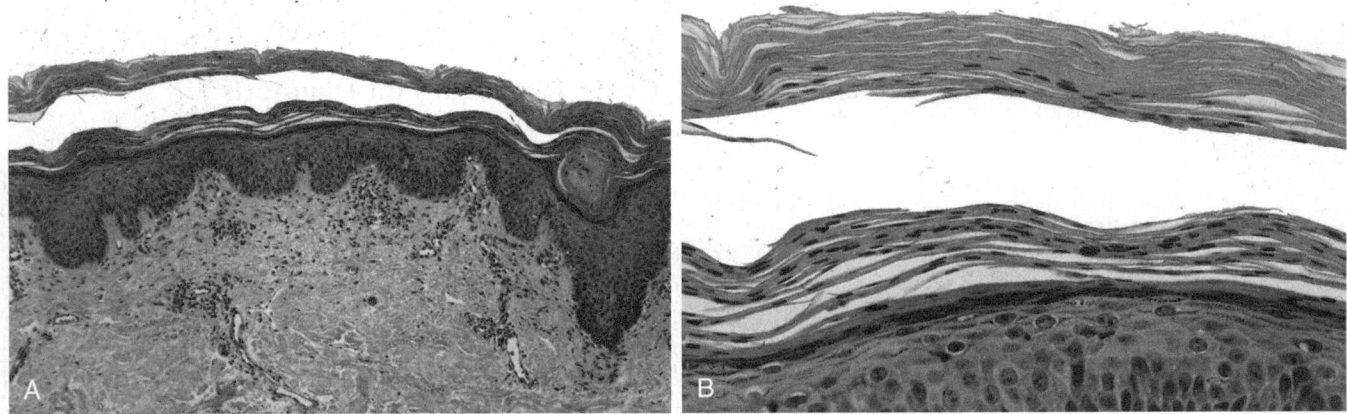

Figure 2-13. Pityriasis rubra pilaris. A, Alternating layers of hyperkeratosis and parakeratosis in both vertical and horizontal patterns, psoriasiform epidermal hyperplasia, and mild superficial perivascular inflammation are seen. **B,** High-power view shows alternating hyperkeratosis and parakeratosis with a normal granular layer.

- Sections of follicular papules show dilated follicular infundibula with follicular plugging

Special Stains and Immunohistochemistry
- Noncontributory

Other Techniques for Diagnosis
- Noncontributory

Differential Diagnosis
- Psoriasis
  - Pityriasis rubra pilaris resembles psoriasis clinically
  - Characteristic histologic changes of psoriasis such as parakeratosis with neutrophils, hypogranulosis, regular epidermal hyperplasia, and thin suprapapillary plates are not seen in pityriasis rubra pilaris

PEARLS

- *A familial form of pityriasis rubra pilaris inherited as an autosomal dominant trait is recognized*

SELECTED REFERENCES

Barr RJ, Young EM Jr: Psoriasiform and related papulosquamous disorders. J Cutan Pathol 12:412-425, 1985.
Klein A, Landthaler M, Karrer S: Pityriasis rubra pilaris: a review of diagnosis and treatment. Am J Clin Dermatol 11:157-170, 2010.
Mobini N, Toussaint S, Kamino H: Noninfectious erythematous, papular, and squamous diseases. In Elder DE, Elenitsas R, Johnson BL Jr, et al (eds): Lever's Histopathology of Skin, 10th ed. Philadelphia, Lippincott Williams & Wilkins, 2008, p 169.
Piamphongsant T, Akaraphant R: Pityriasis rubra pilaris: a new proposed classification. Clin Exp Dermatol 19:134-138, 1994.

SUPERFICIAL AND DEEP PERIVASCULAR DERMATITIS

Dermatitis with Minimal Epidermal Changes

LYMPHOCYTES PREDOMINANT
POLYMORPHOUS LIGHT ERUPTION
Clinical Features
- Pruritic papules and plaques that typically occur in young women mostly during summer, induced by ultraviolet radiation (UVR)

- Eruption starts a few minutes to a few hours after exposure and lasts for hours to days
- Extensor aspects of arms and upper chest are most frequently involved

Histopathology
- Epidermis is mostly unremarkable or shows small foci of spongiosis
- Prominent papillary dermal edema with occasional subepidermal separation and extravasated red cells
- Superficial and deep perivascular, predominantly lymphocytic infiltrate (Figure 2-14)

Special Stains and Immunohistochemistry
- Noncontributory

Other Techniques for Diagnosis
- Lupus band test is negative

Differential Diagnosis
- Cutaneous Lupus Erythematosus
  - Typically the subacute and tumid forms should be considered in the differential diagnosis

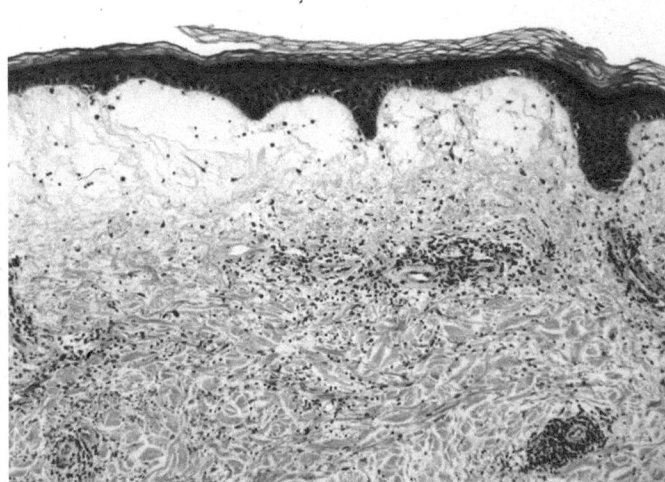

Figure 2-14. Polymorphous light eruption. A superficial and deep perivascular lymphocytic infiltrate is associated with marked papillary dermal edema.

- Polymorphous light eruption lacks changes at the dermoepidermal junction, has less prominent periadnexal infiltrate, and lacks interstitial mucin deposits, features typically seen in cutaneous lupus
- Papillary dermal edema is more prominent in polymorphous light eruption than in subacute cutaneous lupus erythematosus
- Jessner Lymphocytic Infiltrate
  - Shows changes similar to tumid form of lupus erythematosus and may be related

PEARLS

- *Treatment is mostly prophylactic*
- *Limitation of UVR exposure, proper clothing, and application of sunscreens during exposure are helpful*

SELECTED REFERENCES

Boonstra HE, van Weelden H, Toonstra J, van Vloten WA: Polymorphous light eruption: a clinical, photobiologic, and follow-up study of 110 patients. J Am Acad Dermatol 42:199-207, 2000.

Hasan T, Ranki A, Jansen CT, Karvonen J: Disease associations in polymorphous light eruption: a long-term follow-up study of 94 patients. Arch Dermatol 134:1081-1085, 1998.

Lipsker D, Mitschler A, Grosshans E, Cribier B: Could Jessner's lymphocytic infiltrate of the skin be a dermal variant of lupus erythematosus? An analysis of 210 cases. Dermatology 213:15-22, 2006.

EOSINOPHILS PREDOMINANT
INSECT BITE REACTION (PAPULAR URTICARIA)
Clinical Features

- An allergic reaction induced by bites from mosquitoes, fleas, and bedbugs
- Papules and papulovesicles that are intensely pruritic and often become excoriated

Histopathology

- Epidermis and cornified layer may show changes of excoriation
- A superficial and deep perivascular and interstitial mixed inflammatory cell infiltrate containing frequent eosinophils and arranged in a V- or wedge-shaped pattern is the characteristic finding (Figure 2-15A and B)

Special Stains and Immunohistochemistry
- Noncontributory

Other Techniques for Diagnosis
- Noncontributory

Differential Diagnosis
- The histologic changes may be similar in hypersensitivity reactions caused by some drugs and scabies

PEARLS

- *In the case of tick bites, parts of the tick mouthparts may be found in the dermis*
- *A dense chronic lymphoid response (persistent arthropod bite reaction) and lymphoid hyperplasias can be seen with insect bites*

SELECTED REFERENCES

Ackerman AB, Chongchitnant N, Sanchez J, et al: Histologic Diagnosis of Inflammatory Skin Diseases: An Algorithmic Method Based on Pattern Analysis, 2nd ed. Baltimore, Williams & Wilkins, 1997, p 202.

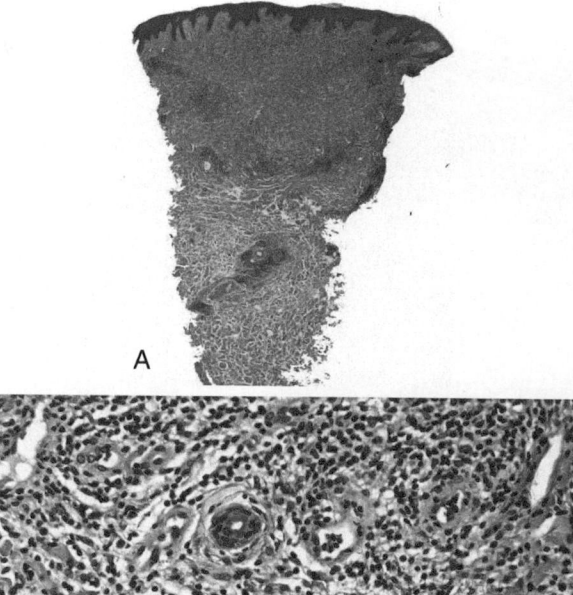

Figure 2-15. Insect bite reaction. A, A superficial and deep perivascular and interstitial infiltrate is arranged in a wedge shape. **B,** High-power view shows frequent eosinophils within the infiltrate.

Gilliam AC, Wood GS: Cutaneous lymphoid hyperplasias. Semin Cutan Med Surg 19:133-141, 2000.

Howard R, Frieden IJ: Papular urticaria in children. Pediatr Dermatol 13:246-249, 1996.

Kain KC: Skin lesions in returned travelers. Med Clin N Am 83:1077-1102, 1999.

Interface Dermatitis
PITYRIASIS LICHENOIDES
Clinical Features

- Self-limited cutaneous eruption of unknown cause that affects young adults and children
- Two forms are recognized:
  - Pityriasis lichenoides et varioliformis acuta
    - An acute, more severe form also known as Mucha-Habermann disease, seen in children and young adults
  - Pityriasis lichenoides chronica
    - Chronic, milder form seen in adults
  - Occasional transitional forms with changes between the two extremes occur
- In pityriasis lichenoides et varioliformis acuta, a papular, papulonecrotic, and occasionally vesiculopustular eruption occurs on trunk and proximal extremities and usually resolves in a few weeks; crops of new lesions can continue to appear, and the disease process itself may have a chronic course
- In pityriasis lichenoides chronica, recurrent crops of reddish brown papules with adherent scales occur on trunk and extremities and resolve in a few weeks

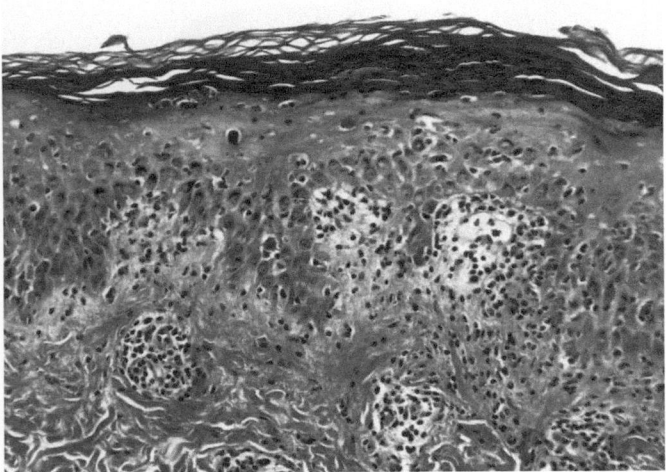

Figure 2-16. Pityriasis lichenoides acuta. Parakeratosis containing collections of neutrophils, vacuolar alteration of the basal cell layer, and patchy lichenoid and perivascular lymphocytic inflammation are seen. Scattered necrotic keratinocytes and extravasated red cells are present.

Histopathology
- Parakeratosis and a scale crust with neutrophils in severe cases (Figure 2-16)
- Epidermal spongiosis and necrotic keratinocytes with eventual erosion and ulceration
- Vacuolar alteration of the basal cell layer
- Papillary dermal edema and extravasated red cells
- Superficial and deep perivascular, predominantly lymphocytic infiltrate that also obscures the dermoepidermal junction
- In pityriasis lichenoides chronica, hyperkeratosis, parakeratosis, mild epidermal hyperplasia, and interface changes are seen; there is superficial perivascular lymphohistiocytic infiltrate with extravasated red cells
- In ulceronecrotic variant of pityriasis lichenoides et varioliformis acuta, there may be lymphocytic vasculitis

Special Stains and Immunohistochemistry
- Noncontributory

Other Techniques for Diagnosis
- Noncontributory

Differential Diagnosis
- Lymphomatoid Papulosis
  - May show histologic overlap with pityriasis lichenoides
  - Atypical lymphoid cells that are CD30 positive are the hallmark of lymphomatoid papulosis
- Vesicular Insect Bite Reactions
  - Can be differentiated from pityriasis lichenoides et varioliformis acuta by the presence of frequent eosinophils in the inflammatory cell infiltrate
  - A spongiotic vesicle may be present at the site of the bite

PEARLS

- *Inflammatory cell infiltrate consists mostly of lymphocytes with a predominance of CD8-positive T-lymphoid cells*

SELECTED REFERENCES

Bowers S, Warshaw EM: Pityriasis lichenoides and its subtypes. J Am Acad Dermatol 55:557-572, 2006.
Ersoy-Evans S, Greco MF, et al: Pityriasis lichenoides in childhood: a retrospective review of 124 patients. J Am Acad Dermatol 56:205, 2007.
Kempf W, Kazakov DV, Palmedo G, et al: Pityriasis lichenoides et varioliformis acuta with numerous CD30(+) cells: a variant mimicking lymphomatoid papulosis and other cutaneous lymphomas: a clinicopathologic, immunohistochemical, and molecular biological study of 13 cases. Am J Surg Pathol 36:1021-1029, 2012.
Magro CM, Morrison C, Kovatich A, et al: Pityriasis lichenoides is a cutaneous T-cell dyscrasia: a clinical, genotypic, and phenotypic study. Hum Pathol 33:788, 2002.

FIXED DRUG ERUPTION
Clinical Features
- Well-defined, circumscribed patches occur at the same site in response to repeated intake of the drug
- Lesions are slightly edematous and erythematous and may develop dusky centers and become bullous
- Lesions heal with pigmentation

Histopathology
- Vacuolar alteration of the basal cell layer and scattered necrotic keratinocytes; changes identical to those in erythema multiforme (Figure 2-17)
- Bullae result from full-thickness epidermal necrosis, similar to that seen in toxic epidermal necrolysis
- Superficial and deep perivascular and occasionally lichenoid inflammatory cell infiltrate with lymphocytes, neutrophils, and eosinophils
- Melanophages in upper dermis

Special Stains and Immunohistochemistry
- Noncontributory

Other Techniques for Diagnosis
- Noncontributory

Differential Diagnosis
- Erythema Multiforme and Toxic Epidermal Necrolysis
  - May have histologic changes similar to those of fixed drug eruption
  - Clinical information is essential

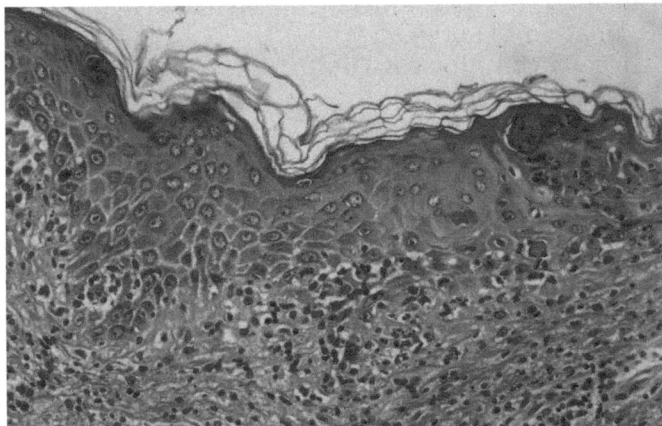

Figure 2-17. Fixed drug eruption. Necrotic keratinocytes in the epidermis, vacuolar alteration of the basal cell layer, and patchy lichenoid inflammatory cell infiltrate that obscures the dermoepidermal junction are seen. Histologic changes are similar to those seen erythema multiforme.

- Deeper perivascular inflammatory cell infiltrate with lymphocytes, neutrophils, and eosinophils, when present, favor fixed drug eruption

PEARLS

- *Fixed drug eruptions occur most commonly with trimethoprim-sulfamethoxazole, acetylsalicylic acid, and phenolphthalein*
- *Increasing number of lesions can occur with each successive administration of the offending drug*

SELECTED REFERENCES

Crowson AN, Magro CM: Recent advances in the pathology of cutaneous drug eruptions. Dermatol Clin 17:537-560, viii, 1999.
Roujeau JC: Neutrophilic drug eruptions. Clin Dermatol 18:331-337, 2000.
Sehgal VN, Srivastava G: Fixed drug eruption (FDE): changing scenario of incriminating drugs. Int J Dermatol 45:897-908, 2006.
Shiohara T, Mizukawa Y: Fixed drug eruption: a disease mediated by self-inflicted responses of intraepidermal T cells. Eur J Dermatol 17:201-208, 2007.

LYMPHOMATOID PAPULOSIS

Clinical Features

- Presents as multiple, small papules that are most often short lived but usually recurrent

Histopathology

- Superficial and deep mixed cell infiltrate that is wedge shaped and also lichenoid
- In addition to neutrophils, eosinophils, and plasma cells, a significant number of atypical lymphocytes, including Reed Sternberg-like cells (type A), are present
- Surface ulceration may be present
- Atypical lymphocytes with cerebriform nuclei in a lichenoid pattern and resembling mycosis fungoides (type B) are seen in some examples
- Rarely, dense monomorphous infiltrate of atypical lymphocytes resembling anaplastic large cell lymphoma (type C) can be seen in association with typical clinical features of lymphomatoid papulosis (Figure 2-18)

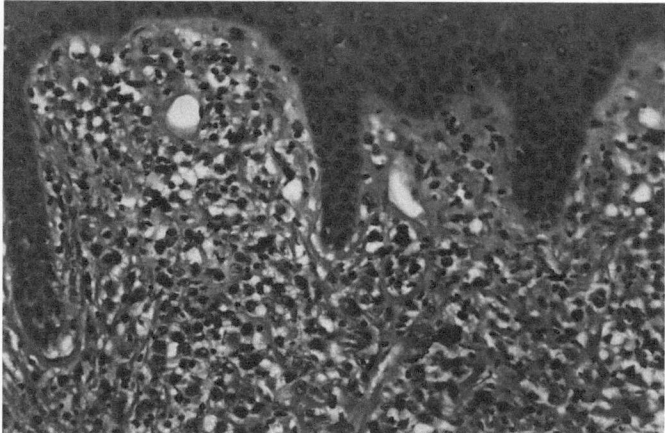

Figure 2-18. Lymphomatoid papulosis. Section shows a dense perivascular and interstitial infiltrate consisting predominantly of lymphocytes. A significant number of the lymphocytes are large and contain enlarged hyperchromatic and irregular nuclei.

Special Stains and Immunohistochemistry

- The atypical lymphocytes are positive for CD30

Other Techniques for Diagnosis

- Clonal rearrangement of T-cell receptor gene may be present

Differential Diagnosis

- Insect Bite Reaction
  - Activated lymphocytes may be present
  - Atypical cells that are CD30 positive are characteristic of lymphomatoid papulosis
- Pityriasis Lichenoides Acuta
  - Histologic patterns of both conditions may be similar
  - Demonstration of CD30-positive lymphoid cells in lymphomatoid papulosis is helpful in the differential diagnosis

PEARLS

- *CD30 positive cells may be present in reactive conditions such as insect bites, drug eruption, and viral infections; clinical correlation is essential*
- *Progression of lymphomatoid papulosis to large cell anaplastic lymphoma (CD30 positive) can occur, suggesting that lymphomatoid papulosis may represent the benign end in the spectrum of CD30-positive T cell lymphoproliferative disorders*

SELECTED REFERENCES

Cerroni L: Lymphomatoid papulosis, pityriasis lichenoides et varioliformis acuta, and anaplastic large-cell (Ki-1+) lymphoma. J Am Acad Dermatol 37:287, 1997.
Demierre MF, Goldberg LJ, Kadin ME, Koh HK: Is it lymphoma or lymphomatoid papulosis? J Am Acad Dermatol 36:765-772, 1997.
Guitart J, Querfeld C: Cutaneous CD30 lymphoproliferative disorders and similar conditions: a clinical and pathologic prospective on a complex issue. Semin Diagn Pathol 26:131-140, 2009.
LeBoit PE: Lymphomatoid papulosis and cutaneous CD30+ lymphoma. Am J Dermatopathol 18:221-235, 1996.
Wang HH, Myers T, Lach LJ, et al: Increased risk of lymphoid and non-lymphoid malignancies in patients with lymphomatoid papulosis. Cancer 86:1240-1245, 1999.
Werner B, Massone C, Kerl H, Cerroni L: Large CD30-positive cells in benign, atypical lymphoid infiltrates of the skin. J Cutan Pathol 35:1100-1107, 2008.

Psoriasiform Dermatitis

SECONDARY SYPHILIS

Clinical Features

- Hematogenous dissemination of causative organism, *Treponema pallidum*, results in cutaneous eruption that can be macular, papular, papulosquamous, or, rarely, pustular
- Associated constitutional symptoms such as fever and lymphadenopathy may be present; other manifestations include condyloma lata, syphilis cornee, lues maligna, and alopecia

Histopathology

- Patchy or confluent parakeratosis containing neutrophils
- Regular (psoriasiform) epidermal hyperplasia with focal spongiosis (Figure 2-19A)
- Epidermal hyperplasia is least in macular lesions and most in condylomata lata

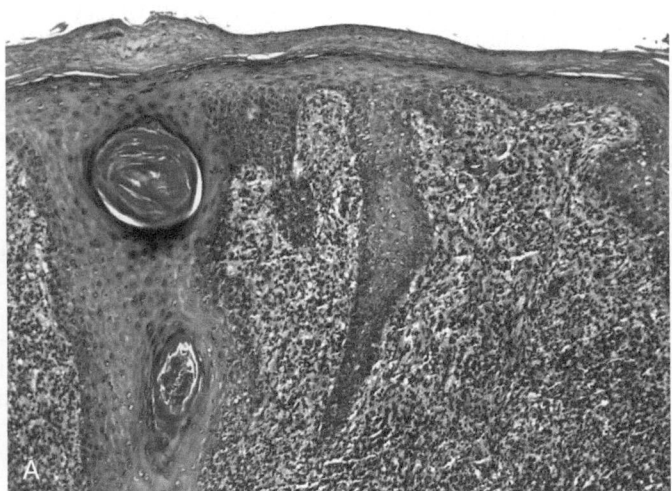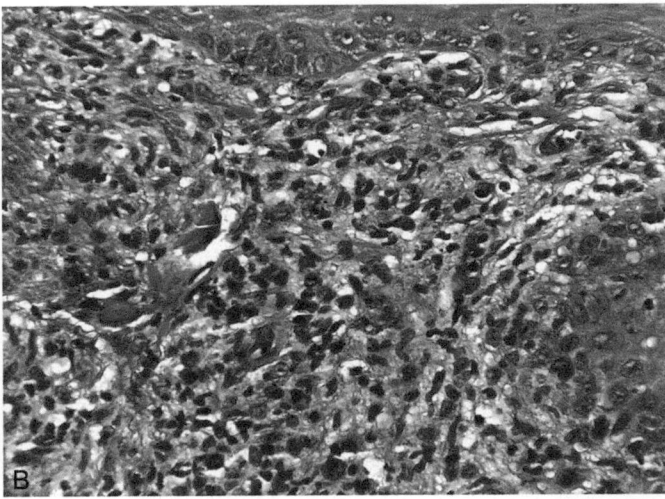

Figure 2-19. Secondary syphilis. A, Histologic section shows parakeratosis with neutrophils, epidermal hyperplasia, and a dense bandlike inflammatory cell infiltrate that obscures the dermoepidermal junction. **B,** On high-power view, the infiltrate contains a large number of plasma cells.

- Vacuolar alteration of the basal cell layer, occasional necrotic keratinocytes, and edema of papillary dermis
- Superficial and deep perivascular and periadnexal lymphoplasmacytic infiltrate that can also be lichenoid with obscuring of the dermoepidermal junction; plasma cells may be present around nerves (Figure 2-19B)
- Infiltrate can be lymphocytic, lymphoplasmacytic, or lymphohistiocytic with rare granuloma formation

Special Stains and Immunohistochemistry
- Silver stain (Warthin-Starry) may show spirochetes within the epidermis in one third of cases
- Immunohistochemistry with monoclonal antibody to *T. pallidum* yields better detection rates

Other Techniques for Diagnosis
- PCR

Differential Diagnosis
- Mycosis Fungoides
  - Shows psoriasiform lichenoid pattern similar to syphilis; however, in mycosis fungoides, atypical lymphoid cells are present within the dermal infiltrate and in the mildly spongiotic epidermis
  - Plasma cells are not frequent
- Subacute and Chronic Spongiotic Dermatitis, Including Photoallergic Dermatitis
  - May show some psoriasiform hyperplasia and spongiosis
  - In general, plasma cells are not prominent
- Pityriasis Lichenoides
  - Can simulate secondary syphilis but shows predominantly a lymphocytic infiltrate without plasma cells
- Psoriasis and Psoriasiform Drug Eruption
  - Inflammatory infiltrate is not deep
  - Suprapapillary plate thinning is not a feature of secondary syphilis
- Sarcoid and Other Conditions with a Prominent Granulomatous Pattern
  - May appear similar to the granulomatous pattern of secondary syphilis

PEARLS
- *An unusual variant of secondary syphilis is lues maligna, an ulcerative form characterized by thrombotic endarteritis of vessels in the deep dermis resulting in ischemic necrosis*
- *Serologic tests are the most common method of diagnosing syphilis*

SELECTED REFERENCES
Abell E, Marks R, Wilson Jones E: Secondary syphilis: a clinicopathological review. Br J Dermatol 93:53, 1975.
Goens JL, Janniger CK, De Wolf K: Dermatologic and systemic manifestations of syphilis. Am Fam Physician 50:1013-1020, 1994.
Hoang MP, High WA, Molberg KH: Secondary syphilis: a histologic and immunohistochemical evaluation. J Cutan Pathol 31:595-599, 2004.
Jeerapaet P, Ackerman AS: Histologic patterns of secondary syphilis. Arch Dermatol 107:373, 1973.
Müller H, Eisendle K, Bräuninger W, Kutzner H, et al: Comparative analysis of immunohistochemistry, polymerase chain reaction and focus-floating microscopy for the detection of Treponema pallidum in mucocutaneous lesions of primary, secondary and tertiary syphilis. Br J Dermatol 165:50-60, 2011.

NODULAR AND DIFFUSE DERMATITIS

Neutrophils Predominant
SWEET SYNDROME

Clinical Features
- Acute febrile neutrophilic dermatosis, or Sweet syndrome, is characterized by fever, leukocytosis, and a cutaneous eruption that consists of violaceous plaque-like lesions involving the extremities, face, and trunk
- It is chiefly a disease of adults and seen occasionally in children
- An underlying myeloproliferative disorder, most commonly acute myeloid leukemia or inflammatory disease and rarely solid tumors may be present
- Sweet syndrome–like eruption is reported with many drugs

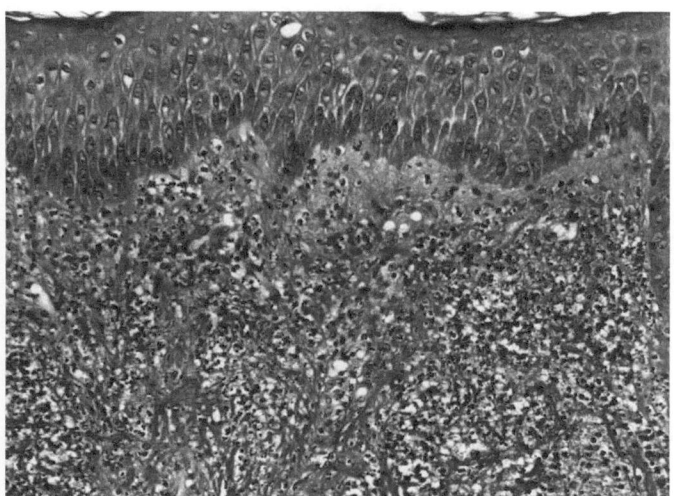

Figure 2-20. Sweet syndrome. Histologic section shows a diffuse dermal infiltrate consisting predominantly of neutrophils and extravasated red blood cells. Intact blood vessels help to differentiate this from leukocytoclastic vasculitis.

Histopathology
- Dense, diffuse, upper dermal infiltrate of predominantly neutrophils and neutrophilic nuclear dust with scattered lymphocytes, histiocytes, and eosinophils
- Edema of the papillary dermis (Figure 2-20)
- Dilated blood vessels with plump endothelial lining and extravasated red blood cells

Special Stains and Immunohistochemistry
- Special stains for microorganisms to exclude an infectious etiology

Other Techniques for Diagnosis
- Noncontributory

Differential Diagnosis
- Leukocytoclastic Vasculitis
  - Vascular damage with fibrin deposition in the vessel wall seen in leukocytoclastic vasculitis is not a feature of Sweet syndrome
- Pyoderma Gangrenosum
  - Inflammatory infiltrate (predominately neutrophilic) is deeper and denser than in Sweet syndrome
  - Surface ulceration and secondary vasculitis may be present

PEARLS
- *Sweet syndrome is believed to be a hypersensitivity reaction of unknown etiology*
- *Potential infectious etiology should be considered and excluded in all cases of neutrophilic dermatoses*

SELECTED REFERENCES

Buck T, González LM, Lambert WC, Schwartz RA: Sweet's syndrome with hematologic disorders: A review and reappraisal. Int J Dermatol 47:775-782, 2008.
Cohen PR, Kurzrock R: Sweet's syndrome: a neutrophilic dermatosis classically associated with acute onset and fever. Clin Dermatol 18:265-282, 2000.
Huang W, McNeely MC: Neutrophilic tissue reactions. Adv Dermatol 13:33-64, 1997.
Raza S, Kirkland RS, Patel AA, et al: Insight into Sweet's syndrome and associated-malignancy: a review of the current literature. Int J Oncol; 42:1516, 2013.
Roujeau JC: Neutrophilic drug eruptions. Clin Dermatol 18:331-337, 2000.
Sweet RD: Acute febrile neutrophilic dermatosis. Br J Dermatol 74:349, 1964.
Uihlein LC, Brandling-Bennett HA, Lio PA, Liang MG: Sweet syndrome in children. Pediatr Dermatol 29:38, 2012.

PYODERMA GANGRENOSUM
Clinical Features
- Idiopathic ulceronecrotic skin disease that begins as follicular papules and pustules that eventually ulcerate
- Lower extremities and trunk are often involved
- Fully developed lesions show necrotic center with a raised, undermined border with a dusky-purple hue
- Pyoderma gangrenosum may be the cutaneous manifestation of underlying systemic diseases such as inflammatory bowel disease, connective tissue disease, hematopoietic malignancies, and liver diseases

Histopathology
- Features are nonspecific and vary according to the area biopsied
- The center of the lesion shows ulcer with necrosis, dense diffuse neutrophilic infiltrate, and occasionally secondary vasculitis (Figure 2-21)
- Biopsy of the undermined border shows mixed inflammatory cell infiltrate in addition to neutrophils
- Periphery of the lesions shows primarily a lymphocytic and histiocytic reaction

Special Stains and Immunohistochemistry
- Special stains and microbiologic cultures help to exclude an infectious etiology

Other Techniques for Diagnosis
- Noncontributory

Differential Diagnosis
- Sweet Syndrome
  - Neutrophilic infiltrate is typically more superficial and less dense
- Bacterial Cellulitis
  - Should always be considered in the differential diagnosis
  - Requires demonstration of bacteria by special stains or microbiologic cultures

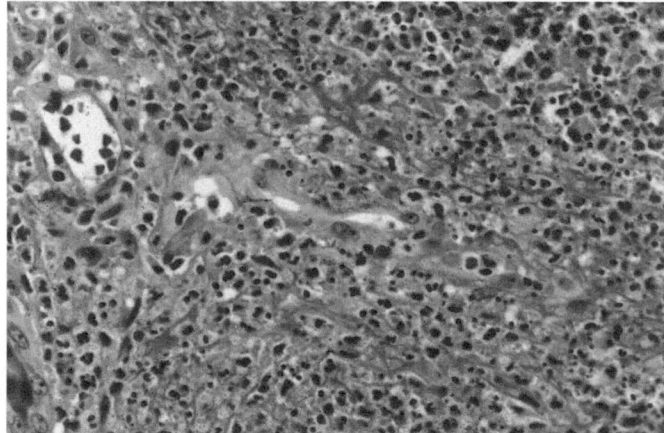

Figure 2-21. Pyoderma gangrenosum. Histologic section shows a dense diffuse dermal infiltrate of predominantly neutrophils. Blood vessels show plump endothelial lining. The infiltrate is generally denser than that seen in Sweet syndrome.

SELECTED REFERENCES

Binus AM, Qureshi AA, Li VW, Winterfield LS: Pyoderma gangrenosum: a retrospective review of patient characteristics, comorbidities and therapy in 103 patients. Br J Dermatol 165:1244. 2011.
Callen JP: Pyoderma gangrenosum. Lancet 351:581-585, 1998.
Powell FC, Collins S: Pyoderma gangrenosum. Clin Dermatol 18:283-293, 2000.
Ruocco E, Sangiuliano S, Gravina AG, et al: Pyoderma gangrenosum: an updated review. J Eur Acad Dermatol Venereol 23:1008, 2009.
Su WP, Schroeter AL, Perry HO, et al: Histopathologic and immunopathologic study of pyoderma gangrenosum. J Cutan Pathol 13:323, 1986.

EOSINOPHILS PREDOMINANT

Eosinophilic Cellulitis

Clinical Features

• Eosinophilic cellulitis (Wells syndrome) is a rare, recurrent dermatosis of uncertain pathogenesis, characterized by sudden onset of erythematous patches that evolve into painful plaques
• May be idiopathic or associated with insect bites, parasitosis, infections, myeloproliferative disorders, and drug reactions
• Associated with peripheral blood eosinophilia in at least 50% of the patients

Histopathology

• Spongiotic intraepidermal vesicles may be present
• Diffuse and dense dermal infiltrate of eosinophils occasionally extending into the subcutaneous tissue
• Eosinophil degranulation is more prominent in older lesions and may impregnate the collagen bundles (flame figures)
• Palisading histiocytes with central necrobiosis may be seen in florid lesions

Special Stains and Immunohistochemistry

• Noncontributory

Other Techniques for Diagnosis

• Noncontributory

Differential Diagnosis

• Consider other dermal hypersensitivity reactions, including reactions to insect bites, parasites, and drugs

SELECTED REFERENCES

Caputo R, Marzano AV, Vezzoli P, Lunardon L: Wells syndrome in adults and children: a report of 19 cases. Arch Dermatol 142:1157, 2006.
Falagas ME, Vergidis PI: Narrative review: diseases that masquerade as infectious cellulitis. Ann Intern Med 142:47, 2005.
Fujii K, Tanabe H, Kanno Y, et al: Eosinophilic cellulitis as a cutaneous manifestation of idiopathic hypereosinophilic syndrome. J Am Acad Dermatol 49:1174-1177, 2003.
McCalmont TH, Altemus D, Maurer T, Berger TG: Eosinophilic folliculitis: the histologic spectrum. Am J Dermatopathol 17:439, 1995.

SCABIES

Clinical Features

• Scabies is a contagious, pruritic, papulovesicular, and pustular eruption caused by the mite Sarcoptes scabiei
• The eruption constitutes an hypersensitivity reaction and is most pronounced on the abdomen, buttocks, and anterior axillary folds
• Burrows are produced by the female mite and typically involve the palms, web spaces between fingers, and male genitalia
• Persistent pruritic nodules or nodular scabies involving most commonly the scrotum can be seen up to several months after treatment

Histopathology

• Sections taken from the burrow show a tunnel-like space between layers of parakeratosis; the mite or its products such as eggshells and fecal deposits need to be demonstrated for a definite diagnosis (Figure 2-22)
• Spongiosis and vesiculation may be present in the epidermis
• Superficial and deep dermal infiltrate containing varying numbers of eosinophils
• Persistent nodular lesions show dense, diffuse, mixed inflammatory cell infiltrate containing eosinophils, thick-walled blood vessels, and occasionally atypical mononuclear cells; pseudolymphomatous pattern may also be seen (the mite is generally absent in these lesions)

Special Stains and Immunohistochemistry

• Noncontributory

Other Techniques for Diagnosis

• A suspected burrow can be shaved, placed on a glass slide, and examined under oil immersion

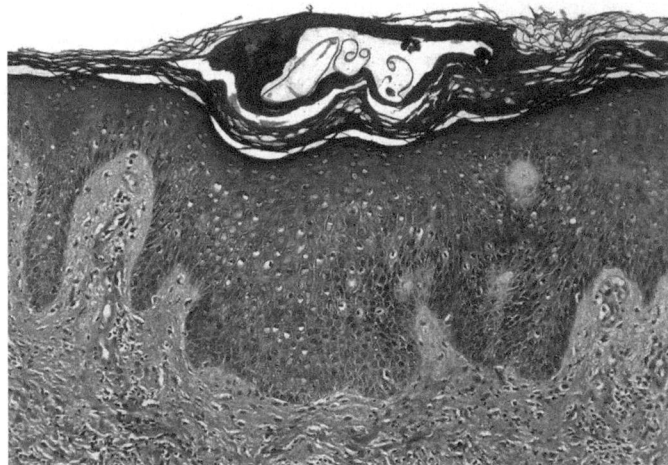

Figure 2-22. Scabies. Histologic section shows a parakeratotic burrow containing body parts of the mite of scabies. The dermal inflammatory cell infiltrate typically contains frequent eosinophils.

Differential Diagnosis

- In the absence of the mite or its products in the cornified layer, the histologic changes cannot be distinguished from other hypersensitivity reactions such as those caused by arthropod bites

PEARLS

- *Norwegian scabies is a rare variant in which an immeasurable number of mites is present within the cornified layer; generally seen in patients with congenital or iatrogenic impairment of immune responses, the mentally deficient, and physically debilitated patients*

SELECTED REFERENCES

Angel TA, Nigro J, Levy ML: Infestations in the pediatric patient. Pediatr Clin N Am 47:921-935, 2000.

Brites C, Weyll M, Pedroso C, et al: Severe and Norwegian scabies are strongly associated with retroviral (HIV-1/HTLV-1) infection in Bahia, Brazil. AIDS 16:1292, 2002.

Chosidow O: Scabies and pediculosis. Lancet 355:819-826, 2000.

Fernandez N, Torres A, Ackerman AB: Pathological findings in human scabies. Arch Dermatol 113:320, 1977.

Fuller LC. Epidemiology of scabies. Curr Opin Infect Dis 26:123, 2013.

Histiocytes Predominant
XANTHOGRANULOMA
Clinical Features

- Benign non-Langerhans cell histiocytosis that most commonly occurs during infancy (within first 6 months of life) but can be seen occasionally in adults
- About 20% are congenital
- Usually presents as single or multiple tan to pink-red nodules that almost always regress over time to a tan macule or depression
- Occasionally found in the deep soft tissue
- Infrequent association with neurofibromatosis and urticaria pigmentosa (mastocytosis)

Histopathology

- Well-defined or focally infiltrative margins
- Characterized by uniform-appearing histiocytes with an eosinophilic, vacuolated, or xanthomatous cytoplasm
- Touton giant cells are typically seen (Figure 2-23)
- Admixture of neutrophils, eosinophils, and lymphocytes is commonly present
- Resolving lesion resembles dermatofibroma

Special Stains and Immunohistochemistry

- Oil red O highlights intracytoplasmic neutral lipids
- CD68 and factor XIIIa positive
- CD1a negative; S-100 protein usually negative

Other Techniques for Diagnosis

- Noncontributory

Differential Diagnosis

- Langerhans Cell Histiocytosis (Eosinophilic Granuloma)
  - Characterized by the presence of histiocytes and eosinophils
  - Histiocytes positive for CD1a and S-100 protein
  - Electron microscopy demonstrates Birbeck granules
- Fibrous Histiocytoma (Dermatofibroma)
  - Found in adults (usually third to fifth decades)

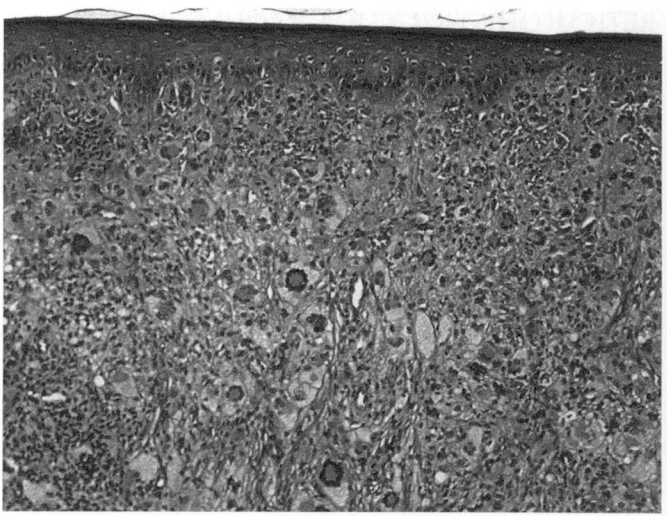

Figure 2-23. Xanthogranuloma. Histologic section shows dermal infiltrate of predominantly histiocytes, including multinucleated histiocytes containing foamy cytoplasm and nuclei arranged at the periphery in a wreathlike pattern (Touton giant cells). Lymphocytes are present in the background.

  - Composed of spindle-shaped fibroblasts and histiocytic cells arranged in a storiform pattern
  - Typically lacks Touton giant cells
- Xanthoma
  - Typically associated with hyperlipidemia
  - Composed of sheets of histiocytes containing abundant intracytoplasmic lipid
  - Cholesterol clefts and multinucleated giant cells are typical

PEARLS

- *Pathogenesis remains uncertain; believed to be a reactive rather than neoplastic process*
- *Not associated with a lipid abnormality*
- *Skin lesions almost always regress with time and ultimately appear as a slight depression on the skin surface*
- *Overall prognosis is excellent*
- *Disseminated disease has been reported to be associated with juvenile chronic myeloid leukemia*

SELECTED REFERENCES

Burgdorf WH, Zelger B: JXG, NF1, and JMML: alphabet soup or a clinical issue? Pediatr Dermatol 21:174, 2004.

Dehner LP: Juvenile xanthogranulomas in the first two decades of life: a clinicopathologic study of 174 cases with cutaneous and extracutaneous manifestations. Am J Surg Pathol 27:579, 2003.

Freyer DR, Kennedy R, Bostrom BC, et al: Juvenile xanthogranuloma: forms of systemic disease and their clinical implications. J Pediatr 129:227-237, 1996.

Hernandez-Martin A, Baselga E, Drolet BA, Esterly NB: Juvenile xanthogranuloma. J Am Acad Dermatol 36:355-367; quiz, 368-369, 1997.

Janssen D, Harms D: Juvenile xanthogranuloma in childhood and adolescence: a clinicopathologic study of 129 patients from the Kiel pediatric tumor registry. Am J Surg Pathol 29:21, 2005.

Raygada M, Arthur DC, Wayne AS, et al: Juvenile xanthogranuloma in a child with previously unsuspected neurofibromatosis type 1 and juvenile myelomonocytic leukemia. Pediatr Blood Cancer 54:173, 2010.

RETICULOHISTIOCYTIC GRANULOMA

Clinical Features
- Typically occurs in adults
- Most frequently presents as red-brown cutaneous nodules
- Typically well-circumscribed nodule with a red-brown to yellow cut surface
- May present as localized (giant cell reticulohistiocytoma) or systemic disease (multicentric reticulohistiocytosis)
- Cutaneous reticulohistiocytoma (localized form)
  - May present as single or multiple skin lesions
  - Clinical features similar to xanthogranuloma
- Multicentric reticulohistiocytosis (systemic form)
  - Rare condition
  - May involve lymph nodes, heart, bone, and joints in addition to widespread skin involvement
  - Patients may present with progressive erosive arthritis, fever, and weight loss
  - Association with hyperlipidemia, internal malignancies, and autoimmune diseases

Histopathology
- Essentially similar features in both localized and systemic forms
- Well-defined infiltrate of multinucleated, uniform epithelioid histiocytes with abundant eosinophilic, "glassy" cytoplasm (Figure 2-24)
- Infrequent mitotic activity
- Scattered chronic inflammatory cells

Special Stains and Immunohistochemistry
- CD68 positive
- S-100 protein and CD1a negative

Other Techniques for Diagnosis
- Noncontributory

Differential Diagnosis
- Malignant Fibrous Histiocytoma (Pleomorphic Sarcoma)
  - Deep-seated, cellular tumor composed of pleomorphic tumor cells arranged in a storiform pattern
  - High mitotic rate often with many atypical forms
  - Areas of hemorrhage and necrosis common
- Malignant Melanoma

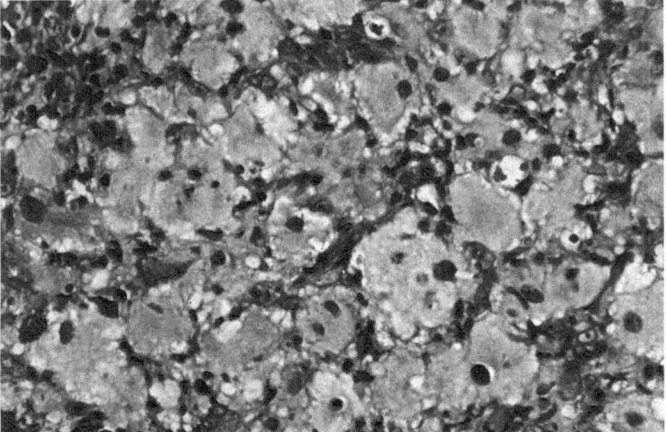

Figure 2-24. Reticulohistiocytic granuloma. The dense dermal infiltrate consists of lymphocytes and histiocytes. The cytoplasm of the histiocytes shows characteristic ground-glass appearance.

- Large, pleomorphic cells with large nuclei and prominent nucleoli
- High mitotic rate often seen
- Melanin pigment may be seen
- Positive for S-100 protein and Melan-A

PEARLS
- *Solitary form of reticulohistiocytoma and xanthogranuloma may be regarded as part of a spectrum*
- *Disseminated reticulohistiocytosis is associated with various malignancies (carcinoma of the breast, colon, or lung) or systemic disease (tuberculosis, diabetes, hypothyroidism)*
- *Polyarthritis seen in the disseminated form is due to infiltrate of similar histiocytic cells found in skin around the joints*

SELECTED REFERENCES
Jung HD, Kim HS, Lee JY, et al: Multicentric reticulohistiocytosis. Acta Derm Venereol 93:124-125, 2013.

Luz FB, Gaspar AP, Ramos-e-Silva M, et al: Immunohistochemical profile of multicentric reticulohistiocytosis. Skinmed 4:71, 2005.

Miettinen M, Fetsch JF: Reticulohistiocytoma (solitary epithelioid histiocytoma): a clinicopathologic and immunohistochemical study of 44 cases. Am J Surg Pathol 30:521, 2006.

Snow JL, Muller SA: Malignancy-associated multicentric reticulohistiocytosis: a clinical, histological, and immunophenotypic study. Br J Dermatol 133:71-76, 1995.

Tajirian AL, Malik MK, Robinson-Bostom L, et al: Multicentric reticulohistiocytosis. Clin Dermatol 24:486, 2006.

PALISADING AND NECROBIOTIC GRANULOMAS
GRANULOMA ANNULARE
Clinical Features
- Benign granulomatous process of unknown etiology
- Occurs most commonly in children and young adults; females more commonly affected than males
- Predilection for areas of trauma and exposure, typically the dorsal surface of the hands and feet, ankles, knees, and elbows
- Single or multiple annular dermal plaques with central clearing and raised erythematous borders
- Spontaneous regression of the lesions occurs, but they occasionally recur

Histopathology
- Histiocytes in the dermis in an interstitial pattern or as palisades surrounding zones of degenerating collagen with mucin; patterns between the two extremes can occur (Figure 2-25)
- Typically involves upper and middle dermis; occasionally only the upper or deep dermis
- Multinucleated histiocytes, some of which contain elastic fibers in the cytoplasm
- Perivascular infiltrates of lymphocytes; eosinophils in varying numbers may be present
- Occasional neutrophils and nuclear fragmentation in areas of mucinous degeneration

Special Stains and Immunohistochemistry
- Colloidal iron stain highlights mucin

Other Techniques for Diagnosis
- Noncontributory

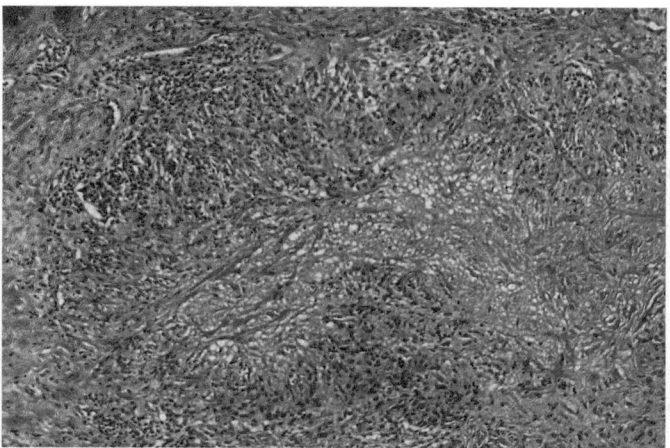

Figure 2-25. Granuloma annulare. Histologic section shows palisade of histiocytes surrounding zones of myxoid degeneration of collagen. The granulomas are typically located in the upper dermis.

Differential Diagnosis
- Rheumatoid Nodule
  - Zone of necrobiosis is usually highly eosinophilic, occasionally resembling fibrin and no mucinous deposits
  - Involvement of subcutaneous tissue is typical
- Necrobiosis Lipoidica
  - Biopsy specimens are usually rectangular
  - Basophilic degeneration of collagen is stratified between layers of inflammatory cell infiltrate
  - Plasma cells are frequently present in the inflammatory cell infiltrate
  - Involvement of deep dermis is typical

PEARLS

- *A subcutaneous variant of granuloma annulare (pseudorheumatoid nodule) typically presents in children with deep-seated nodules in the dermis or subcutaneous fat in which histologic differentiation from rheumatoid nodule can be difficult*
- *A well-known diagnostic pitfall is diagnosing epithelioid sarcoma as granuloma annulare, and vice versa*

SELECTED REFERENCES

Barren DF, Cootauco MH, Cohen BA: Granuloma annulare: a clinical review. Prim Care Pract 1:33-39, 1997.
Güneş P, Göktay F, Mansur AT, et al: Collagen-elastic tissue changes and vascular involvement in granuloma annulare: a review of 35 cases. J Cutan Pathol 36:838, 2009.
Ko C, Glusac E, Shapiro P: Noninfectious granulomas. In Elder DE, Elenitsas R, Johnson BL Jr, et al (eds): Lever's Histopathology of Skin, 10th ed. Philadelphia, Lippincott Williams & Wilkins, 2008, p 361.
Magro CM, Crowson AN, Regauer S: Granuloma annulare and necrobiosis lipoidica tissue reactions as a manifestation of systemic disease. Hum Pathol 27:50-56, 1996.

NECROBIOSIS LIPOIDICA
Clinical Features
- Degenerative cutaneous disease of unknown etiology
- Three times more common in women than men
- Typically seen in diabetic patients in their fifth and sixth decades and in nondiabetic patients between the ages of 20 and 40 years
- Characteristically affects the anterior tibial surface but also has a predilection for the thighs, popliteal areas, and dorsum of the feet and arms
- Indurated yellow-brown oval plaques with a violaceous border
- Center of the plaque may later become atrophic with a distinctive yellow waxy hue

Histopathology
- Rectangular contour of biopsy sample
- Epidermal atrophy and superficial dermal telangiectasia
- Alternating horizontal layers of basophilic degeneration of collagen and palisades consisting of histiocytes, lymphocytes, and plasma cells (Figure 2-26)
- Zones of dermal sclerosis
- Sarcoidal type granulomas are seen on occasion

Special Stains and Immunohistochemistry
- Noncontributory

Other Techniques for Diagnosis
- Noncontributory

Differential Diagnosis
- Rheumatoid Nodule

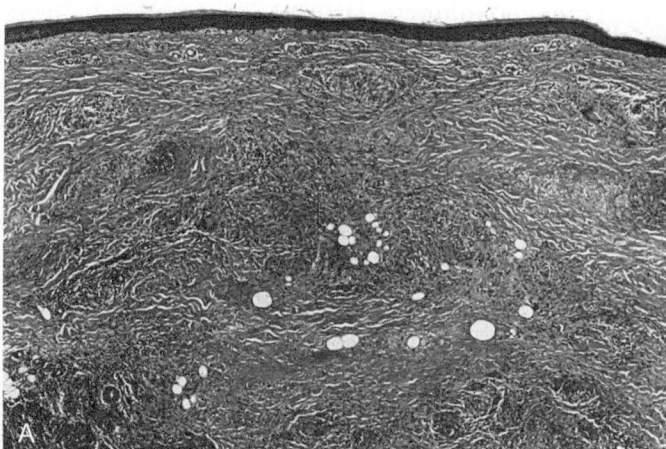
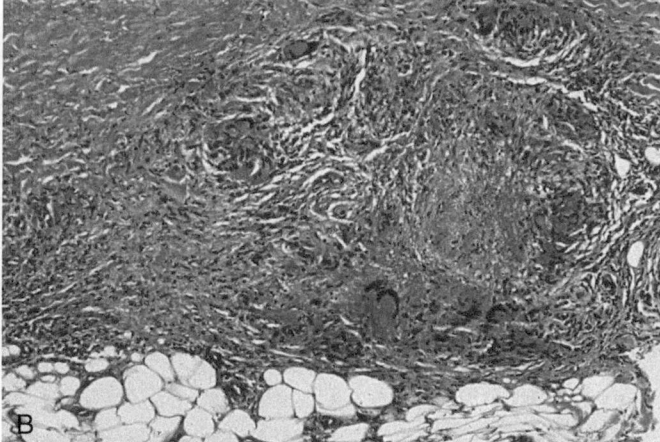

Figure 2-26. Necrobiosis lipoidica. A, Low-power view shows zones of granulomas alternating with those of fibrosis and extending into deep dermis. **B,** High-power view shows histiocytes, including multinucleated giant cells surrounding zones of collagen degeneration in the deep dermis.

- Areas of fibrinoid degeneration are typically sharply demarcated and involve subcutaneous tissue
- Granuloma Annulare
  - Demarcated zones of necrobiosis with mucin, typically in the upper half of the dermis
  - Late sclerotic lesions may resemble morphea

PEARLS

- *Less than 1% of the patients with diabetes develop necrobiosis lipoidica*
- *Cases of squamous cell carcinoma (SCC) developing in lesions of necrobiosis are reported*

SELECTED REFERENCES

Imtiaz KE, Khaleeli AA: Squamous cell carcinoma developing in necrobiosis lipoidica. Diabetic Med 18:325-328, 2001.

Lowitt MH, Dover JS: Necrobiosis lipoidica. J Am Acad Dermatol 25:735-748, 1991.

Magro CM, Crowson AN, Regauer S: Granuloma annulare and necrobiosis lipoidica tissue reactions as a manifestation of systemic disease. Hum Pathol 27:50-56, 1996.

O'Toole EA, Kennedy U, Nolan JJ, et al: Necrobiosis lipoidica: only a minority of patients have diabetes mellitus. Br J Dermatol 140:283-286, 1999.

Reid SD, Ladizinski B, Lee K, et al: Update on necrobiosis lipoidica: a review of etiology, diagnosis, and treatment options. J Am Acad Dermatol 69:783-791, 2013.

RHEUMATOID NODULE

Clinical Features

- Chronic deeply seated inflammatory nodules that occur in patients with rheumatoid arthritis and occasionally in patients with systemic lupus erythematosus
- Rheumatoid nodules are seen during the disease course in 30% to 40% of patients with rheumatoid arthritis
- Predilection for areas subject to mechanical trauma, typically in para-articular locations, including metacarpophalangeal and proximal interphalangeal joints
- Solitary or multiple, firm, nontender, freely mobile, large subcutaneous nodules

Histopathology

- Central areas of homogeneous eosinophilic degeneration of collagen surrounded by peripheral palisade of histiocytes and lymphocytes (Figure 2-27)
- Located in the subcutaneous tissue and deep dermis
- Occasional vascular proliferation associated with fibrosis in the surrounding stroma

Special Stains and Immunohistochemistry

- Noncontributory

Other Techniques for Diagnosis

- Serologic evaluation for rheumatoid factor

Differential Diagnosis

- Subcutaneous Granuloma Annulare
  - Areas of necrobiosis typically contain mucin
- Necrobiosis Lipoidica
  - Typically seen on the anterior tibial surface
  - Layers of necrobiosis are stratified with inflammatory cell infiltrates

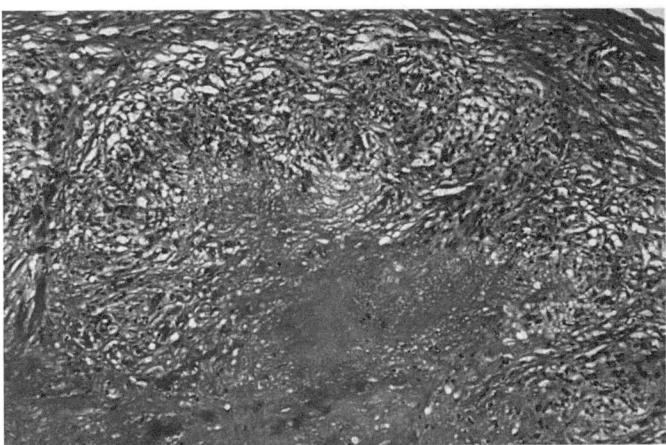

Figure 2-27. Rheumatoid nodule. Palisading granulomas surrounding zones of fibrinoid degeneration of collagen are present within the subcutaneous tissue.

PEARLS

- *Rheumatoid nodules are almost always associated with high titer of rheumatoid factor*

SELECTED REFERENCES

Dubois EL, Friou GJ, Chandor S: Rheumatoid nodules and rheumatoid granulomas in systemic lupus erythematosus. JAMA 220:515, 1972.

Sayah A, English JC 3rd: Rheumatoid arthritis: a review of the cutaneous manifestations. J Am Acad Dermatol 53:191, 2005.

Veys EM, De Keyser F: Rheumatoid nodules: differential diagnosis and immunohistological findings. Ann Rheum Dis 52:625, 1993.

NECROBIOTIC XANTHOGRANULOMA

Clinical Features

- Rare disorder often associated with paraproteinemia and seen in middle age-elderly patients
- Presents as discrete papules and large, yellow indented nodular plaques with atrophy
- Most commonly involves the periorbital region but may also occur on trunk, neck, and extremities

Histopathology

- Granulomatous inflammation in the deep dermis and subcutaneous tissue composed of histiocytes, including many foam cells, Touton giant cells, and lymphoid infiltrate (Figure 2-28)
- Intervening broad zones of necrobiosis
- Cholesterol clefts
- Lymphoid follicles are sometimes present

Special Stains and Immunohistochemistry

- Noncontributory

Other Techniques for Diagnosis

- Serum protein electrophoresis shows IgG monoclonal gammopathy in most patients

Differential Diagnosis

- Necrobiosis Lipoidica
  - Characteristically affects the anterior tibial surface but also has a predilection for the thighs, popliteal areas, and dorsum of the feet and arms
  - Alternating horizontal layers of basophilic degeneration of collagen and palisades consisting of histiocytes, lymphocytes, and plasma cells
  - Foam cells not prominent

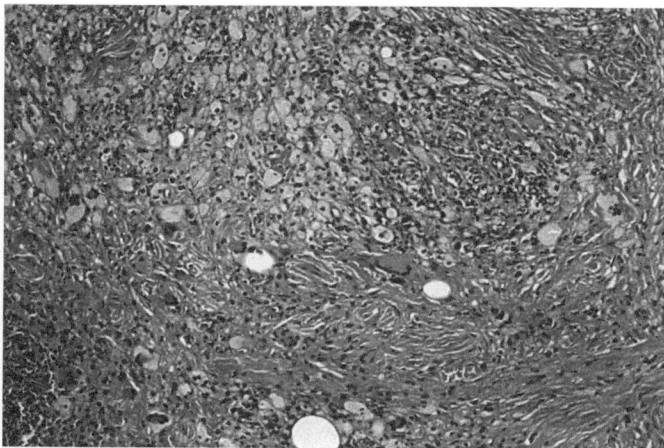

Figure 2-28. Necrobiotic xanthogranuloma. Histologic section shows a dense dermal infiltrate composed of histiocytes and lymphocytes associated with degenerated collagen. Many of the histiocytes have foamy cytoplasm, and some are multinucleated.

- Subcutaneous Granuloma Annulare
  - May be differentiated by the presence of mucinous degeneration and lack of foam cells
- Xanthomas and Xanthogranulomas
  - Do not have areas of necrobiosis

PEARLS

- *In some patients with necrobiotic xanthogranuloma, an underlying multiple myeloma is present*

SELECTED REFERENCES

Cornblath WT, Dotan SA, Trobe JD, Headington JT: Varied clinical spectrum of necrobiotic xanthogranuloma. Ophthalmology 99:103-107, 1992.
Finan MC, Winkelmann RK: Histopathology of necrobiotic xanthogranuloma with paraproteinemia. J Cutan Pathol 14:92-99, 1987.
Mehregan DA, Winkelmann RK: Necrobiotic xanthogranuloma. Arch Dermatol 128:94-100, 1992.
Wood AJ, Wagner MV, Abbott JJ, Gibson LE: Necrobiotic xanthogranuloma: a review of 17 cases with emphasis on clinical and pathologic correlation. Arch Dermatol 145:279-284, 2009.

SARCOIDAL GRANULOMAS
SARCOIDOSIS
Clinical Features

- Systemic granulomatous disease of unknown etiology, possibly secondary to activation of an unknown antigen
- Overall, a relatively uncommon disease; usually seen in females living in the north temperature zone (e.g., Scandinavians); in the United States, it is more common in blacks
- Cutaneous involvement is seen in one fourth of patients with systemic sarcoidosis, whereas cutaneous lesions are the only manifestation in about one fourth of patients with sarcoidosis
- Maculopapular eruption with predilection for the face, posterior neck and shoulders, and extensor surfaces of extremities
- Lesions typically appear as small (< 1 cm), erythematous to violaceous papules; occasional cutaneous and subcutaneous nodules

- Lesions tend to coalesce into yellow to brown plaques with occasional development of central clearing to form annular lesions
- Other cutaneous manifestations:
  - Lupus pernio presents with violaceous or erythematous papules, plaques, or nodules predominantly involving the central facial skin and associated with increased risk of pulmonary involvement
  - Lofgren syndrome is characterized by acute onset and the triad of hilar adenopathy, acute polyarthritis, and erythema nodosum and is typically self-limiting

Histopathology

- Superficial and deep dermal coalescent noncaseating granulomas (Figure 2-29)
- Granulomas contain multinucleated eosinophilic epithelioid histiocytes with minimal peripheral lymphocytic infiltrates ("naked" tubercles)
- Multinucleated epithelioid histiocytes may contain asteroid bodies (eosinophilic stellate inclusions)
- Involvement of subcutaneous fat may result in lobular pattern of panniculitis due to noncaseating granulomas

Special Stains and Immunohistochemistry

- Special stains for organisms (GMS, PAS, and acid-fast bacilli) to rule out an infectious etiology

Other Techniques for Diagnosis

- Kveim test has 80% sensitivity
- Chest radiograph: variable bilateral involvement ranging from hilar lymphadenopathy to interstitial pulmonary infiltrates

Differential Diagnosis

- Tuberculoid Leprosy
  - Acid-fast stain reveals the presence of bacilli within the histiocytes of granulomas
  - Granulomas follow nerves
- Fungal Infection
  - There may be a neutrophilic component to the inflammation
  - PAS and GMS stains reveal the presence of fungal organisms

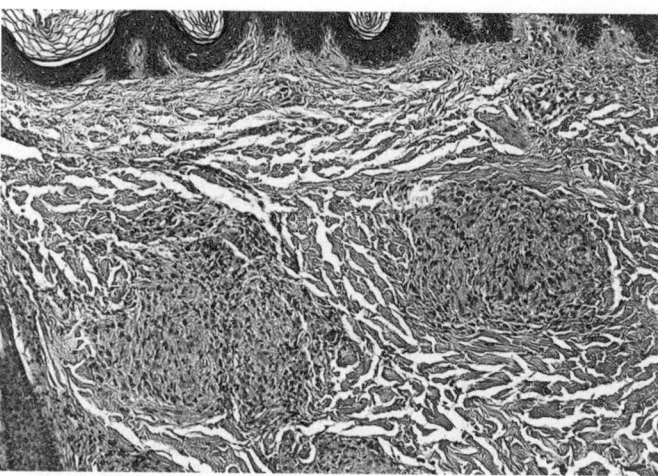

Figure 2-29. Sarcoidosis. Histologic section shows noncaseating granulomas within the dermis. The granulomas are composed of histiocytes with only a sparse lymphocytic component (naked tubercles).

- Foreign-Body Granuloma
  - Polarized light reveals the presence of birefringent foreign material in giant cells
  - Sarcoidal type granulomas can be seen as a reaction to foreign body material

PEARLS

- *Cutaneous lesions of sarcoidosis may localize in previous scars, such as those caused by herpes zoster and tattoos*
- *Diagnosis of systemic sarcoidosis requires biopsy confirmation*

SELECTED REFERENCES

Ball NJ, Kho GT, Martinka M: The histologic spectrum of cutaneous sarcoidosis: a study of twenty-eight cases. J Cutan Pathol 31:160-168, 2004.

Hanno R, Needelman A, Eiferman RA, et al: Cutaneous sarcoidal granulomas and the development of systemic sarcoidosis. Arch Dermatol 117:203, 1981.

Mangas C, Fernández-Figueras MT, Fité E, et al: Clinical spectrum and histological analysis of 32 cases of specific cutaneous sarcoidosis. J Cutan Pathol 33:772, 2006.

Olive KE, Kataria YP: Cutaneous manifestations of sarcoidosis. Arch Intern Med 145:1811, 1985.

Walsh NM, Hanly JG, Tremaine R, Murray S: Cutaneous sarcoidosis and foreign bodies. Am J Dermatopathol 15:203-207, 1993.

FOREIGN-BODY GRANULOMAS

Clinical Features

- Immune reaction to a foreign body implanted within the viable layers of the skin
- Commonly seen lesion with no age or gender predilection
- Predilection for hands, feet, and other sites subject to trauma
- Erythematous subcutaneous nodules, typically less than 1 cm

Histopathology

- Early lesions present as a neutrophilic abscess
- Localized granuloma usually surrounding birefringent foreign material or keratin (Figure 2-30)
- Multinucleate histiocytes with centrally located nuclei (foreign-body giant cells)
- Occasional histiocytes filled with cytoplasmic vacuoles of varying diameter (Swiss cheese pattern)
- Sarcoidal type granulomas are typically seen with silica, beryllium, and zirconium

Special Stains and Immunohistochemistry

- Noncontributory

Other Techniques for Diagnosis

- Noncontributory

Differential Diagnosis

- Infectious Granuloma
  - Foreign-body giant cells are typically absent
  - Acid-fast, Gram, PAS, and GMS stains highlight causative organisms

PEARLS

- *Materials capable of producing a foreign-body granuloma include vegetable spines, metals, wooden splinters, silk or nylon sutures, paraffin, silicone, silica, urates, oils, keratinous material, and neoplasms*

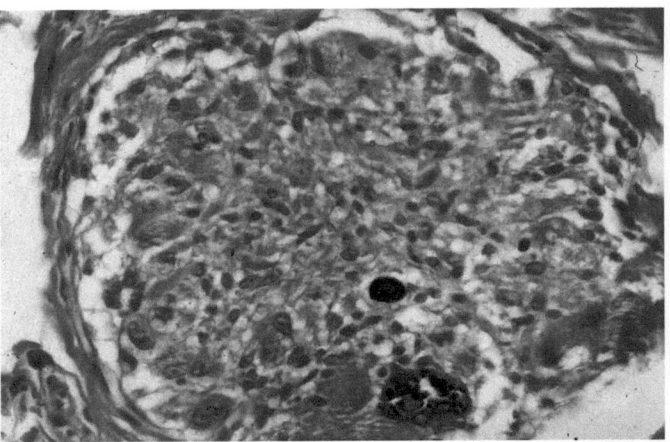

Figure 2-30. Foreign-body granuloma. The granulomas may resemble those of sarcoidosis. However, some of the histiocytes contain foreign-body material.

SELECTED REFERENCES

Montemarano AD, Sau P, Johnson FB, James WD: Cutaneous granulomas caused by an aluminum-zirconium complex: an ingredient of antiperspirants. J Am Acad Dermatol 37(3 Pt 1):496-498, 1997.

Walsh NM, Hanly JG, Tremaine R, Murray S: Cutaneous sarcoidosis and foreign bodies. Am J Dermatopathol 15:203-207, 1993.

INFECTIOUS GRANULOMAS
LEPROSY

Clinical Features

- An endemic disease of tropical and subtropical countries including the Indian subcontinent and Southeast Asia
- Caused by *Mycobacterium leprae* and predominantly involves the skin and peripheral nerves
- Shows an immunopathologic spectrum with minimal to marked host response and resulting clinicopathologic spectrum consisting of tuberculoid leprosy with maximal host response at one end to lepromatous leprosy with minimal response at the other end; borderline leprosy shows features intermediate between the two
- Tuberculoid Leprosy
  - Lesions are scant and consist of hypopigmented papules and plaques associated with anesthesia
- Lepromatous Leprosy
  - Multiple symmetrical macules, papules, or nodules are present
  - Involvement of the face (leonine facies) and ulnar, radial, and common peroneal nerves can occur
- Borderline Leprosy
  - Lesions are less numerous and less symmetrical than in lepromatous leprosy

Histopathology

- Tuberculoid Leprosy
  - Large, elongated epithelioid granulomas with peripheral lymphocytic infiltrate arranged along neurovascular bundles
- Lepromatous Leprosy
  - Diffuse dermal infiltrate composed predominantly of foam cells, with few lymphocytes and plasma cells
- Borderline Leprosy

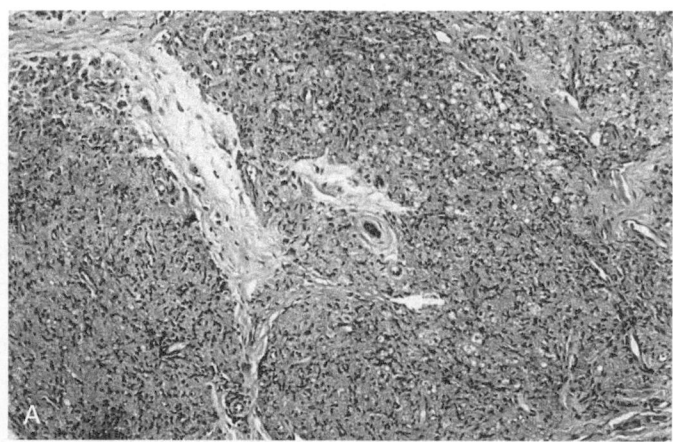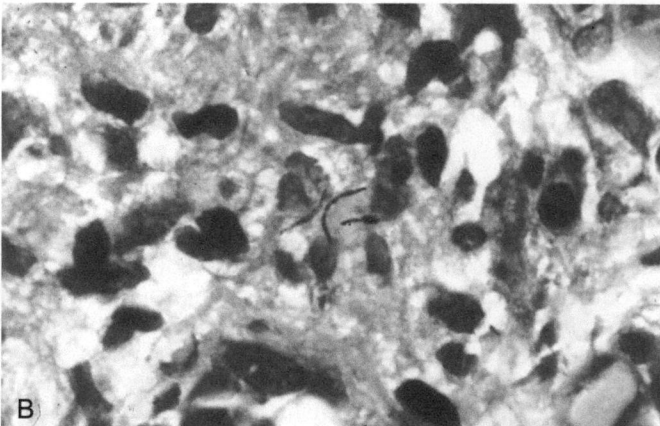

Figure 2-31. Leprosy. A, Hematoxylin and eosin–stained section shows poorly formed granulomas within the dermis. Some of the histiocytes have foamy cytoplasm. **B,** Acid-fast bacillus stain demonstrates the acid-fast bacilli within the cytoplasm of some of the histiocytes.

- Admixture of foamy macrophages and epithelioid histiocytes that are not arranged as well-formed granulomas; lymphocytes in significant numbers (Figure 2-31A)

Special Stains and Immunohistochemistry
- Acid-fast bacilli can be demonstrated within the cytoplasm of the histiocytes; maximal numbers are present in lepromatous leprosy and the least in tuberculoid leprosy (Figure 2-31B)
- Organisms can be identified in the nerves and hair erector muscles

Other Techniques for Diagnosis
- PCR techniques for infectious agent

Differential Diagnosis
- Abundant foam cells in lepromatous leprosy may invoke a xanthomatous pattern and require demonstration of the acid-fast bacilli for definite diagnosis
- Tuberculoid granulomas of tuberculoid leprosy may resemble sarcoidosis and occasionally foreign-body granulomas

PEARLS

- *Histioid leprosy is a variant of lepromatous leprosy that histologically resembles a histiocytoma but shows a high number of bacilli*

SELECTED REFERENCES

Abulafia J, Vignale RA: Leprosy: pathogenesis updated. Int J Dermatol 38:321-334, 1999.
Britton WJ, Lockwood DNJ: Leprosy. Lancet 363:1209-1219, 2004.
Choudhuri K: The immunology of leprosy: unravelling an enigma. Int J Lepr 63:430, 1995.
De Wit MYL, Faber WR, Krieg SR, et al: Application of a polymerase chain reaction for the detection of *Mycobacterium leprae* in skin tissues. J Clin Microbiol 29:906, 1991.
Whitty CJ, Lockwood DN: Leprosy-new perspectives on an old disease. J Infect 38:2-5, 1999.

PRIMARY CUTANEOUS TUBERCULOSIS: LUPUS VULGARIS

Clinical Features
- Lupus vulgaris is a form of secondary or reactivation tuberculosis developing in previously infected and sensitized persons

- Usually results from hematogenous spread from an old, reactivated focus in the lung or from lymphatic extension from a tuberculous cervical lymphadenitis
- One or more well-demarcated, reddish brown patches typically involving the skin of nose and adjacent areas of face
- Chronic course with peripheral extension of the lesions
- Over time, the affected areas become atrophic and occasionally ulcerate

Histopathology
- Most commonly involves the upper half of dermis
- Tuberculoid granulomas characterized by epithelioid and multinucleated histiocytes; scattered lymphocytes in the background
- Giant cells are of both Langerhans and foreign-body type; central caseation is minimal or absent
- In older lesions, extensive fibrosis replaces the granulomas
- Depending on the stage, the overlying epidermis may be atrophic, ulcerated, or hyperplastic; pseudo-epitheliomatous epidermal hyperplasia can be seen at the edge of ulcers

Special Stains and Immunohistochemistry
- Special stains may only rarely demonstrate tubercle bacilli because they are typically present in small numbers

Other Techniques for Diagnosis
- PCR detection of mycobacterial DNA is valuable in confirming the diagnosis

Differential Diagnosis
- Other infectious and noninfectious causes of granulomatous inflammation should be considered

PEARLS

- *Squamous cell carcinoma and basal cell carcinoma have been reported to develop in long standing lesions of lupus vulgaris*

SELECTED REFERENCES

Haim S, Friedman-Birnbaum R: Cutaneous tuberculosis and malignancy. Cutis 21:643, 1978.
Kate MS, Dhar R, Borkar DB, Ganbavale DR: Longstanding lupus vulgaris with basal cell carcinoma. Indian J Pathol Microbiol 52:588-590, 2009.

Marcoval J, Servitje O, Moreno A, et al: Lupus vulgaris: clinical, histopathologic, and bacteriologic study of 10 cases. J Am Acad Dermatol 26:404-407, 1992.

Negi SS, Basir SF, Gupta S, et al: Comparative study of PCR, smear examination and culture for diagnosis of cutaneous tuberculosis. J Commun Dis 37:83-92, 2005.

DEEP FUNGAL INFECTIONS

Clinical Features

- Deep mycosis can be primarily a cutaneous fungal infection or be part of systemic infections such as those involving the respiratory system or reticuloendothelial system, especially in immunocompromised hosts
- Primary cutaneous and subcutaneous mycoses are often caused by saprophytic organisms and include sporotrichosis, chromoblastomycosis, histoplasmosis, coccidiomycosis, blastomycosis, and cryptococcosis

Histopathology

- Characteristic histologic pattern is pseudoepitheliomatous hyperplasia with extensive suppurative and granulomatous inflammation in the dermis (Figure 2-32A)
- Small neurophilic abscesses are surrounded by varying numbers of lymphocytes, plasma cells, epithelioid histiocytes, and multinucleated giant cells
- Involvement of the subcutaneous fat generally results in a lobular pattern of panniculitis that is also suppurative and granulomatous
- Causative fungal organisms can be found in the cytoplasm of the histiocytes or within the abscesses
- Size and morphology of fungal organisms can further help in identification of the specific organisms
  - Blastomycosis: 8- to 15-μm thick-walled spores with single broad-based buds
  - Paracoccidioidomycosis: 6- to 20-μm spores with narrow-necked buds ("mariner's wheels")
  - Chromoblastomycosis: 6- to 12-μm thick-walled dark-brown spores in clusters ("copper pennies")
  - Cryptococcosis: 4- to 12-μm spores with wide capsule in gelatinous background or 2- to 4-μm spores in granulomatous areas; narrow-based buds
  - Histoplasmosis: 2- to 4-μm round or oral spores with clear halo, located in the cytoplasm of histiocytes
  - Sporotrichosis: 4- to 6-μm round to oval spores, intraepidermal abscesses may be present

Special Stains and Immunohistochemistry

- Special stains, PAS, and GMS stains are invaluable in locating and identifying the causative fungal organisms (Figure 2-32B)
- Mucicarmine is used to differentiate *Cryptococcus* species from other fungi such as *Blastomyces* species

Other Techniques for Diagnosis

- Microbiologic cultures to isolate the organisms
- PCR techniques are becoming available for various fungi

Differential Diagnosis

- In addition to deep fungal infections, atypical mycobacterial infections and halogenodermas should be considered in the differential diagnosis of suppurative and granulomatous inflammation with pseudoepitheliomatous hyperplasia
- Subcutaneous Phaeohyphomycosis (Phaeohyphomycotic Cyst)
  - Presents as deep coalescing suppurative granulomas surrounded by a fibrous capsule
  - Suppurative inflammation may also be caused by bacterial and mycobacterial organisms

PEARLS

- *Necrotizing skin lesions with vasculitis and granulomas can be seen in disseminated aspergillosis, mucormycosis, and* Fusarium *species infections*
- *Cryptococcosis can present with a xanthomatous pattern, especially in immunocompromised hosts*
- *Host response may be minimal in immunocompromised hosts such as patients with cancer and requires high degree of suspicion to evaluate for infectious agents*

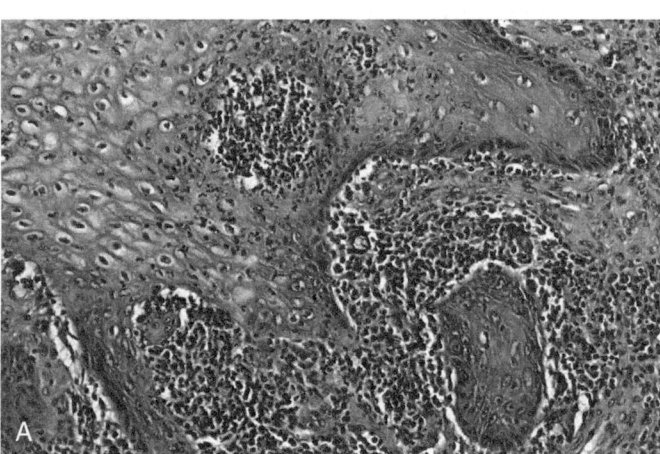
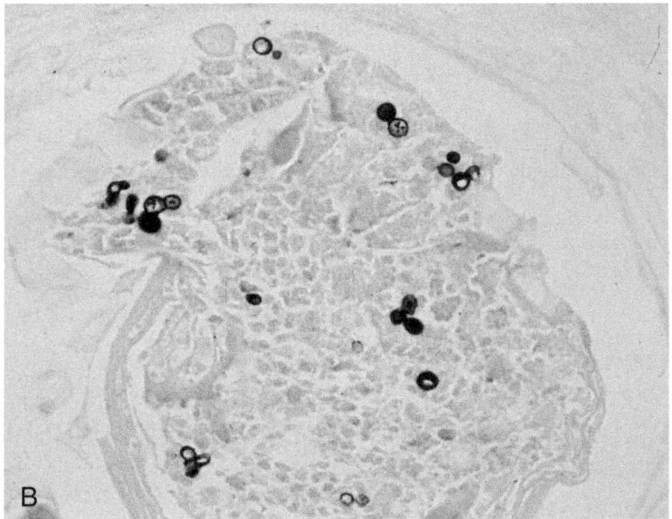

Figure 2-32. Blastomycosis. A, Hematoxylin and eosin–stained section shows epidermal hyperplasia associated with suppurative and granulomatous inflammation. **B,** Gomori methenamine silver stain demonstrates yeast forms of blastomycosis, some of which show characteristic broad-based budding.

SELECTED REFERENCES

Body BA: Cutaneous manifestations of systemic mycoses. Dermatol Clin 14:125-135, 1996.

Chapman SW, Daniel CR 3rd: Cutaneous manifestations of fungal infection. Infect Dis Clin N Am 8: 879-910, 1994.

Ogawa H, Summerbell RC, Clemons KV, et al: Dermatophytes and host defence in cutaneous mycoses. Med Mycol 36(suppl 1):166-173, 1998.

Rivitti EA, Aoki V: Deep fungal infections in tropical countries. Clin Dermatol 17:171-190, 1999.

LEISHMANIASIS

Clinical Features

- Leishmaniasis is a protozoan disease transmitted by the sandfly
- Manifests as localized or diffuse cutaneous, mucocutaneous, and visceral disease
- Two forms of cutaneous leishmaniasis are recognized
  - American cutaneous leishmaniasis
    - Caused by *Leishmania braziliensis* complex or *Leishmania mexicana* complex
    - Occurs in the American continent
  - Oriental cutaneous leishmaniasis
    - Caused by *Leishmania tropica*
    - Occurs in parts of Europe, Middle East, Asia, and Africa
  - In both forms, the cutaneous lesions occur as single or multiple erythematous papules on exposed skin several weeks after the bite of infected sandfly
- Papules may enlarge to form nodules that can ulcerate

Histopathology

- Dense diffuse infiltrate of histiocytes with scattered lymphocytes and plasma cells is present in the dermis (Figure 2-33)
- In early lesions, numerous parasites are noted within the cytoplasm of the histiocytes
- A smear from an early lesion can be positive for the parasites
- Late lesions are characterized by tuberculoid-type granulomas and lymphocytes

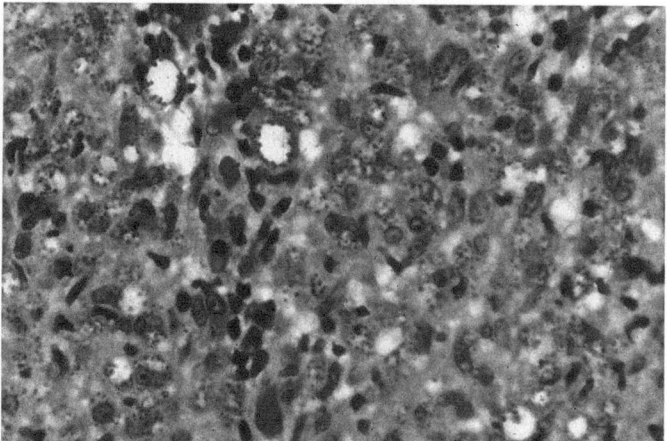

Figure 2-33. Leishmaniasis. High-power view shows an infiltrate of plasma cells and histiocytes. Within the cytoplasm of the histiocytes, there are organisms that are 2 to 4 μm in size. A Giemsa stain can also be used to highlight the organisms.

Special Stains and Immunohistochemistry

- Giemsa stain is helpful in identifying the parasite, which is 2 to 4 μm

Other Techniques for Diagnosis

- PCR is a specific diagnostic tool

Differential Diagnosis

- Rhinoscleroma
  - Histiocytes (Mikulicz cells) are larger than the histiocytes in leishmaniasis
  - Caused by *Klebsiella pneumoniae rhinoscleromatis*, which is 2 to 3 μm
  - Plasma cells and Russell bodies are more prominent
- Histoplasmosis
  - Generally associated with necrosis
  - Organisms are 2 to 4 μm, round to oval, and surrounded by a clear halo
  - Best seen with GMS and PAS stains
- Granuloma Inguinale
  - Histiocytic infiltrate is admixed with neutrophilic abscesses
  - Causative organism is *Calymmatobacterium granulomatis*
  - Histiocytes contain Donovan bodies, which are encapsulated round to oval bodies measuring 1 to 2 μm

PEARLS

- *Mucocutaneous leishmaniasis may involve upper respiratory tract and nasopharynx and is seen in the American forms*
- *Visceral leishmaniasis includes kala-azar produced by* Leishmania donovani, *which occurs in Africa, Asia, and parts of Brazil; the Mediterranean kala-azar is seen in parts of Europe and Latin American countries*
- *Cutaneous leishmaniasis can occur as localized form, mucocutaneous form, chronic or verrucous form, relapse form, or diffuse form*
- *Localized and diffuse forms are at opposite ends of the spectrum and reflect the strength of immune response of the host to the parasite*

SELECTED REFERENCES

Bogdan C: Leishmaniasis in rheumatology, haematology and oncology: epidemiological, immunological and clinical aspects and caveats. Ann Rheum Dis 71(suppl 2):i60-i66, 2013.

Choi CM, Lerner EA: Leishmaniasis as an emerging infection. J Invest Dermatol Symp Proc 6:175, 2001.

Dedet JP, Pratlong F, Lanotte G, Ravel C: Cutaneous leishmaniasis: the parasite. Clin Dermatol 17:261-268, 1999.

Mehregan DR, Mehregan AH, Mehregan DA: Histologic diagnosis of cutaneous leishmaniasis. Clin Dermatol 17:297-304, 1999.

Reithinger R, Dujardin JC. Molecular diagnosis of leishmaniasis: current status and future applications. J Clin Microbiol 45:21, 2007.

VASCULITIS

LEUKOCYTOCLASTIC VASCULITIS

Clinical Features

- Many underlying diseases can manifest clinically as palpable purpuric lesions and histologically as leukocytoclastic vasculitis

- Immune complex–mediated diseases such as IgA vasculitis (Henoch-Schönlein purpura), connective tissue diseases, autoimmune diseases, and drug-induced and infectious etiologies are among the most common causes of leukocytoclastic vasculitis
- Microscopic polyangiitis involving skin may show changes of leukocytoclastic vasculitis

Histopathology
- Characteristic pattern is a neutrophilic small-vessel vasculitis typically involving the postcapillary venules in the superficial dermis (Figure 2-34)
- Leukocytoclasis, or fragmentation of the neutrophilic nuclei into dust; the inflammatory cell infiltrate may also contain eosinophils and lymphocytes
- Damage to the vessel wall results in extravasation of red cells
- Deposits of fibrin may be seen around the involved vessels
- In severe cases, luminal occlusion with resulting ischemic necrosis of the epidermis

Special Stains and Immunohistochemistry
- Gram, PAS, and GMS stains are helpful in diagnosing infectious causes
- In leukocytoclastic vasculitis caused by *Neisseria meningitides*, organisms can be demonstrated within the endothelial cells and neutrophils

Other Techniques for Diagnosis
- Immunofluorescence studies demonstrate IgM, C3, and fibrinogen surrounding the dermal vessels; IgA is present in Henoch-Schönlein purpura
- Serologic studies are essential in excluding autoimmune-mediated leukocytoclastic vasculitis

Differential Diagnosis
- Other causes of neutrophilic dermatosis such as Sweet syndrome
- May be considered especially in early lesions, where the vascular damage is not easily seen

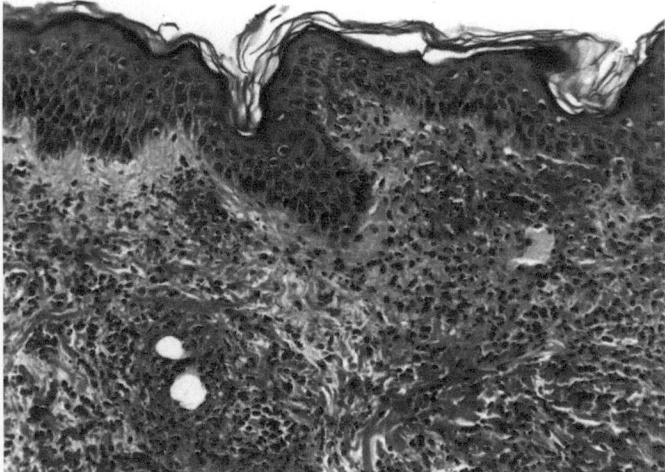

Figure 2-34. Leukocytoclastic vasculitis. Histologic section shows perivascular infiltrate of neutrophils, neutrophilic nuclear dust, and extravasated red blood cells. Deposits of fibrin are present in and around the damaged blood vessels.

- Erythema Elevatum Diutinum
  - Represents a chronic form of leukocytoclastic vasculitis
  - Characterized by red to violaceous papules typically involving extensor surfaces of extremities
- Granuloma Faciale
  - Another chronic form of leukocytoclastic vasculitis typically presenting as brown-red papules or plaques almost always involving the face
- Livedo Vasculitis
  - Typically involves lower legs
  - Histologic changes include deposition of fibrinoid material within the vessel walls with resulting luminal occlusion and ulceration of epidermis
  - Inflammatory cell infiltrate is generally sparse
- Septic Vasculitis
  - Generally associated with thrombi in the vascular lumina, in addition to acute leukocytoclastic vasculitis; there may be intraepidermal pustules

PEARLS

- *A true lymphocytic vasculitis of the small blood vessels is only rarely documented and is reported to occur in collagen vascular disease, pityriasis lichenoides, and lymphomatoid papulosis*
- *Noninflammatory small-vessel vasculitis histologically characterized by deposits of homogeneous pink material within and around vascular lumina can be seen in monoclonal cryoglobulinemia, thrombotic thrombocytopenic purpura (TTP), and warfarin (Coumadin)- or heparin-induced vasculitis*

SELECTED REFERENCES

Claudy A: Pathogenesis of leukocytoclastic vasculitis. Eur J Dermatol 8:75-79, 1998.
Gibson LE, Su WP: Cutaneous vasculitis. Rheum Dis Clin N Am 21:1097-1113, 1995.
Kawakami T, Kawanabe T, Saito C, et al: Clinical and histopathologic features of 8 patients with microscopic polyangiitis including two with a slowly progressive clinical course. J Am Acad Dermatol 57:840-848, 2007.
Niiyama S, Amoh Y, Tomita M, et al: Dermatological manifestations associated with microscopic polyangiitis. Rheumatol Int 28:593-595, 2008.
Szer IS: Henoch-Schönlein purpura. Curr Opin Rheumatol 6:25-31, 1994.

SUPERFICIAL MIGRATORY THROMBOPHLEBITIS
Clinical Features
- Typically presents as multiple, tender erythematous nodules on lower legs
- New lesions erupt as older lesions resolve
- May be a manifestation of Behçet disease, hypercoagulable states, and malignancy

Histopathology
- Affected vessel is typically a small or medium-sized vein situated in deep dermis or subcutaneous tissue of lower extremity (Figure 2-35)
- Vascular lumen is completely occluded by thrombus
- An inflammatory cell infiltrate composed of neutrophils, lymphocytes, and histiocytes extends between the muscle bundles of the vein
- Recanalization and resorption of thrombus occurs with granulomatous reaction

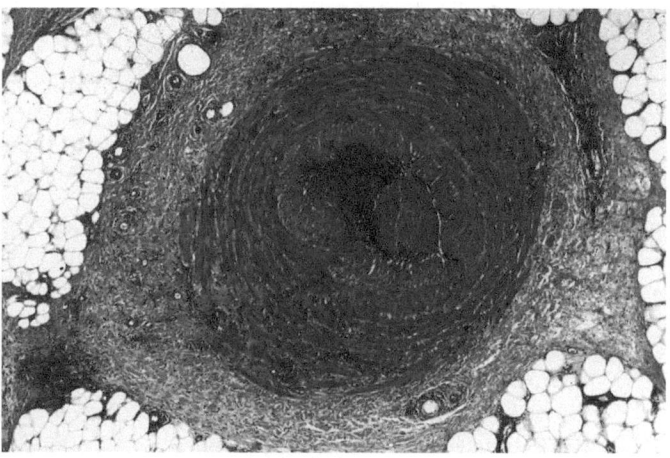

Figure 2-35. Thrombophlebitis. A large blood vessel located in the subcutaneous tissue shows inflammatory cell infiltrate in the wall and an organizing thrombus within the lumen.

Special Stains and Immunohistochemistry
- Elastic tissue stain is helpful to highlight elastic lamina of vessel wall

Other Techniques for Diagnosis
- Noncontributory

Differential Diagnosis
- Subcutaneous Polyarteritis Nodosa
  - Can present as nodules on the legs
  - Histologic findings are those of a neutrophilic vasculitis of medium-sized arteries with fibrinoid necrosis
  - Elastic tissue stain may be helpful in distinguishing the arteries of polyarteritis nodosa from the veins of thrombophlebitis
- Nodular Vasculitis
  - Can resemble thrombophlebitis clinically
  - Histologic changes include lymphohistiocytic infiltrates in the vessel wall with intimal thickening and thrombosis
  - Small and medium-sized arteries and veins of the subcutaneous fat are typically involved
  - An associated lobular panniculitis (erythema induratum) is generally present with granulomatous inflammation surrounding zones of fat necrosis
- Wegener Granulomatosis
  - Although most patients with Wegener granulomatosis typically present with leukocytoclastic vasculitis, true granulomatous inflammation and necrotizing vasculitis can occur in subcutaneous tissue
  - Assays for antineutrophil cytoplasmic antibody (ANCA) may be helpful in the diagnosis of Wegener granulomatosis

PEARLS

- *As a result of stasis and venous hypertension, veins of the legs can show an increase in elastic tissue and smooth muscle in their walls, which can pose a problem in differentiating veins from arteries*
- *Recurrent migratory phlebitis is associated with adenocarcinoma, especially of the pancreas (Trousseau syndrome)*

SELECTED REFERENCES

Hall LD, Dalton SR, Fillman EP, et al: Re-examination of features to distinguish polyarteritis nodosa from superficial thrombophlebitis. Am J Dermatopathol 35:463-471, 2013.
Luis Rodríguez-Peralto J, Carrillo R, Rosales B, et al: Superficial thrombophlebitis. Semin Cutan Med Surg 26:71-76, 2007.
Sakane T, Takeno M, Suzuki N, Inaba G: Behçet's disease. N Engl J Med 341:1284-1291, 1999.
Samlaska CP, James WD, Simel D: Superficial migratory thrombophlebitis and factor XII deficiency. J Am Acad Dermatol 22:939-943, 1990.

VESICULOBULLOUS DERMATOSES

SUBCORNEAL PUSTULAR DERMATOSIS (SNEDDON-WILKINSON DISEASE)

Clinical Features
- Chronic dermatosis, characterized by sterile pustules typically involving flexural surfaces and axillary and inguinal folds
- Pustules may be arranged in annular or serpiginous patterns

Histopathology
- *Subcorneal* collection of neutrophils and rare eosinophils (Figure 2-36)
- Mild epidermal spongiosis with neutrophils may be present
- Superficial perivascular infiltrate of neutrophils, rare eosinophils, and lymphocytes
- Occasional acantholytic keratinocytes may be seen

Special Stains and Immunohistochemistry
- Gram and PAS/GMS stains to exclude infectious etiology

Other Techniques for Diagnosis
- Immunofluorescence studies to exclude autoimmune bullous disorders

Differential Diagnosis
- Bullous Impetigo
  - Histologic changes in bullous impetigo are identical to those of subcorneal pustular dermatosis
  - Bullous impetigo is caused in most cases by group A streptococci

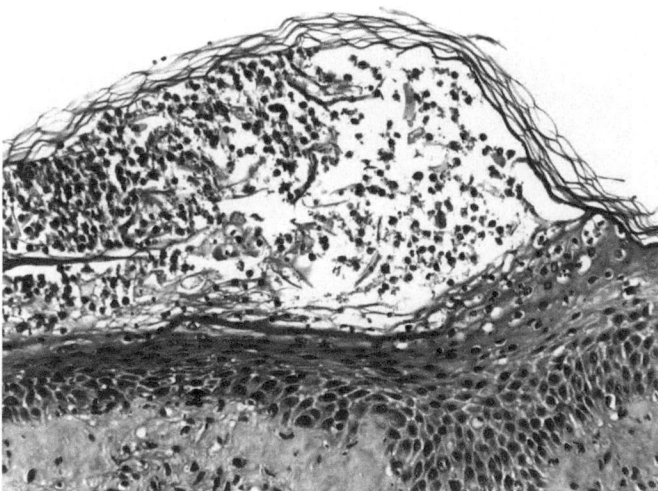

Figure 2-36. Subcorneal pustular dermatosis. There are neutrophilic aggregates underneath the cornified layer. Acantholytic keratinocytes may be seen in addition to neutrophils.

- Demonstration of bacteria by Gram stain or cultures is diagnostic
- Dermatophytosis
  - Can occasionally present as subcorneal pustules
  - PAS and GMS stains are useful in demonstrating the fungal organisms
- Pemphigus Foliaceus, Pemphigus Erythematosus, and IgA Pemphigus
  - Can present with subcorneal pustules with acantholysis
  - In general, acantholytic cells are more frequent in pemphigus than in subcorneal pustular dermatosis
  - For definitive diagnosis, immunofluorescence studies are essential
- Psoriasis
  - Can present with subcorneal pustules
  - Presence of spongiosis (spongiform pustules) in pustular psoriasis helps in the differential diagnosis
- Pustular Drug Eruption/Acute Exanthematous Pustular Dermatosis (AGEP)
  - Presents with subcorneal or intraepidermal pustules
  - Presence of epidermal spongiosis and eosinophils in the dermal inflammatory cell infiltrate is helpful

PEARLS

- *Subcorneal pustular dermatosis may be associated with monoclonal gammopathy, most commonly IgA paraproteinemia*
- *Acantholysis in subcorneal pustular dermatosis is most likely due to the effect of proteolytic enzymes in the pustules*

SELECTED REFERENCES

Cheng S, Edmonds E, Ben-Gashir M, Yu RC: Subcorneal pustular dermatosis: 50 Years on. Clin Exp Dermatol 33:229-233, 2008.

Reed J, Wilkinson J: Subcorneal pustular dermatosis. Clin Dermatol 8: 301-313, 2000.

Tsuruta D, Ishii N, Hamada T, et al: IgA pemphigus. Clin Dermatol 29:437, 2011.

Yasuda H, Kobayashi H, Hashimoto T, et al: Subcorneal pustular dermatosis type of IgA pemphigus: demonstration of autoantibodies to desmocollin-1 and clinical review. Br J Dermatol 143:144-148, 2000.

PEMPHIGUS
Clinical Features

- Pemphigus is a group of autoimmune vesicular dermatoses that includes pemphigus vulgaris and pemphigus vegetans, pemphigus foliaceus and pemphigus erythematosus (superficial forms), IgA pemphigus, and paraneoplastic pemphigus
- Generally affects middle-aged and older patients and presents as large, flaccid bullae that break easily
- Positive Nikolsky sign is seen when lateral pressure on vesicles causes "sliding off" of the epithelium
- Sites of predilection include scalp, periocular region, sternum, middle back, umbilicus, and groin
- Oral lesions are present in most cases and may be the presenting symptom in some cases

Histopathology

- Characteristic histologic pattern is that of an intraepidermal acantholytic vesicular dermatosis (Figure 2-37A)
- Acantholysis results in clefts and blisters that are typically suprabasal in location
- Basal keratinocytes are attached to the dermis (tombstone-like)
- Blister cavity contains acantholytic keratinocytes that appear rounded with condensed cytoplasm and have enlarged nuclei with prominent nucleoli
- Acantholysis can extend to epithelium of follicles
- Variable amounts of superficial dermal inflammation often with eosinophils
- Early lesions are characterized only by epidermal spongiosis with eosinophils
- Superficial forms of pemphigus show acantholysis in the upper part of the epidermis, close to the granular layer
- Concomitant interface dermatitis is present in paraneoplastic pemphigus
- IgA pemphigus shows a histologic pattern similar to that of subcorneal pustular dermatosis

Special Stains and Immunohistochemistry

- Noncontributory

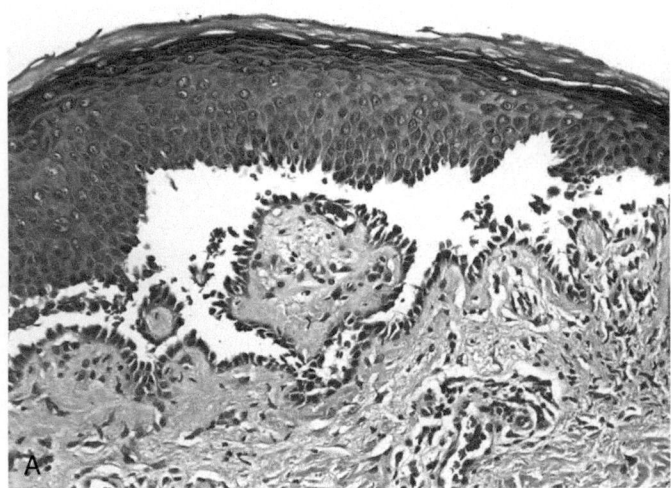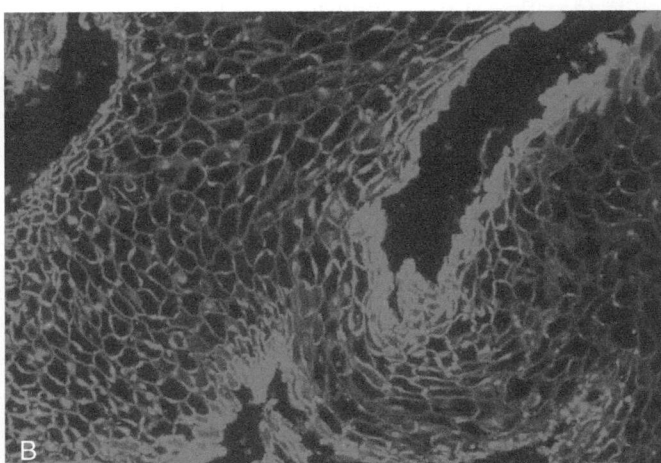

Figure 2-37. Pemphigus. A, Histologic section shows intraepidermal vesicle with prominent suprabasal acantholysis. **B,** Immunofluorescence studies show intercellular pattern of staining for IgG in the epidermis.

Other Techniques for Diagnosis

- Direct immunofluorescence studies show an intercellular pattern with IgG in pemphigus vulgaris, and IgA in IgA pemphigus (Figure 2-37B); granular deposits of IgG or IgM at the dermoepidermal junction in addition to the characteristic intercellular pattern may be seen in paraneoplastic pemphigus
- Indirect immunofluorescence studies and Enzyme-linked immunosorbent assay (ELISA) to detect circulating antibodies against intercellular antigens
- Tzanck preparation is helpful in demonstration of acantholytic keratinocytes in the blisters of pemphigus

Differential Diagnosis

- Hailey-Hailey Disease (Benign Familial Pemphigus)
  - Inherited as an autosomal dominant trait
  - Characterized histologically by acantholysis and epidermal hyperplasia
  - In contrast to pemphigus, Hailey-Hailey disease shows full-thickness acantholysis (dilapidated brick wall pattern)
  - Involvement of hair follicles is not present
- Grover Disease (Transient Acantholytic Dermatosis)
  - Presents clinically as a pruritic, papular, and papulovesicular eruption involving chest, back, and thighs of middle-aged and elderly patients
  - Acantholysis is limited to small foci as opposed to widespread acantholysis seen in pemphigus
  - Acantholysis can also show a histologic pattern similar to that seen in Darier disease and Hailey-Hailey disease; foci of spongiosis may be present
  - Presence of more than one pattern in a single specimen aids in the diagnosis
- Darier Disease (Keratosis Follicularis)
  - Transmitted as an autosomal dominant trait
  - Presents as persistent, slowly progressive hyperkeratotic papules in a follicular distribution
  - Histologic features include suprabasal acantholysis with formation of clefts or lacunae and dyskeratosis resulting in formation of corps ronds and grains
  - Corps ronds and grains are helpful in distinguishing Darier disease from pemphigus
- Herpesvirus Infection
  - Acantholytic pattern associated with necrotic keratinocytes
  - Presence of multinucleated cells with characteristic viral changes helps in the differential diagnosis
- Staphylococcal Scalded Skin Syndrome
  - Few acantholytic cells may be present in staphylococcal scalded skin syndrome
  - A cleavage plane in the granular layer is helpful in the diagnosis

PEARLS

- *Pemphigus vegetans is a variant of pemphigus vulgaris in which the lesions heal with verrucous vegetations*
- *Immunofluorescence studies are critical in definite diagnosis of pemphigus*
- *Biopsy of perilesional skin or edge of the blister with surrounding intact skin should be done for best results*

SELECTED REFERENCES

Amagai M: Pemphigus. In Bolognia JL, Jorizzo JL, Schaffer JV, et al (eds): Dermatology, 3rd ed. Philadelphia, Elsevier, vol 1, 2012, p 461.

Amagai M: Pemphigus: Autoimmunity to epidermal cell adhesion molecules. Adv Dermatol 11:319-352; discussion, 353, 1996.

Benchikhi H, Ghafour S, Disky A, et al: Pemphigus: analysis of 262 cases. Int J Dermatol 47:973-975, 2008.

Calvanico NJ, Robledo MA, Diaz LA: Immunopathology of pemphigus. J Autoimmun 4:3-16, 1991.

Grando SA: Pemphigus autoimmunity: hypotheses and realities. Autoimmunity 45:7, 2012.

Nguyen VT, Ndoye A, Bassler KD, et al: Classification, clinical manifestations, and immunopathological mechanisms of the epithelial variant of paraneoplastic autoimmune multiorgan syndrome: a reappraisal of paraneoplastic pemphigus. Arch Dermatol 137:193-206, 2001.

Robinson ND, Hashimoto T, Amagai M, Chan LS: The new pemphigus variants. J Am Acad Dermatol 40:649-671; quiz, 672-673, 1999.

BULLOUS PEMPHIGOID

Clinical Features

- Bullous pemphigoid is an autoimmune blistering disorder that affects elderly patients and presents as large, tense bullae involving trunk, extremities, and intertriginous areas
- Nikolsky sign is negative
- Oral lesions are present in about one third of the patients

Histopathology

- *Subepidermal* vesicle often filled with eosinophils is the characteristic feature (Figure 2-38A)
- Superficial perivascular mixed inflammatory cell infiltrate rich in eosinophils
- In the cell-poor variant, only scant inflammatory cell infiltrate is present
- Early (prebullous/urticarial) lesions may present with epidermal spongiosis with eosinophils (eosinophilic spongiosis) and superficial dermal infiltrate of eosinophils

Special Stains and Immunohistochemistry

- Noncontributory

Other Techniques for Diagnosis

- Direct immunofluorescence studies show a linear deposition of C3 and IgG at the dermoepidermal junction (Figure 2-38B)
- Salt-split skin immunofluorescence shows that the pemphigoid antibodies are localized to the roof of the blister in most cases

Differential Diagnosis

- Herpes Gestationis
  - Presents as intensely pruritic lesions on the abdomen and extremities of pregnant women in second and third trimesters
  - Histologic changes and immunofluorescence findings may be indistinguishable from bullous pemphigoid
  - However, in herpes gestationis, more neutrophils and basal cell necrosis may be seen
  - Clinical information is invaluable
- Epidermolysis Bullosa Acquisita
  - Presents as blisters developing on acral areas that heal with scarring
  - Histologic and immunofluorescence changes may be identical to that of bullous pemphigoid
  - Eosinophils are fewer in number, and lymphocytes and neutrophils may predominate

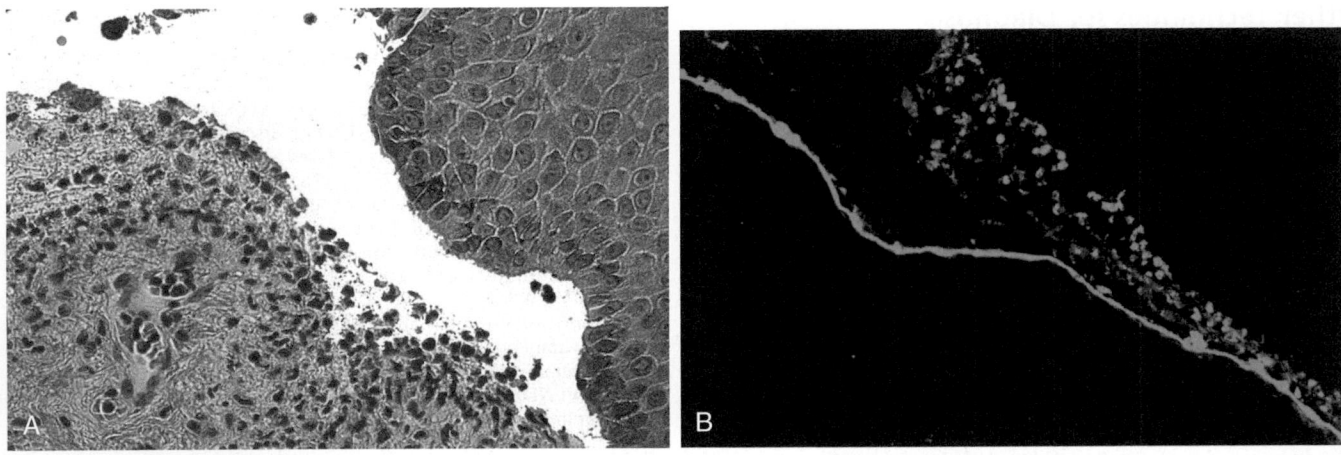

Figure 2-38. Bullous pemphigoid. A, Histologic section shows subepidermal blister containing eosinophils and some neutrophils. **B,** Immunofluorescence studies show linear staining at the dermoepidermal junction for IgG (and C3).

- Immunofluorescence of salt-split skin shows the localization of IgG antibodies to the floor of the blister
- Porphyria Cutanea Tarda
  - Subepidermal blister with minimal inflammatory cell infiltrate
  - The dermal papillae extend into the blister cavity with a festooning appearance
  - PAS-positive eosinophilic deposits around the blood vessels of the papillary dermis are characteristic

PEARLS

- *Cicatricial pemphigoid (benign mucosal pemphigoid) typically presents as blisters involving mucous membranes that erode, ulcerate, and heal with scarring*
- *Mucous membranes of mouth, conjunctiva larynx, nose, and anus can be affected*

SELECTED REFERENCES

Engineer L, Bhol K, Ahmed AR: Pemphigoid gestationis: a review. Am J Obstet Gynecol 183:483-491, 2000.

Gammon WR, Kowalewski C, Chorzelski TP, et al: Direct immunofluorescence studies of sodium chloride-separated skin in the differential diagnosis of bullous pemphigoid and epidermolysis bullosa acquisita. J Am Acad Dermatol 22:664, 1990.

Kasperkiewicz M, Zillikens D, Schmidt E: Pemphigoid diseases: pathogenesis, diagnosis, and treatment. Autoimmunity 45:55, 2012.

Nousari HC, Anhalt GJ: Pemphigus and bullous pemphigoid. Lancet 354:667-672, 1999.

Olasz EB, Yancey KB: Bullous pemphigoid and related subepidermal autoimmune blistering diseases. Curr Dir Autoimmun 10:141-166, 2008.

Schmidt E, della Torre R, Borradori L: Clinical features and practical diagnosis of bullous pemphigoid. Dermatol Clin 29:427, 2011.

DERMATITIS HERPETIFORMIS

Clinical Features

- Young to middle-aged males are usually affected
- Lesions are pruritic, symmetrical, grouped papulovesicles involving elbows, knees, back, buttocks, and scalp

Histopathology

- *Subepidermal* bullae filled with neutrophils and varying numbers of eosinophils characterize a fully evolved vesicle

- Neutrophilic aggregates (microabscesses) are present at the tips of the dermal papillae, at the edge of the blister, and in papular lesions (Figure 2-39A)
- Moderate amount of superficial perivascular lymphocytic, neutrophilic, and eosinophilic infiltrate may be present in the dermis

Special Stains and Immunohistochemistry

- Noncontributory

Other Techniques for Diagnosis

- Direct immunofluorescence studies show granular deposits of IgA within the dermal papillae of normal skin and lesional skin (Figure 2-39B)
- Serologic tests often detect elevated levels of IgA tissue transglutaminase antibodies, IgA epidermal transglutaminase antibodies, and IgA endomysial antibodies

Differential Diagnosis

- Linear IgA Dermatosis
  - Can be indistinguishable from dermatitis herpetiformis on histology
  - However, in linear IgA dermatosis, the neutrophils are often seen in a linear array at the dermoepidermal junction
  - Direct immunofluorescence shows a linear pattern of IgA deposition at basement membrane zone
- Bullous Systemic Lupus Erythematosus
  - Shares histologic features with dermatitis herpetiformis and linear IgA dermatosis
  - Immunofluorescence findings of granular band-like deposits of IgG and C3 at basement membrane zone are characteristic of bullous systemic lupus erythematosus

PEARLS

- *Dermatitis herpetiformis is associated with gluten-sensitive enteropathy and shows celiac sprue–like changes on jejunal biopsy and the skin lesions respond to gluten-free diet*
- *High frequency of HLA DQ2 or HLA DQ8 is seen in patients with dermatitis herpetiformis*

SELECTED REFERENCES

Ahmed AR, Hameed A: Bullous pemphigoid and dermatitis herpetiformis. Clin Dermatol 11:47-52, 1993.Hull CM, Zone JJ: Dermatitis herpetiformis and linear IgA bullous dermatosis. In Bolognia JL,

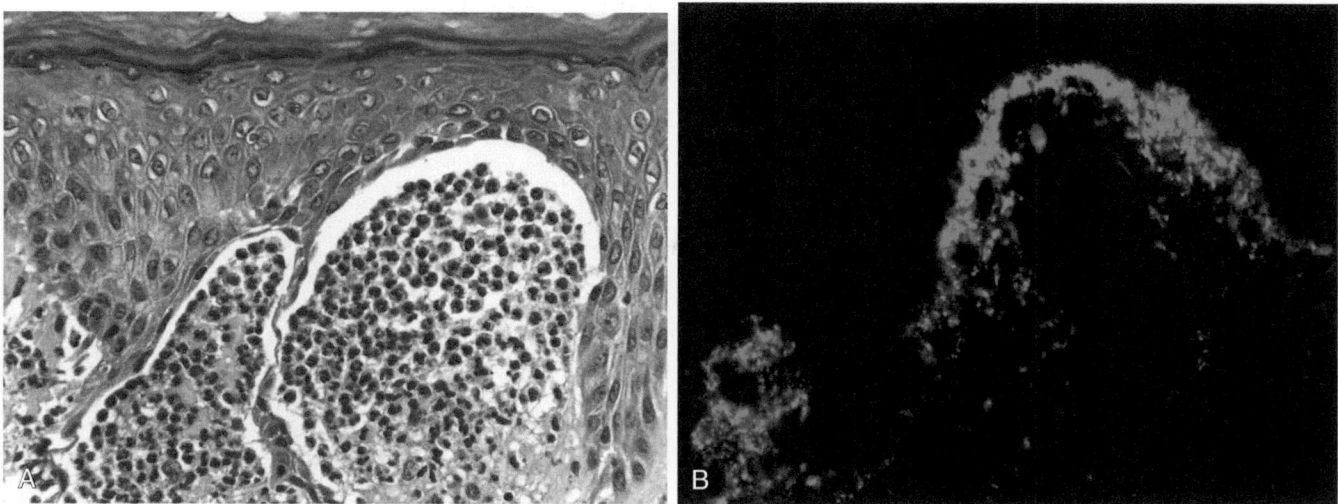

Figure 2-39. Dermatitis herpetiformis. A, Histologic section shows separation at the dermoepidermal junction associated with aggregates of neutrophils, especially at the tips of the dermal papillae (papillary microabscesses). **B,** Immunofluorescence studies show granular deposits of IgA at the tips of dermal papillae

Jorizzo JL, Schaffer JV, et al. (eds): Dermatology, 3rd ed, vol 1. Philadelphia, Elsevier, 2012, p 491.

Kárpáti S: Dermatitis herpetiformis. Clin Dermatol 30:56-59, 2012.

Smith EP, Zone JJ: Dermatitis herpetiformis and linear IgA bullous dermatosis. Dermatol Clin 11:511-526, 1993.

FOLLICULITIS

ACNE VULGARIS

Clinical Features

- Common disease of adolescents and young adults
- Manifests as open and closed comedones and inflammatory nodules on the face and anterior and posterior trunk
- Nodulocystic acne and acne conglobata are severe expressions of acne vulgaris

Histopathology

- Comedones show dilated follicular infundibulum that is plugged by keratin, lipid, and microorganisms
- Rupture of the follicular wall results in an intense inflammatory reaction with neutrophils (Figure 2-40A)

in the early stages and foreign-body-type granulomatous reaction in later stages

- Healing takes place by scarring

Special Stains and Immunohistochemistry

- PAS and GMS stains are helpful in excluding infectious etiology

Other Techniques for Diagnosis

- Noncontributory

Differential Diagnosis

- Histologic differential diagnoses of folliculitis and perifolliculitis include various infectious processes such as herpesvirus infection and fungal infection
  - Multinucleated cells with viral inclusions are present in the follicular epithelium in herpesvirus folliculitis
  - GMS and PAS stains are helpful to rule out fungal infection involving follicles
  - Granulomatous rosacea
  - Granulomatous perifollicular inflammation and dilated blood vessels; the follicles are generally intact

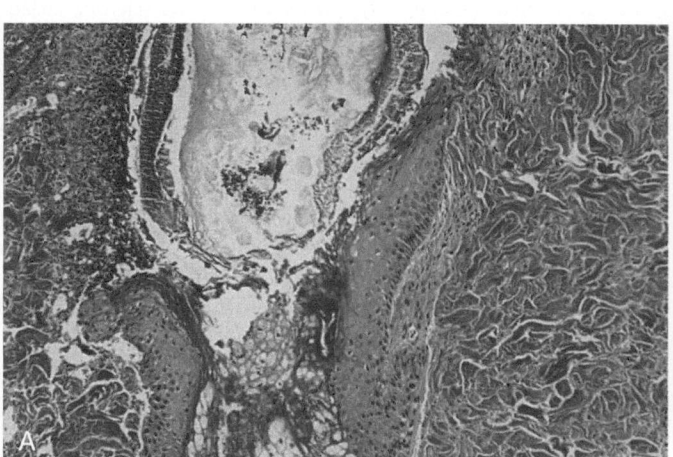

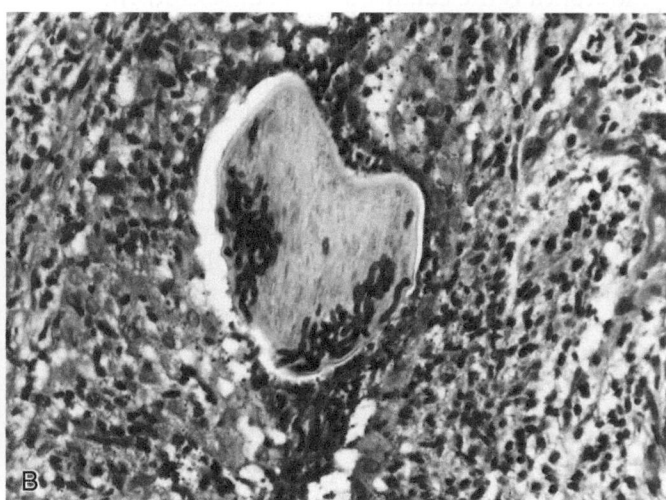

Figure 2-40. A, Acne vulgaris. Histologic section shows a disrupted follicle and neutrophilic infiltrate. **B,** Majocchi granuloma. PAS stain shows fungal forms in the hair shaft and surrounding dense inflammatory cell infiltrate.

- Eosinophilic Pustular Folliculitis
  - Typically seen in infants and in association with immunocompromised states
  - Can be differentiated by the presence of spongiosis with eosinophils, subcorneal pustule with eosinophils, and perifollicular infiltrate rich in eosinophils
- Majocchi Granuloma
  - Nodular folliculitis and perifolliculitis caused most frequently by *Trichophyton rubrum*
  - PAS stain demonstrates spores and hyphae within hairs and hair follicles and in the dermal inflammatory cell infiltrate (Figure 2-40B)

PEARLS

- *Follicular occlusion triad—which includes hidradenitis suppurativa, acne conglobata, and perifolliculitis capitis abscedens et suffodiens—represents a chronic, deep-seated folliculitis resulting in abscesses and sinus tract formation that heals with scarring*
- *Folliculitis barbae, folliculitis decalvans, and folliculitis keloidalis nuchae represent types of chronic deep folliculitis that heal with scarring*

SELECTED REFERENCES

Cunliffe WJ, Holland DB, Clark SM, Stables GI: Comedogenesis: some new aetiological, clinical and therapeutic strategies. Br J Dermatol 142:1084-1091, 2000.

Fujiyama T, Tokura Y: Clinical and histopathological differential diagnosis of eosinophilic pustular folliculitis. J Dermatol 40:419-423, 2013

Goodman GJ: Postacne scarring: a review of its pathophysiology and treatment. Dermatol Surg 26:857-871, 2000.

Ilkit M, Durdu M, Karakaş M: Majocchi's granuloma: a symptom complex caused by fungal pathogens. Med Mycol 50:449-457, 2012.

FIBROSING DERMATOSES

MORPHEA AND SCLERODERMA

Clinical Features

- Scleroderma is a connective tissue disease of unknown etiology characterized by thickening and sclerosis of skin
- Morphea is the cutaneous form of scleroderma without associated systemic involvement; lesions can be plaquelike, linear, segmental, or generalized
- Lesions are round to oval, indurated with a smooth surface, and ivory colored; a violaceous border may be present
- Morphea may occur in younger patients and may present with more circumscribed and well-demarcated lesions than will occur with systemic scleroderma
- Sites of predilection include face, distal extremities, and trunk

Histopathology

- Biopsies of early inflammatory lesions representing the violaceous border of actively enlarging lesions show a perivascular and interstitial infiltrate of lymphocytes and plasma cells associated with thickening of collagen bundles in the reticular dermis
- Septa in the subcutaneous fat show marked thickening and inflammatory cell infiltrate; newly formed collagen is seen as fine wavy fibers (Figure 2-41A,B)

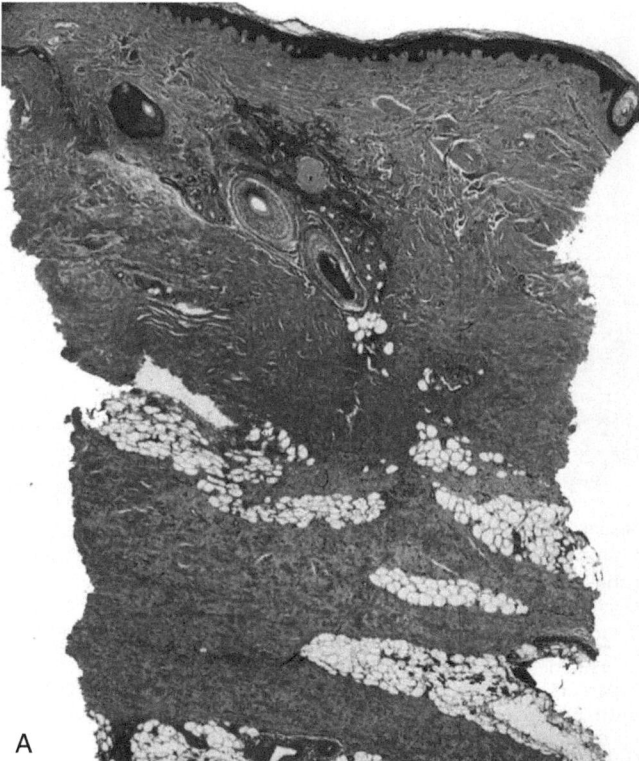

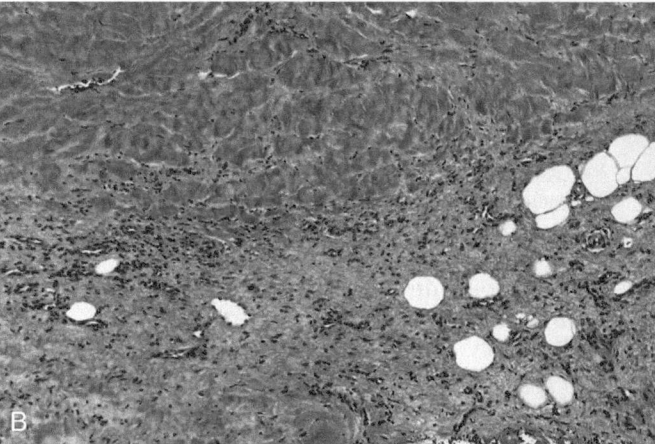

Figure 2-41. Morphea. A, Low-power view shows marked thickening of the dermis with sclerotic bands of collagen extending into the subcutaneous fat. **B,** High-power view shows sclerotic collagen extending into the subcutaneous fat associated with lymphocytic inflammation.

- Fully evolved sclerotic lesions show closely packed collagen bundles in the reticular dermis with only minimal inflammatory cell infiltrate
- Eccrine glands appear atrophic and are placed higher in the dermis; there is progressive sclerotic destruction of capillaries and adnexal structures
- Underlying fascia and occasionally skeletal muscle tissue may also show fibrosis and sclerosis

Special Stains and Immunohistochemistry

- Noncontributory

Other Techniques for Diagnosis

- Up to 90% of patients with systemic scleroderma and 50% with localized scleroderma have a positive antinuclear antibody (ANA) but the significance is unclear

- More than 90% have anticentromere antibody, which correlates with morphea/limited cutaneous systemic sclerosis or CREST syndrome (associated with a better prognosis)
- About 20% to 40% have antibodies to Scl 70 (antitopoisomerase), which correlates with systemic sclerosis

Differential Diagnosis

- Scleredema
  - Presents as diffuse, nonpitting swelling and induration of skin and shows clinical and histologic similarities to scleroderma
  - Collagen bundles may be thickened but are not hyalinized
  - Widened spaces between collagen bundles are present
  - Special stains can be used to demonstrate the presence of hyaluronic acid in these spaces
- Lichen Sclerosus
  - Histologic changes show significant overlap with morphea and coexistence of the two is not uncommon
  - Presence of epidermal atrophy, follicular plugging, vacuolar change of basal cell layer, edema/homogenization of papillary dermis and absence of elastic fibers in the sclerotic areas favors a diagnosis of lichen sclerosus
- Chronic Radiation Dermatitis
  - Dermal collagen bundles are swollen and often hyalinized, showing some similarities to morphea
  - Epidermal atrophy, large bizarre fibroblasts with pleomorphic nuclei, inflammation, and telangiectasia in the superficial dermis occur
  - Additionally, fibrous thickening of the blood vessels, especially of the deep dermis, is seen
- Nephrogenic Systemic Fibrosis
  - Systemic disorder seen in patients with renal impairment and characterized by thickening of skin of trunk and extremities
  - Histologic sections show thickened collagen bundles and spindled fibroblasts that extend into subcutaneous septae and subjacent fascia
  - Immunohistochemical studies show the spindled cells to be CD34 positive
  - Differentiation from scleroderma and other fibrosing dermatitis may require clinical and laboratory evidence of renal impairment

PEARLS

- *A subset of scleroderma known as* CREST *syndrome presents with Raynaud phenomenon in all affected patients; the manifestations include calcinosis cutis, Raynaud phenomenon, esophageal involvement, sclerodactyly, and telangiectasis*
- *Eosinophilic fasciitis (Shulman syndrome) is a disorder characterized by involvement of deep fascia by sclerosis and eosinophilic infiltrate and most likely represents a deep form of morphea*

Selected References

Canady J, Karrer S, Fleck M, Bosserhoff AK: Fibrosing connective tissue disorders of the skin: molecular similarities and distinctions. J Dermatol Sci 70:151-158, 2013.

Cowper SE, Boyer PJ: Nephrogenic systemic fibrosis: an update. Curr Rheumatol Rep 8: 151-157, 2006.
Kreuter A, Wischnewski J, Terras S, et al: Coexistence of lichen sclerosus and morphea: a retrospective analysis of 472 patients with localized scleroderma from a German tertiary referral center. J Am Acad Dermatol 67:1157-1162, 2012.
Tyndall A, Fistarol S: The differential diagnosis of systemic sclerosis. Curr Opin Rheumatol 25:692-699, 2013
Uitto J, Santa Cruz DJ, Bauer EA, et al: Morphea and lichen sclerosus et atrophicus: clinical and histopathologic studies in patients with combined features. J Am Acad Dermatol 3:271, 1980.
Wigley FM: Clinical aspects of systemic and localized scleroderma. Curr Opin Rheumatol 6:628-636, 1994.

PANNICULITIS

ERYTHEMA NODOSUM

Clinical Features

- Acute form generally presents with sudden onset of symmetrical, tender, erythematous subcutaneous nodules on the extensor aspects of lower legs
- Associated fever, malaise, and arthropathy may be present
- Chronic form, also known as *erythema nodosum migrans*, presents as unilateral nodules on lower legs that resolve and recur in other sites

Histopathology

- A granulomatous fibrosing septal panniculitis is the characteristic finding (Figure 2-42A,B)
- Early lesions are characterized by a mixed inflammatory cell infiltrate of lymphocytes, eosinophils, and neutrophils, more intense at the periphery of the lobule
- Later lesions show widening of the septa with increasing number of macrophages in the infiltrate; well-formed granulomas are often in the septa; this feature is more prominent in late stages of acute erythema nodosum and chronic erythema nodosum

Special Stains and Immunohistochemistry

- Special stains and microbiologic cultures to exclude an infectious etiology

Other Techniques for Diagnosis

- Noncontributory

Differential Diagnosis

- Erythema Induratum and Nodular Vasculitis
  - A mixed lobular and septal pattern of inflammation
  - Vasculitis and zones of fat necrosis
- Subcutaneous Sarcoidosis
  - Noncaseating granulomas in the overlying dermis in addition to those in the subcutaneous fat help in differentiating sarcoidosis from erythema nodosum
- Infectious Panniculitis
  - Presence of neutrophilic infiltrate and granuloma formation should raise the possibility of an underlying infection, in particular subcutaneous tuberculosis
  - Special stains and cultures are necessary

PEARLS

- *Streptococcal pharyngitis is the most common among the known associations of erythema nodosum*
- *Crohn disease and sarcoidosis are also known to be associated with erythema nodosum*

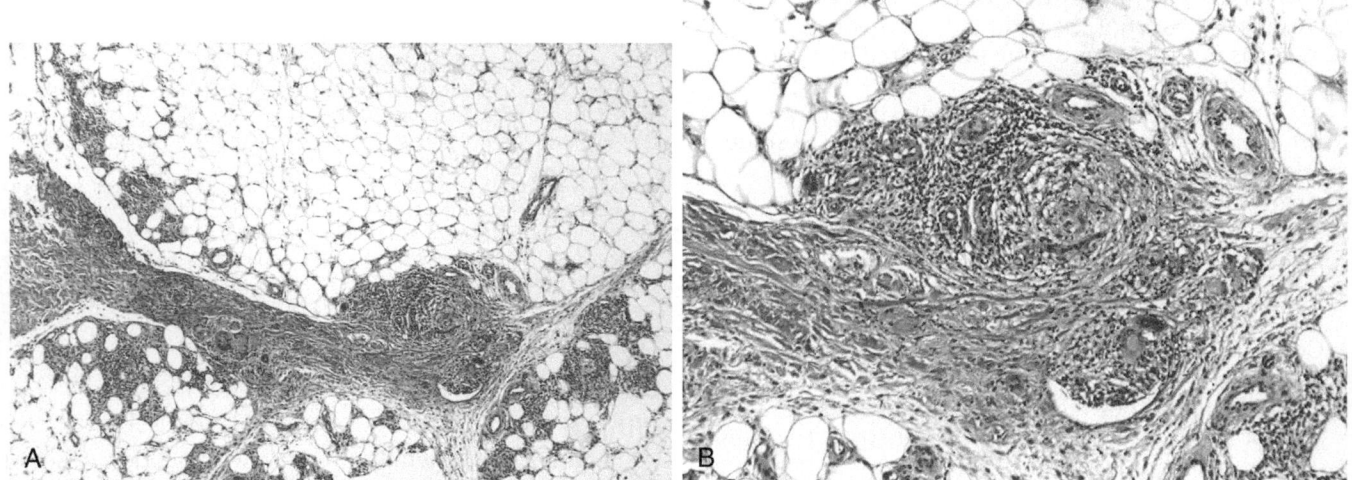

Figure 2-42. Erythema nodosum. A, Low-power view shows a predominantly septal involvement by a fibrosing process. **B,** High-power view shows broadening of the septa of the subcutaneous fat by fibrosis and granulomatous inflammation.

SELECTED REFERENCES

Cribier B, Caille A, Heid E, Grosshans E: Erythema nodosum and associated diseases: a study of 129 cases. Int J Dermatol 37:667-672, 1998.
Meyerson MS: Erythema nodosum leprosum. Int J Dermatol 35:389-392, 1996.
Requena L, Sanchez Yus E: Panniculitis. Part I. Mostly septal panniculitis. J Am Acad Dermatol 45:163-183, 2001.
White WL, Hitchcock MG: Diagnosis: erythema nodosum or not? Semin Cutan Med Surg 18:47-55, 1999.

SUBCUTANEOUS FAT NECROSIS OF THE NEWBORN

Clinical Features

- Uncommon, painless, self-limited disease that affects full-term and postterm infants
- Presents at 1 to 6 weeks of age as asymptomatic, firm nodules on cheeks, shoulders, back, buttocks, and thighs
- Hypercalcemia and less commonly, thrombocytopenia are reported complications in these patients

Histopathology

- Predominantly lobular pattern of inflammation with foci of fat necrosis, surrounded by macrophages and multinucleated giant cells (Figure 2-43A)
- Cytoplasm of the macrophages and giant cells contains needle-shaped crystals of lipid arranged in radial array (Figure 2-43B)
- Deposits of calcium may be seen

Special Stains and Immunohistochemistry

- Noncontributory

Other Techniques for Diagnosis

- Noncontributory

Differential Diagnosis

- Sclerema Neonatorum
  - Usually affects premature, ill newborns
  - Presents as rapidly spreading diffuse hardening of subcutaneous tissue of back, shoulders, and buttocks
  - Lobular pattern of panniculitis with cells containing needle-shaped crystals arranged in radial array similar to subcutaneous fat necrosis
  - Minimal to absent inflammation in the background in sclerema neonatorum is helpful in the differential diagnosis
- Poststeroid Panniculitis
  - May show similar changes with needle-shaped crystals in fat cells
  - Clinical history of steroid treatment is essential
- Pancreatic Fat Necrosis
  - Can present as lobular panniculitis; however, foci of fat necrosis are associated with ghostlike fat cells with thick borders and calcifications
  - Crystals in radial array are not a feature
- Lipodystrophy
  - Lobular panniculitis with predominantly histiocytic infiltrate
  - No needle-shaped clefts in the histiocytes

PEARLS

- *Subcutaneous fat necrosis is a self-limited disease of unknown etiology*

SELECTED REFERENCES

Friedman SJ, Winkelmann RK: Subcutaneous fat necrosis of the newborn: light, ultrastructural and histochemical microscopic studies. J Cutan Pathol 16:99-105, 1989.
Mahé E, Girszyn N, Hadj-Rabia S, et al: Subcutaneous fat necrosis of the newborn: a systematic evaluation of risk factors, clinical manifestations, complications and outcome of 16 children. Br J Dermatol 156:709, 2007.
Requena L, Sanchez Yus E: Panniculitis. Part II. Mostly lobular panniculitis. J Am Acad Dermatol 45:325-361, 2001.
Tran JT, Sheth AP: Complications of subcutaneous fat necrosis of the newborn: a case report and review of the literature. Pediatr Dermatol 20:257, 2003.
Zeb A, Darmstadt GL: Sclerema neonatorum: a review of nomenclature, clinical presentation, histological features, differential diagnoses and management. J Perinatol 28:453, 2008.

CYSTS, PROLIFERATIONS, AND NEOPLASMS

CYSTS

EPIDERMAL INCLUSION CYST (INFUNDIBULAR CYST)

Clinical Features

- Typically results from progressive cystic ectasia of the infundibulum of the hair follicle following mechanical occlusion of the orifice

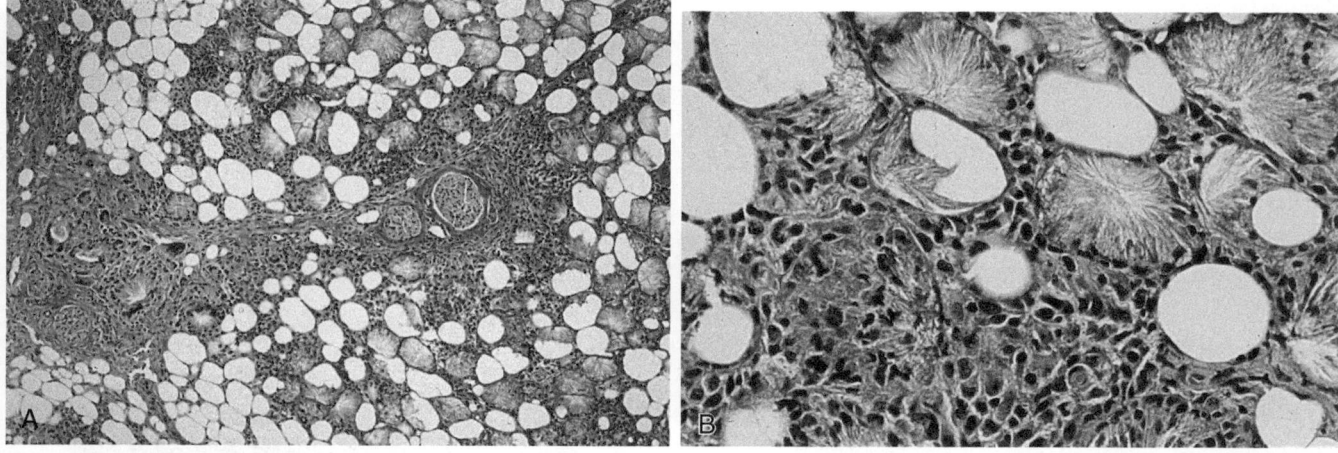

Figure 2-43. Subcutaneous fat necrosis. A, Low-power view shows a predominantly lobular pattern of inflammation. **B,** High-power view shows the lobules containing areas of fat necrosis and a moderately dense mixed inflammatory cell infiltrate, including lymphocytes and histiocytes. Multinucleated histiocytes containing needle-shaped crystals in radial array are a characteristic finding.

- Predilection for the head, neck, and trunk
- One or more freely movable, dermal, skin-colored, firm nodules less than 5 cm in diameter

Histopathology
- Rounded dermal cyst filled with laminated keratin that tends to fall out during processing of tissue (Figure 2-44A)
- Cyst lining resembles epidermis or infundibular epithelium with prominent granular layer
- Rupture of the cyst into the dermis produces a granulomatous reaction with foreign-body giant cells
- Pseudocarcinomatous hyperplasia may ensue from the remnants of the cyst wall, which can be mistaken for SCC

Special Stains and Immunohistochemistry
- Noncontributory

Other Techniques for Diagnosis
- Noncontributory

Differential Diagnosis
- Trichilemmal Cyst
  - Benign cyst occurring most commonly on the scalp as multiple cystic nodules
  - Cyst contents consist of compact keratin, and the lining resembles the isthmus of hair follicle; abrupt keratinization with absent granular layer is characteristic (Figure 2-44B)
  - Calcifications are frequently found
  - Proliferating trichilemmal cystic neoplasm: a low-grade neoplasm characterized by lobules of eosinophilic epithelial cells (isthmic) and infiltrative growth pattern
- Steatocystoma
  - Most commonly occurs as multiple nodules on presternal skin, upper arms, axillae, and scrotum; inherited in an autosomal dominant pattern
  - Occasionally may be seen in solitary form
  - Histologic sections show a collapsed cystic space in the dermis lined by squamous epithelium, with the innermost layer composed of homogeneous keratin with an undulating or crenulated appearance (Figure 2-44D)
  - Mature sebaceous lobules are present in the vicinity, and hair shafts may be seen in the lumen

- Dermoid Cyst
  - Usually present at birth
  - Occurs most commonly on the head around the eyes as a result of sequestration of skin along lines of closure
  - Cyst lining is composed of epidermis with associated mature adnexal structures; hair follicles contain hair shafts that project into the lumen
- Hidrocystoma
  - Usually occurs on the face as a translucent nodule with a bluish hue
  - Lining is composed of a row of secretory cells surrounded by elongated myoepithelial cells (Figure 2-44C)
  - "Decapitation" secretions when present point toward the apocrine nature of the cyst (apocrine hidrocystoma)
- Infectious Granuloma
  - Granulomatous reaction surrounding a ruptured epidermal inclusion cyst may raise the possibility of an infectious process
  - Gram and PAS stains may be necessary to demonstrate the organisms

PEARLS

- *Incomplete excision often leads to recurrences*
- *Multiple epidermal inclusion cysts occur on the face and scalp in patients with Gardner syndrome*

SELECTED REFERENCES

Pariser RJ: Benign neoplasms of the skin. Med Clin N Am 82:1285-1307, 1998.
Perniciaro C: Gardner's syndrome. Dermatol Clin 13:51-56, 1995.
Vicente J, Vazquez-Doval FJ: Proliferations of the epidermoid cyst wall. Int J Dermatol 37:181-185, 1998.

EPIDERMAL PROLIFERATIONS AND NEOPLASMS

SEBORRHEIC KERATOSIS
Clinical Features
- Occurs characteristically in middle-aged and elderly individuals

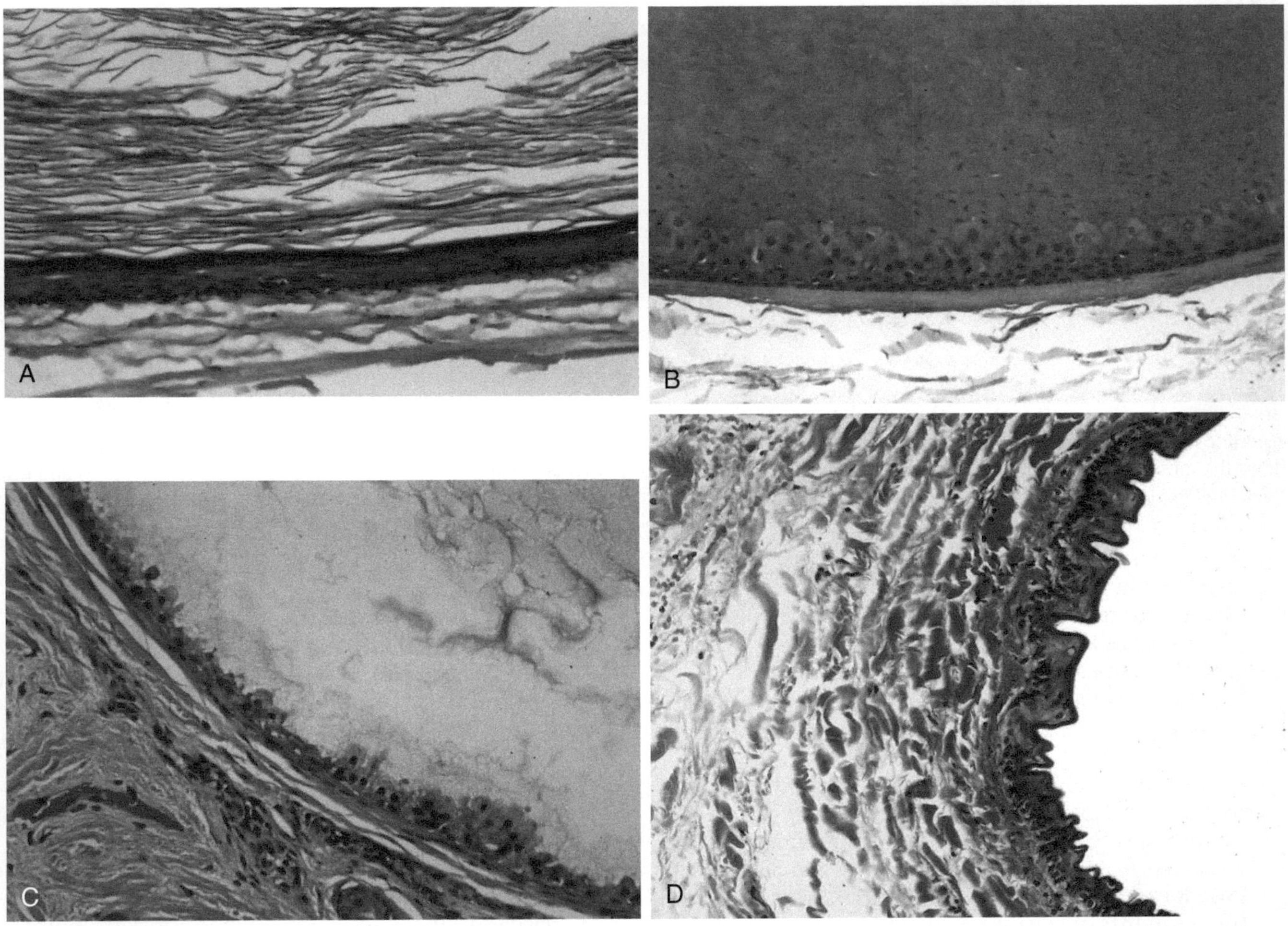

Figure 2-44. A, Epidermal inclusion cyst. Histologic section shows a cyst filled with laminated keratin and lined by stratified squamous epithelium with granular layer. **B,** Trichilemmal cyst. The presence of compact keratin in the lumen of this cyst lined by stratified squamous epithelium with no granular layer distinguishes it from an epidermal inclusion cyst. **C,** Hidrocystoma. This cyst, lined by only two layers of cells, an inner luminal row with decapitation secretion, and outer myoepithelial cells, is easily differentiated from an epidermal inclusion cyst. The cyst lumen contains secretions rather than the laminated keratin seen in epidermal inclusion cyst. **D,** Steatocystoma. The thin epithelial lining of this cyst is covered by an undulating keratin layer.

- Predilection for the trunk with common involvement of the extremities, head, and neck
- Round, variably sized plaques with stuck-on appearance
- Plaques are usually tan to dark brown
- Small, porelike ostia impacted with keratin

Histopathology
- Hyperkeratosis
- Proliferation of uniform squamous and basaloid cells in the epidermis (Figure 2-45)
- Presence of keratin-filled cysts (horn cysts) that occasionally communicate with the overlying skin (pseudohorn cysts)
- Other histologic variants include adenoid, reticulated, clonal, and inverted follicular keratosis types

Special Stains and Immunohistochemistry
- Noncontributory

Other Techniques for Diagnosis
- Noncontributory

Differential Diagnosis
- Epidermal Nevus and Acanthosis Nigricans

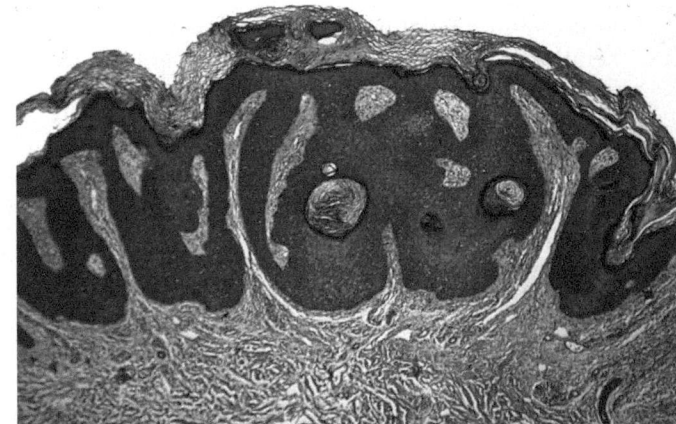

Figure 2-45. Seborrheic keratosis. Histologic section shows an epidermal proliferation composed of monomorphous keratinocytes. Laminated hyperkeratosis and pseudohorn cysts are characteristic features.

- May be indistinguishable from seborrheic keratosis on histologic grounds alone
- Verruca Vulgaris
  - Papillomatous changes in seborrheic keratosis can resemble a verruca vulgaris
  - In verruca, the tips of the papillae are covered by columns of parakeratosis, often with hemorrhages in the cornified layer
- Clonal pattern of seborrheic keratosis can mimic an intraepidermal poroma or even squamous cell carcinoma in situ; however, cytologic atypia, dyskeratosis, and mitotic figures are generally absent in seborrheic keratosis.
- SCC
  - Irritated or inverted follicular keratosis variant has scattered "squamous eddies" that may resemble keratin pearls of SCC; however, squamous eddies are simply whorls of keratinocytes and do not contain central parakeratosis, which is characteristic of keratin pearls

PEARLS

- *Sign of Leser-Trélat: sudden onset of hundreds of seborrheic keratoses related to internal malignancy*
- *Dermatosis papulosa nigra: multiple lesions appearing on the face of patients of African descent with histologic features identical to those of seborrheic keratosis*

SELECTED REFERENCES

Eads TJ, Hood AF, Chuang TY, et al: The diagnostic yield of histologic examination of seborrheic keratoses. Arch Dermatol 133:1417-1420, 1997.
Schwartz RA: Sign of Leser-Trélat. J Am Acad Dermatol 35:88-95, 1996.
Soyer HP, Kenet RO, Wolf IH, et al: Clinicopathological correlation of pigmented skin lesions using dermoscopy. Eur J Dermatol 10:22-28, 2000.
Toussaint S, Salcedo E, Kamino H: Benign epidermal proliferations. Adv Dermatol 14:307-357, 1999.

CLEAR CELL ACANTHOMA

Clinical Features

- Commonly affects middle-aged and older individuals
- Predilection for lower extremities
- Lesions grow slowly but frequently ulcerate and have an oozing, erythematous surface
- Small (< 2 cm), solitary nodule or plaque that is sharply delineated

Histopathology

- Overlying parakeratotic cornified layer, often containing neutrophils (Figure 2-46)
- Abrupt intraepidermal proliferation of squamoid cells with pale to clear cytoplasm
- Elongated rete ridges with well-vascularized dermal papillae
- Presence of neutrophils within intercellular spaces of the involved epidermis
- Decreased or absent melanin in affected cells

Special Stains and Immunohistochemistry

- PAS stain highlights the abundant glycogen in the pale cells

Other Techniques for Diagnosis

- Noncontributory

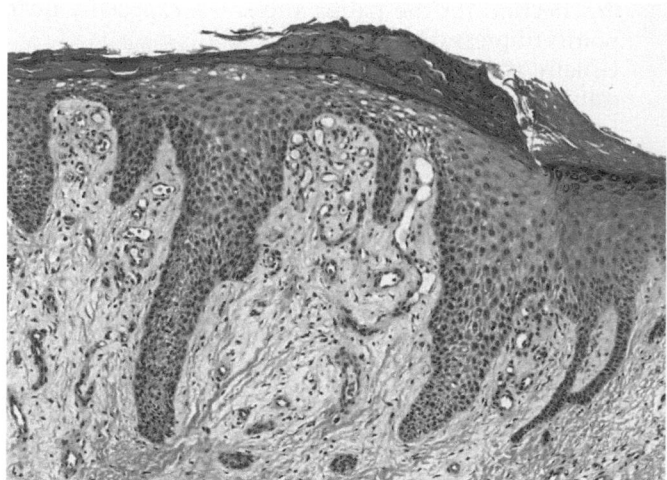

Figure 2-46. Clear cell acanthoma. Histologic section shows a sharply demarcated epidermal proliferation composed of keratinocytes with pale cytoplasm. Parakeratosis and neutrophils in the parakeratosis and among the clear cells are typical findings.

Differential Diagnosis

- Eccrine Poroma
  - Sheetlike down-growth of monomorphous epithelial cells
  - Keratinization and early erosion and ulceration present on the surface of epidermis
  - Richly vascular stroma with dilated, tortuous vessels
  - Small foci of spiraling cuboidal cells lining eccrine ducts may be present in epithelium
- Psoriasis
  - Parakeratosis with neutrophils associated with regular epidermal hyperplasia
  - Cytoplasm of the keratinocytes is not pale or clear

PEARLS

- *Clinically, clear cell acanthomas appear stuck on like seborrheic keratosis and vascular similar to pyogenic granuloma*

SELECTED REFERENCES

Brownstein MH: The benign acanthomas. J Cutan Pathol 12:172-188, 1985.
Langer K, Wuketich S, Konrad K: Pigmented clear cell acanthoma. Am J Dermatopathol 16:134-139, 1994.
Pariser RJ: Benign neoplasms of the skin. Med Clin N Am 82:1285-1307, v-vi, 1998.
Toussaint S, Salcedo E, Kamino H: Benign epidermal proliferations. Adv Dermatol 14:307-357, 1999.

VERRUCAE (VERRUCA VULGARIS, PLANTAR WARTS, VERRUCA PLANA)

Clinical Features

- Benign epidermal proliferation due to infection with varying strains of human papillomavirus (HPV)
- Verruca Vulgaris
  - Associated with HPV-1, -2, -4, -7, -49
  - Most common type of wart
  - Predilection for the dorsal aspect of the hands and feet
  - Circumscribed, papillomatous, flesh-colored nodules
- Palmoplantar Warts
  - Associated with HPV-1, -2, -3, -4, -27, -29, -57

- Predilection for the palms and soles, especially near points of pressure
- Usually painful and surrounded by a thick reactive callus
- Hyperkeratotic nodules appearing on the dorsum of the foot surrounded by a thick reactive callus
- Verruca Plana
  - Associated with HPV-3, -10, -28, -49
  - Predilection for the face and dorsal aspect of the hands
  - Multiple, flesh-colored papules
  - Typically distributed in a linear fashion

Histopathology

- Verruca Vulgaris
  - Flame-shaped tongues of epidermis with overlying hyperkeratosis and parakeratosis (Figure 2-47)
  - Epithelial cells contain enlarged coarse keratohyalin granules, cytoplasmic pallor, and clearing
  - HPV particles cause nuclear pallor and dispersion of chromatin, imparting a steel-gray appearance
  - Koilocytes (cells with pyknotic nuclei surrounded by cytoplasmic vacuolation)
- Palmoplantar Warts
  - Endophytic epithelial down-growths covered with dense hyperkeratotic and parakeratotic scale
  - Epithelial cells with viral changes similar to those found in verruca vulgaris
  - Uppermost viable epithelial cells also contain irregular eosinophilic cytoplasmic inclusions
- Verruca Plana
  - Multiple blunt epidermal papillae with parakeratosis and minimal hyperkeratosis
  - Epithelial cells with viral changes similar to those found in verruca vulgaris

Special Stains and Immunohistochemistry

- Noncontributory

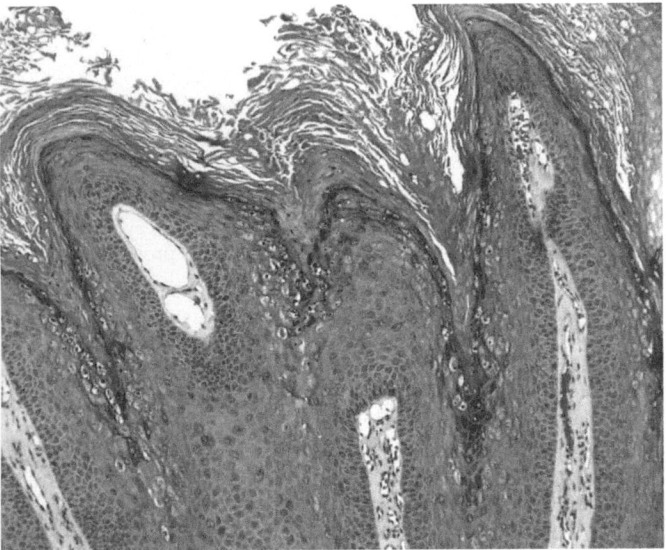

Figure 2-47. Verruca vulgaris. Histologic section shows papillomatous proliferation of epidermal keratinocytes covered by parakeratosis. Hypergranulosis, presence of vacuolated keratinocytes (koilocytes), and dilated blood vessels in the papillary dermis are additional findings.

Other Techniques for Diagnosis

- PCR and ISH techniques may be used to type the HPV

Differential Diagnosis

- Molluscum Contagiosum
  - Cytoplasmic inclusions are typically round to ovoid and eosinophilic
- Epidermodysplasia Verruciformis
  - Shows histologic changes similar to verruca plana
- Keratoacanthoma
  - Typically has a central crater filled with cornified material
  - Large keratinocytes with abundant glassy cytoplasm surround the crater
  - Neutrophilic microabscesses within the epithelial nests

PEARLS

- *Verrucous carcinoma may be included in the differential diagnosis of single large lesions involving the plantar aspect of the foot; a superficial biopsy may show changes indistinguishable from verruca plantaris (clinical suspicion and a deep biopsy are critical in arriving at the correct diagnosis)*

SELECTED REFERENCES

Beutner KR: Nongenital human papillomavirus infections. Clin Lab Med 20:423-430, 2000.
Brentjens MH, Yeung-Yue KA, Lee PC, et al: Human papillomavirus: a review. Dermatol Clin 20:315, 2002.
Nuovo GJ, Ishag M: The histologic spectrum of epidermodysplasia verruciformis. Am J Surg Pathol 24:1400, 2000.
Tyring SK: Human papillomavirus infections: epidemiology, pathogenesis, and host immune response. J Am Acad Dermatol 43:S18-S26, 2000.
Xu X, Erickson L, Chen L, Elder D: Diseases caused by viruses. In Elder DE, Elenitsas R, Johnson BL Jr, et al (eds): Lever's Histopathology of Skin, 10th ed. Philadelphia, Lippincott Williams & Wilkins, 2008, p 637.

ACTINIC KERATOSIS

Clinical Features

- Lesions typically affect middle-aged to older patients
- Predilection for sun-exposed skin of individuals with light skin color
- Lesions are typically multiple and present as small (< 1 cm), erythematous papules with adherent scale; occasionally pigmented

Histopathology

- Alternating columns of orthokeratosis and parakeratosis (Figure 2-48)
- Orthokeratotic sparing corresponds to the opening of follicular infundibula
- Budding of basal cell epithelium and keratinocytic atypia
- Solar elastosis

Special Stains and Immunohistochemistry

- Noncontributory

Other Techniques for Diagnosis

- Noncontributory

Differential Diagnosis

- SCC in Situ
  - Confluent parakeratosis with no intervening areas of orthokeratosis
  - Full-thickness keratinocytic atypia with complete lack of maturation

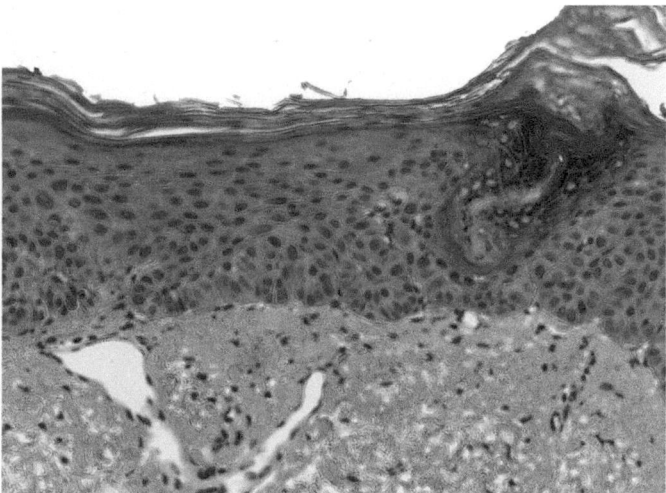

Figure 2-48. Actinic keratosis. Histologic section shows areas of parakeratosis associated with hypogranulosis that spares the openings of the adnexal structures. Budding of the basal cells, keratinocytic atypia, and solar elastosis is present.

PEARLS

- *Actinic cheilitis: actinic keratosis of the vermillion border of the lower lip presenting as zones of discoloration and pallor*
- *Actinic keratosis can progress into SCC and may represent an incipient SCC*

SELECTED REFERENCES

Cockerell CJ: Histopathology of incipient intraepidermal squamous cell carcinoma ("actinic keratosis"). J Am Acad Dermatol 42:11-17, 2000.

Cohn BA: From sunlight to actinic keratosis to squamous cell carcinoma. J Am Acad Dermatol 42:143-144, 2000.

Schwartz RA: The actinic keratosis: a perspective and update. Dermatol Surg 23:1009-1019; quiz, 1020-1021, 1997.

SQUAMOUS CELL CARCINOMA

Clinical Features

- Malignant epithelial tumor of the epidermal keratinocytes
- Commonly affects men older than 60 years
- Risk factors include solar irradiation, radiation therapy, immunosuppression, local carcinogens such as tars and oils, and hereditary diseases such as xeroderma pigmentosa and albinism
- Tumors typically favor sun-exposed areas, including the upper face, ears, lower lip, and dorsum of hands
- Generally presents as solitary, slowly enlarging, indurated nodule that may develop central ulceration
- Variations include verrucous, papillary, and acantholytic forms

Histopathology

- Moderate and confluent parakeratosis
- Epidermal proliferation with cytologic atypia, keratin pearl formation, and invasive pattern (Figure 2-49A)
- Neoplastic cells are characterized by moderate amounts of eosinophilic cytoplasm, nuclear enlargement, and hyperchromasia
- Lower part of the neoplasm may show an infiltrative pattern; perineural invasion may be present in deeply invasive neoplasms
- Acantholytic pattern seen in some examples
- Degree of differentiation is generally assessed by the degree of keratin pearl formation

Special Stains and Immunohistochemistry

- Cytokeratin positivity is useful in differentiating poorly differentiated SCC from other neoplasms

Other Techniques for Diagnosis

- Noncontributory

Differential Diagnosis

- Squamous Cell Carcinoma in Situ (Bowen Disease)
  - Variant of SCC in situ occurring on sun-exposed and non-sun-exposed skin
  - Histologic changes include confluent parakeratosis and full thickness atypia of the epidermal keratinocytes with frequent mitoses and dyskeratotic cells (Figure 2-49B)
  - Bowenoid papulosis is a clinical entity characterized by multiple papules in the genital area but histologically indistinguishable from Bowen disease; the recent Lower Anogenital Squamous Terminology (LAST) standardization project for HPV-related lesions recommended that each of these lesions be reported as a "high grade squamous intraepithelial lesion" with Bowenoid papulosis further suggested in parentheses or comment when clinically appropriate
- Keratoacanthoma
  - Best regarded as a variant of well-differentiated SCC with a potential for spontaneous regression
  - Presents as symmetrical cup-shaped lesions filled with orthokeratotic cornified layer and surrounded by lips of epidermal proliferation (Figure 2-49C)
  - Epithelial cells typically contain abundant glassy eosinophilic cytoplasm and only mild cytologic atypia
  - Neutrophilic microabscesses are a characteristic feature
- Verrucous Carcinoma
  - Plantar verrucous carcinoma can be easily misdiagnosed as verruca if the biopsy is superficial
  - Surface shows hyperkeratosis, parakeratosis, and epidermal hyperplasia
  - Deeper biopsy shows broad bands of epidermal proliferation filled with parakeratotic centers; the bases of the proliferation are large and bulbous and invade the deep dermis in a pushing manner (Figure 2-49D)
- Spindle Cell SCC versus Atypical Fibroxanthoma
  - Presence of intercellular bridges in SCC
  - Cytokeratin positivity in SCC
- Inverted Follicular Keratosis
  - Shows features of an irritated seborrheic keratosis or verruca with squamous eddies
  - No keratin pearls
- Pseudocarcinomatous Epidermal Hyperplasia
  - Occurs most often at the edges of ulcers, deep fungal infections, pyodermas, and other proliferative inflammatory processes
  - Presence of granulomas and neutrophilic microabscesses suggests an inflammatory process

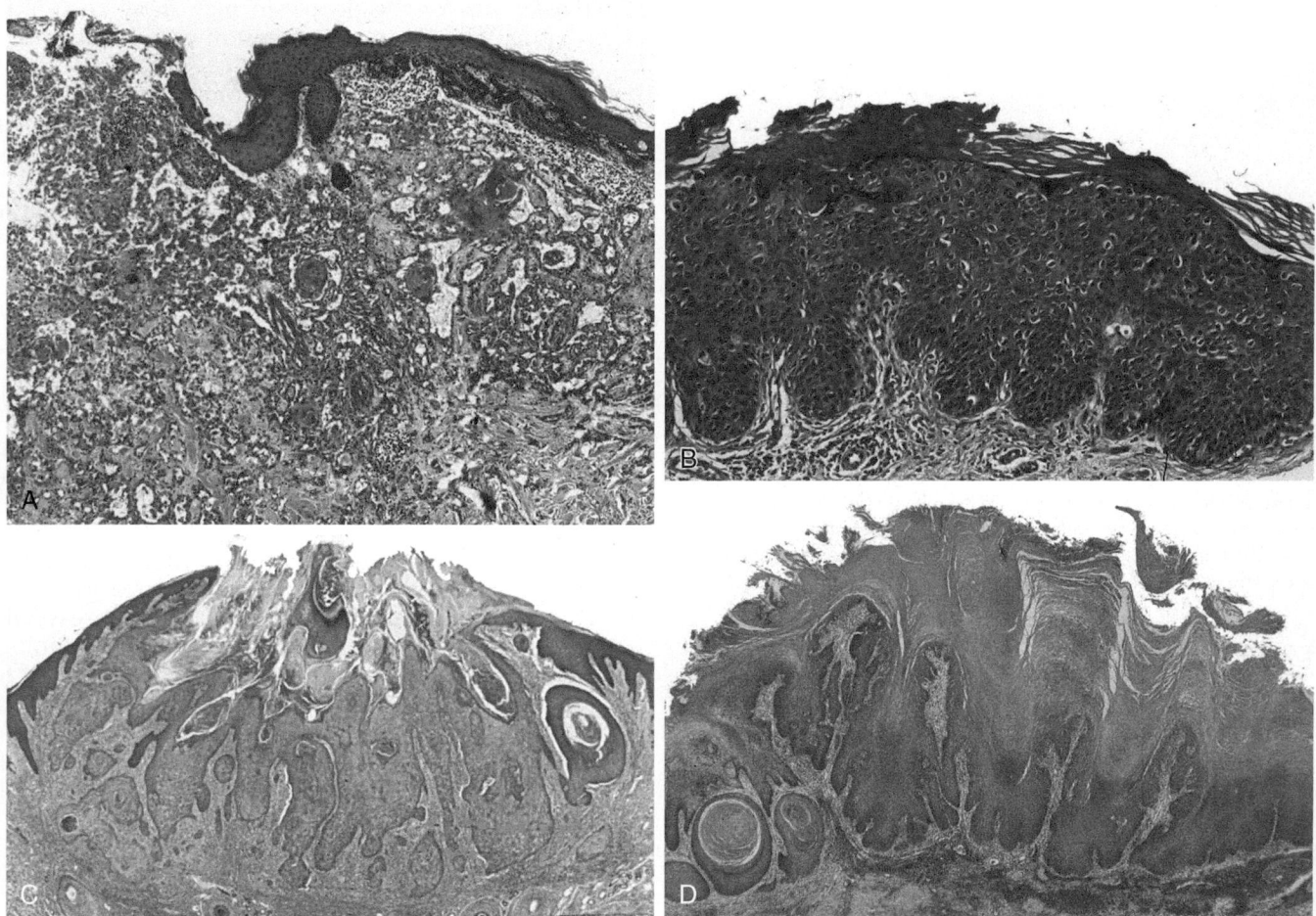

Figure 2-49. A, Squamous cell carcinoma. Histologic section shows an irregular proliferation of atypical keratinocytes. Acantholytic pattern is present. Keratin pearls composed of parakeratosis surrounded by atypical keratinocytes are characteristically seen in well-differentiated and moderately differentiated squamous cell carcinoma. **B,** Squamous cell carcinoma in situ (Bowen disease). Confluent parakeratosis and increased thickness of epidermis are present. The epidermis contains atypical keratinocytes with pleomorphic nuclei, dyskeratotic cells, and frequent mitotic figures above the basal cell layer. The changes are confined to the epidermis, and therefore this lesion is considered a form of squamous cell carcinoma in situ. **C,** Keratoacanthoma. The characteristic architecture of this exoendophytic neoplasm with a central cup-shaped crater surrounded by proliferation of large keratinocytes with abundant glassy cytoplasm and minimal cytologic atypia differentiates this form of squamous cell carcinoma from the conventional squamous cell carcinoma. Neutrophilic microabscesses may be seen at the base of the neoplasm. **D,** Verrucous carcinoma. The epidermal proliferation shows tunnel-like invaginations filled with parakeratosis. The neoplasm infiltrates as bulbous expansions of the rete.

PEARLS

- Marjolin ulcer *refers to SCC arising at the periphery of a longstanding ulcer or scar*
- *SCC arising on sun-damaged skin has low potential for metastasis*

SELECTED REFERENCES

Brand D, Ackerman AB: Squamous cell carcinoma, not basal cell carcinoma, is the most common cancer in humans. J Am Acad Dermatol 42:523-526, 2000.

Darragh TM, Colgan TJ, Cox T, et al: The Lower Anogenital Squamous Terminology Standardization Project for HPV-Associated Lesions: background and consensus recommendations from the College of American Pathologists and the American Society for Colposcopy and Cervical Pathology. Arch of Pathol Lab Med 136:1266-1297, 2012.

Maguire B, Smith NP: Histopathology of cutaneous squamous cell carcinoma. Clin Dermatol 13:559-568, 1995.

Roth JJ, Granick MS: Squamous cell and adnexal carcinomas of the skin. Clin Plast Surg 24:687-703, 1997.

Salasche SJ: Epidemiology of actinic keratoses and squamous cell carcinoma. J Am Acad Dermatol 42:4-7, 2000.

FOLLICULAR NEOPLASMS

TRICHOEPITHELIOMA

Clinical Features

- Trichoepithelioma can occur in either a solitary or multiple form
- Solitary lesions frequently affect adults and have a predilection for the face
- Multiple lesions often present during childhood, with a predilection for the upper trunk, neck, scalp, and face, especially the nasolabial folds and preauricular regions; transmitted as an autosomal dominant trait
- Solitary lesions appear as pale, small to medium (< 2 cm), skin-colored papules

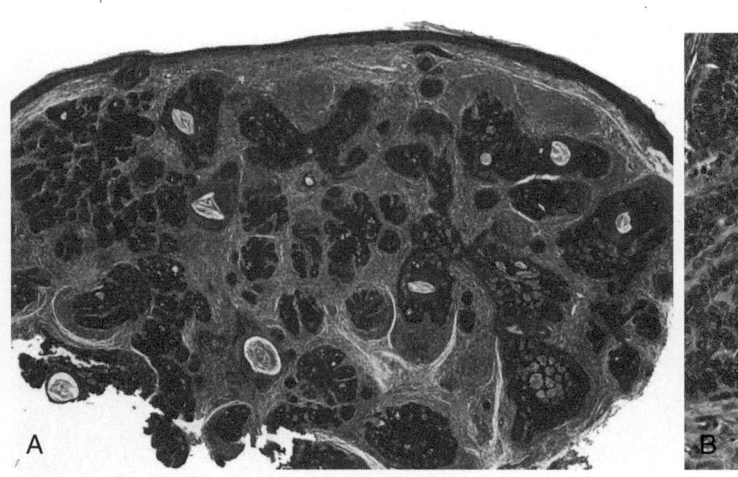
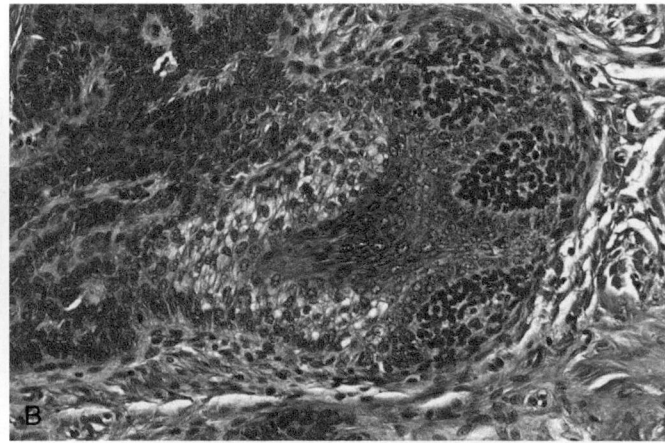

Figure 2-50. Trichoepithelioma. A, Low-power view shows a well-circumscribed dermal proliferation of basaloid cells embedded in a cellular stroma and containing keratinous cysts. **B,** High-power view shows follicular differentiation in the form of bulbs and papillae.

- Multiple lesions appear as small (< 1 cm), flesh-colored papules

Histopathology
- Well-circumscribed, symmetrical lesion composed of basaloid and eosinophilic cells in small or large nodules within a variably cellular stroma; they may also show retiform or cribriform patterns (Figure 2-50A)
- Basaloid cells are encircled by fibroblasts resembling follicular germs and bulbs with associated papillae (signs of follicular differentiation) (Figure 2-50B)
- Retraction artifacts, if present, are within the fibrotic stroma rather than around the basaloid cells
- Multiple infundibulocystic structures filled with keratin are present within the epithelial islands

Special Stains and Immunohistochemistry
- Noncontributory

Other Techniques for Diagnosis
- Noncontributory

Differential Diagnosis
- Basal Cell Carcinoma (BCC)
  - Multiple nests of basaloid cells that emanate from the undersurface of the epidermis
  - Nests show peripheral palisading and presence of a mucinous stroma with retraction artifacts
  - Immunohistochemistry: CD10 is positive in the stromal cells but not the epithelial cells in trichoepithelioma and is positive in the epithelial cells of BCC
- Syringoma
  - Contains ductal structures filled with proteinaceous material
- Microcystic Adnexal Carcinoma (Sclerosing Sweat Duct Carcinoma)
  - Extends deep into the dermis with neoplastic nests getting smaller toward the base
  - Keratin-filled cysts and ductal structures are present
  - Infiltrative borders and perineural invasion may be present
- Trichoadenoma
  - Characterized by numerous infundibulocystic structures surrounded by eosinophilic cells resembling those of follicular infundibulum; germinative cells are sparse

PEARLS

- *Desmoplastic trichoepithelioma is a distinct variant of trichoepithelioma that is characterized by narrow strands and columns of germinative epithelial cells, infundibulocystic structures filled with keratin, and a fibrotic stroma*
- *Giant solitary trichoepithelioma is a variant of trichoepithelioma that measures several centimeters in size and is typically located in the deep dermis and subcutaneous tissue*
- *Trichoblastoma and trichoepithelioma constitute different morphologic patterns of a benign neoplasm composed of follicular germinative cells*

SELECTED REFERENCES

Ackerman AB, Reddy VB, Soyer HP: Neoplasms with Follicular Differentiation. New York, Ardor Scribendi, 2001.
Brownstein MH, Shapiro L: Desmoplastic trichoepithelioma. Cancer 40:2979-2986, 1977.
Centurion SA, Schwartz RA, Lambert WC: Trichoepithelioma papulosum multiplex. J Dermatol 27:137-143, 2000.
Matt D, Xin H, Vortmeyer AO, et al: Sporadic trichoepithelioma demonstrates deletions at 9q22.3. Arch Dermatol 136:657-660, 2000.
Pham TT, Selim MA, Burchette JL Jr, et al: CD10 expression in trichoepithelioma and basal cell carcinoma. J Cutan Pathol 33:123-128, 2006.

PILOMATRICOMA (PILOMATRIXOMA, CALCIFYING EPITHELIOMA OF MALHERBE)

Clinical Features
- Most common in children and adolescents
- Sites of predilection include the face, neck, and upper extremities
- Firm, solitary, deep-seated nodules between 0.5 and 3 cm in diameter

Histopathology
- Sharply demarcated, well-circumscribed proliferation of dark-staining aggregates of matrical and supramatrical cells (Figure 2-51A)
- Pale-staining cells that exhibit a ghost of nucleus ("ghost" or "shadow" cells) (Figure 2-51B)
- Granulomatous inflammation with foreign-body giant cells adjacent to shadow cells

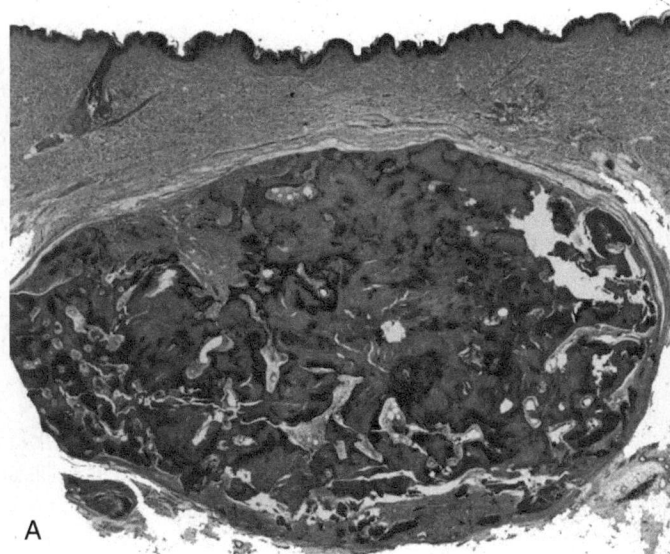

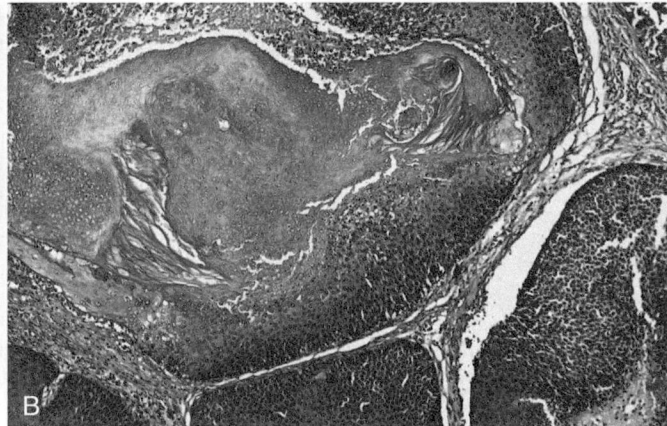

Figure 2-51. Pilomatricoma. A, Low-power view shows a well-circumscribed dermal nodule composed of basaloid cells, shadow cells, and areas of calcifications. **B,** High-power view shows basaloid cells and shadow cells with distinct cell borders but only an outline of nucleus. Areas of granulomatous inflammation can be present.

- Mitotic figures may be present in the small basophilic cells, but nuclear atypia and infiltrative growth are uncommon
- Early lesions: cystic cavity surrounded by rows of matrical cells
- Older lesions: preponderance of ghost or shadow cells with dystrophic calcification, ossification, and granulomatous inflammation

Special Stains and Immunohistochemistry
- Noncontributory

Other Techniques for Diagnosis
- Noncontributory

Differential Diagnosis
- Calcified Trichilemmal Cyst
  - Absence of shadow or ghost cells
  - Cyst lined by epithelial cells with abundant eosinophilic cytoplasm
- Malignant Pilomatricoma (Matrical Carcinoma)
  - Rare entity
  - Infiltrative growth pattern
  - Striking nuclear atypia, frequent abnormal mitoses, and necrosis en masse

PEARLS

- *Multiple lesions and familial patterns linked to myotonic dystrophy*
- *Shadow cells represent faulty attempts of the matrical cells to form hair shafts*

Selected References

Ackerman AB, Reddy VB, Soyer HP: Neoplasms with Follicular Differentiation. New York, Ardor Scribendi, 2001.
Berberian BJ, Colonna TM, Battaglia M, Sulica VI: Multiple pilomatricomas in association with myotonic dystrophy and a family history of melanoma. J Am Acad Dermatol 37:268-269, 1997.
Hardisson D, Linares MD, Cuevas-Santos J, et al: Pilomatrix carcinoma: a clinicopathologic study of six cases and review of the literature. Am J Dermatopathol 23:394-401, 2001.
Julian CG, Bowers PW: A clinical review of 209 pilomatricomas. J Am Acad Dermatol 39:191-195, 1997.
Kaddu S, Soyer HP, Hodl S, Kerl H: Morphological stages of pilomatricoma. Am J Dermatopathol 18:333-338, 1996.
Sherrod QJ, Chiu MW, Gutierrez M. Multiple pilomatricomas: cutaneous marker for myotonic dystrophy. Dermatol Online J 14:22, 2008.

TRICHILEMMOMA
Clinical Features
- Predilection for the nose, cheek, and upper lip
- Lesions are usually solitary
- Presents as verrucous or smooth, small (< 1 cm), flesh-colored papule

Histopathology
- The lesion has the silhouette of a verruca
- Vertically oriented bulbous hyperplasia of infundibular epithelium that contains cells with clear or pale cytoplasm (Figure 2-52)

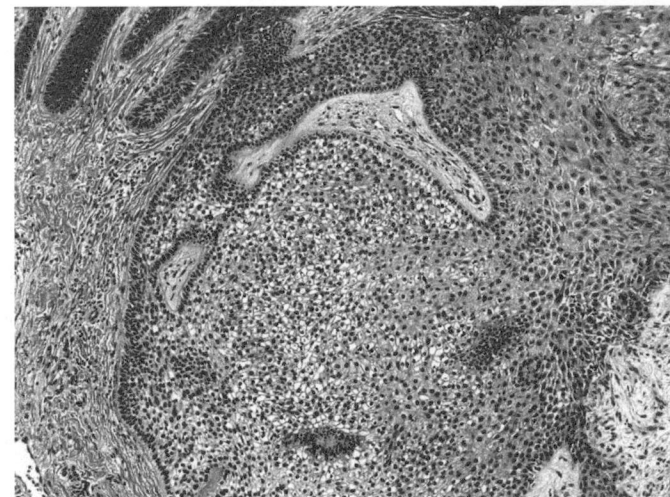

Figure 2-52. Trichilemmoma. Histologic section shows a sharply defined proliferation of cells with clear cytoplasm resembling the outer root sheath of a hair follicle.

- The columnar clear cells are arranged in a palisade at the periphery similar to those seen in the outer root sheath of a normal hair follicle
- The epithelial proliferation is surrounded by a thick hyalinized basement membrane
- Dilated tortuous blood vessels may be present in the papillary dermis
- Desmoplastic trichilemmoma: shows irregular extensions of clear cells into a sclerotic dermis simulating an invasive carcinoma; the upper part of the lesion shows typical features of trichilemmoma

Special Stains and Immunohistochemistry
- PAS stain demonstrates glycogen in the clear cells

Other Techniques for Diagnosis
- Noncontributory

Differential Diagnosis
- Verruca
  - Most trichilemmomas have architectural and cytologic features of verruca in the process of involution
  - Atypical verruca lacks the epithelial cells with clear cytoplasm (trichilemmal differentiation)
- Inverted Follicular Keratosis
  - Similar silhouette of verruca and trichilemmoma
  - Additionally, there are squamous eddies within the hyperplastic infundibular epithelium

PEARLS

- *Cowden disease: autosomal dominant disorder presenting with multiple trichilemmomas associated with a variety of malignancies (breast, gastrointestinal, thyroid, and reproductive organs)*

SELECTED REFERENCES

Brownstein MH, Shapiro L: Trichilemmoma: analysis of 40 new cases. Arch Dermatol 107:866-869, 1973.
Kanitakis J: Adnexal tumours of the skin as markers of cancer-prone syndromes. J Eur Acad Dermatol Venereol 24:379-87, 2010.
Lloyd KM, Denis M: Cowden's disease: a possible new symptom complex with multiple system involvement. Ann Intern Med 58:136-142, 1963.

BASAL CELL CARCINOMA
Clinical Features
- Typically affects older individuals
- Predilection for sun-exposed skin (face, hands)
- Small, well-circumscribed, pearly tan-gray papule devoid of scale
- Lesions enlarge with time and tend to ulcerate (rodent ulcers)

Histopathology
- Nests and islands of basaloid cells attached to the undersurface of epidermis and extending into the dermis (Figure 2-53A)
- Peripheral palisading of basaloid cells of the nests (Figure 2-53B)
- Basaloid cells are typically uniform with frequent mitotic activity and abundant apoptotic cells
- Characteristic retraction artifact between the palisading cells and the normal stroma
- Areas of squamous differentiation and perineural invasion are seen in aggressive (infiltrative) forms
- Variants of basal cell carcinoma: pigmented, morphealike or sclerosing, superficial, nodular, keratotic, adenoid, micronodular, and fibroepithelial types

Special Stains and Immunohistochemistry
- Noncontributory

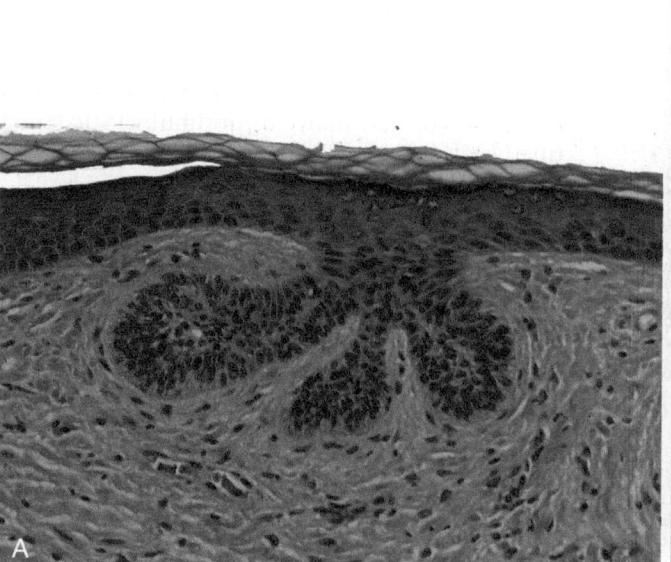
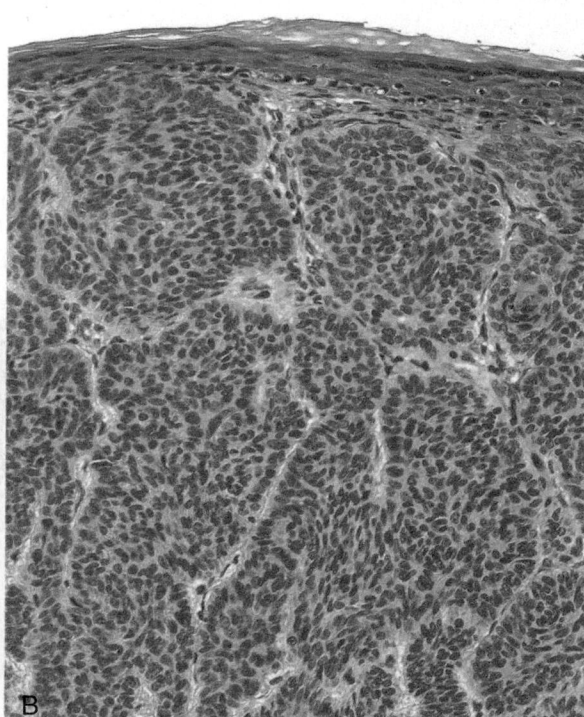

Figure 2-53. A, Basal cell carcinoma, superficial. Histologic section shows small nests of basaloid cells with peripheral palisading. **B,** Section shows a nodular proliferation of basaloid cells with peripheral palisading.

Other Techniques for Diagnosis
* Noncontributory

DIFFERENTIAL DIAGNOSIS
* Trichoepithelioma and Trichoblastoma
  * Nests of basaloid cells usually without mitotic activity, individual cell necrosis, or separation artifacts
  * Abundant fibrotic stroma
  * Retraction artifacts within a cellular stroma rather than around the epithelial nests
  * Evidence of follicular differentiation in the form of germs, bulbs, and papillae is more common
  * CD10-positive stroma

PEARLS

* *Basal cell nevus syndrome: multiple basaloid hamartomas on the cutaneous surface associated with palmar keratotic pits, jaw cysts, and basal cell carcinomas in non–sun-exposed locations*
* *BCCs rarely metastasize; when they do, the primary lesion is usually advanced*

SELECTED REFERENCES

Ackerman AB, Reddy VB, Soyer HP: Neoplasms with Follicular Differentiation. New York, Ardor Scribendi, 2001.

Goldberg LH: Basal cell carcinoma. Lancet 347:663-667, 1996.

Maloney ME: Histology of basal cell carcinoma. Clin Dermatol 13:545-549, 1995.

Mason JK, Helwig EB, Graham JH: Pathology of the nevoid basal cell carcinoma syndrome. Arch Pathol 79:401, 1965.

Mehregan AH: Aggressive basal cell epithelioma on sunlight-protected skin. Am J Dermatopathol 5:221, 1983.

Rippey JJ: Why classify basal cell carcinomas? Histopathology 32:393-398, 1998.

Strutton GM: Pathological variants of basal cell carcinoma. Aust J Dermatol 38(suppl 1):S31-S35, 1997.

ECCRINE AND APOCRINE NEOPLASMS

SYRINGOMA

Clinical Features
* Commonly affects females, usually at the onset of puberty
* Predilection for the face, eyelids, neck, and upper anterior chest but can occur at other sites including penis and vulva
* Multiple small (1 to 3 mm), yellowish, firm papules

Histopathology
* Symmetrical, well-circumscribed lesions with an eosinophilic fibrous stroma
* Confined to the upper half of the dermis
* Elongated aggregates of epithelial cells of varying shapes and tubules in a markedly fibrotic stroma
* Cords and nests of epithelial cells often continuous with tubules (likened to comma shapes or tadpoles) (Figure 2-54)
* Epithelial cells may have scant cytoplasm or abundant pale-staining cytoplasm
* Ductal lumina may contain eosinophilic PAS-positive material

CLEAR CELL SYRINGOMA
* Contains mostly nests of clear cells with occasional tubules

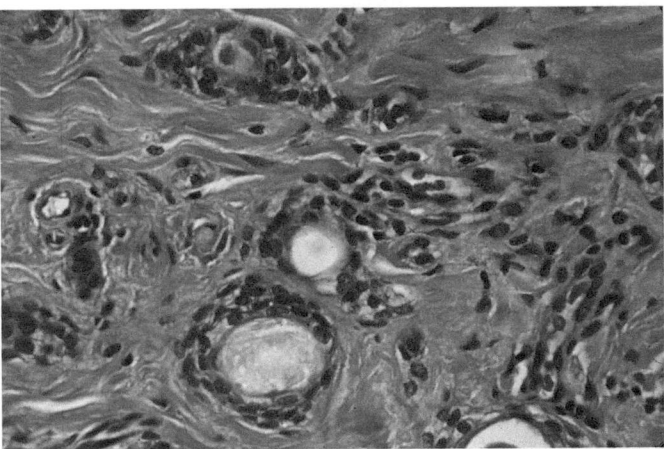

Figure 2-54. Syringoma. Histologic section shows nests, strands, and ducts composed of monomorphous epithelial cells. The ductal structures are lined two layers of cells, and some have elongated contours (tadpole-like).

CHONDROID SYRINGOMA (MIXED TUMOR)
* Composed of syringomatous ductal structures surrounded by a blue-gray mucinous stroma with occasional areas of cartilage formation, similar to a mixed tumor of the salivary gland

Special Stains and Immunohistochemistry
* PAS: ductal lumina may contain eosinophilic PAS-positive material
* Carcinoembryonic antigen (CEA) and epithelial membrane antigen (EMA) highlight the ductal lumina
* Clear cell syringoma: cytoplasmic glycogen highlighted with PAS

Other Techniques for Diagnosis
* Noncontributory

Differential Diagnosis
* BCC (Sclerosing and Keratotic)
  * Predilection for sun-exposed skin, typically face and hands
  * Multiple nests of basaloid cells with peripheral palisading infiltrating between a sclerotic stroma
* Trichoepithelioma
  * Nests of cells that typically do not show ductal lumina but contain many infundibulocystic structures filled with keratin
* Microcystic Adnexal Carcinoma (Sclerosing Sweat Duct Carcinoma)
  * Clinically presents as a solitary lesion that is typically larger (1 to 3 cm)
  * Deeply infiltrative histologic pattern
  * Perineural invasion

PEARLS

* *Syringoma is believed to show differentiation toward the intraepidermal portion of the eccrine sweat duct*

SELECTED REFERENCES

Feibelman CE, Maize JC: Clear-cell syringoma: a study by conventional and electron microscopy. Am J Dermatopathol 6:139-150, 1984.

Goyal S, Martins CR: Multiple syringomas on the abdomen, thighs, and groin. Cutis 66:259-262, 2000.

Karam P, Benedetto AV: Syringomas: new approach to an old technique. Int J Dermatol 35:219-220, 1996.

POROMA

Clinical Features

- Benign adnexal tumor related to the eccrine sweat duct
- Predilection for the palms and soles (60%), trunk, head, and neck
- Lesions have a tendency to crust and ulcerate
- Present as small (2 to 3 cm), firm to rubbery, painless nodules

Histopathology

- Sheetlike down-growth of monomorphous dark (poroid) cells and tubules lined by pale (cuticular) cells (Figure 2-55)
- Intracytoplasmic vacuolization and necrosis en masse may be present
- Cystic spaces and foci of keratinization may be present
- Early erosion and ulceration of the superficial epidermis
- Richly vascular stroma with dilated, tortuous vessels
- Variants: intraepidermal poroma (hidroacanthoma simplex), dermal duct tumor, and poroid hidradenoma

Special Stains and Immunohistochemistry

- Noncontributory

Other Techniques for Diagnosis

- Noncontributory

Differential Diagnosis

- Clear Cell Acanthoma
  - Overlying parakeratotic cornified layer often containing neutrophils
  - Abrupt acanthotic proliferation of pale squamoid cells
  - Elongated rete ridges with well-vascularized dermal papillae
  - Presence of neutrophils within intercellular spaces of the involved epidermis
- Seborrheic Keratosis
  - Characteristic horn and pseudohorn cysts
  - Stroma is not vascular
- Porocarcinoma

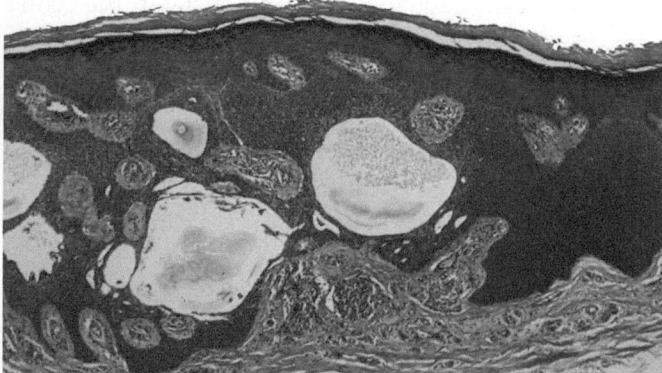

Figure 2-55. Poroma. Histologic section shows a sharply demarcated intraepidermal proliferation of monomorphous cuboidal cells with scattered ductal lumina. The stroma is vascular.

- Asymmetrical, poorly circumscribed proliferation of cords and lobules of polygonal cells with marked nuclear atypia, frequent mitosis, and necrosis

PEARLS

- *Poromas display differentiation toward eccrine ducts*
- *Eccrine poromatosis: multiple lesions affecting the palms and soles*

SELECTED REFERENCES

Hamanaka S, Otsuka F: Multiple malignant eccrine poroma and a linear epidermal nevus. J Dermatol 23:469-471, 1996.

Lee NH, Lee SH, Ahn SK: Apocrine poroma with sebaceous differentiation. Am J Dermatopathol 22:261-263, 2000.

Mousawi A, Kibbi AG: Pigmented eccrine poroma: a simulant of nodular melanoma. Int J Dermatol 34:857-858, 1995.

Pena J, Suster S: Squamous differentiation in malignant eccrine poroma. Am J Dermatopathol 15:492-496, 1993.

Robson A, Greene J, Ansari N, et al: Eccrine porocarcinoma (malignant eccrine poroma): a clinicopathologic study of 69 cases. Am J Surg Pathol 25:710-720, 2001.

SPIRADENOMA

Clinical Features

- Benign proliferation of eccrine ductal and secretory structures
- Lesions typically occur in children and young to middle-aged adults
- Predilection for the trunk and extremities
- Lesions are typically solitary and painful but can occur as multiple lesions infrequently
- Small (1 to 2 cm), dome-shaped, skin-colored nodules

Histopathology

- Relatively well circumscribed neoplasm with solid and tubular components (Figure 2-56A)
- Solid component has up to three types of cells
  - Large cells with ovoid nuclei and pale cytoplasm, located within the centers of the nodules of neoplastic cells (Figure 2-56B)
  - Small dark cells with hyperchromatic nuclei and scant cytoplasm, located at the periphery of the aggregations
  - Mature lymphocytes scattered among the small and large neoplastic epithelial cells
- Tubules resembling dilated ducts and lined by large, pale epithelial cells
- Richly vascular stroma
- Evenly distributed globules of eosinophilic basement membrane material within the epithelial aggregates

Special Stains and Immunohistochemistry

- Noncontributory

Other Techniques for Diagnosis

- Noncontributory

Differential Diagnosis

- Cylindroma
  - Low-power view reveals multiple nests of basaloid cells that appear to fit together like pieces of a jigsaw puzzle
- Benign Vascular Tumors
  - Lack nodular aggregates of epithelial cells

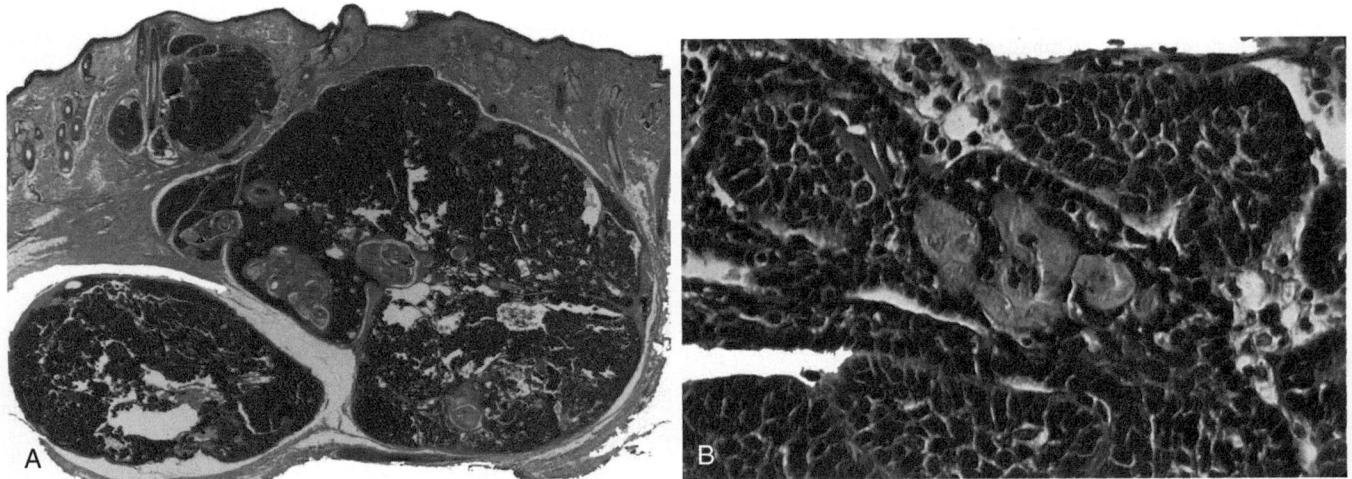

Figure 2-56. Spiradenoma. A, Low-power view shows a well-circumscribed dermal nodule with occasional ductal lumina. **B,** High-power view shows sheets of larger cells with pale cytoplasm and smaller cells with scant cytoplasm. Globules of hyaline basement membrane–like material are present within the aggregations.

PEARLS

- *Painful nature of spiradenoma is related to the numerous unmyelinated axons in the stroma*
- *Malignant transformation, although uncommon, has been reported*

SELECTED REFERENCES

Argenyi ZB, Nguyen AV, Balogh K, et al: Malignant eccrine spiradenoma: a clinicopathologic study. Am J Dermatopathol 14:381-390, 1992.

Bedlow AJ, Cook MG, Kurwa A: Extensive naevoid eccrine spiradenoma. Br J Dermatol 140:154-157, 1999.

Cooper PH, Frierson HF Jr, Morrison AG: Malignant transformation of eccrine spiradenoma. Arch Dermatol 121:1445-1448, 1985.

Mambo NC: Eccrine spiradenoma: clinical and pathologic study of 49 tumors. J Cutan Pathol 10:312-320, 1983.

Yoshida A, Takahashi K, Maeda F, Akasaka T: Multiple vascular eccrine spiradenomas: a case report and published work review of multiple eccrine spiradenomas. J Dermatol 37: 990-994, 2010.

CYLINDROMA

Clinical Features

- Benign adnexal neoplasm with apocrine differentiation
- May occur as a solitary lesion or multiple lesions
- Multiple form is inherited in a dominant pattern and presents in females at an earlier age as multiple dome-shaped nodules on the scalp; other sites of involvement include face and, rarely, trunk and extremities
- Nodules vary in size from a few millimeters to several centimeters
- Over time, the scalp nodules coalesce to larger nodules and may resemble a turban (hatlike growth)

Histopathology

- Well-circumscribed dermal nodules composed of islands of epithelial cells that fit together like pieces of jigsaw puzzle and are separated from each other only by thick hyaline sheaths (Figure 2-57)
- Two types of cells are present in the epithelial islands
  - Cells with small, dark-staining nuclei at the periphery of the islands

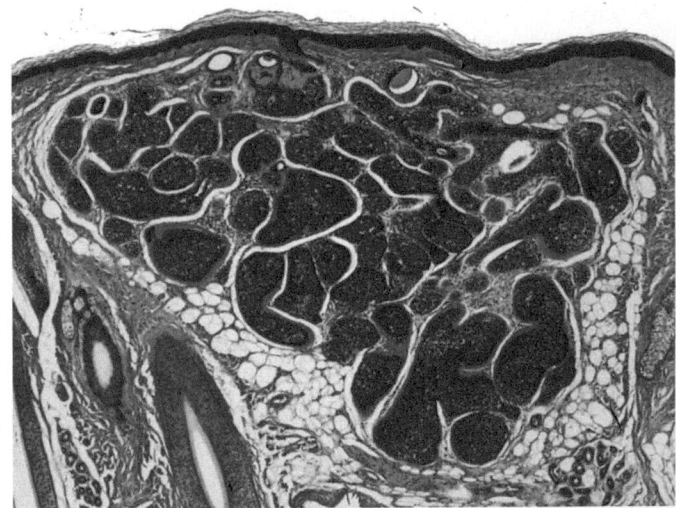

Figure 2-57. Cylindroma. Histologic section shows a well-circumscribed dermal nodule composed of epithelial islands that are separated by thick hyaline sheaths and fit together like pieces of a puzzle.

  - Cells with large light-staining nuclei in the center of the islands
- Tubular lumina lined by ductal cells and filled with amorphous material are often present
- Drops of eosinophilic hyaline material can be present within the epithelial islands

Special Stains and Immunohistochemistry

- Hyaline sheaths are PAS positive and diastase resistant
- Ductal structures can be highlighted with EMA, CEA, and PAS

Other Techniques for Diagnosis

- Familial cylindromatosis (turban tumor syndrome) is associated with mutations in the *CYLD* gene on chromosome 16q12.1

Differential Diagnosis

- Malignant Cylindroma

- In rare instances, malignant change characterized by cytologic and nuclear pleomorphism, atypical mitotic figures, loss of hyaline sheaths, and infiltrating pattern can be seen
- Areas of spiradenoma can coexist within cylindromas

PEARLS

- *Multiple cylindromas may be associated with multiple trichoepitheliomas and perhaps represent different expressions of the same genetic disorder*
- *Hyaline sheaths are synthesized by the neoplastic cells and are believed to represent basement membrane–like material*

SELECTED REFERENCES

Blake, PW, Toro, JR: Update of cylindromatosis gene (CYLD) mutations in Brooke-Spiegler syndrome: novel insights into the role of deubiquitination in cell signaling. Hum Mutat 30:1025-1036, 2009.

Lee MW, Kelly JW: Dermal cylindroma and eccrine spiradenoma. Aust J Dermatol 37:48-49, 1996.

Meybehm M, Fischer HP: Spiradenoma and dermal cylindroma: comparative immunohistochemical analysis and histogenetic considerations. Am J Dermatopathol 19:154-161, 1997.

Van der Putte SC: The pathogenesis of familial multiple cylindromas, trichoepitheliomas, milia, and spiradenomas. Am J Dermatopathol 17:271-280, 1995.

Young AL, Kellermayer R, Szigeti R, et al: CYLD mutations underlie Brooke-Spiegler, familial cylindromatosis, and multiple familial trichoepithelioma syndromes. Clin Genet 70:246-249. 2006.

CLEAR CELL HIDRADENOMA (NODULAR HIDRADENOMA)

Clinical Features

- Generally presents as solitary dermal nodule 0.5 to 2 cm in diameter
- May have a cystic component
- Synonyms include *nodular hidradenoma, solid-cystic hidradenoma,* and *eccrine acrospiroma*

Histopathology

- Well-circumscribed, lobulated dermal nodule that may extend into the subcutaneous fat (Figure 2-58A)
- Lobules contain masses of cells with clear cytoplasm; some cells are polyhedral, and others are fusiform with elongated nuclei (Figure 2-58B)

- Occasional lumina lined by cuboidal cells or columnar cells with decapitation secretions
- Cystic spaces filled with eosinophilic homogeneous material, which most likely results from degeneration of neoplastic cells
- Stroma between the nodules is characteristically eosinophilic and hyalinized

Special Stains and Immunohistochemistry

- PAS stain demonstrates glycogen in the clear cells
- Immunohistochemical studies show positivity for cytokeratin; EMA, CEA highlight the ducts

Other Techniques for Diagnosis

- Noncontributory

Differential Diagnosis

- Trichilemmoma
  - Also contains clear cells; however, cystic spaces and tubular lumina characteristic of clear cell hidradenoma are not present
- Malignant Nodular Hidradenoma
  - Cytologic pleomorphism and high mitotic rate suggest aggressive behavior
  - Zonal or diffuse necrosis in addition to infiltrative, poorly circumscribed borders in an asymmetrical nodular neoplasm should suggest a diagnosis of malignant nodular hidradenoma
  - Typically arise de novo rather than in association with preexisting benign lesions

PEARLS

- *Nodular hidradenomas may occasionally recur; recurrent tumors show frequent mitoses or nuclear pleomorphism and should be completely excised*

SELECTED REFERENCES

Hashimoto K, DiBella RJ, Lever WF: Clear cell hidradenoma: histological, histochemical, and electron microscopic studies. Arch Dermatol 96:18-38, 1967.

Nandeesh BN, Rajalakshmi T: A study of histopathologic spectrum of nodular hidradenoma. Am J Dermatopathol 34:461-470, 2012.

Waxtein L, Vega E, Cortes R, et al: Malignant nodular hidradenoma. Int J Dermatol 37:225-228, 1998.

Winkelmann RK, Wolff K: Solid-cystic hidradenoma of the skin: clinical and histopathologic study. Arch Dermatol 97:651-661, 1968.

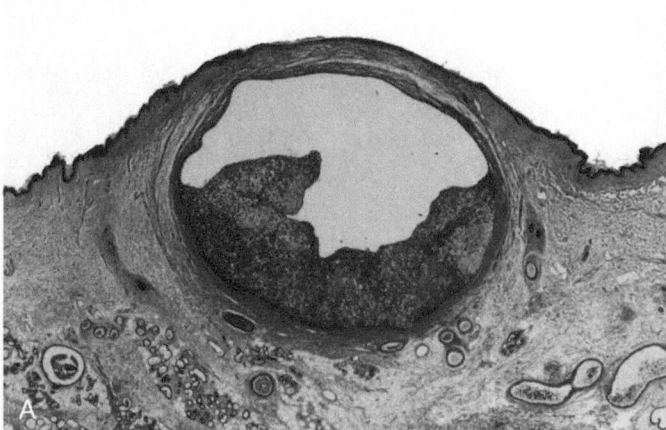
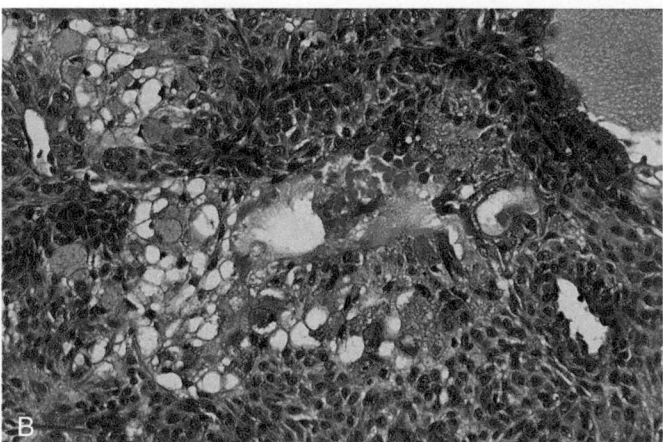

Figure 2-58. Clear cell (nodular) hidradenoma. **A,** Low-power view shows a well-circumscribed, lobulated, and partly cystic dermal nodule. **B,** High-power view shows lobules of cells with clear cytoplasm and ductal lumens lined by cells with decapitation secretions and cystic spaces filled with eosinophilic material.

SYRINGOCYSTADENOMA PAPILLIFERUM

Clinical Features

- Occurs most often on scalp or face, presenting at birth or in early childhood as a single papule or multiple papules or as a solitary plaque
- Occurs near puberty in a preexisting nevus sebaceus on the scalp in one third of the cases

Histopathology

- Epidermis shows papillomatous hyperplasia
- One or multiple invaginations extend down from the epidermis
- Upper part of the invaginations is lined by epidermis, whereas the lower part is lined by papillary projections extending into the luminal aspect (Figure 2-59A)
- Papillary projections are lined by two rows of epithelial cells; the luminal row consists of columnar cells with oval nuclei and occasionally with decapitation secretions; the outer row consists of small cuboidal cells with scant cytoplasm and small, round nuclei (Figure 2-59B)
- Within the stroma, a dense plasma cell infiltrate is present
- Apocrine sweat glands are often noted at the base of the lesion

Special Stains and Immunohistochemistry

- Apocrine differentiation is supported by the demonstration of gross cystic disease fluid protein (GCDFP) in some cases

Other Techniques for Diagnosis

- Noncontributory

Differential Diagnosis

- Hidradenoma Papilliferum
  - Occurs on labia majora, perineum, and perianal regions of women
  - Presents as a dermal nodule measuring a few millimeters to 2 cm

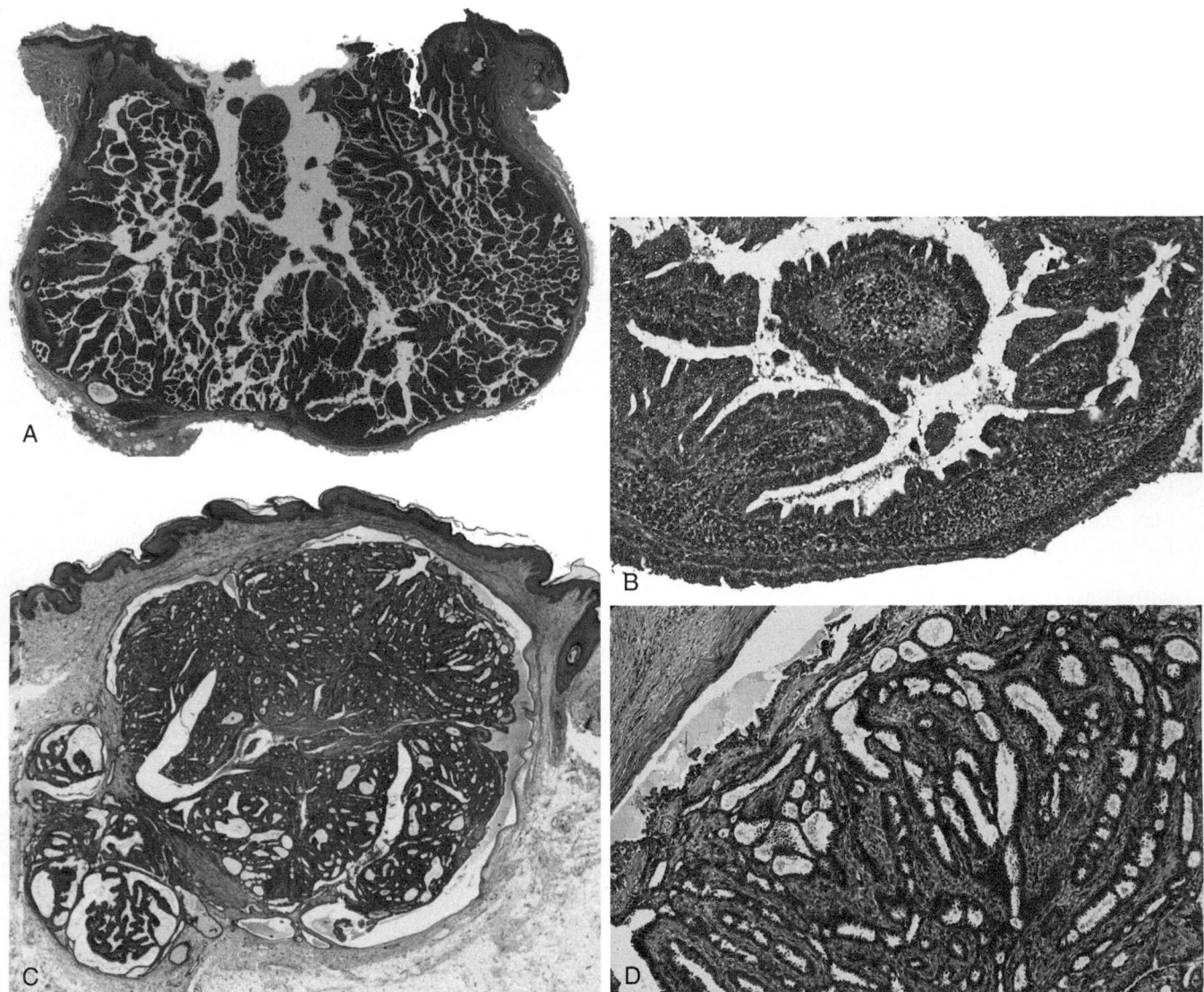

Figure 2-59. A, Syringocystadenoma papilliferum. Histologic section shows cystic epidermal invagination into which papillary structures project. **B,** Syringocystadenoma papilliferum. High-power view shows that the papillae are lined by two rows of cells: the luminal row is composed of columnar cells with decapitation secretions. Plasma cells are present within the stroma. **C,** Hidradenoma papilliferum. In contrast to syringocystadenoma, this is a predominantly dermal nodule with a cystic appearance. **D,** Hidradenoma papilliferum. High-power view shows complex papillary fronds lined by columnar cells with decapitation secretions.

- Histologically, it is a well-circumscribed nodule that is cystic with no connection to the surface (Figure 2-59C)
- Papillary fronds lined by a single row of columnar cells showing decapitation secretions project into the cystic space (Figure 2-59D)
- Tubular lumina lined by secretory cells surrounded by myoepithelial cells are also present
- Tubular apocrine adenoma
  - Generally contains numerous, irregularly shaped tubular structures lined by two rows of cells
  - Some may contain papillary projections and resemble syringocystadenoma papilliferum; however, the lesion does not connect to the overlying epidermis

PEARLS

- *Features of both eccrine and apocrine differentiation can be seen in some examples of syringocystadenoma papilliferum*

SELECTED REFERENCES

Kazakov DV, Requena L, Kutzner H, et al: Morphologic diversity of syringocystadenocarcinoma papilliferum based on a clinico-pathologic study of 6 cases and review of the literature. Am J Dermatopathol 32:340-347, 2010.

Mazoujian G, Margolis R: Immunohistochemistry of gross cystic disease fluid protein (GCDFP-15) in 65 benign sweat gland tumors of the skin. Am J Dermatopathol 10:28-35, 1988.

Numata M, Hosoe S, Itoh N, et al: Syringadenocarcinoma papilliferum. J Cutan Pathol 12:3-7, 1985.

Toribio J, Zulaica A, Peteiro C: Tubular apocrine adenoma. J Cutan Pathol 14:114-117, 1987.

MICROCYSTIC ADNEXAL CARCINOMA (SCLEROSING SWEAT DUCT CARCINOMA)

Clinical Features

- Locally aggressive neoplasm that invades deeply but generally does not metastasize
- Characteristic site of involvement is the upper lip; other sites include chin, nasolabial fold, and cheek

Histopathology

- Poorly circumscribed infiltrating dermal lesion that extends deep into the subcutaneous tissue and skeletal muscle (Figures 2-60A and B)
- Continuity with the epidermis is generally not seen

- Islands of epithelial cells with formation of keratin-filled cysts in a desmoplastic stroma are characteristic; in other areas, ductal structures lined by two cell layers are seen
- Cysts are not detected in all tumors; may be composed entirely of ductlike structures
- Ducts typically become smaller as they infiltrate into deeper tissue
- May have only minimal cytologic atypia, and mitotic figures are often difficult to find
- Perineural invasion is often seen

Special Stains and Immunohistochemistry
- Noncontributory

Other Techniques for Diagnosis
- Noncontributory

Differential Diagnosis
- Syringoma
  - May be indistinguishable, especially if the deeply infiltrative nature of microcystic adnexal carcinoma cannot be appreciated owing to the superficial nature of the biopsy
  - Lacks infiltrative pattern and perineural invasion
- Desmoplastic Trichoepithelioma
  - Generally confined to the upper half of the dermis
  - May contain cysts but lacks ductal structures
- Sclerosing Basal Cell Carcinoma
  - Infiltrative pattern of strands and nests of basaloid cells associated with stromal sclerosis
  - No cysts or ductlike structures present

PEARLS

- *The possibility of microcystic adnexal carcinoma should always be considered in assessment of trichoepitheliomatous and syringomatous neoplasms extending to the base of the specimen*

SELECTED REFERENCES

Cook TF, Fosko SW: Unusual cutaneous malignancies. Semin Cutan Med Surg 17:114-132, 1998.

Friedman PM, Friedman RH, Jiang SB, et al: Microcystic adnexal carcinoma: collaborative series review and update. J Am Acad Dermatol 41:225-231, 1999.

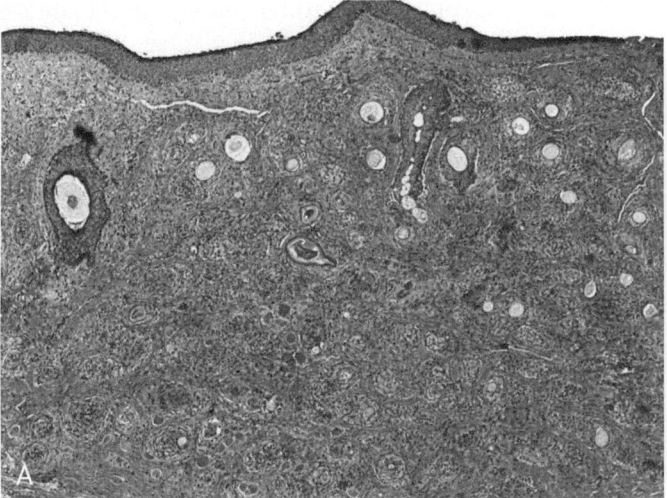
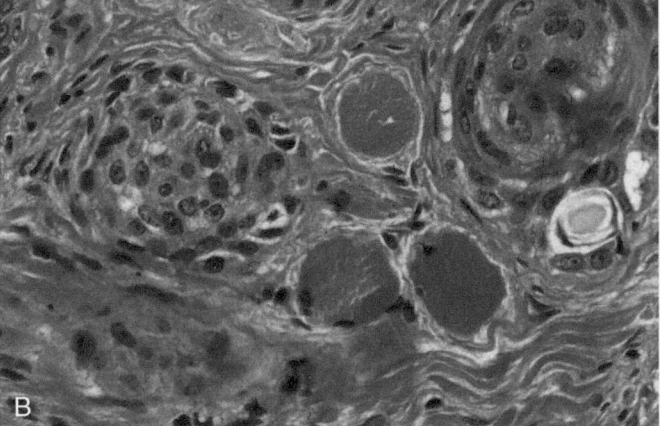

Figure 2-60. Microcystic adnexal carcinoma. A, Low-power view shows a deeply infiltrative neoplasm composed of ductal structures and keratin-filled cysts. **B,** High-power view shows rather monomorphous epithelial islands infiltrating between the skeletal muscle fibers.

Goldstein DJ, Barr RJ, Santa Cruz DJ: Microcystic adnexal carcinoma: a distinct clinicopathologic entity. Cancer 50:566-572, 1982.

Nelson BR, Lowe L, Baker S, et al: Microcystic adnexal carcinoma of the skin: a reappraisal of the differentiation and differential diagnosis of an underrecognized neoplasm. J Am Acad Dermatol 29:840-845, 1993.

Wetter R, Goldstein GD: Microcystic adnexal carcinoma: a diagnostic and therapeutic challenge. Dermatol Ther 21:452-458, 2008.

SEBACEOUS PROLIFERATIONS AND NEOPLASMS

NEVUS SEBACEUS

Clinical Features

- Presents at birth on the scalp or face as a single, yellowish, slightly raised, hairless plaque
- In childhood, it may have a linear configuration; at puberty, the lesions appear verrucous and nodular
- Some patients may present with extensive nevus sebaceus as part of neurocutaneous syndrome

Histopathology

- Sebaceous glands in nevus sebaceus show the same developmental pattern as normal sebaceous glands
  - At birth, ebaceous lobules are prominent (a result of the effect of maternal hormones)
  - After infancy, ebaceous lobules are small and decreased in number
- At puberty
  - Large numbers of mature sebaceous glands are seen
  - Associated epidermal changes include papillomatous hyperplasia (Figure 2-61)
  - Malformed follicular germs resembling basal cell carcinoma can be present
  - Apocrine glands located deep in the dermis are present in most cases
  - In adulthood, various adnexal neoplasms, the most common being trichoblastoma and syringocystadenoma papilliferum, can develop in nevus sebaceus

Special Stains and Immunohistochemistry

- Noncontributory

Other Techniques for Diagnosis

- Noncontributory

Differential Diagnosis

- Diagnosis of nevus sebaceus can be missed if the biopsy specimen is taken at a stage at which sebaceous lobules are small and few

- Epidermal Nevus
  - Lacks sebaceous lobules
- Sebaceous Gland Hyperplasia
  - Single enlarged sebaceous gland that opens into a dilated duct

PEARLS

- *BCC and rarely SCC and adnexal carcinomas can develop in nevus sebaceus*
- *Trichoblastoma is the most common adnexal neoplasm developing in nevus sebaceus*
- *Small biopsy of nevus sebaceus may show only prominent sebaceous lobules and can be misinterpreted as sebaceous gland hyperplasia*

SELECTED REFERENCES

Cribier B, Scrivener Y, Grosshans E: Tumors arising in nevus sebaceus: a study of 596 cases. J Am Acad Dermatol 42:263-268, 2000.

Jaqueti G, Requena L, Sanchez Yus E: Trichoblastoma is the most common neoplasm developed in nevus sebaceus of Jadassohn: a clinicopathologic study of a series of 155 cases. Am J Dermatopathol 22:108-118, 2000.

Miller CJ, Ioffreda MD, Billingsley EM: Sebaceous carcinoma, basal cell carcinoma, trichoadenoma, trichoblastoma, and syringocystadenoma papilliferum arising within a nevus sebaceus. Dermatol Surg 30:1546-1549, 2004.

Morioka S: The natural history of nevus sebaceus. J Cutan Pathol 12:200, 1985.

Steffen C, Ackerman AB (eds): Nevus sebaceus. In Steffen C, Ackerman AB (eds): Neoplasms with Sebaceous Differentiation. Philadelphia, Lea & Febiger, 1996, p 89.

SEBACEOMA (SEBACEOUS EPITHELIOMA)

Clinical Features

- Occurs more commonly in middle-aged and older individuals
- Predilection for the facial skin and scalp
- Occasionally bleeds or ulcerates
- Small (< 1 cm), solitary, tan-yellow circumscribed papule or ill-defined plaque

Histopathology

- Well-circumscribed lesion
- Admixture of lipidized and basaloid cells (Figure 2-62)

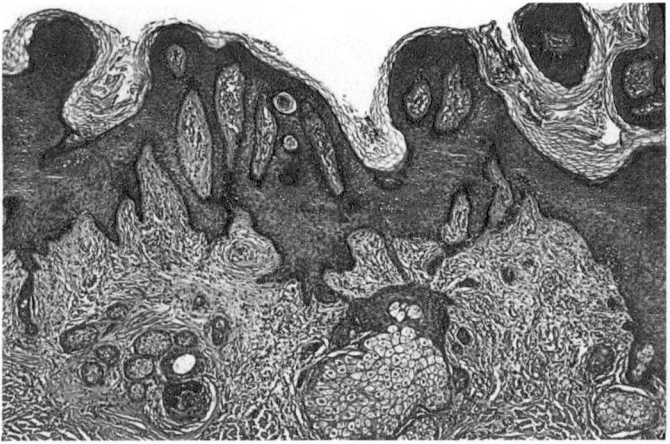

Figure 2-61. Nevus sebaceus. Histologic section shows papillomatous epidermal hyperplasia associated with prominent sebaceous lobules and poorly formed follicular units.

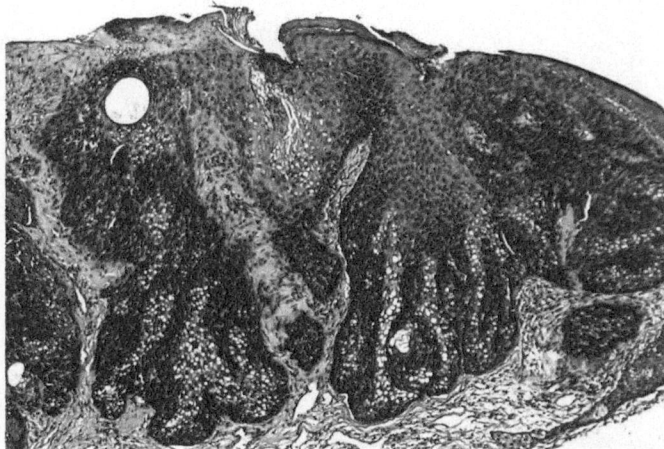

Figure 2-62. Sebaceoma (Sebaceous epithelioma). Well-circumscribed proliferation of an admixture of basaloid cells and cells with abundant vacuolated cytoplasm characteristic of sebaceous differentiation is seen.

- Basaloid cells tend to occur at the periphery of the lesion
- No nuclear atypia; however, mitotic figures may be present
- Rippled pattern sebaceoma: shows a unique arrangement of small, monomorphous, cigar-shaped basaloid cells in linear rows parallel to one another, resembling Verocay bodies; this arrangement of cells produces the rippled pattern; scattered cells and ducts with sebaceous differentiation are seen

Special Stains and Immunohistochemistry
- Oil red O (fresh tissue) highlights the lipid in the sebocytes
- Positive for EMA

Other Techniques for Diagnosis
- Noncontributory

Differential Diagnosis
- Sebaceous Hyperplasia
  - Single enlarged sebaceous gland
  - Lobules are composed of mostly mature sebaceous cells and open into a single dilated duct
- Sebaceous Adenoma
  - Sharply demarcated lobules composed of undifferentiated basaloid cells and mature sebaceous cells
  - Smaller and more superficial than sebaceoma
  - May represent the mature end of the spectrum of sebaceoma

PEARLS

- *Sebaceous neoplasms may be associated with Muir-Torre syndrome, a phenotypic subtype of Lynch syndrome that is associated with inherited defects in DNA mismatch repair genes and visceral malignancies*
- *Immunohistochemical stains for loss of mismatch repair proteins (MSH2/MLH1) should be considered in sebaceous neoplasms*

SELECTED REFERENCES

Dinneen AM, Mehregan DR: Sebaceous epithelioma: a review of twenty-one cases. J Am Acad Dermatol 34:47-50, 1996.

Kiyohara T, Kumakiri M, Kuwahara H, et al: Rippled-pattern sebaceoma: a report of a lesion on the back with a review of the literature. Am J Dermatopathol 28:446-448, 2006.

Lee BA, Yu L, Ma L, et al: Sebaceous neoplasms with mismatch repair protein expressions and the frequency of co-existing visceral tumors. J Am Acad Dermatol 67:1228-1234, 2012.

Misago N, Narisawa Y: Sebaceous neoplasms in Muir-Torre syndrome. Am J Dermatopathol 22:155-161, 2000.

Roberts ME, Riegert-Johnson DL, Thomas BC, et al: Screening for Muir-Torre syndrome using mismatch repair protein immunohistochemistry of sebaceous neoplasms. J Genet Couns 22:393-405, 2013.

Steffen C, Ackerman AB: Sebaceoma. In Steffen C, Ackerman AB (eds): Neoplasms with Sebaceous Differentiation. Philadelphia, Lea & Febiger, 1994, p 385.

SEBACEOUS CARCINOMA

Clinical Features
- Rare malignant sebaceous gland neoplasm
- Affects women more often than men
- Predilection for the eyelids in association with the meibomian gland and the gland of Zeis

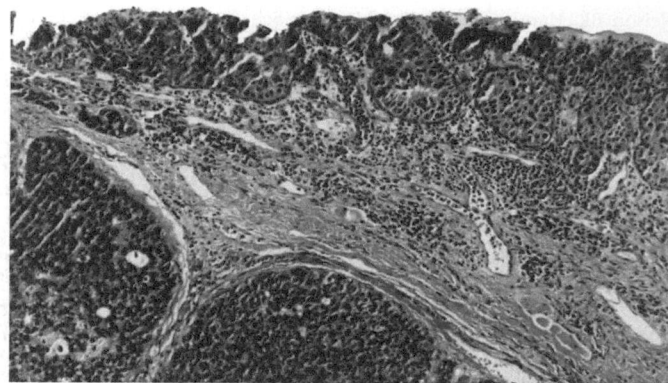

Figure 2-63. Sebaceous carcinoma. Histologic section shows irregular lobules of pleomorphic basaloid cells with scattered mature sebocytes. Pagetoid spread into the overlying epithelium; mitotic figures and individually necrotic cells are present.

- Related to irradiation and other neoplastic growths, including
  - BCC
  - SCC
  - Keratoacanthoma
  - Visceral carcinomas (Muir-Torre syndrome)
- Presents as asymptomatic, firm, ill-defined nodule, usually less than 1 cm in diameter; may be ulcerated

Histopathology
- Irregular lobules of varying sizes composed of many undifferentiated basaloid cells with some cells showing sebaceous differentiation, usually in the middle of the lobule (Figure 2-63)
- Some lobules may contain squamoid areas resembling SCC
- Sebaceous carcinoma of eyelid typically shows pagetoid spread to the overlying conjunctival epithelium or epidermis

Special Stains and Immunohistochemistry
- Positive for EMA, cytokeratins 7/8, androgen receptor and adipophilin

Other Techniques for Diagnosis
- Noncontributory

Differential Diagnosis
- Sebaceous Epithelioma (Sebaceoma)
  - Generally circumscribed and symmetrical
  - No necrosis or surface ulceration

PEARLS

- *Sebaceous carcinoma is an aggressive neoplasm with potential for metastasis and mortality; features associated with a poor prognosis include size greater than 1 cm, poor differentiation, multicentricity, extensive tissue infiltration, and lymphovascular invasion*
- *Sebaceous carcinomas occurring in Muir-Torre syndrome are much less likely to metastasize*

SELECTED REFERENCES

Ansai S, Takeichi H, Arase S, et al: Sebaceous carcinoma: an immunohistochemical reappraisal. Am J Dermatopathol 33:579-587, 2011.

Dasgupta T, Wilson LD, Yu JB: A retrospective review of 1349 cases of sebaceous carcinoma. Cancer 115:158-165, 2009.

Nelson BR, Hamlet KR, Gillard M, et al: Sebaceous carcinoma. J Am Acad Dermatol 33:1-15, 1995.

Rao NA, Hidayat AA, McLean IW, et al: Sebaceous carcinomas of the ocular adnexa: a clinicopathologic study of 104 cases, with five-year follow-up data. Hum Pathol 13:113-122, 1982.

Wick MR, Goellner JR, Wolfe JT 3rd, et al: Adnexal carcinomas of the skin. II. Extraocular sebaceous carcinomas. Cancer 56:1163-1172, 1985.

MELANOCYTIC PROLIFERATIONS AND NEOPLASMS

CONGENITAL MELANOCYTIC NEVUS

Clinical Features

- Presents at birth or shortly thereafter as variably sized pigmented lesion
- Size varies from 1.5 cm to more than 20 cm (giant congenital nevus)
- Bathing trunk–type congenital nevus is characterized by an uneven verrucous surface, variations of shades of brown and blue, and increased hair growth throughout the lesion
- Large congenital nevi show mild variation in color and epidermal hyperplasia
- Small congenital nevi are seen as solitary light-tan to brown, uniformly pigmented macules
- Congenital nevi change with age and develop darker areas, nodules, and coarse hair
- Giant congenital nevi of head and neck region may be associated with leptomeningeal melanocytosis and neurologic disorders

Histopathology

- Like acquired nevi, congenital nevi may be junctional, compound, or intradermal
- Broad lesions, characterized by nests of monomorphous melanocytes at the dermoepidermal junction and in the dermis (Figure 2-64)
- Dermal nests show marked adnexocentricity and angiocentricity, in addition to infiltrating between the collagen bundles
- Deep infiltration into the reticular dermis and extension along the septa of the subcutaneous fat are seen in giant congenital nevi

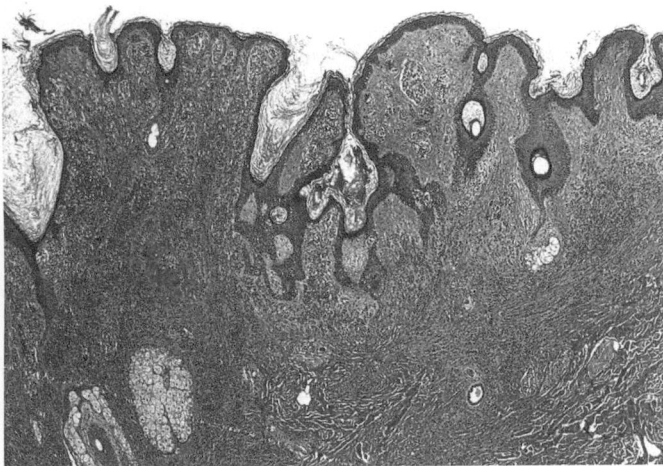

Figure 2-64. Congenital melanocytic nevus. Low-power view shows a broad proliferation of monomorphous melanocytes arranged as nests extending deep into the dermis, where they surround the adnexal structures.

- Cellular proliferative nodules with occasional mitotic figures may occur in the dermal component of some congenital nevi

Special Stains and Immunohistochemistry
- Noncontributory

Other Techniques for Diagnosis
- Noncontributory

Differential Diagnosis
- Diagnosis based on clinical and histopathologic findings is generally not problematic
- Small congenital nevi when taken by a shave biopsy may show features similar to Clark's dysplastic nevus

PEARLS

- *Giant congenital nevi when associated with leptomeningeal melanosis may be complicated by the development of malignant melanoma and other primitive malignancies such as rhabdomyosarcoma, with an estimated risk of 4% to 12%*
- *Risk for developing melanoma in giant congenital nevi is reported to be as high as 1000 times greater than in the normal population*

SELECTED REFERENCES

Marghoob AA, Schoenbach SP, Kopf AW, et al: Large congenital melanocytic nevi and the risk for the development of malignant melanoma: a prospective study. Arch Dermatol 132:170-175, 1996.

Mark GJ, Mihm MC Jr, Liteplo MG, et al: Congenital melanocytic nevi of the small and garment type: clinical, histologic, and ultrastructural studies. Hum Pathol 4: 395-418, 1973.

Phadke PA, Rakheja D, Le LP, et al: Proliferative nodules arising within congenital melanocytic nevi: a histologic, immunohistochemical, and molecular analyses of 43 cases. Am J Surg Pathol 35:656-669, 2011.

Swerdlow AJ, English JS, Qiao Z: The risk of melanoma in patients with congenital nevi: a cohort study. J Am Acad Dermatol 32:595-599, 1995.

Swerdlow AJ, Green A: Melanocytic naevi and melanoma: an epidemiological perspective. Br J Dermatol 117:137-146, 1987.

Vourc'h-Jourdain M, Martin L, Barbarot S, et al: Large congenital melanocytic nevi: therapeutic management and melanoma risk: a systematic review. J Am Acad Dermatol 68:493-8.e1-e14, 2013.

Walton RG, Jacobs AH, Cox AJ: Pigmented lesions in newborn infants. Br J Dermatol 95:389-396, 1976.

Yamazaki F, Osumi T, Kosaki K, et al: Large congenital melanocytic nevi with atypical teratoid/rhabdoid tumor. Pediatr Blood Cancer 60:1240-1241, 2013.

ACQUIRED MELANOCYTIC NEVI

Clinical Features

- Most acquired melanocytic nevi appear within the first two decades of life
- Nevi begin as small, tan-brown macules and progress to become papules
- Acquired melanocytic nevi are characterized by small size, uniform color, and well-defined borders

Histopathology

- Symmetrical, well-circumscribed proliferation of monomorphous melanocytes arranged as well-formed nests at the dermoepidermal junction or in the dermis (Figure 2-65A)
- Junctional nests are evenly distributed
- Nests of melanocytes in the dermis show maturation with progressive descent

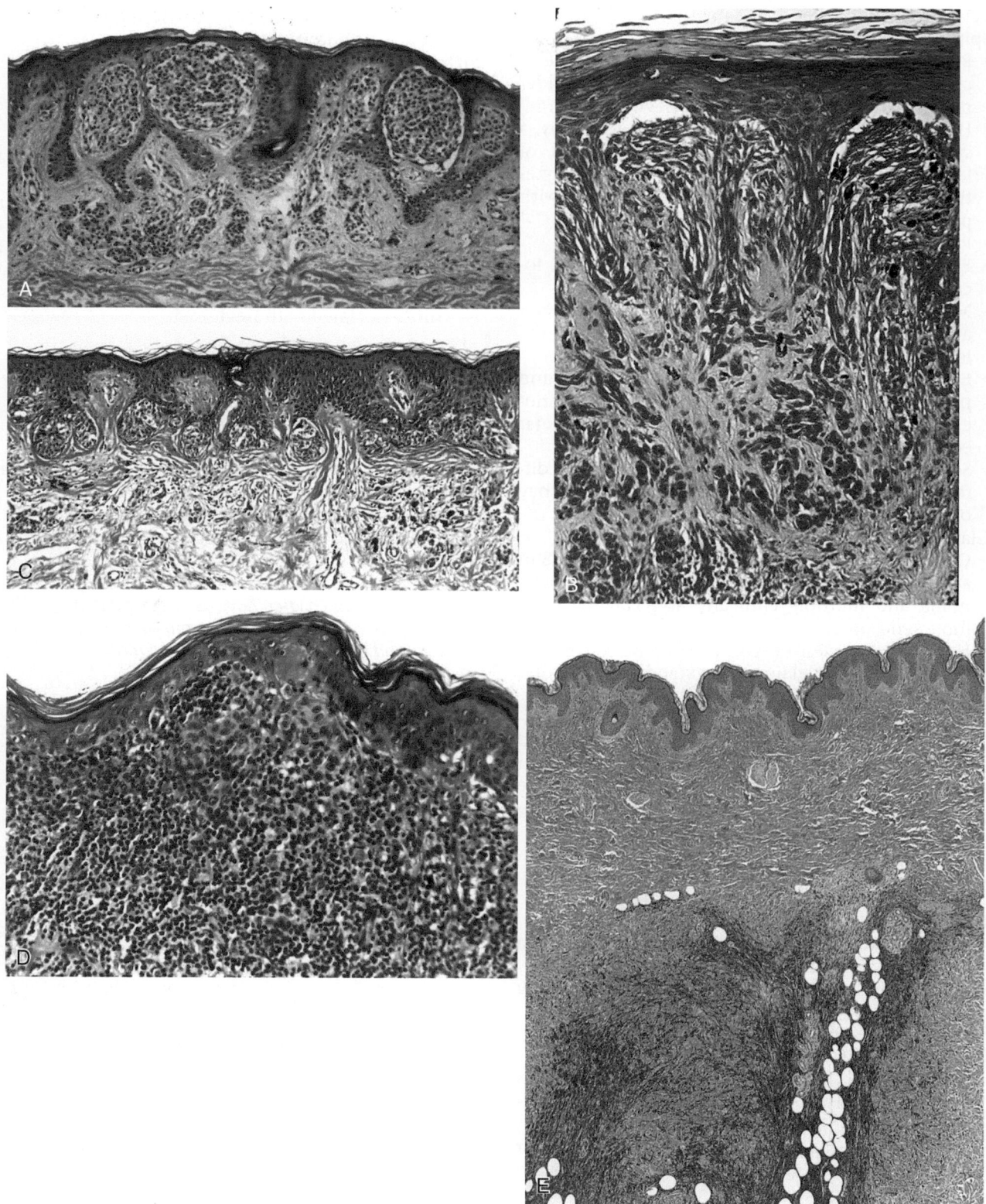

Figure 2-65. A, Acquired (compound) melanocytic nevus. Section shows nests of monomorphous melanocytes at the dermoepidermal junction and within the dermis, where they show maturation with progressive descent. **B,** Spitz nevus. Hyperkeratosis and parakeratosis, epidermal hyperplasia and a proliferation of spindle and epithelioid melanocytes are seen at the dermoepidermal junction and within the dermis. Clefts around the nests and eosinophilic globules are characteristic findings. **C,** Compound nevus, Clark's dysplastic type. Section shows junctional nests of melanocytes with bridging between the adjacent rete and associated concentric and lamellar fibroplasia. The melanocytes are slightly large and contain melanin-laden cytoplasm. The dermal nests are surrounded by inflammatory cell infiltrate and melanophages. **D,** Halo nevus. Section shows nests of melanocytes at the dermoepidermal junction and within the dermis, where they are surrounded by a dense infiltrate of lymphocytes. **E,** Blue nevus. Section shows a deep dermal proliferation of spindle-shaped melanocytes containing abundant melanin.

- Special variants of melanocytic nevi
  - Spitz nevus
    - Presents as solitary, small (< 1 cm), pink papule in children younger than 14 years; can occur in older patients and also as a congenital nevus
    - Histologically, Spitz nevi are characterized by a symmetrical, well-circumscribed proliferation of large spindle-shaped and epithelioid melanocytes that are uniform from side to side and mature with progressive descent (Figure 2-65B)
    - Pagetoid spread can be seen
    - Eosinophilic hyaline globules (Kamino bodies) located at the dermoepidermal junction
    - Mitotic figures may be present but usually are not atypical and are not present at the base of the lesion
    - Epidermal hyperplasia with hyperkeratosis and parakeratosis, patchy perivascular lymphohistiocytic inflammation, and papillary dermal vascular ectasia are features characteristic of Spitz nevi
    - Some examples of Spitz nevi may be difficult to differentiate from melanomas, especially when they occur in older patients
  - Clark dysplastic nevus
    - Originally described by Clark and others in 1978 in a subgroup of patients with family history of melanoma and multiple clinically atypical nevi (B-K mole syndrome)
    - Histologically, these nevi are broad, with the nests at the dermoepidermal junction extending far beyond the dermal component (shoulders) (Figure 2-65C)
    - Nests at the junction show bridging between adjacent rete and are surrounded by concentric and lamellar fibroplasia
    - Some of the melanocytes at the junction are large with enlarged nuclei and contain dusty melanin-laden cytoplasm; pagetoid spread is not present
    - Mild perivascular lymphocytic infiltrate and increased vascularity may be present in the papillary dermis
  - Halo nevus
    - Characterized clinically by the appearance of a zone of depigmentation surrounding a nevus
    - Most occur on the back of children and young adults
    - Complete regression can occur, leaving a depigmented macule
    - Histologically, halo nevus is a compound nevus with a dense lymphocytic inflammation that results in destruction of melanocytes (Figure 2-65D)
    - In the earlier stages, the melanocytes may appear large and atypical; later stages are characterized by complete disappearance of melanocytes
  - Blue nevus
    - Clinically presents as a blue-gray papule
    - Histologically, dendritic melanocytes with melanin pigment are present as nests and fascicles within the dermis (Figure 2-65E)
    - In cellular blue nevi, cellular islands of large oval melanocytes with pale cytoplasm extend deep in the dermis
    - Some blue nevi may be congenital

Special Stains and Immunohistochemistry
- Noncontributory

Other Techniques for Diagnosis
- Noncontributory

Differential Diagnosis
- Malignant Melanoma
  - Acquired melanocytic nevi should be differentiated from malignant melanoma
  - In general, the architectural and cytologic features of nevi are distinct from those of melanoma and include small size, symmetry, circumscription, and evenly spaced junctional nests
  - Maturation of dermal nests is a helpful histologic feature associated with nevi

PEARLS

- *Melanocytic nevi on scalp, periauricular area, acral skin, genitalia, breast, and periumbilical location ("nevi on special sites") may simulate malignant melanoma*
- *Recurrent melanocytic nevus has many histologic features similar to malignant melanoma*
- *Spitzoid melanomas are melanomas that simulate Spitz nevi and pose a challenge to accurate histopathologic diagnosis*
- *Spitzoid (childhood type) melanomas occurring in prepubescent children have architectural and cytopathologic features distinct from those that occur in adults and generally have a better prognosis*

SELECTED REFERENCES

Clark WH Jr, Reimer RR, Greene M, et al: Origin of familial malignant melanoma from heritable melanocytic lesions. Arch Dermatol 14:732, 1978.
Elder DE: Precursors to melanoma and their mimics: nevi of special sites. Mod Pathol 19(suppl 2):S4-S20, 2006.
Fabrizi G, Pagliarello C, Parente P, et al: Atypical nevi of the scalp in adolescents. J Cutan Pathol 34:365-369, 2007.
Mones JM, Ackerman AB: Melanomas in prepubescent children: review comprehensively, critique historically, criteria diagnostically, and course biologically. Am J Dermatopathol 25:223-238, 2003.
Mooi WJ, Krausz T: Spitz nevus versus spitzoid melanoma: diagnostic difficulties, conceptual controversies. Adv Anat Pathol 13:147-156, 2006.
Rapini RP: Spitz nevus or melanoma? Semin Cutan Med Surg 18:56-63, 1999.
Spitz S: Melanomas of childhood. Am J Pathol 24:591, 1948.
Xu X, Murphy G, Elenitsas R, Elder D: Benign pigmented lesions and malignant melanoma. In Elder DE, Elenitsas R, Johnson BL Jr, et al (eds): Lever's Histopathology of Skin, 10th ed. Philadelphia, Lippincott Williams & Wilkins, 2008, p 699.

MALIGNANT MELANOMA

Clinical Features
- Most melanomas arise de novo and present as asymmetrical, irregularly pigmented lesions with ill-defined borders
- Generally measure more than 4 mm in diameter
- Clinically, melanomas occurring on sun-damaged skin of the face and presenting as large, irregularly pigmented patches have been referred to as *lentigo maligna (melanoma)*
- Those occurring on acral skin are known as *acral lentiginous melanoma*
- *Superficial spreading melanoma* refers to the histologic pattern of a prominent pagetoid spread

- *Nodular melanoma* refers to a thick, more advanced melanoma
- Up to 20% of melanomas originate in association with nevi, which include congenital nevi and Clark dysplastic nevi

Histopathology
- Broad, poorly circumscribed, asymmetrical proliferation of large atypical melanocytes appearing as single cells and nests at the dermoepidermal junction (Figure 2-66A)
- Single melanocytes extend into the overlying epidermis in a pagetoid pattern (Figure 2-66B)
- Nests of melanocytes are not distributed evenly at the dermoepidermal junction
- Dermal nests, when present, do not show maturation with progressive descent (Figure 2-66C)
- Mitotic figures, including atypical ones and necrosis, may be present (Figure 2-66D)
- Clark levels
  - Level 1: melanoma in situ
  - Level 2: extension into papillary dermis
  - Level 3: neoplastic cells fill the papillary dermis and extend up to reticular dermis
  - Level 4: extension into reticular dermis
  - Level 5: extension into subcutaneous fat

Special Stains and Immunohistochemistry
- When a malignant neoplasm is poorly differentiated, melanocytic markers such as S-100 protein, Melan-A, and HMB-45 may be useful in confirming the diagnosis of melanoma

Other Techniques for Diagnosis
- Genes believed to be associated with melanoma in a background of multiple dysplastic nevi include the following (10% of cases):
  - *CMM1* gene on chromosome 1p36
  - Tumor suppressor gene *p16* (chromosome 9p)
  - Cyclin-dependent kinase gene (*CDK4*) located on chromosome 12q
- Comparative genomic hybridization and other molecular techniques are being developed to aid in differentiating nevi from melanoma
- Mutations in genes encoding proteins in the MAPK pathway such as BRAF, NRAS, and MEK (MAPK kinase p) are implicated in melanoma biology

Differential Diagnosis
- Malignant melanoma can be differentiated from non-melanocytic neoplasms such as Paget disease and pagetoid Bowen disease by immunohistochemical methods
- Differentiation from melanocytic nevi is best achieved using histologic criteria based on architectural and

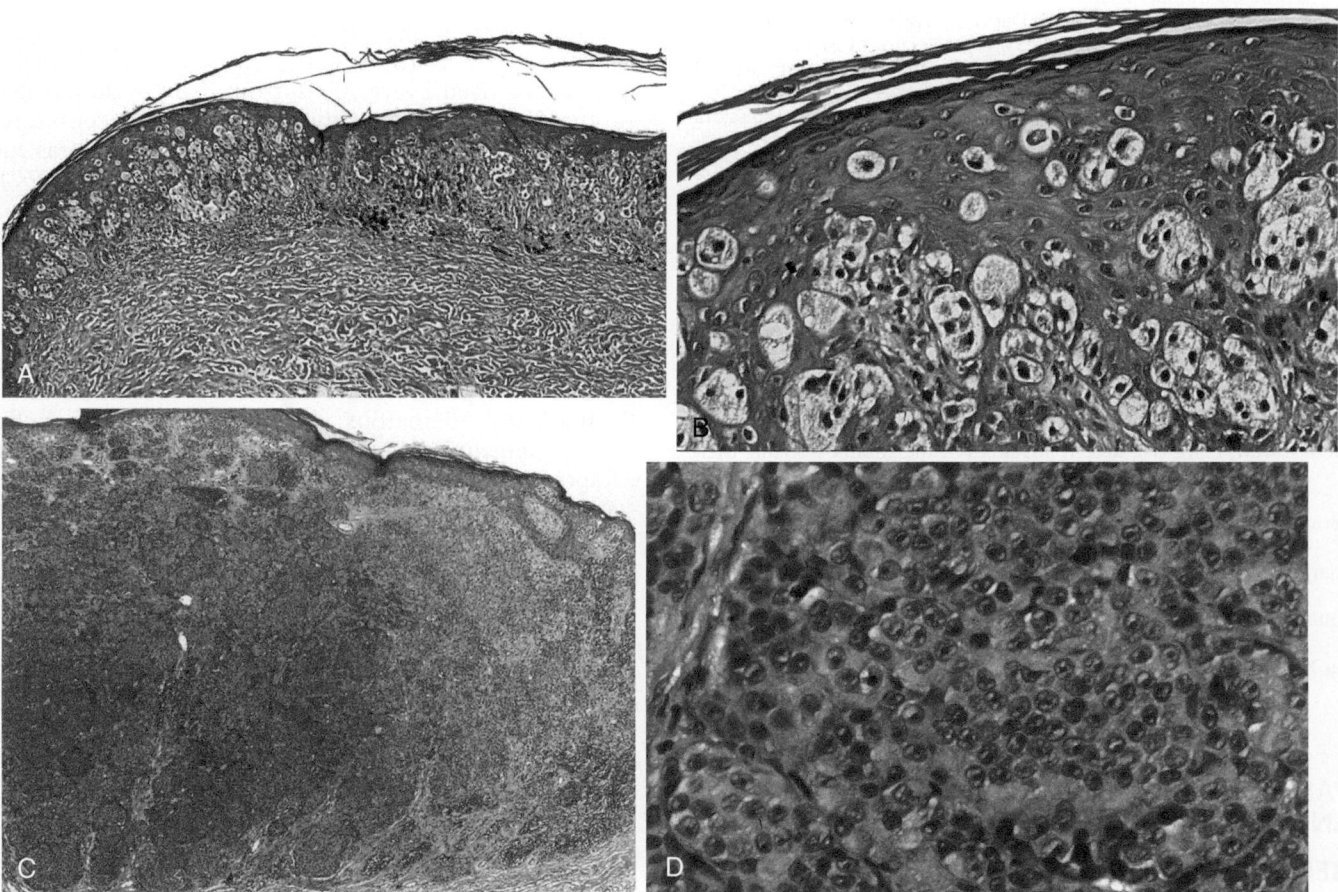

Figure 2-66. A, Malignant melanoma, superficial spreading. Low-power view shows a broad proliferation of large atypical melanocytes arranged in poorly formed nests at the dermoepidermal junction and within the dermis. **B,** Malignant melanoma, superficial spreading. High-power view shows pagetoid melanocytes in a pagetoid pattern involving all levels of epidermis. **C,** Malignant melanoma, nodular. Low-power view shows nodular proliferation of atypical melanocytes arranged as confluent nests and sheets. **D,** Malignant melanoma, nodular. High-power view shows markedly atypical melanocytes with pleomorphic nuclei and prominent nucleoli. Mitotic figures are present.

cytologic features in concert with clinical features; molecular methods hold some promise for the future
- Spitz nevus versus spitzoid melanoma continues to be a challenging differential diagnosis: all Spitz and Spitz-like lesions require complete excision

PEARLS

- *Desmoplastic and neurotropic malignant melanoma is a variant characterized by the presence of spindle-shaped melanocytes that may be mistaken for fibroblastic proliferation*
- *Breslow thickness (the thickness of melanoma measured from the granular layer of the epidermis), the presence or absence of ulceration, and mitotic rate provide useful prognostic information*
- *Melanoma in situ, when diagnosed and treated early, is associated with a 100% cure rate*
- *About 10% of melanomas are found to run in families and are associated with multiple atypical nevi*
- *Targeted therapies such as BRAF or MEK inhibitors for BRAF mutated melanomas are becoming available for advanced stage melanomas*

SELECTED REFERENCES

Bauer J, Bastian BC: Distinguishing melanocytic nevi from melanoma by DNA copy number changes: comparative genomic hybridization as a research and diagnostic tool. Dermatol Ther 19:40-49, 2006.

Botton T, Yeh I, Nelson T, Vemula SS, et al: Recurrent BRAF kinase fusions in melanocytic tumors offer an opportunity for targeted therapy. Pigment Cell Melanoma Res 26:845-851, 2013.

Clark WH Jr, Elder DE, Guerry DIV, et al: A study of tumor progression: the precursor lesions of superficial spreading and nodular melanoma. Hum Pathol 15:1147-1165, 1984.

Edwards SL, Blessing K: Problematic pigmented lesions: approach to diagnosis. J Clin Pathol 53:409-418, 2000.

Greene MH, Clark WH Jr, Tucker MA, et al: The high risk of melanoma in melanoma prone families with dysplastic nevi. Ann Intern Med 102:458, 1985.

Harvell JD, Kohler S, Zhu S, et al: High-resolution array-based comparative genomic hybridization for distinguishing paraffin-embedded Spitz nevi and melanomas. Diagn Mol Pathol 13:22-25, 2003.

Kanzler MH, Mraz-Gernhard S: Primary cutaneous malignant melanoma and its precursor lesions: diagnostic and therapeutic overview. J Am Acad Dermatol 45:260-276, 2001.

Menzies AM, Long GV: Recent advances in melanoma systemic therapy: BRAF inhibitors, CTLA4 antibodies and beyond. Eur J Cancer 49:3229-3241, 2013.

Perniciaro C: Dermatopathologic variants of malignant melanoma. Mayo Clin Proc 72:273-279, 1997.

Sharpless E, Chin L: The INK4a/ARF locus and melanoma. Oncogene 22:3092-3098, 2003.

Solus JF, Kraft S: Ras, Raf, and MAP kinase in melanoma. Adv Anat Pathol 20:217-226, 2013.

Xu X, Murphy G, Elenitsas R, Elder D: Benign pigmented lesions and malignant melanoma. In Elder DE, Elenitsas R, Johnson BL Jr, et al (eds): Lever's Histopathology of Skin, 10th ed. Philadelphia, Lippincott Williams & Wilkins, 2008, p 699.

VASCULAR PROLIFERATIONS AND NEOPLASMS

HEMANGIOMAS (CAPILLARY HEMANGIOMA AND CAVERNOUS HEMANGIOMA, ANGIOKERATOMA)

Clinical Features
- Acquired or congenital lesion consisting of dilated dermal vessels

- Capillary Hemangioma
  - Typically affects people in the first decade of life and spontaneously regresses
  - Small (< 1 cm), strawberry-red lesions
- Cavernous Hemangioma
  - Commonly observed as acquired lesions on the face, neck, and trunk of middle-aged and older individuals
  - Small (< 1 cm), bright-red, symmetrical, dome-shaped papules

Histopathology
- Capillary Hemangioma
  - Well-circumscribed proliferation of small vessels lined by flattened endothelial cells (Figure 2-67A)
  - Congenital lesions are typically lobulated and have numerous vessels
  - Acquired lesions typically develop luminal ectasia with age
- Cavernous Hemangioma
  - Poorly circumscribed collections of large ectatic vessels
  - Vessels have thicker walls and occasionally contain intraluminal thrombi
- Angiokeratoma
  - Numerous dilated thin-walled capillaries in the papillary dermis associated with epidermal hyperplasia and hyperkeratosis (Figure 2-67B)
  - May be seen in Fabry disease
- Glomus and Glomangioma
  - Solitary or multiple painful nodules histologically characterized by vessels surrounded by glomus cells (uniform rounded eosinophilic cells with central nuclei) that show immunohistochemical and ultrastructural features of smooth muscle cells (Figure 2-67C)

Special Stains and Immunohistochemistry
- Noncontributory

Other Techniques for Diagnosis
- Noncontributory

Differential Diagnosis
- Pyogenic Granuloma
  - Lesions typically show superficial ulceration and a markedly edematous stroma with a mononuclear and neutrophilic infiltrate
- Kaposi Sarcoma
  - Composed of slitlike vascular spaces and surrounding stroma infiltrated with lymphocytes and plasma cells
  - Extravasated red blood cells
  - Positive for HHV-8

PEARLS

- *Maffucci syndrome: association of cavernous hemangiomas with multiple enchondromas*
- *Kasabach-Merritt syndrome: association of cavernous hemangiomas with a consumptive coagulopathy secondary to intralesional thrombosis*
- *Blue rubber bleb nevus syndrome: association of cavernous hemangiomas with gastrointestinal tract vascular proliferations*

SELECTED REFERENCES

Esterly NB: Cutaneous hemangiomas, vascular stains and malformations, and associated syndromes. Curr Probl Dermatol 7: 6, 1995.

Fishman SJ, Mulliken JB: Hemangiomas and vascular malformations of infancy and childhood. Pediatr Clin N Am 40:1177-1200, 1993.

Frieden IJ: Which hemangiomas to treat—and how? Arch Dermatol 133:1593-1595, 1997.

Mulliken JB, Fishman SJ, Burrows PE: Vascular anomalies. Curr Probl Surg 37:517-584, 2000.

Schiller PI, Itin PH: Angiokeratomas: an update. Dermatology 193:275, 1996.

PYOGENIC GRANULOMA (LOBULAR CAPILLARY HEMANGIOMA)

Clinical Features

- Reactive, proliferating capillary hemangioma usually in response to localized trauma
- Commonly affects children
- Predilection for sites of minor trauma, including the face and distal extremities
- Lesions typically enlarge rapidly and have a tendency to bleed with minor trauma
- Friable, small (< 1 cm), erythematous papule; often pedunculated
- Lesions are initially finely lobulated and raspberry in color but become yellow, brown, or black with time

Histopathology

- Superficial ulceration typically present in early lesions (Figure 2-68)
- Proliferation of capillary-sized vessels surrounded by an epidermal collarette
- Vessels typically lined by swollen endothelial cells
- Markedly edematous stroma, which fibroses with time
- Inflammatory infiltrate composed of neutrophils and mononuclear cells

Special Stains and Immunohistochemistry

- Noncontributory

Other Techniques for Diagnosis

- Noncontributory

Differential Diagnosis

- Capillary or Cavernous Hemangioma
  - Lesions typically contain dilated vascular channels without significant stromal edema or inflammatory infiltrate
- Bacillary Angiomatosis

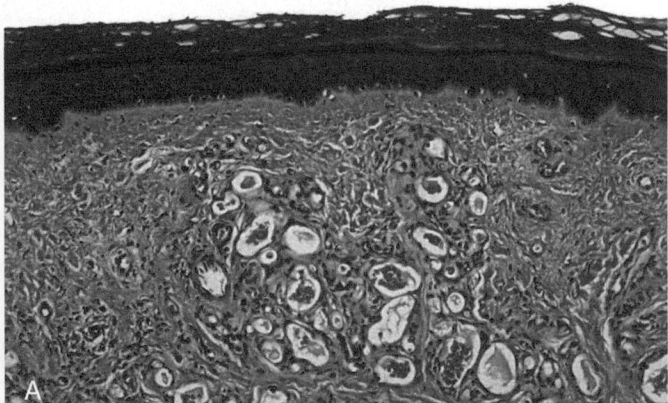
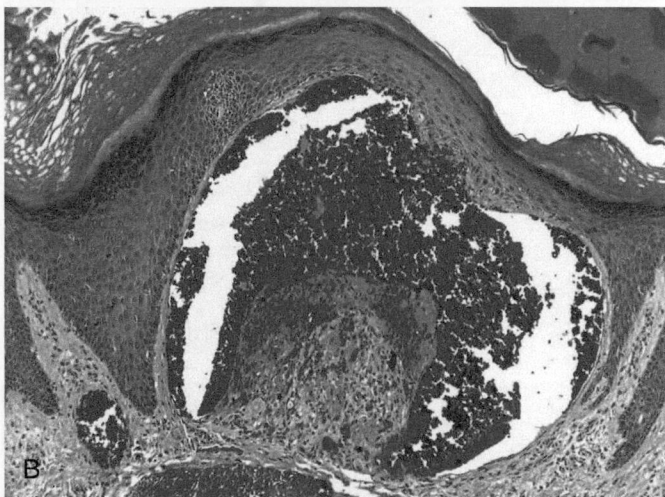
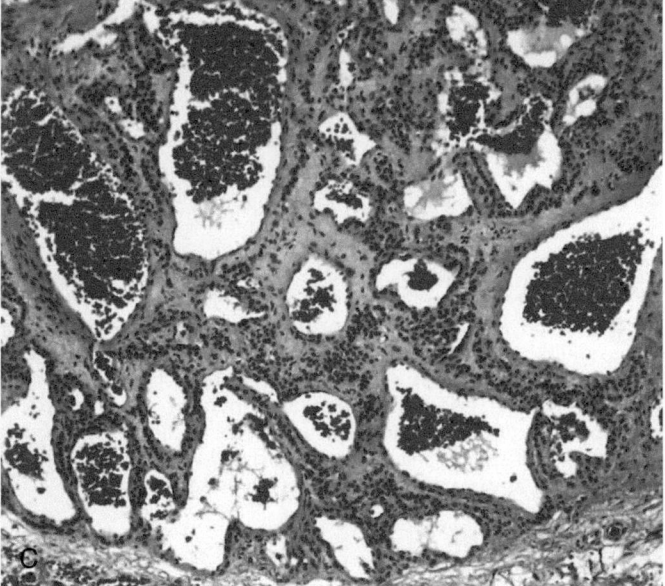

Figure 2-67. A, Hemangioma. Histologic section shows well-formed vascular spaces in the dermis filled with red blood cells. **B,** Angiokeratoma. Section shows epidermal hyperplasia, hyperkeratosis, and markedly dilated vascular spaces extending into the epidermis. **C,** Glomangioma. Section shows dilated blood vessels surrounded by a monomorphous population of round to oval cells.

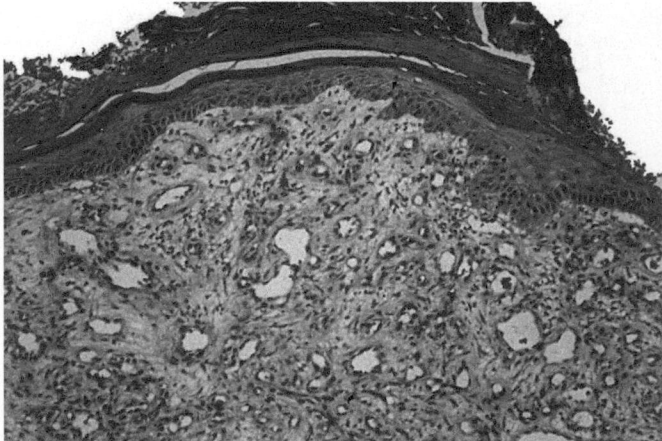

Figure 2-68. Pyogenic granuloma. Histologic section shows focal epidermal ulceration covered by neutrophilic scale crust and a lobular proliferation of vascular spaces associated with stromal edema and inflammatory cell infiltrate, including neutrophils.

- Infectious angiomatosis often seen in HIV-infected patients and caused by *Rochalimaea henselae* or *Rochalimaea quintana*, small gram-negative rods belonging to *Bartonella* species
- Clumps of granular basophilic material that shows bacilli with Warthin-Starry or Giemsa stain are characteristically present in association with neutrophilic infiltrates

PEARLS

- *Pyogenic granuloma of the gingiva occurring in pregnant women is known as* epulis

SELECTED REFERENCES

Chian CA, Arrese JE, Pierard GE: Skin manifestations of Bartonella infections. Int J Dermatol 41:461, 2002.

Fortna RR, Junkins-Hopkins JM: A case of lobular capillary hemangioma (pyogenic granuloma), localized to the subcutaneous tissue and a review of the literature. Am J Dermatopathol 29:408, 2007.

Park YH, Houh D, Houh W: Subcutaneous and superficial granuloma pyogenicum. Int J Dermatol 35:205-206, 1996.

Patrice SJ, Wiss K, Mulliken JB: Pyogenic granuloma (lobular capillary hemangioma): a clinicopathologic study of 178 cases. Pediatr Dermatol 8:267, 1994.

Plettenberg A, Lorenzen T, Burtsche BT, et al: Bacillary angiomatosis in HIV-infected patients: an epidemiological and clinical study. Dermatology 201:326, 2000.

Requena L, Sangueza OP: Cutaneous vascular proliferation. Part II. Hyperplasias and benign neoplasms. J Am Acad Dermatol 37:887-919, 1997.

KAPOSI SARCOMA

Clinical Features

- Slowly progressive multifocal vasoproliferative lesion of low-grade malignancy
- Four forms are recognized
  - Classic Kaposi sarcoma
    - Affects mainly males of Eastern European and Mediterranean descent
    - Presents as slowly developing nodules and plaques primarily affecting lower extremities
  - Endemic Kaposi sarcoma
    - Occurs among native blacks in Central Africa
    - Affects younger patients and children
  - Epidemic Kaposi sarcoma
    - Occurs in immunocompromised states associated with HIV infection
    - Typically involves trunk and mucosal surfaces
  - Kaposi sarcoma associated with iatrogenic immunosuppression
    - Immunosuppressed states, associated with the treatment for transplant rejection, greatly increase the risk for Kaposi sarcoma

Histopathology

- Histopathologic findings are similar in all forms of Kaposi sarcoma
- Early patch stage
  - Characterized by slitlike spaces between the collagen bundles that often follow adnexal structures and preexisting blood vessels that appear to protrude into newly formed blood vessels (promontory sign) (Figure 2-69A)
  - Extravasated red blood cells and plasma cells may be present

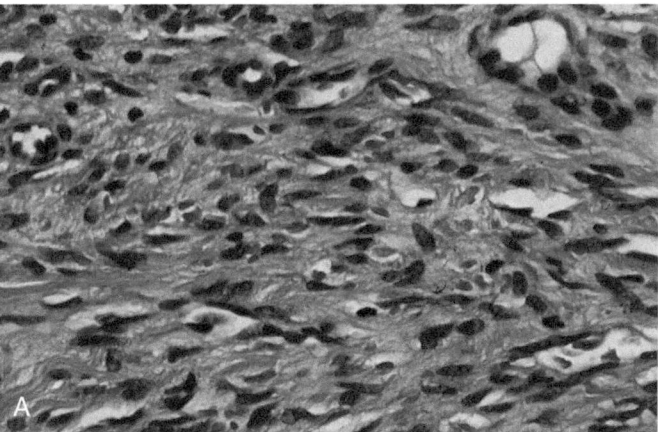

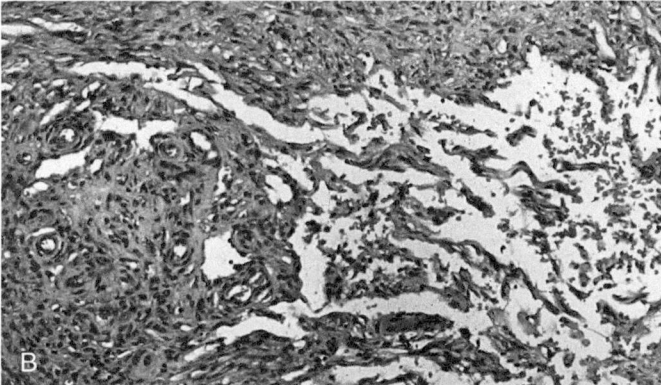

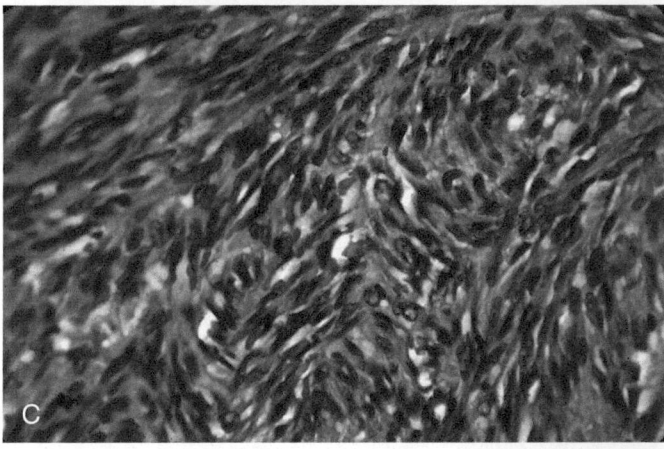

Figure 2-69. A, Kaposi sarcoma, patch stage. Histologic section shows slitlike spaces between the collagen bundles and extravasated red blood cells. **B,** Kaposi sarcoma, plaque stage. Histologic section shows a spindle cell proliferation and irregular vascular spaces. **C,** Kaposi sarcoma, nodular stage. Histologic section shows a solid proliferation of spindle-shaped cells associated with extravasated red cells. Nuclear atypia and mitotic figures are present.

- Plaque stage
  - Characterized by a proliferation of spindle-shaped cells arranged as short fascicles and a diffuse proliferation of blood vessels (Figure 2-69B)
  - Intracytoplasmic hyaline globules may be seen
- Nodular stage
  - Well-defined nodules of vascular spaces and spindle-shaped cells replace the dermis (Figure 2-69C)
  - Hemosiderin-laden macrophages are noted in the vicinity

- Intracellular and extracellular hyaline globules are easily seen
- Late aggressive lesions of Kaposi sarcoma have features of an aggressive sarcoma with greater degree of cytologic atypia and high mitotic rate

Special Stains and Immunohistochemistry

- Hyaline globules are PAS positive and diastase resistant
- Vascular nature of Kaposi sarcoma may be confirmed by immunostains CD31 and CD34
- Immunohistochemical stain for HHV-8 in all forms of Kaposi sarcoma and helps in the differentiation from other vascular proliferations

Other Techniques for Diagnosis

- Noncontributory

Differential Diagnosis

- Early lesions need to be differentiated from benign vascular proliferations such as targetoid hemosiderotic hemangioma and fibrous histiocytoma
- Late aggressive forms need to be differentiated from other aggressive sarcomas and require immunohistochemical stains
- Angiosarcoma
  - Asymmetrical collection of angulated, irregular vessels infiltrating between collagen bundles
  - Vascular lumina lined by endothelial cells that contain hyperchromatic irregular nuclei and prominent nucleoli

PEARLS

- *Natural course of Kaposi sarcoma varies widely depending on the clinical setting*
  - *At presentation, the classic form is typically restricted to the surface of the body and has a relatively indolent course (associated with long survival)*
  - *Endemic and epidemic subsets are typically more widespread at presentation and may have an aggressive clinical course*

SELECTED REFERENCES

Antman K, Chang Y: Kaposi sarcoma. N Engl J Med 342:1027-1038, 2000.

Cheuk W, Wong KO, Wong CS, et al: Immunostaining for human herpesvirus 8 latent nuclear antigen-1 helps distinguish Kaposi's sarcoma from its mimics. Am J Clin Pathol 121:335, 2004.

Dittmer DP, Damania B: Kaposi sarcoma associated herpesvirus pathogenesis (KSHV): an update. Curr Opin Virol 3:238-244, 2013.

Friedman-Kien AE, Saltzman BR: Clinical manifestations of classical, endemic African, and epidemic AIDS-associated Kaposi's sarcoma. J Am Acad Dermatol 22:1237, 1990.

Iscovich J, Boffetta P, Franceschi S, et al: Classic Kaposi sarcoma: epidemiology and risk factors. Cancer 88:500-517, 2000.

ANGIOSARCOMA

Clinical Features

- Malignant proliferation of endothelial cells
- Commonly affects elderly (sixth to seventh decades) males
- Can also occur after lymphedema (postmastectomy) and radiation therapy
- Predilection for the face, scalp, and neck
- Lesions typically progress rapidly, leading to ulceration and hemorrhage
- Present as dusky irregular erythematous plaques, which are often ulcerated

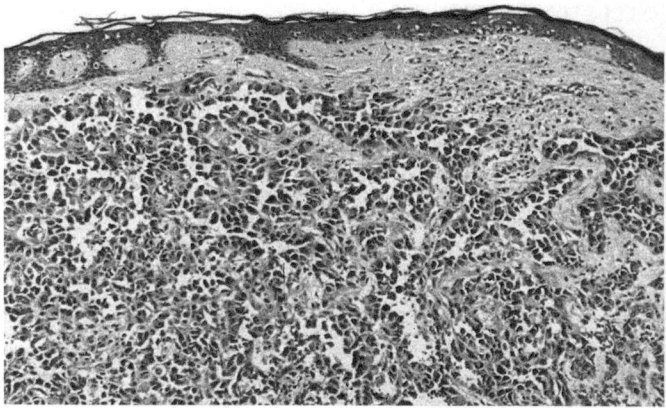

Figure 2-70. Angiosarcoma. Histologic section shows irregularly shaped vascular spaces lined by highly atypical endothelial cells with marked nuclear pleomorphism.

Histopathology

- Asymmetrical collection of angulated, irregular vascular spaces infiltrating between collagen bundles (Figure 2-70)
- Endothelial cells lining the vascular spaces have hyperchromatic irregular nuclei and prominent nucleoli; high mitotic rate
- In epithelioid angiosarcoma, the neoplastic cells are large and pleomorphic with abundant eosinophilic cytoplasm and a large nucleus with a prominent nucleolus
- Adjacent lymphatic spaces are often dilated
- Infiltrate of lymphocytes

Special Stains and Immunohistochemistry

- ERG, CD31, and CD34 highlight endothelial cells
- D2-40 staining in tumors of lymphatic origin

Other Techniques for Diagnosis

- Electron microscopy: Weibel-Palade bodies (rod-shaped lysosome-like structures) characteristic of endothelial cells

Differential Diagnosis

- Epithelioid Hemangioma
  - Lesions are typically symmetrical and contain plump endothelial cells without nuclear atypia
- Kaposi sarcoma
  - Capillary spaces are typically slitlike
  - Associated inflammatory infiltrate is composed of plasma cells and lymphocytes
- Intravascular Papillary Endothelial Hyperplasia
  - Lesions typically contain papillary fronds with no endothelial cell atypia; most likely represents an organizing thrombus
- Epithelial and Melanocytic Neoplasms
- Epithelioid angiosarcoma may lack distinct vascular spaces and simulate epithelial or melanocytic neoplasms
- Immunohistochemical studies are necessary for accurate diagnosis

PEARLS

- *Stewart-Treves syndrome: angiosarcoma arising in the upper extremities of patients who have undergone radical mastectomy with axillary lymph node dissection*
- *A rare variant of angiosarcoma is an entity known as* malignant endovascular papillary angioendothelioma, *or Dabska tumor*

SELECTED REFERENCES

Billings SD, McKenney JK, Folpe AL, et al: Cutaneous angiosarcoma following breast-conserving surgery and radiation: an analysis of 27 cases. Am J Surg Pathol 28:781, 2004.

McKay KM, Doyle LA, Lazar AJ, et al: Expression of ERG, an Ets family transcription factor, distinguishes cutaneous angiosarcoma from histiocytic mimics. Histopathology 61:989-991, 2012.

Mendenhall WM, Mendenhall CM, Werning JW, et al: Cutaneous angiosarcoma. Am J Clin Oncol 29:524, 2006.

Requena L, Sangueza OP: Cutaneous vascular proliferations. Part III. Malignant neoplasms, other cutaneous neoplasms with significant vascular component, and disorders erroneously considered as vascular neoplasms. J Am Acad Dermatol 38:143-175, 1998.

Schwartz RA, Dabski C, Dabska M: The Dabska tumor: a thirty-year retrospect. Dermatology 201:1-5, 2000.

SMOOTH MUSCLE NEOPLASMS

LEIOMYOMAS (ARRECTOR PILI MUSCLE TYPE, ANGIOLEIOMYOMA, DARTOIC LEIOMYOMA)

Clinical Features

- Benign dermal and subcutaneous tumors composed of smooth muscle
- Arrector pili muscle hamartomas are painful lesions commonly affecting persons during the second and third decades of life
- Predilection for the face, anterior aspect of the trunk, and extensor surfaces of the extremities
- Typically present as small (typically < 1 cm), smooth, firm, cutaneous nodules
- Nodules are usually pink to yellow or brown and translucent or waxy in appearance
- Angioleiomyomas usually occur as painful solitary subcutaneous lesions affecting the extremities especially the lower extremities
- Dartoic leiomyomas occur as solitary, painless, flesh-colored lesions affecting the genitalia, including the scrotum, labia majora, and areola

Histopathology

- Arrector Pili Muscle Type
  - Symmetrical proliferation of smooth muscle within the superficial and deep dermis (Figure 2-71A)
  - Interlacing fascicles of smooth muscle cells containing eosinophilic cytoplasm and cigar-shaped nuclei
- Angioleiomyoma
  - Well-circumscribed nodule of interlacing bundles of smooth muscle (Figure 2-71B)
- Admixture of small branching vessels, typically venules
- Dartoic Leiomyomas
  - Similar in appearance to arrector pili muscle hamartomas

Special Stains and Immunohistochemistry

- Smooth muscle actin (SMA), desmin and calponin positive

Other Techniques for Diagnosis

- Noncontributory

Differential Diagnosis

- Leiomyosarcoma
  - Asymmetrical tumor with infiltrative fascicles of smooth muscle cells with coarse nuclei and numerous mitoses
- Neurofibroma
  - Well-circumscribed, unencapsulated dermal mass of nerve sheath cells and fibroblasts
  - Epidermal atrophy with indistinct rete ridges
  - Spindle cells appear as wavy fibers with bland nuclei
  - Characteristic presence of mast cells in the background
- Dermatofibroma
  - Well-circumscribed but unencapsulated proliferation of fibroblasts with entrapped collagen bundles
  - Characteristic hyperplasia of the overlying epidermis with basal cell hyperpigmentation
  - Thick bundles of collagen are present at the periphery of the lesion

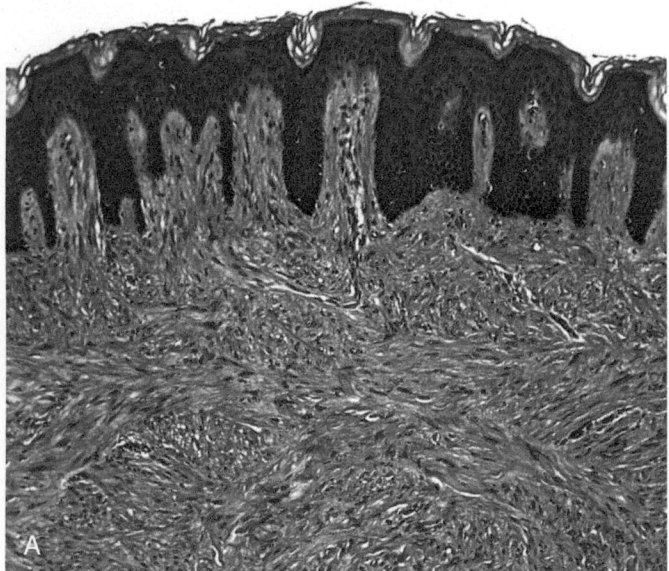
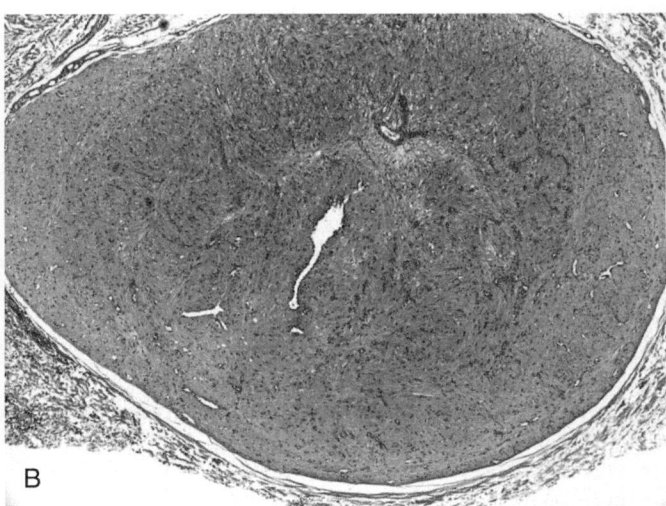

Figure 2-71. A, Leiomyoma, arrector pili muscle type. Fascicles of smooth muscle cells are seen within the upper part of the dermis. **B,** Leiomyoma, vascular type. A deep, dermal, well-circumscribed nodule composed of smooth muscle cells that surround and merge with the vessels walls.

* *Multiple pilar-type leiomyomas are the commonest type*

SELECTED REFERENCES

Calonje E, Fletcher CD: New entities in cutaneous soft tissue tumours. Pathologica 85:1-15, 1993.
Heffernan MP, Smoller BR, Kohler S: Cutaneous epithelioid angioleiomyoma. Am J Dermatopathol 20:213-217, 1998.
Kawagishi N, Kashiwagi T, Ibe M, et al: Pleomorphic angioleiomyoma. Am J Dermatopathol 22:268-271, 2000.
Sajben FP, Barnette DJ, Barrett TL: Intravascular angioleiomyoma. J Cutan Pathol 26:165-167, 1999.
Spencer JM, Amonette RA: Tumors with smooth muscle differentiation. Dermatol Surg 22:761-768, 1996.

CUTANEOUS LEIOMYOSARCOMA

Clinical Features
* Malignant proliferation of smooth muscle cells typically with features of arrector pili muscles
* Lesions commonly affect persons during the second and third decades of life
* Typically widely distributed with no appreciable site predilections
* Bleeding and ulceration of lesions commonly occur
* Firm dermal nodules typically less than 2 cm in diameter with discolored or depressed overlying skin

Histopathology
* Asymmetrical infiltrative fascicles of smooth muscle
* Intermixed zones of hypercellularity and better-differentiated zones
* Nuclei are hyperchromatic and have coarsely clumped chromatin (Figure 2-72)
* High mitotic rate

Special Stains and Immunohistochemistry
* May be helpful in differentiating leiomyosarcoma from other spindle cell tumors
* Cells of leiomyosarcoma typically show positivity for desmin and SMA

Other Techniques for Diagnosis
* Noncontributory

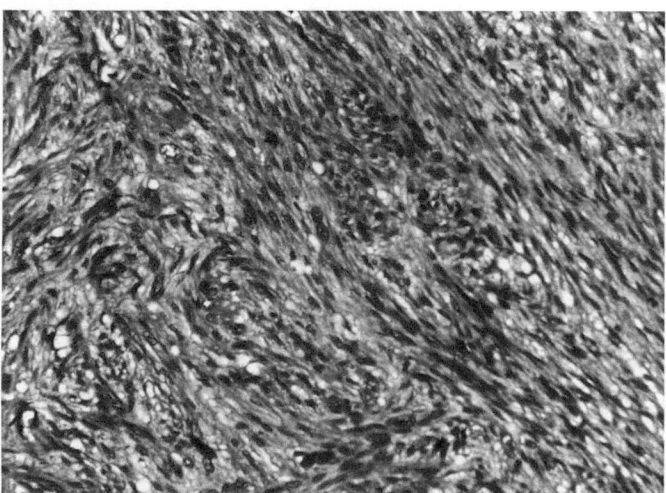

Figure 2-72. Leiomyosarcoma. Histologic section shows spindle-shaped cells with enlarged and hyperchromatic nuclei. Mitotic figures are present.

Differential Diagnosis
* Leiomyoma
  * Well-circumscribed proliferation of smooth muscle cells that typically form fascicles
  * Cells are uniform and lack nuclear atypia
* Dermatofibrosarcoma Protuberans (DFSP)
  * Characterized by a storiform pattern and infiltration into the underlying subcutaneous fat
  * Positive for CD34

* *Leiomyosarcomas typically metastasize through the bloodstream after invasion through the dermis*

SELECTED REFERENCES

Cook TF, Fosko SW: Unusual cutaneous malignancies. Semin Cutan Med Surg 17:114-132, 1998.
Diaz-Cascajo C, Borghi S, Weyers W: Desmoplastic leiomyosarcoma of the skin. Am J Dermatopathol 22:251-255, 2000.
Fish FS: Soft tissue sarcomas in dermatology. Dermatol Surg 22:268-273, 1996.
Kaddu S, Beham A, Cerroni L, et al: Cutaneous leiomyosarcoma. Am J Surg Pathol 21:979-987, 1997.
Lin JY, Tsai RY: Subcutaneous leiomyosarcoma on the face. Dermatol Surg 25:489-491, 1999.
Sidbury R, Heintz PW. Beckstead JH, White CR Jr: Cutaneous malignant epithelioid neoplasms. Adv Dermatol 14:285-306, 1999.
Spencer JM, Amonette RA: Tumors with smooth muscle differentiation. Dermatol Surg 22:761-768, 1996.

FIBROBLASTIC PROLIFERATIONS AND NEOPLASMS

KELOID

Clinical Features
* Scar that has grown beyond its initial margins
* Usually presents as a well-defined, round to linear elevation of the skin
* Tends to occur more often in females than males
* Dark-skinned individuals are more commonly affected
* Common sites include the earlobe following ear piercing
* Typically associated with trauma or surgery

Histopathology
* Characterized by accumulation of thick, hyalinized collagen fibers arranged in a haphazard pattern (Figure 2-73)
* Prominent myxoid matrix
* Early lesions are more vascular, whereas older lesions are predominantly fibrous

Special Stains and Immunohistochemistry
* Noncontributory

Other Techniques for Diagnosis
* Noncontributory

Differential Diagnosis
* Hypertrophic Scar
  * Scar is limited to the area of injury
  * Also shows thickened collagen fibers, but shows a smaller amount of myxoid matrix

* *Treated by various modes of therapy ranging from tropical steroid injections to surgical excision*
* *Unknown etiology; may be familial*

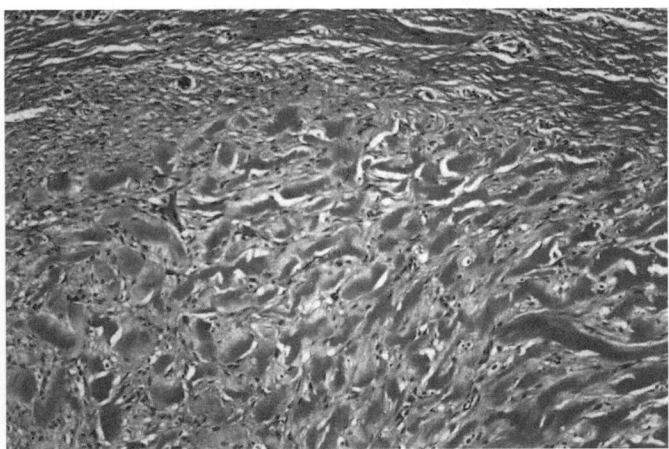

Figure 2-73. Keloid. Histologic section shows a nodular proliferation of fibroblasts associated with irregularly thickened bundles of collagen.

SELECTED REFERENCES

English RS, Shenefelt PD: Keloids and hypertrophic scars. Dermatol Surg 25:631-638, 1999.

Niessen FB, Spauwen PH, Schalkwijk J, Kon M: On the nature of hypertrophic scars and keloids: a review. Plast Reconstruct Surg 104:1435-1458, 1999.

Sahl WJ Jr, Clever H: Cutaneous scars: part I. Int J Dermatol 33:681-691, 1994.

Sahl WJ Jr, Clever H: Cutaneous scars: part II. Int J Dermatol 33:763-769, 1994.

DERMATOFIBROMA

Clinical Features

- Reactive hyperplasia of fibroblasts, histiocytes, and vascular elements
- Common lesion that affects mostly young or middle-aged adults, with slightly higher incidence in females
- Predilection for the arms and legs and other areas exposed to trauma
- Slow-growing, painless, usually single lesions that expand in a symmetrical fashion
- Typically small (< 1 cm), freely mobile, and tan to brown colored

Histopathology

- Well-circumscribed but unencapsulated proliferation of fibroblasts with entrapped collagen bundles (Figure 2-74A)
- Characteristic hyperplasia of the overlying epidermis with basal cell hyperpigmentation
- Thick bundles of collagen are present at the periphery of the lesion
- Occasional xanthomatous features with admixed histiocytes, foam cells, and multinucleated giant cells (lipidized variant) (Figure 2-74B)
- Occasional vascular proliferation with hemosiderin deposition (aneurysmal variant)
- Other histologic variants: epithelioid, palisading
- Cellular dermatofibroma: densely cellular and increased mitotic activity

Special Stains and Immunohistochemistry

- Negative for CD34; cellular dermatofibroma shows positivity at the periphery of lesion
- Positive for factor XIIIa

Other Techniques for Diagnosis

- Noncontributory

Differential Diagnosis

- DFSP
  - Lesions have a characteristic storiform pattern
  - Typically infiltrates the subcutaneous fat in a lacelike pattern
  - Foci of hypercellularity and mitoses are usually present
- Neurofibroma
  - Well-circumscribed, unencapsulated dermal mass of nerve sheath cells and fibers
  - Epidermal atrophy with indistinct rete ridges
  - Spindle cells appear as wavy fibers with bland nuclei
  - Characteristic presence of mast cells in the background
- Basal cell Carcinoma
  - Follicular induction seen in dermatofibromas may resemble basal cell carcinoma
  - Predilection for sun-exposed skin, typically face and hands

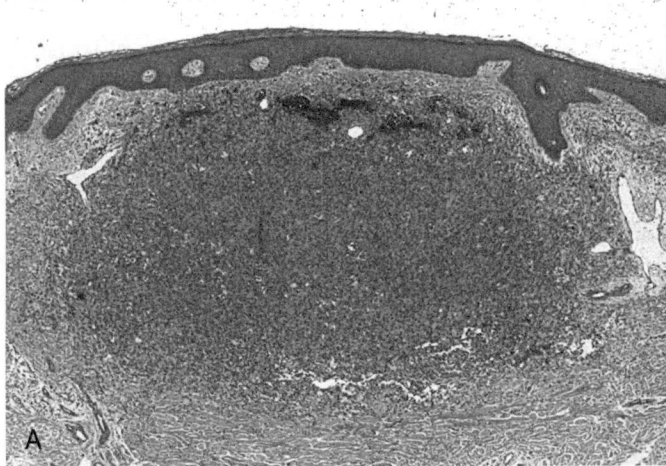
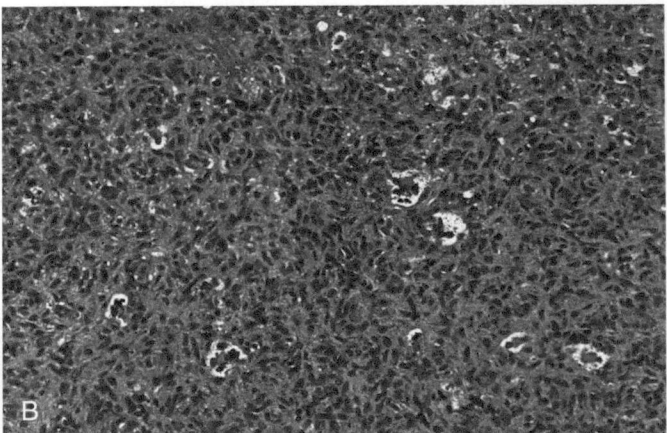

Figure 2-74. Dermatofibroma. A, Histologic section shows a well-defined dermal nodule of fibroblasts and histiocytes. **B,** High-power view shows fibroblasts and multinucleated histiocytes with foamy cytoplasm and hemosiderin pigment.

- Multiple nests of basaloid cells with peripheral palisading and presence of a mucinous stroma with retraction artifacts
- Basaloid cells are typically uniform and have frequent mitotic activity and abundant apoptosis

PEARLS

- *Dermatofibromas rarely present with hyperesthesia and minor pain*
- *Fitzpatrick sign: application of centripetal compression results in central dimpling of the dermatofibromas due to tethering of the mass to the deep dermis*

SELECTED REFERENCES

Calonje E, Mentzel T, Fletcher CD: Cellular benign fibrous histiocytoma: clinicopathologic analysis of 74 cases of a distinctive variant of cutaneous fibrous histiocytoma with frequent recurrence. Am J Surg Pathol 18:668-676, 1994.

Cohen PR, Rapin RP, Farhood AI: Dermatofibroma and dermatofibrosarcoma protuberans: differential expression of CD34 and factor XIIIa. Am J Dermatopathol 16:573-574, 1994.

De Unamuno P, Carames Y, Fernandez-Lopez E, et al: Congenital multiple clustered dermatofibroma. Br J Dermatol 142:1040-1043, 2000.

Gleason BC, Fletcher CD: Deep "benign" fibrous histiocytoma: clinicopathologic analysis of 69 cases of a rare tumor indicating occasional metastatic potential. Am J Surg Pathol 32:354-362, 2008.

DERMATOFIBROSARCOMA PROTUBERANS

Clinical Features

- Locally invasive fibroblastic tumor
- Uncommon lesion typically seen in males during the third and fourth decades
- Predilection for the trunk and occasionally the proximal extremities
- Initially slow-growing, single lesion that accelerates in growth after a period of quiescence
- Initially presents as firm, freely mobile, tan to brown cutaneous nodule
- With time, lesions enlarge to form a blue-red, multilobular nodules

Histopathology

- Asymmetrical, diffuse, deep dermal to subcutaneous lesion (Figure 2-75A)
- Proliferation of bland spindle cells in a typical cartwheel or storiform pattern
- Neoplastic cells infiltrate into the subcutaneous fat in lacelike pattern (Figure 2-75B)
- Few mitotic figures; rare atypical mitoses, necrosis, or multinucleated giant cells
- Overlying epidermis is typically thinned

Special Stains and Immunohistochemistry

- CD34 positive

Other Techniques for Diagnosis

- Cytogenetics: characteristic chromosomal translocation t(17;22) with resulting COL1A1-PDGFB fusion in most cases

Differential Diagnosis

- Dermatofibroma
  - Well-circumscribed but unencapsulated proliferation of fibroblasts with entrapped collagen bundles
  - Characteristic hyperplasia of the overlying epidermis with basal cell hyperpigmentation
  - Thick bundles of collagen are present at the periphery of the lesion

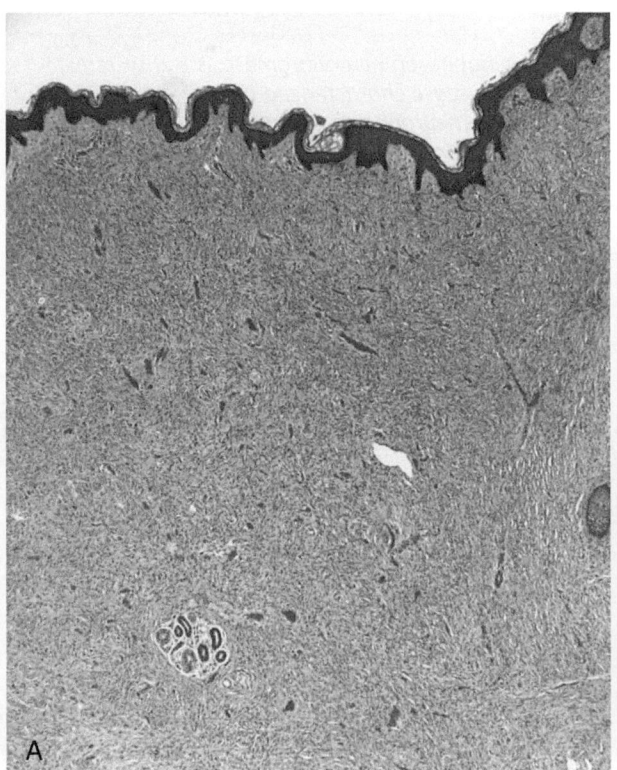
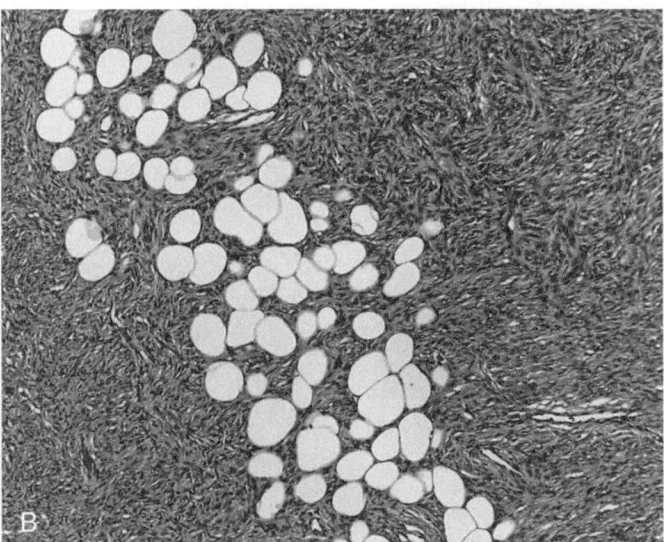

Figure 2-75. Dermatofibrosarcoma protuberans. A, Low-power view shows a deeply infiltrative proliferation of spindle-shaped cells. **B,** High-power view shows the slender spindle-shaped cells infiltrating and replacing the subcutaneous fat.

- Neurofibroma
  - Well-circumscribed, unencapsulated dermal mass of nerve sheath cells and nerve fibers
  - Epidermal atrophy with indistinct rete ridges
  - Spindle cells appear as wavy fibers with bland nuclei
  - Presence of mast cells in the background

PEARLS

- *Surgical removal of a DFSP is often followed by a recurrence due to the infiltrative nature of the tumor*
- *Bednar variant contains spindle-shaped cells with melanin pigment*

SELECTED REFERENCES

Cohen PR, Rapini RP, Farhood AI: Dermatofibroma and dermatofibrosarcoma protuberans: differential expression of CD34 and factor XIIIa. Am J Dermatopathol 16:573-574, 1994.

Llombart B, Serra-Guillén C, Monteagudo C, et al: Dermatofibrosarcoma protuberans: a comprehensive review and update on diagnosis and management. Semin Diagn Pathol 30:13-28, 2013.

Patel KU, Szabo SS, Hernandez VS, et al: Dermatofibrosarcoma protuberans COL1A1-PDGFB fusion is identified in virtually all dermatofibrosarcoma protuberans cases when investigated by newly developed multiplex reverse transcription polymerase chain reaction and fluorescence in situ hybridization assays. Hum Pathol 39:184-193, 2008.

Zelger B, Sidoroff A, Stanzl U, et al: Deep penetrating dermatofibroma versus dermatofibrosarcoma protuberans: a clinicopathologic comparison. Am J Surg Pathol 18:677-686, 1994.

NEURAL NEOPLASMS

NEUROFIBROMA

Clinical Features

- Benign tumors of perineural supporting cells
- Lesions tend to be solitary and unassociated with any particular age or gender group except when associated with von Recklinghausen neurofibromatosis
- Can involve any site, but lesions tend to avoid palms and soles
- Present as small (< 1 cm), soft, tan papules or nodules, occasionally larger or pedunculated

Histopathology

- Well-circumscribed, unencapsulated dermal mass of nerve sheath cells and fibroblasts
- Epidermal atrophy with indistinct rete ridges
- Spindle cells with wavy and bland nuclei (Figure 2-76A)
- Characteristic presence of mast cells in the background

Special Stains and Immunohistochemistry

- S-100 protein positive

Other Techniques for Diagnosis

- Noncontributory

Differential Diagnosis

- Palisaded and Encapsulated Neuroma
  - Well-circumscribed superficial dermal nodule resembling schwannoma
  - Spindle-shaped cells with elongated nuclei arranged in palisades (Figure 2-76B)
- Dermatofibroma
  - Well-circumscribed but unencapsulated proliferation of fibroblasts and histiocytes in varying numbers
  - Characteristic hyperplasia of the overlying epidermis with basal cell hyperpigmentation
  - Thick bundles of collagen may be present at the periphery of the lesion
- Schwannoma
  - Typically consists of an encapsulated spindle cell proliferation with distinct zones
    - Antoni A zones (hypercellular and composed predominantly of spindle cells)
    - Antoni B zones (hypocellular areas composed of spindle cells with abundant mucinous background)
    - Verocay bodies (parallel arrangements of nuclei)

PEARLS

- *Von Recklinghausen neurofibromatosis is a systemic hereditary disease characterized by café-au-lait spots and multiple neurofibromas composed of cellular and hypertrophied nerve trunks that usually develop after birth but before puberty*
- *Spindle cell elements of neurofibromas are primarily composed of Schwann cells*

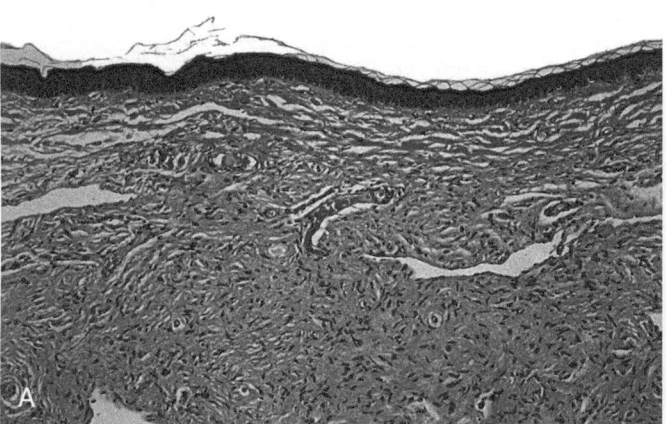
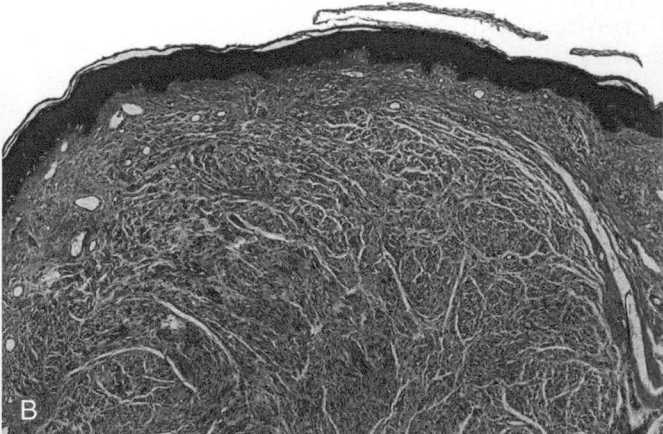

Figure 2-76. A, Neurofibroma. Histologic section shows a dermal proliferation of spindle-shaped cells with wavy nuclei and a loose myxoid stroma. Mast cells are typically present in the background. **B,** Palisaded and encapsulated neuroma. Histologic section shows a well-circumscribed nodule of spindle-shaped cells with elongated nuclei and a palisaded arrangement.

SELECTED REFERENCES

Argenyi ZB, Santa-Cruz D, Bromley C: Comparative light-microscopic and immunohistochemical study of traumatic and palisaded and encapsulated neuromas of the skin. Am J Dermatopathol 14:504, 1992.

Murphy GF, Elder DE: Atlas of Tumor Pathology: Non-Melanocytic Tumor of the Skin. Third Series, Fascicle 1. Washington, DC, Armed Forces Institute of Pathology, 1990.

Riccardi VM: Von Recklinghausen neurofibromatosis. N Engl J Med 305:1617, 1981.

MERKEL CELL CARCINOMA (CUTANEOUS NEUROENDOCRINE CARCINOMA)

Clinical Features

- Uncommon neoplasm with neuroendocrine differentiation
- Most common sites of involvement are head and extremities
- Presents most commonly as a solitary nodule and rarely as multiple nodules
- Lesions are pink, firm, and nodular and typically range in size from 0.8 to 4 cm
- Skin ulceration is uncommon

Histopathology

- Dermal nodule composed of small, round, blue cells with scant cytoplasm and irregular nuclei with uniformly distributed chromatin (Figure 2-77A)
- Neoplastic cells are arranged in sheets or trabeculae and may form pseudorosettes
- Nucleoli are inconspicuous, and nuclear molding may be present (Figure 2-77B)
- Frequent mitotic figures and individually necrotic tumor cells are common
- Stroma between the nests of neoplastic cells is scant
- Neoplastic cells may extend into the overlying epidermis in a pagetoid pattern
- Overlying epidermis may show varying degrees of atypia and occasionally SCC

Special Stains and Immunohistochemistry

- Neuron-specific enolase (NSE) and neurofilament positive
- Chromogranin, synaptophysin positive
- Cytokeratin 20 positive (Figure 2-77C)

Other Techniques for Diagnosis

- Electron microscopy shows membrane-bound dense-core granules and perinuclear bundles or whorls of intermediate filaments

Differential Diagnosis

- Metastatic Small Cell Carcinoma
  - Immunohistochemical stain for cytokeratin 20 negative
  - Primary site specific markers such as TTF-1 for lung are positive
- Malignant Lymphoma
  - Immunohistochemical stains CD45 and T- and B-cell markers are helpful
- Other primitive neuroectodermal tumors such as Ewing sarcoma and neuroblastoma should be considered

PEARLS

- *Divergent differentiation consisting of squamous, adnexal, and melanocytic areas can be seen in neuroendocrine carcinoma of the skin*
- *Merkel cell polyomavirus (MCPyV) is detected in significant number of cases*

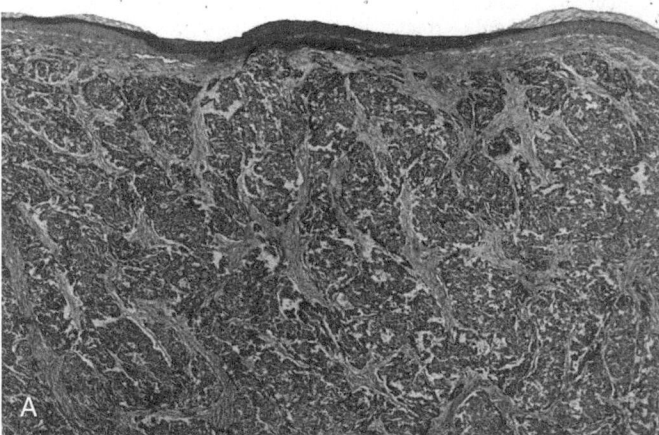
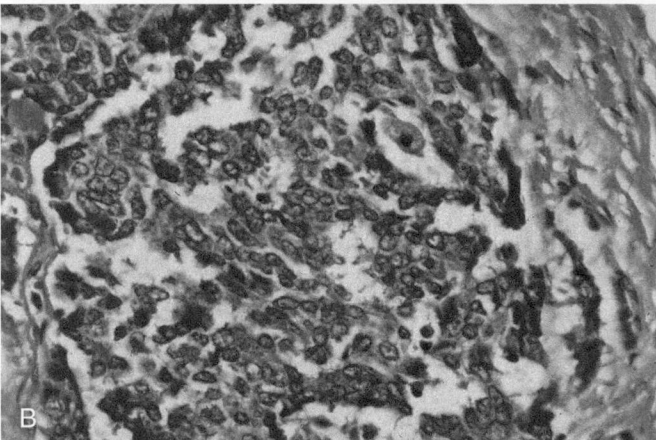
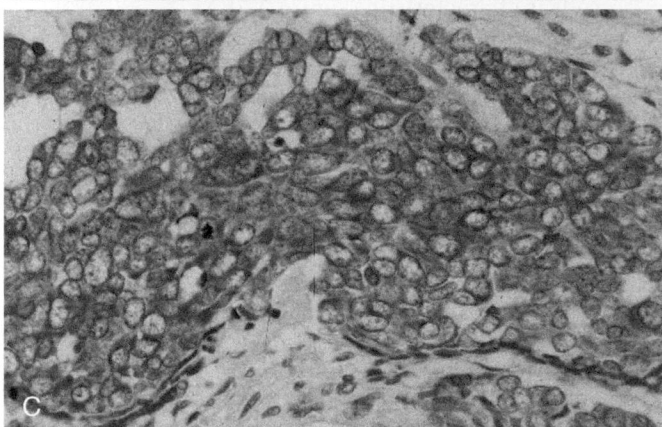

Figure 2-77. Merkel cell carcinoma. A, Low-power view shows a dermal nodule of small blue cells arranged in sheets and trabeculae. **B,** High-power view shows cells with scant cytoplasm and irregular nuclei. Nucleoli are inconspicuous. Mitotic figures and individually necrotic cells are present. **C,** Cytokeratin stain shows perinuclear dotlike positivity of the neoplastic cells.

SELECTED REFERENCES

Amber K, McLeod MP, Nouri K: The Merkel cell polyomavirus and its involvement in Merkel cell carcinoma. Dermatol Surg 39:232-238, 2013.

Daoud MA, Mete O, Al Habeeb A, Ghazarian D: Neuroendocrine carcinoma of the skin: an updated review. Semin Diagn Pathol 30:234-244, 2013.

Haneke E: Electron microscopy of Merkel cell carcinoma from formalin-fixed tissue. J Am Acad Dermatol 12:487, 1985.

Isimbaldi G, Sironi M, Taccagni GL, et al: Tripartite differentiation (squamous, glandular, and melanocytic) of a primary cutaneous neurocrine carcinoma: an immunocytochemical and ultrastructural study. Am J Dermatopathol 15:260, 1993.

Ratner D, Nelson BR, Brown MD, Johnson TM: Merkel cell carcinoma. J Am Acad Dermatol 29:143, 1993.

Smith KJ, Skelton HG 3rd, Holland TT, et al: Neuroendocrine (Merkel cell) carcinoma with an intraepidermal component. Am J Dermatopathol 15:528, 1993.

HEMATOPOIETIC PROLIFERATIONS AND NEOPLASMS

URTICARIA PIGMENTOSA

Clinical Features
- Can present in four forms
  - Arising in infancy and childhood without associated systemic lesions
  - Arising in adolescence or adulthood without associated systemic lesions
  - Systemic mast cell disease
  - Mast cell leukemia
- Cutaneous lesions can take many forms
  - Maculopapular: can occur in infantile and adult forms
  - Nodular and plaquelike: can occur in infantile and adult forms
  - Solitary nodule: seen in infancy
  - Diffuse erythroderma: always starts in infancy
  - Telangiectasia macularis eruptive perstans: occurs in adults

Histopathology
- Nodules and plaques
  - Dense, diffuse dermal infiltrate composed of mast cells is characteristic (Figure 2-78A)
  - Infiltrate may extend into subcutis
  - Mast cells contain metachromatic granules in the cytoplasm
- Maculopapular type and telangiectasia macularis eruptive perstans
  - Mast cells are distributed in a perivascular pattern in the upper dermis
  - Erythrodermic urticaria pigmentosa
  - Mast cells are arranged in a dense bandlike pattern in the upper dermis

- Eosinophils are present in varying numbers; especially if biopsy is taken after urtication
- Subepidermal bullae may be noted in some cases (bullous mastocytosis)
- Increased pigment in the basal cell layer of epidermis and melanophages in the dermis are responsible for the pigmentation of the lesions clinically

Special Stain and Immunohistochemistry
- Metachromatic granules in mast cells are best seen with Giemsa, toluidine blue, and Leder stains
- Immunohistochemical stain for mast cell tryptase and CD117 positive (Figure 2-78B)

Other Techniques for Diagnosis
- Noncontributory

Differential Diagnosis
- Langerhans Cell Histiocytosis
  - Can be differentiated by the presence of aggregates of histiocytes in the epidermis that are positive for CD1a and S-100 protein
- Inflammatory Dermatoses
  - In sparsely cellular examples of urticaria pigmentosa, special stains are essential to demonstrate mast cells and differentiate from other dermatitis
  - Mast cells have a distinct appearance and are easy to differentiate from other cellular infiltrates in the dermis in most cases

PEARLS

- *Mast cells stimulate the melanocytes of the epidermis to produce more melanin*
- *In systemic mast cell disease, mostly seen in adults, massive infiltration of the bones may cause collapse of vertebrae and fractures of large bones*
- *Systemic mast cell disease can also involve lymph nodes, liver, spleen, gastrointestinal tract, and central nervous system*

SELECTED REFERENCES

Briley LD, Phillips CM: Cutaneous mastocytosis: a review focusing on the pediatric population. Clin Pediatr (Phila) 47:757-761, 2008.

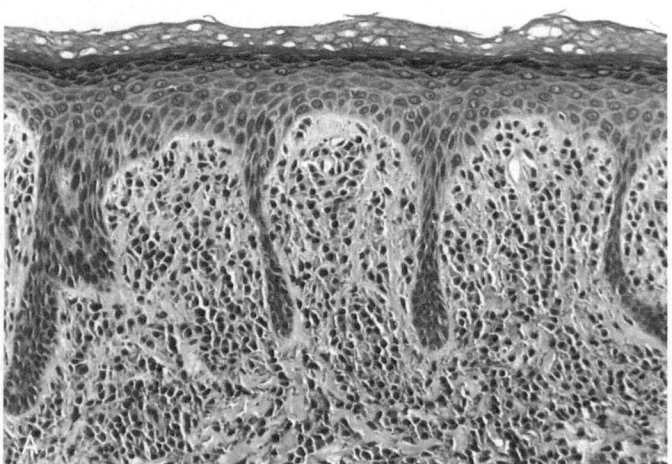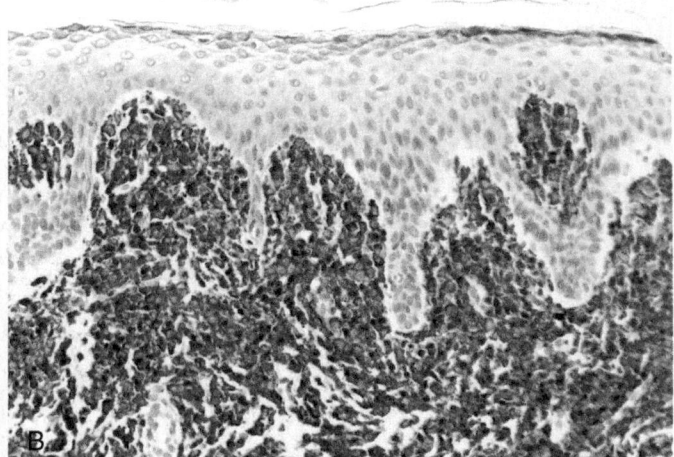

Figure 2-78. Urticaria pigmentosa. **A,** Hematoxylin and eosin–stained section shows a dense, diffuse dermal infiltrate of mast cells. **B,** Immunohistochemical stain for mast cell tryptase highlights the mast cells.

Leaf FA, Jaecks EP, Rodriguez DR: Bullous urticaria pigmentosa. Cutis 58:358-360, 1996.

Mihm MC, Clark WH, Reed RJ, et al: Mast cell infiltrates of the skin and the mastocytosis syndrome. Hum Pathol 4: 231, 1973.

Topar G, Staudacher C, Geisen F, et al: Urticaria pigmentosa: a clinical, hematopathologic, and serologic study of 30 adults. Am J Clin Pathol 109:279-285, 1998.

LANGERHANS CELL HISTIOCYTOSIS (LETTERER-SIWE DISEASE, HAND-SCHÜLLER-CHRISTIAN DISEASE, EOSINOPHILIC GRANULOMA)

Clinical Features
- A histiocytic proliferative disorder of unknown etiology composed of three separate clinical entities
- Letterer-Siwe Disease (Acute Disseminated Form)
  - Rare disease usually seen in male infants between 3 months and 3 years of age
  - Patients commonly present with constitutional signs, extraosseous lesions, hepatosplenomegaly, lymphadenopathy, and cutaneous lesions
  - Predilection of the cutaneous lesions for the scalp, face, mouth, neck, trunk, and buttocks
  - Scaling, yellow-brown, purpuric, papular eruptions
- Hand-Schüller-Christian Disease (Chronic Multifocal Form)
  - Rare disease usually seen in toddlers between 2 and 6 years of age
  - Patients commonly present with chronic otitis media and portions of the classical triad of cranial bone defects, exophthalmos, and diabetes insipidus as well as cutaneous lesions
  - Predilection of the cutaneous lesions for the chest, axillae, and groin
  - Similar to Letterer-Siwe disease with occasional red-brown papulopustular or papulonodular lesions
- Eosinophilic Granuloma (Chronic Focal Form)
  - Rare disease usually seen in toddlers between 2 and 5 years of age
  - Patients commonly develop osteolytic, pulmonary, cutaneous, and occasionally cranial lesions
  - Predilection of cutaneous lesions for the scalp, face, oral cavity, and groin

- Multiple ulcerative crusted papules or multiple subcutaneous nodules

Histopathology
- The histologic picture is essentially similar in all clinical forms and is characterized by the presence of Langerhans cells in an appropriate context
- Characteristic Langerhans cells are large and rounded with indistinct cell membranes and clearly demarcated lobulated or folded nuclei
- Langerhans cells are variably present throughout the dermis and frequently found in the epidermis (Figure 2-79A)
- Prominent infiltrate of eosinophils may be present in the background

Special Stains and Immunohistochemistry
- S-100 protein: Langerhans cells, melanocytes, and activated histiocytes are positive
- CD1a and Langerin: Langerhans cells are positive (Figure 2-79B)

Other Techniques for Diagnosis
- Electron microscopy: presence of tennis racquet–shaped Birbeck granules within Langerhans cells

Differential Diagnosis
- Xanthogranuloma
  - Lesions contain multinucleated cells with peripheral vacuolization of the cytoplasm (Touton giant cells)
- Reticulohistiocytoma
  - Lesions contain multinucleated cells with red-purple granular cytoplasm (ground-glass giant cells)
- Congenital Self-Healing Reticulohistiocytosis
  - Scattered papules and nodules are present at birth or appear shortly after
  - Ground-glass giant cells on histology
  - Lesions begin to involute in 2 to 3 months and completely regress within 1 year
- Cutaneous T-Cell Lymphoma
  - Composed of atypical lymphoid cells
  - Positive for leukocyte common antigen (LCA) and T-cell markers

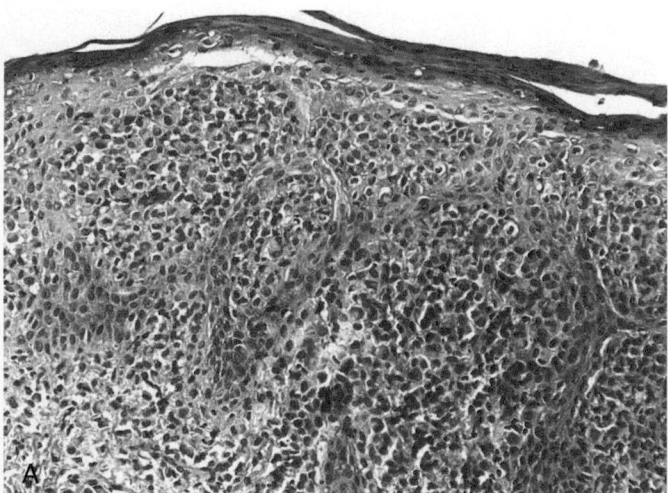
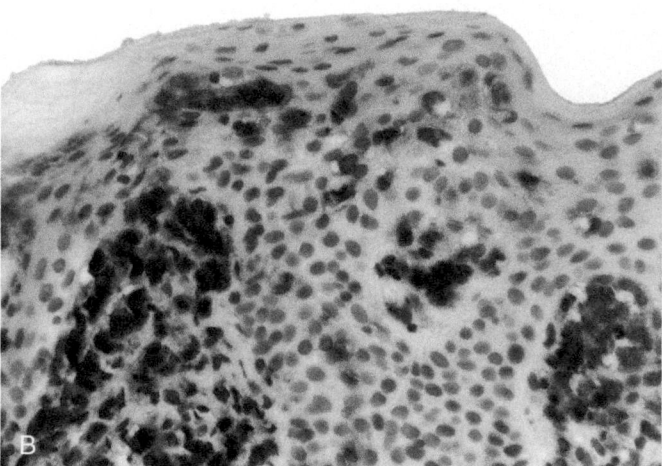

Figure 2-79. Langerhans cell histiocytosis. A, Histologic section shows dermal infiltrate of histiocytic cells with abundant cytoplasm and irregular lobulated nuclei; many of the cells extend into the overlying epidermis. **B,** Immunohistochemical stain for CD1a shows strong positivity of the histiocytic cells.

PEARLS

- *Langerhans cells may occasionally appear vacuolated and multinucleated, giving a xanthomatous appearance*
- *Prognosis and clinical course depend on the age of the patient and the extent of organ involvement*
- *Activating BRAF mutations are reported*

Selected References

Badalian-Very G, Vergilio JA, Fleming M, Rollins BJ: Pathogenesis of Langerhans cell histiocytosis. Annu Rev Pathol 8:1-20, 2013.

Howarth DM, Gilchrist GS, Mullan BP, et al: Langerhans cell histiocytosis: diagnosis, natural history, management, and outcome. Cancer 85:2278, 1999.

Kapur P, Erickson C, Rakheja D, et al: Congenital self-healing reticulohistiocytosis (Hashimoto-Pritzker disease): ten-year experience at Dallas Children's Medical Center. J Am Acad Dermatol 56:290, 2007.

Minkov M, Prosch H, Steiner M, et al: Langerhans cell histiocytosis in neonates. Pediatr Blood Cancer 45:802, 2005.

CUTANEOUS T-CELL LYMPHOMA (MYCOSIS FUNGOIDES)

Clinical Features

- Mycosis fungoides is the most common form of primary cutaneous lymphoma
- It may present as a patch, plaque, or nodule or tumor
- Patches of mycosis fungoides are erythematous and scaly and affect trunk and proximal extremities
- Lesions typically vary in size from 1 cm to several centimeters
- Plaques are usually well defined and occasionally annular
- Nodules and tumors represent advanced disease and are indistinguishable from other aggressive cutaneous lymphomas; lesions are reddish brown and firm and are often ulcerated
- All forms may be seen in the same patient at the same time

Histopathology

- Patch stage
  - Patchy lichenoid infiltrate of lymphocytes in markedly thickened papillary dermis and in small collections within a minimally spongiotic epidermis (Figure 2-80A,B)
  - Epidermis may show psoriasiform hyperplasia
- Plaque stage
  - Features are similar to those seen in patch stage, but the infiltrate is denser and more bandlike
  - Lymphocytes may be cytologically atypical
- Tumor stage
  - Diffuse dermal infiltrate of atypical lymphocytes with convoluted nuclei
  - Increase in the number of medium to large lymphoid cells
  - Large cell transformation: large cells >25% or discrete nodule of large cells

Special Stains and Immunohistochemistry

- Typical phenotype: CD3, CD4, and CD5 positive and CD8 negative; CD8 positive variants occur in younger patients presenting as hypopigmented lesions
- Diminished or loss of CD7 expression
- CD30 positive large cells in large cell transformation

Other Techniques for Diagnosis

- Gene rearrangement studies for T-cell receptor

Differential Diagnosis

- Spongiotic Dermatitis
  - Early lesions of mycosis fungoides may be difficult to differentiate from spongiotic dermatitis
  - Papillary dermal collagen changes and intraepidermal collections of lymphocytes with only minimal spongiosis favor mycosis fungoides
  - Nodules of mycosis fungoides need to be differentiated from other cutaneous lymphomas

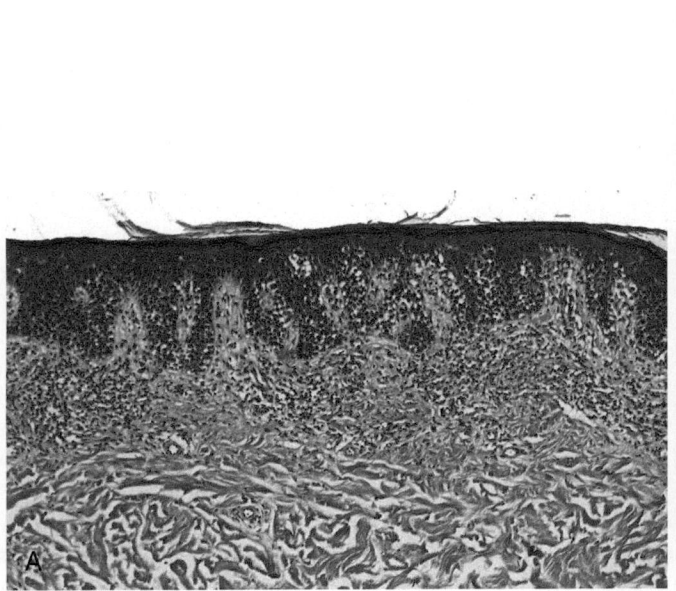
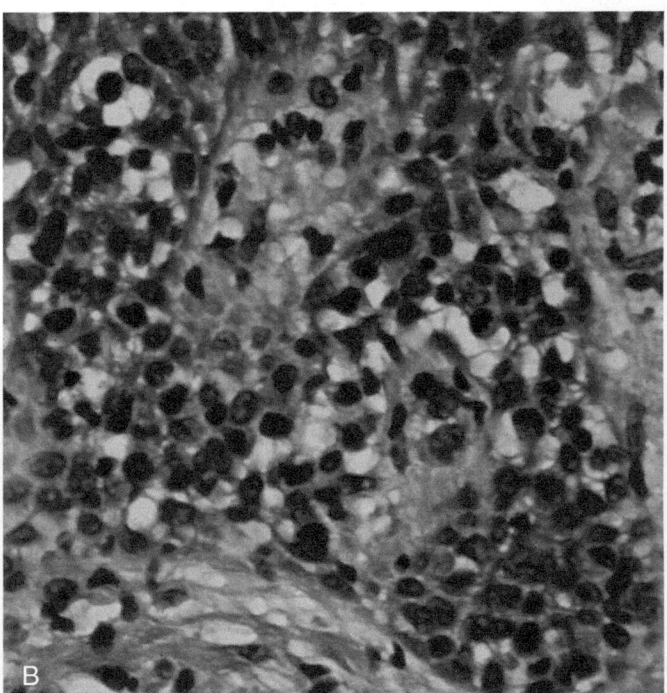

Figure 2-80. Mycosis fungoides. A, Psoriasiform epidermal hyperplasia and a bandlike infiltrate of lymphoid cells within a thickened papillary dermis are seen. **B,** Collections of atypical lymphoid cells are seen in the epidermis (epidermotropism, Pautrier microabscesses).

- Immunohistochemical studies to confirm T-cell phenotype are helpful in differentiating from B-cell lymphomas and lymphoid hyperplasias

PEARLS

- *Sézary syndrome represents an erythrodermic form of mycosis fungoides with neoplastic cells populating the peripheral blood*
- *Follicular mucinosis may be a feature in some cases of mycosis fungoides*

SELECTED REFERENCES

Dalton JA, Yag-Howard C, Messina JL, Glass LF: Cutaneous T-cell lymphoma. Int J Dermatol 36:801-809, 1997.

Reddy K, Bhawan J: Histologic mimickers of mycosis fungoides: a review. J Cutan Pathol 34:519-525, 2007.

Siegel RS, Pandolfino T, Guitart J, et al: Primary cutaneous T-cell lymphoma: review and current concepts. J Clin Oncol 18:2908-2925, 2000.

Willemze R, Jaffe E, Burg G, et al: WHO-EORTC classification for cutaneous lymphomas. Blood 105:3768-3785, 2005.

PRIMARY CUTANEOUS CD30-POSITIVE T-CELL LYMPHOMA (ANAPLASTIC LARGE CELL LYMPHOMA)

Clinical Features

- Represents the malignant end in the spectrum of related diseases that include lymphomatoid papulosis
- Characterized by the presence of atypical lymphoid cells expressing CD30 antigen
- Presents as one or multiple large nodules
- Frequently ulcerated
- Patients of any age: systemic involvement more common in children

Histopathology

- Dense dermal infiltrate of large atypical lymphocytes with abundant cytoplasm and irregular vesicular nuclei with coarse chromatin (Figure 2-81A and B)
- Multinucleated cells often seen
- Mitotic figures may be present
- Infiltrate may extend into the subcutaneous tissue

Special Stains and Immunohistochemistry

- Anaplastic lymphoid cells are positive for CD30
- Most of the neoplastic cells are CD4 positive

Other Techniques for Diagnosis

- Gene rearrangement studies show clonal rearrangement of the T-cell receptor gene
- ALK-1 positivity indicates possible cutaneous involvement by systemic anaplastic large cell lymphoma

Differential Diagnosis

- Lymphomatoid Papulosis
  - Presents clinically as multiple small lesions
  - Histologically, the infiltrate is mixed, and fewer atypical lymphoid cells are present
- Hodgkin Disease
  - Cutaneous involvement is secondary to extension from involved lymph nodes; very rare
  - Characterized by presence of Reed-Sternberg or lacunar cells (positive for CD15 and CD30)

PEARLS

- *CD30-positive cells are also seen in late-stage (transformed) mycosis fungoides and pleomorphic T-cell lymphoma*
- *CD30 expression is also seen in carcinomas such as embryonal carcinoma*
- *Primary cutaneous anaplastic large cell lymphoma should be differentiated from secondary cutaneous involvement of primary systemic lymphoma and other high-grade lymphomas that are associated with significantly worse prognosis*

SELECTED REFERENCES

Bekkenk MW, Geelen FA, van Voorst Vader PC, et al: Primary and secondary cutaneous CD30(+) lymphoproliferative disorders: a report from the Dutch Cutaneous Lymphoma Group on the long-term follow-up data of 219 patients and guidelines for diagnosis and treatment. Blood 95:3653-3661, 2000.

Kummer JA, Vermeer MH, Dukers D, et al: Most primary cutaneous CD30-positive lymphoproliferative disorders have a CD4-positive cytotoxic T-cell phenotype. J Invest Dermatol 109:636-640, 1997.

Leboit PE: Lymphomatoid papulosis and cutaneous CD30+ lymphoma. Am J Dermatopathol 18:221, 1996.

Murphy GF, Hsu M: Cutaneous lymphomas and leukemias. In Elder DE, Elenitsas R, Johnson BL Jr, et al (eds): Lever's Histopathology of Skin, 10th ed. Philadelphia, Lippincott Williams & Wilkins, 2008, p 911.

Paulli M, Berti E, Rosso R, et al: CD30/Ki-1-positive lymphoproliferative disorders of the skin: clinicopathologic correlation and statistical analysis of 86 cases. A multicentric study from the European Organization for Research and Treatment of Cancer. Cutaneous Lymphoma Project Group. J Clin Oncol 13:1343, 1995.

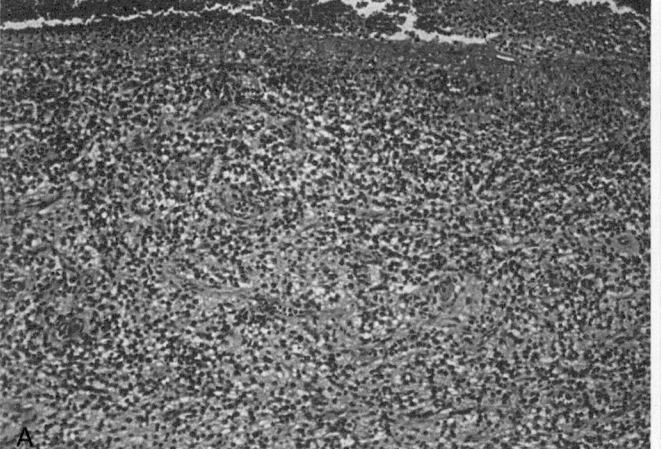 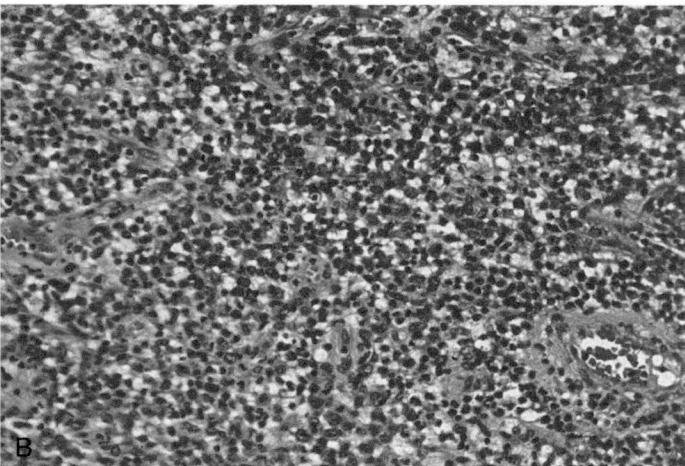

Figure 2-81. Primary cutaneous anaplastic large cell lymphoma. A, Histologic section shows epidermal ulceration and a dense dermal infiltrate of lymphoid cells. **B,** High-power view shows highly atypical lymphoid cells with irregular vesicular nuclei and coarse chromatin. These cells are typically positive for CD30.

Chapter 3
Head and Neck

MICHELLE D. WILLIAMS • ADEL K. EL-NAGGAR

CHAPTER OUTLINE

THYROID GLAND

GRANULOMATOUS THYROIDITIS (de QUERVAIN THYROIDITIS)

Clinical Features

- Also called subacute thyroiditis
- Presents with clinically marked tenderness of thyroid, fever, sore throat, and malaise most likely related to systemic viral illness
- Most commonly affects middle-aged women
- Majority of cases show complete resolution; initial phase often is hyperthyroid (elevated thyroxine [T_4] and triiodothyronine [T_3] levels); may lead to hypothyroidism, usually euthyroid on resolution
- Rarely comes to surgery; treated with aspirin, steroids

Gross Pathology

- Asymmetrically enlarged, firm thyroid
- Nodular process involving entire gland

Histopathology

- Nodular process, variable fibrosis
- Mixed inflammatory infiltrate: lymphoplasmacytic, giant cells, neutrophils with microabscesses (early), and foamy histiocytes
- Giant cells contain ingested extravasated colloid material (Figure 3-1)
- Centered around follicles, which are lost in later stage

Special Stains and Immunohistochemistry

- May need acid-fast bacillus (AFB) stain and Gomori methenamine silver (GMS) stain to evaluate for infectious etiology

Other Techniques for Diagnosis

- Noncontributory

Differential Diagnosis

ACUTE THYROIDITIS

- Neutrophilic infiltration within thyroid gland parenchyma
- Microabscesses and necrosis common, possible vasculitis
- No granuloma formation
- Caused by bacterial, fungal, or viral infections

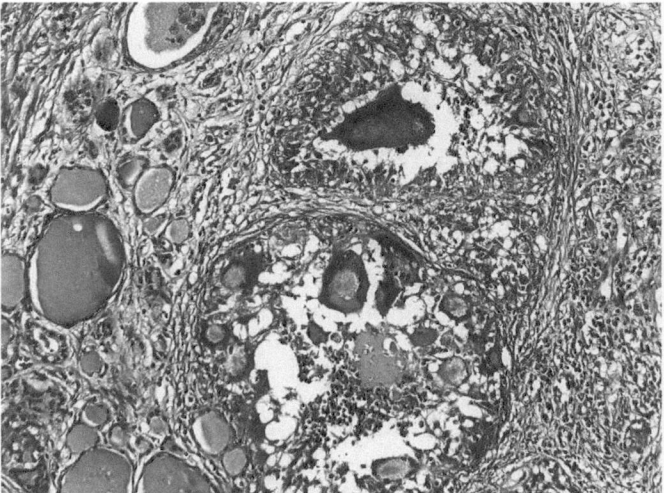

Figure 3-1. Subacute thyroiditis (de Quervain thyroiditis). Section shows foreign-body giant cell granulomas. The giant cells contain ingested colloid material.

GRANULOMATOUS DISEASES

- Sarcoidosis: granulomas (noncaseating) in interstitial location
- Tuberculosis: caseating granulomas (AFB stain)
- Fungal: usually acute and necrotizing, less likely granulomatous (GMS stain)

RIEDEL THYROIDITIS

- Diffuse fibrotic process involving the thyroid obliterating the thyroid architecture
- Fibrosis extends to soft tissue outside the thyroid
- Giant cells are absent

HASHIMOTO THYROIDITIS

- Lymphocytic thyroiditis with germinal center formation and oxyphilic change of the follicular epithelium
- May have extensive fibrosis with follicular loss and architectural distortion

PALPATION THYROIDITIS

- Result of minor trauma to thyroid tissue
- Usually an incidental finding
- Scattered small foci of histiocytes, few lymphocytes, and rare giant cells within thyroid follicles (no neutrophils)

PEARLS

- *Associated with systemic viral infection, usually self-limited, ending euthyroid*
- *Neutrophilic inflammation only seen in initial or early stage of disease*

SELECTED REFERENCES

Benbassat CA, Olchovsky D, Tsvetov G, Shimon I: Subacute thyroiditis: clinical characteristics and treatment outcome in fifty-six consecutive patients diagnosed between 1999 and 2005. J Endocrinol Invest 30:631-635, 2007.

Duininck TM, van Heerden JA, Fatourechi V, et al: De Quervain's thyroiditis: surgical experience. Endocrine Pract 8:255-258, 2002.

Kojima M, Nakamura S, Oyama T, et al: Cellular composition of subacute thyroiditis: an immunohistochemical study of six cases. Pathol Res Pract 198:833-837, 2002.

CHRONIC LYMPHOCYTIC THYROIDITIS (HASHIMOTO THYROIDITIS)

Clinical Features

- Immune-mediated inflammatory disease
- Autoantibodies detected in serum: antithyroglobulin, antithyroid peroxidase, antithyroid microsomal antibodies
- Marked female predominance (5:1); peak in middle-aged women
- Higher incidence in high-iodine areas (United States, Japan)
- Clinically hypothyroid with diffuse, firm, enlarged thyroid
- Familial cases; associations with human leukocyte antigen (HLA)-DR3 and HLA-DR5
- Higher incidence in Turner and Down syndromes and familial Alzheimer disease
- May coexist with other autoimmune diseases (Sjögren syndrome, diabetes, others)
- Increased risk for primary thyroid lymphoma
- IgG4 may be related to a subset with fibrosis

Gross Pathology

- Firm, diffusely enlarged thyroid
- Cut surface is pale tan-yellow and nodular (Figure 3-2A)

Histopathology

- Marked lymphoplasmacytic infiltration with germinal center formation (Figure 3-2B)
- Follicles are small with scant colloid
- Oncocytic metaplasia (Hürthle cell change) with enlarged, hyperchromatic nuclei of follicles may show proliferation (dominant nodules)
- Squamous metaplasia is common
- Fibrosis varies; marked in fibrous variant
- Nodularity of follicles and inflammation may extend into adjacent soft tissue (do not mistake for metastasis in lymph node)
- Optically clear and enlarged follicular nuclei often present

Special Stains and Immunohistochemistry

- Rarely necessary—inflammation is mixed B (CD20) and T (CD3, CD4, CD8) cells, plasma cells polyclonal (κ and λ cells)

Other Techniques for Diagnosis

- Clinical evaluation for antibodies

Differential Diagnosis

EXTRANODAL MARGINAL ZONE B-CELL LYMPHOMA (MUCOSA-ASSOCIATED LYMPHOID TISSUE [MALT] LYMPHOMA)
- Rapid enlargement with sheets of lymphocytic infiltrate
- Increased risk in Hashimoto thyroiditis

ASSOCIATED PAPILLARY THYROID CARCINOMA
- Look for architectural distortion, fibrosis, invasive nests
- Cellular proliferation with strict nuclear criteria of papillary carcinoma
- Optically clear and enlarged nuclei may accompany lymphocytic thyroiditis

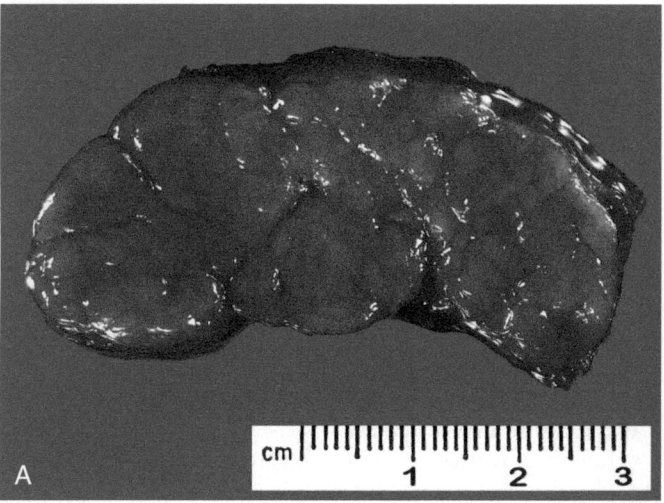
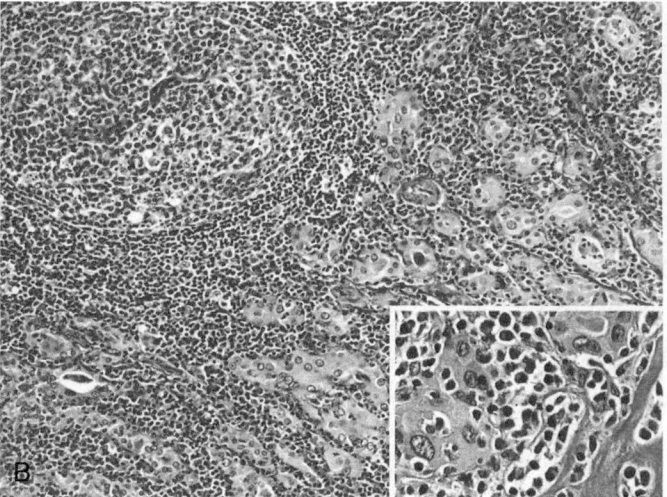

Figure 3-2. Hashimoto thyroiditis. **A,** Gross photograph showing thyroid enlargement with a pale lobulated cut surface. **B,** Marked lymphocytic infiltration with germinal center formation; *inset* shows follicular atrophy, marked plasma cell infiltrate, and fibrosis.

FOLLICULAR NEOPLASM

- Well-circumscribed lesion with capsule
- Define based on capsular breach and lymphovascular invasion

NONSPECIFIC LYMPHOCYTIC THYROIDITIS

- Scattered, patchy chronic inflammation, occasional germinal center
- Lacking oncocytic changes
- Minimal fibrosis

PEARLS

- *May coexist with other thyroid neoplasms (especially papillary thyroid carcinoma); follicular nuclear changes may overlap*
- *Rare malignant transformation into lymphoma (MALT, diffuse large B-cell lymphoma)*
- *Benign follicles and lymphocytes may form nodules separated from the gland (parasitic nodule) in soft tissue*

SELECTED REFERENCES

Deshapande V, Huck A, Ooi E, et al: Fibrosing variant of Hashimoto thyroiditis is an IgG4 related disease. J Clin Pathol 65:725-728, 2012.

MacDonald L, Yazdi HM: Fine needle aspiration biopsy of Hashimoto's thyroiditis: sources of diagnostic error. Acta Cytol 43:400-406, 1999.

Nguyen GK, Ginsberg J, Crockford PM, Villanueva RR: Hashimoto's thyroiditis: cytodiagnostic accuracy and pitfalls. Diagn Cytopathol 16:531-536, 1997.

RIEDEL THYROIDITIS

Clinical Features

- Also called Riedel struma, fibrous thyroiditis
- Very rare; predilection for women (5:1) with peak in fifth decade
- Clinically appears as an ill-defined, extremely firm, painless goiter
- May present with dyspnea as a result of tracheal compression
- One third of patients will develop a process in other sites: mediastinal or retroperitoneal fibrosis, sclerosing cholangitis (regarded as a manifestation of the idiopathic inflammatory fibrosclerosis disorders)

Gross Pathology

- Diffuse enlargement of thyroid gland, hard, stonelike with adherent soft tissue
- Cut surface white, fibrotic, and "woody"

Histopathology

- Prominent finding is fibrosis extending into soft tissue and muscle (greater than inflammation)
- Scattered mixed chronic inflammatory infiltrate (lymphocytes, plasma cells, neutrophils, monocytes, eosinophils) (Figure 3-3)
- "Occlusive phlebitis" with infiltration of veins by lymphocytes and plasma cells; vessels have thickened wall and myxoid change
- Giant cells or germinal centers are not present

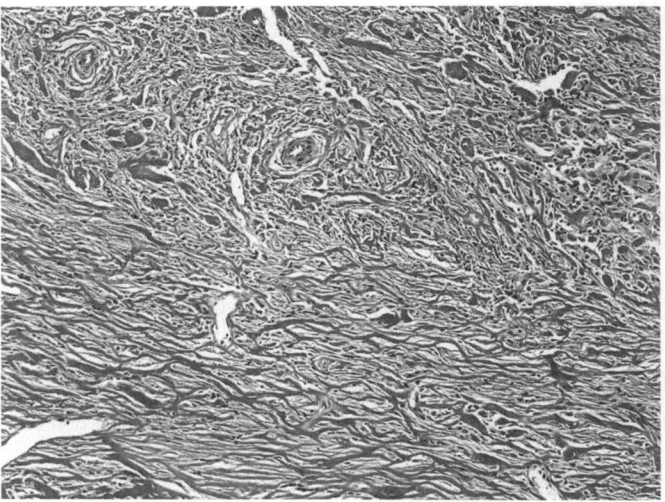

Figure 3-3. Riedel thyroiditis. Diffuse fibrosis is present with scattered inflammatory cells.

Special Stains and Immunohistochemistry

- Noncontributory

Other Techniques for Diagnosis

- Noncontributory

Differential Diagnosis

HASHIMOTO THYROIDITIS (FIBROUS VARIANT)

- Characterized by lobulated, follicular epithelium with oncocytic change, giant cells, lymphocytes with germinal center formation, and plasma cells
- Eosinophils not identified

UNDIFFERENTIATED THYROID CARCINOMA

- Scattered malignant cells (spindle, epithelioid, or pleomorphic) within fibrosis
- Cytokeratin may assist in identification of tumor cells within fibrosis and outside of the thyroid gland

GRANULOMATOUS (SUBACUTE) THYROIDITIS

- Asymmetrical enlargement of the thyroid gland
- Granulomas with giant cells involving follicles, neutrophils at early stage

PEARLS

- *Clinically may be mistaken for malignancy*
- *Treatment with corticosteroid or tamoxifen therapy; surgery for compression*
- *Benign: self-limited (almost half develop hypothyroidism)*

SELECTED REFERENCES

Harigopal M, Sahoo S, Recant WM, DeMay RM: Fine-needle aspiration of Riedel's disease: report of a case and review of the literature. Diagn Cytopathol 30:193-197, 2004.

Schwaegerle SW, Bauer TW, Esselstyn CB: Riedel's thyroiditis. Am J Clin Pathol 90:715-722, 1988.

Yasmeen T, Khan S, Patel SG, et al: Clinical case seminar. Riedel's thyroiditis: report of a case complicated by spontaneous hypoparathyroidism, recurrent laryngeal nerve injury, and Horner's syndrome. J Clin Endocrinol Metab 87:3543-3547, 2002.

GRAVES DISEASE (DIFFUSE TOXIC GOITER)

Clinical Features

- Autoimmune thyroid disease; thyroid-stimulating immunoglobulin (TSI)
- Peak in third to fourth decade; marked predominance in woman at least 5:1
- Strong association with HLA-DR3 and HLA-B8
- Clinically presents with thyrotoxicosis: muscle weakness, weight loss, exophthalmos, tachycardia, and goiter
- Suppressed thyroid-stimulating hormone (TSH), increased T_4 and T_3

Gross Pathology

- Diffuse enlargement of the thyroid, usually symmetrical (Figure 3-4A)
- Diffusely beefy-red cut surface

Histopathology

- Hyperplastic thyroid follicles with papillary infoldings (Figure 3-4B)
- Follicular nuclei remain round and basally located, may be clear
- Colloid is typically decreased; when present, shows prominent peripheral scalloping
- Colloid increases after treatment
- Lymphocytic inflammation patchy in stroma (varies)
- Nuclear atypia and stromal fibrosis may be seen after radioactive iodine therapy

Special Stains and Immunohistochemistry

- Noncontributory

Other Techniques for Diagnosis

- Clinical evaluation for antibodies and thyroid levels

Differential Diagnosis

ADENOMATOID NODULE, NODULAR HYPERPLASIA

- Follicles of varying sizes with occasional Sanderson polsters (groups of small, active follicles at one pole)
- Nonencapsulated

PAPILLARY THYROID CARCINOMA

- Complete nuclear features are absent in Graves disease (overlapping, grooving)
- Invasive pattern when present is helpful

PEARLS

- *Treatment is drug therapy or radioactive iodine; surgery if uncontrolled*
- *Morphologic appearance cannot predict the patient's current functional status*
- *Radioactive iodine causes nuclear atypia in follicular cells of no significance*

SELECTED REFERENCES

LiVolsi VA: The pathology of autoimmune thyroid disease: a review. Thyroid 4:333-339, 1994.

Lloyd RV, Douglas BR, Young WF: Endocrine diseases. In King DW (ed): Atlas of Nontumor Pathology. Washington, ARP Press, 2002, pp 125-133.

Takamatso J, Takeda K, Katayama S, et al: Epithelial hyperplasia and decreased colloid content of the thyroid gland in triiodothyronine predominant Graves disease. J Endocrinol Metab 75:1145-1150, 1992.

MULTINODULAR GOITER

Clinical Features

- Also known as adenomatoid goiter, adenomatous hyperplasia
- Incidence of 3% to 5% in general population; endemic in iodine-deficient areas
- Probably caused by impairment of hormone production
- Adult females predominate over adult males (8:1)
- Clinically often asymptomatic; may cause discomfort, compression
- May grow to massive size in neck or mediastinum
- Number and size of nodules varies; dominant nodule leads to workup

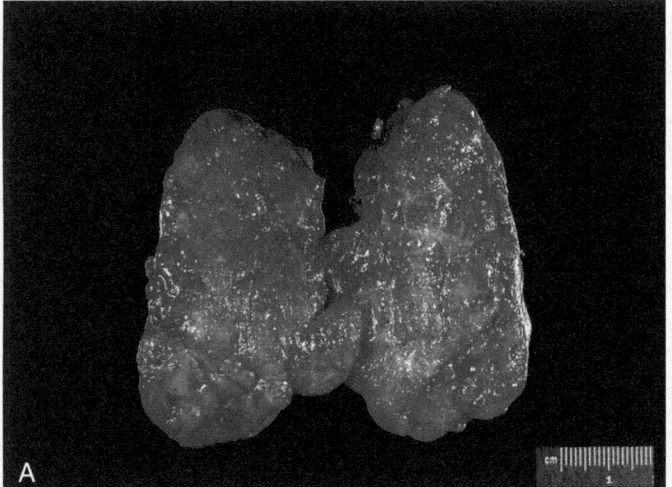
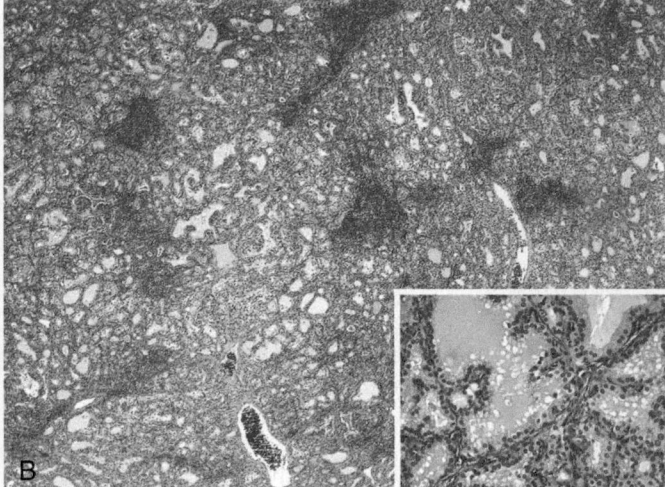

Figure 3-4. Graves disease. A, Gross photograph of a diffusely enlarged pale thyroid. **B,** Low-power view shows scant colloid in hyperplastic follicles with papillary formations and inflammatory infiltrate; *inset* shows bland nuclei, papillary growth pattern, and scalloped colloid.

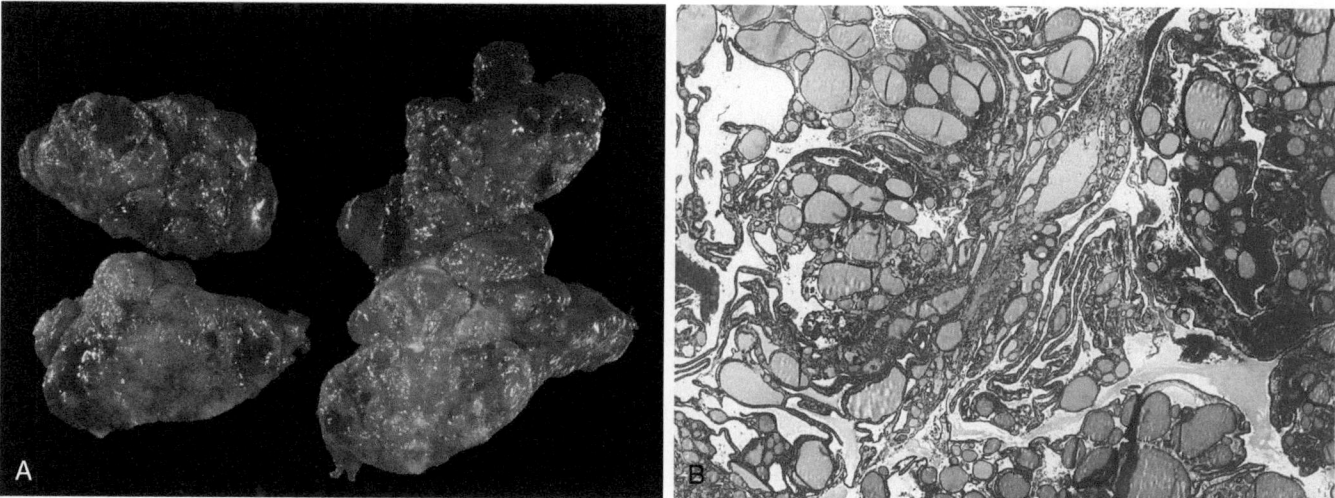

Figure 3-5. Goiter. A, Gross photograph of an enlarged thyroid with nodularity, fibrosis, and hemorrhage. **B,** Thyroid follicles vary in size and are often dilated with colloid accumulation.

Gross Pathology

- Enlarged, nodular thyroid gland, may be asymmetrical (Figure 3-5A)
- Cut surface shows various-sized nodules, often with colloid
- Variegated appearance from hemorrhage to cystic degeneration and calcification

Histopathology

- Heterogeneous, unencapsulated, medium to large distended follicles (Figure 3-5B)
- May have scattered, solid, microfollicular nodules; papillary hyperplasia; or oncocytic changes
- Surrounding thyroid follicles are usually not compressed by nodules
- Background of hemorrhage, fibrosis, calcification
- Parasite nodules (nodules separated from the main gland) are common

Special Stains and Immunohistochemistry

- Noncontributory

Other Techniques for Diagnosis

- Noncontributory

Differential Diagnosis

FOLLICULAR ADENOMA

- Typically solitary
- Composed of uniform small follicles or macrofollicles
- Distinct fibrous capsule surrounds nodular proliferation
- Compression of adjacent thyroid tissue

GRAVES DISEASE

- Gross examination: diffuse, beefy-red, less nodular than multinodular goiter
- Hyperplastic thyroid follicles with papillary infoldings
- Vacuolated cytoplasm of follicular cells, and colloid with scalloped borders
- Laboratory tests indicate hyperthyroidism

AMYLOID GOITER

- Diffusely enlarged thyroid; waxy, pale cut surface

- Amyloid deposits around vessels and intercellular between follicles
- Secondary follicle atrophy and squamous metaplasia
- Congo red stain with polarization to detect birefringent apple-green amyloid
- Clinical history, evaluation for cause (e.g., myeloma, rheumatologic diseases)

PEARLS

- *Cellular hyperplastic nodules can be difficult to distinguish from follicular neoplasms by fine-needle aspiration (FNA)*
- *Most common cause of sudden increase in size of hyperplastic nodules is hemorrhage and cystic degeneration*
- *Extensive nodularity and enlargement may extend to mediastinum and cause detached nodules (parasitic thyroid nodules)*

SELECTED REFERENCES

Kotwal A, Priya R, Qadeer I: Goiter and other iodine deficiency disorders: a systematic review of epidemiological studies to deconstruct the complex web [erratum in: Arch Med Res 38:366, 2007]. Arch Med Res 38:1-14, 2007.

Krohn K, Führer D, Bayer Y, et al. Molecular pathogenesis of euthyroid and toxic multinodular goiter. Endocr Rev 26:504-524, 2005.

Ríos A, Rodríguez JM, Canteras M, et al: Risk factors for malignancy in multinodular goitres. Eur J Surg Oncol 30:58-62, 2004.

DYSHORMONOGENETIC GOITER

Clinical Features

- Rare genetic disorder of defects in thyroid hormone synthesis pathway, most commonly cannot incorporate iodine
- Patients are usually hypothyroid, frequently with enlarged thyroid
- May present with congenital hypothyroidism; mean age, 16 years
- Slight female predominance
- Rare cases of associated carcinoma; predominately follicular carcinomas
- Surgery in children or young adult for dominant nodule or compression

Gross Pathology

- Enlarged for age, frequently nodular, lacking colloid

Histopathology

- Nodular arrangement of small follicles with scant colloid separated by fibrous trabeculae; may show papillary areas (Figure 3-6)
- Often hypercellular with marked cellular pleomorphism (thyroid cancer is not diagnosed by pleomorphism)
- Follicles may extend to involve adjacent soft tissue; not a sign of malignancy

Special Stains and Immunohistochemistry

- Noncontributory

Other Techniques for Diagnosis

- Clinical evaluation for underlying genetic defect

Differential Diagnosis

NODULAR HYPERPLASIA

- Bland follicular cells forming nonencapsulated nodules
- Frequently follicles enlarged with colloid

FOLLICULAR ADENOMA, CARCINOMA

- Uniform, small follicles (unlike atypical cytology of background follicles in dyshormonogenetic goiter)
- Nodule surrounded by fibrous capsule
- Vascular invasion or capsular invasion must be present to make a diagnosis of follicular carcinoma

GRAVES DISEASE

- Hyperplastic thyroid follicles with papillary infoldings
- Follicular cells with granular cytoplasm
- Scant colloid; when present, apical vacuolation leads to scalloping of colloid
- Laboratory tests indicating hyperthyroidism

POSTRADIOACTIVE IODINE THERAPY

- Cytologic atypia
- Various degrees of fibrosis

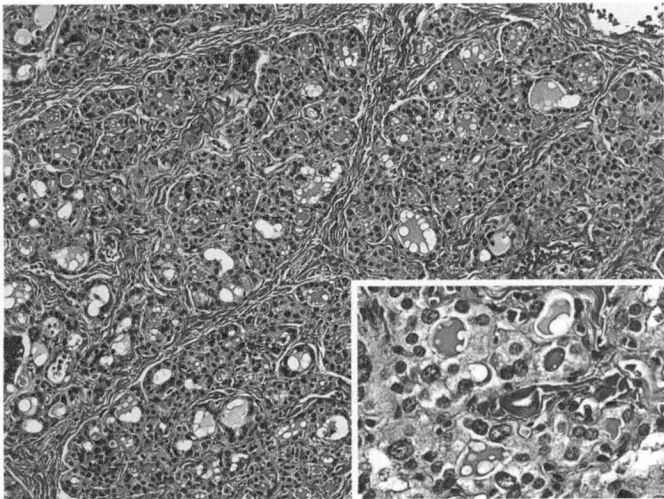

Figure 3-6. Dyshormonogenetic goiter. Small thyroid follicles with scant colloid composed of follicular cells with atypical nuclei (*inset*) and surrounded by dense fibrosis.

- Clinical history of prior therapy
- Frequently an older patient group

PEARLS

- *Histology is diagnostic, although clinical history should also be noted; frequently patient is young*
- *Caution in diagnosing cancer in this setting, requires characteristic nuclear features to diagnosis papillary carcinoma (presence of papillary architecture is not sufficient); diagnosis of follicular carcinoma requires capsular or vascular invasion*
- *Nuclei of the follicular neoplasm are frequently more uniform than the background dyshormogenetic thyroid*

SELECTED REFERENCES

Deshpande AH, Bobhate SK: Cytological features of dyshormonogenetic goiter: case report and review of the literature. Diagn Cytopathol 33:252-254, 2005.

Ghossein RA, Rosai J, Heffess C: Dyshormonogenetic goiter: a clinicopathologic study of 56 cases. Endocr Pathol 8:283-292, 1997.

Kennedy JS: The pathology of dyshormonogenetic goitre. J Pathol 99:251-264, 1969.

THYROGLOSSAL DUCT CYST

Clinical Features

- Congenital persistence of the thyroid developmental tract
- Midline, from foramen cecum (tongue) to hyoid bone, to pyramidal lobe or isthmus
- May fistulize to skin
- Moves on swallowing
- Most often detected during childhood or young adulthood
- Associated thyroid tissue may develop well-differentiated thyroid carcinomas

Gross Pathology

- Cystic lesion in soft tissue, middle third of hyoid bone, skin if fistula present

Histopathology

- Cyst is lined by respiratory or squamous epithelium (Figure 3-7)
- Secondary inflammation and granulation tissue if infected; lining may be lost
- Underlying stroma contains mucus glands and thyroid follicles (50% of cases)

Special Stains and Immunohistochemistry

- Thyroid epithelium is positive for thyroid transcription factor-1 (TTF-1) and thyroglobulin

Other Techniques for Diagnosis

- Noncontributory

Differential Diagnosis

BRANCHIAL CLEFT CYST

- Located in the lateral neck
- Cyst lined by squamous, columnar, or ciliated epithelium or, if ulcerated, by granulation tissue

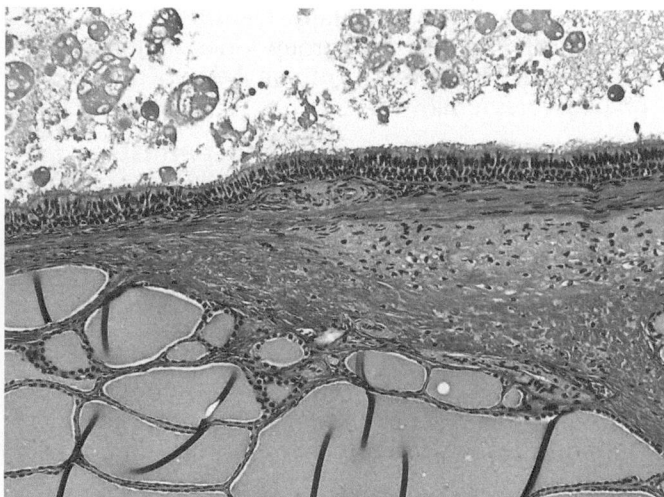

Figure 3-7. Thyroglossal duct cyst. Respiratory epithelium-lined cyst in the midline, often with thyroid follicles in the wall.

- Prominent lymphoid infiltrate in cyst wall
- Cyst may contain anucleated squamous cells, histiocytes, or cholesterol clefts
- Epithelium is thyroglobulin negative (differentiate from metastatic papillary carcinoma)

ADENOMATOID, COLLOID NODULE
- May occur in isthmus or pyramidal lobe, leading to midline mass
- Squamous metaplasia can occur, but squamous debris is rare; colloid is typically abundant
- Lacks ciliated cells

PEARLS

- *Malignancy may occur in the thyroid tissue (most cases involve papillary carcinoma); medullary carcinoma is not seen (different route of embryologic development)*
- *Ciliated cells are occasionally seen on FNA of thyroid gland nodules near the trachea from "tracheal aspirates" if the needle enters the trachea (patient usually coughs when this occurs)*

SELECTED REFERENCES

Allard RH: The thyroglossal cyst. Head Neck Surg 5:134-146, 1982.
Mondin V, Ferlito A, Muzzi E, et al: Thyroglossal duct cyst: personal experience and literature review. Auris Nasus Larynx 35:11-25, 2008.
Shahin A, Burroughs FH, Kirby JP, Ali SZ: Thyroglossal duct cyst: a cytopathologic study of 26 cases. Diagn Cytopathol 33:365-369, 2005.

BRANCHIAL CLEFT CYST

Clinical Features

- Anterolateral neck mass, multiple locations based on which pouch is affected
- Derived from first, second, third, or fourth branchial pouches
- Congenital, identified in children and young adults (be wary in older adults)

Gross Pathology
- Mostly unilocular cysts with slightly granular inner surface due to presence of numerous lymphoid follicles
- May be associated with a fistula tract

Histopathology
- Cyst and fistula tracts are lined by squamous, columnar, or ciliated epithelium
- Subepithelial stroma contains abundant lymphoid tissue
- Lining contains mucinous and serous or even sebaceous glands, particularly when located in lower neck area
- Cyst may contain anucleated squames, histiocytes, and cholesterol clefts (Figure 3-8)

Special Stains and Immunohistochemistry
- Noncontributory

Other Techniques for Diagnosis
- Noncontributory

Differential Diagnosis

SQUAMOUS CELL CARCINOMA (SCC) METASTATIC TO LYMPH NODE WITH SECONDARY CYSTIC CHANGE
- Must be considered in all adult patients with neck mass
- Aggregates of malignant squamous cells forming cyst in lymph node
- May at times appear cytologically bland
- Squamous pearl formation may be seen
- Sights of primary tumor are frequently in Waldeyer ring (tonsils, base of tongue) and are not apparent at time of presentation (image and biopsy for primary)

CYSTIC PAPILLARY THYROID CARCINOMA METASTATIC TO LYMPH NODE
- Cystic lining may be flattened without overt nuclear changes
- Adequate sections usually show papillary architecture and nuclear features
- Thyroglobulin level on FNA fluid diagnostic
- Lateral neck location of thyroid tissue equals metastasis
- TTF-1 and thyroglobulin will be positive

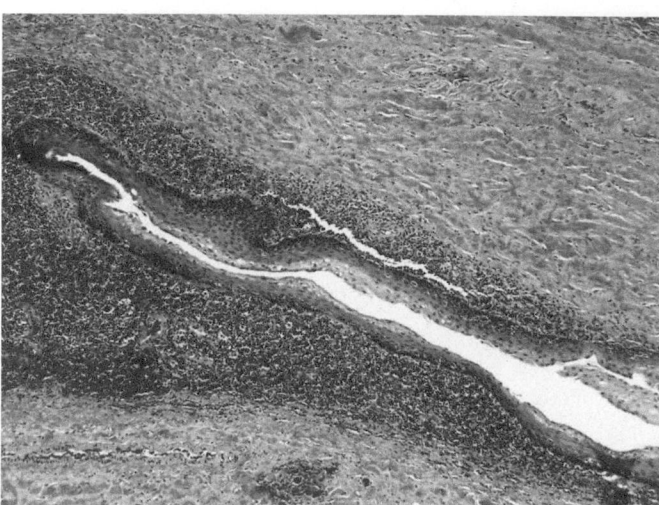

Figure 3-8. Branchial cleft cyst. Epithelium-lined cystic space has associated lymphoid stroma; the cyst is often lined by respiratory epithelium but may be squamous, as in this case.

SELECTED REFERENCES

Al-Khateeb TH, Al Zoubi F: Congenital neck masses: a descriptive retrospective study of 252 cases. J Oral Maxillofac Surg 65:2242-2247, 2007.

Burgess KL, Hartwick RWJ, Bedard YC: Metastatic squamous cell carcinoma presenting as a neck cyst: differential diagnosis from inflamed branchial cleft cyst in fine-needle aspirates. Acta Cytol 37:494-498, 1993.

Firat P, Ersoz C, Uguz A, Onder S: Cystic lesions of the head and neck: cytohistological correlation in 63 cases. Cytopathology 18:184-190, 2007.

TERATOMA

Clinical Features

- Very rare primary thyroid neoplasm with trilineage differentiation
- Reported in newborn patients to those in their 50s; same incidence in males and females
- Teratomas are classified as benign (mature), immature, and malignant
- Teratomas of infants: > 90% benign, often contain immature components
- Teratomas in adolescents and adults: 50% malignant

Gross Pathology

- Variable with multiloculated cysts, soft glial tissue, gritty bone or cartilage (Figure 3-9)

Histopathology

- Mixture of mature or immature tissues (ectoderm, endoderm, and mesoderm)

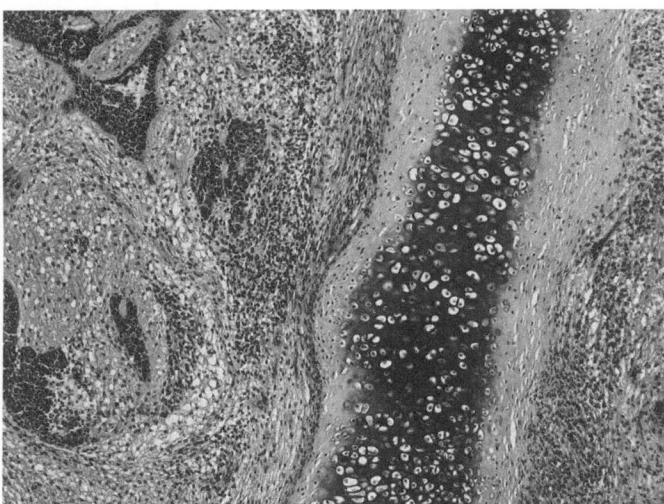

Figure 3-9. Thyroid teratoma. Trilineage cellular components are present—mature cartilage, glial tissue, and a malignant epithelial component.

- Thyroid parenchyma should be identified
- Maturation of neural tissue determines grade
- Frank malignant component may be present (i.e., embryonal carcinoma)

Special Stains and Immunohistochemistry

- Various stains to highlight lineages

Other Techniques for Diagnosis

- Noncontributory

Differential Diagnosis

THYROGLOSSAL DUCT CYST
- Cyst lined by respiratory or squamous epithelium
- May be associated with chronic inflammation
- Clinically correlate with anatomic region (anterior, midline)

LYMPHOMA
- Single population of atypical small cells
- Other tissue types are not identified
- Immunohistochemistry (IHC) to identify cell type

RHABDOMYOSARCOMA
- Single population of tumor cells without other lineages
- Rhabdomyoblasts may be found in teratomas

SELECTED REFERENCES

Nishihara E, Miyauchi A, Hirokawa M, et al: Benign thyroid teratomas manifest painful cystic and solid composite nodules: three case reports and a review of the literature. Endocrine 30:231-236, 2006.

Thompson LD, Rosai J, Heffess CS: Primary thyroid teratomas: a clinicopathologic study of 30 cases. Cancer 88:1149-1158, 2000.

HYALINIZING TRABECULAR TUMOR

Clinical Features

- Follicular neoplasm of debated classification
- Females affected more than males; patients are usually in their 50s and 60s

Gross Pathology

- Solitary, well-circumscribed nodule

Histopathology

- Trabecular and insular growth patterns (Figure 3-10)
- Large elongated cells with oval nuclei
- Nuclear grooves and intranuclear cytoplasmic inclusions
- Intracytoplasmic bodies and perinuclear halos are common

Special Stains and Immunohistochemistry

- TTF-1 and thyroglobulin positive

Other Techniques for Diagnosis

- *RET/PTC* gene rearrangements in some suggest link to papillary thyroid carcinoma

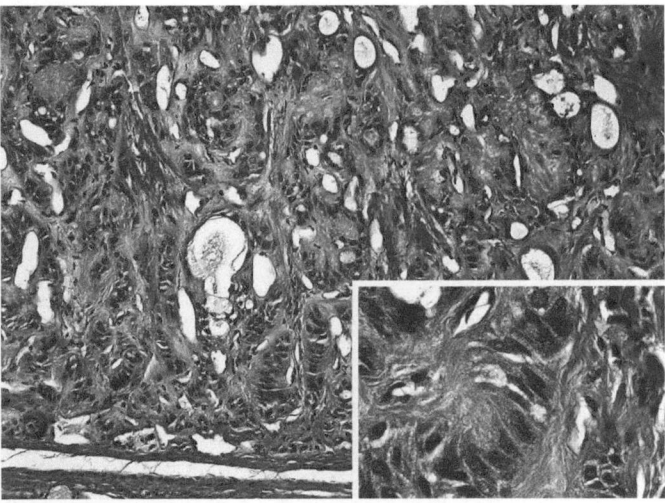

Figure 3-10. Hyalinizing trabecular tumor. Trabeculae and nests of elongated cells with prominent grooves and pseudonuclear inclusions (*inset*).

Differential Diagnosis

PAPILLARY THYROID CARCINOMA
- Shares overlapping nuclear features, including clearing and grooves
- Invasive growth pattern is helpful
- Lymphovascular invasion is often identified

FOLLICULAR ADENOMA
- Nuclei in general are bland and round, lacking clearing and grooving
- Lacks intracytoplasmic bodies

PARAGANGLIOMA
- Rare tumor in thyroid; cells forming nests
- Nuclear features are bland and round, lacking clearing and grooves
- Positive for chromogranin, synaptophysin
- Negative for TTF-1 and thyroglobulin

MEDULLARY THYROID CARCINOMA
- Overlapping nuclear features of grooving and elongation
- Overlapping growth patterns (trabecular)
- Amyloid helpful when present
- Thyroglobulin negative
- Both express TTF-1

PEARLS

- *Unclear if biologically capable of metastasis*
- *Suggested relationship to papillary thyroid carcinoma*
- *Conservative treatment recommended*

SELECTED REFERENCES

Baloch ZW, LiVolsi VA: Cytologic and architectural mimics of papillary thyroid carcinoma: diagnostic challenges in fine-needle aspiration and surgical pathology specimens. Am J Clin Pathol 125:S135-S144, 2006.

Casey MB, Sebo TJ, Carney JA: Hyalinizing trabecular adenoma of the thyroid gland: cytologic features in 29 cases. Am J Surg Pathol 28:859-867, 2004.

Galgano MT, Mills SE, Stelow EB: Hyalinizing trabecular adenoma of the thyroid revisited: a histologic and immunohistochemical study of thyroid lesions with prominent trabecular architecture and sclerosis. Am J Surg Pathol 30:1269-1273, 2006.

LiVolsi VA: Hyalinizing trabecular tumor of the thyroid: adenoma, carcinoma, or neoplasm of uncertain malignant potential? Am J Surg Pathol 24:1683-1684, 2000.

FOLLICULAR ADENOMA

Clinical Features

- Benign tumor more common (about 5:1) than follicular carcinoma
- Usually solitary lesion; mainly affects lobes of thyroid, rare in isthmus
- Predilection for middle-aged women; clinically euthyroid
- Associated with iodine deficiency and Cowden disease (hamartomas, *PTEN* gene)

Gross Pathology

- Solitary, well-circumscribed, round to oval nodule, thin capsule (Figure 3-11A)

Histopathology

- Encapsulated follicular proliferation; variable amount of colloid (Figure 3-11B)
- Thin fibrous capsule may contain small blood vessels; thinner than in follicular carcinoma
- Various architectural patterns: trabecular or solid, microfollicular, and macrofollicular, which have no clinical significance
- Central area may be hypocellular with loose and edematous stroma
- Uniform polygonal follicle cells with round or oval nuclei
- Absent or minimal mitotic activity
- Occasionally bizarre nuclei do not indicate malignancy
- Papillary or pseudopapillary structures without nuclear changes
- Follicular adenoma variants
  - Adenoma with oncocytic (Hürthle) cells
    - Follicular cells with ample eosinophilic cytoplasm with round nuclei and prominent nucleoli
    - More susceptible to infarction, especially after FNA
    - No clinical significance
  - Atypical adenoma, follicular lesion of uncertain malignant potential
    - May show necrosis, infarction, mitoses
    - Thickened capsule with irregularity and partial capsule invasion
    - Lacks lymphovascular invasion
    - Worrisome features without meeting criteria for carcinoma
  - Toxic adenoma (rare)
    - Also called Plummer adenoma
    - Solitary, hyperfunctioning nodule causing hyperthyroidism
    - Cytologic features within nodule mimics Graves disease

Special Stains and Immunohistochemistry

- Thyroglobulin and TTF-1 positive

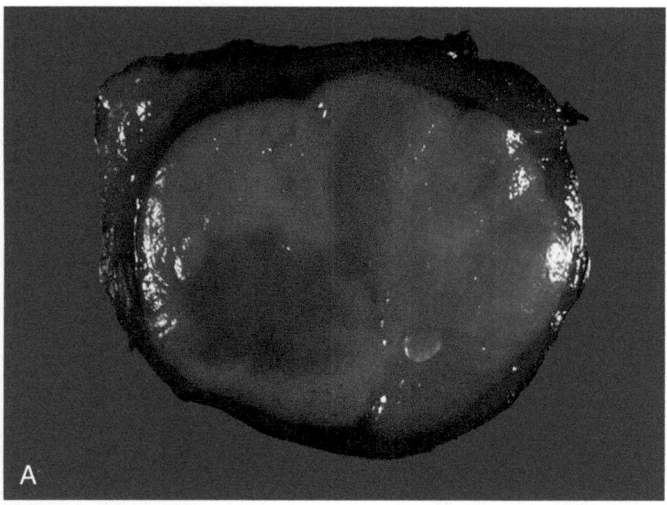
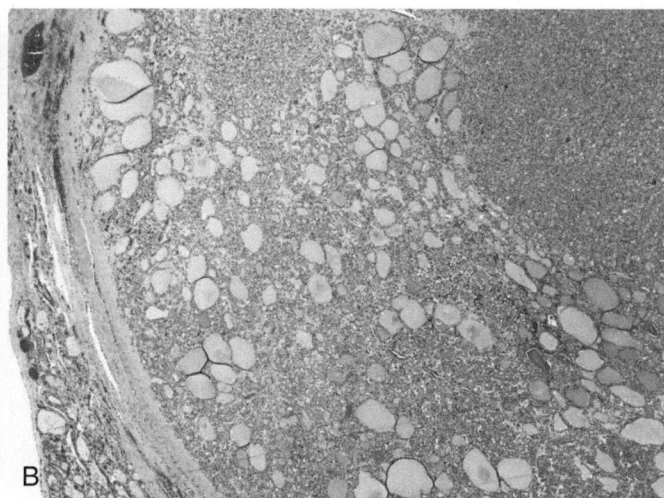

Figure 3-11. Follicular adenoma. A, Gross photograph of a thyroid lobe with a well-defined nodule without a prominent capsule. **B,** The cellular proliferation is well circumscribed with a thin capsule.

- Cytokeratin positive
- Chromogranin and calcitonin negative

Other Techniques for Diagnosis

- One fourth of cases are aneuploid; however, this does not correlate clinically with malignant behavior or recurrence
- Some reports of *Ras* mutations and *PAX/PPARgamma* rearrangements (see "Follicular Carcinoma")

Differential Diagnosis

HYPERPLASTIC NODULE
- Typically multiple; mixture of microfollicles and macrofollicular, marked colloid
- Incomplete fibrous capsule; does not compress surrounding thyroid tissue

FOLLICULAR CARCINOMA
- Follicular proliferation with thick capsule and evidence of vascular invasion or full-thickness capsular invasion by neoplastic follicles

ENCAPSULATED FOLLICULAR VARIANT OF PAPILLARY CARCINOMA
- Characterized by follicular architecture with cytologic features of classic papillary carcinoma, including enlarged, cleared nuclei, and intranuclear cytoplasmic pseudoinclusions
- May have microfollicles or macrofollicles

MEDULLARY THYROID CARCINOMA, NODULAR C-CELL HYPERPLASIA
- Not encapsulated
- Isochromatic cytoplasm versus eosinophilic cytoplasm in follicular cells
- Calcitonin positive; also frequently expresses TTF-1

INTRATHYROIDAL PARATHYROID (NORMAL) OR PARATHYROID ADENOMA
- Well circumscribed, may or may not have intercellular fat
- Small, hyperchromatic nuclei in nests, which may have cytoplasmic clearing

- Parathyroid hormone positive
- Calcitonin and TTF-1 negative

PEARLS

- *FNA shows follicular lesion or follicular neoplasm; treatment is lobectomy or subtotal thyroidectomy*
- *Frozen sections are of little value and are discouraged*
- *Thorough examination of the follicular capsule is warranted*

SELECTED REFERENCES

Baloch ZW, Fleisher S, LiVolsi VA, Gupta PK: Diagnosis of "follicular neoplasm": a gray zone in thyroid fine-needle aspiration cytology. Diagn Cytopathol 26:41-44, 2002.
Baloch ZW, LiVolsi VA: Follicular-patterned lesions of the thyroid: the bane of the pathologist. Am J Clin Pathol 117:143-150, 2002.
Baloch ZW, LiVolsi VA: Our approach to follicular-patterned lesions of the thyroid. J Clin Pathol 60:244-250, 2007.
Suster S: Thyroid tumors with a follicular growth pattern: problems in differential diagnosis. Arch Pathol Lab Med 130:984-988, 2006.

FOLLICULAR CARCINOMA

Clinical Features

- Malignant epithelial tumor with follicular cell differentiation and no features of the other distinctive types of thyroid malignancy
- Constitutes about 5% of thyroid cancers
- In iodine-deficient areas, it comprises between 25% and 40% of thyroid cancers
- Not associated with prior radiation therapy
- Predilection for women
- Patients present with a solitary nodule that is typically "cold" on isotopic scan
- Patients are usually euthyroid

Gross Pathology

- Solid, round tumor with fibrous capsule that is thicker and more irregular than in adenomas, usually larger than 1 cm (Figure 3-12A)

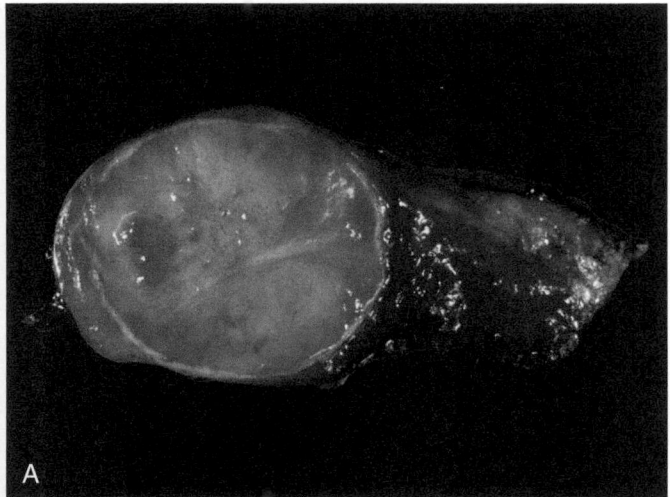

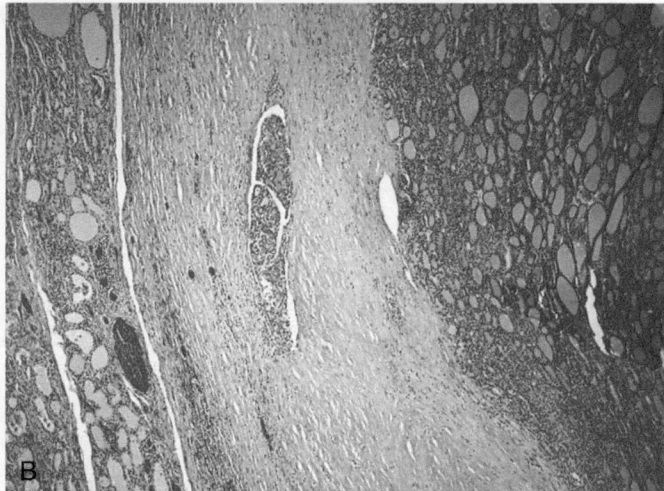

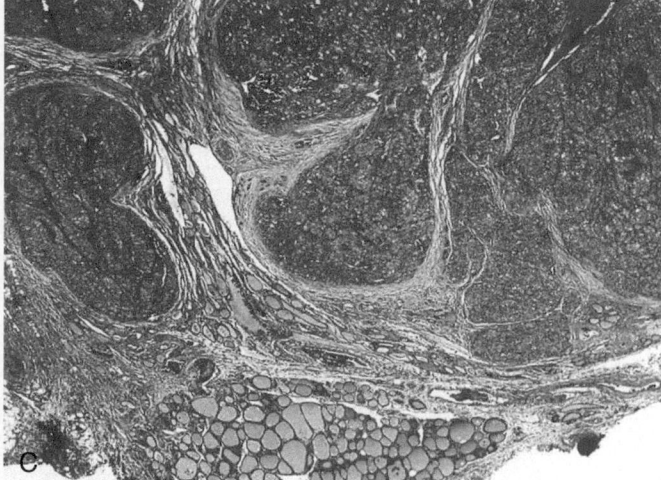

Figure 3-12. Follicular carcinoma. A, Gross photograph of a circumscribed thyroid mass with thickened capsule and gross invasion of the capsule at the superior left aspect of the image. **B,** Lymphovascular invasion is present within the markedly thickened capsule. **C,** Widely invasive follicular carcinoma with nodules extending into the adjacent thyroid parenchyma.

- Cut surface is light-tan and solid; secondary changes such as cystic degeneration, hemorrhage, and fibrosis
- Mahogany-colored nodule corresponds to Hürthle cell morphology

Histopathology (Figures 3-12B and C)

- Frequently divided into (1) minimally invasive and (2) widely invasive, although these definitions are variably used
- Cells similar to those of follicular adenoma: round or oval nuclei in follicular cells
- Various architectural patterns: solid, trabecular, microfollicular, macrofollicular (not clinically significant)
- Diagnosis depends on demonstration of full-thickness capsular or vascular invasion
- Capsular invasion
  - Penetration of entire thickness of capsule is required (mere presence of follicular cell clusters within capsule is not regarded as capsular invasion)
  - Caution of FNA defects in capsule with associated hemorrhage and reactive changes
- Vascular invasion (also termed *angioinvasive follicular carcinoma*)
  - Vessel should be located within or outside the capsule; frequently of large caliber
  - Tumor cells should be within the vascular lumen and must be at least focally attached to the vessel wall (not pushing beneath the vessel)
  - Some require endothelial growth over a portion of the tumor or fibrin deposition

Special Stains and Immunohistochemistry

- Thyroglobulin positive
- No currently available marker to distinguish adenoma from carcinoma

Other Techniques for Diagnosis

- Translocation of *PAX8/PPARgamma* t(2;3) seen in approximately 35% of follicular carcinomas
- Identification of *Ras* mutations (*K-ras, N-ras,* or *H-ras* in 40% to 50%) (also seen in adenomas and follicular variants of papillary carcinoma)

Differential Diagnosis

FOLLICULAR ADENOMA

- Thin fibrous capsule without evidence of vascular invasion

ATYPICAL ADENOMA OR FOLLICULAR LESION OF UNCERTAIN MALIGNANT POTENTIAL

- Cellular follicular lesion with thickened capsule
- Cells may partially invade capsule
- Lymphovascular invasion is not identified

DOMINANT NODULE OF NODULAR HYPERPLASIA

- Background of multiple, variably sized nodules
- No fibrous capsule

FOLLICULAR VARIANT OF PAPILLARY CARCINOMA

- Nuclear features of papillary carcinoma present: overlapping and clearing of nuclei, pseudoinclusions, and nuclear grooves in most of the lesion (not just focally)

FOLLICULAR VARIANT OF MEDULLARY CARCINOMA

- Calcitonin positive and thyroglobulin negative

- Polygonal cells with abundant eosinophilic to clear cytoplasm and coarsely clumped chromatin with inconspicuous nucleoli; may have plasmacytoid appearance

PEARLS

- *Vascular invasion is a more reliable sign of malignancy than capsular invasion*
- *FNA cannot distinguish between follicular lesions (i.e., adenoma from carcinoma), requiring surgical excision for diagnosis*
- *FNA can produce WHAFFT ("worrisome histologic alterations following FNA of the thyroid") (including artifactual capsular invasion)*
- *Typically metastasize via hematogenous route, most commonly to lung and bone*

SELECTED REFERENCES

D'Avanzo A, Treseler P, Ituarte PH, et al: Follicular thyroid carcinoma: histology and prognosis. Cancer 100:1123-1129, 2004.

Kroll TG: Molecular events in follicular thyroid tumors. Cancer Treat Res 122:85-105, 2004.

Leteurtre E, Leroy X, Pattou F, et al: Why do frozen sections have limited value in encapsulated or minimally invasive follicular carcinoma of the thyroid? Am J Clin Pathol 115:370-374, 2001.

LiVolsi VA, Baloch ZW: Follicular neoplasms of the thyroid: view, biases, and experiences. Adv Anat Pathol 11:279-287, 2004.

Rosai J, Kuhn E, Carcangiu ML: Pitfalls in thyroid tumour pathology. Histopathology 49:107-120, 2006.

Thompson LD, Wieneke JA, Paal E, et al: A clinicopathologic study of minimally invasive follicular carcinoma of the thyroid gland with a review of the English literature. Cancer 91:505-524, 2001.

PAPILLARY THYROID CARCINOMA

Clinical Features

- Most common type of thyroid cancer (80%) in the United States
- More common in women (4:1)
- Well-documented association with radiation exposure (after Chernobyl and Hiroshima)
- Relative incidence is higher in areas of high iodine intake compared with follicular carcinoma
- Prognostic features include age and gender (worse when > 45 years of age and male)
- Regional lymph node metastasis is common (50% of cases at presentation); does not adversely affect long-term prognosis

Gross Pathology

- Variable, from well circumscribed to diffusely involving lobe or multifocal
- White-gray, firm, granular cut surface; may have small papillary structures (Figure 3-13A)
- Calcifications may be present

Histopathology (Figures 3-13B and C)

- Complex branching true papillae (contain fibrovascular stalks)
- Papillae lined by neoplastic epithelial cells with characteristic enlarged optically clear, empty "Orphan Annie eye" nuclei (formalin fixation only), nuclear grooves (usually parallel to long axis), cytoplasmic pseudoinclusions, and overlapping nuclei

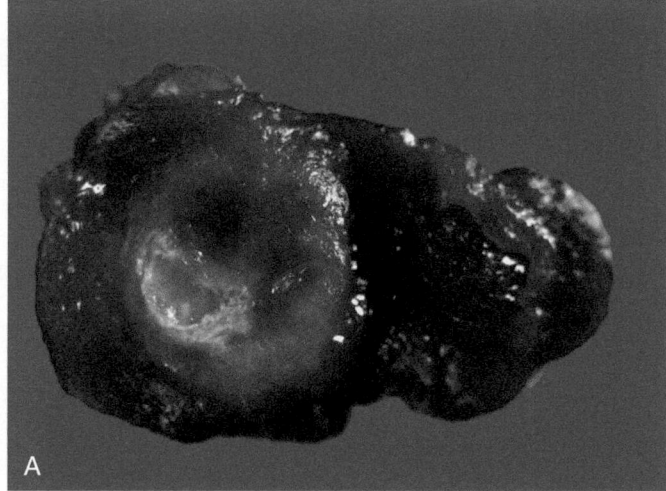

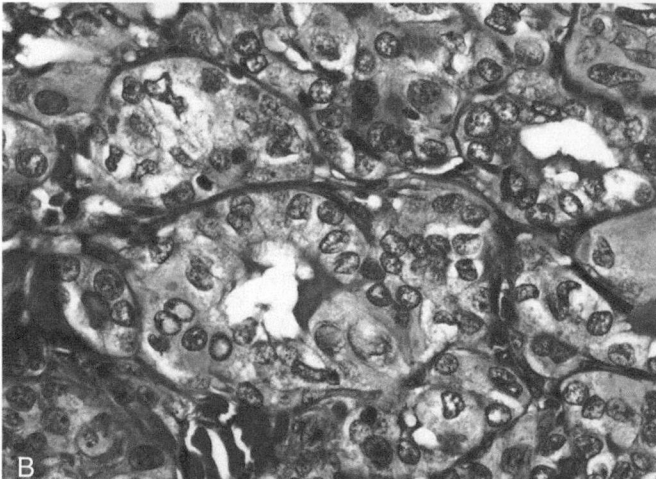

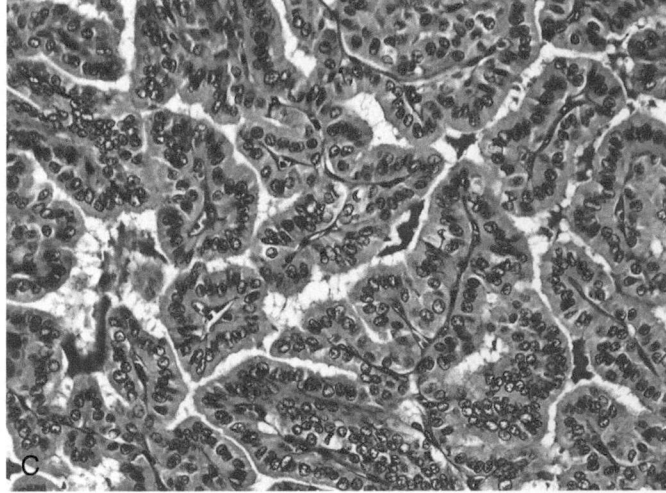

Figure 3-13. Papillary thyroid carcinoma. A, Gross photograph of a thyroid with a partially calcified tumor. **B,** Papillary thyroid carcinoma growing in microfollicles consistent with the follicular variant. **C,** Papillary architecture with fibrovascular cores. The nuclei are clear, elongated, and grooved.

- Psammoma bodies seen in up to 50% of cases
- Cystic growth pattern is commonly present in lymph nodes with flattened nuclei
- Solid areas, squamous metaplasia, are not infrequently seen

- Colloid is thick and dark eosinophilic with bubblegum-like quality
- Stroma is often abundant, and fibrous lymphatic invasion is common
- Multicentricity is common compared with follicular neoplasms
- Histologic variants
  - Microcarcinoma
    - Microscopic tumor less than 1 cm in diameter
    - Subcapsular region and scar growth pattern is common
    - Common at autopsy
    - Most do not require additional treatment
  - Follicular variant of papillary carcinoma
    - Microfollicular or macrofollicular
    - May mimic adenoma or adenomatous nodule
    - Nuclear features must show enlargement, clearing, and grooves throughout most of the lesion
    - Focal papillae may be found if multiple sections are taken
    - Prognosis is similar to that for classic papillary carcinoma
  - Diffuse sclerosing variant
    - Often, diffusely involves both lobes
    - Extensive fibrosis, squamous metaplasia, lymphocytic infiltrate, and psammoma bodies
    - Solid or papillary growth with extensive lymphovascular spread
    - Higher incidence of cervical lymph node and pulmonary metastases
  - Oncocytic variant
    - Distinct Hürthle cell features (abundant eosinophilic cytoplasm) with classic papillary thyroid carcinoma nuclei often with papillary architecture
    - Nuclei frequently do not overlap secondary to ample cytoplasm
    - May be associated with lymphoid stoma in chronic lymphocytic thyroiditis
    - Degenerative changes after FNA are common
  - Tall or columnar cell variant
    - More common in older patients
    - Often greater than 5 cm, extrathyroidal extension and vascular invasion are more frequent
    - Tall cell nuclei at base with cells that are three times as tall as wide and have abundant eosinophilic cytoplasm
    - Columnar nuclei are pseudostratified and luminal with basal cytoplasmic vacuoles and squamous metaplasia
    - Stage for stage, similar to conventional papillary thyroid carcinoma

Special Stains and Immunohistochemistry

- Noncontributory—although high-molecular-weight cytokeratins (CK19), galectin-3, and HBME-1 are noted to be expressed in papillary thyroid carcinoma, lack of sensitivity, and specificity limits their use

Other Techniques for Diagnosis

- Oncogene alterations
  - Point mutation *BRAF*, exon 15 (up to 60%)
  - Translocations of *RET* proto-oncogene with multiple different genes (*RET/PTC* gene rearrangements),

30% more often in children and those with radiation exposure
- *N-ras* mutations particularly follicular variant (10%)
- *TRK* gene rearrangements with multiple genes (10%)
- New tyrosine kinase inhibitors affect the *BRAF* and *RET* pathways and may provide targeted therapy for patients with aggressive disease or distant metastases

Differential Diagnosis

Papillary Hyperplasia in Graves Disease and Adenomatous Goiter

- Classic nuclear features of papillary carcinoma are absent

Follicular Adenoma and Carcinoma

- Most commonly exhibits a microfollicular pattern with fibrous capsule
- Large-vessel vascular invasion frequently seen in follicular carcinoma
- Lack characteristic nuclear features such as enlargement and overlapping of cleared-out nuclei

Medullary Carcinoma

- Spindle and plasmacytoid features; may be follicular or papillary growth pattern
- Amyloid frequently present in stroma (Congo red positive)
- Calcitonin positive and thyroglobulin negative

PEARLS

- *All variants of papillary carcinoma, irrespective of architecture, must have characteristic nuclear features (hypochromasia, elongated nucleus with grooves, and intranuclear pseudoinclusions)*
- *Prognosis correlates with clinical factors (age, sex, stage)*
- *Clear "Orphan Annie eye" nuclei are an artifact of formalin fixation and are not seen in frozen sections and cytologic preparations*
- *Psammoma bodies are not pathognomonic*

Selected References

Akslen LA, LiVolsi VA: Prognostic significance of histologic grading compared with subclassification of papillary thyroid carcinoma. Cancer 88:1902-1908, 2000.

Al-Brahim N, Asa SL: Papillary thyroid carcinoma: an overview. Arch Pathol Lab Med 130:1057-1062, 2006.

DeLellis RA: Pathology and genetics of thyroid carcinoma. J Surg Oncol 94:662-669, 2006.

Michels JJ, Jacques M, Henry-Amar M, Bardet S: Prevalence and prognostic significance of tall cell variant of papillary thyroid carcinoma. Hum Pathol 38:212-219, 2007.

Sanders EM Jr, LiVolsi VA, Brierley J, et al: An evidence-based review of poorly differentiated thyroid cancer. World J Surg 31:934-945, 2007.

Trovisco V, Soares P, Sobrinho-Simoes M: BRAF mutations in the etiopathogenesis, diagnosis, and prognosis of thyroid carcinomas. Hum Pathol 37:781-786, 2006.

MEDULLARY THYROID CARCINOMA

Clinical Features

- Malignant tumor composed of neural crest–derived C cells
- Accounts for up to 5% of thyroid malignancies
- Can be sporadic (80%) or hereditary (20%); more common in women

- Lymph nodes common at presentation (about 50%)
- Elevated serum calcitonin; can be used to monitor residual, recurrent, or metastatic disease postoperatively; carcinoembryonic antigen (CEA) elevation is usually a late finding in progressive disease
- Hereditary types include familial medullary thyroid carcinoma and multiple endocrine neoplasia (MEN) IIA and IIB and are caused by different germline mutations in *RET* proto-oncogene
  - Sporadic type
    - Occurs in middle-aged adults, some show *RET* mutations in the tumors
    - Solitary tumor mass
  - Familial medullary thyroid carcinoma
    - Medullary carcinoma without other endocrine abnormalities, onset in adults
  - MEN IIA
    - Medullary carcinoma, pheochromocytoma, parathyroid adenoma or hyperplasia
    - Mean age at diagnosis in MEN IIA cases is in the third decade
    - Often multicentric and involve both thyroid lobes
  - MEN IIB
    - All patients develop medullary thyroid carcinoma, with onset in childhood or young adult
    - Same possible endocrinopathies as MEN IIA, plus gastrointestinal and ocular ganglioneuromas and skeletal abnormalities

Gross Pathology

- Often circumscribed
- Cut section is tan-yellow with soft to firm consistency (Figure 3-14A)
- Tumors arise in upper and middle third of lobe, corresponding to the area in which C cells predominate
- May have multifocal nodules in hereditary types

Histopathology

- Wide spectrum of histologic patterns, including solid, lobular, trabecular, insular, and sheetlike
- Tumor cells are round, polygonal, or spindle shaped; frequently mixed cell types
- Polygonal cells have abundant amphophilic to clear cytoplasm, and nuclei often have a plasmacytoid appearance (Figure 3-14B)
- Cytoplasmic pseudoinclusions and grooves can be seen
- Nuclear chromatin is coarsely clumped (i.e., salt-and-pepper like) with inconspicuous nucleoli
- Binucleated cells are commonly seen
- Necrosis, hemorrhage, and mitoses are rare features
- Bizarre nuclear atypia can occur
- Variants (have no clinical significance)
  - Follicular or trabecular, papillary, paraganglioma-like, amphicrine, small cell, giant cell, clear cell, encapsulated, oncocytic, melanotic (melanin pigment present), and squamous types have been described
- Stromal amyloid is present in up to 80% of cases; amyloid can induce foreign-body giant cell reaction
- Stroma may contain calcifications or rarely psammoma bodies

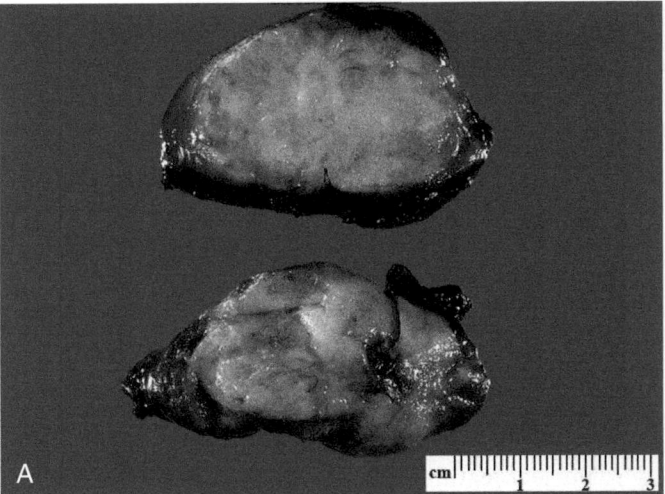
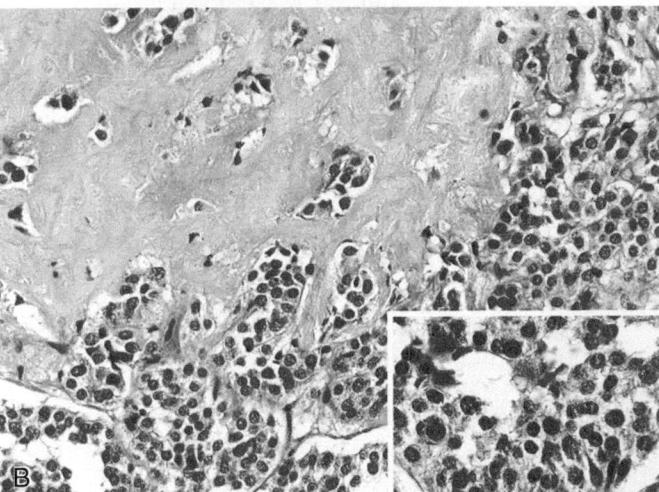
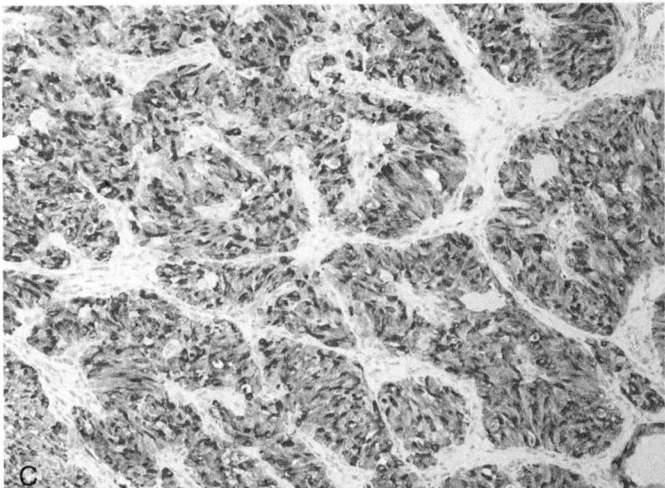

Figure 3-14. Medullary thyroid carcinoma. A, Gross photograph of a pale-tan tumor replacing the thyroid parenchyma. **B,** Nests of neuroendocrine cells are associated with dense amorphous stroma (amyloid). Higher-power magnification (*inset*) of tumor cells shows the amphophilic cytoplasm and the round nuclei with salt-and-pepper chromatin. **C,** Immunohistochemical stain for calcitonin is positive in a medullary thyroid carcinoma with spindled morphology.

- Can be diagnosed preoperatively by FNA but should be supported by immunocytochemistry; use caution because nuclear changes include grooving and pseudonuclear inclusions

Special Stains and Immunohistochemistry

- Calcitonin positive (Figure 3-14C)
- Chromogranin and synaptophysin positive
- Carcinoembryonic antigen (CEA) positive in tumor cells and serum; may have prognostic value
- Congo red positive in amyloid material (polarizes: birefringence apple-green)
- TTF-1 usually positive
- Thyroglobulin negative

Other Techniques for Diagnosis

- Germline mutations in *RET* proto-oncogene are present in all hereditary forms
- *RET* mutations are identified in some sporadic cases (20% to 80%)
- Genetic testing for germline mutations should be offered to all patients diagnosed with medullary thyroid carcinoma regardless of age at diagnosis

Differential Diagnosis

C-Cell Hyperplasia, Reactive
- Lacks fibrosis
- Proliferations of C cells may surround follicles, mimicking invasion
- Scattered cells are often appreciated only by immunostaining

C-Cell Hyperplasia, Nodular (Preneoplastic)
- Greater than 50 cells per cluster
- Identified on hematoxylin and eosin stain, confirmed by immunostaining
- Lacks fibrosis, infiltration
- Nodular proliferation considered preneoplastic
- Difficult to separate from or define microscopic medullary thyroid carcinoma

Follicular Carcinoma
- Stroma does not contain amyloid
- Thyroglobulin positive and calcitonin negative

Papillary Carcinoma
- Characteristic nuclear features of papillary thyroid carcinoma
- Thyroglobulin positive and calcitonin negative
- Pseudoinclusions and grooving may be seen in both papillary and medullary carcinoma

Poorly Differentiated Thyroid Carcinoma
- Islands of tumor cells that typically grow in a solid fashion but may form small follicles
- Stroma does not contain amyloid (negative for Congo red)
- Thyroglobulin positive and calcitonin negative

Plasmacytoma (Extramedullary)
- Plasmacytoid form of medullary carcinoma can resemble a plasmacytoma
- Immunoglobulin light-chain restriction can be demonstrated by kappa and lambda staining, negative for calcitonin

Paraganglioma
- Lobular, nested growth pattern (Zellenballen)

- Nuclei are round with fine granular chromatin
- Rare in this location
- Negative for calcitonin and TTF-1

Hyalinizing Trabecular Tumor
- Well circumscribed
- Lacks amyloid
- Thyroglobulin positive and calcitonin negative

Spindle Cell Tumor with Thymus-Like Differentiation (SETTLE)
- Occurs in young patients (teens to 20s)
- Well circumscribed
- Biphasic tumor of spindled and epithelial cells in glands, tubules, and sheets
- TTF-1, thyroglobulin, and calcitonin negative

PEARLS

- *Medullary carcinoma can mimic a variety of benign and malignant thyroid neoplasms*
- *TTF-1 is positive in most medullary thyroid carcinomas*
- *Presence of C-cell hyperplasia suggests hereditary or germline mutation, as does bilateral and associated endocrine abnormalities (i.e., parathyroid)*
- *Incidental finding of C-cell hyperplasia (> 50 cells in aggregate, often seen bilaterally) should be reported*
- *Survival correlates with stage; familial non-MEN-related type has best overall prognosis of hereditary forms*
- *Radioactive iodine plays no role in treatment*

Selected References

Guyetant S, Josselin N, Savagner F, et al: C-cell hyperplasia and medullary thyroid carcinoma: clinicopathological and genetic correlations in 66 consecutive patients. Mod Pathol 16:756-763, 2003.

Leboulleux S, Baudin E, Travagli JP, Schlumberger M: Medullary thyroid carcinoma. Clin Endocrinol (Oxf) 61:299-310, 2004.

Massoll N, Mazzaferri EL: Diagnosis and management of medullary thyroid carcinoma. Clin Lab Med 24:49-83, 2004.

Simpson NE, Kidd KK, Goodfellow PJ, et al: Assignment of multiple endocrine neoplasia type IIA to chromosome 10 by linkage. Nature 328:528-529, 1987.

POORLY DIFFERENTIATED THYROID CARCINOMA

Clinical Features

- Poorly differentiated carcinoma arising from follicular cells (insular or trabecular pattern)
- May arise from follicular carcinoma or papillary carcinoma
- Rare in the United States (2% to 3% of thyroid carcinomas)
- Mean age at diagnosis is in the fifth and sixth decades
- Slightly more common in women
- Viewed by the World Health Organization (WHO) classification as a morphologic variant of follicular carcinoma
- Intermediate behavior between well-differentiated and anaplastic thyroid carcinomas

Gross Pathology

- Typically greater than 5 cm
- Cut surface is gray-white and solid with areas of necrosis
- Usually extrathyroidal extension with gross invasion into adjacent soft tissue

Histopathology

- Tumor cells with round to oval hyperchromatic nuclei and scant cytoplasm forming a nested pattern (insulae) (Figure 3-15)
- May be defined by the presence of convoluted nuclei; mitotic activity > 3/10 high-power fields (hpff); or tumor necrosis
- Infiltrative growth pattern with invasion into surrounding tissue

Special Stains and Immunohistochemistry

- Pax8 positive in the majority of tumors
- Thyroglobulin and TTF-1 often focally or weakly positive
- Cytokeratin positive
- Calcitonin negative (if positive classify as medullary)

Other Techniques for Diagnosis

- See "Papillary Thyroid Carcinoma" and "Follicular Carcinoma" for current expression patterns

Differential Diagnosis

MEDULLARY CARCINOMA

- Round to oval, spindled, or plasmacytoid
- Amyloid in stroma (Congo red positive)
- Calcitonin positive and thyroglobulin negative
  ### UNDIFFERENTIATED (ANAPLASTIC) CARCINOMA
- Pleomorphic cellular features may also show giant, spindled, or squamous cells
- Lacks architectural growth pattern (insulae)

CARCINOMA SHOWING THYMUS-LIKE DIFFERENTIATION (CASTLE)

- Occurs in adults, fifth decade

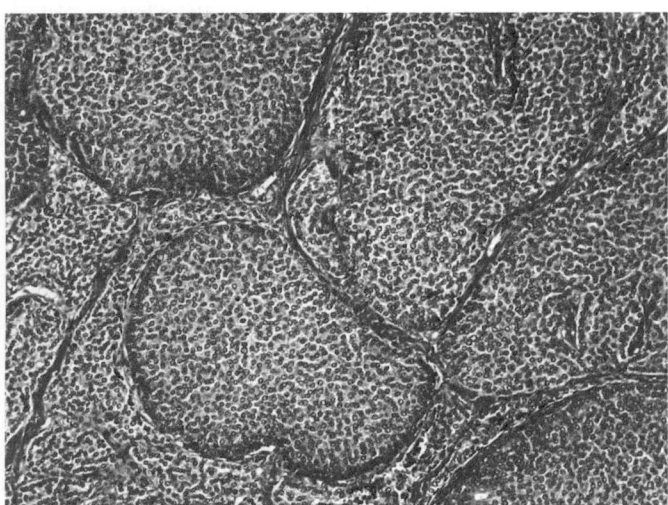

Figure 3-15. Poorly differentiated thyroid carcinoma. Solid nests of follicular cells with scant cytoplasm lacking the nuclear features of papillary thyroid carcinoma.

- One third develop metastatic disease
- Invasive growth in sheets and nests with dense fibrosis; moderately pleomorphic cells
- TTF-1, thyroglobulin, and calcitonin negative
- Tumor positive for CD5

PEARLS

- *May originate from papillary or follicular carcinoma, clinically aggressive*
- *Not viewed as a distinct tumor but in the spectrum from well-differentiated to anaplastic or undifferentiated thyroid carcinoma*
- *If calcitonin is positive, classify as medullary thyroid carcinoma*

SELECTED REFERENCES

Hiltzik D, Carlson DL, Tuttle RM, et al: Poorly differentiated thyroid carcinomas defined on the basis of mitosis and necrosis: a clinicopathologic study of 58 patients. Cancer 106:1286-1295, 2006.

Sanders EM Jr, LiVolsi VA, Brierley J, et al: An evidence-based review of poorly differentiated thyroid cancer. World J Surg 31:934-945, 2007.

Volante M, Collini P, Nikiforov YE, et al: Poorly differentiated thyroid carcinoma: the Turin proposal for the use of uniform diagnostic criteria and an algorithmic diagnostic approach. Am J Surg Pathol 31:1256-1264, 2007.

Volante M, Landolfi S, Chiusa L, et al: Poorly differentiated carcinomas of the thyroid with trabecular, insular, and solid patterns: a clinicopathologic study of 183 patients. Cancer 100:950-957, 2004.

UNDIFFERENTIATED (ANAPLASTIC) CARCINOMA

Clinical Features

- Less than 5% of thyroid neoplasms; also called *pleomorphic carcinoma*
- Highly malignant tumor, totally or partially undifferentiated by microscopy
- Mean age at diagnosis is sixth to seventh decades; slightly more common in women
- Presents as a rapidly enlarging neck mass in the thyroid region associated often with compression signs, including dyspnea, dysphagia, and hoarseness
- High likelihood of cervical lymph node metastases at presentation
- Fatal in most cases within 6 months regardless of treatment
- Most of the anaplastic carcinomas arise from a preexisting tumor, usually a papillary carcinoma

Gross Pathology

- Widely invasive tumor, often with spread beyond the thyroid (Figure 3-16A)
- Variegated appearance with necrotic and hemorrhagic areas

Histopathology

- Three patterns may be seen: squamoid, spindle cell, and giant cell (often more than one pattern within a tumor) (Figure 3-16B)
  - Squamoid pattern (WHO classifies as SCC)
    - Resembles nonkeratinizing SCC; rarely, squamous pearls are present

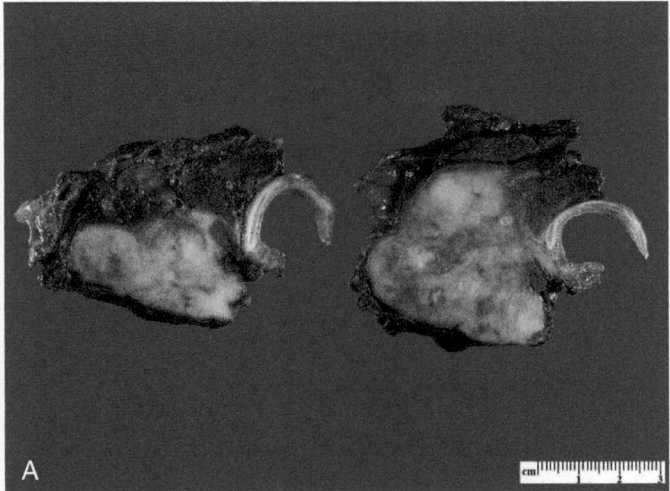

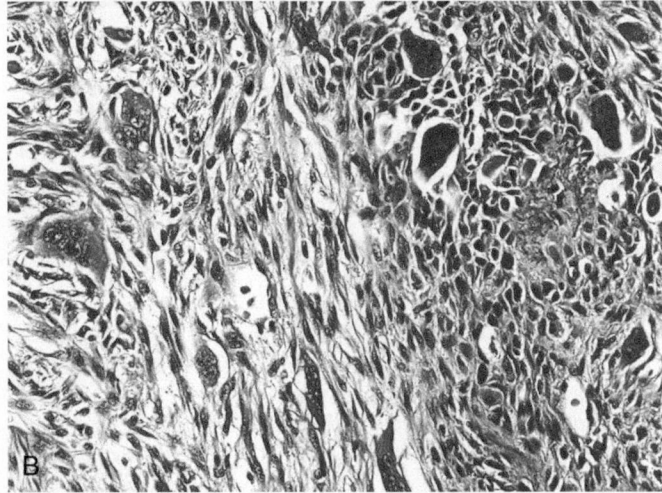

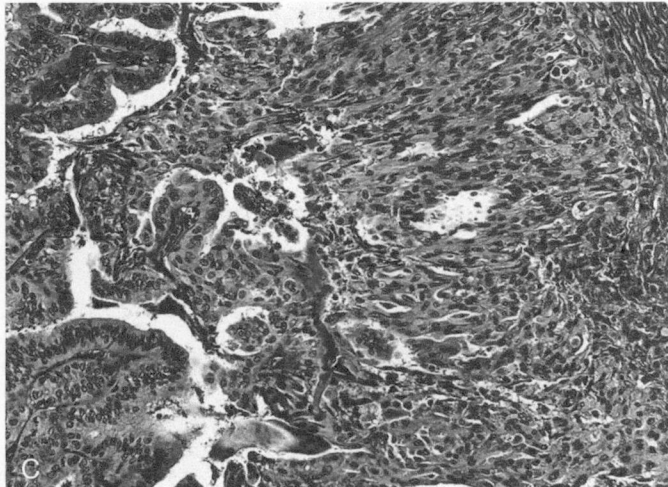

Figure 3-16. Undifferentiated (anaplastic) carcinoma. A, Gross photograph of the tumor invading trachea and soft tissue. **B,** Anaplastic spindled and giant cells are present. **C,** Papillary thyroid carcinoma (*left side*) merging with an anaplastic thyroid carcinoma with spindled morphology.

- Exclude direct extension from aerodigestive tract primary
- Squamous metaplasia in papillary thyroid carcinoma lacks atypia

- Spindle cell pattern
  - Resembles a sarcoma (fibrosarcoma, malignant fibrous histiocytoma, or angiosarcoma)
  - May have sharply demarcated foci of necrosis, myxoid change, or prominent vascularity
- Giant cell pattern
  - Markedly pleomorphic cellular features, including many tumor giant cells with bizarre nuclei, usually solid growth pattern
- Scattered inflammatory cells, high mitotic activity, necrosis, and infiltrative growth pattern are typically seen in all three patterns
- Rarely heterologous elements are seen, such as neoplastic cartilage and bone (most common in spindle cell type)
- Metastases resemble primary morphology
- Background well-differentiated component (most often papillary) may be identified, confirming thyroid origin of anaplastic carcinoma (Figure 3-16C)

Special Stains and Immunohistochemistry

- Cytokeratin (particularly low molecular weight) and epithelial membrane antigen (EMA) patchy positive
- Vimentin positive
- Frequently thyroglobulin and TTF-1 negative; may identify focal weak expression to confirm tumor origin
- If calcitonin is positive, more likely to be an anaplastic variant of medullary carcinoma

Other Techniques for Diagnosis

- Most tumors have complex chromosomal alterations
- Strong association with *TP53* mutations

Differential Diagnosis

POORLY DIFFERENTIATED CARCINOMA
- Nests of uniform, small, round tumor cells
- Aggressive, but prognosis better than for anaplastic

MEDULLARY CARCINOMA
- Round to oval, spindled, or plasmacytoid features
- Amyloid stroma (Congo red positive)
- Calcitonin positive and thyroglobulin negative

PAPILLARY CARCINOMA, SOLID VARIANT
- Characteristic nuclear features such as cleared-out nuclei, nuclear pseudoinclusions, grooves, and overlapping of nuclei
- Thyroglobulin positive (stronger and more uniform than anaplastic)

TRUE SARCOMA OF THE THYROID
- Rare
- Does not have recognizable foci of epithelial differentiation or various patterns
- Vimentin positive and cytokeratin negative

METASTATIC CARCINOMA TO THE THYROID
- Well-circumscribed, usually multiple nodules, or intralymphatic
- Does not show as much cytologic pleomorphism
- Clinical history important to rule out metastasis

MALIGNANT LYMPHOMA
- Source of diagnostic error
- Leukocyte common antigen (LCA) positive; cytokeratin negative

PEARLS

- *Highly aggressive tumor, usually with extrathyroidal extension at the time of diagnosis*
- *Surgical resection rarely alters tumor progression, which is rapidly fatal even if surgically resected (frequently only a biopsy is performed)*
- *Coexisting papillary thyroid carcinoma when present aids in confirming thyroid origin*

SELECTED REFERENCES

Kebebew E, Greenspan FS, Clark OH, et al: Anaplastic thyroid carcinoma: treatment outcome and prognostic factors. Cancer 103:1330-1335, 2005.

Venkatesh YS, Ordonez NG, Schultz PN, et al: Anaplastic carcinoma of the thyroid: a clinicopathologic study of 121 cases. Cancer 66:321-330, 1990.

Wiseman SM, Loree TR, Rigual NR, et al: Anaplastic transformation of thyroid cancer: review of clinical, pathologic, and molecular evidence provides new insights into disease biology and future therapy. Head Neck 25:662-670, 2003.

LYMPHOMA

Clinical Features

- Up to 5% of thyroid tumors; malignant tumor is composed of lymphoid cells
- More common in women; peak incidence is in the seventh decade
- Rapidly enlarging, firm, hard thyroid; compression symptoms are common
- Considered primary when the thyroid gland is the predominant or exclusive site of involvement
- The thyroid is involved in 5% of systemic lymphoma or leukemia
- Primary thyroid lymphoma is rare (about 2% of all thyroid malignancies)
- Primary thyroid lymphoma is often associated with autoimmune thyroiditis (Hashimoto or lymphocytic thyroiditis); causal relationship is widely accepted

Gross Pathology

- Solid, homogeneous, tan mass with a fish-flesh appearance
- Unencapsulated tumor with a poorly defined tumor-gland interface
- No necrosis or hemorrhage

Histopathology

NON-HODGKIN LYMPHOMA
- Most common
- Thyroid is considered to be a MALT site, and low-grade and high-grade lymphomas can occur
- Most are of B-cell origin, large cell type
- Diffuse pattern of growth with entrapped thyroid follicles (Figure 3-17)
- Extends into skeletal muscle and fat
- Lymphoma cells may accumulate within follicular lumens

T-CELL LYMPHOMA
- Extranodal involvement by mycosis fungoides can affect the thyroid

HODGKIN DISEASE
- Rarely involves the thyroid gland
- Usually nodular sclerosing type

Special Stains and Immunohistochemistry

- LCA positive
- Cytokeratin and thyroglobulin highlight entrapped follicular structures
- For subtyping, refer to Chapter 14

Other Techniques for Diagnosis

- For subtyping, refer to Chapter 14

Differential Diagnosis

HASHIMOTO THYROIDITIS, CHRONIC LYMPHOCYTIC THYROIDITIS
- Infiltrate of mature small lymphocytes without atypia
- Lymphoid follicles with germinal centers common
- Expansion and effacing of germinal centers are not seen

PEARLS

- *Although patients with chronic lymphocytic thyroiditis are at increased risk, primary lymphomas of the thyroid are still rare*
- *Accumulation of lymphoid cells is seen within follicular lumens (a histologic feature usually not seen in thyroiditis and Graves disease)*
- *Prognosis depends on the classification and stage of the tumor*
- *Plasmacytomas of the thyroid are believed to represent a variant of MALT with plasma cell differentiation*

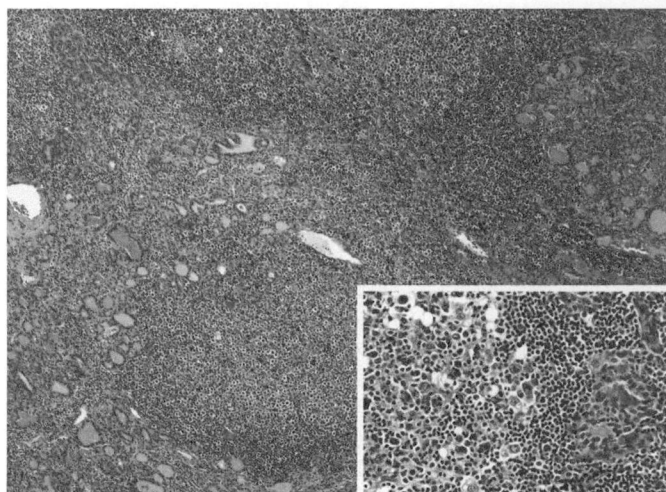

Figure 3-17. Lymphoma, follicular grade 3. Atypical lymphoid infiltrate surrounds and replaces thyroid follicles. At high power (*inset*), the nuclear atypia and discohesive nature of the lymphoma cells are noted.

SELECTED REFERENCES

Belal AA, Allam A, Kandil A, et al: Primary thyroid lymphoma: a retrospective analysis of prognostic factors and treatment outcome for localized intermediate and high grade lymphoma. Am J Clin Oncol 24:299-305, 2001.

Derringer GA, Thompson LD, Frommelt RA, et al: Malignant lymphoma of the thyroid gland: a clinicopathologic study of 108 cases. Am J Surg Pathol 24:623-639, 2000.

Thieblemont C, Mayer A, Dumontet C, et al: Primary thyroid lymphoma is a heterogeneous disease. J Clin Endocrinol Metab 87:105-111, 2002.

Widder S, Pasieka JL: Primary thyroid lymphomas. Curr Treat Options Oncol 5:307-313, 2004.

TUMORS METASTASIZING TO THE THYROID GLAND

Clinical Features

- Direct extension from carcinomas of the head and neck area (pharynx, larynx, trachea, esophagus); occurs most frequently with SCCs
- Hematogenous metastasis to the thyroid occurs in patients with widespread disease
- Common tumors metastasizing to the thyroid are malignant melanoma and carcinomas of the lung, gastrointestinal tract, breast, kidney, and head and neck area
- Clinically present as thyroid enlargement

Gross Pathology

- Often multiple nodules
- Appearance varies with primary lesion; may be very vascular in the case of renal cell carcinoma

Histopathology

- Varies with the histology of the primary tumor (Figure 3-18)
- Metastatic renal cell carcinoma is markedly vascular with clear cytoplasm
- Nuclear atypia may favor metastasis because thyroid carcinomas (well differentiated) have bland nuclear features

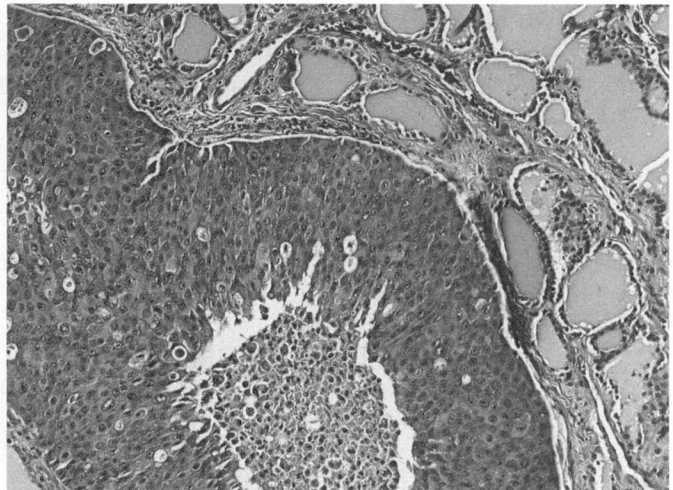

Figure 3-18. Metastasis to thyroid. High-grade adenocarcinoma with comedo necrosis. Tumor nests are present in lymphatic spaces.

Special Stains and Immunohistochemistry

- Thyroglobulin negative in all metastatic tumors
- See "Differential Diagnosis"

Other Techniques for Diagnosis

- Noncontributory

Differential Diagnosis

MALIGNANT MELANOMA
- Variable cytology, often large polygonal cells with prominent nucleoli
- S-100 protein, HMB-45, melan-A, tyrosinase positive

RENAL CELL CARCINOMA
- Cells with abundant clear cytoplasm and surrounding delicate vascularity
- Cytokeratin and vimentin positive (also seen in papillary thyroid carcinomas)

CARCINOID TUMOR
- Typically has a nested architecture
- Uniform cells with round nuclei and neuroendocrine-type chromatin
- Chromogranin, synaptophysin, and cytokeratin positive; rarely expresses calcitonin
- Clinical history required to differentiate from primary medullary carcinoma

BREAST CARCINOMA
- Glandular or solid growth pattern typically with marked cytologic atypia and desmoplastic stroma
- Mucin stains may be positive (mucin may be seen in papillary thyroid carcinomas)

PEARLS

- *Always obtain a good clinical history so that any previous malignancy is revealed*
- *If something does not fit into a known primary thyroid tumor, use select immunohistochemical stains and obtain clinical correlation*

SELECTED REFERENCES

Chen H, Nicol TL, Udelsman R: Clinically significant, isolated metastatic disease to the thyroid gland. World J Surg 23:177-180, 1999.

Heffess CS, Wenig BM, Thompson LD: Metastatic renal cell carcinoma to the thyroid gland: a clinicopathologic study of 36 cases. Cancer 95:1869-1878, 2002.

Wood K, Vini L, Harmer C: Metastases to the thyroid gland: the Royal Marsden experience. Eur J Surg Oncol 30:583-588, 2004.

PARATHYROID GLANDS

PARATHYROID CYST

Clinical Features

- Rare lesions, more common in the neck than mediastinum
- Clinically often mistaken for cystic thyroid nodule, may be palpable
- Can result from degeneration of an adenomatous or hyperplastic parathyroid gland

- Usually nonfunctioning; minority are functioning and associated with hyperparathyroidism
- More common in women than men
- Peak incidence in fourth to sixth decades

Gross Pathology

- Can measure up to 10 cm
- Thin-walled, unilocular cyst
- Cyst fluid is thin and watery, occasionally hemorrhagic
- May appear to distend from the surface of the thyroid gland but is loosely attached

Histopathology

- Cyst is lined by flattened to cuboidal epithelium with small, basally located nuclei and clear cytoplasm
- Cyst wall consists of fibrous connective tissue
- Entrapped parathyroid chief cells can be seen in wall in cases resulting from degeneration of adenoma, hyperplasia

Special Stains and Immunohistochemistry

- Parathyroid hormone (PTH) and cytokeratin positive
- Thyroglobulin and TTF-1 negative
- FNA of cyst fluid may be sent for PTH and thyroglobulin levels to confirm diagnosis

Other Techniques for Diagnosis

- Noncontributory

Differential Diagnosis

THYROID CYST

- Fluid on FNA positive for thyroglobulin, negative for PTH
- Lining cells positive for TTF-1 and thyroglobulin

DEGENERATED PARATHYROID ADENOMA OR HYPERPLASIA

- Cystic degeneration may occur in either adenoma or hyperplasia
- Background cells are those of adenomatous or hyperplastic parathyroid tissue
- Entrapped parathyroid chief cells can be seen in wall in cases resulting from degeneration of adenoma or hyperplasia

CYSTIC PARATHYROID ADENOMA

- May be associated with hyperparathyroidism–jaw tumor (HPT-JT) syndrome
- Higher risk for parathyroid carcinoma

THIRD PHARYNGEAL POUCH CYSTS

- Mediastinal cysts that contain both parathyroid and thymic tissue

BRANCHIAL CLEFT CYST

- Located in the lateral neck
- Cyst lined by squamous, columnar, or ciliated epithelial lining
- Abundant lymphoid stroma in cyst wall

PEARLS

- *FNA is the best "first" test to evaluate neck nodules*
- *When FNA of a neck nodule yields clear fluid, a parathyroid cyst should be in the differential diagnosis, and the fluid should be sent for PTH assay because microscopic examination is nonspecific (histiocytes and a few epithelial cells that may be mistaken for follicular thyroid epithelium)*

SELECTED REFERENCES

Ippolito G, Palazzo FF, Sebag F, et al: A single-institution 25-year review of true parathyroid cysts. Langenbecks Arch Surg 391:13-18, 2006.

Layfield LJ: Fine needle aspiration cytology of cystic parathyroid lesions: a cytomorphologic overlap with cystic lesion of the thyroid. Acta Cytol 35:447-450, 1991.

Ujiki MB, Nayar R, Sturgeon C, Angelos P: Parathyroid cyst: often mistaken for a thyroid cyst. World J Surg 31:60-64, 2007.

PARATHYROID HYPERPLASIA

Clinical Features

- Hyperplasia of parathyroid tissue that involves more than one gland, usually all four
- *Primary hyperparathyroidism* (result of parathyroid hyperplasia in about 15% of cases)
  - Patients have increased PTH, hypercalcemia, and hypophosphatemia
- Secondary hyperparathyroidism
  - Typically secondary to chronic renal failure, which causes hypocalcemia and hyperphosphatemia leading to increased PTH levels
- Hyperplasia of chief cells may be associated with multiple MEN syndromes (I, IIA, and IIB)

Gross Pathology

- Typically all glands are enlarged, but they may be unequally enlarged (normal glands weigh up to 40 mg)
- Cut section appears homogeneous but may be nodular or have cystic changes

Histopathology

- Proliferation of chief cells, oncocytic cells, transitional cells, or clear cells, which are frequently mixed (Figure 3-19A)
- Nodular pattern of cellular growth within the gland
- Cellular growth pattern may be solid, follicular (glandlike), or in cords
- Occasionally mitotic figures may be identified
- Involved glands have decreased intracytoplasmic fat content and decreased intercellular fat (Figure 3-19B)

Special Stains and Immunohistochemistry

- Oil red O on frozen section will demonstrate decreased intracytoplasmic fat (also seen in adenomas)

Other Techniques for Diagnosis

- MEN *menin* gene on chromosome 11q
- MEN II *Ret* proto-oncogene on chromosome 10q

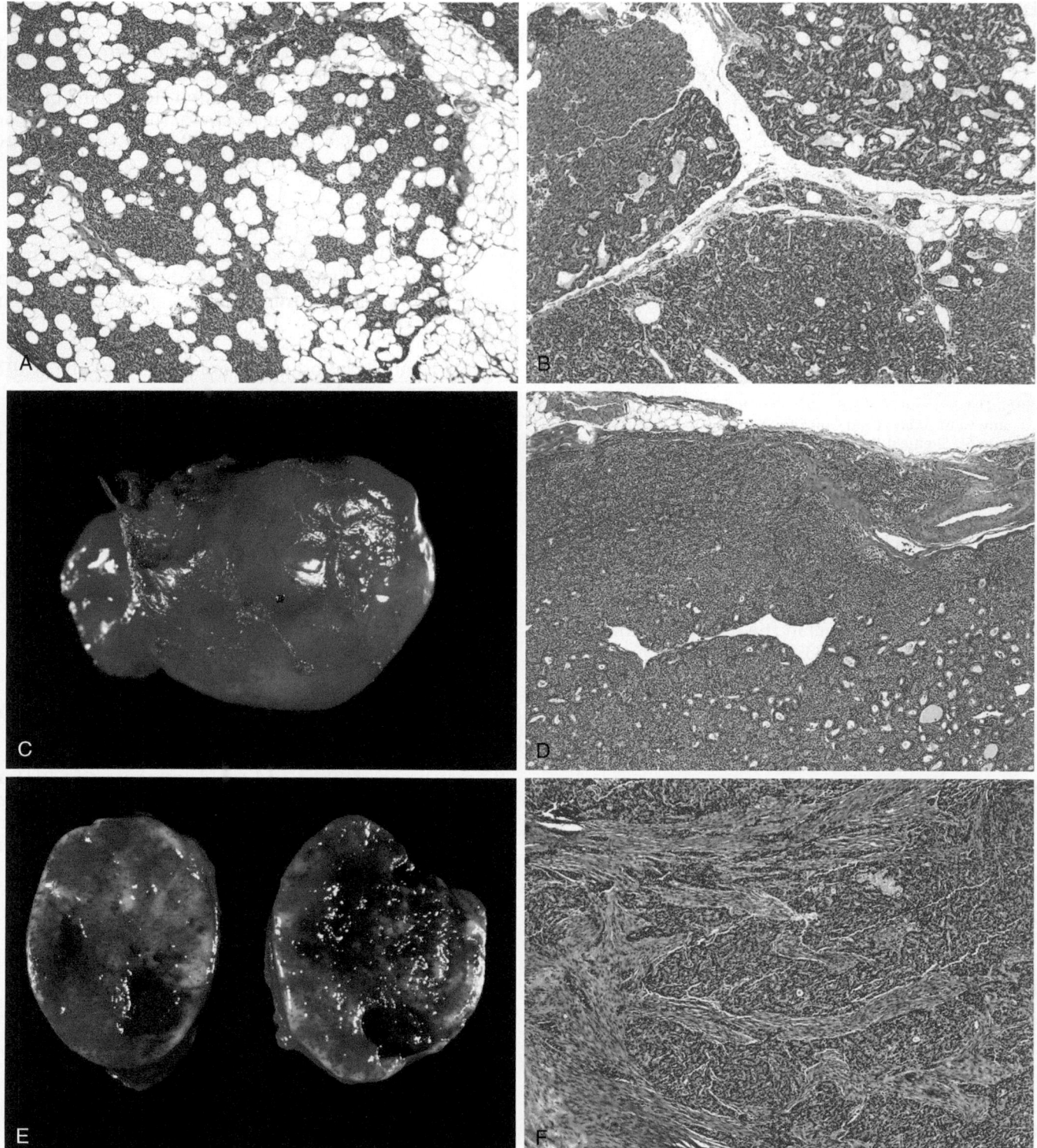

Figure 3-19. A, Normal parathyroid. Note the cellularity of the gland showing nests of chief cells with intercellular adipose tissue. **B,** Hyperplastic parathyroid. Multiple lobulated nests of parathyroid cells show loss of intercellular adipose tissue. **C,** Parathyroid adenoma. Gross photograph shows a smooth, well-circumscribed, enlarged gland. **D,** Parathyroid adenoma. Low-power view shows an expansile nodule (adenoma); note a small, compressed rim of normal parathyroid at top of nodule. **E,** Parathyroid carcinoma. Gross photograph of a parathyroid carcinoma with necrosis. **F,** Parathyroid carcinoma. Low-power view shows infiltrating uniform tumor cells in a dense stromal reaction.

Differential Diagnosis

PARATHYROID ADENOMA

- Typically only one enlarged gland; two adenomas are rare
- Rim of compressed parathyroid tissue, but otherwise normal parathyroidal tissue is often present

PEARLS

- *Intraparenchymal fat will be reduced in both hyperplasia and adenomas*
- *Treatment is subtotal parathyroidectomy (i.e., removal of 3½ glands)*

SELECTED REFERENCES

Elliott DD, Monroe DP, Perrier ND: Parathyroid histopathology: is it of any value today? J Am Coll Surg 203:758-765, 2006.

Johnson SJ, Sheffield EA, McNicol AM: Best practice no. 183: examination of parathyroid gland specimens. J Clin Pathol 58:338-342, 2005.

PARATHYROID ADENOMA

Clinical Features

- Benign neoplasm composed of chief cells
- Most commonly occurs in the fifth and sixth decades, female predominance (3:1)
- Most are single adenomas involving one gland
- May occur in various sites such as within the thyroid, mediastinum, or retroesophageal area
- Single most common cause of primary hyperparathyroidism (about 80% of cases)
- Patients may present with signs of hypercalcemia ("stones, moans, psychiatric overtones"), or elevated serum calcium is incidentally found during routine blood tests
- Evaluate by ultrasound, sestamibi scan, or computed tomography
- May be associated with MEN I and II or HPT-JT syndrome (also associated with parathyroid carcinoma)

Gross Pathology

- Single enlarged gland; two adenomas are rare
- Round to oval with thin capsule (Figure 3-19C)
- Reddish brown on cut sectioning, usually homogeneous, may on occasion show cystic changes and hemorrhage
- Typically weigh more than 300 mg and up to several grams

Histopathology

- Well circumscribed; cellular proliferation of chief cells that may have clear or oncocytic changes
- Adjacent rim of compressed normal parathyroid tissue is seen in about half of cases and is not required for diagnosis (Figure 3-19D)
- Stromal fat content, although minimal to absent in adenoma, is not reliable in separating adenoma from hyperplasia

- Cells with bizarre nuclei may be seen (endocrine atypia), not a sign of malignancy
- Mitoses are usually absent; high mitotic rate should raise suspicion for malignancy
- Growth pattern is solid, nested, follicular, or pseudopapillary; follicular cystic structures may contain colloid-like periodic acid–Schiff (PAS)–positive material
- Variants
  - Atypical adenoma
    - Lacks unequivocal evidence of malignancy
    - May show thickened capsule, dense fibrotic bands without lymphovascular invasion or invasion into adjacent structures (i.e., thyroid, esophagus, larynx)
  - HPT-JT
    - Familial, autosomal dominant, involving *HRPT2* gene, which encodes parafibromin
    - Cystic change common
    - Associated with parathyroid carcinoma in 10% to 15%

Special Stains and Immunohistochemistry

- Cytokeratin, chromogranin, and PTH positive
- Thyroglobulin and TTF-1 negative
- Follicle or cyst contents is PAS positive and thyroglobulin negative

Other Techniques for Diagnosis

- Frequent loss of chromosome 11q (location of MEN I) not seen in carcinomas
- Cyclin D1/PRAD1 oncogene activated by clonal rearrangement (40%)
- Sestamibi scan can localize most parathyroid adenomas preoperatively, and rapid intraoperative PTH assay allows for a minimally invasive parathyroidectomy (MIP), which is a small incision with removal of only the affected gland, avoiding neck exploration and identification of all four glands

Differential Diagnosis

PARATHYROID HYPERPLASIA

- May be primary or secondary, frequently as a result of renal failure
- If primary, may be associated with MEN I and II
- All glands are enlarged, often asymmetrically

PARATHYROID CARCINOMA

- Ill-defined, infiltrative mass with extension into adjacent structures

THYROID NODULES

- Follicular nodules: thyroglobulin and TTF-1 positive and PTH negative
- Medullary thyroid carcinoma: calcitonin and CEA positive; negative for PTH

ONCOCYTIC NODULES IN PARATHYROIDS OF ELDERLY PATIENTS

- Oncocytic cells within the parathyroid gland increase with age and may form small nodules

- *Most parathyroid adenomas are functionally active*
- *Treatment is surgical resection of adenoma—preoperative localization and use of intraoperative PTH assay allows for limited surgical exploration with identification and resection of only the affected gland, resulting in less morbidity*
- *Thyroid lesions may coexist*

SELECTED REFERENCES

Absher KJ, Truong LD, Khurana KK, Ramzy I: Parathyroid cytology: avoiding diagnostic pitfalls. Head Neck 24:157-164, 2002.
Carling T: Molecular pathology of parathyroid tumors. Trends Endocrinol Metab 12:53-58, 2001.
Grimelius L, Johansson H: Pathology of parathyroid tumors. Semin Surg Oncol 13:142-154, 1997.

PARATHYROID CARCINOMA

Clinical Features

- Malignant tumor derived from the chief cells of the parathyroid gland
- Rare cause of hyperparathyroidism (accounts for < 1% of cases)
- High probability of local recurrence and late metastasis to lymph nodes, distant sites
- Age range is 45 to 55 years, 10 years younger than adenomas; no sex predilection
- Usually marked hypercalcemia (higher than in patients with adenomas) at presentation, leading to increased renal and bone disease
- May be associated with HPT-JT syndrome

Gross Pathology

- Ill-defined, infiltrative mass with extension into muscle, thyroid, esophagus, or trachea (Figure 3-19E)
- Cut section firm and gray-white
- Mean size, 3 cm; mean weight, 6 g
- Lymph nodes usually not involved at time of surgery
- Surgeons report adherent and difficult-to-remove mass

Histopathology

- Histology is frequently mild to moderate variation in chief cells resembling adenomas; rarer cases have marked pleomorphism and macronucleoli
- Various architectural patterns include solid (most often), glandular, and trabecular (Figure 3-19F)
- Thick acellular fibrous bands and thick capsule (60% of cases) are common
- For diagnosing carcinoma, invasion should extend into adjacent structures (esophagus, larynx, muscle)
- Necrosis is worrisome for carcinoma
- Vascular invasion (10% to 15% of cases) is defined as attachment to the wall within a vessel located outside the tumor (diagnostic of carcinoma)
- Capsule in carcinoma is generally thicker than in adenoma
- Mitoses are seen in about 50% of cases but can also be seen in adenoma or hyperplasia

Special Stains and Immunohistochemistry

- Cytokeratin and chromogranin positive
- TTF-1 and thyroglobulin negative
- Parafibromin loss (in 75%) may be secondary to sporadic or germline alteration in HRPT2 gene

Other Techniques for Diagnosis

- Recurrent loss of chromosome 13q (region of retinoblastomas and *BRCA2* tumor suppressor genes)
- Hyperparathyroidism-jaw tumor syndrome involving *HRPT2* gene (1q25), which encodes parafibromin (germ-line alteration)

Differential Diagnosis

PARATHYROID HYPERPLASIA
- Well-defined growth pattern without extension into adjacent structures
- Multiple parathyroid glands enlarged

PARATHYROID ADENOMA
- Well-defined mass with a distinct, thin fibrous capsule; lacks infiltrative growth pattern
- Lacks capsular and vascular invasion

ATYPICAL ADENOMA
- May have some features associated with parathyroid carcinoma, such as adherence to soft tissue, broad fibrous bands, and capsular invasion
- The term *atypical adenoma* is used if some of these features are present, but the tumor lacks unequivocal evidence of malignancy, including vascular invasion or invasion into muscle or adjacent structures

PRIMARY NEOPLASMS OF THE THYROID
- Lack clinical hyperparathyroidism (hypercalcemia)
- Papillary and follicular tumors are positive for thyroglobulin and negative for chromogranin; medullary carcinoma is positive for calcitonin and frequently positive for TTF-1

- *Treatment is surgical en bloc resection; if local recurrence happens, it is usually during first 3 years after surgery*
- *Most common sites of metastases are cervical lymph nodes, lung, and liver; metastases typically occur late*
- *No scientific basis for progression from hyperplasia to adenoma to carcinoma*

SELECTED REFERENCES

Clayman GL, Gonzalez HE, El-Naggar A, Vassilopoulou-Sellin R: Parathyroid carcinoma: evaluation and interdisciplinary management. Cancer 100:900-905, 2004.
DeLellis RA: Parathyroid carcinoma: an overview. Adv Anat Pathol 12:53-61, 2005.
Evans HL: Criteria for the diagnosis of parathyroid carcinoma: a critical study. Surg Pathol 4:244-265, 1991.

TUMORS METASTASIZING TO THE PARATHYROID GLANDS

Clinical Features

- Metastases to the parathyroid glands are relatively rare

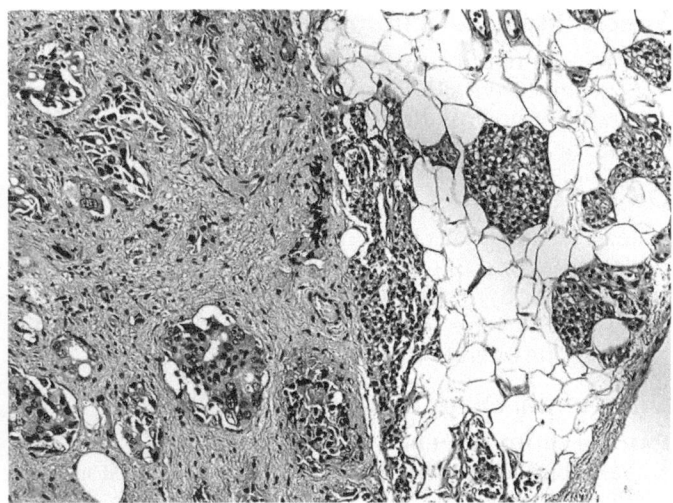

Figure 3-20. Metastasis to parathyroid gland. Prostatic adenocarcinoma with large nuclei infiltrating fibrous tissue between parathyroid follicles as seen on frozen section.

- Most common sites of origin are breast, skin, lung, soft tissue, and involvement by leukemia
- Rarely the destruction of parathyroid tissue by the metastases may lead to clinical presentation of hypoparathyroidism

Gross Pathology and Histopathology

- Depends on the primary site of malignancy (Figure 3-20)

Special Stains and Immunohistochemistry

- Staining for PTH and other epithelial markers may be helpful

Other Techniques for Diagnosis

- Depends on primary tumor

Differential Diagnosis

- Depends on cell type and pattern
- Clinical history is essential

PEARLS

- *Parathyroids may be involved by direct extension of tumors from adjacent structures (thyroid, larynx) or from distant sites (metastatic spread)*

SELECTED REFERENCES

De la Monte SM, Hutchins GM, Moore GW: Endocrine organ metastases from breast carcinoma. Am J Pathol 114:131-136, 1984.
Venkatraman L, Kalangutkar A, Russell CF: Primary hyperparathyroidism and metastatic carcinoma within parathyroid gland. J Clin Pathol 60:1058-1060, 2007.

SALIVARY GLANDS

SIALADENITIS

Clinical Features

- May present as acute, chronic, and granulomatous forms
- Causative agents include viral (paramyxovirus, Epstein-Barr virus [EBV], coxsackievirus, influenza A, parainfluenza virus) and bacterial (*Staphylococcus aureus*, *Streptococcus* species, gram-negative bacteria) organisms
- Chronic sialadenitis may be associated with rheumatoid arthritis
- Predisposing conditions include dehydration, malnutrition, immunosuppression, and sialolithiasis
- Etiology of granulomatous subtype is tuberculosis, mycosis, sarcoidosis, duct obstruction
- Male predilection; mean age, 40 years

Gross Pathology

- Sialolith (stone) may be present (more common in extraglandular secretory ducts than in gland)
- Firm to hard; gland consistency depends on the extent of fibrosis

Histopathology

- Varies depending on the causative agent (viral versus bacterial), underlying condition (sialolithiasis, obstruction), and age of lesion (acute or chronic)
- Variable atrophic changes, fibrosis, and acute and chronic inflammatory features (Figure 3-21)
- Interlobular variation of the extent of inflammatory and fibrotic changes
- Chronic sclerosing sialadenitis of the submandibular gland is unilateral and characterized by lymphocytic and plasmacytic inflammation encasing ducts

Special Stains and Immunohistochemistry

- Noncontributory

Other Techniques for Diagnosis

- Noncontributory

Differential Diagnosis

BENIGN LYMPHOEPITHELIAL LESION
- Epimyoepithelial islands within lymphoid stroma
- Parenchymal atrophy

BENIGN LYMPHOEPITHELIAL CYST ALMOST ALWAYS IN PAROTID GLAND
- Often bilateral
- Irregular luminal surface with lymphoid infiltrate in wall of cyst
- Often associated with HIV infection

NECROTIZING SIALOMETAPLASIA
- Reactive inflammatory condition with lobular coagulative necrosis of acini
- Squamous metaplasia and pseudoepitheliomatous hyperplasia of overlying mucosal epithelium
- May resemble neoplasia if unilateral
- Can affect any site (palate is common), probably related to ischemia
- FNA yields mostly ductal elements and some chronic inflammatory cells

PEARLS

- *Clinically, sialadenitis can be confused with malignancy*

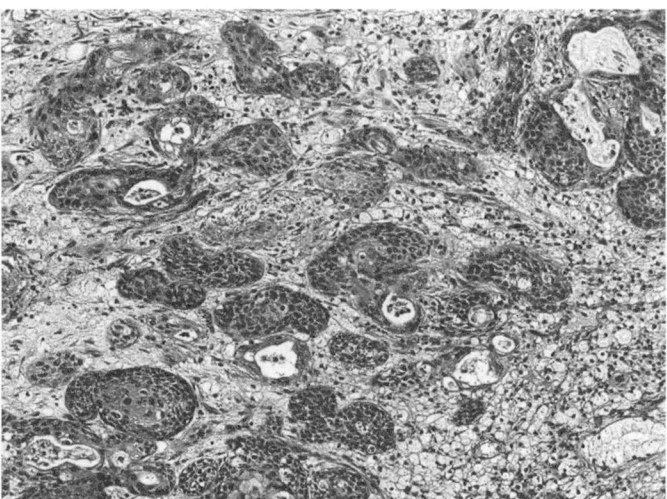

Figure 3-21. Chronic sialadenitis, sialometaplasia. Retained lobular architecture with fibrosis and marked squamous metaplasia of the ducts.

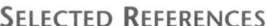

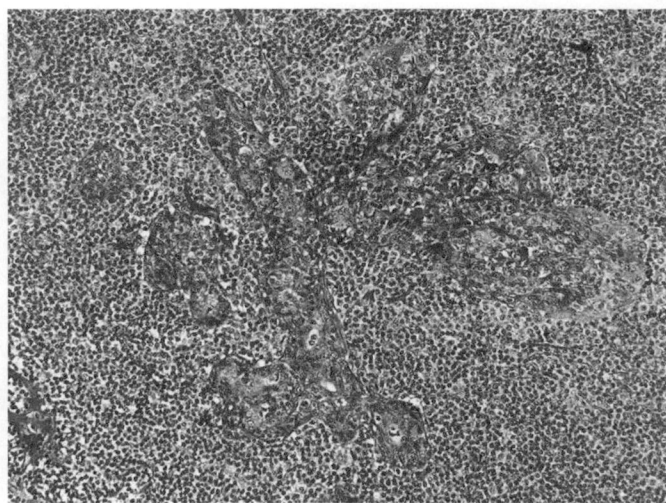

Figure 3-22. Benign lymphoepithelial lesion. High-power view shows a vaguely defined epimyoepithelial island surrounded by small lymphoid cells.

SELECTED REFERENCES

Brook I: Diagnosis and management of parotitis. Arch Otolaryngol Head Neck Surg 118:469-471, 1992.

O'Brien CJ, Murrant BJ: Surgical management of chronic parotitis. Head Neck 15:445-449, 1993.

Richardson MS: Non-neoplastic lesions of the salivary glands. In Thompson LDR, Goldblum JR (eds): Head and Neck Pathology. Philadelphia, Elsevier, 2006, pp 283-286.

Van der Walt JD, Leake J: Granulomatous sialadenitis of the major salivary glands: a clinicopathological study of 57 cases. Histopathology 11:131-144, 1987.

BENIGN LYMPHOEPITHELIAL LESION (MIKULICZ DISEASE)

Clinical Features

- Most common cause of diffuse bilateral enlargement of salivary and lacrimal glands
- Clinically, slowly increasing bilateral and symmetrical swelling of salivary glands
- One manifestation of Sjögren syndrome
- Systemic autoimmune disease; develop small clonal expansions; can evolve into lymphoma

Gross Pathology

- Multiple small, tan nodules may diffusely replace gland

Histopathology

- Epimyoepithelial islands are solid nests of mainly basal epithelial cells and myoepithelial cells; typically permeated by monocytoid B cells of MALT; they can also be seen in low-grade MALT lymphoma (Figure 3-22)
- Lymphoid infiltrate can contain well-formed germinal centers; polyclonal and composed predominantly of T cells
- Intercellular hyaline material resembling basal lamina is deposited

Special Stains and Immunohistochemistry

- B- and T-cell markers and kappa and lambda stains on paraffin or frozen tissues

Other Techniques for Diagnosis

- Flow cytometry to evaluate clonality
- Gene rearrangement studies to exclude lymphoma, if indicated

Differential Diagnosis

MALIGNANT LYMPHOEPITHELIAL CARCINOMA

- Undifferentiated carcinoma with lymphoid stroma
- Most in salivary location, EBV associated

PEARLS

- *Increased risk for developing malignant lymphoma in both salivary and extrasalivary locations*
- *Lymphomas are mostly B-cell phenotype; large cell lymphoma or MALT type*
- *Features that indicate development of lymphoma include prominent aggregations of monomorphic medium-sized lymphoid cells with abundant pale cytoplasm and uniform nuclei (monocytoid B cells); involvement of adjacent fat and connective tissue, immunohistochemical evidence of monoclonality*

SELECTED REFERENCES

Batsakis JG: Pathology consultation: carcinoma ex lymphoepithelial lesion. Ann Otol Rhinol Laryngol 92:657-658, 1983.

MacLean H, Ironside JW, Cullen JF, Butt Z: Mikulicz syndrome and disease: 2 case reports highlighting the difference. Acta Ophthalmol 71:136-141, 1993.

McCurley TL, Collins RD, Ball E, Collins RD: Nodal and extranodal lymphoproliferative disorders in Sjögren syndrome: a clinical and immunopathologic study. Hum Pathol 482-492, 1990.

Peel RL: Diseases of the salivary glands. In Barnes L (ed): Surgical Pathology of the Head and Neck. New York, Marcel Dekker, 2001, pp 635-642.

LYMPHOEPITHELIAL CYST

Clinical Features

- Present in the parotid or upper cervical lymph nodes
- Similar to a salivary duct cyst

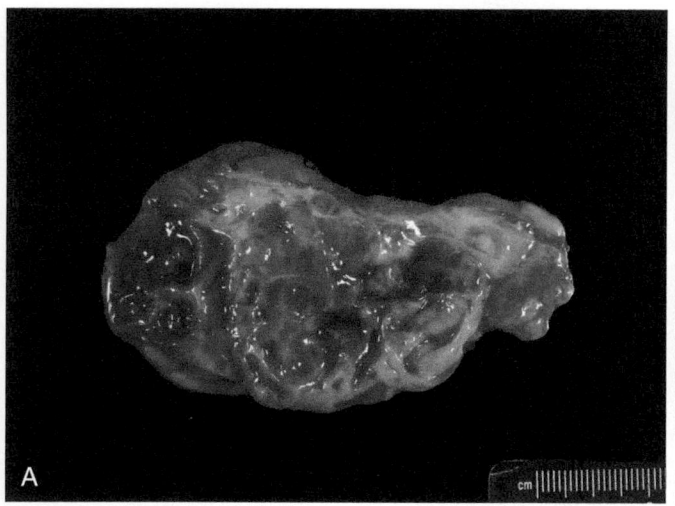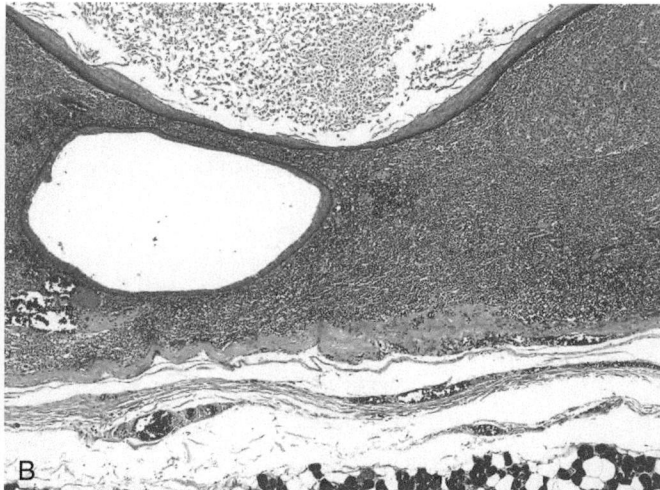

Figure 3-23. Lymphoepithelial cyst. A, Gross photograph of multiple lymphoepithelial cysts within the parotid gland. **B,** Low-power view shows a cyst lined by epithelium and a prominent lymphoid infiltrate in the cyst wall.

- Etiology
  - Originates from remnant of branchial apparatus and is similar to a branchial cleft cyst
  - Cystic formation of salivary gland nests in intraparotid or periparotid lymph node
- Some cases associated with HIV infection, often bilateral

Gross Pathology

- Multiloculated cysts on cut surface (Figure 3-23A)
- Solid, tan homogeneous areas in the cyst wall represent lymphoid tissue

Histopathology

- Multilocular cysts covered by glandular or squamous epithelium surrounded by hyperplastic lymphoid follicles with germinal center formation (Figure 3-23B)
- HIV-associated cases
  - Multifocal
  - Occur early and associated with florid lymphoid hyperplasia

Special Stains and Immunohistochemistry

- Noncontributory

Other Techniques for Diagnosis

- Noncontributory

Differential Diagnosis

Cystic Warthin Tumor
- Lymphoid follicle formation with oncocytic epithelium

Branchial Cleft Cyst
- Lateral location is in neck near sternocleidomastoid muscle
- Cyst is lined by squamous, columnar, or ciliated epithelium
- Cyst wall has prominent lymphoid stroma
- Cyst may contain anucleated keratinized epithelium, histiocytes, or cholesterol clefts

PEARLS

- *HIV infection show marked increase in dendritic reticular cells and intrafollicular CD8-positive lymphocytes*
- *FNA can be diagnostic and therapeutic; can be the first indication that the patient should be tested for HIV*

Selected References

Cleary KR, Batsakis JG: Lymphoepithelial cysts of the parotid region: a new face on an old lesion. Ann Otol Rhinol Laryngol 99:162-164, 1990.

Mandel L, Reich R: HIV parotid gland lymphoepithelial cysts: review and case reports. Oral Surg Oral Med Oral Pathol 74:273-278, 1992.

Richardson MS: Non-neoplastic lesions of the salivary glands. In Thompson LDR, Goldblum JR (eds): Head and Neck Pathology. Philadelphia, Elsevier, 2006, pp 288-290.

Terry JH, Loree TR, Thomas MD, Marti JR: Major salivary gland lymphoepithelial lesions and the acquired immunodeficiency syndrome. Am J Surg 162:324-329, 1991.

SALIVARY DUCT CYST

Clinical Features

- Cystic dilatation of a salivary duct due to ductal obstruction
- Majority occur in parotid

Gross Pathology

- Well-circumscribed, unilocular cyst with smooth lining
- Cyst contains thin, watery to viscous fluid

Histopathology

- Cyst wall consists of dense fibroconnective tissue with mild to moderate infiltrate of chronic inflammatory cells and lined by stratified squamous epithelium P (Figure 3-24)
- Goblet-type mucinous or oncocytic cells may be present in the epithelium
- Surrounding parenchyma of parotid is atrophic as a result of compression
- Mild sialadenitis and duct ectasia may be seen

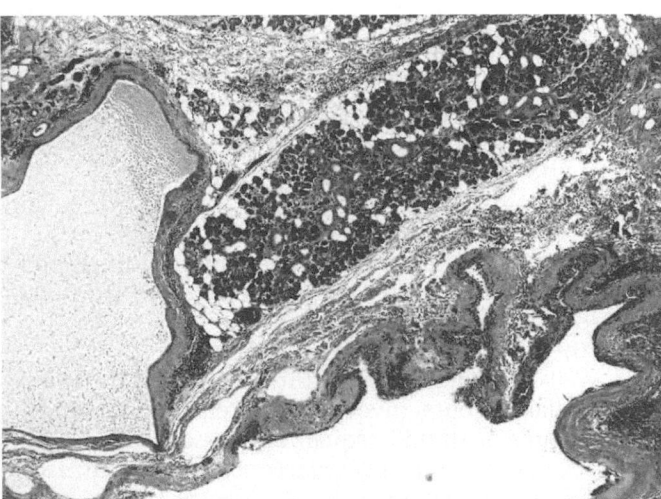

Figure 3-24. Salivary duct cyst. Low-power view shows a cyst lined by a single layer of epithelium. Notice the adjacent salivary gland tissue and marked fibrosis of the wall.

Special Stains and Immunohistochemistry

- Noncontributory

Other Techniques for Diagnosis

- Noncontributory

Differential Diagnosis

MUCUS RETENTION CYST (RANULA)

- More common in minor salivary glands, lower lip
- Lack of cystic wall
- Pools of mucin in fibrous tissue

CYSTIC WARTHIN TUMOR

- Cyst wall lined by oncocytic cuboids or columnar epithelium with underlying dense lymphoid stroma

PEARLS

- *Surgical excision is curative*

SELECTED REFERENCES

Cohen MN, Rao U, Shedd DP: Benign cysts of the parotid gland. J Surg Oncol 27:85-88, 1984.

Peel RL: Diseases of the salivary glands. In Barnes L (ed): Surgical Pathology of the Head and Neck. New York, Marcel Dekker, 2001, pp 651-653.

MUCOCELE (RANULA)

Clinical Features

- Most common non-neoplastic lesion of the salivary glands (4% to 9%)
- Two types of mucoceles: extravasation type and retention type
  - Extravasation-type mucocele
    - Results from extravasation of secreted salivary fluid into surrounding tissue; peak incidence in third decade
- Lip most common location
  - Retention-type mucocele (plunging ranula)
  - Mucus pools within epithelium-lined cysts (partially obstructed excretory ducts with cystic dilatation or congenital or acquired weakness of duct wall)
- Occurs in all ages; peak incidence in seventh decade
- Clinically may fluctuate in size; can develop within hours to days

Gross Pathology

- Small, dome-shaped swelling of mucosa ranging in size from 0.2 to 1 cm
- Consistency is soft and fluctuant

Histopathology

- Extravasation type
  - Pool of mucin often with scattered inflammation surrounded by granulation tissue (Figure 3-25)
- Retention type
  - Mucin pool surrounded by cuboidal to stratified squamous epithelial lining and fibrotic cyst wall

Special Stains and Immunohistochemistry

- Noncontributory

Other Techniques for Diagnosis

- Noncontributory

Differential Diagnosis

SALIVARY DUCT CYST

- True epithelium-lined cyst with chronic inflammation in wall
- Compression of surrounding parenchyma, which has atrophic changes

LYMPHOEPITHELIAL CYST

- Multilocular cyst with marked lymphoid tissue in wall

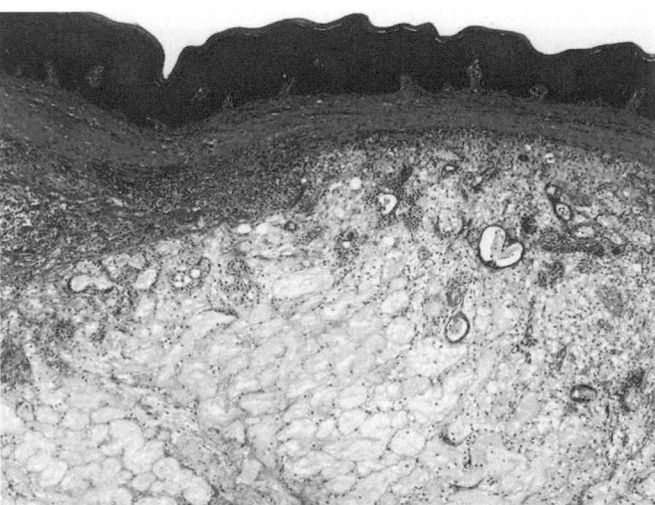

Figure 3-25. Mucocele (extravasation type). Low-power view shows pools of mucoid material surrounded by inflammation and minor salivary glands.

SELECTED REFERENCES

Das S, Das AK: A review of pediatric oral biopsies from a surgical service in a dental school. Pediatr Dent 15:208-211, 1993.

Richardson MS: Non-neoplastic lesions of the salivary glands. In Thompson LDR, Goldblum JR (eds): Head and Neck Pathology. Philadelphia, Elsevier, 2006, pp 279-283.

MIXED TUMOR (PLEOMORPHIC ADENOMA)

Clinical Features

- Benign tumor that manifests both epithelial and mesenchymal elements
- Most common neoplasm of salivary gland origin; constitutes about 30% of all parotid neoplasms and 60% of benign tumors from all salivary gland sites
- Most common salivary gland tumor in children and adolescents; higher incidence in women
- Most common intraoral site is the palate, followed by the upper lip and buccal mucosa
- Usually solitary, most common associated tumor is Warthin tumor
- Peak incidence is in fourth decade
- Typically presents as a slow-growing, asymptomatic, discrete, mobile, often multinodular, firm mass; may become large if untreated
- Often occurs in the lower pole of the superficial lobe; facial paralysis may occur only as result of extrinsic compression of facial nerve, not invasion

Gross Pathology

- Round to ovoid mass with smooth surface
- Most tumors are encapsulated (incomplete fibrous capsule); tumors that originate from minor salivary glands are often unencapsulated
- Cut surface is homogeneous or variegated, tan to white, with shiny, translucent zones that represent myxochondroid or cartilaginous areas; often lobulated, especially when larger than 1 cm (Figure 3-26A)
- Occasionally, hemorrhage and infarction occur secondary to surgical or FNA biopsy

Histopathology

- Shows both epithelial and mesenchymal differentiation; proportions are variable and heterogeneous cellular composition
  - Epithelial component
    - Well-formed ductal structures formed of inner epithelial and outer myoepithelial cells associated with features of spindle, squamous, basaloid, cuboidal, oncocytoid, mucous, sebaceous, round, plasmacytoid, polygonal, or clear cells (Figure 3-26B)
    - Squamous differentiation with keratin pearls can occur
    - Cytologic features of epithelial cells are bland; rare, if any, mitotic activity
  - Mesenchymal component
    - Myxoid, hyaline, cartilaginous, or osseous differentiation
- Several variants
  - Cellular type: epithelial element predominates; constitutes more than 80% of tumor in only 12% to 15% of cases
  - Myxoid type: myxochondromatous mesenchymal element predominates (most tumors have a myxoid component that makes up about 30% of tumor)
- Thickness of fibrous capsule varies; often absent in predominantly myxoid tumors and in tumors arising in minor salivary glands

Special Stains and Immunohistochemistry

- Noncontributory

Other Techniques for Diagnosis

- Cytogenetic studies often show clonal chromosomal rearrangements, 8q12 and 12q13-15

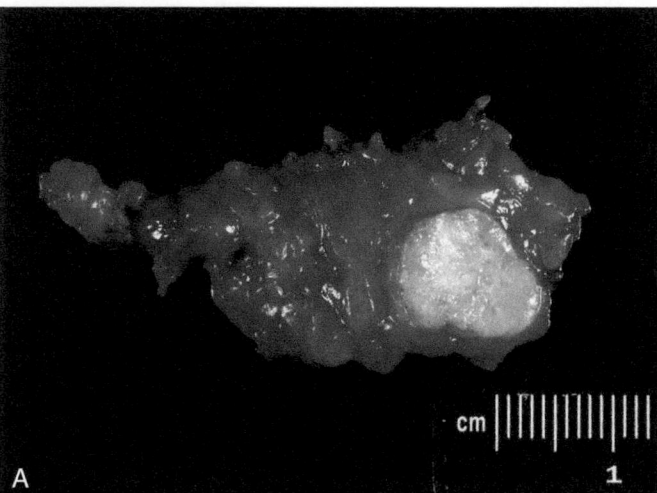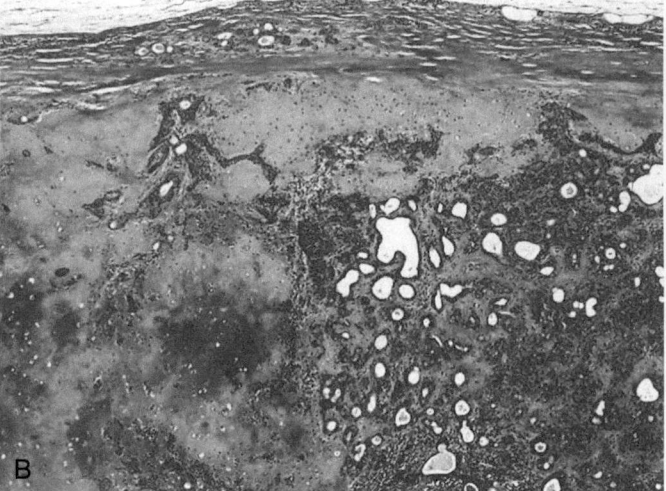

Figure 3-26. Benign mixed tumor (pleomorphic adenoma). A, Gross photograph shows a well-circumscribed, gray-white nodule. **B,** A cellular tumor composed of ducts and myoepithelial cells (*right*) is adjacent to the hypocellular cartilaginous areas (*left*).

- Patients with 8q12 abnormalities are typically younger
- No correlation between cytogenetic findings and prognosis

Differential Diagnosis

POLYMORPHOUS LOW-GRADE ADENOCARCINOMA (PARTICULARLY IN MINOR SALIVARY GLAND)
- Frequently shows perineural growth and is infiltrative into periglandular tissue
- Forms small tubular structures or single-file cords of cells at the periphery

CARCINOMA EX PLEOMORPHIC ADENOMA
- Malignant tumor arising in a background of a mixed tumor

SELECTED REFERENCES

Brachtel EF, Pilch BZ, Khettry U, et al: Fine-needle aspiration biopsy of a cystic pleomorphic adenoma with extensive adnexa-like differentiation: differential diagnostic pitfall with mucoepidermoid carcinoma. Diagn Cytopathol 28:100-103, 2003.

Bullerdiek J, Wobst G, Meyer-Bolte K, et al: Cytogenetic subtyping of 220 salivary gland pleomorphic adenomas: correlation to occurrence, histological subtype, and in vitro cellular behavior. Cancer Genet Cytogenet 65:27-31, 1993.

Das DK, Anim JT: Pleomorphic adenoma of salivary gland: to what extent does fine needle aspiration cytology reflect histopathological features? Cytopathology 16:65-70, 2005.

Glas AS, Hollema H, Nap RE, Plukker JT: Expression of estrogen receptor, progesterone receptor, and insulin-like growth factor receptor-1 and of MIB-1 in patients with recurrent pleomorphic adenoma of the parotid gland. Cancer 94:2211-2216, 2002.

Lee PS, Sabbath-Solitare M, Redondo TC, Ongcapin EH: Molecular evidence that the stromal and epithelial cells in pleomorphic adenomas of salivary gland arise from the same origin: clonal analysis using human androgen receptor gene (HUMARA) assay. Hum Pathol 31:498-503, 2000.

MYOEPITHELIOMA

Clinical Features

- Benign tumor composed entirely of myoepithelial cells
- May represent the end of the pleomorphic adenoma spectrum
- About 2% to 5% of benign salivary gland tumors
- Sites: parotid (50%) and minor salivary glands (40%)
- Men and women affected equally
- Peak incidence in third decade
- Typically presents as an asymptomatic mass

Gross Pathology

- Well circumscribed and may be encapsulated
- Cut surface is solid, tan, or yellow-tan and glistening

Histopathology (Figure 3-27)

- Three characteristic histologic growth patterns
  - Spindle cell variant
    - Composed of interlacing fascicles of uniform spindle cells that have elongated nuclei and eosinophilic cytoplasm
    - May manifest clusters of polygonal or round epithelial or clear cells
    - Minimal formation of myxoid stoma
  - Plasmacytoid cell variant
    - Cells show plasmacytoid features, most common subtype

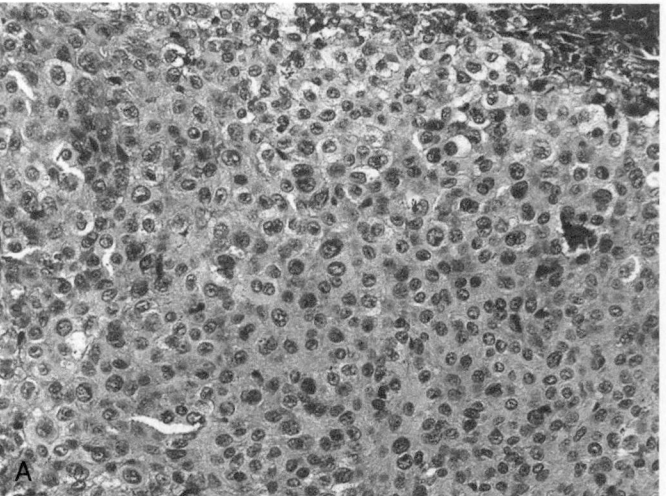

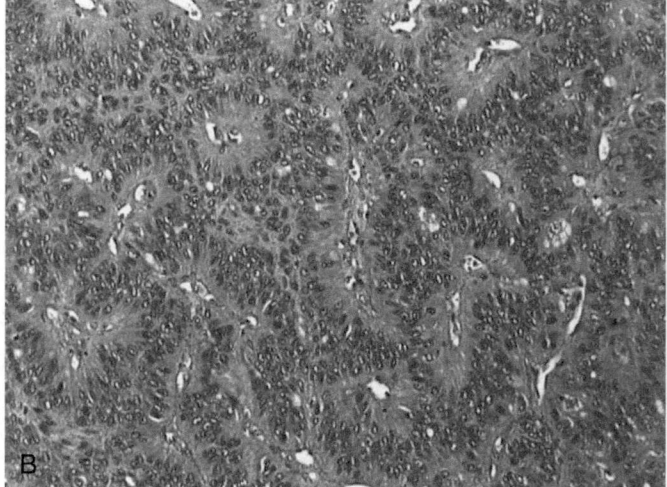

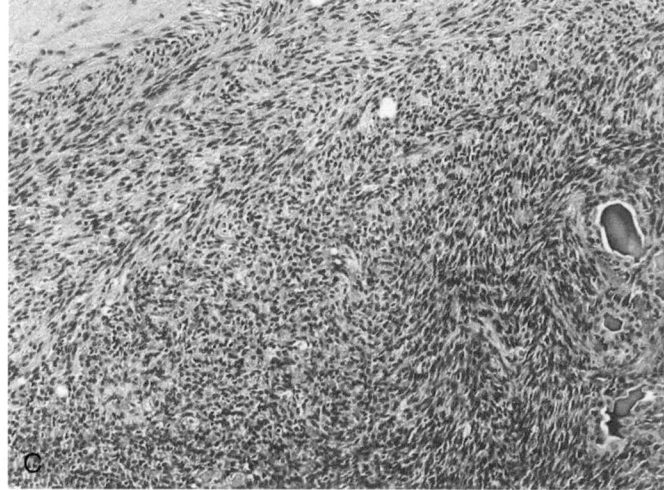

Figure 3-27. Myoepithelioma. A, Solid sheets of round myoepithelial cells. **B,** Myoepithelial cells are forming trabeculae with a rosette-like pattern. **C,** Marked spindling of the myoepithelial cells.

- Epithelioid variant
  - Tumors are composed of epithelioid cells with round to oval vesicular nuclei, inconspicuous nucleoli, and eosinophilic cytoplasm
  - Few spindle and plasmacytoid cells may be present

- Occasionally microcystic architecture with mucoid stroma
- Stroma, when present, shows hyaline or myxoid features

Special Stains and Immunohistochemistry

- Cytokeratin, muscle-specific actin (MSA), glial fibrillary acidic protein (GFAP), calponin, and S-100 protein: variable reactivity

Other Techniques for Diagnosis

- Noncontributory

Differential Diagnosis

MYOEPITHELIAL-RICH MIXED TUMOR (PLEOMORPHIC ADENOMA)

- Areas of conventional of benign mixed tumor

MYOEPITHELIAL CARCINOMA

- Infiltrative borders with and without cellular features of malignancy
- Slightly older; mean age, 50 years; same incidence in males and females
- Most arise in parotid
- Unencapsulated, multinodular
- Morphologic cellular variability (spindled, stellate, epithelioid, plasmacytoid)
- Cytologically, often bland-appearing adenoma but locally invasive
- Also designate carcinoma when perineural or lymphovascular invasion is identified

SPINDLE CELL TUMORS (RARE IN THE MAJOR AND MINOR SALIVARY GLANDS)

- Nerve sheath tumors: schwannoma
  - Cytokeratin negative, S-100 protein positive
- Fibrous histiocytomas: cytokeratin negative
- Nodular fasciitis: cytokeratin negative
- Monophasic spindle cell synovial sarcoma
  - Often has high-grade histology
  - May be positive for cytokeratin, epithelial or mixed forms

METASTATIC RENAL CELL CARCINOMA (DIFFERENTIATE FROM CLEAR CELL MYOEPITHELIOMA)

- History is important
- Distinct delicate vascularity surrounds tumor cells

PEARLS

- *Differentiate adenoma from carcinoma by circumscription verses invasion*
- *Histologically, myoepithelial cells are diverse in appearance*

SELECTED REFERENCES

Hungermann D, Roeser K, Buerger H, et al: Relative paucity of gross genetic alterations in myoepitheliomas and myoepithelial carcinomas of salivary glands. J Pathol 198:487-494, 2002.
Nagao T, Sugano I, Ishida Y, et al: Salivary gland malignant myoepithelioma: a clinicopathologic and immunohistochemical study of ten cases. Cancer 83:1292-1299, 1998.
Savera AT, Sloman A, Huvos AG, Klimstra DS: Myoepithelial carcinoma of the salivary glands: a clinicopathologic study of 25 patients. Am J Surg Pathol 24:761-774, 2000.
Simpson RH, Jones H, Beasley P: Benign myoepithelioma of the salivary glands: a true entity? Histopathology 27:1-9, 1995.

WARTHIN TUMOR (PAPILLARY CYSTADENOMA LYMPHOMATOSUM)

Clinical Features

- Second most common benign salivary tumor
- Most occur in parotid gland
- Unusually low frequency in black patients
- More common in males
- Presents as a painless, sometimes fluctuant swelling (usually 2 to 4 cm in diameter)
- May present as multifocal or bilateral lesions

Gross Pathology

- Well-circumscribed, fluctuant mass
- Cut surface shows brown mucoid and turbid materials in cystic spaces and small granular tissue excrescences; cystic areas are tan to nodular foci and may be hemorrhagic (Figure 3-28A)

Histopathology

- Thin capsule, usually sharply demarcated from surrounding parenchyma
- Epithelial component composed of tall columnar and basaloid oncocytic cells lining cysts and forming prominent papillae
- Cystic spaces lined by papillary proliferation of oncocytic epithelium with lymphoid stroma; can show lymphoid follicles (Figure 3-28B)
- Cyst contents include cellular debris and laminated bodies resembling corpora amylacea, and calcifications
- Squamous metaplasia may be present

Special Stains and Immunohistochemistry

- Noncontributory

Other Techniques for Diagnosis

- Noncontributory

Differential Diagnosis

ONCOCYTOMA

- Typically a solid proliferation of oncocytic cells; may occasionally be cystic
- Lacks lymphoid component

PAPILLARY ONCOCYTIC CYSTADENOMA

- Lacks lymphoid component

LYMPHOEPITHELIAL CYSTS IN HIV PATIENTS

- Often bilateral
- Lack oncocytes

LYMPHADENOMA

- Lacks oncocytic cell component

PAROTID DUCT CYST

- Lacks dense lymphoid stroma

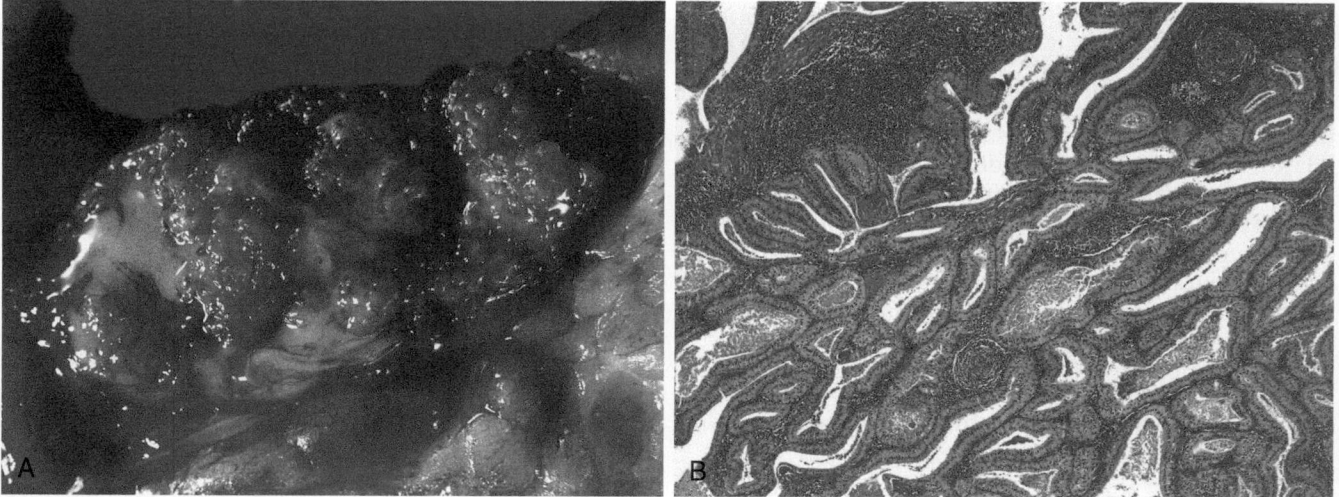

Figure 3-28. Warthin tumor. A, Gross photograph of a parotid mass shows a partially cystic mass with a fine nodular, papillary surface. **B,** Section shows a cystic tumor composed of uniform, bland oncocytic epithelium surrounded by lymphoid cells.

PEARLS

- *Pathogenesis uncertain; possibly two forms: reactive (non-neoplastic) characterized by multifocality and bilaterality, and neoplastic characterized by a single site with rare association with mucoepidermoid carcinoma and oncocytic carcinoma*
- *May arise in an intraparotid lymph node*
- *FNA findings (amorphous background, lymphoid cells, oncocytes, and necrosis) can raise the differential diagnosis of branchial cleft cyst, oncocytoma, cystic SCC*

SELECTED REFERENCES

Lewis PD, Baxter P, Paul Griffiths A, et al: Detection of damage to the mitochondrial genome in the oncocytic cells of Warthin's tumour. J Pathol 191:274-281, 2000.

Maiorano E, Lo Muzio L, Favia G, Piattelli A: Warthin's tumour: a study of 78 cases with emphasis on bilaterality, multifocality and association with other malignancies. Oral Oncol 38:35-40, 2002.

Schwerer MJ, Kraft K, Baczako K, Maier H: Cytokeratin expression and epithelial differentiation in Warthin's tumour and its metaplastic (infarcted) variant. Histopathology 39:347-352, 2001.

Webb AJ, Eveson JW: Parotid Warthin's tumour Bristol Royal Infirmary (1985-1995): a study of histopathology in 33 cases. Oral Oncol 38:163-171, 2002.

ONCOCYTOMA

Clinical Features

- Rare benign epithelial neoplasm composed of onco-cytic (mitochondria-rich) cells
- Predominant site is the parotid gland
- Typically occurs in older population
- Presents as swelling, and mass effect may rarely be painful
- Recurrence rate ranges from 0% to 30%

Gross Pathology

- Single, well-defined and encapsulated tan to red-brown mass (Figure 3-29A)

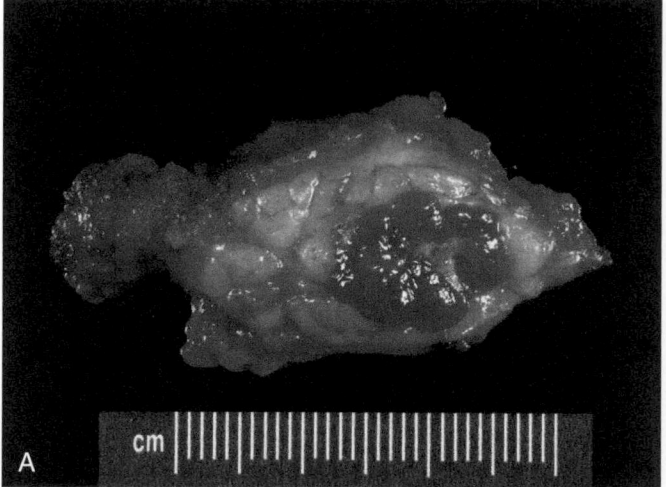

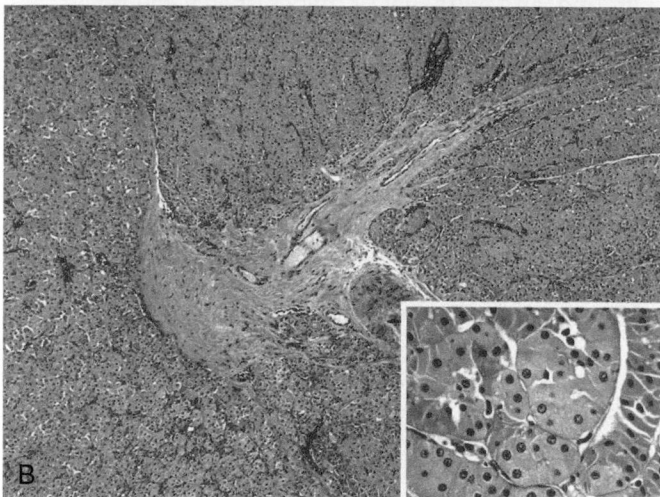

Figure 3-29. Oncocytoma. A, Gross photograph shows a lobular mahogany nodule with central scar within the parotid tissue. **B,** Low-power view shows a solid tumor composed of uniform cells with abundant granular eosinophilic cytoplasm and central scar. High-power view (*inset*) shows uniform round nuclei often with prominent nucleoli and granular cytoplasm.

• Usually solid, but cysts can be present occasionally

Histopathology

• Sheets of relatively large, oncocytic cells (strongly eosinophilic cells with abundant finely granular cytoplasm) with distinct cell borders that contain centrally placed nuclei with fine chromatin and a single conspicuous nucleolus (Figure 3-29B)
• Often arranged in an organoid pattern or in clusters with surrounding thin fibrous bands and capillaries
• Variably sized cystic spaces are present, occasionally with lymphoid infiltrate
• May manifest clear cell features

Special Stains and Immunohistochemistry

• Noncontributory

Other Techniques for Diagnosis

• Noncontributory

Differential Diagnosis

Oncocytic Metaplasia in Salivary Gland

• Normal salivary gland with focal oncocytic cell overgrowth
• May be multifocal; occasionally diffuse
• Oncocytes increase in numbers with increasing age of the patient (most likely due to internal cellular derangement or demand on the respiratory pathway cycle of mitochondria)

Warthin Tumor

• Papillary cystic architecture and lymphoid stroma
• Squamous metaplasia is a common finding but is rarely seen in oncocytomas

Pleomorphic Adenoma with Oncocytic Metaplasia

• Varied architectural patterns, chondromyxoid background, and epithelial or myoepithelial cell types

Mucoepidermoid Carcinoma

• May arise or occur within Warthin tumor and show oncocytic features
• Invasive, multinodular pattern of growth

Metastatic Renal Cell Carcinoma, Granular and Clear Cell Types

• High-grade cellular and nuclear features
• History of renal cell carcinoma

Clear Cell Carcinoma, Not Otherwise Specified (NOS)

• Unencapsulated and infiltrative
• Nuclei eccentric, often with small nucleoli

Clear Cell Acinic Cell Carcinoma

• Invasive, multilobular pattern
• Clear cells in this entity will be negative for PAS granules
• Oncocytic nuclei are not a feature

PEARLS

• *Neither nuclear atypia nor tumor infiltration correlates with biologic behavior*
• *Recurrence rates are higher if tumor is multifocal or if incompletely excised*
• *Excision is the primary treatment because radiation therapy has been linked to malignant transformation*

SELECTED REFERENCES

Brandwein MS, Huvos AG: Oncocytic tumors of major salivary glands: a study of 68 cases with follow-up of 44 patients. Am J Surg Pathol 15:514-528, 1991.
Coli A, Bigotti G, Bartolazzi A: Malignant oncocytoma of major salivary glands: report of a post-irradiation case. J Exp Clin Cancer Res 17:65-70, 1998.
Ito K, Tsukuda M, Kawabe R, et al: Benign and malignant oncocytoma of the salivary glands with an immunohistochemical evaluation of Ki-67. ORL J Otorhinolaryngol Relat Spec 62:338-341, 2000.
Paulino AF, Huvos AG: Oncocytic and oncocytoid tumors of the salivary glands. Semin Diagn Pathol 16:98-104, 1999.

CYSTADENOMA

Clinical Features

• Rare benign cystic epithelial tumor
• Occurs predominantly in parotid and minor salivary glands (lip and buccal mucosa)

Gross Pathology

• Encapsulated, well-circumscribed mass
• Multiple small cystic spaces within salivary gland

Histopathology

• A single cyst or variably sized cysts with variable intraluminal papillary proliferation lined by cuboidal or columnar epithelium (Figure 3-30)
• Lumens contain eosinophilic fluid with epithelial and inflammatory cells; calcifications and crystals are rarely seen
• Occasionally, gland formation may be seen
• May display oncocytic cellular and squamous metaplastic features

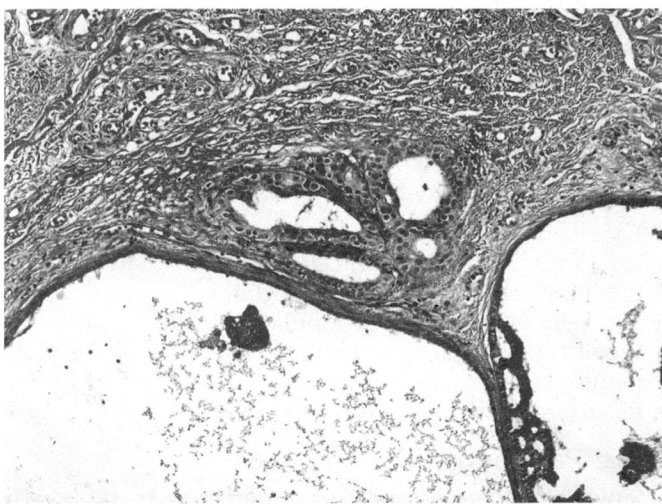

Figure 3-30. Cystadenoma. Cystic lesion lined by bland epithelium.

Special Stains and Immunohistochemistry
- Noncontributory

Other Techniques for Diagnosis
- Noncontributory

Differential Diagnosis
WARTHIN TUMOR
- More common in parotid gland
- Composed of bilayered oncocytic epithelium and marked lymphoid hyperplasia in surrounding stroma

CONGENITAL POLYCYSTIC DISEASE
- Developmental malformation of ductal system
- Multicystic mass with luminal spheroliths and apocrine-like lining epithelium
- Mainly in infants and young children

DUCT ECTASIA WITH FOCAL EPITHELIAL PROLIFERATION SECONDARY TO OBSTRUCTION
- Associated changes include acinar atrophy, chronic inflammation, and fibrosis
- No epithelial cell proliferation

INTRADUCTAL PAPILLOMA
- Always unicystic and occur in dilated salivary gland duct
- Intraluminal papillary fronds are more numerous and complex

LOW-GRADE PAPILLARY CYSTADENOCARCINOMA
- Must have an invasive growth pattern with infiltration into adjacent tissue
- Cytologic atypia can be minimal
- Exclude low-grade mucoepidermoid carcinoma

PEARLS
- *Treatment is conservative but complete resection*
- *Differential includes both benign and malignant entities*

SELECTED REFERENCES
Danford M, Eveson JW, Flood TR: Papillary cystadenocarcinoma of the sublingual gland presenting as a ranula. Br J Oral Maxillofac Surg 30:270-272, 1992.
Nakagawa T, Hattori K, Iwata N, Tsujimura T: Papillary cystadenocarcinoma arising from minor salivary glands in the anterior portion of the tongue: a case report. Auris Nasus Larynx 29:87-90, 2002.

HEMANGIOMA

Clinical Features
- May be capillary or cavernous
- Occurs in adults and adolescents
- About 80% of cases affect females
- Juvenile hemangiomas occur in patients younger than 1 year; most occur in parotid gland (previously called *benign infantile hemangioendothelioma*)
- Often congenital and present as a bluish discoloration of overlying skin
- Can extend into hypopharynx and intracranially
- Rapid enlargement suggests malignancy

Gross Pathology
- No distinctive mass
- Dark red-purple parenchyma

Histopathology
- Juvenile hemangioma
  - Closely packed sheets of cells within salivary gland parenchyma
  - Small capillary channels and larger, thin-walled vessels at periphery
  - Variable mitotic rate
- Adult-type hemangioma
  - Larger, thin-walled vascular channels lined by plump endothelial cells (Figure 3-31)
  - Variable mitotic rate
  - Minimal cellular features of malignancy

Special Stains and Immunohistochemistry
- CD31 positive in endothelial cells

Other Techniques for Diagnosis
- Noncontributory

Differential Diagnosis
LYMPHANGIOMA
- Dilated lymphatic spaces lined by uniform, flattened endothelial cells
- Absence of luminal red blood cells

ANGIOSARCOMA
- High-grade tumor with irregular vascular spaces lined by pleomorphic, atypical cells
- Typically has a high mitotic rate

PEARLS
- *Progressive interstitial fibrosis and infarction of tumors often occur over time*
- *Treatment may include excision, embolization, alcohol injection, steroid therapy, laser therapy, and radiation; propranolol may also be effective*

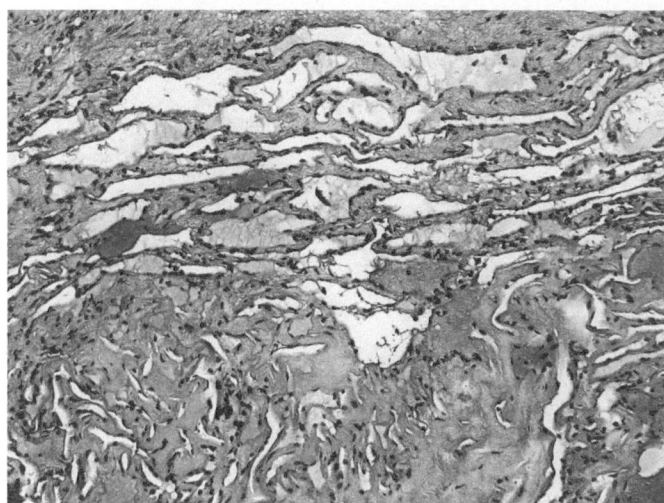

Figure 3-31. Hemangioma (cavernous). Thin-walled dilated vessels lined by bland endothelial cells.

- *By age 7 years, 70% to 90% of hemangiomas will have involuted spontaneously*
- *Presence of high cellularity and mitotic activity does not make the lesion malignant; be cautious before making a diagnosis of malignancy in children*

SELECTED REFERENCES

Livesey JR, Soames JV: Cystic lymphangioma in the adult period. J Laryngol Otol 106:566-568, 1992.

Mantravadi J, Roth LM, Kafrawy AH: Vascular neoplasms of the parotid gland: parotid vascular tumors. Oral Surg Oral Med Oral Pathol 75:70-75, 1993.

Peel RL: Diseases of the salivary glands. In Barnes L (ed): Surgical Pathology of the Head and Neck. New York, Marcel Dekker, 2001, pp 684-688.

BASAL CELL ADENOMA

Clinical Features

- A monomorphic adenoma composed of basal cells
- Most commonly involving parotid gland (70%), usually superficial aspect
- Peak incidence in sixth and seventh decades; extremely rare in children; female predominance
- Clinically, presents as a single, well-defined movable nodule; membranous subtype tends to be multifocal

Gross Pathology

- Sharply circumscribed or multinodular mass
- Vary in size
- Cut section shows a homogeneous, gray to tan mass; usually solid, occasionally cystic

Histopathology

- Monotonous cellular growth lacking the myxochondroid stroma of mixed tumors
- Characterized by uniform small cells with round to oval, hyperchromatic nuclei, pale eosinophilic to amphophilic cytoplasm, and indistinct cell borders (basaloid cells) (Figure 3-32)

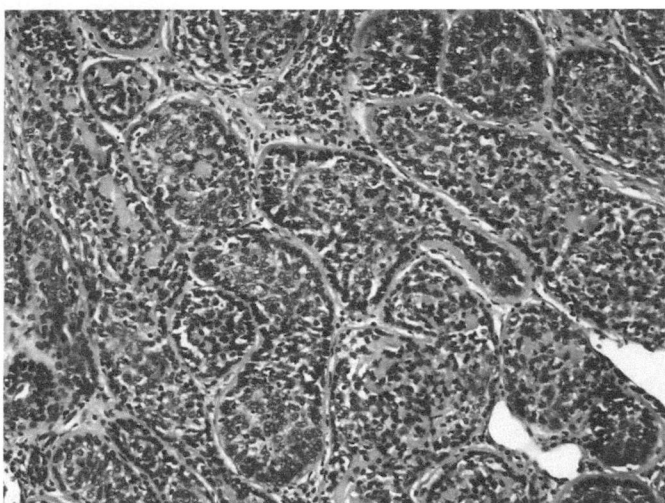

Figure 3-32. Basal cell adenoma. A neoplasm composed of nests of uniform, small basaloid cells with dense basement membrane between nests.

- Squamous and squamoid features may be seen
- Four recognized subtypes: trabecular, solid, tubular, and membranous (often have mixed patterns)
  - Trabecular type
    - Interlacing narrow bands of basaloid cells
    - May have variable proportion of ductal lumens
    - Loose fibrous stroma surrounding trabeculae
  - Solid type
    - Variably sized aggregates of epithelial tumor cells with scant surrounding dense collagenous stroma
    - Palisading nuclei at border of epithelial cell islands and stroma (stromal interface)
    - Foci of squamous whorls and "eddies" may be seen
  - Tubular type
    - Predominance of ductal differentiation
    - Lumens bordered by cuboidal ductal cells that may show palisading; resembles canalicular adenoma
  - Membranous type
    - Prominent hyaline material or basal lamina forms thick bands surrounding the islands of basal cells

Special Stains and Immunohistochemistry

- Noncontributory

Other Techniques for Diagnosis

- Noncontributory

Differential Diagnosis

MIXED TUMOR (PLEOMORPHIC ADENOMA)

- Characteristic chondromyxoid stroma is the most helpful distinguishing feature
- Epithelial cells "blend" with mesenchymal (stromal) component (lacks sharp interface)
- Often GFAP positive

ADENOID CYSTIC CARCINOMA

- Cribriform architecture
- Tumor cells have irregular, hyperchromatic, angulated nuclei
- Infiltrative growth pattern
- Often have perineural invasion

CANALICULAR ADENOMA

- Occurs predominantly in the upper lip
- Composed of branching and anastomosing cords two cell layers thick, which are often separate and form small cystic spaces (beads-on-a-string appearance)
- Surrounding loose stroma

BASAL CELL ADENOCARCINOMA (MALIGNANT COUNTERPART TO BASAL CELL ADENOMA)

- Infiltrative growth pattern
- Tumor cells have bland cytologic features
- May have perineural or vascular invasion

BASAL CELL CARCINOMA OF SKIN ORIGIN

- Clinical history of locally invasive skin primary
- May be metastasis from skin of face and scalp
- Invasive growth pattern
- May show mitoses and more irregular, hyperchromatic nuclei

- *Overall excellent prognosis with low recurrence rates following surgical excision, except for membranous subtype, which may recur in up to 25% of cases owing to tendency to be multifocal and unencapsulated*
- *Membranous basal cell adenomas histologically resemble dermal cylindromas*
- *Rare reports of malignant transformation; higher rates in membranous subtype*

Selected References

Batsakis JG, Luna MA, el-Naggar AK: Basaloid monomorphic adenomas. Ann Otol Rhinol Laryngol 100:687-690, 1991.

Choi HR, Batsakis JG, Callender DL, et al: Molecular analysis of chromosome 16q regions in dermal analogue tumors of salivary glands: a genetic link to dermal cylindroma? Am J Surg Pathol 26:778-783, 2002.

Daley TD, Gardner DG, Smout MS: Canalicular adenoma: not a basal cell adenoma. Oral Surg Oral Med Oral Pathol Oral Radiol Endodontol 57:181-188, 1984.

Ferreiro JA: Immunohistochemistry of basal cell adenoma of the major salivary glands. Histopathology 24:539-542, 1994.

SEBACEOUS LYMPHADENOMA

Clinical Features

- Rare benign tumor (< 1% of all adenomas of the major salivary glands)
- Mean age, sixth decade
- Slightly more common in men
- Almost exclusively found in parotid gland
- Presents as a slow-growing, firm mass

Gross Pathology

- Sharply circumscribed and encapsulated
- Usually solid, occasionally cystic
- Gray-white to yellow-gray cut surface
- Usually 1 to 3 cm in diameter

Histopathology

- Composed of cells that form solid nests of variable size and cystic areas surrounded by fibrous, often hyalinized stroma and lymphoid stroma
- Sebaceous and squamous differentiation is focal; no or only minimal cytologic atypia (Figure 3-33)
- Foreign-body giant cell reaction and histiocytes may be present

Special Stains and Immunohistochemistry

- Noncontributory

Other Techniques for Diagnosis

- Noncontributory

Differential Diagnosis

SEBACEOUS CARCINOMA
- Infiltrative growth pattern and high-grade cellular features

METASTATIC SQUAMOUS CARCINOMA WITH CLEAR CELL FEATURES
- May have areas of necrosis
- Often infiltrates surrounding tissue

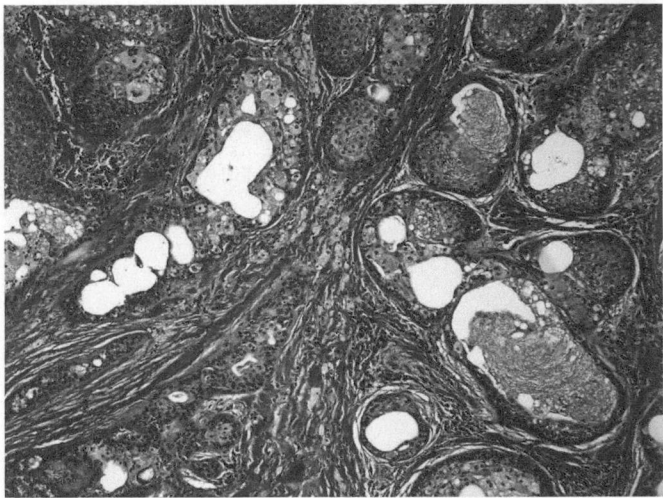

Figure 3-33. Sebaceous adenoma. Nests of cells with various levels of vacuolization of the cytoplasm corresponding to sebaceous differentiation.

- *Benign behavior; no recurrences or malignant degeneration*
- *Treatment is typically local excision*

Selected References

Cramer SF, Gnepp DR, Kiehn CL, Levitan J: Sebaceous differentiation in adenoid cystic carcinoma of the parotid gland. Cancer 46:1405-1410, 1980.

Gnepp DR, Brannon R: Sebaceous neoplasms of salivary gland origin: report of 21 cases. Cancer 53:2155-2170, 1984.

Merwin WH Jr, Barnes L, Myers EN: Unilocular cystic sebaceous lymphadenoma of the parotid gland. Arch Otolaryngol Head Neck Surg 111:273-275, 1985.

Peel RL: Diseases of the salivary glands. In Barnes L (ed): Surgical Pathology of the Head and Neck. New York, Marcel Dekker, 2001, pp 728-731.

ADENOID CYSTIC CARCINOMA

Clinical Features

- Constitutes about 10% of all salivary gland tumors
- Most common malignancy of the submandibular gland
- May occur in any site with salivary tissue
- All ages, peak in fourth to sixth decades; slightly more common in females
- Presents as a slow-growing, sometimes painful mass; patients often have a long clinical course
- May present with facial nerve paralysis

Gross Pathology

- May appear well-circumscribed, but is deceptively infiltrative; tumor extends well beyond visible and palpable limits of grossly evident tumor
- Solid, gray-white mass with marked propensity to grow along nerves (Figure 3-34A)

Histopathology

- Three major growth patterns: cribriform (classic), tubular, and solid; most tumors have mixtures of cytoarchitectural patterns

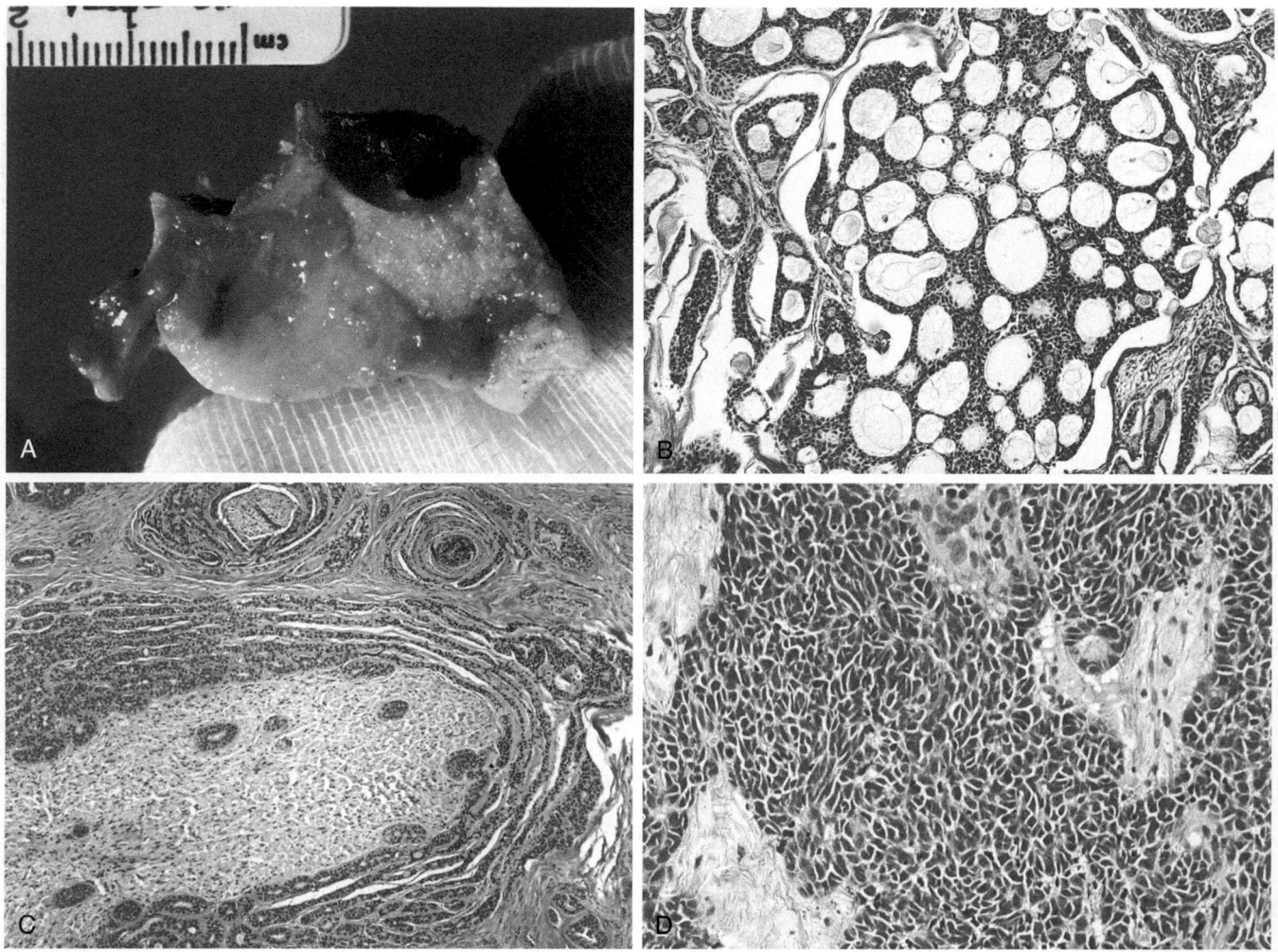

Figure 3-34. Adenoid cystic carcinoma. A, Maxillectomy specimen with a tan-white tumor of the palate replacing bone. **B,** Proliferation of tumor cells with a cribriform growth pattern. **C,** Tumor cells in a tubular pattern showing marked perineural and intraneural invasion. **D,** High-power view of a solid adenoid cystic carcinoma showing increased pleomorphism and mitotic figures.

- Cribriform pattern (classic)
  - Constitutes about 50% of cases
  - Composed of small cylindrical structures (i.e., sievelike appearance with pseudocystic spaces) that are encased by tumor cells (Figure 3-34B)
  - Cylindrical structures contain eosinophilic material (basal lamina) or basophilic substance (glycosaminoglycans)
  - Tumor cells are small, pale to clear, and round to oval with angulated, hyperchromatic nuclei, small nucleoli, nuclear-cytoplasmic (N/C) ratio of 1:1
- Tubular pattern
  - Found in 20% to 30% of cases
  - Tubules lined by cuboidal epithelial cells (Figure 3-34C)
- Solid or basaloid pattern
  - Least frequent, 10% to 15% of cases
  - Solid proliferation of monotonous basaloid cells
  - May show necrosis and high-grade malignant cellular features (Figure 3-34D)
  - Focal areas, cribriform or tubular patterns must be present
- Stroma is eosinophilic, hyalinized, or collagenous

- Propensity for perineural invasion is found in greater than 50% of cases

Special Stains and Immunohistochemistry
- p63 positive in myoepithelial-like component; negative in solid pattern
- CD117 (Ckit) positive in 90% of tumors (not specific for this salivary gland entity)

Other Techniques for Diagnosis
- Cytogenetics: may have chromosome structural or balanced translocation involving 6q regions

Differential Diagnosis
POLYMORPHOUS LOW-GRADE ADENOCARCINOMA (PLGA)
- Occurs mainly in minor salivary glands
- Wide variety of architectural patterns, but cribriform architecture is typically not prominent
- Perineural invasion is common

BASALOID SCC (SOLID TYPE)
- Predilection for hypopharynx, base of tongue, and larynx

- Small hyperchromatic cells in lobules and cords
- Squamous component (dysplasia or carcinoma) in mucosal epithelium

EPITHELIAL-MYOEPITHELIAL CARCINOMA
- No cribriform pattern
- Both tumors may produce basal lumina and have hyalinized stroma
- Composed of bicellular ductal proliferation
- Outer cell is prominent with clear cytoplasm; inner cell is ductal cells

PEARLS

- *Characterized by a lengthy clinical course with multiple recurrences and late metastasis*
- *Adenoid cystic carcinomas with tubular or cribriform growth patterns have better prognosis than solid tumors*
- *Unlike most other salivary gland carcinomas, distant metastases are far more common than regional lymph node metastases (usually metastasizes by hematogenous route)*
- *Lung is the most common site for metastases; may remain stable for many years*
- *Overall has 35% to 60% 5-year survival rate*
- *Surgical resection with or without radiation is typical treatment; neck dissection if clinically positive*

SELECTED REFERENCES

Cheuk W, Chan JK, Ngan RK: Dedifferentiation in adenoid cystic carcinoma of salivary gland: an uncommon complication associated with an accelerated clinical course. Am J Surg Pathol 23:465-472, 1999.

Edwards PC, Bhuiya T, Kelsch RD: C-kit expression in the salivary gland neoplasms adenoid cystic carcinoma, polymorphous low-grade adenocarcinoma, and monomorphic adenoma. Oral Surg Oral Med Oral Pathol Oral Radiol Endodontol 95:586-593, 2003.

Martins C, Fonseca I, Roque L, et al: Cytogenetic similarities between two types of salivary gland carcinomas: adenoid cystic carcinoma and polymorphous low-grade adenocarcinoma. Cancer Genet Cytogenet 128:130-136, 2001.

Stallmach I, Zenklusen P, Komminoth P, et al: Loss of heterozygosity at chromosome 6q23-25 correlates with clinical and histologic parameters in salivary gland adenoid cystic carcinoma. Virchows Arch 440:77-84, 2002.

ACINIC CELL CARCINOMA

Clinical Features

- Constitutes about 2% of all salivary gland tumors and 10% to 15% of malignant tumors
- Up to 90% occur in parotid gland; remainder are found in submandibular and minor salivary glands
- Peak incidence is in fourth and fifth decades; more common in women
- Presents as slow-growing, solitary, mobile mass; may occasionally be painful or fixed to adjacent muscle or skin

Gross Pathology

- Usually single, well-circumscribed nodule; occasionally multiple or bilateral
- Typically 1 to 3 cm
- Cut surface is gray to maroon with lobular and solid-cystic features

Histopathology

- Malignant neoplasm in which neoplastic cells demonstrate acinar differentiation
- Four growth patterns: solid, microcystic, papillary-cystic, and follicular; often have mixed pattern; solid and microcystic are most common and often are intermixed (Figure 3-35)
- Cells may show acinar, intercalated duct, vacuolated, and clear features
- Classic acinic cell carcinoma shows sheets of large, polygonal cells with uniform, round, eccentric nuclei and coarsely granular to vacuolated cytoplasm
- Usually minimal cytologic atypia in all cellular and architectural patterns; mitotic rate is variable
- Most tumors have infiltrative margins (may only be identified at microscopic level)
- Stroma is sparse, may contain marked lymphoid reaction with germinal centers

Special Stains and Immunohistochemistry

- PAS highlights cytoplasmic granularity (diastase resistant)

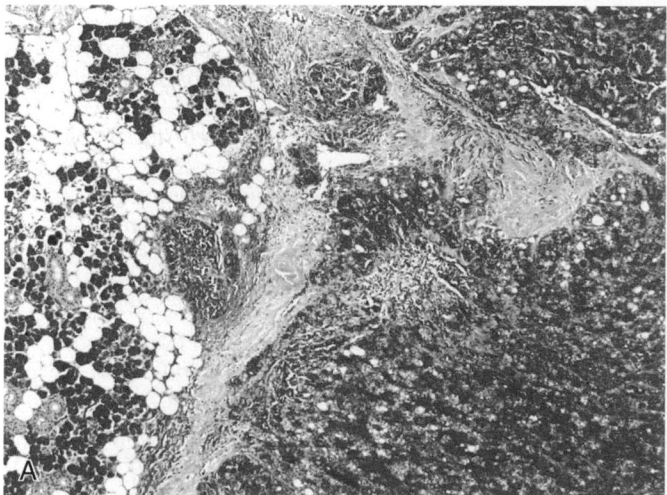

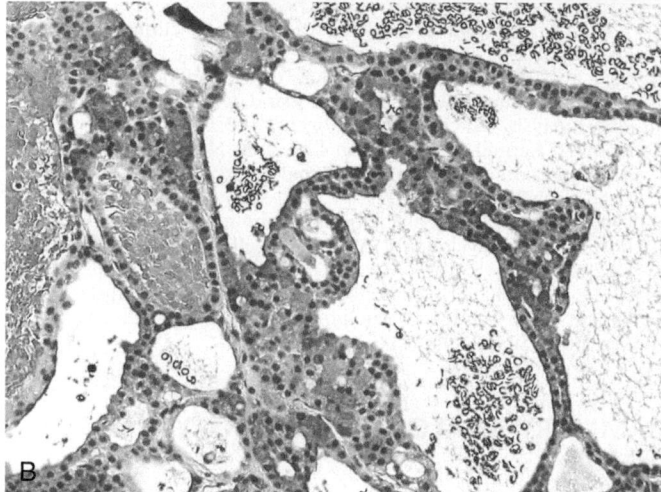

Figure 3-35. Acinic cell carcinoma. A, Low-power view shows a basophilic, granular neoplasm with solid growth involving the parotid. **B,** Prominent cystic growth pattern is present with macrocysts and microcysts composed of granular basophilic tumor cells.

Other Techniques for Diagnosis

- Noncontributory

Differential Diagnosis

PAPILLARY CYSTADENOCARCINOMA OF SALIVARY GLAND

- Uncommon tumors
- Presence of mucous cells (mucicarmine positive) favors cystadenocarcinoma
- Usually does not show microcystic pattern and lacks serous acinar differentiation

MUCOEPIDERMOID CARCINOMA

- Lacks serous acinar cell differentiation
- Clear cell and oncocytic types

METASTATIC GRANULAR RENAL CARCINOMA

- Lacks serous acinar cell differentiation
- History of renal cell carcinoma

PEARLS

- *Difficult to predict biologic behavior based on histology alone*
- *Aggressive behavior associated with solid pattern, necrosis, large size, hyalinization of stroma, infiltrative borders, high mitotic rate, and cellular atypia; favorable findings include encapsulation and lack of intratumoral vascular permeation*
- *About 20% of tumors recur locally; may metastasize to regional lymph nodes*
- *Tumors arising in the minor salivary glands and those with lymphocyte-rich stroma are associated with a favorable clinical outcome*
- *Papillary-cystic architecture is associated with an aggressive course*
- *FNA biopsy findings should be distinguished from normal salivary gland acini, which will contain fat and ductal epithelium*

SELECTED REFERENCES

Ellis GL, Corio RL: Acinic cell adenocarcinoma: a clinicopathologic analysis of 294 cases. Cancer 52:542-549, 1983.

El-Naggar AK, Abdul-Karim FW, Hurr K, et al: Genetic alterations in acinic cell carcinoma of the parotid gland determined by microsatellite analysis. Cancer Genet Cytogenet 102:19-24, 1998.

Hoffman HT, Karnell LH, Robinson RA, et al: National Cancer Data Base report on cancer of the head and neck: acinic cell carcinoma. Head Neck 21:297-309, 1999.

Jin C, Jin Y, Hoglund M, et al: Cytogenetic and molecular genetic demonstration of polyclonality in an acinic cell carcinoma. Br J Cancer 78:292-295, 1998.

Laskawi R, Rodel R, Zirk A, Arglebe C: Retrospective analysis of 35 patients with acinic cell carcinoma of the parotid gland. J Oral Maxillofac Surg 56:440-443, 1998.

MAMMARY ANALOGUE SECRETORY TUMOR

Clinical Features

- Defined by molecular alteration – translocation involving ETV6 gene
- Majority arise in the parotid gland
- Mean age 40s, slight male predominance
- Low-grade behavior (similar to acinic cell carcinoma with occasional lymph node metastases)

Gross Pathology

- Uncircumscribed to multinodular
- Pale to white

Histopathology

- Uniform cells with bland vesicular nuclei
- Growth patterns: tubular, multicystic, and solid
- Vaguely acinar

Special Stains and Immunohistochemistry

- S-100 protein diffusely positive (not specific for this salivary entity)
- Mammaglobin positive
- PAS with diastase: negative for granules

Other Techniques for Diagnosis

- Fluorescence in situ hybridization (FISH) for translocation of genes ETV6 with NTRK3 (t12;15) (p13;q25)

Differential Diagnosis

ACINIC CELL CARCINOMA

- Acini, microcystic, macrocystic and solid patterns
- PAS positive

MUCOEPIDERMOID CARCINOMA

- Typically biphasic; mucinous and epidermoid/intermediate cells
- Clear cell and oncocytic types
- May carry distinct translocation CRTC1-MAML2

POLYMORPHOUS ADENOCARCINOMA

- Arise in minor salivary glands
- Varied growth patterns; solid, tubular, papillary, whirling
- Majority S100 positive

PEARLS

- *New salivary gland entity based on chromosomal translocation*
- *Morphologically and behaviorally close to acinic cell carcinoma*
- *May arise in minor salivary glands (uncommon for acinic cell carcinoma)*
- *Dedifferentiation has been described*

SELECTED REFERENCES

Chiosea SI, Griffith C, Assaad A, Seethala RR: Clinicopathological characterization of mammary analogue secretory carcinoma of salivary glands. Histopathology 61:387-394, 2012.

Skálová A, Vanecek T, Majewska H, et al: Mammary analogue secretory carcinoma of salivary glands with high-grade transformation: report of 3 cases with the ETV6-NTRK3 gene fusion and analysis of TP53, β-catenin, EGFR, and CCND1 genes. Am J Surg Pathol 2013 Oct 18. [Epub ahead of print].

Skálová A, Vanecek T, Sima R, et al: Mammary analogue secretory carcinoma of salivary glands, containing the ETV6-NTRK3 fusion gene: a hitherto undescribed salivary gland tumor entity. Am J Surg Pathol 34:599-608, 2010.

POLYMORPHOUS LOW-GRADE ADENOCARCINOMA

Clinical Features

- Also called *terminal duct carcinoma* (histogenetic origin)
- Occurs predominantly in the intraoral minor salivary glands, especially at the junction of the hard and soft palates
- May occur in the parotid gland
- Wide age range; peaks in fifth and sixth decades
- Female predominance (2:1)
- Frequently presents as a firm, nontender swelling; can erode underlying bone

Gross Pathology

- Polypoid tumor usually with intact mucosal covering; rarely ulcerated
- Circumscribed, unencapsulated, firm mass with tan, homogeneous cut surface
- Typically ranges from 1 to 5 cm

Histopathology

- Well circumscribed, but lacks a capsule and shows peripheral infiltration into surrounding tissue (often infiltrates in single-file pattern)
- Patterns include solid, tubular, trabecular, and ductular (cribriform, cystic, and papillary-cystic may be focally seen); mixed patterns account for the polymorphous appearance (Figure 3-36)
- May show a single-file pattern, narrow ductlike structures; may display a characteristic concentric whirling pattern at the periphery
- Composed of uniform, cytologically bland, cuboidal to columnar to spindle-shaped cells with round to ovoid nuclei and inconspicuous to obvious nucleoli; scant, eosinophilic to clear cytoplasm and indistinct cell borders
- Nuclear clearing that may mimic papillary thyroid carcinoma
- Variable collagenous or hyaline stroma; tyrosine crystals are rarely seen
- Mitotic figures and necrosis are rare
- Infiltrative growth pattern; may invade adjacent bone
- Propensity for perineural invasion, vascular invasion is less frequent
- Wide surgical resection is treatment of choice; resection of adjacent bone necessary if bony infiltration is present

Special Stains and Immunohistochemistry

- S-100 often positive

Other Techniques for Diagnosis

- Noncontributory

Differential Diagnosis

ADENOID CYSTIC CARCINOMA

- Occurs mostly in parotid, whereas PLGA occurs mostly in minor salivary glands
- Characteristic cribriform architecture with nuclei that are hyperchromatic and angulated

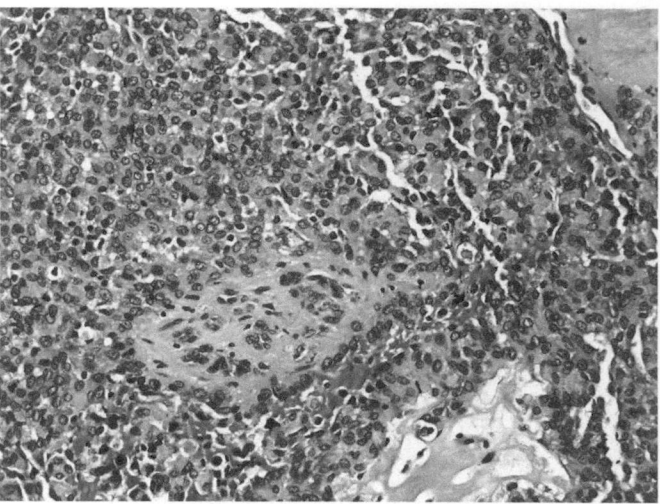

Figure 3-36. **Polymorphous low-grade adenocarcinoma.** Histologic section shows a tumor composed of monomorphous tumor cells growing in sheets and nests.

MONOMORPHIC ADENOMA

- Well circumscribed without invasion into surrounding tissue
- Monomorphous architectural pattern
- No perineural invasion

PEARLS

- *Most occur in minor salivary glands*
- *Recognition aided by combination of architectural features and bland cytology*
- *Mixed growth patterns lead to polymorphous appearance*
- *Although termed* low grade, *perineural invasion is common and may lead to local recurrences*

SELECTED REFERENCES

Anderson C, Krutchkoff D, Pederson C, et al: Polymorphous low grade carcinoma of minor salivary gland: a clinicopathologic and comparative immunohistochemical study. Mod Pathol 3:76-82, 1990.

Kemp BL, Batsakis JG, El-Naggar AK, et al: Terminal duct adenocarcinomas of the parotid gland. J Laryngol Otol 109:466-468, 1995.

Perez-Ordonez B, Linkov I, Huvos AG: Polymorphous low-grade adenocarcinoma of minor salivary glands: a study of 17 cases with emphasis on cell differentiation. Histopathology 32:521-529, 1998.

Simpson RH, Pereira EM, Ribeiro AC, et al: Polymorphous low-grade adenocarcinoma of the salivary glands with transformation to high-grade carcinoma. Histopathology 41:250-259, 2002.

MUCOEPIDERMOID CARCINOMA

Clinical Features

- Constitutes about 5% of all salivary gland tumors; most common malignant tumor of the salivary glands
- Most arise in parotid gland (about 60% of cases); remainder in minor salivary glands
- Slightly more common in women; peak age is in fifth decade
- Wide age distribution, most common malignant salivary gland tumor in children
- Typically presents as solitary, painless mass; variable involvement of facial nerve depending on tumor grade

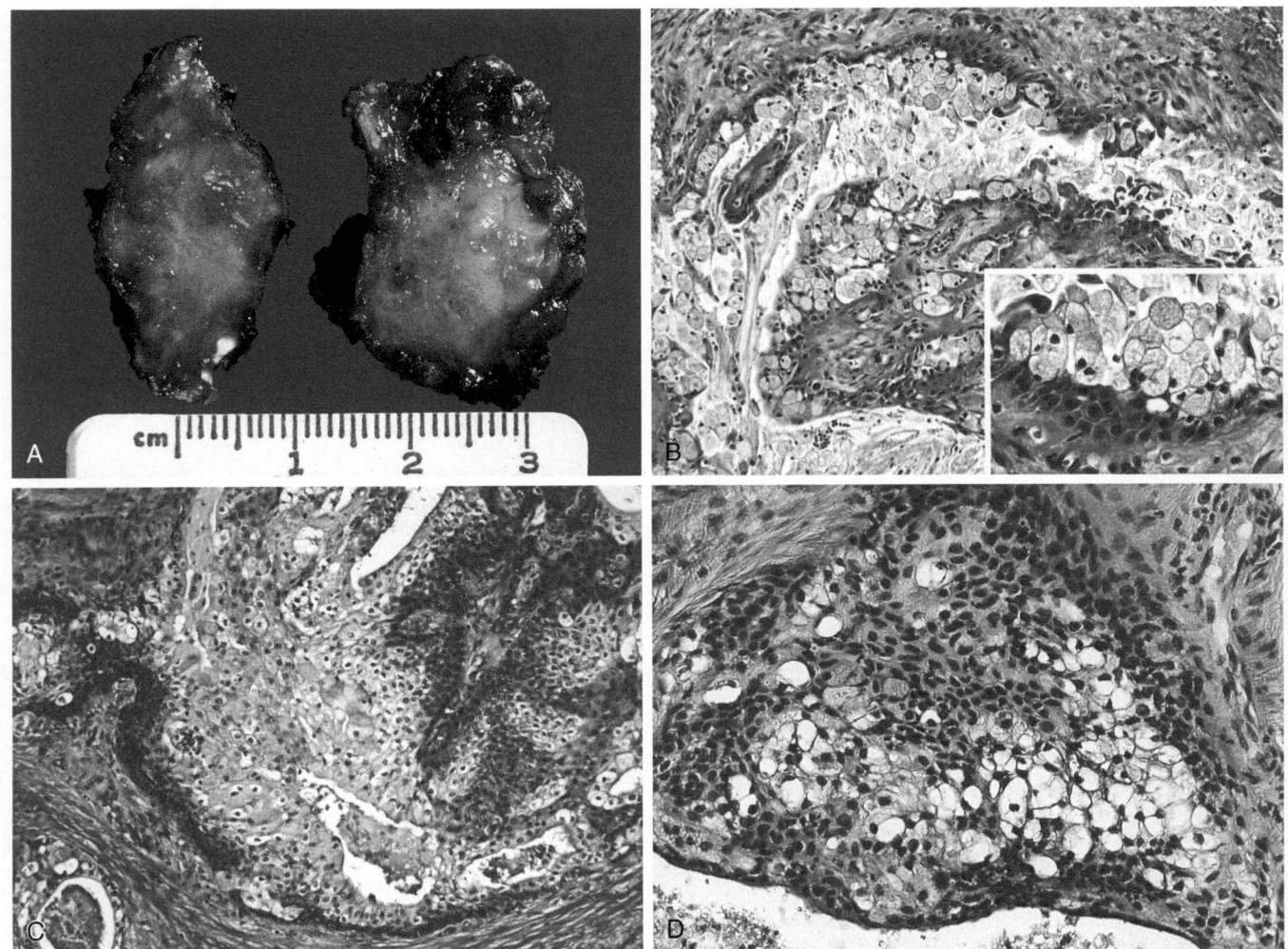

Figure 3-37. Mucoepidermoid carcinoma. A, Gross photograph of a solid, ill-defined mass corresponding to an intermediate-grade tumor. **B,** Low-grade mucoepidermoid carcinoma consisting of prominent mucinous cells surrounding cystic spaces. High-power view (*inset*) shows mucin cells and underlying intermediate cells. **C,** Characteristic features include smaller, basaloid intermediate cells, larger eosinophilic epithelioid cells (central in nests), scattered mucous cells, and cystic spaces. **D,** High-power view showing intermediate, epithelioid, and clear cell changes.

- Increased risk after exposure to radiation
- May be associated with Warthin tumor

Gross Pathology

- Partially encapsulated and sometimes circumscribed tumors with lobulated, firm, gray-tan cut surface
- On cut sectioning, tumor is variably solid and cystic, with cysts containing viscid mucoid material (Figure 3-37A)
- Average size 2 to 5 cm

Histopathology

- Composed of varying proportions of mucous, epidermoid, and intermediate-type cells
  - Mucous cells
    - Neoplastic cells that are columnar and have foamy cytoplasm; may resemble goblet cells or clear cells (Figure 3-37B)
    - Found in clusters or interspersed around the epidermoid or intermediate cells
    - Typically line cystic spaces
    - Usually a minor component of the tumor
    - May need mucin stain to identify this component
  - Epidermoid cells
    - Found in clusters; may form a partial lining of the cystic areas
  - Intermediate-type cells
    - Most common cell type
    - Variably sized cells ranging from basaloid cells up to larger cells with more abundant cytoplasm (Figure 3-37C)
    - Often form islands or grow in sheets
- May also have clear cells, which are usually a minor component; clear cytoplasm is due mainly to glycogen and less often to mucin (Figure 3-37D)
- Architecture is cystic or papillary cystic with lumens filled with mucin; often have pools of extravasated mucin in surrounding tissue
- Grading
  - Grade 1 (low): largely cystic with focal cellular proliferation
  - Grade 2 (intermediate): focal cystic areas with intervening cellular proliferation and invasive features
  - Grade 3 (high): solid cellular proliferation with high-grade cellular features

- In general, higher-grade tumors have few cystic spaces and more solid areas, whereas lower-grade tumors are predominantly cystic

Special Stains and Immunohistochemistry

- Mucicarmine: mucous cells are positive
- IHC is noncontributory
- Translocation of (11;19) and resultant fusion gene transcript, *CTRC1/MAML2*

Other Techniques for Diagnosis

- Noncontributory

Differential Diagnosis

SIALOMETAPLASIA (FROM LOW-GRADE MUCOEPIDERMOID CARCINOMA)

- Reactive condition often secondary to nonspecific inflammation
- Proliferation of squamous cells with occasional mucous cells; squamous metaplasia often seen following FNA
- Squamous nests are admixed with ductal epithelium
- No intermediate-type cells or cystic areas
- Squamous carcinoma with clear or dyskeratotic features

CYSTADENOCARCINOMA

- Cystic or papillary-cystic architecture
- Lacks infiltrative growth pattern
- Cysts lined by columnar or cuboidal, monomorphic cells (less variation in cell types)

PEARLS

- *Prognosis depends on clinical stage and tumor grade*
- *May rarely be associated with other benign salivary gland tumors (Warthin tumor)*
- *Local recurrence is common if not completely excised*
- *Low-grade tumors rarely metastasize; high-grade tumors may metastasize to lung, bone, and brain*
- *Treatment is typically wide excision with free margins*

SELECTED REFERENCES

Auclair PL, Goode RK, Ellis GL: Mucoepidermoid carcinoma of the salivary glands: evaluation and application of grading criteria in 143 cases. Cancer 69:2021-2030, 1992.

Brandwein MS, Ivanov K, Wallace DI, et al: Mucoepidermoid carcinoma: a clinicopathologic study of 80 patients with special reference to histological grading. Am J Surg Pathol 25:835-845, 2001.

Gibbons MD, Manne U, Carroll WR, et al: Molecular differences in mucoepidermoid carcinoma and adenoid cystic carcinoma of the major salivary glands. Laryngoscope 111:1373-1378, 2001.

Guzzo M, Andreola S, Sirizzotti G, Cantu G: Mucoepidermoid carcinoma of the salivary glands: clinicopathologic review of 108 patients treated at the National Cancer Institute of Milan. Ann Surg Oncol 9:688-695, 2002.

EPITHELIAL-MYOEPITHELIAL CARCINOMA

Clinical Features

- Rare low-grade malignant tumor
- Constitutes less than 1% of salivary gland tumors
- Most common in major salivary glands, particularly parotid gland
- Peak incidence is in sixth decade; slight female predominance
- Patients typically present with a localized, painful swelling

Gross Pathology

- Typically well circumscribed and multilobular
- Firm, solid, gray-white cut surface (Figure 3-38A)
- Occasionally hemorrhage and necrosis are seen
- Typically 2 to 3 cm
- Recurrent tumors often have irregular borders

Histopathology

- Biphasic tumors composed of myoepithelial cells and minor component of ductal cells (Figure 3-38B)
  - Myoepithelial cells
    - Relatively large, polygonal to spindle-shaped cells with clear cytoplasm and eccentrically located nuclei
    - Located peripherally and surround the ductal cells
  - Ductal cells
    - Smaller, uniform cuboidal cells with eosinophilic cytoplasm and round nuclei

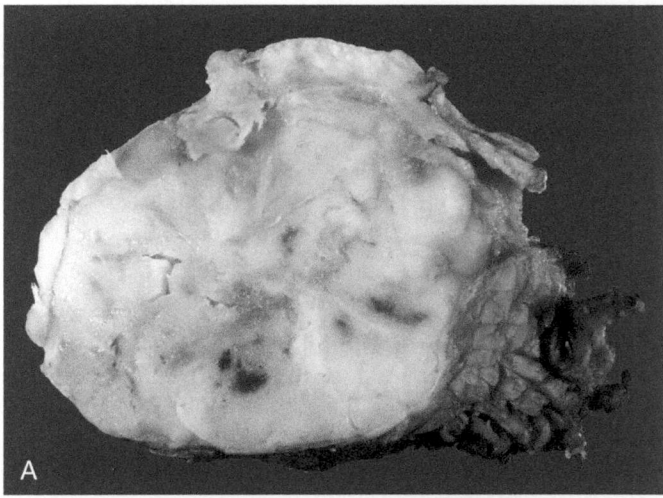

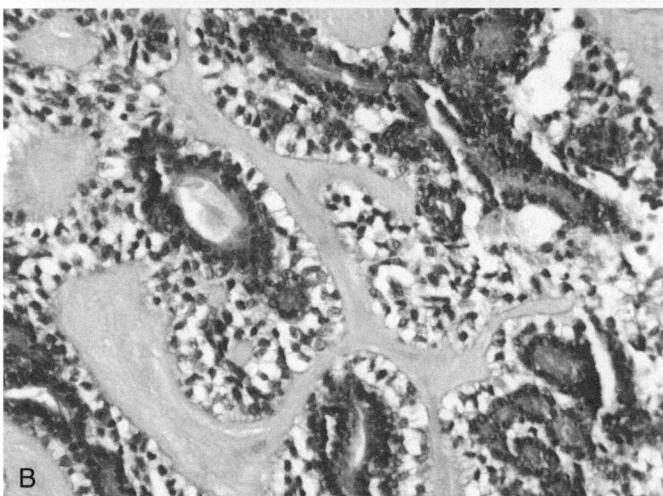

Figure 3-38. Epithelial-myoepithelial carcinoma. A, Gross photograph of a large, white-tan mass with focal hemorrhage replacing the parotid. **B,** Histologic section shows nests of ductlike structures (central in nests and more basophilic) surrounded by myoepithelial cells with pale to clear cytoplasm.

- Form the lining of small ducts that contain eosinophilic proteinaceous material
- Cytologic atypia is usually mild; ductal cells are uniform; variable atypia in myoepithelial cells may be seen
- May have clear myoepithelial cells arranged in an organoid pattern, in sheets or in nests; in these cases, ductal cells may be inconspicuous
- Stroma varies from loose and myxoid to collagenous and hyalinized; occasionally, hyaline basement membrane–like material surrounds tumor nests
- Often have distinct fibrous bands of stroma surrounding tumor lobules
- Variably sized cystic spaces are frequently present
- Occasionally has infiltrative growth pattern or perineural invasion

Special Stains and Immunohistochemistry

- Not essential for diagnosis
- Cytokeratin: ductal cells are positive; myoepithelial cells may be positive
- S-100 protein and smooth muscle actin (SMA): myoepithelial cells are positive; ductal cells are negative
- Calponin and p63: myoepithelial cells are positive

Other Techniques for Diagnosis

- Noncontributory

Differential Diagnosis

BENIGN MIXED TUMOR (PLEOMORPHIC ADENOMA)
- Mesenchymal element (not just myxoid areas)
- Well circumscribed, noninvasive

MYOEPITHELIAL CARCINOMA
- Most arise in parotid
- Unencapsulated, multinodular, invasive
- Cytologically often bland with morphologic cellular variability (spindled, stellate, epithelioid, plasmacytoid)
- Duct formation is not a component of this tumor

ADENOID CYSTIC CARCINOMA
- Characteristic ductal and small cribriform architecture
- Ductal cells often inconspicuous and smaller with more hyperchromatic, angulated nuclei
- More commonly has infiltrative growth pattern and perineural invasion

PLGA
- Occurs mainly in minor salivary glands
- Composed of a uniform population of bland-appearing cells
- Infiltrative growth, often in single-file pattern
- Myoepithelial component is usually not prominent

PEARLS

- *Low-grade malignant neoplasm with recurrence rate of about 30%; recurrences may develop many years after initial diagnosis*
- *May metastasize to regional lymph nodes and occasionally to distant organs; rarely results in death*
- *No correlation has been established between histology and prognosis*

SELECTED REFERENCES

Batsakis JG, el-Naggar AK, Luna MA: Epithelial-myoepithelial carcinoma of salivary glands. Ann Otol Rhinol Laryngol 101:540-542, 1992.

Lee HM, Kim AR, Lee SH: Epithelial-myoepithelial carcinoma of the nasal cavity. Eur Arch Otorhinolaryngol 257:376-378, 2000.

Miliauskas JR, Orell SR: Fine-needle aspiration cytological findings in five cases of epithelial-myoepithelial carcinoma of salivary glands. Diagn Cytopathol 28:163-167, 2003.

Seethala RR, Barnes EL, Hunt JL: Epithelial-myoepithelial carcinoma: a review of the clinicopathologic spectrum and immunophenotypic characteristics in 61 tumors of the salivary glands and upper aerodigestive tract. Am J Surg Pathol 31:44-57, 2007.

SALIVARY DUCT CARCINOMA

Clinical Features

- High-grade ductal carcinoma morphologically resembling breast adenocarcinoma
- About 9% of malignant salivary tumors; more than 90% of cases in major glands
- Wide age distribution (22 to 91 years), peak in sixth to seventh decades
- Male predominance
- Presents as a rapidly enlarging mass; may ulcerate and cause facial nerve dysfunction
- May arise in longstanding stable lesion with rapid growth (carcinoma ex pleomorphic adenoma)

Gross Pathology

- Solid, white-gray with necrosis; hemorrhage is common

Histopathology

- Glandular or ductal structures with infiltrative growth pattern characteristically seen; variety of other patterns, including solid areas, cords, nests, or small cystic spaces (Figure 3-39)
- Large ducts with "Roman bridges" and comedo necrosis
- Often oncocytic cytoplasm
- Perineural and perivascular invasion common
- Lymph node metastases also common

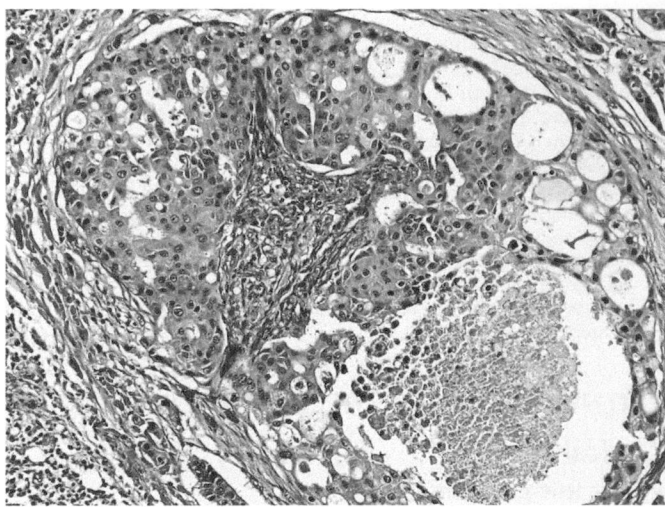

Figure 3-39. Salivary duct carcinoma. High-grade eosinophilic cells with prominent nucleoli forming glands and nests with comedo necrosis.

Special Stains and Immunohistochemistry

- Most express androgen receptor
- *EGFR* expression in half of cases
- *HER-2* overexpression (secondary to amplification) in a subset

Other Techniques for Diagnosis

- Noncontributory

Differential Diagnosis

SCC

- Poorly differentiated from skin or metastasis; morphologically may overlap
- Keratinization if present is helpful
- Acantholysis may mimic duct formation

ADENOCARCINOMA, NOS

- A diagnosis of exclusion; tumors must lack morphologic criteria of a more specific salivary gland carcinoma before this diagnosis is made
- Low-grade tumors have minimal pleomorphism and low mitotic rate

METASTATIC ADENOCARCINOMA

- Medical history and clinical evaluation provide important data

PEARLS

- *Salivary duct carcinoma is a high-grade carcinoma with a poor prognosis*
- *Local recurrence, regional and distant metastases are common*
- *Rarely may express breast and prostate immunohistochemical markers; clinical history is important to differentiate from metastases*

SELECTED REFERENCES

Dagrada GP, Negri T, Tamborini E, et al: Expression of HER-2/neu gene and protein in salivary duct carcinomas of parotid gland as revealed by fluorescence in-situ hybridization and immunohistochemistry. Histopathology 44:301-302, 2004.

Jaehne M, Roeser K, Jaekel T, et al: Clinical and immunohistologic typing of salivary duct carcinoma: a report of 50 cases. Cancer 103:2526-2533, 2005.

Nasser SM, Faquin WC, Dayal Y: Expression of androgen, estrogen, and progesterone receptors in salivary gland tumors: frequent expression of androgen receptor in a subset of malignant salivary gland tumors. Am J Clin Pathol 119:801-806, 2003.

Williams MD, Roberts D, Blumenschein GR Jr, et al: Differential expression of hormonal and growth factor receptors in salivary duct carcinomas: biologic significance and potential role in therapeutic stratification of patients. Am J Surg Pathol 31:1645-1652, 2007.

CARCINOMA EX MIXED TUMOR (CARCINOMA EX PLEOMORPHIC ADENOMA)

Clinical Features

- Malignant transformation of benign mixed tumor occurs in less than 10%
- Most common in the parotid gland (> 75% of cases)
- Rare in patients younger than 30 years; more common in women
- Many patients have a longstanding or recurrent parotid mass with recent, rapid growth; typically painless

Gross Pathology

- Poorly circumscribed and often with infiltrative margins
- Cut section is tan-gray with hemorrhage, necrosis, and cystic degeneration
- Variable size

Histopathology

- Diagnosis requires presence of benign mixed tumor areas (either concomitantly or as recurrence from previously excised tumor) in addition to malignant carcinomatous component
- Epithelial component is malignant; most commonly classified as adenocarcinoma NOS and salivary duct carcinoma (e.g., undifferentiated carcinoma, polymorphous low-grade adenocarcinoma, epithelial myoepithelial carcinoma) (Figure 3-40)
- Malignant component often infiltrates capsule and extends into adjacent soft tissue; tumor may be localized without capsular involvement (designated as encapsulated, in situ, or noninvasive carcinoma ex mixed tumor)
- High-grade cellular features; perineural and vascular invasion often seen
- Necrosis and hemorrhage are common but seen more frequently in high-grade tumors

Special Stains and Immunohistochemistry

- Depends on the type of salivary gland carcinoma present; see under specific entities

Other Techniques for Diagnosis

- Noncontributory

Differential Diagnosis

SALIVARY DUCT CARCINOMA

- History and thorough sampling of the tumor will identify benign mixed tumor component

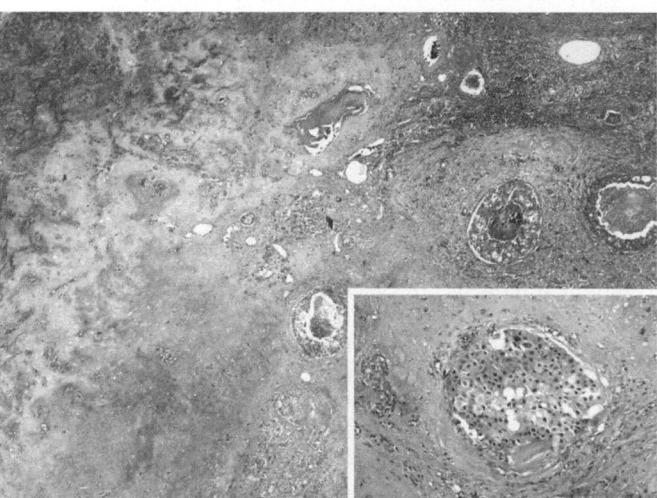

Figure 3-40. Carcinoma ex mixed tumor. Low-power view shows a biphasic tumor with a mixed tumor on the left with chondroid matrix and a carcinoma on the right. High-grade ductal carcinoma with eosinophilic cytoplasm and glandular spaces (*inset*).

CARCINOSARCOMA
- Both epithelial and heterologous mesenchymal malignant components

PEARLS

- *Local recurrence indicates poorer prognosis and is commonly seen before distant metastases (lung, bone, brain, liver)*
- *In cases of encapsulated, in situ, or noninvasive carcinoma ex mixed tumor, the prognosis of completely excised tumors equals that of benign mixed tumors*

SELECTED REFERENCES

Duck SW, McConnel FM: Malignant degeneration of pleomorphic adenoma—clinical implications. Am J Otolaryngol 14:175-178, 1993.

El-Naggar AK, Callender D, Coombes MM, et al: Molecular genetic alterations in carcinoma ex-pleomorphic adenoma: a putative progression model? Genes Chromosomes Cancer 27:162-168, 2000.

Felix A, Rosa-Santos J, Mendonca ME, et al: Intracapsular carcinoma ex pleomorphic adenoma: report of a case with unusual metastatic behaviour. Oral Oncol 38:107-110, 2002.

Lewis JE, Olsen KD, Sebo TJ: Carcinoma ex pleomorphic adenoma: pathologic analysis of 73 cases. Hum Pathol 32:596-604, 2001.

LiVolsi VA, Perzin KH: Malignant mixed tumors arising in salivary glands. I. Carcinomas in benign mixed tumors: a clinicopathologic study. Cancer 39:2209-2230, 1977.

CARCINOSARCOMA

General Features

- Rare
- True malignant mixed tumor with both carcinomatous and sarcomatous components
- Most arise in parotid gland
- Most patients are older than 50 years
- Patients usually present with relatively rapid growth of a parotid mass with pain, facial nerve paralysis, and skin ulceration

Gross Pathology

- Often large; usually greater than 3 cm
- Unencapsulated with a solid, gray-tan cut surface
- Often have areas of necrosis, hemorrhage, and calcification

Histopathology

- Composed of carcinomatous and sarcomatous components; sarcomatous component usually predominates and usually consists of chondrosarcoma; osteosarcoma, fibrosarcoma, malignant fibrous histiocytoma (MFH), and liposarcoma have been reported (Figure 3-41)
- Carcinomatous component is most commonly high-grade ductal adenocarcinoma, but squamous cell carcinoma, undifferentiated carcinoma, and other salivary gland carcinomas have been reported
- Sarcomatous and carcinomatous components are usually intermixed but may be distinctly separate

Special Stains and Immunohistochemistry

- Carcinomatous component positive for cytokeratin, EMA, and often S-100 protein

Other Techniques for Diagnosis

- Noncontributory

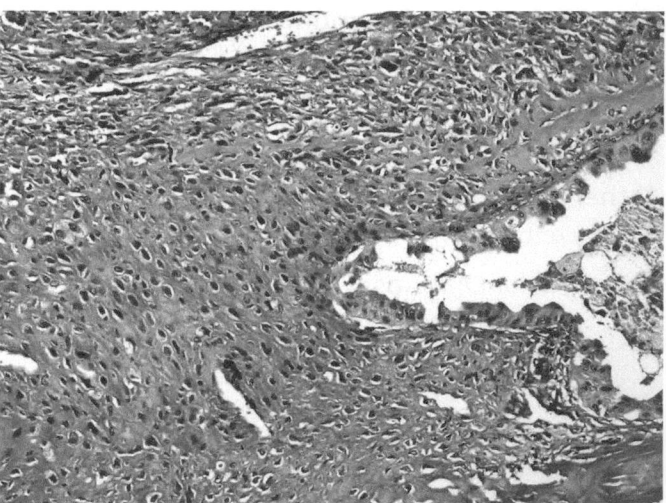

Figure 3-41. Carcinosarcoma. High-power view shows a neoplasm composed of pleomorphic epithelial cells and malignant mesenchymal elements (osteoid differentiation).

Differential Diagnosis

SARCOMATOID CARCINOMA (SPINDLE CELL CARCINOMA)

- Presence of cytokeratin in both components would favor this classification
- Spindled and epithelial components are carcinoma (derived from epithelium)

SARCOMA OF THE SALIVARY GLANDS

- Chondrosarcoma is more likely a component of a carcinosarcoma than a pure chondrosarcoma
- Lack distinct carcinomatous component
- Typically negative for cytokeratin

SYNOVIAL SARCOMA

- Rare tumor of salivary glands
- Biphasic tumor composed of fascicles of uniform spindle cells admixed with epithelioid cells, often showing focal glandular architecture
- Less cytologic atypia
- Immunostains are typically not helpful because both tumors show variable positivity for cytokeratin and vimentin

PEARLS

- *Metastases and recurrences may consist of both carcinomatous and sarcomatous components and only sarcomatous component*
- *High-grade, aggressive neoplasm with predilection for hematogenous spread rather than spread by lymphatics*
- *Most common metastatic site is the lung*

SELECTED REFERENCES

Bleiweiss IJ, Huvos AG, Lara J, Strong EW: Carcinosarcoma of the submandibular gland: immunohistochemical findings. Cancer 69:2031-2035, 1992.

Kwon MY, Gu M: True malignant mixed tumor (carcinosarcoma) of parotid gland with unusual mesenchymal component: a case report and review of the literature. Arch Pathol Lab Med 125:812-815, 2001.

Toynton SC, Wilkins MJ, Cook HT, Stafford ND: True malignant mixed tumor of a minor salivary gland. J Laryngol Otol 108:76-79, 1994.

UNDIFFERENTIATED NEUROENDOCRINE (SMALL CELL) CARCINOMA

Clinical Features

- Rare tumor (< 1% of all salivary gland tumors)
- May involve areas in the head and neck, including the salivary glands, nasal cavity, hypopharynx, larynx, and trachea
- Within the salivary glands, most common in the parotid
- Peak incidence in fifth to seventh decades; much more common in males
- Presents as a rapidly growing, painless mass; patients often have enlarged cervical lymph nodes at the time of presentation

Gross Pathology

- Poorly circumscribed with infiltrative margins
- Often multilobulated with a solid, gray-tan cut surface

Histopathology

- Infiltrative growth pattern with extension into adjacent salivary gland and soft tissue
- Solid sheets, nests, or cords of small, hyperchromatic, uniform cells with inconspicuous to small nucleoli and finely granular chromatin; nuclear molding and marked crush artifact is typical (Figure 3-42)
- High mitotic rate and frequent tumor necrosis
- Nests or sheets of tumors cells surrounded by hyalinized, fibrous stroma
- Some tumors demonstrate focal ductal differentiation or have partially formed glandular spaces
- Vascular invasion often present

Special Stains and Immunohistochemistry

- Cytokeratin positive (characteristic perinuclear staining pattern)
- Synaptophysin, chromogranin, and neuron-specific enolase (NSE) positive
- Vimentin occasionally positive S-100 protein and HMB-45 negative

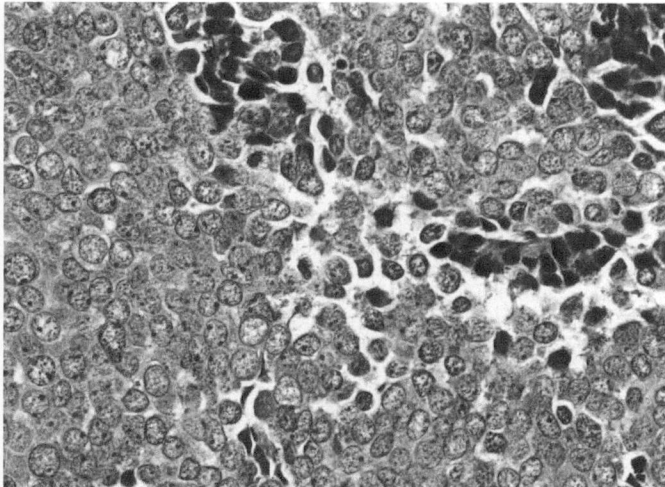

Figure 3-42. Undifferentiated neuroendocrine carcinoma. High-power view of poorly defined tumor cells with scant cytoplasm and variable nuclear chromatin.

Other Techniques for Diagnosis

- Noncontributory

Differential Diagnosis

ADENOID CYSTIC CARCINOMA (SOLID VARIANT)

- Solid sheets or nests of small cells with hyperchromatic nuclei and a high mitotic rate
- Lacks nuclear molding
- Negative for synaptophysin, chromogranin, and NSE

NON-HODGKIN LYMPHOMA

- More solid growth pattern; does not form nests or cords
- Often infiltrate around normal salivary gland ducts and acini
- Positive for LCA
- Negative for cytokeratin

METASTATIC NEUROENDOCRINE CARCINOMA

- History is important
- Small cell carcinoma of the lung usually TTF-1 positive (not specific)
- Merkel cell carcinoma may metastasize to periparotid lymph node; CK20 positive, dot-like; TTF-1 negative

PEARLS

- *High-grade malignant neoplasm*
- *Overall, better prognosis than in patients with small cell carcinomas of the lung*
- *Less than 50% 5-year survival rate*
- *Primary treatment is surgical excision followed by radiation or chemotherapy; neck dissection is often performed, especially with clinically positive lymph nodes*

SELECTED REFERENCES

Cameron WR, Johansson L, Tennvall J: Small cell carcinoma of the parotid: fine needle aspiration and immunohistochemical findings in a case. Acta Cytolog 34:837-841, 1990.

Gnepp DR, Wick MR: Small cell carcinoma of the major salivary glands: an immunohistochemical study. Cancer 66:185-192, 1990.

Nagao T: Small cell carcinoma. In Barnes L, Eveson JW, Reichart P, Sidransky D (eds): World Health Organization Classification of Tumours: Pathology and Genetics: Head and Neck Tumours. Lyon, IARC Press, 2005, pp 247-248.

LYMPHOEPITHELIAL CARCINOMA

Clinical Features

- Also called *malignant lymphoepithelial lesion* or *undifferentiated carcinoma with lymphoid stroma*
- Rare tumor, making up less than 1% of salivary tumors
- Marked predilection for Eskimos and Arctic inhabitants and Inuits
- Wide age range with a slight female predominance
- Most occur in the parotid gland (>75% of cases)
- May occur in association with or subsequent to a benign lymphoepithelial lesion
- Like nasopharyngeal lymphoepithelial carcinoma, this is also associated with EBV
- Usually presents as a painful mass; patients may have facial nerve paralysis
- Frequently have positive cervical lymph nodes at presentation

Gross Pathology

- Infiltrative margins with involvement of adjacent salivary gland and soft tissue
- Lobulated and firm with a solid, tan cut surface

Histopathology

- Undifferentiated carcinoma associated with abundant lymphoid stroma and often germinal centers
  - Epithelial component
    - Irregular nests of malignant epithelial cells that are round to polygonal to slightly spindle shaped and have large, atypical, vesicular nuclei, one to many prominent nucleoli, eosinophilic cytoplasm, and indistinct cell borders (Figure 3-43)
    - Epithelial component may consist of small nests, syncytial aggregates, cords, or trabeculae or appear as isolated cells
    - Usually high but variable mitotic rate
  - Lymphoid component
    - Surrounding lymphoid stroma is often dense and consists of uniform small lymphocytes admixed with plasma cells and histiocytes
    - Typically have well-formed germinal centers
- Occasional benign epimyoepithelial islands with associated lymphoid stroma admixed with the malignant component
- Marked histologic similarity between salivary gland and nasopharyngeal lymphoepithelial carcinoma

Special Stains and Immunohistochemistry

- Cytokeratin: epithelial cells are positive
- LCA: highlights lymphoid component

Other Techniques for Diagnosis

- EBV genomes can be detected by in situ hybridization in malignant epithelial cells; elevated titers of serum immunoglobulin A (IgA) against EBV capsid antigen or IgG against EBV nuclear antigen

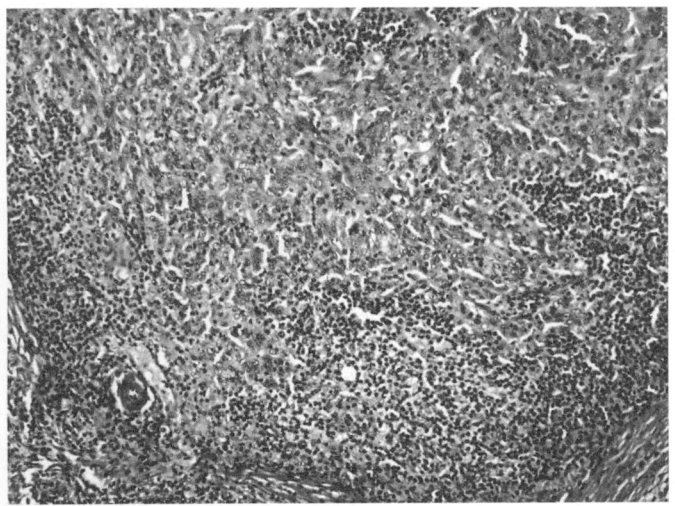

Figure 3-43. Lymphoepithelial carcinoma. High-power view shows a poorly differentiated carcinoma (larger cells, *top half*) surrounded by small uniform lymphoid elements.

Differential Diagnosis

METASTATIC AMELANOTIC MELANOMA
- Typically lacks dense lymphoid stroma and germinal centers
- S-100 protein and HMB-45 positive
- Cytokeratin negative

LARGE CELL LYMPHOMA
- Lymphocytic markers positive

BENIGN LYMPHOEPITHELIAL LESION
- Well-defined mass without infiltration into adjacent tissue
- Epithelial component is composed of benign cells with a low mitotic rate
- Similar-appearing lymphoid component

LARGE CELL UNDIFFERENTIATED CARCINOMA
- Malignant component of lymphoepithelial carcinoma has cytologic features similar to those of large cell undifferentiated carcinoma
- Lacks lymphoid stroma

METASTATIC NASOPHARYNGEAL LYMPHOEPITHELIAL CARCINOMA
- Cannot be reliably distinguished based on histology, IHC, and electron microscopy
- Careful clinical history and examination are essential
- Parotid is an uncommon site for metastasis of nasopharyngeal lymphoepithelial carcinoma

PEARLS

- *Considered an undifferentiated carcinoma but has an overall better prognosis than large cell undifferentiated carcinoma*
- *Factors indicating a poor prognosis are high mitotic rate, anaplasia, and necrosis*
- *Most important prognostic factor is clinical stage*
- *Treatment is typically surgical excision combined with radiation therapy*

SELECTED REFERENCES

Albeck H, Nielson NH, Hansen HE: Epidemiology of nasopharyngeal and salivary gland carcinoma in Greenland. Arctic Med Res 51:189-195, 1992.

Bialas M, Sinczak A, Choinska-Stefanska A, Zygulska A: EBV-positive lymphoepithelial carcinoma of salivary gland in a woman of a non-endemic area: a case report. Pol J Pathol 53:235-238, 2002.

Hamilton-Dutoit SJ, Therkildsen MH, Nielsen NH, et al: Undifferentiated carcinoma of the salivary gland in Greenlandic Eskimos: demonstration of Epstein-Barr virus DNA by in situ nucleic acid hybridization. Hum Pathol 22:811-815, 1991.

Leung SY, Chung LP, Yuen ST, et al: Lymphoepithelial carcinoma of the salivary gland: in situ detection of Epstein-Barr virus. J Clin Pathol 48:1022-1027, 1995.

LYMPHOMA

Clinical Features

- May be primary or secondary; considered secondary if patient has noncontiguous positivity involving multiple sites

- May be nodal or extranodal because parotid gland contains intraparenchymal lymph nodes
- Common tumor of salivary glands; many studies have shown lymphoma to be the fourth or fifth most common tumor involving this location; typically involves the parotid gland
- Most lymphomas are non-Hodgkin lymphomas; Hodgkin disease involving salivary glands is rare
- Increased risk for developing lymphoma in patients with autoimmune disease, particularly Sjögren syndrome
- Most major salivary gland lymphomas arise de novo
- More common in females, especially those with an autoimmune disease
- In young males with salivary gland lymphoma, HIV infection should be ruled out

Gross Pathology

- Firm, solid mass, with a tan, homogeneous cut surface
- May show infiltrative margins with involvement of surrounding tissue

Histopathology

- Most lymphomas are non-Hodgkin lymphomas of B-cell type
- Dense proliferation of lymphoid cells infiltrates and grows around normal salivary gland ducts and acini, resulting in distortion of the normal salivary gland architecture
- Most common lymphomas include follicular small cleaved, follicular mixed, and diffuse large cell lymphomas
- Tumor often infiltrates surrounding soft tissue
- Plasmacytoid lymphocytes, which are common in chronic lymphocytic lymphoma (CLL), may show Dutcher bodies (intranuclear inclusions consisting of immunoglobulin)
- Prominent crush artifact is common
- MALT-type lymphomas show characteristic epimyoepithelial islands and a mixture of small to medium-sized lymphocytes and monocytoid B cells (Figure 3-44)

- Hodgkin lymphoma usually is confined to intraparenchymal lymph node tissue; most frequent histologic types are nodular sclerosing and lymphocyte predominant
- Salivary gland non-MALT, non-Hodgkin lymphomas have similar prognosis as their nodal counterpart

Special Stains and Immunohistochemistry

- LCA (CD45) positive
- Most salivary gland lymphomas are of B-cell type and thus are positive for pan-B-cell markers
- Cytokeratin: epimyoepithelial islands in MALT lymphomas are positive
- See Chapter 14 for immunohistochemical staining patterns of specific lymphomas

Other Techniques for Diagnosis

- Refer to Chapter 14 for specific diagnostic techniques

Differential Diagnosis

SIALADENITIS

- Mixture inflammatory infiltrate consisting of lymphocytes, plasma cells, and occasionally neutrophils
- Germinal center formation sometimes seen
- IHC demonstrates a mixed population of T and B cells; often a predominance of T cells

HIV-ASSOCIATED LYMPHADENOPATHY

- Lymphoid infiltrate is often atypical, and florid follicular hyperplasia may be seen; tingible body macrophages in germinal centers are typically seen
- Commonly have squamous lined cysts and small epithelial nests within lymphoid proliferation
- Often bilateral
- MALT-type salivary gland lymphomas are low-grade, indolent lymphomas; they can transform to more aggressive large cell lymphomas
- Hodgkin disease is rare in salivary glands but occurs most often in the parotid gland; male predominance with a bimodal age distribution

PEARLS

- *FNA with morphologic and flow-cytometric analysis for diagnosis*
- *Lymphomas of the salivary glands may involve intraparotid nodes or the parenchyma*
- *Higher risk in patients with autoimmune disease (Sjögren syndrome)*

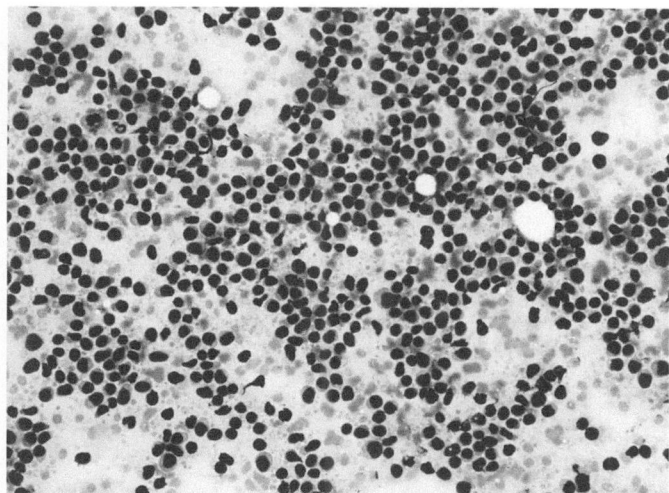

Figure 3-44. Lymphoma, B-cell extranodal marginal zone. Fine-needle aspiration shows discohesive lymphoid cells with an immunophenotype of a MALT lymphoma involving the parotid.

SELECTED REFERENCES

Chan ACL, Chan JKC, Abbondanzo SL: Haematolymphoid tumours. In Barnes EL, Eveson JW, Reichart P, Sidransky D (eds): World Health Organization Classification of Tumours: Pathology and Genetics: Head and Neck Tumours. Lyon, IARC Press, 2005, pp 277-280.

Ioachim HL, Ryan JR, Blaugrund SM: Salivary gland lymph nodes: the site of lymphadenopathies and lymphomas associated with human immunodeficiency virus infection. Arch Pathol Lab Med 112:1224-1228, 1988.

Masaki Y, Sugai S: Lymphoproliferative disorders in Sjögren's syndrome. Autoimmun Rev 3:175-182, 2004.

Royer B, Cazals-Hatem D, Sibilia J, et al: Lymphomas in patients with Sjögren's syndrome are marginal zone B-cell neoplasms, arise in diverse extranodal sites, and are not associated with viruses. Blood 90:766-767, 1997.

TUMORS METASTASIZING TO THE SALIVARY GLANDS

Clinical Features

- Most metastases to the salivary glands are found in the intraparotid or submandibular lymph nodes
- May mimic a primary tumor of the salivary gland
- Most common metastatic tumors are SCCs of the head and neck or skin, malignant melanoma, or carcinomas from the lung, kidney, and breast; less commonly from the prostate and gastrointestinal tract

Gross Pathology

- Depends on the primary tumor
- Metastatic malignant melanoma may be pigmented (Figure 3-45)

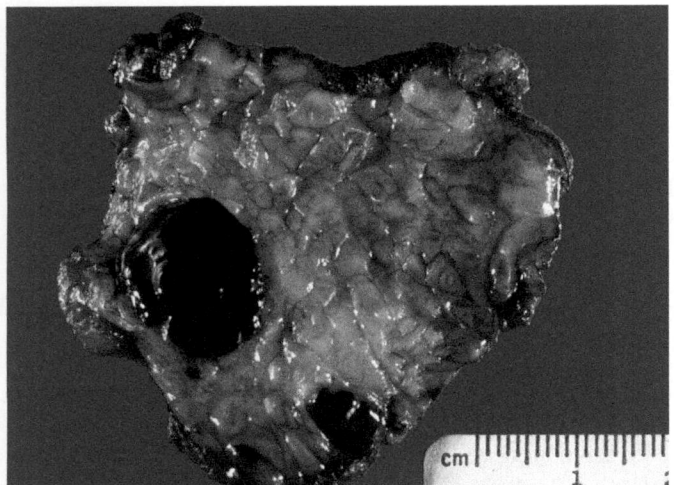

Figure 3-45. Metastasis (melanoma) to parotid. Pigmented nodules corresponding to metastatic melanoma to intraparotid lymph nodes are present on gross examination.

Histopathology

- Histopathologic features resemble those of the primary tumor

Special Stains and Immunohistochemistry

- A battery of epithelial, melanocytic and neuroendocrine markers

Other Techniques for Diagnosis

- Noncontributory

Differential Diagnosis

- Depends on cell type and growth pattern

PEARLS

- *History is necessary*
- *Peculiar features for a primary tumor—think possible metastasis*
- *SCCs in this region are most often metastases from skin*

SELECTED REFERENCES

Hrebinko R, Taylor SR, Bahnson RR: Carcinoma of prostate metastatic to parotid gland. Urology 41:272-273, 1993.

Seifert G, Hennings K, Caselitz J: Metastatic tumors to the parotid and submandibular glands: analysis and differential diagnosis of 108 cases. Pathol Res Pract 181:684-692, 1986.

PARANASAL SINUSES AND NASOPHARYNX

- See Tables 3-1 and 3-2
- See Figure 3-46

ACUTE AND CHRONIC SINUSITIS

Clinical Features

- Common, occurring in 20% of the population
- Purulent and nonpurulent types
- Most commonly involves the maxillary sinus

TABLE 3-1 IMMUNOHISTOCHEMICAL MARKERS USEFUL IN THE DIFFERENTIAL DIAGNOSIS OF UNDIFFERENTIATED SINONASAL AND SKULL-BASE NEOPLASMS

Marker	Olfactory Neuroblastoma	Ewing Sarcoma, PNET	RMS	Lymphoma	NEC	Melanoma
Keratin	–/Focal	–	– (Alveolar +/–)*	–	+	Rare
Synaptophysin, chromogranin	+++	+	– (Alveolar +/–)*	–	+++	Rare
HMB-45	–	–	–	–	++	+++
CD99	–	+++	+/–	–	–	–
Desmin	–	–	+++	–	–	–
Myogenin/MyD1	–	–	+++	–	–	–
S-100	Focal	–	–	–	Focal	++
CD45	–	–	–	+++	–	–
Other techniques		t(11:22)	t(2;13)†	EBV+‡		CD117 10%-15% BRAF 5%

NEC, neuroendocrine carcinoma; PNET, peripheral neuroectodermal tumor; RMS, rhabdomyosarcoma.
*Alveolar RMS: Keratin positivity in up to 50% and 40% positivity for synaptophysin or chromogranin.
†Translocation in the alveolar subset of rhabdomyosarcomas.
‡NK/T-cell lymphoma associated with Epstein-Barr virus (EBV) test by Epstein-Barr–encoded RNA (EBER) in situ hybridization.

TABLE 3-2 CLINICOPATHOLOGIC COMPARISONS OF SINONASAL AND NASOPHARYNGEAL SPINDLED LESIONS

	Nasopharyngeal Angiofibroma	Hemangiopericytoma	Lobular Capillary Hemangioma	Solitary Fibrous Tumor	Kaposi Sarcoma
Age	15-25 years	50-60 years most common	Any age; male teens, women in their 30s	Broad range, 30-60 years	Non-HIV elderly, HIV+ in fourth decade
Sex	M	M+F	M+F	M+F	M >> F
Location	Nasopharynx	Sinus, nasal cavity	Septum > other	Any	Skin, mucosa
Symptoms	Epistaxis	Congestion, epistaxis	Congestion, epistaxis	Congestion, epistaxis	Asymptomatic
Histology	Stellate stroma	Spindled, epithelioid proliferation	Lobular growth	Variably cellular, spindled cells, ropey collagen	Spindled cells, extravasated red blood cells
Vasculature	Haphazard vessels	Thin, slitlike, irregular branching vessels	Capillary proliferation	Irregular, branching vessels	Irregular, angulated vessels
IHC	Vessels CD34+, SMA partially around vessels	SMA+	Vessels CD34+	Stromal cells CD34+	CD31+, HHV-8+

F, female; HIV, human immunodeficiency virus; HHV-8, human herpesvirus type 8; IHC, immunohistochemistry; M, male; SMA, smooth muscle actin.

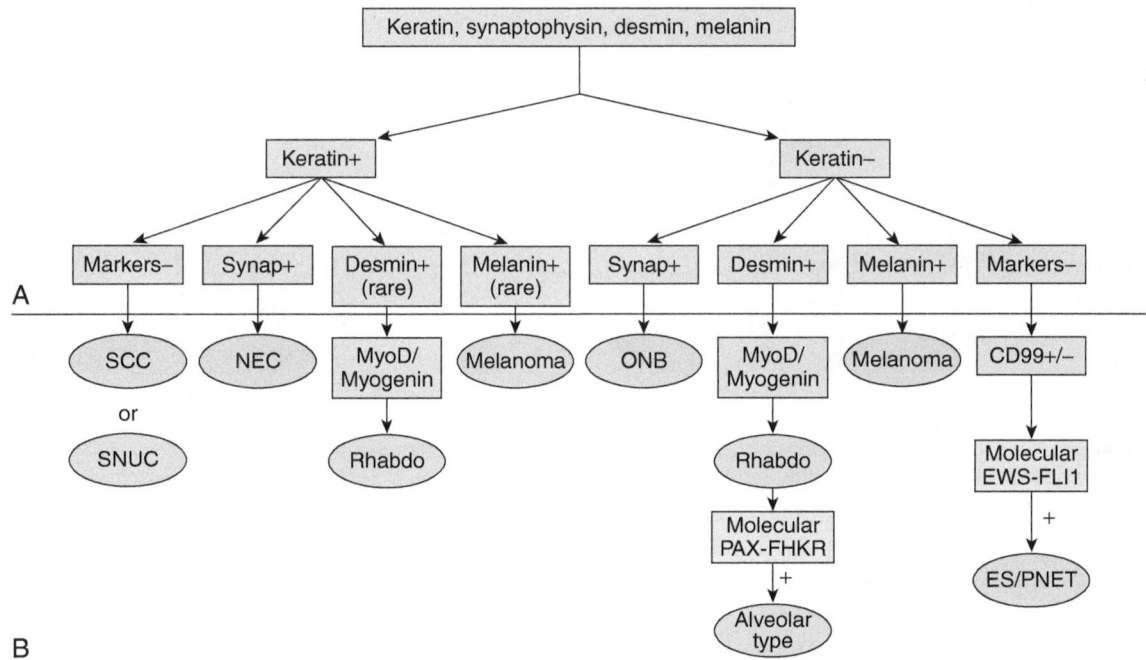

Figure 3-46. Diagnostic algorithm for immunohistochemical evaluation of undifferentiated skull-base tumors. An initial panel **(A)** of keratin, synaptophysin (Synap), desmin, and melanin markers allows for the classification of most neoplasms. Panel **B** includes confirmatory, ancillary markers and molecular studies for rhabdomyosarcoma (Rhabdo), myoD or myogenin, and PAX-FKHR for the alveolar type, and Ewing sarcoma or peripheral neuroectodermal tumor (ES/PNET), CD99, and EWS-FLI1. NEC, neuroendocrine carcinoma; ONB, olfactory neuroblastoma; SCC, squamous cell carcinoma; SNUC, sinonasal undifferentiated carcinoma.

- Acute may be postviral
- Chronic secondary to fungal or bacterial organisms

Gross Pathology
- Edematous, reddish to gray, soft tissue

Histopathology
- Respiratory mucosa with mixed inflammatory infiltrate, edema, glandular hyperplasia, basement membrane thickening, and squamous metaplasia (Figure 3-47A)
- Eosinophils may be present
- Underlying bone may show remodeling and thickening

Special Stains and Immunohistochemistry
- Fungal infection should be excluded by GMS and PAS staining

Other Techniques for Diagnosis
- Noncontributory

Differential Diagnosis
ALLERGIC FUNGAL SINUSITIS (NONINVASIVE)
- Most common in third to seventh decade; same incidence in males and females
- Thick, putty-like secretions (Figure 3-47B)

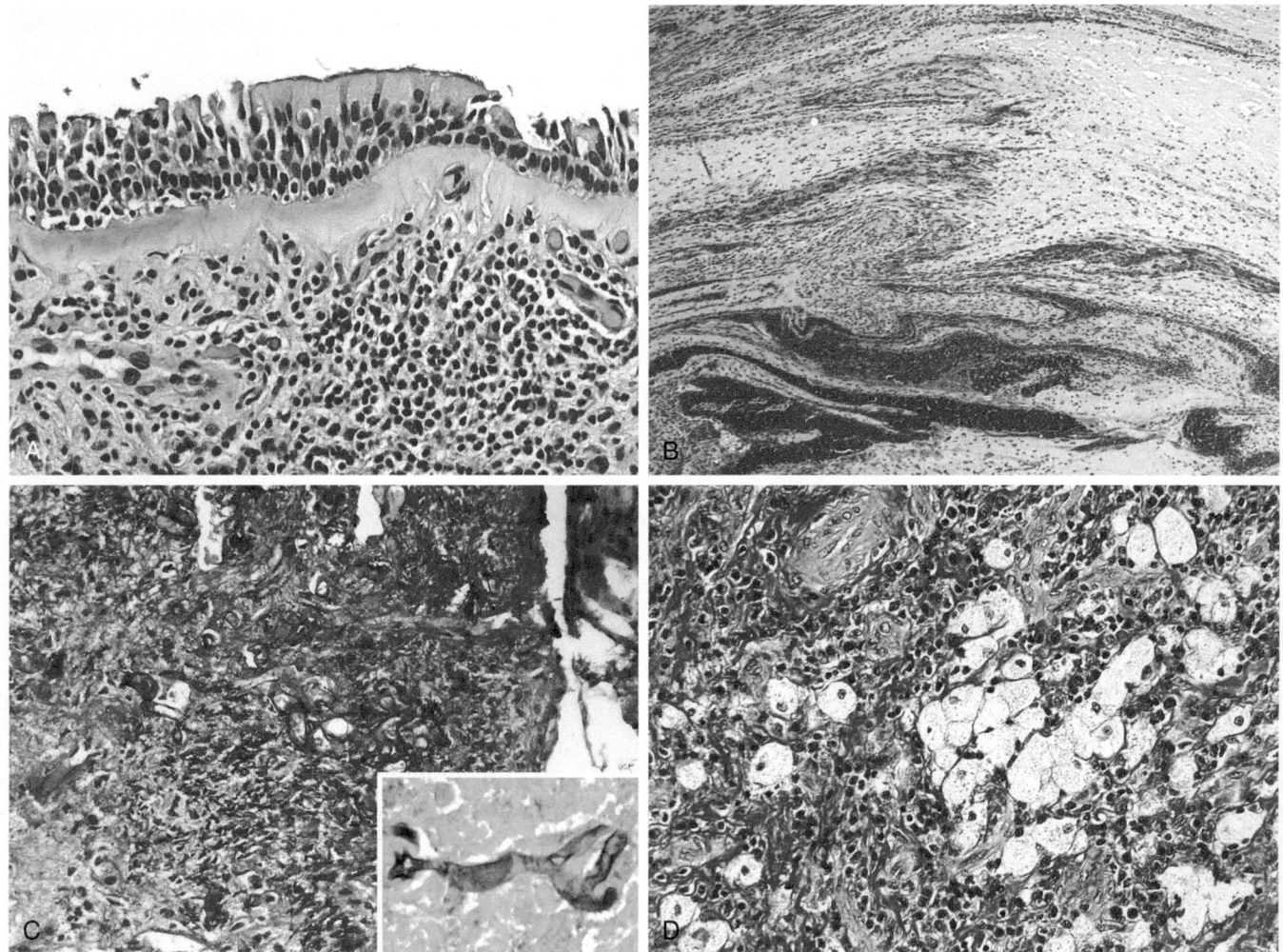

Figure 3-47. A, Chronic sinusitis. A thickened basement layer is present beneath the respiratory epithelium, and chronic inflammation fills the submucosa. **B,** Allergic fungal sinusitis. Thick secretions show layering of mucous and inflammatory cells, a characteristic finding of "tidal waves." **C,** Invasive fungal sinusitis. Marked tissue necrosis and inflammation with fungal hyphae are identified. Gomori methenamine silver stain highlights the fungal wall (*inset*). **D,** Rhinoscleroma. Large vacuolated histocytes (Mikulicz cells) are filled with microorganisms.

- Pools of eosinophilic mucin with abundant eosinophils (layered secretions)
- Charcot-Leyden crystals often present
- Fungal hyphae not associated with tissue (*Aspergillus, Curvularia,* and other species) speciation done by culture

INVASIVE FUNGAL SINUSITIS
- Usually associated with diabetes mellitus or immune compromise
- Spreads rapidly; treatment is surgical débridement
- Fungal organisms invade blood vessels and cause thrombosis and necrosis (Figure 3-47C)
- Thick, twisted, ribbon-like, nonseptate hyphae (zygomycoses)

MYOSPHERULOSIS
- Iatrogenically induced by packing the nose with petroleum-based ointments
- Characterized by large spaces (pseudocysts) with brown spherules that represent altered erythrocytes surrounded by a thin membrane

RHINOSCLEROMA
- Lymphoplasmacytic inflammation with large vacuolated macrophages (Mikulicz cells), may be polypoid (Figure 3-47D)
- Caused by *Klebsiella* species; identified on Warthin-Starry stain
- Endemic in Central America, India, and other countries

PEARLS

- *Complication of chronic sinusitis involving maxillary sinus is mucocele (pseudocyst), which can cause destruction of bone and be clinically mistaken for a malignant process*
- *Cultures required for speciation if microorganisms are suspected*

SELECTED REFERENCES

Batsakis JG, El-Naggar AK: Rhinoscleroma and rhinosporidiosis. Ann Otol Rhinol Laryngol 101:879-882, 1992.
Granville L, Chirala M, Cernoch P, et al: Fungal sinusitis: histologic spectrum and correlation with culture. Hum Pathol 35:474-481, 2004.

Polzehl D, Moeller P, Riechelmann H, Perner S: Distinct features of chronic rhinosinusitis with and without nasal polyps. Allergy 61:1275-1279, 2006.

Taxy JB: Paranasal fungal sinusitis: contributions of histopathology to diagnosis: a report of 60 cases and literature review. Am J Surg Pathol 30:713-720, 2006.

NASAL POLYP

Clinical Features

- Stromal and epithelial proliferation of uncertain pathogenesis
- Usually bilateral and multiple
- Uncommon under 20 years of age; develops in 10% to 20% of children with cystic fibrosis
- Etiologic factors are inflammation, allergy, and muco-viscidosis (cystic fibrosis)
- May also develop as part of mucopolysaccharidosis (Hurler syndrome)
- Choanal polyps arising from the paranasal sinuses are morphologically similar
- Local recurrence is common

Gross Pathology

- Variably sized, soft, fleshy, gray-pink, polypoid masses
- Cut surface often translucent and edematous
- May fill entire nasal cavity and extend into sinuses

Histopathology

- Loose myxoid stroma and seromucous glands covered by respiratory epithelium with occasional foci of squamous metaplasia
- Thickened basement membrane and submucosal hyalinization
- Mixed acute and chronic inflammatory infiltrate including eosinophils; called *allergic polyp* if eosinophils predominate (Figure 3-48A)
- May show a pseudoangiomatous appearance of dilated vascular channels
- May become fibrotic

Special Stains and Immunohistochemistry

- Noncontributory

Other Techniques for Diagnosis

- Noncontributory

Differential Diagnosis

Respiratory Epithelial Adenomatoid Hamartoma

- Often polypoid mass (Figure 3-48B)
- Increased glands composed of bland pseudostratified ciliated epithelium surrounded by a thick basement membrane separated by stroma
- Glands and ducts often connect to the surface
- Rare; males affected more than females, in sixth decade
- Differentiate from papillomas and adenocarcinomas

Rhinosporidiosis

- Hyperplastic polypoid lesions in nasal cavity
- Numerous globular cysts measuring up to 300 μm in diameter containing numerous endospores (2 to 9 μm) of *Rhinosporidium seeberi* highlighted by silver stain, PAS, or mucicarmine
- Marked lymphoplasmacytic infiltrate

Glial Heterotopia

- Congenital malformation without connection to the central nervous system
- Intranasal (30%) or extranasal (60%) manifestations
- Mature glial elements and fibrosis
- Astrocytes may show gemistocytic change
- Encephalocele would connect to the central nervous system and may reveal meninges

Rhabdomyosarcoma

- Usually more cellular with small primitive cells
- Botryoid variant may be polypoid
- Atypical spindle cells; positive for desmin, myogenin, and MyoD1

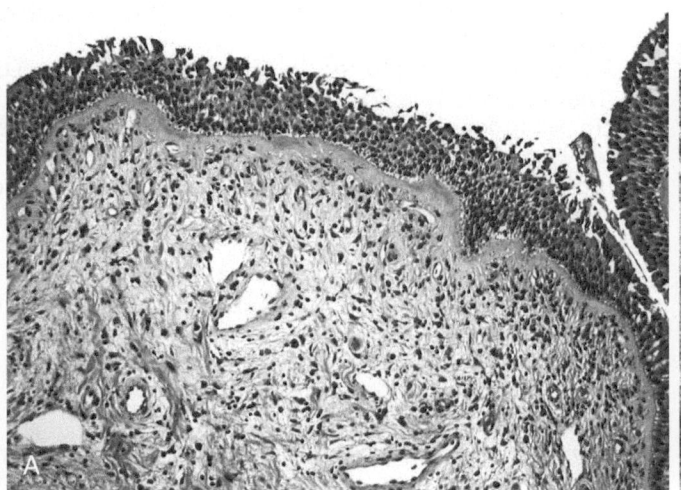
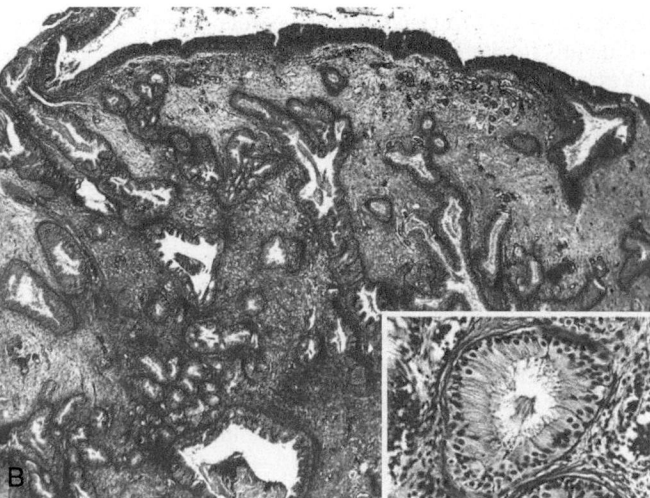

Figure 3-48. A, Nasal polyp—inflammatory. Edematous stroma is admixed with inflammatory cells and increased vasculature. **B,** Respiratory epithelial adenomatoid hamartoma. Low-power view shows a polypoid mass with prominent glands within the stroma. At higher power (*inset*), the glands are bilayered and lined by a ciliated epithelium and a surrounding prominent basement membrane.

ANGIOFIBROMA

- Almost exclusively found in males aged 10 to 25 years
- Arise in nasopharynx
- Haphazardly arranged small, thin-walled blood vessels of varying sizes
- Stroma frequently collagenous with stellate fibroblasts

PEARLS

- *Clinical presentation of "polyps" may represent other pathologic diagnoses*
- *Presence of eosinophils is not restricted to allergic polyps*

SELECTED REFERENCES

Barnes L: Schneiderian papillomas and nonsalivary glandular neoplasms of the head and neck. Mod Pathol 15:279-297, 2002.

Garavello W, Gaini RM: Histopathology of routine nasal polypectomy specimens: a review of 2,147 cases. Laryngoscope 115:1866-1868, 2005.

Graeme-Cook F, Pilch BZ: Hamartomas of the nose and nasopharynx. Head Neck 14:321-327, 1992.

Mortuaire G, Pasquesoone X, Leroy X, Chevalier D: Respiratory epithelial adenomatoid hamartomas of the sinonasal tract. Eur Arch Otorhinolaryngol 264:451-453, 2007.

NASOPHARYNGEAL ANGIOFIBROMA

Clinical Features

- Occurs almost exclusively in young males between the ages of 6 and 29 years (peak, 15 years)
- Arises from fibrovascular stroma in posterolateral wall or roof of the nasopharynx or posterior nasal cavity
- Patients typically present with nasal obstruction and epistaxis
- Locally aggressive, may extend into sinuses or base of skull

Gross Pathology

- Well-circumscribed, unencapsulated, polypoid mass
- Tan-gray and fibrous cut surface may show spongy composition from vasculature

Histopathology

- Haphazardly arranged blood vessels lined by endothelial cells for various sizes, often thin walled
- Vessels are various sizes, often slitlike; larger vessels may have incomplete muscular wall (Figure 3-49)
- Stroma varies from loose and edematous to dense, acellular, and collagenous
- May have stellate, spindled, or angulated stromal cells
- Frequent mast cells, rare mitotic activity
- Postembolization inflammation, foreign body giant cells, and foreign material

Special Stains and Immunohistochemistry

- Beta-catenin positive nuclear expression in > 70% (usually not required for diagnosis)
- CD31, CD34 positive in endothelial cells lining vascular spaces
- Androgen receptor positive in 75% of cases within endothelial cells
- Stromal cells positive for vimentin; negative for smooth muscle markers and CD34

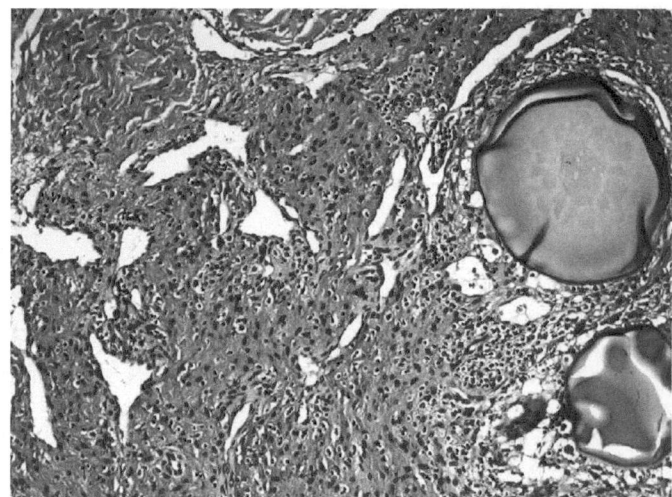

Figure 3-49. Nasopharyngeal angiofibroma. Prominent vessels are surrounded by small, elongated stromal cells in a fibrous background. Embolization material is noted on the *right* with surrounding inflammation.

Other Techniques for Diagnosis

- Beta-catenin mutations in 70% (usually not required for diagnosis)

Differential Diagnosis

LOBULAR CAPILLARY HEMANGIOMA (PYOGENIC GRANULOMA)

- In the respiratory tract, almost always involves the nasal cavity, frequently the septum (60%)
- Vascular tumor with a lobular arrangement
- Large central vessel surrounded by tightly packed capillaries

HEMANGIOPERICYTOMA (GLOMANGIOPERICYTOMA)

- Rare; has been described in all age groups; slight female predilection
- Cellular tumor characterized by staghorn-shaped irregular vascular spaces may be hyalinized (Figure 3-50A)
- Spindle, round cells with rare mitotic activity (Figure 3-50B)
- Spindle cells positive for SMA and negative for CD34 (Figures 3-50C and D)
- Often indolent, without recurrence if completely resected
- Increased mitotic rate and high cytologic atypia associated with aggressive behavior

SOLITARY FIBROUS TUMOR

- Mixture of hyalinized stroma, ropey collagen, spindle cells, and vessels
- Stromal cells are positive for CD34

KAPOSI SARCOMA

- Typically in immunocompromised patients, most commonly HIV
- Slitlike vascular spaces with extravasated red blood cells and hyaline globules
- Positive for human herpesvirus-8 (HHV-8)

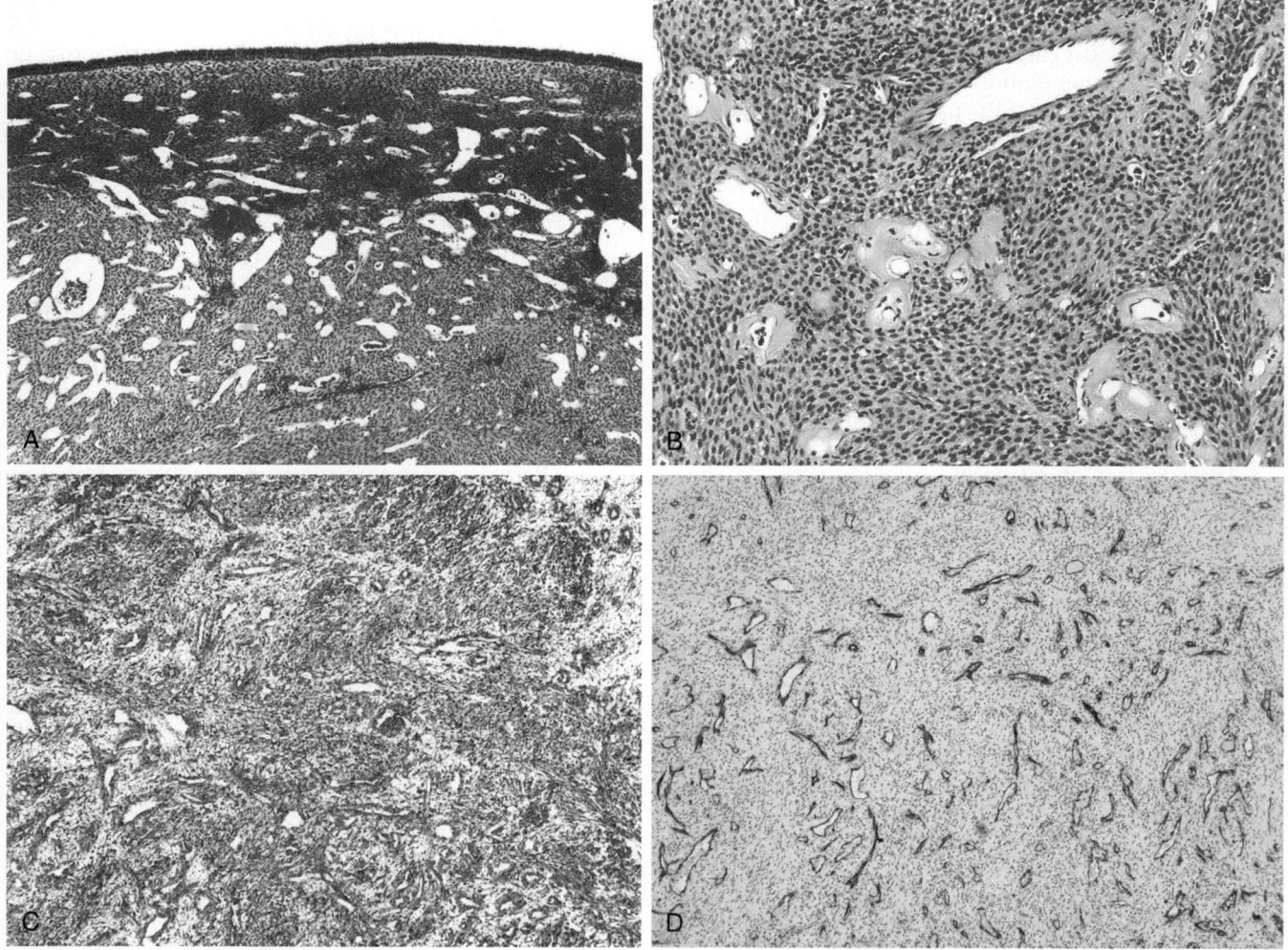

Figure 3-50. Hemangiopericytoma. A, Low power shows a marked vascular and spindled proliferation within the submucosa. **B,** High power shows the bland oval to spindled cells and scattered vessels. **C,** Smooth muscle actin immunohistochemical stain is diffusely positive in the spindled cells. **D,** CD34 immunohistochemical stain highlights only the background vessels.

ANGIOSARCOMA

- Rare in nasopharynx
- Characterized by anastomosing, irregularly shaped vascular spaces lined by atypical endothelial cells
- High mitotic rate
- Tumor cells are positive for vascular markers (CD31, CD34, factor VIII-rel antigen)

PEARLS

- *As a vascular tumor, presurgical embolization is common, with embolization material frequently seen in resected specimens*
- *Clinical correlation is useful regarding age and sex of patient*
- *Malignant transformation (rare) is possibly associated with radiation treatment*

SELECTED REFERENCES

Abraham SC, Montgomery EA, Giardiello FM, Wu TT: Frequent beta-catenin mutations in juvenile nasopharyngeal angiofibromas. Am J Pathol 158:1073-1078, 2001.

Glad H, Vainer B, Buchwald C, et al: Juvenile nasopharyngeal angiofibromas in Denmark 1981-2003: diagnosis, incidence, and treatment. Acta Otolaryngol 127:292-299, 2007.

Puxeddu R, Berlucchi M, Ledda GP, et al: Lobular capillary hemangioma of the nasal cavity: a retrospective study on 40 patients. Am J Rhinol 20:480-484, 2006.

Thompson LD, Miettinen M, Wenig BM: Sinonasal-type hemangiopericytoma: a clinicopathologic and immunophenotypic analysis of 104 cases showing perivascular myoid differentiation. Am J Surg Pathol 27:737-749, 2003.

Wyatt ME, Finlayson CJ, Moore-Gillon V: Kaposi's sarcoma masquerading as pyogenic granuloma of the nasal mucosa. J Laryngol Otol 112:280-282, 1998.

SINONASAL PAPILLOMA (SCHNEIDERIAN PAPILLOMA)

Clinical Features

- Benign neoplasms of the respiratory mucosa subtypes: inverted, fungiform, and cylindrical cell papillomas
- Typically found in the nasal cavity and paranasal sinuses; rare in the nasopharynx
- Most common in adult men (male-to-female ratio, 2:1), occasionally seen in children

- Typically affect patients ages 30 to 50 years
- Clinically present as nasal obstruction or epistaxis
- Unilateral in most cases
- Some studies have demonstrated human papillomavirus (HPV) DNA in certain papillomas (exophytic and inverted)
- Inverted papilloma
  - Most common of the subtypes
  - Arises in the lateral nasal wall and paranasal sinuses
  - Likely to recur if incompletely excised
  - About 10% to 15% of cases may develop malignant transformation
- Exophytic papilloma
  - Also called *fungiform papilloma*
  - Arise on the nasal septum
- Cylindrical cell papilloma (least common)
  - Also called *oncocytic papilloma*
  - Arises in the lateral nasal wall, less often paranasal sinuses
  - May be associated with squamous carcinoma or other carcinomas

Gross Pathology

- Soft tan-white tissue often with small papillae or invaginations

Histopathology

- Most of the nasal cavity is lined by ciliated columnar epithelium (schneiderian), except the nasal vestibule, which is lined by stratified squamous epithelium
- Mixed morphology can occur
- Inverted papilloma
  - Deeply invaginated nests of benign squamous epithelium (5 to 30 cells thick) with intact smooth basement membrane, stroma without desmoplasia
  - Surface epithelium is usually squamous or transitional but may be ciliated, columnar, or mucinous
  - Neutrophils and mixed inflammatory infiltrate are seen (Figure 3-51A)

- Dysplasia may be present and should be reported and graded (low or high grade)
- May coexist with a frankly invasive carcinoma, most often squamous carcinoma
- Exophytic papilloma
  - Exophytic architecture with well-defined papillae showing fibrovascular cores
  - Surface epithelium is usually squamous, transitional
  - Surface keratinization is absent except in areas of irritation
- Cylindrical cell papilloma
  - Multilayered tall, cytologically bland columnar cells may be oncocytic
  - Surface epithelium is often ciliated and typically two to eight cells thick
  - Frequently contain mucous cells, inspissated mucin, and mucin pools
  - Microabscesses with neutrophils within epithelium
  - Inflammatory infiltrate in stroma is common
  - May show an exophytic or endophytic growth pattern (Figure 3-51B)

Special Stains and Immunohistochemistry

- Cytokeratin positive
- Mucicarmine highlights goblet cells

Other Techniques for Diagnosis

- In situ hybridization or polymerase chain reaction (PCR) detects HPV types 6 and 11 in many cases (some fungiform and inverted papillomas)

Differential Diagnosis

SQUAMOUS PAPILLOMA

- Arises from the squamous epithelium near the nasal vestibule
- Polypoid mass lined by mature squamous epithelium with keratinization
- Lacks microabscesses, mucin cells

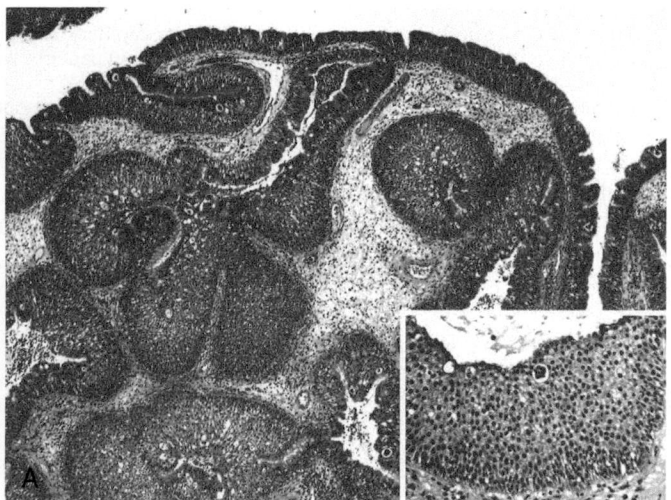
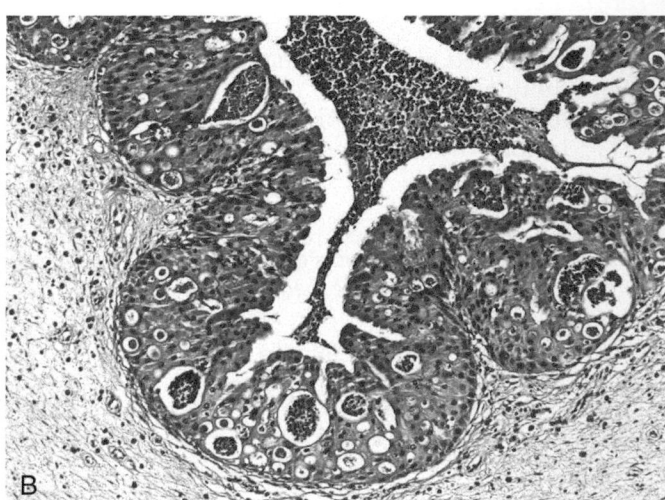

Figure 3-51. Schneiderian papilloma. A, Inverted type. Well-circumscribed nests of transitional epithelium push into the stroma. At high power (*inset*), an intact basement membrane is present with maturation of the epithelium and associated inflammation with intraepithelial cyst formation. **B,** Cylindrical cell type. The surface epithelium is replaced by cells with prominent eosinophilic cytoplasm (oncocytic change) with microcysts filled with neutrophils.

SQUAMOUS CARCINOMA, NONKERATINIZING

- Infiltrative growth pattern with stromal invasion and desmoplastic response
- Pleomorphic cells with large, hyperchromatic nuclei and prominent nucleoli; high mitotic rate often with atypical mitoses
- May coexist with or arise from an inverted papilloma

INFLAMMATORY POLYP

- Multiple and usually bilateral; involves both the nasal cavity and paranasal sinuses
- Associated with chronic rhinitis and asthma
- Mucous glands within fibroblastic stroma associated with mixed acute and chronic inflammation
- Epithelium lacks histologic features described previously

RESPIRATORY EPITHELIAL ADENOMATOID HAMARTOMA (REAH)

- Increased glands composed of multilayered, columnar cells with cilia surrounded by a thick, prominent basement membrane
- Glands are separated by stroma and often connect to surface
- Rare; males affected more than females, in sixth decade
- Lacks microabscesses

SINONASAL ADENOCARCINOMA (NONENTERIC TYPE)

- Proliferation of cytologically low-grade, back-to-back glands filling stroma
- In the differential of a cylindrical cell papilloma

RHINOSPORIDIOSIS

- Hyperplastic polypoid lesions in nasal cavity
- Numerous globular cysts measuring up to 300 µm in diameter containing numerous endospores (2 to 9 µm) of *Rhinosporidium seeberi* highlighted by silver stain, PAS, or mucicarmine
- Cysts also present in stroma (cylindrical papilloma "cysts" only in epithelium)

PAPILLARY SQUAMOUS CARCINOMA

- Exophytic proliferation with fibrovascular cores
- Epithelium shows full-thickness dysplastic cells
- Invasion may be difficult to identify

PEARLS

- *Inverted schneiderian papillomas are the most commonly encountered*
- *Carcinoma may be associated with inverted and cylindrical papillomas*
- *No current criteria to predict which papillomas will develop carcinoma*
- *Recurrence is common with incomplete excision*

SELECTED REFERENCES

Barnes L: Schneiderian papillomas and nonsalivary glandular neoplasms of the head and neck. Mod Pathol 15:279-297, 2002.
Batsakis JG, Suarez P: Schneiderian papillomas and carcinomas: a review. Adv Anat Pathol 8:53-64, 2001.
Kaufman MR, Brandwein MS, Lawson W: Sinonasal papillomas: clinicopathologic review of 40 patients with inverted and oncocytic schneiderian papillomas. Laryngoscope 112:1372-1377, 2002.
Syrjänen KJ: HPV infections in benign and malignant sinonasal lesions. J Clin Pathol 56:174-181, 2003.

SQUAMOUS CELL CARCINOMA OF THE SINONASAL REGION

Clinical Features

- SCC of the sinonasal area is rare (about 3% of all head and neck neoplasms)
- More than half of paranasal SCCs occur in the maxillary antrum, about 30% in the nasal cavity, 10% in the ethmoid
- Increased risk related to cigarette smoking and nickel exposure; also related to exposure to chromium, isopropyl alcohol, and radium
- Male predominance (2:1); typically in sixth and seventh decades
- Presenting symptoms include nasal obstruction, epistaxis, pain, and alterations in voice

Gross Pathology

- Cut surface is tan-white with areas of necrosis and hemorrhage
- Infiltrative growth pattern

Histopathology

- Most are easily recognized intermediate- to high-grade tumors with obvious squamous differentiation and often focal keratinization; nonkeratinizing carcinomas do occur (Figure 3-52)
- Less common histologic subtypes include verrucous carcinoma, basaloid carcinoma, and spindle cell (sarcomatoid) carcinoma
- Desmoplastic stroma present
- Dysplastic squamous epithelium is seen at the edges of early lesions
- Lymph node involvement in 15%; increases with extension outside of nasal cavity

Special Stains and Immunohistochemistry

- Cytokeratin positive
- Synaptophysin and chromogranin negative

Other Techniques for Diagnosis

- Noncontributory

Differential Diagnosis

SINONASAL UNDIFFERENTIATED CARCINOMA (SNUC)

- Nests, trabeculae, or sheets of poorly differentiated cells with high mitotic rate and necrosis; lacks squamous differentiation; lacks keratinization
- Moderate-sized cells, frequently with prominent nucleoli

SCHNEIDERIAN PAPILLOMAS

- Inverted growth pattern has intact basement membrane without desmoplasia
- Epithelium is uniform; may show dysplasia
- May accompany and give rise to sinonasal squamous carcinoma

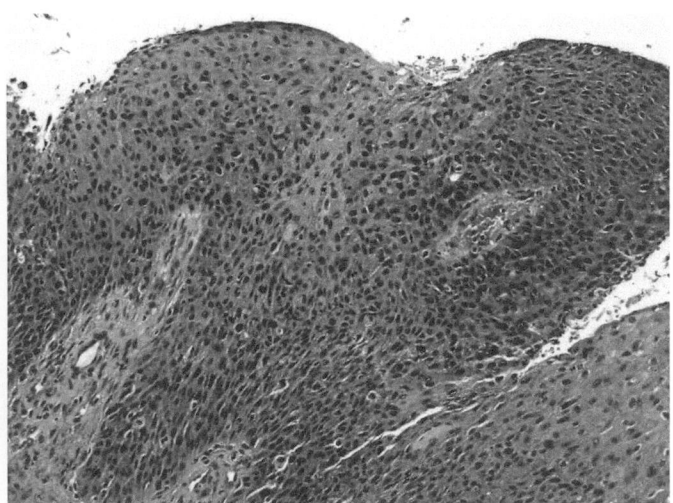

Figure 3-52. Squamous cell carcinoma arising in the maxillary sinus. Morphologically similar to squamous cell carcinomas in other head and neck sites, full-thickness pleomorphic cells with hyperchromatic nuclei are seen.

PEARLS

- *Recurrences are common regardless of mode of treatment*
- *Death typically due to local spread (60% 5-year survival rate)*
- *High frequency of second primary squamous carcinomas of the oral cavity and larynx and other sites (lung and esophagus)*

SELECTED REFERENCES

Dulguerov P, Jacobsen MS, Allal AS, et al: Nasal and paranasal sinus carcinoma: are we making progress? A series of 220 patients and a systematic review. Cancer 92:3012-3029, 2001.

Pilch BZ, Bouqout J, Thompson LDR: Squamous cell carcinoma. In Barnes EL, Evenson JW, Reichart P, Sidransky D (eds): World Health Organization Classification of Tumours: Pathology and Genetics: Head and Neck Tumours. Lyon, IARC Press, 2005, pp 15-17.

Thompson LDR: Malignant neoplasms of the nasal cavity, paranasal sinuses and nasopharynx. In Thompson LDR, Goldblum JR (eds): Head and Neck Pathology. Philadelphia, Churchill Livingstone, 2006, pp 155-160.

Wieneke JA, Thompson LD, Wenig BM: Basaloid squamous cell carcinoma of the sinonasal tract. Cancer 85:841-854, 1999.

MIDLINE-NUT CARCINOMA

Clinical Features

- Recently defined probable poorly differentiated subtype of squamous carcinoma
- Defined by recurrent translocation of the nuclear protein in testis (NUT) gene
- Highly aggressive malignancy with mean survival 7 months
- Wide age range, first recognized in children/adolescence
- Common in midline including sinonasal region though not exclusively

Gross Pathology

- *Ill-defined, infiltrative tumor*

Histopathology

- Predominately high-grade undifferentiated cells and necrosis
- May show areas of squamatization with keratinization (helpful)
- Highly infiltrative and destructive

Special Stains and Immunohistochemistry

- NUT protein overexpression identified by immunohistochemistry

Other Techniques for Diagnosis

- Rearrangement of the nuclear protein in testis (NUT) gene on Chr 15q14 detected by fluorescence in situ hybridization (FISH)

Differential Diagnosis

SQUAMOUS CARCINOMA, NONKERATINIZING

- Infiltrative growth pattern with stromal invasion and desmoplastic response
- Pleomorphic cells with large, hyperchromatic nuclei and prominent nucleoli; high mitotic rate often with atypical mitoses
- Negative for NUT translocation/overexpression

SINONASAL UNDIFFERENTIATED CARCINOMA (SNUC)

- Nests, trabeculae, or sheets of poorly differentiated cells with high mitotic rate and necrosis; lacks squamous differentiation; lacks keratinization
- Moderate sized cells, frequently with prominent nucleoli
- Negative for NUT translocation/overexpression

PEARLS

- *May account for high grade carcinomas in young patients*
- *Often portends a rapid clinical course*
- *Diagnosis made by identifying the molecular alteration in the NUT protein*
- *Antibody to test for overexpression by immunohistochemistry is now available*

SELECTED REFERENCES

Bauer DE, Mitchell CM, Strait KM, et al: Clinicopathologic features and long-term outcomes of NUT midline carcinoma. Clin Cancer Res 18:5773-5779, 2012.

Bishop JA, Westra WH: NUT midline carcinomas of the sinonasal tract. Am J Surg Pathol 36:1216-1221, 2012.

Haack H, Johnson LA, Fry CJ, et al: Diagnosis of NUT midline carcinoma using a NUT-specific monoclonal antibody. Am J Surg Pathol 33:984-991, 2009.

SINONASAL UNDIFFERENTIATED CARCINOMA

Clinical Features

- Rare high-grade undifferentiated carcinoma of unclear etiology
- More common in males (3:1); mean age, sixth decade
- Patients present with nasal obstruction, facial pain, proptosis, or epistaxis

- One third develop cervical lymphatic node metastases
- Poor survival; median survival, 18 months

Gross Pathology

- Large irregular mass with bone invasion

Histopathology

- Tumor grows in sheets, trabeculae, or nests (Figure 3-53)
- Moderate-sized hyperchromatic cells with poorly defined cell borders and high N/C ratio
- Prominent single nucleoli
- Frequent mitoses
- Prominent tumor necrosis
- Keratinization not identified
- Lymphocytic infiltrate not identified (differentiates from nasopharyngeal)

Special Stains and Immunohistochemistry

- Positive for pan-cytokeratin, frequently cytokeratin 7
- Negative for cytokeratin 5/6
- Rare, focal synaptophysin, chromogranin

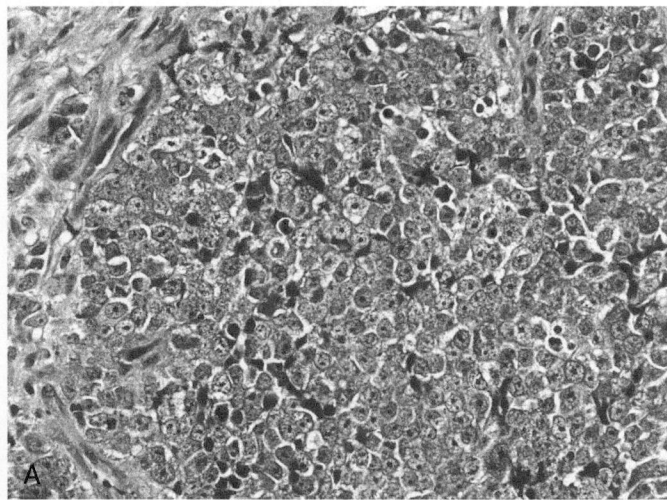

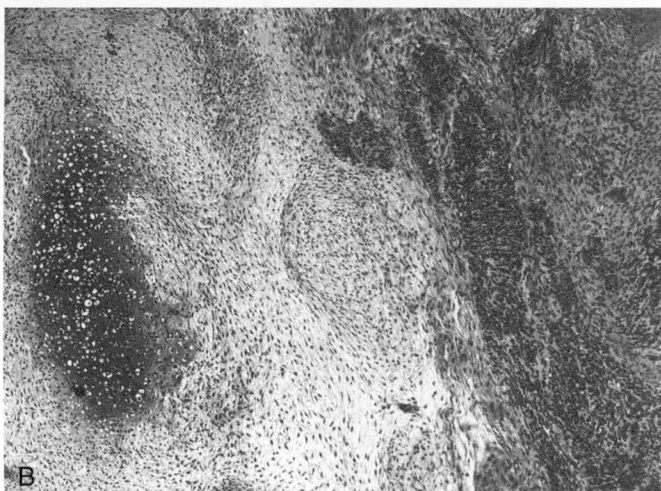

Figure 3-53. A, Sinonasal undifferentiated carcinoma. Nests of undifferentiated cells with prominent nucleoli and apoptotic figures are seen. **B,** Teratocarcinoma. Mixed cell lineages are identified within the tumor from primitive neuroblastoma (*right*) and cartilage (*left*).

Other Techniques for Diagnosis

- Noncontributory

Differential Diagnosis

NASOPHARYNGEAL CARCINOMA (UNDIFFERENTIATED TYPE)

- Site of tumor aids in differential
- Accompanying lymphoid infiltrate (absent in SNUC)
- EBV frequently positive (negative in SNUC)

SCC

- Keratinization usually identified (absent in SNUC)
- Grade based on degree of differentiation and keratinization
- Basaloid SCC shows focal abrupt keratinization

ADENOCARCINOMA

- Hyperchromatic large cells in glands and nests
- Intestinal type shows intracellular mucin

SMALL, ROUND BLUE CELL TUMORS IN THE SINONASAL REGION

- Neuroblastoma, rhabdomyosarcoma, Ewing sarcoma, lymphoma, melanoma
- IHC panel of markers aids in classification
  - Pan-cytokeratin, CD45, desmin, synaptophysin, chromogranin, S-100, pan-melanin markers

PEARLS

- *Highly aggressive neoplasm with mean survival less than 2 years*
- *Strong or diffuse neuroendocrine markers not identified in SNUC*
- *Differentiation from nasopharyngeal carcinoma difficult in large tumors involving both regions*

SELECTED REFERENCES

Cerilli LA, Holst VA, Brandwein MS, et al: Sinonasal undifferentiated carcinoma: immunohistochemical profile and lack of EBV association. Am J Surg Pathol 25:156-163, 2001.

Ejaz A, Wenig BM: Sinonasal undifferentiated carcinoma: clinical and pathologic features and a discussion on classification, cellular differentiation, and differential diagnosis. Adv Anat Pathol 12:134-143, 2005.

Franchi A, Moroni M, Massi D, et al: Sinonasal undifferentiated carcinoma, nasopharyngeal-type undifferentiated carcinoma, and keratinizing and nonkeratinizing squamous cell carcinoma express different cytokeratin patterns. Am J Surg. Pathol 26:1597-1604, 2002.

Jeng YM, Sung MT, Fang CL, et al: Sinonasal undifferentiated carcinoma and nasopharyngeal-type undifferentiated carcinoma: two clinically, biologically, and histopathologically distinct entities. Am J Surg Pathol 26:371-376, 2002.

NASOPHARYNGEAL CARCINOMA

Clinical Features

- Squamous carcinoma arising in the nasopharynx with features that distinguish it from features of oral cavity and oropharynx SCC by epidemiology
- Adverse prognostic factors: older age, high stage, male sex, bony invasion of skull base, and cranial nerve paralysis

- Divided into keratinizing and nonkeratinizing types (includes undifferentiated carcinoma)
- Nasopharyngeal carcinoma, keratinizing type
  - SCC, graded by degree of differentiation (well, moderately, or poorly differentiated)
  - Keratinization identified
  - Less commonly associated with EBV
  - Occurs in older patients
  - Less radiosensitive, poor outcome
- Nasopharyngeal carcinoma, nonkeratinizing type
  - Recent World Health Organization tumor classification groups nonkeratinizing squamous carcinoma with the undifferentiated type because both are strongly associated with EBV
  - Prevalent in Southeast Asia and Northern Africa, rare in United States and Europe
  - Peak incidence, 40 to 60 years of age; more common in males (3:1)
  - Most common presentation is unilateral cervical lymphadenopathy; patients also commonly have nasal and middle-ear symptoms
  - Environmental factors: diet high in nitrosamines-salted fish, smoking, formaldehyde, and EBV infection
  - Etiologic factors include genetic predisposition (familial occurrence), associated with specific HLA loci, which are prognostic in Chinese patients

Gross Pathology

- Tumor may be difficult to detect clinically; usually "blind" biopsies
- Frozen sections used to direct number of biopsies for diagnostic material

Histopathology

- Undifferentiated nasopharyngeal carcinoma (lymphoepithelial carcinoma)
  - Two growth patterns
    - Regaud type: well-defined tumor nests separated by fibrous stroma with inflammatory cells (Figure 3-54A)
    - Schmincke type: sheets or syncytia of tumor cells infiltrated by inflammatory cells (masking tumor cells); can mimic malignant lymphoma

- Nuclei are characteristically vesicular with a smooth outline and large eosinophilic nucleolus
- Spindle cells may be present
- Mitoses are easily identified; necrosis may be extensive
- In situ component is identified in a minority of cases
- Occasionally, eosinophils can be the predominant inflammatory component
- Desmoplastic stroma is uncommon
- Stromal amyloid deposition is occasionally seen
- SCC nonkeratinizing
  - Infiltrative growth pattern with stromal invasion and desmoplasia
  - Pleomorphic cells with large, hyperchromatic nuclei and prominent nuclei; high mitotic rate often with atypical mitoses
- Keratinizing nasopharyngeal carcinomas
  - SCC with associated desmoplasia and keratin pearls

Special Stains and Immunohistochemistry

- Cytokeratin positive, highlights malignant cells within lymphoid stroma
- High-molecular-weight cytokeratins positive (CK5/6, 34βE12)
- EBV latent membrane protein-1 (LMP-1) by IHC weak and positive in only one-third of tumors (in situ Epstein-Barr–encoded RNA (EBER) is more sensitive) (Figure 3-54B)

Other Techniques for Diagnosis

- In situ hybridization demonstrates specific viral mRNA of EBV in tumor cell nuclei (EBER)
- Detection of IgG antibody (directed against early EBV antigen) and IgA antibody (against capsid viral antigen) in serum used in the United States for presumptive diagnosis of nasopharyngeal carcinoma

Differential Diagnosis

NON-HODGKIN (LARGE CELL) LYMPHOMA

- Variably large nuclei may morphologically overlap
- Immunohistochemical panel of lymphoid and epithelial markers for lineage

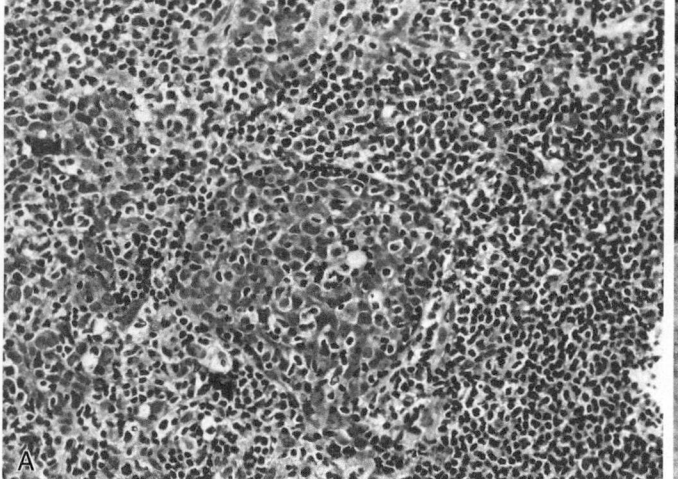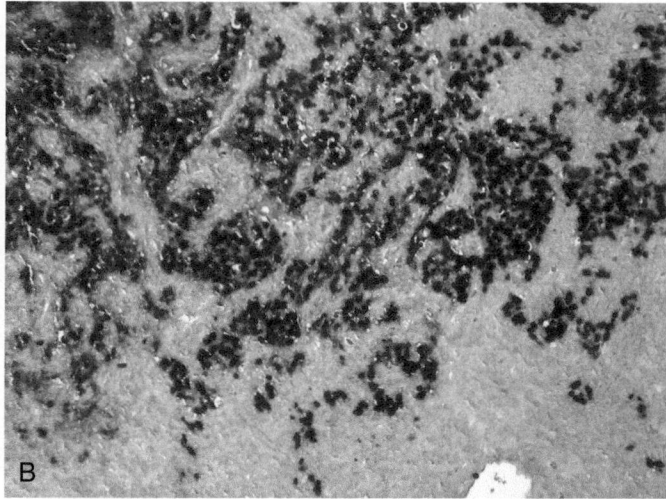

Figure 3-54. Nasopharyngeal carcinoma. A, Undifferentiated type. Large neoplastic cells are present admixed with a lymphocytic stroma. **B, Epstein-Barr virus.** Tumor cell nuclei are positive for Epstein-Barr virus-encoded RNA (EBER) by in situ hybridization.

SINUS HISTIOCYTOSIS

- Histiocytic cells with small nuclei and low N/C ratio
- Rare or absent mitotic activity
- Positive for CD68; negative for cytokeratin

SNUC

- Tumor bulk should be located in the sinonasal region but may extend to involve nasopharynx
- EBV negative
- No keratinization or lymphocytic infiltrate

PEARLS

- *Lymphoid tissue is not neoplastic; the term* lymphoepithelial *is a misnomer*
- *Cervical lymphadenopathy is the most common mode of presentation*
- *Radiation is typical treatment because EBV-positive tumors are sensitive; chemotherapy is frequently added*
- *Survival is worse for keratinizing SCC, probably secondary to lack of EBV association and radiotherapy resistance*

SELECTED REFERENCES

Lo KW, To KF, Huang DP: Focus on nasopharyngeal carcinoma. Cancer Cell 5:423-428, 2004.
Shi W, Pataki I, MacMillan C, et al: Molecular pathology parameters in human nasopharyngeal carcinoma. Cancer 94:1997-2006, 2002.
Viguer JM, Jimenez-Heffernan JA, Lopez-Ferrer P, et al: Fine-needle aspiration cytology of metastatic nasopharyngeal carcinoma. Diagn Cytopathol 32:233-237, 2005.
Wei WI, Sham JS: Nasopharyngeal carcinoma. Lancet 365:2041-2054, 2005.
Wenig BM: Nasopharyngeal carcinoma. Ann Diagn Pathol 3:374-385, 1999.

SQUAMOUS CELL CARCINOMA OF THE TONSIL OR OROPHARYNX

Clinical Features

- Tonsil is the most common site in the oropharynx for SCC
- More common in men, in fifth and sixth decades, associated with tobacco use
- Also seen in nonsmokers, men and women, usually in fourth and fifth decades, associated with high-risk HPV
- Clinically, 30% initially present with neck mass (metastasis)
- Other clinical signs are difficulty swallowing, sore throat, and ear pain

Gross Pathology

- Endophytic tan-pink tumor; may enlarge tonsil
- May be small, poorly visualized in crypts (submit tonsils in entirety for examination in adults)
- Firm white on cut sections

Histopathology

- Most are easily recognized intermediate- to high-grade tumors with obvious squamous differentiation and at least focal keratinization (Figure 3-55A)

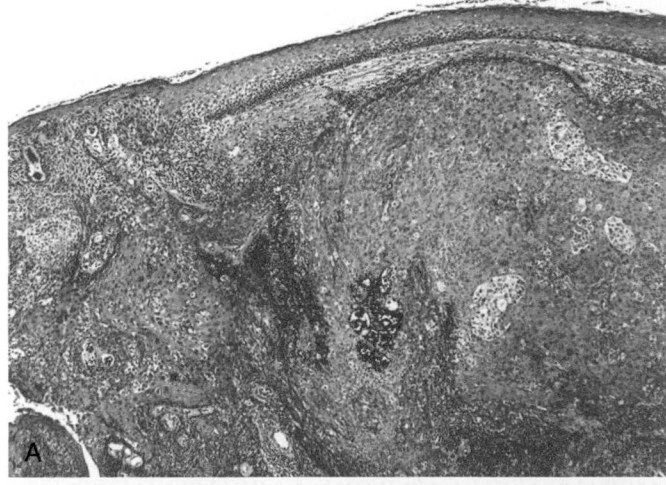

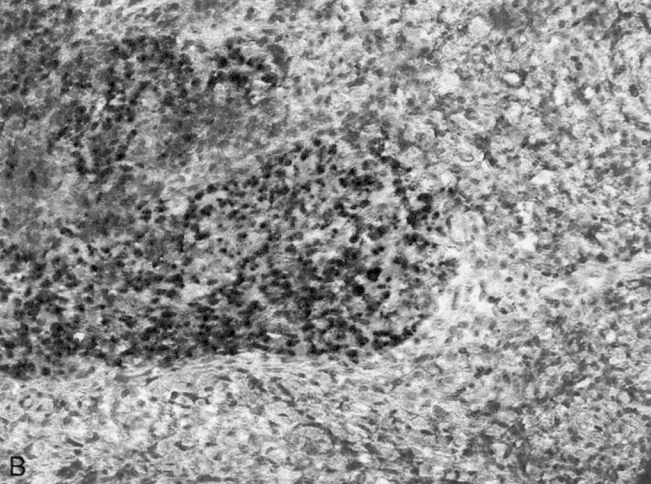

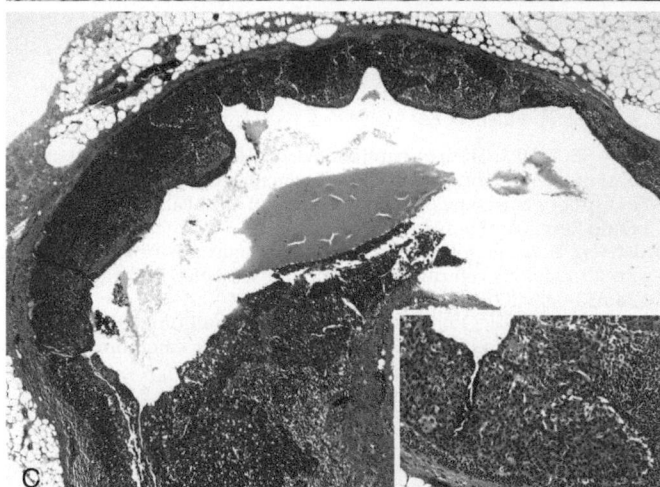

Figure 3-55. A, Tonsil squamous cell carcinoma. Atypical squamous epithelium with invasion into the submucosa is present forming irregular nests with variable keratinization. **B,** Tonsil squamous cell carcinoma, human papillomavirus (HPV) positive. In situ hybridization for HPV-16 is positive within the tumor nuclei. **C,** Metastatic cystic squamous cell carcinoma. A prominent cystic space is present surrounded by a neoplastic lining within a cervical lymph node. At high power (*inset*), the epithelium is hyperchromatic and haphazard (neoplastic).

- Often, nonkeratinizing/low keratinizing SCC is frequently HPV associated (Figure 3-55B)
- Less common histologic subtypes include verrucous carcinoma, basaloid carcinoma, and spindle cell carcinoma

Special Stains and Immunohistochemistry

- Cytokeratin positive

Other Techniques for Diagnosis

- HPV testing for high-risk types (in situ hybridization)
- HPV positivity seen in 30% to 70% of oropharyngeal squamous carcinomas and associated with a better prognosis
- p16 by IHC overexpressed in HPV-positive tumors

Differential Diagnoses

NASOPHARYNGEAL CARCINOMA, UNDIFFERENTIATED CARCINOMA

- Composed of groups of undifferentiated large cells with vesicular nuclei associated with prominent lympho-plasmacytic reaction
- EBV often positive (EBER detected by in situ hybridization)

PEARLS

- *Patients often present with cystic metastasis to the neck (not branchial cleft cysts) (Figure 3-55C)*
- *Treatment is often with radiation therapy to primary site and neck (tonsillectomy or biopsy for diagnosis)*
- *Increased risk for developing a second primary malignancy elsewhere in the head and neck*
- *HPV positivity is often identified in nonsmokers and associated with a better prognosis (more radiosensitive)*

SELECTED REFERENCES

El-Mofty SK, Patil S: Human papillomavirus (HPV)-related oropharyngeal nonkeratinizing squamous cell carcinoma: characterization of a distinct phenotype. Oral Surg Oral Med Oral Pathol Oral Radiol Endodont 101:339-345, 2006.
Goldenberg D, Sciubba J, Koch WM: Cystic metastasis from head and neck squamous cell cancer: a distinct disease variant? Head Neck 28:633-638, 2006.
Li W, Thompson CH, O'Brien CJ, et al: Human papillomavirus positivity predicts favourable outcome for squamous carcinoma of the tonsil. Int J Cancer 106:553-558, 2003.
Syrjänen S: HPV infections and tonsillar carcinoma. J Clin Pathol 57:449-455, 2004.
Thompson LD, Heffner DK: The clinical importance of cystic squamous cell carcinomas in the neck: a study of 136 cases. Cancer 82:944-956, 1998.

SINONASAL ADENOCARCINOMA

Clinical Features

- Arise from either the respiratory epithelium or seromucinous glands
- Tumors may arise in the nasal cavity or sinus region
- Clinical symptoms include obstruction and epistaxis
- Three distinct types of adenocarcinomas: enteric type, nonenteric type, and salivary type

- Enteric type (intestinal type)
  - Associated with woodworking (hardwood exposure), leather, some chemical manufacturing
  - Arises from schneiderian surface mucosa involving ethmoids, then nasal, then maxillary
  - Prominent male predominance (9:1), often in the sixth decade
- Nonenteric type (nonintestinal type)
  - Classified as low- or high-grade nonenteric seromucinous adenocarcinomas
  - Arise from seromucinous glands
  - Wide age range; low-grade median 50 years, high-grade median 60 years
  - No known environmental causes
- Salivary type
  - Morphologically identical to those in the salivary gland region
  - Adenoid cystic carcinoma is the most frequent type
  - Essentially any salivary histology may be seen

Gross Pathology

- Enteric type (intestinal type)
  - Fungating mass may show ulceration, hemorrhage
  - Friable gray mass with mucoid material
- Nonenteric type (nonintestinal type)
  - Varies based on grade
- Salivary type
  - Submucosal mass with infiltration

Histopathology

- Enteric type (intestinal type)
  - Hyperchromatic, atypical columnar epithelium (Figure 3-56A)
  - Invasion with desmoplasia present
  - Mucin and frequently goblet cells present
  - Intestinal metaplasia of schneiderian mucosa without atypia may be present
  - Intermediate- to high-grade tumors
- Nonenteric type (nonintestinal type)
  - Low grade
    - Relatively cytologically bland proliferation of seromucinous glands
    - Small glands are back to back, or papillary growth (Figure 3-56B)
    - Can be difficult to distinguish from hyperplastic glands and to identify invasion
    - Atypical mitoses and necrosis generally absent
  - High grade
    - Solid growth pattern is common
    - Moderate to marked pleomorphism
    - High mitotic rate, prominent necrosis
- Salivary type
  - Morphologies include those in the salivary regions (refer to "Salivary Glands" for features)
    - Pleomorphic adenoma, adenoid cystic carcinoma, acinic cell carcinoma (Figure 3-56C)
    - Polymorphous low-grade carcinoma
    - Other morphologic entities

Special Stains and Immunohistochemistry

- Enteric type (intestinal type)
  - Cytokeratin positive, may express CK7 and CK20

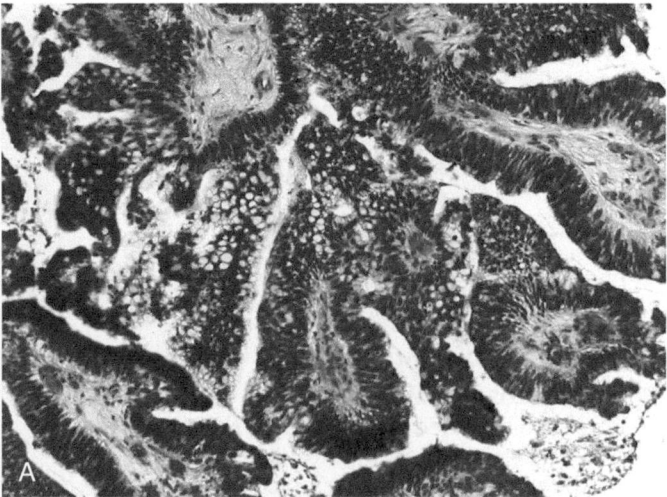

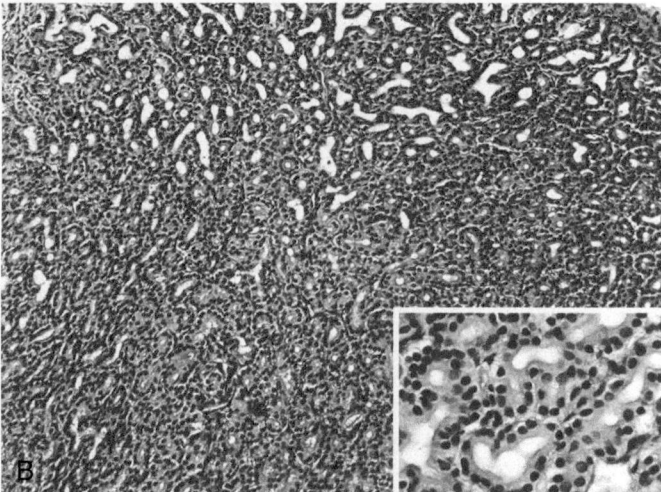

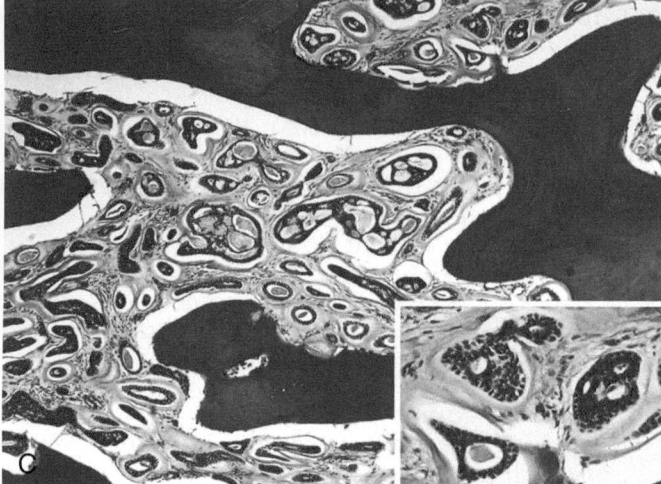

Figure 3-56. Sinonasal adenocarcinoma. A, Enteric (intestinal) type. Elongated hyperchromatic nuclei form glandular structures reminiscent of colonic adenocarcinoma. **B,** Nonenteric type. Back-to-back, uniform glands composed of cytologically bland cells fill the stroma (*inset*). **C,** Salivary type. Tubules and cribriform patterns of adenoid cystic carcinoma are invading bone. *Inset,* Higher-power view of the neoplastic cells.

- CDX2 often positive (nuclear)
- As the morphology resembles intestinal-like mucosa, gains marker expression like colon

---

- Markers cannot be used to distinguish primary from metastasis (clinical correlate required)
- Nonenteric type (nonintestinal type)
  - Cytokeratin 7 positive
  - May express S-100 protein
- Salivary type
  - Cytokeratin 7 positive
  - May express S-100 protein

Other Techniques for Diagnosis

- Enteric type (intestinal type)
  - *Ras* mutations (15%)
  - *TP53* mutations (18% to 44%)

Differential Diagnosis

- Clinical history of exposures is helpful

SNUC
- High-grade tumor with prominent necrosis
- Tumor cells with prominent nucleoli without differentiation
- Mucinous cells and intracellular mucin not identified

SCHNEIDERIAN PAPILLOMA-CYLINDRICAL CELL TYPE INVERTED GROWTH PATTERN HAS INTACT BASEMENT MEMBRANE WITHOUT DESMOPLASIA
- Epithelium is uniform with cilia identified
- Microabscesses are present within epithelium

NASOPHARYNGEAL PAPILLARY ADENOCARCINOMA
- Described in children and adults; same incidence in males and females
- Papillary growth and nest of uniform tumor cells in nasopharynx
- Nuclei mimic papillary thyroid carcinoma: enlarged, oval, clear, and folds
- TTF-1 is positive in this entity; thyroglobulin is negative
- Low-grade malignancy with resection being curative

TERATOCARCINOSARCOMA
- Mixture of several tumor lineages, high-grade carcinoma, neuroblastoma, sarcoma, and occasionally germ cell tumors
- Large friable mass with extensive necrosis
- More common in males
- Poor prognosis

PEARLS

- *Diverse histologies occur from low- to high-grade tumors*
- *IHC cannot separate primary from metastatic disease for intestinal-type adenocarcinoma and requires clinical correlation*

SELECTED REFERENCES

Barnes L: Schneiderian papillomas and nonsalivary glandular neoplasms of the head and neck. Mod Pathol 15:279-297, 2002.
Cathro HP, Mills SE: Immunophenotypic differences between intestinal-type and low-grade papillary sinonasal adenocarcinomas: an immunohistochemical study of 22 cases utilizing CDX2 and MUC2. Am J Surg Pathol 28:1026-1032, 2004.

Franchi A, Gallo O, Santucci M: Clinical relevance of the histological classification of sinonasal intestinal-type adenocarcinomas. Hum Pathol 30:1140-1145, 1999.

Neto AG, Pineda-Daboin K, Luna MA: Sinonasal tract seromucous adenocarcinomas: a report of 12 cases. Ann Diagn Pathol 7:154-159, 2003.

Pineda-Daboin K, Neto A, Ochoa-Perez V, Luna MA: Nasopharyngeal adenocarcinomas: a clinicopathologic study of 44 cases including immunohistochemical features of 18 papillary phenotypes. Ann Diagn Pathol 10:215-221, 2006.

OLFACTORY NEUROBLASTOMA (ESTHESIONEUROBLASTOMA)

Clinical Features

- Malignant neuroendocrine neoplasm, 5% of sinonasal tumors
- Wide age range, bimodal peaks around ages 15 and 55 years; no sex predilection
- Most often located at roof of nasal cavity
- Presenting symptoms include nasal obstruction and hemorrhage

Gross Pathology

- Reddish gray, vascular, polypoid mass with soft consistency

Histopathology

- Lobular nests of uniform, relatively small monomorphic cells with round nuclei, fine and course chromatin, scant cytoplasm, and indistinct cell membrane (Figure 3-57)
- Nests surrounded by fibrovascular cores and sustentacular cells
- Fibrillary stroma corresponds to neuronal processes seen ultrastructurally
- Ganglion cells are rarely seen but when present are diagnostic
- Homer-Wright pseudorosettes seen in 30% of cases (annular arrays of cells surrounding central aggregates of cytoplasmic fibrils) or Flexner-type rosettes (glandular lumen) seen in 5% of cases
- Higher-grade tumors are less uniform, with more mitoses and pleomorphism

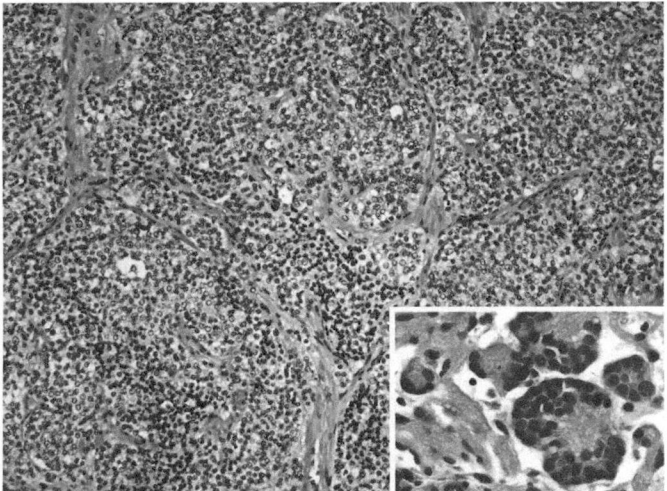

Figure 3-57. Olfactory neuroblastoma. Neoplastic small blue cells infiltrate into the submucosa as single cells and in nests. Neurofibrillary stroma is present, and rosettes are occasionally identified (*inset*).

Special Stains and Immunohistochemistry

- Synaptophysin, chromogranin, neuron-specific enolase, neurofilament positive
- S-100 protein positive in sustentacular cells surrounding some nests of tumor
- Cytokeratin occasionally focally positive
- CEA and EMA negative

Other Techniques for Diagnosis

- Electron microscopy: numerous cytoplasmic dense core neurosecretory granules

Differential Diagnosis

RHABDOMYOSARCOMA

- Round to spindled cells, possible rhabdomyoblasts
- Lacks rosette formation and fibrillary background
- Positive for muscle differentiation markers; desmin (cytoplasmic) and MyoD1 and myogenin (nuclear)

SNUC

- Nests, ribbons, or trabeculae of polygonal cells with round, hyperchromatic nuclei; large, prominent nucleoli; moderate eosinophilic cytoplasm
- High mitotic rate and prominent individual cell or central necrosis
- Vascular or lymphatic invasion often seen
- No rosettes or fibrillar background
- Positive for cytokeratin and may show focal synaptophysin or chromogranin
- Worse prognosis

SINONASAL MELANOMA

- Primitive, often round tumor cells may show prominent nucleoli
- Discohesive with pseudopapilla
- Expresses S-100 protein or melan-A, HMB-45, tyrosinase
- Pagetoid spread occasionally seen
- Clinically, nasal obstruction may mimic nasal polyps

PERIPHERAL NEUROECTODERMAL TUMOR (PNET), EWING SARCOMA

- Can resemble SNUC, neuroblastoma, or rhabdomyosarcoma
- Neuroendocrine markers not helpful
- Positive for CD99 (nonspecific)
- Characteristic t(11;22) in 90% of tumors; paraffin sections can be analyzed by fluorescence in situ hybridization (FISH) analysis to confirm diagnosis

PITUITARY ADENOMA

- Ectopic origin or direct extension into paranasal sinuses (sphenoid)
- Positive for cytokeratin and chromogranin; variable positivity for pituitary hormones

MALIGNANT LYMPHOMA

- Diffuse infiltrate of discohesive cells with large nuclei and clumped chromatin
- Lacks rosettes and fibrillary background
- LCA positive

SMALL CELL NEUROENDOCRINE CARCINOMA

- Same histologic features as pulmonary small cell carcinoma

- Small cells with hyperchromatic nuclei, nuclear molding, and scant cytoplasm
- Necrosis and high mitotic rate
- Positive for neuroendocrine markers and cytokeratin

PEARLS

- *Differential is broad, must consider multiple other tumors in this location*
- *Local recurrence common secondary to invasion (sinuses, orbit, base of skull)*
- *Most common sites of metastases are cervical lymph nodes and lung*
- *Postoperative radiation given to improve local control*

SELECTED REFERENCES

Diaz EM Jr, Johnigan RH 3rd, Pero C, et al: Olfactory neuroblastoma: the 22-year experience at one comprehensive cancer center. Head Neck 27:138-149, 2005.

Ingeholm P, Theilgaard SA, Buchwald C, et al: Esthesioneuroblastoma: a Danish clinicopathological study of 40 consecutive cases. Acta Pathol Microbiol Immunol Scand 110:639-645, 2002.

Mahooti S, Wakely PE Jr: Cytopathologic features of olfactory neuroblastoma. Cancer 108:86-92, 2006.

Windfuhr JP: Primitive neuroectodermal tumor of the head and neck: incidence, diagnosis, and management. Ann Otol Rhinol Laryngol 113:533-543, 2004.

RHABDOMYOSARCOMA

Clinical Features

- Most common sarcoma arising in the head and neck; accounts for 45% of head and neck sarcomas
- Embryonal type most common in children, alveolar type in adults; pleomorphic variant rare
- Patients present with a soft tissue mass, sinus symptoms, or both
- Nasopharynx more common than sinuses

Gross Pathology

- Poorly circumscribed, fleshy, polypoid (mimicking polyps)
- Cut surface is gray-red with a soft consistency

Histopathology

- Embryonal rhabdomyosarcoma
  - Makes up 80% of rhabdomyosarcoma of the head and neck
  - Hyperchromatic round to spindled cells; rhabdomyoblasts are larger with eosinophilic cytoplasm (Figure 3-58A)
  - Cross-striations are rare
  - Stroma may be myxoid
  - Subtypes of embryonal rhabdomyosarcoma include botryoid and spindled (Figure 3-58B)

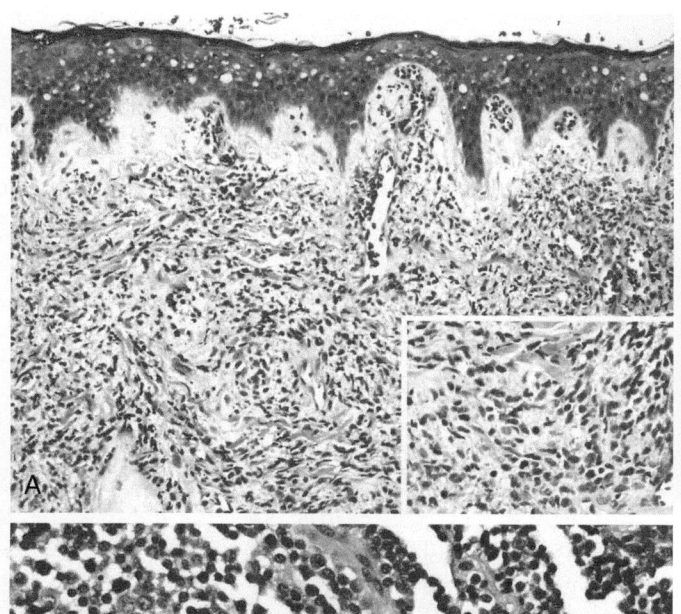

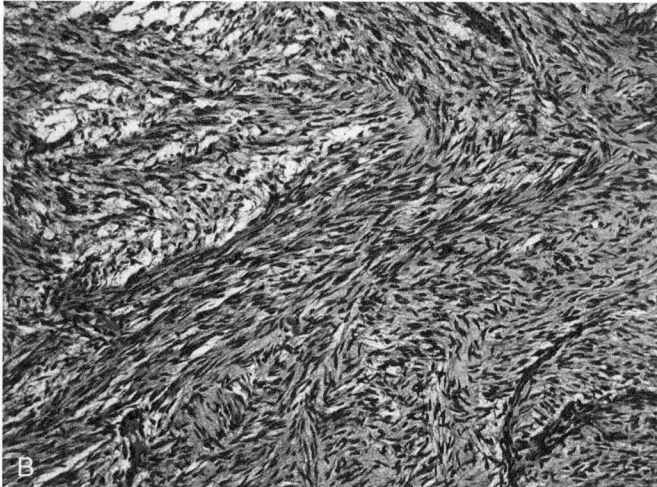

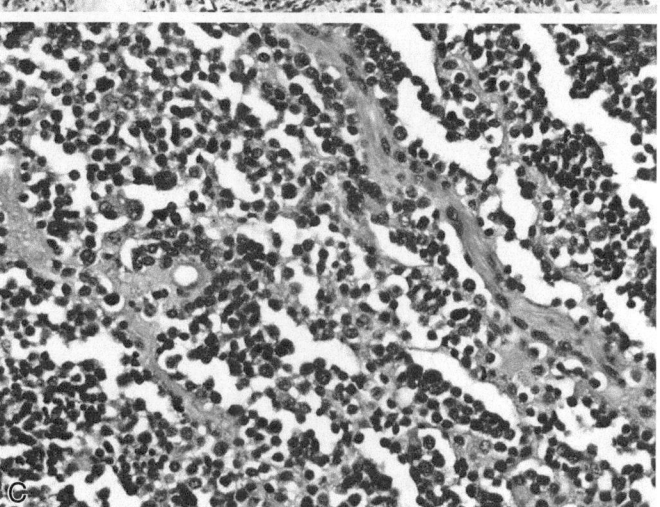

Figure 3-58. Rhabdomyosarcoma. A, Embryonal type. Small hyperchromatic neoplastic cells infiltrate the stroma. Desmin, by immunohistochemical analysis, is positive in the cytoplasm of tumor cells (*inset*). **B,** Spindled type. In this variant of embryonal type, the neoplastic cells form elongated fascicles. Myogenin, by immunohistochemical analysis, is positive in the nucleus of tumor cells (*inset*). **C,** Alveolar type. Hyperchromatic tumor cells are discohesive, leaving "alveolar-like" spaces.

- Botryoid type
  - Small blue cells in abundant myxoid stroma
  - Cambium layer composed of more compact cells below epithelial surface
- Spindled type
  - Fairly uniform spindled cells, rare rhabdoid cells, occasional striations (Figure 3-58B)
- Alveolar rhabdomyosarcoma
  - Nests of small, discohesive round to oval hyperchromatic tumor cells separated by fibrous tissue (Figure 3-58C)
  - Mitotic figures are common
  - Multinucleated giant cells may be present
  - Solid growth and clear cell morphology have been described
- Pleomorphic rhabdomyosarcoma
  - Large, pleomorphic cells rarely showing cross-striations
  - Need immunohistochemical evidence of skeletal muscle differentiation or cytoplasmic cross-striations

Special Stains and Immunohistochemistry

- Positive for desmin, myoglobin, myosin, and MSA (nonspecific)
- Positive for MyoD1 (nuclear expression; regulatory protein in skeletal muscle differentiation)—confirmatory marker
- Myogenin (nuclear expression; regulatory protein in skeletal muscle differentiation)—confirmatory marker
- May rarely express cytokeratin (alveolar subtype up to 50% positive)
- Alveolar subtype may have aberrant synaptophysin or chromogranin (40%)

Other Techniques for Diagnosis

- Embryonal rhabdomyosarcoma has characteristic 11pLOH
- Alveolar rhabdomyosarcoma has characteristic t(2;13); occasionally, t(1;13) *PAX2* or *PAX3* translocated with *FKHR* may have prognostic significance
- FISH can be performed for these translocations on paraffin sections

Differential Diagnosis

- Same as for olfactory neuroblastoma (as listed previously)

PEARLS

- *Differential diagnosis includes all of the small round blue cell tumors, and evaluation should incorporate morphology and IHC*
- *A useful initial battery of immunohistochemical stains for differential diagnosis of a small round blue cell tumor in the head and neck includes cytokeratin, LCA, S-100, synaptophysin, desmin, and melanoma marker*

SELECTED REFERENCES

Bahrami A, Gown AM, Baird GS, et al: Aberrant expression of epithelial and neuroendocrine markers in alveolar rhabdomyosarcoma: a potentially serious diagnostic pitfall. Mod Pathol 21:795-806, 2008.

Folpe AL: MyoD1 and myogenin expression in human neoplasia: a review and update. Adv Anat Pathol 9:198-203, 2002.

Nascimento AF, Fletcher CD: Spindle cell rhabdomyosarcoma in adults. Am J Surg Pathol 29:1106-1113, 2005.

Parham DM: Pathologic classification of rhabdomyosarcomas and correlations with molecular studies. Mod Pathol 14:506-514, 2001.

Sorensen PH, Lynch JC, Qualman SJ, et al: PAX3-FKHR and PAX7-FKHR gene fusions are prognostic indicators in alveolar rhabdomyosarcoma: a report from the children's oncology group. J Clin Oncol 20:2672-2679, 2002.

Xia SJ, Pressey JG, Barr FG: Molecular pathogenesis of rhabdomyosarcoma. Cancer Biol Therapy 1:97-104, 2002.

SINONASAL MELANOMA

Clinical Features

- Uncommon (< 5%) sinonasal tumor
- Less than 1% of all melanoma cases
- Equal incidence in males and females in fifth to eighth decades
- Higher incidence in Japanese
- Patients present with sinus symptoms, obstruction, or epistaxis
- Generally poor prognosis, less than 50% survival rate at 5 years

Gross Pathology

- Varies from gray to tan, can be pigmented brown or black
- Often polypoid and friable

Histopathology

- Sheets or nests of small to medium-sized epithelioid, rhabdoid, spindled, or pleomorphic cells; may show nucleoli (Figure 3-59)
- Discohesiveness leads to pseudopapillary structure of tumor around vessels
- Mitoses present
- Intracytoplasmic melanin may be present
- Melanocytes at junction of surface respiratory epithelium or pagetoid spread may be noted

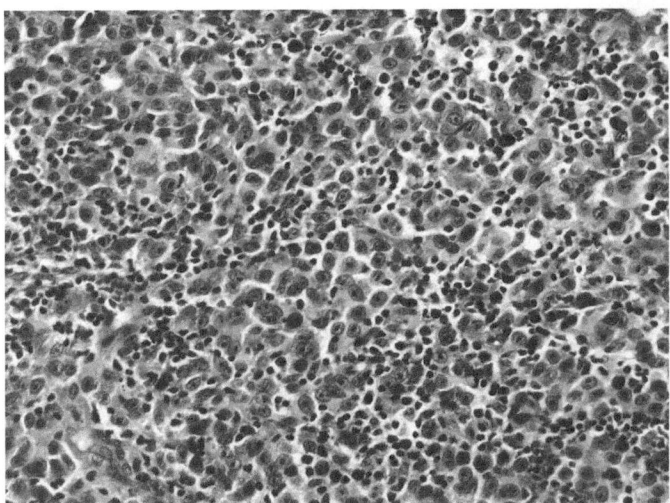

Figure 3-59. Sinonasal melanoma. Relatively homogeneous tumor cells with prominent nucleoli are present without identifiable pigment.

Special Stains and Immunohistochemistry

- Positive for S-100 and melanocyte markers (melan-A, HMB-45, tyrosinase)
- No markers to distinguish primary from metastasis (clinical correlate required)

Other Techniques for Diagnosis

- Although rarely performed, electron microscopy will show premelanosomes and melanosomes

Differential Diagnosis

OLFACTORY NEUROBLASTOMA

- Growth patterns may be similar
- Rosette formation and fibrillary background
- Cells with clumped hyperchromatic chromatin
- Positive for synaptophysin, chromogranin (occasionally in melanoma)

RHABDOMYOSARCOMA

- Hyperchromatic round to spindled cells; rhabdomyoblasts may be seen
- Striations when present are helpful
- Positive for muscle differentiation markers; desmin, MyoD1, and myogenin

SNUC

- Nests, ribbons, or trabeculae of polygonal cells with round, hyperchromatic nuclei; large, prominent nucleoli; and moderate eosinophilic cytoplasm
- High mitotic rate and prominent individual cell or central necrosis
- Vascular or lymphatic invasion often seen
- Cytokeratin positive

PNET, EWING SARCOMA

- High N/C ratio
- Fine nuclear chromatin and small nucleoli
- Positive for CD99 (nonspecific)
- Characteristic t(11;22) in 90% of tumors; paraffin sections can be analyzed by FISH analysis to confirm diagnosis

MALIGNANT LYMPHOMA

- Diffuse infiltrate of discohesive lymphoid cells with large nuclei and clumped chromatin
- LCA positive
- May be EBV positive depending on type

PEARLS

- *Distinct molecular profile compared to cutaneous melanoma, CD117 mutations (10% to 15%) and lower BRAF mutations (5%)*
- *Morphologically, sinonasal melanoma mimics other primary small round blue cell tumors of this region*
- *A useful initial battery of immunohistochemical stains for differential diagnosis of a small round blue cell tumor in the head and neck includes cytokeratin, LCA, S-100, synaptophysin, desmin, and a melanoma marker (melan-A)*
- *Clinical correlation is required to exclude metastasis to sinonasal region (1% of cases); other metastases are usually present with metastatic presentation*

SELECTED REFERENCES

Batsakis JG, Suarez P, El-Naggar AK: Mucosal melanomas of the head and neck. Ann Otol Rhinol Laryngol 107:626-630, 1998.

Beadling C, Jacobson-Dunlop E, Hodi FS, et al: KIT gene mutations and copy number in melanoma subtypes. Clin Cancer Res. 14:6821-6828, 2008.

Prasad ML, Jungbluth AA, Iversen K, et al: Expression of melanocytic differentiation markers in malignant melanomas of the oral and sinonasal mucosa. Am J Surg Pathol 25:782-787, 2001.

Thompson LD, Wieneke JA, Miettinen M: Sinonasal tract and nasopharyngeal melanomas: a clinicopathologic study of 115 cases with a proposed staging system. Am J Surg Pathol 27:594-611, 2003.

LYMPHOMA

Clinical Features

- Extranodal natural killer (NK) cell and T-cell lymphoma (angiocentric)
  - Endemic in some Asian countries (Japan, Taiwan), parts of Latin America; less common in Western countries
  - Peaks in sixth decade, more common in males (3:1)
  - Clinical symptoms of obstruction, epistaxis, and septal perforation
  - Most often affecting nasal cavity
  - EBV positive
- Other lymphomas
  - All types of non-Hodgkin lymphomas have been described in this location
  - Most common is diffuse large cell lymphoma involving sinuses
  - B-cell lymphomas, although rare, affect nasopharynx, oropharynx, and sinuses
  - Phenotypically, most Western hemisphere cases are B-cell type (Asian and South American cases are T-cell type)
  - Clinical features are nonspecific and related to obstruction or hemorrhage

Gross Pathology

- Extranodal NK/T-cell lymphoma (angiocentric)
  - Ulcerated lesions often reach large size
- Other lymphomas
  - Typically present as a polypoid mass

Histopathology

- Extranodal NK/T-cell lymphoma (angiocentric)
  - Usually exuberant inflammation
  - Variable cytologic atypia of mostly small to medium-sized lymphocytes; nucleoli are inconspicuous (Figure 3-60A)
  - Prominent necrosis and karyorrhexis
  - Vascular invasion and angiocentricity (viable cells seen cuffing a residual blood vessel) may not be demonstrable in all cases
- Other lymphomas (Figure 3-60B)
  - Varies with subtype; refer to Chapter 14

Special Stains and Immunohistochemistry

- Extranodal NK/T-cell lymphoma (angiocentric)
  - Lymphocytes are positive for CD2, CD43, and NK cell antigen CD56; negative for CD3, CD57, and CD11
- Other lymphomas

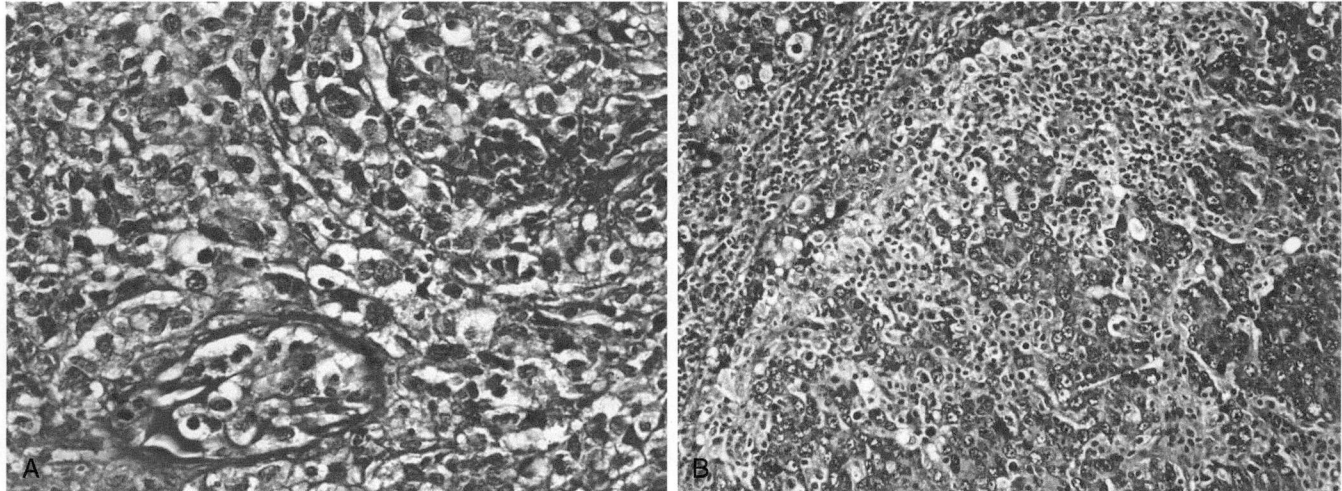

Figure 3-60. A, Extranodal NK/T-cell lymphoma. An atypical lymphoid infiltrate shows large pleomorphic cells. **B,** Diffuse large B-cell lymphoma. There is infiltration of tissue by large atypical cells with open chromatin and background of small, scattered lymphocytes.

- LCA positive
- Cytokeratin negative
- B-cell (CD20) and T-cell (CD3) markers should be done for phenotyping
- EMA and CD30 may be positive in anaplastic large cell lymphomas and true histiocytic lymphomas

Other Techniques for Diagnosis

- Extranodal NK/T-cell lymphoma (angiocentric)
  - T-cell receptor rearrangements are usually absent and clonality is difficult to demonstrate
  - EBV positive by in situ hybridization
- Other lymphomas
  - Varies with subtype (refer to Chapter 14)

Differential Diagnosis

NASOPHARYNGEAL CARCINOMA

- Nuclei are characteristically vesicular with a smooth outline and a single large eosinophilic nucleolus
- Location of nasopharynx
- Cytokeratin-positive tumor in dense lymphocytic infiltrate
- Often EBV positive (not helpful because EBV is often present in nasal lymphomas)

OLFACTORY NEUROBLASTOMA

- Rosette formation and fibrillary background may be identified
- Cells with clumped hyperchromatic chromatin
- Positive for synaptophysin, chromogranin

WEGENER GRANULOMATOSIS

- Varying stages of vasculitis involving arterioles, small arteries, and veins can be difficult to find
- A neutrophilic infiltrate and fibrinoid necrosis
- Giants cells scattered
- Areas of geographic necrosis usually predominate
- Clinical workup shows cytoplasmic antineutrophil cytoplasmic antibodies (c-ANCA) against proteinase-3 (PR3)

COCAINE ABUSE

- Shows necrosis and nonspecific inflammation of epithelium and stroma
- No vasculitis

PEARLS

- *The term lethal midline granuloma is outdated and should not be used as a pathologic diagnosis*
- *Extranodal NK/T-cell lymphoma is EBV positive and negative for T-cell receptor monoclonal rearrangements*
- *In Western countries, B-cell lymphomas are more common; T-cell lymphomas are more common in Asia and Latin America*

SELECTED REFERENCES

Heffner DK: Wegener's granulomatosis is not a granulomatous disease. Ann Diagn Pathol 6:329-333, 2002.

Kim GE, Koom WS, Yang WI, et al: Clinical relevance of three subtypes of primary sinonasal lymphoma characterized by immunophenotypic analysis. Head Neck 26:584-593, 2004.

Li CC, Tien HF, Tang JL, et al: Treatment outcome and pattern of failure in 77 patients with sinonasal natural killer/T-cell or T-cell lymphoma. Cancer 100:366-375, 2004.

Li S, Feng X, Li T, et al: Extranodal NK/T-cell lymphoma, nasal type: a report of 73 cases at MD Anderson Cancer Center. Am J Surg Pathol 37:14-23, 2013.

Seyer BA, Grist W, Muller S: Aggressive destructive midfacial lesion from cocaine abuse. Oral Surg Oral Med Oral Pathol Oral Radiol Endodont 94:465-470, 2002.

TUMORS METASTASIZING TO THE PARANASAL SINUSES AND NASOPHARYNX

Clinical Features

- Metastases to the paranasal sinuses and nasopharynx are rare
- Most common are renal cell carcinoma, melanoma, and breast carcinoma

Gross Pathology

- Depends on location and tumor type

Histopathology

- Renal cell carcinoma
  - Clear cell type mistaken for alveolar rhabdomyosarcoma, clear cell variant
  - Characteristic arborizing vascular pattern surrounds tumor cells
- Malignant melanoma
  - Estimated 1% risk for metastasis to this region
  - Most melanomas encountered are primary sinonasal; however, clinically must exclude metastasis
- Breast carcinoma
  - Infiltrating ductal carcinoma has pleomorphic cells with high mitotic rate
  - Lobular carcinoma can have bland-appearing cells

Special Stains and Immunohistochemistry

- Renal cell carcinoma
  - Cytokeratin and vimentin positive
  - Clear cells contain glycogen
- Malignant melanoma
  - No markers distinguish primary from metastatic
- Breast carcinoma
  - Estrogen receptor and progesterone receptor variably positive
  - *HER-2* may be positive (correlate with primary tumor expression)

Other Techniques for Diagnosis

- Noncontributory

Differential Diagnosis

- Clinical history is essential

PEARLS

- *Always obtain clinical history when histology is not definitive for primary tumor*

Selected References

Lee HM, Kang HJ, Lee SH: Metastatic renal cell carcinoma presenting as epistaxis. Eur Arch Otorhinolaryngol 262:69-71, 2005.

Marchioni D, Monzani D, Rossi G, et al: Breast carcinoma metastases in paranasal sinuses, a rare occurrence mimicking a primary nasal malignancy. Acta Otorhinolaryngol Ital 24:87-91, 2004.

Mickel RA, Zimmerman MC: The sphenoid sinus—a site for metastasis. Otolaryngol Head Neck Surg 102:709-716, 1990.

Simo R, Sykes AJ, Hargreaves SP, et al: Metastatic renal cell carcinoma to the nose and paranasal sinuses. Head Neck 22:722-727, 2000.

Wanamaker JR, Kraus DH, Eliacher I, Lavertu P: Manifestations of metastatic breast carcinoma to the head and neck. Head Neck 15:257-262, 1993.

ORAL CAVITY

LEUKOPLAKIA

Clinical Features

- A clinical term to describe a white patch or plaque that either is localized or has geographic distribution
- Occurs predominantly in older individuals, slightly more common in males
- A subset considered premalignant (4% to 20% may undergo malignant transformation)
- Most common in the buccal mucosa
- Highest incidence of dysplasia in leukoplakia involving the floor of the mouth and ventrolateral aspect of the tongue and lip
- Hairy leukoplakia
  - Occurs predominantly in patients with HIV infection
  - Common site, the lateral borders of tongue

Gross Pathology

- White to grayish yellow plaques on surface epithelium with wrinkled, rough surface (Figure 3-61A)

Histopathology

- Hyperkeratosis, parakeratosis, or both
- Acanthosis and hyperplasia of the squamous epithelium
- Mild or moderate (lichenoid) chronic inflammation may be seen in submucosa
- Dysplastic changes may be present (enlarged, hyperchromatic nuclei; loss of maturation); can extend to

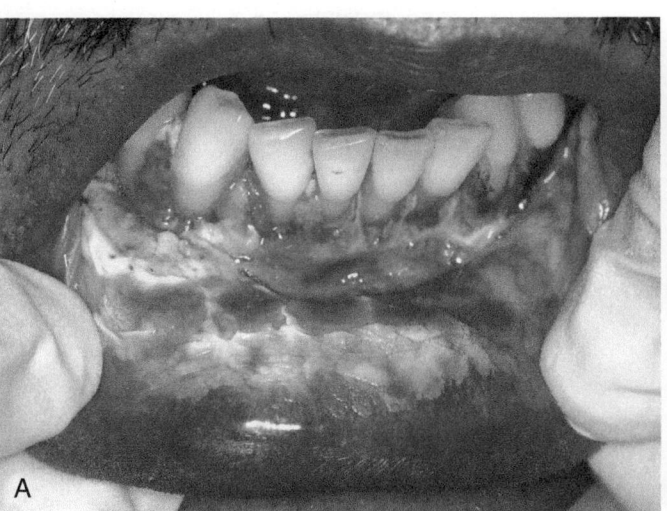
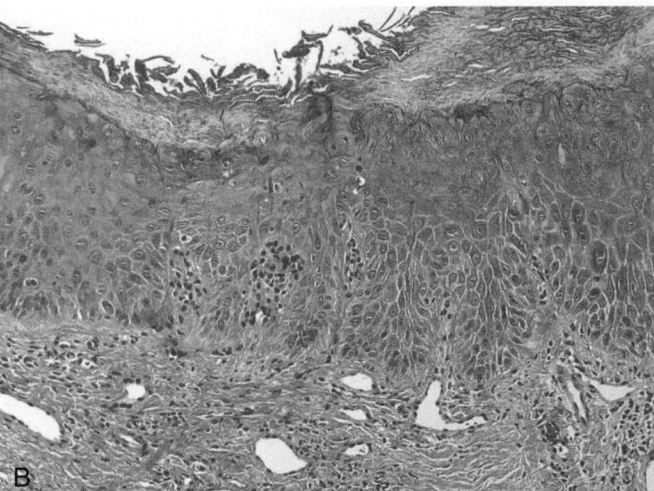

Figure 3-61. Leukoplakia. A, Clinical photograph shows extensive white patches or plaques of the lower lip and gingiva. **B,** Histologically, the squamous mucosa shows marked hyperkeratosis and parakeratosis and underlying dysplasia.

ducts of minor salivary glands; graded as mild, moderate, or severe (Figure 3-61B)
• Often superinfection with *Candida* species

Special Stains and Immunohistochemistry
• Noncontributory

Other Techniques for Diagnosis
• Noncontributory

Differential Diagnosis

SQUAMOUS DYSPLASIA (MILD TO SEVERE)
• May appear grossly white or red-granular (erythroplastic)
• In situ SCC: full-thickness cytologic atypia, disarray of epithelium and intact basement membrane (appears thinned on staining for type IV collagen and laminin)

LICHEN PLANUS
• Less common than leukoplakia
• Bandlike lymphocytic infiltration of the subepithelium, with spongiotic changes in basal cells
• Sawtooth rete ridges

ACTINIC CHEILITIS
• Same morphology and pathogenesis as actinic keratosis of the skin
• Biopsy is mandatory because of the lack of reliable clinical signs predicting malignancy; erythematous, granular plaque is worrisome

PEARLS

• Leukoplakia *is a clinical term with variation in pathologic findings*
• *Leukoplakia may show only hyperkeratosis or be preneoplastic with squamous dysplasia*

SELECTED REFERENCES

Devaney KO, Rinaldo A, Zeitels SM, et al: Laryngeal dysplasia and other epithelial changes on endoscopic biopsy: what does it all mean to the individual patient? J Otorhinolaryngol Relat Spec 66:1-4, 2004.

Fernandez JF, Benito MAC, Lizaldez EB, Monatañés MA: Oral hairy leukoplakia: a histopathologic study of 32 cases. Am J Dermatopathol 12:571-578, 1990.
Muller S, Waldron CA: Premalignant lesions of the oral cavity. In Barnes L (ed): Surgical Pathology of the Head and Neck. New York, Marcel Dekker, 2001, pp 343-360.
Southam JC, Felix DH, Wray D, Cubie HA: Hairy leukoplakia: a histological study. Histopathology 19:63-67, 1991.

SQUAMOUS PAPILLOMA

Clinical Features
• Most common oral neoplasm
• Affects all ages, usually seen in adults
• Etiologic factors are viruses (HPV types 2, 4, 6, 11, 13, and 32) and mechanical irritation
• Preferred sites are palate, tongue, gingiva, and lips
• May occur as a component of Cowden syndrome
• Usually single but may be multiple

Gross Pathology
• Painless, exophytic, white to pink mass with warty or papillary surface (Figure 3-62A)
• Usually smaller than 1 cm

Histopathology
• Broad papillary projections composed of hyperplastic stratified squamous epithelium around a scant fibrovascular core (Figure 3-62B)
• May have varying amounts of parakeratosis, hyperkeratinization, ulceration, inflammation, or superficial *Candida* species infection

Special Stains and Immunohistochemistry
• Noncontributory

Other Techniques for Diagnosis
• In situ hybridization for HPV

Differential Diagnosis

SCC WITH PAPILLARY GROWTH
• Marked cytologic atypia, full thickness
• Infiltrative growth pattern

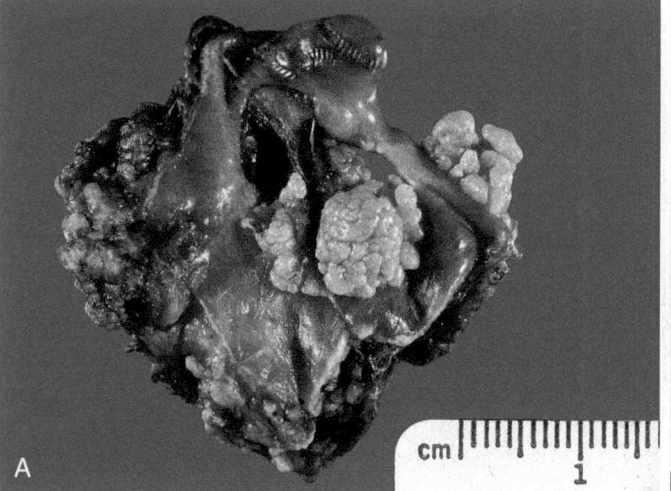
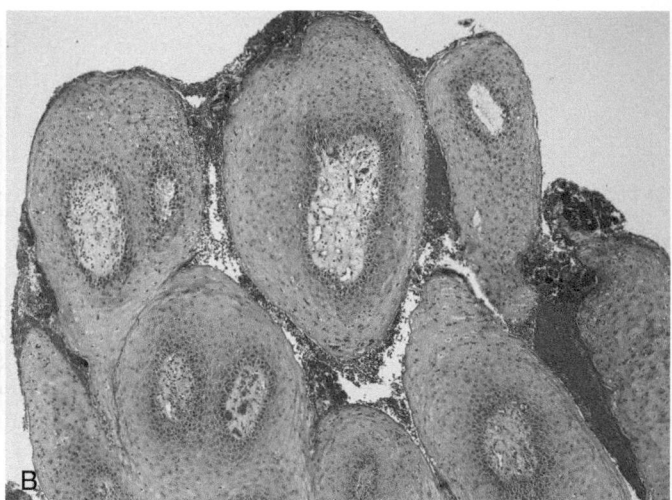

Figure 3-62. Squamous papilloma. A, Gross evaluation shows exophytic tan-white nodular masses of the oral mucosa. **B,** Low-power view shows papillary fronds covered by stratified squamous epithelium with marked hyperkeratosis.

VERRUCA VULGARIS (COMMON WART)
- Uncommonly involves mouth
- Large basophilic inclusions in epithelial cells

CONDYLOMA ACUMINATUM
- Squamous dysplasia with HPV effect (koilocytic atypia)
- Clusters of coalescing exophytic masses
- Fronds broader and blunter than papillomas

PEARLS

- *Squamous atypia and basal cell hyperplasia may occur; dysplasia is rare*
- *Recurrences are infrequent but may happen after incomplete excision*

SELECTED REFERENCES

Abby LJ, Page DG, Sawyer DR: The clinical and histopathologic features of a series of 464 oral squamous cell papillomas. Oral Surg Oral Med Oral Pathol 49:419-428, 1980.

Jenson AB, Lancaster WD, Hartmann DP, Shaffer EL Jr: Frequency and distribution of papillomavirus structural antigens in verrucae, multiple papillomas, and condylomata of the oral cavity. Am J Pathol 107:212-218, 1982.

Westra W: Benign neoplasms of the oral cavity and oropharynx. In Thompson LDR, Goldblum JR (eds): Head and Neck Pathology. Philadelphia, Churchill Livingstone, 2006, pp 243-246.

PYOGENIC GRANULOMA (LOBULAR CAPILLARY HEMANGIOMA)

Clinical Features

- Also called *lobular capillary hemangioma*
- Etiology: infection, trauma, hormonal stimulation (pregnancy)
- May occur at any age; more common in females
- Most common mass of the gingiva

Gross Pathology

- Sharply circumscribed, elevated, dark red, soft nodule

- Often ulcerated (Figure 3-63A)
- Sessile or pedunculated, usually friable and hemorrhagic

Histopathology

- Proliferation of small blood vessels arranged in a lobular growth pattern (mass of granulation tissue) (Figure 3-63B)
- Fibromyxoid or edematous stroma with acute and chronic inflammation
- Overlying squamous epithelium may be atrophic or ulcerated

Special Stains and Immunohistochemistry
- Noncontributory

Other Techniques for Diagnosis
- Noncontributory

Differential Diagnosis

HEMANGIOMA OR LYMPHANGIOMA
- Occurs mostly in the tongue
- Composed of larger vascular or lymphatic channels

KAPOSI SARCOMA OF ORAL CAVITY
- Palate is most common location
- Characterized by slitlike vascular channels with extravasated red blood cells
- Typically associated with HIV-positive patients
- Cells are HHV-8 positive

PERIPHERAL GIANT CELL GRANULOMA
- Nonencapsulated mass of granulation tissue with numerous osteoclast-like giant cells
- Varying degrees of hemorrhage, hemosiderin, and acute and chronic inflammation; metaplastic bone may be seen

PEARLS

- *May regress completely; can fibrose and resemble fibroepithelial polyp*
- *Recurrence rate after surgical treatment is 16%*
- *Treatment is local excision*

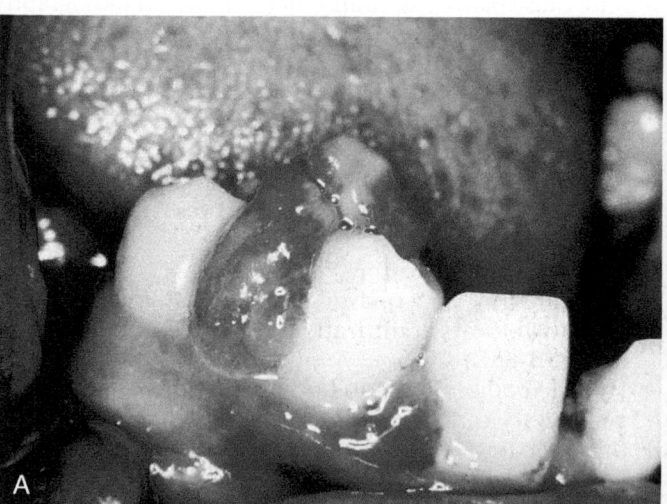
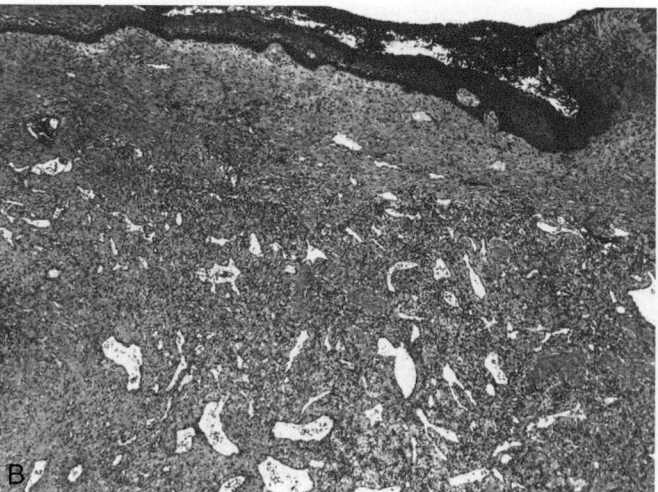

Figure 3-63. Pyogenic granuloma (lobular capillary hemangioma). A, Clinical photograph showing a polypoid mass extending from the gingiva with a ragged erythematous or ulcerated surface. **B,** Low-power view shows a polypoid lesion covered by stratified squamous epithelium and partial ulceration. Note the lobular architecture of the vascular proliferation.

SELECTED REFERENCES

Bodner L, Dayan D: Intravascular papillary endothelial hyperplasia of the mandibular mucosa. Int J Oral Maxillofac Surg 20:263-274, 1991.

Kapadia SB, Heffner DK: Pitfalls in the histopathologic diagnosis of pyogenic granuloma. Eur Arch Otorhinolaryngol 249:195-200, 1992.

Verbin RS, Guggenheimer J, Appel BN: Benign neoplastic and non-neoplastic lesions of the oral cavity and oropharynx. In Barnes L (ed): Surgical Pathology of the Head and Neck. New York, Marcel Dekker, 2001, pp 263-266.

GRANULAR CELL TUMOR

Clinical Features

- Can occur anywhere in the oral cavity; most common on the tongue
- Typically presents as a painless submucosal nodule
- No age preference in adults; rare in children; more common in females
- Uncertain etiology

Gross Pathology

- Firm, submucosal nodule
- Typically small, may measure up to 5 cm

Histopathology

- Overlying squamous epithelium shows pseudoepitheliomatous hyperplasia (Figure 3-64)
- Characterized by sheets, nests, or cords of large, polyhedral cells with granular acidophilic cytoplasm and small hyperchromatic nuclei

Special Stains and Immunohistochemistry

- S-100 protein, Leu-7, and myelin basic protein of the granular cell are positive
- Granules are PAS positive and contain lysosomes

Other Techniques for Diagnosis

- Noncontributory

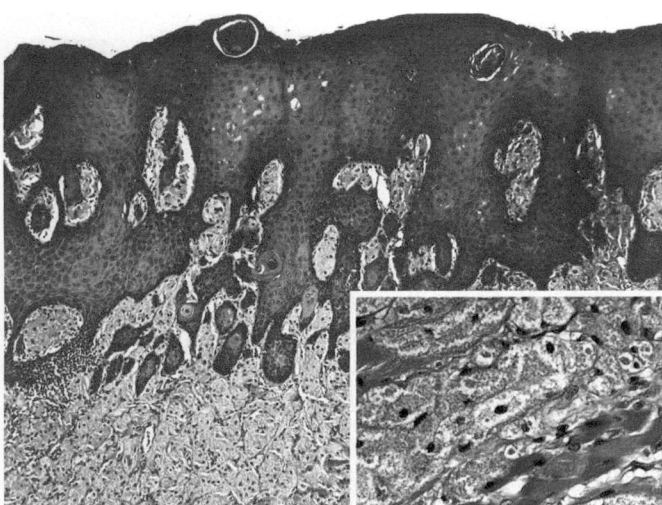

Figure 3-64. Granular cell tumor. Section shows a hyperplastic pseudoepitheliomatous squamous epithelium with marked irregularity of the nests at the basement membrane. The submucosa is replaced by eosinophilic granular cells with small hyperchromatic nuclei (*inset*).

Differential Diagnosis

METASTATIC GRANULAR RENAL CELL CARCINOMA

- Clinical history helpful
- Greater cytologic atypia
- Positive for cytokeratin and vimentin

PEARLS

- *Pseudoepitheliomatous hyperplasia can be mistaken for SCC*
- *About 10% of patients have multiple tumors*
- *Histogenesis believed to be of neural or Schwann cell origin*
- *Most are benign; rare cases of malignant behavior are seen*
- *Features of malignancy: high mitotic activity, necrosis, nuclear pleomorphism, and high cellularity; definitive criterion for malignancy is metastasis*
- *Can occur in nerves (supporting the Schwann cell origin theory)*

SELECTED REFERENCES

Kapadia SB: Tumors of the nervous system. In Barnes L (ed): Surgical Pathology of the Head and Neck. New York, Marcel Dekker, 2001, pp 813-817.

Muzur MT, Shultz JJ, Myers JL: Granular cell tumor: immunohistochemical analysis of 21 benign tumors and one malignant tumor. Arch Pathol Lab Med 114:692, 1990.

RADICULAR CYST

Clinical Features

- Also called *periapical cyst*
- Accounts for 10% of all inflammatory cysts in the oral mucosa
- Cyst formation caused by infection of the dental pulp by caries or trauma
- Most often involves the root of maxillary incisors and mandibular molars; typically no destruction or displacement of teeth
- Seldom associated with deciduous teeth
- May cause pain or be found incidentally on radiography
- Radiographically shows a round or flask-shaped radiolucency with prominent radiopaque margin (Figure 3-65A)

Gross Pathology

- Fragments of glistening or granular soft tissue; rarely is the tooth removed with the cyst intact; cyst lining may or may not be appreciated (Figure 3-65B)

Histopathology

- Cyst lined by hyperplastic stratified squamous epithelium with focal keratinization; goblet cells are common (Figure 3-65C)
- Hyaline bodies (Rushton bodies) are unique to odontogenic cysts and are seen in about 10% of lesions; helpful in separating odontogenic from fissural cysts
- Cyst wall has chronic inflammation, cholesterol clefts, and foamy histiocytes

Special Stains and Immunohistochemistry

- Noncontributory

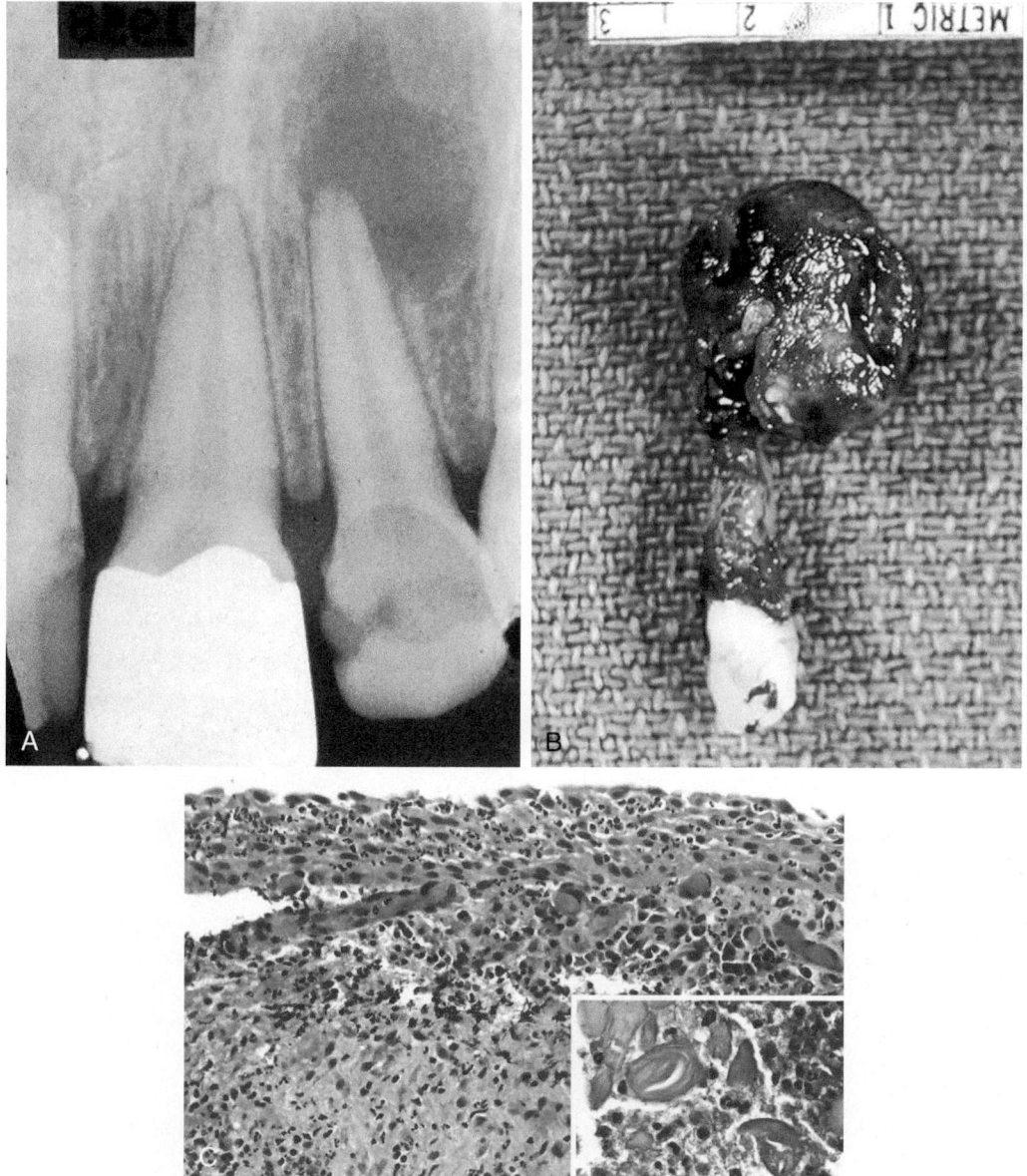

Figure 3-65. Radicular cyst. A, Radiograph showing a radiolucent region associated with the tooth root. **B,** Corresponding resection specimen with mass associated with the tooth root. **C,** The mass consists of a cyst with a squamous epithelial lining with marked inflammation. Associated hyaline (Rushton) bodies may be identified (*inset*).

Other Techniques for Diagnosis

- Noncontributory

Differential Diagnosis

ODONTOGENIC KERATOCYST

- Radiographically, a unilocular or multilocular radiolucency in posterior mandible or maxilla
- Keratinizing squamous epithelium with fibrous, noninflammatory cyst wall
- No Rushton bodies

DENTIGEROUS CYST

- Atypical cyst of unerupted permanent tooth
- Lined by stratified squamous epithelium without cyst wall inflammation

PEARLS

- *Radicular cysts have no potential to differentiate along odontogenic tumor cell lines as do the odontogenic keratocyst and dentigerous cysts*
- *May rarely undergo neoplastic transformation to SCC, ameloblastoma, or mucoepidermoid carcinoma*

SELECTED REFERENCES

High AS, Hirschman PN: Age changes in residual radicular cysts. J Oral Pathol 15:524-528, 1986.

Rushton MA: Hyaline bodies in the epithelium of dental cysts. Proc R Soc Med 48:407-409, 1955.

Verbin RS, Barnes L: Cysts and cyst-like lesions of the oral cavity, jaws and neck. In Barnes L (ed): Surgical Pathology of the Head and Neck. New York, Marcel Dekker, 2001, pp 1464-1468.

DENTIGEROUS CYST

Clinical Features

- Encases the crown of an unerupted permanent tooth
- May clinically present as a missing tooth
- Most often involves third molars
- May be asymptomatic or cause bony expansion and displacement of teeth
- Radiographically, a unilocular radiolucency (Figure 3-66A)

Gross Pathology

- Enlarged, swollen soft tissue with cystic formation (Figure 3-66B)

Histopathology

- Cyst lined by stratified squamous epithelium in direct continuity with enamel epithelium, which covers the crown of the unerupted tooth (Figure 3-66C)
- No inflammation unless superinfected

Special Stains and Immunohistochemistry

- Noncontributory

Other Techniques for Diagnosis

- Noncontributory

Differential Diagnosis

RADICULAR CYST

- Associated with root of tooth

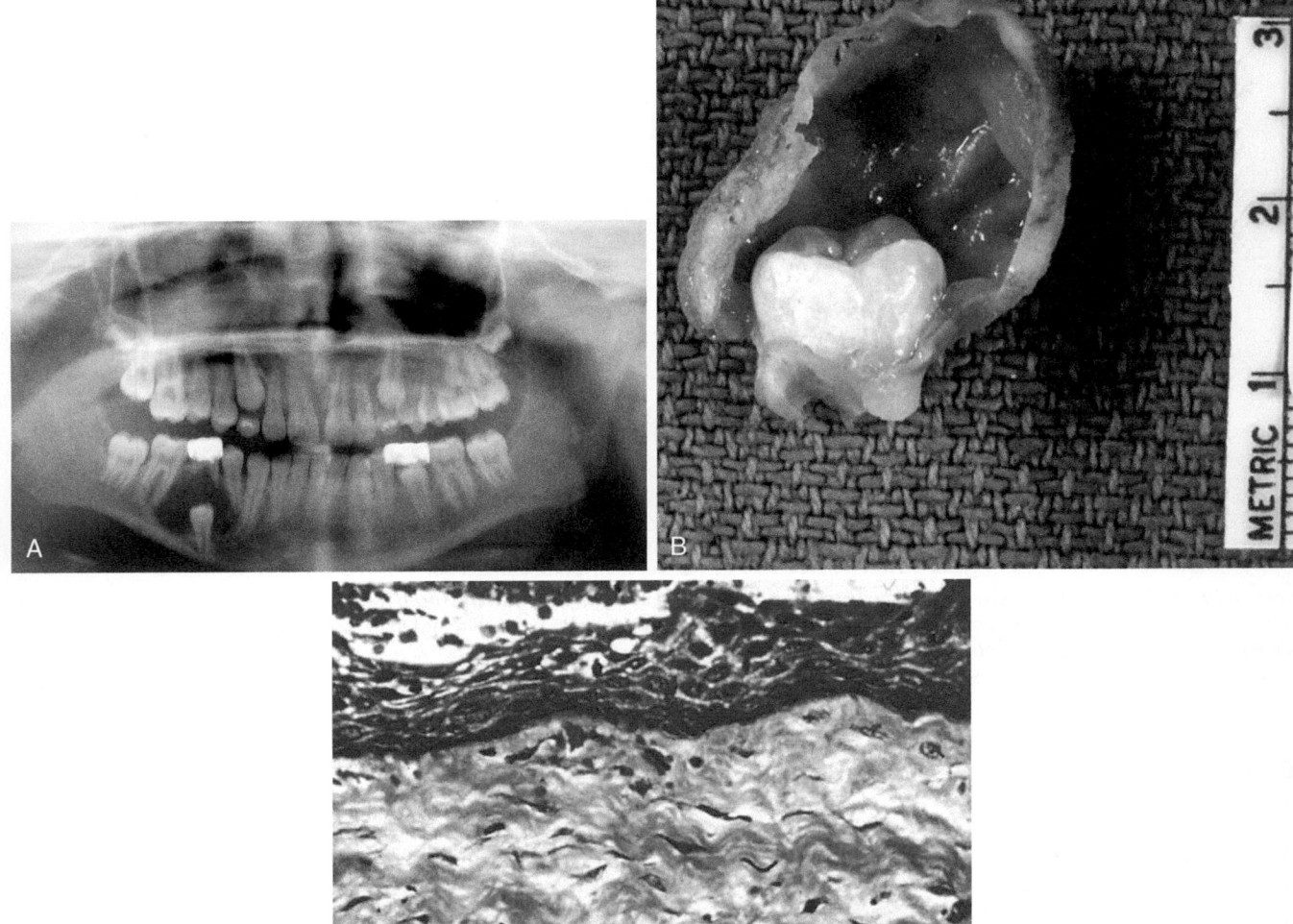

Figure 3-66. Dentigerous cyst. **A,** Radiograph. **B,** Gross photo of the cyst surrounding the crown of an unerupted tooth. **C,** The cyst lining is bland stratified squamous epithelium without inflammation of the cyst wall.

- Cyst wall contains chronic inflammatory cells
- Hyaline bodies (Rushton bodies) are characteristic but are seen in only about 10% of cases

KERATOCYSTIS ODONTOGENIC TUMOR

- Radiographically, unilocular or multilocular radiolucency in posterior mandible or maxilla
- Lined by keratinizing squamous epithelium with fibrous, noninflammatory cells

PEARLS

- *Correlate pathologic findings with radiographic imaging (i.e., Panorex)*
- *Determine location and association with an unerupted tooth*

SELECTED REFERENCE

Eversole LR, Sabes WR, Rovin S: Aggressive growth and neoplastic potential of odontogenic cysts: with special reference to central epidermoid and mucoepidermoid carcinomas. Cancer 35:270-282, 1975.

KERATOCYSTIC ODONTOGENIC TUMOR
(Figure 3-67)

Clinical Features

- Radiographically, unilocular or multilocular radiolucency
- Most occur in the posterior mandible or maxilla

Gross Pathology

- Unilocular or more frequently multilocular cyst with creamy fluid representing cytokeratin debris

Histopathology

- Thin keratinizing stratified squamous epithelium with fibrotic cyst wall lacking inflammation

Special Stains and Immunohistochemistry

- Noncontributory

Other Techniques for Diagnosis

- Noncontributory

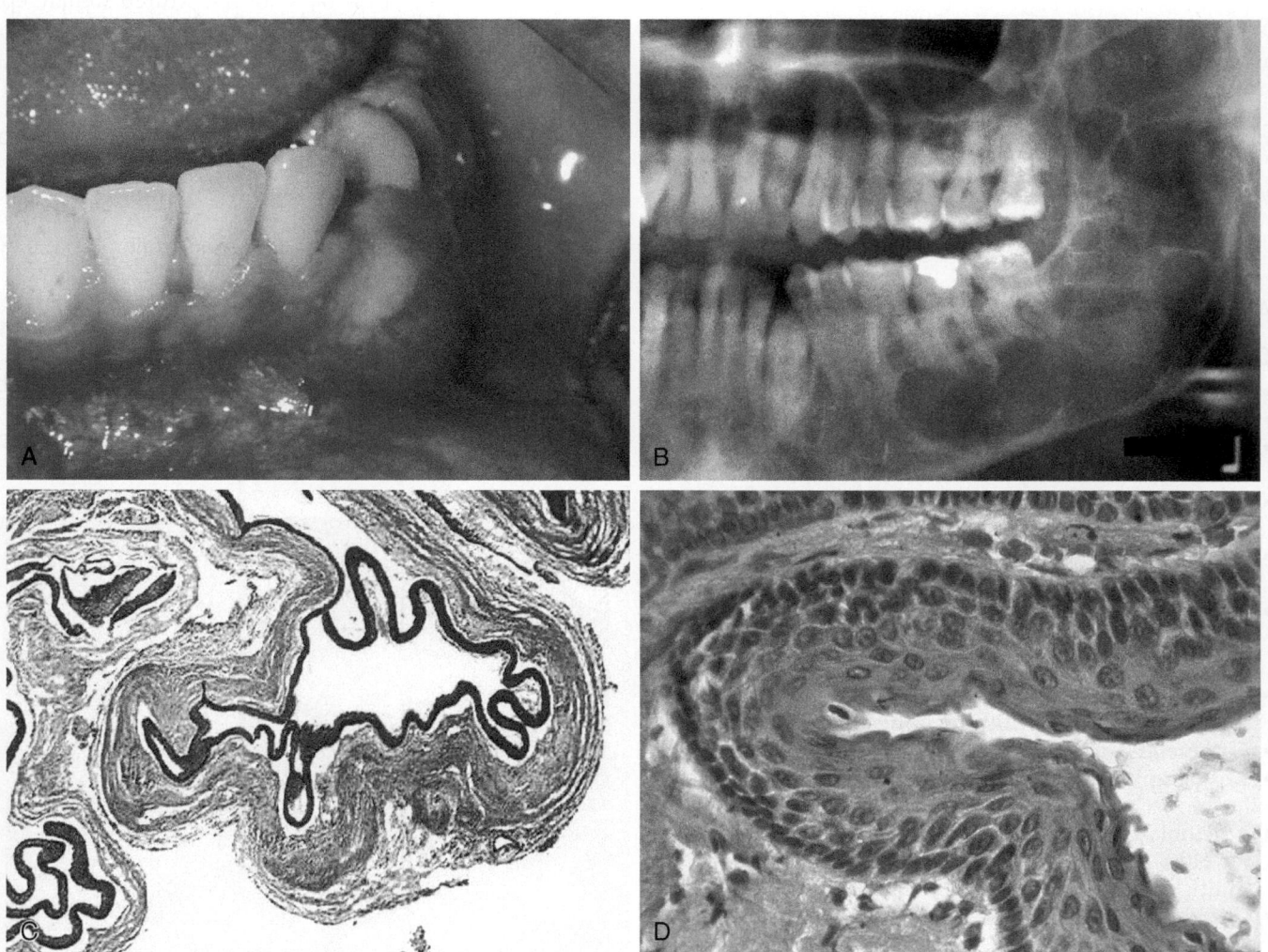

Figure 3-67. Odontogenic keratocyst. A, Clinical photograph of a mandibular mass with intact overlying mucosa. **B,** Corresponding radiograph of a translucent, cystic mass extending up the mandibular ramus. **C,** Low-power image shows an epithelial lined cyst with fibrous wall generally without inflammation. **D,** High-power view of the epithelial cyst wall composed of bland stratified squamous epithelium often with a corrugated surface.

Differential Diagnosis

RADICULAR CYST
- Associated with root of tooth
- Cyst wall contains chronic inflammatory cells
- Hyaline bodies (Rushton bodies) are characteristic but are seen in only about 10% of cases

DENTIGEROUS CYST
- Atypical cyst of unerupted permanent tooth
- Lined by stratified squamous epithelium without cyst wall inflammation

PEARLS
- *Potential for destructive growth and tendency for recurrence*
- *May be associated with nevoid basal cell carcinoma syndrome (autosomal dominant condition characterized by keratocysts of jaw, multiple basal cell carcinomas of the skin, skeletal anomalies, palmar and plantar dyskeratosis, ectopic soft tissue calcifications, and ovarian fibromas)*

SELECTED REFERENCES

Areen RG, McClatchey KD, Baker HL: Squamous cell carcinoma developing in an odontogenic keratocyst: report of a case. Arch Otolaryngol Head Neck Surg 107:568-569, 1981.

Blanas N, Freund B, Schwartz M, Furst IM: Systematic review of the treatment and prognosis of the odontogenic keratocyst. Oral Surg Oral Med Oral Pathol Oral Radiol Endodontol 90:553-558, 2000.

Verbin RS, Barnes L: Cysts and cyst-like lesions of the oral cavity, jaws and neck. In Barnes L (ed): Surgical Pathology of the Head and Neck. New York, Marcel Dekker, 2001, pp 1452-1460.

AMELOBLASTOMA

Clinical Features
- Most common odontogenic neoplasm
- Males and females equally affected
- Occurs more frequently in whites, followed by blacks and Asians (especially Chinese)
- Average age is 33 years; unicystic lesions occur a decade earlier
- Location: mandible is affected more than maxilla (ratio 4:1), typically posterior mandible
- Many occur in association with impacted third molars; some arise from the epithelial lining of dentigerous cysts
- Typically grows slowly and is asymptomatic until large; may resorb teeth or infiltrate bone and soft tissue
- Can metastasize (rarely)
- Radiographically, multiloculated, "soap-bubble" radiolucency
- Ameloblastomas of sinonasal region show predilection for older men (more than 80% are infiltrating, solid, or multicystic)
- Clinicopathologic forms: multicystic, unicystic, and peripheral
  - Unicystic and multicystic
    - Occur in younger patients
    - Noninfiltrating form; low recurrence rate after conservative treatment (10% to 15%)
    - May recur as the infiltrating multicystic type
  - Peripheral
    - Least common; more common in older adults
    - Extraosseous location

Gross Pathology
- Cut surface reveals solid and cystic areas
- Solid areas are white to gray with little hemorrhage and no necrosis
- Variably sized cysts that contain clear to yellow fluid

Histopathology
- Follicular and plexiform pattern cellular; other patterns are acanthomatous, granular cell, basaloid, desmoplastic, and keratoameloblastoma-like (exceptionally rare)
  - Follicular pattern (resembles dental follicle)
    - Variably sized islands of odontogenic epithelium whose peripheral palisading tall columnar cells display reverse nuclear polarity and subnuclear vacuoles (Figure 3-68)
    - Fibrous connective tissue stroma surrounds epithelial islands
    - Nuclei are uniform with no mitotic activity
    - Centers of islands have loose-textured stellate epithelial cells, often with microcyst formation
  - Plexiform pattern
    - Broad anastomosing sheets of cells with stellate epithelium at center; peripheral cells are tall columnar with reverse nuclear polarity and subnuclear vacuoles
    - Stroma is looser and can have cyst formation
  - Acanthomatous pattern
    - Follicular islands show squamous metaplasia or cytokeratin production
- All ameloblastomas, except for the desmoplastic variant, have mature fibrous stroma; in desmoplastic variant, stromal osteoid production is seen
- Most important prognostic feature is presence or absence of infiltration
- Histologic subtypes do not influence treatment or prognosis

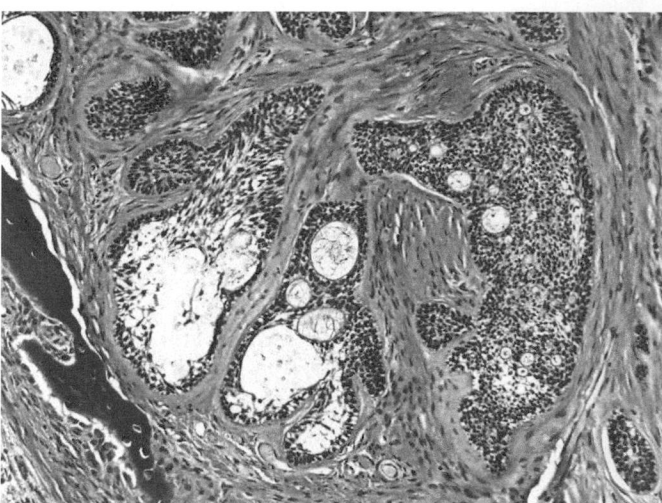

Figure 3-68. Ameloblastoma. Low-power view shows epithelial nests with peripheral palisading, loose stellate centers, and microcysts growing in a dense stroma adjacent to thinned bone.

Special Stains and Immunohistochemistry

- Noncontributory

Other Techniques for Diagnosis

- Noncontributory

Differential Diagnosis

AMELOBLASTIC FIBROMA

- Benign mixed tumor of epithelial-mesenchymal odontogenic neoplasm
- Connective tissue resembles dental papilla
- Epithelial nests of cuboidal to columnar cells with stellate reticulum
- Well-defined basement membrane
- Most in posterior mandible

SCC

- Markedly atypical squamous cells with an infiltrative growth pattern
- Mitoses frequently identified

BASAL CELL CARCINOMA

- Desmoplastic stroma
- Often history of prior skin cancer
- Mitoses may be noted

SALIVARY-TYPE ADENOCARCINOMAS

- Rarely primary intraosseous
- Reverse polarization of epithelium not usually seen

PEARLS

- *Recurrence rate of infiltrating ameloblastomas treated surgically by curettage is high (up to 90%); important to excise with adequate bone margin*
- *Grows slowly; recurrences may take several years to become radiographically apparent; can recur many years after treatment*

SELECTED REFERENCES

Chen Y, Wang JM, Li TJ: Ameloblastic fibroma: a review of published studies with special reference to its nature and biological behavior. Oral Oncol 43:960-969, 2007.

Feinberg SE, Steinberg B: Surgical management of ameloblastoma: current status of the literature. Oral Surg Oral Med Oral Pathol 81:383-388, 1996.
Melrose RJ: Benign epithelial odontogenic tumors. Semin Diagn Pathol 16:271-287, 1999.
Reichart PA, Philopsen HP, Sommer S: Ameloblastoma: biologic profile of 3677 cases. Eur J Cancer 31B:86-99, 1995.

CALCIFYING EPITHELIAL ODONTOGENIC TUMOR (PINDBORG TUMOR)

Clinical Features

- Presents as a slow-growing mass with few symptoms; jaw swelling or resorption of teeth may be seen
- Usual age is between 30 and 50 years
- No gender predilection
- Most occur in posterior mandible, 25% in the maxilla
- May rarely be extraosseous
- Association with impacted tooth in about 50% of cases
- Radiographically, a poorly demarcated, multilocular radiolucency (Figure 3-69A)

Gross Pathology

- Generally a solid mass with variable amount of calcification
- Cortical thinning of bone, but rarely invasion beyond periosteum

Histopathology

- Sheets of large polyhedral epithelial cells often displaying intercellular bridges (Figure 3-69B)
- Cells have abundant eosinophilic cytoplasm, pleomorphic nuclei with prominent nucleoli, and intranuclear pseudoinclusions; cells may be binucleated
- No mitosis, necrosis, or inflammation
- Characteristic concentric ring calcifications (Liesegang rings)
- Occasionally pink, amorphous, amyloid-like material present, typically scant stromal fibrosis

Special Stains and Immunohistochemistry

- Congo red positive (amyloid-like material has apple-green birefringence under polarized light)

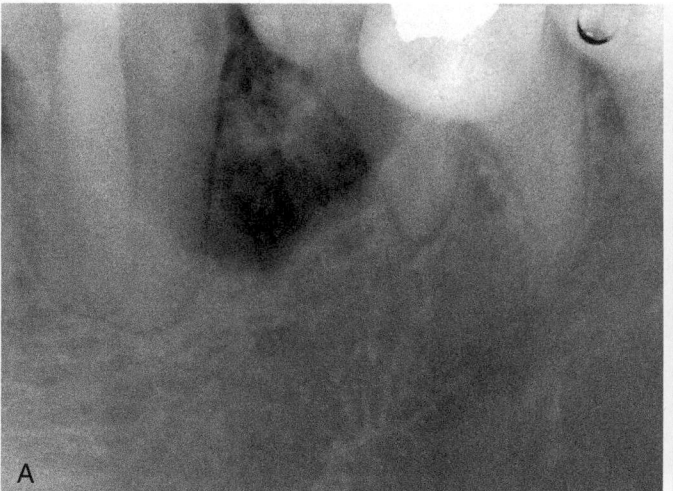
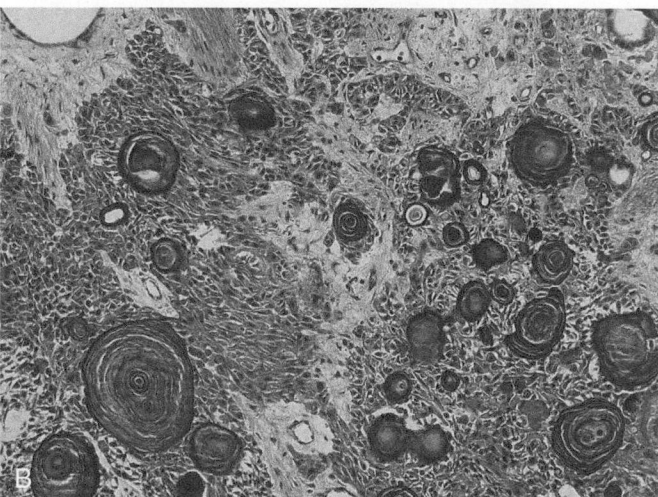

Figure 3-69. **Calcifying epithelial odontogenic tumor. A,** Radiograph of radiolucent mass with fine granular opacifications between two teeth. **B,** Histologic section shows sheets of epithelial cells and calcifications.

Other Techniques for Diagnosis

• Noncontributory

Differential Diagnosis

SCC

• Invasive growth pattern
• Cells show cytologic features of malignancy; associated squamous dysplasia in adjacent squamous epithelium is often seen

PEARLS

• *Even small tumors are infiltrating*
• *Surgical resection should have adequate bone margin of at least 1 cm*
• *Recurrence rate is 14%; recurrences are slow growing, and long follow-up is recommended*

SELECTED REFERENCES

Franlin CD, Pindborg JJ: The calcifying epithelial odontogenic tumor: a review and analysis of 113 cases. Oral Surg Oral Med Oral Pathol 42:753-765, 1976.

Philipsen HP, Reichart PA: Calcifying epithelial odontogenic tumour: biological profile based on 181 cases from the literature. Oral Oncol 36:17-26, 2000.

Veness MJ, Morgan G, Collins AP, Walker DM: Calcifying epithelial odontogenic (Pindborg) tumor with malignant transformation and metastatic spread. Head Neck 23:692-696, 2001.

ADENOMATOID ODONTOGENIC TUMOR

Clinical Features

• Uncommon benign lesion
• Typically found in second decade of life
• Female-to-male ratio of 2:1
• Twice as common in maxilla as in mandible
• Predilection for anterior part of both jaws; canine location accounts for about 60% of cases
• Most cases are associated with an impacted tooth; rarely extraosseous

• Radiographically, well-demarcated radiolucency with or without associated impacted tooth (Figure 3-70A)

Gross Pathology

• Thick fibrous capsule with abundant gray to white tissue in the center
• Small calcifications give cut surface a gritty feel
• May present as a thick-walled cyst with small amount of fluid and a soft, shaggy surface

Histopathology

• Thick fibrous capsule surrounds variably sized nodular areas of epithelium composed of cuboidal or low columnar cells with virtually no connective tissue stroma
• Dystrophic calcification is often associated with the epithelial cell nodules
• Ductlike spaces within epithelial cell nodules contain an amorphous eosinophilic material that does not stain for amyloid but may be an abortive enamel-like product (Figure 3-70B)

Special Stains and Immunohistochemistry

• Noncontributory

Other Techniques for Diagnosis

• Noncontributory

Differential Diagnosis

AMELOBLASTOMA

• More commonly found in the posterior mandible (80%)
• Different radiologic appearance
• Typically has a follicular architecture characterized by islands of odontogenic epithelium in a fibrous connective tissue stroma

PEARLS

• *Prognosis is excellent*
• *Conservative surgical excision (enucleation) is curative; recurrence is exceptionally rare*

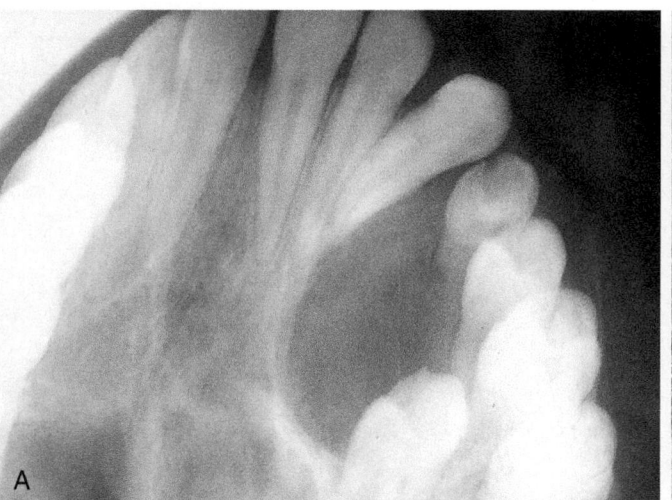 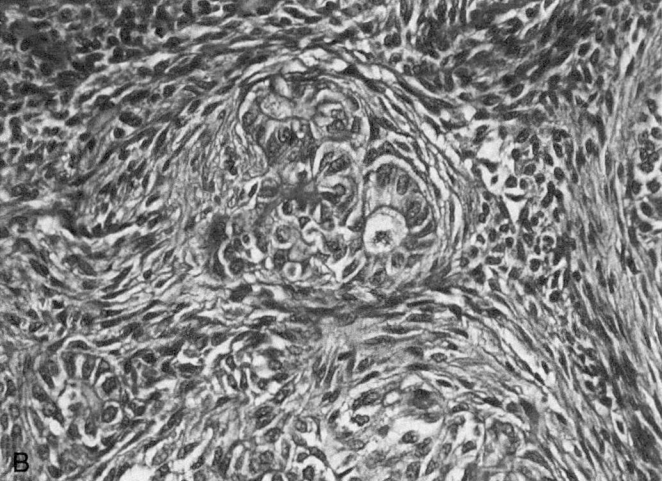

Figure 3-70. Adenomatoid odontogenic tumor. A, Radiograph of well-demarcated translucent area of the maxilla with associated impacted tooth. **B,** Microscopic examination shows a neoplasm composed of ductlike spaces in epithelial nests surrounded by solid areas of ameloblast-like fibroblasts.

SELECTED REFERENCES

Philipsen HP, Reichart PA: Adenomatoid odontogenic tumor: facts and figures. Oral Oncol 35:125-131, 1998.

Rick GM: Adenomatoid odontogenic tumor. Oral Maxillofac Surg Clin N Am 16:333-354, 2004.

BENIGN CEMENTOBLASTOMA

Clinical Features

- Rare benign mesenchymal odontogenic tumor
- Slow growing and can reach a large size
- Intimately associated with roots of teeth
- Mostly affects young adults, but may occur at any age
- Most commonly mandibular first molar and premolars
- Typically presents with pain (reminiscent of osteoblastoma)
- Radiographically, well-defined radiopaque mass obliterating the root of the involved tooth and with a peripheral thin radiolucent zone (Figure 3-71A)

Gross Pathology

- Calcified mass adherent to the root of affected tooth

Histopathology

- Calcified cemental tissue deposition on a tooth root (Figure 3-71B)
- Thick trabeculae of cementum strongly basophilic with numerous irregular reversal lines resembling Paget

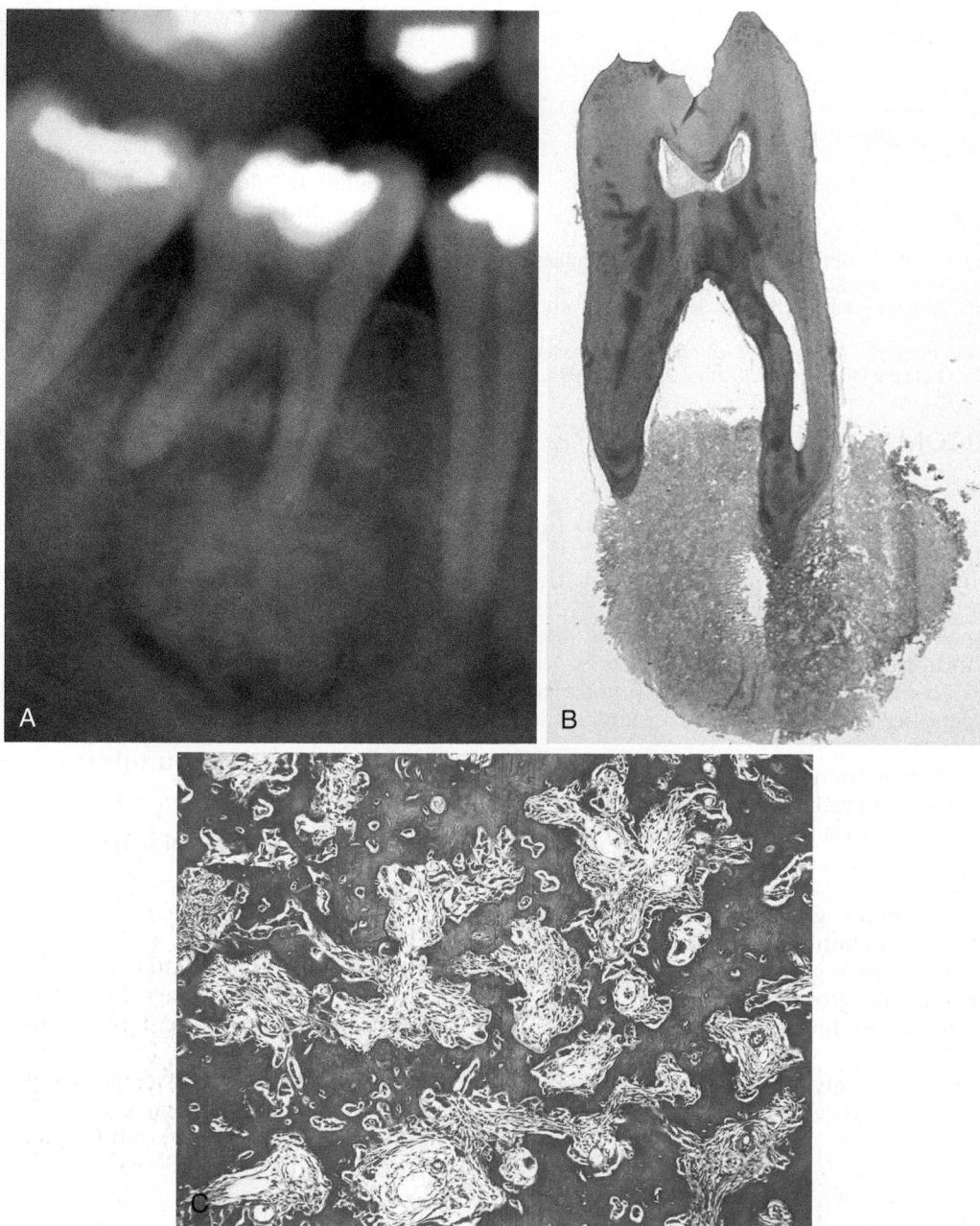

Figure 3-71. Benign cementoblastoma. A, Radiograph showing a well-defined mass with a peripheral radiolucent zone associated with the tooth root. **B,** Whole-mount section of the corresponding resected specimen with tooth and mass at the root. **C,** Histologic section shows dense bony trabeculae with intervening proliferative fibrovascular tissue.

bone; trabeculae rimmed with active cementoblasts (Figure 3-71C)
- Periphery shows radiating columns of cementoid with interspersed fibrovascular tissue
- Dilated vascular spaces and osteoclast-like giant cells are occasionally seen

Special Stains and Immunohistochemistry

- Noncontributory

Other Techniques for Diagnosis

- Noncontributory

Differential Diagnosis

OSTEOBLASTOMA OF THE JAW

- May envelop roots of teeth but does not originate from the cementum of the root surface

PEARLS

- *Treatment is surgical excision with extraction of affected tooth*

SELECTED REFERENCES

El-Mofty SK: Cemento-ossifying fibroma and benign cementoblastoma. Semin Diagn Pathol 16:302-307, 1999.

Melrose RJ: Benign epithelial odontogenic tumors. Semin Diagn Pathol 16:271-287, 1999.

Ulmansky M, Hansen EH, Praetorius F: Benign cementoblastoma: a review and five new cases. Oral Surg Oral Med Oral Pathol 77:48-55, 1994.

CHONDROSARCOMA

Clinical Features

- Most common site is the pelvis, but also affects the proximal femur and humerus
- Rarely occurs in the jaw but has predilection for the maxilla and skull base
- Chondrosarcomas may be primary or secondary (arising from enchondromas or osteochondromas)
- Classified into central, peripheral, or juxtacortical tumors depending on location and radiographic characteristics
- More common in men than women (2:1); peak incidence in third to sixth decades, two decades earlier for secondary chondrosarcomas

Gross Pathology

- Central chondrosarcomas grow intramedullary and may extend into cortical bone
- Peripheral chondrosarcomas grow from the cortex of the bone into soft tissue; may grow into medullary cavity
- Cut surface is white to bluish gray depending on amount of cartilage
- May be cystic and have myxoid or gelatinous areas; hemorrhage, necrosis, and calcification may be seen

Histopathology

- Composed of conventional, mesenchymal, and dedifferentiated subtypes
- Variable histology depending on amount of chondroid matrix
  - Conventional

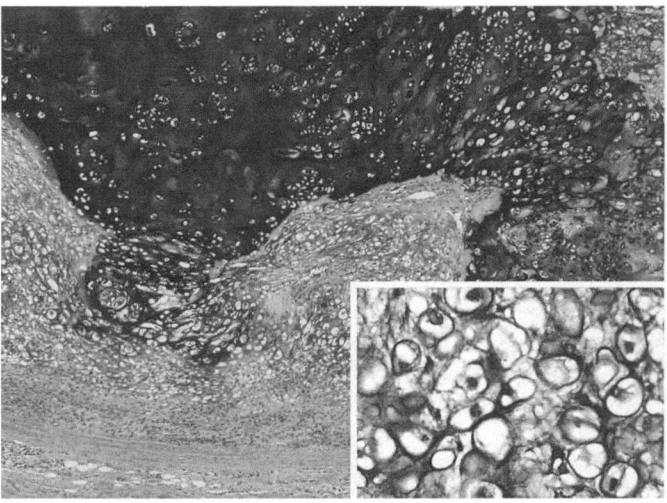

Figure 3-72. Chondrosarcoma. Section shows a lobulated mass composed of variably cellular neoplastic chondrocytes. At high power (*inset*), the chondrocytes have open, large nuclei.

- Irregular lobules of cartilage separated by fibrous strands and invade bone; higher cellularity at the periphery of the lobules (Figure 3-72)
- Chondrocytes in clusters; atypia varies from slight nuclear enlargement to large, bizarre nuclei
- Multinucleated chondrocytes may be seen
- Higher-grade tumors have increased cytologic atypia; grade 3 findings of peripheral spindling or > 2 mitoses/10 hpf
- Mitotic activity is not present in grade tumors
- Mesenchymal
  - Spindle cells or small blue cells intermixed with hyaline cartilage
  - Rare subtype, third decade
  - Propensity for jawbones
- Dedifferentiated
  - Two distinct tumor components: chondrosarcoma component (often grade 1) and dedifferentiated malignant spindle cell areas that mimic fibrosarcoma or osteosarcoma

Special Stains and Immunohistochemistry

- Noncontributory

Other Techniques for Diagnosis

- Noncontributory

Differential Diagnoses

CHONDROBLASTIC OSTEOSARCOMA

- May have areas of cartilage but also has atypical osteoblasts and abnormal osteoid formation (irregular, lacelike)
- May be confused with osseous metaplasia or reactive osteoid within a chondrosarcoma
- Pure hyaline (without myxoid) frequently in chondrosarcomas, less in osteosarcoma

CHONDROMA

- Should be distinguished from grade 1 chondrosarcoma
- Does not have bony or fibrous trabeculae or islands of bone within cartilage

CHORDOMA

- Strong predilection for the axial skeleton, particularly the spheno-occipital region
- Peak incidence in third to fifth decades
- Radiographically, appears as an expansible, destructive mass, often extending outside of the bone
- Microscopically, lobules and cords of large cells with low N/C ratio and characteristic vacuolated cytoplasm (physaliferous cells) within myxoid matrix
- Chondroid type chordoma can be differentiated based on immunohistochemical characteristics: positive for cytokeratin, EMA, Brachyury (notochord) origin marker, and S-100 protein

PEARLS

- *Metastatic sites are lungs, skin, and soft tissue*
- *Complete surgical excision should be performed; prognosis depends on stage and histologic grade; metastases are uncommon for grade 1 chondrosarcomas, but about 70% of grade 3 chondrosarcomas metastasize; recurrences are often of a higher histologic grade*
- *Radiologic correlation is crucial*

SELECTED REFERENCES

Jeffrey PB, Biava CG, Davis RL: Chondroid chordoma: a hyalinized chordoma without cartilaginous differentiation. Am J Clin Pathol 103:271-279, 1995.

Pellitteri PK, Ferlito A, Fagan JJ, et al: Mesenchymal chondrosarcoma of the head and neck. Oral Oncol 43:970-975, 2007.

Saito K, Unni KK, Wollan PC, Lund BA: Chondrosarcoma of the jaw and facial bones. Cancer 76:1550-1558, 1995.

Thompson LD, Gannon FH: Chondrosarcoma of the larynx: a clinico-pathologic study of 111 cases with a review of the literature. Am J Surg Pathol 26:836-851, 2002.

OSTEOSARCOMA

Clinical Features

- Rare tumor in the jaw region, constitutes about 5% of all osteosarcomas
- May have predilection for the mandible or equal to maxilla
- Maxillary tumors occur, particularly at alveolar ridge
- Most cases are de novo; may be associated with radiation, Paget disease, and fibrous dysplasia (secondary osteosarcomas)
- Most tumors arise from the medullary cavity or, rarely, periosteum of the jaws (juxtacortical osteosarcomas)
- Osteosarcomas of the jaw occur at an older age (third to fourth decades), and swelling, pain, and paresthesias are typical
- Radiographic presentation ranges from radiolucent to radiopaque with classic sunburst pattern
- Jaw osteosarcomas tend to be better differentiated (grade 2 to 3) than appendicular osteosarcomas
- Genetic predisposition to osteosarcomas in children with familial bilateral retinoblastoma

Gross Pathology

- Cut surface is firm and tan-yellow with bony destruction often into surrounding soft tissue
- Translucent areas (chondroid matrix), hemorrhage, and necrosis may be seen

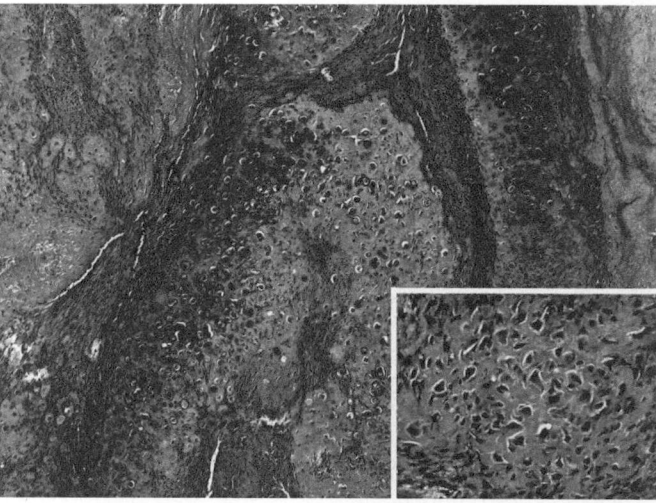

Figure 3-73. Osteosarcoma. Chondroblastic variant with lobules of malignant cartilage. Osteoid is identified within the tumor (*inset*).

Histopathology

- Most osteosarcomas of the jaw are chondroblastic
- All osteosarcoma variants in the jaw have histologic features similar to those of osteosarcomas in the appendicular skeleton
  - Chondroblastic (50% to 60% of cases)
    - Predominance of malignant-appearing chondroid areas with focal osteoid deposition
    - Chondroid differentiation varies in cellularity and lobulation and may be myxoid (Figure 3-73)
  - Fibroblastic (approximately 25% of cases)
    - Malignant spindle cells, variable cellularity; matrix may be scant
    - May mimic fibrosarcoma
  - Osteoblastic (approximately 20% of cases)
    - Predominance of malignant osteoid, which is irregular with a lacelike filigree pattern
    - Variable mineralization of the osteoid
  - Telangiectatic (rare)
    - Composed of dilated blood-filled spaces separated by cellular septa containing malignant cells with a high mitotic rate
    - Haphazard distribution of osteoid deposition

Special Stains and Immunohistochemistry

- Noncontributory

Other Techniques for Diagnosis

- Noncontributory

Differential Diagnoses

CHONDROSARCOMA

- May be difficult to differentiate from chondroblastic variant
- Less common in mandible
- Tumor-forming osteoid is absent

MYXOID AND SALIVARY NEOPLASMS

- Relationship to bone should be considered; radiographic correlation
- Keep chondroblastic osteosarcoma in differential
- Search for osteoid is warranted

OSSIFYING FIBROMA

- Often hypercellular, composed of uniform cells lacking nuclear pleomorphism
- Radiologic features are classic and reliably distinguish these entities

OSTEOBLASTOMA

- Well-defined mass characterized by irregular trabeculae of osteoid and woven bone with vascularized stroma
- Lacks nuclear pleomorphism
- Cartilaginous areas are rare

PEARLS

- *Jaw osteosarcomas are most often chondroblastic*
- *May mimic myxoid or salivary neoplasms*
- *Treatment of osteosarcoma of the jaw is surgery; role of chemotherapy is unclear*
- *Radiologic correlation is of paramount importance in the diagnosis of both cartilaginous and bony lesions*

SELECTED REFERENCES

Kassir RR, Rassekh CH, Kinsella JB, et al: Osteosarcoma of the head and neck: meta-analysis of nonrandomized studies. Laryngoscope 107:56-61, 1997.
Garrington GE, Scofield HH, Cornyn J, Hooker SP: Osteosarcoma of the jaws: analysis of 56 cases. Cancer 20:377-391, 1996.
Mark RJ, Sercarz JA, Tran L, et al: Osteogenic sarcoma of the head and neck: the UCLA experience. Arch Otolaryngol Head Neck Surg 117:761-766, 1991.
Sturgis EM, Potter BO: Sarcomas of the head and neck region. Curr Opin Oncol 15:239-252, 2003.

SQUAMOUS CELL CARCINOMA

Clinical Features

- Predisposing factors are smoking, tobacco, immunosuppression (in organ transplant recipients), mechanical irritation, and sun exposure
- Predominantly affects men older than 50 years, but incidence in younger patients and women is increasing
- Other high-risk areas are floor of mouth and ventrolateral tongue
- Patients have 100-fold increased risk for developing a second primary in the region
- May be multiple; if so, tongue is most commonly affected
- HIV infection: oropharyngeal and tonsillar cancer

Gross Pathology

- Irregular mucosal surface with red granular areas
- Cut surface is tan-white with occasional areas of necrosis or hemorrhage (Figure 3-74A)

Histopathology

- Aggressive features: finger-like invasive fronts
- Similar to SCCs in other locations: usually moderately to poorly differentiated (Figure 3-74B)
- Epithelium adjacent to invasive tumor often shows carcinoma in situ or varying degrees of squamous dysplasia (field cancerization)
- Perineural invasion

Special Stains and Immunohistochemistry

- Cytokeratin positive: express CK5/6, CK8, and CK19 but are CK20 negative
- Overexpression of *TP53* oncogene in 30% to 50% of cases

Other Techniques for Diagnosis

- Nondiploid tumors are typically more advanced clinically than diploid tumors
- In multiple tumors, TP53 expression is similar, and they are also clonal by karyotypic and FISH analysis
- Loss of heterozygosity (LOH) of TP53 by PCR in 70% of tumors

Differential Diagnosis

VERRUCOUS CARCINOMA

- Low-grade variant of SCC
- Most common in oral cavity (buccal mucosa and lower gingiva)
- Elderly men more commonly affected
- Associated with chewing tobacco
- Grossly large soft papillary tumor

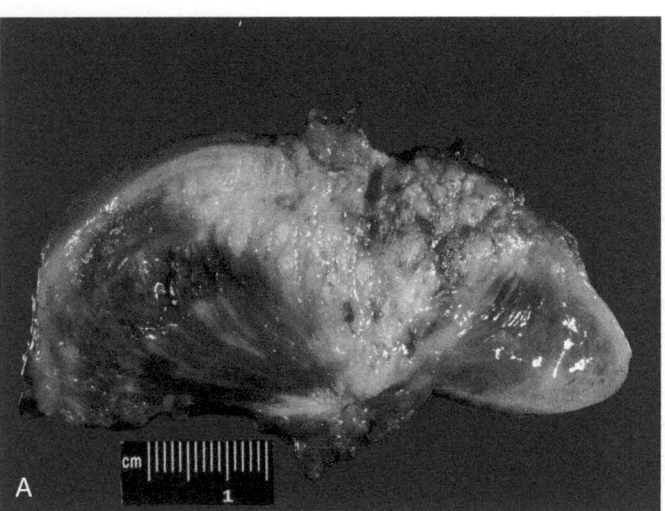

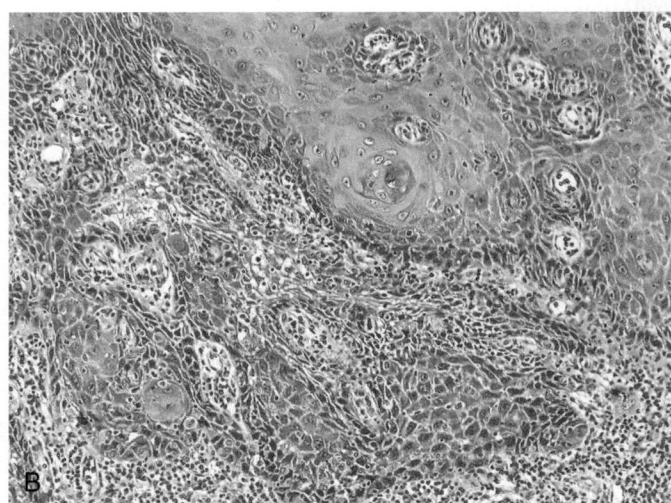

Figure 3-74. **Squamous cell carcinoma. A,** Gross examination of a hemiglossectomy specimen shows a large tumor ulcerating the mucosa of the tongue and deeply invading into skeletal muscle. **B,** An infiltrating neoplasm is present composed of sheets of keratinizing epithelial cells with hyperchromatic nuclei.

- Locally aggressive but does not metastasize
- Characteristically bland cytologic appearance
- Treatment is surgical because radiation therapy may change the tumor into highly malignant, poorly differentiated, and metastasizing SCC

NASOPHARYNGEAL CARCINOMA
- Rare in United States; SCC arising in the nasopharynx, associated with EBV infection
- Characterized by neoplastic epithelial cells with an intense infiltrate of lymphoid cells

PEARLS

- *Main prognostic factors are stage, location, depth of invasion, and close margins (< 5 mm)*
- *Occasionally, cervical lymph node metastases undergo cystic degeneration or elicit foreign-body giant cell reaction to keratin (can be mistaken for branchial cleft cyst with malignant transformation)*
- *Lymph nodes with extranodal extension increase recurrence and metastases*

SELECTED REFERENCES

Cardesa A, Gale N, Nadal A, et al: Squamous cell carcinoma: verrucous carcinoma: basaloid squamous cell carcinoma. In Barnes EL, Eveson JW, Reichart P, Sidransky D (eds): World Health Organization Classification of Tumours: Pathology and Genetics: Head and Neck Tumours. Lyon, IARC Press, 2005, pp 118-125.

Koch BB, Trask DK, Hoffman HT, et al: National survey of head and neck verrucous carcinoma: patterns of presentation, care, and outcome. Cancer 92:110-120, 2001.

Shah JP, Candela FC, Poddar AK: The patterns of cervical lymph node metastases from squamous carcinoma of the oral cavity. Cancer 66:109-113, 1990.

Suarez PA, Adler-Storthz K, Luna MA, et al: Papillary squamous cell carcinomas of the upper aerodigestive tract: a clinicopathologic and molecular study. Head Neck 22:360-368, 2000.

Wu M, Putti TC, Bhuiya TA: Comparative study in the expression of p53, EGFR, TGF-alpha, and cyclin D1 in verrucous carcinoma, verrucous hyperplasia, and squamous cell carcinoma of head and neck region. Appl Immunohistochem Mol Morphol 10:351-356, 2002.

TUMORS METASTASIZING TO THE ORAL CAVITY

Clinical Features
- May present as primary intraoral lesions, most commonly involving the gingiva
- Most common primary tumor site is the lung
- Other common primary sites include kidney, breast, skin, prostate, endometrium, and colon

Gross Pathology
- Gingival nodules
- Cut section varies depending on primary tumor: renal cell carcinoma metastasis may be very hemorrhagic; metastatic colonic tumors may have central areas of necrosis (Figure 3-75)

Histopathology
- Depends on the original tumor cell type and grade

Special Stains and Immunohistochemistry
- Carcinomas: cytokeratin positive

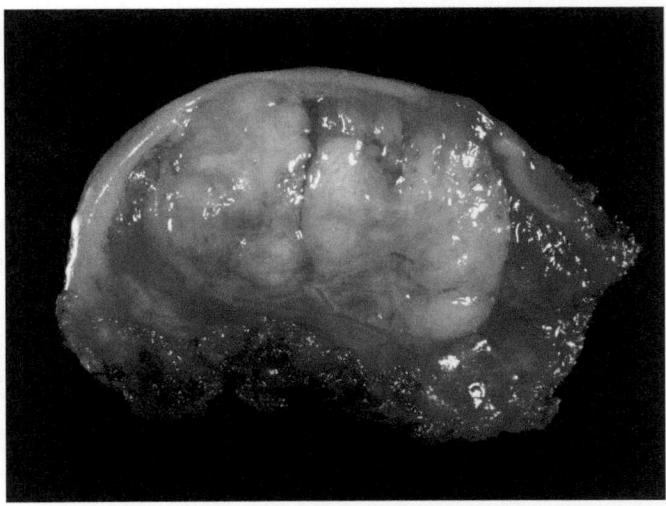

Figure 3-75. Metastasis (renal cell carcinoma) to tongue. Gross photograph shows a submucosal lobulated mass with variable gray translucent to more solid areas.

- Renal cell carcinoma: cytokeratin and vimentin positive, contains intracytoplasmic fat but no glycogen (PAS and D-PAS positive)
- Prostate: prostate-specific antigen (PSA) positive (may be lost with treatment)
- Breast: may be positive for *HER-2-neu*, estrogen receptor, progesterone receptor

Other Techniques for Diagnosis
- Noncontributory

Differential Diagnosis
- Metastatic lung, renal cell, colonic, endometrial, breast, prostate carcinoma

METASTATIC MELANOMA
- Large polygonal cells with variably pleomorphic nuclei and prominent nucleoli
- Positive for S-100 protein and HMB-45

PEARLS

- *Unusual cell type or growth pattern should suggest possibility of a metastasis*

SELECTED REFERENCES

Baden E, Duvillard P, Micheau C: Metastatic papillary endometrial carcinoma of the tongue: case report and review of the literature. Arch Pathol Lab Med 116:965-968, 1992.

Hirshberg A, Shnaiderman-Shapiro A, Kaplan I, Berger R: Metastatic tumours to the oral cavity: pathogenesis and analysis of 673 cases. Oral Oncol 44:743-752, 2008.

LARYNX

LARYNGEAL (VOCAL CORD) NODULE OR POLYP

Clinical Features
- Also called *singers' nodule*
- Typically develops after prolonged misuse or overuse of voice

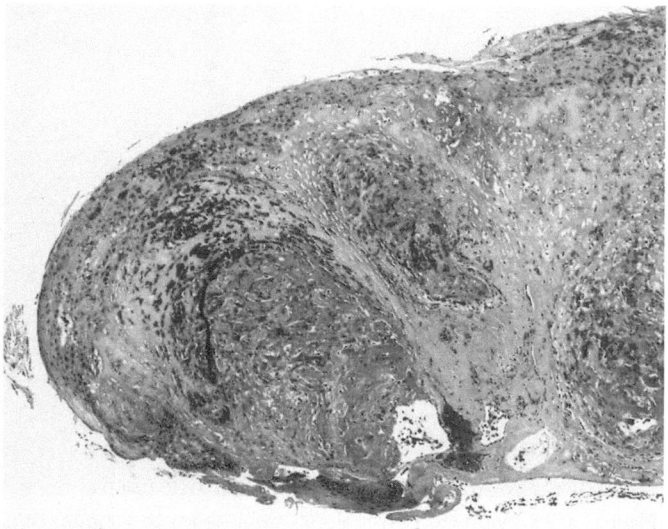

Figure 3-76. Vocal cord nodule. Squamous mucosa is present with underlying hyalinized and vascular stroma.

- Occurs most commonly in adult men as well as singers and smokers
- Most common on anterior third of vocal cord
- Patients present with hoarseness

Gross Pathology

- Round, polypoid, often pedunculated whitish nodule on the vocal cord

Histopathology

- Classified as telangiectatic or gelatinous polyps
  - Telangiectatic form
    - Numerous thin-walled vessels in a loose, collagenous stroma (Figure 3-76)
    - Mixed chronic inflammatory exudate in stroma
  - Gelatinous form
    - Nodule composed of scattered fibroblasts, fibrin, and loose, edematous stroma with less obvious thin-walled vessels
- Both are polypoid nodules covered by an intact overlying stratified squamous epithelium
- Hemosiderin deposition is common in long-standing lesions

Special Stains and Immunohistochemistry

- Noncontributory

Other Techniques for Diagnosis

- Noncontributory

Differential Diagnosis

JUVENILE LARYNGEAL PAPILLOMAS
- Papillary squamous papillomas with or without koilocytosis
- Immunohistochemical or molecular tests for HPV
- Propensity for recurrence

CONTACT ULCER, GRANULOMATOUS ULCER
- Typically affects the posterior commissure of vocal cord

- Exuberant granulation tissue and ulceration of overlying squamous epithelium

PEARLS

- *Florid papillary endothelial hyperplasia can be mistaken for angiosarcoma*
- *Eosinophilic, proteinaceous material may resemble amyloid but negative staining for Congo red*
- *Small lesions may regress with voice rest; larger ones often need to be surgically excised*
- *No association with subsequent development of carcinoma*

SELECTED REFERENCES

Barnes L: Diseases of the larynx, hypopharynx, and esophagus. In Barnes L (ed): Surgical Pathology of the Head and Neck. New York, Marcel Dekker, 2001, pp 128-132.

Kleinsasser O: Pathogenesis of vocal cord polyps. Ann Otol Rhinol Laryngol 91:378-381, 1982.

Wenig BM, Heffner DK: Contact ulcers of the larynx: a re-acquaintance with the pathology of an often under-diagnosed entity. Arch Pathol Lab Med 114:825-828, 1990.

LARYNGEAL PAPILLOMA

Clinical Features

- Papillary exophytic squamous epithelial proliferation of the true vocal cords; may also occur in the larynx, oropharynx, and trachea
- Two types: juvenile and adult type
  - Juvenile type
    - Presents in children or adolescents
    - Typically multiple and occurs on true vocal cords
    - Tends to spread to epiglottic and subglottic area, rarely trachea and bronchi
  - Adult type
    - Male predominance
    - Typically solitary
    - Infrequently recurrent
- Etiology: HPV, particularly types 6 and 11

Gross Pathology

- Polypoid soft lesions, variably sized (Figure 3-77A)

Histopathology

- Squamous cell papillary proliferation with fibrovascular core, acanthosis, and koilocytosis (HPV effect) (Figure 3-77B)
- Mild chronic inflammation and hyperemia of submucosa
- Epithelial atypia may be seen; grade dysplasia if present

Special Stains and Immunohistochemistry

- Noncontributory

Other Techniques for Diagnosis

- In situ and PCR-based techniques for HPV

Differential Diagnosis

SCC
- Invasive growth pattern, desmoplastic stroma
- Cytologic atypia, dyskeratosis

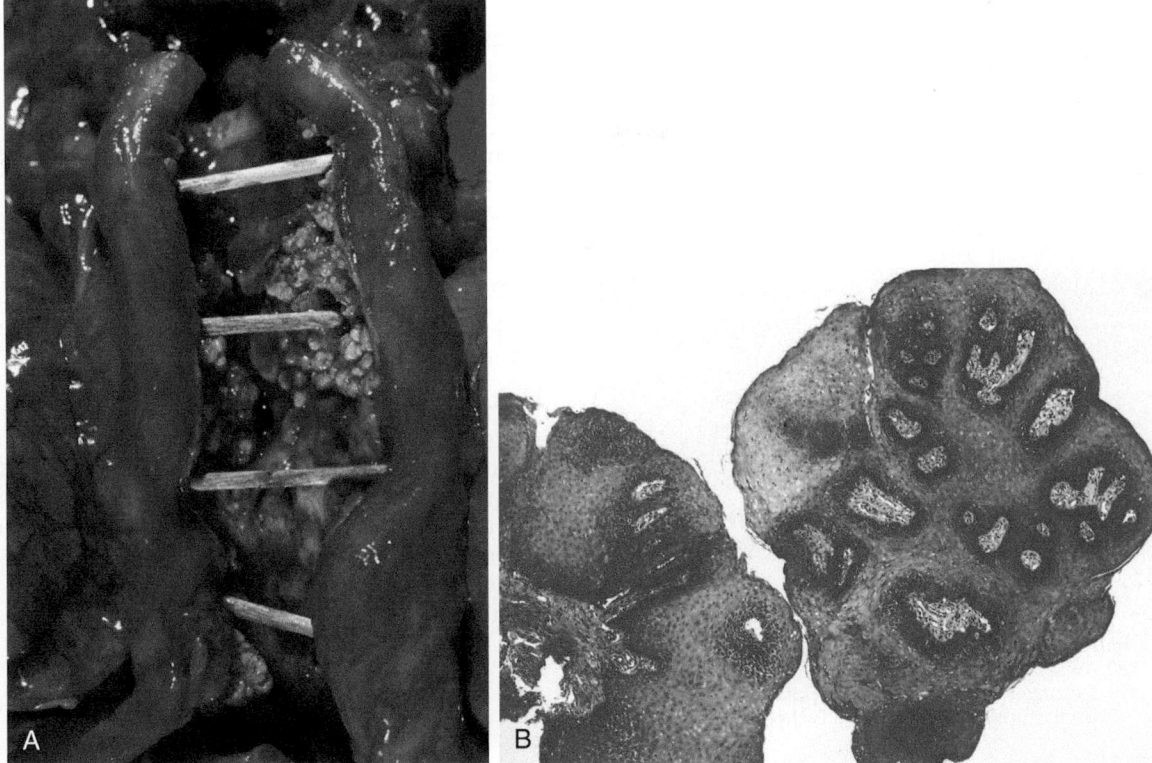

Figure 3-77. Respiratory papillomatosis. A, Specimen photograph of extensive exophytic growths (papillomas) covering the laryngeal and tracheal surfaces. **B,** Histologic section shows squamous epithelium with hyperplasia in broad sheets with fibrovascular cords.

PEARLS

- *Papillomas with dysplasia or solitary lesions should be followed closely or surgically excised to rule out invasive carcinoma*
- *Respiratory papillomas (juvenile and adult) are multiple with propensity for recurrences and a small but definite risk for developing SCC*
- *Risk for SCC is strongly linked to previous radiation*

SELECTED REFERENCES

Lele SM, Pou AM, Ventura K, et al: Molecular events in the progression of recurrent respiratory papillomatosis to carcinoma. Arch Pathol Lab Med 126:1184-1188, 2002.

Lindeberg H, Elbrond O: Laryngeal papillomas: clinical aspects in a series of 231 patients. Clin Otolaryngol 14:333-342, 1989.

Penaloza-Plascencia M, Montoya-Fuentes H, Flores-Martinez SE, et al: Molecular identification of 7 human papillomavirus types in recurrent respiratory papillomatosis. Arch Otolaryngol Head Neck Surg 126:1119-1123, 2000.

Rimell F, Maisel R, Dayton V: In situ hybridization and laryngeal papillomas. Ann Otol Rhinol Laryngol 101:119-126, 1992.

AMYLOIDOSIS OF THE LARYNX

Clinical Features

- Uncommon; less than 1% of benign nodules of the larynx
- Most often false cord; may be bilateral or involve true cords
- Usually localized disease: may be familial, secondary, or part of systemic disease
- Laryngeal amyloid in most cases consists of immunoglobulin light chains and is classified as a fibril type similar to primary amyloid
- Hoarseness is often the presenting clinical symptom

Gross Pathology

- Cut surface: firm, translucent, homogeneous tan to redbrown nodule

Histopathology

- Submucosal amorphous, acellular, eosinophilic material; often perivascular and periglandular (Figure 3-78)
- Chronic inflammatory infiltrate, including plasma cells, histiocytes, and few giant cells

Special Stains and Immunohistochemistry

- Congo red: amyloid displays apple-green birefringence with polarized light

Other Techniques for Diagnosis

- Noncontributory

Differential Diagnosis

VOCAL CORD NODULE
- Amyloid stains are negative

SELECTED REFERENCES

Cohen SR: Ligneous conjunctivitis: an ophthalmic disease with potentially fatal tracheobronchial obstruction: laryngeal and tracheobronchial features. Ann Otol Rhinol Laryngol 90:509-518, 1990.

Ferrara G, Boscaino A: Nodular amyloidosis of the larynx. Pathologica 87:94-96, 1995.

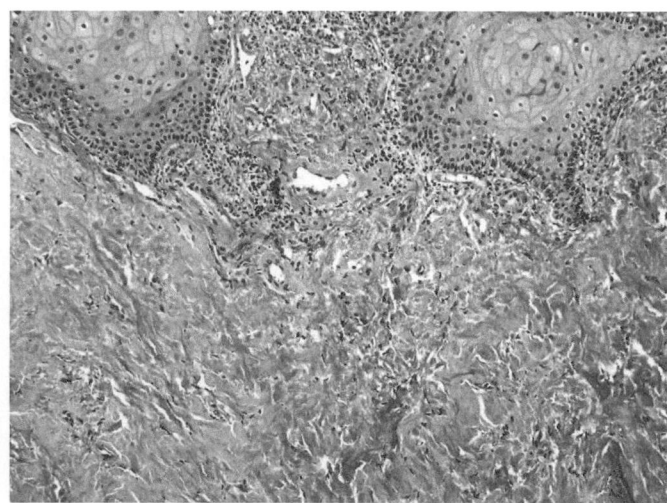

Figure 3-78. Amyloidosis of larynx. Section shows squamous mucosa with submucosal deposits of amorphous eosinophilic material (amyloid).

Richards SH, Bull PD: Lipoid proteinosis of the larynx. J Laryngol Otol 87:187-190, 1973.

Thompson LDR, Derringer GA, Wenig BM: Amyloidosis of the larynx: a clinicopathologic study of 11 cases. Mod Pathol 13:528-535, 2000.

SQUAMOUS CELL CARCINOMA OF THE LARYNX

Clinical Features

- Accounts for 0.4% and 1.3% of carcinomas in women and men, respectively
- Risk factors: smoking and alcohol abuse
- HPV may be associated with a very small number of cases (< 5%)
- Locations: supraglottic, glottic, and subglottic sites (different lymphatic drainage)
- Glottic carcinomas (two-thirds), most arise anteriorly on the mobile portion of the vocal cord; least common is the subglottic location
- Clinically, hoarseness, mass cause pain, dysphagia, and hemoptysis

Gross Pathology

- Exophytic, fungating lesions of variable sizes, often ulcerated and necrotic (Figure 3-79A)

Histopathology

- Premalignant epithelial lesions may border the tumor
- Graded: well, moderately, and poorly differentiated squamous carcinoma based on the degree of cytologic atypia, mitotic activity, and presence of keratin pearl formation (Figure 3-79B)
- Most are moderately differentiated
- Subtypes include
  - Nonkeratinizing SCC
    - Often seen in the supraglottic location
    - More often has pushing rather than infiltrative margins
  - Verrucous SCC
    - Markedly keratinized, well-differentiated tumor that is wartlike on low power
    - Cytologic features are bland, but tumor is locally destructive
    - Parakeratosis is abundant; orthokeratotic squamous cells
    - Broad and sharply demarcated base with bland-appearing squamous epithelium (Figure 3-80)

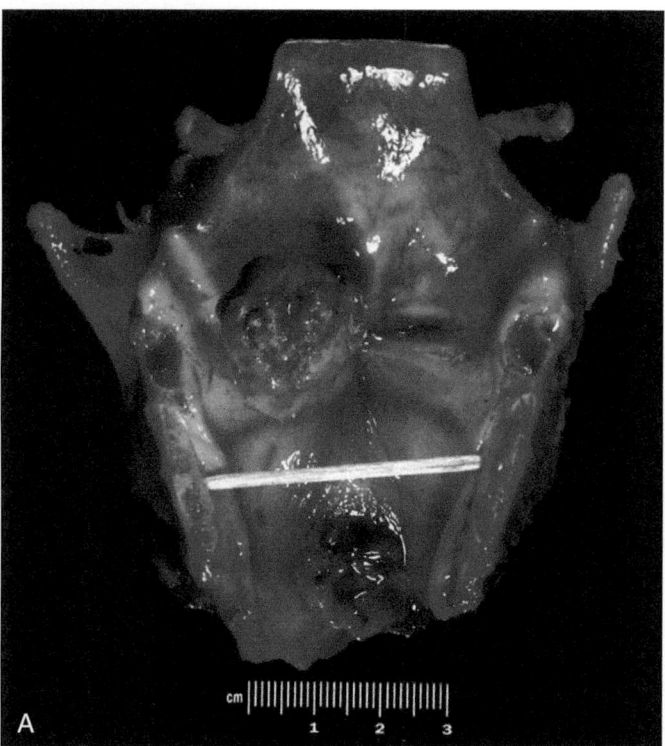

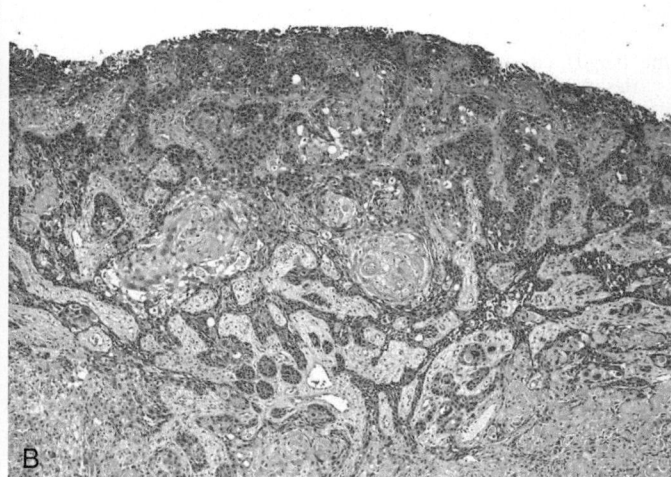

Figure 3-79. Squamous cell carcinoma of larynx. A, Gross photograph of an exophytic and ulcerated glottic tumor. **B,** Histologic section shows an infiltrating neoplasm composed of nests and anastomosing cords of invasive atypical squamous cells with focal keratin pearl formation.

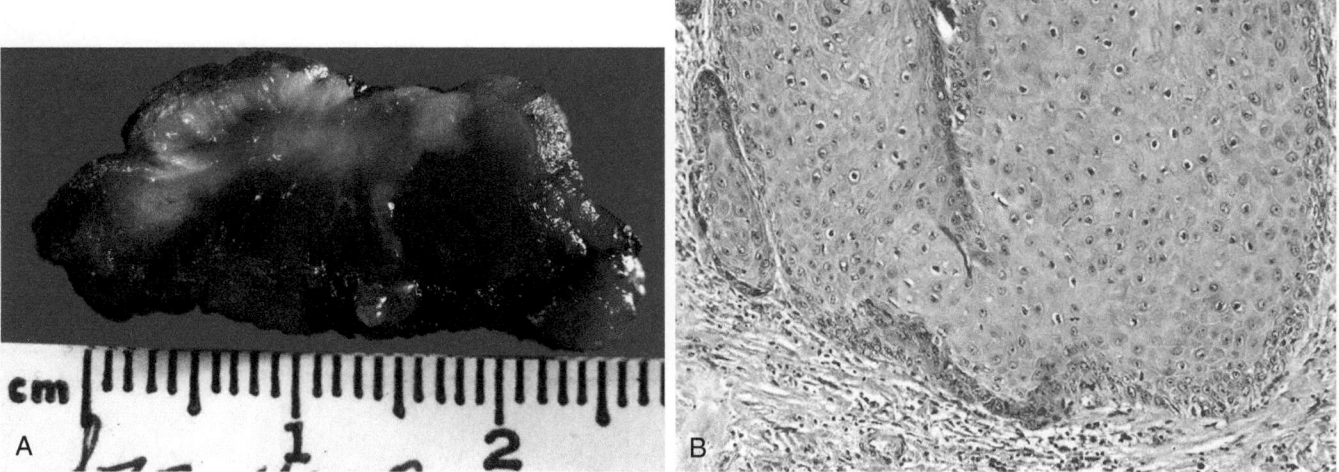

Figure 3-80. Verrucous squamous cell carcinoma. A, Gross photograph of a broad exophytic epithelial proliferation. **B,** Broad pushing base of squamous epithelium with maturation.

- Limited metastatic potential
- Basaloid SCC
  - Basaloid cells in nests and cords (Figure 3-81)
  - Hyaline basement membrane
  - Often with central necrosis
  - Minor and localized abrupt keratinization
- Spindle cell SCC (sarcomatoid carcinoma)
  - Rare variant
  - Prominent spindle cell, sarcoma-like with associated minor component of conventional squamous carcinoma (Figure 3-82A)
  - May show metaplastic features and heterologous elements

Special Stains and Immunohistochemistry

- Cytokeratin, for sarcomatoid variant, positive (may be weak or focal in basaloid variant) (Figure 3-82B)

Other Techniques for Diagnosis

- Noncontributory

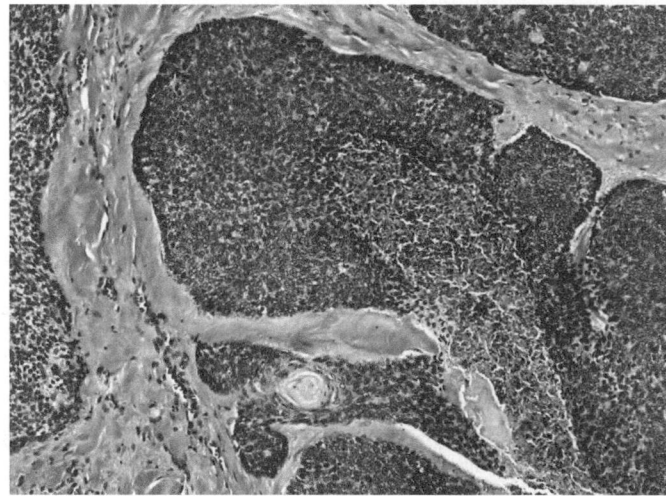

Figure 3-81. Basaloid squamous cell carcinoma. Nests of basaloid epithelial cells often with central necrosis and occasional abrupt keratin formation.

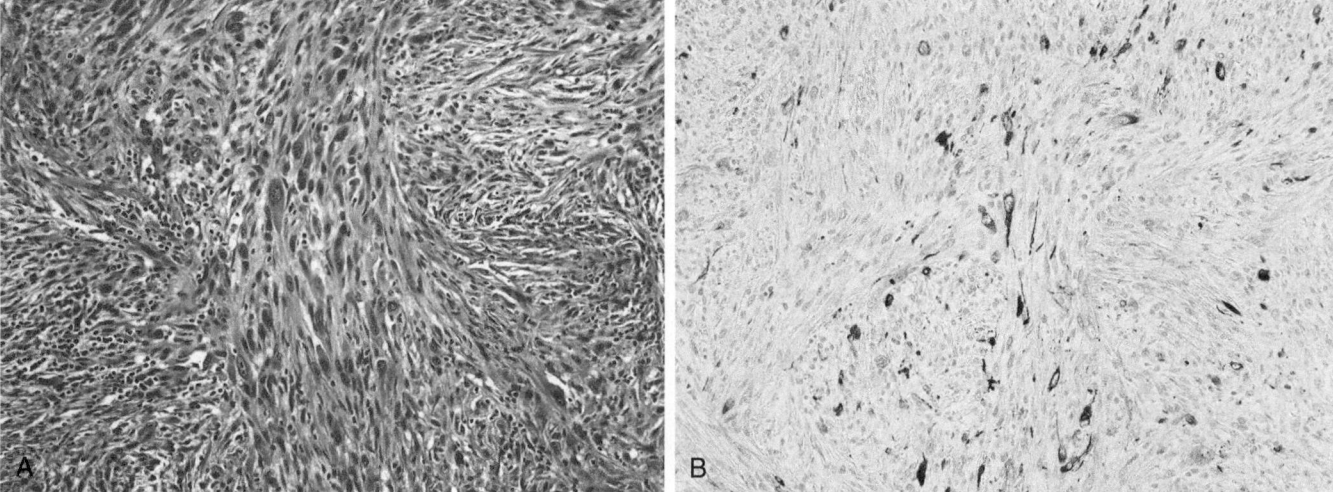

Figure 3-82. Spindle cell squamous cell carcinoma (sarcomatoid carcinoma). A, Histologic section showing a cellular spindled neoplasm with cellular atypia and nuclear hyperchromasia. **B,** Cytokeratin immunohistochemical stain highlights some of the tumor cells supporting epithelial origin.

Differential Diagnoses

VERRUCOUS HYPERPLASIA
- Exophytic, noninvasive
- Rete ridges broad
- Stroma may have chronic inflammatory cells
- Cytologic features of squamous epithelium are bland and well-differentiated

SQUAMOUS PAPILLOMA
- Noninvasive, papillary, proliferation of mature squamous cells with or without acanthosis and koilocytosis (HPV effect) overlying thin fibrovascular cores
- Fibrovascular cores are covered by an orderly, stratified squamous epithelium

PEARLS

- *Prognosis varies with*
  - *Location: best for glottic, then supraglottic, and worst for subglottic tumors*
  - *Size: if larger than 2 cm, 40% chance of metastasis*
  - *Grade: worse prognosis with high-grade tumors*
  - *Tumor margin: the farther away the surgical margin is from the tumor, the higher the survival rate*
- *Increased risk for developing other secondary malignancies (often elsewhere in the head and neck or respiratory tract)*
- *Nonkeratinizing SCC occurs more often in the supraglottic location and spreads along the mucosal surface*
- *Basaloid SCC typically has poor prognosis and is often at an advanced stage when detected*

SELECTED REFERENCES

Jovanovic A, van der Tol IG, Schulten EA, et al: Risk of multiple primary tumors following oral squamous cell carcinoma. Int J Cancer 56:320-323, 1994.

Thompson LD, Wenig BM, Heffner DK, Gnepp DR: Exophytic and papillary squamous cell carcinomas of the larynx: a clinicopathologic series of 104 cases. Otolaryngol Head Neck Surg 120:718-724, 1999.

Thompson LD, Wieneke JA, Miettinen M, Heffner DK: Spindle cell (sarcomatoid) carcinomas of the larynx: a clinicopathologic study of 187 cases. Am J Surg Pathol 26:153-170, 2002.

Wiernik G, Millard PR, Haybittle JL: The predictive value of histological classification into degrees of differentiation of squamous cell carcinoma of the larynx and hypopharynx compared with survival of patients. Histopathology 619:411-417, 1991.

NEUROENDOCRINE CARCINOMA OF THE LARYNX

Clinical Features

- Classified into carcinoid, atypical carcinoid, and neuroendocrine carcinoma
- Rare (make up less than 1% of all laryngeal malignancies)
- Typically found in men in sixth and seventh decades
- Occurs more often in smokers
- Patients typically present with hoarseness

Gross Pathology

- Submucosal, polypoid mass usually 2 to 4 cm
- Often ulcerated if large

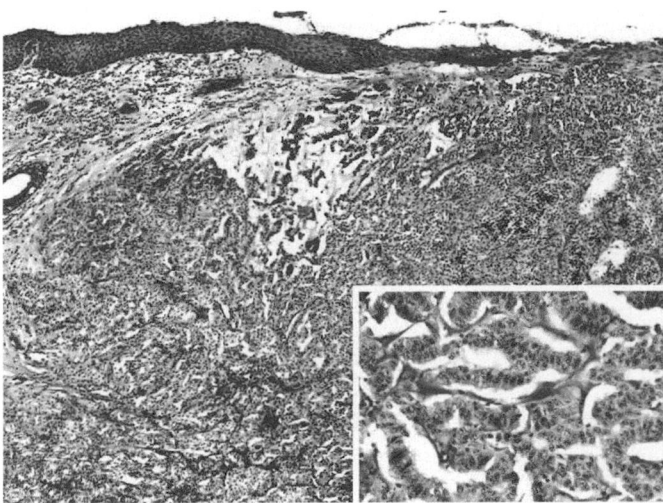

Figure 3-83. Atypical carcinoid (neuroendocrine carcinoma) of the larynx. An infiltrating cellular mass is present with a trabecular pattern. At higher power (*inset*), nuclei with speckled chromatin is appreciated.

Histopathology

- Carcinoid
  - Tumor cells arranged in nests and cords surrounded by delicate fibrovascular stroma
  - Uniform cytologic features with moderate eosinophilic, finely granular cytoplasm and nuclei with finely granular chromatin
  - Low mitotic rate and no necrosis
- Atypical carcinoid
  - More common in the larynx than typical carcinoid (Figure 3-83)
  - Similar architecture to carcinoid but has higher mitotic activity (2 to 10/10 hpf) and small foci of necrosis
- Neuroendocrine carcinoma
  - Diffuse pattern of growth consisting of small to intermediate-sized cells with hyperchromatic nuclei, inconspicuous nucleoli, scant cytoplasm, and ill-defined cytoplasmic borders; prominent nuclear molding
  - High mitotic rate (more than 10/10 hpf) and often extensive necrosis

Special Stains and Immunohistochemistry

- Neuroendocrine markers (synaptophysin, chromogranin) positive
- Cytokeratin positive

Other Techniques for Diagnosis

- Noncontributory

Differential Diagnosis

MALIGNANT MELANOMA
- Other melanoma markers (melan-A, HMB-45) should be used because S-100 protein can be positive in neuroendocrine carcinomas

METASTATIC OR LOCALLY INVASIVE MEDULLARY CARCINOMA
- History of primary medullary carcinoma

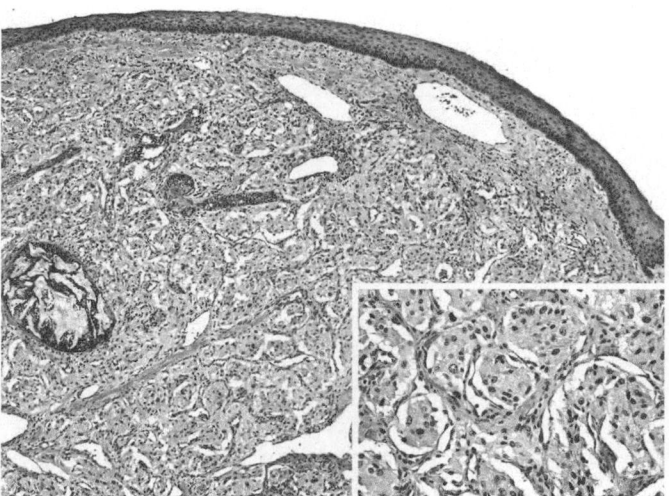

Figure 3-84. Paraganglioma of the larynx. Rare in this location, paragangliomas show classic nested (Zellenballen) growth pattern of neuroendocrine cells (*inset*) surrounded by delicate fibrovascular septae. Focal embolization material is present (*left*).

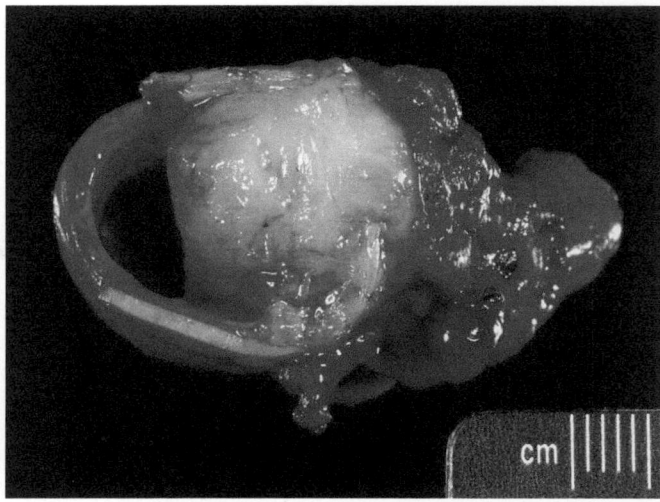

Figure 3-85. Squamous cell carcinoma of trachea. Gross photograph of a squamous cell carcinoma filling the tracheal lumen.

- Serum calcitonin elevation
- TTF-1 usually expressed in medullary (thyroid origin)

PARAGANGLIOMA
- S-100 protein positive sustentacular cells
- Keratin is negative
- Positive for neuroendocrine markers (Figure 3-84)

PEARLS

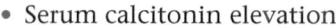

- *Biologic behavior of small cell neuroendocrine tumor is similar to that in the lung*
- *Poor prognostic features include lymph node metastases, vascular invasion, and positive margins*
- *Carcinoids are treated surgically*
- *Neuroendocrine carcinoma multimodality therapy*

SELECTED REFERENCES

Batsakis JG, El-Naggar AK, Luna MA: Neuroendocrine tumors of larynx. Ann Otol Rhinol Laryngol 101:710-714, 1992.

Gillenwater A, Lewin J, Roberts D, El-Naggar AK: Moderately differentiated neuroendocrine carcinoma (atypical carcinoid) of the larynx: a clinically aggressive tumor. Laryngoscope 115:1191-1195, 2005.

Hirsch MS, Faquin WC, Krane JF: Thyroid transcription factor-1, but no p53, is helpful in distinguishing moderately differentiated neuroendocrine carcinoma of the larynx from medullary carcinoma of the thyroid. Mod Pathol 17:631-636, 2004.

Soga J, Osaka M, Yakuwa Y: Laryngeal endocrinomas (carcinoids and relevant neoplasms): analysis of 278 reported cases. J Exp Clin Cancer Res 21:5-13, 2002.

TRACHEA

CLASSIFICATION OF TRACHEAL MALIGNANCIES

- SCC most common in the lower third; poor prognosis

- Salivary-type carcinoma (adenoid cystic carcinoma) arising in the upper third is second in frequency (Figure 3-85)
- Small cell carcinoma, carcinoid tumor, and adenocarcinoma are rare

SQUAMOUS CELL CARCINOMA

Gross Pathology
- Variably sized, exophytic, ulcerated lesions (Figure 3-86)

Histopathology
- Similar to squamous carcinomas at other sites

Special Stains and Immunohistochemistry
- Noncontributory

Other Techniques for Diagnosis
- Noncontributory

Differential Diagnoses

PAPILLOMA AND PAPILLOMATOSIS OF THE TRACHEA
- Microscopic features are similar to lesions seen in the larynx
- In general, those associated with laryngeal papillomatosis begin in childhood and have a lower incidence of malignant transformation than those cases with only bronchial and tracheal involvement

NONSQUAMOUS LESIONS
- Minor salivary tumors
- Metastases

PEARLS

- *Tumors involving the larynx may also arise as primary tumors of the trachea*
- *Predominately SCCs and then salivary gland tumors; other entities are rare*

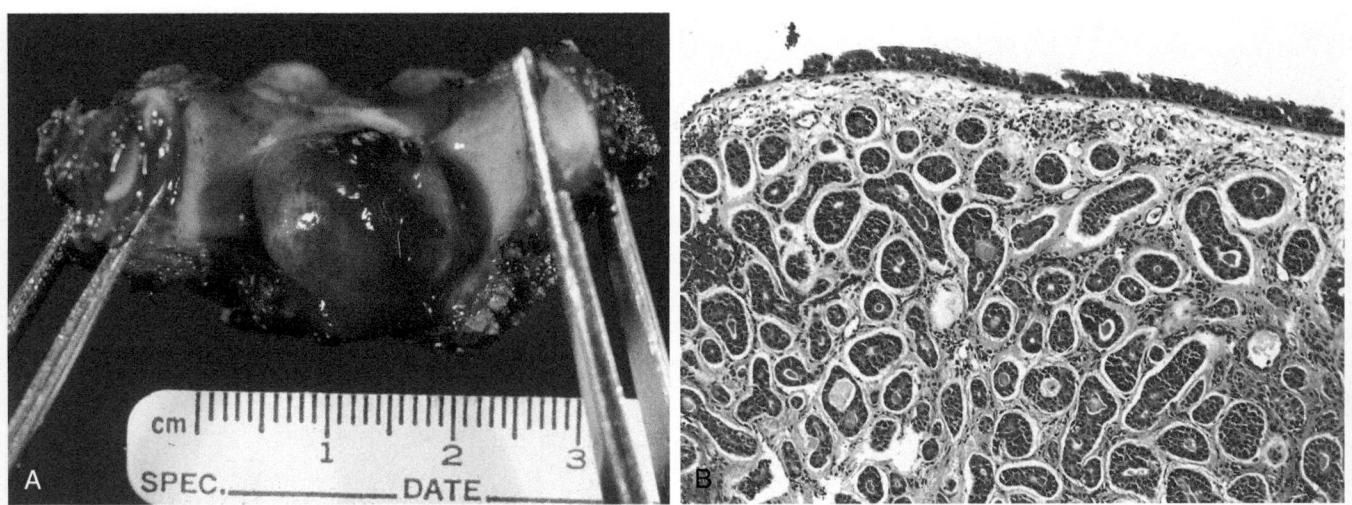

Figure 3-86. Adenoid cystic carcinoma of trachea. **A,** Gross photograph of a polypoid submucosal mass in the trachea. **B,** The tumor cells are growing in tubules beneath the respiratory mucosa.

SELECTED REFERENCES

Allen M: Malignant tracheal tumors. Mayo Clin Proc 68:680-684, 1993.

Fechner RE, Fitz-Hugh GS: Invasive tracheal papillomatosis. Am J Surg Pathol 4:79-86, 1980.

Heffner DK: Diseases of the trachea. In Barnes L (ed): Surgical Pathology of the Head and Neck. New York, Marcel Dekker, 2001, pp 601-625.

Horinouchi H, Ishihara T, Kawamura M, et al: Epithelial myoepithelial tumour of the tracheal gland. J Clin Pathol 46:185-187, 1993.

Chapter 4
Lung and Pleura

ALIYA N. HUSAIN

CHAPTER OUTLINE

NON-NEOPLASTIC CONDITIONS

Pediatric and Congenital Diseases
CONGENITAL PULMONARY AIRWAY MALFORMATION (CPAM)

Clinical Features

- Uncommon developmental anomaly predominantly seen in infants that has features of both immaturity and malformation of the airways and distal lung parenchyma (formerly congenital cystic adenomatoid malformation [CCAM])
- Often detected by antenatal ultrasound during the second trimester
- Reported incidence ranges from 1 in 25,000 to 35,000 pregnancies
- About 60% of lesions show variable, spontaneous regression during gestation
- Postnatal diagnosis of CPAM
    - About 66% present in the neonatal period either as an infant with respiratory distress (cyanosis, grunting, tachypnea) or as a stillborn infant with anasarca
    - The remaining patients present later during childhood with recurrent pneumonia, cough, dyspnea, or cyanosis

Gross Pathology

- Masses of maldeveloped lung tissue composed of cystic or adenomatous overgrowth of terminal bronchioles and air spaces
- CPAM makes direct communication with the tracheobronchial tree through abnormal connecting bronchi

Histopathology

CPAM Type 0

- Small lungs with finely nodular surface in infants who are often less than 50% of expected weight for gestational age; lesions appear solid grossly
- Disorganized proximal airways form the bulk of the lesion; distal components of the normal tracheobronchial tree are rarely present
- Mesenchymal cells and collagen—along with thick-walled arteries, large vascular channels, collections of basophilic debris, and foci of extramedullary hematopoiesis—form the prominent intervening tissue

CPAM Type 1

- Medium and large interconnecting cysts (1 to 10 cm) usually limited to one lobe
- Cyst walls composed of bronchial epithelium, often with clusters of mucous cells and smooth muscle bands with vascular connective tissue

CPAM Type 2

- Back-to-back, dilated bronchiolar-like cysts (0.5 to 2 cm) that blend with normal parenchyma
- Cysts separated by alveolar ductlike structures and small arterioles and venules and sometimes skeletal muscle (Figure 4-1)
- Associated with other severe anomalies in 50% of cases (sirenomelia, renal agenesis or dysgenesis, diaphragmatic hernia, and cardiovascular anomalies)

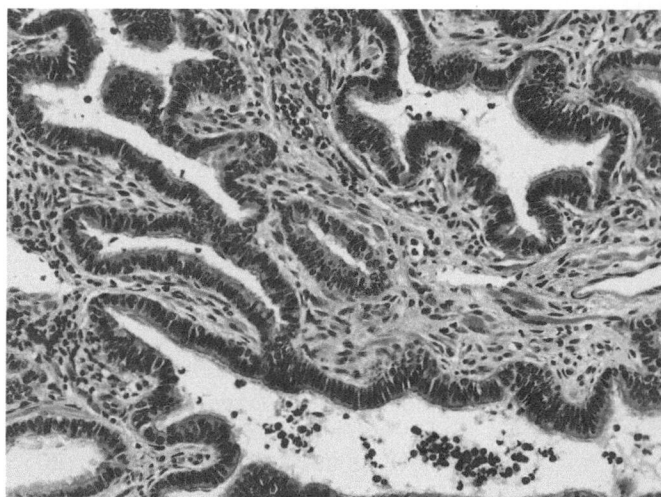

Figure 4-1. Congenital pulmonary airway malformation. Intermediate-power photomicrograph of H&E-stained section shows cysts lined by a single layer of ciliated columnar epithelial cells. The stroma contains cells with skeletal muscle differentiation (congenital pulmonary airway malformation, type 2).

CPAM Type 3

- Original type of CPAM described in 1949 that occurs almost exclusively in males and is associated with maternal polyhydramnios in 80% of cases
- Lesion that forms a solid mass involving the lobe or even entire lung resulting in mediastinal shift and compression with subsequent hypoplasia of adjacent lung
- Composed of randomly arranged glandlike structures, less than 0.2 cm, resembling bronchioalveolar ducts lined with low cuboidal epithelium

CPAM Type 4

- Variable sized cysts are distributed peripherally and can involve more than one lobe
- Walls of larger cysts can be thick (0.1 to 0.3 cm) with muscular arteries
- Lined by single layer of pneumocytes
- Capillary beds are located beneath epithelial lining

Special Stains and Immunohistochemistry

- Thyroid transcription factor-1 (TTF-1) and surfactant protein A and B label the epithelial lining of CPAM type 4 lesions

Other Techniques for Diagnosis

- Noncontributory

Differential Diagnosis

Pulmonary Sequestration

- Pulmonary sequestration has a systemic rather than a pulmonic blood supply and does not communicate with the tracheobronchial tree
- CPAM type 2 is seen within up to 50% of extralobar pulmonary sequestrations

Pleuropulmonary Blastoma (PPB)

- CPAM type 1 does not have a subepithelial or septal mesenchymal spindle cell component (with or without cartilage)
- CPAM type 4 is lined by type 2 alveolar cells instead of the cuboidal or columnar cells seen in PPB

Consider congenital diaphragmatic hernia, bronchogenic cyst, congenital lobar emphysema.

PEARLS

- *Diagnosis of CPAM cannot be made in the presence of chronic inflammation and fibrosis*
- *CPAM is reported to be rarely associated with the development of bronchioloalveolar carcinoma (BAC) and rhabdomyosarcoma (RMS) in adolescent or adult patients*
- *Presence of mucinous epithelium and completeness of resection should be assessed to assist with follow-up*

SELECTED REFERENCES

Mani H, Shilo K, Galvin JR, et al: Spectrum of precursor and invasive neoplastic lesions in type 1 congenital pulmonary airway malformation: case report and review of the literature. Histopathology 51:561-565, 2007.

Stocker JT: Cystic lung disease in infants and children. Fetal Pediatr Pathol 28:155-184, 2009.

Stocker JT, Mani H, Husain AN: The respiratory tract. In Stocker JT, Dehner LP, Husain AN (eds), Stocker and Dehner's Pediatric Pathology, 3rd ed. Philadelphia, Lippincott Williams & Wilkins, 2011, pp 464-469.

BRONCHOPULMONARY SEQUESTRATION

Clinical Features

- Rare congenital malformation involving a segment of lung with no connection to the normal tracheobronchial tree and with anomalous systemic blood supply
- Two types: intralobar sequestration (ILS) and extralobar sequestration (ELS)

Gross Pathology

INTRALOBAR SEQUESTRATION

- About 98% are in lower lobe, lack pleural covering, and are sharply demarcated from adjacent lung parenchyma
- Pedicle or hilus containing vascular structures may be present
- Numerous cysts of variable size within a solid, fibrotic mass

ENTRALOBAR SEQUESTRATION

- Most common on left side; may be subdiaphragmatic, oval or pyramidal, circumscribed, pink to gray-white mass (0.5 to 15 cm)
- Covered with visceral pleura and separate from the normal lung

Histopathology

INTRALOBAR SEQUESTRATION

- Marked chronic inflammation with mucus accumulation and microcyst formation
- Remnants of bronchi and bronchioles within a dense fibrotic stroma with numerous lymphocytes

ENTRALOBAR SEQUESTRATION (Figure 4-2)

- Irregular, enlarged (two to five times) bronchi, bronchioles, and alveoli
- If present, bronchial structures range from normal to irregular lumens lined with pseudostratified columnar epithelium
- No significant inflammatory or fibrotic component is present
- Dilated subpleural lymphatics may be severe
- Areas of CPAM type 2 are present in up to half the cases

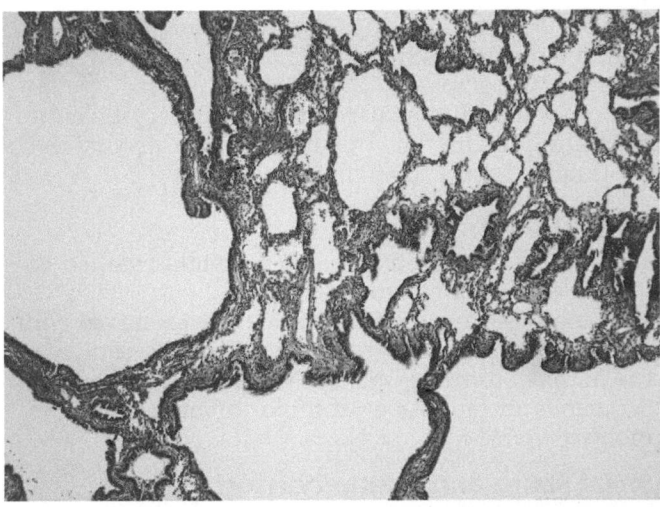

Figure 4-2. Bronchopulmonary sequestration. In this extralobar sequestration, there are too many dilated bronchioles (congenital pulmonary airway malformation) and normal-appearing lung. No cartilage was identified within the lesion.

Special Stains and Immunohistochemistry

- Noncontributory

Other Techniques for Diagnosis

- Noncontributory

Differential Diagnosis

- CPAM: communicates with the tracheobronchial tree and has normal pulmonary arterial supply
- Consider bronchogenic cyst, congenital lobar emphysema, primary lung abscess

PEARLS

- *ELS is frequently associated with CPAM type 2*
- *ELS is associated with other congenital anomalies, which determine the prognosis*
- *Ultrasound-detected lesions can partially or completely resolve before delivery*

SELECTED REFERENCES

Andrade CF, Ferreira HP, Fischer GB: Congenital lung malformations. J Bras Pneumol 37:259-271, 2011.

Desai S, Dusmet M, Ladas G, et al: Secondary vascular changes in pulmonary sequestrations. Histopathology 57:121-127, 2010.

BRONCHOGENIC CYST

Clinical Features

- Cystic lesion arising from anomalous budding of the tracheobronchial anlage of the primitive foregut during development
- Mostly located within the mediastinum, or less frequently at any point along tracheobronchial tree, but does not communicate with it
- Occasionally found peripherally in the lung parenchyma or within the cervical, intrapleural, or suprasternal cutaneous regions or occasionally below the diaphragm or pericardium

Gross Pathology

- Round to oval mass that molds around adjacent structures on radiograph
- Smooth-walled, unilocular or multilocular cystic lesion containing viscous fluid that may form an air-fluid level
- Cysts range from 1 to 10 cm (Figure 4-3A)

Histopathology

- Thin-walled cyst lined by ciliated pseudostratified columnar epithelium (Figure 4-3B)
- Wall composed of smooth muscle fascicles mixed with cartilage islands and seromucinous glands similar to the normal bronchus, without alveoli
- Squamous metaplasia or chronic inflammation commonly present

Special Stains and Immunohistochemistry

- Noncontributory

Modern Techniques for Diagnosis

- Noncontributory

Differential Diagnosis

- CPAM: alveolar tissue can be present
- Mediastinal cysts: esophageal cyst (absence of cartilage, double muscular wall layer), enteric cyst (lined by gastric mucosa), thymic cyst, cystic teratoma, pericardial cyst
- Consider pulmonary sequestration, abscess, cystic bronchiectasis, postinfarction cyst, interstitial emphysema, pleuropulmonary blastoma

PEARLS

- *Inflamed cysts may be difficult to definitively diagnose*
- *Malignant degeneration occurs very rarely in cystic lesions*

Selected References

Chang YC, Chang YL, Chen SY, et al: Intrapulmonary bronchogenic cysts: computed tomography, clinical and histopathologic correlations. J Formos Med Assoc 106:8-15, 2007.
Correia-Pinto J, Gonzaga S, Huang Y, et al: Congenital lung lesions—underlying molecular mechanisms. Semin Pediatr Surg 19:171-179, 2010.

CONGENITAL LOBAR EMPHYSEMA (CLE)

Clinical Features

- Hyperinflation of one or more lobes of the lung, often diagnosed on computed tomography (CT)
- Rare, with estimated prevalence of 1 in 20,000 to 30,000
- Males affected more than females (3:1)
- Most patients present within first 6 months of life with tachypnea, cyanosis, wheezing, and increased labor of breathing
- Recurrent pneumonia and failure to thrive can occur

Gross Pathology

- Hyperinflated lobe leads to compression of adjacent normal lung and mediastinal shift
- Upper lobes are involved in virtually all cases, with the left upper lobe being affected more commonly
- Enlarged lobe maintains appropriate shape

Histopathology

- Overinflation of the lobe with alveolar distention without fibrosis

SPECIAL STAINS AND IMMUNOHISTOCHEMISTRY

- Noncontributory

OTHER TECHNIQUES FOR DIAGNOSIS

- Noncontributory

Differential Diagnosis

- Pneumothorax: radiologically lacks the linear bronchovascular and alveolar markings of CLE; treatments aimed at pneumothorax can worsen patient's actual CLE
- Consider localized interstitial emphysema, CPAM, pulmonary sequestration, bronchogenic cyst, congenital diaphragmatic hernia

PEARLS

- *Most cases are idiopathic*
- *Either intrinsic or extrinsic obstruction of the bronchus supplying the developing lobe is seen in 25% of CLE patients, leading to air trapping within the affected lobe*

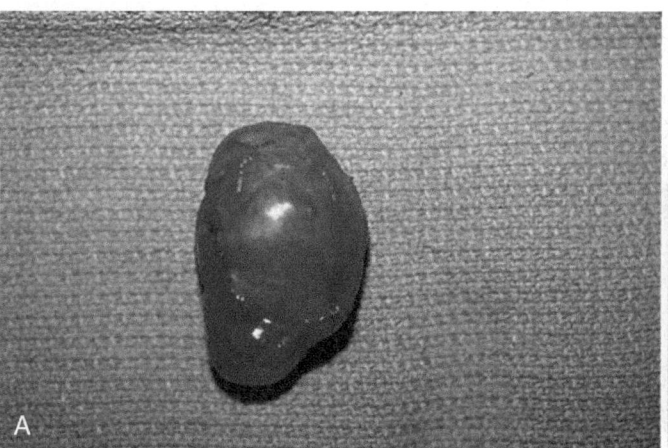
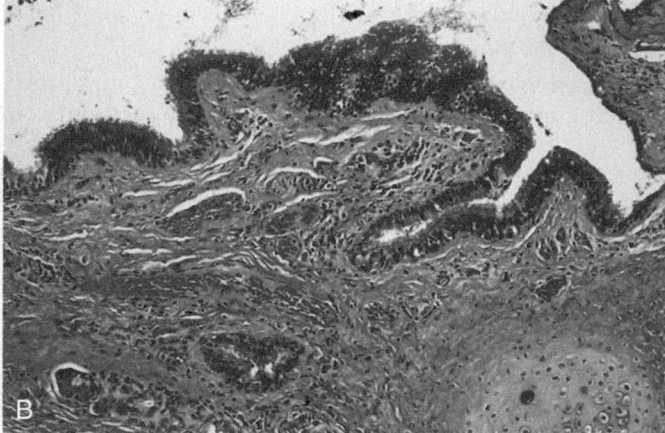

Figure 4-3. Bronchogenic cyst. A, Gross picture of a bronchogenic cyst that is smooth walled and unilocular. **B,** Microscopic picture of a 6-cm mediastinal cystic mass demonstrates respiratory epithelial lining, seromucinous glands, and cartilage.

- *Intrinsic obstruction is often secondary to defects in bronchial wall (e.g., decreased bronchial cartilage), whereas extrinsic obstruction is often caused by vascular malformations or intrathoracic masses (tumor, cyst)*
- *Cardiovascular anomalies are present in 14% of CLE patients*

SELECTED REFERENCES

Guidry C, McGahren ED: Pediatric chest I: Developmental and physiologic conditions for the surgeon. Surg Clin North Am 92:615-643, 2012.
Shanti CM, Klein MD: Cystic lung disease. Semin Pediatr Surg 17:2-8, 2008.

OBSTRUCTIVE LUNG DISEASES

Large Airway Diseases
CHRONIC BRONCHITIS

Clinical Features

- Clinically defined as a productive cough of unknown cause occurring on most days for 3 or more months for at least 2 successive years
- Chronic bronchitis and emphysema share extensive overlap clinically and are often referred to as chronic obstructive pulmonary disease (COPD)
- Most common in cigarette smokers and those exposed to dust or irritating fumes
- Affects 5% of the U.S. population

Gross Pathology

- Increased mucus in the airways due to mucus hypersecretion
- Thickened bronchial wall due to mucous gland enlargement

Histopathology

- Mucus hypersecretion due to increased submucosal glands and goblet cell hyperplasia
- Enlargement and dilation of gland ducts
- Reid index is the ratio of gland thickness to bronchial wall thickness; Reid index greater than 0.5 is consistent with chronic bronchitis
- Chronic inflammation is mild and does not correlate with mucous gland enlargement
- Respiratory bronchiolitis is typically present in cigarette smokers

Special Stains and Immunohistochemistry

- Noncontributory

Other Techniques for Diagnosis

- Noncontributory

Differential Diagnosis

- Asthma: associated with eosinophils and sub-basement membrane fibrosis

PEARLS

- *Diagnosis of chronic bronchitis requires exclusion of other causes of chronic cough, including lung carcinoma, bronchiectasis, cystic fibrosis (CF), congestive heart failure, and tuberculosis*

SELECTED REFERENCE

Travis WD: Non-neoplastic disorders of the lower respiratory tract. In Atlas of Non-tumor Pathology. First Series, Fascicle 2. Washington, DC, American Registry of Pathology: Armed Forces Institute of Pathology; Universities Associated for Research and Education in Pathology, 2002.

ASTHMA
Clinical Features

- Chronic inflammatory disorder of the airways in which mast cells, eosinophils, T lymphocytes, neutrophils, and epithelial cells play a pathophysiologic role
- Clinical diagnosis: episodic symptoms of airflow obstruction that is at least partially reversible, and alternative diagnoses ruled out
- Status asthmaticus is acute respiratory failure due to refractory bronchospasms with inflammation of the airway, mucus plugging, and edema

Gross Pathology

- Plugging of bronchioles and medium and small bronchi with thick, tenacious mucus
- Hyperinflated lungs and secondary saccular bronchiectasis

Histopathology

- Mucus plugging of bronchi and bronchioles mixed with eosinophils, epithelial cells, and Charcot-Leyden crystals
- Curschmann spirals (mucus plugs) and creola bodies (whorls of desquamated epithelial cells) seen in sputum cytology
- Sub-basement membrane fibrosis with patchy desquamated or denuded epithelium (Figure 4-4)
- Goblet cell hyperplasia and occasional squamous metaplasia
- Thickened airway walls due to edema, smooth muscle hyperplasia, and submucosal gland hyperplasia
- Eosinophilic infiltration of medium and small bronchi

Special Stains and Immunohistochemistry

- Noncontributory

Other Techniques for Diagnosis

- Noncontributory

Differential Diagnosis

- Chronic bronchitis: histologically similar but has few or no eosinophils

PEARLS

- *Atopy is the strongest predisposing factor to developing asthma*
- *Eosinophilic inflammation is the hallmark of asthma but paucicellular asthma also occurs*
- *Can be complicated by allergic bronchopulmonary aspergillosis*

SELECTED REFERENCE

Husain AN: The lung. In Kumar V, Abbas AK, Aster JC (eds), Robbins and Cotran Pathologic Basis of Disease, 9th ed. Philadelphia, Saunders, 2014 (in press).

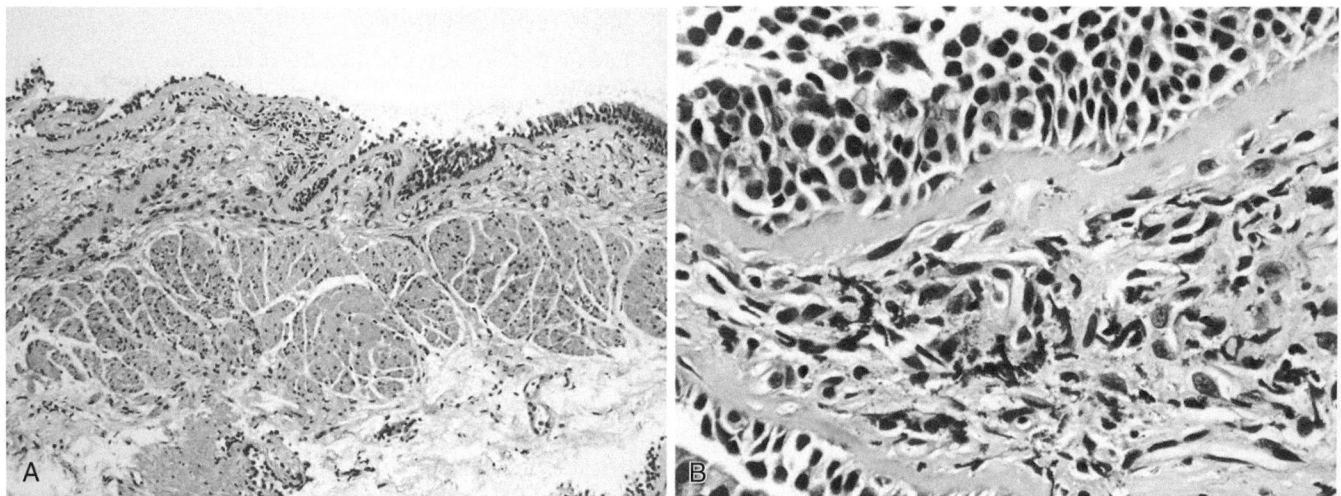

Figure 4-4. Asthma. A, This endobronchial biopsy from a treated asthmatic patient shows sub-basement membrane fibrosis and prominent smooth muscle bundles. **B,** High-power photomicrograph shows submucosal eosinophils and chronic inflammation.

BRONCHIECTASIS

Clinical Features

- Historically, most cases of bronchiectasis were secondary to infection; antibiotic therapy has led to a marked decrease in the incidence of abnormal irreversible bronchial dilation
- Causes of bronchiectasis include cystic fibrosis, primary ciliary dyskinesia, immunodeficiency, rheumatoid arthritis, inflammatory bowel disease and graft-versus-host disease; 30% are idiopathic
- Patients present with persistent cough and large amounts of foul-smelling sputum
- High-resolution CT is the procedure of choice for non-invasive diagnosis
- Disease is radiologically classified into cylindrical, varicose, and saccular or cystic bronchiectasis

Gross Pathology

- Slightly less than 50% of cases are bilateral
- By definition, bronchiectasis is present when the diameter of the bronchus exceeds the diameter of the accompanying bronchial artery, ranging from mild to massive dilation
- Dilated bronchi are filled with yellow-green mucopurulent secretions
- Grossly dilated bronchi can extend out to the pleural surface

Histopathology

- Dilated bronchi filled with mucopurulent exudate or necrotic debris
- Mucosa shows varying degrees of necrosis or sloughing, inflammation, and reparative or metaplastic changes
- Chronic inflammation of bronchial wall with fibrosis is seen
- Follicular bronchiectasis describes cases with lymphoid hyperplasia
- Secondary pneumonia and bronchiolitis obliterans are often associated

Special Stains and Immunohistochemistry

- Noncontributory

Other Techniques for Diagnosis

- Screen for known causes of bronchiectasis, such as CF, immotile cilia syndrome

Differential Diagnosis

POSTINFECTIOUS BRONCHIAL DAMAGE

- Commonly associated organisms: *Pseudomonas aeruginosa, Mycobacterium avium-intracellulare*, gram-negative bacilli, *Haemophilus influenzae, Streptococcus pneumoniae, Staphylococcus aureus*, β-hemolytic streptococcus

CYSTIC FIBROSIS

- CF is the most common cause of bronchiectasis in children and is invariably present among bronchiectasis patients older than 6 months
- Widespread bronchiectasis with mucus plugging of large and small airways, pleural adhesions or fibrosis, abscess, and cystic changes (Figure 4-5)

PRIMARY CILIA DYSKINESIS

- Immotile cilia, Kartagener syndrome, Young syndrome, secondary cilia dyskinesis
- About 1.5% of patients with bronchiectasis have primary cilia dyskinesia
- Ultrastructural abnormalities affect virtually all cilia and are characterized by loss of dynein arms, absence of radial spokes, microtubule transposition, absence of microtubules, compound cilia, or disorientated cilia

CONGENITAL

- α_1-Protease inhibitor deficiency, unilateral hyperlucent lung (Swyer-James syndrome), tracheobronchomegaly, congenital cartilage deficiency, and pulmonary sequestration

MIDDLE LOBE SYNDROME

- Recurrent or permanent atelectasis of right middle lobe or lingula, with chronic inflammation
- Strong association with lymphadenopathy and malignancy

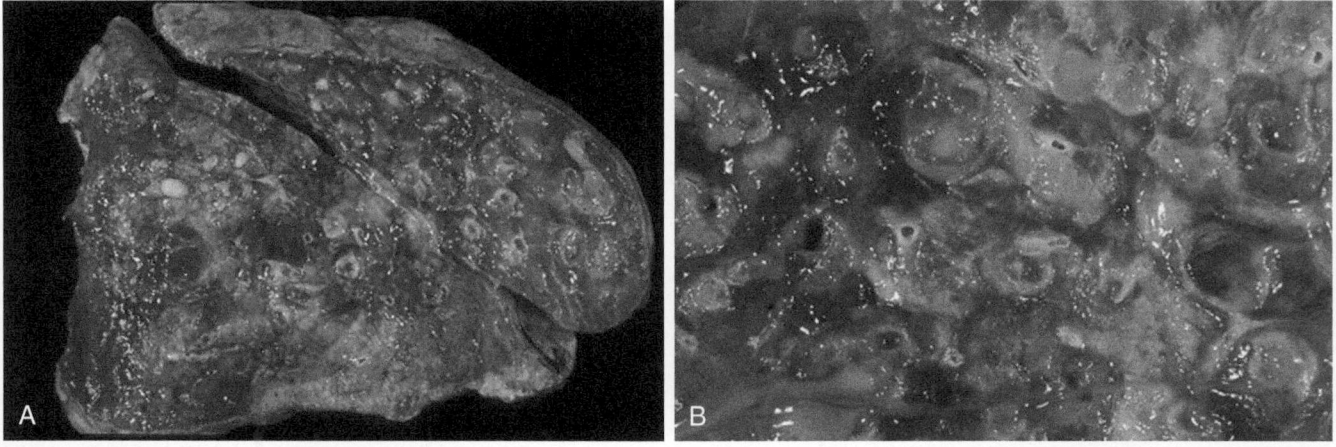

Figure 4-5. Cystic fibrosis. A, Gross picture of the cut surface of the explanted lung shows dilated bronchi throughout. **B,** The dilated bronchi are thick walled and filled with green-yellow mucoid material.

PEARLS

- *Predisposing factors for the development of bronchiectasis include bronchopulmonary infection, bronchopulmonary obstruction, congenital anatomic defect, immunodeficiency states, hereditary abnormalities, and other rare miscellaneous factors*
- *Antibiotic therapy and prophylaxis for pediatric infections has resulted in a steep decline in the number of cases of bronchiectasis, with many cases in developed countries now due to an underlying disorder*
- *Can be complicated by allergic bronchopulmonary aspergillosis*

SELECTED REFERENCE

Barbareschi M, Cavazza A, Leslie KO: Non-neoplastic pathology of the large and small airways. In Leslie KO, Wick MR (eds), Practical Pulmonary Pathology: A Diagnostic Approach, 2nd ed. Philadelphia, Elsevier, 2011, pp 277-310.

Small Airway Diseases and Emphysema
SMALL AIRWAY DISEASES

- See Table 4-1

EMPHYSEMA

Clinical Features

- Emphysema is often present in patients with moderate or severe COPD, often with chronic bronchitis; less commonly, some patients have asthma associated with these disorders
- Onset typically occurs during midlife years with slowly progressive shortness of breath in patients with a long smoking history

Gross Pathology

- Proximal acinar or centrilobular emphysema is most often seen in cigarette smokers
- Panacinar or panlobular emphysema is seen in patients with α_1-antitrypsin deficiency
- Distal acinar or paraseptal emphysema is characteristically found in the subpleural areas of the upper lobes and posterior aspects of the lower lobes, and it may be related to bullous disease or idiopathic spontaneous pneumothorax
- Irregular or scar emphysema is found at the periphery of scars, adjacent to healed granulomas, or in association with interstitial lung disease

Histopathology

- *Emphysema* is a pathologic term used to describe abnormal, permanent enlargement of air spaces distal to the terminal bronchioles due to destruction of the walls without fibrosis
- All forms of emphysema have a similar underlying histologic pattern of large, dilated alveoli, many with club-shaped septa projecting into the air spaces (Figure 4-6)
- No interstitial fibrosis is present, except for some peribronchial fibrosis associated with pigmented macrophages and chronic inflammation seen in smokers
- Secondary hypertensive changes are commonly present

Special Stains and Immunohistochemistry

- Noncontributory

Other Techniques for Diagnosis

- Noncontributory

Differential Diagnosis

INTERSTITIAL EMPHYSEMA

- Air dissects out of the alveolar spaces and into the loose connective tissue of the interlobular septa, the subpleural region, and around bronchovascular bundles forming clear cystic spaces

PEARLS

- *There is too much air for the amount of lung parenchyma, even in atelectatic areas*
- *Inflating emphysematous lungs with formalin before taking histologic sections is recommended*

TABLE 4-1 CLINICAL AND PATHOLOGIC FEATURES OF SMALL AIRWAY DISEASES

	Constrictive Bronchiolitis	Acute Bronchiolitis	Diffuse Bronchiolitis	Respiratory Bronchiolitis	Mineral Dust Bronchiolitis	Follicular Bronchiolitis
General features	Mainly involves terminal conducting airway Associated with obstructive airway disease	Children and infants with wheezing and associated viral infection	Rare form affecting Asian adults, particularly Japanese	Common in cigarette smokers	Restrictive lung disease due to parenchymal fibrosis (pneumoconiosis)	Obstructive lesions due to external compression of the bronchioles
Histopathology	Peribronchiolar and submucosal fibrosis Incomplete or complete luminal obliteration Chronic inflammation Epithelial metaplasia Smooth muscle hyperplasia	Intense acute and chronic inflammation of small bronchioles Associated epithelial necrosis and sloughing Edema Inflammatory exudate in bronchiole lumen	Infiltration of lymphocytes, plasma cells, and foamy macrophages Prominent intraluminal neutrophils Organization of exudate with polypoid plugs	Inflammatory infiltrate within respiratory bronchiole interstitium and adjacent alveoli Smooth muscle hypertrophy Mild fibrosis Prominent pigmented alveolar macrophages	Deposits of inhaled dust primarily around respiratory bronchioles Increased fibrosis Luminal narrowing	1- to 2-mm peribronchial nodules Lymphoid hyperplasia and reactive germinal centers Hyperplasia of bronchus-associated lymphoid tissue (BALT)
Associated conditions	CVD Infection (viral) Inhalation injury CHP Drugs Organ transplantation IBD Neuroendocrine cell hyperplasia Multiple carcinoid tumorlets	Viral infection Bacterial infection	Associated with human leukocyte antigen Bw54 Increased cold agglutinins, ESR, and leukocytosis	Inhalation of asbestos, iron oxide, aluminum oxide, talc, mica, silica, silicate, coal	N/A	CVD (rheumatoid arthritis, Sjögren syndrome) Immunodeficiency (AIDS) Infection (mycoplasma, tuberculosis) Hypersensitivity reaction Cystic fibrosis Bronchiectasis Chronic aspiration

CHP, chronic hypersensitivity pneumonia; CVD, collagen vascular disease; ESR, erythrocyte sedimentation rate; IBD, inflammatory bowel disease.

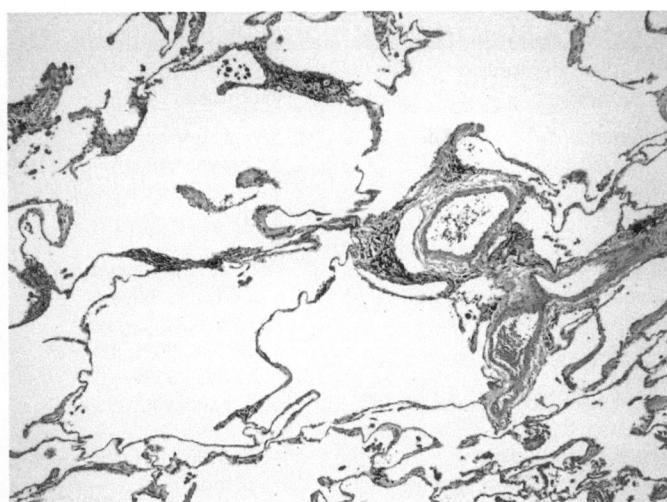

Figure 4-6. Emphysema. The alveolar spaces are markedly enlarged with only minimal interstitial fibrosis. Note anthracosis and the club-shaped alveolar walls projecting into the spaces.

SELECTED REFERENCE

Barbareschi M, Cavazza A, Leslie KO: Non-neoplastic pathology of the large and small airways. In Leslie KO, Wick MR (eds), Practical Pulmonary Pathology: A Diagnostic Approach, 2nd ed. Philadelphia, Elsevier, 2011, pp 282-307.

RESTRICTIVE AND INTERSTITIAL LUNG DISEASES

Interstitial Pneumonias

DIFFUSE ALVEOLAR DAMAGE (DAD), ACUTE RESPIRATORY DISTRESS SYNDROME (ARDS), AND ACUTE INTERSTITIAL PNEUMONIA (AIP)

Clinical Features

- Acute lung injury (ALI): form of lung injury which varies from noncardiogenic pulmonary edema to ARDS, caused by sepsis, shock, hypoxia, direct damage by inhalants, other organs not involved
- ARDS: severe fulminant form of acute lung injury often with multiorgan involvement
- AIP: lung injury with no known etiology
- DAD: pathologic correlate of ARDS and AIP (Table 4-2)

Gross Pathology

- Rigid, heavy, hemorrhagic lungs in exudative phase
- Firm, consolidated, pale-gray lungs in proliferative phase
- Spongy, cystic, pale-gray lungs in fibrotic phase

Histopathology

- DAD is bilateral and patchy (*diffuse* refers to the whole alveolus, not the whole lung) with an early or exudative phase followed by a proliferative or organizing phase (but combinations can be seen) and a late fibrotic phase (in a minority of patients)

EXUDATIVE PHASE (FIRST WEEK AFTER INJURY)

- Type 1 pneumocyte necrosis, inflammatory exudate, hyaline membranes, partial alveolar collapse with interstitial edema (Figure 4-7)
- Endothelial injury with congestion, neutrophil aggregates, and minimal microthrombi

PROLIFERATIVE PHASE (SECOND WEEK AFTER INJURY)

- Florid fibroblastic and myofibroblastic proliferation within interstitium and alveolar air spaces with type 2 pneumocyte proliferation
- Remnants of hyaline membranes occasionally seen within air spaces or incorporated into the interstitium
- Occasional squamous metaplasia with atypia
- Intimal proliferation, medial hypertrophy, and thrombi in small pulmonary arteries

FIBROTIC PHASE (LATE)

- Thick interstitial fibrosis and microcyst formation

Special Stains and Immunohistochemistry

- Noncontributory

Other Techniques for Diagnosis

- Noncontributory

Differential Diagnosis

INFECTION

- Granulomas, viral inclusions (e.g., cytomegalovirus [CMV]), foci of necrosis, neutrophil aggregates or microabscess formation

USUAL INTERSTITIAL PNEUMONIA (UIP) OR ACCELERATED UIP

- Fibrotic areas shows temporal heterogeneity in UIP, whereas histopathologic changes in DAD are relatively uniform from field to field
- Fibrosis encountered in DAD contains more fibroblasts and myofibroblasts, more edematous stroma, and less collagen deposition

DAD IN PATIENTS WITH COLLAGEN VASCULAR DISEASE

- Dermatomyositis, polymyositis, scleroderma, and rheumatoid arthritis may present with DAD pattern
- Acute lupus pneumonitis, Takayasu arteritis, polyarteritis nodosa, Behçet syndrome, and microscopic polyarteritis can present with an AIP-like clinical picture

PEARLS

- *Hyaline membranes are a histologic hallmark of DAD and are seen in ARDS/AIP but are not present in UIP, nonspecific interstitial pneumonia (NSIP), or cryptogenic organizing pneumonia (COP)*
- *Diagnosis of AIP is considered in patients presenting with severe community-acquired pneumonia who fail to respond to appropriate antibiotic therapy and in whom no other causative etiology is identified*
- *The clinical course of AIP is rapidly progressive, with more than 78% (range, 60% to 100%) of patients dying within 6 months due to respiratory failure and right heart failure*
- *Most patients who recover from ALI/ARDS have near-normal lung function*

TABLE 4-2	CLINICAL, RADIOLOGIC, AND PROGNOSTIC FEATURES OF IDIOPATHIC INTERSTITIAL PNEUMONIAS			
Clinical Diagnosis	Histologic Pattern	Duration of Illness	Distribution and Typical Computed Tomography Findings	Prognosis
IPF	UIP	Chronic (>12 months)	Subpleural predominance Honeycombing Reticular opacities Traction bronchiectasis Ground-glass opacities	5-year survival, 20% (2-3 year mean)

NSIP	NSIP	Subacute to chronic (months to years)	Subpleural, basal, symmetrical
			  peribronchovascular ground-glass opacities
			Reticular opacities
			Lower lobe volume loss
			Rare honeycombing
				Cellular NSIP: 10-year
				  survival, > 90%
				Fibrotic NSIP: 5-year
				  survival, 90%; 10-year
				  survival, 35%

COP	OP	Subacute (<3 months)	Subpleural, peribronchial patchy consolidation, nodularity	5-year survival, >95%
ARDS, ALI, AIP	DAD	Acute (1-2 weeks)	Lower zone, peripheral consolidation Ground-glass opacities with lobular sparing	40%-60% mortality rate in <6 months
DIP	DIP	Subacute (weeks to months)	Subpleural predominance Ground-glass opacities Thin-walled cysts Reticular opacities Rare honeycombing	5-year survival, > 95%
RB-ILD	RB	Subacute (weeks to months)	Diffuse bronchial wall thickening Centrilobular nodules Patchy ground-glass opacity	No deaths reported

AIP, acute interstitial pneumonia; ALI, acute lung injury; ARDS, acute respiratory distress syndrome; COP, cryptogenic organizing pneumonia; DAD, diffuse alveolar damage; DIP, desquamative interstitial pneumonia; IPF, idiopathic pulmonary fibrosis; NSIP, nonspecific interstitial pneumonia; OP, organizing pneumonia; RB, respiratory bronchiolitis; RB-ILD, respiratory bronchiolitis–associated interstitial lung disease; UIP, usual interstitial pneumonia.

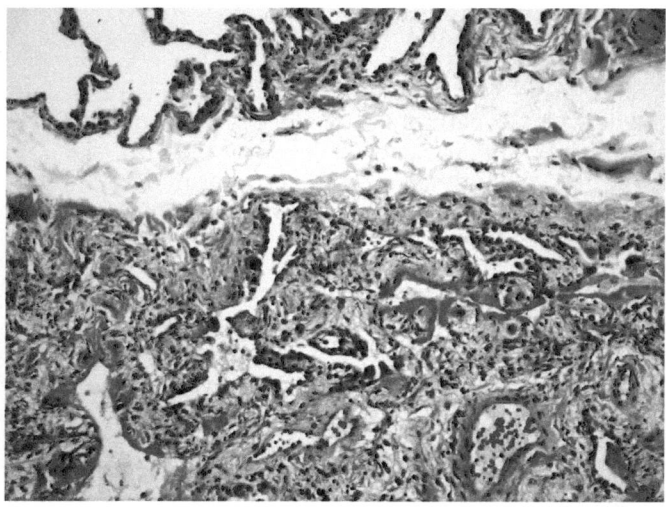

Figure 4-7. Acute interstitial pneumonia. This photomicrograph of the exudative phase shows patchy widening of interstitium due to hyaline membranes, edema, and a sparse inflammatory infiltrate in the lobule seen in the lower part of the picture, whereas the upper lobule is spared.

Selected References

Beasley MB: The pathologist's approach to acute lung injury. Arch Pathol Lab Med 134:719-727, 2010.

Obadina ET, Torrealba JM, Kanne JP: Acute pulmonary injury: high-resolution CT and histopathological spectrum. Br J Radiol 86:20120614, 2013. Epub 2013 May 9.

Mukhopadhyay S, Parambil JG: Acute interstitial pneumonia (AIP): relationship to Hamman-Rich syndrome, diffuse alveolar damage (DAD), and acute respiratory distress syndrome (ARDS). Semin Respir Crit Care Med 33:476-485, 2012.

CRYPTOGENIC ORGANIZING PNEUMONIA (COP)

Clinical Features

- Mean age of onset is 55 years
- No known etiology; cigarette exposure is not a predisposing factor
- Patients present with subacute illness (median, 3 months) consisting of cough and dyspnea, often associated with weight loss, sweats, chills, fever, and myalgia
- Most patients recover after steroid therapy; however, there is a significant relapse rate 1 to 3 months after cessation of therapy

Gross Pathology

- See Table 4-2

Histopathology

- Intraluminal plugs (Masson bodies) composed of fibroblasts and myofibroblasts embedded in loose connective tissue that invariably occlude alveoli, alveolar ducts, and less frequently the bronchioles (bronchiolar component may be minor or absent) (Figure 4-8)
- Patchy, bronchiolocentric distribution of Masson bodies, with extension into adjacent alveoli through the intra-alveolar pores of Kohn, giving a butterfly pattern
- Within the intraluminal plugs are small clusters of lymphocytes, plasma cells, histiocytes, and endothelial proliferation, resembling granulation tissue
- Mild chronic interstitial inflammation with foci of foamy macrophages

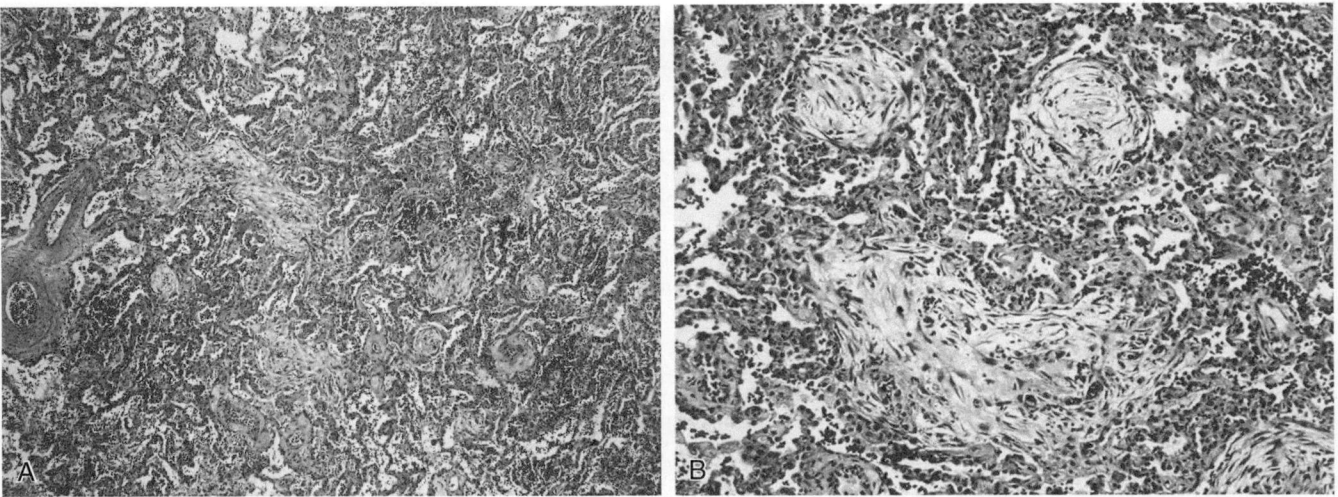

Figure 4-8. Cryptogenic organizing pneumonia. A, Lower-power photomicrograph shows nodules of myxoid loose fibrous tissue filling alveolar spaces and streaming from one space to another. **B,** Nodules of young fibrous tissue (Masson bodies) are seen distending some alveolar spaces. The adjacent lung parenchyma is compressed and the alveolar walls are relatively normal.

- Pertinent negatives: honeycombing, dense interstitial fibrosis, granulomas, neutrophils or abscess formation, necrosis, hyaline membranes or air space fibrin, predominant eosinophilic infiltrates, and vasculitis

Special Stains and Immunohistochemistry

- Loose connective tissue stains green with the Movat stain compared with the yellow staining pattern characteristic of dense fibrosis

Other Techniques for Diagnosis

- Noncontributory

Differential Diagnosis

USUAL INTERSTITIAL PNEUMONIA

- Chronic clinical course
- Extensive, temporally heterogeneous pattern of fibrosis with dense scarring, honeycombing, and architectural destruction
- Fibroblastic foci of UIP adjacent to areas of dense fibrosis, in contrast to the polypoid intraluminal location of connective tissue seen in COP

NONSPECIFIC INTERSTITIAL PNEUMONIA

- Mild to moderate chronic interstitial inflammation or fibrosis without Masson bodies

DESQUAMATIVE INTERSTITIAL PNEUMONIA

- Intra-alveolar finely pigmented smoker's macrophages without Masson bodies

ARDS/DIFFUSE ALVEOLAR DAMAGE

- Patients are acutely ill
- Depending on time of biopsy, there is interstitial edema, hyaline membranes, type 2 pneumocyte hyperplasia, and organized fibrosis within alveolar walls and, occasionally, alveolar spaces

PEARLS

- *COP is a distinct clinicopathologic diagnosis of exclusion employed when all other underlying causes of organizing pneumonia are excluded*

SELECTED REFERENCE

Roberton BJ, Hansell DM: Organizing pneumonia: a kaleidoscope of concepts and morphologies. Eur Radiol 21:2244-2254, 2011.

USUAL INTERSTITIAL PNEUMONIA (UIP)

Clinical Features

- UIP is a histologic pattern of lung disease that occurs in a variety of clinical settings; when no underlying disease is identified, the clinical diagnosis of idiopathic pulmonary fibrosis (IPF) is made
- Patients present with progressive, chronic exertional dyspnea associated with nonproductive cough
- Incidence of 7.4 to 10.7 cases per 100,000 and prevalence of 13 to 20 per 100,000 make UIP the most common type of idiopathic interstitial pneumonia (47% to 62%)
- Average age of onset is 67 years, with median survival of 3 years
- More common in males and smokers
- Associated clinical conditions include IPF, collagen vascular disease, drug toxicity, chronic hypersensitivity pneumonia, asbestosis, familial IPF, Hermansky-Pudlak syndrome

Gross Pathology

- See Table 4-2

Histopathology

- Patchy fibrosis with subpleural and paraseptal distribution (Figure 4-9)
- Areas of fibrosis adjacent to normal-appearing lung parenchyma creating a variegated appearance on low power (variation in intensity)
- Dense, pink fibrosis, which represents chronic scarring adjacent to pale, light blue, myxoid fibroblastic foci, which represent acute or active wound repair (temporal heterogeneity)
- Fibroblastic foci composed of parallel palisades of fibroblasts and connective tissue beneath hyperplastic type 2 pneumocytes or bronchiolar epithelium

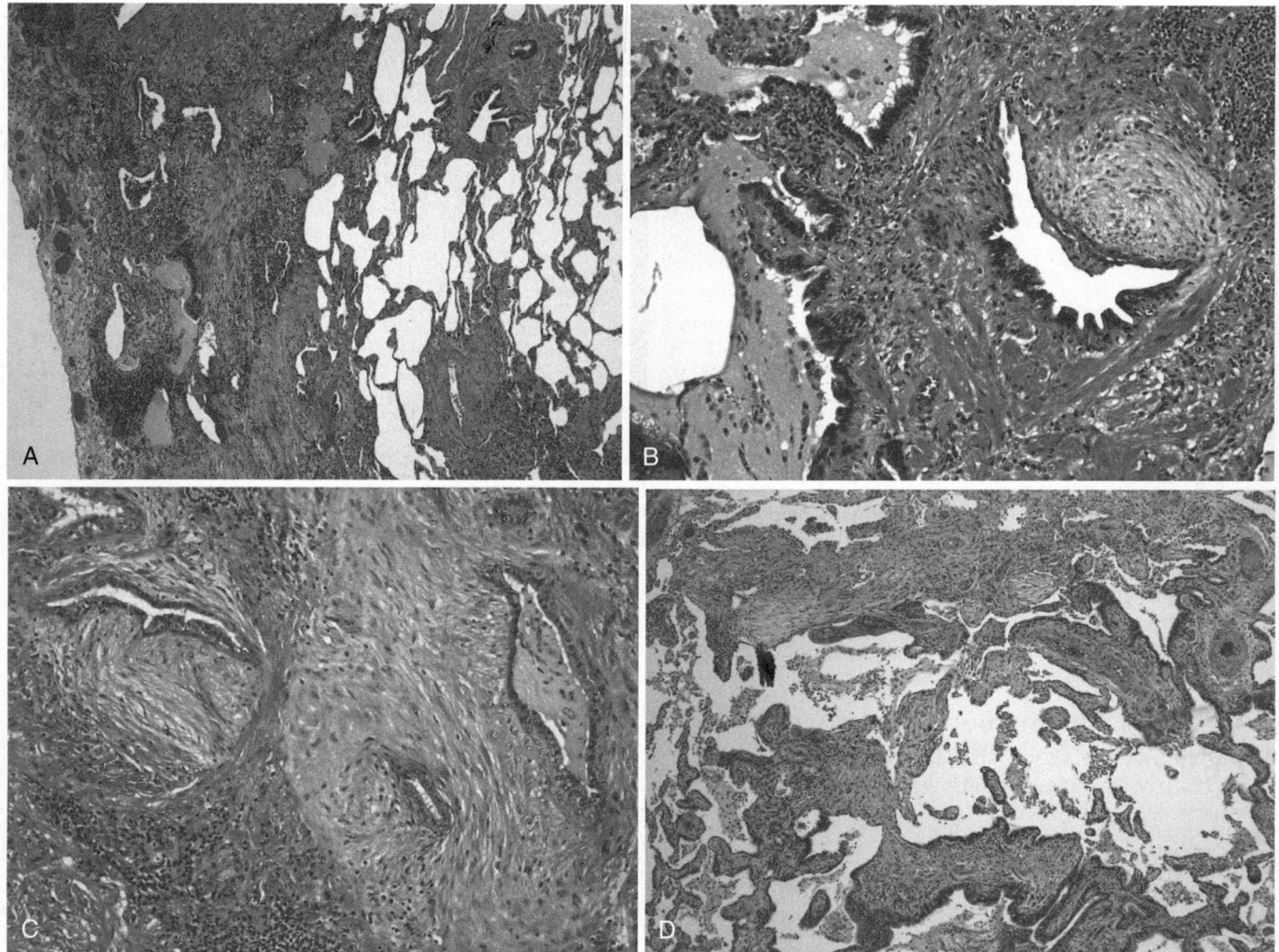

Figure 4-9. Usual interstitial pneumonia (UIP). A, Patchy fibrosis is seen in the subpleural region, which is extending into deeper lung parenchyma, whereas some alveolar walls are not involved (variation in intensity). **B,** Fibroblastic focus is present in the submucosa of a small bronchiole *(center right)* in an area of honeycombing (fibrosis causing destruction of alveolar architecture with remaining air spaces lined by bronchiolar epithelium). **C,** Very large fibroblastic foci are seen here. Fibroblastic focus is a subepithelial area of young fibrosis with abundant myxoid intercellular matrix and fibroblasts running parallel to the airspace. Older *(pink)* collagen is seen adjacent to the fibroblastic foci (variation in time). **D,** Bronchiolar metaplasia and foci of acute and chronic inflammation, as seen here, are common in UIP.

- Little to no interstitial inflammation away from areas of fibrosis
- Honeycomb change is often present and is an important diagnostic feature
- Cystically dilated bronchioles lined by ciliated columnar respiratory epithelium within areas of fibrosis that replace normal alveoli
- Secondary traction bronchiectasis and peribronchiolar fibrosis with associated epithelial hyperplasia (peribronchiolar metaplasia) can also occur
- Lower lobes are most severely affected

Special Stains and Immunohistochemistry

- Noncontributory

Other Techniques for Diagnosis

- High-resolution CT scans often diagnostic in the appropriate clinical setting

Differential Diagnosis

CHRONIC HYPERSENSITIVITY PNEUMONIA WITH FIBROSIS

- Predominantly bronchocentric and mostly involves upper lobes
- Poorly formed granulomas or scattered giant cells
- More cellular, less subpleural fibrosis, and less honeycomb change

LANGERHANS CELL HISTIOCYTOSIS

- Stellate configuration and bronchiolocentric distribution of nodules
- Emphysematous changes prominent in longstanding cases
- Fibroblastic foci are rare

ORGANIZING PNEUMONIA

- Lack of fibrosis or interstitial pneumonia away from intraluminal fibrosis
- Little or no architectural distortion

- *Diagnosis of UIP is confounded by inadequate sampling, microscopic findings resembling other conditions (e.g., DIP-like areas), and the fact that UIP-like fibrosis occurs in other conditions*
- *American Thoracic Society/European Respiratory Society (ATS/ERS) guidelines define IPF as a distinct type of chronic fibrosing interstitial pneumonia of unknown cause limited to the lungs and associated with a surgical specimen showing a histologic UIP pattern*
- *If in addition to UIP, other histologic patterns of other interstitial lung disease are present (e.g., NSIP), the final diagnosis is based on the worst area seen and hence remains UIP*
- *Clinician should identify cases of UIP associated with an underlying collagen vascular disease because of the markedly better clinical course*
- *Cigarette smoking confers a 1.6- to 2.3-fold increased risk for developing UIP*
- *Fibroblastic foci are not specific to UIP but are always present in UIP and are a key feature for diagnosis*
- *Combined findings of UIP and DAD, capillaritis, infection, or organizing pneumonia with extensive fibroblastic proliferation are associated with an accelerated or acute phase of IPF and often represent the terminal phase of the illness*

Selected References

Cipriani NA, Strek M, Noth I, et al: Pathologic quantification of connective tissue disease-associated versus idiopathic usual interstitial pneumonia. Arch Pathol Lab Med 136:1253-1258, 2012.
Popper HH: Interstitial lung diseases-can pathologists arrive at an etiology-based diagnosis? A critical update. Virchows Arch 462:1-26, 2013.
Takemura T, Akashi T, Kamiya H, et al: Pathological differentiation of chronic hypersensitivity pneumonitis from idiopathic pulmonary fibrosis/usual interstitial pneumonia. Histopathology 61:1026-1035, 2012.

NONSPECIFIC INTERSTITIAL PNEUMONIA (NSIP)

Clinical Features

- Characterized by varying degrees of fibrosis and inflammation (cellular and fibrotic subtypes) and does not meet the criteria for other forms of idiopathic interstitial pneumonia
- Second most common subtype of idiopathic interstitial pneumonia that accounts for 14% to 36% of all idiopathic interstitial pneumonia
- Commonly recognized pattern in patients with collagen vascular diseases, hypersensitivity pneumonia, drug toxicity, and immunodeficiency
- Patients present with a subacute illness with dyspnea, cough, or fever and typically have a history of cigarette smoking
- Cellular NSIP: average age of diagnosis is 39 years; 5- and 10-year survival rates approach 100%
- Fibrotic NSIP: average age of diagnosis is 51 years; 5- and 10-year survival rates are 90% and 35%, respectively

Gross Pathology

- See Table 4-2

Histopathology

- Pertinent negatives: dense fibrosis, honeycombing, fibroblastic foci, granulomas, eosinophils, neutrophils, organisms, necrosis

CELLULAR NSIP

- Diffuse interstitial lymphoplasmacytic infiltrate with no significant fibrosis and preservation of lung architecture
- Type 2 pneumocyte hyperplasia
- Minor features: focal organizing pneumonia, lymphoid aggregates, alveolar macrophages

FIBROTIC NSIP

- Loose to dense interstitial fibrosis causing uniform thickening of alveolar walls with preservation of lung architecture (Figure 4-10)
- Fibrosis lacks temporal heterogeneity of UIP (fibroblastic foci are inconspicuous or insignificant in number) and no honeycombing
- Mild to moderate chronic inflammation
- Minor features: organizing pneumonia, lymphoid aggregates, alveolar macrophages, bronchial metaplasia, metaplastic calcifications or bone formation

Special Stains and Immunohistochemistry

- Noncontributory

Other Techniques for Diagnosis

- Noncontributory

Differential Diagnosis

UIP VERSUS NSIP

- Underlying lung architecture is preserved in NSIP
- Fibrosis is heterogenous in UIP and homogeneous in NSIP (fibrotic type)

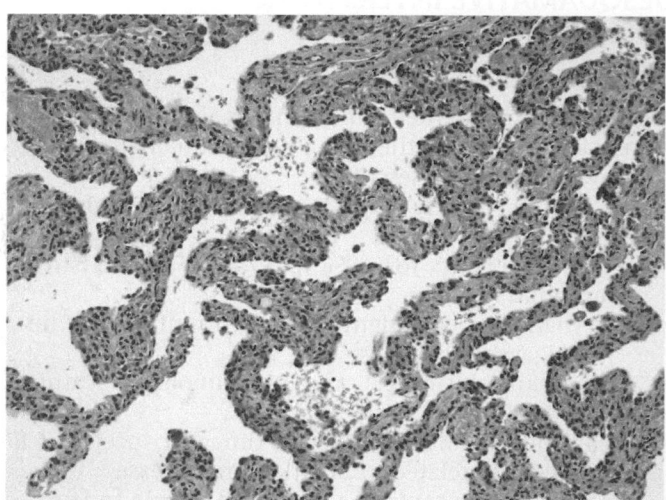

Figure 4-10. Nonspecific interstitial pneumonia. The alveolar walls are uniformly thickened by mild fibrosis and mature small lymphocytes.

- Fibroblastic foci and honeycomb fibrosis are rare or inconspicuous in NSIP
- Inflammation is relatively more abundant in NSIP (cellular type)

HYPERSENSITIVITY PNEUMONITIS
- Scattered, poorly formed granulomas and intraluminal fibrosis, which is bronchiolocentric in hypersensitivity pneumonitis
- More diffuse pattern in NSIP

LYMPHOID INTERSTITIAL PNEUMONIA
- Extensive, chronic alveolar septal inflammation with architectural distortion in lymphoid interstitial pneumonia versus mild, patchy inflammation in NSIP (cellular type)

ORGANIZING PNEUMONIA
- Intraluminal plugs of fibrotic tissue within distal airways and alveoli

PEARLS

- *NSIP is a diagnosis of exclusion; it lacks the features of UIP, DIP, COP, and DAD*
- *NSIP is the most common histologic pattern of lung damage observed in patients with collagen vascular disease*
- *Extensive lymphoid follicles or plasmacytic differentiation within interstitial infiltrates is suggestive of associated collagen vascular disease*

SELECTED REFERENCES

Glaspole I, Goh NS: Differentiating between IPF and NSIP. Chron Respir Dis 7:187-195, 2010.
Husain AN: Nonspecific interstitial pneumonia. In Thoracic Pathology. Philadelphia, Elsevier, 2012, pp 69-70.
Poletti V, Romagnoli M, Piciucchi S, Chilosi M: Current status of idiopathic nonspecific interstitial pneumonia. Semin Respir Crit Care Med 33:440-449, 2012.

DESQUAMATIVE INTERSTITIAL PNEUMONIA (DIP)

Clinical Features

- Clusters of pigmented macrophages within the distal air spaces that were thought to be desquamated pneumocytes when first described
- Uncommon disease, which along with respiratory bronchiolitis–associated interstitial lung disease (RB-ILD), accounts for 10% to 17% of all interstitial pneumonias
- More than 90% of patients report current or past history of cigarette smoking
- Shares many histologic and epidemiologic features with RB-ILD
- DIP and RB-ILD likely represent different spectra of a single smoking-related interstitial lung disease
- Average age of onset is 46 years, with a male-to-female ratio of 2:1
- Subacute illness lasting weeks to months with dyspnea, cough, or chest pain

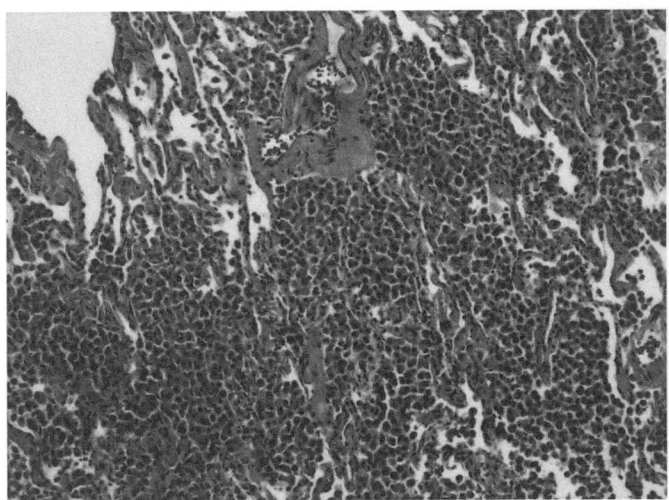

Figure 4-11. Desquamative interstitial pneumonitis. The alveolar spaces are filled with finely pigmented macrophages in a patient who also has emphysema (enlarged alveoli).

Gross Pathology
- See Table 4-2

Histopathology
- Even, uniform filling of distal air spaces by cohesive clusters of pigmented alveolar macrophages with finely granular brown pigment within abundant cytoplasm (Figure 4-11)
- Subtle to mild uniform interstitial fibrosis with hyperplasia of type 2 pneumocytes
- Scattered lymphoid aggregates, often with germinal centers
- Blue bodies (intra-alveolar laminated basophilic concretions) sometimes present
- Medial and intimal thickening of vascular structures
- Mild bronchiolar fibrosis with minimal inflammation
- Pleural inflammation and fibrosis sometimes present along with dilated pleural lymphatics
- Negative findings: architectural remodeling, dense fibrosis, honeycombing, fibroblastic foci

Special Stains and Immunohistochemistry
- Prussian blue stain for iron demonstrates finely granular pigment within macrophages that contrasts with coarse brown hemosiderin granules associated with pulmonary hemorrhage

Other Techniques for Diagnosis
- Noncontributory

Differential Diagnosis
RB-ILD
- Bronchiolocentric accumulation of macrophages with sparing of distal air spaces in RB-ILD, whereas DIP has more extensive and diffuse changes
- RB-ILD associated with more benign clinical course

UIP
- DIP lacks the architectural distortion and honeycombing seen in UIP
- Fibrous component of DIP (if present) is mild and without fibroblastic foci

NSIP

- Cellular NSIP: increased interstitial inflammation, few alveolar macrophages
- Fibrosing NSIP: interstitial fibrosis, few alveolar macrophages

FOCAL, NONSPECIFIC DIP-LIKE REACTIONS

- Likely represent RB-ILD and often seen around scar, tumor, or infarction

PEARLS

- *DIP-like condition described in infants with mutations in the SP-C gene coding for surfactant protein C*
- *DIP and RB-ILD lesions can persist for long periods of time after smoking cessation*
- *Reported association of DIP with sirolimus therapy*

SELECTED REFERENCES

Flores-Franco RA, Luevano-Flores E, Gaston-Ramirez C: Sirolimus-associated desquamative interstitial pneumonia. Respiration 74:237-238, 2007.

Godbert B, Wissler MP, Vignaud JM: Desquamative interstitial pneumonia: an analytic review with an emphasis on aetiology. Eur Respir Rev 22:117-123, 2013.

Kawabata Y, Takemura T, Hebisawa A, et al: Desquamative Interstitial Pneumonia Study Group: desquamative interstitial pneumonia may progress to lung fibrosis as characterized radiologically. Respirology 17:1214-1221, 2012.

LYMPHOID INTERSTITIAL PNEUMONIA (LIP)

Clinical Features

- True idiopathic LIP is extremely rare
- Historically, most cases previously diagnosed as LIP were actually low-grade B-cell lymphomas, typically marginal zone B-cell lymphoma of the mucosa-associated lymphoid tissue (MALT) type (discussed later)
- In children, LIP is a common manifestation of HIV infection and establishes the diagnosis of AIDS
- In adults, LIP can be associated with HIV, AIDS, or other immunocompromised states
- Clinical presentation in children includes recurrent bacterial and viral infections, failure to thrive, parotiditis, and occasionally respiratory failure
- Chest radiograph
  - In children, bilateral miliary reticulonodular infiltrates
  - In adults, patchy areas of alveolar consolidation as well as miliary-type infiltrates

Gross Pathology

- Scattered nodular solid areas

Histopathology

- Extensive diffuse interstitial chronic inflammation, comprised of mainly mature lymphocytes, plasma cells, and histiocytes (Figure 4-12)
- Minimal to mild interstitial fibrosis and germinal centers may be present

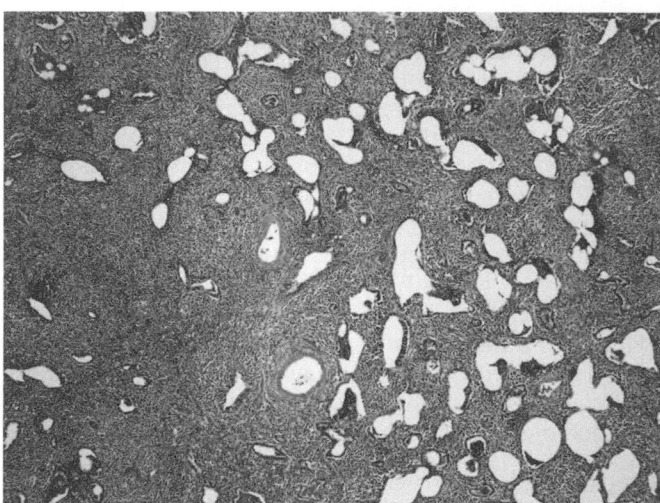

Figure 4-12. Lymphoid interstitial pneumonia. There is a marked mononuclear cell infiltrate in the alveolar septa and around blood vessels and airways partially obliterating lung architecture in this 5-year-old with AIDS.

Special Stains and Immunohistochemistry

- Not monoclonal, stains for fungi and bacteria are negative

Other Techniques for Diagnosis

- Epstein-Barr virus (EBV) can be detected in most cases by in situ hybridization

Differential Diagnosis

- Viral pneumonitis: may need to be determined by serologic testing

PEARLS

- *Pathogenesis of LIP is unknown and presumably caused by the direct effects of HIV on the lung tissue*
- *EBV plays a cofactor in triggering the lymphoproliferative response; however, EBV is not isolated from all patients with the disease*
- *LIP does not progress to interstitial fibrosis of the lung in children or adults*

SELECTED REFERENCES

Fukuoka J, Leslie KO: Chronic diffuse lung diseases. In Leslie KO, Wick MR (eds), Practical Pulmonary Pathology: A Diagnostic Approach, 2nd ed. Philadelphia, Elsevier, 2011, pp 229-231.

Tian X, Yi ES, Ryu JH: Lymphocytic interstitial pneumonia and other benign lymphoid disorders. Semin Respir Crit Care Med 33:450-461, 2012.

HYPERSENSITIVITY PNEUMONITIS (HP)

Clinical Features

- Bilateral, interstitial granulomatous lung disease representing an immune-mediated reaction to inhaled organic antigens or chemicals, with upper lobe predominance
- More than 200 different organic antigens are associated with HP, with thermophilic actinomycetes and avian proteins responsible for most cases

- Prevalence ranges from 5% to 15% of the population exposed to known inciting antigens
- Acute HP: onset within 4 to 8 hours of exposure to high levels of antigen and resolves within 24 to 48 hours
- Subacute HP: continuous or intermittent exposure to low levels of antigen; symptoms can resolve following steroid treatment and removal of offending antigen
- Chronic HP: similar to subacute HP, but fibrosis is present, and long-term prognosis is worse

Gross Pathology

- Patchy to diffuse ground-glass opacities on CT
- Poorly defined centrilobular nodules corresponding to cellular bronchiolitis, organizing pneumonia, or peribronchiolar interstitial pneumonitis

Histopathology

- Acute phase: biopsy rarely done
- Subacute phase
  - Small, poorly formed, noncaseating granulomas with occasional multinucleated giant cells and a patchy mononuclear cell infiltration consisting of lymphocytes and plasma cells adjacent to respiratory or terminal bronchioles (Figure 4-13)
  - Large histiocytes with foamy cytoplasm present in the alveoli and the interstitium
- Chronic phase: HP has three distinct histologic patterns
  - UIP-like pattern: subpleural, patchy, pauci-cellular fibrosis and architectural distortion; fibroblastic foci; focal areas of subacute HP pattern
  - Fibrotic NSIP-like pattern: homogeneous, linear fibrosis with preservation of lung architecture
  - Irregular peribronchiolar pattern: peribronchiolar fibrosis; additional UIP-like pattern of subpleural fibrosis

Special Stains and Immunohistochemistry

- Negative fungal and acid-fast bacilli (AFB) stains

Other Techniques for Diagnosis

- Noncontributory

Differential Diagnosis

NSIP

- Granulomas and giant cells are not features of NSIP
- NSIP may be the sole histologic lesion of HP, and careful exposure history potentially is the best method to distinguish NSIP from HP in these cases

UIP

- Giant cells and granulomas are not features of UIP
- Peribronchiolar fibrosis and upper lobe predominance favor HP
- UIP is most severe in lower lobes with subpleural distribution

LIP

- More prominent interstitial lymphoid infiltrate with extensive alveolar septal involvement
- Granulomas and intraluminal fibrosis are less common in LIP (5% in LIP versus 67% in HP)

SARCOIDOSIS

- Granulomas are well-formed, tightly packed, and sharply delineated with a hyalinized rim and are distributed along bronchovascular bundles and pleura
- Intraluminal fibrosis and UIP-like or NSIP-like component absent in sarcoidosis

PEARLS

- *Best diagnosed by wedge biopsy*
- *The chronic form of HP is the type that will eventually be biopsied*
- *Chronic hypersensitivity pneumonitis has a fibrotic component that resembles UIP*
- *Presence of fibrosis on lung biopsy is an important poor prognostic factor*
- *If a known history of exposure exists, but the biopsy shows only NSIP-like or UIP-like fibrosis, the possibility of chronic HP should be considered*
- *About 95% of HP cases occur in nonsmokers*

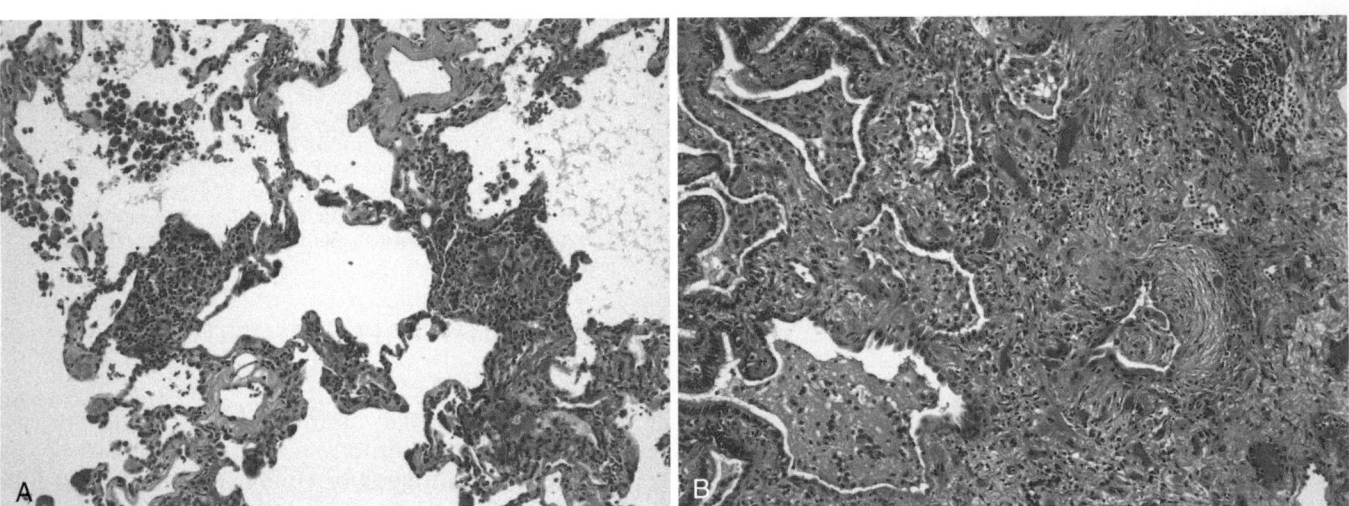

Figure 4-13. Hypersensitivity pneumonitis. A, Poorly formed granulomas with multinucleated giant cells are seen in centrilobular location (adjacent to small arteries) in this patient with subacute HP. There are macrophages and lymphocytes but, typically, no eosinophils. **B,** Chronic HP shows the typical UIP pattern with fibrosis, fibroblastic foci, and honeycombing.

SELECTED REFERENCES

Myers JL: Hypersensitivity pneumonia: the role of lung biopsy in diagnosis and management. Mod Pathol 25(suppl 1):S58-S67, 2012.

Ohshimo S, Bonella F, Guzman J, et al: Hypersensitivity pneumonitis. Immunol Allergy Clin North Am 32:537-556, 2012.

Selman M, Pardo A, King TE Jr: Hypersensitivity pneumonitis: insights in diagnosis and pathobiology. Am J Respir Crit Care Med 186:314-324, 2012.

EOSINOPHILIC LUNG DISEASES

Clinical Features

- Eosinophilic lung diseases are classified into three major categories
  - Eosinophilic lung disease of unknown etiology
    - Simple pulmonary eosinophilia/Löffler syndrome (SEP)
    - Acute eosinophilic pneumonia (AEP), onset < 1 month
    - Chronic eosinophilic pneumonia (CEP), onset > 1 month
  - Eosinophilic lung disease of determined cause
    - Allergic bronchopulmonary aspergillosis (ABPA)
    - Bronchocentric granulomatosis (BG)
    - Parasitic infections
    - Drug reaction
  - Eosinophilic vasculitis
    - Allergic angiitis
    - Churg-Strauss syndrome

ACUTE EOSINOPHILIC PNEUMONIA

- Acute onset of respiratory distress in an otherwise healthy person, mimicking infectious pneumonia
- Diagnostic criteria include high eosinophil percentage on bronchoalveolar lavage (BAL) (> 25%), but peripheral blood eosinophil percentages usually normal at time of presentation (rises in a few days)
- Associated with cigarette smoke (in two thirds) and dust exposure
- Bilateral patchy areas of ground-glass opacities with interstitial thickening on CT
- Histologic appearance similar to acute phase of diffuse alveolar damage but with alveolar and interstitial eosinophilic infiltrates (Figure 4-14)
- Hypertrophic, detached type 2 pneumocytes without disruption of the basal lamina
- Prompt and complete clinical response to corticosteroid therapy

CHRONIC EOSINOPHILIC PNEUMONIA

- Peripheral eosinophilia ranging from mild to severe
- Elevated IgE in 7% of patients
- Peripheral consolidation, most commonly involving the middle and lower zones (reversed pulmonary edema pattern on CT)
- Eosinophils, lymphocytes, and deeply eosinophilic macrophages (forming pseudogranulomas) in the intra-alveolar air spaces and interstitium; eosinophilic microabscesses
- Damage to the basal lamina with subsequent interstitial and intra-alveolar fibrosis in 50% of patients

Special Stains and Immunohistochemistry

- Noncontributory

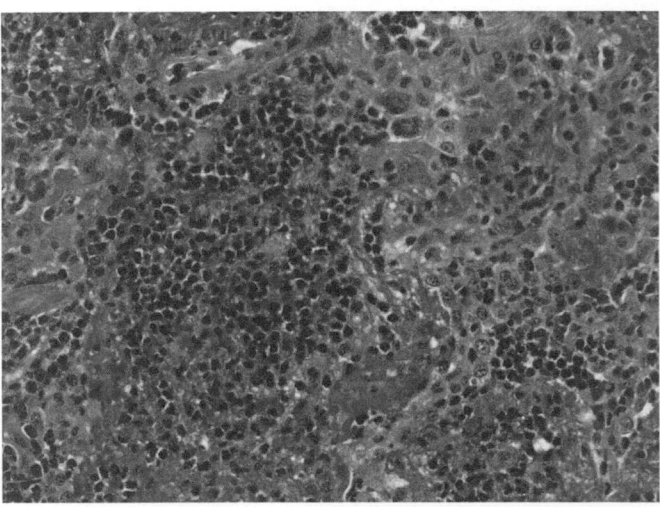

Figure 4-14. Eosinophilic pneumonia. Marked eosinophilic infiltration is seen both in the interstitium and in the alveolar spaces with eosinophilic abscess, fibrinous exudate, and reactive type 2 pneumocytes. The presence of occasional giant cells raises the differential of Langerhans cell histiocytosis.

Other Techniques for Diagnosis

- Noncontributory

Differential Diagnosis

- Asthma, drug reaction, Churg-Strauss syndrome
- Some fungal infections (e.g., aspergillosis, coccidioidomycosis)
- Parasite infestation
  - Allergic reaction: *Entamoeba, Toxocara* species; *Clonorchis sinensis*
  - Direct invasion: *Ascaris lumbricoides* infection (strong association with SEP), schistosomiasis, Paragonimus westermani, Ancylostoma duodenale infection
  - Others: dirofilariasis, *Strongyloides stercoralis, Wuchereria bancrofti,* and *Brugia malayi* infection

PEARLS

- *The diagnosis of eosinophilic lung disease can be made if any of the following are present: pulmonary opacities with peripheral eosinophilia, biopsy-proven tissue eosinophilia, or increased eosinophils in BAL*
- *CEP can be histologically differentiated from AEP based on the greater extent of interstitial and alveolar fibrosis and fewer eosinophils in chronic disease*
- *White blood cell differential count is a crucial aspect of the evaluation because most eosinophilic lung diseases manifest with peripheral eosinophilia*
- *Charcot-Leyden crystals are bipyramidal crystals that may be present in sputum or tissue and are a hallmark of eosinophil-related disease*

SELECTED REFERENCES

Akuthota P, Weller PF: Eosinophilic pneumonias. Clin Microbiol Rev 25:649-660, 2012.

Cottin V, Cordier JF: Eosinophilic lung diseases. Immunol Allergy Clin North Am 32:557-586, 2012.

Leslie KO, Gruden JF, Parish JM, Scholand MB: Transbronchial biopsy interpretation in the patient with diffuse parenchymal lung disease. Arch Pathol Lab Med 131:407-423, 2007.

SARCOIDOSIS

Clinical Features

- Chronic, multisystem granulomatous disorder of unknown etiology
- Occurs most commonly in young adults (20 to 40 years old) with slight female predominance
- In United States, higher incidence in African Americans; also common in Scandinavians and Irish
- The lung is involved in 90% to 95% of patients
- Patients present with either an abrupt, acute illness showing a better prognosis or with a chronic, insidious illness and a persistent, progressive disease course
- Angiotensin-converting enzyme (ACE) serum levels can be elevated during active phases

Gross Pathology

- Irregular, well-circumscribed nodules (2 to 5 mm) have a perilymphatic distribution and are most numerous along the bronchi and pulmonary vessels

- Late-stage sarcoidosis shows interstitial fibrosis and cavitary lesions
- About 5% of cases have a single or multiple large nodules (nodular sarcoidosis)

Histopathology

- Interstitial noncaseating granulomas distributed along lymphatic routes: pleura, interlobular septa, and bronchovascular bundles (Figure 4-15)
- Granulomas composed of epithelioid histiocytes with or without multinucleated giant cells
- Granulomas are tightly clustered, well-formed, and often surrounded by concentric fibrosis, which over time becomes hyalinized with a lamellar appearance
- Necrosis is usually absent; however, a minority of cases demonstrates small, punctate foci of necrosis
- Granulomas directly involve vessels (67% of cases) and pleura (10% of cases)
- Variety of inclusions, some of which may be confused for microorganisms

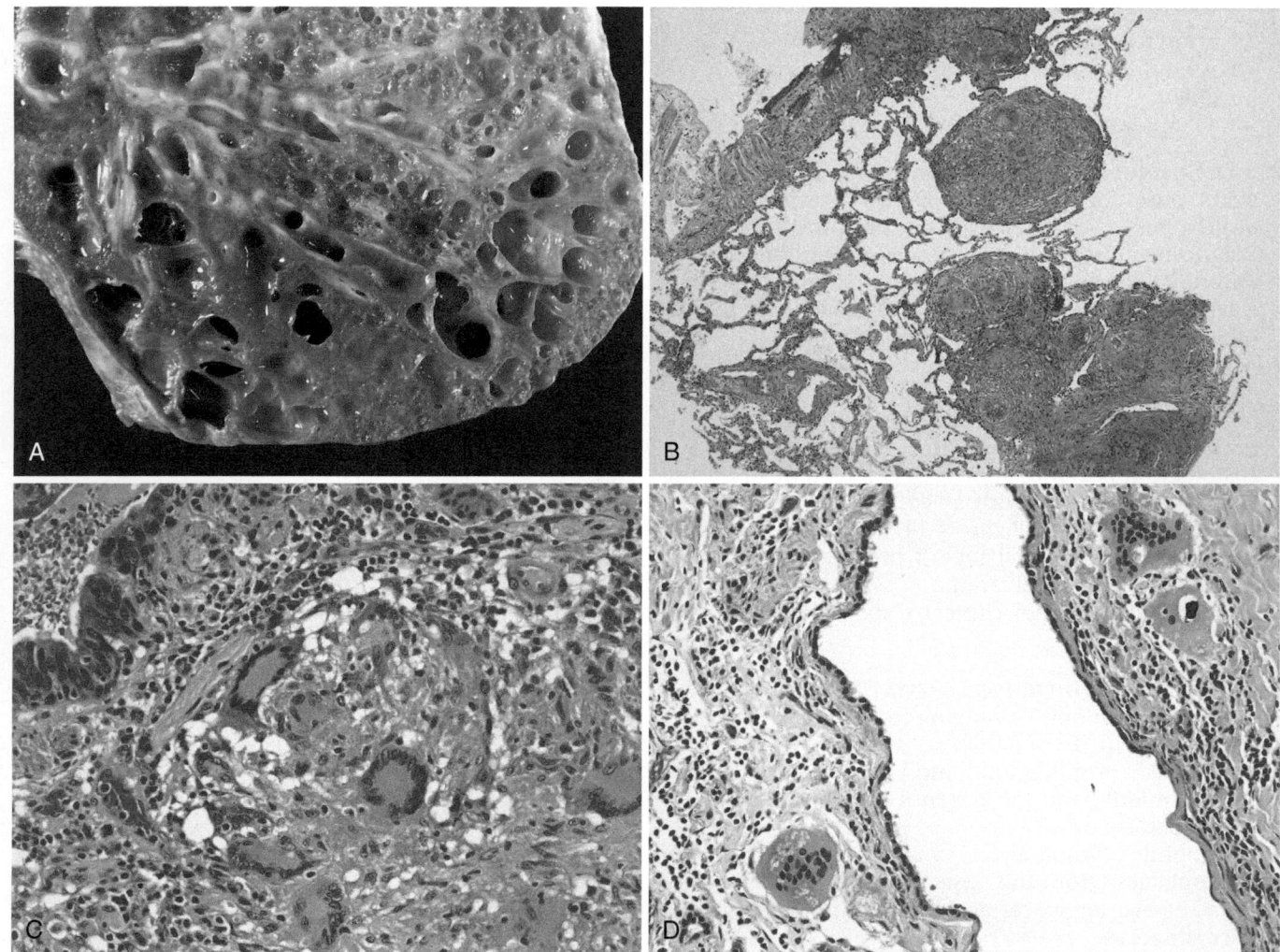

Figure 4-15. Sarcoidosis. **A,** Gross photograph of the cut surface of lung in end stage sarcoidosis shows marked fibrosis and distortion of lung architecture (honeycombing). **B,** Low-power photomicrograph shows characteristic well-formed non-necrotizing granulomas in this transbronchial biopsy. **C,** The sarcoid granuloma is formed by histiocytes and few lymphocytes. Langerhans-type giant cells, with peripheral horseshoe arrangement of nuclei, are present. Note submucosal location of the granuloma. **D,** Various inclusions (asteroid body in the lower left and Schumann body in the upper right) can be seen within the cytoplasm of the giant cells, which are characteristic, but not diagnostic, for sarcoidosis.

- Asteroid bodies (2% to 9%)
- Schaumann bodies, conchoidal bodies (70%)
- Hamazaki-Wesenberg bodies (GMS stain positive, Ziehl-Neelsen acid fast, misinterpreted for fungi)
- Microcalcifications, birefringent calcium oxalate, and calcium carbonate (mistaken for fungi or *Pneumocystis jiroveci*)
- Small number of patients progress to end-stage fibrosis and honeycombing, with an associated risk for cavitation, *Aspergillus* species infection, and subsequent hemoptysis

Special Stains and Immunohistochemistry

- GMS, periodic acid–Schiff (PAS), AFB stains negative for microorganisms

Other Techniques for Diagnosis

- Noncontributory

Differential Diagnosis

INFECTION

- Special stains to exclude fungal (e.g., histoplasmosis) and mycobacterial infection
- *Mycobacterium avium-intracellulare*: granulomas are distributed around airways (bronchocentric) and may fill bronchiolar lumen, along with a granulomatous vasculitis component

HYPERSENSITIVITY PNEUMONITIS

- Granulomas are not as well formed or as sharply delineated
- More prominent interstitial chronic inflammation

REACTION TO INHALED SUBSTANCES (e.g., TALC, ALUMINUM, BERYLLIUM)

- Consider exposure history and beryllium lymphocyte stimulation test

CONDITIONS ASSOCIATED WITH SARCOID-LIKE DISORDERS

- Malignancies (lymphoma, lung carcinoma, carcinoid tumors, testicular germ cell tumors)
- Collagen vascular disease (systemic lupus erythematosus [SLE], Sjögren syndrome, primary biliary cirrhosis)

PEARLS

- *Sarcoidosis is a clinical diagnosis, and the pathologic diagnosis of non-necrotizing (or noncaseating) granulomatous inflammation, etiology undetermined, with comments regarding the negative results of special stains for microorganisms is appropriate*
- *Hemoptysis suggests the presence of mycetoma*

SELECTED REFERENCES

El-Zammar OA, Katzenstein AL: Pathological diagnosis of granulomatous lung disease: a review. Histopathology 50:289-310, 2007.

Gupta D, Agarwal R, Aggarwal AN, et al: Sarcoidosis and tuberculosis: the same disease with different manifestations or similar manifestations of different disorders. Curr Opin Pulm Med 18:506-516, 2012.

Leslie KO, Gruden JF, Parish JM, Scholand MB: Transbronchial biopsy interpretation in the patient with diffuse parenchymal lung disease. Arch Pathol Lab Med 131:407-423, 2007.

Hemorrhagic Diseases
IDIOPATHIC PULMONARY HEMOSIDEROSIS

Clinical Features

- Recurrent, diffuse alveolar hemorrhage with no known etiology
- Occurs almost exclusively in children and adolescents with an equal sex distribution
- Patients present with an insidious onset of productive cough, hemoptysis, iron deficiency anemia, and weight loss
- Spontaneous remissions and exacerbations are common
- Coexists with several other diseases: IgA nephropathy, celiac disease, and dermatitis herpetiformis
- Radiographic studies reveal bilateral alveolar and reticulonodular infiltrates

Gross Pathology

- Marked increase in lung weight with areas of red-brown consolidation

Histopathology

- Dense aggregates of hemosiderin-laden macrophages with mild septal fibrosis to severe intra-alveolar hemorrhage (Figure 4-16)
- Degeneration, sloughing, and hyperplasia of alveolar epithelial cells

Special Stains and Immunohistochemistry

- Prussian blue positive

Other Techniques for Diagnosis

- Noncontributory

Differential Diagnosis

OTHER PULMONARY HEMORRHAGIC SYNDROMES

- Goodpasture syndrome: circulating antibasement membrane antibodies
- Vasculitis-associated angiitis, Wegener granulomatosis, and SLE

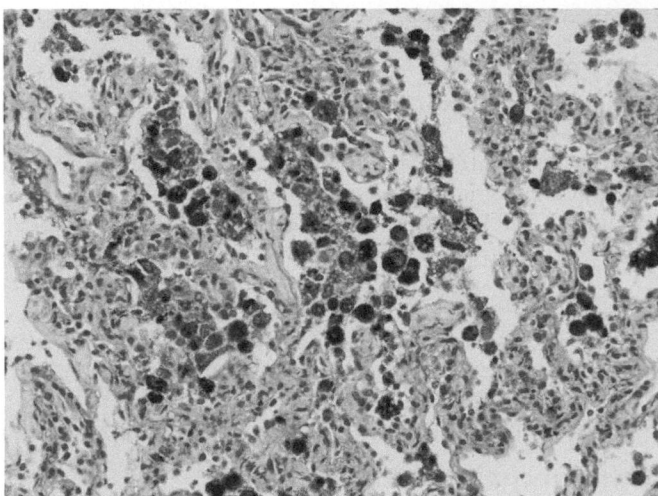

Figure 4-16. Idiopathic pulmonary hemosiderosis. Prussian blue staining is positive for iron within intra-alveolar macrophages containing hemosiderin.

PEARLS

- *Biopsy specimens should be assessed for immune complex or immunoglobulin deposition using immunofluorescence or immunohistochemistry because these findings are inconsistent with Idiopathic pulmonary hemosiderosis (IPH)*
- *Biopsies should not demonstrate any specific pathologic findings such as granulomas, vasculitis or capillaritis, pulmonary infarction, or infection*
- *Outcome has improved dramatically after implementation of immunosuppressive therapy, leading to the presumption that this is an immune-mediated disease*

SELECTED REFERENCES

Nuesslein TG, Teig N, Rieger CH: Pulmonary haemosiderosis in infants and children. Paediatr Respir Rev 7:45-48, 2006.

Poggi V, Lo Vecchio A, Menna F, et al: Idiopathic pulmonary hemo-siderosis: a rare cause of iron-deficiency anemia in childhood. J Pediatr Hematol Oncol 33:e160-e162, 2011.

GOODPASTURE SYNDROME AND ANTIBASEMENT MEMBRANE ANTIBODY DISEASE (ABMABD)

Clinical Features

- Autoimmune disorder caused by antibodies that react with glomerular and pulmonary basement membranes
- Rare disease with an incidence of 0.9 per million persons per year
- Typically affects young white males or elderly women with renal disease
- Younger patients frequently present with pulmonary symptoms (e.g., hemoptysis) before manifesting renal symptoms, whereas older patients develop glomerulo-nephritis and renal failure before the onset of pulmonary problems
- Hemoptysis ranges from mild to life threatening

Gross Pathology

- Diffusely consolidated lungs with areas of red-brown consolidation

Histopathology

- Lung biopsy is useful in cases with limited renal involvement
- Extensive intra-alveolar hemorrhage and numerous hemosiderin-laden macrophages (Figure 4-17)
- Fibrous thickening of alveolar septa with pneumocyte hyperplasia

Special Stains and Immunohistochemistry

- Immunofluorescence studies: linear staining of basement membrane along alveolar septa for IgG, IgM, or IgA and complement
- Circulating autoantibodies can be detected by serology

Other Techniques for Diagnosis

- Electron microscopy: widened gaps between endothelial cells and fragmentation of capillary basement membranes

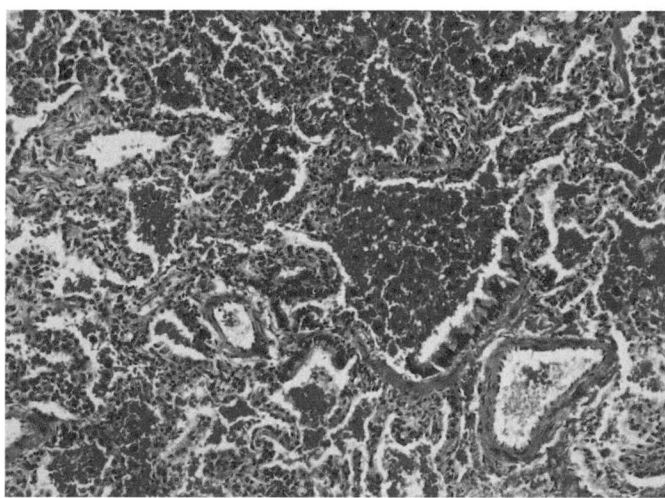

Figure 4-17. Goodpasture syndrome. H&E-stained section shows recent hemorrhage and hemosiderin-laden intra-alveolar macrophages, indicating old hemorrhage as well as a mild interstitial chronic inflammation.

Differential Diagnosis

IDIOPATHIC PULMONARY HEMOSIDEROSIS

- No renal involvement
- Antibasement membrane antibodies are not identified

WEGENER GRANULOMATOSIS

- PR3-ANCA (c-ANCA) in serum
- Necrotizing capillaritis and granulomas are prominent features

SLE

- Antinuclear antibody (ANA) positive
- Necrotizing capillaritis is a prominent feature

PEARLS

- *One third of patients have positive serum c-ANCA or p-ANCA in addition to ABMABD*
- *Antibodies of ABMABD target the noncollagenous domain of the α_3 chain of type IV collagen, and antibody titer correlates with disease severity*
- *About 90% of patients have HLA-DR2*
- *Diagnosis is often established from kidney biopsy specimens*

SELECTED REFERENCES

Bazari H, Guimaraes AR, Kushner YB: Case records of the Massachusetts General Hospital. Case 20-2012. A 77-year-old man with leg edema, hematuria, and acute renal failure. N Engl J Med 366:2503-2515, 2012.

Fishbein GA, Fishbein MC: Lung vasculitis and alveolar hemorrhage: pathology. Semin Respir Crit Care Med 32:254-263, 2011.

Pneumoconioses
SILICOSIS

Clinical Features

- Chronic lung disease is distinguished by parenchymal nodules and interstitial fibrosis due to inhalation of dust containing crystalline silicon dioxide

- Roughly 1500 cases are diagnosed annually in the United States
- Acute silicosis: patients develop symptoms within 3 years of exposure
- Classic or chronic silicosis: disease develops at least 20 years after exposure
- Accelerated silicosis: similar to acute silicosis, but symptoms develop later, typically within 3 to 10 years of exposure
- Simple silicosis: nodules 10 mm or less
- Progressive massive fibrosis: nodules are greater than 1 cm

Gross Pathology

- Firm, spherical, slate-gray to tan hyalinized nodules
- Nodules may coalesce to form irregular masses predominantly in the upper lobes

Histopathology

ACUTE SILICOSIS

- Pulmonary edema and interstitial inflammation
- Alveoli become filled by a granular, eosinophilic, PAS-positive lipoproteinaceous substance with prominent cholesterol clefts (pulmonary alveolar proteinosis)

CLASSIC SILICOSIS

- Firm, rounded, sharply demarcated nodules, from a few millimeters to several centimeters in diameter, predominantly localized to upper lobes and subpleural regions
- Nodules are composed of an amorphous center surrounded by whorls of mature, dense, lamellar collagen showing varying degrees of calcification and necrosis
- A peripheral zone of particle-laden macrophages, lymphocytes, and fibroblasts cuffs the nodule
- Weakly birefringent silicate crystals can be identified with polarized light

SILICOTUBERCULOSIS

- Tuberculosis is a common complication of silicosis and occurs in 25% of patients with acute or classic silicosis
- Silicotic nodules demonstrate central necrosis and epithelioid granulomatous reaction

Special Stains and Immunohistochemistry

- Elastic stain can facilitate the identification of obliterated vessels within the lesions

Other Techniques for Diagnosis

- Noncontributory

Differential Diagnosis

PULMONARY ALVEOLAR PROTEINOSIS (PAP)

- Resembles acute silicosis
- Eosinophilic material is present within alveolar spaces, alveolar ducts, and bronchioles (Figure 4-18)
- The intra-alveolar material stains with surfactant apoprotein antibodies
- Little inflammation or fibrosis is present
- Secondary infection with *Nocardia* infection, fungi, viruses, mycobacteria, or *Pneumocystis jiroveci* pneumonia (PCP) can occur
- PAP can be associated with hematologic malignancy, inorganic dust exposure, or immunodeficiency

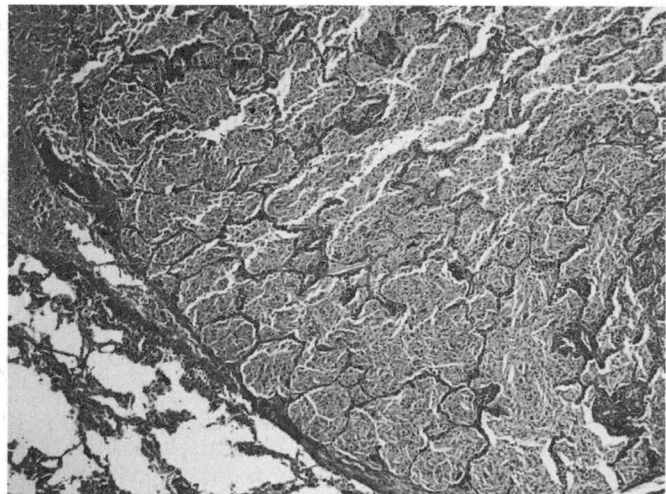

Figure 4-18. Pulmonary alveolar proteinosis. Pink granular proteinaceous material is seen filling the alveolar spaces with only minimal inflammation.

PEARLS

- *Silicosis, coal worker pneumoconiosis, asbestosis are the most common types of pneumoconioses*
- *Pneumoconiosis can be clinicopathologically classified as*
  - *Fibrotic: focal nodularity or diffuse fibrosis—silicosis, coal worker pneumoconiosis, asbestosis, berylliosis, and talcosis*
  - *Nonfibrotic: particle-laden macrophages with minimal or no fibrosis—siderosis (iron oxide), stannosis (tin oxide), baritosis (barium sulfate)*
- *A small but definite association between silicosis and lung cancer has been described in the literature*

SELECTED REFERENCES

Lee S, Hayashi H, Maeda M, et al: Environmental factors producing autoimmune dysregulation—chronic activation of T cells caused by silica exposure. Immunobiology 217:743-748, 2012.
Leung CC, Yu IT, Chen W: Silicosis. Lancet 379:2008-2018, 2012.
Petsonk EL, Rose C, Cohen R: Coal mine dust lung disease: new lessons from old exposure. Am J Respir Crit Care Med 187:1178-1185, 2013.

ASBESTOSIS

Clinical Features

- Asbestosis is primarily associated with four settings in developed countries
  - Older workers exposed to asbestos years ago
  - Workers managing existing sources (building or facility managers)
  - Asbestos abatement procedures
  - Renovation or demolition of asbestos-containing structures
- Asbestosis typically occurs 15 to 20 years after exposure
- Inhaled asbestos fibers are deposited deep in the lungs and reach the pleura through lymphatic channels in macrophages or through direct penetration
- Patients present with dyspnea, clubbing, and restrictive lung disease

Gross Pathology

- Fibrosis is predominantly distributed in the lower lobes
- Pleural fibrosis, calcifications, and honeycombing are common findings

Histopathology

- Asbestos fibers or asbestos bodies accompanied by interstitial fibrosis
- Diffuse interstitial fibrosis with chronic inflammation and type 2 pneumocyte hyperplasia
- Alveolar epithelial cells often contain eosinophilic material that resembles Mallory hyaline
- Asbestos bodies are straight or curved, 10- to 100-μm fibers with a central clear core and diffusely beaded pattern surrounded by a gold to yellow coating with terminal bulbs or knobs (Figure 4-19)
- Ferruginous bodies: similar to asbestos bodies but lack a clear central core

Special Studies and Immunohistochemistry

- Electron microscopy: facilitates the identification and characterization of asbestos fibers

Other Techniques for Diagnosis

- Amount of asbestos can be quantified in tissue by mass spectrometry

Differential Diagnosis

NSIP
- Lacks asbestos fibers

UIP
- Patchy fibrosis with temporal heterogeneity that is more pronounced in the lower lobes
- Lacks asbestos bodies

PEARLS

- *Transbronchial biopsy specimens are usually too small for analysis for asbestos bodies; BAL can be more useful to identify asbestos bodies*

- *Asbestos is a heterogenous group of hydrated magnesium silicate materials that typically separate into fibers when crushed*
- *An important implication for significant asbestos exposure is the associated increased risk for malignancy (e.g., lung cancer or mesothelioma)*
- *Asbestos exposure is the largest single cause of occupational cancer in the United States; it is also a significant cause of morbidity from nonmalignant disease*
- *However, most patients with asbestosis (lung fibrosis) do not develop cancer*

SELECTED REFERENCES

Lazarus AA, Philip A: Asbestosis. Dis Mon 57:14-26, 2011.
Liu G, Cheresh P, Kamp DW: Molecular basis of asbestos-induced lung disease. Annu Rev Pathol 8:161-187, 2013.

Iatrogenic Diseases
RADIATION PNEUMONITIS

Clinical Features

- Clinical symptoms of acute radiation pneumonitis (dyspnea on exertion and nonproductive cough) usually develop 6 weeks to 6 months after completion of therapy
- The likelihood of a patient developing an adverse response to radiation therapy depends on (1) individual susceptibility, (2) amount of radiation, (3) dose rate, (4) duration of therapy, and (5) and the volume of lung irradiated
- Several factors add to the toxic effects of radiation, including (1) concomitant chemotherapy, (2) prior history of irradiation, and (3) infection

Gross Pathology

- Noncontributory

Histopathology

- Acute pneumonitis: similar to acute or organizing DAD with hyaline membranes, type 2 pneumocyte hyperplasia, and interstitial fibroblast proliferation (Figure 4-20)

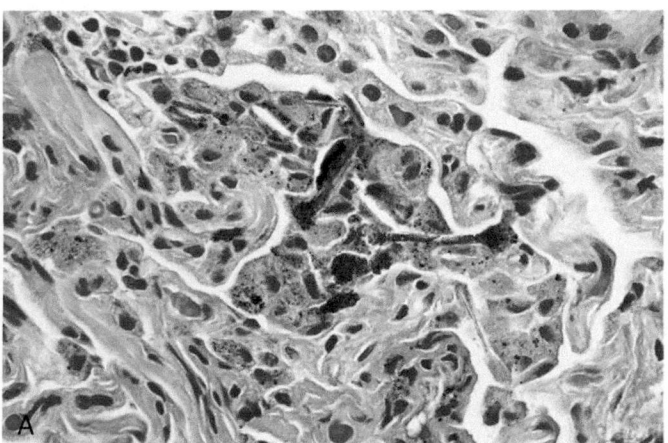
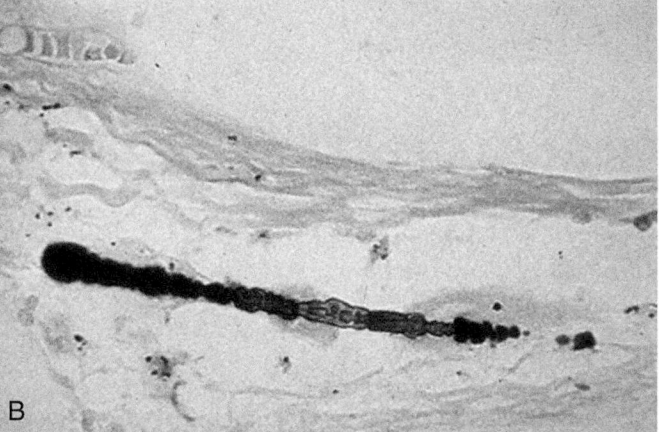

Figure 4-19. Asbestosis. A, Asbestos bodies appear brown on H&E stain because they are covered with protein containing hemosiderin. **B,** This high-power photomicrograph of a Prussian blue reaction shows an asbestos body with a bulbous end and beads along its length. The other bulbous end is not present, presumably because of the plane of sectioning.

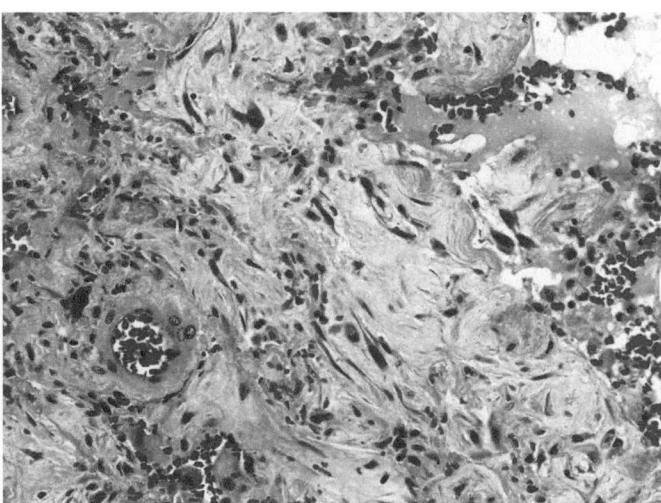

Figure 4-20. Radiation pneumonitis. High-power photomicrograph shows reactive atypical fibroblasts with enlarged nuclei in a background of young fibrosis.

- Fibrotic stage: may follow clinically apparent acute radiation pneumonitis or may develop insidiously without a previous acute illness and is similar to nonspecific fibrosis with hyperplasia and cytologic atypia of type 2 pneumocytes
- Regardless of the process, the presence of foam cells and interstitial atypical stromal cells (radiation fibroblasts) is relatively distinctive for radiation injury
- Foam cells are lipid-rich modified macrophages and smooth muscle cells similar to the cells that accumulate in fatty streaks and atheromatous plaques and may be found in the intima of arterioles of any irradiated organ
- Atypical stromal cells have abundant, usually basophilic cytoplasm and enlarged hyperchromatic nuclei with or without prominent nucleoli; mitotic figures are rare

Special Stains and Immunohistochemistry

- CT scan is sensitive in detecting radiographic evidence of pneumonitis

Other Techniques for Diagnosis

- Noncontributory

Differential Diagnosis

- Consider other causes of DAD

PEARLS

- *Foam cells and atypical stromal cells are distinctive features of radiation injury*
- *The injury is largely confined to the radiation field; however, it has been reported in contralateral nonirradiated lung*
- *Acute radiation pneumonitis is usually responsive to corticosteroid therapy*
- *Radiation-induced carcinomas usually have an induction period of more than 10 years*

SELECTED REFERENCES

Graves PR, Siddiqui F, Anscher MS, Movsas B: Radiation pulmonary toxicity: from mechanisms to management. Semin Radiat Oncol 20:201-207, 2010.

Krasin MJ, Constine LS, Friedman DL, et al: Radiation-related treatment effects across the age spectrum: differences and similarities or what the old and young can learn from each other. Semin Radiat Oncol 20:21-29, 2010.

BLEOMYCIN TOXICITY

Clinical Features

- Bleomycin is an antitumor antibiotic isolated from *Streptomyces verticillus*
- Incidence of bleomycin toxicity is less than 5%
- The sensitivity of lungs to bleomycin is attributed to hydrolase, an enzyme that inactivates the drug; bleomycin is concentrated in the lung, which is relatively deficient in the enzyme
- Patients present with insidious onset of dry cough, dyspnea, and fever

Gross Pathology

- Noncontributory

Histopathology

- DAD is present, usually in acute or organizing phase, with hyperplasia of type II pneumocytes
- Pneumocyte atypia is a characteristic feature but is not specific
- Some cases progress to fibrotic phase with interstitial scarring; the fibrosis tends to be nonuniform, focal, or nodular (Figure 4-21)

Special Stains and Immunohistochemistry

- Noncontributory

Other Techniques for Diagnosis

- Noncontributory

Differential Diagnosis

- DAD, acute interstitial pneumonia
- Amiodarone toxicity (Figure 4-22)
  - Amiodarone causes DAD, possibly through direct toxic effect, in about one third of patients

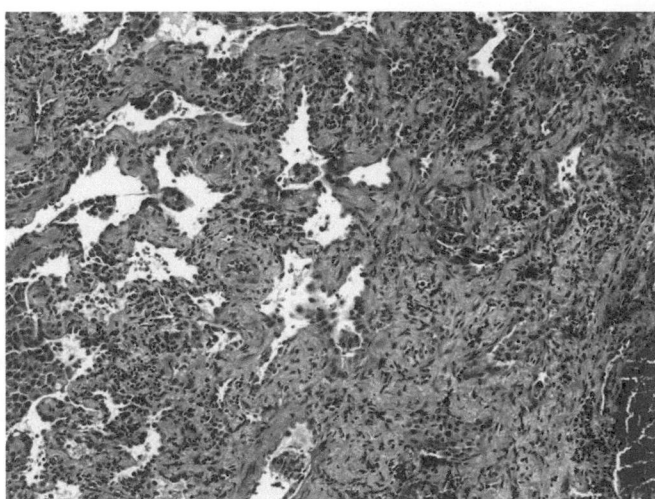

Figure 4-21. Bleomycin toxicity. There is interstitial fibrosis with mild chronic inflammation. The pneumocytes are hyperplastic with reactive atypia.

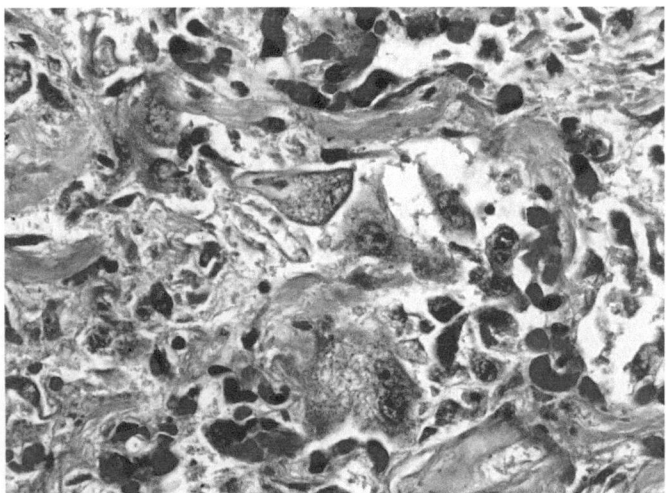

Figure 4-22. Amiodarone toxicity. Finely vacuolated cytoplasm is seen both in the alveolar macrophages and in the reactive pneumocytes.

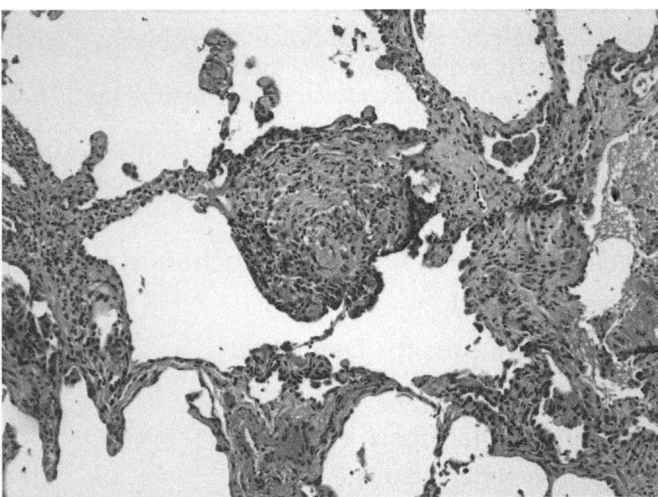

Figure 4-23. Methotrexate pneumonitis. Poorly formed granulomas and a mixed inflammatory infiltrate, including eosinophils, are seen.

- In addition to interstitial inflammation and hyperplasia of type II pneumocytes, there is an accumulation of foamy histiocytes in air spaces
- Electron microscopy shows lamellar inclusions in alveolar macrophages
- Methotrexate toxicity (Figure 4-23)

PEARLS

- *Toxicity of bleomycin is dose related; toxicity tends to increase by concomitant use of oxygen, drugs (e.g., cyclophosphamide), and radiation therapy*
- *Bleomycin is one of the drugs suggested to elicit the radiorecall phenomenon—that is, a phenomenon in which previous irradiation appears to cause latent damage that may be unmasked later (e.g., by use of bleomycin)*

SELECTED REFERENCES

Huang TT, Hudson MM, Stokes DC, et al: Pulmonary outcomes in survivors of childhood cancer: a systematic review. Chest 140:881-901, 2011.

Kasper M, Barth K: Bleomycin and its role in inducing apoptosis and senescence in lung cells: modulating effects of caveolin-1. Curr Cancer Drug Targets 9:341-353, 2009.

VASCULAR CONDITIONS

VASCULITIDES

- See Figure 4-24 and Table 4-3

SELECTED REFERENCES

Fishbein GA, Fishbein MC: Lung vasculitis and alveolar hemorrhage: pathology. Semin Respir Crit Care Med 32:254-263, 2011.
Martín-Suñé N, Ríos-Blanco JJ: Pulmonary affectation of vasculitis. Arch Bronconeumol 48:410-418, 2012.
Nachman PH, Henderson AG: Pathogenesis of lung vasculitis. Semin Respir Crit Care Med 32:245-253, 2011.

PULMONARY HYPERTENSION

Clinical Features

- See Table 4-4 for the Revised Clinical Classification of Pulmonary Hypertension (2009)
- Idiopathic pulmonary arterial hypertension (IPAH) is a rare disease with an incidence of 2 to 3 cases per 1 million persons per year and a prevalence of 15 cases per 1 million persons
- IPAH is three times more common in women than men
- Other forms of PAH are much more common
  - About 8% to 60% of all patients with scleroderma
  - Up to 20% of patients with rheumatoid arthritis, 5% to 15% of patients with SLE
  - About 20% to 40% of patients with sickle cell disease
- Most patients with pulmonary hypertension present with dyspnea, fatigue, anginal chest pain, syncope, nonproductive cough, peripheral edema, and rarely hemoptysis
- The most common cause of pulmonary hypertension is left heart failure
- Pulmonary systolic pressure is greater than 25 mm Hg owing to a decrease in the cross-sectional area of the pulmonary vascular bed

Gross Pathology

- Atherosclerotic plaques, usually small, develop in large pulmonary arteries

Histopathology

- See Table 4-5
- Grading scheme applies only to IPAH and APAH (associated with pulmonary arterial hypertension) secondary to congenital heart disease and some drugs (e.g., phenytoin)
- Only grades I, II, and III are seen in secondary pulmonary hypertension
- Plexiform lesions (present in severe disease) (Figure 4-25)
- Areas of dilation due to thinning of arterial walls
- Within dilated vessels, glomeruloid plexus of slitlike vascular channels

Special Stains and Immunohistochemistry

- Trichrome and elastic von Gieson stains highlight the vascular lesions

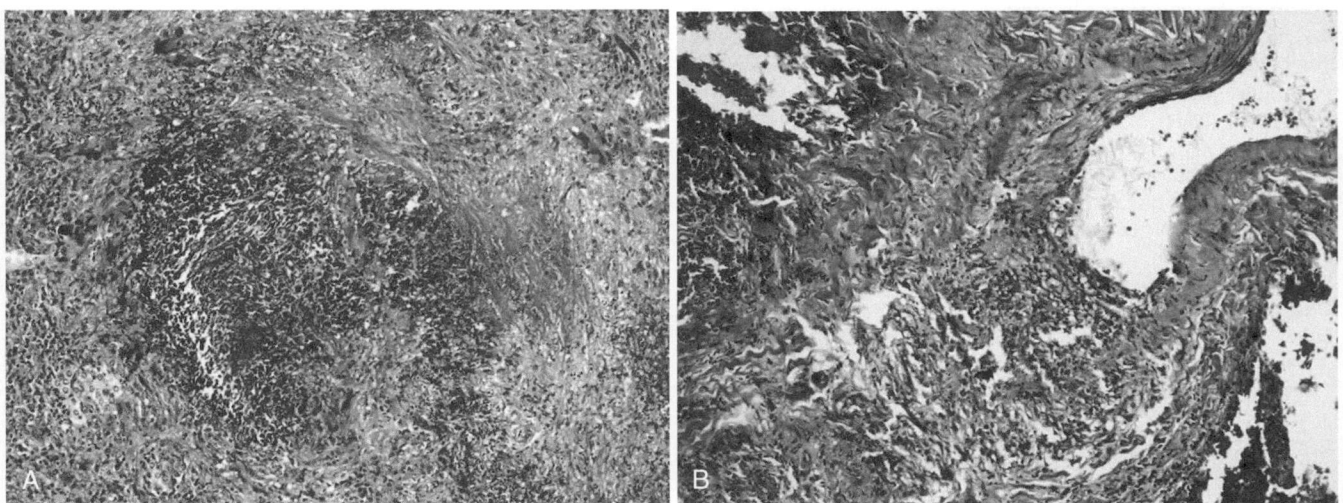

Figure 4-24. Wegener granulomatosis. A, Low-power photomicrograph shows a granuloma with geographic basophilic necrosis, which is characteristic of Wegener granulomatosis. **B,** High-power photomicrograph shows granulomatous vasculitis.

TABLE 4-3	**CLINICAL AND PATHOLOGIC FEATURES OF WEGENER GRANULOMATOSIS (GRANULOMATOSIS WITH POLYANGIITIS) AND CHURG-STRAUSS SYNDROME**	
	Wegener Granulomatosis	**Churg-Strauss Syndrome**
General	Triad of upper airway involvement (e.g., sinusitis), lower respiratory tract involvement, and glomerulonephritis	Multisystem disorder with asthma, rhinitis, peripheral eosinophilia, and systemic vasculitis
Target organs	Head and neck, lungs, renal	Lungs, skin, heart, central nervous system, joints, gastrointestinal system, kidneys
ANCA	c-ANCA (> 90%) Usually PR3-ANCA	p-ANCA (40%-60%) Usually MPO-ANCA Occasionally PR3-ANCA
Gross findings	Multiple nodules (0.5-10 cm) 50% demonstrate cavitation Lower lobe predominance	Multifocal parenchymal consolidations Eosinophilic pleural effusions (30%) Stellate-shaped peripheral pulmonary arteries Rare cavitations
Histologic findings	Parenchymal necrosis (microscopic or geographic) Small vessel vasculitis (arteritis, venulitis, capillaritis) Elastic lamina destruction Granulomatous inflammation Microabscess Palisading histiocytes Scattered giant cells Poorly formed granulomas	Asthmatic bronchitis Eosinophilic pneumonia Occasional pleural and septal inflammation Extravascular granuloma with palisading histiocytes and MNGC surrounding central necrosis ("allergic granuloma") Vasculitis with chronic inflammatory cells, eosinophils, epithelioid cells, MNGC, or neutrophils Diffuse hemorrhage
Differential diagnosis	Lymphoma Churg-Strauss syndrome Sarcoidosis Necrotizing sarcoid granulomatosis Granulomatous infection Rheumatoid nodules DPHS	Wegener granulomatosis EP (no systemic vasculitis) ABPFD (no systemic vasculitis) Parasites (*Strongyloides stercoralis, Toxocara canis*) Fungal infection Hodgkin disease Drug-induced vasculitis (carbamazepine)
Pearls	Tissue and peripheral eosinophilia, < 10% Asthma is rare Cardiac disease is rare Severe renal disease Severe, destructive sinus disease	Tissue and peripheral eosinophilia typical Asthma is typical Cardiac disease is common Mild renal disease Mild sinus involvement, typically allergic rhinitis Consider in patients with difficult-to-control asthma who develop significant cardiac, gastrointestinal, or neurologic disease

ABPFD, allergic bronchopulmonary fungal disease; ANCA, antineutrophil cytoplasmic antibody; DPHS, diffuse pulmonary hemorrhage syndrome; EP, eosinophilic pneumonia; MNGC, multinucleated giant cells.

TABLE 4-4 REVISED CLINICAL CLASSIFICATION OF PULMONARY HYPERTENSION (VENICE 2003)

Pulmonary Arterial Hypertension (PAH)
- Idiopathic (IPAH)
- Familial (FPAH)
- Associated with (APAH)
Collagen vascular disease
Congenital systemic-to-pulmonary shunts
Portal hypertension
HIV infection
Drugs and toxins
Other (thyroid disorders, glycogen storage disease, Gaucher disease, hereditary hemorrhagic telangiectasia, hemoglobinopathies, myeloproliferative disorders, splenectomy)
- Associated with significant venous or capillary involvement
- Pulmonary veno-occlusive disease (PVOD)
- Pulmonary capillary hemangiomatosis (PCH)

Pulmonary Hypertension with Left Heart Disease
- Left-sided atrial or ventricular heart disease
- Left-sided valvular heart disease

Pulmonary Hypertension Associated with Lung Disease and Hypoxemia
- Chronic obstructive pulmonary disease (COPD)
- Interstitial lung disease
- Sleep-disordered breathing and alveolar hypoventilation disorders
- Chronic exposure to high altitude
- Developmental abnormalities

Pulmonary Hypertension Due to Chronic Thrombotic or Embolic Disease
- Thromboembolic obstruction of proximal pulmonary arteries
- Thromboembolic obstruction of distal pulmonary arteries
- Nonthrombotic pulmonary embolism (tumor, parasites, foreign material)

Miscellaneous
- Sarcoidosis, histiocytosis X, lymphangiomatosis, compression of pulmonary vessels (adenopathy, tumor, fibrosing mediastinitis)

From Simonneau G, Galie N, Rubin LJ, et al: Clinical classification of pulmonary hypertension. J Am Coll Cardiol 43(suppl S):5S-12S, 2004.

TABLE 4-5 GRADING SCHEME FOR IDIOPATHIC PULMONARY ARTERIAL HYPERTENSION AND DISEASE ASSOCIATED WITH PULMONARY ARTERIAL HYPERTENSION

Grade	Reversible	Histologic Features
I	Yes	Medial hypertrophy of pulmonary arteries
		Extension of muscle into the wall of pulmonary arterioles
II	Yes	Muscle hypertrophy plus proliferation of intimal cells in arterioles and small muscular arteries
III	Yes	Muscle hypertrophy plus subendothelial fibrosis
		Concentric masses of fibrous tissue and reduplicated internal elastic lamina with vascular lumen occlusion of small arteries and arterioles
		Large elastic arteries show atherosclerosis
IV	No	Muscle hypertrophy is less apparent
		Progressive dilation of small arteries, particularly vessels with intimal fibrous occlusion
		Plexiform lesions occur
V	No	Plexiform and angiomatoid lesions
		Intra-alveolar hemosiderin-filled macrophages
VI	No	Necrotizing arteritis with thrombosis
		Fibrinoid necrosis of the arterial wall with transmural neutrophilic and eosinophilic infiltrates

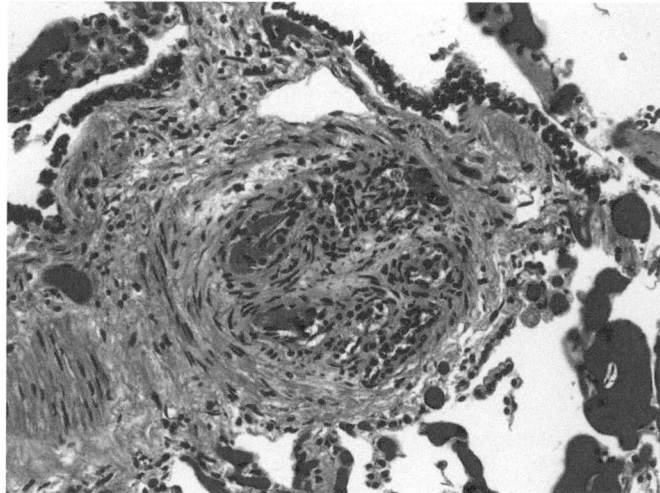

Figure 4-25. Pulmonary hypertension. H&E-stained section shows a plexiform lesion within a pulmonary artery branch.

Other Techniques for Diagnosis
- Noncontributory

Differential Diagnosis

PULMONARY VENO-OCCLUSIVE DISEASE (PVOD)
- Rare cause of pulmonary hypertension, with estimated annual incidence of 0.1 cases per million persons and occurring more commonly in children and young adults
- Extensive and diffuse occlusion of pulmonary venules and small veins in lobular septa by intimal fibrosis; involvement of larger veins is rare
- Media of the veins may become arterialized with increased elastic fibers
- Pulmonary arterioles demonstrate moderate to severe medial hypertrophy in about half of the cases
- Alveolar capillaries may become dilated and tortuous such that PVOD can be confused with pulmonary capillary hemangiomatosis
- Hemosiderin may be prominent and confused with idiopathic pulmonary hemosiderosis
- Arteritis and plexiform lesions are usually absent

PULMONARY HYPERTENSION DUE TO CHRONIC THROMBOTIC OR EMBOLIC DISEASE
- Little or no medial hypertrophy in pulmonary arteries and arterioles
- Recent organizing and organized thrombi possible
- Eccentric intimal fibrosis that focally obliterates the lumen
- Recanalization of thrombi is common

PULMONARY CAPILLARY HEMANGIOMATOSIS (PCH)
- Extremely rare disorder with dense proliferation of capillaries within the alveolar septa causing thickening of the alveolar walls

- *The terms* primary *and secondary* pulmonary hypertension *are no longer used in the clinical medicine literature*
- *Familial pulmonary arterial hypertension (FPAH) as well as a subset of sporadic idiopathic PAH is linked to mutations in the BMPR2 gene on 2q33-q34*

SELECTED REFERENCES

Montani D, Günther S, Dorfmüller P, et al: Pulmonary arterial hypertension. Orphanet J Rare Dis 8:97, 2013.
Task Force for Diagnosis and Treatment of Pulmonary Hypertension of European Society of Cardiology (ESC); European Respiratory Society (ERS); International Society of Heart and Lung Transplantation (ISHLT), Galiè N, Hoeper MM, Humbert M, et al: Guidelines for the diagnosis and treatment of pulmonary hypertension. Eur Respir J 34:1219-1263, 2009.

INFECTIOUS DISEASES

Viral
CYTOMEGALOVIRUS (CMV) PNEUMONIA

Clinical Features

- CMV infects healthy individuals in whom it remains dormant in white cells; it reactivates in immunocompromised hosts
- In addition to pneumonia, CMV causes hepatitis, esophagitis, colitis, meningoencephalitis, chorioretinitis, and congenital and neonatal infections

Gross Pathology

- High-resolution CT demonstrates micronodules, consolidations, ground-glass opacities, and irregular reticular opacities in transplant recipients
- One- to 3-cm nodular masses in AIDS patients

Histopathology

- Based on its characteristic cytopathic changes in lung tissue specimens (Figure 4-26) CMV is the most commonly recognized pneumonia-causing virus by pathologists
- CMV infects endothelial cells, respiratory epithelial cells, fibroblasts, and macrophages
- Infected cells with CMV inclusions vary in number from few to numerous

Special Stains and Immunohistochemistry

- Immunohistochemistry usually highlights more viral inclusions than seen on hematoxylin and eosin (H&E) and also stains nuclei that are infected but do not show cytopathic effects yet

Other Techniques for Diagnosis

- Noncontributory

Differential Diagnosis

- See Table 4-6

- *In the nonimmunocompromised host, with little or no histopathologic reaction, rare CMV inclusions may represent an incidental finding*
- *Ganciclovir therapy induces morphologic changes to the intranuclear inclusions such that they become globular and eosinophilic*
- *CMV immunohistochemistry or in situ hybridization is helpful for identifying rare, occult inclusions as well as early infection before cytopathic changes develop*
- *Additional infectious agents may be present in immunocompromised patients, particularly* Pneumocystis jiroveci *in AIDS patients*
- *If the clinical, histologic, and radiologic findings are inconsistent with pneumonia, positive CMV BAL cultures and serum polymerase chain reaction (PCR) should be interpreted conservatively*

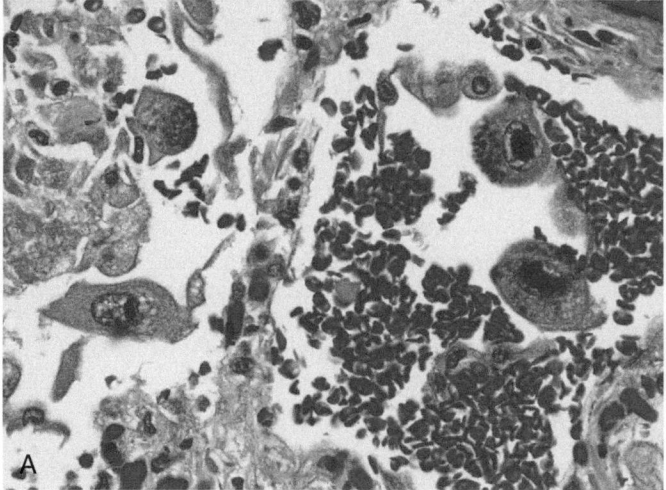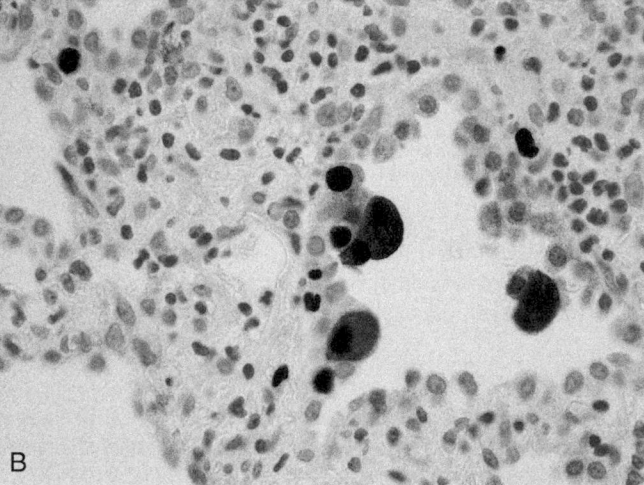

Figure 4-26. Cytomegalovirus (CMV) pneumonia. A, Enlarged cells with diagnostic intranuclear (single) and cytoplasmic (multiple smaller) inclusions are present. The cytoplasmic inclusions resemble toxoplasmosis and may be the only finding in a small biopsy. **B,** Immunoperoxidase stain using antibody mixture against immediate-early and early nuclear antigens demonstrates infected normal-sized nuclei (upper left and middle) that are not yet showing the cytopathic effect of CMV as well as classically enlarged nuclei. This allows for early diagnosis of CMV when diagnostic inclusions are not present in the biopsy.

TABLE 4-6 DIAGNOSTIC FEATURES OF VIRAL PNEUMONIAS

Virus	Inclusions Nuclear	Inclusions Cytoplasmic	Cytologic Features	Histopathologic Features
Cytomegalovirus (CMV)	Yes	Yes	**Nuclear features:** Single 20-μm inclusion with halo, thickened nuclear membrane, rounded clump of chromatin extending into halo **Cytoplasmic features:** multiple, 1- to 3-μm inclusions	Miliary pattern, inflammation, and necrosis Diffuse interstitial pneumonitis Hemorrhagic pneumonia CMV inclusions with minimal inflammation
Herpes simplex virus	Yes	No	Squamous cells with dense, eosinophilic inclusions surrounded by clear halo and marginated, bead chromatin at the periphery; best found at interface between viable and necrotic lung Rare multinucleated cells with nuclear inclusions	Necrotizing tracheobronchitis with ulceration Necrotizing bronchiolocentric pneumonia Interstitial pneumonitis resembling diffuse alveolar damage
Measles	Yes	Yes	Very large (100-μm diameter), multinucleated giant cells with nuclear and large eosinophilic cytoplasmic inclusions	Necrotizing bronchiolitis Giant cell pneumonia
Adenovirus	Yes	No	Smudge cells with basophilic inclusion with smudgy nuclear membrane often filling entire nucleus *or* Densely eosinophilic nuclear inclusions	Necrotizing bronchitis, bronchiolitis Interstitial pneumonia with necrosis, hemorrhage, and diffuse alveolar damage-like features
Influenza	No	No	N/A	Squamous metaplasia
Respiratory syncytial virus	No	Yes	Multinucleated syncytial cells in airway walls Eosinophilic cytoplasmic inclusions	Bronchiolitis with focal epithelial ulceration Interstitial pneumonia
Parainfluenza virus	No	Yes	Multinucleated giant cells with small cytoplasmic inclusions	Giant cell pneumonia with genotypes 2 and 3
Hantavirus	No	No	Virus is identified by immunohistochemistry or polymerase chain reaction	Marked alveolar edema Immature leukocytes within alveolar capillaries

Data from Travis WD: *Non-neoplastic Disorders of the Lower Respiratory Tract. Atlas of Non-tumor Pathology. First Series, Fascicle 2. Washington, DC, American Registry of Pathology: Armed Forces Institute of Pathology; Universities Associated for Research and Education in Pathology, 2002.*

SELECTED REFERENCE

Cunha BA: Cytomegalovirus pneumonia: community-acquired pneumonia in immunocompetent hosts. Infect Dis Clin North Am 24:147-158, 2010.

Bacterial
LEGIONELLA PNEUMONIA

Clinical Features

- The gram-negative bacteria *Legionella* species are believed to cause 1% of all pulmonary infections and 15% of pneumonia in hospitalized patients
- *Legionella* causes two diseases: *Legionella* pneumonia and the milder Pontiac fever

Gross Pathology

- Focal and nodular pattern of lung involvement
- Rounded lesions occasionally seen

Histopathology

- A neutrophilic infiltrate, a monocyte, and macrophage infiltrate, or a combined neutrophil, monocyte, and macrophage infiltrate is present
- Intra-alveolar fibrin and hemorrhage are common
- Prominent nuclear debris creates a dusty or dirty appearance
- Occasional vasculitic component is present

Special Stains and Immunohistochemistry

- Tissue silver stains (Warthin-Starry, Steiner, and Dieterle stains) demonstrate the bacteria
- Immunofluorescence methods on tissue sections are available

Other Techniques for Diagnosis

- Electron microscopy demonstrates bacteria within macrophages and neutrophils

Differential Diagnosis

- Bronchopneumonia and lobar pneumonia due to other bacterial infections

PEARLS

- Legionella *is a relatively common cause of both community-acquired and hospital-acquired pneumonia*
- *The major disadvantage of the urinary antigen test is that it is specific for* Legionella pneumophila, *serogroup 1 only*

NOCARDIOSIS

Clinical Features

- Rare lung infection caused by the gram-positive bacilli *Nocardia* species (*Nocardia asteroides* accounts for more than 80% of cases), with an incidence of 500 to 1000 cases per year in the United States

- Inhalation of the saprophytic organisms in decaying organic matter and soil is the main route of infection
- Chronic immunosuppression is secondary to AIDS, Cushing disease, corticosteroid therapy, lymphoma, and chronic granulomatous disease
- At the time of diagnosis, 50% of cases of pulmonary nocardiosis have disseminated to other organs (e.g., skin, bone, kidney, and brain)

Gross Pathology

- Numerous, often coalescent abscesses that may contain thick, green pus

Histopathology

- *Nocardia* species are long, thin, beaded bacterial filaments 1 μm in thickness that branch at right angles (Chinese character pattern) (Figure 4-27)
- Neutrophils form microabscesses, leading to necrotizing pneumonia in acute nocardiosis
- Organisms are best seen in areas of necrosis or suppuration
- *Nocardia* species form a ball-like mass within cavitary spaces in rare instances
- In immunocompromised patients, there are small, poorly formed granulomas with few neutrophils

Special Stains and Immunohistochemistry

- *Nocardia* species are difficult to identify, so a high index of suspicion and knowledge of the morphology increase the chances of positive identification
- GMS, Brown and Brenn, and Brown and Hopps stains demonstrate the organisms
- Coates-Fite, Kinyoun, and Fite-Faraco stains show the weakly acid-fast organisms

Other Techniques for Diagnosis

- PCR methods are available to identify *Nocardia* species from BAL or tissue biopsy specimens

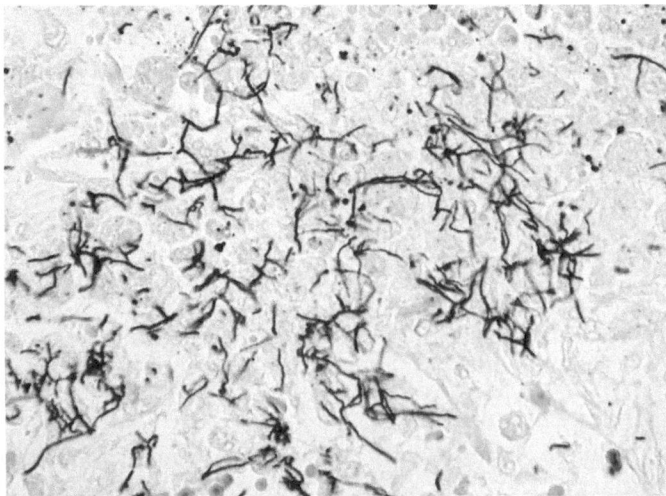

Figure 4-27. Nocardiosis. Branching thin filamentous bacteria are best visualized on GMS stain.

Differential Diagnosis

ACTINOMYCOSIS

- Uncommon pulmonary infection caused by the anaerobic filamentous *Actinomyces* species
- Gram-positive, beaded, branching, filamentous bacteria that branch at right angles
- Sulfur granule formation, often accompanied by the Splendore-Hoeppli phenomenon, is a feature of *Actinomyces* but not *Nocardia* species

PEARLS

- *Organisms are difficult to recognize; silver stains are most helpful, but molecular or immunohistochemical methods may be needed to establish the diagnosis*

MYCOBACTERIUM TUBERCULOSIS

Clinical Features

- Tuberculosis is a chronic infection caused by the bacillus *Mycobacterium tuberculosis*
- In the United States, tuberculosis most often occurs in homeless, incarcerated, impoverished, elderly, and immunosuppressed individuals
- Primary tuberculosis is transmitted through the inhalation of 1- to 5-μm airborne droplets containing the bacillus
- Secondary tuberculosis is due to reactivation of primary infection or, less likely, reinfection
- Miliary tuberculosis reflects hematogenous spread of the organism, causing systemic tuberculosis

Gross Pathology

- Ghon lesion: round, 1- to 2-cm, gray-white pulmonary parenchymal nodule with a necrotic center, usually close to the pleura in the lower upper lobe or upper lower lobe
- Ghon complex: Ghon lesion associated with enlarged hilar lymph nodal involvement
- Ranke complex: in 95% of cases, cell-mediated immunity controls the infection, and the Ghon complex undergoes progressive fibrosis and calcification

Histopathology

- Necrotizing granulomas containing mycobacterial organisms (4-μm, slim, beaded rods) are present within the lung parenchyma and mediastinal lymph nodes
- Granulomas are bordered by palisading histiocytes and contain epithelioid cells, which often fuse to form Langerhans-type multinucleated giant cells (Figure 4-28)
- Severe pulmonary complications include
  - Enlargement of necrotizing granuloma into cavitary lesion
  - Rupture of necrotizing granuloma into pleura, vascular structure, or bronchus with subsequent empyema, embolization, and bronchopneumonia, respectively

Special Stains and Immunohistochemistry

- Ziehl-Neelsen acid-fast stain is the optimal staining method for identification
- Other staining methods are auramine-rhodamine fluorescent, Fite, and Kinyoun stains

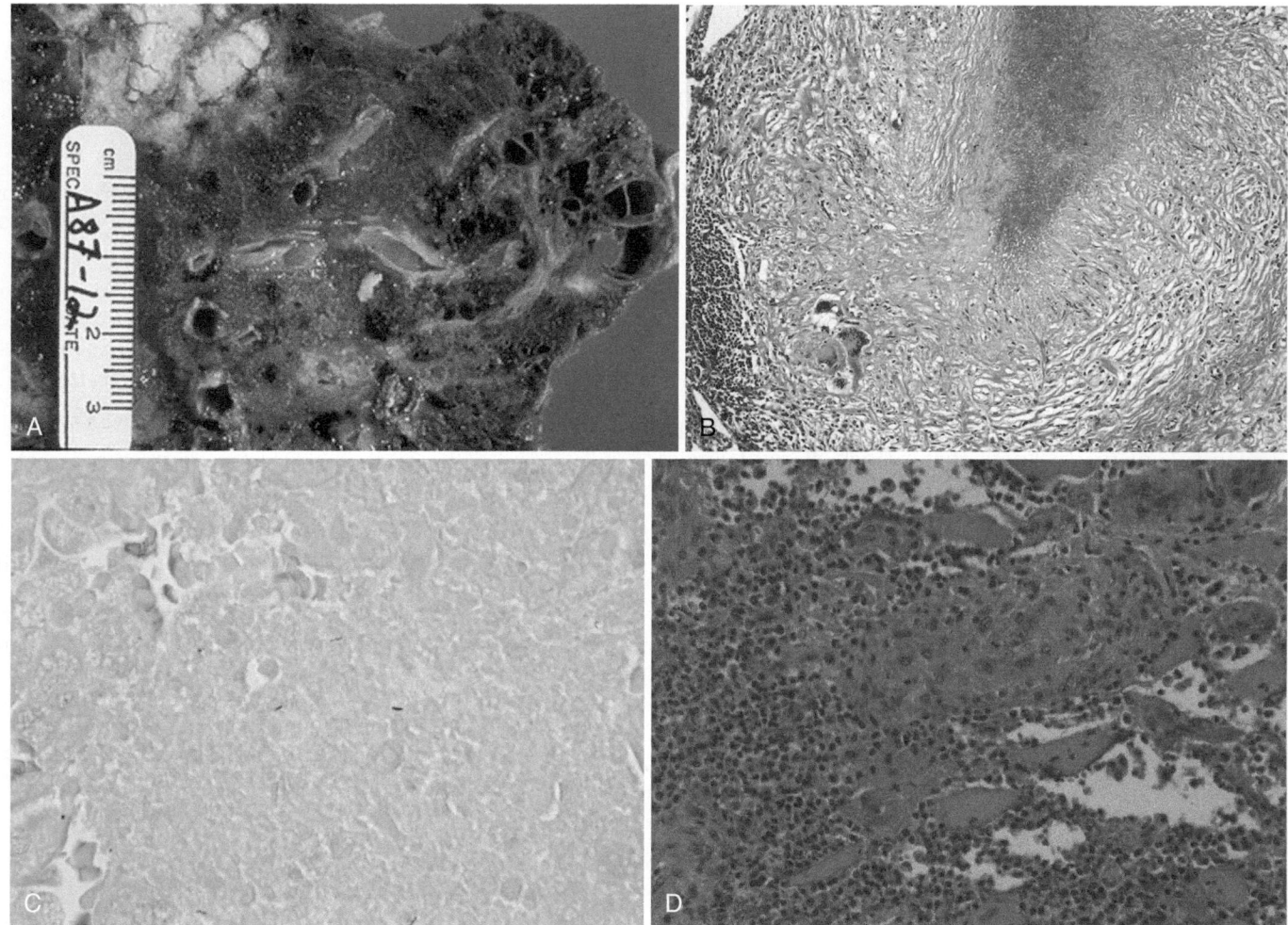

Figure 4-28. Tuberculosis. A, Gross picture of the cut surface of a lung shows caseating granulomas (cheesy white appearance). **B,** H&E-stained section shows a granuloma with central necrosis (*left side*) and Langerhans-type giant cells (peripherally arranged nuclei). **C,** Acid-fast bacillus stain shows few acid-fast bacilli (pink rods) in this nonimmunocompromised patient. **D,** Occasionally superimposed bacterial infection can cause diagnostic confusion as in this patient finally diagnosed with tuberculosis who presented with an abscess and neutrophilic inflammation.

Other Techniques for Diagnosis

- PCR-based identification is faster than culture and is useful in cases in which specimen was not obtained for culture

Differential Diagnosis

- Nontuberculosis mycobacterial pneumonia, fungal pneumonia, Wegener granulomatosis, sarcoidosis, *Nocardia* species

PEARLS

- *About 1×10^4 to 10^6 organisms/mL are needed for a positive Ziehl-Neelsen acid-fast stain*
- *The diagnosis of most cases of* Mycobacterium tuberculosis *pneumonia is based on clinical presentation, history, physical signs and symptoms, and sputum culture*
- *Virulence is attributed to particular cell envelope components (peptidoglycan, arabin galactan, and mycolic acids), the lipopolysaccharide lipoarabinomannan (LAM), and mycobacterial cell entry protein (Mcep) encoded by mce1A*

ATYPICAL MYCOBACTERIAL PNEUMONIA

Clinical Features

- Atypical mycobacterial infection is important in AIDS and other immunosuppressed patients, older persons with or without underlying lung disease, and patients with CF
- The most common atypical mycobacterial agent of human infection is *Mycobacterium avium* complex (MAC)
- MAC infections tend to occur late in the course of AIDS
- The portal of entry is most likely the gastrointestinal tract
- MAC can be cultured from lungs, lymph nodes, spleen, liver, bone marrow, and gastrointestinal tract

Gross Pathology

- Cavitary lesions in the upper lobes, similar to pulmonary tuberculosis, are seen in about 90% of HIV patients with *Mycobacterium kansasii* infection and in perhaps 50% of HIV patients with MAC infection

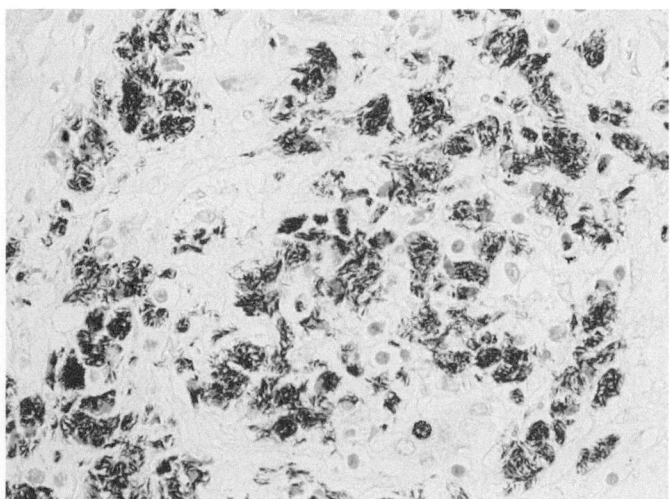

Figure 4-29. Atypical mycobacterial pneumonia. Acid-fast stain demonstrates numerous bright pink intracellular organisms, which can be easily seen in this biopsy specimen from an AIDS patient.

- About 50% patients with MAC lung disease have nodules associated with bronchiectasis, which occur most frequently in the right middle lobe and lingula

Histopathology

- Similar to that seen in ordinary tuberculosis, necrotizing granulomatous inflammation is the most common feature
- Non-necrotizing granulomas are often present as well
- In AIDS and other immunocompromised patients, there may be a nonspecific inflammatory reaction composed of poorly organized histiocytic infiltrates, acute and chronic inflammation, fibrosis, and organizing pneumonia

Special Stains and Immunohistochemistry

- Organisms appear as long, thin, beaded, red bacilli on acid-fast stains (Figure 4-29)
- Immunohistochemical methods using antibody for *Mycobacterium tuberculosis* are sensitive and specific

Other Techniques for Diagnosis

- Auramine-rhodamine fluorescent stain outlines the organisms in sputum and tissue

Differential Diagnosis

- Other granulomatous infections, sarcoidosis

PEARLS

- *The ATS diagnostic criteria for nontuberculous mycobacterial infections include both imaging studies consistent with pulmonary disease and recurrent isolation of mycobacteria from sputum or bronchial wash in a symptomatic patient*
- *Other* Mycobacterium *species that cause lung disease include* M. abscessus, M. fortuitum, M. xenopi, M. malmoense, M. szulgai, M. simiae, *and* M. asiatica
- *Pulmonary disease due to rapidly growing mycobacteria (RGM) is predominantly due to* M. abscessus *(80% of cases) and* M. fortuitum *(15% of cases)*

SELECTED REFERENCES (BACTERIAL PNEUMONIA)

American Thoracic Society; Infectious Diseases Society of America: Guidelines for the management of adults with hospital-acquired, ventilator-associated, and healthcare-associated pneumonia. Am J Respir Crit Care Med 171:388-416, 2005.

Marrie TJ, Costain N, La Scola B, et al: The role of atypical pathogens in community-acquired pneumonia. Semin Respir Crit Care Med 33:244-256, 2012.

Nair GB, Niederman MS: Community-acquired pneumonia: an unfinished battle. Med Clin North Am 95:1143-1161, 2011.

Wunderink RG, Niederman MS: Update in respiratory infections 2011. Am J Respir Crit Care Med 185:1261-1265, 2012.

Fungal
ASPERGILLOSIS

- See Table 4-7

Clinical Features

- Pulmonary aspergillosis is usually caused by *Aspergillus fumigatus*, *Aspergillus niger*, or *Aspergillus flavus*
- Hemoptysis is frequently reported and can be so massive as to be life threatening
- Patterns of pulmonary aspergillosis
  - Colonization of preexisting cavities in the lung (fungus ball)
  - Hypersensitivity reaction: allergic bronchopulmonary aspergillosis, eosinophilic pneumonia, bronchocentric granulomatosis, and hypersensitivity pneumonia
  - Invasive: acute invasive aspergillosis, necrotizing pseudomembranous tracheobronchitis, chronic necrotizing aspergillosis, bronchopleural fistula

Gross Pathology

- Areas of hemorrhage and necrosis with consolidation or cavitation

TABLE 4-7	**DIFFERENTIAL DIAGNOSIS OF HYPHAL FUNGI**			
	Aspergillus Species	*Zygomycetes Species*	*Fusarium Species*	*Pseudalleschera boydii*
Width	3-6 μm	5-25 μm	3-8 μm	2-5 μm
Outline	Parallel	Irregular	Parallel	Parallel
Branching pattern	Dichotomous* Acute angle	Haphazard, > 90-degree angle	Right angle, occasionally 45 degrees	Haphazard
Septation	Frequent	Inconspicuous	Frequent	Frequent

*Dichotomous indicates that the daughter branch is the same width as the parental branch.

- Fungal balls are friable, brown to red lesions ranging in size from 1 to 7 cm that are loosely associated with the cavity wall
- Target lesion: nodular pulmonary infarct with central pale necrotic zone surrounded by a hemorrhagic rim or infarct

Histopathology

- Usual form is hyphae; conidial heads form rarely where organism is exposed to air
- Splendore-Hoeppli phenomenon: radiating eosinophilic material at edges of fungal masses
- Classic tissue reaction is in the form of a hemorrhagic infarct with sparse inflammatory infiltrate that evolves into necrotizing pneumonia
- Fungal hyphae are found invading blood vessel walls and permeating alveolar septae (Figure 4-30)
- Fungal emboli can completely occlude vessels, causing the so-called target lesion

Special Stains and Immunohistochemistry

- Gomorri-methanamine silver (GMS) and periodic acid Schiff (PAS) highlight fungal structures

Other Techniques for Diagnosis

- PCR methods available in reference laboratories for identification

Differential Diagnosis

- Other fungal infections: zygomycosis and *Candida, Fusarium,* and *Penicillium* species
- Allergic bronchopulmonary aspergillosis
  - Hypersensitivity reaction that occurs mostly in patients with CF or asthma due to colonization with *Aspergillus* species
  - Mucoid impaction of the bronchi and eosinophilic pneumonia
- Bronchocentric granulomatosis (BCG)
  - BCG represents a histopathologic pattern of injury secondary to infectious or noninfectious etiology (e.g., allergy)

- Necrotizing granulomatous inflammation destroys the walls of small bronchi and bronchioles
- Palisading histiocytic reaction replaces the airway wall

ZYGOMYCOSIS

Clinical Features

- Uncommon opportunistic fungal infection is most commonly due to *Rhizopus* species acquired through spore inhalation
- Patients present with fever, cough, chest pain, dyspnea, and hemoptysis, which can be massive
- Infection begins in the nasal turbinates and then spreads to the orbits, brain, or lungs
- Mortality rate due to infection or hemoptysis usually exceeds 50%
- Almost all cases of zygomycosis occur in the presence of some underlying condition: diabetes mellitus, hematologic malignancies (neutropenia), organ transplantation (immunosuppressive therapy), broad-spectrum antibiotic therapy, severe malnutrition, and skin or mucosal lesions secondary to burns, trauma, or surgical incisions

Gross Pathology

- Diffuse pneumonia with infarction and necrosis
- Direct extension to the mediastinum, pericardium, and heart

Histopathology

- Cross-sectioned hyphae are round or oval with clear centers
- Rare chlamydoconidium forms when the organism is exposed to air
- Zygomycetes are angioinvasive, and infarcts are a hallmark of infection
- Granulomatous vasculitis is occasionally present

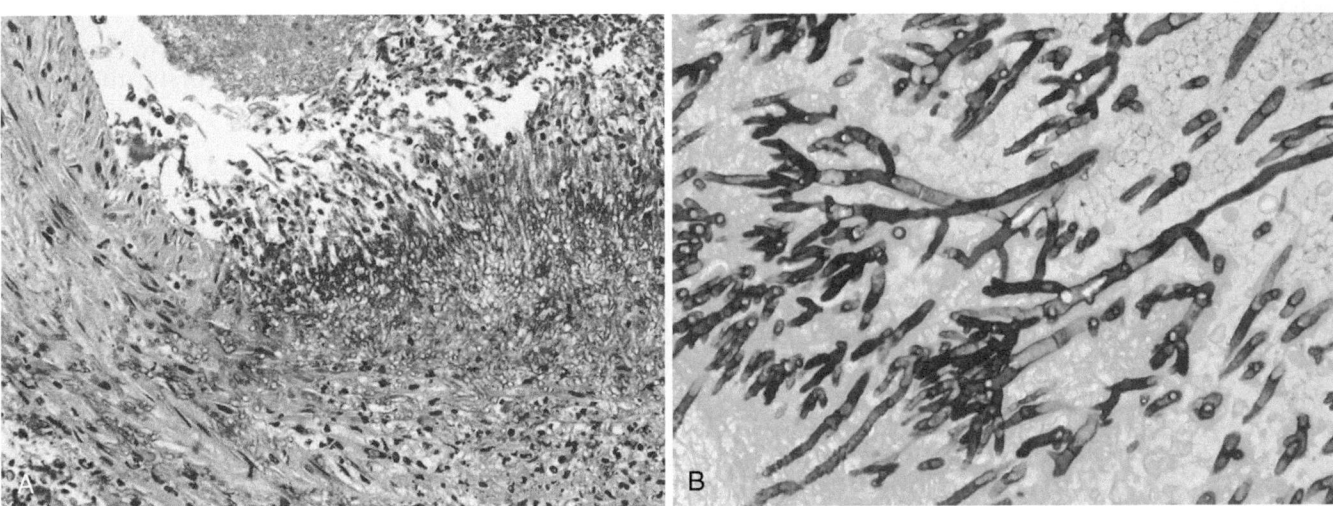

Figure 4-30. Aspergillosis. A, Radiating arrangement of fungal hyphae invading through arterial wall can be easily seen on H&E stain. **B,** GMS stain shows characteristic septate hyphae with parallel walls and acute angle branching.

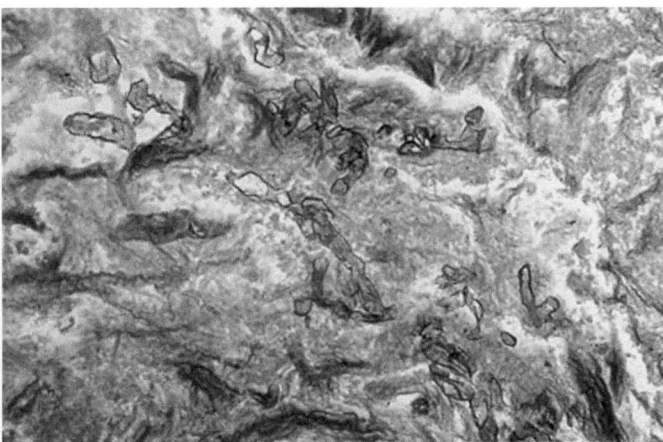

Figure 4-31. Zygomycosis. GMS stain shows broad wavy ribbon-like hyphae, some with 90-degree branching.

Special Stains and Immunohistochemistry

- Organisms can be identified with GMS and PAS stains (Figure 4-31)

Other Techniques for Diagnosis

- PCR methods available in reference laboratories for identification

Differential Diagnosis

- See Table 4-7

PEARLS

- *The term* zygomycosis *is more precise than the commonly used term* mucormycosis *because other members of this class of fungi cause infection*
- *Ketone reductase is produced by the organism and allows it to survive in high-glucose, acidic conditions (e.g., diabetic ketoacidosis)*
- *Iron availability is crucial for the growth of Zygomycetes species, and paradoxically, deferoxamine increases susceptibility to zygomycosis—perhaps by functioning as a siderophore for the fungi*
- *Rhinocerebral and pulmonary zygomycosis is acquired through spore inhalation*

HISTOPLASMOSIS

- See Table 4-8

Clinical Features

- Dimorphic, soil-dwelling fungus
- Most infected persons show few or no symptoms
- Acute pulmonary histoplasmosis
  - Self-limited illness in young children exposed to the fungus for the first time
  - Acute, severe pulmonary infection following exposure to a large inoculum of *Histoplasma capsulatum* with clinical manifestations similar to ARDS
- Disseminated histoplasmosis
  - Frequently occurs in patients with underlying immune dysfunction (infants; patients with AIDS, hematologic malignancy, immunosuppressive therapy, congenital T-cell deficiency)
- Chronic pulmonary histoplasmosis
  - Most patients are adults with some form of underlying lung disease (e.g., emphysema)
  - Patients can develop chronic, cavitary lesions

Gross Pathology

- Pathology varies from chronic fibrocavitary lesions with hilar lymphadenopathy to circumscribed, solitary fibrocaseous nodules with concentric, calcified lamellae (tree-barking) to miliary nodules (buckshot appearance)

Histopathology

- Narrow-based budding yeast with one blunt end and one pointed end (i.e., pear-shaped), often found in clusters
- Budding forms are relatively difficult to find, and hyphal forms are incredibly rare
- Necrotizing granulomatous inflammation occurs in the setting of chronic infection
- Granulomas are well circumscribed with a thick fibrous capsule, are not infrequently calcified (Figure 4-32A), and have necrotic central areas, which are the best place to find organisms
- Clusters of organisms are found within foamy macrophages in the immunocompromised

TABLE 4-8	**DIFFERENTIAL DIAGNOSIS OF YEASTLIKE FUNGI**					
	Coccidioides immitis	*Histoplasma capsulatum*	*Cryptococcus neoformans*	*Blastomyces dermatitidis*	*Candida Species*	*Torulopsis glabrata*
Size	Spherules: 30-100 μm Endospores: 2-5 μm	2-4 μm	2-20 μm	8-15 μm	2-6 μm	2-5 μm
Shape	Round to oval	Round to oval, pear-shaped	Round to oval	Round to oval	Round to oval	Round to oval
Budding	Endosporulation	Single, narrow based	Single to multiple, narrow based	Single, broad based	Single, chains, narrow based	Single, narrow based
Cell wall	Thin	Thin	Thick mucinous capsule	Thick, refractile	Thin	Thin
Hyphae, pseudohyphae	Rare	Rare	Rare	Rare	Pseudohyphae and rare true hyphae	None
Nuclei	Single	Single	Single	Multiple	Single	Single
Mucicarmine staining	Negative	Negative	Positive	Negative	Negative	Negative

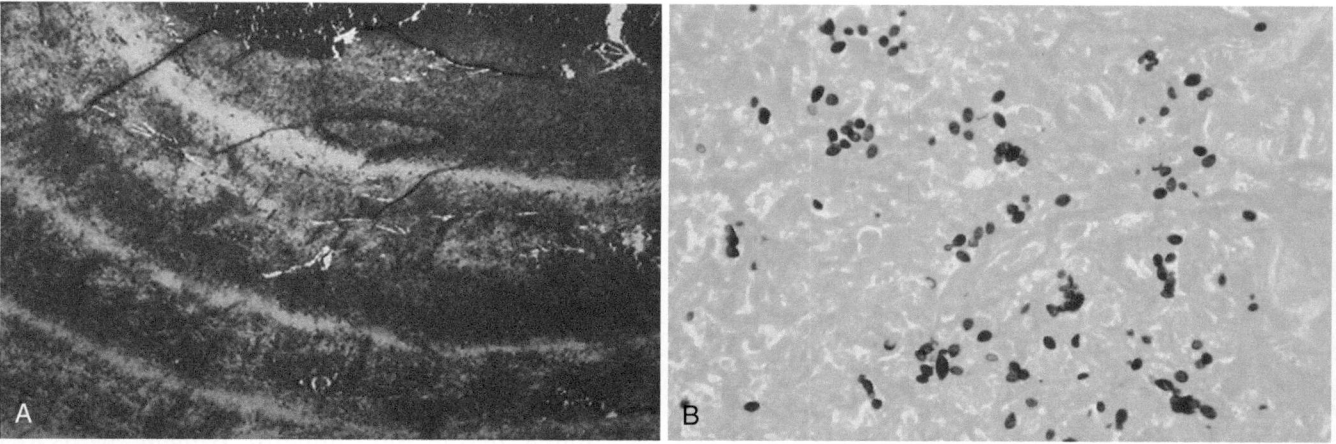

Figure 4-32. Histoplasmosis. A, Low-power photomicrograph of an H&E-stained section shows circular deposits of calcium in the granuloma (tree-bark appearance). **B,** GMS stain shows small pear-shaped yeasts that are pointed at one end and rounded at the other. Occasional budding yeasts can also be seen.

Special Stains and Immunohistochemistry

- GMS is the best stain to identify *Histoplasma* species (Figure 4-32B)

Other Techniques for Diagnosis

- Direct immunofluorescence on histologic sections can assist with the diagnosis

Differential Diagnosis

- See Table 4-8 and (Figure 4-33)

PEARLS

- *In the United States, histoplasmosis is most common in the Midwest within the Ohio and Mississippi River valleys, where more than 80% of young adults have been previously infected*
- *Histoplasmosis has a predilection for elderly patients, likely because of the association of histoplasmosis with emphysema*

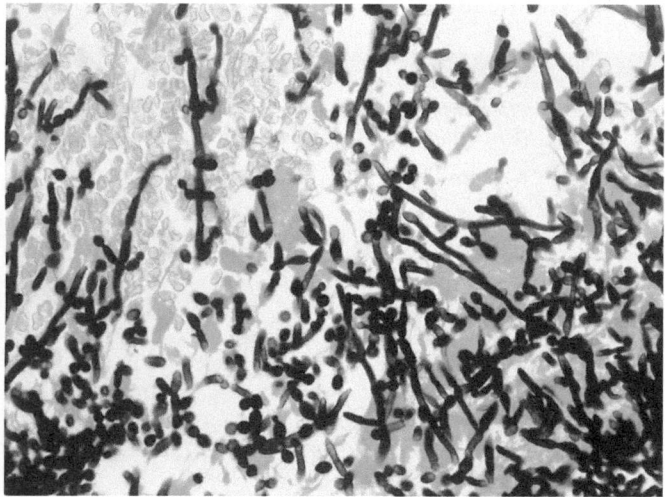

Figure 4-33. Candidiasis. GMS stain shows budding yeasts and pseudohyphae. Note sausage-link appearance caused by pinching in of the wall.

- *Granulomatous mediastinitis is a complication of pulmonary infection with massive enlargement of multiple nodes that are often matted and undergo caseous necrosis*
- *Mediastinal fibrosis is a rare, frequently lethal complication of pulmonary histoplasmosis affecting younger patients 20 to 40 years old*
- *Pericarditis, pleural disease, and broncholithiasis are additional rare complications*

COCCIDIOIDOMYCOSIS

Clinical Features

- Dimorphic fungus is endemic to the southwestern United States and Central America and causes granulomatous disease in humans
- Primary pulmonary coccidioidomycosis is usually asymptomatic, subclinical, and self-limited
- Patients who develop clinically apparent pulmonary disease show a range of pathologic findings: acute pneumonia; eosinophilic pneumonia; solitary pulmonary nodule; chronic progressive infection with fibrocavitary lesions, bronchopleural fistula, or empyema
- Disseminated disease shows miliary or extrapulmonary dissemination

Gross Pathology

ACUTE COCCIDIOIDOMYCOSIS

- Patchy, unilateral parenchymal consolidations that are often perihilar or in lower lobes
- Multifocal, peripheral, subpleural nodules or masses

PERSISTENT PULMONARY COCCIDIOIDOMYCOSIS

- Pulmonary nodules typically develop in areas of previous consolidation
  - Single, peripheral, spherical, and well-delineated
- Single, thin-walled cavitary lesions occur in a subset of patients
  - Upper lobe predominance
  - May rupture into pleural cavity, resulting in bronchopleural fistula or pneumothorax

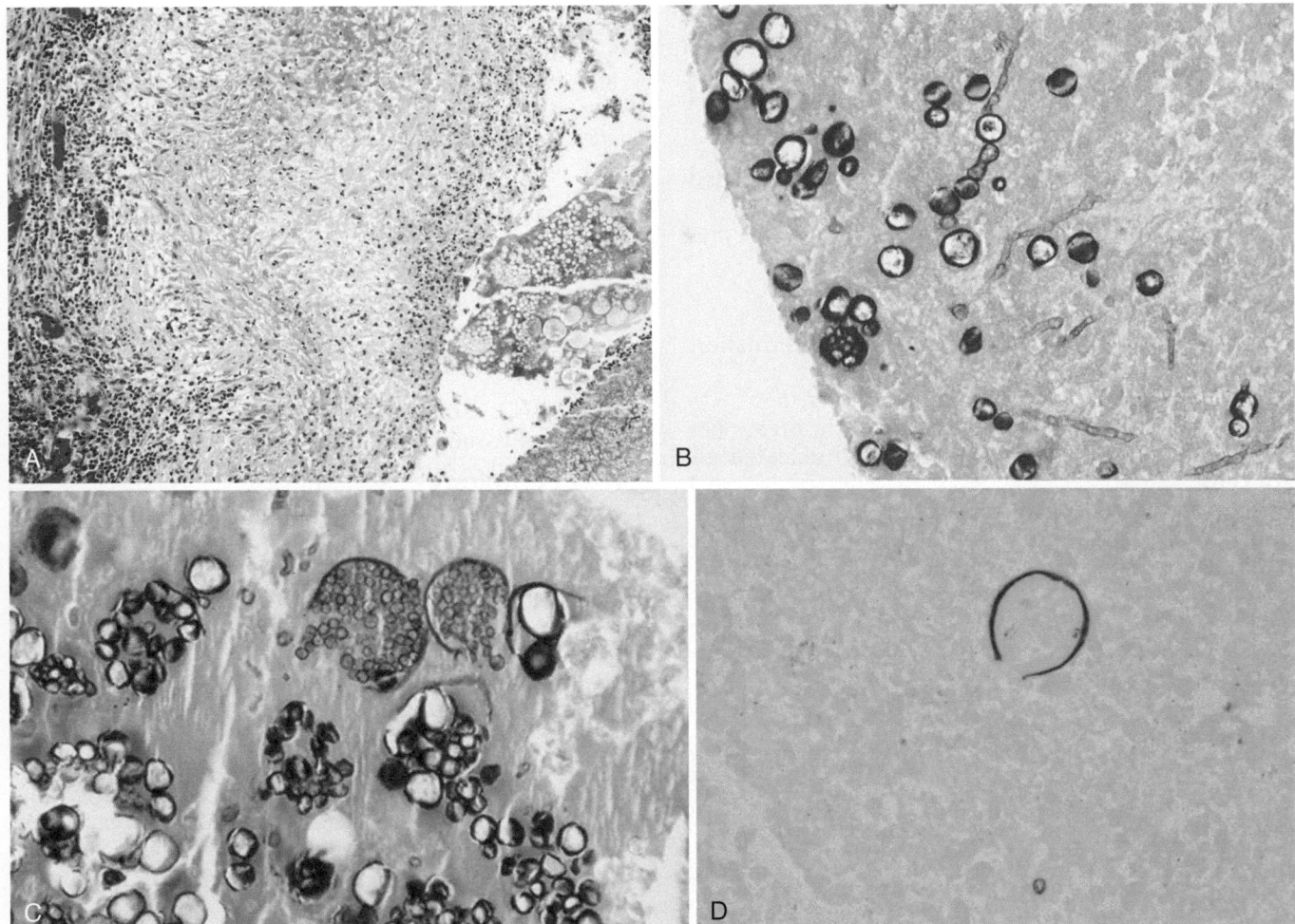

Figure 4-34. Coccidioidomycosis. **A,** A necrotizing granuloma with multiple organisms (*right side*) is seen in this medium-power photomicrograph of an H&E-stained section. **B,** On periodic acid–Schiff stain, large spherules and hyphae are stained pink. **C,** On GMS stain, large spherules and numerous endospores are stained black. **D,** GMS stain showing only the ruptured spherule.

CHRONIC PROGRESSIVE COCCIDIOIDOMYCOSIS
- Unilateral or bilateral apical consolidations with occasional cavitation

Histopathology
- Grossly apparent pulmonary nodules typically correspond with necrotizing granulomas (Figure 4-34)
- Organisms likely to be found within neutrophilic infiltrates or necrotic zones
- Immature spherules, mature spherules, and endospores are present in the biopsy tissue
- Immature spherules lack endospores and are PAS positive
- Mature spherules possess a thick, refractile wall that is either lined or filled with endospores (diagnostic feature)
- Endospores are mononuclear with punctate, PAS-positive, cytoplasmic inclusions
- Mycelia can be observed in aerated cavitary lesions or bronchopleural fistulas

Special Stains and Immunohistochemistry
- PAS and GMS stains help identify the organisms

Other Techniques for Diagnosis
- Noncontributory

Differential Diagnosis
- See Table 4-8

PEARLS

- *Cutaneous manifestations of pulmonary coccidioidomycosis include erythema nodosum and erythema multiforme and occur in about 20% of patients, typically young white women*

BLASTOMYCOSIS

Clinical Features
- Blastomycosis occurs predominantly in the Mississippi, Missouri, and Ohio River valleys, as well as the Great Lakes region and the southeastern United States
- Patients present with no history of antecedent infection, or blastomycosis can develop months to years after an episode of acute pulmonary blastomycosis

- Patients present with cough, high temperature, arthralgias, and myalgias
- Extrapulmonary spread to bone and skin can occur
- It is much more common in immunosuppressed patients

Gross Pathology

- Pleural involvement is common and often associated with pleural effusions
- Bilateral, patchy parenchymal consolidations have predilection for posterior lower lobes

Histopathology

- Intense neutrophilic infiltrates with abscess formation is the initial response (Figure 4-35A)
- Necrotizing granulomatous inflammation ensues
- Organisms can be identified in necrotic areas, between the inflammation, and in multinucleated giant cells
- Large aggregates of organisms form in cases of disseminated infection, forming so-called yeast lakes, with minimal associated inflammation

Special Stains and Immunohistochemistry

- GMS and PAS stains adequately demonstrate the organisms (Figure 4-35B)

OTHER TECHNIQUES FOR DIAGNOSIS

- Noncontributory

Differential Diagnosis

- See Table 4-8

PEARLS

- *Pulmonary blastomycosis can present virtually identically to bacterial pneumonia, tuberculosis, histoplasmosis, ARDS, or lung carcinoma*
- *Blastomycosis can form nodules or masses that are radiographically indistinguishable from primary*

- *pulmonary malignancy, particularly if hilar or mediastinal lymphadenopathy is present*
- *Blastomycoses dermatitidis can take 4 to 5 weeks to culture, so prompt histologic diagnosis can have a big effect on patient management*

CRYPTOCOCCOSIS

Clinical Features

- Pulmonary lesions of cryptococcosis are usually clinically and radiographically silent
- Severe disease occurs only in immunosuppressed patients
- Diagnosis is established by culture or histologic examination of tissue or BAL fluid

Gross Pathology

- Focal parenchymal consolidation with a gelatinous cut surface

Histopathology

- Capsule-deficient forms are typically encountered in immunocompetent hosts
- Histologic reaction can be minimal with organisms filling in alveolar spaces
- Fibrohistiocytic reaction accompanies numerous, densely packed organisms, mimicking lipoid pneumonia
- Granulomatous inflammation with fibrosis occurs in immunocompetent patients with organisms found within giant cells and macrophages

Special Stains and Immunohistochemistry

- GMS stain identifies all forms of the organism
- Mucicarmine, Alcian blue, and PAS (diastase resistant) stain the mucinous capsule (Figure 4-36)

Other Techniques for Diagnosis

- PCR methods available in reference laboratories for identification

---

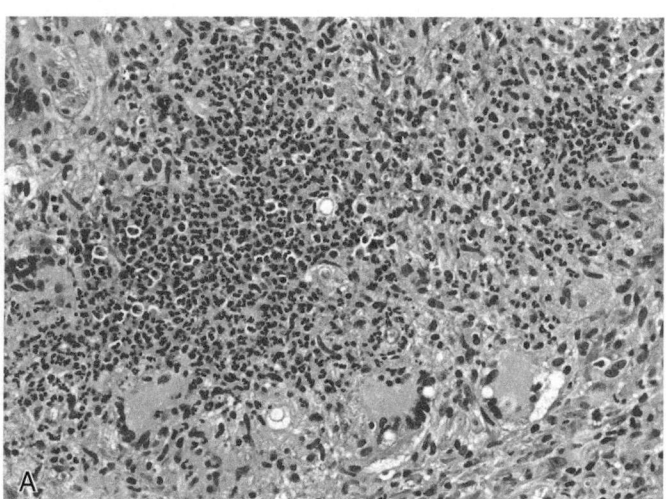 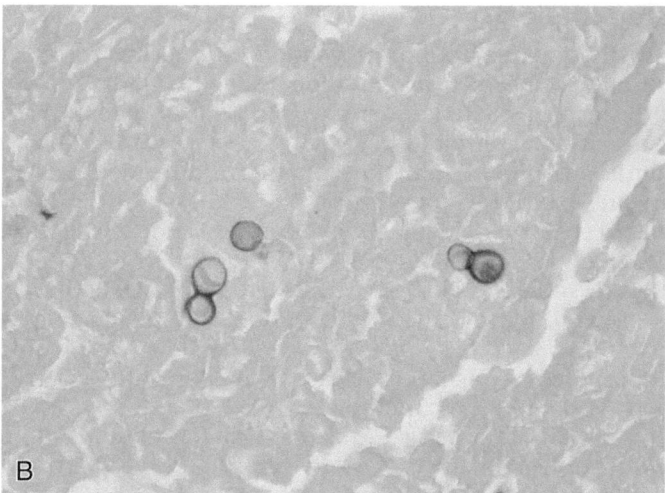

Figure 4-35. Blastomycosis. A, Within the mixed inflammatory infiltrate (granulomatous and neutrophilic), large budding yeasts can be seen on H&E. **B,** GMS stain shows broad-based budding yeasts.

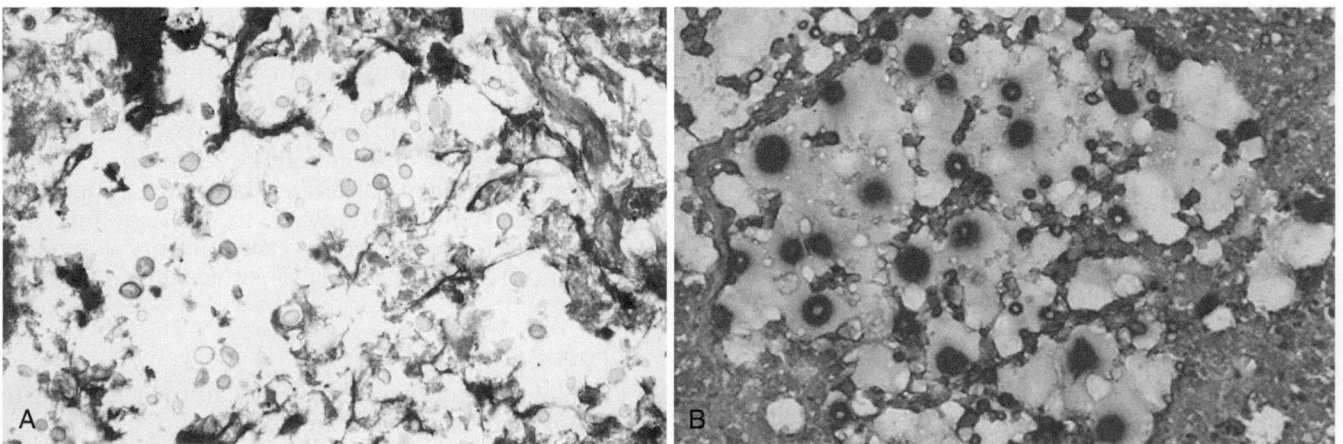

Figure 4-36. Cryptococcosis. A, H&E stain of this endobronchial biopsy shows numerous yeasts with no inflammatory response. **B,** Mucicarmine stain demonstrates thick mucinous capsules, which stain bright red.

Differential Diagnosis

• See Table 4-8

PEARLS

• *Although the lung is the most likely initial portal of entry and infection, disseminated foci with a normal chest radiograph can be seen*

PNEUMOCYSTIS JIROVECI PNEUMONIA (PCP OR PJP)

Clinical Features

• Pneumocystis is one of the major causes of opportunistic fungal pneumonia in immunocompromised patients
• Four clinical forms: asymptomatic infections, infantile pneumonia, pneumonia in immunocompromised hosts, and extrapulmonary infections
• Infantile pneumonia typically presents as an epidemic in malnourished or premature children
• Extrapulmonary infections result from dissemination from lungs to other organs, such as lymph nodes, spleen, bone marrow, liver, kidneys, heart, brain, pancreas, and skin

Gross Pathology

• Bilateral alveolar and interstitial infiltrates radiating out from the hilum on CT

Histopathology

• Alveoli are filled with frothy, acellular, eosinophilic, proteinaceous material
• The material is composed of masses of cysts and trophozoites, desquamated alveolar cells, alveolar macrophages, and few inflammatory cells (Figure 4-37)
• Multiple morphologic forms of *Pneumocystic jiroveci*
  ○ Trophozoites are pleomorphic, measure 2 to 4 μm, and conjugate to produce a diploid zygote that develops into a cyst
  ○ Cysts are spherical when they contain sporozoites; empty cysts are indented or cup shaped
  ○ Up to eight intracystic sporozoites measuring 1 to 2 μm develop within the cysts and are subsequently released and go on to develop into trophic forms
• Less common reactions to *Pneumocystis* species include granulomas, infarcts, giant cells, interstitial fibrosis, and interstitial plasma cell infiltrates

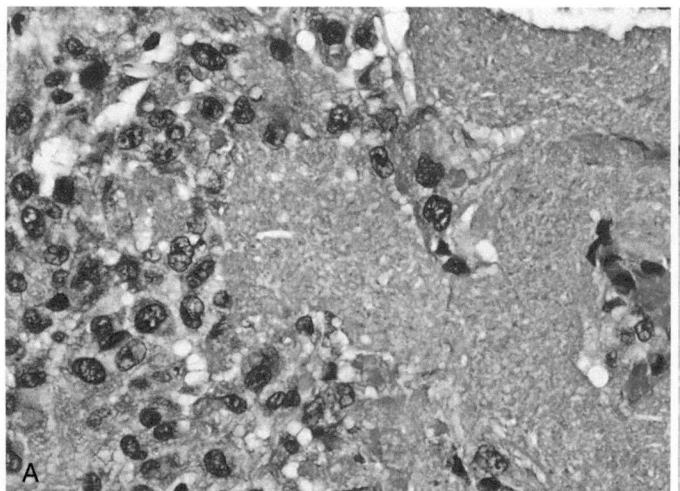
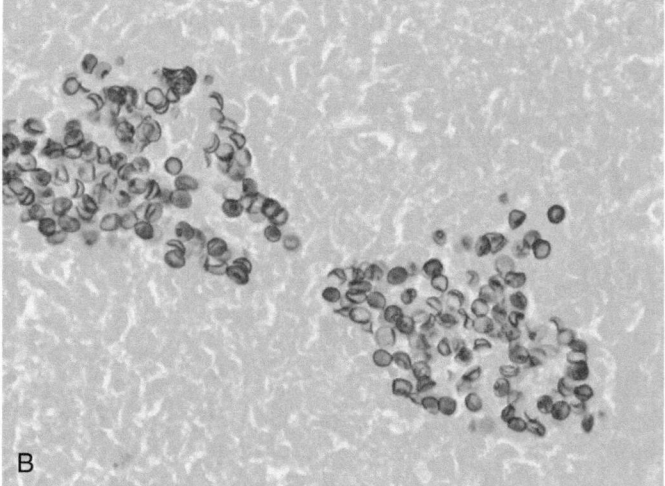

Figure 4-37. Pneumocystis jiroveci pneumonia. A, H&E-stained section shows eosinophilic frothy acellular intra-alveolar exudate characteristic of *Pneumocystis* pneumonia. **B,** GMS stains the cysts black. Some cysts are round to oval with dotlike structures, and some are helmet-shaped.

Special Stains and Immunohistochemistry

- GMS stain is most useful to demonstrate the cyst forms, which stain black or brown; cysts often contain dark bodies or dots, which correspond to focal thickening of cyst wall and should not be confused with sporozoites
- Toluidine blue stains the cyst wall blue and also stains fungal elements
- Giemsa, Wright, and Wright-Giemsa (Diff-Quik) dyes stain the trophozoites and intracystic sporozoites pale blue with a punctate red nucleus; these dyes do not stain the cyst forms

Other Techniques for Diagnosis

- Monoclonal immunofluorescent antibodies recognize the cyst wall and have increased specificity compared with other staining methods
- PCR targets include mitochondrial 23S rRNA (mtLSUrRNA) and internal transcribed spacers (ITS), which have higher sensitivity than methods targeting cytoplasmic 5S rRNA and dihydrofolate reductase (DHFR) regions

Differential Diagnosis

- DAD
- Histoplasmosis

PEARLS

- *Coinfection with other organisms (e.g., CMV) occurs, particularly in immunosuppressed patients*
- *Pneumocystis microbes are classified as fungi on the basis of rRNA and mitochondrial sequence homologies*
- *Pneumocystis jiroveci is the organism that infects humans and causes PCP, whereas Pneumocystis carinii is found in rats*
- *PCP is the most common cause of pneumothorax in patients with HIV*
- *Highest incidence of PCP in HIV-infected children is in the first year of life, with peak incidence at ages 3 to 6 months and often accompanied by a significant lymphoplasmacytic interstitial infiltrate*

SELECTED REFERENCES (FUNGAL PNEUMONIA)

Gigliotti F, Wright TW: Pneumocystis: where does it live? PLoS Pathog 8:e1003025, 2012.

Husain AN: Fungal pneumonia. In Thoracic Pathology. Philadelphia, Elsevier, 2012, pp 181-198.

Limper AH, Knox KS, Sarosi GA, et al: American Thoracic Society Fungal Working Group. An official American Thoracic Society statement: Treatment of fungal infections in adult pulmonary and critical care patients. Am J Respir Crit Care Med 183:96-128, 2011.

SURGICAL COMPLICATIONS

LUNG TRANSPLANTATION

Clinical Features

- Early complications include acute rejection, bacterial infection, pulmonary edema, acute respiratory distress syndrome (ARDS), diffuse alveolar hemorrhage
- Patients are evaluated for these complications with transbronchial biopsy and BAL

- Acute cellular rejection typically occurs within the first 3 to 6 months; however, the earliest manifestations of rejection can occur within the first week or years later
- More than 80% of lung transplant recipients experience an episode of acute cellular rejection
- It can be difficult to differentiate acute cellular rejection from infection owing to overlapping clinical findings; reduction of forced expiratory volume in 1 second (FEV_1) is the most sensitive clinical finding for rejection

Gross Pathology

- Radiologic findings range from normal to interstitial pulmonary edema and are nonspecific

Histopathology

- See Table 4-9
- Transbronchial biopsy should yield at least three to five tissue fragments, and ideally more than 100 alveoli and one bronchiole should be present
- Acute rejection
  - Lymphoid infiltration of the airways often accompanies acute rejection in the form of lymphocytic bronchitis and bronchiolitis (Figure 4-38)
  - However, lymphocytic bronchitis or bronchiolitis can occur in the absence of parenchymal acute rejection
- Airway inflammation
- Bronchiolitis obliterans (BO, chronic rejection): deposition of bland fibrous tissue within the submucosa of bronchioles in either a concentric or eccentric fashion; consequently, the airway lumen becomes narrowed
- Usually develops at the end of the first year or later; 50% of patients show evidence of bronchiolitis obliterans at 5 years

Special Stains and Immunohistochemistry

- CMV stain is most helpful; GMS and AFB stains are used when histology suggests infection
- Elastic or trichrome stains may be helpful in the workup of chronic rejection

Other Techniques for Diagnosis

- Noncontributory

Differential Diagnosis

- Infection
  - Perivascular lymphoid infiltrates also occur in the setting of CMV and *Pneumocystis* species infection
- Posttransplantation lymphoproliferative disorder

PEARLS

- *Minimal acute rejection is treated only when the patient is symptomatic, whereas mild rejection is treated regardless of symptoms*
- *BO is the hallmark of chronic rejection; however, biopsy is not required for diagnosis of bronchiolitis obliterans syndrome, which is based on irreversible deterioration of lung function tests*

TABLE 4-9	**GRADING SCHEME FOR TRANSPLANT REJECTION**
Rejection Grade	**Histologic Findings**
A0	No evidence of mononuclear leukocyte infiltration, hemorrhage, or necrosis
A1	Perivascular or perivenular lymphoid cuffing
	Difficult to observe at low-power microscopy
	Density of lymphoid cells should be at least two cell layers thick
A2	Perivascular infiltrate expands and becomes easier to detect at low-power microscopy (more than three cell layers)
	Rare eosinophils, but not neutrophils, may be seen
A3	Expansion of the mononuclear infiltrate into perivascular and peribronchiolar alveolar interstitium
	Neutrophils may be apparent
	Endothelialitis, a subendothelial infiltration along with reactive or hyperplastic endothelial changes, is occasionally present
A4	Diffuse infiltrates extending from the perivascular areas to the pulmonary interstitium
	Diffuse alveolar damage with hyaline membranes, parenchymal necrosis, and hemorrhage
	Neutrophils may be seen in small numbers
B0	No airway inflammation
B1	Minimal airway inflammation
B2	Circumferential band of mononuclear cells with occasional eosinophils within the submucosa of bronchi or bronchioles
B3	Expansion of the infiltrate into a dense, bandlike process composed of mononuclear leukocytes, activated lymphocytes, and eosinophils
	Satellitosis of lymphocytes and epithelial cell necrosis
B4	Severe airway inflammation composed of dense bands of mononuclear leukocytes with ulceration of the airway epithelium
	Fibropurulent exudates containing neutrophils and necrotic debris

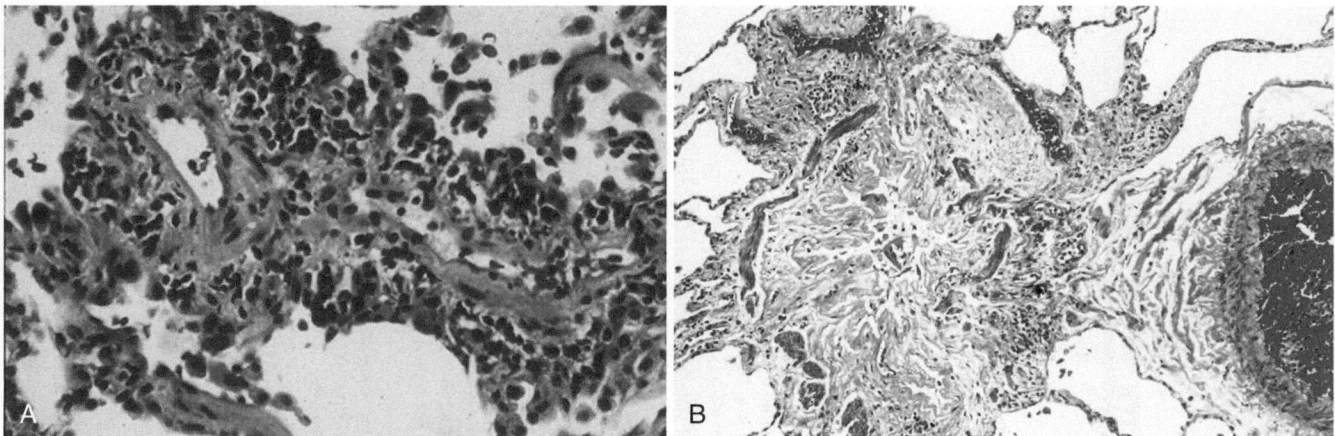

Figure 4-38. A, Acute rejection in lung transplantation. There is a complete cuff of inflammatory cells (predominantly lymphocytes) more than three layers thick around the pulmonary arteriole (grade A2). **B,** Chronic rejection in lung transplantation. There is near-total occlusion of the bronchiole by submucosal fibrosis. Note the residual discontinuous smooth muscle of the bronchiole in contrast to the adjacent artery.

SELECTED REFERENCE

Husain AN: Lung transplantation. In Thoracic Pathology. Philadelphia, Elsevier, 2012, pp 208-214.

NEOPLASTIC CONDITIONS

BENIGN EPITHELIAL TUMORS

- See Table 4-10

Preinvasive Epithelial Lesions
SQUAMOUS DYSPLASIA (SD) AND SQUAMOUS CARCINOMA IN SITU (SCIS)

Clinical Features

- Relatively common, centrally localized lesion occurs in large airways of patients with history of cigarette smoke exposure

- SD/SCIS is almost always asymptomatic
- Most patients have a previous high-grade preinvasive lesion, a history of lung or head and neck cancer, or synchronous lung cancer

Gross Pathology

- Difficult to detect grossly or bronchoscopically
- Detection is facilitated by autofluorescence bronchoscopy (AFB)
- About 75% of lesions are flat or superficial; 25% are nodular or polypoid
- CIS usually arises near bifurcations in segmental bronchi

Histopathology

- Often multifocal lesions ranging from 1 to 3 mm (SD) to 4 to 12 mm (SCIS)
- Four histologic grades: mild, moderate, and severe dysplasia, and SCIS

TABLE 4-10	DIAGNOSTIC FEATURES OF BENIGN EPITHELIAL NEOPLASMS				
	Juvenile Laryngotracheal Papillomatosis and Squamous Cell Papilloma (Figure 4-39)	Alveolar Adenoma	Papillary Adenoma	Mucous Gland Adenoma	Mucinous Cystadenoma
Clinical features	Rare primary lung tumor (<0.5%) Associated with human papillomavirus- 6 and -11 Obstructive symptoms	Rare Most cases are asymptomatic	Rare Most cases are asymptomatic	Extremely rare Patients complain of obstructive symptoms	Extraordinarily rare
Gross findings	Arise from main bronchus Exophytic, cauliflower-like papillary projection into lumina, 0.7 to 9 cm (mean, 1.5 cm)	Most tumors are peripheral or subpleural, 0.7 to 6 cm Well-demarcated, smooth, lobulated, multicystic, yellow-tan lesions	Well-defined, soft, spongy to firm, gray-white to brown lesion, 1 to 4 cm	White-pink to tan, smooth, gelatinous, mucoid, solid or cystic, cut surface, 0.7 to 7.5 cm	Unilocular, mucus-filled cyst, 1 to 5 cm Thin cyst walls (0.1 cm)
Histology	Loose fibrovascular cores covered by stratified squamous epithelium 20% show koilocyte-like cytologic atypia	Unencapsulated, multicystic lesions Lined by bland, flattened, cuboidal, and hobnailed cells Cystic spaces are larger centrally and filled with eosinophilic fluid and periodic acid–Schiff–positive granular debris Squamous metaplasia	Well-circumscribed Papillary growth with fibrovascular cores lined by cuboidal or columnar cells Ciliated or oxyphilic cells can also be found Intracellular mucin, atypia, and mitoses are rare to absent	Circumscribed, exophytic nodules Mucin-filled cystic spaces, microacini, glands, tubules, and papillae Cysts lined by bland flat, cuboidal or columnar mucus-producing cells	Mucinous cystic lesion lined by discontinuous layer of cuboidal or columnar mucinous cells Basal, hyperchromatic nuclei Multinucleated giant cell associated with extravasated mucin
Differential diagnosis	Squamous cell carcinoma shows invasion and malignant cytology Juvenile laryngotracheal papillomatosis rarely involves the lower respiratory tract	Lymphangioma Sclerosing hemangioma Adenocarcinoma Bronchioloalveolar carcinoma Primary or metastatic spindle cell tumor	Sclerosing hemangioma Alveolar adenoma Papillary adenocarcinoma Primary lung Metastatic thyroid	Low-grade mucoepidermoid carcinoma Mucinous cystadenoma Adenocarcinoma	Mucinous cystadenocarcinoma, adenocarcinoma, colloid bronchioloalveolar carcinoma, mucinous congenital pulmonary airway malformation Bronchogenic cyst

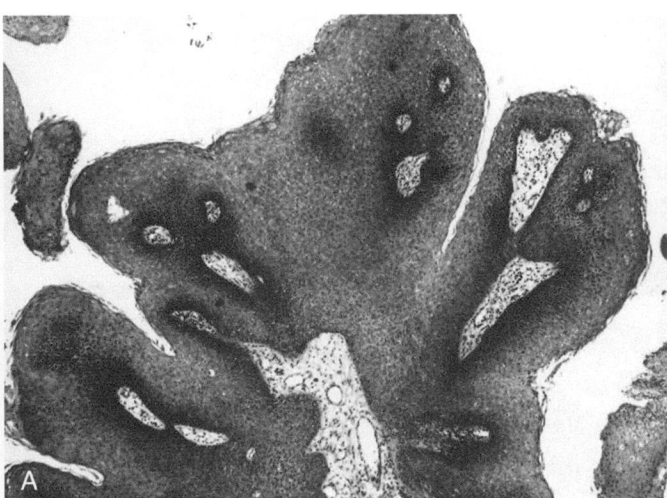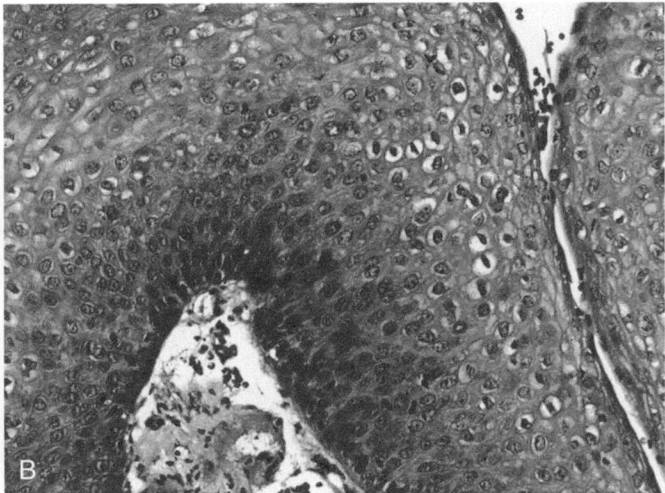

Figure 4-39. Squamous papilloma. A, Low-power photomicrograph shows a papillary lesion composed of acanthotic squamous epithelium with fibrovascular cores. **B,** At higher power, human papillomavirus–related changes (koilocytes) are seen in the upper layers of the squamous epithelium (*right side*).

- Severe dysplasia shows cytologic atypia (increased cell size and pleomorphism) and mitoses extending to the upper third of the epithelium
- SCIS shows extreme atypia without maturation extending to the surface and replacing the entire thickness of the epithelium

Special Stains and Immunohistochemistry

- Noncontributory

Other Techniques for Diagnosis

- Noncontributory

Differential Diagnosis

BASAL CELL HYPERPLASIA (BCH)
- BCH shows more than three layers of basal cells in otherwise normal pseudostratified columnar respiratory-type epithelium

SQUAMOUS METAPLASIA (SM)
- SM likely arises from BCH
- Found in chronic inflammatory conditions

REACTIVE ATYPIA OF INFLAMMATION, INFECTION, AND CHEMORADIATION
- Reactive lesions show hypercellularity but lack the cytologic dysplasia

INVASIVE CARCINOMA IN TRANSBRONCHIAL BIOPSY SPECIMENS
- Free, detached fragments of SCIS are difficult to distinguish from invasive carcinoma, and helpful clues favoring SCIS include straight to curvilinear fragment edges, a flat superficial epithelial surface, and a straight to undulating basement membrane
- Endobronchial papillary squamous cell carcinoma (SCC) can be difficult to diagnose

PEARLS

- *The progression is thought to be from basal cell hyperplasia to squamous metaplasia to SD to SCIS and finally to invasive SCC*
- *The follow-up behavior of severe SD/SCIS lesions varies by study: some authors show invariable progression to invasive cancer, others show that only a minority of high-grade SD/SCIS progresses*
- *The risk for low-grade SD progressing to invasive cancer is minimal*
- *Two additional subtypes of bronchial epithelial dysplasia have recently been described: columnar cell dysplasia (CCD) and bronchial epithelial dysplasia with transitional differentiation (TD type)*

SELECTED REFERENCE

Lantuéjoul S, Salameire D, Salon C, Brambilla E: Pulmonary preneoplasia: sequential molecular carcinogenetic events. Histopathology 54:43-54, 2009.

ATYPICAL ADENOMATOUS HYPERPLASIA (AAH)

Clinical Features

- A peripheral lesion found in the centriacinar region close to respiratory bronchioles that arises from bronchioloalveolar epithelium
- Almost always found as an incidental histologic finding in lungs with existing adenocarcinoma or adenocarcinoma in situ (AIS)
- About 50% of cases show between two and six AAH lesions

Gross Pathology

- AAH appears as a gray to yellow discrete nodule ranging from 1 to 5 mm, with most being smaller than 3 mm

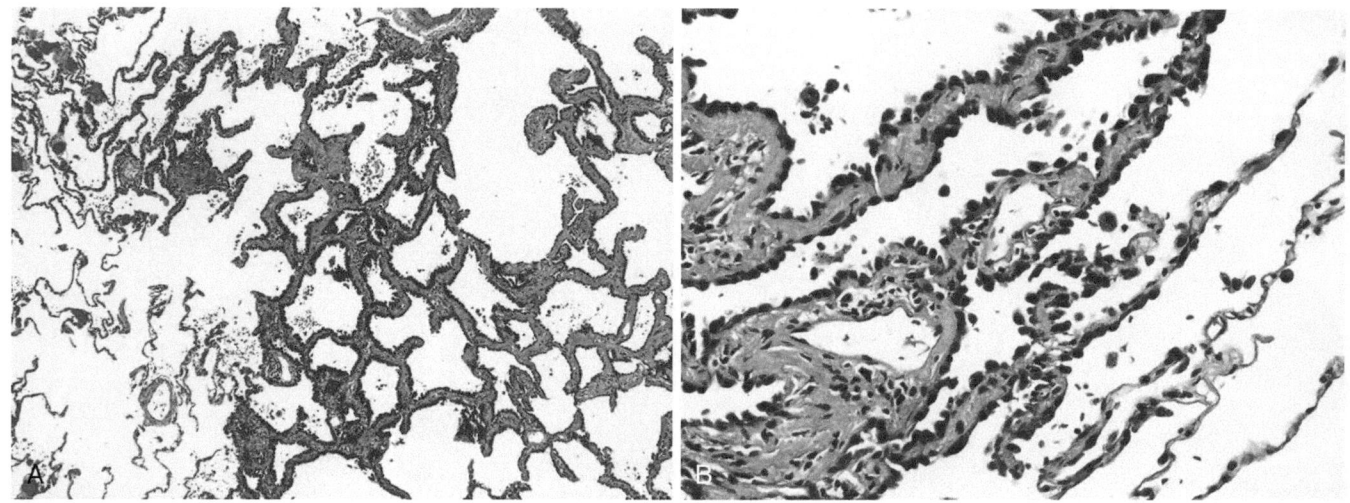

Figure 4-40. Atypical adenomatous hyperplasia. A, Low-power photomicrograph shows a distinct small lesion with atypical pneumocytes lining alveolar septa with mild fibrosis. **B,** High power shows atypical pneumocytes with a hobnail appearance.

Histopathology

- Lesions stand out at scanning-power magnification
- Alveolar walls are thickened by fibrosis and lined by a heterogeneous population of cells including cuboidal cells, peg cells, and flat type 1 pneumocytes (Figure 4-40)
- Large gaps can exist between cells conferring an interrupted appearance
- Occasional large or multinucleated cells are present
- Intranuclear inclusions that stain positive for surfactant apoprotein A (PE10) are present in up to 25% of the cells
- Ciliated and mucous cells are virtually absent, and mitoses are rare
- Cellularity and cytologic atypia are variable

Special Stains and Immunohistochemistry

- Noncontributory

Other Techniques for Diagnosis

- Noncontributory

Differential Diagnosis

LOCALIZED NONMUCINOUS AIS

- Alveolar architecture is preserved in both AAH and AIS
- AIS is usually more than 10 mm in diameter, with a more homogeneous cell population; larger AIS shows central collapse with fibrosis or scar (an important area to look for evidence of invasion)
- AIS shows three or more of the following: marked cell stratification, high cell density with nuclear overlap, coarse nuclear chromatin with prominent nucleoli, some mitoses, and increased cell height; AAH rarely displays more than one of those features

DIFFUSE INTERSTITIAL LUNG DISEASE

- AAH occurs in the absence of underlying interstitial inflammation or fibrosis

PERIBRONCHIOLAR METAPLASIA

- Centriacinar lesion composed of ciliated bronchiolar-type cells with fibrosis

PAPILLARY ADENOMA

- About 1- to 4-cm, well-demarcated tumor with papillary architecture
- True papillae are not a feature of AAH

ALVEOLAR ADENOMA

- Peripheral, well-circumscribed tumor smaller than 6 cm
- Composed of variably sized spaces lined with cuboidal cells overlying a spindle cell–rich stroma with focal myxoid changes

MICRONODULAR PNEUMOCYTE HYPERPLASIA

- Extremely rare lesion associated with tuberous sclerosis or lymphangioleiomyomatosis (LAM)
- Well-demarcated lesion several millimeters in diameter composed of uniform cuboidal cells arranged in a more solid pattern than AAH

PEARLS

- *AAH is thought to be the precursor of nonmucinous AIS and invasive adenocarcinoma; it is also seen in patients with squamous cell carcinoma (field effect)*
- *Similar to invasive adenocarcinoma, AAH shows mutations in the Kras and EGFR genes, but the invasive potential of Kras mutations is not clearly demonstrated*

SELECTED REFERENCE

Noguchi M: Stepwise progression of pulmonary adenocarcinoma: clinical and molecular implications. Cancer Metastasis Rev 29:15-21, 2010.

ADENOCARCINOMA IN SITU (AIS, FORMERLY BRONCHIOLOALVEOLAR CARCINOMA)

Clinical Features

- Precursor lesion of adenocarcinoma, less than 3 cm but more than 0.5 cm
- Often peripheral and asymptomatic; incidental finding on radiology

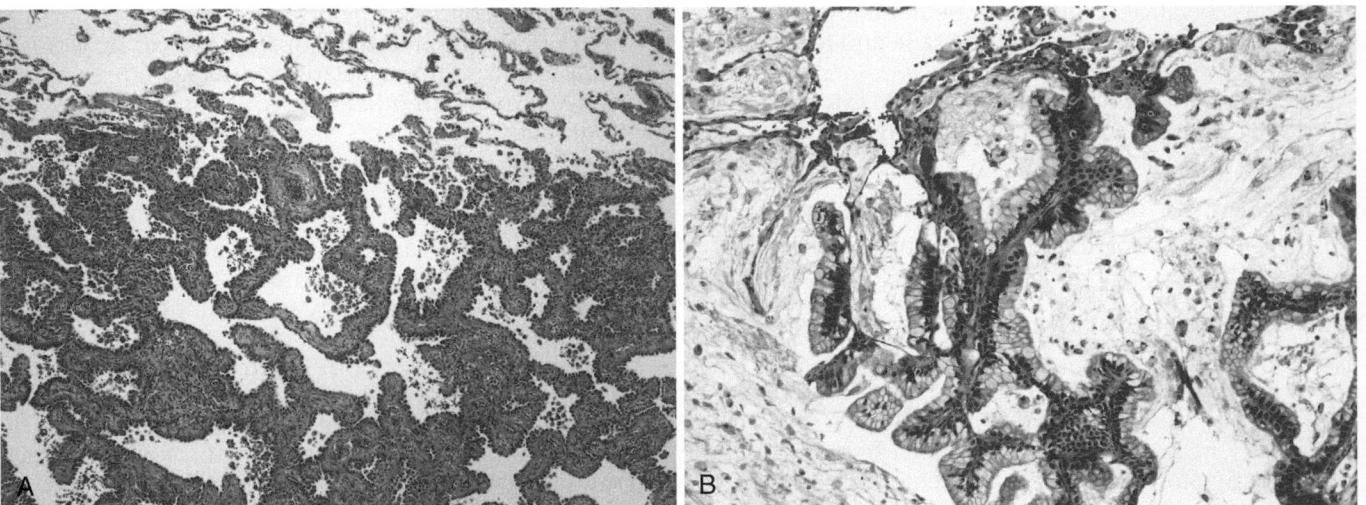

Figure 4-41. Adenocarcinoma in situ. **A,** This low-power photograph from a 1.2-cm lesion shows atypical nonmucinous cells lining preexisting alveoli, without invasion. **B,** In contrast, this in situ tumor has mucinous cells growing along pre-existing alveolar septae.

Gross Pathology

- AIS is usually seen as a single peripheral nodule that is soft and poorly circumscribed; rarely mucinous

Histopathology

- Tumor cells grow along preexisting alveolar septae without invasion into stroma, blood vessels, or pleura with no gaps between them (in contrast to AAH) (Figure 4-41)
- Alveolar walls may be thickened slightly by fibrosis, but there is no desmoplasia
- Usually low grade with relatively uniform nuclei and small nucleoli; there are few mitoses and necrosis is absent; occasionally the tumor cells are larger with more atypia and prominent nucleoli
- Subdivided into nonmucinous (most common) and nonmucinous

Special Stains and Immunohistochemistry

- Noncontributory

Other Techniques for Diagnosis

- Noncontributory

Differential Diagnosis

AAH

- Alveolar architecture is preserved in both AAH and AIS and morphology may be quite similar
- By definition, AAH is equal to or less than 0.5 mm whereas AIS is more than 5 mm, usually more than 10 mm in diameter

PERIBRONCHIOLAR METAPLASIA

- Centriacinar lesion composed of ciliated bronchiolar-type cells with fibrosis

ADENOCARCINOMA, WELL-DIFFERENTIATED

- Focus of invasion may be difficult to identify, but that is what separates it from AIS; thus, the diagnosis of AIS can only be made on a complete resection

PEARLS

- *AIS (formerly bronchioloalveolar carcinoma) is thought to be the precursor of invasive adenocarcinoma, both nonmucinous and mucinous*
- *When seen on a biopsy, should be reported as lepidic pattern; may represent AIS or adenocarcinoma*
- *Similar to invasive adenocarcinoma, AIS shows mutations in the* Kras *and* EGFR *genes*

SELECTED REFERENCE

Travis WD, Brambilla E, Noguchi M, et al: International association for the study of lung cancer/American Thoracic Society/European Respiratory Society international multidisciplinary classification of lung adenocarcinoma. J Thorac Oncol 6:244-285, 2011.

DIFFUSE IDIOPATHIC PULMONARY NEUROENDOCRINE CELL HYPERPLASIA (DIPNECH)

Clinical Features

- Extremely rare lesion that gives rise to low-grade, peripheral carcinoid tumor

Gross Pathology

- As lesions progress to carcinoid tumorlets and carcinoid tumors they appear as small, well-demarcated, gray-white nodules resembling miliary bodies

Histopathology

- Widespread proliferation of pulmonary neuroendocrine cells manifesting as increased numbers of individual cells, small groups, or nodular aggregates or nests in the bronchial or bronchiolar epithelium
- Nodules of neuroendocrine cells can protrude into airway lumens and occasionally cause an occlusion

- As lesions advance, pulmonary neuroendocrine cells break through the basement membrane and form 2- to 5-mm carcinoid tumorlets
- Marked fibrosis is often associated with carcinoid tumorlets and carcinoid tumor (lesions larger than 5 mm are classified as carcinoids)

Special Stains and Immunohistochemistry

- Positive for chromogranin, synaptophysin, and cytokeratin 8/18

Other Techniques for Diagnosis

- Noncontributory

Differential Diagnosis for DIPNECH

- Pulmonary neuroendocrine cell (PNEC) hyperplasia in fibroinflammatory disease (e.g., bronchiectasis), incidental PNEC hyperplasia, minute meningothelial nodules

PEARLS

- *DIPNECH may be a precursor lesion of a subset of carcinoid tumors that are invariably low grade and peripheral; the precursor to centrally localized, high-grade carcinoid tumors has not yet been clearly identified*

SELECTED REFERENCE

Gosney JR, Williams IJ, Dodson AR, et al: Morphology and antigen expression profile of pulmonary neuroendocrine cells in reactive proliferations and diffuse idiopathic pulmonary neuroendocrine cell hyperplasia (DIPNECH). Histopathology 59:751-762, 2011.

Malignant Epithelial Tumors
ADENOCARCINOMA

Clinical Features

- Most common type of lung cancer, accounting for about 40% of all cases of invasive lung cancer in the United States; increasing incidence since the early 2000s

- Roughly 75% of lung adenocarcinomas are peripheral
- The most common variant of lung cancer in women and nonsmokers; its association with cigarette smoking is weaker than with other types of lung carcinoma
- About half the patients have metastases to lymph nodes, brain, bone, or adrenal glands at presentation

Gross Pathology

- Disease classically arises as a single peripheral mass, less likely as multiple synchronous tumors, of variable size; may arise centrally in the hilum or perihilar bronchus
- Tumors are gray-tan and firm with variable amounts of necrosis
- Less common growth patterns include endobronchial adenocarcinoma, pneumonia-like consolidation, pseudomesotheliomatous carcinoma and multifocal bilateral disease
- Penetration of the pleura leads to dissemination within the pleural cavity, pleural effusions, and occasionally chest wall invasion

Histopathology

- Tumor is characterized by gland formation or mucin production (Figure 4-42)
- Intracytoplasmic mucin or mucin within glandular lumina is a key feature
- Glands are usually surrounded by desmoplastic stroma
- Minimally invasive adenocarcinoma (MIA) is used to define tumors that are > 3 cm with an invasive component that is > 5 mm; these may be nonmucinous or mucinous
- A spectrum of morphology is usually seen within a single tumor; the percentage of major growth pattern should be reported with the minor pattern(s) in 5% increments:
  - Acinar pattern
    - Acini and tubules formed by cuboidal or columnar cells resembling bronchial glands with mucin production, most common pattern

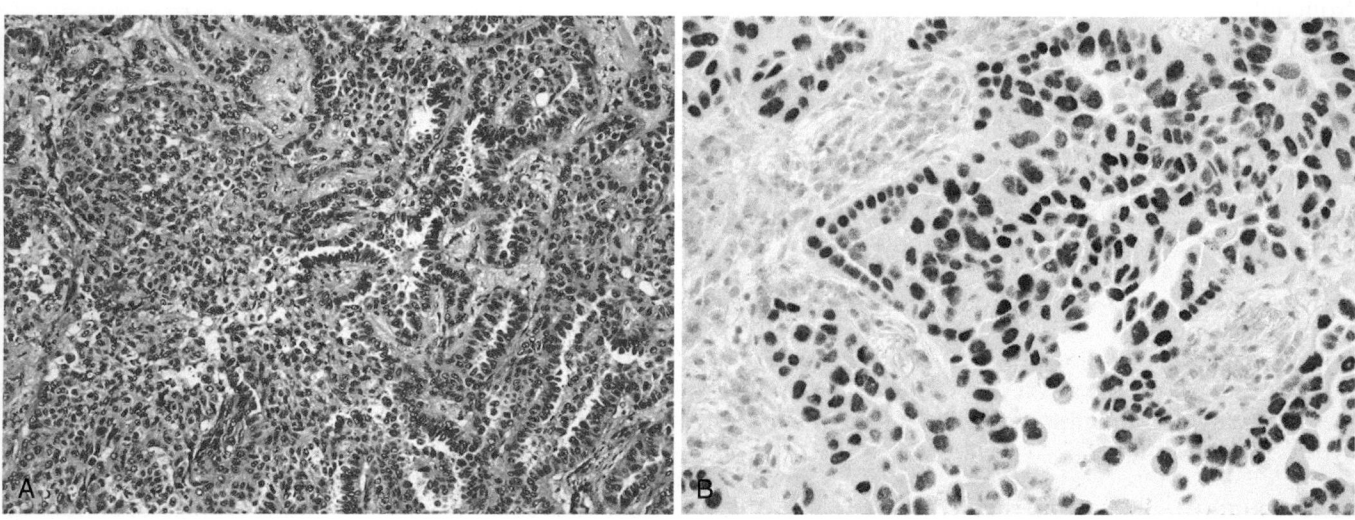

Figure 4-42. Adenocarcinoma. A, This photomicrograph shows a mixed pattern with solid areas and gland formation in this moderately to poorly differentiated adenocarcinoma. **B,** TTF-1 stain is strongly positive in adenocarcinoma; note residual small pneumocytes (middle left), which should normally be positive and serve as an internal control.

- Papillary pattern
  - Central fibrovascular cores lined by large, atypical cells with enlarged, hyperchromatic nuclei, prominent nucleoli, and frequent mitoses
  - Papillae often show secondary and tertiary branching patterns
  - Psammoma bodies can be present
- Micropapillary pattern
  - Small papillary tumor clusters without microvascular cores
- Lepidic pattern
  - Composed of tumor cells growing along preexisting alveolar walls
  - Often seen at the periphery of an otherwise invasive adenocarcinoma, which may be acinar, or one of the other patterns
- Solid pattern
  - Lacks papillae, tubules, and acini and is composed of nests and sheets of polygonal cells
- Signet-ring pattern
  - Tumor cells contain large intracytoplasmic mucin vacuoles with peripherally displaced nuclei
  - Solid pattern with more than 10% signet ring is more likely to have the *EML4-ALK* mutation
- Clear cell pattern
  - Clear cells may be a part of any pattern and are usually focal; there is no clinical or prognostic significance to this pattern
  - When extensive, needs to be differentiated from metastatic renal cell carcinoma
- Histologic variants
  - Mucinous adenocarcinoma (formerly mucinous BAC)
    - Larger than 3 cm, invasive focus >5 mm, or multifocal or uncircumscribed tumor of any size with miliary spread into adjacent lung
    - Tall cells with basal nuclei, abundant intracytoplasmic mucin
    - TTF-1 usually negative, may be CK7 negative; thus, difficult to differentiate from metastatic gastrointestinal carcinoma
  - Colloid adenocarcinoma
    - Dissecting pools of mucin with islands of often bland tumor cells
  - Fetal adenocarcinoma
    - Composed of tubules with columnar cells resembling fetal lung and endometrioid adenocarcinoma
  - Clear cell adenocarcinoma: rule out metastatic renal cell carcinoma

Special Stains and Immunohistochemistry

- Mucin production can be demonstrated with mucicarmine, PAS, or Alcian blue stains
- Tumor cells are positive for the epithelial markers: CAM5.2, pancytokeratin AE1/AE3, epithelial membrane antigen (EMA), carcinoembryonic antigen (CEA), CD15, Ber-Ep4, and B72.3/BRST-3/TAG-72
- Adenocarcinomas usually express CK7 and are negative for CK20
- TTF-1 (nuclear) or Napsin A are expressed in >90% of lung adenocarcinomas, which allow for differentiation from squamous cell carcinoma in high-grade tumors

Other Techniques for Diagnosis

- *EGFR* mutations seen in less than 10% to 20% of patients allow for targeted therapy
- *KRAS* mutations are present in 30% and *EML4-ALK* in 4%

Differential Diagnosis

METASTATIC ADENOCARCINOMA
- Presentation with multiple lung masses favors metastasis
- Metastatic colonic adenocarcinoma is typically CK7 negative and CK20 positive
- CDX2 is positive in gastrointestinal carcinomas, but some pulmonary mucinous adenocarcinomas may also be positive
- Estrogen and progesterone receptors and gross cystic disease fluid protein-15 are often positive in breast carcinomas
- Prostate-specific antigen and prostatic acid phosphatase are positive in metastatic prostate carcinoma
- TTF-1 is positive in primary lung and metastatic thyroid carcinoma; thyroglobulin is positive in the latter, and mucin staining is positive in the former

MESOTHELIOMA
- IHC panel should include TTF-1, two epithelial markers (MOC 31, BG8, or CEA), and two mesothelial markers (calretinin, CK5/6, WT-1, or D2-40)

BRONCHIOLAR METAPLASIA
- Bronchiolar metaplasia often occurs in fibrotic processes such as UIP
- Papillary or invasive growth patterns or intracytoplasmic mucin production favors adenocarcinoma

PEARLS

- The pathologic diagnosis should include the histologic subtypes, for example, "adenocarcinoma, with acinar (60%), papillary (20%), and lepidic (20%) patterns"
- Minimally invasive adenocarcinomas with invasive area of 5 mm or less within lepidic growth areas (total tumor diameter of 3 cm or less) have excellent prognosis
- Micropapillary pattern is associated with higher risk of lymph node metastases
- Incidence of intrapulmonary metastasis is most common in adenocarcinoma
- Molecular analysis of adenocarcinoma suggests two differing pathways involving either the K-ras gene or the EGFR gene
- K-ras mutations in codons 12, 13, or 61 are present in 30% of adenocarcinomas, are particularly common in smokers, and are occasionally present in SCC
- Activating mutations in EGFR are clustered in exons 18 to 21 and associated with female sex, never-smoked status, adenocarcinoma histology, and Asian ethnicity

SELECTED REFERENCES

Couraud S, Zalcman G, Milleron B, et al: Lung cancer in never smokers: a review. Eur J Cancer 48:1299-1311, 2012.
Kadara H, Kabbout M, Wistuba II: Pulmonary adenocarcinoma: a renewed entity in 2011. Respirology 17:50-65, 2012.
Raparia K, Villa C, DeCamp MM, et al: Molecular profiling in non-small cell lung cancer: a step toward personalized medicine. Arch Pathol Lab Med 137:481-491, 2013.

Travis WD, Brambilla E, Noguchi M, et al: International association for the study of lung cancer/American Thoracic Society/European Respiratory Society international multidisciplinary classification of lung adenocarcinoma. J Thorac Oncol 6:244-285, 2011.

Travis WD, Brambilla E, Riely GJ: New pathologic classification of lung cancer: relevance for clinical practice and clinical trials. J Clin Oncol 31:992-1001, 2013.

SQUAMOUS CELL CARCINOMA (SCC)

Clinical Features

- Accounts for roughly 20% of all invasive lung cancer
- Strong association with cigarette smoking
- Small minority of patients presenting with signs of obstruction (e.g., recurrent infection, hemoptysis, cough)

Gross Pathology

- About 75% of cases are centrally located, arising from proximal bronchi
- Tumor forms a firm gray-white mass with desmoplastic stromal reaction
- Areas of necrosis and cavitation can be present
- Endobronchial growth may occlude the airway lumen, leading to bronchiectasis, infection, or bronchopneumonia

Histopathology

- Tumor cells display squamous cell differentiation in the form of keratinization, pearl formation, and intercellular bridges (Figure 4-43)

PAPILLARY VARIANT

- Exophytic, papillary, and endobronchial growth pattern
- Most patients present with low-stage disease and a relatively good prognosis with greater than 60% 5-year survival

CLEAR CELL VARIANT

- Rare (< 0.3% of all lung cancer)
- Tumor is composed almost entirely of large, polygonal cells with clear cytoplasm; note, clear cell change is common, and up to one third of all primary lung cancers have foci of clear cell change composing 10% to 20% of the tumor

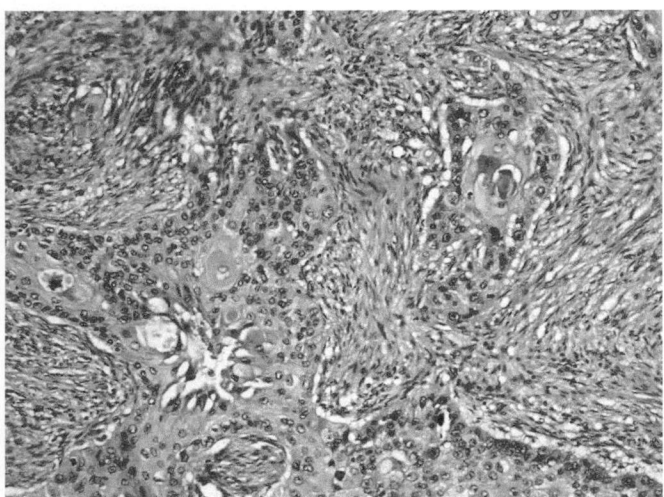

Figure 4-43. Squamous cell carcinoma. This moderately well-differentiated squamous cell carcinoma shows focal keratinization with formation of keratin pearls. Marked desmoplastic reaction is present.

- Resembles metastatic renal clear cell carcinoma, metastatic thyroid carcinoma, adenocarcinoma with clear cell change, and large cell carcinoma

SMALL CELL VARIANT

- Poorly differentiated carcinoma with small cells, hyperchromatic, irregular nuclei, prominent nucleoli, moderate cytoplasm, and distinct cell-cell boundaries
- Focal squamous differentiation
- Lacks the even, homogeneous, salt-and-pepper chromatin pattern and nuclear molding seen in small cell lung carcinoma (SCLC) and stains negative for chromogranin and synaptophysin

BASALOID VARIANT

- Nests of poorly differentiated tumor cells with prominent palisading peripheral nuclei
- Differential diagnosis of this variant of SCC includes adenoid cystic carcinoma, which occurs in younger patients and has a better prognosis

NONKERATINIZING VARIANT

- Resembles urothelial carcinoma

Special Stains and Immunohistochemistry

- SCC express high-molecular-weight keratin 34βE12, CK5/6, CEA, p40/p63, and low-molecular-weight keratin (35βH11)
- SCC is negative for TTF-1 and Napsin A, which together with positivity for p40 is useful for making the diagnosis in undifferentiated tumors

Other Techniques for Diagnosis

- Gain of the chromosomal locus 3q26 through either 3q26 amplification or polysomy is the most common genomic abnormality in SCC
- Expression of *p53* gradually increases in dysplastic squamous epithelium

Differential Diagnosis

SCC VERSUS SCLC

- SCLC is p40 negative and often TTF-1 positive, whereas SCC is generally p40 positive and TTF-1 negative

PEARLS

- *Five-year survival rate for SCC is generally better than that of adenocarcinoma*
- *In addition to 3q26 amplification, other cytogenetic features of SCC include loss on 3p, 9p, and 8p, and p53 mutation*
- *Loss of p16INK4A correlates with significantly worse survival in NSCLC, particularly for SCC*
- *Targeted therapy is on the horizon with identification of amplifications of PIK3CA, SOX2, and DDR2 mutations and amplifications of BRF2*

SELECTED REFERENCES

Drilon A, Rekhtman N, Ladanyi M, Paik P: Squamous-cell carcinomas of the lung: emerging biology, controversies, and the promise of targeted therapy. Lancet Oncol 13:e418-e426, 2012.

Sereno M, Esteban IR, Zambrana F, et al: Squamous-cell carcinoma of the lungs: is it really so different? Crit Rev Oncol Hematol 84:327-339, 2012.

SMALL CELL LUNG CARCINOMA (SCLC)

Clinical Features

- SCLC occurs almost exclusively in smokers
- It accounts for about 13% of lung cancer cases in the United States
- In general, SCLC initially responds to chemotherapy and therefore needs to be separated from non–small cell lung carcinoma (NSCLC)
- Combined small cell carcinoma variant displays classic SCLC features, with an additional component consisting of any histologic subtype of NSCLC
- Because SCLC is a high-grade tumor with widespread dissemination at presentation, it used to be staged as limited disease versus extensive disease; however, now the TNM system is used

Gross Pathology

- White-tan, soft, friable perihilar mass with extensive necrosis and frequent nodal metastases
- Tumor spreads along bronchi in a submucosal and circumferential pattern with usual lymphatic invasion
- About 5% of cases present as peripheral coin-shaped lesions

Histopathology

- Tumor cells are generally smaller than the size of three resting lymphocytes
- Tumor cells have scant cytoplasm and may have round, oval, or spindle-shaped nuclei
- Cell borders are indistinct, and molding is a common feature
- In a better preserved biopsy and surgical resections, the cells appear larger than in a crushed biopsy; chromatin pattern is salt-and-pepper, and more cytoplasm can be seen than one would expect (Figure 4-44)
- An important diagnostic feature is the absence of nucleoli; however, larger tumor cells can occasionally display a few inconspicuous nucleoli
- Mitotic rates are high, averaging more than 60 mitoses/10 hpf, and necrosis is often extensive
- Growth patterns include nesting, trabeculated, peripheral palisading, and rosette formation—similar to other neuroendocrine tumors; sheetlike growth without a neuroendocrine pattern is also common
- Combined SCLC represents less than 3% of SCLC cases and is the only variant of SCLC recognized by the 2004 World Health Organization (WHO) classification
  - Non–small cell component is usually squamous cell, adenocarcinoma, or large cell carcinoma; less commonly, spindle cell or giant cell carcinoma
  - The non–small cell component needs to be specified in the diagnosis

Special Stains and Immunohistochemistry

- Virtually all SCLC stain with cytokeratin (including CK7) and EMA
- About 90% of SCLC cells express TTF-1
- About 90% of SCLC cells stain positive for one or more of the neuroendocrine markers; less than 10% of SCLC cases are negative for all neuroendocrine markers
- In a small biopsy, high mitotic index (Ki-67 positivity of over 50% but often up to 90%) in SCLC is helpful in distinguishing it from a lower grade neuroendocrine tumor (carcinoid)

Other Techniques for Diagnosis

- Deletion of chromosome 3p is a consistent finding in SCLC, and this region may include the fragile histidine triad gene (*FHIT*) located at 3p14.2
- About 20% of SCLCs show mutations in the *Rb* gene
- About 70% to 95% of SCLCs show *Bcl-2* expression
- SCLC shows the highest rate of *p53* mutation of all lung carcinomas, and consequently a strong nuclear p53 staining pattern in greater than 10% to 20% of cells is strongly suggestive of a *p53* mutation; however, none of the molecular abnormalities have led to any specific therapy as yet

Differential Diagnosis

LYMPHOCYTIC INFILTRATE

- In a small biopsy sample, crushed lymphocytes can be difficult to distinguish from SCLC without IHC analysis (LCA, keratin AE1/AE3, and CAM5.2)

ATYPICAL CARCINOID

- SCLC displays relatively more necrosis, karyorrhexis, and mitoses (high mitotic index) than atypical carcinoid
- Carcinoid tumors generally show more extensive and robust staining for chromogranin

PEARLS

- *The diagnosis of SCLC is made by light microscopy, and negative staining for neuroendocrine markers does not exclude the diagnosis*
- *SCLC shows a tendency to crush in forceps and bronchial biopsies*
- *DNA from necrotic tumor cells can get deposited in the walls of vessels and connective tissue (the Azzopardi phenomenon)*
- *Infrequently, patients produce autoantibodies that bind to SCLC cells and non-neoplastic cells of the central nervous system or neuromuscular junction, resulting in cerebellar degenerative syndromes or Lambert-Eaton myasthenic syndrome*
- *SCLC cells can also produce a number of polypeptide hormones, including adrenocorticotropic hormone and vasopressin, resulting in various paraneoplastic and ectopic hormonal syndromes*
- *The Rb gene has been reported to be deleted in more than 90% of SCLCs and in 15% of NSCLCs*

SELECTED REFERENCES

Jones CD, Cummings IG, Shipolini AR, McCormack DJ: Does surgery improve prognosis in patients with small-cell lung carcinoma? Interact Cardiovasc Thorac Surg 16:375-380, 2013.

Joshi M, Ayoola A, Belani CP: Small-cell lung cancer: an update on targeted therapies. Adv Exp Med Biol 779:385-404, 2013.

Travis WD: Update on small cell carcinoma and its differentiation from squamous cell carcinoma and other non-small cell carcinomas. Mod Pathol 25(suppl 1):S18-S30, 2012.

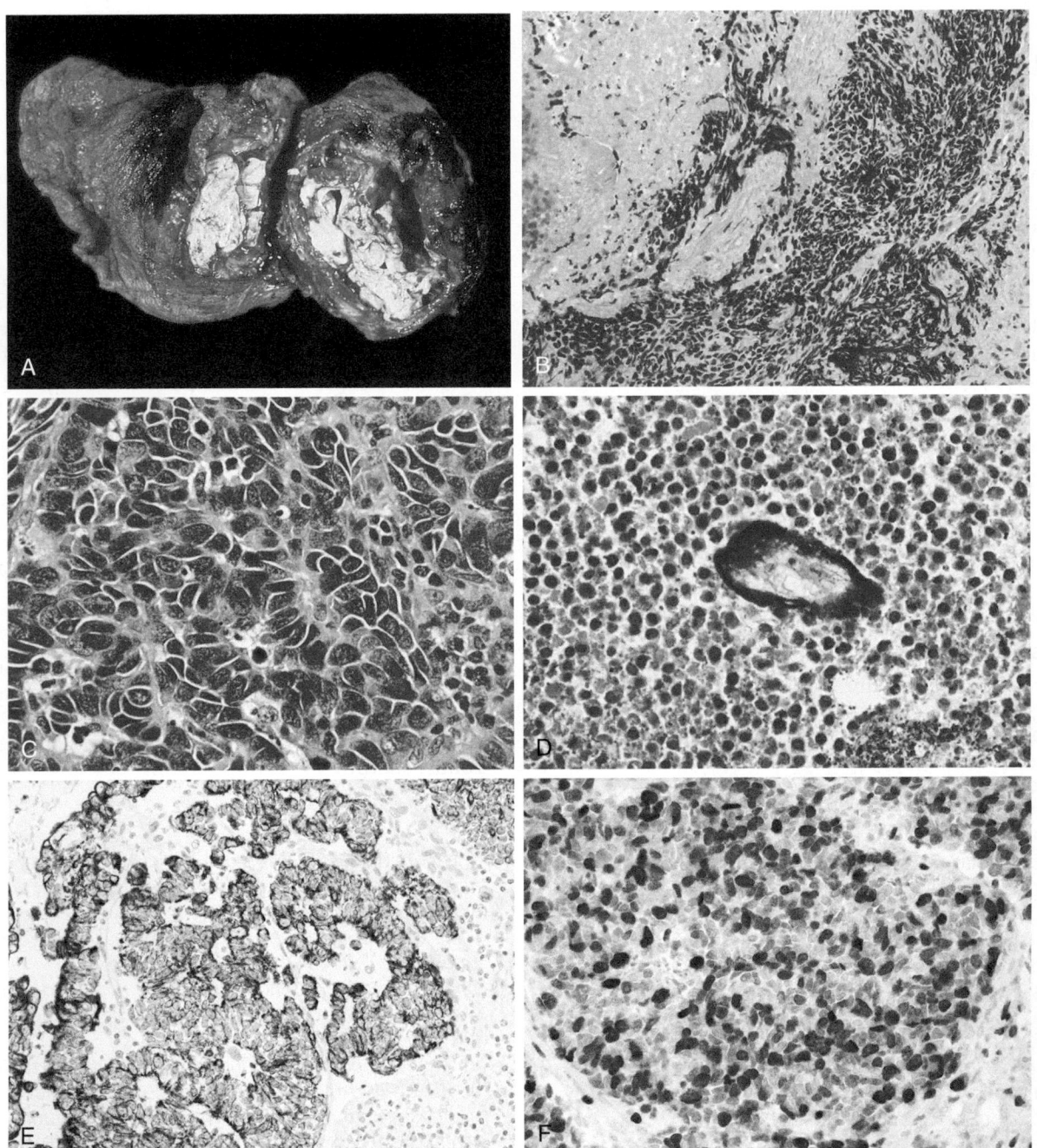

Figure 4-44. Small cell carcinoma. A, Grossly, all lung carcinomas tend to have a similar appearance. In this resection specimen, a large irregular tan-white tumor mass is seen in the lung. **B,** Low-power photomicrograph shows nests of crushed cells and large areas of necrosis, typical of transbronchial biopsies. **C,** This photomicrograph of a resected tumor shows well-preserved intermediate-sized tumor cells forming pseudorosettes with mitoses, salt-and-pepper chromatin, and rare inconspicuous nucleoli. **D,** Azzopardi effect is seen with crushed DNA around a blood vessel in this largely necrotic tumor. **E,** Immunoperoxidase stain for keratin CAM5.2 can be helpful in distinguishing carcinoma from lymphocytes. **F,** Ki-67 stain shows nuclear staining in the majority of tumor cells, which is helpful in distinguishing it from carcinoid tumor.

LARGE CELL CARCINOMA

Clinical Features

- Undifferentiated tumor lacks the diagnostic features of squamous cell carcinoma, adenocarcinoma, or small cell carcinoma with the use of an IHC stain panel
- Represents 1% to 2% of all lung cancers

Gross Pathology

- Usually is a large central or peripheral tumor with a fleshy, pink-tan cut surface
- Foci of tumor necrosis are common
- Invasion through the pleura into the chest wall or adjacent structures frequently occurs

Histopathology

- A diagnosis of exclusion after adenocarcinoma, squamous cell carcinoma, and small cell carcinoma have been ruled out
- Tumor cells possess large vesicular nuclei with prominent nucleoli, moderate amounts of cytoplasm, and well-defined cell-cell borders (Figure 4-45)
- Tumor cells are arranged in sheets or nests

Special Stains and Immunohistochemistry

- TTF-1, p40, and neuroendocrine markers (synaptophysin, chromogranin, CD56) are negative

Differential Diagnosis

ADENOCARCINOMA, SOLID TYPE
- Mucin is focally positive and TTF-1 is almost always positive

SQUAMOUS CELL CARCINOMA
- p40 is positive

PEARLS

- *The diagnosis of large cell carcinoma is now infrequent due to use of specific IHC stains (TTF-1 and p40)*

LARGE CELL NEUROENDOCRINE CARCINOMA (LCNEC)

- LCNEC represents 3% of lung cancers
- Has organoid nesting, trabecular growth, rosette formation, and perilobular palisading patterns of growth
- Tumor cells are large with abundant cytoplasm
- Prominent nucleoli help differentiate from small cell carcinoma
- Mitotic activity is robust (>10 mitoses/10 hpf; average, 66 mitoses/10 hpf), and large zones of necrosis are common

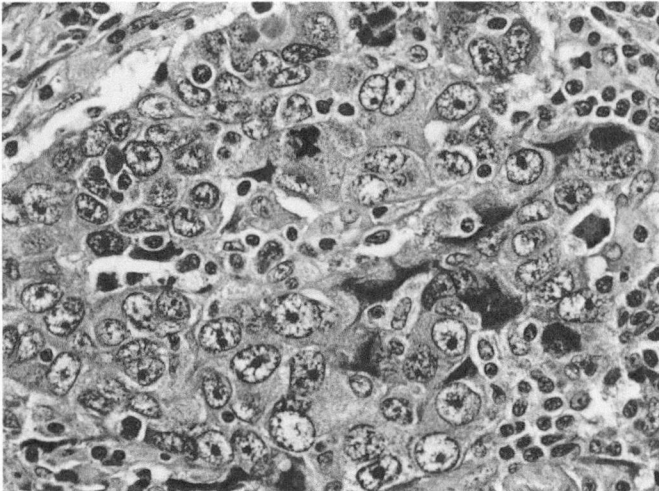

Figure 4-45. Large cell carcinoma. Clusters of highly atypical large cells (compare size to normal lymphocytes) are seen within fibrous tissue. Nucleoli are prominent.

Special Stains and Immunohistochemistry

- Staining with neuroendocrine markers is often patchy and relatively weak, similar to SCLC and in stark contrast to the robust, diffuse staining seen in carcinoids
- Diffusely positive for keratin and CEA; 50% of LCNEC tumors express TTF-1

Differential Diagnosis

POORLY DIFFERENTIATED SQUAMOUS CELL CARCINOMA
- Foci of intercellular bridges and keratin formation are present in SCC

BASALOID CARCINOMA VERSUS BASALOID VARIANT OF SQUAMOUS CELL CARCINOMA
- Presence of squamous differentiation, even if focal, favors the basaloid variant of squamous cell carcinoma; p40 is strongly positive

SOLID TYPE OF ADENOCARCINOMA
- Minimum of 5 mucin droplets/2 hpf; TTF-1 is usually positive

ATYPICAL CARCINOID
- From 2 to 10 mitoses/10 hpf and punctate necrosis

PEARLS

- *Large cell carcinoma may be difficult to diagnose on a small transbronchial biopsy; neuroendocrine markers should be done if the histologic pattern suggests neuroendocrine differentiation*
- *LCNEC is an aggressive, rare tumor with dismal prognosis that is treated with chemotherapy drugs similar to those used for small cell carcinoma*

SELECTED REFERENCES

Swarts DR, Ramaekers FC, Speel EJ: Molecular and cellular biology of neuroendocrine lung tumors: evidence for separate biological entities. Biochim Biophys Acta 1826:255-271, 2012.

Travis WD: Advances in neuroendocrine lung tumors. Ann Oncol 21(suppl 7):vii, 65-71, 2010.

CARCINOID TUMOR

Clinical Features

- Carcinoid tumors are low-grade malignancies that make up 1% to 2% of all primary lung cancers
- Mean age of diagnosis for typical and atypical carcinoid tumors is 45 and 55 years, respectively
- Atypical carcinoid is associated with cigarette smoking
- Young adults, adolescents, and children can get carcinoid tumors
- Carcinoid tumors arise at numerous sites in the body, with lung being the second most common site after the gastrointestinal tract
- Bronchial carcinoid may present with obstructive symptoms due to mass effect: cough, wheezing, dyspnea, chest pain, hemoptysis, and recurrent pneumonia; peripheral carcinoid tumors are usually asymptomatic

Gross Pathology

- Most tumors (70%) arise centrally in the main or major bronchi and are frequently endobronchial; 30% are peripheral, arising in segmental bronchi or beyond
- Tumors are firm, well-demarcated, yellow-tan, nodular masses with a glistening cut surface and usually measure less than 2 cm
- The overlying mucosa may be intact or ulcerated

Histopathology

- Carcinoid tumors are part of the spectrum of neuroendocrine lung tumors that includes large cell neuroendocrine carcinoma, small cell carcinoma, and typical and atypical carcinoid tumors
- Carcinoid tumors are composed of a uniform population of polygonal cells with fine, granular cytoplasm, inconspicuous nucleoli, and scanty cytoplasm (Figure 4-46)
- Nuclear atypia and pleomorphism may be marked, but these features do not distinguish between typical and atypical carcinoid
- Growth patterns suggestive of neuroendocrine differentiation include organoid, trabecular, spindle cell, papillary, pseudoglandular, rosette, and follicular
- True gland formation is rare, and spindling of tumor cells can be significant—particularly in peripherally localized carcinoid tumors
- The stroma is typically vascular, or less often, hyalinized with cartilage or metaplastic bone formation
- Typical carcinoid (80% to 90% of pulmonary carcinoids): greater than 0.5 cm in diameter, 1 mitosis/10 hpf, and no evidence of necrosis
- Atypical carcinoid (10% to 20% of pulmonary carcinoids): focal necrosis or 2 to 10 mitoses/10 hpf

Special Stains and Immunohistochemistry

- About 80% of carcinoid tumors stain with cytokeratin antibodies
- Typical carcinoid tumors are strongly positive for neuroendocrine markers (chromogranin, synaptophysin, and CD56)
- Atypical carcinoid tumors show modestly reduced staining for neuroendocrine markers; however, the difference does not distinguish atypical from typical carcinoid
- Sustentacular cells express S-100 protein
- Most carcinoid tumors express CD99

Other Techniques for Diagnosis

- Noncontributory

Differential Diagnosis

OTHER NEUROENDOCRINE TUMORS

- SCLC and LCNEC show fewer positive cells with less intense staining for neuroendocrine markers
- Carcinoid and large cell neuroendocrine tumors make up less than 3% of all lung cancers, whereas small cell lung cancer is more common, accounting for 13% of all lung cancers
- Carcinoid tumorlets resemble typical carcinoid and are less than 5 mm in diameter

LARGE CELL NEUROENDOCRINE CARCINOMA (LCNEC)

- Greater than 10 mitoses/10 hpf (median, 70/10 hpf)
- Relatively more necrosis
- Larger cell size with vesicular, coarse, or fine chromatin, visible nucleoli, and lower nuclear-to-cytoplasmic ratio than atypical carcinoid

Small Cell Lung Carcinoma (SCLC)

- High mitotic rates (median, 80/10 hpf)
- Frequent, extensive necrosis
- Fine granular chromatin, absent or faint nucleoli, scanty cytoplasm, and nuclear molding

PULMONARY CARCINOID VERSUS INTESTINAL OR PANCREATIC CARCINOID TUMORS

- About 80% to 95% of pulmonary carcinoid tumors are TTF-1 positive, whereas intestinal and pancreatic carcinoids do not express TTF-1

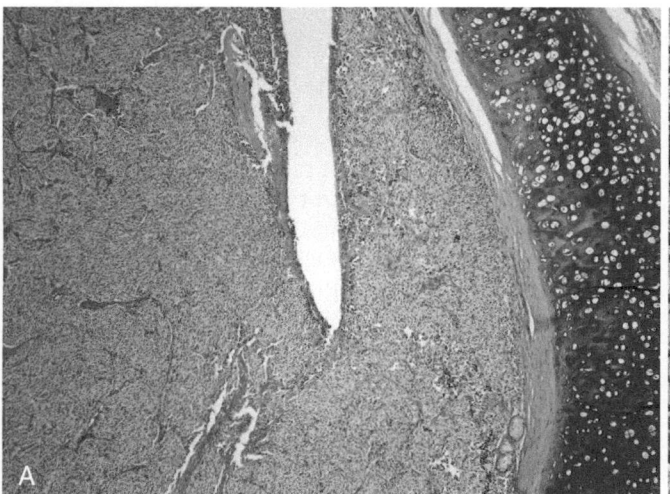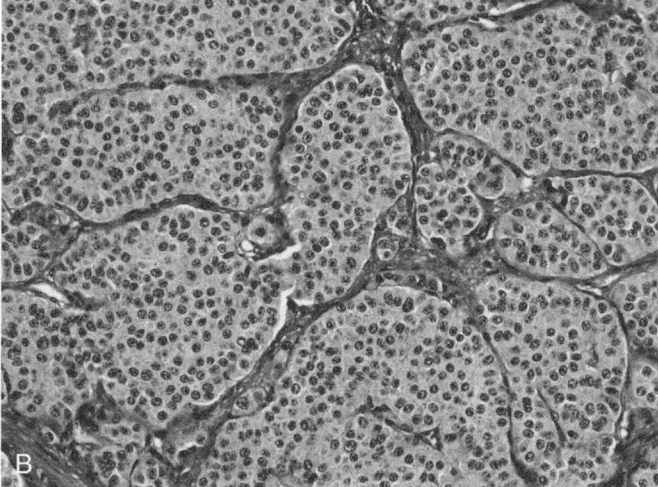

Figure 4-46. Carcinoid tumor. A, A polypoid lesion with a uniform appearance is seen protruding into the lumen of the bronchus. **B,** At high power, an organoid pattern is seen. The cells are uniform, with abundant cytoplasm, round to oval nuclei, and salt-and-pepper chromatin.

ADENOCARCINOMA AND OTHER CARCINOMAS

- Pseudoglandular growth patterns may mimic adenocarcinoma, mucoepidermoid, or acinic cell carcinoma
- Adenocarcinoma displays more atypia, more mucin production, and less expression of neuroendocrine markers than carcinoid tumors

PEARLS

- *Typical carcinoid tumors rarely metastasize and have a good prognosis (about 90% 5-year survival rate after complete resection)*
- *Atypical carcinoid tumors show a greater propensity for metastasis, and 5-year survival rate is about 50%*
- *Typical and atypical carcinoid tumors can occur in patients with multiple endocrine neoplasia type I syndrome (MEN I)*
- *Gene mutations in p53, Rb, and cyclin D1 are much more common in LCNEC and SCLC than in carcinoid tumors*
- *Carcinoid syndrome, Cushing syndrome, and synthesis of ectopic growth hormone–releasing hormone is rare in pulmonary carcinoid tumor*

SELECTED REFERENCES

Bertino EM, Confer PD, Colonna JE, et al: Pulmonary neuroendocrine/carcinoid tumors: a review article. Cancer 115:4434-4441, 2009.

Travis WD: Advances in neuroendocrine lung tumors. Ann Oncol 21(suppl 7):vii, 65-71, 2010.

Mesenchymal Tumors
PULMONARY HAMARTOMA

Clinical Features

- About 5% to 8% of all solitary pulmonary nodules and 75% of all benign lung tumors
- Most hamartomas are discovered between the ages of 50 and 60 years, and men are affected 2 to 3 times more frequently than women
- Most patients have a history of cigarette smoke exposure
- Most peripheral lesions are clinically silent, whereas endobronchial lesions may cause obstructive symptoms

Gross Pathology

- About 90% of tumors are located in the lung periphery, whereas 10% are located centrally
- Gray-white, sharply demarcated, firm, lobulated nodule ranging in size from 1 to 9 cm with mean diameter of 1.5 cm

Histopathology

- Benign neoplasm containing a mixture of epithelial and mesenchymal tissues
- The tumor is composed of a haphazard arrangement of cartilage, fibromyxoid tissue, fat, smooth muscle, or bone (Figure 4-47)
- Nodules are separated by clefts lined with non-neoplastic, ciliated, or nonciliated respiratory epithelium
- All components are well-differentiated, and fat is present in more than half of all specimens

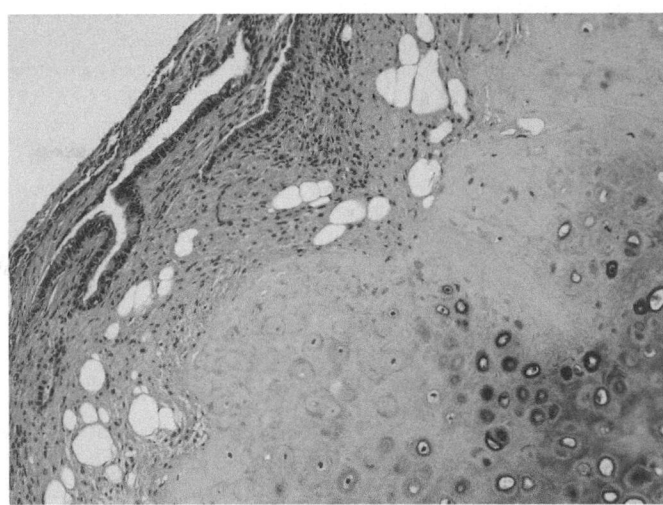

Figure 4-47. Hamartoma. Benign cartilage, fat, and bronchial epithelium are seen in this low-power photomicrograph.

Special Stains and Immunohistochemistry

- Noncontributory

Other Techniques for Diagnosis

- Noncontributory

Differential Diagnosis

CARNEY TRIAD

- Rare disorder that predominantly affects women and often presents during teenage years, with epithelioid gastrointestinal stromal tumors (GISTs) and extra-adrenal paragangliomas
- Pulmonary chondromas, often multiple and lacking cleftlike spaces, lined by respiratory epithelium

LEIOMYOMA

- Leiomyomas do not contain fat or cartilage

LIPOMA

- Typically found in central bronchi, more often left-sided, and can present with obstructive symptoms (wheezing, recurrent pneumonia, or bronchiectasis)
- Smooth-walled polypoid lesion projecting into bronchus lumen
- Mature adipose tissue with occasional giant cells
- Lacks other mesenchymal elements

PEARLS

- *Cartilage is the most common type of tissue in pulmonary hamartomas*
- *Chromosomal regions 12q15 and 6p21, corresponding to high mobility group (HMG) loci, are often involved in many benign tumors, including pulmonary hamartoma and lipoma*
- *The presence of both fat and calcification on high-resolution CT is a specific combination for hamartomas, particularly in tumors smaller than 2.5 cm in diameter*
- *Malignant transformation is very rare*

Selected References

Mondello B, Lentini S, Buda C, et al: Giant endobronchial hamartoma resected by fiberoptic bronchoscopy electrosurgical snaring. J Cardiothorac Surg 6:97-100, 2011.

Trahan S, Erickson-Johnson MR, Rodriguez F, et al: Formation of the 12q14-q15 amplicon precedes the development of a well-differentiated liposarcoma arising from a nonchondroid pulmonary hamartoma. Am J Surg Pathol 30:1326-1329, 2006.

Zhu H, Huang S, Zhou X: Mesenchymal cystic hamartoma of the lung. Ann Thorac Surg 93:e145-e147, 2012.

LYMPHANGIOLEIOMYOMATOSIS (LAM)

Clinical Features

- Diffuse, extensive proliferation of smooth muscle–like spindle cells (LAM cells) frequently associated with cystic changes primarily occurring in women during their reproductive years (sporadic disease) and occurring in both sexes when associated with tuberous sclerosis
- Rare disease; estimated incidence of 1 case per 100,000 persons per year
- LAM is now considered to be a low-grade, destructive metastasizing tumor, involving the lungs; axillary, thoracic, and retroperitoneal lymph nodes (where it manifests as fluid-filled cystic structures known as *lymphangioleiomyomas*); renal angiomyolipomas; hamartomas; and uterine leiomyomas
- Patients typically present with progressive dyspnea, cough, chylous pleural effusions, recurrent pneumothoraces, and hemoptysis
- Ten-year survival rate is more than 90%

Gross Pathology

- High-resolution CT shows numerous bilateral, 2- to 5-mm thin-walled cysts, which in the clinical context of pneumothorax or chylothorax, as well as obstructive pulmonary function tests and impaired diffusion capacity, is diagnostic for LAM
- Hyperaerated lungs with extensive, diffuse cysts measuring 0.5 to 2 cm in diameter affecting both lungs and distorting the pleural surfaces

Histopathology

- Two major lesions in LAM
  - Disorderly proliferation of benign-appearing smooth muscle cells in peribronchial, perivascular, and perilymphatic regions throughout the lung (Figure 4-48)
  - Variably sized, air-filled cysts lined by plaquelike or nodular aggregates of smooth muscle bundles
- Two types of LAM cells
  - Small spindle cells that react with proliferating cell nuclear antigen (PCNA; discussed later) and likely represent a more proliferative state
  - Larger epithelioid cells that react with HMB-45 and likely represent a more differentiated state
- LAM cells have no significant atypia or mitotic activity; however, over time, these cells proliferate and destroy lung parenchyma
- Secondary to hemorrhage, hemosiderin-laden macrophages or a foreign-body granulomatous reaction may be present

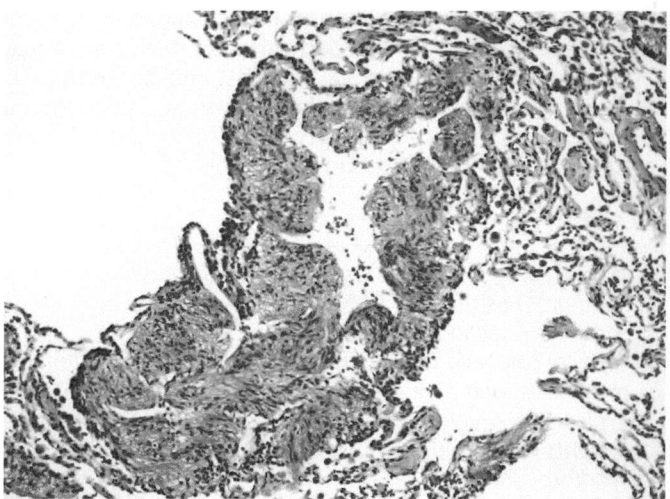

Figure 4-48. Lymphangioleiomyomatosis. There is an abnormal proliferation of bland uniform spindle cells with eosinophilic cytoplasm (smooth muscle cells).

- LAM histology score (LHS) corresponds with prognosis and may be quantified by the extent of replacement of normal lung tissue with cystic lesions and LAM cell nodules
  - LHS-1: < 25%
  - LHS-2: 25% to 50%
  - LHS-3: > 50%

Special Stains and Immunohistochemistry

- Desmin, smooth muscle actin, and vimentin expression is present, consistent with smooth muscle differentiation
- Smooth muscle bundles stain positive for HMB-45, estrogen receptor, bcl-2, and, often, D2-40

Other Techniques for Diagnosis

- Molecular analysis demonstrates the loss of heterozygosity and somatic mutations in the gene *TSC2* (16p13), a tumor suppressor gene that codes for tuberin

Differential Diagnosis

Benign Metastasizing Leiomyoma

- Lacks the delicate, thin-walled cysts seen in LAM
- Patient history of uterine leiomyoma
- Smooth muscle bundles typically form nodular arrangements
- HMB-45 negative

Leiomyosarcoma

- No diffuse cystic changes
- Cellular atypia, mitoses, and necrosis
- Negative for HMB-45

Peribronchiolar Smooth Muscle Hyperplasia in Honeycomb Fibrosing Lesions

- Reactive smooth muscle hyperplasia and cystic changes are common findings in pulmonary fibrosis; however, extensive, diffuse interstitial fibrosis and remodeled lung architecture with some inflammation are absent in LAM
- HMB-45 negative

PEARLS

- *A spectrum of mutations in the TSC2 gene have been identified in patients with LAM*
- *Some studies suggest that LAM cells migrate or metastasize to the lung from angiomyolipomas or lymph nodes*
- *Women with LAM appear to have a high prevalence of meningiomas*
- *An inverse relationship exists in LAM smooth muscle cells between immunoreactivity for HMB-45 and for PCNA, suggesting that LAM cells represent a population of smooth muscle cells in variable states of differentiation*

SELECTED REFERENCES

Badri KR, Gao L, Hyjek E, et al: Exonic mutations of TSC2/TSC1 are common but not seen in all sporadic pulmonary lymphangioleiomyomatosis. Am J Respir Crit Care Med 187:663-665, 2013.

McCormack FX, Travis WD, Colby TV, et al: Lymphangioleiomyomatosis: calling it what it is: a low-grade, destructive, metastasizing neoplasm. Am J Respir Crit Care Med 186:1210-1212, 2012.

Meraj R, Wikenheiser-Brokamp KA, Young LR, et al: Utility of transbronchial biopsy in the diagnosis of lymphangioleiomyomatosis. Front Med 6:395-405, 2012.

INFLAMMATORY MYOFIBROBLASTIC TUMOR (IMT)

Clinical Features

- IMT is most common in the lung, but it can be found in most major organs, the retroperitoneum, the mesentery, the mediastinum, the dura, and the abdominal cavity
- IMT can affect individuals of any age (range, 9 days to 87 years), but most patients are children or young adults (mean age, 30 years) with an equal male-to-female ratio
- IMT accounts for more than 50% of pulmonary tumors in children
- Some cases are associated with human herpesvirus-8 (HHV-8); EBV is associated with splenic and nodal-based but not pulmonary IMT
- Reported rates of recurrence range from 25% to 40% and are more common with extrapulmonary IMT

Gross Pathology

- Generally solitary, unencapsulated, round, rubbery masses sharply demarcated from the adjacent lung parenchyma
- Cut surface varies from yellow-grey, to tan, to white
- Size ranges from 1 to 6 cm (mean, 3 cm); they can become as large as 36 cm
- Penetration of the pleura is common, and polypoid endobronchial protrusions occasionally occur

Histopathology

- Composed of spindle cells with fibroblastic and myofibroblastic differentiation arranged in a fascicular or storiform pattern mixed with inflammatory cells in a myxoid, fibrotic, or hyalinized stroma (Figure 4-49)
- Lesions often obliterate the underlying lung architecture

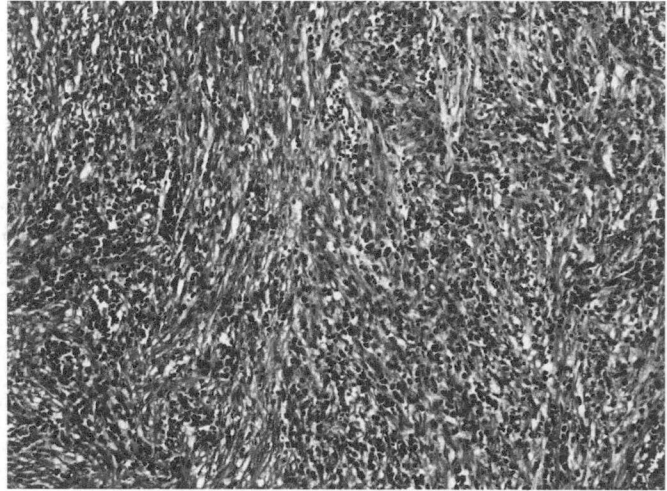

Figure 4-49. Inflammatory myofibroblastic tumor. This photomicrograph shows a cellular lesion composed of bland spindle cells admixed with inflammatory cells (plasma cells and lymphocytes).

- Variable proportions of cellular elements from predominantly myofibroblastic to predominantly plasmacytic
- Spindle cells have oval nuclei, fine chromatin, inconspicuous nucleoli, and abundant eosinophilic cytoplasm
- Nuclear atypia is minimal to none, but occasional spindle cells have large vesicular nuclei with prominent nucleoli resembling ganglion cells or Reed-Sternberg cells
  - These rare atypical cells often display granular, cytoplasmic overexpression of the ALK protein
- Mitoses are generally scanty (0 to 2/10 hpf) but can be as numerous as 15/10 hpf
- A robust inflammatory component composed of plasma cells, lymphocytes, macrophages, foamy histiocytes, occasional Touton-type giant cells, and small numbers of eosinophils or neutrophils is present and may be so prominent as to obscure the spindle cells
- Invasion of small vessels, the chest wall, or hilar soft tissue occasionally occurs

Special Stains and Immunohistochemistry

- Spindle cells express vimentin (> 95%), smooth muscle actin (86%), muscle-specific actin (82%), and focally desmin (41%)
- ALK-1 and p80 expression occurs in about 45% of cases
- Cytokeratin immunoreactivity likely represents entrapped epithelial elements
- Spindle cells are negative for CD117/c-KIT, S-100, myogenin, and myoglobin

Other Techniques for Diagnosis

- Noncontributory

Differential Diagnosis

FIBROUS HISTIOCYTOMA OF SOFT TISSUE
- Shares a similar storiform histologic pattern with IMT

PLASMACYTOMA
- Rarely involves the lungs
- Composed of atypical, monoclonal plasma cells with numerous mitotic figures and little to no fibrosis

PULMONARY AMYLOIDOSIS

- Waxy, hard irregular nodules
- Congo red stain is useful to differentiate amyloid tumor from IMT

PULMONARY HYALINIZING GRANULOMA

- Multiple lesions with extensive hyalinization and mild lymphocytic infiltrate
- Lamellar collagen arranged in storiform or whorled arrays

INFLAMMATORY FIBROSARCOMA

- Low-grade sarcoma composed of fascicles or whorls of fibroblastic or myofibroblastic cells mixed with plasma cells and collagen
- Spindle cells show prominent nuclear atypia and can invade large vessels or the pleura

PEARLS

- *The current consensus is that the spindle cell component is neoplastic in most cases of IMT*
- *Research suggests that the spindle cells are derived from fibroblastic reticulum cells (FBRCs), which are a subtype of accessory immune cells that interact with lymphocytes and their progeny during immune responses*
- *The presence of chromosomal abnormalities is consistent with a clonal origin and can help to explain, in part, the spectrum of aggressive behavior of these lesions*
- *A subset of IMT occurring in the lung or abdomen during the first decade of life has been shown to possess a chromosomal rearrangement involving the ALK locus at 2p23; these tumors may show more aggressive behavior and increased recurrence rates*
- *Complete excision is recommended if possible to minimize the rate of recurrence*

SELECTED REFERENCES

Kovach SJ, Fischer AC, Katzman PJ, et al: Inflammatory myofibroblastic tumors. J Surg Oncol 94:385-391, 2006.
Mano H: ALKoma: a cancer subtype with a shared target. Cancer Discov 2:495-502, 2012.
Maurya V, Aditya Gupta U, et al: Spontaneous resolution of an inflammatory pseudotumour of the lung subsequent to wedge biopsy. Arch Bronconeumol 49:31-34, 2013.
Siminovich M, Galluzzo L, López J, et al: Inflammatory myofibroblastic tumor of the lung in children: anaplastic lymphoma kinase (ALK) expression and clinico-pathological correlation. Pediatr Dev Pathol 15:179-186, 2012.

PLEUROPULMONARY BLASTOMA (PPB)

Clinical Features

- Rare childhood tumor arising in the lung parenchyma in association with the pleura or in the mediastinum
- Mean age of patients is 2.5 years, but occasionally older children and adolescents are affected
- Three morphologic subtypes represent a continuum of histologic and biologic progression
  - Type I is the least common, accounting for less than 15% of PPB cases, and affects the youngest group of patients (median age, 10 months)
  - Type II accounts for 40% to 50% of all PPB and affects somewhat older children than type I (median age, 34 months)
  - Type III accounts for 40% of PPB cases and occurs in older patients (median age, 44 months)

Gross Pathology

- The neoplasms appear cystic, solid, or mixed and are subtyped accordingly
  - Type I: purely cystic
  - Type II: combined cystic and solid pattern
  - Type III: well-circumscribed, solid, mucoid, tan-white, partially friable or necrotic mass with pleural attachments, involving either one lobe or the entire lung

Histopathology

- Malignant cells are a biphasic mixture of (Figure 4-50)
  - Primitive, small, elliptical, undifferentiated blastemal cells with scanty cytoplasm and solitary,

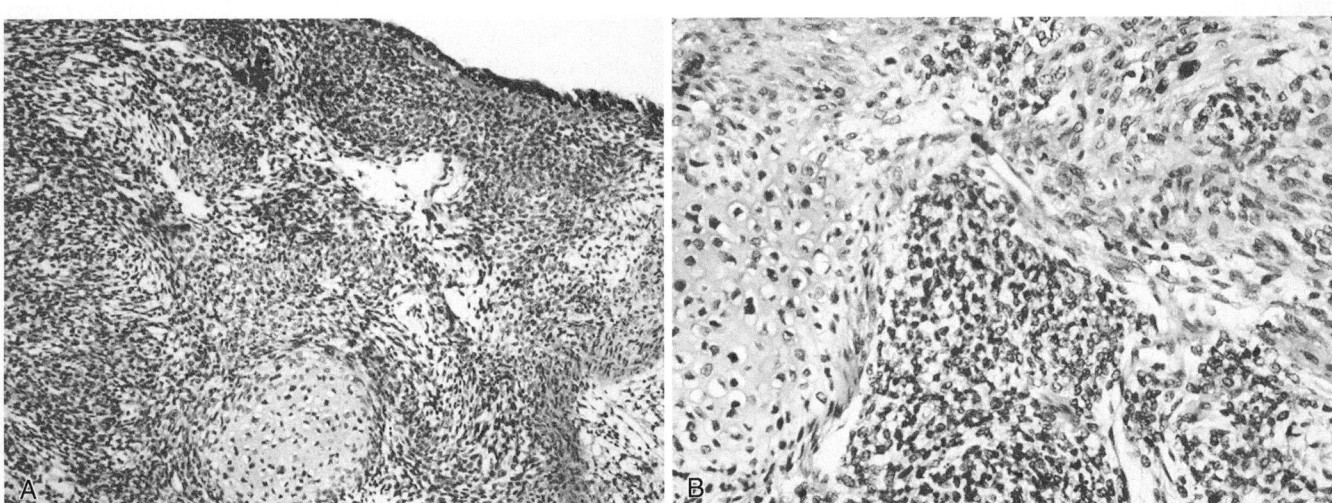

Figure 4-50. Pleuropulmonary blastoma. A, Epithelial lining is present in the *upper right-hand corner.* The solid portion of the tumor is composed of solid and loose sarcomatous tissue and nodules of malignant cartilage. **B,** High-power photomicrograph shows high-grade undifferentiated blastomatous and chondrosarcomatous components.

spherical hyperchromatic nuclei with occasional distinct nucleoli
  - Larger, spindle-shaped, often rhabdomyoblastic cells
- Epithelial cells are not a component of the neoplasm and when present represent entrapped mesothelial or epithelial elements
- Focal rhabdomyosarcomatous differentiation, either as individual or groups of strap cells with cross striations, is present in most cases

Special Stains and Immunohistochemistry

- Blastemal cells and proliferating spindle cells react with vimentin; they are negative for cytokeratin and epithelial membrane antigen
- Neoplastic cells displaying differentiation often react with desmin, smooth muscle actin, and muscle-specific actin
- Cartilaginous nodules express S-100

Other Techniques for Diagnosis

- PPB families harbor heterozygous germline mutations in DICER1, a gene encoding an endoribonuclease critical to the generation of small noncoding regulatory RNAs; expression of DICER1 protein was undetectable in the epithelial component of PPB tumors but was retained in the malignant mesenchyme (sarcoma); it is hypothesized that loss of DICER1 in the epithelium of the developing lung alters the regulation of diffusible factors that promote mesenchymal proliferation

Differential Diagnosis

CPAM

- CPAM and type I PPB affect infants and young children
- Type I PPB shows the presence of dense subepithelial or septal spindle cells with or without foci of immature cartilage

METASTATIC WILMS TUMOR

- PPB is negative for cytokeratin, whereas epithelial component of Wilms tumor is positive
- Wilms tumor is positive for WT-1 (nuclear)

PRIMARY PULMONARY SARCOMAS OF CHILDREN

- Rhabdomyosarcoma and leiomyosarcoma show monophasic myogenous differentiation

ADULT PULMONARY BLASTOMA (APB)

- Despite its similar nomenclature, APB is an altogether separate entity considered to be a sarcomatoid carcinoma
- Relative to other rare lung tumors, APB is relatively common and usually presents as a well-defined peripheral lung mass in adults with a female predominance
- APB is a biphasic tumor composed of malignant, fetal-type tubular epithelial structures and an immature mesenchymal stroma, whereas the epithelial structures in PPB are entrapped, nonmalignant components
- The tubules and stroma of APB resemble fetal lung between 10 and 16 weeks' gestation (the pseudoglandular stage of lung development)
- Tubules in APB contain nonciliated, pseudostratified columnar cells with an endometrioid appearance and PAS-positive subnuclear or supranuclear vacuoles

- The stroma in APB has a blastema-like morphology composed of small, oval- to spindle-shaped cells in a myxoid matrix with occasional foci of differentiated sarcomatous elements (i.e., rhabdomyosarcoma, chondrosarcoma, and osteosarcoma)
- The stroma shows a tendency to condense around the malignant glands in APB
- Morulas are seen at the bases of glands in close to half of APB

PEARLS

- *Roughly 25% of PPB cases are associated with familial cancer syndrome: thyroid tumors, cystic nephroma, ovarian teratoma, multiple intestinal polyps, and other tumors*
- *It is believed that PPB progresses from type I to type III over time, and definitive surgery before progression from type I to either type II or type III is the key to successful management of PPB*

SELECTED REFERENCES

Hill DA, Ivanovich J, Priest JR, et al: DICER1 mutations in familial pleuropulmonary blastoma. Science 325:965, 2009.

Hill DA, Jarzembowski JA, Priest JR, et al: Type I pleuropulmonary blastoma: pathology and biology study of 51 cases from the international pleuropulmonary blastoma registry. Am J Surg Pathol 32:282-295, 2008.

Priest JR, Williams GM, Hill DA, et al: Pulmonary cysts in early childhood and the risk of malignancy. Pediatr Pulmonol 44:14-30, 2009.

Lymphoproliferative Disorders
MARGINAL ZONE B-CELL LYMPHOMA OF THE MUCOSA-ASSOCIATED LYMPHOID TISSUE (MALT) TYPE

Clinical Features

- Primary pulmonary lymphoma is rare, representing 0.5% to 1% of primary pulmonary malignancies
- Pulmonary MALT lymphoma accounts for 70% to 90% of primary lung lymphoma, making it a "common rare tumor"
- Presentation in patients younger than 50 years is rare unless some underlying immunosuppression is present (i.e., autoimmune disease, HIV)
- An associated monoclonal gammopathy is present in 30% of cases
- Pleural effusions are rare to absent

Gross Pathology

- Consolidated, yellow-tan mass

Histopathology

- Lymphoid infiltrates composed of a monomorphic population of malignant cells with centrocyte-like morphology consisting of slightly irregular nuclei with scanty cytoplasm surrounding reactive follicles (Figure 4-51)
- Follicles may be obscured by an exuberant lymphoma infiltrate (follicular colonization or mantle zone colonization)

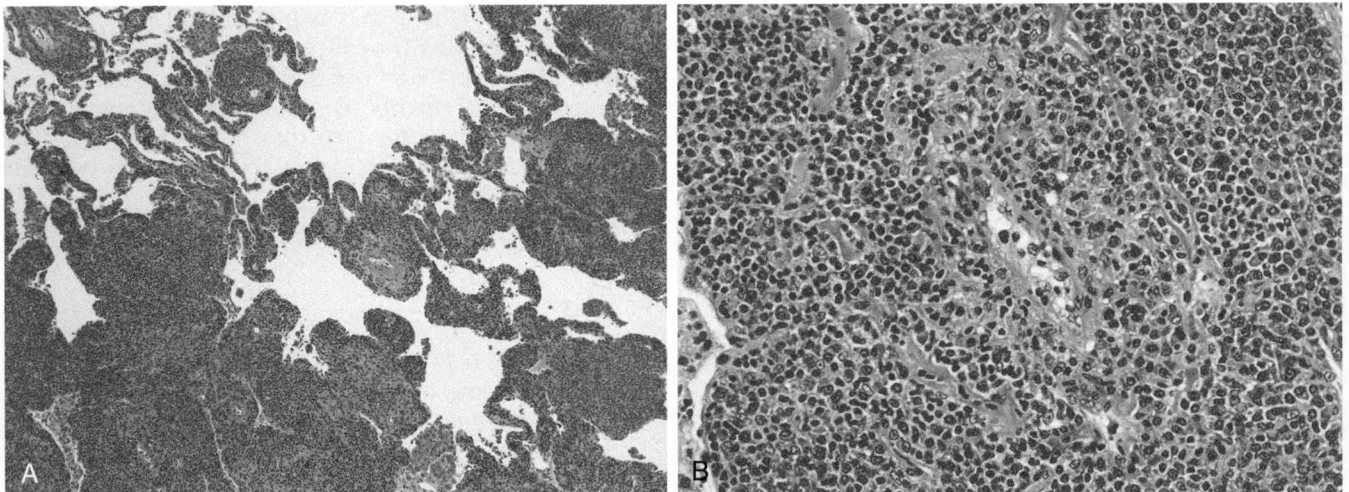

Figure 4-51. Mucosa-associated lymphoid tissue (MALT) lymphoma. A, The malignant cells form nodules and infiltrate alveolar septa. **B,** High-power photomicrograph shows the malignant lymphoid cells infiltrating a blood vessel wall.

- There is a lymphangitic pattern of growth along interlobular septa and bronchovascular bundles creating a nodular interstitial infiltrate
- Expansion of the nodules into solid masses effaces and obliterates the underlying lung architecture
- Lymphoepithelial lesions are formed as lymphoma cells infiltrate the bronchial epithelium and are a common finding
- Plasmacytoid lymphocytes, plasma cells with intranuclear Dutcher bodies, small normal lymphocytes, and large transformed cells may be present
- Central necrosis and giant lamellar bodies are occasional features

Special Stains and Immunohistochemistry

- Tumor cells express CD20, CD43, bcl-2, PAX5, and CD79
- Tumor cells are negative for CD5, CD10, CD21, CD23, bcl-6, and cyclin D1
- Follicular dendritic cells can be identified with CD21, CD23, and CD35

Other Techniques for Diagnosis

- About 60% to 70% of tumors show clonal rearrangements of the JH region of the immunoglobulin heavy chain
- Roughly two thirds of MALT lymphomas display trisomy 3
- About 20% to 50% of MALT lymphomas show t(11;18) (q21;q21)
- Translocations t(14;18)(q32;q21) and t(1;14)(p22;q32) are also present in some MALT lymphomas and may function by up-regulating NF-κ B signaling

Differential Diagnosis

FOLLICULAR BRONCHITIS OR BRONCHIOLITIS

- Lymphoepithelial lesions can occur in reactive conditions and lymphoma
- MALT lymphoma displays an expanded B-cell infiltrate beyond the follicles
- Reactive lymphocytic infiltrates form small aggregates of B cells
- Clonality can be demonstrated by light-chain restriction in MALT lymphoma cells

LYMPHOID INTERSTITIAL PNEUMONIA (LIP)

- Seen in immunocompromised patients, especially pediatric AIDS patients
- Not monoclonal

CHRONIC LYMPHOCYTIC LYMPHOMA (CLL)

- CLL infiltrates are limited to the bronchovascular bundles without infiltration and destruction of the lung architecture
- CLL is positive for CD20, PAX5, CD79a, CD5, CD43, and bcl-2; it is negative for CD10, CD23, and bcl-6

PEARLS

- *MALT is absent from the lung in physiologic conditions and becomes apparent during chronic antigenic stimulation*
- *No antigens have been identified, but certain autoimmune disorders (e.g., SLE, multiple sclerosis, Hashimoto thyroiditis, and Sjögren syndrome) may play a role in MALT lymphoma*

SELECTED REFERENCES

Arnaoutakis K, Oo TH: Bronchus-associated lymphoid tissue lymphomas. South Med J 102:1229-1233, 2009.
Guinee DG Jr: Update on nonneoplastic pulmonary lymphoproliferative disorders and related entities. Arch Pathol Lab Med 134:691-701, 2010.
William J, Variakojis D, Yeldandi A, et al: Lymphoproliferative neoplasms of the lung: a review. Arch Pathol Lab Med 137:382-391, 2013.

PULMONARY LANGERHANS CELL HISTIOCYTOSIS (PLCH)

Clinical Features

- Occurs in young adults, most commonly between the ages of 30 and 50 years
- Strong association with cigarette smoking in adults
- Uncommon in African Americans and Asians

- Patients present with dyspnea, cough, and occasionally pneumothorax (10% to 15%)
- In children (non-smoking-related neoplastic disorder), multisystem disease of bone, pituitary, skin, and lymph nodes, which may involve the lung sometimes

Gross Pathology

- Early stages: multiple small nodules (1 to 5 mm) in a centrilobular distribution with middle and upper zone predominance
- Later stages: larger, irregular, tan-gray nodules with central lucency due to cavitation or bronchiolar dilation
- Disease becomes progressively cystic with irregular, bizarre shapes

Histopathology

- Characteristic low-magnification pattern of multiple nodular infiltrates with stellate borders centered around small airways
- Nodules can have a Medusa-head appearance due to tendrils of cellular infiltrates extending into the surrounding alveolar interstitium
- A distinctive form of cicatricial change occurs as nodules interconnect with adjacent nodules
- Infiltrate is composed of uniform sheets of Langerhans cells with varying numbers of eosinophils, lymphocytes, and plasma cells
- Langerhans cells have moderate amounts of eosinophilic cytoplasm and pale nuclei with prominent nuclear grooves (Figure 4-52)
- PLCH lesions progress from cellular nodules to intermediate cellular-fibrotic nodules to fibrotic scars, and biopsy specimens often show a spectrum of these changes
- End-stage nodules are paucicellular, are fibrotic, and lack Langerhans cells yet retain the stellate pattern facilitating the diagnosis of PLCH
- Nodular lesions can invade vascular structures, causing vasculopathy and abnormal pulmonary hemodynamics
- Smoking associated respiratory bronchiolitis is invariably present in adjacent lung tissue

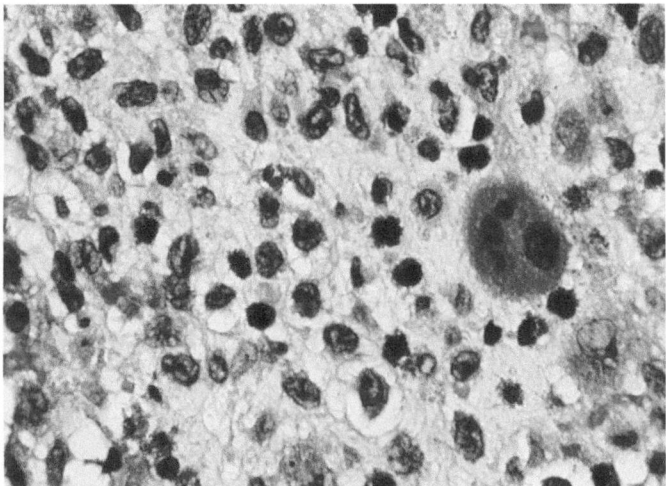

Figure 4-52. Pulmonary Langerhans cell histiocytosis. High-power photomicrograph shows histiocytes with characteristic grooved nuclei. The same nuclei are present in the multinucleated giant cell. Eosinophils are also present, although not required for diagnosis.

Special Stains and Immunohistochemistry

- Langerhans cells stain positive for S-100, CD1a, and Langerin and are negative for CD68
- Various studies examining clonality favor the notion that Langerhans cells are a reactive, polyclonal proliferation secondary to chronic antigenic stimulation due to cigarette smoking

Other Techniques for Diagnosis

- Electron microscopy: Birbeck granules within the Langerhans cells

Differential Diagnosis

RESPIRATORY BRONCHIOLITIS

- Weakly brown pigmented alveolar macrophages adjacent to respiratory bronchioles
- Lacks the cellular and nodular interstitial lesions

CHRONIC EOSINOPHILIC PNEUMONIA (CEP)

- Intra-alveolar eosinophils in CEP without Langerhans cells

UIP

- Fibrotic scars in PLCH retain a stellate shape with a bronchiolocentric distribution and lack UIP-like temporal heterogeneity

REACTIVE EOSINOPHILIC PLEURITIS

- Nonspecific pleural reaction occurring in the setting of pneumothorax
- Restricted to the pleura
- Prominent eosinophils mixed with proliferating mesothelial cells and chronic inflammation

PEARLS

- *Histology of PLCH in children is essentially identical to that in adults*
- *High-resolution CT studies demonstrate that PLCH lesions evolve in the following sequence: nodules, cavitated nodules, cysts, and eventually confluent cysts*
- *PLCH is regarded as a reactive proliferative disease of Langerhans cells, in contrast to the extrapulmonary forms of Langerhans cell histiocytosis, which are neoplastic processes*
- *Pulmonary lesions show abundant expression of transforming growth factor-β_1 and granulocyte-macrophage colony-stimulating factor*

SELECTED REFERENCES

Nagarjun Rao R, Moran CA, Suster S: Histiocytic disorders of the lung. Adv Anat Pathol 17:12-22, 2010.
Vassallo R: Diffuse lung diseases in cigarette smokers. Semin Respir Crit Care Med 33:533-542, 2012.

POSTTRANSPLANTATION LYMPHOPROLIFERATIVE DISORDER (PTLD)

Clinical Features

- A morphologically heterogeneous group of EBV-driven lymphoid proliferations
- Occurs more frequently with solid organ transplantation (3% to 5% of heart and lung transplantations)

- A localized or multifocal lymphoproliferative process in which the transplanted lung is often involved
- Proliferations are composed of polyclonal to monoclonal populations of cells

Gross Pathology

- Single or multifocal well-defined solid nodules or diffuse consolidations of lung parenchyma

Histopathology

- Abnormal lymphocytic proliferation occurring in the setting of chronic immunosuppression for organ transplantation that is associated with EBV
- Lymphoid cell populations range from a mixed lymphocytic hyperplasia composed of polyclonal B cells and other polymorphic cell types to monomorphic, monoclonal lymphoplasmacytoid, immunoblastic, or large B-cell lymphomas (Figure 4-53)
- Hence, PTLD encompasses a spectrum of lesions that range from histologically benign lymphoid proliferations to frankly malignant lymphoma, as follows:
  - Plasmacytic hyperplasia
    - Underlying lung architecture is maintained
    - Small polyclonal T and B lymphocytes, plasma cells, and occasional immunoblasts are present
    - EBV can be detected in most cases
    - Most common pattern to occur in children and young adults
  - Polymorphic lymphoproliferative disorder
    - Lymphoid infiltrate distorts the underlying lung architecture
    - Mixture of lymphocytes, plasmacytoid cells, and occasional immunoblasts, which may resemble Reed-Sternberg cells
    - The lymphoid cells are generally clonal and contain EBV
  - Malignant lymphoma or multiple myeloma
    - Monotonous population of lymphocytes or plasma cells that resemble lymphoma or multiple myeloma
    - Most tumors are diffuse large B-cell lymphomas and contain EBV

Special Stains and Immunohistochemistry

- EBV, CD45, B-cell markers, and T-cell markers permit further characterization
- Flow cytometry is useful for phenotype analysis of the proliferating lymphocytes

Other Techniques for Diagnosis

- Gene rearrangement studies useful in establishing clonality

Differential Diagnosis

- Lymphoid interstitial pneumonia (LIP)

PEARLS

- *In bone marrow transplantations, PTLD is usually of donor origin, whereas in solid organ transplantation, it is usually of recipient origin*
- *Interval between transplantation and development of PTLD is 1 month to 4 years*
- *Regression or resolution commonly occurs after reduction in immunosuppressive therapy on PTLD occurring in the first year after transplantation*

Other Neoplastic Conditions
MALIGNANT MESOTHELIOMA

Clinical Features

- Rare tumor showing a male predominance and a strong association with asbestos exposure but with a long latent period
- Most patients are between 50 and 70 years old
- Associated with a poor prognosis, with average survival of less than 1 year; epithelioid mesothelioma has a somewhat better survival
- Smoking does not increase the risk for malignant mesothelioma; however, the combination of smoking and asbestos exposure greatly increases the risk for lung carcinoma

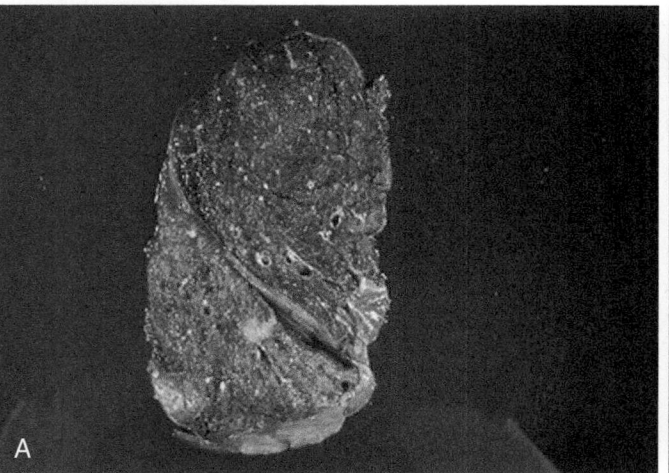
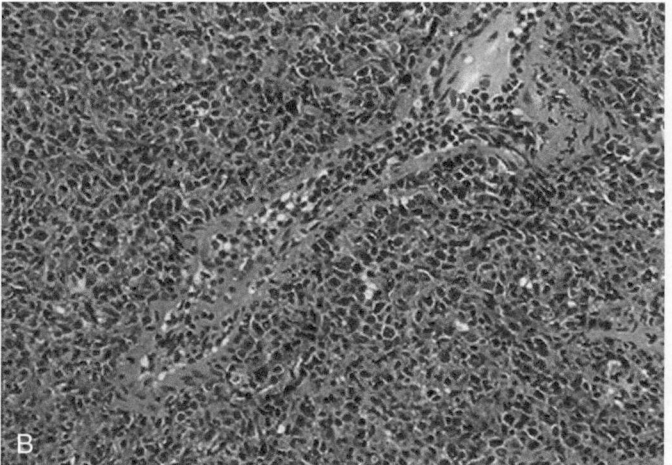

Figure 4-53. Posttransplantation lymphoproliferative disorder. A, Gross picture of cut surface of lung at autopsy in this lung transplant recipient shows tan-white nodules. **B,** Highly atypical lymphocytes are seen infiltrating the lung parenchyma and blood vessel wall.

Gross Pathology

- Malignant mesothelioma encases the lungs and extends diffusely through the pleural space

Histopathology

- A malignant tumor of mesothelial cells with a diffuse growth pattern involving the visceral and parietal pleura and, less commonly, the peritoneum (Figure 4-54)
- Three histologic categories: epithelioid, sarcomatoid, and biphasic
  - Epithelioid variant
    - Represents 65% to 70% of malignant mesothelioma
    - Growth patterns are tubulopapillary, glandular or acinar, solid, or micropapillary (most often a mixture of these patterns is present)
    - Neoplastic cells are usually bland and cytologically homogeneous with round nuclei, vesicular chromatin with prominent nucleoli, and a moderate amount of eosinophilic cytoplasm
  - Sarcomatoid variant
    - Pleomorphic spindle cells growing in short fascicles, typically with a storiform pattern, within a fibrous stroma
    - Desmoplastic mesothelioma, a subtype of the sarcomatoid variant representing roughly 10% of all cases of mesothelioma, shows a dense, collagenous stroma separating the neoplastic cells
  - Biphasic variant
    - Tumors contain both epithelioid and sarcomatous components in which the minor component exceeds 10% of the tumor

Special Stains and Immunohistochemistry

- Positive for keratin AE1/AE3, CAM5.2, and CK7; specific mesothelial markers include calretinin, CK5/6, WT-1, D2-40

Other Techniques for Diagnosis

- Cytogenetics: homozygous deletion of the CDKN2A/ARF locus at 9p21, which codes for the tumor suppressor genes p16INK4a and p14ARF, is a common finding and helps to differentiate mesothelioma from reactive lesions

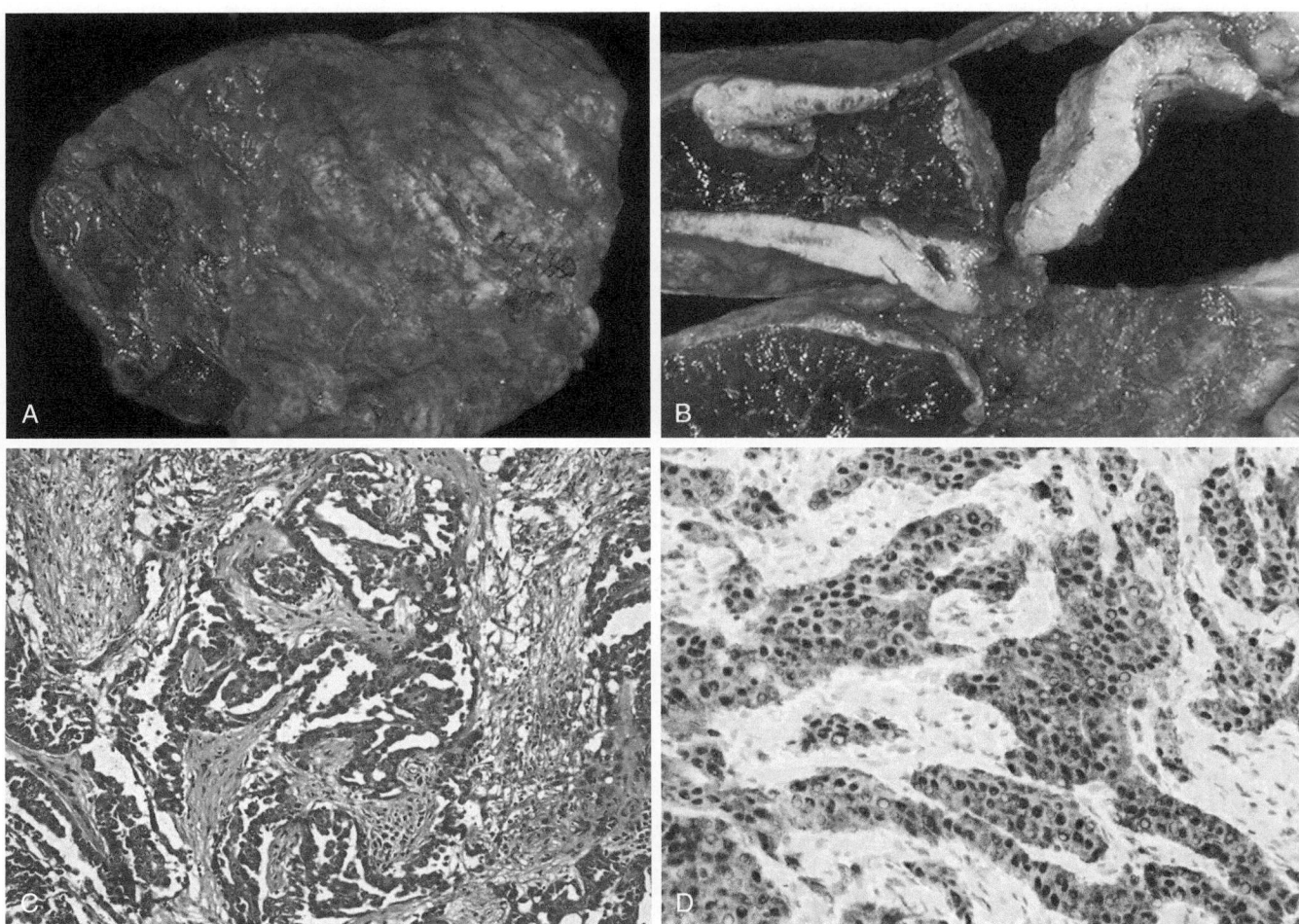

Figure 4-54. Malignant mesothelioma. A, Gross photograph of the pneumonectomy specimen shows tumor encasing the lung. **B,** Gross photograph of cut surface shows malignant mesothelioma growing along the pleura and encasing the dark-red lung parenchyma. **C,** H&E-stained section shows glandular and papillary patterns of epithelioid malignant mesothelioma. **D,** Calretinin stain shows both nuclear and cytoplasmic staining in most epithelioid tumors.

Differential Diagnosis

ADENOCARCINOMA

- A panel of immunohistochemical stains that includes at least two mesothelial markers and at least two markers for adenocarcinoma
- Adenocarcinoma markers include MOC-31, BG8, CEA, CD15, Ber-Ep4, B72.3, TTF-1, and estrogen and progesterone receptors for breast and gynecologic carcinomas
- Calretinin is the most useful mesothelial marker and demonstrates strong and diffuse staining of the cytoplasm and nuclei of both benign and malignant mesothelial cells; nuclear staining must be present to make the diagnosis of malignant mesothelioma
- CK5/6 is expressed in the cytoplasm of mesothelial and squamous cells; it is rarely expressed by adenocarcinoma
- WT-1 shows a nuclear expression pattern in mesothelioma as well as in serous carcinomas of the ovary

REACTIVE MESOTHELIAL HYPERPLASIA

- Invasion of mesothelioma cells into the adipose tissue of the parietal pleura is evidence of malignancy
- Cytoplasmic desmin staining is more consistent with reactive mesothelial hyperplasia, whereas diffuse, linear membranous EMA, strong p53, and GLUT1 staining supports malignant epithelioid mesothelioma

DESMOPLASTIC MESOTHELIOMA VERSUS CHRONIC FIBROSING PLEURITIS

- Mesothelial markers are not helpful, and both desmoplastic mesothelioma and reactive mesothelial cells express cytokeratins and vimentin
- Cytokeratin antibody cocktails help to identify invasion into adjacent adipose tissue
- Cytokeratin cocktails also demonstrate the disordered growth pattern of desmoplastic mesothelioma
- In contrast, reactive mesothelial cells in chronic fibrosing pleuritis are arranged in a more orderly manner parallel to the pleural surface

SOLITARY FIBROUS TUMOR

- Most commonly involves pleura as a slow-growing, localized mass
- Grossly, firm with white cut surface; focal necrosis, cystic degeneration may be present
- Proliferation of uniform spindle-shaped cells in a collagenous background
- Hemangiopericytoma-like vascular pattern with alternating hypocellular and hypercellular areas
- CD34, CD99, and bcl-2 positivity in most cases, negative for cytokeratins

PEARLS

- *Calretinin stains both nucleus and cytoplasm with stronger nuclear staining, which is a helpful feature of mesothelial cells*
- *Invasion is the best indication of malignant mesothelioma*
- *Patients with purely epithelioid mesothelioma show the longest survival, whereas the shortest survival occurs with sarcomatoid histology—yet the difference between the two survival rates is only a matter of months*

SELECTED REFERENCE

Husain AN, Colby T, Ordonez N, et al: International Mesothelioma Interest Group. Guidelines for pathologic diagnosis of malignant mesothelioma: 2012 update of the consensus statement from the International Mesothelioma Interest Group. Arch Pathol Lab Med 137:647-667, 2013.

Chapter 5
Thymus and Mediastinum

SAUL SUSTER • CESAR A. MORAN

CHAPTER OUTLINE

THYMIC CYST

Clinical Features

- Uncommon; constitutes less than 10% of mediastinal cysts
- May be congenital or acquired
- Found in the anterior mediastinum, but may occur in ectopic locations such as neck, pleura, and posterior mediastinum
- Invariably benign
- Age range: 20 to 50 years, often asymptomatic; larger cysts can present with cough, dyspnea, and chest pain
- Acquired thymic cysts are associated with inflammatory processes and have been found in association with mediastinal Hodgkin lymphoma or its treatment, occasionally non-Hodgkin lymphoma, germinoma, yolk sac tumor, thymoma, thymic carcinoma, Langerhans cell granulomatosis, congenital syphilis, or prior thoracotomy for other diseases
- Radiologic findings: well-circumscribed mass in the anterior mediastinum measuring up to 18 cm in diameter

Gross Pathology

- Typically presents as a large encapsulated mass attached directly to thymic remnant or attached by a pedicle
- Calcifications may be present in the cyst wall

- Two types
  - Unilocular (congenital): thin-walled cyst filled with serous fluid
  - Multilocular (acquired): thick-walled cyst filled with thick, turbid hemorrhagic fluid

Histopathology

- Unilocular cysts usually have a flat or cuboidal lining; thymic remnants are not usually appreciated in their walls (Figure 5-1)
- Multilocular cysts have a lining that is usually flattened but may be stratified squamous, cuboidal, columnar, or ciliated
- Cyst lining is often in continuity with thymic remnants in the wall of the cyst and may be traced to dilated Hassall corpuscles
- Inflammatory infiltrate present in the walls of the cysts, often with hyperplastic follicles with prominent germinal centers
- Cholesterol cleft granulomas
- No cartilage, smooth muscle, or other differentiated mesenchymal tissue

Special Stains and Immunohistochemistry

- Cytokeratin may highlight the epithelium and demonstrate thymic tissue in the wall

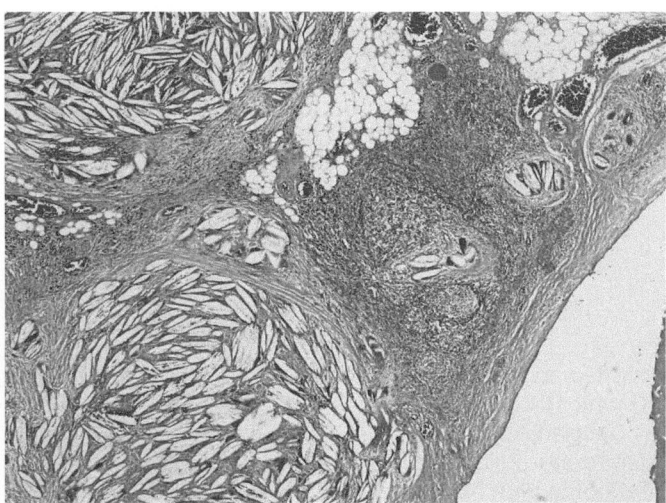

Figure 5-1. Thymic cyst. Cyst wall lined by simple cuboidal epithelium. The cyst wall contains lymphocytic infiltrate and cholesterol cleft granulomas.

Other Techniques for Diagnosis

- Noncontributory

Differential Diagnosis

PARATHYROID CYST
- Typically found in anterior-superior mediastinum
- Thin-walled cyst lined by attenuated parathyroid endocrine cells and filled with clear fluid

CYSTIC HYGROMA (LYMPHANGIOMA)
- Most common in childhood
- Composed of nonencapsulated complex cavernous spaces lined by flattened endothelium and filled with clear fluid and occasional small lymphocytes
- Embedded in collagenous fibroblastic tissue with sparse lymphoid infiltrate
- No epithelial elements present

ESOPHAGEAL CYST
- Usually in continuity with the esophagus in the middle mediastinum
- Cyst wall shows alternating layers of smooth muscle
- No thymic tissue identifiable in the wall, usually with few or no lymphocytes

BRONCHIAL CYST
- Attached to trachea or major bronchi
- Lined by ciliated columnar (respiratory) epithelium but may occasionally undergo metaplastic changes
- Smooth muscle and cartilage in cyst wall
- No thymic tissue in wall

CYSTIC TERATOMA
- Cysts are lined by any type of epithelium and may contain sebaceous glands and hair follicles

- Other common components include neural tissue, gastrointestinal tract elements, cartilage, and respiratory structures
- Monodermal teratoma may show only epithelial elements and prominent granulomatous foreign body–type response

CYSTIC THYMOMA
- May present as a discrete area of thickening or nodularity in the wall of a multilocular cyst
- Expansile nodule showing biphasic population of small T lymphocytes and thymic epithelial cells devoid of normal thymic architecture

CYSTIC DEGENERATION IN HODGKIN LYMPHOMA
- Represents cystic degeneration of thymic tissue within or adjacent to the tumor
- Solid foci showing a mixed population of lymphocytes with atypical lymphoid cells
- Demonstration of Reed-Sternberg cells by immunohistochemical staining with appropriate markers (e.g., CD15, CD30)

SELECTED REFERENCES

Suster S, Barbuto D, Carlson G, Rosai J: Multilocular thymic cysts with pseudoepitheliomatous hyperplasia. Hum Pathol 22:455-460, 1991.
Suster S, Rosai J: Multilocular thymic cyst: an acquired reactive process. Study of 18 cases. Am J Surg Pathol 15:388-398, 1991.

FOREGUT CYSTS OF THE MEDIASTINUM: BRONCHIAL (BRONCHOGENIC) CYST, ESOPHAGEAL CYST, ENTERIC DUPLICATION CYST*

Clinical Features
- These foregut cysts of the mediastinum are believed to represent congenital developmental anomalies
- Bronchial and esophageal cysts may be asymptomatic or present with cough, dyspnea, pain, or dysphagia due to compression

BRONCHIAL CYST
- Usually in adults
- Moves with respiration

ESOPHAGEAL CYST (ESOPHAGEAL DUPLICATION)
- Presents in childhood or adolescence
- Male predominance

ENTERIC DUPLICATION CYST
- Also known as foregut duplication cyst or enterogenous cyst
- Usually presents in infancy or childhood
- Strong male predominance
- Patients may have cough, pain, dysphagia, dyspnea, failure to thrive; rarely presents with massive hemoptysis

---

*Cystic neoplasms are discussed with the corresponding tumor types.

- May be associated with other congenital malformations, including vertebral abnormalities, intestinal atresia or malrotation, and congenital cardiac malformations

Gross Pathology
- Round and usually unilocular
- Size varies from a few millimeters up to 15 cm

BRONCHIAL CYST
- Attached to trachea or major bronchus
- Mucinous contents

ESOPHAGEAL CYST
- Typically located at the level of the midesophagus; may be attached to or within wall of esophagus
- Mucinous contents

ENTERIC CYST
- Mostly confined to posterior mediastinum
- Predilection for children and adolescents
- Usually attached to the vertebral column
- Thin wall
- May present with dysphagia if there is compression of the esophagus

Histopathology
BRONCHIAL CYST
- Epithelium is typically respiratory columnar but may undergo squamous metaplasia (Figure 5-2)
- Cartilage and smooth muscle are present in the cyst wall

ESOPHAGEAL CYST
- Epithelium is typically squamous but may be columnar

- Two discrete layers of smooth muscle are present at least focally in the cyst wall
- No cartilage

ENTERIC CYST
- Epithelium may be of gastric type (including parietal cells), intestinal, colonic, or squamous
- Cyst lining has a lamina propria, muscularis mucosae, and muscularis propria
- Cyst wall may contain ganglion cells
- Particularly with gastric mucosa, ulceration and hemorrhage may be present because of the effects of acid production

Special Stains and Immunohistochemistry
- Noncontributory

Other Techniques for Diagnosis
- Noncontributory

Differential Diagnosis
THYMIC CYST
- Lining epithelium is usually squamous
- Lymphocytes and true thymic tissue in the wall
- No well-defined smooth muscle layers
- No cartilage

MESOTHELIAL CYST
- Distinctive mesothelial lining
- Filled with clear thin fluid
- Lacks well-developed muscle bundles and lamina propria

CYSTIC TERATOMA
- Generally located in the anterior mediastinum
- Typically has focal solid areas
- Additional tissue types foreign to the site of origin are common and often consist of neural elements, cartilage, and pancreatic islets
- Not attached to bronchus, esophagus, or vertebral column

FOREGUT CYSTS
- Some cysts show overlap features between different types of cysts in this section; these represent partial duplication of structures derived from the foregut but cannot be subclassified into one of the three types described here and are generically termed *foregut cysts*

PEARLS
- *Computed tomography (CT) and magnetic resonance imaging can define the anatomic relationships and the cystic nature of the lesion*
- *Surgical resection is curative*

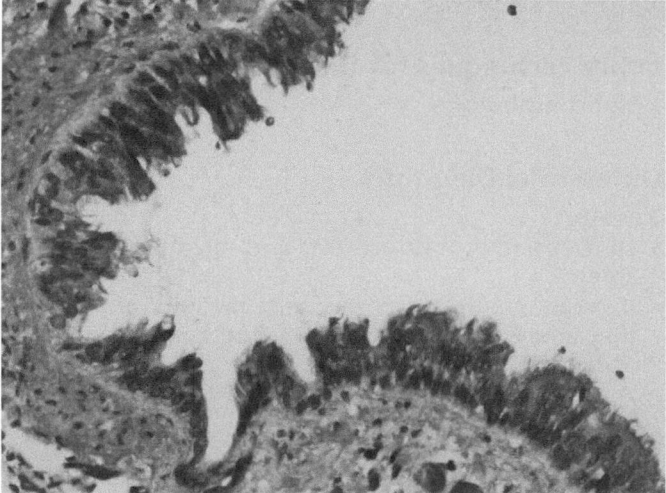

Figure 5-2. Foregut cyst. The lining is composed of tall, pseudostratified columnar ciliated epithelium.

SELECTED REFERENCES

Strollo DC, Rosado-de-Christenson ML, Jett JR: Primary mediastinal tumors: part II. Tumors of the middle and posterior mediastinum. Chest 112:1344-1357, 1997.

Wick MR: Cystic lesions of the mediastinum. Semin Diagn Pathol 22:241-253, 2005.

MESOTHELIAL CYST

Clinical Features

- Typically found at the costophrenic angle; may occur in the mediastinum
- Affects men and women of all ages; more common in adults than children
- When attached to pericardium, they are designated as pericardial cysts

Gross Pathology

- Thin-walled cyst filled with clear serous fluid
- Typically unilocular
- Pericardial cysts may have mucoid contents

Histopathology

- Typically has an attenuated mesothelial lining with fibrous tissue within the cyst wall
- Lacks smooth muscle, specialized epithelium, or cholesterol granulomas

Special Stains and Immunohistochemistry

- Noncontributory

Other Techniques for Diagnosis

- Noncontributory

Differential Diagnosis

THYMIC CYST.
- Located in the anterior mediastinum; more superior than pericardial and mesothelial cysts
- Residual thymic tissue is found in the wall on careful examination
- Epithelium is sometimes hyperplastic

LYMPHANGIOMA
- Typically found in anterior mediastinum
- More common in childhood
- Usually multiloculated with fibrous walls lined by attenuated cells
- Cyst lining cells are cytokeratin negative, but may express one or more antigens of endothelial cells (CD31 or CD34)

PEARLS

- *Mesothelial cysts are most often asymptomatic and found as incidental radiologic findings*
- *Differentiation between mesothelial and pericardial cysts is based on anatomic location*
- *Cysts attached to the pericardium are pericardial cysts*
- *Mesothelial-lined cysts elsewhere in the mediastinum are mesothelial cysts*
- *Careful gross and histologic examination may be necessary to exclude thymic tissue or elements of a foregut cyst*
- *Always benign*
- *Drainage under radiologic guidance may be an alternative to surgical resection*

SELECTED REFERENCES

Strollo DC, Rosado-de-Christenson ML, Jett JR: Primary mediastinal tumors: part II. Tumors of the middle and posterior mediastinum. Chest 112:1344-1357, 1997.

Wick MR: Cystic lesions of the mediastinum. Semin Diagn Pathol 22:241-253, 2005.

TRUE THYMIC HYPERPLASIA

Clinical Features

- Seen in children and occasionally in adults after chemotherapy for malignancy
- May be associated with hyperthyroidism, myasthenia gravis, or other autoimmune disease

Gross Pathology

- Thymic enlargement with increase in volume and normal weight of the gland

Histopathology

- Normal lobular architecture with normal distribution of lymphocytes and epithelial cells
- Preservation of corticomedullary differentiation

Special Stains and Immunohistochemistry

- Noncontributory

Other Techniques for Diagnosis

- Noncontributory

Differential Diagnosis

THYMOMA
- Differentiation into cortex and medulla is usually absent
- If areas resembling cortex and medulla are present, they are not arranged normally and do not display the normal lobulation

THYMIC FOLLICULAR HYPERPLASIA
- Well-formed lymphoid follicles with germinal centers
- CD20-positive B lymphocytes are present within germinal centers

SELECTED REFERENCES

Carmosino L, Di Benedetto A, Feffer S: Thymic hyperplasia following successful chemotherapy: a report of two cases and review of the literature. Cancer 56:1526-1528, 1985.

Steinmann GG: Changes in the human thymus during aging. In Müller-Hermelink HK (ed): The Human Thymus: Histophysiology and Pathology. Berlin, Springer-Verlag, 1986, pp 43-88.

Suster S, Rosai J: The thymus. In Mill SE (ed): Histology for Pathologists, 3rd ed. Philadelphia, Lippincott Williams & Wilkins, 2006, pp 505-526.

THYMIC FOLLICULAR HYPERPLASIA

Clinical Features

- Associated with myasthenia gravis, rheumatoid arthritis, systemic lupus erythematosus, and other autoimmune disorders

Gross Pathology

- Thymus is of normal size and weight in most cases

Histopathology

- Thymic hyperplasia characterized by numerous follicles with germinal centers

Special Stains and Immunohistochemistry

- Follicles are composed of normal B cells and will show reactivity with CD20

Other Techniques for Diagnosis

- Flow cytometry or molecular diagnostic techniques—that is, gene rearrangement—can rule out clonality if lymphoma is in the differential

Differential Diagnosis

FOLLICULAR LYMPHOMA

- Patients usually have widespread systemic disease
- Uncommon in young adults
- More uniform population of lymphoid cells
- Few or no tingible body macrophages
- Flow cytometry and molecular diagnostic techniques demonstrate monoclonal population of B cells
- B cells in follicles strongly express bcl-2 protein

NORMAL THYMUS WITH PROMINENT CORTICOMEDULLARY DIFFERENTIATION

- Normal thymic lobules show sharp angles; follicles are round

- Hassall corpuscles are seen in thymic medulla, not in germinal centers
- Thymic medulla contains cytokeratin-positive epithelial cells, which are not seen in germinal centers

SELECTED REFERENCES

Kornstein MJ, Brooks JJ, Anderson AO, et al: The immunohistology of the thymus in myasthenia gravis. Am J Pathol 117:184-194, 1984.

Loning T, Caselitz, Otto HF: The epithelial framework of the thymus in normal and pathological conditions. Virchows Archiv 329:7-20, 1981.

Moran C, Suster S, Gil J, Jagirdaar J: Morphometric analysis of germinal centers in the thymuses of nonthymomatous patients with myasthenia gravis. Arch Pathol Lab Med 114:689-691, 1990.

Okabe H: Thymic lymph follicles: a histopathological study of 1,356 autopsy cases. Acta Pathol Japonica 16:109-130, 1966.

THYMOLIPOMA

Clinical Features

- Rare tumor
- Peak incidence in young adults
- Often large, and patients are symptomatic (dyspnea, cough) as a result of compression of adjacent structures

Gross Pathology

- Thymus gland is enlarged but soft, with preserved lobulation
- Yellow cut surface with whitish fibrous strands

Histopathology

- Mature adipose tissue interspersed with strands of unremarkable thymic tissue
- Thymic component may be well populated with lymphocytes

Special Stains and Immunohistochemistry

- Noncontributory

Other Techniques for Diagnosis

- Noncontributory

Differential Diagnosis

INVOLUTION OF THYMUS GLAND
- Involuted thymus is of normal size or smaller than normal for age

THYMOMA
- Contains little or no fat

LIPOMA
- Occurs mostly in middle-aged to older adults
- Occurs anywhere in mediastinum but rarely within the thymus
- Does not contain thymic tissue

PEARLS

- *Appearance on CT may suggest a cyst*
- *Probably a hamartoma*
- *Rare associations include Graves disease, Hodgkin lymphoma, and myasthenia gravis*

SELECTED REFERENCES

Moran CA, Rosado-de-Christenson ML, Suster S: Thymolipoma: Clinicopathologic review of 33 cases. Mod Pathol 8:741-744, 1995.

Rosado-de-Christenson ML, Pugatch RD, Moran CA, Galobardes J: Thymolipoma: analysis of 27 cases. Radiology 193:121-126, 1994.

THYMOMA

Clinical Features

- Most commonly found in adults; peak incidence in the fifth decade
- Most common solid primary neoplasm of the mediastinum
- Typically located in anterior-superior mediastinum; may also arise from thymic rests: pleura, pulmonary hilum, pericardium, posterior or middle mediastinum, and thyroid
- Radiograph shows a lobulated mass that is occasionally calcified
- Clinical associations
  - Myasthenia gravis
  - Lambert-Eaton syndrome
  - Pure red cell aplasia
  - Hypogammaglobulinemia
- Other associations
  - Systemic lupus erythematosus
  - Rheumatoid arthritis
  - Scleroderma
  - Polymyositis
- Prognosis and staging: thymomas exhibit a range of biologic behavior from noninvasive, encapsulated tumors to aggressive infiltrative tumors
  - Most noninvasive tumors are cured by surgical resection
  - Most important predictor of clinical course is the presence and extent of invasion into other mediastinal structures
- Staging system used for thymomas reflects this range of behavior (modified Koga et al, 1994)
  - Stage I: completely encapsulated (including microscopic invasion into the capsule)
  - Stage IIa: microscopic invasion through the capsule
  - Stage IIb: macroscopic invasion into surrounding fatty tissue or pleura/pericardium
  - Stage III: macroscopic invasion of neighboring organs (pericardium, great vessels, or lung)
  - Stage IVa: pericardial or pleural implants
  - Stage IVb: Hematogenous or lymphatic dissemination

Gross Pathology

- Most are lobulated and encapsulated with a solid, gray-white cut surface
- Larger tumors may show extensive cystic changes

Histopathology

- Thymomas exhibit a range of histologic features
- Generally encapsulated with a distinct fibrous capsule
- Dual cell population composed of neoplastic proliferation of thymic epithelial cells admixed with variable numbers of non-neoplastic T lymphocytes
- Majority of T lymphocytes are of cortical type (immature)
- Most thymomas display organotypic morphology, meaning that the tumors show features distinctive of the normal thymus, including the following:
  - Fibrous bands forming angulated tumor lobules
  - Variable numbers of immature T lymphocytes
  - Proliferation of bland-appearing thymic epithelial cells
  - Perivascular spaces
  - Foci of so-called medullary differentiation (rounded areas with lower lymphocyte density)
  - No significant cytologic atypia or pleomorphism
- Neoplastic epithelial cells may be of two types
  - Oval or spindled cells with bland nuclei and dispersed chromatin and occasional small chromocenters
  - Round or polygonal (epithelioid) cells with abundant lightly eosinophilic or amphophilic cytoplasm and distinct round eosinophilic nucleolus
- Histologic classification is still a matter of debate; most commonly accepted scheme is the one proposed by the World Health Organization (Travis et al, 2004)
  - WHO thymoma type A: composed primarily of benign-appearing spindle cells (Figure 5-3)
  - WHO thymoma type AB: composed of small spindle cells (type A) admixed with abundant lymphocytes
  - WHO thymoma type B: composed of round or polygonal epithelial cells with varying amounts of immature and mature T lymphocytes (Figure 5-4); this group is subdivided into three types (B1 to B3) based on progressive decrease in the proportion of lymphocytes to epithelial cells and progressive increase in cytologic atypia of neoplastic epithelial cells
    - Type B1: large number of T lymphocytes containing few, isolated, scattered round or polygonal thymic epithelial cells with minimal cytologic atypia (Figure 5-5)

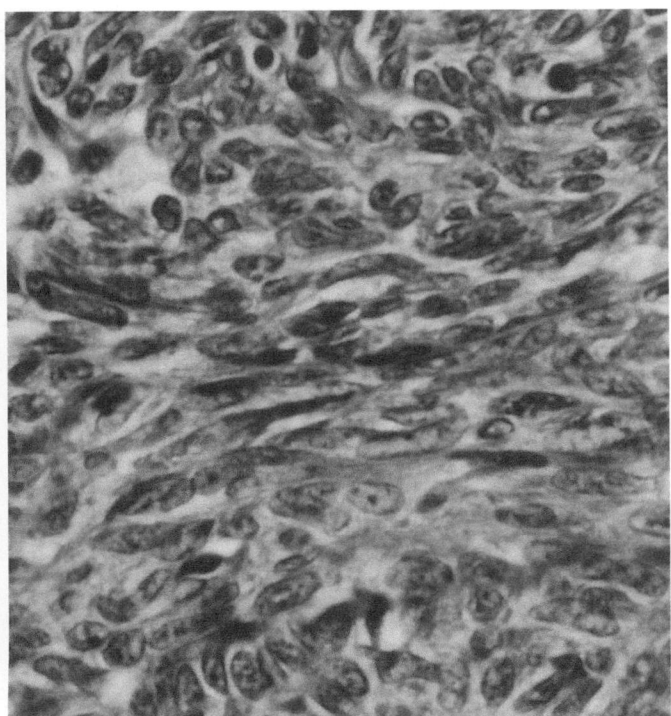

Figure 5-3. Thymoma type A. The tumor cells are elongated and spindled with scant cytoplasm.

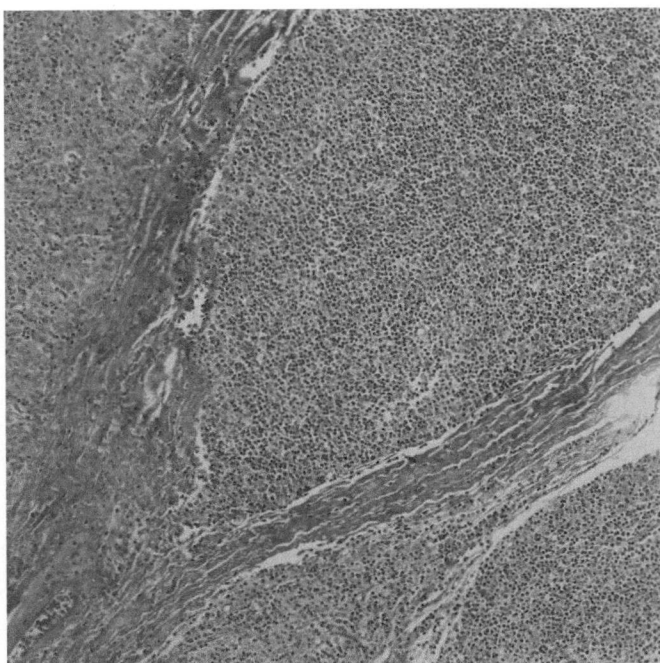

Figure 5-5. Thymoma type B1. Scanning magnification shows a predominant population of small lymphocytes with scant epithelial cells separated by broad bands of fibrous connective tissue.

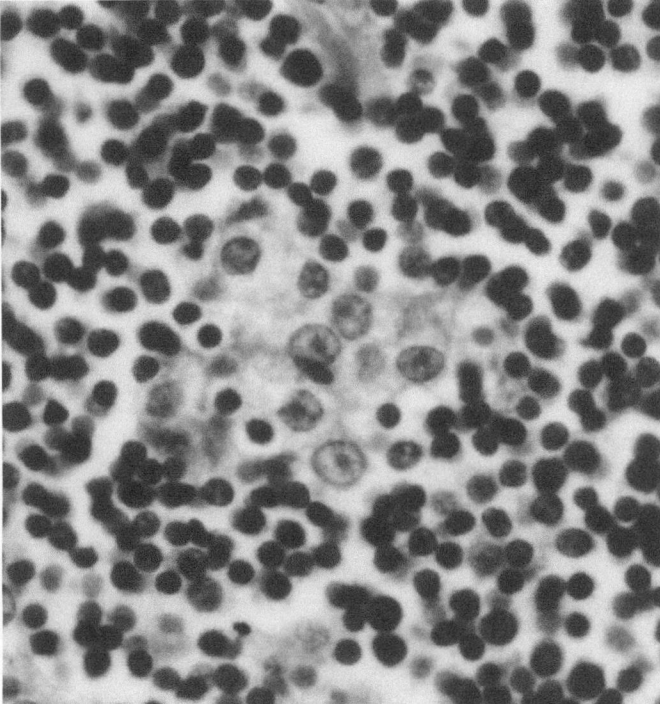

Figure 5-4. Thymoma type B. The tumor is composed predominantly of lymphocytes with a background containing round epithelial cells with vesicular nuclei and abundant cytoplasm.

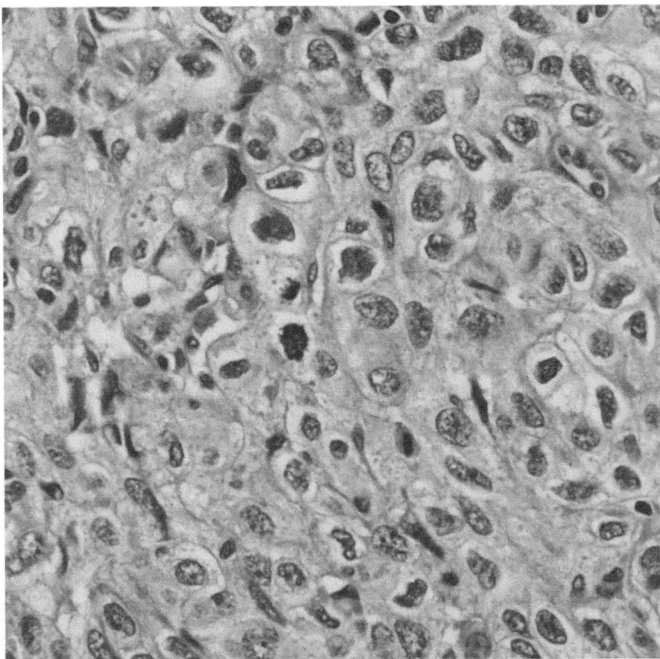

Figure 5-6. Thymoma type B3. The tumor is composed predominantly of large epithelioid cells with enlarged and hyperchromatic nuclei and sharp cell borders. Rare mitotic figures can be seen (*center*).

- Type B2: about equal number of T lymphocytes and thymic epithelial cells showing mild to minimal cytologic atypia
- Type B3: large number of polygonal epithelial cells admixed with few lymphocytes; the epithelial cells

show enlarged nuclei with increased chromatin pattern, occasional prominent nucleoli, and rare mitotic figures and contain abundant eosinophilic cytoplasm with sharp cell borders (Figure 5-6)
- WHO thymomas of special types, including micronodular thymoma, metaplastic thymoma, microscopic thymoma, thymoma with anaplasia, and thymic carcinoma

- Limitations of above scheme include difficulties in interobserver reproducibility, overlap in cytologic features for the various categories due to tumor heterogeneity, conflicting results of clinical survival studies for the various categories, lack of a biologic substrate for the classification, and the existence of numerous morphologic variants that do not fit into any of the standard categories
- Unusual morphologic variants include thymomas with clear cells, glandlike structures, cribriform areas, macrocystic and microcystic structures, papillary structures, rhabdomyomatous cells, heavy plasma cell stromal infiltration, extensive areas of infarction and necrosis, starry-sky pattern, storiform pattern (in spindle cell thymoma), hemangiopericytic pattern (in spindle cell thymoma), rosette-like structures (in spindle cell thymoma), spindle cell pseudosarcomatous stroma, massive stromal sclerosis, and others
- Classification of thymomas
  - There has been considerable controversy regarding which (if any) of these histologic features predict clinical behavior or reflect the differentiation of the tumor cells
  - Table 5-1 shows the numerous classification schemes for thymoma
- Features used for classification
  - Type of epithelial cell (spindle versus round or polygonal)
  - Organotypic organization
  - Relative proportion of epithelial cells and lymphocytes
  - Degree of epithelial atypia
- Features predictive of invasion or metastatic potential include the following:
  - Predominance of polygonal epithelial cells
  - Epithelial pleomorphism and atypia
  - Loss of organotypic features
- Thymic tumors with overtly malignant epithelium are called *thymic carcinomas* (see under "Thymic Carcinoma")

Special Stains and Immunohistochemistry

- Limited role in diagnosis
- Cytokeratin: highlights epithelial cells, particularly in lymphocyte-rich tumors
- P63 and PAX8: nuclear positivity in thymic epithelial cells
- CD3: highlights T-cell population
- CD1a/CD99: highlight immature T lymphocytes
- CD20: may be positive in epithelial cells of some thymomas

Other Techniques for Diagnosis

- Electron microscopy: very limited role; can demonstrate tonofilaments, tight intercellular junctions, desmosomes, elongated cytoplasmic processes, and basal lamina of epithelial cells; high potential for sampling error
- Flow cytometry: can be misleading in cases of lymphocyte-rich thymoma by showing an immature terminal deoxynucleotidyl transferase (TdT)-positive lymphoblastic population that can lead to an erroneous diagnosis of lymphoblastic lymphoma
- Gene rearrangement studies: no clonality is found in the lymphocytes of thymoma
- Other molecular studies: no role identified yet for diagnosis

Differential Diagnosis

THYMIC HYPERPLASIA VERSUS LYMPHOCYTE-RICH THYMOMA

- Thymic tissue maintains normal thymic architecture in hyperplasia; architecture and cortical or medullary proportions are distorted in thymoma
- Cases with lymphoid follicular hyperplasia contain follicles with active germinal centers

LYMPHOMA VERSUS LYMPHOCYTE-RICH THYMOMA

- Most likely lymphoid neoplasms to be confused for thymoma are lymphoblastic, Burkitt, and Hodgkin lymphoma

LYMPHOBLASTIC LYMPHOMA

- Most often seen in children and adolescents
- Patients often have leukemia with blasts in peripheral blood
- Medium-sized lymphoid cells with fine chromatin and absence of nucleoli; mitoses typically numerous
- Most often of T-cell lineage; expresses TdT and other early T-cell antigens

TABLE 5-1	**COMPARISON OF CLASSIFICATIONS OF THYMOMA**		
World Health Organization (Travis, 2004)	Traditional (Bernatz et al, 1961)	Histogenetic (Marino and Müller-Hermelink, 1985)	Suster and Moran (1999)
Type A	Spindle cell thymoma	Medullary thymoma	Thymoma, well differentiated
Type AB	—	Mixed thymoma	Thymoma, well differentiated
Type B1	Lymphocyte-rich thymoma	Cortical thymoma	Thymoma, well differentiated
Type B2	Lymphoepithelial thymoma	Predominantly cortical	Thymoma, well differentiated
Type B3	Epithelial-rich thymoma	Well-differentiated thymic carcinoma	Atypical thymoma (moderately differentiated)
Thymic carcinoma (formerly thymoma type C)	Thymic carcinoma	Thymic carcinoma	Thymic carcinoma (poorly differentiated thymic epithelial neoplasm)

- May reflect the pattern of antigen expression seen on normal and mature cortical or medullary thymocytes; therefore, flow cytometry must be interpreted with caution
- Molecular diagnostics (gene rearrangement studies) may be needed to rule out a clonal T-cell process
- Most important stain for diagnosis is cytokeratin; shows scattered keratin-positive thymic epithelial cells admixed with the immature lymphoid cell population in lymphocyte-rich thymoma

Burkitt Lymphoma

- Clonal B-cell process that can be demonstrated by flow cytometry
- Sheets of primitive lymphoid cells with multiple small nucleoli
- Can be confused with lymphocyte-rich thymoma owing to starry-sky pattern
- Cytokeratin demonstrates no epithelial cell component
- Ki-67 shows virtually 100% positivity of the lymphoid cells

Nodular Sclerosing Hodgkin Lymphoma

- Reed-Sternberg and lacunar cells may be identified immunohistochemically (positive for CD15 and CD30; negative for CD3, CD45, and CD20), whereas the atypical epithelial cells of thymoma demonstrate cytokeratin staining
- Hodgkin lymphoma is often associated with cystic changes of the thymus

Castleman Disease

- Characteristic follicles with hyalinized vessels and sclerotic germinal centers surrounded by concentrically arranged layers of lymphocytes in the mantle zone (onion-skinning)

Spindle Cell Sarcoma versus Spindle Cell Thymoma

- Both can show a storiform pattern
- Spindle cells in spindle cell sarcomas are reactive for vimentin and negative for cytokeratin
- Spindle cell thymoma can resemble solitary fibrous tumors due to prominent hemangiopericytic growth pattern; cells are positive for cytokeratin in thymoma

PEARLS

- *Thymomas are tumors of the epithelial component of the thymus; associated lymphocytes in the background are benign*
- *Thymomas have a strong association with myasthenia gravis and other autoimmune disorders*
- *Primary treatment is surgical excision*
- *Classification is still controversial*
- *Invasion of adjacent mediastinal structures remains the most widely accepted predictor of aggressive behavior*

SELECTED REFERENCES

Bernatz PE, Harrison EG, Claggett OT: Thymoma: a clinicopathologic study. J Thorac Cardiovasc Surg 42:424-444, 1961.

Koga K, Matsuno Y, Noguchi M, et al: A review of 79 thymomas: modification of staging system and reappraisal of conventional division into invasive and non-invasive thymoma. Pathol Int 44:359-367, 1994.

Kornstein MJ, Curran WJ Jr, Turrisi AT III, Brooks JJ: Cortical versus medullary thymomas: a useful morphologic distinction? Hum Pathol 19:1335-1339, 1988.

Marino M, Müller-Hermelink HK: Thymoma and thymic carcinoma: relation of thymoma epithelial cells to the cortical and medullary differentiation of the thymus. Virch Arch 407:119-149, 1985.

Pan CC, Wu HP, Yang CF, et al: The clinicopathological correlation of epithelial subtyping in thymoma: a study of 112 consecutive cases. Hum Pathol 25:893-899, 1994.

Suster S, Moran CA: Classification of thymoma: the WHO and beyond. Hematol Oncol Clin NA 22:381-392, 2008.

Suster S, Moran CA: Primary thymic epithelial neoplasms: spectrum of differentiation and histological features. Semin Diagn Pathol 16:2-17, 1999.

Suster S, Moran CA: Problem areas and inconsistencies in the WHO classification of thymoma. Semin Diagn Pathol 22:188-197, 2005.

Suster S, Moran CA: Thymoma classification: current status and future trends. Am J Clin Pathol 125:542-554, 2006.

Suster S, Moran CA: Thymoma, atypical thymoma and thymic carcinoma: a novel conceptual approach to the classification of thymic epithelial neoplasms. Am J Surg Pathol 111:826-833, 1999.

Travis WD, Brambilla E, Muller-Hermelink HK, Harris CC: Pathology and genetics of tumors of the lung, pleura, thymus and heart. In World Health Organization Classification of Tumours. Lyon, IARC Press, 2004.

THYMIC CARCINOMA

Clinical Features

- Thymic epithelial neoplasm with cellular atypia and aggressive clinical course
- No association with paraneoplastic syndromes of thymoma such as myasthenia gravis or pure red cell aplasia
- May arise from malignant progression in a longstanding, preexisting thymoma
- Predominantly found in middle age to late adulthood
- Patients may present with chest pain, dyspnea, or superior vena cava syndrome
- Primary thymic carcinomas are rare; secondary invasion of the thymus by primary carcinoma of the lung or metastatic tumor in mediastinal lymph nodes is more common
- Thymic carcinoma is a diagnosis of exclusion; extensive clinical and radiologic studies must be undertaken to rule out the possibility of an occult or late metastasis from another organ before rendering this diagnosis

Gross Pathology

- Usually not encapsulated
- Gray-white tumor with a hard, gritty cut surface often showing hemorrhage and necrosis
- Stroma may be desmoplastic, but these tumors do not have the broad fibrous septa seen in thymoma
- Some variants may have prominent cystic changes

Histopathology

- Differs from thymoma by having overt histologic features of a malignancy and complete loss of organotypic features of thymic differentiation
- Lymphocytes are of B-cell type instead of immature T lymphocytes
- Numerous microscopic subtypes; they essentially resemble a variety of carcinomas arising in other organs
- Can be divided into histologically low-grade and high-grade tumors (Table 5-2)

KERATINIZING SQUAMOUS CELL CARCINOMA OF THE THYMUS

- Resembles invasive squamous cell carcinoma seen elsewhere; must rule out early massive mediastinal spread from an occult bronchial primary by bronchoscopy

POORLY DIFFERENTIATED (LYMPHOEPITHELIOMA-LIKE) NONKERATINIZING SQUAMOUS CELL CARCINOMA (FIGURE 5-7)

- Histologic features similar to lymphoepithelioma-like carcinoma of the nasopharynx
- Comedo-like central areas of necrosis are a distinctive and constant feature
- Lymphocytes in the stroma may or may not be present
- Rarely related to Epstein-Barr virus (EBV) as seen in nasopharyngeal carcinomas

MUCOEPIDERMOID CARCINOMA

- Resembles that seen in salivary glands; may be low grade (well-differentiated) and high grade (moderately and poorly differentiated) (Figure 5-8)
- Can be associated with prominent cystic changes
- Mucicarmine stain is helpful for highlighting cytoplasmic mucin in the tumor cells

CLEAR CELL CARCINOMA

- Composed of clear cells containing abundant glycogen with surrounding delicate stroma
- May resemble clear cell carcinoma of the kidney or may result from clear cell changes in well-differentiated squamous cell carcinoma

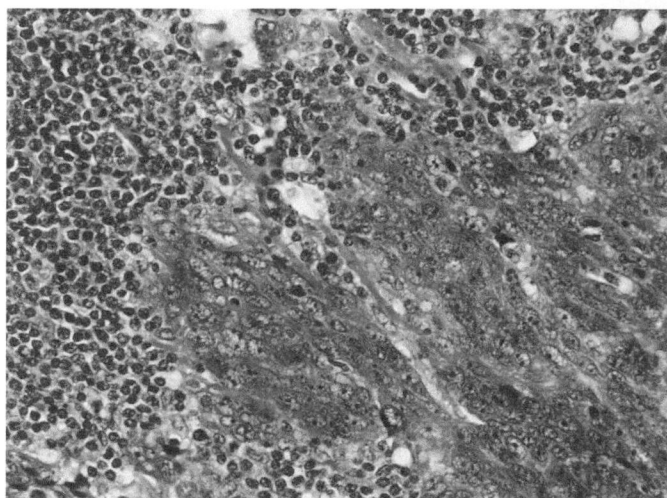

Figure 5-7. Thymic carcinoma, poorly differentiated, nonkeratinizing squamous cell type (lymphoepithelioma-like carcinoma). The tumor is composed of sheets of large cells with vesicular nuclei and prominent eosinophilic nucleoli with a scant and indistinct rim of cytoplasm. Notice the adjacent dense lymphoid stroma.

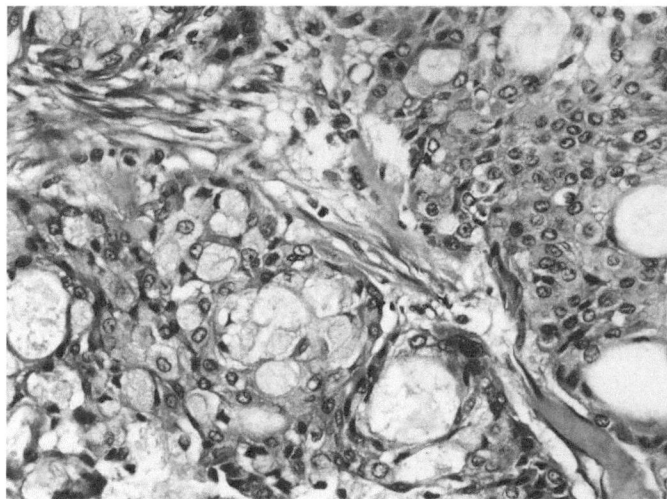

Figure 5-8. Thymic carcinoma, mucoepidermoid type. The tumor is composed of sheets of squamoid intermediate cells admixed with mucocytes and cystic spaces filled with mucin.

TABLE 5-2 COMPARISON OF LOW-GRADE AND HIGH-GRADE THYMIC CARCINOMAS

Low-Grade	High-Grade
Well-differentiated squamous cell carcinoma	Moderate to poorly differentiated (lymphoepithelioma-like) nonkeratinizing squamous cell carcinoma
Well-differentiated mucoepidermoid carcinoma	
Basaloid carcinoma	Moderate to poorly differentiated mucoepidermoid carcinoma
Papillary carcinoma	
Well-differentiated mucinous adenocarcinoma	Spindle cell carcinoma and thymic carcinosarcoma
	Clear cell carcinoma
	Anaplastic carcinoma

BASALOID CARCINOMA

- Composed of nests of basaloid cells showing peripheral palisading (Figure 5-9)
- Can present in association with prominent cystic changes

SPINDLE CELL (SARCOMATOID) CARCINOMA

- Spindle and pleomorphic cells with hyperchromatic nuclei, prominent nucleoli, and numerous mitoses
- Spindle cells are cytokeratin positive
- Often associated with preexisting spindle cell thymoma
- When associated with clear-cut sarcomatous elements, is designated thymic carcinosarcoma

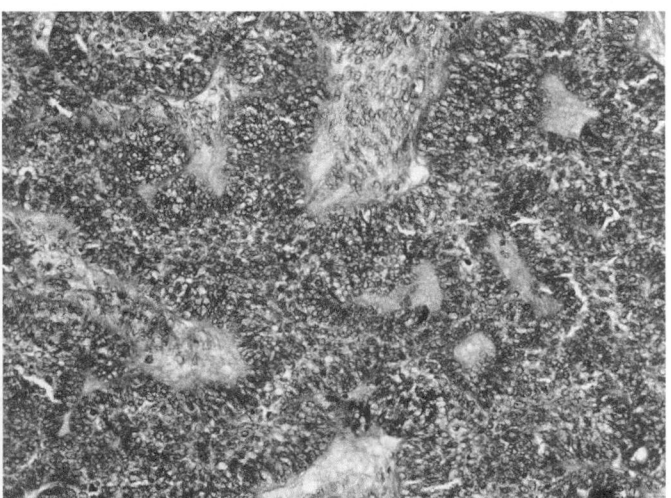

Figure 5-9. Thymic carcinoma, basaloid type. The tumor is composed of a monotonous proliferation of hyperchromatic cells showing striking peripheral palisading of nuclei.

Special Stains and Immunohistochemistry

- Periodic acid-Schiff (PAS) and mucicarmine stains may be useful in clear cell carcinoma and mucoepidermoid carcinoma to identify intracytoplasmic glycogen and mucin, respectively
- Universally express cytokeratin and may react with other epithelial markers such as carcinoembryonic antigen (CEA), epithelial membrane antigen (EMA), and MOC31
- May also show positivity for CD5 or CD117

Other Techniques for Diagnosis

- Noncontributory

Differential Diagnosis

METASTATIC CARCINOMA

- Clinical history is important; possibility of metastasis from occult primary elsewhere must be ruled out first

EPITHELIOID HEMANGIOENDOTHELIOMA

- May closely resemble carcinoma
- Cells contain abundant cytoplasm with prominent cytoplasmic vacuoles
- Cells are positive for FVIII-RA and CD31 in epithelioid hemangioendothelioma
- Caveat: some cases of epithelioid hemangioendothelioma can be keratin positive; must always add vascular markers to distinguish from carcinoma

GERM CELL TUMORS

- Positive for placental alkaline phosphatase (PLAP), human chorionic gonadotropin (HCG), or α-fetoprotein (AFP)
- Serum AFP or HCG is often elevated

LYMPHOMA

- Positive for leukocyte common antigen (LCA) and other lymphoid markers (e.g., CD3, CD20, CD30) and negative for cytokeratin
- Flow cytometry and gene rearrangement studies helpful to document monoclonality

PEARLS

- *Careful history and clinical and radiologic evaluation are needed to diagnose a carcinoma in the thymus as a primary thymic carcinoma*
- *Variants that may be cured by surgical excision include well-differentiated squamous cell, mucoepidermoid, and basaloid carcinoma; other variants have generally poor prognosis*

SELECTED REFERENCES

Moran CA, Suster S: Mucoepidermoid carcinoma of the thymus: clinicopathologic study of six cases. Am J Surg Pathol 19:826-834, 1995.

Suster S: Thymic carcinoma: update of current diagnostic criteria and histologic types. Semin Diagn Pathol 22:188-197, 2005.

Suster S, Moran CA: Primary thymic epithelial neoplasms showing combined features of thymoma and thymic carcinoma: clinic pathologic study of 22 cases. Am J Surg Pathol 20:1469-1480, 1996.

Suster S, Moran CA: Spindle cell carcinoma of the thymus: clinicopathologic and immunohistochemical study of 15 cases of a novel form of thymic carcinoma. Am J Surg Pathol 23:691-700, 1999.

Suster S, Moran CA: Thymic carcinoma: spectrum of differentiation and histologic types. Pathology 30:111-122, 1998.

Suster S, Rosai J: Thymic carcinoma: clinicopathologic study of 60 cases. Cancer 67:1025-1032, 1991.

Wick MR, Scheithauer BW, Weiland LH, Bernatz PE: Primary thymic carcinomas. Am J Surg Pathol 6:613-630, 1982.

NEUROENDOCRINE NEOPLASMS OF THE THYMUS

Clinical Features

- Most common in middle-aged adults
- Strong male predominance
- Histologic spectrum from well-differentiated tumors (carcinoid) to poorly differentiated carcinomas histologically similar to small cell carcinoma of the lung; histologic features and clinical behavior correlate
- Carcinoids arising in the mediastinum are most often of thymic origin
- Thymic carcinoid
  - Typically more aggressive than bronchial carcinoid
  - May be locally invasive or can metastasize
  - May recur after a long disease-free interval
  - Paraneoplastic syndromes are found in one third of these patients and include Cushing syndrome, syndrome of inappropriate antidiuretic hormone (SIADH), and Lambert-Eaton syndrome
  - No expression of the full carcinoid syndrome
- Up to one third of low-grade tumors occur in association with multiple endocrine neoplasia (MEN) types I or II and tend to follow a more aggressive course

Gross Pathology

- Unencapsulated, firm mass with a gray-pink, gritty texture due to fine calcifications
- Focal hemorrhage and necrosis are common
- No fibrous septa or lobulation (in contrast to thymoma)

Histopathology

- Classification based on histologic grade
  - Well-differentiated
    - Fewer than three mitoses/10 high-power fields (hpf)
    - Minimal atypia
    - Classic organoid pattern
    - No more than pinpoint, small foci of necrosis
  - Moderately differentiated
    - Intermediate features between well-differentiated and poorly differentiated tumors
    - Organoid architecture is generally not present
    - Moderate cytologic atypia with prominent nucleoli
    - Moderate mitotic activity (3 to 10 mitoses/10 hpf)
  - Poorly differentiated (high-grade) neuroendocrine carcinoma
    - More than 10 mitoses/10 hpf
    - Marked atypia or areas of small cell carcinoma
    - Extensive necrosis
    - Total loss of organoid architecture
    - Some tumors may show admixtures of differing histologic grades
- Histologic features
  - Low-grade tumors
    - Uniform polygonal cells with oval nucleus, stippled chromatin, and granular cytoplasm (Figure 5-10)
    - Cells arranged in nests, trabeculae, ribbons, and cords; may have pseudorosette formation
    - Nests may show focal central areas of comedo-like necrosis and calcification
    - Artifactual clefts between nests of tumor cells and surrounding stroma

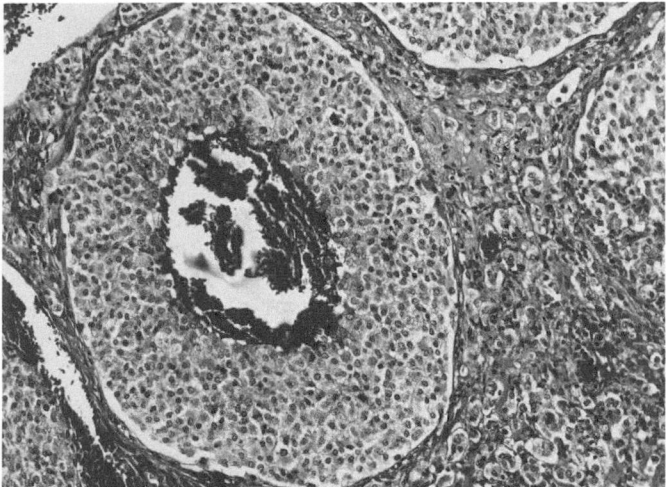

Figure 5-10. Well-differentiated neuroendocrine carcinoma of the thymus (thymic carcinoid). The tumor shows a monotonous population of tumor cells with small nuclei and dispersed chromatin pattern (salt-and-pepper). Some of the tumor cells form balls with central, comedo-like areas of necrosis and artifactual retraction from the surrounding stroma.

- Variant morphologic findings
  - Amyloid-like stroma associated occasionally with calcitonin production
  - Spindle cell morphology
  - Oncocytic cytoplasmic features
  - Pigmentation: melanin, lipofuscin
- Moderate- to high-grade tumors
  - Diffuse, lymphoma-like architecture
  - Histology similar to small cell (oat cell) neuroendocrine carcinoma of the lung
  - Pulmonary neuroendocrine carcinomas can have widespread metastases from a small primary lesion; thorough clinical and radiologic evaluation is necessary to prove that such a tumor in the thymus is a primary thymic carcinoma
  - Small cells with nuclear moulding and scant cytoplasm
  - Fine salt-and-pepper, stippled chromatin
  - A large cell variant of poorly differentiated neuroendocrine carcinoma has also been described
  - Prominent crush artifact and apoptosis
  - Cases showing transitions between low-grade (well-differentiated) and high-grade (poorly differentiated) neuroendocrine carcinoma have also been described

Special Stains and Immunohistochemistry

- Neoplastic cells are reactive for cytokeratin, chromogranin, synaptophysin, and CD56
- May express neuropeptides: adrenocorticotropic hormone (ACTH), serotonin, somatostatin, gastrin, and others

Other Techniques for Diagnosis

- Electron microscopy: cells contain cytoplasmic dense core neurosecretory granules

Differential Diagnosis

LARGE CELL LYMPHOMA
- Diffuse growth pattern; no ribbons, festoons, or trabecular pattern
- Tumor cells have vesicular nuclei
- Mitotic and apoptotic figures are numerous
- Positive for LCA and CD20

METASTATIC MALIGNANT MELANOMA
- Cells are generally more pleomorphic and have more abundant cytoplasm and prominent macronucleoli
- Positive for S-100 protein, Melan-A and HMB-45
- Cytokeratin negative

MEDULLARY CARCINOMA OF THYROID GLAND
- Neuroendocrine carcinoma of the thymus can also have scattered cells reactive for calcitonin
- Neoplastic C cells are reactive for carcinoembryonic antigen (CEA) and calcitonin

PARAGANGLIOMA
- Prominent atypia (nucleomegaly) in the absence of mitotic activity
- Negative for cytokeratin

Metastatic Carcinoid or Neuroendocrine Carcinoma
- Careful clinical and radiologic evaluations are the only tools to differentiate primary from secondary thymic involvement

PEARLS

- *Neuroendocrine neoplasms of the thymus are best considered as a spectrum from low-grade tumors (carcinoid) to high-grade carcinomas similar to small cell carcinoma of the lung*
- *Metastasis or extension from the lung to the thymus of small cell carcinoma of pulmonary origin is more common than a thymic primary*
- *Low-grade tumors (carcinoid)*
  - *Any thymic carcinoid has the potential for metastasis*
  - *Poorer prognosis when associated with MEN syndromes or with ACTH production*
  - *Treated with surgical excision; tumor is resistant to chemotherapy and radiation*
  - *May recur after long intervals (e.g., 10 years)*
- *High-grade neuroendocrine carcinoma*
  - *Treatment approach is generally the same as for a pulmonary tumor of similar histology*

Selected References

Klemm KM, Moran CA: Primary neuroendocrine carcinomas of the thymus. Semin Diagn Pathol 16:32-41, 1999.
Moran CA: Primary neuroendocrine carcinomas of the mediastinum: review of current criteria for histopathologic diagnosis and classification. Semin Diagn Pathol 22:223-229, 2005.
Moran CA, Suster S: Neuroendocrine carcinomas (carcinoid tumor) of the thymus: a clinicopathologic analysis of 80 cases. Am J Clin Pathol 114:100-110, 2000.
Moran CA, Suster S: Thymic neuroendocrine carcinomas with combined features ranging from well-differentiated (carcinoid) to small cell carcinoma: a clinicopathologic and immunohistochemical study of 11 cases. Am J Clin Pathol 113:345-350, 2000.
Rosai J, Higa E: Mediastinal endocrine neoplasm, of probable thymic origin, related to carcinoid tumor: clinicopathologic study of 8 cases. Cancer 29:1061-1074, 1972.
Suster S, Moran CA: Neuroendocrine neoplasms of the mediastinum. Am J Clin Pathol 115(S1):17-27, 2001.
Wick MR, Danney JA, Bernatz PE, Brown LR: Primary mediastinal carcinoid tumors. Am J Surg Pathol 6:195-205, 1982.
Wick MR, Scheithauer BW: Thymic carcinoid: a histologic, immunohistochemical, and ultrastructural study of 12 cases. Cancer 53:475-484, 1984.

CHRONIC MEDIASTINITIS

Clinical Features

- Generally affects anterior-superior mediastinum; often just anterior to the carina
- Occurs at any age; most common in young adult years
- Female predominance is seen
- About half the cases are associated with fungal infection (commonly histoplasmosis, also *Aspergillus)* and *Nocardia* species and mycobacteria; also following methysergide treatment
- About half the cases are idiopathic
- Delayed cell-mediated hypersensitivity response is the postulated mechanism in the infectious cases
- Radiologic appearance is an asymmetrical widening of the mediastinum
- The most common non-neoplastic cause of superior vena cava syndrome
- Can cause pulmonary vein compression and thrombosis

Gross Pathology

- Firm, white, densely fibrotic tissue
- Generally compresses rather than invades mediastinal structures

Histopathology

- Dense, hypocellular, hypovascular fibrohyaline tissue
- Entrapped lymphocytes
- Granulomas (caseating or noncaseating)
- May see infectious organisms

Special Stains and Immunohistochemistry

- PAS and Grocott methenamine silver (GMS): help identify fungal organisms
- Acid-fast stain for mycobacteria

Other Techniques for Diagnosis

- Microbiology: Gram stain, cultures, and serology
- Polymerase chain reaction (PCR) may be useful for rapid detection of mycobacteria or fungi

Differential Diagnosis

Solitary Fibrous Tumor.
- Well-defined neoplasm composed of haphazardly arranged bland spindle cells in a dense, well-vascularized collagenous stroma
- Positive for CD34 and bcl-2

Hodgkin Lymphoma, Nodular Sclerosing
- Relatively acellular fibrous bands separate highly cellular nodules containing a mixed infiltrate
- Characterized by scattered atypical cells consisting of Hodgkin cells, Reed-Sternberg cells, or lacunar cells
- Inflammatory infiltrate includes lymphocytes, plasma cells, and eosinophils
- Granulomas may be present

Large Cell Lymphoma with Sclerosis
- Numerous atypical large lymphoid cells in a fibrous tissue background
- Highly proliferative tumor with mitoses and apoptotic bodies
- Large cells are CD20 positive

PEARLS

- *Special stains should be performed to rule out microorganisms*
- *Some authors consider sclerosing mediastinitis and chronic mediastinitis as separate entities; others believe this process is a reaction pattern that may occur in response to infection or drugs, or as an autoimmune-type reaction*
- *Sclerosing mediastinitis is reportedly more cellular than chronic mediastinitis and is composed of fibroblasts, lymphocytes, plasma cells, and eosinophils*
- *At later stages, the lesion becomes hypocellular and hypovascular with dense collagenous fibrosis*
- *Treated with excision and corticosteroids*

SELECTED REFERENCE

Flieder DB, Moran C, Suster S: Idiopathic fibroinflammatory (fibrosing/sclerosing) lesions of the mediastinum: a study of 30 cases with emphasis on morphologic heterogeneity. Mod Pathol 12:257-264, 1999.

HODGKIN LYMPHOMA

Clinical Features

- Most common malignant tumor of the mediastinum
- Occurs predominantly in the anterior compartment
- Lymph nodes and thymus may be involved
- Young women in their 20s and 30s are most commonly affected
- Often presents with B symptoms, including fever, night sweats, weight loss, and fatigue

Gross Pathology

- Fleshy mass with sclerotic bands
- With thymic involvement, cystic degeneration is common

Histopathology

- Nodular sclerosing variant is the most common type
- Type is best determined by lymph node analysis, as the diagnostic features may not be represented in extranodal sites
- When extranodal, such as in the thymus, Hodgkin disease generally forms a discrete mass
  - Collagenous fibrosis and the typical background cells (small lymphocytes, plasma cells, and eosinophils) are present
  - Classic Reed-Sternberg cells in a background consistent with Hodgkin lymphoma are needed to establish a new diagnosis of Hodgkin lymphoma in an extranodal site
  - In a patient with an established diagnosis of Hodgkin lymphoma, mononuclear cells with the other features of Reed-Sternberg cells (Hodgkin cells) in the background of collagen and cells typical of Hodgkin lymphoma are sufficient to diagnose involvement of an extranodal site (Figure 5-11)

Special Stains and Immunohistochemistry

- Immunohistochemical confirmation is often desirable, even if the histology is characteristic
- Reed-Sternberg cells and their lacunar variants are reactive with CD15 and CD30 antibodies
- Hodgkin and Reed-Sternberg cells are usually negative for CD45
- Occasionally Reed-Sternberg cells and their variants are positive for CD20 or T-cell marker CD45RO (UCHL 1) antibody

Other Techniques for Diagnosis

- Negative for T- or B-cell gene rearrangements

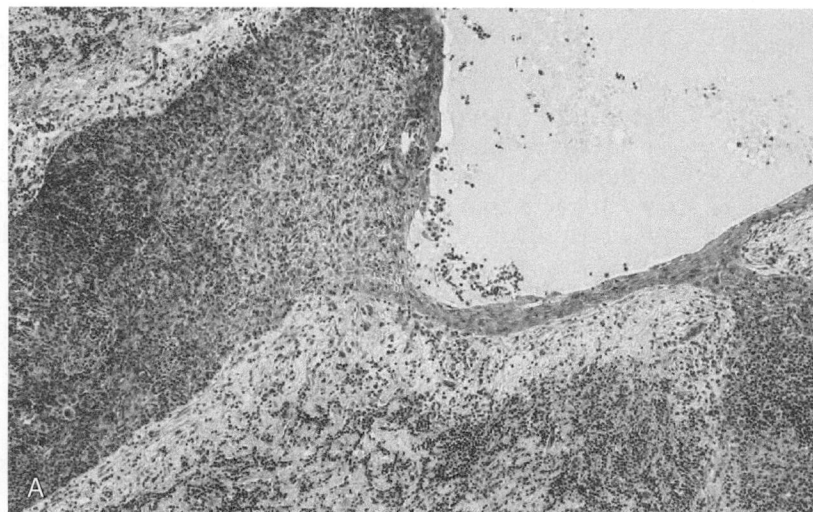 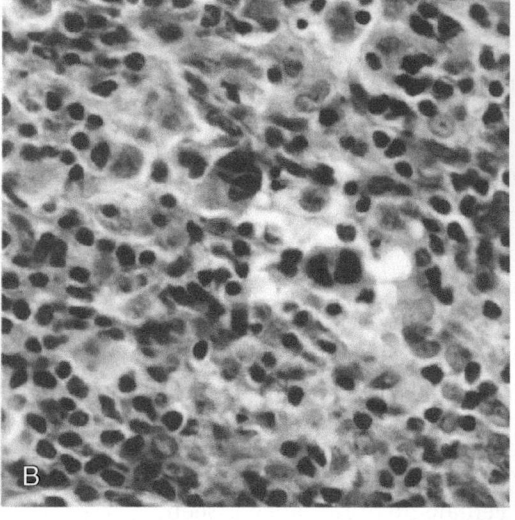

Figure 5-11. Hodgkin lymphoma with cystic changes. A, Low magnification shows cystically dilated thymic epithelium infiltrated by a dense lymphoid cell population. **B,** Higher magnification shows large binucleated and mononuclear forms of Hodgkin cells.

Differential Diagnosis

THYMOMA

- Low-power view can mimic Hodgkin disease because of sclerosis forming well-defined nodules composed of large and small cells; nodules are generally angulated rather than round in thymoma
- No atypical lymphoid cells (Hodgkin cells)
- Eosinophils and plasma cells are rare
- Thymoma cells are positive for epithelial markers (cytokeratin)

THYMIC CYST

- Cyst has an epithelial cell lining
- No atypical lymphoid cells are seen
- Adequate and extensive sampling is required in thymic cysts to rule out Hodgkin disease

SCLEROSING LARGE CELL NON-HODGKIN LYMPHOMA

- Monotonous population of large, atypical lymphoid cells without distinctive milieu of Hodgkin lymphoma (i.e., small lymphocytes, plasma cells, and eosinophils)
- Tumor cells are almost always of B-cell lineage and express CD19, CD20, and CD22
- Negative for CD15, but many cases can be CD30 positive

PEARLS

- *Nodular sclerosing is the most common type of Hodgkin lymphoma seen in the mediastinum*
- *Young women most commonly affected*
- *Can be often cystic—thorough sampling is necessary to identify diagnostic areas*

SELECTED REFERENCES

Burke WA, Burford TH, Dorfman RF: Hodgkin's disease in the mediastinum. J Thorac Cardiovasc Surg 3:287-296, 1967.
Fechner RE: Hodgkin's disease of the thymus. Cancer 23:16-23, 1969.
Katz A, Lattes R: Granulomatous thymoma or Hodgkin's disease of thymus? A clinical and histologic study and a reevaluation. Cancer 23:1-15, 1969.
Kim HC, Nosher J, Haas A, et al: Cystic degeneration of thymic Hodgkin's disease following radiation therapy. Cancer 55:354-356, 1985.

DIFFUSE LARGE CELL LYMPHOMA, B-CELL TYPE

Clinical Features

- Second most common type of lymphoid malignancy of the mediastinum after Hodgkin lymphoma
- Predominantly affects females; peak incidence between 20 and 40 years of age
- Typically found in anterior mediastinum
- Almost always of B-cell lineage
- Usually involves the thymus with or without lymph node involvement
- Signs and symptoms may include superior vena cava syndrome and pleural effusions

Gross Pathology

- Firm mass with foci of necrosis
- Typically shows extensive infiltration into surrounding tissue

Histopathology

- Diffuse growth pattern composed of large atypical lymphoid cells with reniform or multilobated nuclei, vesicular chromatin, and distinct nucleoli
- Large amounts of pale or clear cytoplasm
- Often shows a pattern of stromal sclerosis characterized by compartmentalization of the tumor into discrete nests and islands simulating epithelial malignancy (Figure 5-12)
- Entrapment of thymic and extrathymic fat often seen

Special Stains and Immunohistochemistry

- CD19, CD20, CD22, and CD45 positive
- CD10, CD5, CD43, CD21, and immunoglobulin negative (resembling the phenotype of normal thymic B cells)
- Negative for CD15
- Significant percentage of these cases can be CD30 positive

Other Techniques for Diagnosis

- Flow cytometric or gene rearrangement studies to verify lymphoid B- or T-cell lineage

Differential Diagnosis

GERMINOMA.

- Almost all cases occur in males
- Composed of diffuse population of large cells with abundant cytoplasm and large nuclei with irregular (spiked) nucleoli

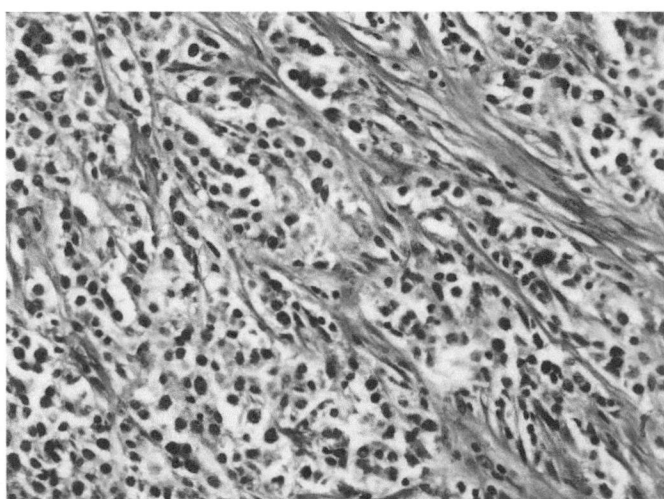

Figure 5-12. Diffuse large cell lymphoma with sclerosis. The tumor is composed of large atypical lymphoid cells showing a compartmentalized appearance owing to fine bands of sclerosis that separate them into small islands.

- Small lymphocytes are concentrated along delicate fibrovascular septa rather than scattered throughout the tumor
- Presence of glycogen in the clear cytoplasm favors the diagnosis of germinoma
- Positive for PLAP, CD117, OCT-4 by immunohistochemistry
- Negative for CD20 and CD45
- Can show striking dotlike paranuclear positivity for low-molecular weight cytokeratin

HODGKIN LYMPHOMA, SYNCYTIAL VARIANT
- Sclerosis is present in broad bands rather than diffusely
- Characterized by large multinucleated tumor cells (Reed-Sternberg cells)
- Large cells are CD15 and CD30 positive
- Large cells are usually negative for CD20 and CD45

LYMPHOBLASTIC LYMPHOMA
- Male predominance
- Patients may have frank leukemia, which is exceptional in mediastinal large cell lymphoma
- Cells with scant cytoplasm and blastic chromatin with absence of nucleoli
- Cells express CD1a, CD3, CD43, TdT, CD99
- Negative for CD20

METASTATIC CARCINOMA
- Sheets or nests of cohesive neoplastic cells
- May form glands or show obvious keratinization
- Tumor cells express cytokeratin; negative for CD20 and CD45

PEARLS

- *Generally affects young women (second to fourth decades)*
- *May involve the thymus*
- *Sclerosis and necrosis are common findings*
- *Almost always of B-cell lineage*
- *Good response to multiagent chemotherapy with consolidation radiation therapy*

SELECTED REFERENCES

Davis RE, Dorfman RF, Warnke RA: Primary large cell lymphoma of the thymus: a diffuse B-cell neoplasm presenting as primary mediastinal lymphoma. Hum Pathol 21:1262-1268, 1990.

Jacobson JO, Aisenberg AC, Lamarre L, et al: Mediastinal large cell lymphoma: an uncommon subset of adult lymphoma curable with combined modality therapy. Cancer 62:1893-1898, 1988.

Menestrina F, Chelosi M, Bonetti F, et al: Mediastinal large cell lymphoma of B-cell type with sclerosis: histopathological and immunohistochemical study of 8 cases. Histopathology 10:589-600, 1986.

Perrone T, Frizzera G, Rosai J: Mediastinal diffuse large cell lymphoma with sclerosis: a clinicopathological study of 60 cases. Am J Surg Pathol 10:176-191, 1986.

Suster S: Primary large-cell lymphomas of the mediastinum. Semin Diagn Pathol 16:51-64, 1999.

LYMPHOBLASTIC LYMPHOMA

Clinical Features
- Predominantly seen in older children and adolescents but can also occur in older adult patients
- Disease shows male predominance (2:1)
- Patients may have a concomitant leukemic phase
- Almost all cases with a mediastinal mass at presentation are of T-cell lineage (see Chapter 14 for discussion on B-lineage lymphoblastic lymphoma)
- Mediastinum is most common location, and thymus is usually involved; with thymic involvement, residual lobules and infiltrated Hassall corpuscles may be seen
- Patients often present with acute onset of respiratory distress owing to the rapidly growing nature of the tumor
- Patients may have central nervous system and gonadal involvement at presentation

Gross Pathology
- Usually solid, infiltrative, and lacks a capsule

Histopathology
- Diffuse growth pattern composed of atypical lymphoid cells with fine chromatin pattern and absent or inconspicuous nucleoli (Figure 5-13)
- Medium-sized cells with high nuclear-to-cytoplasmic ratio
- Cells may have cerebriform nuclear convolutions with finely dispersed chromatin and inconspicuous nucleoli or may be of nonconvoluted type
- Numerous mitotic figures
- Necrosis can be extensive

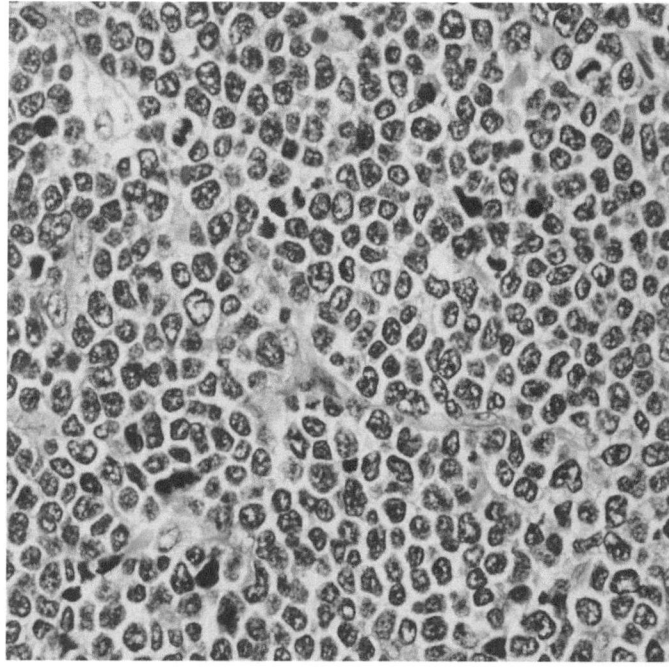

Figure 5-13. Lymphoblastic lymphoma. Atypical lymphoid cells with fine chromatin, inconspicuous nucleoli, and frequent nuclear membrane infoldings are seen.

- Blood vessel invasion and extension into perithymic fibroadipose tissue may be prominent features
- Neoplastic cells can infiltrate the thymus
- May have scattered tingible body macrophages, creating a starry-sky pattern

Special Stains and Immunohistochemistry

- TdT positive in all cases
- LCA positive in 80% of cases
- CD99 positive in most cases
- Tumor cells usually express CD1, CD43, and CD3
- Tumor cells may be positive or negative for CD4 and CD8
- CD45RO expressed in 50% of cases; CD20 is negative

Other Techniques for Diagnosis

- Flow cytometry
  - May be misleading because lymphocytes in lymphocyte-rich thymomas show similar immunophenotype (i.e., immature, blastic T cells)
  - May not always differentiate clonal immature T cells from benign prethymic cells that may be found in thymoma
- Molecular studies: useful to detect gene rearrangement in lymphoblasts to verify clonality
  - Cytogenetics: helps with diagnosis and is related to prognosis; particularly for B-lineage lymphoblastic lymphoma

Differential Diagnosis

THYMOMA.

- Rare in children; however, adults can develop either disease
- Lymphocytic component may be phenotypically indistinguishable from lymphoblastic lymphoma
- Apoptotic lymphocytes may simulate a starry-sky pattern
- Cytokeratin highlights network of epithelial cells throughout the tumor
- Lymphocytes are not clonal

LARGE B-CELL LYMPHOMA

- Tumor cells are larger and have clear cytoplasm, vesicular nuclei, and usually prominent nucleoli; convoluted nuclei are uncommon
- Phenotype is that of a B-cell neoplasm
- Positive for CD20; negative for TdT, CD99, CD1a

Other Small Round Blue Cell Tumors of Childhood

GRANULOCYTIC SARCOMA

- Extremely uncommon
- Search carefully for cells with granular cytoplasm
- Tumor cells positive for myeloperoxidase; negative for TdT
- CD43 and CD45 may be positive and are not helpful in this differential diagnosis

NEUROBLASTOMA

- Typically found in posterior mediastinum
- More commonly seen in younger children
- Composed of smaller round cells with scant cytoplasm forming characteristic rosettes; look for neuropil in the background
- Positive for neuron-specific enolase (NSE), negative for lymphoid markers

EMBRYONAL RHABDOMYOSARCOMA

- Mixture of haphazardly arranged rhabdomyoblasts and undifferentiated primitive cells
- Positive for MyoD1, myogenin, and other markers of muscle differentiation (desmin, actin, and myosin)
- Negative for TdT and lymphoid markers

PRIMITIVE NEUROECTODERMAL TUMOR (PNET)

- Rare in this location
- May have limited neural differentiation (usually positive for synaptophysin and chromogranin)
- Positive for CD99
- Intracytoplasmic glycogen (PAS positive)
- Negative for TdT and lymphoid markers
- Characteristic translocation t(11;22)

SMALL CELL CARCINOMA (NEUROENDOCRINE CARCINOMA, OAT CELL CARCINOMA)

- Mostly in older adults
- May be primary or metastatic
- Small cells with nuclear molding and scant cytoplasm
- Nuclei have fine salt-and-pepper stippled chromatin or smudged chromatin pattern
- Prominent crush artifact and extensive necrosis
- Tumor cells express cytokeratin, chromogranin, and synaptophysin
- Negative for TdT, CD45, and CD3

PEARLS

- *This rapidly growing tumor is seen predominantly in children and adolescents; male predominance*
- *Leukemia and bone marrow involvement is common*
- *Almost all cases presenting with a mediastinal mass are of T-cell lineage*
- *Always include a cytokeratin stain in your panel to make sure you do not miss a lymphocyte-rich thymoma*

SELECTED REFERENCES

Benerjee D, Silva E: Mediastinal mass with acute leukemia: myeloblastoma masquerading as lymphoblastic lymphoma. Arch Pathol 105:126-129, 1981.
Devoe K, Weidner N: Immunohistochemistry of small round cell tumors. Semin Diagn Pathol 17:216-225, 2000.
Ha K, Minded M, Hozumi N, Gelfano EW: Phenotypic heterogeneity at the DNA level in childhood leukemia with a mediastinal mass. Cancer 56:509-513, 1985.
Nathwani BN, Kim H, Rappaport H: Malignant lymphoma, lymphoblastic. Cancer 38:966-983, 1976.

CASTLEMAN DISEASE

Clinical Features

- Reactive condition; also known as angiofollicular lymph node hyperplasia
- Found predominantly involving lymph nodes; occasionally may involve the thymus
- Both sexes may be affected
- Wide age range
- Three types: hyaline vascular, plasma cell, and mixed
  - Hyaline vascular type (about 80% of cases)
    - Usually asymptomatic except for effects of compression by mass
  - Plasma cell type
    - Patients may have anemia, hypergammaglobulinemia, and fever
    - Typically solitary, but multicentric variant does exist
  - Multicentric variant: multiple lymph nodes at multiple sites are involved
- Hepatosplenomegaly
- Hematologic and immunologic abnormalities (pancytopenia, increased erythrocyte sedimentation rate, proteinuria)
- One third of patients develop other malignancies (non-Hodgkin lymphoma [NHL], carcinoma, or Kaposi sarcoma)
- More frequent in patients with human immunodeficiency virus (HIV) infection
- Associated with infection of Kaposi sarcoma–associated herpesvirus (KSHV, human herpesvirus-8 [HHV-8]), especially in HIV-positive patients

Gross Pathology

HYALINE VASCULAR TYPE
- Large single mass
- Well-circumscribed round nodule usually located in the anterior-superior aspect of the mediastinum

PLASMA CELL TYPE
- Forms a mass and more commonly affects multiple lymph nodes

Histopathology

HYALINE VASCULAR TYPE (ABOUT 80% OF CASES)
- Multiple follicles with small germinal centers
- Hyalinized blood vessels penetrate the germinal centers (lollipop sign) (Figure 5-14)
- Germinal centers may show concentric foci of hyalinization resembling Hassall corpuscles
- Small cells of the mantle zone may show distinct concentric layering (onion-skinning)
- Abnormal follicles may contain multiple small germinal centers
- Rich network of capillaries in the interfollicular zone
- Perivascular fibrosis may be seen around interfollicular vessels
- Interfollicular regions are composed primarily of lymphocytes but also contain plasma cells, immunoblasts, and eosinophils

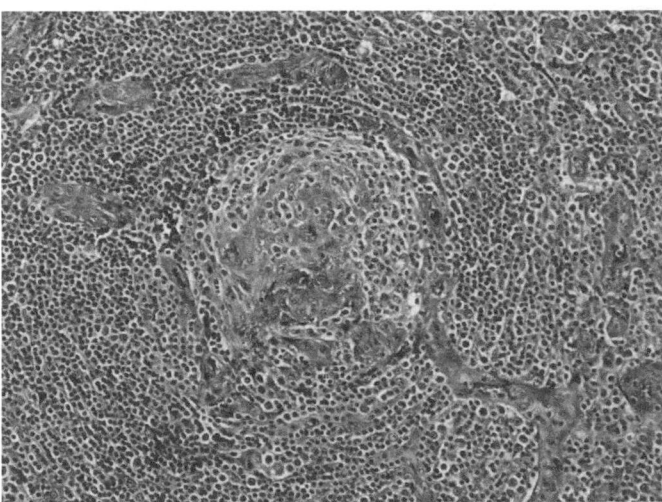

Figure 5-14. Castleman disease. This histologic section shows a germinal center with hyalinized blood vessels and distinct concentric layering.

PLASMA CELL TYPE (10% TO 20%)
- Interfollicular areas contain sheets of plasma cells (diagnostic feature)
- Germinal centers are large and reactive

MIXED (RARE)
- Combination of features from hyaline vascular and plasma cell variants
- Generally asymptomatic unless mass causes compression

Special Stains and Immunohistochemistry

- CD5-positive lymphoid cells are seen at the periphery of the abnormal follicles (suggesting that Castleman disease is a proliferation of CD5-positive lymphocytes stimulated by specific lymphokines)
- Polyclonal population of B lymphocytes and plasma cells

Other Techniques for Diagnosis

- Flow cytometry and gene rearrangement studies: polyclonal

Differential Diagnosis

FOLLICULAR LYMPHOMA
- Monotonous follicles composed of atypical lymphocytes
- Cytologically abnormal cells, most of which have cleaved nuclei (centrocytes)
- Monoclonal B cells
- Positive for CD20 and bcl-2

PLASMACYTOMA
- Pure plasmacytic population composed of clonal plasma cells
- Generally lacks hyalinized germinal centers and onion-skinning of mantle zone

- Must be careful with clonality because several reports have demonstrated a monoclonal plasma cell component in the interfollicular area in Castleman disease

PEARLS

- *Mediastinum is the most common location and most commonly involves lymph nodes*
- *Multicentric type is more common in HIV-positive patients*
- *Multicentric type in HIV-positive patients is associated with HHV-8 infection*

SELECTED REFERENCES

Frizzera G: Atypical lymphoproliferative disorders. In Knowles DM (ed): Neoplastic Hematopathology. Baltimore, Williams & Wilkins, 1992, pp 459-495.

Keller AR, Hochholzer L, Castleman B: Hyaline-vascular and plasma-cell types of giant lymph node hyperplasia of mediastinum and other locations. Cancer 29:670-683, 1972.

O'Reilly PE Jr, Joshi V, Holbrook CT, Weisenburger DD: Multicentric Castleman's disease in a child with prominent thymic involvement: a case report and brief review of the literature. Mod Pathol 6:776-780, 1993.

THYMIC HISTOLOGY IN IMMUNE DEFICIENCIES

Clinical Features

- Thymic histology can be abnormal in a variety of congenital and acquired immune deficiency diseases, particularly in T-lymphocyte deficiencies
- Generally a clinical diagnosis, with patients having characteristic clinical presentation and features of an immune deficiency

Gross Pathology

- DiGeorge syndrome: thymic hypoplasia or aplasia with reduced to absent normal thymic tissue
- Other congenital immune defects: atrophic thymic tissue

Histopathology

DIGEORGE SYNDROME
- Whatever thymic tissue is present is histologically normal or shows variable stress involution

B-CELL IMMUNE DEFECTS
- Features of exaggerated stress involution
- Decreased corticomedullary differentiation
- Decreased number of lymphocytes
- Variable number of Hassall corpuscles

SEVERE COMBINED IMMUNE DEFICIENCY (SCID)
- Pattern is called *thymic dysplasia*
- Small round to oval lobules of spindle to polygonal epithelial cells
- Few or no lymphocytes and absence of Hassall corpuscles
- Patients with less severe forms of deficiency may have a few lymphocytes and Hassall corpuscles

SEVERE ACQUIRED IMMUNE DAMAGE (AIDS AND GRAFT-VERSUS-HOST DISEASE [GVHD])
- Severe lymphocyte depletion
- Hassall corpuscles may disappear
- Apoptotic bodies can be seen
- Apoptosis of thymic epithelial cells has been reported in GVHD

Special Stains and Immunohistochemistry
- Noncontributory

Other Techniques for Diagnosis
- Immunologic studies and lymphocyte function tests used to classify the defect are usually performed on the peripheral blood lymphocytes

Differential Diagnosis

STRESS INVOLUTION
- Clinically important in infants
- Stress involution and immune deficiencies create an overlapping range of histologic and functional alterations in the thymus (differences are those of degree)
- Hassall corpuscles are more often present than in severe thymic dysplasia
- Lobules tend to be triangular rather than rounded
- Apoptotic cells are usually lymphoid

PEARLS

- *Thymus may be a target of attack in GVHD*
- *There may be overlap of histologic features between stress involution and milder forms of thymic dysplasia in congenital immune deficiencies*

SELECTED REFERENCE

Nezelof C: Pathology of the thymus in immunodeficiency states. In Müller-Hermelink HK (ed): The Human Thymus: Histophysiology and Pathology. Berlin, Springer-Verlag, 1986, pp 151-177.

TERATOMA

Clinical Features

- Generally found in early adulthood
- Males and females are affected
- Most common type of mediastinal germ cell tumor

Gross Pathology

- Large, uniloculated or multiloculated cystic mass, often with calcification in the wall
- Greasy or fatty material, hair, and degenerated debris in cysts
- May erode into adjacent structures, including the trachea

Histopathology

- Microscopic appearance is similar to that of cystic teratoma of the ovary

- Cysts are lined by any type of epithelium and may contain sebaceous glands and hair follicles
- Other common components include neural tissue, gastrointestinal tract elements, cartilage, and respiratory structures
- Pancreatic acini are a frequent finding in teratomas in mediastinal location (Figure 5-15)
- Immature teratoma (Figure 5-16)
  - In addition to the components of mature teratoma, immature fetal type epithelial, neural, or mesenchymal elements are present
  - See Chapter 12 for more detailed information

Special Stains and Immunohistochemistry

- Noncontributory

Modern Techniques for Diagnosis

- Noncontributory

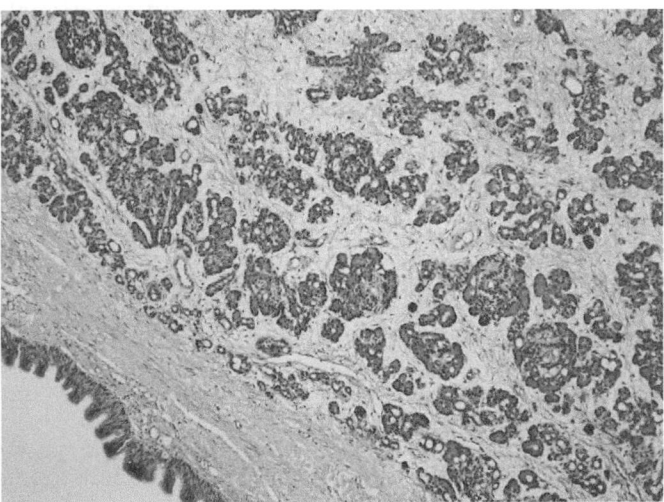

Figure 5-15. Mature teratoma. The tumor shows mature pancreatic tissue in the wall of a cyst.

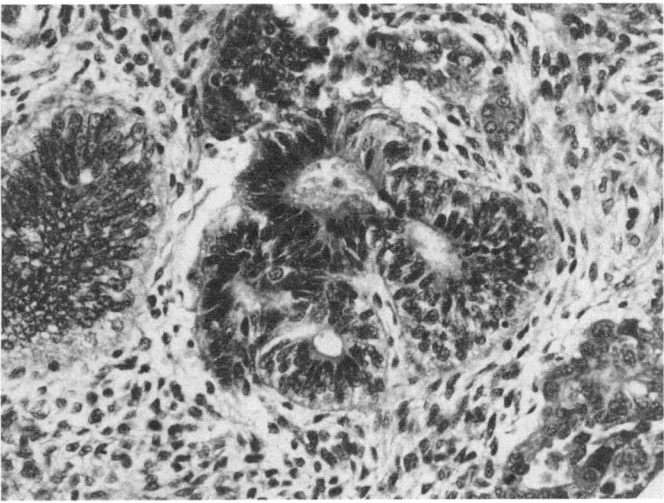

Figure 5-16. Immature teratoma. Histologic section demonstrates immature neural tubules surrounded by immature mesenchymal tissue.

Differential Diagnosis

TERATOMAS WITH ADDITIONAL MALIGNANT COMPONENTS

- Malignant mixed germ cell tumor composed of carcinoma and teratoma, teratoma plus another type of malignant germ cell tumor (such as embryonal carcinoma), and teratoma with a sarcoma

BRONCHIAL CYST

- Connected to bronchus or trachea
- Cyst with epithelial lining, smooth muscle, and cartilage
- Neural or other ectopic elements are absent

FOREGUT CYSTS

- Connected to esophagus or stomach
- Cyst with smooth muscle in wall
- No ectopic elements

PEARLS

- *Benign tumor*
- *Generous sampling of solid areas is advised to rule out immature components and malignant components*
- *Residual mediastinal masses removed after treatment for a malignant germ cell tumor may contain only mature or immature teratoma; thorough sampling is needed to exclude residual malignant components*

SELECTED REFERENCES

Carter D, Bibro MC, Touloukian RJ: Benign clinical behavior of immature mediastinal teratoma in infancy and childhood: report of two cases and review of the literature. Cancer 49:398-402, 1982.

Gonzalez-Crussi F: Extragonadal teratoma. Atlas of Tumor Pathology, 2nd series, Fascicle 18. Washington, DC, Armed Forces Institute of Pathology, 1982.

Moran CA, Suster S: Primary germ cell tumors of the mediastinum. I. Analysis of 322 cases with special emphasis on teratomatous lesions and a proposal for histopathologic classification and clinical staging. Cancer 80:681-690, 1997.

Suster S, Moran CA, Dominguez-Malagon H, Quevedo-Blanco P: Germ cell tumors of the mediastinum and testis: a comparative immunohistochemical study of 120 cases. Hum Pathol 29:737-742, 1998.

TERATOMA WITH ADDITIONAL MALIGNANT COMPONENTS

Clinical Features

- Usually present as large, bulky, and invasive anterior mediastinal masses
- May have elevated levels of HCG or AFP

Gross Features

- Large, fleshy tumors with extensive areas of hemorrhage and necrosis

Histologic Features

- Type I: teratoma with malignant epithelial component (e.g., adenocarcinoma, squamous cell carcinoma)

- Type II: teratoma with additional nonteratomatous germ cell tumor component (e.g., seminoma, choriocarcinoma, yolk sac tumor, embryonal carcinoma)
- Type III: teratoma with sarcomatous components (e.g., liposarcoma, leiomyosarcoma, rhabdomyosarcoma)
- Type IV: teratoma with a combination of any of the preceding features

Special Stains and Immunohistochemistry

- Epithelial markers (e.g., keratin, EMA, CEA): useful for identifying malignant epithelial components
- Specific markers for mesenchymal neoplasms (e.g., smooth muscle actin [SMA], desmin, S-100 protein, myogenin): useful for identifying specific lines of differentiation in sarcomatous components

Other Techniques for Diagnosis

- Noncontributory

SELECTED REFERENCES

Dominguez-Malagon H, Cano-Valdez AM, Moran CA, Suster S: Germ cell tumors with sarcomatous components: a clinicopathologic and immunohistochemical study of 46 cases. Am J Surg Pathol 31:1356-1362, 2007.

Moran CA, Suster S: Germ cell tumors of the mediastinum. Adv Anat Pathol 5: 1-15, 1998.

Moran CA, Suster S: Primary germ cell tumors of the mediastinum. I. Analysis of 322 cases with special emphasis on teratomatous lesions and a new proposal for histopathologic classification and clinical staging. Cancer 80:681-690, 1997.

GERMINOMA (MEDIASTINAL SEMINOMA)

Clinical Features

- Mediastinum is the most common extragonadal site for germ cell tumors
- Usually arises in the thymus
- Marked male predominance, rare in females
- Most commonly found in second through fourth decades
- Patients may present with superior vena cava syndrome and cervical lymphadenopathy

Gross Pathology

- Lobulated, large, soft, solid yellow tumor
- May be cystic in 10% of cases

Histopathology

- Fibrous septa divide tumor into lobules containing nests of neoplastic tumor cells
- Tumor cells have abundant pale cytoplasm, central round nuclei with irregular, spiked nucleoli, and distinct cell borders (Figure 5-17)
- Lymphocytes are mostly located in the fibrous septa
- Tumor cells may be obscured by extensive granulomatous reaction, florid lymphoid follicular hyperplasia, or extensive sclerosis and hyalinization of the stroma
- Spermatocytic and anaplastic variants of seminoma do not occur in the mediastinum

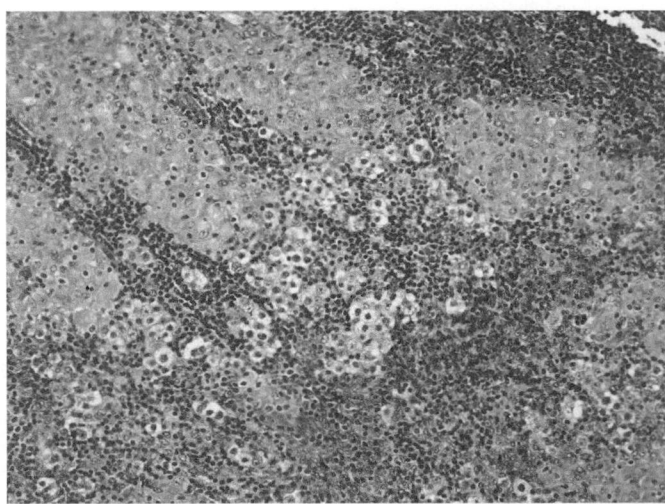

Figure 5-17. Mediastinal seminoma. The tumor is composed of cells with abundant clear cytoplasm, round nuclei, and prominent nucleoli admixed with epithelioid granulomas.

Special Stains and Immunohistochemistry

- Germ cells
  - PLAP positive
  - C-kit (CD117) and OCT-4 positive
  - Cytokeratin positive in 80% of cases with a distinct dotlike, paranuclear pattern
  - PAS: cytoplasmic positivity due to intracytoplasmic glycogen
  - CD30 may be positive in up to 4% of cases
  - LCA negative

Other Techniques for Diagnosis

- Noncontributory

Differential Diagnosis

DIFFUSE LARGE CELL LYMPHOMA WITH SCLEROSIS

- Diffuse large cell population with monotonous compartmentalization due to thin sclerotic bands
- LCA, CD20 positive
- PLAP, CD117 negative

NODULAR SCLEROSING HODGKIN LYMPHOMA, SYNCYTIAL VARIANT

- Relatively acellular fibrous bands separate cellular nodules containing a mixed infiltrate
- Characterized by scattered atypical cells consisting of Hodgkin cells, Reed-Sternberg cells, or lacunar cells
- Inflammatory infiltrate includes lymphocytes, plasma cells, and eosinophils
- Hodgkin cells are positive for CD15 and CD30
- Negative for PLAP

PEARLS

- *Mediastinal seminomas are reportedly more often positive for cytokeratin and vimentin than testicular seminomas*
- *Germinoma is highly sensitive to radiation therapy*

- *Predominantly a male disease*
- *Careful clinical evaluation for a gonadal primary is essential*
- *Thorough sampling and examination for other germ cell elements is necessary*

SELECTED REFERENCES

Burns BF, McCaughey WTE: Unusual thymic seminomas. Arch Pathol Lab Med 110:539-541, 1986.

Hunt RD, Bruckman JE, Farrow GM, et al: Primary anterior mediastinal seminoma. Cancer 49:1658-1663, 1982.

Moran CA, Suster S: Mediastinal seminomas with prominent cystic changes: a clinicopathological study of 10 cases. Am J Surg Pathol 19:1047-1053, 1995.

Moran CA, Suster S, Przygodzki RM, Koss MN: Primary germ cell tumors of the mediastinum: II. Mediastinal seminomas—a clinicopathologic and immunohistochemical study of 120 cases. Cancer 80:691-698, 1997.

Schantz A, Sewall W, Castleman B: Mediastinal germinoma: a study of 21 cases with an excellent prognosis. Cancer 30:1189-1194, 1972.

Suster S, Moran CA, Dominguez-Malagon H, Quevedo-Blanco P: Germ cell tumors of the mediastinum and testis: a comparative immunohistochemical study of 120 cases. Hum Pathol 29:737-742, 1998.

NONSEMINOMATOUS GERM CELL TUMORS (NSGCTs): EMBRYONAL CARCINOMA, YOLK SAC TUMOR (ENDODERMAL SINUS TUMOR), CHORIOCARCINOMA, MIXED GERM CELL TUMOR

Clinical Features

- These tumors occur almost exclusively in males
- Tumors can occur at any age, peak in 20s through 40s
- Patients may present with cough, dyspnea, chest pain, or fatigue
- Gynecomastia at presentation generally indicates a choriocarcinoma component
- Mediastinum is the most common site for extragonadal germ cell tumors
- About 75% or more of mediastinal germ cell tumors are teratomas or seminoma; others are extremely rare
- Tumors have 30 to 40 times greater frequency in patients with Klinefelter syndrome
- At the time of diagnosis, tumors are usually large with invasion into surrounding organs or structures
- Elevated serum AFP in a patient with a germ cell tumor is diagnostic of a nonseminomatous component, usually yolk sac tumor
- Serum HCG may be elevated in any type; HCG above 500 IU indicates a choriocarcinoma component
- Response to therapy and overall survival are worse than for testicular germ cell tumors

Gross Pathology

- Large infiltrative tumors often with hemorrhage and necrosis
- Usually solid but may have cystic areas because of necrosis
- Extensive hemorrhage is characteristic of choriocarcinoma
- Classic rule of thumb for sectioning is to take one block per centimeter of greatest tumor dimension

Histopathology

EMBRYONAL CARCINOMA

- Cohesive clusters of primitive, anaplastic cells arranged in solid or abortive glandular structures
- Large polygonal cells with pleomorphic, round to oval nuclei, prominent nucleoli, and abundant, pale-staining cytoplasm (Figure 5-18)
- High mitotic rate
- Necrosis and hemorrhage are common

YOLK SAC TUMOR

- Variable tumor cytomorphology, ranging from small, round to polygonal monotonous tumor cells with minimal atypia to large, pleomorphic tumor cells
- Reticular or microcystic pattern is characterized by various-sized cystic spaces lined by flattened cells (most common pattern) (Figure 5-19)
- May form tubules and papillary structures

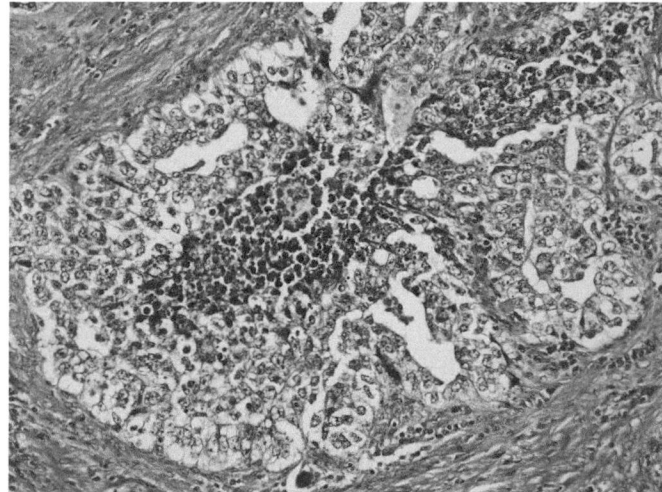

Figure 5-18. Embryonal carcinoma. The tumor shows a solid proliferation of primitive-appearing large cells with oval to round nuclei, prominent nucleoli, and large amounts of pale-staining cytoplasm.

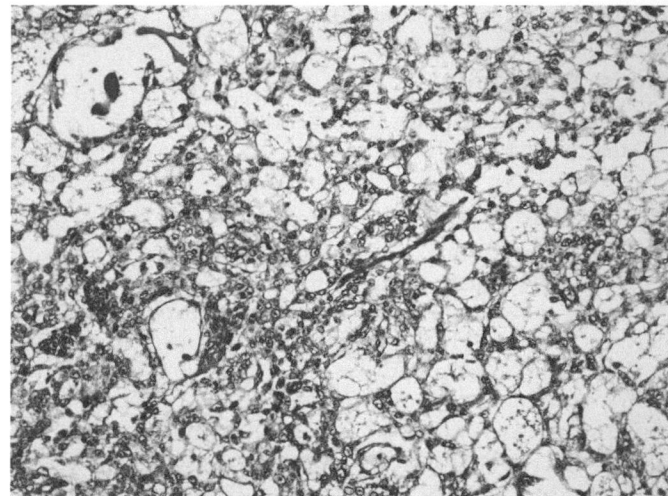

Figure 5-19. Yolk sac tumor (endodermal sinus tumor), reticular pattern. Low-power view shows a reticular pattern with variably sized spaces.

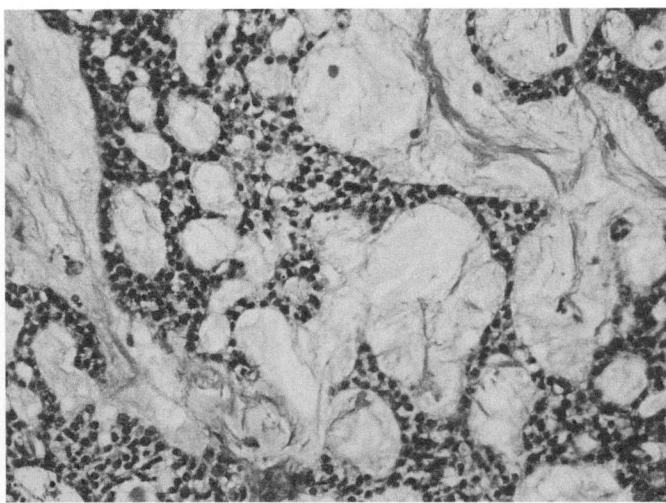

Figure 5-20. Yolk sac tumor with myxoid background. The tumor is characterized by cords of hyperchromatic cells set against a prominent myxoid background.

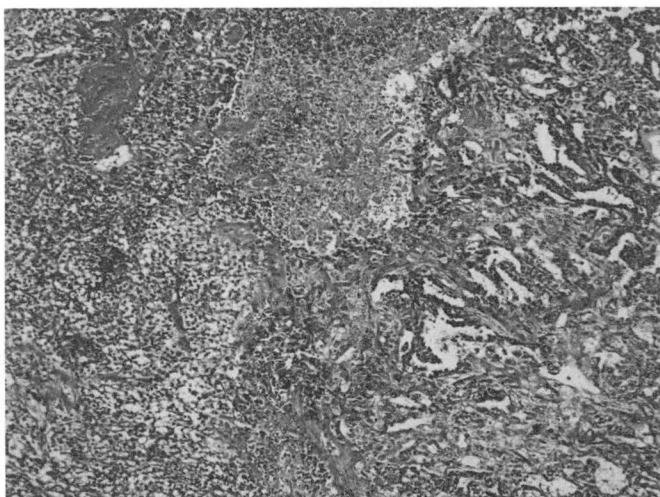

Figure 5-21. Mixed nonteratomatous germ cell tumor. The tumor shows an admixture of seminomatous (*left*) and yolk sac tumor (*right*) components within the same lesion.

- Polyvesicular vitelline pattern is characterized by saclike structures in a background of myxoid or fibrous stroma (Figure 5-20)
- Rarely, hepatoid pattern resembling liver cells in thick plates
- Schiller-Duval bodies (papillary structures with central vascular core covered by neoplastic epithelium) are characteristic but not always present
- Intracellular or extracellular eosinophilic hyaline globules often seen regardless of which pattern predominates
- Sarcomatoid foci may be seen

CHORIOCARCINOMA
- Neoplasm composed of cytotrophoblastic cells admixed with giant syncytiotrophoblastic cells
- Extensive necrosis and hemorrhage common

MIXED NONTERATOMATOUS GERM CELL TUMORS
- Foci with features of different types of germ cell tumor, often including seminoma (Figure 5-21)
- Those with choriocarcinoma and yolk sac components usually show elevated serum levels of both β-HCG and AFP

Special Stains and Immunohistochemistry
- Immunohistochemistry useful in differentiating germ cell tumors from other malignancies in the mediastinum but not for subclassifying NSGCT
- Cytokeratin positive in all nonseminomatous germ cell tumors
- PLAP positive in about 50% of NSGCTs
- AFP positive in about 30% of cases of embryonal carcinoma and in most cases of yolk sac tumor
- HCG positive in giant cells and cytotrophoblastic cells in any germ cell tumor

- Embryonal carcinoma
  - CD30 (Ki-1) often positive
  - CD57 often positive
- Yolk sac tumor
  - Positive for AFP
  - α_1-Antitrypsin positive in hyaline droplets
- Choriocarcinoma
  - β-HCG positive in syncytiotrophoblastic cells and focally in cytotrophoblastic cells
  - Epithelial membrane antigen (EMA) positive in about 50% of cases

Other Techniques for Diagnosis
- Cytogenetics: isochromosome 12p is characteristic

Differential Diagnosis
- Subclassification depends on thorough sampling and meticulous microscopic examination

METASTATIC ADENOCARCINOMA
- Thorough history and clinical-radiologic evaluation is necessary
- Usually negative for AFP (serum and immunohistochemically)
- HCG negative

THYMIC CARCINOMA
- Usually occurs in patients older than 40 years
- May have squamous or neuroendocrine differentiation
- HCG, AFP, and PLAP negative

METASTATIC MELANOMA
- Detailed history is important
- S-100 protein, vimentin, and HMB-45 are generally positive
- Negative for PLAP, HCG, or AFP

PEARLS

- *Almost all cases occur in males*
- *AFP positivity virtually excludes a metastatic adenocarcinoma*
- *Residual mediastinal mass after chemotherapy for a germ cell tumor may be mature teratoma or scar tissue; thorough sampling is necessary to exclude residual malignancy*
- *Most patients have invasion of other organs or distant metastases at time of presentation, and most of these patients die of their disease*
- *Sarcomatous transformation*
- *May have foci of cartilaginous matrix (chondrosarcoma) or skeletal muscle (rhabdomyosarcoma)*
- *Prognosis is extremely poor*
- *Association with hematologic malignancy:*
  - *Seen with yolk sac tumor*
  - *Believed to be due to differentiation of tumor into hematopoietic cells, which migrate to liver, spleen, and bone marrow*
  - *Most are acute myelomonocytic or acute megakaryocytic leukemias*

SELECTED REFERENCES

Grego FA, Oldham RK, Fez MF: The extragonadal germ cell cancer syndrome. Semin Oncol 9:448-455, 1982.

McNeil MM, Leong AS, Sage RE: Primary mediastinal embryonal carcinoma in association with Klinefelter's syndrome. Cancer 47:343-345, 1981.

Moran CA, Suster S: Hepatoid yolk sac tumors of the mediastinum: a clinicopathological and immunohistochemical study of four cases. Am J Surg Pathol 21:1210-1214, 1997.

Moran CA, Suster S: Mediastinal yolk sac tumors associated with prominent multilocular cystic changes of thymic epithelium: a clinicopathologic and immunohistochemical study of five cases. Mod Pathol 10:800-803, 1997.

Moran CA, Suster S: Primary mediastinal choriocarcinomas: a clinicopathologic and immunohistochemical study of 8 cases. Am J Surg Pathol 21:1007-1012, 1997.

Moran CA, Suster S: Yolk sac tumors of the mediastinum with prominent spindle cell features: a clinicopathologic study of three cases. Am J Surg Pathol 21:1173-1177, 1997.

Moran CA, Suster S, Koss MN: Primary germ cell tumors of the mediastinum. III. Yolk sac tumor, embryonal carcinoma, choriocarcinoma, and combined nonteratomatous germ cell tumors of the mediastinum—a clinicopathologic and immunohistochemical study of 64 cases. Cancer 80:699-707, 1997.

Sickels EA, Belliveau RE, Wiernik PH: Primary mediastinal choriocarcinoma in the male. Cancer 33:1196-1203, 1974.

Truong LD, Harris L, Mattioli C, et al: Endodermal sinus tumor of the mediastinum: a report of 7 cases and review of the literature. Cancer 58:730-739, 1986.

NEUROGENIC TUMORS: NEUROBLASTOMA, GANGLIONEUROBLASTOMA, GANGLIONEUROMA

Clinical Features

- Tumors are associated with the sympathetic chain and may be found in the neck, mediastinum, retroperitoneum, and adrenal medulla
- Tumors are categorized as neuroblastoma (NB), ganglioneuroblastoma (GNB), and ganglioneuroma (GN) based on the maturation of the neurons and accompanying Schwann cells
- Tumors in the mediastinum are more likely to show maturation than those in the retroperitoneum or adrenal medulla
- Neuroblastoma is the most common solid tumor of young children
- Ganglioneuroma is the most common in the mediastinum
- Presents with mass effects, including compression of nerve roots and erosion of vertebral bone
- Serum or urine shows elevated catecholamine metabolites homovanillic acid (HMV) and vanillylmandelic acid (VMA)

Gross Pathology

NEUROBLASTOMA

- Large, well-circumscribed mass with a gray, soft cut surface; often has hemorrhage, necrosis, and calcification

GANGLIONEUROBLASTOMA

- Large, well-circumscribed, firm mass with tan-white areas and hemorrhagic areas; focal calcification often seen

GANGLIONEUROMA

- Large, encapsulated tumor with a firm, gray-white, homogeneous cut surface

Histopathology

- See Chapter 9 for more detailed histologic features
- See Table 5-3

NEUROBLASTOMA

- Cellular tumor composed of nodular aggregates of small round blue cells (neuroblasts) separated by delicate fibrovascular septa (Figure 5-22)

TABLE 5-3 COMPARISON OF FEATURES OF NEUROGENIC TUMORS

	Neuroblastoma	Ganglioneuroblastoma	Ganglioneuroma
Age	Young children; 90% < 5 years old	Older children	Older children to adults
Maturation	Minimal to none	Mixed	Mixed to fully mature
Location	Adrenal gland, rarely posterior mediastinum	Posterior mediastinum or retroperitoneum	Posterior mediastinum or retroperitoneum
Behavior	Dismal to excellent depending on stage; average 3-year survival rate of 30%	Overall better prognosis than neuroblastoma	Maturing: favorable Mature: benign

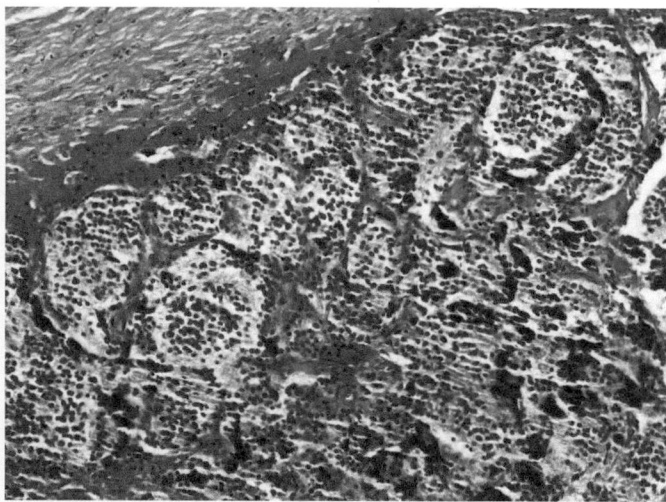

Figure 5-22. Neuroblastoma. The tumor is composed of small round blue cells with scant cytoplasm. Notice the fibrillary background.

- Characterized by Homer-Wright pseudorosettes (round spaces surrounded by palisading peripheral nuclei and filled with a faintly eosinophilic fibrillary matrix)

GANGLIONEUROBLASTOMA
- Similar histology to neuroblastoma except ganglion cell differentiation is seen (admixture of ganglion cells and undifferentiated cells)
- Developing or mature ganglion cells make up more than half the cell population
- Small undifferentiated cells make up a minority of the tumor

GANGLIONEUROMA
- Spindle cell tumor resembling neurofibroma but with numerous ganglion cells (Figure 5-23)

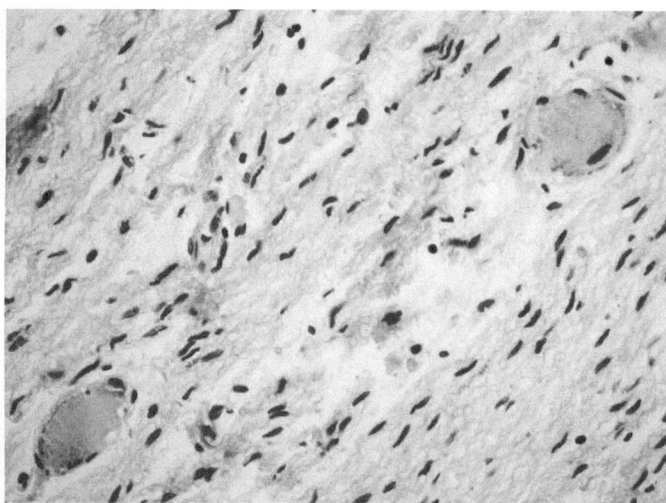

Figure 5-23. Ganglioneuroma. Histologic section shows a tumor composed of spindle cells with wavy nuclei and scattered mature ganglion cells.

- Maturing tumors are composed of differentiating neuroblasts, ganglion cells, and neuropil
- Mature tumors are composed of sheets of Schwann cells admixed with clusters of mature ganglion cells in a loose myxoid background

Special Stains and Immunohistochemistry
- Neuroblastoma and ganglion cells are reactive for
  - Neurofilament
  - Synaptophysin
  - Chromogranin
  - NSE (caution: NSE has broad cross-reactivity with other cell types)
- Stromal cells (Schwann cells) are reactive for
  - S-100 protein
  - Glial fibrillary acidic protein (GFAP)
  - Myelin basic protein

Other Techniques for Diagnosis
- Electron microscopy: neuroblastoma is composed of undifferentiated small cells with round nuclei and scant cytoplasm; neurofilaments, neurosecretory granules, or both may be present
- Cytogenetics (neuroblastoma): may be associated with deletion of chromosome 1p

Differential Diagnosis: Neuroblastoma
EWING SARCOMA, PNET
- Generally found in long bones or occasionally in soft tissue; rare in mediastinum
- Tumor cells may have clear cytoplasm containing glycogen (positive for PAS)
- Positive for CD99
- Characteristic translocation t(11;22)

EMBRYONAL RHABDOMYOSARCOMA
- Admixture of small primitive blue cells and scattered larger cells with abundant eosinophilic cytoplasm (rhabdomyoblasts)
- Positive for muscle markers such as desmin, myogenin, MyoD1, and muscle-specific actin (MSA)
- Negative for neural markers

LYMPHOBLASTIC LYMPHOMA
- Positive for TdT, CD3, and CD45
- Usually clonal T-cell population; rarely clonal B-cell population
- Caution: also positive for CD99

SMALL CELL CARCINOMA
- Typically found in older adults
- Lung primary far more common than mediastinal primary
- Positive for low-molecular-weight cytokeratins; negative for NSE

GANGLIONEUROBLASTOMA AND GANGLIONEUROMA
- Malignant melanoma
  - Positive for HMB-45, melan-A, and S-100 protein
- Paraganglioma
  - Zellballen pattern with surrounding sustentacular cells
  - Sustentacular cells positive for S-100 protein
  - Positive for chromogranin and synaptophysin
- Schwannoma and malignant schwannoma
  - Typically show Antoni A and B areas and Verocay bodies
  - Absent ganglion cells
- Neurofibroma
  - Spindle cell tumor with no ganglion cells

PEARLS

- *Neuroblastoma: prognosis is related to disease stage, which is a complex scheme based on age at diagnosis and cytogenetic and histologic findings*
- *Stages I and II (good prognosis) are associated with specific cytogenetic findings (chromosome 1 deletion), no amplification of N-myc gene, and greater than 95% 3-year survival rate*
- *Stages III and IV (poor prognosis) have from less than 5% to about 50% survival rate (Table 5-4)*

SELECTED REFERENCES

Adam A, Hochholzer L: Ganglioneuroblastoma of the posterior mediastinum: a clinicopathologic review of 80 cases. Cancer 47:373-381, 1981.

Ambros PF, Ambros IM, Strehl S, et al: Regression and progression in neuroblastoma. Does genetics predict tumor behavior? Eur J Cancer 31A:510-515, 1995.

Brodeur GM: Molecular basis for heterogeneity in human neuroblastomas. Eur J Cancer 31A:505-510, 1995.

Devoe K, Weidner N: Immunohistochemistry of small round cell tumors. Semin Diagn Pathol 17:216-224, 2000.

Joshi VV: Peripheral neuroblastic tumors: Pathologic classification based on recommendations of international neuroblastoma pathology committee (modification of Shimada classification). Pediatr Dev Pathol 3:184-199, 2000.

Young DG: Thoracic neuroblastoma/ganglioneuroma. J Pediatr Surg 18:37-41, 1983.

SCHWANNOMA

Clinical Features

- Most common tumor in the posterior mediastinum
- Generally a single mass; multiple schwannomas may be associated with von Recklinghausen disease (neurofibromatosis type I)
- May be asymptomatic or present with pain, cough, or symptoms related to nerve involvement or compression
- No sex predilection
- Peak incidence in third and fourth decades

Gross Pathology

- Round to oval encapsulated tumor
- Usually attached to a nerve trunk
- About 10% have an intravertebral tumor and are dumbbell shaped
- Firm, solid tumor with a tan to yellow cut surface
- Cystic changes and myxoid areas may be seen

Histopathology

- Well-formed fibrous capsule
- Spindle cell tumor composed of Antoni A and B patterns (hypercellular and hypocellular areas, respectively)
- Verocay bodies are characteristic and consist of palisading nuclei with central hypocellular area
- Blood vessels are hyalinized and thick walled
- Focal collections of foamy histiocytes
- Osseous and cartilaginous metaplasia can be seen
- Cystic changes may be seen
- Ancient schwannoma
  - Atypical nuclei
  - Stromal sclerosis
  - Little or no mitotic activity
- Cellular schwannoma
  - Encapsulated, but can erode adjacent structures
  - Highly cellular spindle cell proliferation with predominance of Antoni A areas and no Antoni B areas
  - Variable nuclear atypia
  - Low mitotic activity
  - Strong S-100 protein positivity

Special Stains and Immunohistochemistry

- S-100 protein positive (more often in benign tumors)
- CD57 positive
- GFAP: some schwannomas may be positive

Other Techniques for Diagnosis

- Electron microscopy: spindle cells show numerous long-spaced (130-nm periodicity) collagen fibrils referred to as *Luse bodies* and reduplication of the basal lamina; pigment, if present, is neuromelanin and is not in melanosomes; long, slender cytoplasmic prolongations are characteristic

Differential Diagnosis

NEUROFIBROMA
- Stronger association with neurofibromatosis
- Lacks thick fibrous capsule
- Grows within and enlarges nerve
- Hypocellular, myxoid areas without hypercellular areas
- Absence of Antoni A and B areas and Verocay bodies
- Silver stain may reveal nerve fibers within the tumor

TABLE 5-4	PROGNOSTIC FACTORS FOR NEUROGENIC TUMORS	
Good Prognosis	**Poor Prognosis**
Near triploid or hyperdiploid (aneuploid)	Tetraploid or near diploid
Presence of 1p36 tumor suppressor gene	Loss of heterozygosity
No amplification of *N-myc*	Amplification of *N-myc* (> 10 copies)
No expression of TRKA factor receptor	

LEIOMYOMA
- Less common in this location
- Negative for S-100 protein
- Positive for SMA

PEARLS

- *Multiple schwannomas may be associated with von Recklinghausen disease*
- *Well-formed fibrous capsule with typical histologic features, including Verocay bodies and Antoni A and Antoni B areas*
- *Excellent prognosis; surgical excision of solitary tumors is curative*

SELECTED REFERENCES

Ackerman LV, Taylor FH: Neurogenous tumors within the thorax: a clinical pathologic evaluation of 48 cases. Cancer 4: 669-691, 1951.
Dickersin GR: The electron microscopic spectrum of nerve sheath tumors. Ultrastruct Pathol 11:103-146, 1987.
Marchevsky AM: Mediastinal tumors of peripheral nervous system origin. Semin Diagn Pathol 16:65-78, 1999.
Weiss SW, Langloss JM, Enzinger FM: Value of S-100 protein in the diagnosis of soft tissue tumors with particular reference to benign and malignant Schwann cell tumors. Lab Invest 49:299-308, 1983.

METASTATIC TUMORS

Clinical Features

- Both small cell and non-small cell carcinomas of the lung can metastasize early to the mediastinum
- Large mediastinal mass and small lung primary may be seen
- Other tumors arising in neighboring structures, including esophagus, trachea, chest wall, pleura, and vertebrae, may also appear to be arising in the mediastinum
- Tumors metastasizing to mediastinal lymph nodes may expand and appear as thymic primary tumors on gross and microscopic examination (particularly breast, thyroid, kidney, prostate, testis, and malignant melanoma)
- Clinical history and radiologic findings are important

Gross Pathology

- Noncontributory

Histopathology

- Histologic features are those seen in primary malignancies

Special Stains and Immunohistochemistry

- Often not helpful because many metastatic carcinomas are cytokeratin positive but have no other specific staining characteristics

- S-100 protein, Melan-A and HMB-45 are useful in the diagnosis of malignant melanoma
- Prostatic-specific antigen (PSA) and prostatic acid phosphatase (PSAP) may be useful in diagnosing a metastasis from a prostatic primary
- BRST2 or GCDFP15 positive in breast carcinoma
- Thyroid transcription factor-1 (TTF-1) positive in lung and thyroid gland tumors
- Synaptophysin and chromogranin positive in small cell carcinomas from lung or other primary site
- LCA positive in lymphoma

Other Techniques for Diagnosis

- As per suspected primary tumor

Differential Diagnosis

- Clinical history is essential when evaluating malignant mediastinal neoplasms

THYMIC CARCINOMA
- Diagnosis of exclusion

GERMINOMA
- Positive for PLAP

YOLK SAC TUMOR
- Positive for AFP; may be positive for PLAP

EMBRYONAL CARCINOMA
- Positive for PLAP and CD30 (Ki-1); may be positive for AFP

LYMPHOMA
- Positive for CD45
- Anaplastic lymphoma positive for CD30 (Ki-1)
- Flow cytometry or gene rearrangements to demonstrate clonal lymphoid population

PEARLS

- *Metastatic tumors account for most epithelial malignancies in the mediastinum*
- *Most common primary sites include trachea, bronchi, lung parenchyma, and esophagus*
- *Immunohistochemical staining is important when evaluating metastatic tumors in this location*

SELECTED REFERENCES

McLoud TC, Kalisher L, Stark P, Green R: Intrathoracic lymph node metastases from extrathoracic neoplasms. Am J Radiol 131:403-407, 1978.
McLoud TC, Meyer JE: Mediastinal metastasis. Radiol Clin North Am 20:453-468, 1982.
Middleton G: Involvement of the thymus by metastatic neoplasms. Br J Cancer 20:41-46, 1966.

Chapter 6

Gastrointestinal System

ROBERT E. PETRAS

CHAPTER OUTLINE

ESOPHAGUS

CONGENITAL AND ACQUIRED ESOPHAGEAL ABNORMALITIES

Clinical Features

ESOPHAGEAL ECTOPIAS
- Gastric
  - Affects up to 20% of population
  - Found in cervical esophagus; referred to as *inlet patch* (Figure 6-1)
  - May produce peptic symptoms in older patients
  - Rare examples of dysplasia or carcinoma reported complicating inlet patches
- Sebaceous: so-called Fordyce granules
- Pancreatic
  - Rare in esophagus
  - Can be seen with trisomy 18 or trisomy 13
  - More often seen as a metaplasia in reflux

ESOPHAGEAL ATRESIA
- Complete atresia is found in about 1 in 3000 live births
- Associated with tracheoesophageal fistula in about 1 in 1000 live births
- Risk factors include male sex, low birth weight, premature birth, and twin gestation (monozygotic)
- Classic presentation includes choking in a newborn infant and excessive drooling; affected patients have a propensity to aspirate or develop respiratory distress
- Atresia is associated with Down syndrome (10% of atresias), single umbilical artery, and other syndromes involving the heart, urogenital tract, and skeleton
- May be associated with VATER syndrome (vertebral anomalies, anal atresia, tracheoesophageal fistula, renal defects)

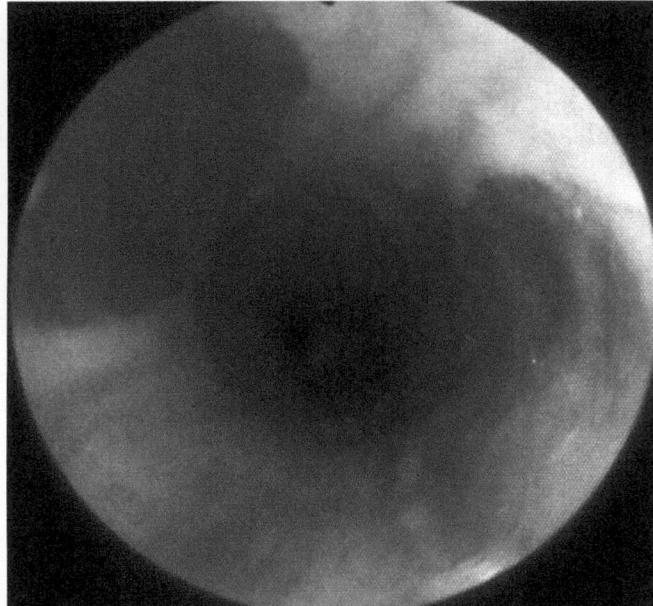

Figure 6-1. Endoscopic photograph of inlet patch in the cervical esophagus. Areas of erythematous gastric-type mucosa are surrounded by gray-white glistening squamous mucosa.

CONGENITAL ESOPHAGEAL DUPLICATION
- Manifests most commonly as cysts, but diverticula or tubular malformations can also be seen
- Cysts occur as a result of partial arrest during early development (< 8 weeks), when esophagus is lined by columnar epithelium; lined by gastric epithelium if lesion persists into adulthood
- Symptoms include dysphagia, anorexia, dyspnea, and pain

ESOPHAGEAL DIVERTICULA
- Saccular protrusions of the esophagus
- Zenker diverticulum is most common (70%); located immediately above the upper esophageal sphincter (associated with cricopharyngeal motor dysfunction)
- Less commonly, diverticula develop at the midpoint of the esophagus or immediately proximal to the lower esophageal sphincter (epiphrenic) (so-called traction diverticulum)
- Typically present in elderly patients
- Produce a repository for swallowed food; complicated by dysphagia and halitosis

ESOPHAGEAL WEBS AND RINGS
- Webs
  - Congenital and acquired constrictions caused by diaphragm-like sleeve of mucosa (at right angle to long axis of esophagus)
  - Often symptomatic and typically cause dysphagia
  - Upper esophageal webbing associated with iron deficiency anemia, glossitis, and cheilosis is called *Plummer-Vinson syndrome* and in many patients also includes autoimmune disorders (thyroid disorders, Sjögren syndrome, and inflammatory bowel disease); predisposes to squamous cell carcinoma of the upper esophagus
  - Webs associated with Plummer-Vinson syndrome are proximal, arise anteriorly, and are up to 0.2-cm thick; may occasionally be circumferential
- Rings
  - Developmental constrictions secondary to chronic disease states, which may include reflux or scleroderma
  - May be mucosal or muscular; muscular rings are almost always associated with hiatal hernia
  - Called *Schatzki rings* if located at or immediately above the gastroesophageal junction
  - Rings and corrugations (so-called feline esophagus) can be a manifestation of eosinophilic esophagitis (see "Eosinophilic Esophagitis")

ESOPHAGEAL HERNIA (DIAPHRAGMATIC HERNIA)
- Generally an acquired condition
- Displacement of the distal esophagus from normal (subdiaphragm) intra-abdominal location into thoracic cavity
- May move caudad to cephalad (sliding) or incarcerate in the anterior mediastinum (paraesophageal)

Gross and Endoscopic Pathology

ESOPHAGEAL ECTOPIAS
- Gastric
  - Discrete pink to red area in cervical esophagus surrounded by gray-white squamous mucosa
  - Variable sizes (several millimeters to large enough to encircle esophagus)

- Sebaceous
  - Small, light-yellow plaques
- Pancreatic
  - Smooth, well-defined submucosal mass resembling leiomyoma or lipoma, sometimes with central dimple

ESOPHAGEAL ATRESIA (TRACHEOESOPHAGEAL FISTULA)
- Type I: blind proximal esophagus with no fistula
- Type II: proximal fistula with completely interrupted distal esophagus
- Type III: blind proximal esophagus with distal tracheoesophageal fistula arising at tracheal bifurcation (most common)
- Type IV: esophagus with both proximal and distal communications with trachea

ESOPHAGEAL DUPLICATION
- Commonly seen as posterior cysts
- May be within esophageal wall or extramural

ESOPHAGEAL DIVERTICULA
- Zenker diverticulum
  - Saccular protrusion immediately above the upper esophageal sphincter
  - May be several centimeters

ESOPHAGEAL WEBS AND RINGS
- Webs
  - Often produce strictures
- Rings
  - Encircle esophagus and generally occur at the esophagogastric junction (Schatzki ring)
  - Muscular rings arise at the phrenoesophageal membrane attachment

ESOPHAGEAL HERNIA (DIAPHRAGMATIC HERNIA)
- Intrathoracic portion tends to dilate and undergo ischemic changes
- May lead to ischemic necrosis (rare)

Histopathology

ESOPHAGEAL ECTOPIAS
- Gastric
  - Foveolar mucosa with specialized glands, complete with parietal, chief, and endocrine cells
  - May resemble specialized columnar epithelium of Barrett esophagus with mucin-producing goblet cells
  - May contain *Helicobacter pylori* (rare)
- Sebaceous
  - Mucosal and submucosal sebaceous glands
- Pancreatic
  - Typically pancreatic acinar tissue; may also contain islet cells

ESOPHAGEAL DUPLICATION
- Intramural or extramural cysts lined by respiratory, gastric, intestinal, or squamous mucosa
- Should have a duplicated muscularis externa

ESOPHAGEAL DIVERTICULA
- Zenker diverticulum
  - Squamous-lined sac displaying variable acanthosis, chronic inflammation, and ulceration
  - May have thin muscular layer

ESOPHAGEAL WEBS AND RINGS
- Webs
  - Thin sleeve of fibrovascular connective tissue covered by squamous mucosa on both sides
  - Gastric mucosa may line distal side
  - Inflammation often present
  - Muscle layer is absent
- Rings
  - Mucosal rings are similar to webs except they have a few fibers of muscularis mucosae (squamous epithelium covering a thin sleeve of connective tissue) and are often covered by gastric mucosa distally
  - Muscular rings have a prominent muscle component
  - Those associated with eosinophilic esophagitis show an increase in the squamous basal cell layer with papillomatosis and increased (> 15 per high-power field [hpf]) intraepithelial eosinophils (see "Eosinophilic Esophagitis")

ESOPHAGEAL HERNIA (DIAPHRAGMATIC HERNIA)
- Variable degrees of chronic inflammation, fibromuscular proliferation in the lamina propria, and regenerative epithelial changes

Special Stains and Immunohistochemistry
- Noncontributory

Other Techniques for Diagnosis
- Noncontributory

Differential Diagnosis

ESOPHAGEAL ECTOPIAS
- Generally must be differentiated from benign and malignant esophageal tumors; requires biopsy
- Rare examples of proximal esophageal adenocarcinoma arising in gastric heterotopia are described

ESOPHAGEAL ATRESIA
- Relatively straightforward clinical diagnosis
- May overlap clinically with respiratory conditions, particularly if associated with tracheoesophageal fistula

BRONCHOGENIC CYSTS AND ESOPHAGEAL DUPLICATION
- May be difficult to distinguish
- Bronchogenic cysts are typically anterior, contain cartilage, and are lined by respiratory mucosa
- Cyst wall containing cartilage and bronchial glands without a muscularis mucosae is best interpreted as a bronchogenic cyst

PEARLS

- *A posterior cyst with two muscular layers, no cartilage, and attachment to esophagus is most likely an esophageal duplication*
- *Ectopias, atresia, and duplication are congenital conditions; diverticula, rings, webs, and diaphragmatic hernias are acquired conditions*

SELECTED REFERENCES

Borhan-Manesh F, Farnum JB: Incidence of heterotopic gastric mucosa in the upper oesophagus. Gut 32:968-972, 1991.

Dantas RO, Villanova MG: Esophageal motility impairment in Plummer-Vinson syndrome: correction by iron treatment. Dig Dis Sci 38:968-971, 1993.

Hocking M, Young DG: Duplication of the alimentary tract. Br J Surg 68:92-96, 1981.

Quan L, Smith DW: The VATER association: vertebral defects, anal atresia, tracheoesophageal fistulas with esophageal atresia, radial and renal dysplasia. A spectrum of associated defects. J Pediatr 82:104-107, 1973.

Tang P, McKinley MJ, Sporrer M, Kahn E: Inlet patch: prevalence, histologic type and association with esophagitis, Barrett esophagus and antritis. Arch Pathol Lab Med 128:444-447, 2004.

INFECTIOUS ESOPHAGITIS

Clinical Features

- Consists primarily of opportunistic viral and fungal infections in immunocompromised patients, including the following:
  - Patients with acquired immunodeficiency syndrome (AIDS)
  - Patients on steroids or immune modulators (after transplantation)
  - Diabetic patients
  - Debilitated or elderly patients

Gross and Endoscopic Pathology

- Herpesvirus infection: punched-out ulcers (Figure 6-2)
- Cytomegalovirus (CMV): nonspecific ulcer
- *Candida* species: pseudomembranous, gray-white patches
- Pathogenic bacteria: superficial necrosis

Histopathology

HERPES SIMPLEX VIRUS (HSV)

- Biopsies taken from the ulcer edge show acantholysis with multinucleated squamous cells with steel-blue nuclei or Cowdry type A inclusions (Figure 6-3)

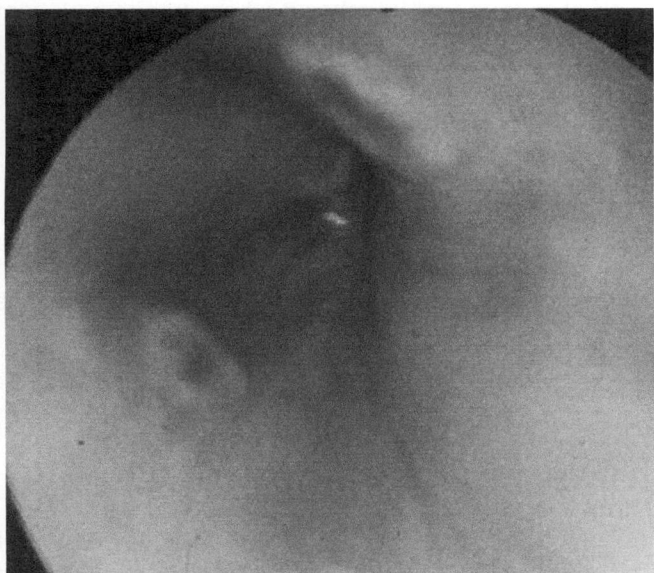

Figure 6-2. Endoscopic photograph of herpes esophagitis demonstrating well-circumscribed ulcers.

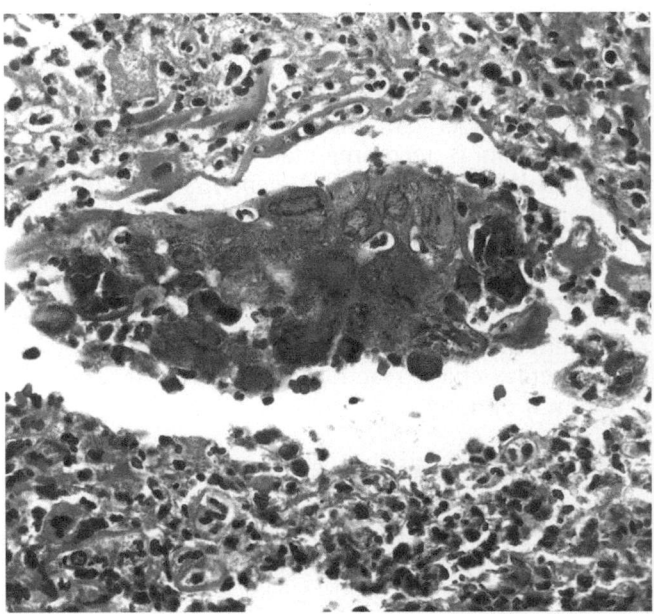

Figure 6-3. Herpes esophagitis. Squamous mucosa adjacent to an ulcer shows multinucleate giant cells with intranuclear inclusions intermingled with fibrinopurulent exudate.

CMV

- Deep biopsies from the ulcer base show classic Cowdry type A inclusions
- Cellular enlargement with granular basophilic intracytoplasmic inclusions and intranuclear inclusions, which are sometimes eosinophilic, large, and targetoid
- Preferentially involves endothelial cells, fibroblasts, or glandular epithelium (rarely infects squamous cells)

FUNGI

- Nonspecific mixed inflammation, ulceration, and granulation tissue with admixed fungal structures
- Pattern of injury associated with Candidiasis includes squamous acantholysis, superficial patchy neutrophils in squamous epithelium, and squamous intraepithelial lymphocytosis
- *Candida*: blastoconidia and pseudohyphae
- *Histoplasma*: small, 1- to 2-μm organisms within histiocyte cytoplasm (rare)
- *Aspergillus*: true hyphae demonstrating dichotomous branching at 45-degree angles (extremely rare in biopsy or surgical specimens)
- *Mucor*: aseptate, folded, ribbon-like hyphae often in an infarcted background (extremely rare in biopsy or surgical specimens)

BACTERIAL

- Bacteria present in esophageal biopsy are generally nonpathogenic
- True bacterial infection is characterized by bacteria present in deeper levels of tissue associated with neutrophilic exudate and necrosis; often part of "black esophagus" (discussed later)

Special Stains and Immunohistochemistry

- Fungal structures are Grocott methenamine silver (GMS) and periodic acid–Schiff (PAS) stain positive
- Alcian blue PAS combination stain with hematoxylin counterstain is recommended for esophageal tissues because it highlights fungal elements and can also be a useful screen for signet ring cell adenocarcinoma and for Barrett esophagus (Figure 6-4)

Other Techniques for Diagnosis

- Immunohistochemistry for HSV and CMV
- Polymerase chain reaction (PCR) for HSV and CMV (rarely, if ever, needed)

Differential Diagnosis

CORROSIVE ESOPHAGITIS

- Acute lesions are similar to infections and are best distinguished by clinical history and the lack of pathologic organisms

REFLUX ESOPHAGITIS

- Can have areas of giant cell change within squamous epithelium in reflux: distinguished from herpetic infection by its lack of characteristic viral inclusions
- Reflux typically causes the characteristic histologic triad involving squamous mucosa
  - Hyperplasia: elongated lamina propria papillae (more than two thirds of thickness of epithelium)
  - Thickened basal layer (more than 15% of epithelial thickness)
  - Increased intraepithelial lymphocytes (with characteristic compressed, irregular nuclear contours) and eosinophils; neutrophils may also be present—although fairly specific for reflux, they occur only in some cases and are therefore not sensitive
- Consistent clinical history
- No organisms identified

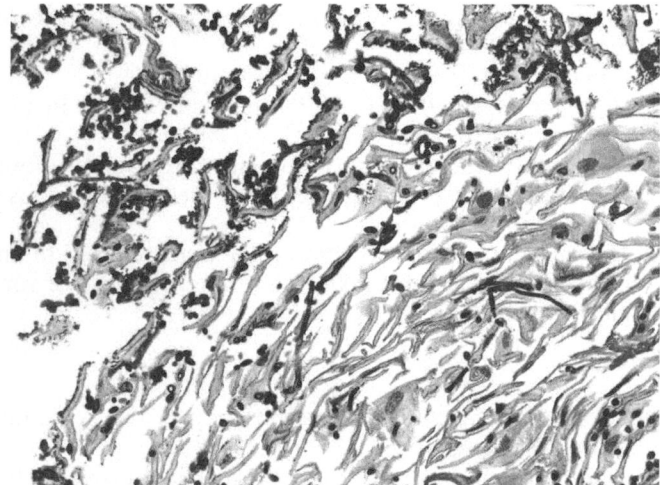

Figure 6-4. Candida esophagitis (Alcian blue and periodic acid-Schiff stains) with budding yeast forms and pseudohyphae among acantholytic squamous cells.

SELECTED REFERENCES

Haulk AA, Sugar AM: Candida esophagitis. Adv Intern Med 36:307-318, 1991.
Knoke M, Bernhardt H: Endoscopic aspects of mycosis in the upper digestive tract. Endoscopy 12:295-298, 1980.
McBane RD, Gross JB Jr: Herpes esophagitis: clinical symptoms, endoscopic appearance and diagnosis in 23 patients. Gastrointest Endosc 37:600-603, 1991.
Myerson D, Hackman RC, Nelson JA, et al: Widespread presence of histologically occult cytomegalovirus. Hum Pathol 15:430-439, 1984.

INJURIOUS ESOPHAGITIS

Clinical Features

CHEMICAL ESOPHAGITIS

- Most severe injury follows suicide attempts (acid, alkali) in adults and accidental ingestion in children

DRUG ESOPHAGITIS

- "Pill" esophagitis: patients report feeling a lump in the throat; can occur after ingestion of any oral medication without adequate hydration
- Some oral medications are particularly corrosive (e.g., alendronate, iron-containing compounds)
- Chemotherapeutic agents are generally directly toxic (rather than by allergic mechanisms)

RADIATION ESOPHAGITIS

- Produces dysphagia and odynophagia
- Location depends on area exposed to the radiation
- May be combined with chemical (chemotherapy) injury

Gross and Endoscopic Pathology

CHEMICAL ESOPHAGITIS

- Affects narrowest esophageal segments (proximal and distal ends and midesophagus where esophagus is compressed by aorta and main-stem bronchus)
- Acute corrosive chemical injury varies from mild erythema to mucosal sloughing, ulceration, or frank necrosis with perforation
- Chronic injury can cause stricture due to fibrosis

DRUG ESOPHAGITIS

- Direct caustic effect of pill produces a localized lesion often in proximal or mid esophagus
- Chemotherapeutic agents may produce diffuse lesions

RADIATION ESOPHAGITIS

- Location depends on area exposed to the radiation
- Typically causes large superficial ulcers

Histopathology

CHEMICAL ESOPHAGITIS

- Variable histologic features range from mild congestion to severe acute inflammation, erosion, ulceration, and granulation tissue reaction
- Lesions heal with submucosal fibrosis

DRUG ESOPHAGITIS

- Pill esophagitis produces discrete, superficial ulceration that is nonspecific
  - Vascular endothelial proliferation can be prominent
- Allergic drug reactions produce eosinophilia
- Chemotherapeutic agents interfere with cell replication, producing basal cell hyperplasia, cytologic atypia

RADIATION ESOPHAGITIS

- Radiation injury is recognized by acanthosis, parakeratosis, necrosis, and stromal cell atypia, including enlarged, stellate fibroblasts and hyalinized blood vessels with enlarged, vesicular endothelial cell nuclei
- All lesions may heal with lamina propria and submucosal fibrosis, leading to stricture

Special Stains and Immunohistochemistry

- Noncontributory

Other Techniques for Diagnosis

- Noncontributory

Differential Diagnosis

REFLUX ESOPHAGITIS

- Location, histologic appearance, and clinical history are usually diagnostic

INFECTIOUS ESOPHAGITIS

- Diagnosed by detection of organisms, sometimes using special stains and immunohistochemical reactions and recognition of cytopathic viral changes

ESOPHAGITIS DISSECANS SUPERFICIALIS ("SLOUGHING ESOPHAGITIS")

- May present with dysphagia; rarely vomiting of tubular cast
- Endoscopy shows whitish strips of peeling mucosa
- Biopsy specimens show detached fragments of squamous mucosa, fungal and bacterial colonies, intraepithelial splitting, necrotic superficial epithelium
- Can be associated with medications (e.g., bisphosphonates), esophageal trauma, stricture, bullous skin disorders, and cigarette smoking

ACUTE ESOPHAGEAL NECROSIS (SO-CALLED BLACK ESOPHAGUS)

- Biopsy specimen contains necrotic tissue, bacterial and fungal colonies
- Appears black on endoscopy; patients present with upper gastrointestinal bleeding
- Usually associated with comorbid conditions such as severe cardiovascular disease with hemodynamic compromise
- High mortality rate (about 30%)

PEARLS

- *Important to have a complete patient clinical history*
- *Consider radiation exposure when bizarre epithelial and stromal cells are encountered*

SELECTED REFERENCES

Abraham SC, Yardley JH, Wu TT: Erosive injury in the upper gastrointestinal tract in patients receiving iron medication: an underrecognized entity. Am J Surg Pathol 23:1241-1247, 1999.

Carmack SW, Vemulapalli R, Spechler SJ, Genta RM: Esophagitis dissecans superficialis ("sloughing esophagitis"): a clinicopathologic study of 12 cases. Am J Surg Pathol 33:1789-1794, 2009.

DeGroen PC, Lubbe DF, Hirsch LJ, et al: Esophagitis associated with the use of alendronate. N Engl J Med 335:1016-1021, 1996.

Gurvits GE, Shapsis A, Lau N, et al: Acute esophageal necrosis: a rare syndrome. J Gastroenterol 42:29-38, 2007.

Misra SP, Dwivedi M: Pill-induced esophagitis. Gastrointest Endosc 55:81, 2002.

Purdy JK, Appelman HD, McKenna BJ: Sloughing esophagitis is associated with chronic debilitation and medications that injure the esophageal mucosa. Mod Pathol 25:767-775, 2012.

INFLAMMATORY ESOPHAGITIS

Clinical Features

DERMATOLOGIC CONDITIONS

- Pemphigus vulgaris
  - Antibody-mediated, blistering skin disorder that may affect skin or squamous mucosa
  - May be induced by drugs
  - May be fatal
  - Peak ages: 40 to 60 years
- Bullous pemphigoid
  - Bullous skin disease affecting mainly elderly patients (fifth to ninth decades)
  - Rarely affects the esophagus
  - Increased incidence in men
- Erythema multiforme
  - Acute eruption of skin and mucosal surfaces
  - Mucosal involvement is termed *Stevens-Johnson syndrome*
- Lichen planus
  - Common inflammatory disorder usually affecting skin and mucosal surfaces but rarely involving the esophagus

GRAFT-VERSUS-HOST DISEASE (GVHD)

- Necrotizing inflammation of mucosa, skin, or glandular epithelia after bone marrow transplantation
- Transplanted T cells attack host

Gross and Endoscopic Pathology

DERMATOLOGIC CONDITIONS

- Pemphigus vulgaris
  - Bleeding and esophageal strictures
- Bullous pemphigoid
  - Esophageal blisters
- Erythema multiforme (Stevens-Johnson syndrome)
  - Resembles reflux or peptic esophagitis
  - Pseudomembranes may form
- Lichen planus
  - Esophageal papules, plaques, or stricture

GVHD

- Typically involves the upper third of the esophagus
- May be focal or diffuse
- Desquamative lesion can cause web formation

Histopathology

DERMATOLOGIC CONDITIONS

- All conditions tend to mirror cutaneous histology
- Pemphigus vulgaris
  - Acantholysis with suprabasal blister formation
  - Conspicuous eosinophilic infiltrate

- Bullous pemphigoid
  - Subepithelial blister formation
  - Conspicuous eosinophilic infiltrate
- Erythema multiforme (Stevens-Johnson syndrome)
  - Focal to diffuse keratinocyte necrosis (forming rounded, eosinophilic bodies)
  - Mixed acute and chronic inflammation
- Lichen planus
  - Bandlike lymphocytic infiltrate in the lamina propria with epithelial lymphocytosis
  - Civatte bodies

GVHD
- Karyorrhexis and apoptosis of epithelial cells
- Variable T-cell infiltrates
- Epithelial atrophy and fibrosis of lamia propria in chronic lesions

Special Stains and Immunohistochemistry
DERMATOLOGIC CONDITIONS
- Pemphigus vulgaris
  - Immunofluorescence studies for antibodies (immunoglobulin G [IgG]) localized to intercellular region of epithelial cells
- Bullous pemphigus
  - Immunofluorescence studies for IgG or IgA localized along basement membranes
- GVHD
  - Immunostains can be used to confirm intraepithelial T lymphocytes but are rarely needed

Other Techniques for Diagnosis
- Immunofluorescence studies performed on esophageal biopsies placed in Michel's fixative

Differential Diagnosis
INFECTIOUS ESOPHAGITIS
- HSV or CMV infection
  - Typically found in immunocompromised hosts
  - Characterized by typical cytopathic changes (viral inclusions)
  - May coexist with GVHD
- Candidiasis
  - "Cheesy" exudates present in immunosuppressed, diabetic, or long-term antibiotic-treated patients
  - Characteristic fungal structures are present
  - May coexist with GVHD

REFLUX ESOPHAGITIS
- Much more common
- Characterized by involvement of lower esophagus near gastroesophageal junction
- Absent history of coexistent skin disorders or bone marrow transplantation

LYMPHOCYTIC ESOPHAGITIS
- Squamous epithelial lymphocytosis can be defined as ≥ 30 lymphocytes per high magnification field (normal < 5)
- Differential includes the following:
  - Reflux esophagitis

- Mucosal candidiasis
- Achalasia
- Pseudoachalasia (malignancy mimicking achalasia clinically)
- Pediatric Crohn disease patients
- Allergic "contact" mucositis
- Lichenoid (interface) mucositis such as lichenoid drug eruptions (e.g., thiazides, anti-hypertensives, nonsteroidal anti-inflammatory drugs [NSAIDs])

PEARLS

- *Primary dermatologic conditions may involve the esophagus because both are composed of squamous epithelium; thus, skin and esophageal histology and immunology are similar*

SELECTED REFERENCES
Cohen S, Saxema A, Waljee AK, et al: Lymphocytic esophagitis: a diagnosis of increasing frequency. J Clin Gastroenterol 46:828-832, 2012.
Haque S, Genta RM: Lymphocytic oesophagitis: clinicopathological aspects of an emerging condition. Gut 61:1108-1114, 2012.
McDonald GB, Sullivan KM, Schuffler MD, et al: Esophageal abnormalities in chronic graft-versus-host disease in humans. Gastroenterology 80:914-921, 1981.
Nielsen JA, Law RM, Fiman KH, Roberts CA: Esophageal lichen planus: a case report and review of the literature. World J Gastroenterol 19:2278-2281, 2013.

EOSINOPHILIC ESOPHAGITIS
Clinical Features
- Can be isolated to esophagus or rarely can be part of a multifocal or diffuse process involving various areas of the gastrointestinal tract (eosinophilic gastroenteritis)
- Can occur in atopic children and young men (male-to-female ratio of 3:1)
- Synchronous eosinophilic gastritis or enteritis is more common in pediatric cases
- Patients may also have peripheral eosinophilia, food sensitivity, asthma, or allergies
- Patients often present with dysphagia

Gross and Endoscopic Pathology
- Patients may develop esophageal strictures or webs/rings usually in the mid- and upper esophagus
- Corrugated appearance (feline esophagus) is commonly observed
- Linear mucosal ulceration may be seen
- White pustules or exudates are also common

Histopathology
- Marked eosinophilic infiltrate (> 15 eosinophils/hpf) of squamous mucosa; intraepithelial eosinophilic abscesses may also develop
- Eosinophils in lamina propria, muscularis mucosae, submucosa, and muscularis propria are less commonly seen
- Elongated rete pegs and marked squamous basal cell hyperplasia are typical

Special Stains and Immunohistochemistry
- Noncontributory

Other Techniques for Diagnosis

- Serum test for eotaxin-3 can be used to confirm diagnosis
- Familial cases associated with a susceptibility locus 5q22 (thymic stromal lymphopoietin [TSLP])

Differential Diagnosis

REFLUX ESOPHAGITIS

- Closely simulates eosinophilic gastroenteritis in some cases; however, reflux generally occurs in the distal esophagus and causes pyrosis and acid regurgitation
- Reflux generally shows fewer than five eosinophils/hpf
- Reflux is no longer an exclusion for diagnosis of eosinophilic esophagitis

PEARLS

- *Esophagus with webs or corrugation with numerous (> 15 eosinophils/hpf) usually indicates eosinophilic esophagitis*
- *Eosinophilic esophagitis often responds to asthma therapy (steroid treatment, fluticasone), oral viscous budesonide, and tends not to respond to proton pump inhibitors (PPI)*
  - *Esophagitis with > 15 eosinophils/hpf responsive to PPIs is now called PPI- responsive esophageal eosinophilia*

SELECTED REFERENCES

Dellon ES, Gonsalves N, Hirano I, et al: ACG clinical guideline: evidenced based approach to the diagnosis and management of esophageal eosinophilia and eosinophilic esophagitis (EoE). Am J Gastroenterol 108:679-692, 2013.

Liacouras CA, Furuta GT, Hirano I, et al: Eosinophilic esophagitis: updated consensus recommendations for children and adults. J Allergy Clin Immunol 128:3-20, 2011.

Mahajau L, Wyllie R, Petras R, et al: Idiopathic eosinophilic esophagitis with stricture formation in a patient with longstanding eosinophilic gastroenteritis. Gastrointest Endosc 46:557-560, 1997.

Vanderheyden AD, Petras RE, DeYoung BR, Mitros FA: Emerging eosinophilic (allergic) esophagitis: increased incidence or increased recognition? Arch Pathol Lab Med 131:777-779, 2007.

Walsh SV, Antonioli DA, Goldman H, et al: Allergic esophagitis in children: a clinicopathologic entity. Am J Surg Pathol 23:390-396, 1999.

REFLUX ESOPHAGITIS AND GASTROESOPHAGEAL REFLUX DISEASE (GERD)

Clinical Features

- Occurs in all ages, including children; most common in adult men older than 40 years
- Patients typically present with dysphagia, heartburn, and acid regurgitation
- Symptoms may be rarely mistaken for angina or myocardial infarction
- Complications include stricture, hemorrhage, and Barrett esophagus (see "Barrett Esophagus")

Gross and Endoscopic Pathology

- One third of patients have normal or slightly erythematous mucosa on endoscopy
- Subset of patients has glandular metaplasia, erosions, or ulcers

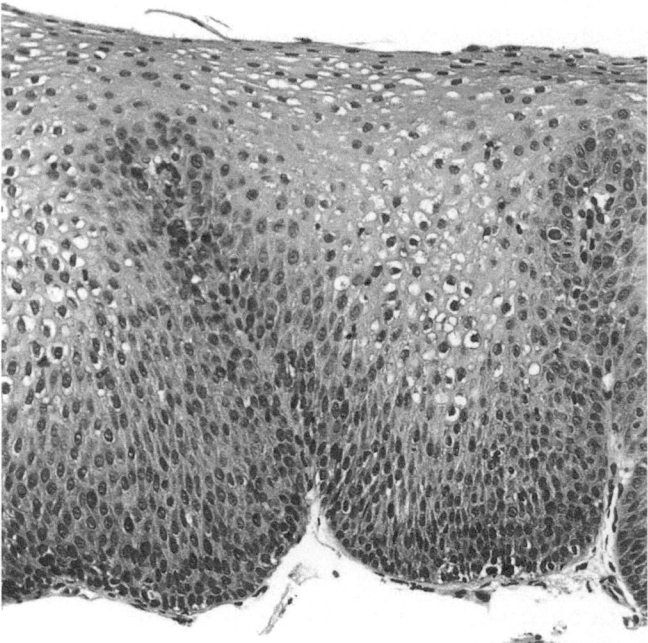

Figure 6-5. Squamous mucosal changes in reflux esophagitis include elongated lamina propria papillae, an increase in the basal cell layer, and scattered intraepithelial eosinophils.

- About 30% of patients with documented abnormal histology have no endoscopic lesion
- Endoscopic grading system (Los Angeles Classification) often used to document severity of esophageal damage
  - Uses four letter (A, B, C, and D) grades: A (the least change) through D (the most severe endoscopic changes)

Histopathology

- Characteristic histologic triad involving squamous mucosa (Figure 6-5)
  - Hyperplasia with elongated or lengthened lamina propria papillae (more than two thirds of thickness of epithelium)
  - Thickened basal layer (more than 15% of epithelial thickness)
  - Increased intraepithelial lymphocytes and eosinophils; neutrophils may also be present but occur only in severe reflux
- Erosive and ulcerated lesions show neutrophilic and eosinophilic exudate over a granulation tissue base
- Barrett esophagus with intestinal metaplasia (goblet cell metaplasia) may be present
- Inflammation of gastric cardia–type mucosa with or without intestinal metaplasia may also be present

Special Stains and Immunohistochemistry

- Combined Alcian blue and PAS staining with hematoxylin counterstain: serves four purposes
  - Defines the relatively PAS-negative, glycogen-free basal layer of the esophagus
  - Detects dark-blue intestinal mucus in goblet cells when intestinal metaplasia is present

- Identifies fungi, if present
- Good screening stain for signet cell adenocarcinoma
- Stains for *Helicobacter pylori* (Warthin-Starry, Diff-Quik, Giemsa, immunohistochemistry) may be helpful when differential includes chronic gastritis and should be done routinely in specimens obtained from the distal esophagus and gastroesophageal junction

Other Techniques for Diagnosis

- Noncontributory

Differential Diagnosis

INFECTIOUS ESOPHAGITIS

- May resemble reflux esophagitis endoscopically, but usually more focal
- Differentiated by the presence of characteristic organisms or cytopathic changes
- Most common organisms:
  - HSV
  - CMV
  - *Candida* species

HELICOBACTER PYLORI GASTRITIS OF CARDIA (CARDITIS) WITH OR WITHOUT INTESTINAL METAPLASIA

- Can be histologically indistinguishable from reflux-related inflammation of gastric cardia type mucosa; *H. pylori* infection typically causes more chronic and active inflammatory cells; *H. pylori* seen on hematoxylin and eosin (H&E) or special stain
- Most cases of chronic inflammation of gastric cardia–type mucosa at the gastroesophageal junction or in lower esophagus are examples of reflux

EOSINOPHILIC ESOPHAGITIS

- Typically in children or young men with an allergic history
- Characterized by numerous intraepithelial eosinophils (> 15 eosinophils/hpf) (Figure 6-6)

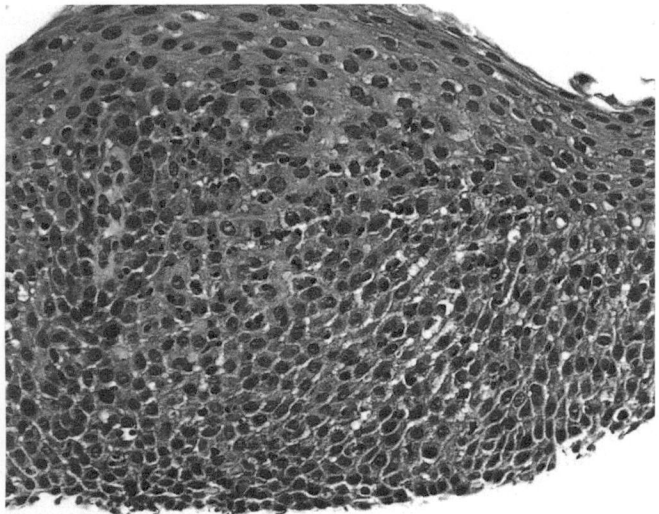

Figure 6-6. Eosinophilic esophagitis. Histologic section shows full-thickness squamous basal cells with numerous (> 15 per high-power field) intraepithelial eosinophils.

- Many cases cannot be reliably separated from reflux esophagitis without clinical history and response to therapy
- Patients with histologic criteria for eosinophilic esophagitis that respond to proton pump inhibitors (clinically and histologically) are now classified as PPI-responsive esophageal eosinophilia, a condition that may be different from reflux

PILL ESOPHAGITIS

- Typically associated with odynophagia (painful swallowing), lump in the throat sensation, and history of consuming oral medications with inadequate amounts of water
- Occurs more proximally in esophagus than do changes caused by reflux
- Nonspecific histology with ulcer

SQUAMOUS DYSPLASIA, SQUAMOUS CELL CARCINOMA

- Less likely than reflux-associated regenerative changes because incidence of esophageal squamous cell carcinoma is declining in the United States
- Dysplasia and carcinoma show
  - Less papillomatosis versus reflux related squamous changes
  - Overlapping, pleomorphic nuclei with high nuclear-to-cytoplasmic ratio
  - Atypical mitoses
  - Single-cell necrosis
  - Paradoxical maturation
  - Squamous pearl formation

PEARLS

- *GERD: classic histologic triad*
  - *Thickened basal layer*
  - *Elongated papillae*
  - *Intraepithelial inflammatory cells, including some eosinophils (generally < 5/hpf)*
- *Always evaluate for the presence of intestinal metaplasia when glandular mucosa is present; routine use of Alcian blue and PAS combination stain, with hematoxylin counterstain recommended*

SELECTED REFERENCES

Black DD, Haggitt RC, Orenstein SR, Whitington PF: Esophagitis in infants: morphometric histological diagnosis and correlation with measures of gastroesophageal reflux. Gastroenterology 98:1408-1414, 1990.

Der R, Tsao-Wei DD, Demeester T, et al: Carditis: a manifestation of gastroesophageal reflux disease. Am J Surg Pathol 25:245-252, 2001.

Haggitt RC: Histopathology of reflux-induced esophageal and supra esophageal injuries. Am J Med 108:109S-111S, 2000.

Katz PO, Gerson LB, Vela MF: Guidelines for the diagnosis and management of gastroesophageal reflux disease. Am J Gastroenterol 108:308-328, 2013.

BARRETT ESOPHAGUS

Clinical Features

- Defined by the American College of Gastroenterology as an endoscopic abnormality (red, velvety mucosa) in the esophagus proved by biopsy to contain intestinal metaplasia

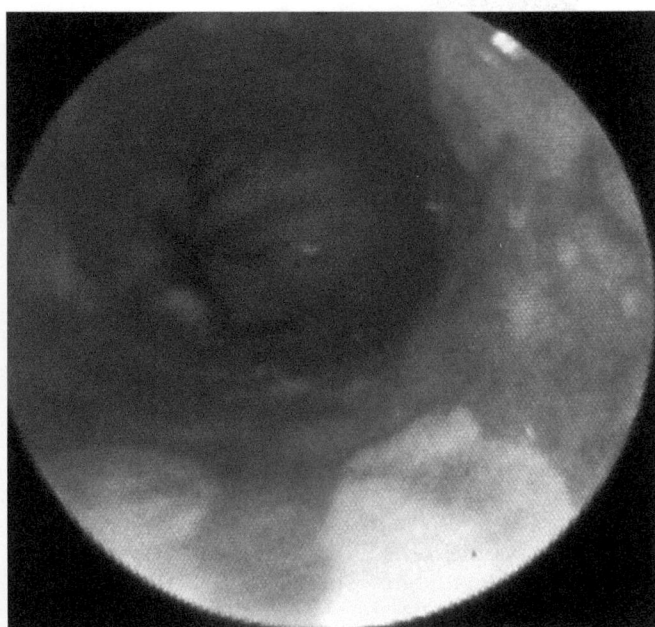

Figure 6-7. Endoscopic photograph of Barrett esophagus. Note the erythematous mucosa that resembles gastric mucosa, which contrasts to the gray-white glistening squamous esophageal mucosa (*foreground*).

- Occurs in up to 45% of patients with chronic gastroesophageal reflux
- Affected patients tend to be white men with reflux symptoms; often have hiatal hernia
- Disease occurs at two age peaks: younger than 15 years and older than 40 years
- Increased risk for adenocarcinoma

Gross and Endoscopic Pathology

- Seen on endoscopy as tongues or islands of flat, red, velvety mucosa or as a circumferential zone of red, velvety mucosa against a pale gray-white esophageal squamous mucosal background (Figure 6-7)

Histopathology

- Esophageal squamous epithelium is replaced by specialized columnar epithelium; columnar epithelium containing goblet cells usually interspersed between cells resembling gastric foveolar epithelium (Figure 6-8)
- To qualify, the goblet cells must have distinct globoid clear cytoplasm on hematoxylin and eosin stain (H&E) stain; verification of goblet cells by positive staining with Alcian blue stain (pH 2.5) is desirable and recommended
- Neither foveolar cells with Alcian blue-negative cytoplasmic vacuoles nor diffuse, "blush" positivity in the regenerative zone of foveolar cells qualifies as intestinal metaplasia
- Careful search must be made for dysplastic glandular epithelium
- Dysplastic glandular cells contain enlarged hyperchromatic, stratified nuclei involving luminal surface
- Dysplasia is categorized as low grade, high grade, or indefinite for dysplasia (see the section on dysplasia under "Barrett Esophagus")

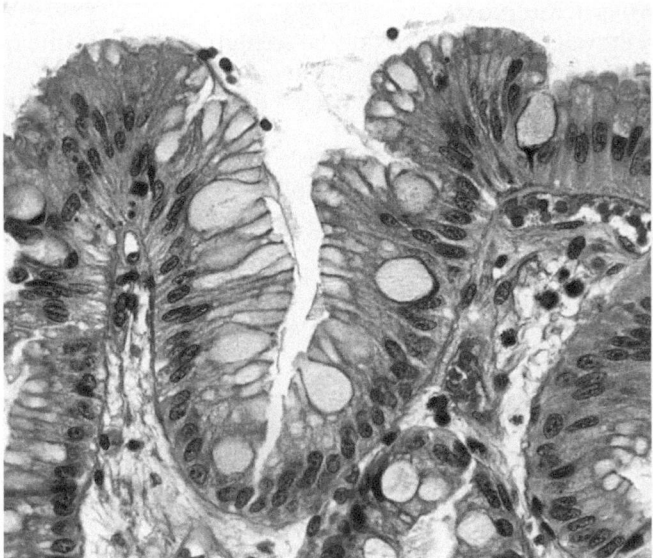

Figure 6-8. Specialized columnar epithelium (intestinal metaplasia) of Barrett esophagus composed of goblet cells interspersed between cells resembling gastric foveolar epithelium.

Special Stains and Immunohistochemistry

- Combined Alcian blue with hematoxylin counterstain and PAS: serves four purposes
  - Defines the PAS-negative, glycogen-free basal layer of the esophagus
  - Detects dark-blue, globoid goblet cells when intestinal metaplasia is present
  - Highlights fungal structures
  - Is a useful screening stain for signet cell adenocarcinoma
- Cytokeratin 7 and 20 profiles can help differentiate gastric cardia intestinal metaplasia from esophageal (Barrett) intestinal metaplasia but are rarely indicated clinically
  - The "Barrett pattern" shows diffuse (superficial and deep) cytokeratin 7 positivity and bandlike superficial cytokeratin 20 positivity; other patterns usually correlate with gastric-type intestinal metaplasia

Other Techniques for Diagnosis

- Use of p53 and Ki-67 staining can improve interobserver agreement on diagnosis of dysplasia
- DNA ploidy studies and use of other markers of cancer risk (e.g., racemase) are reported but are not often used clinically

Differential Diagnosis

CHRONIC GASTRITIS INVOLVING CARDIA-TYPE MUCOSA WITH INTESTINAL METAPLASIA

- Indistinguishable from Barrett esophagus unless seen by the endoscopist in the esophagus
- May be caused by *Helicobacter pylori* infection rather than reflux in a distinct minority of patients

ECTOPIC GASTRIC MUCOSA

- Small foci of gastric mucosa, usually in the cervical esophagus (so-called inlet patch) unassociated with gastroesophageal reflux

ADENOCARCINOMA

- Prevalence is estimated to be as high as 10% at time of diagnosis of Barrett esophagus
- Risk estimates vary widely (30- to 125-fold) in patients with Barrett esophagus
- May be difficult to distinguish intramucosal adenocarcinoma from high-grade dysplasia

PEARLS

- *Generally high-grade dysplasia in a background of Barrett esophagus prompts surgical or endoscopic intervention*

SELECTED REFERENCES

American Gastroenterological Association, Spechler SJ, Sharma P, et al: American Gastroenterological Association medical position statement on the management of Barrett's esophagus. Gastroenterology 140:1084-1091, 2011.

Antonioli DA, Wang HH: Morphology of Barrett's esophagus and Barrett's-associated dysplasia and adenocarcinoma. Gastroenterol Clin North Am 26:495-506, 1997.

Ormsby AH, Goldblum JR, Rice TW, et al: Cytokeratin subsets can reliably distinguish Barrett's esophagus from intestinal metaplasia of the stomach. Hum Pathol 30:288-294, 1999.

Wang KK, Sampliner RE: Updated guidelines 2008 for the diagnosis, surveillance and therapy of Barrett's esophagus 103:788-797, 2008.

DYSPLASTIC LESIONS ASSOCIATED WITH BARRETT ESOPHAGUS

Clinical Features

- Dysplasia is defined as a proliferation of neoplastic cells that are cytologically abnormal yet are still confined within their original basement membrane
- Periodic endoscopic surveillance of patients with Barrett esophagus increases survival (62% versus 20%) over patients without surveillance
- Studies indicate that dysplasia may progress to carcinoma, but estimates of exact pace vary widely (from less than 2 years to up to 10 years)
- Patients harboring low-grade dysplasia are usually treated with antireflux therapy and followed closely; endoscopic eradication is an option
- Patients with high-grade dysplasia confirmed by an expert will be advised to have an intervention such as endoscopic mucosal resection, radiofrequency ablation, photodynamic therapy, cryoablation, laser ablation or surgical excision depending on local expertise, patient age, comorbidities, and patient preference

Gross and Endoscopic Pathology

- Dysplasia usually cannot be grossly or endoscopically distinguished from surrounding Barrett esophagus; sometimes presents as a nodule or plaque

Histopathology

DYSPLASIA

- Consists of a continuous spectrum of architectural and cytologic abnormalities
- Divided into low-grade dysplasia, high-grade dysplasia, and indefinite for dysplasia
- Changes rarely resemble those of an adenoma

- Low-grade dysplasia
  - Slight increase in gland complexity, which consists of branching glands with irregular contours
  - Cytologic atypia consisting of enlarged, pleomorphic, stratified nuclei with surface involvement; abnormal nuclei are generally confined to the basal half of each cell
- High-grade dysplasia
  - Further increase in gland complexity characterized by lateral branching and often back-to-back glands
  - Progressive increase in cytologic atypia
    - Greater nuclear enlargement and pleomorphism
    - Stratified nuclei involving luminal surface haphazardly scattered with nuclei located in apical portion of many cells
    - Atypical cells often with prominent nucleoli and a high nuclear-to-cytoplasmic ratio, high mitotic rate with atypical mitotic figures, and progressive loss of goblet cells (Figure 6-9)
    - Similar cytologic changes to those seen in adenocarcinoma
  - Changes involve surface mucosa as well as crypts
  - Complexity and atypia may be so marked that intramucosal carcinoma (infiltration of carcinoma cells beyond basement membrane into the lamina propria or the muscularis mucosae alone, but not into submucosa) cannot be ruled out
- Indefinite for dysplasia

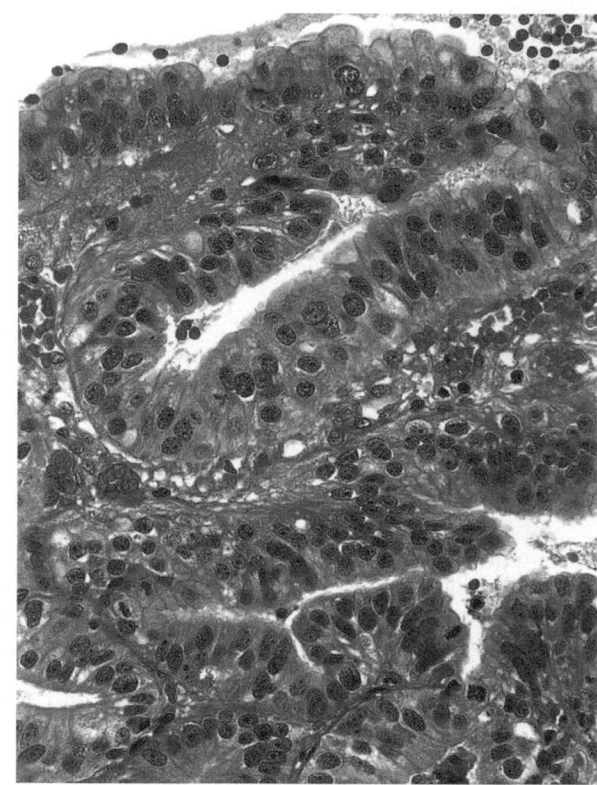

Figure 6-9. High-grade glandular dysplasia arising in Barrett esophagus. There is altered mucosal architecture. The cells demonstrate a high nuclear-to-cytoplasmic size ratio, irregular nuclear crowding, and nuclear stratification.

- Designates changes that have features of dysplasia and regenerative mucosa, usually in an inflamed background, making precise distinction impossible

Special Stains and Immunohistochemistry

- Use of p53, racemase, and Ki-67 staining may aid in difficult cases (e.g., indefinite versus low-grade dysplasia only)
- Several "markers" have been studied (DCC, *C-myc*, and others), but none is of current clinical value

Other Techniques for Diagnosis

- Flow cytometry
  - DNA aneuploidy and elevated S-phase fractions may correlate with progression to carcinoma; experimental only

Differential Diagnosis

REGENERATIVE ATYPIA

- Generally involves areas adjacent to erosions and ulcerations with active inflammation
- Glands may have villiform surface but show normal maturation at surface
- Cells characteristically have equally enlarged cytoplasm and nuclei
- Cytoplasm is typically eosinophilic rather than basophilic
- May be difficult to distinguish from dysplasia; p53 immunohistochemistry can be helpful

DRUG AND IRRADIATION EFFECT

- Covered in detail earlier
- Cytologic changes associated with colchicine toxicity and taxane effect deserve special mention
  - Usually associated with a marked increase in mitotic figures, many with "ring" morphology, which corresponds to metaphase arrest
  - These drugs also cause apoptosis, nuclear stratification, and loss of nuclear polarity that can mimic epithelial dysplasia

ADENOCARCINOMA

- Characterized by individual cell infiltration or desmoplastic reaction
- Intramucosal carcinoma may be difficult to differentiate reliably from high-grade dysplasia

PEARLS

- *Variability of individual nuclei is greater in dysplasia (regenerative atypia is composed of a more uniform population of glands and nuclei)*
- *Regenerative glands generally show mature cells (basal nuclei and abundant mucin) at mucosal surface*
- *Uncertain cases may be legitimately diagnosed as indefinite for dysplasia*
- *Villiform architecture is seen in both regenerative glands and dysplasia*

SELECTED REFERENCES

American Gastroenterological Association, Spechler SJ, Sharma P, et al: American Gastroenterological Association medical position statement on the management of Barrett's esophagus. Gastroenterology 140:1084-1091, 2011.

Daniels JA, Gibson MK, Xu L, et al: Gastrointestinal tract epithelial changes associated with taxanes: marker of drug toxicity versus effect. Am J Surg Pathol 32:473-477, 2008.

Flejou JF, Svrcek M: Barrett's oesophagus: a pathologist's view. Histopathology 50:3-14, 2007.

Iacobuzio-Donahue CA, Lee EL, Abraham SC, et al: Colchicine toxicity: distinct morphologic findings in gastrointestinal biopsies. Am J Surg Pathol 25:1067-1073, 2001.

Lorinc E, Jakobsson B, Landberg G, Veress B: Ki67 and p53 immunohistochemistry reduces interobserver variation in assessment of Barrett's oesophagus. Histopathology 46:642-648, 2005.

Ormsby AH, Petras RE, Henricks WH, et al: Observer variation in the diagnosis of superficial oesophageal adenocarcinoma. Gut 51:671-676, 2002.

Petras RE, Lapinski JE, Bohman KD, Katzin WE: Performance of p53 immunohistochemistry in the setting of glandular atypia versus low-grade dysplasia in a large cohort of patients with Barrett esophagus. Am J Gastroenterol 107:S17-S18, 2012.

Wang KK, Sampliner RE: Updated guidelines 2008 for the diagnosis, surveillance and therapy of Barrett's esophagus 103:788-797, 2008.

ADENOCARCINOMA ASSOCIATED WITH BARRETT ESOPHAGUS

Clinical Features

- Most esophageal adenocarcinomas are associated with Barrett esophagus (Figure 6-10)
- Exact increase in risk posed by Barrett esophagus is unknown; estimates range from 30- to 125-fold increase in risk versus general population
- Occurs in 800 per 100,000 Barrett patients per year
- Present in 10% of patients at initial diagnosis of Barrett esophagus
- Occurs with higher rate in white males
- Risk factors include hiatal hernia, stricture, and chronic reflux
- Most common symptom is dysphagia, but can be asymptomatic

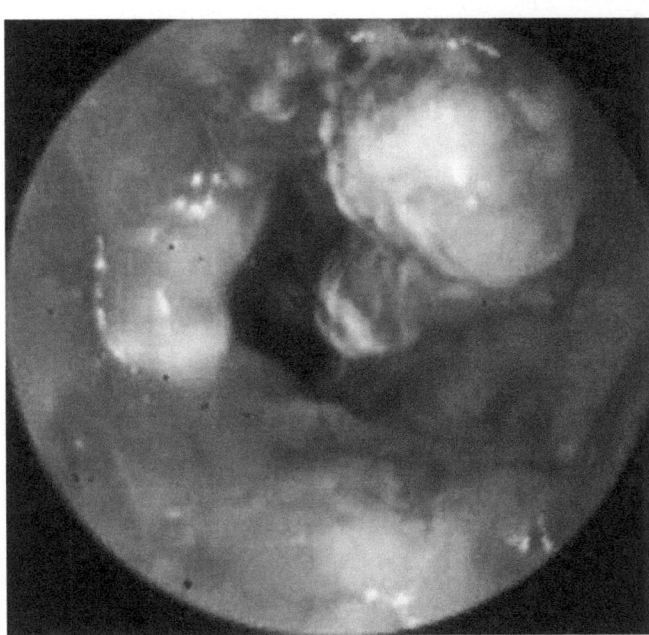

Figure 6-10. Endoscopic photograph of carcinoma complicating Barrett esophagus showing complex intraluminal mass with superficial exudate.

Gross and Endoscopic Pathology

- Tends to occur near gastroesophageal junction
- May form an exophytic mass or can be flat with an infiltrative architecture
- Only 50% are grossly visible endoscopically

Histopathology

- Resembles gastric adenocarcinoma, with both intestinal and diffuse (signet ring cell) types
- Barrett esophagus with dysplasia of varying degree is present in adjacent mucosa

Special Stains and Immunohistochemistry

- Mucin stain positive in adenocarcinoma cells may be helpful in identifying infiltrating carcinoma cells

Other Techniques for Diagnosis

- HER2 analysis by immunohistochemistry and fluorescent in situ hybridization usually done to select patients for trastuzumab therapy

Differential Diagnosis

BARRETT ESOPHAGUS–ASSOCIATED DYSPLASIA
- Characterized by glandular and cytologic atypia without infiltration pattern

GASTRIC CARDIA ADENOCARCINOMA
- May be identical to Barrett esophagus–associated adenocarcinoma
- Staining for CK7 and CK20 can help distinguish Barrett esophagus-related adenocarcinoma (CK7 positive, CK20 negative) from gastric adenocarcinoma

PEARLS

- *A search for goblet cells in glandular epithelium adjacent to any gastroesophageal junction adenocarcinoma helps to identify preexisting Barrett esophagus*
- *Documentation of a squamous proximal mucosal margin is desirable in cases of surgically resected Barrett esophagus–associated adenocarcinoma*
- *Overall prognosis is dismal for invasive adenocarcinoma (15% 5-year survival); prognosis is better for small, well-differentiated adenocarcinoma with fewer than four positive nodes*
- *Follow College of American Pathologists (CAP) cancer protocols in resection specimens*

SELECTED REFERENCES

Bang YJ, Van Cutsem E, Feyereislova A, et al: Trastuzumab in combination with chemotherapy versus chemotherapy alone for treatment of HER2-positive advanced gastric or gastro-oesophageal junction cancer (ToGA): a phase 3, open-label, randomised controlled trial. Lancet 376:687-697, 2010.

Bollschweiler E, Wolfgarten E, Gutschow C, et al: Demographic variations and the rising incidence of esophageal adenocarcinoma in white males. Cancer 92:549-555, 2001.

Drewitz DJ, Sampliner RE, Garewell HS: The incidence of adenocarcinoma in Barrett's esophagus: a prospective study of 170 patients followed 4.8 years. Am J Gastroenterol 92:212-215, 1997.

Ormsby AH, Goldblum JR, Rice TW, et al: The utility of cytokeratin subsets in distinguishing Barrett's-related oesophageal adenocarcinoma from gastric adenocarcinoma. Histopathology 38:307-311, 2001.

BENIGN ESOPHAGEAL LESIONS

Clinical Features

GLYCOGENIC ACANTHOSIS
- Asymptomatic

INFLAMMATORY FIBROID POLYP
- Usually occurs in the stomach and small intestine but may arise in the esophagus
- May produce mild obstructive symptoms

FIBROVASCULAR POLYP
- Rare, slow-growing polyp
- Mild obstructive symptoms may occur
- May rarely prolapse into oral cavity

Gross and Endoscopic Pathology

GLYCOGENIC ACANTHOSIS
- Raised, white plaques
- Usually less than 0.3 cm in diameter

INFLAMMATORY FIBROID POLYP
- Raised, pedunculated, polypoid mass, often with surface ulceration

FIBROVASCULAR POLYP (Figure 6-11)
- Usually attached in upper esophagus
- Polypoid mass; can be extremely large (e.g., 25 cm)
- Smooth surface that may be ulcerated

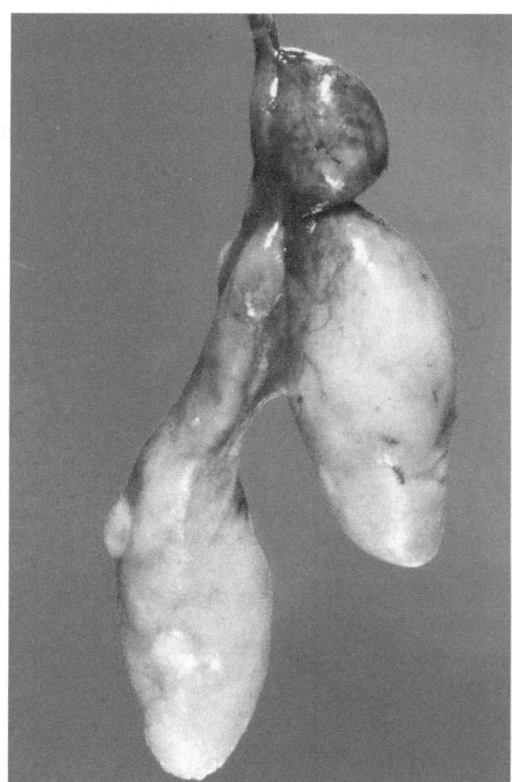

Figure 6-11. Resection specimen of giant fibrovascular polyp of the esophagus. The lobulated intraluminal mass is covered by intact squamous mucosa.

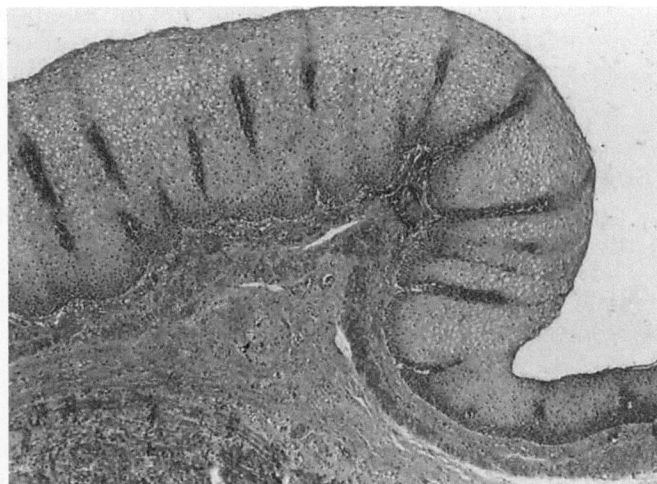

Figure 6-12. Glycogenic acanthosis. Note the marked thickening of the squamous mucosa composed of squamous cells with increased intracellular glycogen.

Histopathology

GLYCOGENIC ACANTHOSIS
- Discrete focus of hyperplastic squamous epithelium containing abundant glycogen (squamous cells with prominent clear cytoplasm) (Figure 6-12)

INFLAMMATORY FIBROID POLYP
- Polypoid mass covered by benign squamous mucosa that may be focally ulcerated
- Stromal component varies in cellularity, edema, and inflammation that is often rich in eosinophils and plasma cells
- Stromal component typically has prominent vascularity with perivascular onion skinning composed of fibroblasts, myofibroblasts, and macrophages (Figure 6-13)
- Occasionally stroma has a pseudosarcomatous appearance

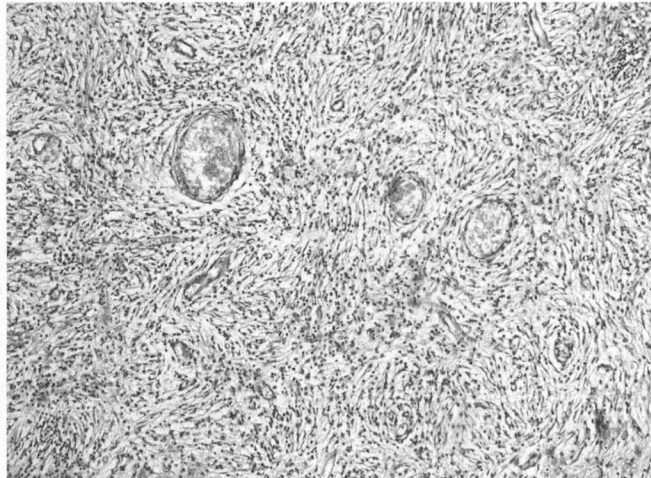

Figure 6-13. Inflammatory fibroid polyp of the esophagus demonstrates edema and inflammatory cells, including plasma cells and eosinophils interspersed between elongate spindle cells and dilated blood vessels.

FIBROVASCULAR POLYPS
- Dense or myxoid fibrovascular core sometimes with adipose tissue covered by benign squamous epithelium

Special Stains and Immunohistochemistry

INFLAMMATORY FIBROID POLYP
- Stromal cells are positive for vimentin and negative for cytokeratin
- CD34 immunostain highlights blood vessels and may stain stromal cells; CD117 is negative

GLYCOGENIC ACANTHOSIS
- PAS-positive epithelium

Other Techniques for Diagnosis
- Inflammatory fibroid polyp often contains somatic mutations of PDGFRA similar to that seen in some gastrointestinal stromal tumors

Differential Diagnosis

Inflammatory fibroid polyp should be differentiated from sarcomatoid carcinoma, sarcoma, and stromal tumors
- Sarcomatoid carcinoma
  - Biphasic histology with both carcinomatous and spindle cell components
  - Typically greater cellularity with increased nuclear pleomorphism
  - Usually positive for cytokeratin, but staining may be focal
- Sarcoma
  - Typically a highly cellular malignant spindle cell neoplasm resembling leiomyosarcoma, fibrosarcoma, or malignant fibrous histiocytoma
- Gastrointestinal stromal tumor
  - Rare in the esophagus
  - Spindle cell or epithelioid neoplasm; CD117 positive, DOG-1 positive

Glycogenic acanthosis should be differentiated from squamous papilloma, condyloma, and fungal esophagitis
- Squamous papilloma
  - Characterized by a greater degree of squamous hyperplasia, papillary structure with a fibrovascular core, and less prominent cytoplasmic glycogenization
- Condyloma
  - Characteristic viral cytopathic changes (koilocytosis), squamous atypia, and hyperkeratosis
- Fungal esophagitis
  - Recognized by detection of fungal organisms; may require use of special stains

PEARLS

- *Careful attention to cytologic characteristics and to the makeup of the inflammatory component and background is important to avoid misdiagnosis of sarcoma and sarcomatous carcinoma*

SELECTED REFERENCES

Avezzano EA, Fleischer DE, Merida MA, et al: Giant fibrovascular polyps of the esophagus. Am J Gastroenterol 85:299-302, 1990.
Nash S: Benign lesions of the gastrointestinal tract that may be misdiagnosed as malignant tumors. Semin Diagn Pathol 7:102-114, 1990.

Liu TC, Lin MT, Montgomery EA, Singhi AD: Inflammatory fibroid polyps of the gastrointestinal tract: spectrum of clinical, morphologic, and immunohistochemistry features. Am J Surg Pathol 37:586-592, 2013.

GRANULAR CELL TUMOR

Clinical Features

- Usually a solitary nodule in the lower esophagus; can be multiple (10% of cases)
- Typically slow growing and generally does not produce symptoms (incidental finding)

Gross and Endoscopic Pathology

- Can be seen throughout the gastrointestinal tract; the esophagus is the preferred site, followed by the large intestine
- Generally small, yellow-white, subepithelial mass
- Typically less than 2 cm; tumors larger than 4 cm may indicate malignancy

Histopathology

- Similar to granular tumors of other sites
- Aggregates of rounded and spindle-shaped cells that resemble smooth muscle with small, round to oval nuclei and granular eosinophilic cytoplasm (Figure 6-14)
- May appear to be arising from nerve or muscle
- Pseudoepitheliomatous hyperplasia of the overlying squamous epithelium is common and can be misinterpreted as squamous carcinoma
  - Malignant granular cell tumor

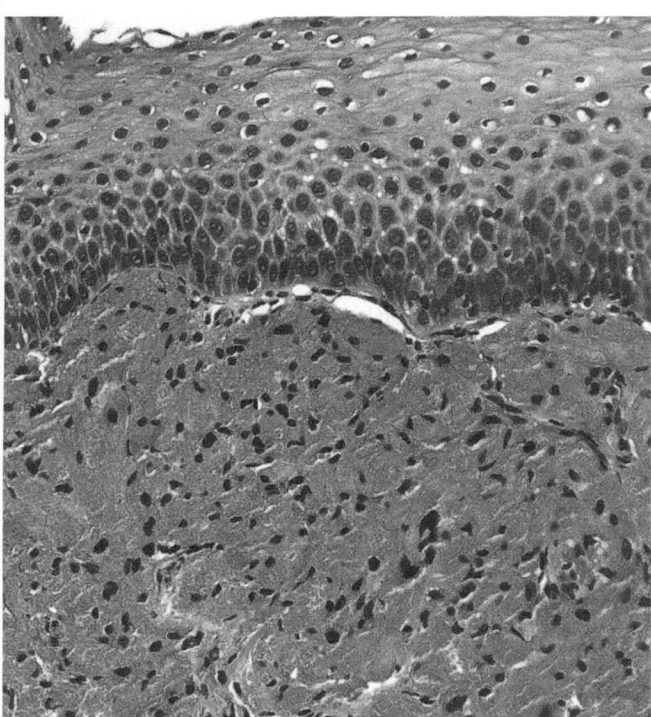

Figure 6-14. Granular cell tumor of the esophagus. Squamous mucosa overlies the uniform population of cells with variably shaped small nuclei, abundant eosinophilic granular cytoplasm, and poorly defined cell borders.

- May be suspected by the presence of increased cellularity, spindle cell areas, nuclear atypia, necrosis, and increased mitotic activity (> 2 per 10 high magnification fields); however, the only definite criterion is metastasis

Special Stains and Immunohistochemistry

- Cytoplasmic positivity for PAS and immunostain positive for S-100 protein

Other Techniques for Diagnosis

- Noncontributory

Differential Diagnosis

SQUAMOUS CELL CARCINOMA

- Especially on small biopsies, granular cell tumors have many times been misdiagnosed as squamous cell carcinoma because of the pseudoepitheliomatous hyperplasia that accompanies the tumor

PEARLS

- *Biopsy and observation may be employed; typically slow growing and cured by local surgical excision; malignant granular cell tumors with metastases have been reported*

SELECTED REFERENCES

Brady PG, Nord HJ, Connar RG: Granular cell tumor of the esophagus: natural history, diagnosis and therapy. Dig Dis Sci 33:1329-1333, 1988.

Goldblum JR, Rice TW, Zuccaro G, et al: Granular cell tumor of the esophagus: a clinical and pathologic study of 13 cases. Ann Thorac Surg 62:860-865, 1996.

SQUAMOUS PAPILLOMA AND CARCINOMA

Clinical Features

- Most symptomatic esophageal tumors are malignant

SQUAMOUS PAPILLOMA

- More common in males (male-to-female ratio is 2.5:1)
- Occurs throughout life
- Two types of squamous papilloma
  - Human papillomavirus (HPV) associated
    - About 30% of esophageal papillomas
    - May coexist with laryngeal papillomatosis; associated with HPV-6 and HPV-11 infections
  - Not HPV associated
    - May be related to reflux esophagitis, eosinophilic esophagitis, or trauma
- Patients typically present with dysphagia and heartburn

SQUAMOUS CELL CARCINOMA

- About 1% of all cancers in the United States
- Risk factors include the following:
  - Male gender (male-to-female ratio is 5:1)
  - Black race
  - Tobacco and ethanol use
  - Low socioeconomic status
  - Diet low in trace elements, minerals, and vitamins or high in hot liquids

- Premalignant conditions include chronic esophagitis and squamous dysplasia or carcinoma in situ and are typically asymptomatic
- Dysphagia is the most common symptom associated with invasive carcinoma; cancer is often advanced at presentation
- Complications of invasive carcinoma include the following:
  - Invasion into adjacent structures (major blood vessel, trachea, laryngeal nerve), causing hemorrhage, aspiration, and hiccups
  - More than half of all patients have positive lymph nodes at diagnosis; many are unresectable
- Most common metastatic sites are liver and lung
- Carcinomas that are considered variants of squamous cell carcinoma include the following:
  - Undifferentiated carcinoma
  - Verrucous carcinoma
  - Spindle cell (sarcomatoid) carcinoma
- Other rare esophageal carcinomas
  - Adenosquamous carcinoma (mucoepidermoid carcinoma)
    - May arise from submucosal glands
    - Can be seen in Barrett esophagus
  - Adenoid cystic carcinoma
    - May arise from submucosal glands

Gross and Endoscopic Pathology

SQUAMOUS PAPILLOMA
- Exophytic, partially pedunculated, soft, pink-tan mass
- About 95% occur in mid- or lower esophagus
- Typically smaller than 1 cm
- Can see endoscopic evidence of coexisting eosinophilic esophagitis (e.g., corrugations)

SQUAMOUS CELL DYSPLASIA AND CARCINOMA
- Dysplasia
  - Often multifocal
  - Dysplastic lesions vary widely in size and may be extensive
  - Most are at least focally erosive
  - Most involve mid- to lower esophagus
- Invasive carcinoma
  - Most (90%) occur in mid- and lower esophagus
  - Most tumors are large, discrete masses projecting into the lumen with variable intramural extension
  - Ulcerating tumors are less common and are typically erosive with infiltration and expansion of esophageal wall (Figure 6-15)
  - Least common is an infiltrating tumor with similar intramural invasion but little or no ulceration
  - Prognosis is generally poor
  - Polypoid tumors have better survival than ulcerative and infiltrative tumors
  - Early lesions (T1) may be multifocal and combined with dysplasia of varying degrees and carcinoma in situ over a wide area

Histopathology

SQUAMOUS PAPILLOMA
- Exophytic and endophytic proliferations of benign squamous epithelium

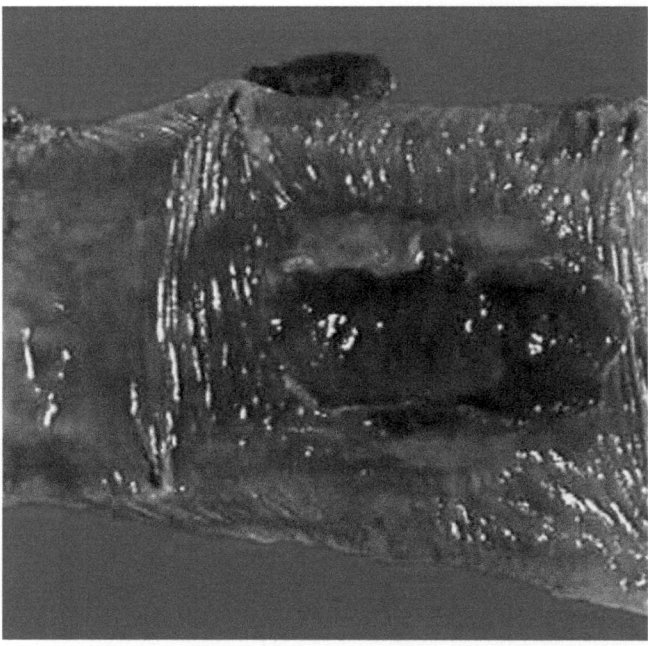

Figure 6-15. Resection specimen of esophageal squamous carcinoma. Note the ulcerated mass lesion.

- Papillary proliferation with fibrovascular core; koilocytosis, hyperkeratosis, and hypergranulosis may occur
- Patterns are often mixed
- Intraepithelial eosinophils sometimes seen

SQUAMOUS CELL DYSPLASIA AND CARCINOMA
- Dysplasia and carcinoma in situ
  - Variable combination of nuclear anaplasia (hyperchromasia, pleomorphism) and disordered maturation
  - As in the cervix, dysplastic lesions are defined as those showing some evidence of maturation and are graded in three or two tiers: mild, moderate, and severe; or low grade and high grade
  - Full-thickness atypia without superficial maturation is termed *carcinoma in situ*
  - Dysplastic cells may extend into metaplastic submucosal glands
- Invasive squamous carcinoma (Figure 6-16)
  - Low-grade carcinomas are characterized by obvious recapitulation of benign counterpart and are composed of syncytial nests of cells with abundant pink cytoplasm, intercellular bridges, and keratin pearls
  - High-grade carcinomas may show only solid nests of cells with pleomorphic nuclei and vague pink cytoplasm
  - Necrosis is often seen in high-grade carcinomas
  - Infiltration is often marked by paradoxical maturation of invading cells with squamous pearl formation and stromal desmoplasia
  - Effects of preoperative radiation include the following:
    - Marked atypia of stromal, endothelial, and squamous metaplasia in the submucosal glandular cells with atypia
    - Postradiation changes include foci of calcified keratinized cells and foreign-body giant cell reaction

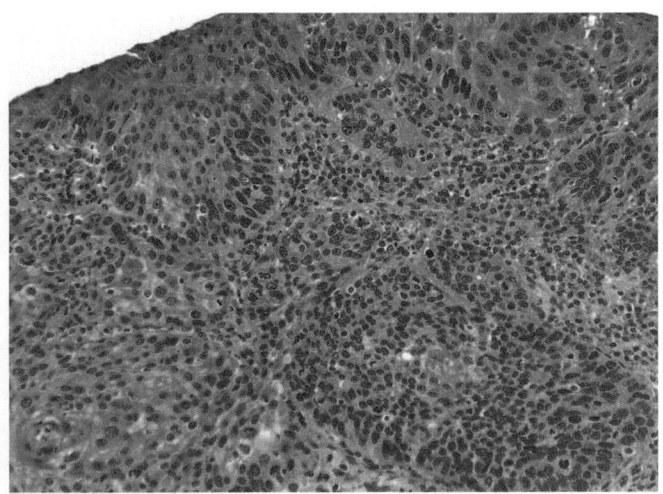

Figure 6-16. Squamous carcinoma of the esophagus characterized by an infiltrative growth pattern and marked cellular atypia.

Special Stains and Immunohistochemistry

SQUAMOUS PAPILLOMA
- Noncontributory

SQUAMOUS CELL CARCINOMA
- Cytokeratin immunostain is positive in virtually all squamous cell carcinomas; exceptions include a minority of high-grade carcinomas; positive in less than 50% of sarcomatoid carcinomas (sarcomatoid areas may react focally with cytokeratin and generally are reactive with vimentin antibodies; antibodies to desmin and muscle-specific actin may be positive)

Other Techniques for Diagnosis

SQUAMOUS PAPILLOMA
- In situ hybridization and PCR to detect and classify HPV

SQUAMOUS CELL CARCINOMA
- Proliferative index with Ki-67 and ploidy status may correlate with prognosis; usually not routinely performed

Differential Diagnosis

ULCERATIVE ESOPHAGITIS
- Usually recognizable endoscopically and typically covers a wide area of distal esophagus
- Biopsies demonstrate regenerative squamous epithelium characterized by basal cell hyperplasia and orderly superficial maturation without significant nuclear pleomorphism
- Keratinization is usually absent

INFECTIOUS ESOPHAGITIS
- Similar histology to ulcerative esophagitis with detection of responsible organism

BARRETT ESOPHAGUS
- Many show inflamed, regenerating squamous epithelium adjacent to diagnostic columnar glands with intestinal metaplasia (goblet cells)

- *Extensive, diffusely ulcerated, flat lesions by endoscopy are most likely benign esophagitis with regenerative atypia*
- *Most squamous cell carcinomas form an exophytic mass with ulceration*
- *Keratinization or keratin pearls, particularly those containing hyperchromatic and atypical cells, are highly suggestive of infiltrating squamous carcinoma*
- *Five-year survival is dictated largely by depth of invasion and lymph node status*
  - *Use CAP cancer protocols to ensure proper staging and grading*
- *Tylosis is an autosomal dominant condition consisting of hyperkeratosis of the palms and soles and oral leukoplakia and is associated with squamous cell carcinoma of the esophagus*

SELECTED REFERENCES

Blot W: Esophageal cancer trends and risk factors. Semin Oncol 21:403-410, 1994.

Iezzoni JC, Mills SE: Sarcomatoid carcinomas (carcinosarcomas) of the gastrointestinal tract: a review. Semin Diagn Pathol 10:176-187, 1993.

Montgomery E, Field JK, Boffetta P, et al: Squamous cell carcinoma of the oesophagus. In Bosman FT, Carneiro F, Hruban RH, Theise ND (eds): World Health Organization Classification of Tumours of the Digestive System. Lyon, IARC Press, 2010, pp 18-24.

Odze R, Antonioli D, Shocket D, et al: Esophageal squamous papillomas: a clinicopathologic study of 38 lesions and analysis for human papillomavirus by the polymerase chain reaction. Am J Surg Pathol 17:803-812, 1993.

Torres CM, Wang HH, Turner JR, et al: Pathologic prognostic factors in esophageal squamous cell carcinoma: a follow-up study of 74 patients with or without preoperative chemoradiation therapy. Mod Pathol 12:961-968, 1999.

SQUAMOUS CELL CARCINOMA VARIANTS

Clinical Features

UNDIFFERENTIATED CARCINOMA
- About 20% of esophageal malignancies
- Highly aggressive

VERRUCOUS CARCINOMA
- Considered a well-differentiated variant of squamous cell carcinoma
- Slow growing but often recurs; low metastatic risk
- Some cases reported after acid ingestion or with achalasia

SARCOMATOID CARCINOMA
- Represents a carcinoma with mesenchymal differentiation
- Rare (< 2% of esophageal malignancies)
- Affects mainly older men (mean age, 62 years)
- Male-to-female ratio is 9:1
- Patients often present with dysphagia and weight loss
- Occasionally arises against a background of Barrett esophagus

Gross and Endoscopic Pathology

UNDIFFERENTIATED CARCINOMA
- Typically large tumor with no distinctive gross features

VERRUCOUS CARCINOMA
- Distinctive warty, exophytic mass

SARCOMATOID CARCINOMA

- Lobulated, large mass (1.5 to 15 cm)
- May be polypoid or pedunculated and usually has a broad attachment to the underlying mucosa
- Minority are flat with an ulcerated surface
- Cut surface is gray and fleshy

Histopathology

UNDIFFERENTIATED CARCINOMA

- As the name implies, the tumor is composed of large, anaplastic cells growing in a nonorganoid pattern
- Tumor cells have pleomorphic, vesicular nuclei with prominent nucleoli and often have prominent eosinophilic cytoplasm (may impart a squamoid appearance)

VERRUCOUS CARCINOMA

- Papillary fronds composed of well-differentiated squamous cells with little cytologic atypia
- Parakeratosis and hyperkeratosis
- Characteristic feature is the "pushing" deep tumor margin (rather than irregular areas of invasion)

SARCOMATOID CARCINOMA

- Although a recognizable invasive or in situ squamous carcinoma is usually present, most of the mass is composed of sarcomatous areas showing variable cellularity
- Biphasic histology has both carcinomatous and spindle cell components
- Spindle cell component is generally hypercellular and malignant-appearing; may resemble malignant fibrous histiocytoma (MFH) or fibrosarcoma
- Chondroid, osseous, and rhabdomyoblastic differentiation may be present
- Epithelial component may be sharply demarcated or admixed and may show squamous, glandular, or undifferentiated morphology
- Metastases may contain any or all components

Special Stains and Immunohistochemistry

UNDIFFERENTIATED CARCINOMA

- Cytokeratin typically positive
- Vimentin negative

VERRUCOUS CARCINOMA

- Noncontributory

SARCOMATOID CARCINOMA

- Carcinomatous elements are generally positive for cytokeratin and may show vimentin positivity
- Sarcomatous elements are strongly positive for vimentin and may show patchy positivity for cytokeratin

Other Techniques for Diagnosis

- Noncontributory

Differential Diagnosis

UNDIFFERENTIATED CARCINOMA VERSUS LYMPHOMA, MELANOMA, AND SARCOMA

- Presents a diagnostic challenge requiring a thorough immunohistochemical workup to demonstrate epithelial differentiation and to rule out anaplastic lymphoma, melanoma, and sarcoma

VERRUCOUS CARCINOMA VERSUS PAPILLOMA AND CONDYLOMA

- Generally have similar histologic features; however, they are best differentiated clinically and with a biopsy specimen large enough to demonstrate the broad pushing deep margin characteristic of verrucous carcinoma

SARCOMATOID CARCINOMA VERSUS SARCOMA, MELANOMA, AND INFLAMMATORY MYOFIBROBLASTIC TUMOR

- Diffuse, strong positivity for smooth muscle actin (SMA) supports diagnosis of leiomyosarcoma (although some leiomyosarcomas are cytokeratin positive, and some sarcomatoid carcinomas are SMA positive)
- Positive staining for cytokeratin, negative S-100 protein, HMB-45, and melan-A immunostaining essentially rule out melanoma
- Tumor composed of stromal cells with a low mitotic rate, no abnormal mitoses, and no significant cytologic anaplasia is typically a benign tumor, and in combination with inflammation, an inflammatory myofibroblastic tumor should be considered

PEARLS

- *Undifferentiated carcinoma is a highly aggressive neoplasm with a poor prognosis*
- *Verrucous carcinoma is a low-grade neoplasm that frequently recurs locally and only rarely metastasizes*
- *Use CAP cancer protocols for proper staging and grading*

SELECTED REFERENCES

Gabbert HE, Nakamura Y, Shimoda T, et al: Squamous cell carcinoma of the oesophagus. In Hamilton SR, Aaltonen LA (ed): World Health Organization Classification of Tumours. Pathology and Genetics: Tumours of the Digestive System. Lyon, IARC Press, 2000, pp 11-19.

Iezzoni JC, Mills SE: Sarcomatoid carcinomas (carcinosarcomas) of the gastrointestinal tract: a review. Semin Diagn Pathol 10:176-187, 1993.

Lewin KJ, Appelman HD: Tumors of the esophagus and stomach. In Atlas of Tumor Pathology, 3rd series, vol 18. Washington, DC, Armed Forces Institute of Pathology, 1996, pp 43-90.

Montgomery E, Field JK, Boffetta P, et al: Squamous cell carcinoma of the oesophagus. In Bosman FT, Carneiro F, Hruban RH, Theise ND (eds): World Health Organization Classification of Tumours of the Digestive System. Lyon, IARC Press, 2010, pp 18-24.

RARE ESOPHAGEAL NEOPLASMS

Clinical Features

- Most esophageal malignancies are squamous cell carcinomas (and variants) and adenocarcinomas; uncommon primary esophageal malignancies include high-grade neuroendocrine carcinoma and melanoma

HIGH-GRADE NEUROENDOCRINE CARCINOMA

- Rare esophageal neoplasm; most are small cell types but rare large cell types as well
- Few cases have been studied; incidence varies depending on country reporting (< 1%, up to 7%)

- Symptoms include dysphagia, weight loss, and chest pain
- Typically presents in older male patients (65 years)
- Tumors reported to secrete adrenocorticotropic hormone (ACTH), calcitonin, vasoactive intestinal polyprotein (VIP), gastrin, and antidiuretic hormone (ADH)
- Associated conditions include Cushing syndrome, hypercalcemia, watery diarrhea, hypokalemia, and achlorhydria

MALIGNANT MELANOMA

- Rare in esophagus (< 1% of esophageal malignancies)
- A primary tumor is less common than metastases from cutaneous melanoma
- Slightly more common in males
- Wide age range, 7 to 80 years (mean, 60 years)
- Symptoms include dysphagia and weight loss

Gross and Endoscopic Pathology

HIGH-GRADE NEUROENDOCRINE CARCINOMA

- May be exophytic, flat, or ulcerative
- May occur in any part of the esophagus
- May erode into tracheobronchial tree, making it difficult to determine the primary site

MALIGNANT MELANOMA

- Often polypoid with a black or gray cut surface
- May arise in any part of the esophagus
- Average size is 7 cm

Histopathology

HIGH-GRADE NEUROENDOCRINE CARCINOMA

- Most are similar to small cell carcinomas elsewhere
  - Composed of small to medium-sized, round to oval cells arranged in sheets, nests, rosettes, or ribbons
  - Tumor cells have densely hyperchromatic nuclei with scant cytoplasm
  - Crush artifact is characteristic (smeared chromatin)
  - High mitotic rate
  - Tumor cell necrosis is typical
  - May occasionally coexist with squamous carcinoma in situ, invasive squamous carcinoma, adenocarcinoma, or carcinoid tumors

MALIGNANT MELANOMA

- Similar to melanomas elsewhere
  - May have epithelioid, spindle, or anaplastic cell morphology
  - Unusual variants include small cell, signet ring cell, and balloon cell types
  - Adjacent squamous mucosa may demonstrate in situ lentiginous melanoma growth pattern, melanosis (increased pigmentation), melanocytosis (proliferation of benign melanocytes), or junctional activity

Special Stains and Immunohistochemistry

HIGH-GRADE NEUROENDOCRINE CARCINOMA

- Variable positivity with chromogranin and synaptophysin antibodies
- Immunostain for thyroid transcription factor-1 (TTF-1) may help identify carcinoma metastatic from lung

MALIGNANT MELANOMA

- Immunoreactivity with S-100 protein, HMB-45, and melan-A supports the diagnosis

Other Techniques for Diagnosis

- Noncontributory

Differential Diagnosis

HIGH-GRADE NEUROENDOCRINE CARCINOMA AND MALIGNANT MELANOMA (METASTATIC VERSUS PRIMARY)

- Both tumors are more common outside the esophagus; therefore, the possibility of a metastasis to the esophagus must be considered
- Other than a careful history, differentiation from metastatic neuroendocrine carcinoma may be impossible; however, this may be irrelevant clinically because high-grade neuroendocrine carcinoma from any site usually presents as a widely disseminated process
- TTF-1 immunohistochemistry may help identify a pulmonary primary
- Diagnostic criteria for primary esophageal melanoma
  - Melanocytosis (proliferation of benign melanocytes) in adjacent squamous mucosa
  - Premalignant melanocytic lesions and melanoma in situ in adjacent epithelium is generally proof of a primary neoplasm

LYMPHOMA

- May be distinguished from high-grade neuroendocrine carcinoma with leukocyte common antigen (LCA) and other lymphoid marker immunostains and by recognizing the discohesive character of the lymphoid cells

PEARLS

- *Always consider metastases when diagnosing an uncommon esophageal malignancy*
- *If the melanoma has overgrown the premalignant changes, it may be impossible to determine whether the neoplasm is a primary tumor or a metastasis*
- *High-grade neuroendocrine carcinoma and primary esophageal melanoma have an extremely poor prognosis*
  - *High-grade neuroendocrine carcinoma: average of 3 months' median survival*
  - *Melanoma: worse prognosis than cutaneous counterpart*

SELECTED REFERENCES

Caldwell CB, Bains MS, Burt M: Unusual malignant neoplasms of the esophagus: oat cell carcinoma, melanoma, and sarcoma. J Thorac Cardiovasc Surg 101:100-107, 1991.

Huang Q, Wu H, Nie L, et al: Primary high-grade neuroendocrine carcinoma of the esophagus: a clinicopathologic and immunohistochemical study of 42 resection cases. Am J Surg Pathol 37:467-483, 2013.

Li B, Lei W, Shao K, et al: Characteristics and prognosis of primary malignant melanoma of the esophagus. Melanoma Res 17:239-242, 2007.

STOMACH

CONGENITAL AND ACQUIRED GASTRIC ABNORMALITIES

Clinical Features

GASTRIC DUPLICATION

- More common in females
- Clinically apparent in first year of life; rarely seen in adults

- One third of patients have other anomalies
- Typically presents as an intrathoracic or intra-abdominal mass
- Complications include ulceration, hemorrhage, rupture, fistula, and rarely malignancy
- Typically fails to be visualized on barium swallow

CONGENITAL PYLORIC STENOSIS
- Incidence is about 3 to 4 per 100 live births
- Typically male neonates and more common in first-born child (three to four times more common in males)
- Presentation
  - Neonatal period
  - Projectile vomiting (nonbilious, postprandial)
  - Abdominal pain
- Abdominal examination classically reveals "pyloric olive"

Heterotopia
- Pancreatic
  - Normal pancreatic tissue entrapped during morphogenesis
  - Represents accessory pancreatic bud

Gross and Endoscopic Pathology
GASTRIC DUPLICATION
- Typically a cystic mass of variable size (10 cm)
- Generally intramural and on the greater curvature of the stomach
- Usually does not communicate with the gastric lumen; if it does, it can be referred to as a *congenital diverticulum*

CONGENITAL PYLORIC STENOSIS
- Progressive hypertrophy and hyperplasia of pyloric sphincter musculature
- Thickness of the pyloric sphincter may be more than 1 cm (two times normal), which results in narrowing of the pyloric channel

Heterotopia
- Pancreatic
  - Presents as a small (< 4 cm), dome-shaped, umbilicated, submucosal mass
  - Central, nipple-like duct
  - Cut surface contains typical lobulated pancreatic parenchyma

Histopathology
GASTRIC DUPLICATION
- May contain normal gastric mucosa; occasionally see small intestinal, respiratory, or pancreas tissue
- Organized muscular wall

Heterotopia
- Pancreatic
  - Most cases contain normal lobulated pancreatic tissue with ducts, acini, and islet cells and variable superimposed inflammation; other changes include the following:
    - Cystic duct dilation
    - Pancreatitis
    - Ductal dysplasia (very rare)
  - Tumors (islet cell, adenocarcinoma)
  - Cases without pancreatic acinar elements or islet cells are classified as adenomyoma

Special Stains and Immunohistochemistry
- Noncontributory

Modern Techniques for Diagnosis
- Pyloric stenosis: may be associated with chromosome 9q duplications

PANCREATIC HETEROTOPIA VERSUS ADENOCARCINOMA
- Heterotopic pancreas and adenomyoma may occasionally produce benign, dilated ducts containing exfoliated cell clusters mimicking carcinoma; however, a benign process is recognized by its orderly lobular arrangement, lack of epithelial anaplasia, and absence of desmoplasia

PEARLS
- *Pancreatic heterotopia: carefully note the normal relationship of ducts, smooth muscle, and lobulated acini to avoid misinterpretation of heterotopia as carcinoma*

SELECTED REFERENCES
Batcup G, Spitz L: A histopathological study of gastric mucosal biopsies in infantile hypertrophic pyloric stenosis. J Clin Pathol 32:625-628, 1979.
Owen DA: The stomach. In Mills SE (ed): Sternberg's Diagnostic Surgical Pathology. Philadelphia, Lippincott Williams & Wilkins, 2010, pp 1279-1312.

XANTHELASMA

Clinical Features
- No association with hyperlipidemia
- Strong association with duodenal reflux, gastritis, or previous gastric surgery

Gross and Endoscopic Pathology
- Single or multiple, flat, discrete, tan-yellow plaques on the gastric mucosa (Figure 6-17)
- Usually 0.1 to 0.2 cm (almost always < 0.5 cm)

Histopathology
- Characterized by sheets of foamy histiocytes (lipid filled) within superficial lamina propria (Figure 6-18)
- Cells have a central, small, benign nucleus and finely vacuolated cytoplasm

Special Stains and Immunohistochemistry
- CD68 positive
- PAS and mucin negative
- Cytokeratin negative

Other Techniques for Diagnosis
- Noncontributory

Differential Diagnosis
SIGNET RING CELL CARCINOMA VERSUS XANTHELASMA
- Signet ring cell carcinoma may contain seemingly bland cells with clear cytoplasm but is also composed of cells with atypical nuclei

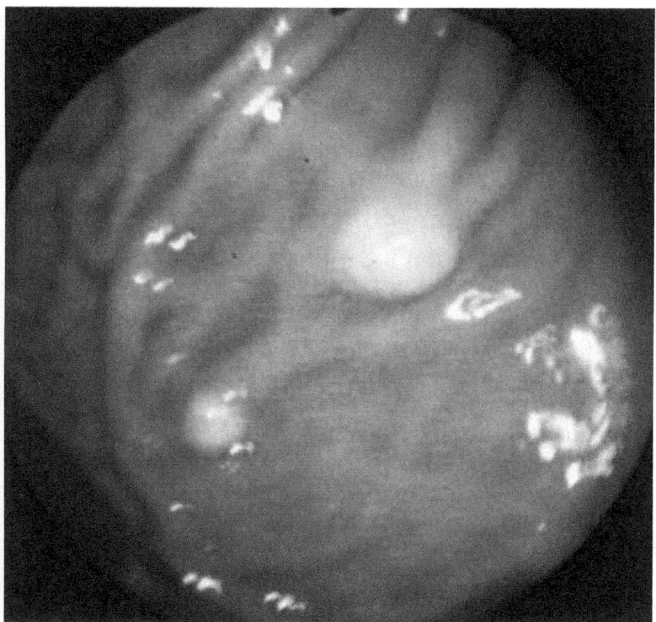

Figure 6-17. Endoscopic view of gastric xanthelasma appearing as two cream-colored to yellow papules.

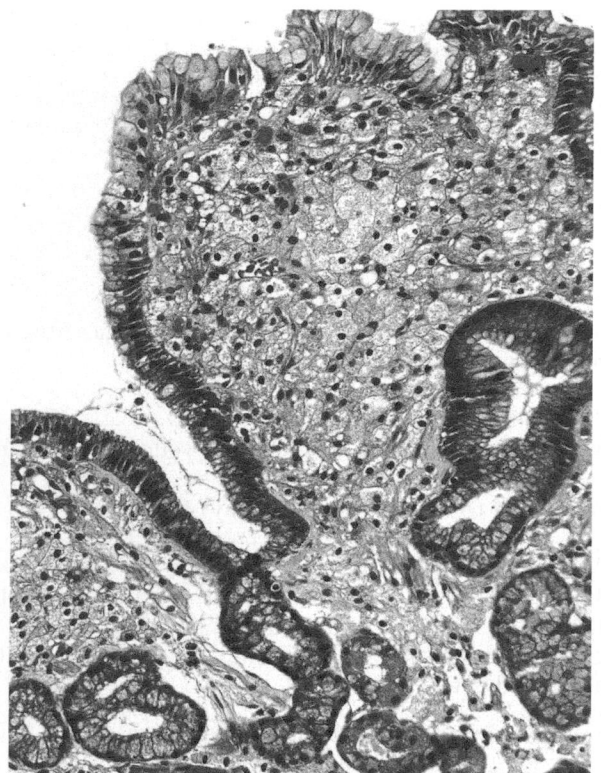

Figure 6-18. Gastric xanthelasma showing aggregates of foamy histiocytes in the lamina propria.

- Mucin stains and cytokeratin immunostains are positive in signet ring cell adenocarcinoma

PEARLS

- *Common incidental finding in autopsy studies and occasionally seen in endoscopic biopsy specimens*

SELECTED REFERENCES

Gencosmanoglu R, Sen-Oran E, Kurtkaya-Yapicier O, Tozun N: Xanthelasmas of the upper gastrointestinal tract. J Gastroenterol 39:215-219, 2004.

Kaiserling E, Heinle H, Itabe H, et al: Lipid islands in human gastric mucosa: morphological and immunohistochemical findings. Gastroenterology 110:369-374, 1996.

ACUTE EROSIVE GASTRITIS

Clinical Features

- Variable symptoms; may be asymptomatic or cause epigastric pain, nausea, vomiting, mild gastrointestinal hemorrhage, or massive hematemesis
- May occasionally cause fatal hematemesis, particularly in alcoholics
- Occurs in significant percentage of patients taking anti-inflammatory medication
- Frequently associated with use of nonsteroidal anti-inflammatory drugs (NSAIDs), particularly aspirin (typically more than eight aspirin tablets/day)
- Also associated with alcohol, heavy smoking, chemotherapy, stress (trauma, burns), and nasogastric intubation

Gross and Endoscopic Pathology

- Varies from mild mucosal hyperemia to mucosal erosion, ulcer, and hemorrhage (acute erosive gastritis)

Histopathology

- Mild: edematous mucosa with scattered neutrophils among superficial epithelial cells or within glands above-basement membrane ("active" gastritis)
- Moderate: mucosal erosion characterized by loss of epithelium and superficial exudate containing hemorrhage, fibrin, and neutrophils (Figure 6-19)

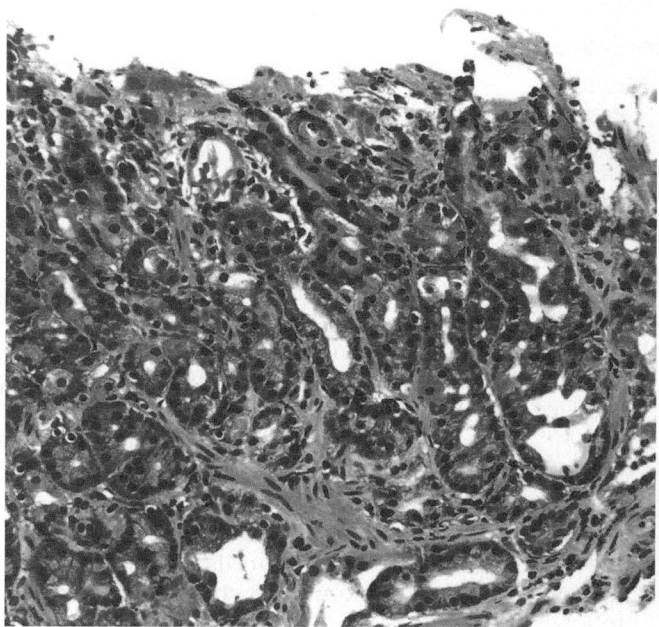

Figure 6-19. Acute erosive gastritis. Note the absence of gastric foveolar epithelium along with the surface eosinophilic change with fibrin, debris, and capillary ectasia.

- Severe: confluent erosions with similar morphology sometimes with ulcer
- All grades are usually accompanied by reactive gastropathy changes (see "Reactive Gastropathy")

Special Stains and Immunohistochemistry

- Stains for *Helicobacter pylori* should be done routinely

Other Techniques for Diagnosis

- Noncontributory

Differential Diagnosis

CHRONIC GASTRITIS

- Characterized by a dense chronic inflammatory infiltrate consisting of both lymphocytes and plasma cells
- Usually lacks mucosal erosions, hemorrhage, and ulceration

PEARLS

- *In fragmented biopsy specimens, look for subtle mix of fibrin, blood, and neutrophils within superficial epithelium*
- *Stain for* Helicobacter pylori *should be performed (Giemsa, Diff-Quik, immunohistochemistry, or silver stain)*

SELECTED REFERENCES

Dixon MF, Genta RM, Yardley JH, et al: Classification and grading of gastritis: the updated Sydney system. Am J Surg Pathol 20:1161-1181, 1996.

Haber MM, Lopez I: Gastric histologic findings in patients with nonsteroidal anti-inflammatory drug-associated gastric ulcer. Mod Pathol 12:592-596, 1999.

Parfitt JR, Driman DK: Pathological effects of drugs on the gastrointestinal tract: a review. Hum Pathol 38:527-536, 2007.

REACTIVE GASTROPATHY

Clinical Features

- Incompletely understood adaptive response to more chronic exposure to many of the factors that are associated with erosive acute gastritis
- Often seen with chronic exposures to ethanol, NSAIDs, steroids, other medicines, stress, and reflux of duodenal contents

Gross and Endoscopic Pathology

- Usually seen as diffuse antral erythema with linear erosions (Figure 6-20)
- Focal mucosal erosion and ulcers can be seen

Histopathology (Figure 6-21)

- Regenerative epithelial changes, including foveolar hyperplasia (elongated, sometimes tortuous gastric pits with serrated luminal border), cytologic atypia (enlarged, mildly hyperchromatic nuclei with prominent nucleoli), and decreased foveolar mucin
- Lamina propria may be congested and have thin strands of connective tissue or smooth muscle
- Inflammation is typically sparse, but scattered chronic inflammatory cells are not uncommon
- Can be associated with mucosal capillary ectasia

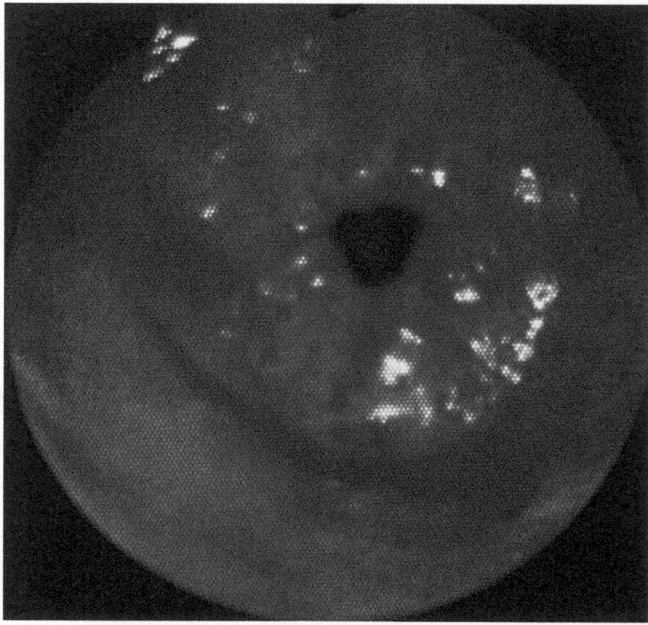

Figure 6-20. Endoscopic photograph of reactive gastropathy with diffusely erythematous gastric antrum.

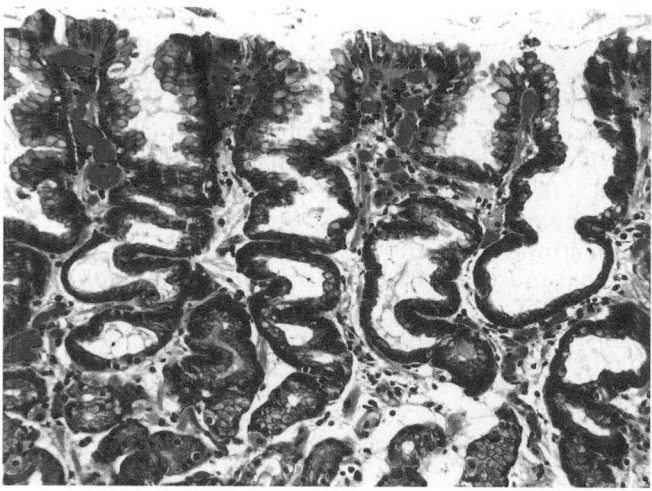

Figure 6-21. Reactive gastropathy with lamina propria edema, fibromuscular proliferation within the superficial mucosa, capillary ectasia, and marked tortuous gastric foveolar hyperplasia. The foveolar epithelium demonstrates reduced intracellular mucus.

Special Stains and Immunohistochemistry

- Noncontributory

Other Techniques for Diagnosis

- Noncontributory

Differential Diagnosis

CHRONIC GASTRITIS AND *HELICOBACTER PYLORI* GASTRITIS

- Diffuse lymphoplasmacytic infiltrate separating gastric pits sometimes containing neutrophils is highly specific for *H. pylori* infection (Figure 6-22)

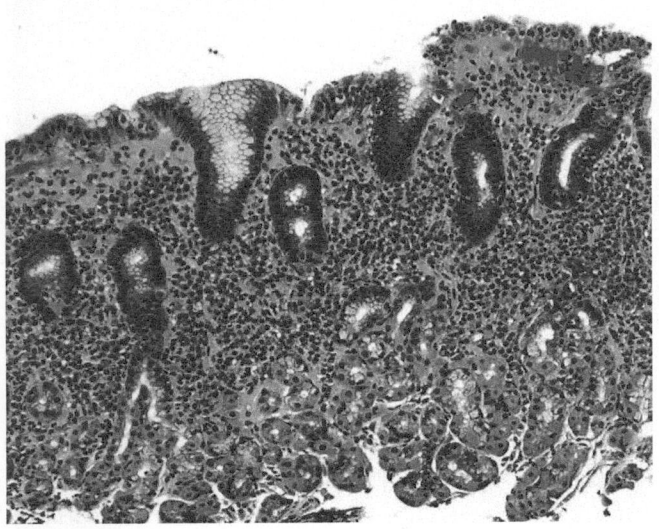

Figure 6-22. Chronic superficial gastritis associated with *Helicobacter pylori* infection.

- Lymphoid aggregates with germinal centers are common
- If numerous, *H. pylori* organisms may be seen on routine stains; organisms are best highlighted with special stains (Giemsa, Diff-Quik, immunohistochemistry or silver stains)

Gastric Antral Vascular Ectasia ("Watermelon Stomach")

- Endoscopy shows nearly parallel erythematous stripes traversing the gastric antrum that resemble the stripes on a watermelon
- Accentuation of reactive gastropathy is seen in patients with atrophic gastritis
- Dilated mucosal capillaries containing fibrin thrombi are present

PEARLS

- *Conceptually, reactive gastropathy represents a mucosal response to injury and is extremely common in the antrum*
- *Sometimes referred to as* chemical gastritis *or* chemical gastropathy

Selected References

Laine L: Nonsteroidal anti-inflammatory drug gastropathy. [Review]. Gastroenterol Endosc Clin North Am 6:489-504, 1996.

Parfitt JR, Driman DK: Pathological effects of drugs on the gastrointestinal tract: a review. Hum Pathol 38:527-536, 2007.

Suit P, Petras R, Bauer T, Petrini J: Gastric antral vascular ectasia: a histologic and morphometric study of "the watermelon stomach." Am J Surg Pathol 11:750-757, 1987.

HELICOBACTER PYLORI–ASSOCIATED GASTRITIS (CHRONIC SUPERFICIAL GASTRITIS AND CHRONIC ANTRAL GASTRITIS)

Clinical Features

- Generally asymptomatic; can have symptoms related to peptic ulcer
- Relationship to nonulcer dyspepsia is controversial
- Affects all populations worldwide; affects nearly 100% of the population in developing countries
- Diffuse antral gastritis commonly affects whites in the United States
- Multifocal atrophic gastritis more common in blacks, Asians, Hispanics, and Scandinavians
- Affects 10% of children and up to half of the adults in the United States
- Affects lower socioeconomic and institutionalized groups at higher rates in all geographic areas
- *H. pylori* is clearly established as the cause of diffuse antral gastritis and is strongly associated with duodenal and gastric ulcers; predisposes certain patients to extranodal marginal zone B-cell lymphoma of mucosa-associated lymphoid tissue (MALT) type or gastric adenocarcinoma
- Most patients with *H. pylori* have chronic antral gastritis or chronic superficial gastritis but are generally asymptomatic

Gross and Endoscopic Pathology

- Classic *H. pylori*–associated chronic gastritis primarily involves the antrum and causes diffuse antral gastritis (DAG)
- Multifocal atrophic gastritis (MAG) typically affects the antral-body junction
- Active lesions may have a reddened, boggy mucosa with thickened rugae, and may mimic an infiltrative disease; chronic lesions may produce a thinned, flat mucosa
- Several studies report no characteristic endoscopic or gross finding; most appear unremarkable at endoscopy
- Correlation between endoscopic impression and histologic findings of gastritis is poor

Histopathology

Diffuse Antral Gastritis

- DAG is characterized by a diffuse lymphoplasmacytic infiltrate that appears to widen the intercryptal and interglandular area and is often accompanied by a neutrophilic component that permeates the epithelium; this chronic active gastritis pattern is associated with *H. pylori* organisms in more than 90% of cases
- Lymphoid aggregates with germinal centers are common with *H. pylori* infection
- May be associated with intestinal metaplasia
- Strong association with duodenal and pyloric ulcers
- *H. pylori* organisms may be seen on H&E staining in many cases; identification is enhanced with special stains
- Gastric body may show chronic superficial gastritis with inflammation limited to the foveolar compartment

Multifocal Atrophic Gastritis

- Thought to occur as sequela of *H. pylori* infection
- Minimal, focal chronic superficial, and deep gastritis with islands of pseudopyloric and intestinal metaplasia
- Active inflammation (neutrophilic) is minimal
- Lymphoid follicles with germinal centers may persist
- Prevalence of *H. pylori* organisms in the lesion is lower
- Association with high gastric ulcers and adenocarcinoma (risk parallels degree of intestinal metaplasia)

- Intestinal metaplasia may be either of the following:
  - Complete (type I): recapitulates true small bowel with goblet cells separated by enterocyte-type absorptive cells
  - Incomplete (type II): "hybrid" mucosa containing goblet cells separated by gastric foveolar cells
- Other changes include glandular atrophy, pseudopyloric metaplasia, regenerative epithelial changes, and, rarely, glandular dysplasia

Special Stains and Immunohistochemistry

- Giemsa, Diff-Quik, immunostain, and silver stains (e.g., Warthin-Starry): all visualize *H. pylori* along the luminal surface of gastric foveolar epithelium; sometimes organisms can be detected in the gastric glands (Figure 6-23)
- Combined Alcian blue and PAS stain with a hematoxylin counterstain best separates intestinal metaplasia (Alcian blue positive) from foveolar gastric cells with prominent vacuoles (PAS positive); this stain is also useful as a cancer screening test and to detect fungi

Other Techniques for Diagnosis

- *Helicobacter pylori* antigen can be detected in stool
- Breath test and *Campylobacter*-like organism (CLO) test exploit urease production by *H. pylori* and can be useful to diagnose or follow up patients

Differential Diagnosis

AUTOIMMUNE GASTRITIS (DIFFUSE CORPORAL ATROPHIC GASTRITIS)

- Affects body and fundus glands including parietal cells, producing atrophy and pyloric metaplasia and areas of intestinal metaplasia
- Hypergastrinemia and autoantibodies to parietal cells or intrinsic factor are present
- Enterochromaffin-like cell hyperplasia and dysplasia and carcinoid tumors may develop as a consequence of hypergastrinemia

ATROPHIC AUTOIMMUNE PANGASTRITIS

- Inflammation and atrophy of body and antrum
- Decreased neuroendocrine cells
- Apoptosis and lymphocytic gastritis sometimes present
- Hypergastrinemia, antibodies to parietal cells, and intrinsic factor not present
- Can be associated with other autoimmune disorders
- May require treatment with prednisone with or without azathioprine

ACUTE EROSIVE GASTRITIS AND REACTIVE GASTROPATHY

- Superficial erosion, hemorrhage, and neutrophilic infiltrate are accentuated over the chronic inflammation of the *H. pylori* gastritis
- Clinical history often detects inciting agent (ethanol, medication, radiation)

HELICOBACTER HEILMANNII GASTRITIS

- Can cause gastritis; is associated with carcinoma and MALT-type lymphoma
- Organism is larger (7 μm) than *H. pylori* and tightly spiraled, resembling a corkscrew (Figure 6-24)
- Treated similarly to *H. pylori* infection

PEARLS

- *In general, a diffuse lymphoplasmacytic infiltrate separating glands containing neutrophils is highly suggestive for* H. pylori *infection*
- H. pylori *is a gram-negative spiral rod about 3.5 μm in size with a flagellum*
- *Diagnosis may be based on breath test and CLO test; however, the gold standard is histologic identification either by H&E alone or by use of special stains (e.g., silver stains or immunohistochemistry) to detect the organism*
- H. pylori–*like inflammation without identifiable organisms can sometimes be explained on the basis of prior antibiotic exposure or migration of* H. pylori *organisms in the setting of proton pump inhibitors; remember to look for organisms in the deep glands*

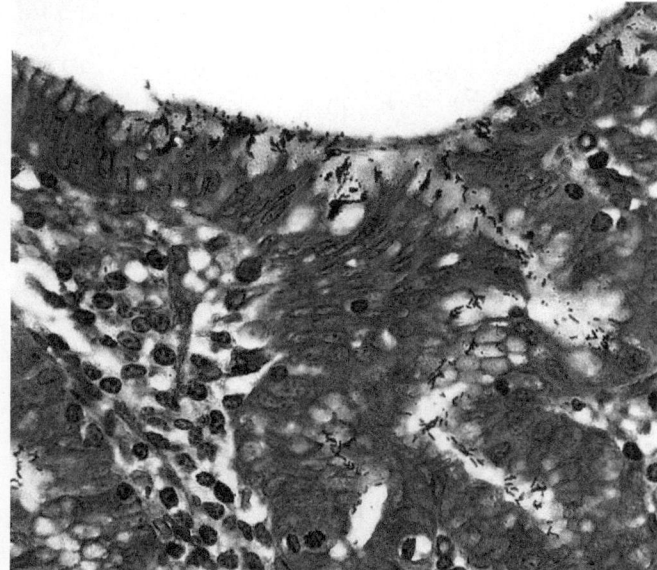

Figure 6-23. *Helicobacter pylori* on Warthin-Starry stain.

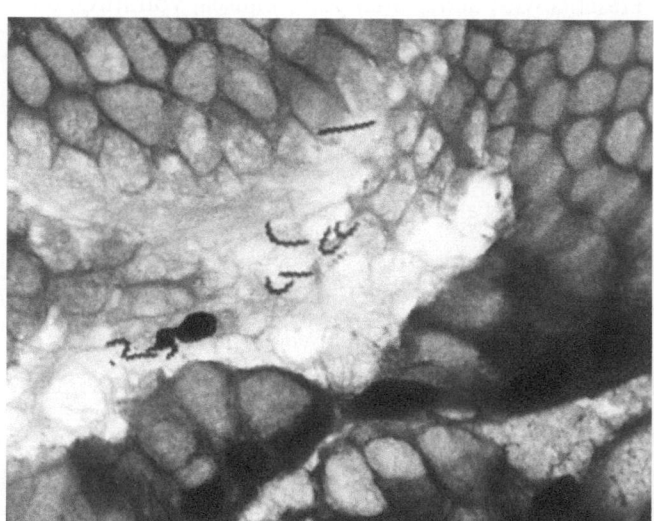

Figure 6-24. *Helicobacter heilmannii* on Giemsa stain. These organisms are larger than *Helicobacter pylori* and are tightly spiraled.

SELECTED REFERENCES

Dixon MF, Genta RM, Yardley J, et al: Classification and grading of gastritis: the updated Sydney system. Am J Surg Pathol 20:1161-1181, 1996.

Fallone CA, Chiba N, Buchan A, et al: Two decades of *Helicobacter pylori*: a review of the fourth western *Helicobacter* congress. Can J Gastroenterol 16:559-563, 2002.

Jevremovic D, Torbenson M, Murray JA, et al: Atrophic autoimmune pangastritis: a distinctive form of antral and fundic gastritis associated with systemic autoimmune disease. Am J Surg Pathol 30:1412-1419, 2006.

SPECIAL TYPES OF GASTRITIS

Lymphocytic Gastritis

- Surface epithelial lymphocytosis (> 25 lymphocytes per 100 gastric foveolar cells) on a background of superficial and deep chronic gastritis
- Associations include past or present *Helicobacter pylori* infection, celiac sprue, lymphocytic colitis, Ménétrier disease-like protein-losing gastropathy, and varioliform (nodular, "octopus sucker") gastritis

Collagenous Gastritis

- Increased (> 15 μm) subepithelial collagen plate, sometimes associated with lymphocytic gastritis
- In children and young adults, may present with anemia and gastric nodules
- In adults, collagenous gastritis can be associated with collagenous colitis and collagenous sprue

Granulomatous Gastritis

- Can be seen with infection (e.g., tuberculosis), Crohn disease, and sarcoidosis, and as a foreign-body giant cell reaction (e.g., so-called cereal granuloma, mucin granuloma)
- In some patients, granulomatous gastritis is considered idiopathic

Eosinophilic Gastritis

- Usually seen in children and adolescents
- Presents with abdominal pain, nausea, vomiting, diarrhea, anemia, and protein loss
- Occasionally linked to food allergy
- Diagnosis requires collections of eosinophils not associated with other inflammatory cells that cause mucosal architectural change or crypt injury; infiltration of muscularis mucosae or deeper layers of the bowel by eosinophils is also considered diagnostic

SELECTED REFERENCES

Haot J, Jouret A, Willette M, et al: Lymphocytic gastritis: perspective study of its interrelationship to varioliform gastritis. Gut 31:283-285, 1990.

Lagorce-Pages C, Fabiani B, Bouvier R: Collagenous gastritis: a report of six cases. Am J Surg Pathol 25:1174-1179, 2001.

Shapiro JL, Goldblum JR, Petras RE: A clinicopathologic study of 42 patients with granulomatous gastritis: is there really "idiopathic" granulomatous gastritis? Am J Surg Pathol 20:462-470, 1996.

Singhal AV, Sepulveda AR: *Helicobacter heilmannii* gastritis: a case study with review of literature. Am J Surg Pathol 29:1537-1539, 2005.

Suerbaum S, Michetti P: *Helicobacter pylori* infection. N Eng J Med 347:1175-1186, 2002.

PEPTIC ULCER DISEASE

Clinical Features

- Affects 4 million people in the United States; 350,000 new cases/year
- Lifetime risk: 10% of men and 4% of women
- Typically occurs in middle-aged or older adults
- Gastric *Helicobacter pylori* is present in 100% of patients with duodenal ulcers and in 80% of patients with gastric ulcers
- Only 10% of patients with *H. pylori* infection develop peptic ulcers
- Symptoms
  - Most patients have epigastric pain
  - Hemorrhage, anemia, or perforation occurs in a minority of patients
  - Pain is worse at night and several hours postprandially; classically relieved by food or antacids
  - Without treatment, ulcers often require years to heal
  - Malignant transformation is rare
  - Complications include bleeding and perforation; bleeding may be massive

Gross and Endoscopic Pathology

- Most occur near pyloric ring (4:1 duodenal)
- Generally smaller than 2 cm; 10% are larger than 4 cm
- Classically discrete, single ulcer with flat margins and a clean base (Figure 6-25)
- No gross or endoscopic feature can reliably distinguish benign from malignant ulcers

Histopathology

- Four levels can be observed in a well-developed ulcer
  - Overlying layer of neutrophils and debris
  - Layer of fibrin and necrotic material

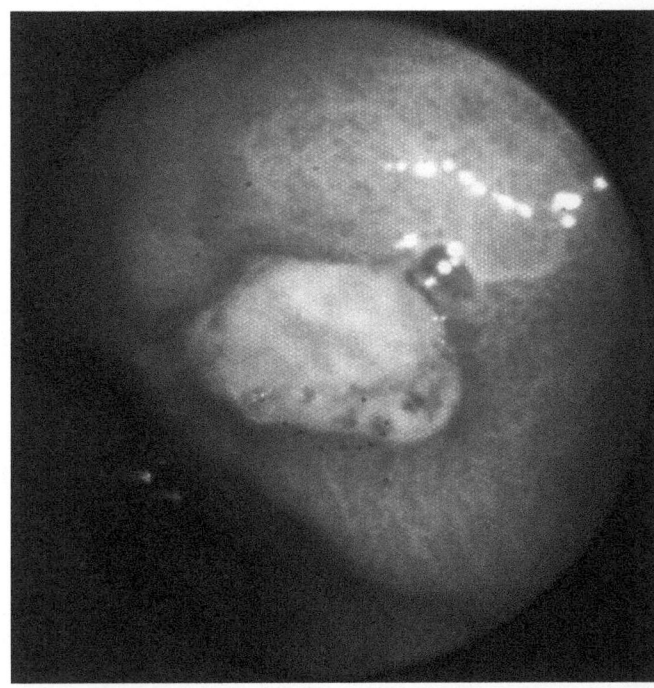

Figure 6-25. Endoscopic view of peptic ulcer of the stomach showing sharply demarcated margins and a clean base.

- Superficial zone of active granulation tissue
- Fibrous scar that by definition interrupts the muscularis mucosae
- Chronic gastritis is present in most patients (unlike with stress ulcers or acute erosive gastritis and reactive gastropathy)

Special Stains and Immunohistochemistry
- Noncontributory

Other Techniques for Diagnosis
- Noncontributory

Differential Diagnosis

GASTRIC CARCINOMA WITH ULCER
- Classically has raised, irregular margins and a necrotic base, but in many cases it is impossible to distinguish based solely on gross and endoscopic appearance
- Histologic features are confirmatory

ACUTE EROSIVE GASTRITIS AND REACTIVE GASTROPATHY
- Similar histology to the ulcer; however, surrounding gastric tissue does not show chronic gastritis and usually demonstrates reactive gastropathy

PEARLS
- *Always consider carcinoma when evaluating biopsies or resections with a clinical diagnosis of peptic ulcer by carefully examining ulcer margins and base for malignant cells; an Alcian blue/PAS combination stain with a hematoxylin counterstain is helpful by showing an abnormal mucin pattern in malignant cells or by highlighting signet ring cells*

SELECTED REFERENCES
Dekigai H, Murakami M, Kita T: Mechanism of *H. pylori*-associated gastric mucosal injury. Dig Dis Sci 40:1332-1339, 1995.
Hersey SJ, Sachs G: Gastric acid secretion. Physiol Rev 75:155-189, 1995.
Makola D, Peura DA, Crowe SE: *Helicobacter pylori* infection and related gastrointestinal diseases. J Clin Gastroenterol 41:548-558, 2007.
Soll AH: Pathogenesis of peptic ulcer and implications for therapy. N Engl J Med 322:909-916, 1990.

HYPERTROPHIC GASTROPATHY

Clinical Features
- Expansion of gastric mucosa results in large rugae
- Either the superficial or the deep gastric epithelial zones may be involved
  - Superficial zone: top half of the mucosa that contains the surface foveolar cells and the "pits" (the upper portion of the tubular epithelium with the mucus neck region)
  - Deep zone: lower portion of the mucosa that contains the glands composed of the differentiated functional cells (parietal, zymogenic, and endocrine)
- Greater than 1- to 1.5-mm-thick mucosa is hypertrophic, which is usually due to epithelial hyperplasia
- Specific syndromes are defined by clinical features (gastrin level and presence of ulcers or protein loss) and gastric architecture (which component is hyperplastic)
- Many gastropathies are described, but two are well characterized: Ménétrier disease and Zollinger-Ellison syndrome
  - Both conditions may mimic an infiltrating carcinoma on radiologic or endoscopic examination
  - High risk for duodenal and jejunal ulcers owing to excessive gastrin secretion and increased acid production in Zollinger-Ellison syndrome

MÉNÉTRIER DISEASE
- Idiopathic condition
- Typically affects males ages 30 to 50 years
- Patients often have abdominal pain, diarrhea, weight loss, and peripheral edema
- Hypersecretion of gastric epithelium leads to hypoproteinemia and edema (protein-losing gastropathy); deep glandular atrophy is associated with hypochlorhydria
- Associations include eosinophilia, pulmonary infections, and thromboses
- Pediatric cases and some cases seen in immunosuppressed patients can occur and are associated with cytomegalovirus infection; in this setting, the hypertrophic gastropathy is often self-limited

ZOLLINGER-ELLISON SYNDROME
- Mucosal hypertrophy due to gastrinoma-driven parietal cell hyperplasia
- Rare disease, fewer than 1 case per 1 million population
- Affects any age from childhood to elderly
- Peak incidence between ages 20 and 50 years
- Affects both genders equally
- Common symptoms include abdominal pain and diarrhea

HELICOBACTER PYLORI–ASSOCIATED GASTROPATHY
- Increased mucosal thickness is due to edema and inflammation; mucosa is not hyperplastic

Gross and Endoscopic Pathology
MÉNÉTRIER DISEASE
- Thick gastric wall with enlarged, cerebriform rugae (Figure 6-26)
- Tends to spare antrum (in adults)

ZOLLINGER-ELLISON SYNDROME
- Similar to Ménétrier disease; giant rugae
- Spares antrum

Histopathology
MÉNÉTRIER DISEASE
- Hyperplasia of superficial foveolar epithelium
- Atrophy of fundic glands
- Superficial pits are elongated and tortuous but are lined by cytologically normal cells
- Hyperplastic foveolar cells secrete excess mucus
- Evolving lesions include the following:
  - Dilated pits producing cysts, which may extend through the muscularis mucosae
  - Expanding pits induce glandular atrophy and hypochlorhydria

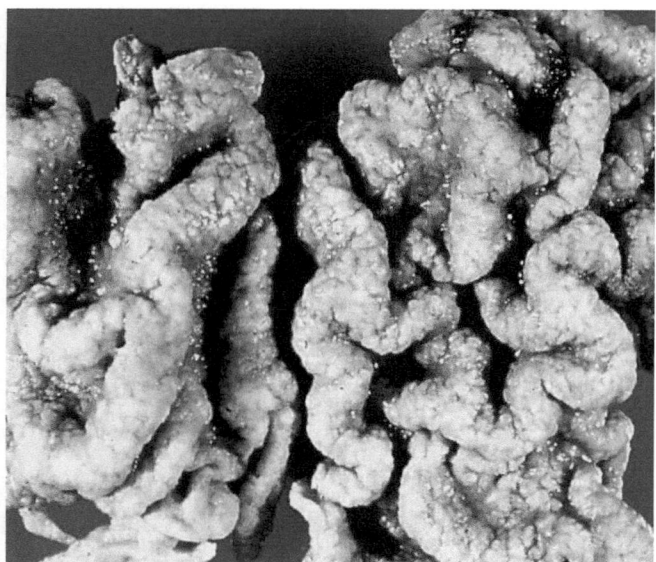

Figure 6-26. Resection specimen of Ménétrier disease with large cerebriform gastric rugae.

- Mixed inflammatory infiltrate
- Hyperplasia of muscularis mucosae with extension upward between glands

ZOLLINGER-ELLISON SYNDROME
- Specialized glands are hyperplastic
- Parietal cells occupy most of the deep portions of the glands and extend high up the neck
- Surface foveolar cells are atrophic
- Most easily identified by recognizing the abnormal pit-to-gland ratio (normal, 1:5)

Special Stains and Immunohistochemistry

- Enterochromaffin-like cell hyperplasia, endocrine cell dysplasia, and carcinoid tumors can arise in the setting of Zollinger-Ellison syndrome and are best seen with immunostain for chromogranin or synaptophysin

Other Techniques for Diagnosis

- Noncontributory

Differential Diagnosis

MÉNÉTRIER DISEASE–LIKE HYPERTROPHIC GASTROPATHY ASSOCIATED WITH LYMPHOCYTIC GASTRITIS
- Associated with giant gastric folds, hypoalbuminemia, and hypochlorhydria
- Background gastritis characterized by large numbers of intraepithelial lymphocytes (> 25 per 100 gastric foveolar cells) (Figure 6-27)

MÉNÉTRIER DISEASE
- Can be histologically indistinguishable from gastric hyperplastic polyp, juvenile polyp, Cronkhite-Canada polyp, or reactive gastropathy in small biopsy specimens
- Careful attention to exact clinical setting and status of adjacent mucosa is critical to accurate diagnosis

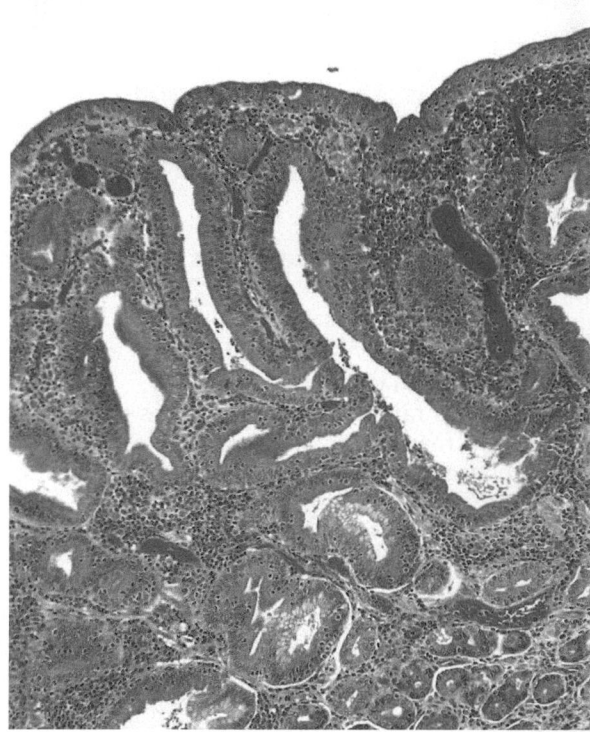

Figure 6-27. Lymphocytic gastritis associated with Ménétrier disease-like gastropathy. Note the foveolar hyperplasia with numerous (> 25 per 100 gastric foveolar cells) intraepithelial lymphocytes.

GASTRITIS GLANDULARIS ET CYSTICA PROFUNDA
- Synonyms include diffuse cystic glandular malformation and diffuse cystic malformation
- Mucosal and submucosal cysts lined by mucus cells, pyloric or Brunner-type glands, or rarely gastric body–type glands enveloped by smooth muscle
- Rare but may be associated with increased risk for gastric carcinoma

ZOLLINGER-ELLISON SYNDROME VERSUS PEPTIC ULCER DISEASE
- Peptic ulcer disease may have surface foveolar hyperplasia but no parietal cell hyperplasia

PEARLS

- *Hypertrophic gastropathy is characterized by giant cerebriform enlargement of the gastric rugae (Figure 6-26)*
- *Ménétrier disease and Zollinger-Ellison syndrome are the most common causes; large folds are less commonly seen with* H. pylori *infection*
- *Most common complication is peptic ulcer, which may cause gastrointestinal hemorrhage; rarely, the hyperplastic mucosa becomes metaplastic and may subsequently undergo malignant transformation*

SELECTED REFERENCES

Haot J, Bogomoletz WV, Jouret A, Manquet P: Ménétrier's disease with lymphocytic gastritis: an unusual association with possible pathogenic implications. Human Pathol 22:379-386, 1991.

Komorowski RA, Caya JG: Hyperplastic gastropathy: clinicopathologic correlation. Am J Surg Pathol 15:577-585, 1991.

Qualman SJ, Hamoudi AB: Pediatric hypertrophic gastropathy (Ménétrier's disease). Pediatr Pathol 12:263-268, 1992.

NON-NEOPLASTIC GASTRIC POLYPS

Clinical Features

HYPERPLASTIC POLYP

- A common polyp in the stomach (accounts for 85% to 90% of gastric polyps in some series); ratio depends on prevalence of familial adenomatous polyposis syndrome patients and the use of proton pump inhibitors in the study group
- Most common in older adults
- Generally occurs in body or antrum
- Associated mainly with chronic gastritis, but also occurs in reactive gastropathy adjacent to ulcers, surgical anastomosis, or gastrostomy sites
- Low malignant potential, but hyperplastic polyps may coexist with adenomas and carcinoma

FUNDIC GLAND POLYP

- May occur sporadically, can be part of familial adenomatous polyposis (FAP) syndromes (FAP, attenuated FAP, and MUTYH-associated polyposis syndrome), and is a common polyp type seen in patients taking proton pump inhibitors
- FAP-associated fundic gland polyps affect one third to one half of all FAP patients and typically occur at a young age (10 to 30 years)
- Sporadic fundic gland polyps are typically found in older women
- Similar polyps seen in patients taking proton pump inhibitors

INFLAMMATORY FIBROID POLYP

- Occurs throughout gastrointestinal tract
- Identical to those described in esophagus
- Typically occurs in adults between 50 and 60 years of age
- Often asymptomatic (incidental finding); large polyps may cause abdominal pain or obstructive symptoms

Gross and Endoscopic Pathology

HYPERPLASTIC POLYP

- Typically small and sessile with a smooth, bosselated surface
- Generally less than 2 cm
- About one third of affected patients have multiple polyps
- Most occur in patients with chronic gastritis or reactive gastropathy

FUNDIC GLAND POLYP

- Small (0.1 to 0.5 cm), nonpedunculated mucosal nodules (Figure 6-28)
- Most involve the fundic mucosa
- Sporadic polyps
  - May be multiple but generally fewer than 20
- Fundic gland polyposis associated with FAP syndrome
  - Characterized by hundreds of polyps covering the gastric mucosa; often many more polyps than in non-FAP–associated fundic gland polyposis; concentrate on greater curvature and usually spares the antrum

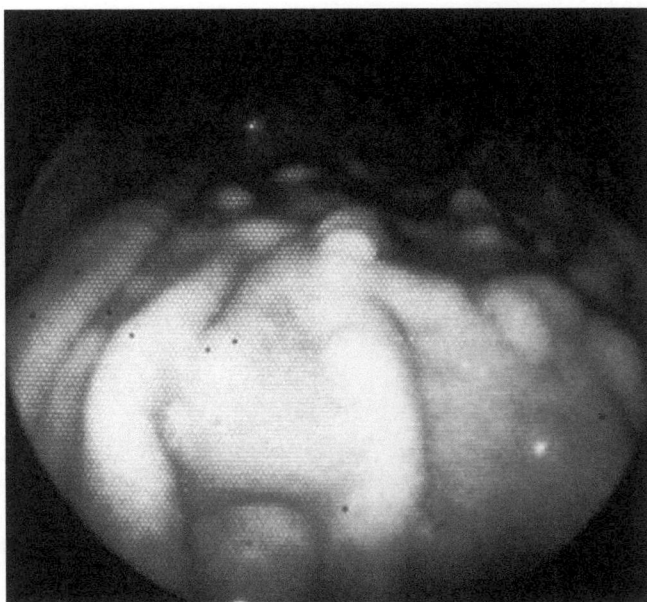

Figure 6-28. Endoscopic photograph of fundic gland polyposis in a patient with familial adenomatous polyposis. Note the small hemispheric polyps on the summit of rugae.

INFLAMMATORY FIBROID POLYP

- Most occur in the antrum
- Most are small (< 2 cm) and usually sessile
- May be single or multiple
- Circumscribed, firm nodules of gray tissue
- Overlying mucosa is often eroded or ulcerated
- Sometimes referred to as *Vanek polyp*

Histopathology

HYPERPLASTIC POLYP (Figure 6-29)

- Elongated, distorted, and branched foveolar pits in a background of edematous and inflamed lamina propria
- Often areas of surface ulceration, granulation tissue, and adjacent regenerative glands
- Glandular lining cells may show intestinal metaplasia; epithelial dysplasia can occur in this setting

FUNDIC GLAND POLYP

- Proliferation of small and dilated (cystic) glands lined by cytologically bland parietal chief cells and sometimes foveolar epithelium
- Occasional polyps show surface epithelial atypia; more commonly seen in FAP syndrome–associated polyps; essentially no malignant potential (Figure 6-30)

INFLAMMATORY FIBROID POLYP

- Appear to arise in the submucosa as a granulation tissue–like reactive phenomenon
- Variable mixture of fibroblasts, myofibroblasts, thin-walled dilated blood vessels, and scattered mixed inflammation (lymphocytes, eosinophils, plasma cells), sometimes with giant cells
- Typically have a hypocellular stroma, but some polyps may be hypercellular
- Predictable evolution
  - Nodular stage: "tissue-culture" fibroblasts and myxoid stroma

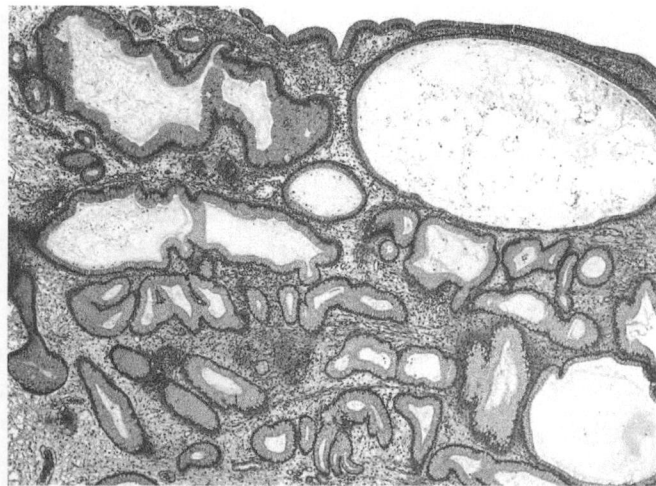

Figure 6-29. Hyperplastic polyp of the stomach showing edematous and inflammatory expansion of the lamina propria associated with mucosal microcyst formation.

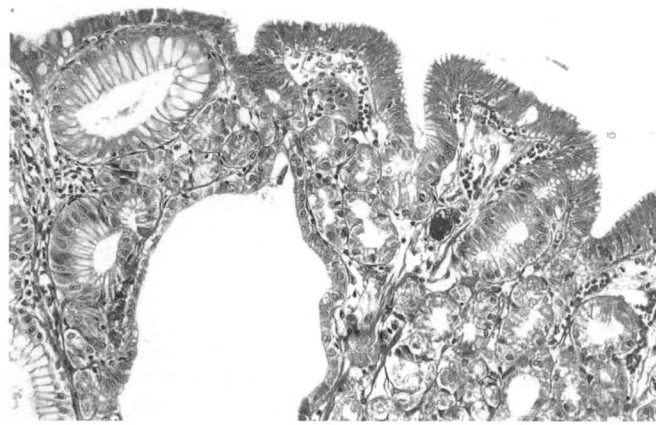

Figure 6-30. Fundic gland polyp associated with familial adenomatous polyposis. In addition to the dilated gastric glands, the surface epithelium shows atypia, a phenotypic marker for familial adenomatous polyposis syndrome-associated fundic gland polyps.

- Fibrovascular stage: vessels within concentric arrays of stromal spindle cells and eosinophils
- Sclerotic: collagenization as final stage

Special Stains and Immunohistochemistry

INFLAMMATORY FIBROID POLYP
- Vimentin and CD34 positive
- Cytokeratin and CD117 negative

Other Techniques for Diagnosis

- Inflammatory fibroid polyps harbor mutations in *PDGFRA* (platelet-derived growth factor receptor alpha) gene

Differential Diagnosis

ADENOMATOUS POLYP VERSUS HYPERPLASTIC POLYP
- Adenomatous polyps are characterized by dysplastic epithelium and typically do not contain as much inflamed stroma or gland dilatation

FUNDIC GLAND POLYP VERSUS SO-CALLED GASTRIC ADENOCARCINOMA WITH CHIEF CELL DIFFERENTIATION (GA-CCD)
- The rare GA-CCD shows an infiltrative growth pattern with irregular anastomosing cords of oxyntic epithelial cells
- The infiltration pattern is usually limited to the mucosa, but atypical cells can rarely be seen within the submucosa
- Some consider these an unusual variant of fundic gland polyp
- Persistence/recurrence has been associated with incomplete endoscopic resection
- Has not been known to metastasize and may be better labeled as "oxyntic gland polyp/adenoma"

GASTROINTESTINAL STROMAL TUMOR (GIST) AND SARCOMA VERSUS INFLAMMATORY FIBROID POLYP
- GIST
  - Composed of interlacing fascicles and whorls of spindle cells with elongated, cigar-shaped nuclei and epithelioid cells
  - Can usually be distinguished based on immunohistochemistry for CD117
  - In light of the *PDGFRA* mutations, inflammatory fibroid polyp may be in fact a benign variant of GIST
- Sarcoma
  - Hypercellular tumors composed of spindle or round cells with nuclear pleomorphism and high mitotic rate

PEARLS

- *Pathogenesis of fundic gland polyps related to mutations of APC and β-catenin genes*
- *Fundic gland polyps essentially occur in three settings (sporadic polyps, PPI-associated polyps, and FAP-associated fundic gland polyposis); best distinguished clinically*
- *On small biopsy specimens, the combination of nonneoplastic, irregular, dilated glands and inflamed stroma is a clue to a hyperplastic polyp*
- *Mixtures of fundic gland polyps and hyperplastic polyps can be seen*

SELECTED REFERENCES

Abraham SC, Nobukawa B, Giardiello FM, et al: Fundic gland polyps in familial adenomatous polyposis: neoplasms with frequent somatic adenomatous polyposis coli gene alterations. Am J Pathol 157:747-754, 2002.

Abraham SC, Park SJ, Mugartegui L, et al: Sporadic fundic gland polyps with epithelial dysplasia: evidence for preferential targeting for mutations in the adenomatous polyposis coli gene. Am J Pathol 161:1735-1742, 2002.

Oberhuber G, Stolte M: Gastric polyps: an update on their pathology and biological significance. Virchows Arch 437:581-590, 2000.

Singhi AD, Lazenby AJ, Montgomery EA. Gastric adenocarcinoma with chief cell differentiation: a proposal for reclassification as oxyntic gland polyp/adenoma. Am J Surg Pathol 36:1030-1035, 2012.

GASTRIC CARCINOMA AND PRECURSOR LESIONS

Clinical Features

- Two distinct clinicopathologic presentations of gastric adenocarcinoma

- Intestinal-type tumors: an exophytic neoplasm similar to colorectal carcinoma
- Diffuse-type tumors: an infiltrative process causing a thickening of the gastric wall
- Each type has separate epidemiologic and predisposing factors
- In the United States, the overall incidence of gastric carcinoma is decreasing (particularly the intestinal type); however, carcinoma of the proximal stomach is increasing
- Certain geographic areas, such as Eastern Asia, Eastern Europe, and Latin America, have a much higher incidence of gastric carcinoma, usually the intestinal type
- Male-to-female ratio is about 2:1, particularly in older patients
- Risk factors include the following:
  - Diet
    - High intake of complex carbohydrates and nitrates
    - Low intake of leafy vegetables, salads, and fresh fruits
    - Consumption of nitrates (or environmental exposure from fertilizer) is deleterious because they are reduced in the stomach to nitrites, which are strong mutagens
    - Salt (used in food preservation) potentiates the carcinogenic effects of nitrites by causing increased cell turnover
  - *Helicobacter pylori*
    - Colonization by *H. pylori* in childhood leads to chronic gastritis, oxidative effects on DNA, and cell proliferation

Precursor Lesions

- Protracted chronic gastritis
  - Produces intestinal metaplasia, which epidemiologically correlates with gastric carcinoma of intestinal type
- Dysplasia: as in Barrett esophagus and ulcerative colitis, the gastric dysplasias include flat dysplasia and polypoid dysplasia (adenomas)
  - Flat dysplasia: classified as low grade or high grade
    - Low-grade dysplasia
      - Slight increase in glandular complexity and cytologic aberrations, including loss of mucinous cells and hyperchromatic, mildly stratified nuclei
    - High-grade dysplasia
      - Marked glandular complexity and frank cytologic anaplasia including regular nuclear stratification, hyperchromasia, and pleomorphism with abnormal mitotic figures and loss of mucinous cells
      - At times the glandular complexity is such that distinction from intramucosal carcinoma is impossible
      - Progression from dysplasia to carcinoma is thought to be slow, and dysplasia may remain stable for years
  - Adenomas
    - Polypoid proliferations; considered to be a localized area of dysplasia
    - Less common than hyperplastic polyps

- Develop in areas of intestinal metaplasia
- Epidemiology is similar to intestinal-type gastric adenocarcinoma
- Estimates of coexistent gastric carcinoma range from 8% to 59%, as do estimates of carcinoma arising in the adenoma (11% to 69%)
- Gastric carcinoma more commonly complicates larger adenomas (> 2 cm)
- Numerous subtypes
  - Tubular, villous, tubulovillous most common
  - Antral-foveolar type, pyloric type much less common
- Ulcers
  - Although one fourth of all gastric carcinomas contain a discrete ulcer, less than 1% arise in a preceding, documented benign ulcer
  - In most cases, it is difficult to determine whether the cancer arose in an ulcer or whether a cancer ulcerated
  - About 5% of clinically and endoscopically presumed benign ulcers are eventually proved to be carcinoma

Gastric Carcinoma

- Common symptoms include early satiety, anorexia, and weight loss
- Like the epithelium from which it arises, gastric carcinoma is a heterogeneous tumor
- Fundamental differences in characteristics of two types of gastric carcinoma
  - Intestinal type
    - More common in elderly men
    - Seen in countries with high gastric cancer risk
    - Associated with dietary and environmental substances
    - Associated with *H. pylori* infection and intestinal metaplasia
    - Arises in a dysplastic precursor
    - Expands centripetally into gastric lumen and wall
    - Better prognosis than diffuse type carcinoma
  - Diffuse type
    - Younger patients and more common in women
    - No identifiable nutritional risk factor
    - May also be associated with *H. pylori* infection
    - Thought to arise from undifferentiated neck cells
    - Type seen with familial cases associated with germline E-cadherin *(CDH1)* gene mutations; these demonstrate a subtle precursor lesion
    - Infiltrates into and expands gastric wall
    - Poor prognosis

Early Gastric Carcinoma

- Superficial malignant tumor that invades the lamina propria, muscularis mucosae and submucosa but has not invaded the muscularis propria
- In large-scale screening programs in countries with a high incidence of gastric carcinoma (Japan), early gastric carcinoma is frequently diagnosed
  - Distinct from other entities, such as high-grade dysplasia, an incipient malignancy still confined within its original glandular basement membrane

Gross and Endoscopic Pathology

PRECURSOR LESIONS

- Flat dysplasia
  - Often associated with chronic gastritis, which is endoscopically diffuse
  - Mucosa may be hyperemic or eroded
  - Usually, flat dysplasia is not endoscopically discernible
- Adenoma
  - Sessile or pedunculated polyp; may be endoscopically indistinguishable from a hyperplastic polyp
- Ulcer
  - Benign form characteristically has discrete, smooth, flat margins and a clean base

GASTRIC CARCINOMA

- May be raised, flat, or ulcerated (Figure 6-31)
- Some tumors are minute (< 0.5 cm)
- Classification of gastric carcinoma by gross or endoscopic features is of little or no value clinically

Histopathology

PRECURSOR LESIONS

- Dysplasia (low and high grade)
  - A spectrum of changes involving increased architectural complexity and cytologic atypia (increased nuclear size, hyperchromasia, pleomorphism, and nuclear stratification)
  - Dysplasia generally resembles adenomas as seen in the colon and small bowel
  - High-grade lesions show increased complexity and cellular atypia
- Adenoma (Figure 6-32)
  - Essentially the same as colorectal adenomas
  - Characterized by variable loss of mucinous cells, nuclear enlargement, pleomorphism, and stratification
  - Can be classified as tubular, villous, and tubulovillous

GASTRIC CARCINOMA

- Expresses a wide variety of histologic phenotypes
- Many histologic classification schemes have been proposed, but none is universally followed or accepted
- Many carcinomas are reminiscent of colorectal malignancies, whereas some retain mucinous features resembling foveolar cells
  - Most investigators and clinicians prefer separation into diffuse and intestinal type of Lauren (Figures 6-33 and 6-34)

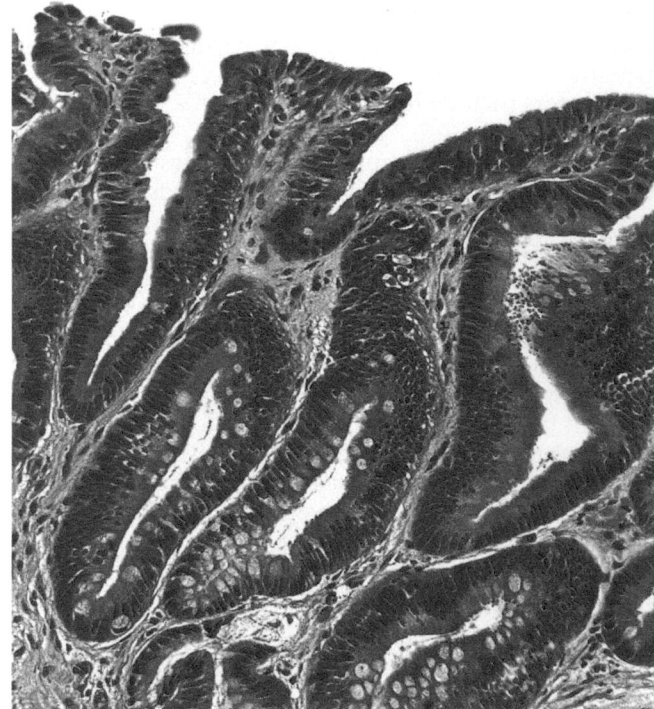

Figure 6-32. Gastric adenoma. The histology is similar to a tubular adenoma seen in the intestines and is arising in intestinal metaplasia.

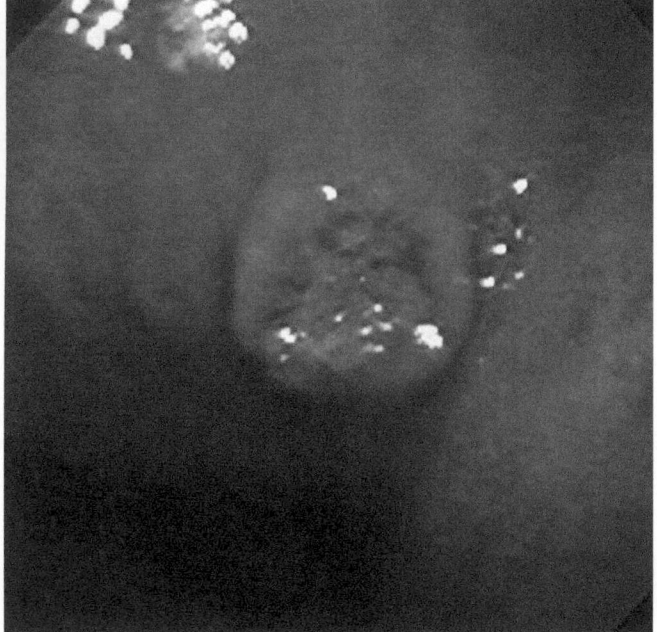

Figure 6-31. Endoscopic photograph of gastric adenocarcinoma demonstrating an irregularly shaped ulcer with undermining infiltrative edges.

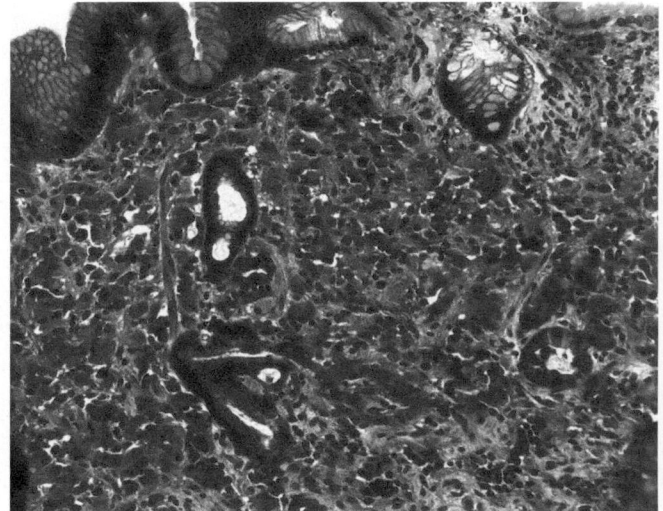

Figure 6-33. Infiltrating gastric adenocarcinoma, mixed intestinal and diffuse type of Lauren with an infiltrative pattern composed of carcinoma cells showing a high nuclear-to-cytoplasmic ratio and some gland formation.

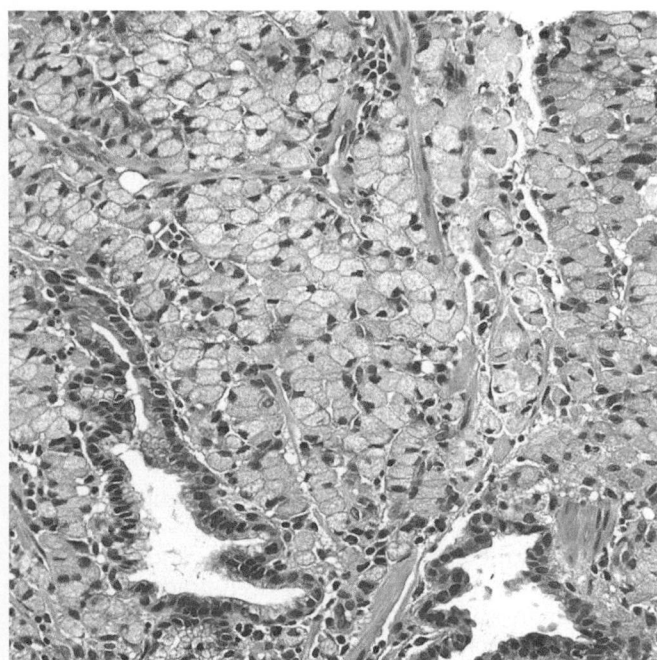

Figure 6-34. Infiltrating poorly differentiated adenocarcinoma, diffuse type of Lauren with signet ring cell differentiation.

- Other rare gastric carcinomas
  - Small cell carcinoma (see "Gastric Neuroendocrine Tumors," presented later), parietal cell carcinoma, hepatoid adenocarcinoma, endodermal sinus tumor and embryonal carcinoma, choriocarcinoma, adenosquamous carcinoma, carcinosarcoma, and spindle cell carcinoma have been described
  - Lymphoepithelioma-like
    - Uncommon undifferentiated carcinoma with dense lymphoid infiltrate; can often find evidence of Epstein-Barr virus infection

Special Stains and Immunohistochemistry

- Cytokeratin: useful stain to confirm poorly differentiated or signet ring cell carcinoma, which may be present within an ulcer base or at ulcer margins or infiltrate between benign glands; requires experience to accurately interpret
- Mucin stains (Alcian blue/PAS combination stain with a hematoxylin counterstain, mucicarmine): serve similar role as cytokeratin, but not all carcinomas are positive; histiocytes may engulf mucin (muciphages), causing confusion with signet ring cells
- Combined Alcian blue and PAS stain with a hematoxylin counterstain: detects intestinal metaplasia (dark blue, globoid goblet cells against magenta foveolar cells); the Alcian blue and PAS stain helps to detect carcinoma cells with abnormal mucin pattern in the lamina propria

Other Techniques for Diagnosis

- Gastric carcinoma, adenocarcinoma of gastric cardia/gastroesophageal junction, and lower esophageal adenocarcinoma are analyzed for HER2 by immunohistochemistry and fluorescence in situ hybridization as a selection criterion for trastuzumab therapy

Differential Diagnosis

CHEMOTHERAPY OR RADIATION EFFECT

- Accentuated atypia mimicking cancer and dysplasia can be seen in the stomach as a complication of regional chemotherapy (e.g., hepatic arterial infusion chemotherapy) and radiation therapy (e.g., SIR-Spheres)
- Radiation and chemotherapy effect are usually associated with preserved mucosal architecture, few mitotic figures, marked cellular enlargement, bizarre atypia, a low nuclear-to-cytoplasmic ratio, and cytoplasmic eosinophilia with vacuolization

CHRONIC GASTRITIS WITH EROSION AND GLANDULAR REGENERATION

- Characterized by maintained architecture, hyperplastic glands containing normal mitotic figures, and enlarged but uniform nuclei (compared with carcinoma or dysplasia)
- Glands mature superficially, and the gland nuclei are not pleomorphic or stratified

ULCER

- Glandular epithelium at ulcer margin demonstrates regeneration
- Foamy histiocytes may be present, but infiltrating single malignant cells, malignant glands, and desmoplasia are absent
- Stroma may contain atypical but reactive fibroblasts, particularly following radiation

INTESTINAL METAPLASIA WITH DYSPLASIA

- Characterized by a background of goblet cells and atypical glands containing cells with stratified, pleomorphic, hyperchromatic nuclei
- Distinction from carcinoma may be difficult but is best made by absence of an infiltrating pattern, frankly malignant cytology, and desmoplasia

PEARLS

- *Overall 5-year survival rate for gastric carcinoma following gastrectomy is 10% to 20%*
  - *Most carcinomas in Western countries present as stage IV (53%)*
  - *Tumor type, size, and grade all have prognostic value*
  - *Single best predictor of survival is depth of invasion; survival is 95% for tumors confined to the submucosa but drops to 50% with involvement through the muscularis propria to the subserosa (T3); T2 lesions have intermediate survival*
- *In gastric biopsies*
  - *If intestinal metaplasia is present, always look for dysplasia and carcinoma*
  - *If the glands appear farther apart than normal, be certain to determine what is separating them; it could be signet ring cell carcinoma, lymphoma, benign lymphoplasmacytic infiltrate, foamy histiocytes, or, rarely, infected histiocytes (fungal or mycobacteria)*
- *Surgical pathology reports for resections should include enough information to determine tumor, node, metastasis (TNM) stage, tumor location, histologic type, degree of differentiation, and presence or absence of tumor at the resection margins; following CAP cancer protocols is recommended*

SELECTED REFERENCES

Abraham SC, Montgomery EA, Singh VK, et al: Gastric adenomas: Intestinal-type and gastric-type adenomas differ in the risk of adenocarcinoma and presence of background mucosal pathology. Am J Surg Pathol 26:1276-1285, 2002.

Bang YJ, Van Cutsem E, Feyereislova A, et al: Trastuzumab in combination with chemotherapy versus chemotherapy alone for treatment of HER2-positive advanced gastric or gastro-oesophageal junction cancer (ToGA): a phase 3, open-label, randomised controlled trial. Lancet 376:687-697, 2010.

Lauren T: The two histologic main types of gastric carcinoma. Acta Pathol Microbiol Scand 64:34, 1965.

Lauwers GY, Franceschi S, Carneiro F, et al: Gastric carcinoma. In Bosman FT, Carneiro F, Hruban RH, Theise ND (eds): World Health Organization Classification of Tumours of the Digestive System. Lyon, IARC Press, 2010, pp 48-58.

Petras R, Hart W, Bukowski R: Gastric epithelial atypia associated with hepatic arterial infusion chemotherapy: Its distinction from early gastric carcinoma. Cancer 56:745-750, 1985.

GASTRIC NEUROENDOCRINE TUMORS (CARCINOID TUMORS AND NEUROENDOCRINE CARCINOMAS)

Clinical Features

- Sometimes divided into four types
  - Type 1: associated with atrophic gastritis (up to 80% of cases)
  - Type 2: associated with Zollinger-Ellison syndrome as part of MEN type 1 (rare)
  - Type 3: sporadic (approximately 15% of cases)
  - Type 4: high-grade neuroendocrine carcinoma
- Dividing lesions into two categories based on pathogenic mechanisms is more useful conceptually
  - Sporadic tumors
    - Typically solitary
    - Can contain immunoreactive gastrin, serotonin, somatostatin, histamine, or bradykinin, but this is rarely important clinically
    - Can behave in an aggressive manner, especially those larger than 2 cm; can be associated with invasion into the gastric wall and metastases to regional lymph nodes and the liver
    - Not associated with endocrine cell hyperplasia in adjacent mucosa
    - No response to antral resection or induction of hypogastrinemia
  - Tumors arising in a background of hypergastrinemia (usually resulting from chronic atrophic gastritis with pernicious anemia)
    - More common type
    - Associated with achlorhydria and hypergastrinemia
    - Arise following progression from hyperplasia of enterochromaffin-like cells to nodular hyperplasia to dysplasia to neoplasia
    - Multiple small mucosal or submucosal nodules, typically smaller than 1 cm
    - Indolent tumors that rarely metastasize
    - May regress following antrectomy (reduction of gastrin secretion)
    - May be seen in patients with Zollinger-Ellison syndrome as part of multiple endocrine neoplasia (MEN) syndrome type 1, or rarely in patients with a primary defect of the proton pump

Gross and Endoscopic Pathology

- Small tumors (several micrometers up to 2 cm); sporadic tumors are usually larger (mean 2 cm) (Figure 6-35)
- Larger lesions are often centrally umbilicated
- Hypergastrinemia related tumors are typically multiple and small (0.1 to 0.3 cm)

Histopathology (Figure 6-36)

- Monomorphic nests, trabeculae, festoons, or glandlike formations
- Tumor cells have central, uniform, rounded nuclei with coarse chromatin pattern and sharply demarcated nuclear membrane and a low mitotic rate
- Typically arise in the deep mucosa and are covered by intact superficial epithelium; can invade the gastric wall and produce desmoplastic reaction
- Hypergastrinemia-associated and sporadic carcinoids can be histologically indistinguishable
- Higher mitotic rates, nuclear anaplasia, and necrosis are components of intermediate or high-grade neuroendocrine carcinoma and predict aggressive behavior
  - Grading scheme proposed by World Health Organization is based on mitosis figures and proportion of tumor nuclei expressing Ki-67
    - Grade 1: < 2 mitoses per 10 high magnification field and percentage of Ki-67 positive cells ≤ 2
    - Grade 2: 2-20 mitoses per 10 high magnification fields and percentage of Ki-67 positive nuclei > 2 to 20
    - Grade 3: > 20 mitoses per 10 high magnification field and percentage of Ki-67 positive nuclei > 20
  - The CAP and World Health Organization (WHO) incorporate grading, tumor size, and topographic information in the following classification
    - A grade 1 tumor < 1 cm in greatest cross dimension limited to mucosa and submucosa is termed "benign well-differentiated neuroendocrine tumor"

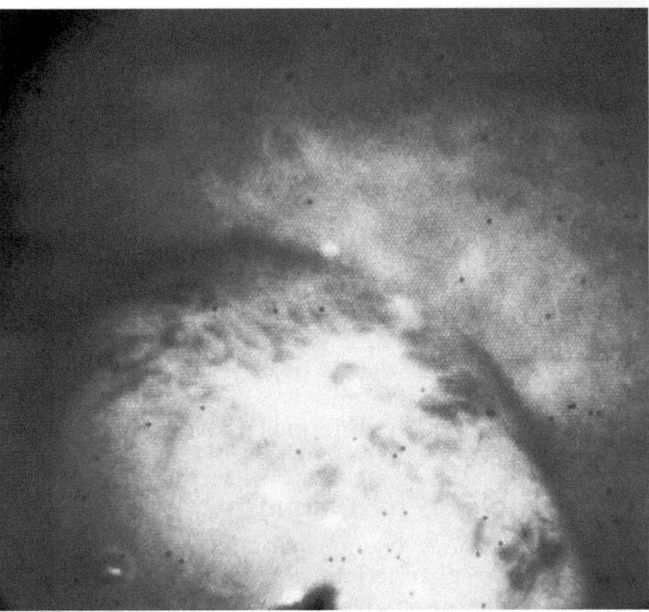

Figure 6-35. Endoscopic photograph of sporadic gastric carcinoid tumor with ulcer (foreground).

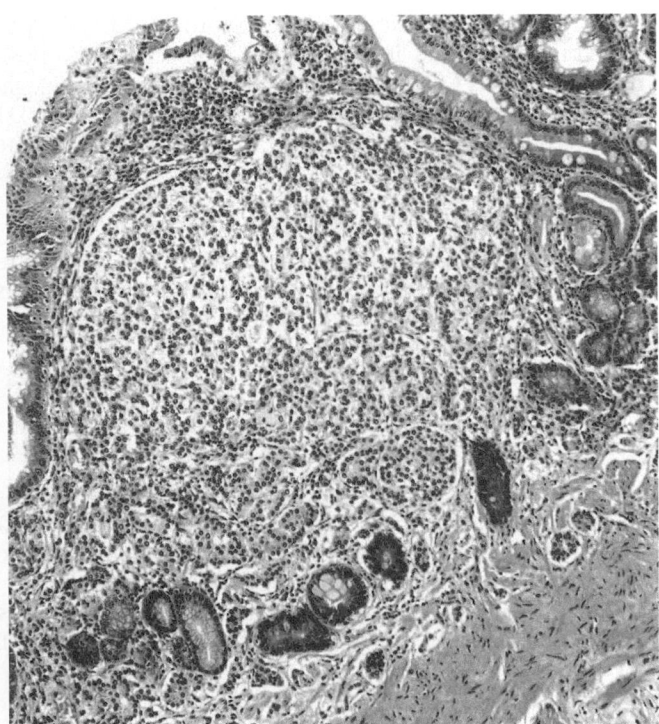

Figure 6-36. Intramucosal gastric carcinoid tumor arising in association with atrophic gastritis and intestinal metaplasia.

- A grade 1 tumor limited to mucosa and submucosa 1 cm to 2 cm in size is called a "well-differentiated neuroendocrine tumor of uncertain malignant potential"
- A grade 1 tumor > 2 cm in size, one invading the muscularis externa or beyond, or a grade 1 tumor associated with metastases is referred to as a "well-differentiated neuroendocrine carcinoma"
- It is implied that high-grade neuroendocrine carcinoma encompasses all tumors that are grade 2 and grade 3

Special Stains and Immunohistochemistry

- Immunoreactive with antibodies to chromogranin and synaptophysin help verify neuroendocrine differentiation and help classify tumors as sporadic (no hyperplasia or dysplasia of enterochromaffin-like cells) or hypergastrinemia related
- Adjacent mucosa in hypergastrinemia-related neuroendocrine tumors can show linear hyperplasia (five or more endocrine cells in a line), nodular hyperplasia (clusters of five or more endocrine cells smaller than 150 μm), endocrine cell dysplasia (growths larger than 150 μm but smaller than 0.5 mm), or neuroendocrine tumors (growths larger than 0.5 mm)
  - Classification of gastric endocrine cell proliferations is only applied to nonantral mucosa; an immunostain for gastrin should be performed to prove that the tissue specimen is not derived from the gastric antrum

Other Techniques for Diagnosis

- Noncontributory

Differential Diagnosis

GASTRIC ADENOCARCINOMA

- Typically forms recognizable glandular elements with a destructive and invasive growth pattern

LYMPHOMA

- Particularly in small biopsies, the small, monomorphic lymphoid cells may superficially resemble those of a neuroendocrine tumor
- Lymphocytic infiltrate is positive for LCA and other lymphoid markers

PEARLS

- *In tumors associated with chronic atrophic (autoimmune) gastritis, lymph node metastases are extremely rare and generally occur only in tumors larger than 1 cm*
- *Some sporadic neuroendocrine tumors and high-grade carcinomas can behave in a more aggressive manner and may prompt more aggressive surgery (complete or partial gastrectomy with lymph node resection)*
- *Remember to exclude melanoma if a tumor resembling a neuroendocrine tumor demonstrates a high Ki-67 labeling index*

SELECTED REFERENCES

Rindi G, Klimstra DS, Arnold R, et al: Nomenclature and classification of neuroendocrine neoplasms of the digestive system. In Bosman FT, Carneiro F, Hruban RH, Theise ND (eds): World Health Organization Classification of Tumours of the Digestive System. Lyon, IARC Press, 2010, pp 13-14.

Solcia E, Arnold R, Capella C, et al: Neuroendocrine neoplasms of the stomach. In Bosman FT, Carneiro F, Hruban RH, Theise ND (eds): World Health Organization Classification of Tumours of the Digestive System. Lyon, IARC Press, 2010, pp 64-68.

Thomas RM, Baybick JH, Elsayed AM, Sobin LH: Gastric carcinoids: an immunohistochemical and clinicopathologic study of 104 patients. Cancer 73:2053-2058, 1994.

Washington MK, Tang LH, Berlin J, et al: Protocol for the examination of specimens from patients with neuroendocrine tumors (carcinoid tumors) of the stomach. Arch Pathol Lab Med 134:187-191, 2010.

Williams GT: Endocrine tumours of the gastrointestinal tract: selected topics. Histopathology 50:30-41, 2007.

GASTRIC LYMPHOMA

Clinical Features

- Gastric lymphoma accounts for 60% to 65% of all gastrointestinal lymphomas
- Diffuse large B-cell lymphoma is most common
- Many gastric lymphomas are derived from mucosa associated lymphoid tissue (MALT)
- Generally affects patients in the fifth and sixth decades of life
- May be asymptomatic or present with an abdominal mass, abdominal pain (related to gastritis or ulcer), weight loss, or less commonly, bleeding
- Clear association between gastric marginal zone B-cell lymphoma of MALT type and *Helicobacter pylori* infection (92% to 100% of cases); treatment of *H. pylori* induces regression in 77% of early lesions (Figure 6-37)
- Indolent behavior and generally an excellent prognosis with marginal zone B-cell lymphoma of MALT type

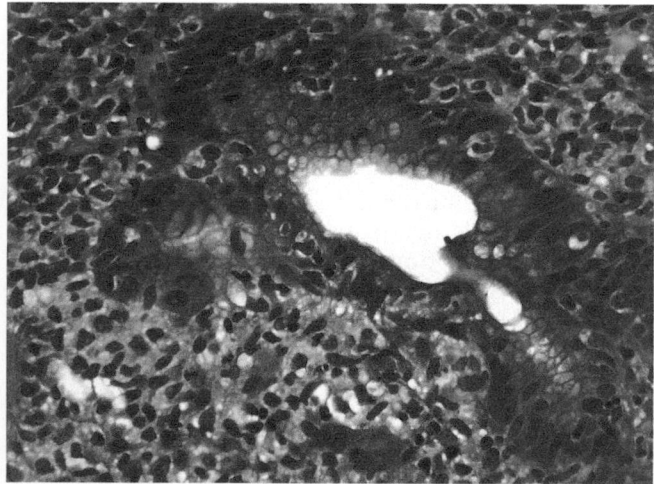

Figure 6-37. Extranodal marginal zone B-cell lymphoma of the mucosa-associated lymphoid tissue involving the stomach. A destructive lymphoepithelial lesion is associated with a proliferation of marginal zone lymphoma cells within the lamina propria.

Gross and Endoscopic Pathology

- Most arise in the antrum
- Early lesions typically form a plaque or small mucosal erosions
- Advanced lesions cause ulcers, diffuse thickening of mucosal folds, or obvious masses

Histopathology

- Marginal zone B-cell lymphoma of MALT type (Figure 6-37)
  - Expansive proliferation of marginal zone lymphocytes at least 150 μm in size with neoplastic lymphocytes can have varying cytologic features ranging from small lymphocytes with round, dark nuclei to small lymphocytes with irregular nuclear contours and pale cytoplasm (centrocyte-like cells) to medium-sized lymphocytes with abundant clear cytoplasm (monocytoid B cells) to plasma cells with Dutcher bodies and scattered large cells (centroblasts or immunoblasts)
  - Three additional characteristic features:
    - Classic feature is the lymphoepithelial lesion (caused by invasion and destruction of gland or cyst by aggregates of neoplastic lymphocytes)
    - Lymphoid follicles often with germinal centers
    - Neoplastic plasma cells
- Diffuse large B-cell lymphoma
  - Confluent, sheetlike proliferations of large transformed cells (centroblasts or immunoblast-like cells)
  - May represent transformation from marginal zone B-cell lymphoma of MALT type; this is suggested by a mixture of low- and high-grade histology in the same tumor and presence of same genotype

Special Stains and Immunohistochemistry

- Large cell lymphoma; confirm B-cell lineage with CD20 immunostain
  - Differentiate germinal center from nongerminal center type using immunostains for CD10, BCL-6, and MUM-1

- Gastric marginal zone B-cell lymphoma of MALT type
  - Workup includes immunostains that should be positive, such as CD20, BCL-2 and CD79a as well as negative staining for CD3, CD5, CD10, CD23, and cyclin D1
  - Aberrant expression of CD43 and CD-5 supports the diagnosis

Other Techniques for Diagnosis

- PCR for B-cell clonality is supportive (with appropriate histology) but may be positive in some cases of gastritis
- Cytogenetics: t(11;18), trisomy 3 and 18 may be seen
- t(11;18) predicts resistance to *H. pylori* therapy
- Flow cytometry positive for CD19, CD20, CD21; negative for CD5, CD10, and CD23

Differential Diagnosis

LYMPHOCYTIC GASTRITIS VERSUS MALT LYMPHOMA

- Gastritis usually lacks lymphoepithelial lesion (cluster of three or more B-cell lymphocytes within gastric glands), which is characteristic of MALT lymphoma
- Intraepithelial lymphocytes are T cells rather than B cells
- Lacks characteristic immunophenotype of MALT lymphoma

PEARLS

- *MALT lymphomas have an excellent prognosis and typically remain confined to the stomach for many years; early lesions often improve with treatment for* H. pylori
- *Biopsy fragments showing diffuse sheets of lymphoplasmacytic cells with lymphoepithelial lesions, particularly in an older patient, suggest MALT lymphoma*

SELECTED REFERENCES

Banks PM: Gastrointestinal lymphoproliferative disorders. Histopathology 50:42-54, 2007.
Chan JK, Ng CS, Isaacson PG: Relationship between high-grade lymphoma and low-grade B-cell mucosa-associated lymphoid tissue (MALToma) of the stomach. Am J Pathol 126:1153-1165, 1990.
Isaacson PG: Gastric lymphoma and *Helicobacter pylori*. N Engl J Med 330:1310-1311, 1994.
Isaacson PG: Lymphomas of mucosa-associated lymphoid tissue (MALT). Histopathology 16:617-619, 1990.
Swerdlow SH, Campo E, Harris NL, et al (eds): WHO Classification of Tumours of Haematopoietic and Lymphoid Tissues. Lyon: IARC, 2008.

LOWER GASTROINTESTINAL TRACT (SMALL AND LARGE INTESTINE)

CONGENITAL ANOMALIES

Clinical Features

MALROTATION

- Varying degrees of malrotation or malfixation are not uncommon
- Results from disturbance of normal counterclockwise rotation of bowel around the superior mesenteric artery
- Occurs in 1 in 6000 live births
- Presenting symptoms are volvulus, obstruction, bilious vomiting, abdominal distention, steatorrhea, and failure to thrive

OMPHALOCELE
- Affects about 1 in 6000 to 1 in 10,000 births
- Results from failure of the intestines to return to the abdominal cavity during the 10th week of development
- May occur as a result of incomplete closure of the abdominal wall during the fourth week of development, which produces a large defect in the anterior abdominal wall (as a result, most of the abdominal viscera remain outside the embryo)
- In both situations, the herniated intestines are contained within a thin membranous sac (composed of peritoneal lining and amnion)
- Up to 50% of affected infants have additional anomalies, including malrotation, Meckel diverticulum, imperforate anus, and cardiovascular defects

GASTROSCHISIS
- Literally means split or open stomach (misnomer because it is the abdominal wall that is split, not the stomach)
- Uncommon, but more common in males
- Incidence is estimated at 1 to 2 cases per 100,000 births
- Presumed to be due to a vascular accident in early embryogenesis (before 12 weeks)
- Results from a defect in the anterior abdominal wall that permits extrusion of the abdominal viscera
- No membranous sac surrounds the extruded viscera

ATRESIA AND STENOSIS
- Rare conditions; found in 1 in 2000 to 1 in 6000 live births
- Duodenal atresia is most common and is associated with other anomalies in 35% of cases
- Higher incidence in twin gestations and in infants of mothers using cocaine
- Colonic atresia virtually never occurs
- Atresia presents in early neonatal period with bilious vomiting

MECKEL DIVERTICULUM
- Failure of the vitelline duct (connects the lumen of the bowel to the yolk sac) to involute produces a Meckel diverticulum
- Generally found within 85 to 100 cm of the ileocecal valve in adults
- About 1% to 4% prevalence
- No gender predilection
- Complications include hemorrhage, peptic ulceration, intussusception, and diverticulitis

INTUSSUSCEPTION
- Telescoping of one intestinal segment into another
- Affects about 2 to 4 per 1000 live births
- Twice as common in males
- Symptoms include abdominal pain, bloody diarrhea, and obstruction
- Complications include bowel infarction and peritonitis
- Children usually have no underlying anatomic abnormalities; intussusception in adults is typically associated with an intraluminal mass

VOLVULUS
- Twisting of a bowel segment around mesentery

- Thought to cause about 10% of all bowel obstructions
- Occurs with or without predisposing causes, including
  - Congenitally long mesentery
  - Meckel diverticulum
  - Congenital band
- Most commonly occurs with redundant loops of sigmoid colon; less common in small intestine, and rarely involves the stomach or transverse colon
- Patients generally present with abdominal pain and obstruction
- Occurs acutely and may produce bowel infarction and peritonitis

Gross and Endoscopic Pathology
MALROTATION
- Intestines occupy abnormal positions
- Generally small bowel appears as a coiled mass of intestine pushed to one side of the abdomen
- Cecum may be on left side of the abdomen
- Fixation band may cause intestinal torsion and infarction

OMPHALOCELE
- Extra-abdominal viscera are covered by a thin membranous sac composed of peritoneum and amnion
- Herniated viscera typically includes intestines; may involve stomach and liver
- Umbilical cord arises from the center of the overlying sac

GASTROSCHISIS
- Abdominal viscera herniate through a defect in the abdominal wall
- Extruded viscera do not have an overlying thin membranous sac
- No involvement of the umbilical cord

ATRESIA AND STENOSIS
- Multiple types of atresias exist and may coexist
  - Imperforate septum across intestinal lumen
  - Bowel segment replaced by a fibrotic cord
  - Bowel segment and associated mesentery completely absent
- Intestinal stenosis is similar to atresia; has a variable reduction of the lumen diameter over a long segment or contains a septum with a central communication; bowel wall layers generally intact

MECKEL DIVERTICULUM (Figure 6-38)
- Antimesenteric ileum is the most common location
- Located 30 cm from ileocecal valve in infants and 85 to 100 cm from the ileocecal valve in adults
- Usually 2 to 15 cm in length

INTUSSUSCEPTION
- Invagination or telescoping of proximal small or large bowel (intussusceptum) into the adjacent distal bowel that encircles it

VOLVULUS
- Segment of bowel may twist around its mesentery
- Involved bowel is ischemic or frankly infarcted (35% to 40% of cases)
- Associated fibrous band or adhesion may be found

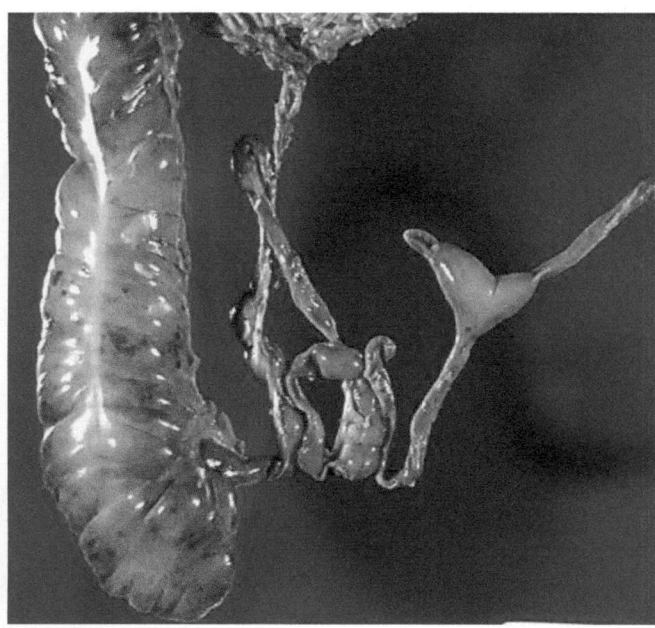

Figure 6-38. Meckel diverticulum (autopsy photograph).

Histopathology

MALROTATION, OMPHALOCELE, AND GASTROSCHISIS
- Normal bowel histology unless complicated by ischemia or peritonitis

ATRESIA AND STENOSIS
- Bowel proximal to the atretic or stenotic area may show ischemic or gangrenous changes (due to dilation of bowel)
- Villous blunting, ulceration, and granulation tissue can be seen; with time, marked submucosal fibrosis and muscularis propria hypertrophy occur
- Blind segment contains meconium, lanugo hair, and mucin

MECKEL DIVERTICULUM
- Usually lined by normal small intestinal mucosa
- May contain ectopic pancreatic or gastric tissue

INTUSSUSCEPTION
- Ischemic changes are common
- Vascular proliferation in lamina propria and deeper bowel layers develops in recurrent cases and can mimic vascular tumors

VOLVULUS
- Variable degrees of ischemia

Special Stains and Immunohistochemistry
- Noncontributory

Other Techniques for Diagnosis
- Noncontributory

Differential Diagnosis
- Malrotation, atresia, Meckel diverticulum, intussusception, and volvulus all are considered in the differential diagnosis in patients with bowel obstruction symptoms

- Combination of clinical, radiographic, and surgical findings is usually diagnostic

PEARLS

- *Meckel diverticulum may contain heterotopic rests of gastric or pancreatic tissue (80% of cases); complications include peptic ulceration, hemorrhage, and diverticulitis*
- *Omphalocele is characterized by a central protrusion of abdominal contents, directly beneath (and with attachment to) the umbilical cord; protruding abdominal organs are covered by a membrane*
- *Omphalocele is typically due to failure of abdominal wall to form rather than to a focal abdominal wall defect, as in gastroschisis*

SELECTED REFERENCES

Dillon PW, Cilley RE: Newborn surgical emergencies: gastrointestinal anomalies, abdominal wall defects. Pediatr Surg 40:1289-1314, 1993.

Dimmick JE, Kalousek DK: Developmental Pathology of the Embryonal Fetus. Philadelphia, JB Lippincott, 1992, p 526.

Rescorla FJ, Shedd FK, Grosfeld JL, et al: Anomalies of intestinal rotation in childhood: analysis of 447 cases. Surgery 108:710-715, 1990.

ENTERIC INFECTIONS IN IMMUNOCOMPETENT HOSTS

Clinical Features

- Populations affected are generally those from underdeveloped countries and immunologically naive travelers to these areas
- Associated with poor sanitation in industrialized nations
- Food- and water-borne illnesses also occur after ingestion of large amounts of bacteria owing to contamination by food handlers or improper preparation or refrigeration and in institutionalized settings

ESCHERICHIA COLI INFECTION
- Pathologic subtypes may not be routinely differentiated from nonpathogenic forms in culture
- May cause prolonged diarrhea; some *E. coli* elaborate an enterotoxin after the bacteria colonize the intestinal epithelium, leading to watery diarrhea and dehydration
- Enterohemorrhagic *E. coli* (e.g., *E. coli* O157:H7) produces a Shiga toxin; this infection is becoming increasingly prevalent in the United States (8% of routine stool cultures); generally occurs in the summer months; severe infection occurs in very young or very old patients who eat contaminated food
- Most infections are mild and self-limited, but hemolytic-uremic syndrome and thrombocytopenic purpura may occur
- At least five other categories of *E. coli* pathogens are recognized
  - Enteroinvasive *E. coli* are associated with a dysentery-like clinical picture
  - Enterotoxigenic, enteropathogenic, enteroaggregative, and diffusely adherent *E. coli* may cause traveler's diarrhea and diarrhea in children

SHIGELLOSIS

- *Shigella* species are virulent invasive gram-negative bacilli that cause bloody diarrhea
- *Shigella dysenteriae* is most common, but infections with *Shigella sonnei* and *Shigella flexneri* are reported
- Associated with fecal contamination of water supply
- Most severe infection seen in infants and children, men who have sex with men (MSM), and malnourished and debilitated individuals

SALMONELLOSIS

- Produces several distinct disease states; the two with primary gastrointestinal involvement are typhoid fever and salmonella gastroenteritis
- Organisms replicate within intracellular vacuoles in enterocytes and macrophages and disseminate systemically
- Typhoid fever
  - Caused by consumption of contaminated food or water
  - Fecal-oral transmission occurs
  - One case per 500,000 people in United States
  - Causes a systemic febrile and diarrheal illness following a 1-week incubation period
  - Complications include massive hemorrhage, peritonitis, and perforation
  - About 15% mortality rate in untreated patients

SALMONELLA GASTROENTERITIS

- Produces febrile diarrheal illness within hours of consumption of food contaminated by one of several types of *Salmonella;* can mimic appendicitis
- Causes 80% of food poisoning incidents
- Strains resistant to multiple antibiotics have arisen as a result of agricultural practices (feed with antibiotic-supplemented grains)

CAMPYLOBACTERIOSIS

- Causes both enteritis and colitis
- Common stool pathogen in infants, teens, and young adults
- Common cause of traveler's diarrhea and illness in hikers who consume untreated mountain water; three times more common than giardiasis in the Rocky Mountains
- *Campylobacter fetus* is a cause of severe systemic illness
- Produces bloody diarrhea up to 1 week after infection
- Complications include meningitis, pseudomembranous colitis, arthropathy, and Guillain-Barré syndrome

CHOLERA

- Produces massive watery diarrhea due to antiabsorptive effect of endotoxin on small intestinal villi
- Incubation period ranges from a few hours to 2 days
- Recovery takes up to 1 week
- Untreated mortality rate of 50% to 75%
- Losses of 15 to 20 L of fluid per day reported (when fluid replacement provided)

YERSINIOSIS

- Can clinically mimic Crohn disease
- Aerobic bacteria present in contaminated food or blood products

- Enterocolitis is the most common clinical manifestation and usually affects young children
- Often associated with mesenteric lymphadenitis
- Fatal infections occur in immunosuppressed patients and patients with iron overload

Gross and Endoscopic Pathology

ESCHERICHIA COLI O157:H7 (ENTEROHEMORRHAGIC E. COLI) (Figure 6-39)

- Hemorrhagic, oozing mucosa, sometimes with ulceration
- Pseudomembranes may be present but are rare
- Generally affects the right side of the colon
- Other *E. coli* pathogens may cause edema or patchy erythema of colon

SHIGELLOSIS

- Typically affects large bowel
- Can see mucosal hemorrhage, ulcer, and occasionally pseudomembranes
- Typical cases show patchy erythema of colonic mucosa

SALMONELLOSIS

- Typhoid fever or *Salmonella* enteritis
  - Longitudinal oval ulcers with elevated edges
  - Ulcers are typically on top of Peyer patches in the terminal ileum
- Nontyphoidal species may cause edema or patchy erythema of colon

CAMPYLOBACTERIOSIS

- Diffuse, hemorrhagic, and focally ulcerative enterocolitis
- Often near ileocecal valve with involvement of Peyer patches

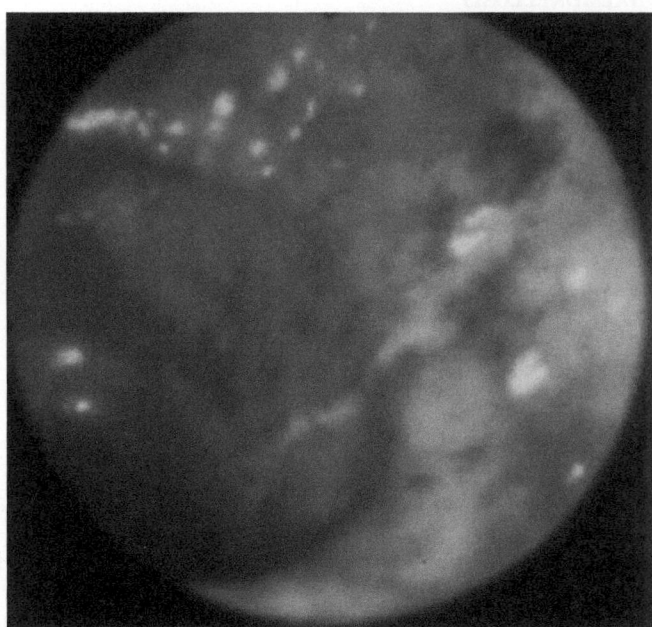

Figure 6-39. *Escherichia coli* **Infection.** A linear shallow ulcer is surrounded by patchy erythematous mucosa.

CHOLERA
- Edematous small bowel mucosa; biopsy rarely done because it adds little to diagnosis or management

YERSINIOSIS
- Diffuse and focal ulcerations and edema in the ileum and colon
- Enlarged mesenteric lymph nodes with foci of necrosis
- Hyperplastic lymphoid follicles in epithelium often with overlying aphthous ulcers

Histopathology

ESCHERICHIA COLI INFECTION INCLUDING E. COLI O157:H7 (ENTEROHEMORRHAGIC E. COLI)
(Figures 6-40 and 6-41)
- Enterohemorrhagic *E. coli* produces both ischemic and infectious colitis (toxin interferes with protein synthesis, causing epithelial and endothelial cell damage)
- Mucosal hemorrhage, infarct, and pseudomembranes can occur
- Focal neutrophilic infiltrates, cryptitis, and crypt abscesses may be present
- Adherent bacteria can be seen in some cases of infection with adherent *E. coli* pathogens

SHIGELLOSIS
- Infective-type pattern of colitis (focal active colitis) characterized by
  - Limited areas of increased inflammatory cells; sometimes seen with focal architectural changes
  - Some areas of biopsy specimen maintain an essentially normal appearance
  - Inflammation is typically acute with patchy cryptitis and neutrophils within the lamina propria without lamina propria plasmacytosis

SALMONELLOSIS
- Typhoid fever or salmonella enteritis
  - Hyperplastic lymphoid follicles with adjacent mucosal hemorrhage, neutrophilic infiltrates, and atrophy and regeneration
  - Progressive hemorrhage and inflammation may produce perforation
  - Can cause focal active colitis pattern of injury

CAMPYLOBACTERIOSIS
- Focal active colitis with neutrophilic infiltrates with cryptitis, hemorrhage, and necrosis

CHOLERA
- Intact mucosa with minimal changes

YERSINIOSIS
- Hyperplastic lymphoid follicles with large germinal centers
- Punctate ulcers with neutrophilic fissures over hyperplastic lymphoid follicles (similar to Crohn disease)
- Suppurative epithelioid granulomas in bowel wall and regional lymph nodes
- Acute cryptitis occurs in colon

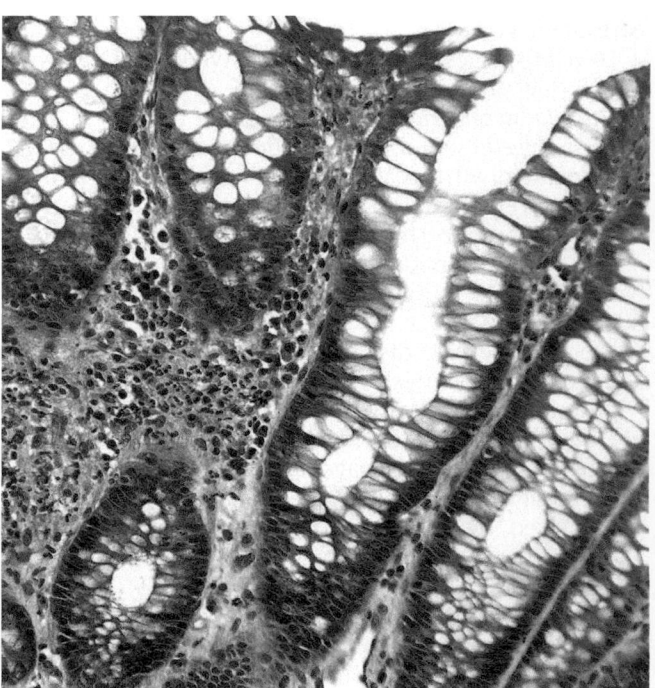

Figure 6-40. Enterohemorrhagic *Escherichia coli* infection showing the infectious pattern of injury with neutrophils loose within the lamina propria.

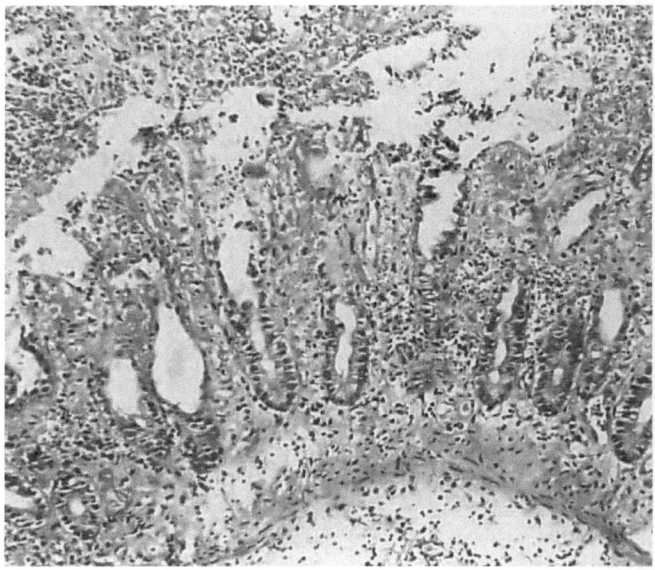

Figure 6-41. Acute ischemic colitis pattern of injury in a patient with enterohemorrhagic *Escherichia coli* infection. There is superficial coagulative necrosis and hemorrhage of the colonic mucosa associated with inflammatory pseudomembrane formation. There is preservation of the deep colonic crypts.

Special Stains and Immunohistochemistry
- Organisms are not reliably detected with histologic stains; Gram-negative organisms can sometimes be seen with yersiniosis

Other Techniques for Diagnosis
- Pathogenic *Escherichia coli*
  - Requires sophisticated techniques such as a serotyping, PCR, or DNA hybridization for diagnosis, although

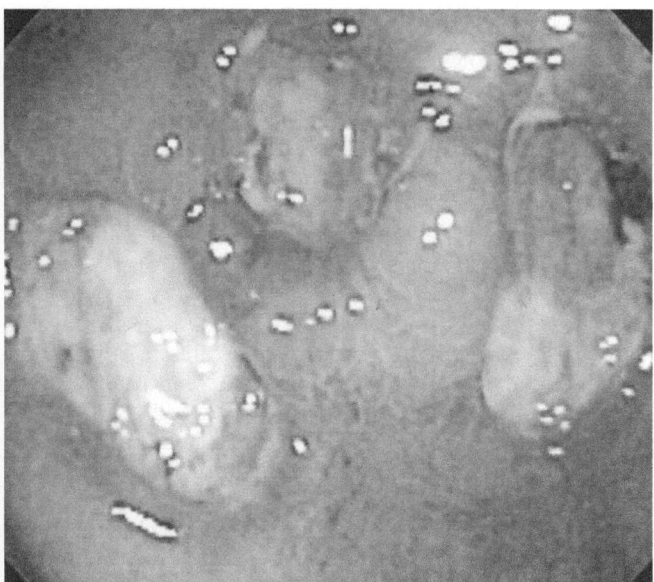

Figure 6-42. Endoscopic photograph of cytomegalovirus-associated colitis showing three well-circumscribed "punched-out" ulcers.

E. coli O157:H7 can be detected from stool culture using selective growth media and serologic techniques
- Pathogenic bacteria are best characterized using microbiologic techniques, serum antibody assays, or occasionally PCR in biopsy specimens

Differential Diagnosis

ENTEROHEMORRHAGIC *ESCHERICHIA COLI*, *CAMPYLOBACTER* SPECIES, AND *SALMONELLA* SPECIES INFECTION VERSUS INFLAMMATORY BOWEL DISEASE, ISCHEMIC COLITIS, AND PSEUDOMEMBRANOUS COLITIS

- Inflammatory bowel disease
  - Characterized by a similar neutrophilic infiltrate but distinguished by a more diffuse involvement, less mucosal hemorrhage, basal plasmacytosis, and greater glandular changes (mucin depletion, gland distortion)
  - Giant cells may be present in any infection, but not the well-formed noncaseating granulomas seen in Crohn disease
  - Suppurative granulomas may be seen with *Campylobacter* species infection
- Ischemic colitis
  - Characterized by superficial necrosis and less acute inflammation than infectious enterocolitis
  - Clinical history and symptoms are often suggestive of ischemia
- Pseudomembranous colitis (*Clostridium difficile*–associated colitis)
  - May be histologically indistinguishable from other causes of infectious colitis
  - Pseudomembrane is composed of desquamated epithelial cells, inflammatory cells, and fibrin material
  - Requires clinical history (i.e., previous antibiotic use) and diagnostic tests for identification
  - Diagnosis is based on detection of toxins (toxin A and toxin B) or nucleic acid amplification tests; culture is not helpful

YERSINIA SPECIES INFECTION VERSUS CROHN DISEASE

- Similar clinical involvement of the terminal ileum with aphthous ulcers
- Crohn disease typically does not produce the extensive suppurative granulomas seen with *Yersinia* species

PEARLS

- Campylobacter *species infection may be complicated by meningitis, Guillain-Barré syndrome, and pseudomembranous colitis*
- Yersinia *species infection is generally associated with mesenteric lymphadenitis*
- Aeromonads, Klebsiella *species, and mycobacterial infection can cause enterocolitis*

SELECTED REFERENCES

Griffin P, Olmstead L, Petras R: *Escherichia coli* O157:H7-associated colitis: a clinical and histologic study of 11 cases. Gastroenterology 99:142-149, 1990.
Lamps LW: Infective disorders of the gastrointestinal tract. Histopathology 50:55-63, 2007.
Nataro JP, Kaper JB: Diarrheogenic *Escherichia coli*. Clin Microbiol Rev 11:142-210, 1998.
Norstrant TT, Kumar NB, Appelman HD: Histopathology differentiates acute self-limited colitis from ulcerative colitis. Gastroenterology 92:318-328, 1987.

INFECTIONS IN IMMUNOCOMPROMISED PATIENTS

Clinical Features

- Enteric infections are common in immunocompromised patients, particularly patients with AIDS; other causes include the following:
  - Transplantation (solid organ and bone marrow)
  - Cancer chemotherapy
  - Autoimmune diseases (treated with steroids)
  - Advanced age
  - Diabetes
  - Long-term antibiotic use
  - Hemodialysis
  - Postoperative complications
  - Indwelling vascular devices
- Infection may occur at any level of the gastrointestinal tract, and symptoms depend on level infected
  - Esophageal infections: dysphagia, odynophagia, chest pain
  - Gastric infections: nausea, vomiting, abdominal pain
  - Intestinal infections: diarrhea
- Complications include bleeding, obstruction, and perforation
- In AIDS patients, about one half of all diarrheal episodes are due to infections; some of the remaining episodes are due to AIDS enteropathy (syndrome characterized by chronic diarrhea, malnutrition, and wasting without evidence of gastrointestinal infection)
  - Fungal, parasitic, bacterial, and viral infections are all common in untreated AIDS and immunocompromised patients

Gross and Endoscopic Pathology

VIRAL INFECTIONS

- CMV: variable, often discrete, ulcers affecting the esophagus, stomach, or intestines (Figure 6-42)
- HSV: painful ulcers or vesicles, often in esophagus, low rectum and anus and perianal skin
- Adenovirus: nonspecific appearance

PARASITIC INFECTIONS

- Giardiasis (*Giardia intestinalis*): nonspecific changes
- Coccidiosis (Cryptosporidium parvum, Isospora belli, and Cyclospora cayetanensis)
  - *Cryptosporidium* and *Isospora* species are most commonly found in patients with AIDS
  - Cyclosporidiosis is more commonly traveler's diarrhea or associated with contaminated food (e.g., imported fruit)
  - All show mild, nonspecific features
- Microsporidiosis (*Enterocytozoon bieneusi* and *Encephalitozoon intestinalis*): mild, nonspecific abnormalities in small bowel

FUNGAL INFECTIONS

- Candidiasis
  - Most common cause of esophagitis in AIDS patients
  - Esophagus is most common site (affects small bowel in disseminated disease)
  - Forms adherent, white-brown plaques with mucosal hyperemia and ulceration
  - May completely denude esophagus
- Aspergillosis
  - Typically involves esophagus, although rare in gastrointestinal tract
  - Often produces necrotic ulcers (due to angioinvasive properties resulting in ischemia)
- Mucormycosis
  - Often produces extensive necrosis (due to angioinvasive properties resulting in ischemia); rarely in gastrointestinal tract
- Histoplasmosis
  - May spread to esophagus and elsewhere from lung
  - Rarely causes esophageal perforation or esophagobronchial fistula

BACTERIAL INFECTIONS

- Bacterial pathogens common to the immunocompromised host include *Salmonella, Shigella,* and *Campylobacter* species (may be difficult to eradicate in AIDS patients)
- Intestinal spirochetosis typically involves the colon diffusely, usually with no endoscopic abnormality; more often seen in immune competent individuals in whom it may be considered a commensal
- Tuberculosis causes shallow ulcers with confluent granulomas; most commonly involves ileocecal region (90%)
- *Mycobacterium avium-intracellulare* (MAI): causes poorly delineated, often plaquelike lesions anywhere in gastrointestinal tract

NONINFECTIOUS AIDS-RELATED ENTEROPATHY

- Often has minimal changes at endoscopy

Histopathology

VIRAL INFECTIONS

- CMV
  - Variable, but often mild mixed inflammation with ulceration and characteristic nuclear or cytoplasmic inclusions typically in endothelial or mesenchymal cells (Figure 6-43)
  - Rarely causes severe disease with vasculitis and intestinal perforation
- HSV
  - In esophageal and perianal lesions, acute inflammation, and necrosis predominate; classic multinucleated cells, acantholysis, and nuclear inclusions in squamous epithelium may be observed
- Adenovirus
  - Mild, nonspecific chronic inflammation in colon with dystrophic goblet cells containing amorphic nuclei and rarely containing diagnostic inclusion bodies

PARASITE INFECTIONS

- Giardiasis
  - Pear-shaped organism similar in size to an enterocyte nucleus (Figure 6-44)
  - Trophozoite has two symmetrical nuclei ("monkey face")
  - Organisms are generally found along the luminal border and induce a variable mucosal inflammatory infiltrate
- Coccidial infections
  - Cryptosporidium parvum (Figure 6-45)
    - Basophilic dotlike organisms (1 to 3 μm) attached to luminal border (brush border) of small intestinal or colonic epithelial cells

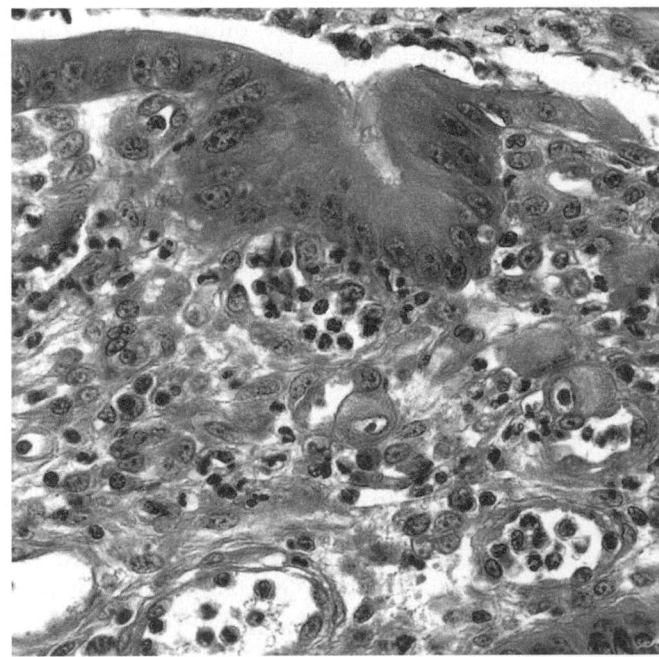

Figure 6-43. Cytomegalovirus-associated colitis showing infected stromal cells with cytomegaly, cytoplasmic inclusions, and prominent intranuclear inclusions with surrounding halo.

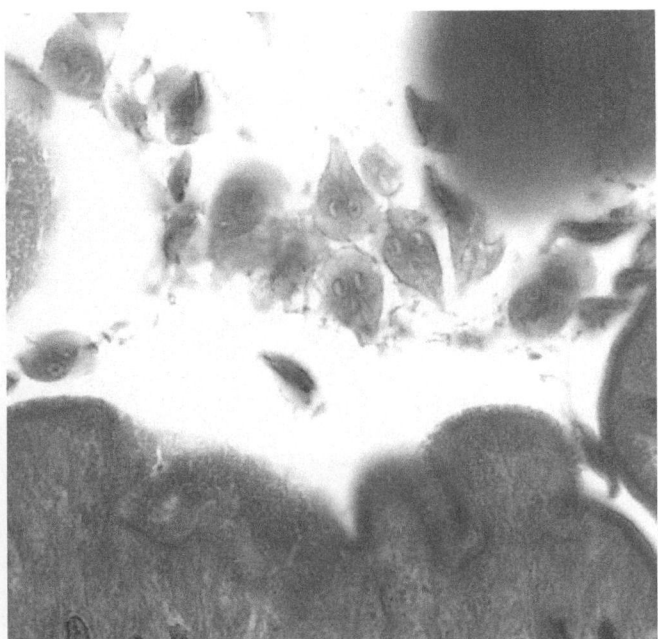

Figure 6-44. Giardiasis. *Giardia lamblia* organisms en face appear pear shaped with paired nuclei.

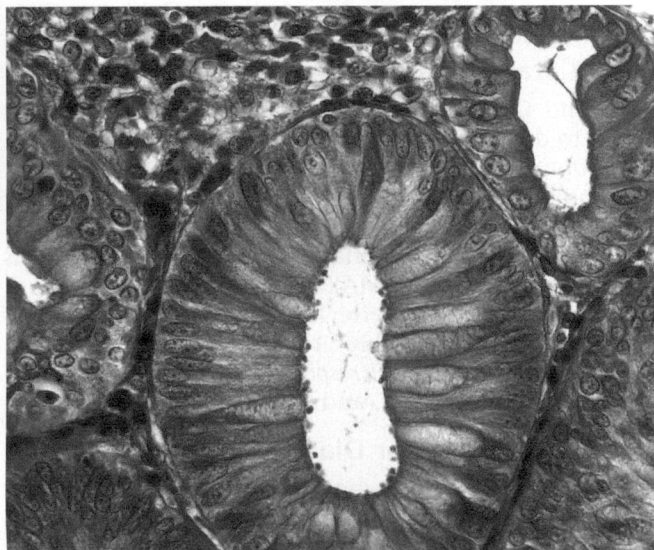

Figure 6-45. Cryptosporidiosis showing developmental forms attached to cell surfaces.

- Usually minimal associated chronic inflammation and variable villous abnormalities; mild villous shortening may be seen
- Isospora belli
  - Coccidia are tiny ovoid structures within the epithelial cells of the intestinal villi (may be difficult to detect); merozoites are banana shaped
- Cyclospora cayetanensis
  - Tiny ovoid structures (2 to 3 μm) in enterocytes (similar to *Isospora* species)
- Microsporidiosis
  - Two forms
    - Mature spores appear as a cluster of dotlike structures (1.5 μm) in the apical cytoplasm of epithelial

cell in the small bowel or colon (often difficult to detect)
- Larger nucleated sporont (3 to 5 μm) is a basophilic structure in epithelial cells near the villus tips; may cause nuclear indentation

FUNGAL INFECTIONS
- Candidiasis
  - Acantholysis with superficial neutrophils within squamous epithelium; can be associated with focal squamous epithelial lymphocytosis
  - Mucosal ulceration with neutrophilic infiltrates in severe cases
  - Yeast and pseudohyphae form within necrotic debris
  - Invasion of submucosa verifies significant disease
  - Invasive disease is characterized by mixture of dimorphic forms, including the 3- to 5-μm blastoconidia (budding oval yeasts) and pseudohyphae (elongated blastoconidia with indentation at pseudosepta representing several separate yeast organisms)
  - True hyphae may form (one elongated organism with parallel walls and no indentation at true septa); branching is absent
- Aspergillosis
  - Often admixed with necrotic or infarcted debris owing to ischemia caused by the angioinvasive properties of the fungus
  - Dichotomous branching at 45-degree angles; 2- to 4-μm-wide hyphae with parallel walls and true septa
  - Rarely seen in surgical or biopsy specimens
- Mucormycosis
  - Wide (10 to 20 μm) aseptate hyphae that are irregularly branched and often create folded, ribbon-like structures
  - Rarely seen in surgical or biopsy specimens
- Histoplasmosis
  - May cause granuloma formation or diffuse collections of histiocytes in the lamina propria
  - Intracellular organisms are 2 to 3 μm
  - Granulomatous inflammation can mimic Crohn disease

BACTERIAL INFECTIONS
- Syphilis and lymphogranuloma venereum
  - Usually a proctitis or anorectal inflammation; can mimic inflammatory bowel disease or neoplasia clinically
  - Associated with intense lymphohistiocytic infiltrate, prominent plasma cells, and lymphoid aggregates without architectural distortion or marked acute inflammation
  - Silver stains and immunohistochemistry for Treponema pallidum not sensitive
  - Diagnosis requires serum testing or special studies on rectal swabs
- Spirochetosis
  - Organisms form a basophilic haze on the luminal surface of colonic biopsy specimens (Figure 6-46)
  - Can be verified with silver stains (e.g., Warthin-Starry) or immunostains for *Treponema* species
- Tuberculosis
  - Ulceration and necrotizing granulomas with Langhans giant cells

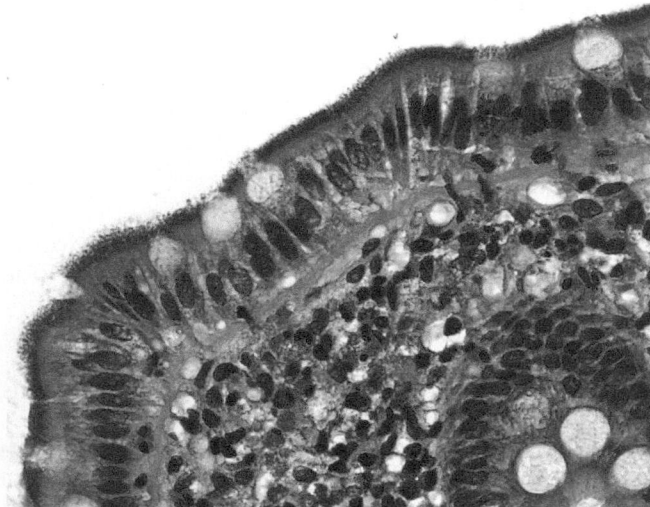

Figure 6-46. Intestinal spirochetosis showing numerous organisms attached to the brushed border.

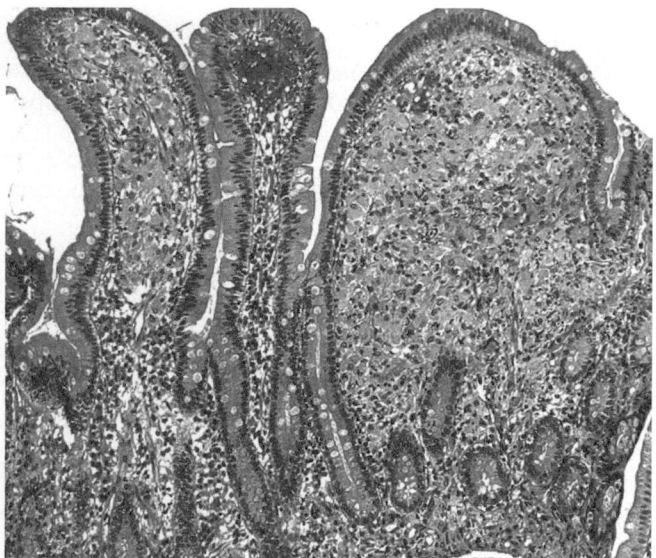

Figure 6-47. *Mycobacterium avium-intracellulare* complex infection involving proximal small intestine. The lamina propria is variably expanded with foamy macrophages.

- MAI
  - Lamina propria contains foamy histiocytes stuffed with acid-fast bacilli (AFB; modified AFB) (Figures 6-47 and 6-48)

AIDS-RELATED ENTEROPATHY
- Nonspecific apoptosis, chronic inflammation, and villous atrophy due to HIV infections of enterocytes and other cells
- Regenerating immature cells have no microvilli
- Noninfectious esophageal ulcers
- Range of histologic features, including focal edema, apoptotic cells, and dense neutrophilic inflammation with erosion
- Erosion may produce large ulcers that are potentially life threatening

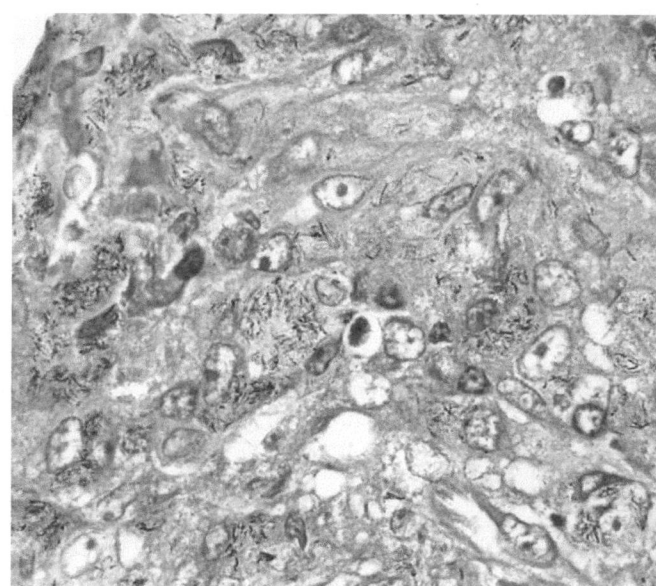

Figure 6-48. *Mycobacterium avium-intracellulare* complex infection (acid-fast stain).

- Electron microscopy reveals viral particles, presumed to be HIV, in mononuclear cells
- Rarely seen since advent of aggressive antiretroviral therapy

Special Stains and Immunohistochemistry
- PAS and GMS: fungal structures are highlighted (best used to detect fungi within ulcerated or necrotic tissue in esophageal and gastric biopsy specimens)
- Giemsa: highlights *Cryptosporidium*, *Isospora*, and *Microsporidium* species
- Trichrome: helps differentiate *Giardia* species from mucus
- Modified AFB: detects MAI infection
- Warthin-Starry or Dieterle: highlights spirochetes
- Immunostains available for CMV (useful), HSV, *Cryptosporidium* and *Microsporidia* species (immunofluorescence), adenovirus, and *Cyclospora* species

Other Techniques for Diagnosis
- PCR available for numerous microorganisms, including CMV and *Microsporidia* species; may work in paraffin blocks
- Diagnosis of parasitic infections is readily made by detecting oocytes or cyst forms in stool specimens; AFB stain detects oocyst of *Cryptosporidia* species in stool samples (not in histologic sections)
- Electron microscopy: may be helpful to identify and speciate some microorganisms (e.g., *Microsporidium* species)

Differential Diagnosis
- Gastrointestinal infection is the foremost consideration in immunocompromised hosts

KAPOSI SARCOMA
- Prevalent in AIDS patients; relatively common in gastrointestinal tract
- Characterized by macular red lesions, composed of a spindle cell proliferation in the lamina propria containing extravasated red blood cells in slitlike spaces
- Immunohistochemistry for HHV-8 diagnostic

WHIPPLE DISEASE

- Closely simulates MAI with PAS-positive foamy histiocytes
- Lacks fat vacuoles and AFB positivity characteristic of MAI infection

PEARLS

- *Even though the patient is immunocompromised, there is usually some inflammation*
- *Consider an opportunistic infection when you see inflammation that you are unable otherwise to account for (even if the patient is not known to be immunocompromised)*
- *Small blue dots in a row on the surface of enterocytes: think of cryptosporidiosis*
- *Small blue dots in the enterocyte: think of microsporidiosis*
- *Blue haze on surface of colonic cells: think of spirochetosis*
- *When mesenchymal cells look too big or there are subtle erosions or inflammation, check mesenchymal cells—particularly endothelial cells—for CMV inclusions*
- *Do not confuse luminal mucin globules for Cryptosporidium species (C. parvum are deeper blue on H&E stain, and generally there are many organisms of equal size along the luminal surface) or for Giardia species (trichrome stain can help)*
- *Giardiasis is common in immune competent patients and is also associated with selective IgA immunodeficiency and common variable immunodeficiency disease (CVID); look for plasma cells and nodular lymphoid hyperplasia; giardiasis can be found in ileal biopsy specimens*
- *Mentally rule out infection in every small bowel biopsy specimen*
- *Consider immunostain for CMV, AFB, and PAS or GMS for gastrointestinal biopsies (unless the tissue is perfectly normal and the endoscopy detected no lesions) in immunocompromised patients*

SELECTED REFERENCES

Arnold CA, Limketkai BN, Illei PB, et al: Syphilitic and lymphogranuloma venereum (LGV) proctocolitis. Am J Surg Pathol 37:38-46, 2013.

Calderaro A, Bommezzadri S, Gorrini C, et al: Infective colitis associated with human intestinal spirochetosis. J Gastroenterol Hepatol 22:1772-1779, 2007.

Greenberg PD, Koch J, Cello JP: Diagnosis of *Cryptosporidium parvum* in patients with severe diarrhea and AIDS. Dig Dis Sci 41:2286-2290, 1996.

Greenson JK, Belitos PC, Yardley JH, Bartlett JG: AIDS enteropathy: occult enteric infections and duodenal mucosal alterations in chronic diarrhea. Ann Intern Med 114:366-372, 1991.

Gutierrez Y: Diagnostic Pathology of Parasitic Infections with Clinical Correlations. Philadelphia, Lea & Febiger, 1990.

Orenstein JM, Chlang J, Steinberg W, et al: Intestinal microsporidiosis as a cause of diarrhea in human immunodeficiency virus-infected patients. Hum Pathol 21:475-481, 1990.

Strom RL, Gruninger RP: AIDS with *Mycobacterium avium-intracellulare* lesions resembling those of Whipple's disease. N Engl J Med 309:1324, 1983.

Varma M, Hester JD, Schaefer FW 3rd, et al: Detection of *Cyclospora cayetanensis* using a quantitative real-time PCR assay. J Microbiol Methods 53:27-36, 2003.

WHIPPLE DISEASE

Clinical Features

- Rare (approximately 30 cases per year worldwide), chronic systemic illness with prominent gastrointestinal symptoms
- Commonly affects white adults between 40 and 60 years of age; strong male predominance
- More common in people of North American and European ancestry
- May involve any organ of the body, most commonly the gastrointestinal tract, joints, and central nervous system
- Common associations
  - Malabsorption and diarrhea
  - Abdominal pain
  - Weight loss
  - Polyarthralgia
  - Peripheral lymphadenopathy
  - Cardiac dysfunction
  - Central nervous system disease (10%)
- Characteristically responsive to antibiotics; often fatal without treatment

Gross and Endoscopic Pathology

- Widespread infiltration of organs by mixed infiltrate consisting of foamy histiocytes, causing the following:
  - Yellowish mucosal plaques in small bowel
  - Occasional shallow ulcers and hemorrhage
  - Thickened bowel wall
  - Enlarged mesenteric and retroperitoneal lymph nodes
  - Hepatosplenomegaly
  - Mesenteric fat and peritoneal plaques

Histopathology

- Lamina propria, muscularis mucosae, and superficial submucosa infiltrated by PAS, diastase-resistant-positive, foamy histiocytes, which contain the Whipple bacillus (Figure 6-49)
- Intestinal villi are blunted by histiocytic infiltrate other than the histiocytes
- Typically minimal or no associated inflammatory infiltrate
- Characteristic large open round spaces in mucosa and submucosa (so-called fat vacuoles), although some represent dilated lymphatics
- Regional lymph nodes may contain foamy histiocytes
- Foreign-body epithelioid granulomas and lipogranulomas are sometimes seen in gastrointestinal mucosa, lymph nodes, spleen, muscles, lung, kidney, and brain
- May simulate organizing fat necrosis in retroperitoneum

Special Stains and Immunohistochemistry

- Diastase-resistant PAS stain: Whipple bacilli within histiocytes are strongly positive; stain is coarsely granular, and bacillary structure cannot be seen (Figure 6-50)
- AFB stain negative
- A specific immunohistochemical stain is available but not widely used

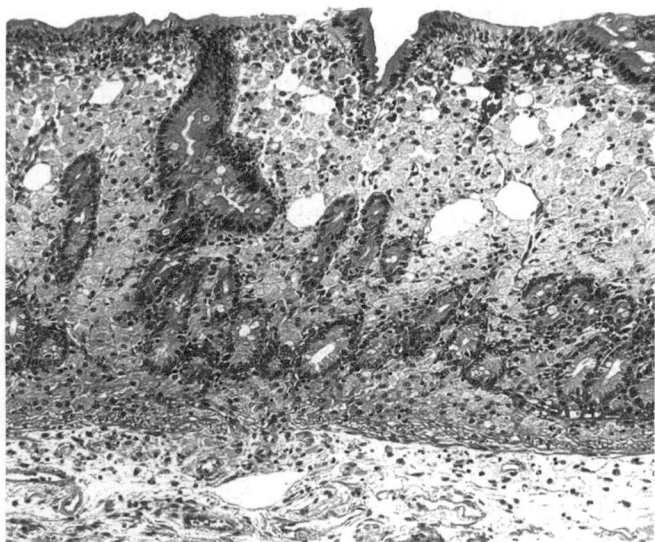

Figure 6-49. Whipple disease within duodenum biopsy specimen. Histologic section shows flattening of the villi and an expansion of the lamina propria by foamy macrophages with fat vacuoles.

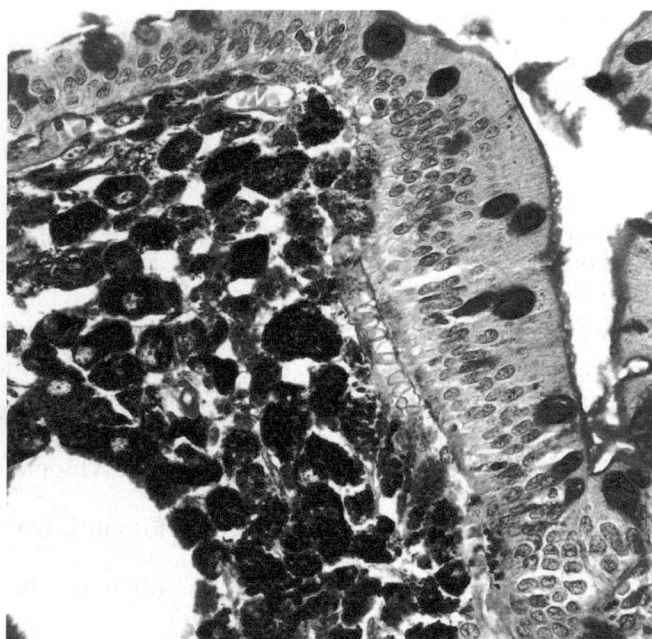

Figure 6-50. Whipple disease. Periodic acid-Schiff stain shows brightly staining, coarsely granular intracytoplasmic inclusions.

Other Techniques for Diagnosis

- PCR: used to sequence the bacterial *16s* ribosomal gene
- Electron microscopy: demonstrates bacterial rods in macrophage cytoplasm
- Has been cultured using special techniques

Differential Diagnosis

MAI INFECTION

- Similar histologic profile with sheets of foamy histiocyte-like cells in the lamina propria
- Differs in the conspicuous absence of fat vacuoles and dilated lymphatics

- Is faintly PAS positive; bacillary shape can still be seen
- More commonly seen in immunocompromised patients

HISTOPLASMOSIS

- Characterized by presence of well-formed granulomas and infiltrates of histiocytes with less "foamy" cytoplasm
- Intracellular, 2- to 3-μm organisms seen with PAS or silver stain

WALDENSTROM MACROGLOBULINEMIA

- Foamy macrophages in lamina propria
- Differs in lack of robust granular staining of macrophages by PAS
- Differs from Whipple disease by showing dilated lymphatics filled with eosinophilic material

PEARLS

- *Whipple disease is caused by a gram-positive bacillus called* Tropheryma whippelii

SELECTED REFERENCES

Arnold CA, Moreira RK, Lam-Himlin D, et al: Whipple disease a century after the initial description: increased recognition of unusual presentations, autoimmune comorbidities, and therapy effects. Am J Surg Pathol 36:1066-1073, 2012.

Baisden BL, Lepidi H, Raoult D, et al: Diagnosis of Whipple disease by immunohistochemical analysis. Am J Clin Pathol 118:742-748, 2002.

Dobbins WO III: Whipple's Disease. Springfield, IL, Charles C. Thomas, 1987.

Relman DA, Schmidt TM, MacDermott RP, Falkow S: Identification of the uncultured bacillus of Whipple's disease. N Engl J Med 327:293-301, 1992.

CELIAC SPRUE

Clinical Features

- Also called gluten-sensitive enteropathy or celiac disease
- Malabsorptive disorder related to immunologic reaction to the toxic component of cereal grains, the gliadin-related proteins in wheat, rye, and barley
- Genetic predisposition in people of Irish and Northern European descent; much more common in whites; prevalence in the United States could be as high as 1%
- Classic presentation includes diarrhea, steatorrhea, flatulence, weight loss, and fatigue; failure to thrive may be seen in infants
- Can also present with iron or folate deficiency, anorexia, bone pain related to osteoporosis, and infertility
- Serologic testing includes IgA antiendomysial and anti-tissue transglutaminase antibody test; both are sensitive and specific; the latter is considered the screening test of choice
- Detecting antibodies against deaminated gliadin peptides (DGP) can help detect celiac sprue in otherwise seronegative patients, especially those with low IgA levels
- Strong association with HLA-DQ2 (more than 98% of cases) and HLA-DQ8 (the other 2%)

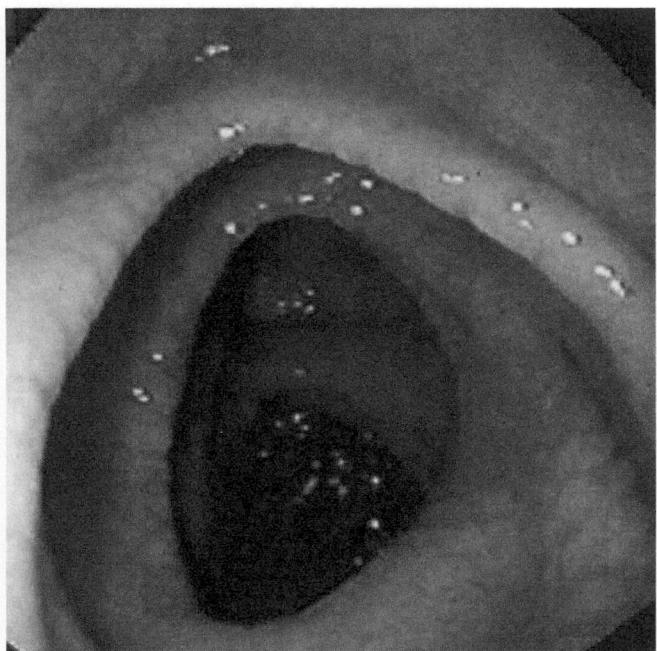

Figure 6-51. Endoscopic photograph of duodenum showing scalloped valvulae conniventes of celiac sprue.

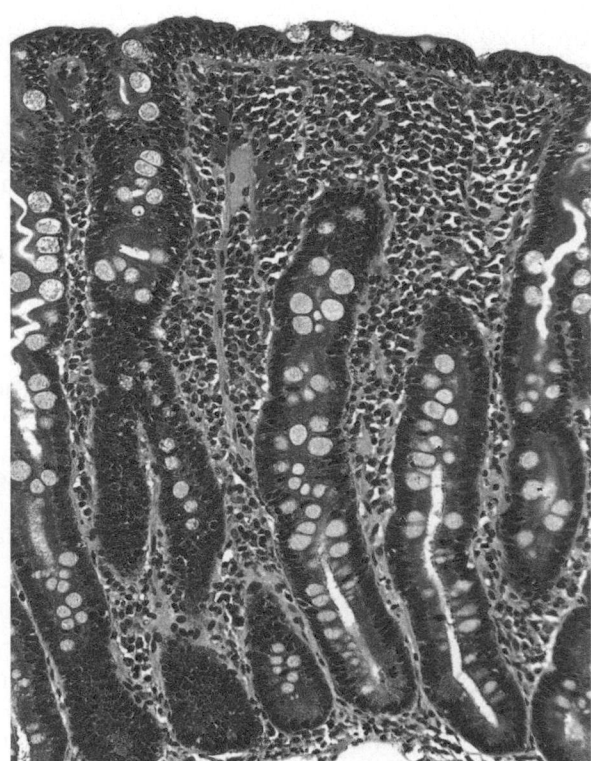

Figure 6-52. Celiac sprue. Histologic section shows a diffuse severe villous abnormality with crypt hyperplasia and epithelial lymphocytosis. The lamina propria is expanded by chronic inflammatory cells, including plasma cells.

Gross and Endoscopic Pathology

- Flattened mucosa typically most prominent in the proximal small intestine; may show scalloping of the valvulae conniventes (Figure 6-51)

Histopathology (Figures 6-52 and 53)

- Characteristic features include shortening of villi and transformation of tall, absorptive enterocytes interspersed with goblet cells and occasional intraepithelial lymphocytes into nonabsorptive low-cuboidal epithelium with nuclear stratification, few goblet cells, and many (>30 per 100 enterocytes but usually >40) intraepithelial lymphocytes
- Surface epithelium shows loss of brush border, and crypts typically show increased mitotic activity
- Secondary features include crypt elongation and hyperplasia
- Lamina propria contains mixed inflammatory infiltrate (T and B lymphocytes, plasma cells, and eosinophils)

Special Stains and Immunohistochemistry

- Immunostain for CD3 can be used to evaluate intraepithelial component and may be helpful in recognizing epithelial lymphocytosis; immunostaining for CD3 is not recommended
- Alcian blue/PAS with a hematoxylin counterstain can be useful to exclude Whipple disease and to detect foveolar metaplasia
- Immunostaining for CD3, CD5, and CD8 should be considered in patients with refractory sprue

Other Techniques for Diagnosis

- Molecular evaluation (e.g., T cell gene rearrangements) should be considered in patients with refractory sprue or in celiac sprue patients developing small intestinal ulcers

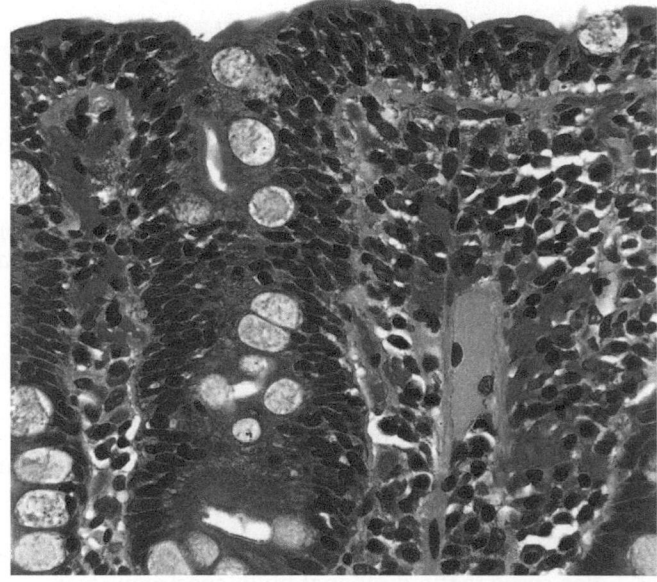

Figure 6-53. Celiac sprue at high magnification emphasizing the intraepithelial lymphocytosis.

Differential Diagnosis

NORMAL MUCOSA

- Malabsorption can be seen with normal small bowel histology (e.g., disaccharidase deficiency)

- Normal villous to crypt ratio of 3:1 to 5:1
- Up to 20 intraepithelial lymphocytes are considered normal

LYMPHOCYTIC ENTEROCOLITIS

- Coexisting lymphocytic colitis and celiac spruelike lesion of the proximal small bowel that is not responsive to gluten withdrawal

REFRACTORY OR UNCLASSIFIED SPRUE

- Refractory to gluten withdrawal for 12 months
  - Refractory sprue type I
    - No atypical lymphocytes
    - Normal surface CD3, CD5, and CD8 intraepithelial lymphocytes
    - Polyclonal T-cell receptor
    - Many respond to azathioprine, prednisone, budesonide, or mesalamine
    - Low rate of progression to enteropathy-associated T-cell lymphoma
  - Refractory sprue type II
    - May have scattered atypical lymphocytes
    - Loss of surface CD3 or CD8 (> 50% of CD3+/CD8−) intraepithelial lymphocytes); aberrant loss of CD5 expression
    - Monoclonal T-cell receptor gene rearrangement (cryptic T-cell lymphoma)
    - Not responsive to azathioprine, prednisone, or interleukin-10 (IL-10)
    - May respond to cladribine, anti-CD52, chemotherapy and stem cell transplantation
    - About 50% fatality rate, with most cases developing enteropathy-associated T-cell lymphoma
- Allergic reaction to protein other than gluten

ENTITIES ASSOCIATED WITH VARIABLE VILLOUS ABNORMALITY WITH INTRAEPITHELIAL LYMPHOCYTOSIS (>30 LYMPHOCYTES PER 100 ENTEROCYTES) (Figure 6-54)

- Latent or partially treated celiac sprue (about 10% of patients)
- Tropical sprue (2% of patients)
  - Occurs in natives and naive visitors to specific tropical locations (e.g., India, Africa, Southeast Asia, Central America, West Indies)
  - Treated with broad-spectrum antibiotics (believed to be infectious etiology) and vitamins
- Dermatitis herpetiformis
- Infectious gastroenteritis and stasis
- Peptic ulceration/*H. pylori* infection
  - Four to six biopsy specimens from the duodenum and duodenal bulb are recommended to rule out celiac sprue
  - Although the most sensitive site for diagnosis of celiac sprue is the duodenal bulb, specimens from this area must be interpreted with caution because the area is prone to peptic injury
  - Alcian Blue/PAS stain with a hematoxylin counterstain can be useful in detecting foveolar metaplasia seen in peptic duodenitis
- Autoimmune diseases (e.g., rheumatoid arthritis, Graves disease, Crohn disease)

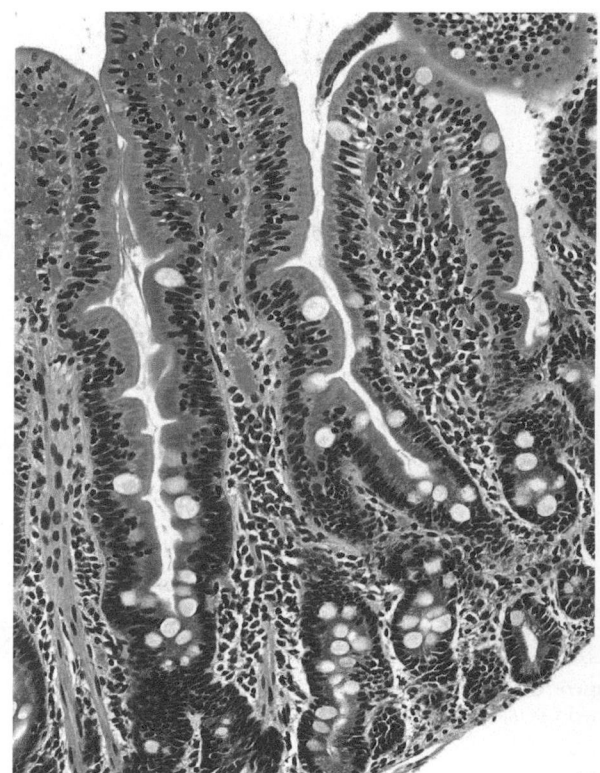

Figure 6-54. Duodenal intraepithelial lymphocytosis. This variable villous abnormality shows villi of near-normal length with increased (> 30 per 100 enterocytes) intraepithelial lymphocytes.

- Drug-related lesions (e.g., NSAIDs, olmesartan)
- Autoimmune enteritis
  - X-linked severe form due to germline mutation of FOXP3 gene can be associated with immune dysregulation and polyendocrinopathy
  - Can have circulating antibodies to enterocytes, goblet cells, parietal cells, and smooth muscle cells
  - Absence of goblet cells and lack of intraepithelial lymphocytosis coupled with a nonresponsiveness to a gluten-free diet can be clues to the diagnosis

ENTITIES ASSOCIATED WITH SEVERE VILLOUS ABNORMALITY AND CRYPT HYPOPLASIA

- Kwashiorkor, marasmus
- Megaloblastic anemia
- Radiation and chemotherapy effect
- Microvillus inclusion disease

ENTITIES ASSOCIATED WITH VARIABLE VILLOUS ABNORMALITY THAT CONTAIN SPECIFIC DIAGNOSTIC CHANGES

- Collagenous sprue
  - Increased subepithelial collagen plate (> 10 μm)
  - Often refractory to gluten withdrawal
  - Can also be associated with drugs (e.g., olmesartan)
- Common variable immune deficiency and selective IgA immunodeficiency
  - Reduced numbers of plasma cells within the lamina propria +/− nodular lymphoid hyperplasia
  - Increased apoptotic bodies
  - May have comorbid giardiasis

- Eosinophilic gastroenteritis
- Parasitic infestation
- Waldenstrom macroglobulinemia
  - Lymphangiectasia with intralymphatic amorphous eosinophilic material
  - Foamy macrophages in lamina propria
- Lymphangiectasia
- Abetalipoproteinemia
  - Enterocytes with intracytoplasmic vacuoles

PEARLS

- *Diagnosis is best made by correlation of clinical history with serology and histologic features (documentation of malabsorption, characteristic histologic features, and improvement of symptoms and resolution of histologic abnormalities on removal of gluten from the diet)*
- *Removal of gluten from the diet is typically curative*
- *Withdrawal of gluten causes a return to normal that progresses from distal to proximal (i.e., duodenum is the last to recover); must consider where biopsy is taken from when evaluating recovery*
- *Fundamental pathology is derived from an immunologic attack on surface enterocytes (transformation to nonabsorptive, low-cuboidal cells with stratified nuclei and numerous interspersed lymphocytes)*
- *Always consider T-cell lymphoma in patients who present with refractory sprue or in celiac sprue patients who have developed small intestinal ulcers (perform immunohistochemistry or PCR)*

SELECTED REFERENCES

Bao F, Green PHR, Bhagat G: An update on celiac disease histopathology and the road ahead. Arch Pathol Lab Med 136:735-745, 2012.

Cellier C, Cerf-Bensussan N: Treatment of clonal refractory celiac disease or cryptic intraepithelial lymphoma: a long road from bench to bedside. Clin Gastroenterol Hepatol 4:1320-1321, 2006.

Freeman HJ, Chopra A, Clandinin MT, Thomson AB: Recent advances in celiac disease. World J Gastroenterol 17:2259-2272, 2011.

Katzin WE, Petras RE: The small intestine. In Mills SE (ed): Histology for Pathologists, 4th ed. Philadelphia, Lippincott, Williams & Wilkins, 2012, pp 647-671.

Petras R, Gramlich T: Non-neoplastic intestinal diseases. In Mills SE (ed): Sternberg's Diagnostic Surgical Pathology, 5th ed. New York, Lippincott, Williams, & Wilkins, 2010, pp 1313-1367.

Rostom A, Murray JA, Kagnoff MF: American Gastroenterological Association (AGA) Institute technical review on the diagnosis and management of celiac disease. Gastroenterology 131:1981-2002, 2006.

Rubio-Tapia A, Hill ID, Kelly CP, et al: ACG clinical guidelines: diagnosis and management of celiac disease. Am J Gastroenterol 108:656-76, 2013.

SMALL INTESTINAL ADENOMA AND ADENOCARCINOMA

Clinical Features

- Can be sporadic and proximal in older patients
- Primary adenomas and adenocarcinomas that occur in the small intestine, especially in younger patients, can be associated with underlying conditions such as the FAP syndromes (FAP, attenuated FAP, and MUTYH-associated polyposis syndrome) and Lynch syndrome
- Adenocarcinoma of the distal small bowel can be a complication of Crohn disease

- More common small bowel malignancies are metastases, lymphoma, and carcinoid tumor

ADENOMA

- Small intestinal adenomas are extremely rare (< 0.05% of all intestinal adenomas)
- Often admixed with adenocarcinoma (65% of all small bowel adenomas)
- Most arise around the major duodenal papilla and present with biliary colic, cholangitis, jaundice, and pancreatitis
- Patients with the familial adenomatous polyposis syndromes have up to a 300 times greater risk for developing carcinoma than nonpolyposis patients

ADENOCARCINOMA

- Far less common than colonic adenocarcinoma
- Risk factors include Lynch syndrome, Peutz-Jeghers syndrome, and Crohn disease
- More common in black men; mean age at diagnosis is 55 years
- Most cases occur in duodenum near major duodenal papilla; Crohn disease–associated adenocarcinoma tends to involve the ileum
- Symptoms include obstruction or bleeding as well as jaundice and pancreatitis

Gross and Endoscopic Pathology

ADENOMA

- Typically multilobulated and soft
- May be pedunculated or sessile
- Tubular adenomas tend to be small (< 3 cm)
- Villous adenomas are more common and are larger (mean, 5 cm)
- Adenomas in patients with FAP associated syndromes are often multiple

ADENOCARCINOMA

- About 25% of lesions are polypoid
- About 75% are ulcerated
- Range in size from less than 2 cm up to 15 cm
- Those described with Crohn disease are often strictured

Histopathology

ADENOMA

- Recapitulates histology of colonic adenomas with tubular, tubulovillous, and villous morphology (Figure 6-55)
- Tubular adenoma
  - Tubelike glands lined by epithelial cells containing hyperchromatic stratified nuclei with mitotic figures at all crypt levels, and few goblet cells, making up 75% to 80% of lesion
  - About 20% of tubular adenomas contain cancer
- Villous adenoma
  - Papillary fronds or leaflike configurations containing central lamina propria cores lined by similar dysplastic epithelium to that seen in tubular adenomas, making up 75% to 80% of lesion
  - Nearly 30% to 60% of villous lesions harbor invasive cancer
- Glandular complexity with complete loss of polarity indicates high-grade dysplasia and carcinoma in situ;

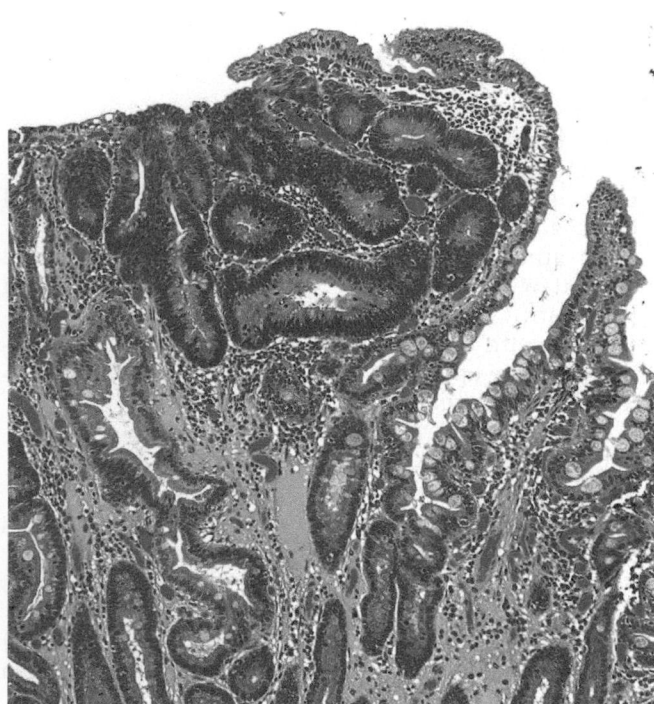

Figure 6-55. Small bowel adenoma in familial adenomatous polyposis. The adenoma resembles colonic tubular adenomas.

glandular fusion or an infiltrative pattern indicates at least intramucosal carcinoma; an infiltration pattern to atypical glands and desmoplasia indicates invasion of at least the submucosa

ADENOCARCINOMA
- Typically arises in association with an adenoma; adenocarcinoma in the setting of Crohn disease often demonstrates adjacent glandular dysplasia
- Malignant histology includes mucinous differentiation, cribriform glands, fused glands, marked stratification, cytologic anaplasia, and, most important, desmoplasia; atypical glands adjacent to large blood vessels, fat, or ganglion cells often accompany submucosal invasion
- Uncommon histology includes papillary adenosquamous carcinoma, signet ring cell carcinoma, and small cell carcinoma

Special Stains and Immunohistochemistry
- Alcian blue/PAS with hematoxylin counterstain very useful in recognizing abnormal mucus in adenomas/adenocarcinomas and foveolar cells in hyperplastic polyp of gastric type

Other Techniques for Diagnosis
- Testing for FAP associated syndromes and Lynch syndrome should be considered in a younger patient

Differential Diagnosis
BRUNNER GLAND NODULES
- Most cases of Brunner gland enlargement are probably hyperplasia because they maintain a normal lobular architecture, demonstrate little mitotic activity, and are histologically mature

- Brunner gland nodules and cysts may produce a mass lesion, but the histology is not dysplastic and can be readily distinguished from intestinal adenoma and adenocarcinoma
- True Brunner gland adenoma and adenocarcinoma are thought to be rare but typically demonstrate transition from normal Brunner glands to adenomatous or adenocarcinomatous tissue

HETEROTOPIC GASTRIC MUCOSA
- Generally small mucosal lesions that are polypoid and are composed of recognizable gastric mucosa with specialized glands (heterotopia) or foveolar epithelium (metaplasia) (Figure 6-56)
- Hyperplastic polyp of gastric type can develop from either; probably the most common proximal small bowel polyp

POLYPS ASSOCIATED WITH VARIOUS POLYPOSIS SYNDROMES
Discussed later in the chapter

PEARLS

- *Many adenomas are complicated by invasive malignancy; specimens require careful examination*
- *When high-grade dysplasia or intramucosal carcinoma is identified in an adenoma, endoscopic mucosal resection or operative resection should be considered because of the high risk for coexisting invasive carcinoma*
- *Carcinoma in the small bowel away from the major duodenal papilla is more likely to be metastatic than primary; get the patient's full clinical history*
- *Ileal small bowel adenocarcinoma can be seen in patients with Crohn disease*
- *Always look for a neuroendocrine tumor even if you may have another reason for a polyp or nodule (e.g., hyperplastic polyp of gastric type, Brunner gland nodule)*

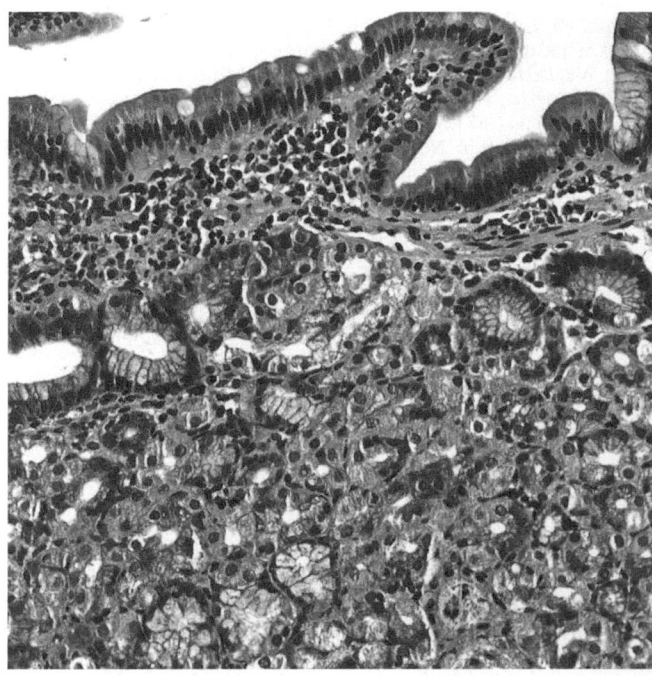

Figure 6-56. Gastric heterotopia. This histologic section shows specialized gastric glands beneath surface duodenal mucosa.

SELECTED REFERENCES

Bjork J, Akerbant H, Iselius L, et al: Periampullary adenomas and adenocarcinomas in familial adenomatous polyposis: cumulative risks and APC gene mutations. Gastroenterology 121:1127-1135, 2001.

Lein GS, Mori M, Enjoji M: Primary carcinoma of the small intestine: a clinicopathologic and immunohistochemical study. Cancer 61:316-323, 1988.

Petras R, Mir-Madjlessi S, Farmer R: Crohn's disease and intestinal carcinoma: a report of 11 cases with emphasis on epithelial dysplasia. Gastroenterology 93:1307-1314, 1987.

Riddell RH, Petras RE, Williams GT, Sobin LH: Tumors of the intestines. Atlas of Tumor Pathology Third Series, Fascicle 32. Washington, DC, Armed Forces Institute of Pathology, 2003.

Sarre R, Frost A, Jagelman D, et al: Gastric and duodenal polyps in familial adenomatous polyposis: a prospective study of the nature and prevalence of upper gastrointestinal polyps. Gut 28:306-314, 1987.

Sigel JE, Petras RE, Lashner BA, et al: Intestinal adenocarcinoma in Crohn's disease: a report of 30 cases with a focus on coexisting dysplasia. Am J Surg Pathol 23:651-655, 1999.

Zollinger RM Jr: Primary neoplasms of the small intestine. Am J Surg 151:654-658, 1986.

NEUROENDOCRINE (CARCINOID) TUMOR OF THE SMALL AND LARGE INTESTINE

Clinical Features

- Carcinoid tumors may be found in any organ in which neuroendocrine cells occur
- About 85% of carcinoid tumors arise in the gastrointestinal tract (constitute about 50% of small intestinal malignancies and less than 2% of colorectal malignancies)
- Most gastrointestinal carcinoid tumors occur in the vermiform appendix, followed by the small intestine (typically ileum), rectum, stomach, and colon
- Most patients are 50 to 70 years old
- May be found incidentally, or patients may present with weight loss, obstruction, or carcinoid syndrome
- Possible secretory products include serotonin, gastrin, somatostatin, VIP, ACTH, and insulin
  - Carcinoid syndrome
    - Occurs in 10% of patients; more common in patients with an ileal carcinoid tumor (Figure 6-58)
    - Usually indicates hepatic metastasis (precluding hepatic degradation of vasoactive amines)

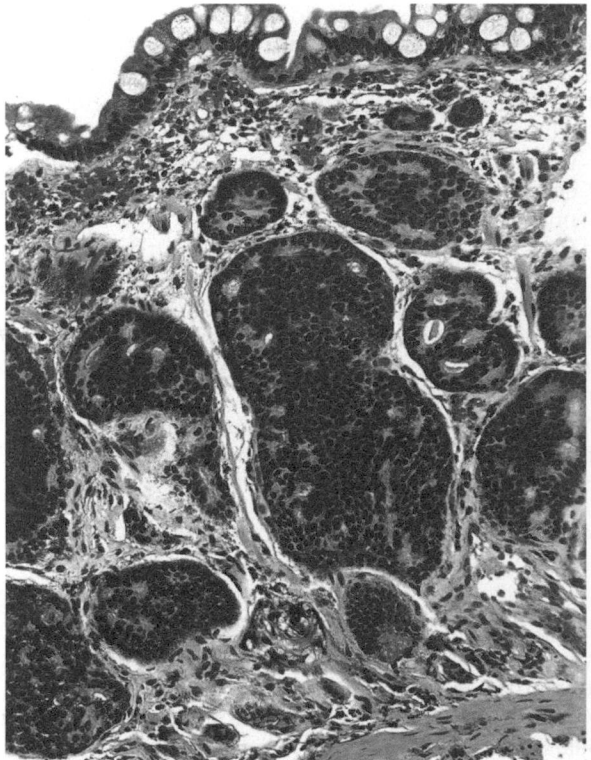

Figure 6-58. Carcinoid tumor of the terminal ileum infiltrating the lamina propria. Note the insular arrangement of carcinoid tumor cells showing pseudoglandular formation.

- Symptoms include flushing, sweating, cardiac symptoms, and diarrhea
- About 50% of patients have endocardial right-sided heart lesion
- Symptoms arise because of increased levels of 5-HT and 5-HIAA

Gross and Endoscopic Pathology

- Location of small and large intestinal carcinoid tumors is as follows: 1% duodenal, 7% jejunal, 80% ileal, and 10% rectal
- Typically small, firm, tan-yellow mucosal or mural nodules that are covered by intact mucosa; sometimes present with mural thickening and stricture (Figure 6-57)
- Rarely larger than 3 cm (often smaller than 1 cm, making them difficult to locate clinically)

Histopathology (Figure 6-58)

- Composed of uniform cells with round, central, monomorphic nuclei showing finely stippled chromatin and scant cytoplasm; faint red cytoplasmic granules can often be seen
- Mitotic rate is low
- Classic architectural patterns include the following:
  - Solid or insular arrangement of cells
  - Ribbons (festoons) or trabeculae
  - Tubules or glands (rosette-like)
- Some tumors may show glandular differentiation
- Typically well-circumscribed but may have an infiltrative growth pattern at the periphery

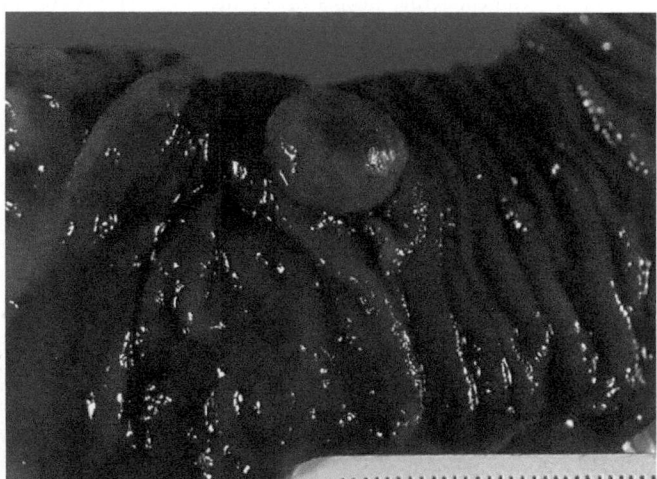

Figure 6-57. Ileal carcinoid in a resection specimen presenting as a polypoid intraluminal lesion.

- Cytologic features and evidence of vascular, lymphatic, or perineural invasion do not predict behavior
- Grade 2 neuroendocrine carcinoma (atypical carcinoid, intermediate-grade neuroendocrine carcinoma)
  - Occasionally tumors show neuroendocrine cellular morphology but are composed of more pleomorphic cells with large, irregular hyperchromatic nuclei and prominent nucleoli
  - Increased mitotic activity (2 to 20 mitoses per 10 hpf; Ki-67 staining percentage > 2 to 20) and single-cell necrosis are common in these tumors
- High-grade neuroendocrine carcinoma, large cell and small cell type, similar to pulmonary primaries can occur
- WHO nomenclature and grading (mitosis and Ki-67 index) is also applied to these neuroendocrine tumors (discussed previously)

Special Stains and Immunohistochemistry

- Chromogranin, synaptophysin positive; hindgut patterns (e.g., rectal) are often chromogranin negative; CD56 and neuron specific enolase immunohistochemistry can also be done; Ki-67 immunohistochemistry recommended
- Virtually all carcinoid tumors contain varying numbers of cells that can be identified with hormonal antibodies including serotonin, somatostatin, gastrin, VIP, ACTH, and insulin, though testing for these is rarely indicated
- Cytokeratin positive in 65% to 70% of cases

Other Techniques for Diagnosis

- DNA content reportedly correlate with survival (not routinely performed)

Differential Diagnosis

GANGLIOCYTIC PARAGANGLIOMA
- Triphasic cellular differentiation
  - Neuroendocrine cells
  - Spindle-shaped cells with Schwann cell differentiation
  - Ganglion cells
- Frequently located in the ampullary region
- Considered a well-differentiated neuroendocrine tumor of uncertain malignant potential

MIXED CARCINOID-ADENOCARCINOMA
- Tends to consist of larger infiltrating tumors
- Mixed histology, including areas of typical carcinoid admixed with carcinomatous areas; carcinoma typically constitutes greater than 50% of the tumor
- Must be distinguished from benign epithelial differentiation within typical carcinoid tumors
- More aggressive behavior; will act like adenocarcinoma

ADENOCARCINOMA
- Invasive growth pattern with glandular differentiation
- Increased cytologic atypia
- Generally lacks neuroendocrine differentiation (i.e., only scattered cells or small groupings)
- Lacks the monomorphic nuclear characteristics of carcinoid tumor

PEARLS

- *Small bowel carcinoids are typically insular in pattern; rectal lesions usually demonstrate a predominant trabecular pattern*
- *Psammoma bodies are commonly found in duodenal neuroendocrine tumors, especially those expressing immunoreactive somatostatin and those associated with neurofibromatosis*
- *Risk for metastasis increases with tumor size*
  - *Less than 1 cm: 2%*
  - *One to 2 cm: 50% (ileal); 15% (rectal)*
  - *More than 2 cm: 80%*
- *All carcinoids are potentially malignant*
- *Clinical evidence of metastases is best method to determine malignant potential; histologic features are generally unreliable*
- *Deep local mural penetration by tumor correlates with decreased survival, as does presence of hepatic and nodal metastasis*
- *Overall (5-year) survival rate for small bowel carcinoid tumors is 90%*
- *Gastrinoma*
  - *Often multiple, but typically small*
  - *Associated with Zollinger-Ellison syndrome and MEN-I syndrome*
  - *Usually malignant behavior*
- *Insulinoma*
  - *May also be associated with MEN-I syndrome and hypoglycemia*
  - *Usually benign behavior*
- *Use CAP protocols for reporting resection specimens*

SELECTED REFERENCES

Capella C, Arnold R, Klimstra DS, et al: Neuroendocrine neoplasms of the small intestine. In Bosman FT, Carneiro F, Hruban RH, Theise ND (eds): World Health Organization Classification of Tumours of the Digestive System. Lyon, IARC Press, 2010, pp 102-107.

Riddell RH, Petras RE, Williams GT, Sobin LH: Tumors of the intestines. Atlas of Tumor Pathology Third Series, Fascicle 32. Washington, DC, Armed Forces Institute of Pathology, 2003.

Rindi G, Klimstra DS, Arnold R, et al: Nomenclature and classification of neuroendocrine neoplasms of the digestive system. In Bosman FT, Carneiro F, Hruban RH, Theise ND (eds): World Health Organization Classification of Tumours of the Digestive System. Lyon, IARC Press, 2010, pp 13-14.

Washington MK, Tang LH, Berlin J, et al: Protocol for the examination of specimens from patients with neuroendocrine tumors (carcinoid tumors) of the colon and rectum. Arch Pathol Lab Med 134:176-180, 2010.

Washington MK, Tang LH, Berlin J, et al: Protocol for the examination of specimens from patients with neuroendocrine tumors (carcinoid tumors) of the small intestine and ampulla. Arch Pathol Lab Med 134:181-186, 2010.

HIRSCHSPRUNG DISEASE (HD)

Clinical Features

- Uncommon disease affecting 1 in 5000 to 30,000 live births
- About 80% of patients are male; 90% present as infants
- Small percentage of patients have other congenital anomalies

- Presenting features include constipation, abdominal obstruction, meconium plug
- Patients with Down syndrome are at increased risk for HD
- Normal anus and anal canal on physical examination

Gross and Endoscopic Pathology

- Classic resected colon consists of a dilated (neurologically normal) proximal segment that narrows (hypoganglionated area) into a contracted (aganglionic) distal segment
- May produce toxic megacolon
- Multiple forms exist
  - Short-segment HD: as little as 3 cm of distal rectum affected (most common form)
  - Long-segment HD: extends beyond sigmoid colon; can involve entire colon and a variable length of small intestine (about 10% of patients)
  - Ultra-short segment HD involves a segment < 2 cm and is diagnosed by manometry
    - Probably more correctly called "internal anal sphincter achalasia"; pathology plays no role in diagnosis

Histopathology

- Absence of ganglion cells from the submucosal and myenteric plexuses
- Hypertrophy of the mural nerves (> 40 μm)
- Hypertrophy of muscularis mucosae and muscularis externa
- Long-segment HD may have normal caliber nerves and false-negative acetylcholinesterase stain (discussed later)

Special Stains and Immunohistochemistry

- Acetylcholinesterase reactions (on frozen tissue): patients with HD demonstrate coarse, irregular nerve fibers extending from the muscularis mucosae up into the lamina propria (normal tissue contains only thin fibers, which are only in muscularis mucosae)
- Neuron-specific enolase (NSE)–positive in ganglion cells; other immunostains (e.g., cathepsin D, PGP9.5, bcl-2) can decorate ganglion cells
- S-100 protein: Schwann cells show perinuclear positivity
- HD shows absent calretinin immunostaining in nerves

Other Techniques for Diagnosis

- Gene mutations detected in 50% of patients include inactivation mutation of *RET* oncogene, mutations in endothelin receptor B; at least nine other gene mutations have been implicated

Differential Diagnosis

HYPOGANGLIONOSIS

- Can cause HD-like syndrome with megacolon
- No accepted definition, but should be diagnosed in patients with a substantial reduction in ganglion cell numbers compared with normal (40 to 80 myenteric neurons per 1 cm of bowel); can be zonal
- Some examples of hypoganglionosis could be similar to idiopathic constipation

INTESTINAL NEURONAL DYSPLASIA

- Clinically mimics HD, and patients typically present with constipation
- Differentiated by presence of hyperplastic plexuses and giant ganglia containing more than eight neurons
- Diagnostic criteria and even the existence of intestinal neuronal dysplasia debated
- Diagnosis should be reserved for florid cases

IDIOPATHIC CONSTIPATION

- Occurs more often in females
- Ganglion cells are present; distinctive abnormalities of the myenteric plexus (e.g., loss of argyrophilic neurons) described with special silver staining techniques; often coexists with melanosis coli
- Reduced volume of interstitial cells of Cajal as demonstrated with immunohistochemistry for CD117 and CD34 reported in some cases

PEARLS

- *Biopsy specimens in actual cases of HD usually contain hypertrophic nerves, but their presence is not diagnostic; calretinin positive nerves rule out Hirschsprung disease*
- *There can be overlap in the histologic changes described in intestinal neuronal dysplasia and neurofibromatosis*
- *The London classification can be useful for categorizing motility disorders (neuropathies, myopathies, abnormalities of interstitial cells of Cajal) that enter into the differential diagnosis*

SELECTED REFERENCES

Guinard-Samuel V, Bonnard A, De Lagausie P, et al: Calretinin immunohistochemistry: a simple and efficient tool to diagnose Hirschsprung disease. Mod Pathol 22:1379-1384, 2009.

Kapur RP: Multiple endocrine neoplasia type 2B and Hirschsprung's disease. Clin Gastroenterol Hepatol 3:423-431, 2005.

Knowles CH, De Giorgio R, Kapur RP, et al: The London classification of gastrointestinal neuromuscular pathology: report on behalf of the Gastro 2009 International Working Group. Gut 59:882-887, 2010.

Puri P, Gosemann JH: Variants of Hirschsprung disease. Semin Pediatr Surg 21:310-318, 2012.

Streutker CJ, Huizinga JD, Campbell F, et al: Loss of CD117 (c-kit) and CD34-positive ICC and associated CD34-positive fibroblasts defines a subpopulation of chronic intestinal pseudo-obstruction. Am J Surg Pathol 27:228-235, 2003.

Toman J, Turina M, Ray M, et al: Slow transit colon constipation is not related to the number of interstitial cells of Cajal. Int J Colorectal Dis 21:527-532, 2006.

DIVERTICULAR DISEASE

Clinical Features

- Most common in societies consuming a Western-style diet (high fat, low fiber)
- In the United States, 50% of adults older than 40 years are affected
- Only 20% of patients have symptoms; particularly obese individuals
- Formation of diverticula is related to weakness in the colonic wall and increased intraluminal pressure
- Symptoms may be related to diverticulitis, which includes lower abdominal pain, rebound tenderness, and fever; symptoms can occur without inflammation

- Patients may have symptoms related to anemia from chronic hemorrhage or have massive acute lower gastrointestinal bleeding
- Complications include obstruction, perforation, peritonitis, hemorrhage, abscess formation, and fistula
- Mucosal prolapse is common in patients with diverticular disease

Gross and Endoscopic Pathology

- Small oval or spherical outpouchings along the large intestine
- About 90% involve the sigmoid colon
- Typically form adjacent to penetrating mural arteries and alongside taeniae coli
- Adjacent muscularis propria may be thickened

Histopathology

- Classic lesion is a protrusion of the mucosa and submucosa through the muscularis propria
- Diverticula may have a flattened or atrophic mucosa and compressed submucosa
- Adjacent tissue, including the muscular propria, is hypertrophied, fibrotic, and chronically inflamed
- Acute inflammation indicates acute diverticulitis; may form peridiverticular abscesses

Special Stains and Immunohistochemistry

- Noncontributory

Other Techniques for Diagnosis

- Noncontributory

Differential Diagnosis

INFLAMMATORY BOWEL DISEASE (PARTICULARLY CROHN DISEASE)

- Both conditions may cause focal mucosal inflammation and thickening of the bowel wall with stricture and fistula; conditions may coexist
- Crohn disease is distinguished by fissural ulcers, ulcers and mucosal inflammation outside of the areas of diverticulitis, transmural inflammation, serosal lymphoid aggregates, superficial aphthous ulcers, and granulomas
- A segmental diverticular disease–associated primary inflammatory bowel disease–like mucosal inflammation is described and is treated similarly to primary inflammatory bowel disease; some patients are eventually proved to have Crohn disease

PEARLS

- *Comprehensive gross examination may be necessary to detect subtle luminal openings of the diverticula in the resected colon*
- *Clinical, radiographic, and even, to some extent, gross features of diverticulosis may mimic carcinoma; however, a mucosal mass is absent*
- *Colovesical and colovaginal fistula can complicate diverticular disease; other fistulas must increase the index of suspicion for coexisting Crohn disease*
- *Diverticula limited to right colon occur more commonly in Hawaii, Japan, and the Orient; the diverticula show all bowel layers in the wall and likely represent congenital maldevelopment*

SELECTED REFERENCES

Goldstein NS, Leon-Armin C, Mani A: Crohn's colitis-like changes in sigmoid diverticulitis specimens is usually an idiosyncratic inflammatory response to the diverticulosis rather than Crohn's colitis. Am J Surg Pathol 24:668-675, 2000.

Imperiali G, Terpin MM, Meucci G, et al: Segmental colitis associated with diverticula: a 7-year follow-up study. Endoscopy 38:610-612, 2006.

Mulhall AM, Mahid SS, Petras RE, Galandiuk S: Diverticular disease associated with inflammatory bowel disease-like colitis: a systematic review. Dis Colon Rectum 52:1072-1079, 2009.

EOSINOPHILIC GASTROENTERITIS

Clinical Features

- Syndrome characterized by gastrointestinal symptoms combined with eosinophilic infiltration of the gastrointestinal tract in the absence of a specific allergen or parasitic infestation, usually seen in children and young adults
- Most patients have peripheral blood eosinophilia (70% of cases)
- Most patients have a history of allergies
- Patients present with variable symptoms ranging from mild nausea and vomiting to an acute abdomen
- Other symptoms include diarrhea, malabsorption, obstruction, or ascites (often depends on level of the bowel wall involved)
- Often have elevation of serum IL-5 levels

Gross and Endoscopic Pathology

- Affects any level of gastrointestinal tract; stomach and small bowel are most common sites; less commonly affects the colon
- Radiographic studies often disclose widened mucosal folds and mural thickening
- Diffuse involvement may occur, producing bowel rigidity and edema

Histopathology

- Three patterns of eosinophilic gastroenteritis described:
  - Mucosal involvement typically causing diarrhea and malabsorption
  - Submucosal involvement associated with intestinal obstruction
  - Mural and serosal involvement leading to ascites and eosinophilic peritonitis
- Diffuse, sheetlike infiltrate of eosinophils typically involving the lamina propria, crypts, or villi
- Often associated with mucosal edema, crypt hyperplasia, or villous atrophy
- Mural fibrosis or muscular hypertrophy can occur
- Serosal involvement may induce subserosal fibrosis

Special Stains and Immunohistochemistry

- Noncontributory

Other Techniques for Diagnosis

- Noncontributory

Differential Diagnosis

- Numerous diseases present with eosinophilic infiltrates; rule out allergies, lymphoma, foreign bodies, systemic vasculitis, drug reaction, and parasitic infestation

COW'S MILK ALLERGY

- Typically affects neonatal or young infants with sensitivity to milk protein; generally responds to prompt switch to soy-based or hydrolysate formula
- Infants present with severe diarrhea, dehydration, and failure to thrive
- Characterized by villous atrophy, neutrophilic infiltrates, and eosinophilic infiltrate
- Overall prognosis is excellent

OTHER FOOD ALLERGIES

- Affects 45% of the population and nearly 10% of children
- Histologically similar to eosinophilic gastroenteritis
- Requires correlation of symptoms with exposure to a specific food

SYSTEMIC MASTOCYTOSIS INVOLVING GASTROINTESTINAL TRACT

- Majority of cases of systemic mastocytosis are confined to the skin; up to 10% may have gastrointestinal involvement
- Associated with D816V kit mutation
- Mast cells in aggregates (> 15 cells) and sheets, pericryptal and beneath luminal surface
- Mast cells may have abnormal morphology such as spindle shapes or elongate cells
- About 80% of cases associated with marked infiltration of eosinophils that can obscure the mast cells
- Abnormal mast cells stain positive for immunostains for CD117, CD2, or CD25

PEARLS

- *Resist the temptation to suggest eosinophilic gastroenteritis at the sight of eosinophils, which are a normal component of the gastrointestinal mucosa*
  - *Collections of eosinophils not associated with other inflammatory cells, groupings of eosinophils associated with mucosal architectural change or injury (e.g., crypt abscesses), and infiltration of the muscularis mucosae and deeper bowel layers are all considered abnormal and in a corroborative clinical setting should be considered diagnostic of eosinophilic gastroenteritis*
- *Whenever collections of eosinophils are seen, it makes sense to check for parasites*
- *Some authors think that > 20 mast cells/hpf as demonstrated by immunohistochemistry for mast cell tryptase or CD117 indicates "mastocytic enterocolitis," an entity that should be treated with antihistamines or mast cell stabilizers*
  - *This controversial study lacked a treatment control group*
  - *It is questionable if mast cell counting is sufficient to assess their role in disease states such as diarrhea predominant irritable bowel syndrome*

SELECTED REFERENCES

Jakate S, Demeo M, John R, et al: Mastocytic enterocolitis: increased mucosal mast cells in chronic intractable diarrhea. Arch Pathol Lab Med 130:362-367, 2006.

Kirsch R, Geboes K, Shepherd NA, et al: Systemic mastocytosis involving the gastrointestinal tract: clinicopathologic and molecular study of five cases. Mod Pathol 21:1508-1516, 2008.

Orenstein SR, Shalaby TM, DiLorenzo C, et al: The spectrum of pediatric eosinophilic esophagitis beyond infancy: a clinical series of 30 children. Am J Gastroenterol 95:1422-1430, 2000.

Petras R, Gramlich T: Non-neoplastic intestinal diseases. In Mills SE (ed): Sternberg's Diagnostic Surgical Pathology, 5th ed. New York: Lippincott, Williams, & Wilkins, 2010, pp 1313-1367.

Steffen RM, Wyllie R, Petras RE, et al: The spectrum of eosinophilic gastroenteritis: report of six pediatric cases and review of the literature. Clin Pediatr 30:404-411, 1991.

Theoharis C, Theoharides MS, Asadi S, et al: Irritable bowel syndrome and elusive mast cells. Am J Gastroenterol 107:727-729, 2012.

GRAFT-VERSUS-HOST DISEASE (GVHD)

Clinical Features

- Characterized by immunologic reaction between (engrafted) donor T lymphocytes and epithelial cells of recipient (host)
- Skin, biliary tract, and gastrointestinal epithelium may be involved
- Most commonly occurs after bone marrow transplantation
- Clinical severity is determined partially by degree of histocompatibility mismatch; however, may also occur in exact major histocompatibility matches, owing to minor histocompatibility antigen mismatch
- Acute GVHD
  - Usually occurs within first 100 days of transplantation
  - Typical gastrointestinal symptoms include diarrhea and abdominal pain
- Recalcitrant cases may progress to chronic GVHD
- Most episodes initially involve skin
- Gastrointestinal tract is involved in 70% of cases

Gross and Endoscopic Pathology

- Variable appearance
- Mucosal erythema and ulcers can be seen endoscopically
- Gross and endoscopic features generally do not correlate well with clinical severity

Histopathology

- Base of crypts shows single epithelial cell necrosis creating lacuna-containing nuclear debris (known as apoptosis) (Figure 6-59)
- May progressively worsen to include many crypts or entire epithelium; may produce crypt abscess and large areas of ulceration and fungal secondary infection
- Chronic or unresolved episodes may contain atrophic, fibrotic, or regenerating epithelium and mucosa

Special Stains and Immunohistochemistry

- Generally unnecessary in the diagnosis of GVHD, but stains for fungi, parasites, and viruses (particularly CMV) may be indicated

Other Techniques for Diagnosis

- Noncontributory

Differential Diagnosis

CHEMOTHERAPY/RADIATION AND DRUG EFFECT

- Chemotherapy and radiation causes apoptosis; these changes last up to 100 days
- Apoptosis is a characteristic injury pattern associated with mycophenolate mofetil/sodium

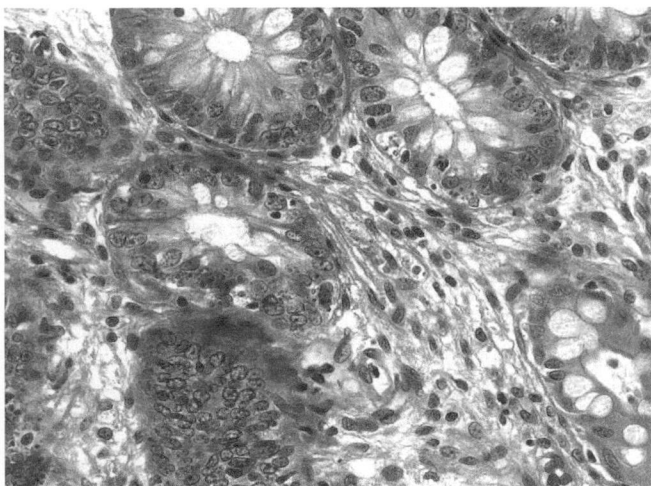

Figure 6-59. Graft-versus-host disease demonstrating numerous apoptotic bodies.

- Mycophenolate-related injury more likely to contain eosinophils (> 15 per 10 hpf) and less likely to have endocrine cell aggregates and apoptotic microabscesses (atrophic and degenerating crypt epithelium with intraluminal necrotic and apoptotic epithelial cells) that are typical for GVHD

OPPORTUNISTIC INFECTION

- Must always be considered along with GVHD in the posttransplantation setting
- Characteristic organisms or cytopathic changes must be recognized for diagnosis

PEARLS

- *Apoptotic cells are present in the skin, bile duct epithelium, and gastrointestinal tract in GVHD*
- *Cytotoxic T cell is the perpetrator*
- *Steroids given for GVHD treatment may predispose to reactivation of CMV infection*
- *Apoptosis can be seen with ischemia, CMV infection, immune deficiency, and bowel preparation*

SELECTED REFERENCES

Asplund S, Gramlich TL: Chronic mucosal changes of the colon in graft-versus-host disease. Mod Pathol 11:513-515, 1998.

Cox G, Matsui S, Lo R, et al: Etiology and outcome of diarrhea after marrow transplantation: a prospective study. Gastroenterology 107:1398-1407, 1994.

Papadimitriou JC, Cangro CB, Lustberg A, et al: Histologic features of mycophenolate mofetil-related colitis: a graft-versus-host disease-like pattern. Int J Surg Pathol 11:295-302, 2003.

Parfitt JR, Jayadumar S, Driman DK: Mycophenolate mofetil-related gastrointestinal mucosal injury: variable injury patterns, including graft-versus-host disease-like changes. Am J Surg Pathol 32:1367-1372, 2008.

Star KV, Ho VT, Wang HH, Odze RD: Histologic features in colon biopsies can discriminate mycophenolate from GVHD-induced colitis. Am J Surg Pathol 37:1319-1328, 2013.

INFLAMMATORY BOWEL DISEASE (IBD)

Clinical Features

- Chronic, recurrent gastrointestinal inflammatory disease of unknown etiology

- Familial predisposition; 10-fold increased risk for first-degree relatives
- Peak incidence in young adults
- Whites are more commonly affected than nonwhites
- Slight female predominance

CROHN DISEASE

- Incidence of 3 per 100,000 people in United States
- Small bowel Crohn disease is associated with IBD-1 gene (*NOD2/CARD15*)
- Usually begins with intermittent episodes of mild diarrhea, fever, and abdominal pain over weeks to months
- About 20% of patients present with severe, acute onset of abdominal pain
- Intestinal complications include strictures, fistula, and malabsorption
- Extraintestinal complications include polyarthritis, ankylosing spondylitis, primary sclerosing cholangitis (uncommon), and uveitis
- Increased risk for small bowel and colonic adenocarcinoma

ULCERATIVE COLITIS

- Incidence of 4 to 12 per 100,000 people in the United States
- Presents with episodic attacks of lower abdominal pain and bloody diarrhea over months, years, or decades
- About 30% require colectomy within 3 years
- Intestinal complications include toxic megacolon and perforation; both can occur during severe episodes
- Extraintestinal complications include polyarthritis, sacroiliitis, ankylosing spondylitis, uveitis, and primary sclerosing cholangitis
- Risk for carcinoma: previous reports have estimated 30% at 35 years after onset; however, estimates now indicate that progression may actually be lower

Gross and Endoscopic Pathology

CROHN DISEASE

- Involves any level of gastrointestinal tract from mouth to anus; classically affects the small bowel
- Mesenteric fat of the involved segment wraps around the bowel surface ("creeping fat" or "fat wrapping") (Figure 6-60)
- Thickened, stiff intestinal wall (stovepipe) with normal-appearing intervening segments (skip lesions)
- Early disease is characterized by aphthous ulcers that progress to discrete ulceration, serpiginous ulcers, linear ulcers, or cobblestoning
- Cobblestoning results from two different ulceration patterns: linear ulcers and small horizontal crevices; the sharp demarcation between edematous but otherwise normal mucosa and surrounding ulcers gives the mucosa a cobblestone appearance (Figure 6-61)
- Ulcers deepen into fissures and can ultimately produce fistulas
- Luminal narrowing often causes characteristic string sign on x-ray

ULCERATIVE COLITIS

- Classically demonstrates involvement of the rectum and variable length of large intestine (without skip lesions) (Figure 6-62)

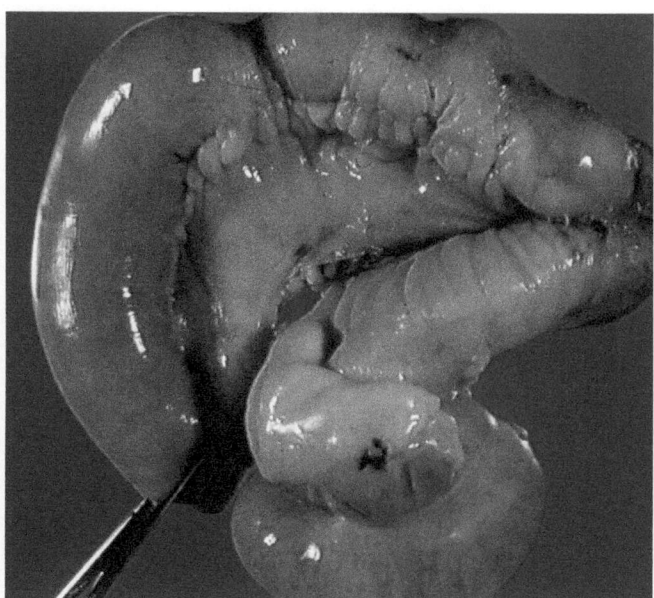

Figure 6-60. Resection specimen of small intestinal Crohn disease with areas of stricture and fat wrapping.

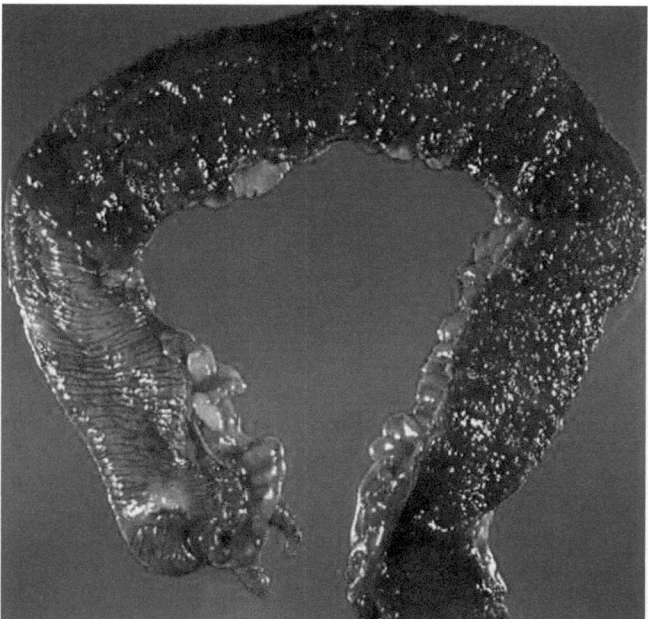

Figure 6-62. Resection specimen of ulcerative colitis. The distal-most margin is involved by the inflammatory process. More proximal involvement is in continuity with the involved rectum.

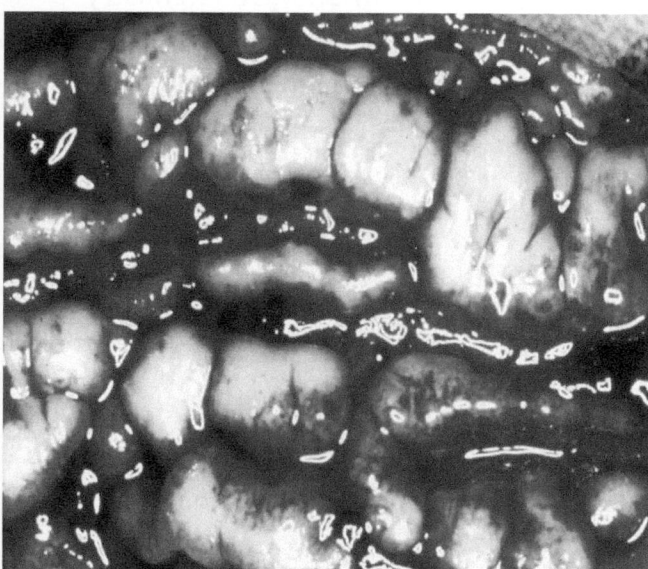

Figure 6-61. Colonic resection specimen of Crohn disease showing cobblestoning. Cobblestoning is created by the combination of two ulcer patterns, longitudinally oriented linear ulcers and small horizontal crevices, which isolate small islands of relatively intact colonic mucosa.

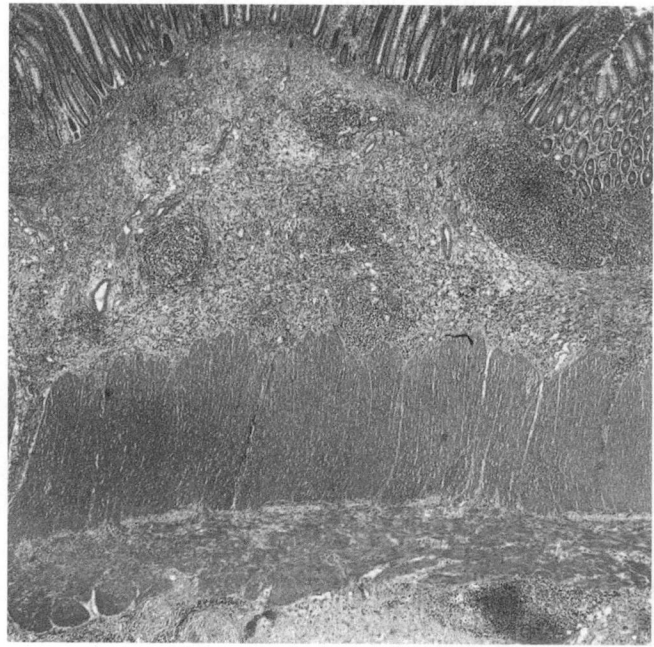

Figure 6-63. Crohn disease of the colon showing transmural lymphoid aggregates in an area not deeply ulcerated.

- Often involves the entire colon (pancolitis) and occasionally spills into ileum (so-called backwash ileitis); in some classification schemes, ileal involvement in the setting of pancolitis is a criterion for inflammatory bowel disease of indeterminate type
- Irregular areas of ulceration, which may be widespread, can surround islands of preserved mucosa (pseudopolyps and inflammatory polyps)
- Deep ulcers extending to the muscularis externa usually correlate with fulminant clinical disease and are a

pathologic criterion for primary inflammatory bowel disease of an indeterminate type in some schemes
- Normal serosa unless complicated by fulminant disease

Histopathology

CROHN DISEASE
- Classic features include patchy, transmural chronic inflammation with intervening normal areas (skip lesions) (Figure 6-63)

- Acute inflammatory fissures can penetrate the muscularis externa
- Associated lymphoid aggregates occur throughout the bowel wall but often along the serosa (rosary bead pattern)
- Granulomas occur in up to 50% cases, both in actively involved and uninvolved tissue
- In chronic disease, Paneth cell and pyloric metaplasia occur
- Neutrophilic infiltrates and crypt abscesses may occur
- Hypertrophied muscularis mucosae, submucosal neural hyperplasia, and mural fibrosis may evolve into strictures
- Difficult to diagnose outside of distal small bowel and large bowel in the absence of granulomas; focally enhanced gastritis in the absence of *H. pylori* can be seen in patients with Crohn disease

ULCERATIVE COLITIS

- Characterized by a dense lymphoplasmacytic and neutrophilic infiltrate generally limited to the mucosa and superficial submucosa (Figure 6-64)
- Inflammatory infiltrate is between widely spaced, regenerating, architecturally distorted glands containing intraepithelial and luminal neutrophils (cryptitis and crypt abscess)
- Inflammation may extend into muscularis propria beneath areas of ulceration in fulminant disease; in some classification schemes, this feature would indicate fulminant primary inflammatory bowel disease of an indeterminate type (Figure 6-65)
- In chronic disease, regenerated glands are distorted and may be branched or shortened (above muscularis mucosae); may contain decreased numbers of goblet cells
- Some patients develop epithelial dysplasia in both flat and elevated lesions (see "Dysplasia in Inflammatory Bowel Disease")

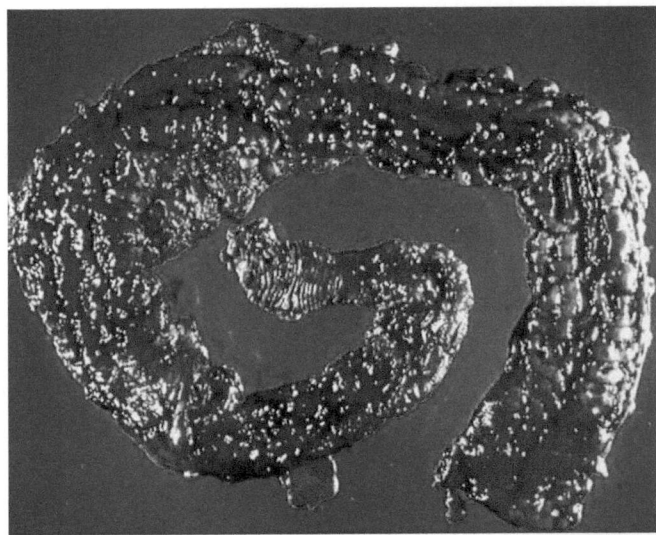

Figure 6-65. Gross photograph of fulminant primary inflammatory bowel disease of an indeterminate type, probably Crohn disease, showing areas of deep ulceration and involvement of the terminal ileum.

Special Stains and Immunohistochemistry

- Noncontributory

Other Techniques for Diagnosis

- Serologic tests such as perinuclear antineutrophil cytoplasmic (pANCA) (for ulcerative colitis) and anti-saccharomyces cerevisiae antibodies (ASCA) (for Crohn disease) can be helpful but are positive in only 50% of patients
- Genetic test for *NOD2/CARD15* mutation associated with small bowel Crohn disease is commercially available

Differential Diagnosis

ACUTE SELF-LIMITED COLITIS

- A self-limited, short-lived (< 6 months) disease presumably due to pathogenic organisms
- Characterized clinically by sudden onset of diarrhea and abdominal pain
- Shows the focal colitis pattern of injury with acute inflammation that predominates over chronic lymphoplasmacytic infiltrates
- Gland alterations are not seen
- Active inflammation associated with little or no mucin depletion
- Neutrophils in the lamina propria

LYMPHOCYTIC COLITIS

- Characterized by a moderate mixed inflammatory infiltrate in the lamina propria especially superficial increase in plasma cells but usually lacking architectural distortion and crypt abscesses; lack of plasma cells could indicate lymphocytic colitis in the setting of immune deficiency (e.g., common variable immunodeficiency syndrome)
- By definition, lymphocytic colitis demonstrates increased intraepithelial lymphocytes (> 15 per 100 surface epithelial cells)

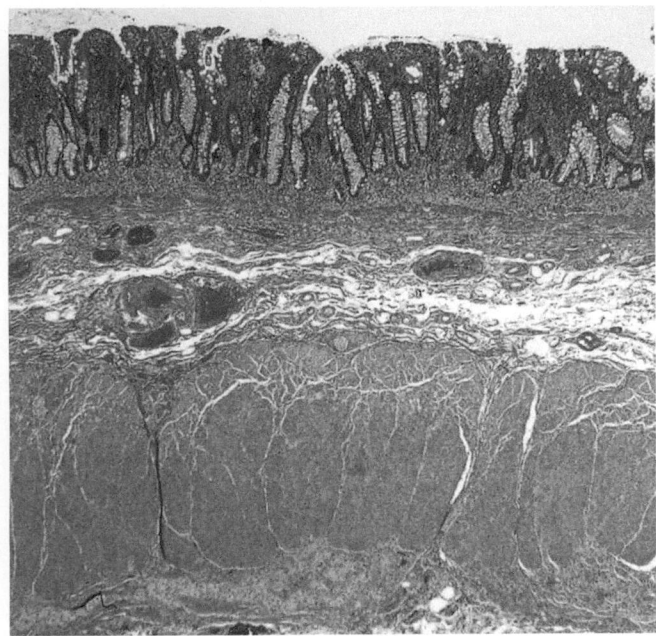

Figure 6-64. Ulcerative colitis in a resection specimen showing architectural and inflammatory changes limited to the mucosa.

- Unlike that in IBD, the clinical setting includes profuse, watery diarrhea and normal colonoscopy
- IBD typically shows greater inflammation, includes more neutrophils, crypt abscesses, architectural distortion (bifid and widely spaced glands), minimal intraepithelial lymphocytes (<6 per 100 colonic epithelial cells), and abnormal endoscopy

COLLAGENOUS COLITIS
- Histologically similar to lymphocytic colitis, but distinguished by presence of a thickened collagen layer beneath the surface basement membrane (>15 μm)
- Feathery strands of collagen extend between glands and displace the inflammatory cells downward
- Presence of Paneth cell metaplasia in collagenous colitis correlates with more severe diarrhea and can cause confusion with IBD
- IBD typically shows greater inflammation, lacks the subepithelial collagen layer, and includes more neutrophils, crypt abscesses, architectural distortion (bifid and widely spaced glands), minimal intraepithelial lymphocytes (<6 per 100 colonic epithelial cells), and abnormal endoscopy

DIVERSION COLITIS
- Occurs in a segment of colon/rectum excluded from the fecal stream; most often a Hartmann pouch constructed at the time of resection of a proximal segment of colon
- About one third of patients are symptomatic with passage of mucous discharge or blood
- Histologic features include prominent lymphoid aggregates and follicles and a dense lymphoid infiltrate in lamina propria
- Scattered neutrophilic infiltrate with foci of cryptitis and rare crypt abscesses may be seen
- Crypt architecture is usually normal if diversion is of short duration
- Often superimposed on changes of ulcerative colitis or Crohn disease in the rectum following colectomy in patients with primary inflammatory bowel disease
- Cured by restoring continuity of the bowel and resumption of fecal stream; can be treated with short-chain fatty acid enemas; some patients require operative excision

INDETERMINATE COLITIS
- Diagnosed when clinical, endoscopic, and biopsy findings have features of both Crohn disease and ulcerative colitis or when resected specimen shows deep ulceration, pseudopolyps, and glandular alterations with ambiguous gross and histologic features (Figure 6-65)
- A diagnosis of ulcerative colitis in a resection specimen requires that inflammation be limited to the large bowel, the rectum must be involved, no skip areas grossly or microscopically, no mural fissures or sinuses, and no granulomas
- Crohn disease in a resection specimen must be corroborated histologically and requires transmural lymphoid aggregates in an area not deeply ulcerated or the presence of non-necrotizing granulomas
- All other cases are best classified as colitis of an indeterminate type

PEARLS
- *IBD is characterized by increased mixed inflammation of the lamina propria, increased basal plasma cells glandular alterations (mucin depletion, branching, shortening, and atrophy) with scattered cryptitis, crypt abscess formation*
- *When acute inflammation predominates without glandular architectural changes, consider acute self-limited colitis*
- *In cases of suspected IBD, it is difficult to confirm a diagnosis of Crohn disease on biopsy; diagnosis may be suggested when granulomas are present, particularly when both normal and inflamed mucosa are identified in biopsies taken during the same colonoscopy*
- *In the absence of a clinical contraindication (e.g., perianal fistula, small bowel disease at operation) patients with a diagnosis of indeterminate colitis are considered suitable for ileal pouch-anal anastomosis*

SELECTED REFERENCES
Bernstein CN, Shanahan F, Anton PA, Weinstein WM: Patchiness of mucosal inflammation in treated ulcerative colitis: a prospective study. Gastrointest Endosc 42:232-237, 1995.

Bonner GF, Petras RE, Cheong DMO, et al: Short- and long-term follow-up of treatment for lymphocytic and collagenous colitis. Inflamm Bowel Dis 6:85-91, 2000.

Farmer M, Petras RE, Hunt LE, et al: The importance of diagnostic accuracy in colonic inflammatory bowel disease. Am J Gastroenterol 95:3184-3188, 2000.

Jenkins D, Balsitis M, Gallivan S, et al: Guidelines for the initial biopsy diagnosis of suspected chronic idiopathic inflammatory bowel disease. British Society of Gastroenterology Initiative. J Clin Pathol 50:93-105, 1997.

Kleer CG, Appleman HD: Ulcerative colitis: patterns of involvement in colorectal biopsies and changes with time. Am J Surg Pathol 22:983-989, 1998.

Martland GT, Shepherd NA: Indeterminate colitis: definition, diagnostic implication and a plea for nosological sanity. Histopathology 50:83-96, 2007.

Rudolph WG, Uthoff SM, McAuliffe TL, et al: Indeterminate colitis: the real story. Dis Colon Rectum 45:1528-1534, 2002

Wang N, Dumot JA, Achkar E, et al: Colonic epithelial lymphocytosis without a thickened subepithelial collagen table: a clinicopathologic study of forty cases supporting a heterogeneous entity. Am J Surg Pathol 23:1068-1074, 1999.

Wehkamp J, Harder J, Weichenthal M, et al: NOD2 (CARD15) mutations in Crohn's disease are associated with diminished alpha-defensin expression. Gut 53:1658-1664, 2004.

BIOPSY OF ILEUM AND POUCHES
- Lymphoid aggregates, pigment, and fibromuscular proliferation within the lamina propria are normally seen in the ileum and should not be misinterpreted as pathologic
  - The pigment is environmental or dietary in origin and deposits in macrophages; it has no clinical significance
  - Pathologic changes in the ileum include inflammation, parasitic infestation, and epithelial lymphocytosis
  - Minimal focal active enteritis can be related to bowel preparation or trauma and prolapse
  - Increased amounts of inflammation with architectural change and pyloric gland metaplasia usually are caused by Crohn disease or can be associated with NSAIDs

• Giardiasis can be seen in terminal ileal biopsy specimens
• Epithelial lymphocytosis can be a manifestation of celiac sprue or lymphocytic enterocolitis

ILEAL RESERVOIRS (POUCHES)

• The term *pouch* is the colloquialism given to the post-colectomy continence restoring operations (continent ileostomy, ileal pouch-anal anastomosis), which are surgical treatments of choice for ulcerative colitis and FAP
• These operations have in common the creation of a pouch or reservoir formed by interconnecting loops of the terminal ileum
• Pouch procedures are not usually done on patients with Crohn disease
• A common late complication of pouch construction is the development of primary inflammation in the pouch, termed *pouchitis*
  • Patients present with increased effluent that can be bloody and foul smelling; patients often have fever and malaise
  • Pouch biopsy is typically done to confirm inflammation and to rule out Crohn disease
    • Pouchitis typically shows ulcers, granulation tissue, architectural change, and depletion or absence of normal lymphoid follicles
    • Afferent limb ulcers and non-necrotizing granulomas should suggest Crohn disease
    • Pyloric gland metaplasia is not usually seen in classic pouchitis and when present suggests Crohn disease, an NSAID-related lesion, or primary refractory pouchitis, a lesion that can be related to colonic change within the pouch
• Dysplasia develops only rarely in a pouch

SELECTED REFERENCES

Lengeling RW, Mitros FA, Brennan JA, Schulze KS: Ulcerative ileitis encountered at ileo-colonoscopy: likely role of nonsteroidal agents. Clin Gastroenterol Hepatol 1:160-169, 2003.

McHugh JB, Appelman HD, McKenna BJ: The diagnostic value of terminal ileal biopsies. Am J Gastroenterol 102:1090-1092, 2007.

Petras R. Role of the pathologist in evaluating chronic pouches. In Bayless TM, Hanauer SB (eds): Advanced Therapy in Inflammatory Bowel Disease, 3rd ed. Shelton, CT, People's Medical Publishing House, 2011, pp 453-456.

Sandborn WJ: Pouchitis following ileal pouch anal anastomosis: definition, pathogenesis, and treatment. Gastroenterology 107:1856-1860, 1994.

Wolf JM, Achkar JP, Lashner BA, et al: Afferent limb ulcers predict Crohn's disease in patients with ileal pouch-anal anastomosis. Gastroenterology 126:1686-1691, 2004.

Wu H, Shen B: Pouchitis and pouch dysfunction. Med Clin North Am 94:75-92, 2010.

DYSPLASIA IN INFLAMMATORY BOWEL DISEASE

Clinical Features

• Dysplasia and carcinoma may occur in both longstanding ulcerative colitis and Crohn disease
• Cancer risk in ulcerative colitis is estimated at up to 20% at 30 years
• Cancer risk in Crohn disease is estimated at 3% at 20 years

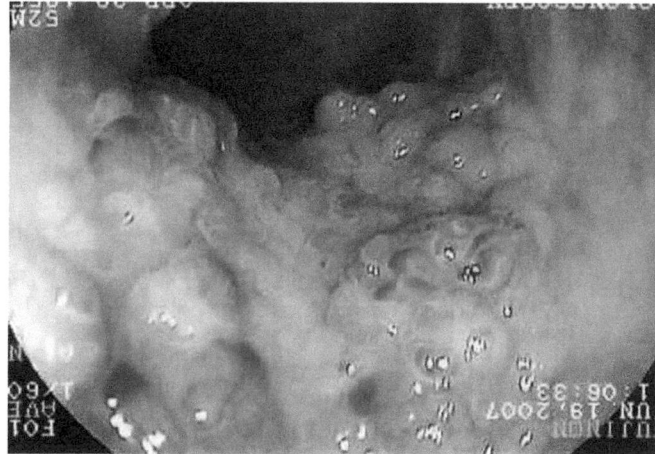

Figure 6-66. Endoscopic photograph of a dysplasia-associated lesion or mass.

• Although imperfect, dysplasia is considered the best marker for cancer risk in inflammatory bowel disease
• Proctocolectomy is advised when dysplasia, especially high-grade dysplasia, is found
• Dysplasia is by nature patchy in distribution and requires multiple biopsy specimens to detect

Gross and Endoscopic Pathology

• Some areas of dysplasia are not grossly distinguishable from adjacent nondysplastic normal or inflamed mucosa (so-called flat dysplasia)
• Many cases are associated with mucosal polyps or plaques (a so-called dysplasia-associated lesion or mass [DALM]) (Figure 6-66)
  • *DALM* is the term used to describe a dysplastic area in longstanding ulcerative colitis associated with a raised or mass lesion (any lesion grossly discernible—a mass, a plaquelike region, a polyp, or a group of polyps)
  • Identifies increased risk for carcinoma, whether high- or low-grade dysplasia is present
  • Often is impossible to distinguish from a sporadic adenoma

Histopathology

• Tissue specimens in IBD are categorized as negative for dysplasia, indefinite for dysplasia, positive low-grade dysplasia, or positive high-grade dysplasia
  • Negative for dysplasia
    • Affected mucosa, although at times inflamed or regenerating, demonstrates normal maturation of the glandular epithelium
    • Mitotic figures and histologic features of regeneration are generally confined to the lower half of the glands
  • Indefinite for dysplasia
    • Used when epithelium has features suggestive of dysplasia, but the changes are insufficient to be unequivocally diagnostic
    • Often occurs in regenerating or inflamed mucosa
    • Also used to describe mucosa with cytologic atypia that differs from that usually seen in dysplasia (e.g., sessile serrated polyp-like change, microvesicular mucinous metaplasia)

- Low-grade dysplasia
  - Characterized by changes similar to those present in an adenomatous polyp, including hyperchromatic, enlarged nuclei with preserved polarity
  - Mucinous differentiation is decreased
  - Dystrophic goblet cells (cytoplasmic vacuole is not in communication with the lumen)
  - Atypia may focally reach the surface
- High-grade dysplasia (Figure 6-67)
  - Prominent nuclear pleomorphism with hyperchromatic, often rounded nuclei that are stratified throughout the cell
  - Atypia extends to the surface
  - Cytologic features resemble those of carcinoma but are confined by a basement membrane

Special Stains and Immunohistochemistry

- Immunostains for p53, β-catenin, CK7, and *bcl*-2 have been investigated but are not often used clinically

Other Techniques for Diagnosis

- Molecular techniques (e.g., loss of heterozygosity) are also described

Differential Diagnosis

INFLAMMATORY ATYPIA

- Characterized by nuclei with prominent nucleoli, but without overt pleomorphism typically associated with dysplasia
- Nuclei tend to have round to oval, smooth external contours, have some uniformity, and are mature toward the luminal surface
- Cryptitis and crypt abscesses are often present

LOW-GRADE VERSUS HIGH-GRADE DYSPLASIA

- Distinction made by the degree of cytologic changes present
- Typically high-grade lesions have marked nuclear pleomorphism, loss of nuclear polarity, and nuclear

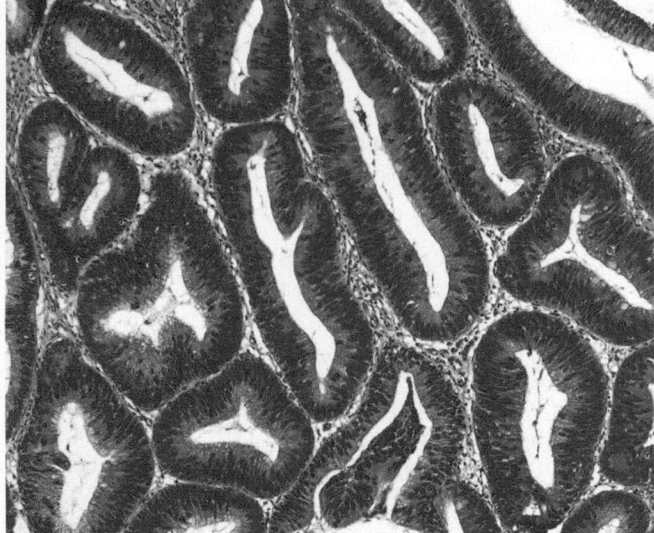

Figure 6-67. High-grade glandular dysplasia in ulcerative colitis. This biopsy specimen from the lesion illustrated in Figure 6-66 shows adenoma-like dysplasia.

stratification that extends to the luminal surface and is readily discernible at low magnification; mitotic figures are often plentiful and may be atypical
- High-grade dysplastic glands have extensive budding, and the surface may have a villiform pattern
- Many surgeons perform total proctocolectomy with ileal pouch–anal anastomosis for low-grade or high-grade dysplasia in a flat mucosa

DALM VERSUS SPORADIC ADENOMA

- Pathologic distinction between these two lesions is not possible
- Characteristics favoring DALM include the following:
  - Patients younger than 40 years with history of ulcerative colitis of long duration (> 10 years)
  - Large lesion (> 1 cm) in an area of proven endoscopic or histologic colitis with dysplasia in the adjacent flat mucosa
  - Positive for p53 (not sensitive or specific enough for clinical use)
  - Negative for bcl-2 (not sensitive or specific enough for clinical use)
  - Chromosome 3p loss of heterozygosity (not generally available)
- Characteristics favoring a sporadic adenoma include the following:
  - Patients older than 40 years with colitis symptoms of shorter duration
  - Small size (< 1 cm)
  - Pedunculated polyp outside proven areas of endoscopic colitis without dysplasia in adjacent mucosa
  - Negative for p53 (not sensitive or specific enough for clinical use)
  - Positive for bcl-2 positivity (not sensitive or specific enough for clinical use)
  - No loss of heterozygosity for chromosome 3p (not generally available)
- Because sporadic adenomas and DALM cannot be separated pathologically, it is better to frame the issue as one of proper patient management; if the raised dysplasia lesion looks adenoma-like endoscopically and histologically and occurs in an area uninvolved endoscopically by colitis, it should be considered a sporadic adenoma and treated by polypectomy alone; if the lesion occurs in an area involved endoscopically by colitis, it is best thought of as an IBD-associated dysplasia
  - "Raised" non-adenoma-like dysplasia lesion
    - Can be defined as a dysplasia lesion that is not endoscopically resectable or dysplasia in a stricture
    - Also includes raised lesions that do not resemble adenomas as seen in non-colitic patients endoscopically or histologically
    - After pathologist confirmation of dysplasia, most investigators advise resection
  - "Raised" adenoma-like dysplasia lesion
    - Endoscopic excision with vigilant follow-up may suffice
    - Many such polypoid dysplasia lesions can be adequately treated by endoscopic polypectomy alone in IBD patients, provided careful patient selection criteria are applied, including the following: the patient is older than 40 years, the lesion is discretely defined endoscopically, excision of the

lesion appears complete to the endoscopist, no other flat dysplasia is identified in the colon (one can use conservative management in patients with multiple adenoma-like dysplasia lesions), and the colon is relatively easy to survey (i.e., compliant patient, no inflammatory polyposis); nevertheless, these patients should receive careful short-term endoscopic surveillance, and colectomy may be appropriate for patients not fulfilling these criteria

SELECTED REFERENCES

Farraye FA, Odze RD, Eaden J, et al: AGA medical position statement on the diagnosis and management of colorectal neoplasia in inflammatory bowel disease. Gastroenterology 138:738-745, 2010.

Farraye FA, Odze RD, Eaden J, Itzkowitz SH: AGA technical review on the diagnosis and management of colorectal neoplasia in inflammatory bowel disease. Gastroenterology 138:746-774, 2010.

Kornbluth A, Sachar DB, Practice Parameters Committee of the American College of Gastroenterology: Ulcerative colitis practice guidelines in adults: American College of Gastroenterology, Practice Parameters Committee. Am J Gastroenterol 105:501-523, 2010.

Odze RD, Farraye FA, Hecht JL, Hornick, JL: Long-term follow-up after polypectomy for adenoma-like dysplastic lesions in ulcerative colitis. Clin Gastroenterol Hepatol 2:534-541, 2004.

Petras R, Mir-Madjlessi S, Farmer R: Crohn's disease and intestinal carcinoma: a report of 11 cases with emphasis on epithelial dysplasia. Gastroenterology 93:1307-1314, 1987.

Petras RE: The significance of adenomas in ulcerative colitis: deciding when a colectomy should be performed. Inflamm Bowel Dis 5:306-308, 1999.

Sigel JE, Petras RE, Lashner BA, et al: Intestinal adenocarcinoma in Crohn's disease: a report of 30 cases with a focus on coexisting dysplasia. Am J Surg Pathol 23:651-655, 1999.

OTHER FORMS OF COLITIS

Clinical Features

INFECTIOUS COLITIS (ACUTE SELF-LIMITED COLITIS)
- Acute onset and short duration (by definition < 6 months)
- Constitutional symptoms, including fever
- History of travel or family members with febrile illness
- Bloody or watery diarrhea

CLOSTRIDIUM DIFFICILE–ASSOCIATED PSEUDOMEMBRANOUS COLITIS
- Recent history of antibiotic administration
- Symptoms include diarrhea and abdominal pain
- Diagnosis is based on identification of *C. difficile* toxin in stool
- Endoscopy reports may describe typical pseudomembranes
- NAP-1 strain causes more serious illness and can be transmitted to otherwise healthy individuals

RADIATION COLITIS
- Usually associated with doses greater than 45,000 cGy
- May be potentiated by presence of diabetes, cardiovascular disease, concurrent chemotherapy
- Acute and chronic forms occur
- Symptoms include diarrhea and abdominal pain; bowel obstruction may occur in the chronic form

ISCHEMIC COLITIS
- Tends to occur in elderly patients with history of cardiovascular or atherosclerotic diseases
- Generally has an acute onset

- Patients may have abdominal pain, nausea, vomiting, diarrhea, or lower gastrointestinal bleeding
- Etiologies include vascular occlusive disease, mechanical obstruction, nonocclusive mesenteric ischemia, drugs that can cause ischemic-type damage (e.g., NSAIDs, oral contraceptives), and infections that can cause ischemic-type change (e.g., enterohemorrhagic *Escherichia coli, Clostridium difficile*)

LYMPHOCYTIC AND COLLAGENOUS COLITIS
- Many cases have unknown pathogenesis; some are related to drugs (e.g., ticlopidine) or infection (e.g., Brainerd diarrhea)
- Patient typically presents with watery diarrhea
- Often patients are older than 50 years
- Collagenous colitis is more common in women
- Associated with immunologic diseases, osteoarthritis, or celiac disease
- Endoscopy is characteristically normal (thus, diagnosis rests solely on microscopic findings)

MUCOSAL PROLAPSE SYNDROMES
- Syndromes include solitary rectal ulcer syndrome, localized colitis cystica profunda, prolapsing mucosal folds in diverticular disease, cap polyposis, and inflammatory cloacogenic polyp
- Many patients show abnormal function of anal and pelvic floor musculature
- Usually middle-aged patients are affected and have constipation, history of difficult defecation, and passage of mucus or blood per rectum

Gross and Endoscopic Pathology

INFECTIOUS COLITIS (ACUTE SELF-LIMITED COLITIS)
- Ranges from mild mucosal edema and erythema to nonspecific ulcerative lesions resembling IBD

CLOSTRIDIUM DIFFICILE–ASSOCIATED PSEUDOMEMBRANOUS COLITIS (ANTIBIOTIC-ASSOCIATED COLITIS) (Figure 6-68)
- Typically segmental involvement with pseudomembranes
- Superficial erosion
- Patchy erythema

RADIATION COLITIS
- Endoscopic findings include dusky mucosa, edema, and loss of superficial vascularity or mucosal capillary ectasia

ISCHEMIC COLITIS
- Depends on severity of ischemia and ranges from mild increase in vascularity and pale, edematous mucosa to dark zones of mucosal hemorrhage to areas of frank green-gray necrosis; ulcers (Figure 6-69)

MICROSCOPIC COLITIS (LYMPHOCYTIC AND COLLAGENOUS COLITIS)
- By definition the endoscopic changes are minimal or absent; patchy erythema

MUCOSAL PROLAPSE SYNDROMES
- Mucosal erythema, ulcer, or polypoid lesion (isolated or multiple, cap polyposis) (Figure 6-70)

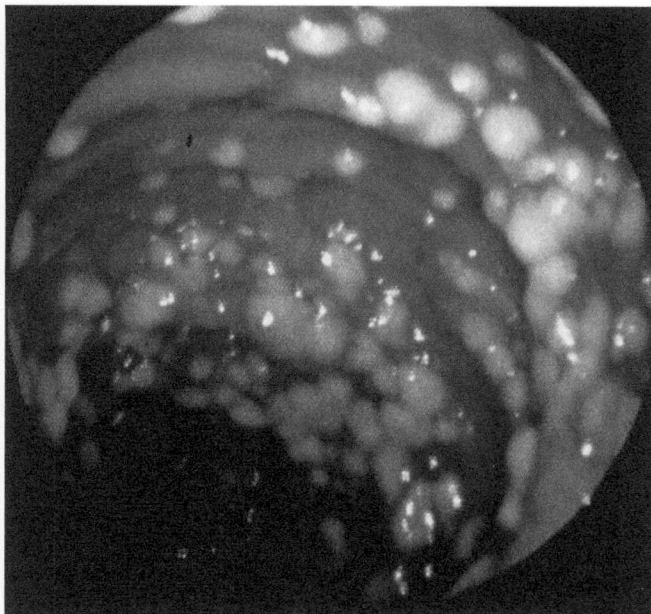

Figure 6-68. *Clostridium difficile-associated* pseudomembranous colitis showing patchy, creamy plaques with intervening erythematous colonic mucosa.

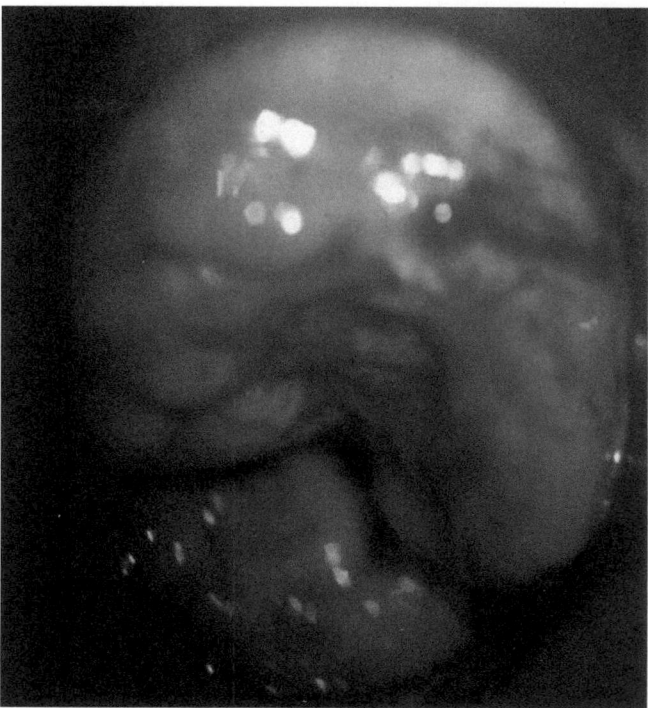

Figure 6-70. Rigid proctoscopic view of solitary rectal ulcer syndrome. The irregularly shaped ulcer is surrounded by heaped-up, firm mucosa.

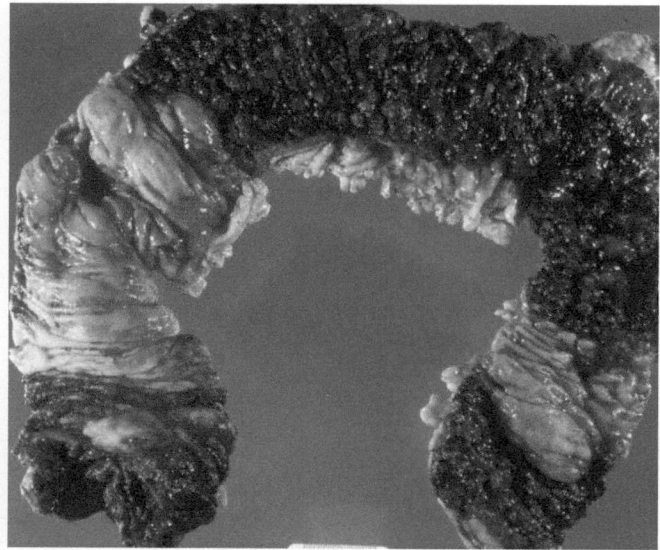
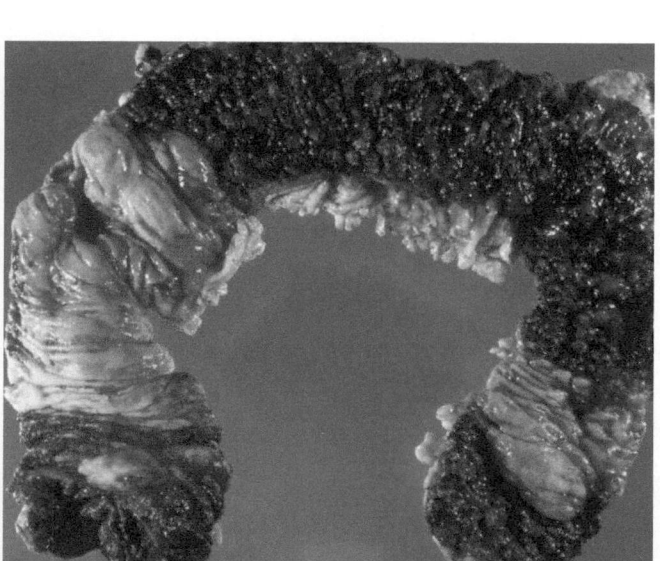

Figure 6-69. Resection specimen of acute ischemic colitis showing patchy areas of ulcer and hemorrhage mimicking Crohn disease.

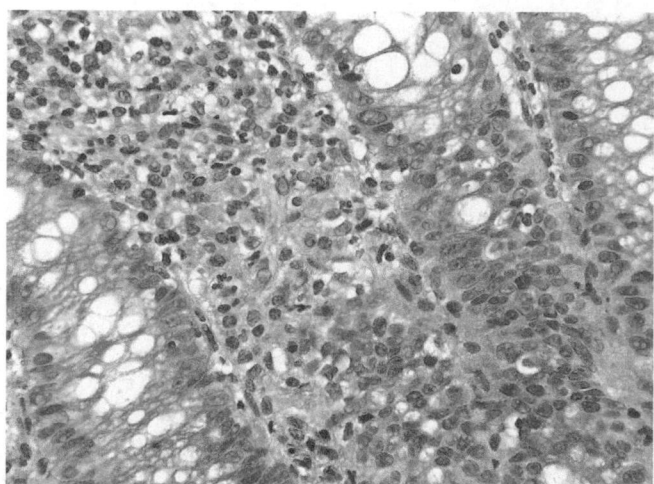

Figure 6-71. The focal active colitis pattern of injury in toxinproved *Clostridium difficile* infection. Note the neutrophils loose within the lamina propria unassociated with increased chronic inflammatory cells.

Histopathology

INFECTIOUS COLITIS (ACUTE SELF-LIMITED COLITIS)

- Typically shows the focal active colitis pattern of inflammation (Figure 6-71)
- Lamina propria hemorrhage and congestion
- Detachment and necrosis of surface epithelium
- Withering of superficial aspects of crypts
- Little glandular distortion or architectural atypia
- Cryptitis and crypt abscesses
- Neutrophils loose in the lamina propria without increased plasma cells

CLOSTRIDIUM DIFFICILE–ASSOCIATED PSEUDOMEMBRANOUS COLITIS

- Classically eruptive acute inflammatory exudate is seen on surface of intact inflamed mucosa (Figure 6-72)
- Superficial erosions may be present
- May show infectious colitis pattern of inflammation (discussed previously)

RADIATION COLITIS

- Acute changes include edema, vascular ectasia, acute cryptitis, and superficial ulceration; usually patchy

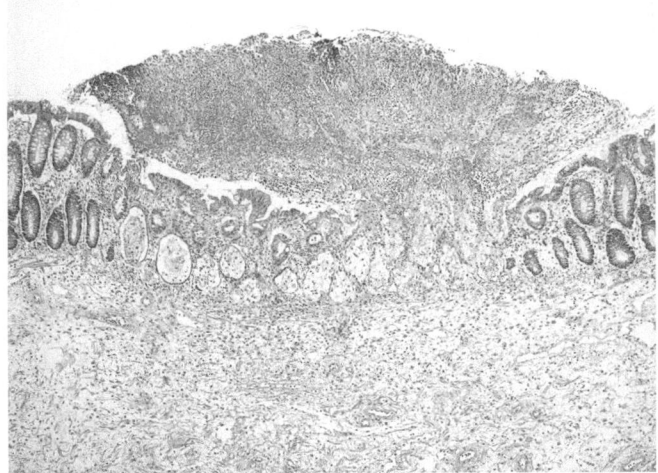

Figure 6-72. *Clostridium difficile*–associated pseudomembranous colitis showing the exploding crypt lesion. The nuclei and karyorrhectic debris are oriented in a curious linear fashion within the inflammatory pseudomembrane.

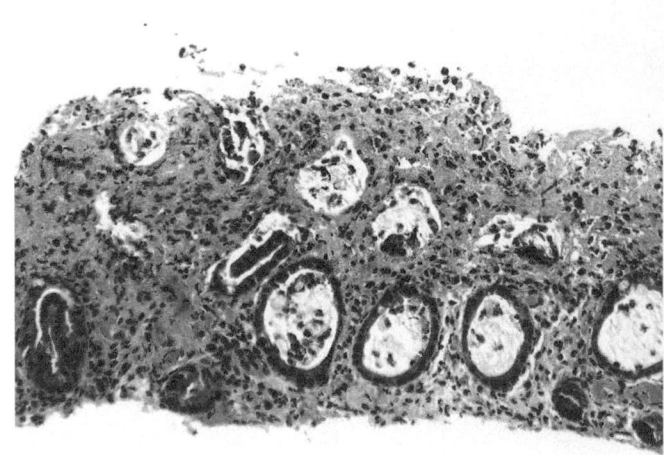

Figure 6-74. Acute ischemic colitis showing coagulative necrosis, mild acute inflammation, and karyorrhectic debris involving the surface with relative preservation of the deep crypt.

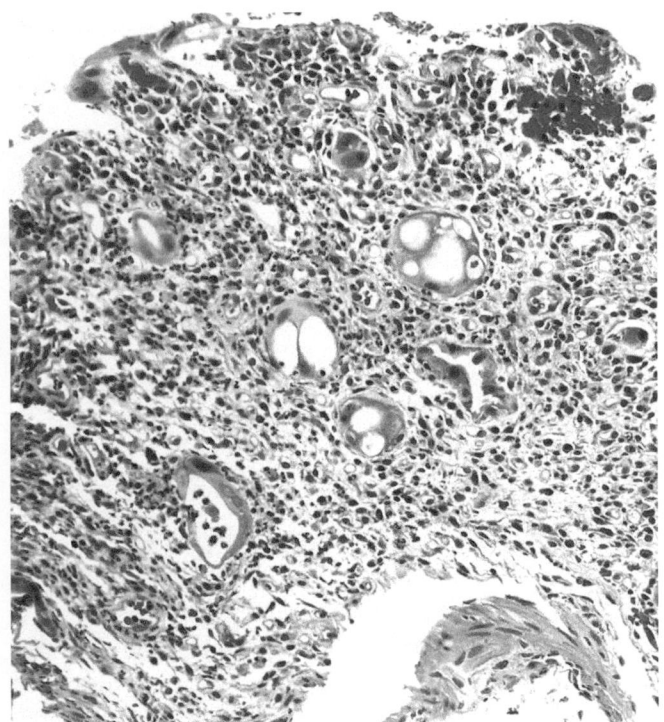

Figure 6-73. Radiation-induced colonic epithelial atypia showing cellular gigantism, a relatively low nuclear-to-cytoplasmic ratio, and cytoplasmic eosinophilia with vacuolization.

- Atypical epithelial cells without an infiltrative pattern, with cellular gigantism, abundant eosinophilic cytoplasm with vacuoles, and possibly emperipolesis in acute forms (Figure 6-73)
- Chronic changes are similar to chronic ischemia and include stromal fibrosis containing atypical fibroblasts and thickened subepithelial collagen, glandular atrophy and distortion, and vascular changes (fibrosis, intimal thickening, and enlarged endothelial cells with vesicular

nuclei); architectural distortion can mimic chronic primary inflammatory bowel disease; packeted midzone lamina propria plasma cells are not uncommon

ISCHEMIC COLITIS (Figure 6-74)
- Mild ischemia is characterized by superficial hemorrhage, patchy mucosal necrosis, dilated vessels, and regenerating crypts producing "decapitated" glands
- Severe ischemic changes include crypt dropout, acute inflammation, acute cryptitis, and coagulative necrosis
- In late lesions, the mucosa ulcerates and is replaced by granulation tissue and eventually fibrous tissue (scarring)

MICROSCOPIC COLITIS (LYMPHOCYTIC AND COLLAGENOUS COLITIS)
- Lymphocytic colitis
  - Characterized by an absolute increase in the chronic inflammatory component in the lamina propria (increase in superficial plasma cells) and increased intraepithelial lymphocytes (> 15 per 100 enterocytes; normal is only 5 to 6 per 100) (Figure 6-75)
- Collagenous colitis
  - Combination of a thickened subepithelial collagen layer (≥15 µm) and increased mixed inflammatory infiltrate of the lamina propria with superficial plasma cells (Figure 6-76)
  - Intraepithelial lymphocytes are often present, and in some areas, subepithelial vacuoles form and the epithelium may be denuded, leaving fragments composed of only "naked" lamina propria

MUCOSAL PROLAPSE SYNDROMES
- Characteristic histology found in polypoid areas or mucosa adjacent to ulcers includes the following:
  - Fibromuscular proliferation and lamina propria (Figure 6-77)
  - Mucosal architectural change
  - Mucosal capillary ectasia

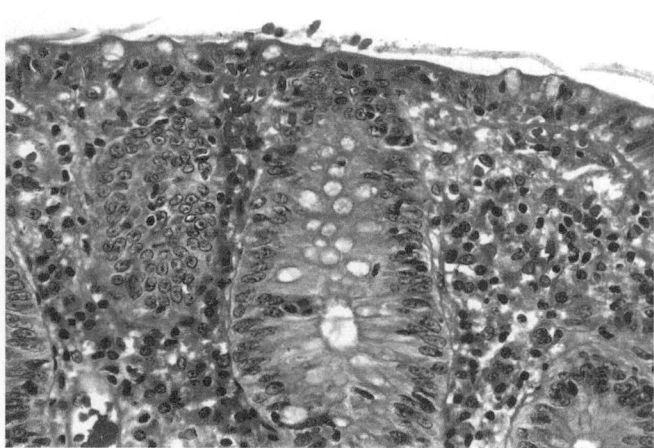

Figure 6-75. Lymphocytic colitis shows an increase in chronic inflammatory cells within the lamina propria and intraepithelial lymphocytosis.

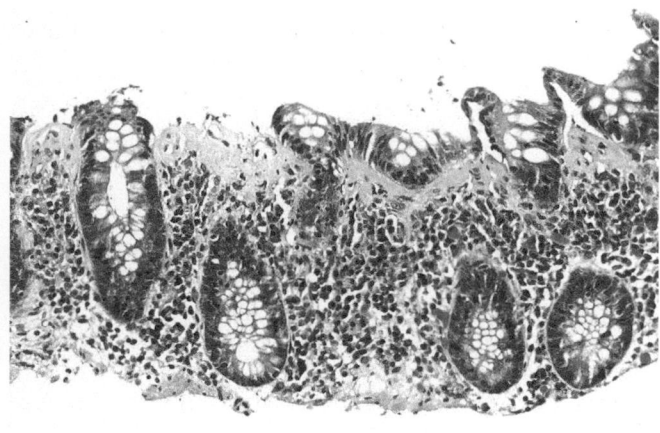

Figure 6-76. Collagenous colitis with increased subepithelial collagen plate, subepithelial vacuoles, and surface epithelial sloughing.

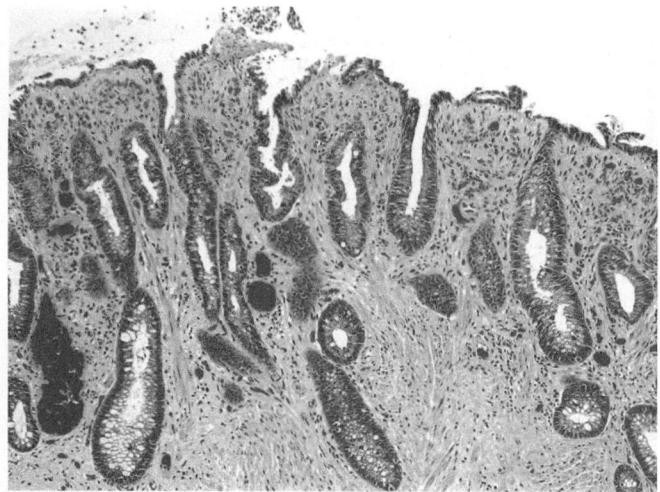

Figure 6-77. Solitary rectal ulcer syndrome. There is architectural distortion accompanied by fibromuscular obliteration of the lamina propria with capillary ectasia.

- May have erosion with inflammatory pseudomembrane
- Misplaced glands in muscularis mucosae or submucosa (so-called localized colitis cystica profunda)

Special Stains and Immunohistochemistry

- Trichrome stain highlights thickened subepithelial collagen band in collagenous colitis; usually not necessary
- Tenascin immunostaining is described in collagenous colitis; not used clinically

Other Techniques for Diagnosis

- Noncontributory

Differential Diagnosis

INFLAMMATORY BOWEL DISEASE

- Clinically patients have repeated bouts of abdominal pain, diarrhea that is often bloody, and fever over months (usually > 6 months)
- Characterized by lymphoplasmacytic infiltrates that reach the crypt bases and by alterations in the glands (branching crypts, mucin depletion, and pyloric and Paneth cell metaplasia)
- Granulomas are sometimes present in Crohn disease

DIVERSION COLITIS AND PROCTITIS

- Occurs in a segment of colon or rectum excluded from the fecal stream; most often a Hartmann pouch constructed at the time of resection of a proximal segment of colon
- Some patients have mucus discharge or diarrhea
- Histologic features include prominent lymphoid aggregates and follicles and a dense lymphoid infiltrate in lamina propria (Figure 6-78)
- Scattered neutrophilic infiltrate with foci of cryptitis and rare crypt abscesses may be seen
- Crypt architecture is usually relatively normal early; diversion of some duration causes glandular atrophy
- Diversion proctitis changes can be superimposed on changes of ulcerative colitis or Crohn disease in patients originally resected for primary inflammatory bowel disease
- Cured by restoration of bowel continuity and resumption of fecal stream; can be treated with short-chain fatty acid enemas

MUCINOUS ADENOCARCINOMA

- The misplaced glands and dissecting mucus in the muscularis mucosae and submucosa seen with localized colitis cystica profunda can closely mimic invasive mucinous adenocarcinoma
- Features that favor mucosal prolapse syndromes include the following:
  - Rounded, pushing external contour to misplaced glands and mucus
  - No epithelium in mucus pools or single discontinuous layer of epithelium at periphery
  - No dysplasia in misplaced epithelium
  - Lack of tumor desmoplasia
  - Presence of hemorrhage and hemosiderin deposits in nearby connective tissues

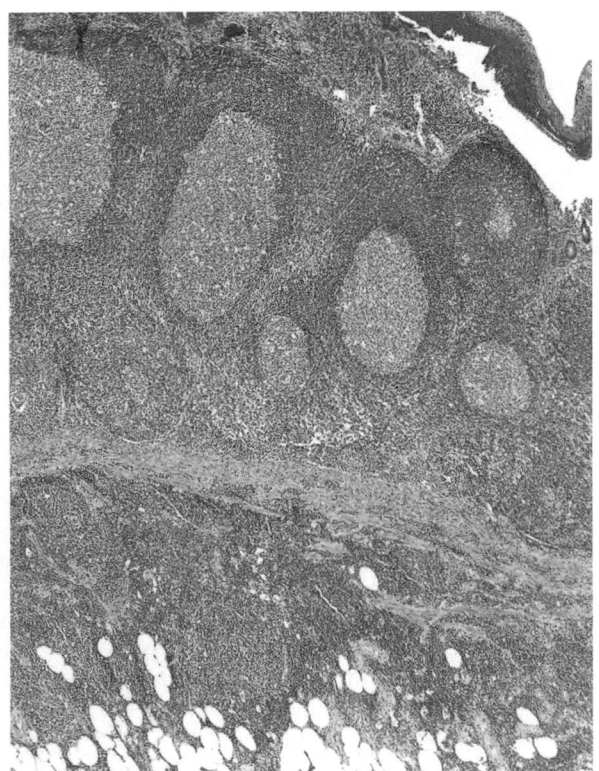

Figure 6-78. Defunctionalized rectum showing marked intramucosal lymphoid hyperplasia associated with surface epithelial atrophy.

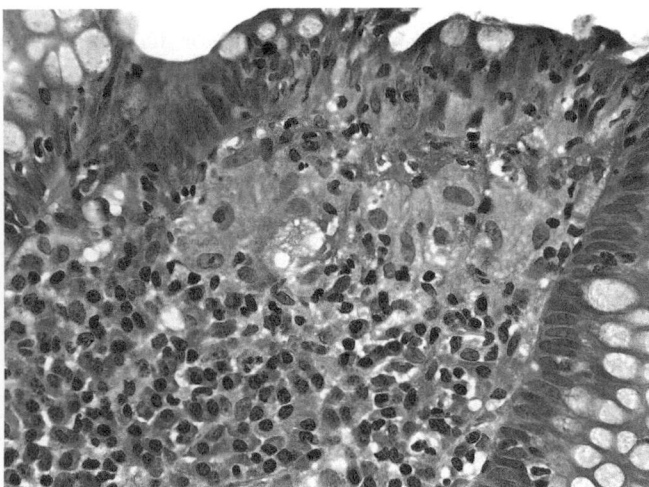

Figure 6-79. Lymphocytic colitis with subepithelial giant cells.

ABERRANT HISTOLOGIC FEATURES IN MICROSCOPIC COLITIS

- Architectural change, subepithelial giant cells, cryptitis, Paneth cell metaplasia, ulcers, or inflammatory pseudomembranes are sometimes seen in cases otherwise typical for lymphocytic colitis or collagenous colitis (Figure 6-79)
- Histology (aberrant or otherwise) generally does not correlate with symptoms, results of treatment, or clinical outcome, with the following exceptions:
  - Cryptitis sometimes correlates with antibiotic use

- Paneth cell metaplasia correlates with severity of diarrhea in collagenous colitis
- Ulcers can be seen with concomitant NSAID use; ulcers may also indicate "fractured" colon in patients with collagenous colitis
  - Colon can fracture during insufflation at endoscopy; this can progress to pneumatosis cystoides intestinalis
- Inflammatory pseudomembranes may indicate comorbid *Clostridium difficile* infection but usually do not
- Lymphocytic colitis with a paucity of plasma cells can be seen in immune deficiencies

CORD COLITIS SYNDROME
- Occurs in approximately 10% of patients undergoing cord-blood stem cell transplantation
- Usually responds to course of antibiotics; may be associated with *Bradyrhizobium enterica*
- Histopathology includes the following:
  - Granulomatous inflammation with mild cryptitis, apoptosis, superficial erosions, and Paneth cell metaplasia
  - Involves upper and lower gastrointestinal (GI) tract
- Knowledge of clinical history imperative

PEARLS

- *Many conditions may mimic IBD; clinical impression is helpful when evaluating colonic biopsies*
- *Colonic biopsies with predominant acute inflammation in the absence of glandular changes generally indicate self-limited colitis rather than IBD*
- *Atypical stromal fibroblasts and associated glandular atrophy with mucosal capillary ectasia are clues to indicate radiation colitis*
- *Subepithelial collagen is abnormal when it is more than 15-μm thick and is diagnostic of collagenous colitis*
- *When cytoplasm is visible under the enterocyte nucleus the section is tangential, do not mistake these for thickened subepithelial collagen (a common trap for the unwary)*
- *Be wary when diagnosing invasive, well-differentiated mucinous adenocarcinoma in the rectum; localized colitis cystica profunda must always be considered and ruled out*
- *Inflammation that is difficult to classify or that shows multiple patterns; think drug effect*

SELECTED REFERENCES

Ayata G, Ithamukkala S, Sapp H, et al: Prevalence and significance of inflammatory bowel disease-like morphologic features in collagenous and lymphocytic colitis. Am J Surg Pathol 26:1414-1423, 2002.

Bhatt AS, Freeman SS, Herrera AF, et al: Sequence-based discovery of *Bradyrhizobium enterica* in cord colitis syndrome. N Engl J Med 369:517-528, 2013.

Griffin P, Olmstead L, Petras R: *Escherichia coli* O157:H7-associated colitis: a clinical and histologic study of 11 cases. Gastroenterology 99:142-149, 1990.

Gupta NK, Masia R: Cord colitis syndrome: a cause of granulomatous inflammation in the upper and lower gastrointestinal tract. Am J Surg Pathol 37:1109-1113, 2013.

Kelly JK: Polypoid prolapsing mucosal folds in diverticular disease. Am J Surg Pathol 15:871-878, 1991.

Libbrecht L, Croes R, Ectors N, et al: Microscopic colitis with giant cells. Histopathology 40:335-338, 2002.

Petras R, Gramlich T: Non-neoplastic intestinal diseases. In Mills SE (ed): Sternberg's Diagnostic Surgical Pathology, 5th ed. New York, Lippincott, Williams & Wilkins, 2010, pp 1313-1367.

Shaz BH, Reddy SI, Ayata G, et al: Sequential clinical and histopathological changes in collagenous and lymphocytic colitis over time. Mod Pathol 17:395-401, 2004.

Sherman A, Ackert JJ, Rajapaksa R, et al: Fractured colon: an endoscopically distinctive lesion associated with colonic perforation following colonoscopy in patients with collagenous colitis. J Clin Gastroenterol 38:341-345, 2004.

AMEBIASIS

Clinical Features

- Worldwide distribution
- Uncommon in the United States, although occurs with increased frequencies in AIDS patients and men who have sex with men
- Most often due to *Entamoeba histolytica*
  - Invasive motile trophozoite
  - Characteristic cyst form (resists gastric acid, chlorination, and room-temperature storage)
- Symptoms vary widely and include the following:
  - Dysentery with diarrhea and rectal bleeding, mimicking IBD
  - Liver abscesses
  - Colonic granulomatous masses that can mimic carcinoma
- Complications include colonic perforation and fistulas or liver abscesses

Gross and Endoscopic Pathology

- Early lesions form small oval ulcers with hyperemic overhanging edges and yellow exudate on base
- Patchy areas of erythema, erosions, and ulceration are especially common in the cecum, appendix, and rectosigmoid (mimics Crohn disease)

Histopathology

- Resected specimens contain ulcers that undermine the adjacent, intact mucosa, producing the characteristic flask shape
- Crypt abscesses and goblet cell depletion
- Biopsy specimens contain only nonspecific inflammation; the focal active colitis pattern of injury can be seen; erosions and ulcers may occur with associated fibrinous exudate, which contains diagnostic organisms (trophozoites); histologic changes mimicking primary inflammatory bowel disease are also described
  - Typical organisms are large (up to 40 µm) oval structures that have a small nucleus with large karyosome and abundant pink, vacuolated cytoplasm (Figure 6-80)
  - Cytoplasm often contains ingested erythrocytes (*Entamoeba histolytica*)

Special Stains and Immunohistochemistry

- Iron hematoxylin in combination with PAS highlights ingested erythrocytes

Other Techniques for Diagnosis

- Serologic tests are available

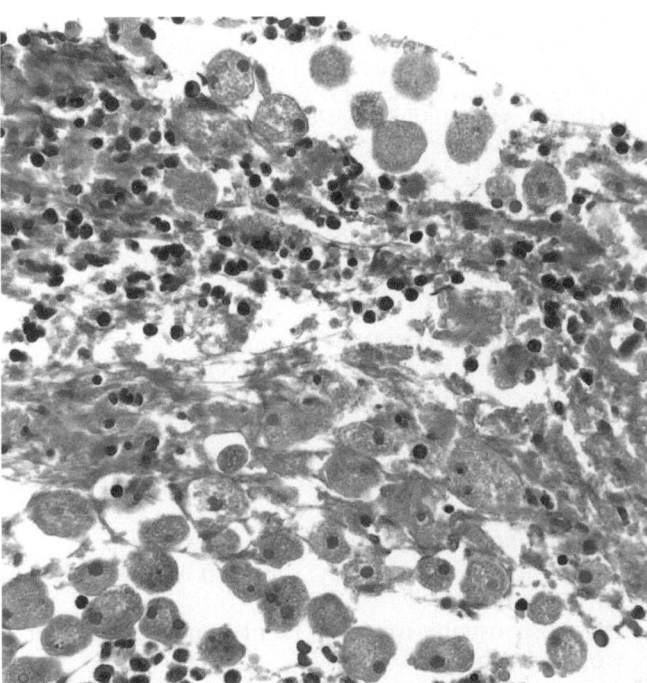

Figure 6-80. Amebiasis. The trophozoites of *Entamoeba histolytica* are larger than histiocytes and show an eccentrically placed circular nucleus. Some of the trophozoites have ingested red blood cells.

Differential Diagnosis

INFLAMMATORY BOWEL DISEASE

- Ulcerative colitis characteristically shows more diffuse colonic involvement with mucosal architectural distortion and lamina propria basal plasmacytosis
- Crohn disease (like amebiasis) may be patchy but is distinguished by fissuring ulcers rather than flask-shaped undermining ulcers; ulcers of Crohn disease tend to have the long axis parallel to the long axis of the bowel; amebic ulcers tend to have the long axis perpendicular to the long axis of the bowel
- IBD lacks fibrinous exudate containing diagnostic organisms
- Biopsy specimens in Crohn disease show focal active colitis pattern of injury, usually with some architectural distortion and increased basal lamina propria plasma cells

PEARLS

- *Always scan the biopsy section for trophozoites when discrete ulcers and fibrinous exudates are present*
- *Trophozoites must be distinguished from histiocytes, which are smaller but have a larger and more irregular nucleus and stain less intensely with PAS*

SELECTED REFERENCES

Allason-Jones E, Mindel A, Sargeunt P, Williams P: Entamoeba histolytica as a commensal intestinal parasite in homosexual men. N Engl J Med 315:353-356, 1986.

Calderaro A, Villanacci V, Bommezzadri S, et al: Colonic amoebiasis and spirochetosis: morphological, ultrastructural and microbiological evaluation. J Gastroenterol Hepatol 22:64-67, 2007.

Connor DH, Neafle RC, Meyers WM: Amebiasis. In Binford CH, Connor DH (eds): Pathology of Tropical and Extraordinary Diseases, vol 1. Washington, DC, Armed Forces Institute of Pathology, 1976.

Merritt RJ, Coughlin E, Thomas DW, et al: Spectrum of amebiasis in children. Am J Dis Child 136:785-789, 1982.

OTHER INTESTINAL PARASITIC INFESTATIONS

Clinical Features

STRONGYLOIDES STERCORALIS

- Diarrhea, malabsorption; autoinfection can be fatal in immunocompromised patients
- Diagnosis usually made by identifying larvae in stool
- Infective form found in soil and can penetrate intact skin

AONCHOTHECA (CAPILLARIA) PHILIPPINENSIS

- Protein-losing enteropathy; found in Asia, Middle East, and Africa
- Diagnosis usually made by identifying eggs, larvae, or worms in stool

TRICHURIS TRICHIURA (WHIPWORM)

- Often asymptomatic but has been associated with abdominal pain and diarrhea; may cause rectal prolapse

ENTEROBIUS VERMICULARIS (PINWORM)

- Nocturnal perianal itching caused by gravid females migrating to perianal skin to deposit eggs

DIPHYLLOBOTHRIUM LATUM (FISH TAPEWORM)

- From raw or undercooked fish
- Usually asymptomatic but may cause intestinal obstruction, vitamin B_{12} deficiency, and pernicious anemia

ANKYLOSTOMA DUODENALE OR NECATOR AMERICANUS (HOOKWORM)

- May have itching at skin site of entry; wheezing and bronchitis when larvae migrates through lungs
- Signs and symptoms of anemia (e.g., pallor, tachycardia)

SCHISTOSOMIASIS

- Can cause colitis or bowel obstruction

Gross and Endoscopic Pathology

STRONGYLOIDES STERCORALIS

- Worms bury themselves in duodenum and jejunum

AONCHOTHECA (CAPILLARIA) PHILIPPINENSIS

- Worms infest jejunum and upper ileum

TRICHURIS TRICHIURA

- Adults are about 4 cm in length and reside in cecum and ascending colon (see Figure 6-83)

ENTEROBIUS VERMICULARIS

- Adults live in cecum; gravid females migrate to anus at night to deposit eggs
- Commonly found in the appendix resection specimen

DIPHYLLOBOTHRIUM LATUM (Figure 6-81)

- Adults can be up to 10 m in length
- Found in small intestine

ANKYLOSTOMA DUODENALE OR NECATOR AMERICANUS

- About 10 mm; live in small intestine

SCHISTOSOMIASIS

- Focal ulcers, stricture, inflammatory polyps

Histopathology

STRONGYLOIDES STERCORALIS

- May see eosinophilic granulomatous reaction

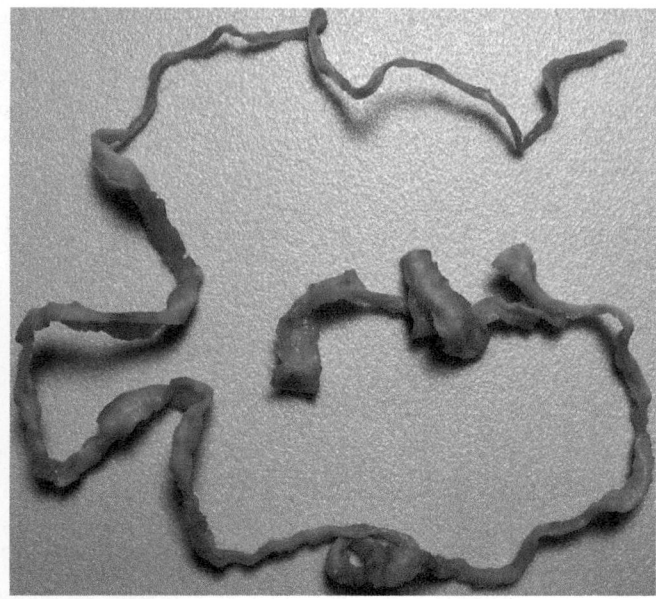

Figure 6-81. Gross photograph of *Diphyllobothrium* species. This worm was removed endoscopically.

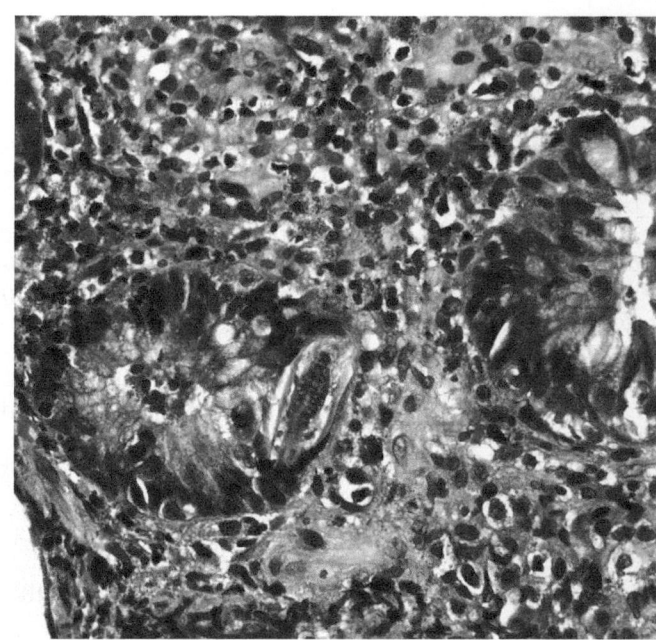

Figure 6-82. Strongyloidiasis with autoinfection. The crypt shows an infiltrating infective filiform larva of *Strongyloides stercoralis*. The lamina propria shows prominent infiltration with eosinophilic leukocytes.

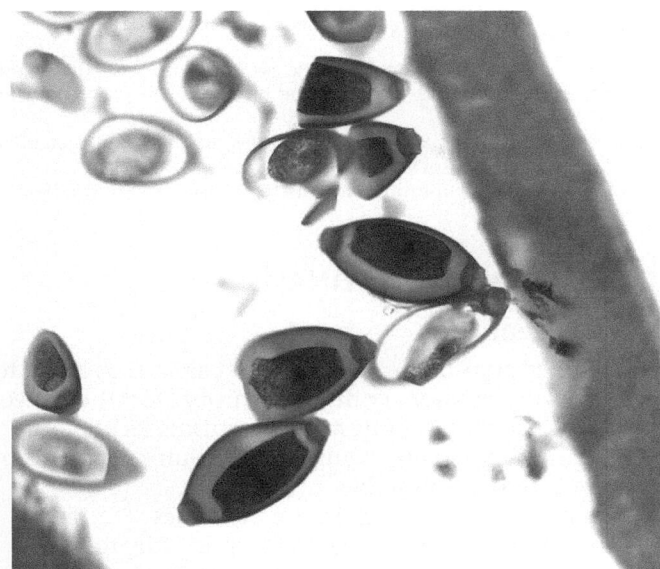

Figure 6-83. *Trichuris trichiura.* Note the characteristic egg morphology in this adult worm removed during endoscopy.

- May see adult female or eggs in small bowel biopsy specimen
- In cases of autoinfection, can see filariform larvae in bowel wall (Figure 6-82)

AONCHOTHECA (CAPILLARIA) PHILIPPINENSIS
- Only rarely described in biopsy specimens
- Morphologic resemblance to those of trichuriasis

TRICHURIS TRICHIURA
- Often extracted at endoscopy; "whip" morphology can be seen on H&E-stained section
- Ova have polar plugs (Figure 6-83)

ENTEROBIUS VERMICULARIS
- Can be seen and extracted at endoscopy
- Lateral alae visible on cross section of worm; eggs with characteristic morphology (Figure 6-84)

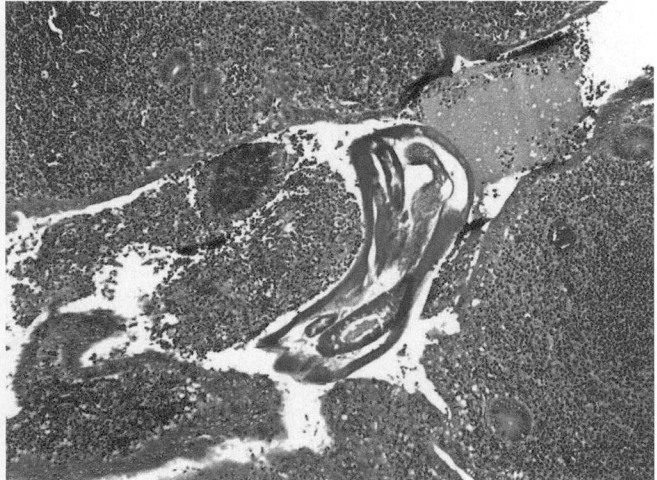

Figure 6-84. *Enterobius vermicularis.* This appendectomy specimen showing acute suppurative appendicitis contains an intraluminal worm with the characteristic lateral alae. Intraluminal bacteria suggestive of *Actinomyces* species are also present.

DIPHYLLOBOTHRIUM LATUM
- Whole mount demonstrates typical morphology; operculate eggs have an abopercular knob

ANKYLOSTOMA DUODENALE OR NECATOR AMERICANUS
- May cause eosinophilic enteritis; diagnosis made usually by identification in stool

SCHISTOSOMIASIS
- Marked inflammatory reaction to eggs

Special Stains and Immunohistochemistry
- Noncontributory

Other Techniques for Diagnosis
- Stool examination

SELECTED REFERENCES
Gutierrez Y: Diagnostic Pathology of Parasitic Infections with Clinical Correlations. Philadelphia, Lea & Febiger, 1990.

Gutierrez Y, Bhatia P, Garbadawala ST, et al: Strongyloides stercoralis eosinophilic granulomatous enterocolitis. Am J Surg Pathol 20:603-612, 1996.

Meyers WM, Neafie RC, Marty AM, Wear DJ (eds): Pathology of Infectious Diseases, vol 1. Helminthiases. Washington, DC, Armed Forces Institute of Pathology, American Registry of Pathology, 2000.

LYMPHANGIECTASIA

Clinical Features
- Primary or secondary forms exist
  - Primary form is typically seen in children and is caused by a congenital obstruction of the lymphatics
  - Secondary form is associated with many conditions, including retroperitoneal fibrosis, pericarditis, pancreatitis, gastrointestinal malignancy, and sarcoidosis
- Symptoms include protein-losing enteropathy, obstruction
- Treatment generally is focused on the underlying condition

Gross and Endoscopic Pathology
- Often form small mucosal elevations that expand the mucosal folds
- Small cysts that may exude milky, chylous fluid
- Small lesions are generally incidental findings

Histopathology
- Primary and secondary forms have same histologic features
- Small multiloculated cysts lined by flat endothelium surrounded by a variable amount of ill-defined supportive stroma
- No red blood cells in the open channels

Special Stains and Immunohistochemistry
- Factor VIII or CD34: lining cells are usually negative but can be positive for immunoreactive D2-40

Other Techniques for Diagnosis
- Noncontributory

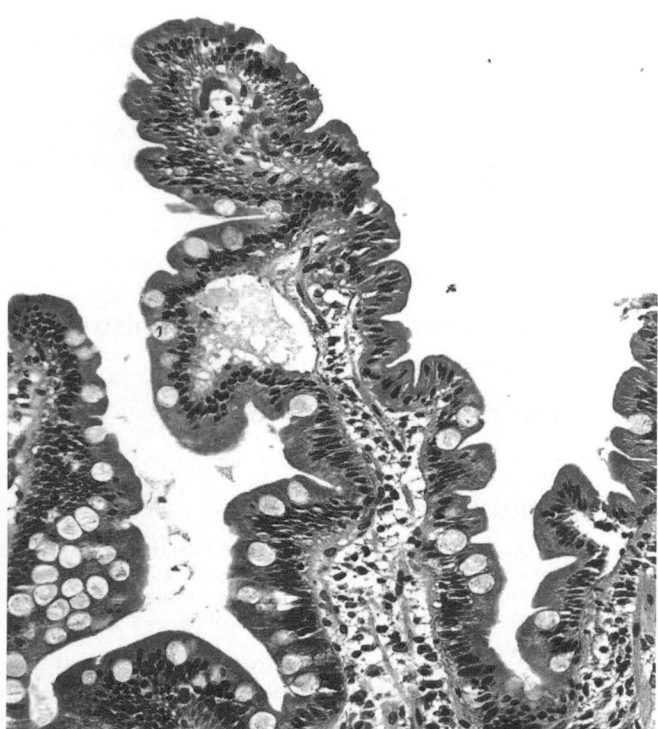

Figure 6-85. Artifact mimicking lymphangiectasia. The surface epithelium has pulled away from the basement membrane, creating an artifactual space mimicking dilated lymphatics.

Differential Diagnosis

- Must be distinguished from fixation-induced separation of basement membrane from surface epithelium, which can produce an artifactual space (Figure 6-85)
- Microscopic dilated mucosal lacteals are of no clinical significance

PNEUMATOSIS INTESTINALIS
- Multiple air-filled cysts, most of which are devoid of an endothelial lining
- Surrounding tissue has wide variability in inflammatory reaction (related to underlying condition); often contains leukocytes, eosinophils, plasma cells, macrophages, and foreign-body giant cells

HEMANGIOMA
- Generally forms a discrete mass
- Can be distinguished from lymphangiectasia by the presence of red cells in the open channels

LYMPHANGIOMA
- Discrete mass lesion composed of microscopic cysts lined by flat endothelium
- Loose, myxoid connective tissue stroma surrounds cysts

PEARLS

- *Primary lymphangiectasis is a rare condition, and protein loss is the predominating clinical presentation*

SELECTED REFERENCES

Kuroda Y, Katoh H, Ohsato K: Cystic lymphangioma of the colon: report of a case and review of the literature. Dis Colon Rectum 27:679-682, 1984.

Vardy PA, Lebenthal E, Shwachman H: Intestinal lymphangiectasia: a reappraisal. Pediatrics 55:842-851, 1975.

Waldmann TA: Protein-losing enteropathy. Gastroenterology 50:422-443, 1966.

PNEUMATOSIS INTESTINALIS

Clinical Features
- Gas-filled cysts in the intestines that are often related to underlying pulmonary disease (chronic form) or infection by gas-forming intestinal organisms (acute form)
- Chronic form more common in adults; acute form more common in infants
- May be found anywhere in the intestines
- Symptoms are usually related to underlying disease
  - Infants: usually coexists with necrotizing enterocolitis, producing severe gastrointestinal complications
  - Adults: diarrhea, flatulence, and excess stool mucus
- Complications include obstruction, volvulus, hemorrhage, and rarely pneumoperitoneum
- Classic radiographic sign is rings of gas in the small or large bowel wall

Gross and Endoscopic Pathology
- Generally a diffuse process but may be localized
- Forms cysts in the mucosa, submucosa, or serosa of small or large intestine (Figure 6-86)
- Cysts are usually near mesenteric border
- Cysts range from 1 mm to several centimeters, often appearing like serosal bubbles
- Submucosal cysts may be imperceptible from the surface but generally cause intestinal crepitance
- Cut surface reveals numerous tiny cysts resulting in a honeycomb appearance

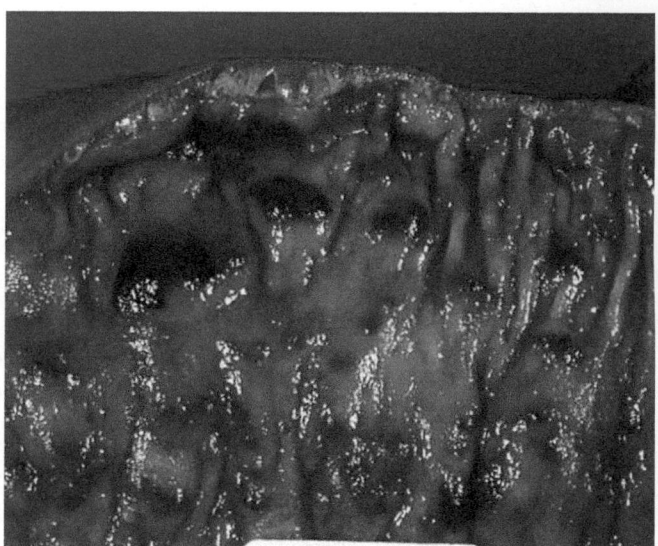

Figure 6-86. Pneumatosis cystoides intestinalis involving sigmoid colon. The surface mucosa shows scattered ischemic changes. The cut section reveals the distended mural gas cysts.

Histopathology

- Multiple air-filled cysts, most of which are devoid of an endothelial lining
- Surrounding tissue has wide variability in inflammatory reaction (related to underlying condition); often contains leukocytes, eosinophils, plasma cells, macrophages, and foreign-body giant cells
- Mucosa can be normal

Special Stains and Immunohistochemistry

- Gram stain rarely detects bacteria around cysts in acute form

Other Techniques for Diagnosis

- Noncontributory

Differential Diagnosis

LYMPHANGIECTASIA

- Microscopic cysts in the small or large intestine with endothelial lining
- Lacks discrete inflammatory component (especially eosinophils and foreign-body giant cells) surrounding cysts

PSEUDOLIPOMATOSIS

- Tiny gas cysts in mucosa and superficial submucosa thought to be caused by insufflation at endoscopy
- No lining; resembles adipose tissue

PEARLS

- *Cysts are thought to form secondary to traumatic rupture of gas into bowel (such as induced by coughing) or to proliferation of gas-forming organisms (such as Clostridium perfringens, Enterobacter aerogenes, and Escherichia coli)*
- *A biopsy specimen can obscure the cysts by collapsing them with only macrophages, giant cells, and eosinophils remaining; care must be taken to avoid misinterpretation as Crohn disease*

SELECTED REFERENCES

Heng Y, Schuffler MD, Haggit RC, Rohrmann CA: Pneumatosis intestinalis: a review. Am J Gastroenterol 90:1747-1758, 1995.
Koreishi A, Lauwers GY, Misdraji J. Pneumatosis intestinalis: a challenging biopsy diagnosis. Am J Surg Pathol 31:1469-1475, 2007.

MELANOSIS COLI

Clinical Features

- Associated with chronic laxative ingestion (anthraquinones, cascara, sagrada, aloes, senna, frangula, rhubarb) and other drugs that induce excessive apoptosis
- Patients generally have a history of constipation

Gross and Endoscopic Pathology

- Dark brown to black mucosal pigmentation (Figure 6-87)
- Primarily involves the right colon
- Severe cases may involve entire colon, appendix, and terminal ileum

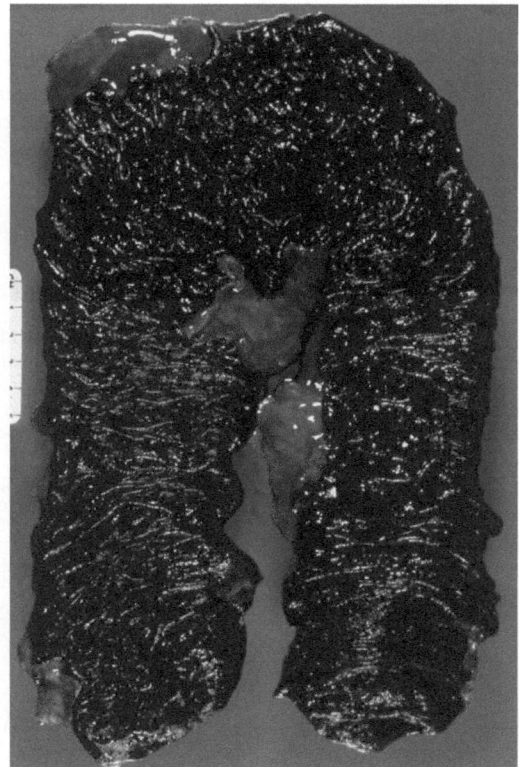

Figure 6-87. Severe melanosis coli (resection specimen).

Histopathology

- Lipofuscin deposits in lamina propria histiocytes
- Pigments are granular, refractile, and golden brown, and form clusters between intact glands
- Draining lymph nodes may contain similar pigments
- Occasionally nonspecific inflammation or microgranulomas (containing pigment) present; the latter can cause confusion with Crohn disease

Special Stains and Immunohistochemistry

- *Melanosis coli* pigment is positive with PAS, AFB, and Fontana-Masson stains
- Perl reaction negative
- Prussian blue (iron) stain negative

Other Techniques for Diagnosis

- Noncontributory

Differential Diagnosis

BROWN BOWEL SYNDROME (CEROIDOSIS)

- Lipofuscin deposits are in the smooth muscle cells of the muscularis mucosae, muscularis propria, and vascular walls rather than in lamina propria histiocytes
- Patients often have vitamin E deficiency (often seen in celiac sprue or cystic fibrosis) and are typically symptomatic (abdominal pain and diarrhea)

PSEUDOMELANOSIS DUODENI

- Deposits of iron in tips of proximal small bowel villi
- Associated with iron containing compounds, hypertension, end-stage renal disease, and diabetes mellitus

PEARLS

- *Presence of the coarse, brown pigments in the lamina propria that are Prussian blue (iron) stain negative and Fontana-Masson stain positive indicates melanosis coli*
- *Hemosiderin deposits in the lamina propria are positive for Prussian blue (iron) stain*
- *Brown granular deposits (lipofuscin) in the smooth muscle cells indicate brown bowel syndrome*

Selected References

Gallager RL: Intestinal ceroid deposition—"brown bowel syndrome": a light and electron microscopic study. Virchows Arch A Pathol Anat Histol 389:143-151, 1980.

Giusto D, Jakate S. Pseudomelanosis duodeni: associated with multiple clinical conditions and unpredictable iron stain ability—a case series. Endoscopy 40:165-167, 2008.

Walker NI, Bennett RE, Axelsen RA: Melanosis coli: a consequence of anthraquinone-induced apoptosis of colonic epithelial cells. Am J Pathol 131:465-476, 1988.

GASTROINTESTINAL POLYPS

Clinical Features

- Typically occur in the colon
- Most common are hyperplastic polyps, inflammatory polyps, and adenomas

HYPERPLASTIC POLYP

- More common in men
- Most common colonic polyp
- In the colon, hyperplastic polyps are 3 to 10 times more common than adenomas
- Almost always asymptomatic

INFLAMMATORY POLYP (PSEUDOPOLYPS)

- Occur in setting of chronic colitis, such as ulcerative colitis, Crohn disease, trauma and prolapse (e.g., near orifice of diverticula), and infectious colitis; may also occur adjacent to mucosal injury (e.g., surgical anastomosis)

ADENOMAS

- Thought to precede development of many carcinomas
- When multiple (> 10), *may* indicate a genetic syndrome (e.g., FAP, attenuated FAP, and MUTYH-associated polyposis syndrome)
- Generally exhibit slow growth with 10-year doubling time
- Prevalence is thought to be around 35% in Western civilizations
- Prevalence increases dramatically after 40 years of age (peak, 60 to 70 years)
- Presence of one adenoma is associated with a 40% to 55% risk for additional adenomas
- Risk for presence of villous architecture and for higher-grade dysplasia increases with multiple adenomas
- Risk for new adenomas is 20% to 60% within 3 to 10 years after initial polypectomy
- Symptoms include the following:
  - Bleeding; however, adenomas smaller than 1 cm are usually asymptomatic, except those in the rectosigmoid area, which may bleed
  - Larger and villous lesions may produce mucinous diarrhea or constipation
  - Ominous signs are obstruction and abdominal pain
- Detection of small sigmoid or rectal adenomas is indication for full colonoscopy

Gross and Endoscopic Pathology

HYPERPLASTIC POLYP

- Usually in sigmoid colon and rectum but can be present throughout the colon; hyperplastic polyps outside of the rectosigmoid colon must be distinguished from sessile serrated polyps (see "Differential Diagnosis")
- Typically smaller than 0.5 cm but rarely larger than 1 cm (larger polyps must be distinguished from sessile serrated polyps; see "Differential Diagnosis") (Figure 6-88)
- Often on crest of mucosal folds
- Often multiple

INFLAMMATORY POLYP

- Small, sessile nodules with smooth surfaces; some with variable shapes
- Often multiple

ADENOMAS (Figure 6-89)

- Most are exophytic, mucosal protrusions
- Three endoscopic types: pedunculated, sessile, and flat/depressed
- Gross architecture is related to histologic type
  - Tubular adenomas are usually small, round, and pedunculated
  - Tubulovillous adenomas are larger
  - Villous adenomas are more likely sessile, flat, or on a short, broad pedicle
- Larger adenomas are more likely to be hemorrhagic
- Flat adenomas are difficult to detect endoscopically and are small, plaquelike mucosal discolorations

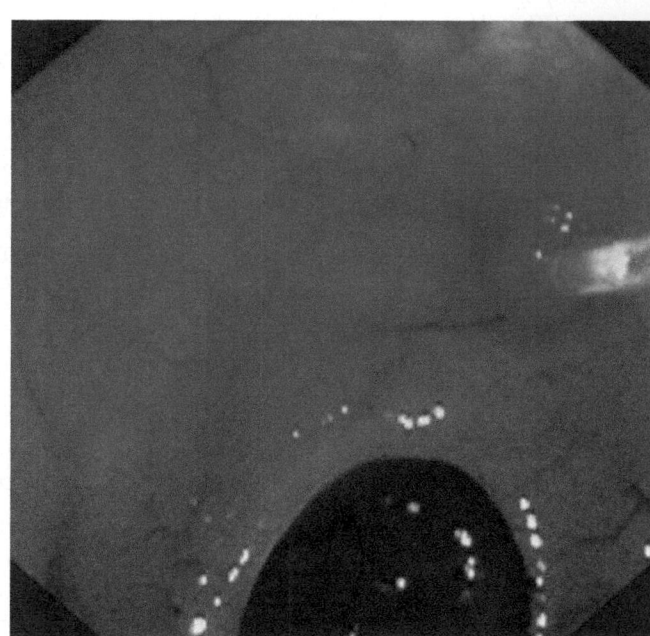

Figure 6-88. Endoscopic view of hyperplastic polyp. Hyperplastic polyps are typically small (<5 mm) and are about the same color as the surrounding colonic mucosa.

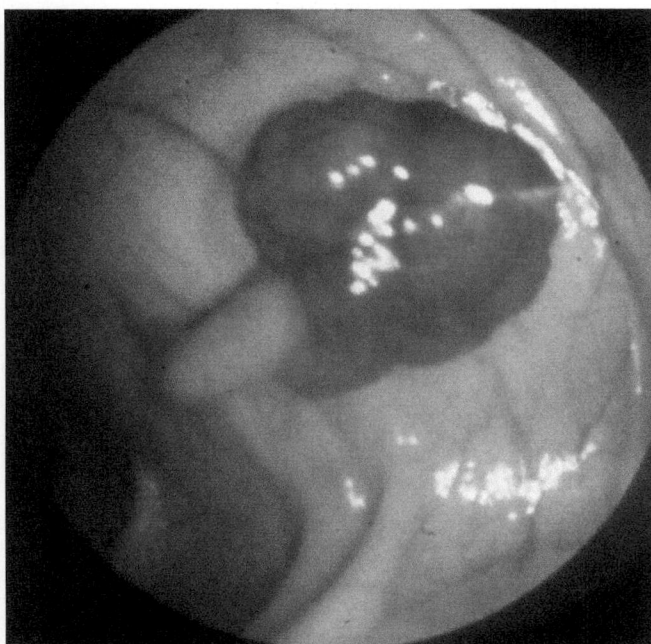

Figure 6-89. Endoscopic view of pedunculated tubulovillous adenoma.

- Estimated 1% of adenomas smaller than 1 cm contain cancer, compared with 45% of adenomas larger than 2 cm

Histopathology

HYPERPLASTIC POLYP
- Characterized by serrated, convoluted (sawtooth pattern) luminal border (due to an increased number of mature colonocytes per unit area) (Figure 6-90)

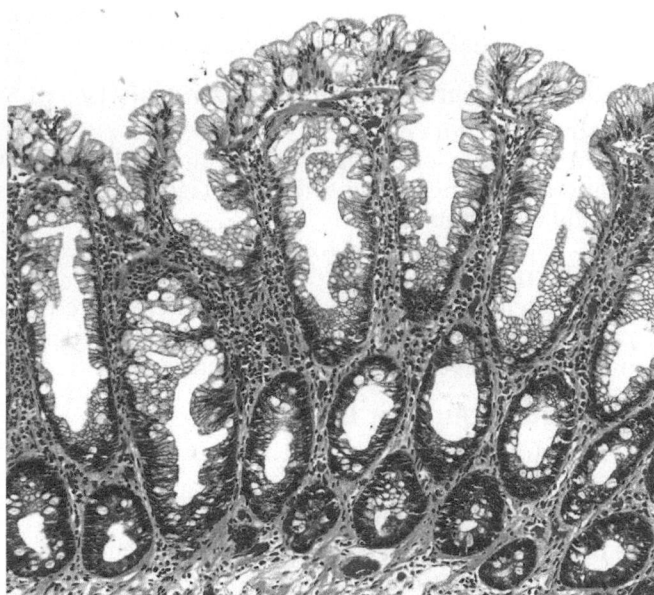

Figure 6-90. Hyperplastic polyp. Histologic section shows elongate crypts lined by evenly distributed goblet cells and absorptive cells. The crypts and surface epithelium have a serrated appearance. The surface basement membrane shows focal hyalinization. Mitotic figures are seen in the crypt base.

- Slight expansion of the mitotically active basal cell zone, limited to the lower half of the crypt (so-called bottom-up atypia)
- Straight crypts that should be wider at the polyp surface
- No dysplasia
- Mixture of absorptive cells and goblet cells

INFLAMMATORY POLYP
- Mixture of inflamed stromal tissue and hyperplastic epithelium in variable proportions
- Sometimes exhibits an ulcerated surface and exuberant granulation tissue reaction containing mixed inflammation
- Dilated epithelial cysts in various stages of degeneration and regeneration—at times simulating adenomatous change
- Those associated with mucosal trauma/prolapse often have smooth muscle in the lamina propria and dilated thick walled blood vessels
- Inflammatory polyp with bizarre stromal cells
  - Designation used for occasional inflammatory polyps that contain large, bizarre spindle or polygonal stromal cells; usually a surface phenomenon and of no clinical significance

ADENOMAS
- Three types: tubular, tubulovillous, villous
- Small, pedunculated adenomas are usually tubular or tubulovillous
- Larger, sessile adenomas usually have a villous component
- All adenomas, by definition, are composed of dysplastic epithelium, characterized by cells with enlarged, hyperchromatic, stratified nuclei and decreased mucin; increased mitotic figures extending to the upper areas of the crypt
- Most adenomas demonstrate some evidence of maturation into mucin-secreting cells called *oligomucous cells*; these cells have variable amounts of mucus, and thus some goblet cells are usually present
- Degree of dysplasia is determined by evidence of maturation
  - Low-grade dysplasia: slightly stratified spindle or oval nuclei with apical cytoplasm (roughly half of the total cell height) and evidence of goblet cell formation
  - High-grade dysplasia: full-thickness, stratified, round nuclei, and little cytoplasm (most nuclei reach the gland lumen) with greater nuclear pleomorphism and little goblet cell differentiation (Figure 6-91)
  - The term *high-grade dysplasia* has been expanded to include more complex cribriform patterns (adenocarcinoma in situ) or cases with infiltration of carcinoma cells into the lamina propria or muscularis mucosae alone (so-called intramucosal adenocarcinoma) that lack submucosal invasion
- Dysplastic epithelium appears first on the superficial surface and eventually replaces the deeper epithelium (so-called top-down atypia)
- Adenomatous epithelium in the submucosa simulating invasive carcinoma (so-called pseudoinvasion) occurs in 2% to 10% of pedunculated polyps, particularly those in the sigmoid colon with long (> 1 cm) stalks;

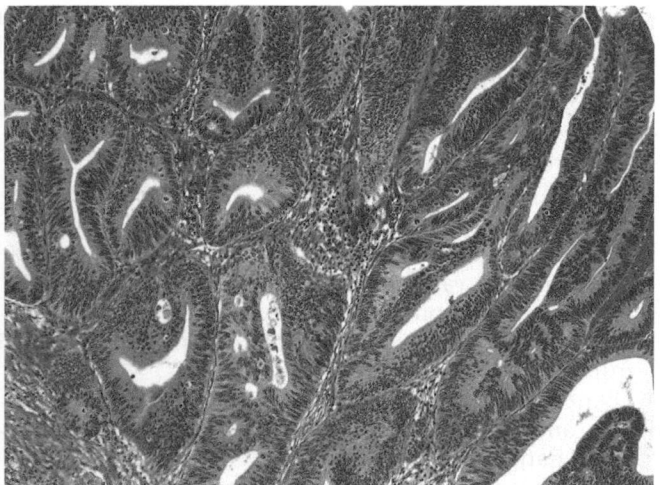

Figure 6-91. Colonic adenoma with high-grade dysplasia demonstrating full-thickness stratification and a focal cribriform pattern.

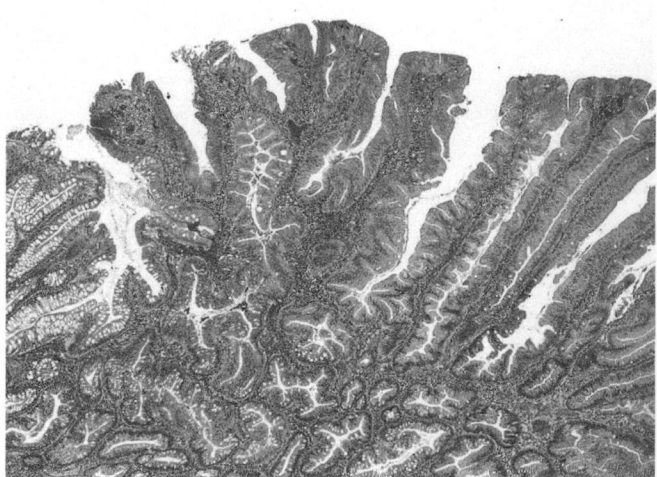

Figure 6-92. Traditionally defined serrated adenoma. These polyps are typically pedunculated, left sided, and demonstrate epithelial dysplasia. The serration imparts a resemblance to hyperplastic polyp. Serrated adenoma typically shows gastric foveolar change and eosinophilic cytoplasmic changes.

thought to arise following torsion resulting in hemorrhage, inflammation, fibrosis, or increased pressure causing herniation of the adenomatous epithelium through defects in the muscularis mucosae
- Pseudoinvasion is recognized by the following conditions:
  - Presence of lamina propria around adenomatous glands or by identifying direct connection to mucosa
  - Hemosiderin deposits and fibrosis rather than desmoplasia
  - Lack of malignant cytology
  - Rounded contours to malpositioned glands without infiltration
- Tubular adenoma
  - Most common (more than 70%)
  - Composed of tubular glands (similar to normal colonic glands), but lined by dysplastic epithelium
  - Tubular architecture constitutes more than 75% to 80% of adenoma
- Villous adenoma
  - Composed of slender, finger-like, or leaflike epithelial fronds and deep crypts extending outward from the muscularis mucosae
  - Fronds contain vascular cores and are lined by dysplastic epithelium
  - Villous architecture composes more than 75% to 80% of adenoma
- Tubulovillous adenoma
  - Mixture of both tubular and villous architecture
  - Villous architecture composes roughly 20% to 25% to 75% to 80% of the adenoma
- Mixed hyperplastic and adenomatous polyp
  - Relatively rare
  - Discrete areas of both hyperplastic and adenomatous histology with a sharp demarcation between the two
  - Most examples likely represent dysplasia in a sessile serrated polyp (see "Differential Diagnosis")
- Traditionally defined serrated adenoma
  - True adenoma (with epithelial dysplasia) characterized by serration; nature of the epithelial atypia is contro-

versial with some experts believing it to be a type of "senescence" rather than true dysplasia (Figure 6-92)
- Lining cells are less mature than in hyperplastic polyps often showing eosinophilic cytoplasm or gastric foveolar metaplasia, and they show superficial mitotic figures, intact nuclear polarity, a high nuclear-to-cytoplasmic ratio, and nuclear pleomorphism; however, the cells have abundant mucin
- May be admixed with areas of hyperplastic polyp, sessile serrated polyp, and classic adenoma
- Usually left sided and pedunculated
- Ectopic crypt formation in which there is budding of proliferating crypts situated perpendicular to the long axis of a filiform or villous structure is touted as the most characteristic histologic feature

Special Stains and Immunohistochemistry

HYPERPLASTIC POLYP
- Trichrome stain or collagen IV immunostain demonstrates a thickened subepithelial collagen zone; this is usually not required

INFLAMMATORY POLYP
- Stromal cells (including bizarre stromal cells) are carcinoembryonic antigen (CEA), cytokeratin, and mucin negative; positive for vimentin and muscle-specific actin

Other Techniques for Diagnosis
- Noncontributory

Differential Diagnosis

SESSILE SERRATED POLYP (SSP) (Figures 6-93 and 6-94)
- Also known by a number of synonyms, including giant or large hyperplastic polyp, polyp with epithelial serrated proliferation, sessile serrated lesion (probably the best term), and sessile serrated adenoma
- Typically right sided, large (> 1 cm), sessile, and often poorly circumscribed

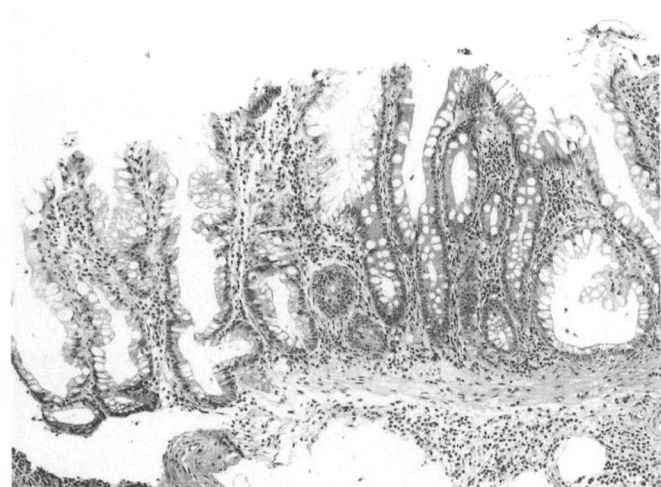

Figure 6-93. Sessile serrated polyp showing branded crypts, deep crypt dilation, horizontal orientation of crypts, and an irregular distribution of goblet cells.

- May mimic enlarged mucosal fold; can show a tenacious mucus cap and peripheral debris endoscopically
- Polyps containing four or more of the following characteristics should be classified as sessile serrated polyp and differentiated from hyperplastic polyp:
  - Basal crypt dilation
  - Crypt branching
  - Horizontal orientation of crypts
  - Inverted histology (glands malpositioned into muscularis mucosae or submucosa)
  - Prominent serration
  - Epithelial-to-stromal ratio exceeding 50%
  - No surface basement membrane thickening

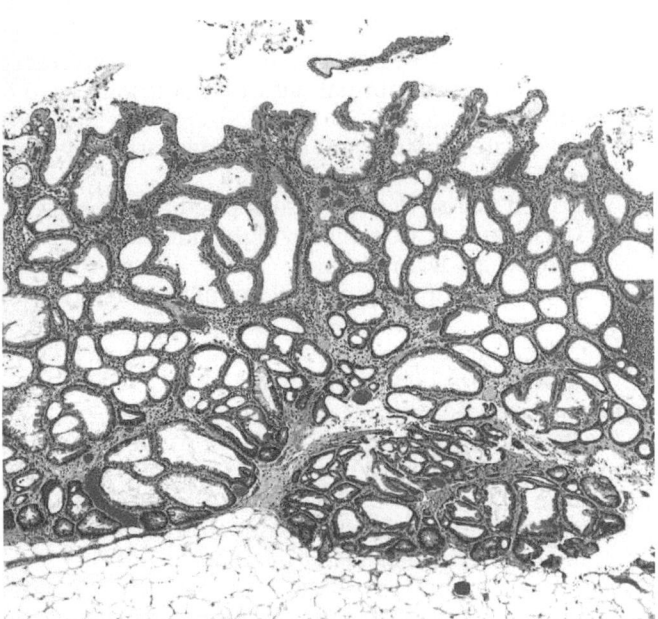

Figure 6-94. Sessile serrated polyp with inverted histology. The regenerative zone of the sessile serrated polyp is enveloped by smooth muscle fibers of the muscularis mucosae; some parts of the polyp have herniated into the submucosa.

- Persistent nuclear enlargement, atypia, and nucleoli in the upper third of crypt
- Mitosis figures in upper third of crypt
- Abnormal patchy distribution of dystrophic goblet cells
- Likely is the specific precursor lesion of sporadic microsatellite instability–high (MSI-H) colorectal carcinoma
- Polyp type seen in serrated polyposis syndrome
- Current recommendations include the following:
  - Endoscopic removal of all serrated lesions proximal to sigmoid colon
  - Surgical resection is rarely necessary but may be appropriate if a serrated lesion cannot be removed by the endoscope or if numerous large serrated lesions are present in the proximal colon (e.g., serrated polyposis syndrome)
  - A sessile serrated polyp with cytologic dysplasia is equivalent to an advanced adenoma
  - Though controversial, an expert panel has concluded that any proximal colonic serrated lesion > 1 cm should be considered a sessile serrated polyp regardless of histology
- Recommendation for postpolypectomy surveillance includes the following:
  - Small (< 10 mm) hyperplastic polyps in rectosigmoid colon: 10 years
  - SSP < 10 mm: 5 years
  - SSP ≥ 10 mm: 3 years
  - SSP with cytologic dysplasia: 3 years
    - Some investigators suggest 1-year surveillance citing that the transition from dysplasia to carcinoma may occur faster in the serrated pathway to colorectal carcinoma
  - Traditionally defined serrated adenoma: 3 years

HAMARTOMATOUS POLYPS
- Discussed later in the chapter

REGENERATIVE CHANGE
- Can be seen with mucosal trauma and prolapse or in inflammatory polyps
- Regenerative epithelium usually shows increased nuclear size, cytoplasmic basophilia, and increased mitoses restricted to the basal half of the crypt with more mature goblet cells and absorptive cells at the surface; usually lacks apoptosis

PEARLS

Inflammatory Polyp

- *To avoid misdiagnosis of neoplasia, carefully evaluate stromal cells (particularly in small biopsies and when the epithelium is atrophic or regenerative), looking for fibromuscular hyperplasia and ectatic capillaries, which are often seen in inflammatory polyps*

Adenomas

- *Biologically, adenomatous growth is thought to progress sequentially, through a continuum: low-grade dysplasia, high-grade dysplasia, carcinoma in situ, intramucosal carcinoma, and invasive carcinoma*

- *Clinically the important distinctions are size, villous component, and presence of high-grade dysplasia or carcinoma*
  - *Carcinoma cells that infiltrate into the lamina propria or muscularis mucosae alone (intramucosal adenocarcinoma) have virtually no risk for metastasis; many advocate classifying these lesions as high-grade dysplasia*
  - *Degree of dysplasia correlates with cancer risk; high-grade dysplasia carries a risk for subsequent advanced adenoma and carcinoma that is several times higher than that of low-grade dysplasia*
  - *Only when the carcinoma cells infiltrate through the muscularis mucosae into the submucosa or beyond are they considered invasive and clinically significant*
  - *Invasion of submucosa is recognized by an infiltrative pattern to the neoplastic glands accompanied by tumor desmoplasia*
  - *Desmoplasia accompanies invasion of at least the submucosa, but it cannot be used to identify the actual depth of invasion in a biopsy specimen*
- *Pathology report should include the following:*
  - *Highest degree of dysplasia present in the biopsy specimen and presence of villous component*
  - *Degree of differentiation and distance from the margin, if invasive carcinoma is present, as well as the presence or absence of vascular and lymphatic invasion*

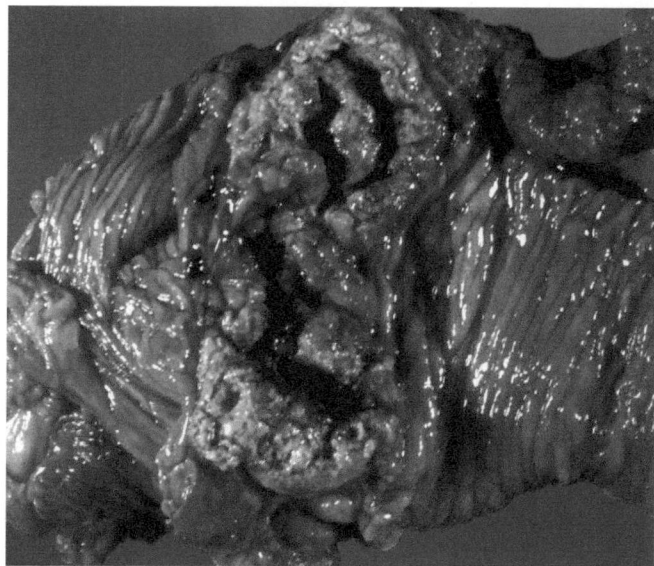

Figure 6-95. Microsatellite instability high colorectal carcinoma.

Selected References

Goldstein NS: Small colonic microsatellite unstable adenocarcinomas and high-grade epithelial dysplasias in sessile serrated adenoma polypectomy specimens: a study of eight cases. Am J Clin Pathol 125:132-145, 2006.

Lieberman DA, Rex DK, Winawer SJ, et al: Guidelines for colonoscopy surveillance after screening and polypectomy: a consensus update by the US Multi-Society Task Force on Colorectal Cancer. Gastroenterology 143:844-857, 2012.

Rex DK, Ahnen DJ, Baron JA, et al: Serrated lesions of the colorectum: review and recommendations from an expert panel. Am J Gastroenterol 107:1315-1329, 2012.

Riddell RH, Petras RE, Williams GT, Sobin LH: Tumors of the intestines. Atlas of Tumor Pathology Third Series, Fascicle 32. Washington, DC, Armed Forces Institute of Pathology, 2003.

Snover DC, Ahnen DJ, Burt RW, Odze RD: Serrated polyps of the colon and rectum and serrated polyposis. In Bosman FT, Carneiro F, Hruban RH, Theise ND (eds): World Health Organization Classification of Tumours of the Digestive System. Lyon, IARC Press, 2010, pp 160-165.

Sweetser S, Smyrk TC, Sinicrope FA: Serrated colon polyps as precursors to colorectal cancer. Clin Gastroenterol Hepatol 11:760-767, 2013.

SPORADIC ADENOMAS AND ADENOCARCINOMA OF THE LARGE INTESTINE

Molecular Classification

- At least five different molecular pathways to colorectal cancer exist based on chromosomal instability (CIN), CpG island methylation (CIMP), microsatellite instability (MSI), and *BRAF* gene status
  - Those thought to have a common adenoma as the precursor lesion include sporadic CIN carcinomas, FAP-related cancers (both with CIN and germline *BRAF*) and the Lynch syndrome–related adenocarcinomas (MSI-high and germline *BRAF*)
  - Those thought to arise from serrated lesions include sporadic MSI-high colorectal cancer (MSI, CIMP, *BRAF* mutated) and a subset of chromosomal instability related carcinoma (CIN, CIMP, microsatellite stable, *BRAF* mutated)
  - A small subset of cancers thought to arise from traditionally defined serrated adenomas as well as common adenomas show CIN, CIMP, MSI-low, and methylation inactivation of MGMT
- Although many molecular pathways to colorectal carcinoma have been described, it is useful to approach colorectal carcinoma with a more simplified strategy
  - About 85% are derived through the chromosomal instability pathway
    - Cancers are often DNA aneuploid by flow cytometry
    - Demonstrate abnormalities of chromosomes 5, 17, and 18
    - FAP-related colorectal carcinomas arise by this pathway
  - About 15% arise in the mutator phenotype pathway
    - These cancers are typically right sided and large
    - Cancers are DNA diploid
    - Cancers demonstrate epiphenomenon referred to as *microsatellite instability*
    - Colorectal carcinoma complicating Lynch syndrome arises by this pathway
- Lynch syndrome
  - Individuals with germline mutations of DNA mismatch repair genes (e.g., *hMLH1, hMSH2, hPMS2, hMSH6*)
  - About 15-fold increased risk for colorectal carcinoma compared with the general population
    - Cancers occur on average in patients 20 years younger than colorectal carcinoma patients from the general population
  - Increased risk for other carcinomas, including endometrium, ovary, stomach, urinary tract, biliary tract, central nervous system, and small bowel

- Can be suspected clinically based on Amsterdam II criteria
  - Three or more relatives with Lynch syndrome–related tumors
  - Colorectal carcinoma in two generations
  - One or more Lynch syndrome–related tumors occurring in a patient younger than 50 years
  - A kindred fulfilling the Amsterdam criteria but without mutation of a known mismatch repair gene is referred to as having *familial colorectal cancer syndrome type X*; some of these patients have mutation in epithelial cell adhesion molecule (EPCAM)

Clinical Features of Colorectal Cancer

- Incidence is about 153,000 new cases and 52,000 deaths/year, accounting for 10% of cancer deaths in the United States
- Peak incidence between 60 to 79 years of age; fewer than 20% occur in patients younger than 50 years of age
- High incidence in populations with diet rich in animal fat and sedentary lifestyle
- Increased risk with chronic inflammatory bowel disease
- Symptoms include the following:
  - Anemia: when present in an elderly male, colon cancer is suspected until proved otherwise
  - Location dependent
    - Right-sided tumors: enlarge without direct symptoms, but bleed easily, thus causing indirect symptoms, including anemia and fatigue
    - Left-sided tumors (where colon caliber is smaller): produce melena, constipation, and diarrhea (change in bowel habits)

Gross and Endoscopic Pathology

ADENOCARCINOMA (Figures 6-95 and 6-96)
- Patulous right colon tends to produce larger exophytic tumors, generally without causing obstruction
- Tumors in the smaller-caliber distal colon evolve into annular "napkin ring" tumors
- Can be fungating, ulcerated, or necrotic masses (Figure 6-96)
- Lynch syndrome and sporadic MSI-H colorectal carcinoma tend to be right sided (75%), can be multiple and tend to be large and bulky

Histopathology

ADENOCARCINOMA
- Histology can be similar regardless of location
- Infiltration of glands of variable differentiation lined by anaplastic epithelial cells
  - Grade I
    - Composed predominantly of well-formed glands in a desmoplastic stroma
  - Grade II
    - Less well-formed glands with focal cribriform architecture
  - Grade III
    - Tumor grows in solid sheets with no distinct gland formation (Figure 6-97)
- Lining cells are fully stratified and have large hyperchromatic nuclei and prominent nucleoli
- Prominent mitotic activity often with atypical forms

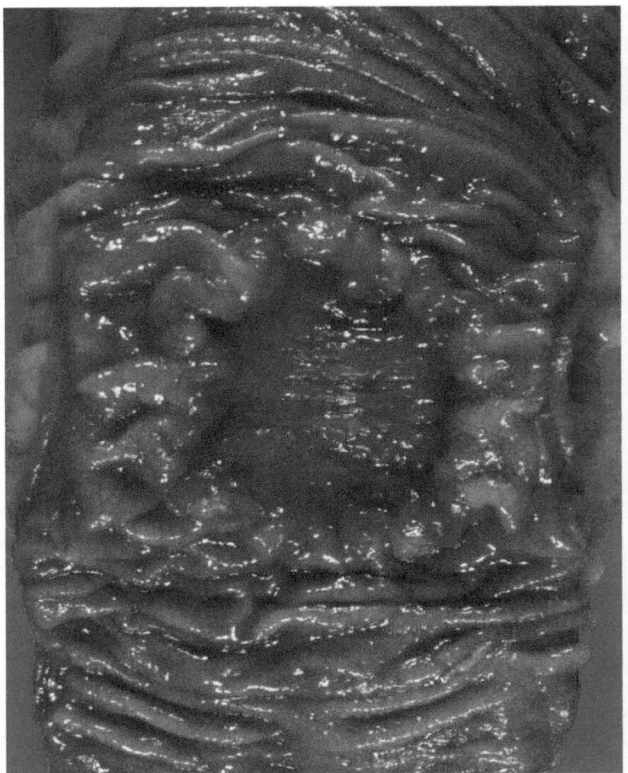

Figure 6-96. Gross resection specimen of ulcerated carcinoma of sigmoid colon.

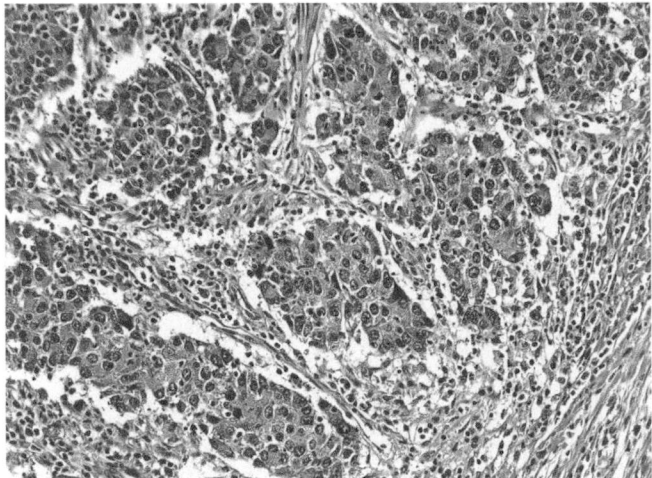

Figure 6-97. Medullary adenocarcinoma. This histologic pattern of colonic carcinoma is characterized by syncytial groups of highly anaplastic epithelial cells without lumen formation. A brisk peritumoral lymphocytic response is present.

- Invasion promotes a characteristic robust desmoplastic tissue reaction, imparting the hard gross consistency

MUCINOUS ADENOCARCINOMA
- Accounts for about 10% of colorectal malignancies
- Production of excess mucin with associated malignant epithelial glands and free-floating, malignant cells

- Generally agreed that 75% to 80% of the tumor area must show extracellular mucus to be linked to a worse prognosis
- Worse prognosis, presumably due to the greater penetration imparted by the mucin

LYNCH SYNDROME AND SPORADIC MSI-H COLORECTAL CANCER

- Can have a prominent lymphoid component, including peritumoral lymphocytes (so-called Crohn-like reaction) and increased intratumoral lymphocytes
- Tend to be poorly differentiated (e.g., undifferentiated or medullary carcinoma) (Figure 6-97)
- Mucinous and signet ring cell histology overrepresented

UNCOMMON TYPES OF COLORECTAL CANCER

- Include high-grade neuroendocrine carcinoma (including small cell and large cell carcinoma), adenosquamous carcinoma, squamous carcinoma, pleomorphic giant cell carcinoma, and carcinosarcoma

Special Stains and Immunohistochemistry

- Immunohistochemistry for mismatch repair gene proteins hMLH1, hMSH2, hPMS2, and hMSH6 is available

Other Techniques for Diagnosis

- PCR tests for microsatellite instability and immunohistochemistry for mismatch repair gene proteins should be performed on cancers fulfilling modified Bethesda criteria, which include the following:
  - Patient younger than 50 years
  - Synchronous or metachronous Lynch syndrome–related tumors regardless of age
  - Colorectal carcinoma with MSI-H histology in a patient younger than 60 years
  - Colorectal carcinoma in a patient with a first-degree relative with a Lynch syndrome–related tumor (< 50 years of age) or first-degree relative with a colorectal adenoma (< 40 years of age)
  - Colorectal carcinoma in a patient with two or more relatives with a Lynch syndrome–related tumor regardless of age
- Microsatellite instability testing and immunohistochemistry for mismatch repair gene proteins probably should be done on all colorectal carcinomas because
  - There is a survival advantage for MSI-H colorectal carcinoma stage for stage compared with MSI-low and MSI stable cancer
  - MSI-H predicts for metachronous carcinomas
  - MSI-H predicts poor response to fluorouracil-based chemotherapy regimens; MSI-H may be associated with a better response to irinotecan-based chemotherapy regimen
  - MSI-H testing aids in the detection of Lynch syndrome because more than 40% of probands patients are older than 50 years, and almost 25% of Lynch syndrome patients do not fulfill Amsterdam or Bethesda guidelines

- Gene sequencing for mismatch repair genes may be indicated in some patients with MSI-H by PCR and some with abnormal immunohistochemistry; this may also be indicated in a kindred with a compelling history regardless of the results of MSI testing or immunohistochemistry

Differential Diagnosis

ENDOMETRIOSIS

- Often involves the colon and rectum (15% to 20% of endometriosis cases); occasionally involves the small intestine
- Typically an incidental finding; generally asymptomatic but occasionally may cause a polyp or bowel obstruction and can mimic carcinoma
- Endometriomas are usually ill-defined masses smaller than 4 or 5 cm; typically involve the serosa and subserosa but may extend through to the mucosa and bulge into the lumen
- Characterized histologically by the presence of endometrial glands and stroma (Figure 6-98)
- Biopsy of the mucosa is often negative unless the mucosa is eroded

METASTATIC CARCINOMA

- No surface component
- Bulk of tumor cells in submucosa
- Immunohistochemistry for CK7 and CK20 can sometimes help differentiate a primary colorectal adenocarcinoma from a metastasis

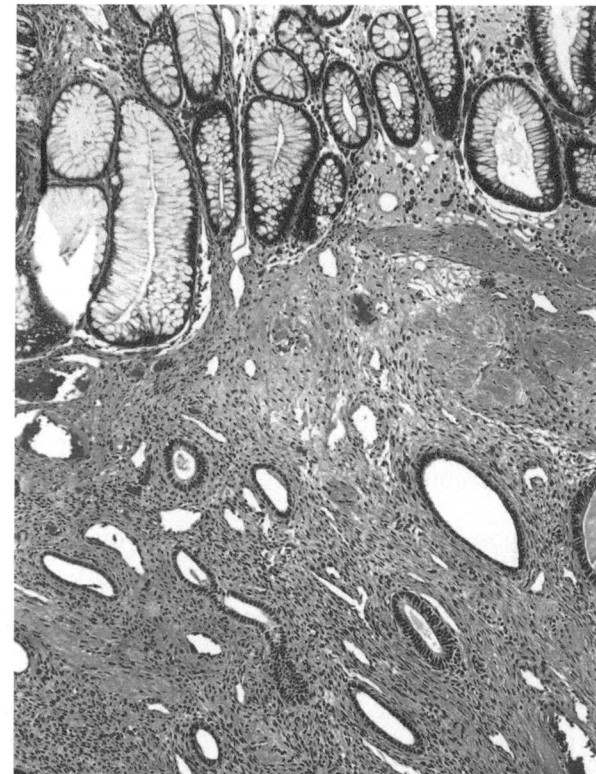

Figure 6-98. Endometriosis involving the sigmoid colon. Note the endometrial glands and stroma within the submucosa.

PEARLS

- *Prognosis: although symptomatic at a smaller size, left-sided neoplasms are more often high stage at diagnosis and thus have poorer prognosis (5-year survival rates are 100%, 80%, 60%, and 10% for stages I, II, III, and IV, respectively)*
- *Weak or absent MSH6 immunostaining is characteristic in Lynch syndrome patients with a germline mutation of MSH2/MSH6; weak or absent MSH6 immunostaining can occasionally be seen in MLH1/PMS2 deficient tumors in which loss of MSH6 is caused by a somatic mutation in the microsatellite within the coding region of MSH6; weak or scanty MSH6 can also be seen in resected cancers that have been treated with preoperative chemotherapy or chemotherapy/radiation therapy in which the mechanism for MSH6 loss is unknown*
- *Use CAP cancer protocols for reporting*

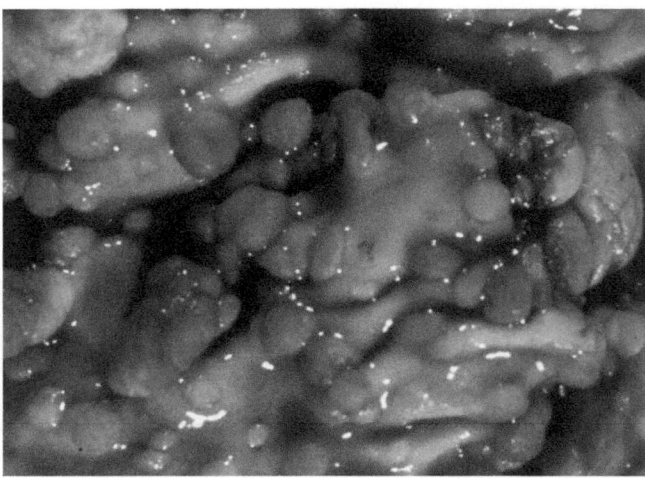

Figure 6-99. Colonic resection specimen from a patient with familial adenomatous polyposis. This close-up view shows numerous adenomas.

SELECTED REFERENCES

Bertagnolli MM, Niedzwiecki D, Compton CC, et al: Microsatellite instability predicts improved response to adjuvant therapy with irinotecan, fluorouracil, and leucovorin in stage III colon cancer: cancer and leukemia group B protocol 89803. J Clin Oncol 27:1814-1821, 2009.

Bosman FT, Carneiro F, Hruban RH, Theise ND (eds): WHO Classification of Tumours of the Digestive System, 4th ed. Lyon, IARC Press, 2010.

Niessen RC, Hoffstra RM, Westers H, et al: Germline hypermethylation of MLH1 and EPCAM deletions are a frequent cause of Lynch syndrome. Genes Chromosomes Cancer 48:737-744, 2009.

Riddell RH, Petras RE, Williams GT, Sobin LH: Tumors of the intestines. Atlas of Tumor Pathology Third Series, Fascicle 32, Washington, DC, Armed Forces Institute of Pathology, 2003.

Shia J, Zhang L, Shike M, et al: Secondary mutation in a coding mononucleotide tract in MSH6 causes loss of immunoexpression of MSH6 in colorectal carcinomas with MLH1/PMS2 deficiency. Mod Pathol 26:131-138, 2013.

Umar A, Boland CR, Terdiman JP, et al: Revised Bethesda Guidelines for hereditary nonpolyposis colorectal cancer (Lynch syndrome) and microsatellite instability. J Natl Cancer Inst 96:261-268, 2004.

POLYPOSIS SYNDROMES

Clinical Features

- Includes syndromes associated with the development of both neoplastic and hamartomatous (non-neoplastic) polyps
  - FAP and variants
  - Peutz-Jeghers syndrome
  - Juvenile polyposis
  - Phosphatase and tensin homologue (PTEN) hamartoma tumor syndrome (e.g., Ruvalcaba-Myhre-Smith syndrome, Cowden syndrome)
  - Cronkhite-Canada syndrome

FAP (Figure 6-99)

- Autosomal dominant transmission with nearly complete penetrance
- Affects about 1 in 7000 to 1 in 30,000 live births
- Adenomas may occur before 1 year of age but usually begin around puberty
- Without colonic resection, development of invasive carcinoma of colon or rectum and death from colorectal carcinoma are inevitable

- FAP-associated gene has been identified on chromosome 5 (5q21), called adenomatous polyposis coli (*APC*) gene
  - Specific mutations within the gene generally correlate with severity of the disease and associated conditions
  - Mutations near the 3′ and 5′ end of the gene and within exon 9 cause a mild form of the disease called *attenuated FAP*
- Associated conditions
  - Congenital hypertrophy of the retinal pigment epithelium
  - Upper gastrointestinal polyps in stomach and small bowel; small bowel adenomas, particularly the periampullary area, can progress to carcinoma (which is the cause of death in more than 20% of patients after colectomy)
  - Mandibular osteomas and other dental and skin lesions and cysts
  - Abdominal desmoid tumors
  - Carcinoma at extraintestinal sites (e.g., papillary thyroid carcinoma and hepatoblastoma)
- Presenting symptoms in patients not in surveillance include bleeding and anemia; symptomatic patients are much more likely to harbor colorectal carcinoma
- No gender preference; all races are affected equally
- Gardner syndrome
  - Variant of FAP characterized by osteomas, fibromatosis, and epidermal cysts
  - High frequency of thyroid and duodenal cancer
- Turcot syndrome
  - Rare variant of FAP coexisting with medulloblastoma
  - Some patients originally thought to have Turcot syndrome have germline mutations of the mismatch repair genes (Lynch syndrome) coexisting with glial neoplasms, usually glioblastoma
- Muir-Torre syndrome
  - Rare autosomal dominant disorder associated with mutations of mismatch repair genes
  - Generally fewer than 100 adenomas, which are frequently in the proximal colon

- Associated with basal cell carcinoma, sebaceous carcinoma, and squamous cell carcinoma
- MUTYH-associated polyposis syndrome
  - Mutation of *mutY* homologue (MYH), a base excision repair gene
  - Autosomal recessive inheritance
  - Afflicted patients acquire somatic mutation of *APC* gene at a high rate
  - Can mimic FAP and attenuated FAP

PEUTZ-JEGHERS SYNDROME
- Genetic disorder characterized by gastrointestinal hamartomas and skin and mucosal hyperpigmentation; diagnostic criteria include the following:
  - Three or more histologically confirmed Peutz-Jeghers polyps
  - Any Peutz-Jeghers polyp with a family history of Peutz-Jeghers syndrome
  - Hyperpigmented lesions of skin and mucous membrane with a family history of Peutz-Jeghers syndrome
  - Any Peutz-Jeghers polyp associated with mucocutaneous pigmentation
- Autosomal dominant with variable penetrance
- Far less common than FAP
- Gastrointestinal polyps and pigmented skin and mucosal lesions present in infancy
- Associated with extraintestinal malignancies, especially involving the pancreas, gonads, and breast; associated with ovarian sex cord tumor with annular tubules and testicular Sertoli cell tumors

JUVENILE POLYPS AND JUVENILE POLYPOSIS SYNDROME
- Isolated juvenile polyps
  - Usually children
  - May have up to five small (< 2 cm) polyps in colon and rectum
  - Prone to autoamputation
- Juvenile polyposis syndrome (Figure 6-100)
  - Defined as six or more juvenile polyps in the colon and rectum, patient with juvenile polyps throughout the gastrointestinal tract, any juvenile polyp in a patient with a positive family history of juvenile polyposis syndrome

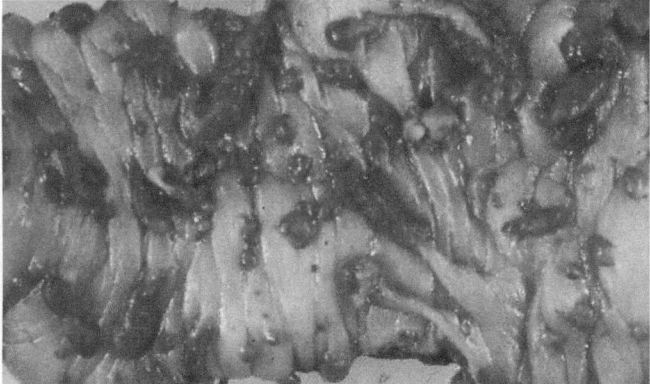

Figure 6-100. Colonic resection specimen from a patient with juvenile polyposis syndrome. Some of the polyps have typical juvenile polyp morphology (pedunculated with a smooth red surface). Some show unusual forms with finger-like multilobulated shapes.

- Familial and nonfamilial forms exist
- Nonfamilial form is associated with other congenital abnormalities in 20% of cases
- Several varieties of familial juvenile polyposis exist with different inheritance patterns, usually autosomal dominant, and involve different areas of the gastrointestinal tract
- Juvenile polyps occur in about 3 in 100,000 patients younger than 10 years
- Patients with juvenile polyposis become symptomatic early in childhood with bleeding (80% of cases) or symptoms of obstruction; polyp may prolapse into anal canal

PTEN HAMARTOMA TUMOR SYNDROME
- Cowden syndrome
  - Rare autosomal dominant disease characterized by hamartomas and neoplasms, mainly of face, thyroid, and gastrointestinal tract
  - Equal sex distribution
  - Most lesions are benign
  - Lesions occur between 20 and 40 years of age
  - Breast carcinoma occurs in up to half of affected patients
- Ruvalcaba-Myhre-Smith syndrome (Bannayan-Riley-Ruvalcaba syndrome)
  - Presents in childhood with macrocephaly, mental deficiency, unusual craniofacial appearance, pigmented macules on the penis, and gastrointestinal polyps

CRONKHITE-CANADA SYNDROME
- Unknown etiology
- Rare adult, nonfamilial (nonhereditary), gastrointestinal polyposis syndrome
- Onset typically occurs in late adulthood
- Associated with alopecia, skin hyperpigmentation, and nail dystrophy; hair loss can be total and usually occurs rapidly
- Symptoms include diarrhea, abdominal pain, and protein and weight loss
- Mortality rate is 60%, due to cachexia

Gross and Endoscopic Pathology
FAP
- In fully developed cases, the colon is carpeted with adenomas (Figure 6-99)
- Sizes range from not grossly visible to larger than 1 cm
- Average number of polyps is generally more than 1000; exceptions include attenuated FAP and MUTYH-associated polyposis syndrome that can demonstrate fewer than 100 polyps

PEUTZ-JEGHERS SYNDROME
- Pigmented lesions resemble freckles; on lips, buccal mucosa, and perianal skin
- Polyps occur throughout the gastrointestinal tract, with small bowel (96% of cases) and colon (30% of cases) most commonly affected
- Usually fewer than 50 polyps
- Polyps range in size from several millimeters to greater than 5 cm

JUVENILE POLYPOSIS SYNDROME

- Six to several hundred polyps most commonly seen in the colon or stomach (Figure 6-100)
- Size ranges from smaller than 1 mm to about 5 cm
- Nearly 90% are within 20 cm of the anus
- Most are pedunculated; unusual shapes; lobulated, globoid, gray-red, mushroom-like masses
- Surface ulceration is common (accounts for bleeding episodes)

PTEN-HAMARTOMA TUMOR SYNDROME

- Cowden syndrome
  - Numerous facial abnormalities occur, including beaked nose, arched palate, and retinal gliomas
  - About 70% of patients have gastrointestinal polyps, which may be anywhere from esophagus to rectum
  - Polyps can resemble hyperplastic or trauma and prolapse-related polyps grossly and endoscopically
  - Facial trichilemmomas, together with gastrointestinal polyps, are considered diagnostic but must be confirmed with gene sequencing
- Ruvalcaba-Myhre-Smith syndrome
  - Pigmented macules on penis
  - Gastrointestinal polyps similar to Cowden syndrome

CRONKHITE-CANADA SYNDROME

- Polyps develop anywhere from esophagus to rectum (Figure 6-101)
- Most polyps are found in the stomach and colon
- Presentation varies from tiny mucosal granularity, which can mimic primary inflammatory bowel disease, to edematous mucosal folds to pedunculated polyps
- Polyps often have gelatinous appearance to cut section because of cyst formation

Histopathology

FAP

- Polyps have histologic features identical to those of sporadic adenomas (tubular, tubulovillous, and villous adenomas)

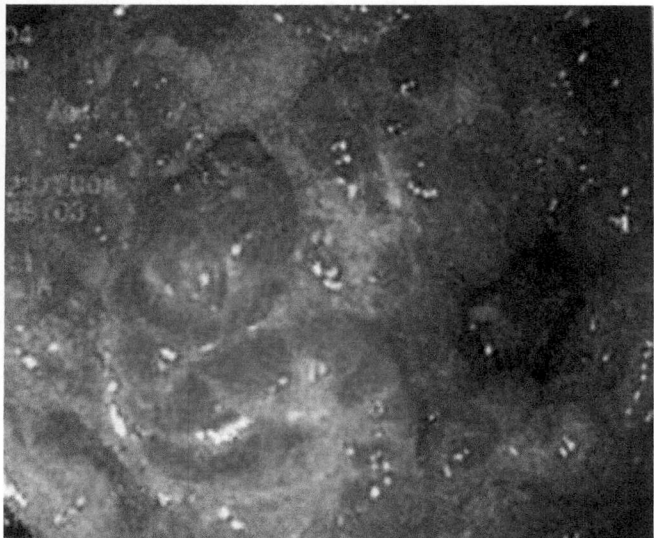

Figure 6-101. Endoscopic photograph of the colon in Cronkhite-Canada syndrome showing diffuse edematous expansion of the colonic mucosa and focal polyp formation with an adherent exudate.

- Earliest lesion consists only of dysplastic epithelium lining one (so-called one-gland adenoma) or several crypts (Figure 6-102)
- Small intestinal polyps are also adenomas composed of dysplastic epithelium; gastric polyps may be adenomas (rare in Western countries) or fundic gland polyps

PEUTZ-JEGHERS SYNDROME

- Represents hamartomatous overgrowth of the muscularis mucosae (Figure 6-103)
- Characterized by an exophytic proliferation composed of epithelium and lamina propria lining intervening treelike or arborizing fascicles of smooth muscle
- Smooth muscle fibers branch out and thin peripherally
- Foci of dysplasia rarely seen
- Mild lamina propria edema with mild mixed inflammatory infiltrate can be present

JUVENILE POLYPOSIS SYNDROME

- Represents hamartomatous overgrowth of the lamina propria (Figure 6-104)

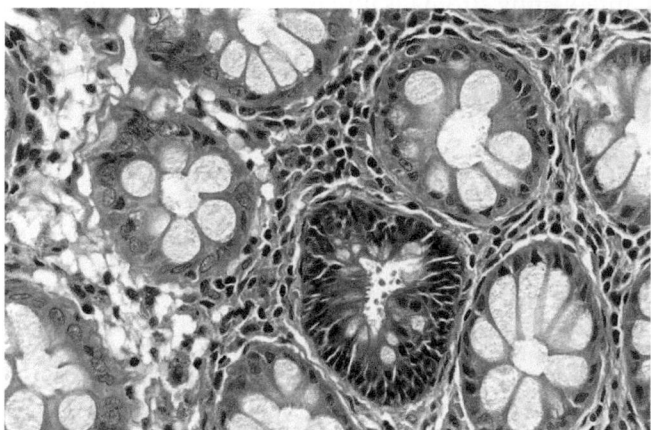

Figure 6-102. One-gland adenoma in familial adenomatous polyposis.

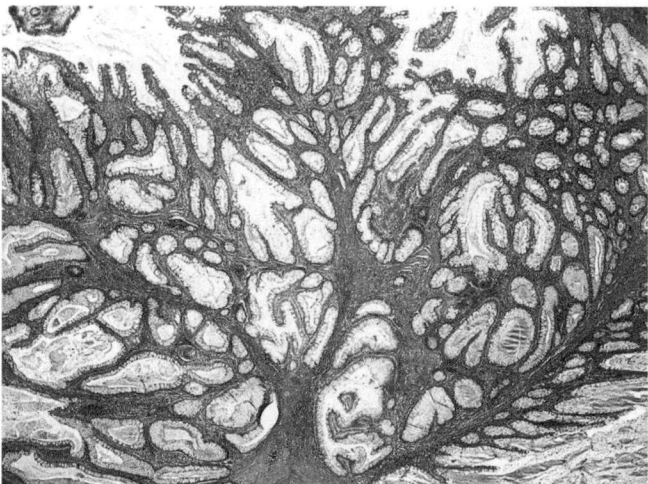

Figure 6-103. Peutz-Jeghers polyp of the colon illustrating the arborizing hamartomatous overgrowth of the muscularis mucosae.

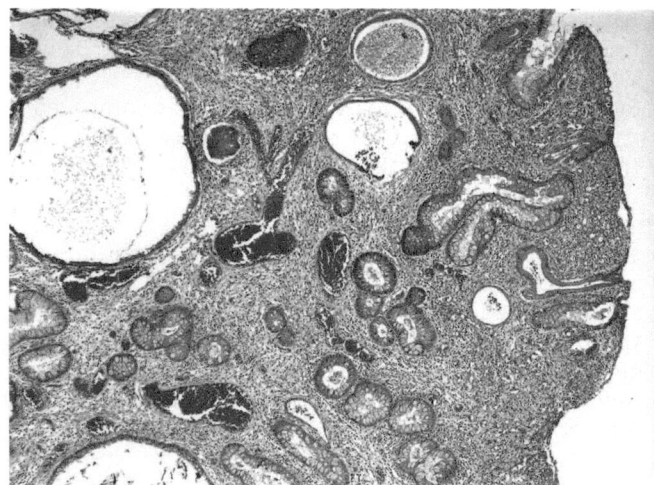

Figure 6-104. Juvenile polyp of the colon demonstrating edematous and inflammatory expansion of the lamina propria associated with mucosal microcyst formation.

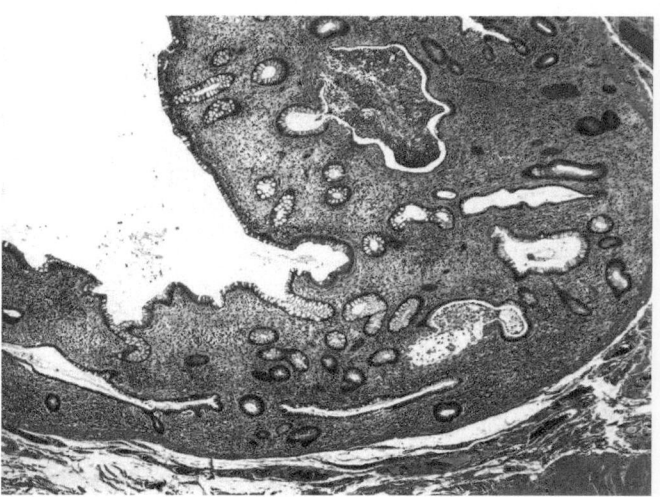

Figure 6-105. Cronkhite-Canada syndrome. The polyp (*center right*) is a localized accentuation of a diffuse mucosal abnormality characterized by edema, chronic inflammation, and microcyst formation.

- Composed of resident benign glands, often focally dilated into cysts, which may be empty or contain mucus; cysts are lined by hyperplastic or atrophic epithelium
- Intervening stroma is inflamed, edematous, and generally devoid of smooth muscle
- Surface is often lined by attenuated glandular epithelium and is often ulcerated or focally replaced by granulation tissue
- Ganglioneuromatous proliferation (ganglion cells and hypertrophic nerves) can occur; there are histologic overlaps with PTEN hamartoma tumor syndrome
- Can have atypical histology with epithelial overgrowth; dysplasia reported in up to 20% of patients and some polyps may even contain malignancy

PTEN HAMARTOMA TUMOR SYNDROMES (COWDEN SYNDROME AND RUVALCABA-MYHRE-SMITH SYNDROME)
- Gastrointestinal polyps may be of the juvenile polyp type; some resemble solitary rectal ulcer syndrome
- Ganglioneuromas and lipomas can be seen

CRONKHITE-CANADA SYNDROME
- Histologic features virtually identical to those of juvenile polyps (Figure 6-105)
- Polyps often have cysts lined by atrophic epithelium
- Rarely, adenomatous change and carcinoma can develop
- Intervening mucosa is abnormal, showing edematous expansion of lamina propria; eosinophils can be prominent

Special Stains and Immunohistochemistry
- Noncontributory

Modern Techniques for Diagnosis
FAP AND GARDNER SYNDROME
- Truncated protein assay is largely replaced by gene sequencing to determine precise location of the mutation within the *APC* gene (5q 21-22)

PEUTZ-JEGHERS SYNDROME
- About 90% linked to mutation in *STK-11* (*LKB1*; 19q13.3)

JUVENILE POLYPOSIS
- Kindred may sometimes link to mutations of *SMAD-4* (*MADH-4*; 18q21.1), some with coexisting hereditary hemorrhagic telangiectasia, and will be linked to mutations of *BMPR1A* (10q22.3)

PTEN-HAMARTOMA TUMOR SYNDROME
- Cowden syndrome linked to mutations of *PTEN* gene (10q22-23) and is definitional
- Ruvalcaba-Myhre-Smith syndrome linked to mutation of *PTEN* gene (10q23.3) and is definitional

Differential Diagnosis
SPORADIC JUVENILE AND PEUTZ JEGHERS POLYPS
- Histologically identical to their nonsyndromatic counterparts
- Diagnosis of the polyposis syndromes requires knowledge of the clinical and family history, the presence of polyps elsewhere in the gastrointestinal tract, and associated conditions

INTESTINAL GANGLIONEUROMATOSIS (Figure 6-106)
- Most ganglioneuromas seen in practice are isolated
- Can be seen in juvenile polyposis syndrome, PTEN hamartoma tumor syndromes, tuberous sclerosis, neurofibromatosis, and MEN-IIB

SERRATED POLYPOSIS SYNDROME (FORMERLY KNOWN AS HYPERPLASTIC POLYPOSIS SYNDROME) (Figure 6-107)
- Defined as five or more serrated polyps proximal to the sigmoid colon, of which two are larger than 1 cm; or any number of serrated polyps proximal to the sigmoid colon in an individual with a first-degree relative with known serrated polyposis syndrome or a patient with more than 20 serrated polyps with any size but distributed throughout the colon
- About half of patients reported with serrated polyposis syndrome have had complicating colorectal carcinoma

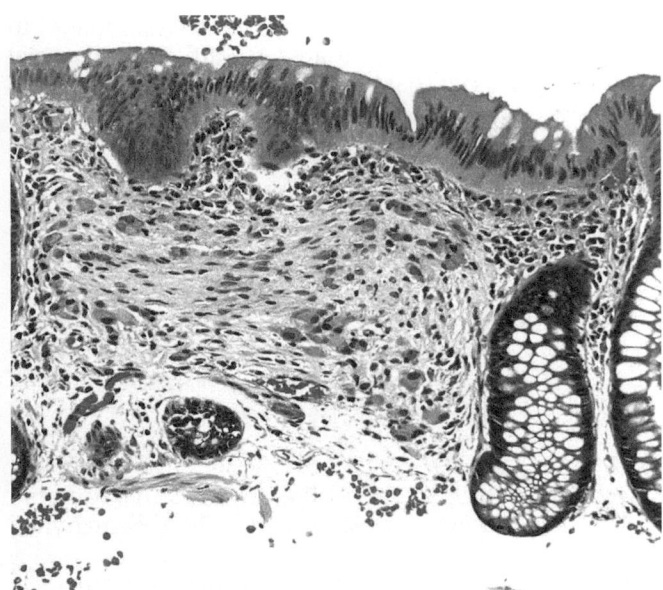

Figure 6-106. Mucosal ganglioneuroma composed of spindle cells and scattered ganglion cells.

- Polyp types vary; typical hyperplastic polyps can be seen; polyps typical of sessile serrated polyp are common, and sessile serrated polyps admixed with areas of dysplasia may occur
- Familial forms may represent an inherited predisposition to DNA hypermethylation
- Some patients with MUTYH-associated polyposis fulfill diagnostic criteria for serrated polyposis syndromes; these patients show both sessile serrated polyps and adenomas

TRADITIONALLY DEFINED SERRATED ADENOMA
- Usually isolated and pedunculated, involving left colon
- Serration may mimic hyperplastic polyp or sessile serrated polyp (Figure 6-92)
- Characterized by gastric metaplasia, eosinophilic cytoplasmic change, and epithelial dysplasia

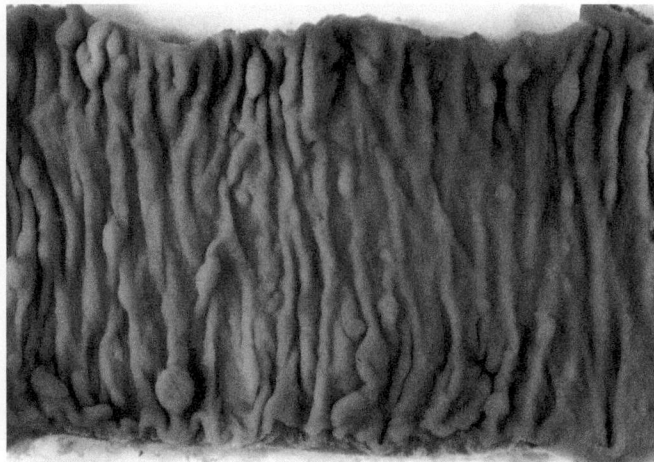

Figure 6-107. Colonic resection specimen from a patient with hyperplastic (serrated) polyposis syndrome. Many polyps have the typical morphology of hyperplastic polyps. Some polyps are large (> 1 cm). Some show unusual morphology, such as plaques or abnormal thickening of mucosal folds.

BENIGN FIBROBLASTIC POLYP/COLORECTAL PERINEURIOMA
- Solitary or multiple; may be found throughout the gastrointestinal tract
- Proliferation of small, tightly packed spindle cells within the lamina propria, often oriented parallel to the muscularis mucosae (Figure 6-108)
- Frequently coexists with hyperplastic polyp-like and sessile serrated polyp-like epithelial changes
- Negative for S-100 protein and other neural markers
- Positive for epithelial membrane antigen but may be immunotechnique sensitive

ELASTOSIS AND ELASTOFIBROMATOUS CHANGE
- Areas of increased elastin fibers in submucosa or muscularis mucosae
- Can cause polyps in the colon and rectum
- Appears as finely granular or fibrillar amphophilic material accompanied by a fibrous component and is often centered around a blood vessel
- Can have scattered eosinophils
- Could be a manifestation of mucosal trauma and prolapse
- Benign and unassociated with a clinical syndrome

MUCOSAL NEUROMA/SCHWANN CELL HAMARTOMA
- Benign spindle cell proliferation in mucosa that expresses immunoreactive S-100 protein and can present as colorectal polyps
- Care must be taken not to overlook ganglion cells, which would indicate a ganglioneuroma
- Can be seen in neurofibromatosis, but the majority occur sporadically and are unassociated with a syndrome

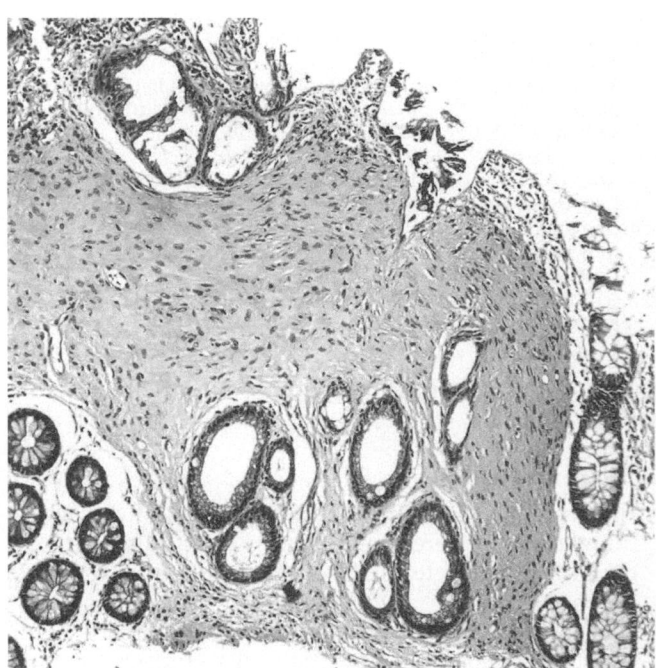

Figure 6-108. Benign fibroblastic polyp (perineurioma) of the colon. The spindle cell proliferation within the lamina propria is associated with hyperplastic polyp-like mucosal changes.

FAP

- *Patients with more than 10 cumulative adenomas should be studied for FAP and related syndromes including MUTYH-associated polyposis*

Juvenile Polyposis Syndrome

- *Biopsies in patients with known history of juvenile polyposis should be carefully screened for dysplasia*
- *Juvenile polyps are usually isolated and sporadic and not part of a polyposis syndrome; they are the most common pediatric gastrointestinal polyps and are prone to autoamputation*

MUTYH-Associated Polyposis

- *Kindred with MUTYH-associated polyposis may sometimes fulfill WHO criteria for serrated polyposis syndrome; they typically have multiple adenomas as well*

SELECTED REFERENCES

Boparai KS, Dekker E, Van Eeden S, et al: Hyperplastic polyps and sessile serrated adenomas as a phenotypic expression of MYH-associated polyposis. Gastroenterology 135:2014-2018, 2008.

Bosman FT, Carneiro F, Hruban RH, Theise ND (eds): WHO Classification of Tumours of the Digestive System, 4th ed. Lyon, IARC Press, 2010.

Giardiello FM, Trimbath JD: Peutz-Jeghers syndrome and management recommendations. Clin Gastroenterol Hepatol 4:408-415, 2006.

Gibson JA, Hornick JL: Mucosal Schwann cell "hamartoma": clinicopathologic study of 26 neural colorectal polyps distinct from neurofibromas and mucosal neuromas. Am J Surg Pathol 33:781-787, 2009.

Hobbs CM, Burch DM, Sobin LH: Elastosis and elastofibromatous change in the gastrointestinal tract: a clinicopathologic study of 13 cases and a review of the literature. Am J Clin Pathol 122:232-237, 2004.

Jass JR: Gastrointestinal polyposes: clinical, pathological and molecular features. Gastroenterol Clin N Am 26:927-946, 2007.

Lipton L, Tomlinson I: The multiple colorectal adenoma phenotype and MYH, a base excision repair gene. Clin Gastroenterol Hepatol 8:633-638, 2004.

Lynch HT, Smyrk T, McGinn T, et al: Attenuated familial adenomatous polyposis (AFAP): a phenotypically and genotypically distinctive variant of FAP. Cancer 76:2427-2433, 1995.

Riddell RH, Petras RE, Williams GT, Sobin LH: Tumors of the intestines. Atlas of Tumor Pathology, Third Series, Fascicle 32. Washington, DC, Armed Forces Institute of Pathology, 2003.

Schreibman IR, Baker M, Amos C, McGarrity TJ: The hamartomatous polyposis syndromes: a clinical and molecular review. Am J Gastroenterol 100:476-490, 2005.

Zamecnik M, Chlumska A: Perineurioma vs. fibroblastic polyp of the colon. Am J Surg Pathol 30:1337-1339, 2006.

GASTROINTESTINAL MESENCHYMAL NEOPLASMS

Clinical Features

- Historically, most spindle cell neoplasms of the gastrointestinal tract were thought to arise from smooth muscle and were thus termed *leiomyoma, leiomyosarcoma,* or *leiomyoblastoma*
- Subsequently, ultrastructural and immunohistochemical studies demonstrated that cells composing these tumors were either undifferentiated or only rarely showed evidence of smooth muscle or neural differentiation, or both

- Currently, most of these stromal tumors are thought to arise from or are differentiated toward the interstitial cell of Cajal, a cell that may control motility (intercalating between autonomic nerves and muscle cells), possibly explaining the prior studies showing neural and muscle differentiation
- Stromal tumors of the gastrointestinal tract are generally split into two groups
  - Recognizable diagnostic entities identical to soft tissue tumors found elsewhere in the body (e.g., schwannoma, leiomyoma)
  - Spindle cell neoplasms, most of which overexpress CD117 (c-Kit) and are referred to as *gastrointestinal stromal tumors (GISTs)*

GIST

- Account for 0.1% to 1% of all gastrointestinal tumors
- Histologic features overlap with other mesenchymal tumors
- Most common in the stomach and small intestine
  - Most patients are older (50 to 70 years of age)
  - About 50% of these tumors ulcerate and bleed
  - The tumor may occur in young women (< 20 years) alone or may be associated with the Carney triad, which includes the following:
    - Epithelioid GIST
    - Pulmonary chondroma
    - Extra-adrenal paraganglioma

Gross and Endoscopic Pathology

GIST

- Both benign and malignant tumors are spherical, well-circumscribed, submucosal or mural tumors that extend into the gastrointestinal lumen; mucosa over lesion may ulcerate (Figure 6-109)
- Cut surface is smooth, pink-white, and firm; may have a lobulated or whorled appearance

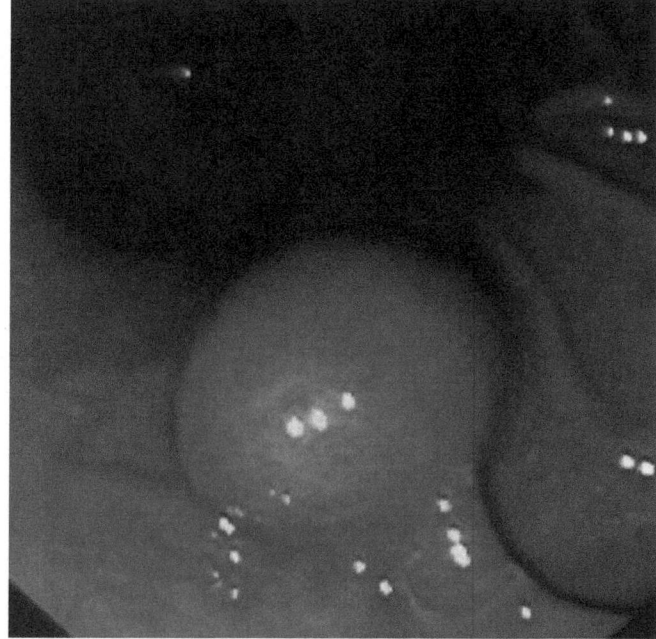

Figure 6-109. Endoscopic view of a gastric gastrointestinal stromal tumor illustrating a spherical mass with intact mucosa.

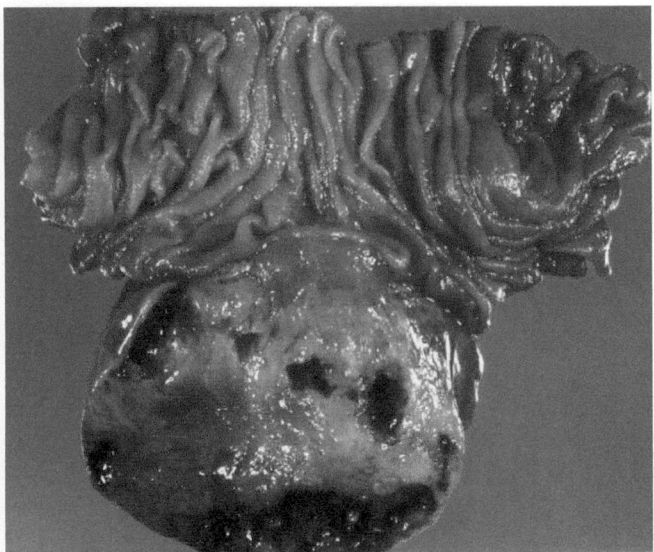

Figure 6-110. Cross section of a resected small intestinal gastrointestinal stromal tumor showing areas of hemorrhagic degeneration.

- Focal areas of hemorrhage, necrosis, or cyst formation may be seen (Figure 6-110)
- Malignant tumors may have fleshy, tan-pink parenchyma with soft, necrotic areas
  - Some tumors may be large with an infiltrative, destructive growth pattern

Histopathology
GIST
- Histologically composed of spindle cells of varying cellularity, hyperchromasia, and nuclear pleomorphism
- May be composed of epithelioid cells (epithelioid GIST) (Figure 6-111)
- Pathologic factors do not necessarily correlate with clinical behavior
- Consensus approach to prognostic groups is recommended
  - Tumors smaller than 2 cm containing fewer than 5 mitoses/50 hpf are considered at very low risk for aggressive behavior

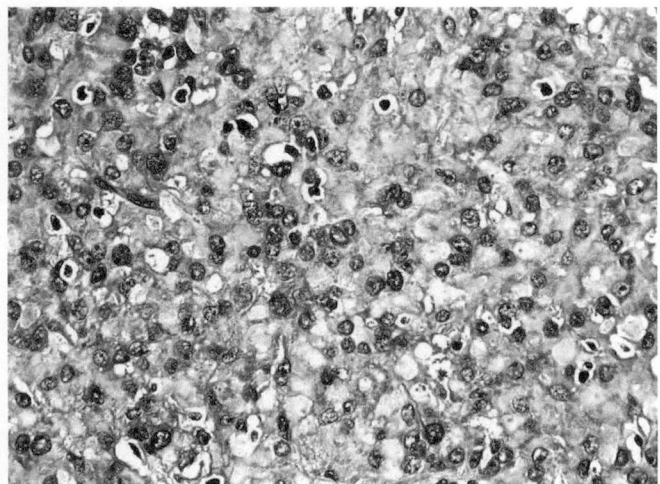

Figure 6-111. Epithelioid gastrointestinal stromal tumors are composed of round cells with peripheral clear cytoplasm.

- Low-risk tumors measure 2 to 5 cm in greatest cross dimension and contain fewer than 5 mitoses/50 hpf
- Intermediate-risk tumors include tumors smaller than 5 cm that have 6 to 10 mitoses/50 hpf and tumors measuring 5 to 10 cm but have fewer than 5 mitoses/50 hpf
- Tumors larger than 5 cm with more than 5 mitoses/10 hpf, any tumor larger than 10 cm, and any tumor with more than 10 mitoses/50 hpf fall into a high-risk group for aggressive behavior
- These consensus risk groups have prognostic significance
  - Risk for an adverse outcome varies with site
    - The proportion of aggressive behavior in gastric tumors ranges from 0% in the very-low-risk group, 1.8% in the low-risk group, 7.3% in the intermediate-risk group, and 45.9% in the high-risk group
    - For small bowel tumors, aggressive behavior had been observed in 0% in the very-low-risk group, 4.3% in the low-risk group, 24.6% in the intermediate-risk group, and 77.2% in the high-risk group
    - Colorectal GISTs are rare, with most patients falling into a high-risk group and with 75% having acted in an aggressive fashion; aggressive behavior has only rarely been observed in colorectal GISTs demonstrating very-low-, low-, or intermediate-risk group characteristics
  - Adjuvant chemotherapy (e.g., imatinib) may be indicated for high-risk GIST

Special Stains and Immunohistochemistry
GIST
- Since introduction of imatinib as effective treatment for metastatic GIST, tumors should be shown to overexpress CD117 (c-Kit) by immunohistochemistry, preferentially as part of an immunohistochemical panel including CD34, desmin, actin, and S-100 protein (or other melanoma markers)
- Scattered cells can be positive for SMA and vimentin
- Spindle cells are positive for CD34 in more than 80% of cases
- Small percentage of GISTs are positive for S-100 protein
- DOG-1 is a very sensitive and specific marker of GISTs; useful in difficult cases with ambiguous or negative CD117 staining

Other Techniques for Diagnosis
- Activating mutations in *KIT* genes are detected in exons 11, 9, 13, and 17, and these may have prognostic significance; about 85% of patients with exon 11 mutation have at least a partial response to imatinib, whereas only half of patients with exon 9 mutations respond; patients with exon 9 mutations may benefit from increased dosage of imatinib; patients with exon 13 or 17 mutations rarely respond to imatinib
- *PDGFRA* mutations (exons 12, 14 and 18) can be seen in cases with wild-type *KIT*; some may respond to imatinib or sunitinib
  - Most common *PDGFRA* mutation (exon 18 D842V) cases are highly resistant to both drugs

Differential Diagnosis

CD117-NEGATIVE GIST
- About 4% of tumors with typical GIST morphology fail to overexpress c-Kit, CD117, or C34 by immunohistochemistry
  - These tumors often show GIST-associated chromosomal abnormalities (monosomy of chromosome 14 or 14q deletion)
  - About 72% show *PDGFRA* mutation
  - About 12% have *KIT* gene mutation
  - Epithelioid GISTs are overrepresented, as are omental and peritoneal GISTs
  - Some patients respond to imatinib
  - DOG-1 immunohistochemistry useful here

SPINDLE CELL CARCINOMA
- Characterized by areas of epithelial differentiation and by cytokeratin immunoreactivity

MALIGNANT FIBROUS HISTIOCYTOMA (MFH)
- May resemble high-grade GIST
- MFH is characterized by presence of storiform architecture and large amounts of collagen (highlighted with trichrome stain)

FIBROMATOSIS
- Characterized by an orderly proliferation of bland, wavy spindle cells, often extending into the mucosa, bowel wall, or mesenteric fat with an infiltrative border; prominent muscular arteries and veins (Figure 6-112)
- Lacks fascicular arrangement of typical smooth muscle tumors
- No cellular atypia
- Can have keloid-like areas
- Usually lacks mitosis figures; no atypical mitoses
- May give false-positive CD117 immunostaining; this varies by immunostaining technique

TRUE SMOOTH MUSCLE TUMOR
- Rare, most often encountered in esophagus or muscularis mucosae of colon and rectum

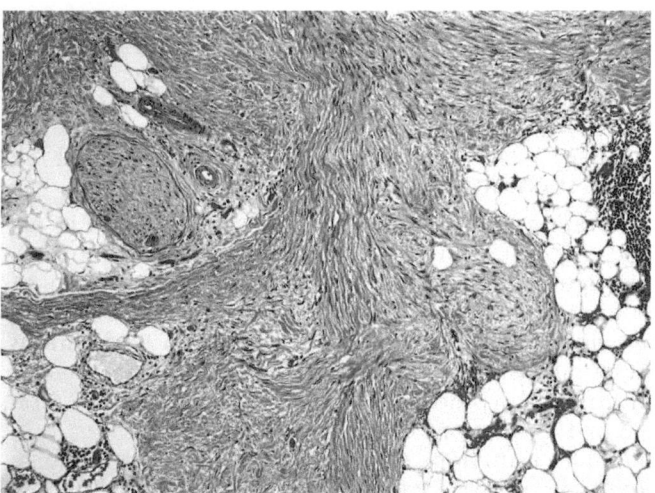

Figure 6-112. Desmoid tumor of the small bowel showing a proliferation of uniform spindle cells without atypia infiltrating the mesenteric adipose tissue.

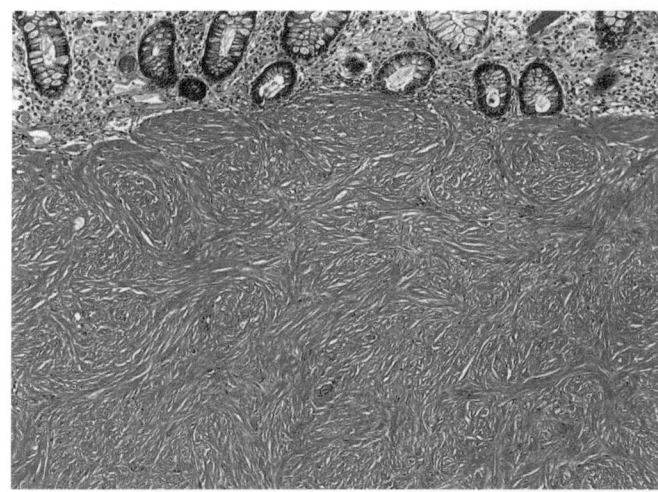

Figure 6-113. Benign leiomyoma of colonic muscularis mucosae showing haphazard intertwining fascicles of plump smooth muscle cells.

- Leiomyomas are typically well-circumscribed with pushing borders; composed of interlacing fascicles of plump spindle cells with cigar-shaped nuclei and minimal mitotic activity (Figure 6-113)
- Leiomyosarcomas are rare but most often described in the stomach, small bowel, or colon
  - Hypercellular tumors with haphazard arrangement of spindle, oval, or rounded cells; bizarre giant cells may be intermixed
  - Infiltrative growth and high mitosis rate
  - Necrosis common
  - Must prove smooth muscle origin (e.g., SMA immunohistochemistry) and must rule out GIST with immunohistochemistry for CD117, CD34, and DOG-1

INFLAMMATORY MYOFIBROBLASTIC TUMOR
- Usually contains admixture of spindle cells and inflammatory cells with plasma cells
- Negative for immunoreactive CD117, CD34, and DOG-1; scattered cells positive for SMA and desmin
- Anaplastic lymphoma kinase is a diagnostic marker for a subset of these cases

SCHWANNOMA
- Typical Antoni A and Antoni B areas with hyalinized blood vessels
- Often demonstrates a prominent cuffing by lymphoid aggregates (Figure 6-114)
- Stains positive for S-100 protein; CD117 and CD34 immunostains variable

SOLITARY FIBROUS TUMOR
- Highly cellular spindle cell tumor associated with deposits of collagen
- CD34 immunostain positive; negative for CD117

GRANULAR CELL TUMOR
- Composed of spindle and epithelioid cells with granular basophilic cytoplasm (Figure 6-115)
- Strong S-100–positive immunostaining; negative for CD117

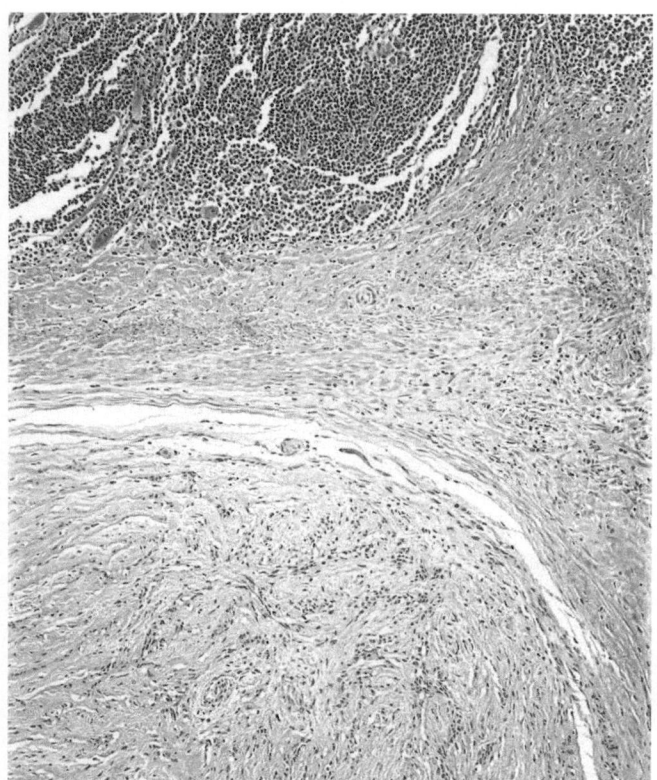

Figure 6-114. Benign schwannoma involving the stomach showing the prominent cuffing of lymphocytes (Crohn-like reaction).

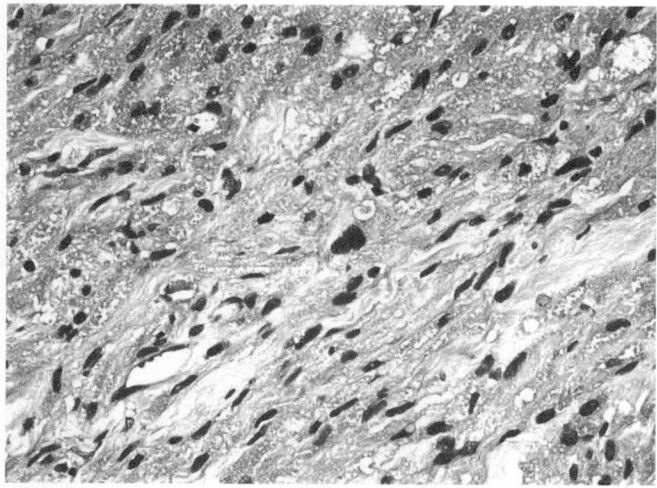

Figure 6-115. Granular cell tumor of the stomach showing round and elongated spindle cells with variably shaped small nuclei and prominent eosinophilic cytoplasmic granules.

GLOMUS TUMOR
- Tumor cells are small and sharply defined, showing solid arrangements around dilated blood vessels (Figure 6-116)
- Robust SMA immunostaining; negative for CD117, CD34, and DOG-1

OSTEOCLAST-RICH TUMOR RESEMBLING CLEAR CELL SARCOMA (MALIGNANT NEUROECTODERMAL TUMOR)
- Can mimic GIST (Figure 6-117)

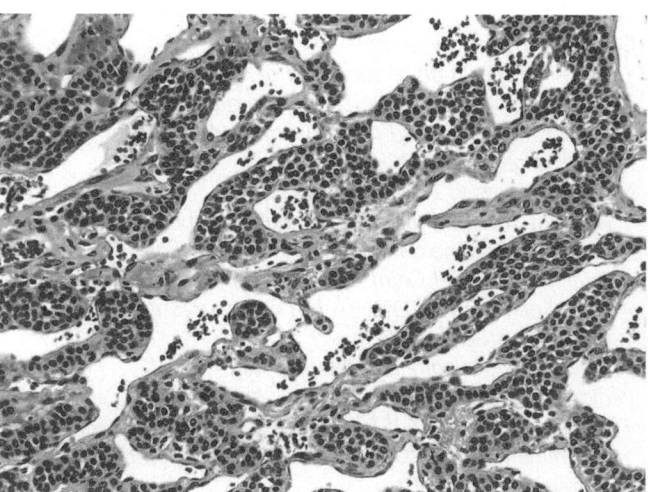

Figure 6-116. Glomus tumor of the stomach is composed of small cells surrounding angulated dilated blood vessels. The glomus tumor cells are round and uniform, with basophilia, cytoplasm, and a centrally placed nucleus. Cellular borders are typically sharply defined.

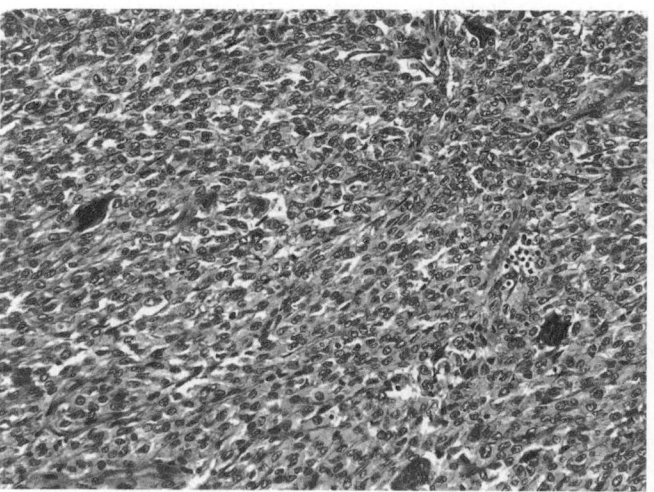

Figure 6-117. Clear cell sarcoma with multinucleated giant cells involving the small intestine. This mimicker of gastrointestinal stromal tumor is composed of highly cellular malignant spindle cells with scattered osteoclast-like giant cells.

- CD117 negative; positive for S-100 protein and stain variably for cytokeratin and melanoma markers (e.g., HMB-45, melan-A)
- Often show *EWSR-CREB1 or EWSR1/ATF1* gene fusions

KAPOSI SARCOMA
- Can be positive for CD34 and CD117 by immunohistochemistry
- Immunohistochemistry for DOG-1 (for GIST) and HHV8 (for Kaposi sarcoma) essential in separating the two

PEARLS
- *Familial and syndromatic GIST exists*
- *Germline mutation in* KIT *and* PDGFRA
  - *Autosomal dominant*
  - *Sometimes associated with perineal hyperpigmentation, nevi, urticaria pigmentosa, systemic mast cell disease*
  - *Indolent clinical course*

- *Carney-Stratakis syndrome*
  - *Germline mutation of succinate dehydrogenase*
  - *Associated with multiple epithelioid gastric GIST, paragangliomas, and pheochromocytoma*
  - *Relative resistance to imatinib*
- *Neurofibromatosis type 1 (NF1)*
  - *Associated with multiple small bowel spindle cell GISTs with skeinoid fibers arising in a background of interstitial cells of Cajal hyperplasia*
  - *Germline KIT and PDGFRA but overexpresses KIT by immunohistochemistry*
  - *Tend to be clinically benign*
- *Pediatric GISTs*
  - *Gastric epithelioid GIST presenting often in females*
  - *Germline KIT and PDGFRA but overexpressed KIT by immunohistochemistry*
  - *Indolent clinical behavior*

SELECTED REFERENCES

Hassan I, You YN, Dozois EJ, et al: Clinical, pathologic, and immunohistochemical characteristics of gastrointestinal stromal tumors of the colon and rectum: implications for surgical management and adjuvant therapies. Dis Colon Rectum 49:609-615, 2006.

Medeiros F, Corless CL, Duensing A, et al: KIT-negative gastrointestinal stromal tumors: proof of concept and therapeutic implications. Am J Surg Pathol 28:889-894, 2004.

Miettinen M, Kopczynski J, Makhlouf HR, et al: Gastrointestinal stromal tumors, intramural leiomyomas, and leiomyosarcomas in the duodenum: a clinicopathologic, immunohistochemical, and molecular genetic study of 167 cases. Am J Surg Pathol 27:625-641, 2003.

Miettinen M, Makhlouf H, Sobin LH, Lasota J: Gastrointestinal stromal tumors of the jejunum and ileum: a clinicopathologic, immunohistochemical, and molecular genetic study of 906 cases before imatinib with long-term follow-up. Am J Surg Pathol 30:477-489, 2006.

Miettinen M, Sobin LH, Lasota J: Gastrointestinal stromal tumors of the stomach: a clinicopathologic, immunohistochemical, and molecular genetic study of 1765 cases with long-term follow-up. Am J Surg Pathol 29:52-68, 2005.

Patil DT, Rubin BP. Gastrointestinal stromal tumor: advances in diagnosis and management. Arch Pathol Lab Med 135:1298-1310, 2011.

Riddell RH, Petras RE, Williams GT, Sobin LH: Tumors of the intestines. Atlas of Tumor Pathology Third Series, Fascicle 32. Washington, DC, Armed Forces Institute of Pathology, 2003.

Rodriguez JA, Guarda LA, Rosai J: Mesenteric fibromatosis with involvement of the gastrointestinal tract: A GIST simulator: a study of 25 cases. Am J Clin Pathol 121:93-98, 2004.

Zambrano E, Reyes-Mugica M, Franchi A, Rosai J: An osteoclast-rich tumor of gastrointestinal tract with features resembling clear cell sarcoma of soft parts: reports of 6 cases of a GIST simulator. Int J Surg Pathol 11:75-81, 2003.

INTESTINAL LYMPHOMA

Clinical Features

- Gastrointestinal tract is most common extranodal site of lymphoma (stomach is most common gastrointestinal site, followed by small intestine and then colon)
- Most are B-cell lymphomas
- By definition, primary intestinal lymphoma lacks superficial lymphadenopathy, shows a normal white blood cell count, has no involvement of liver and spleen while the bulk of disease involves the gastrointestinal tract
- Patients present with abdominal pain, weight loss, intestinal obstruction, acute abdomen

FOLLICULAR LYMPHOMA
- Rarely primary in the gastrointestinal tract; sometimes an incidental finding
- Can present as a polyp or lymphomatous polyposis (Figure 6-118)
- Composed of small cleaved (follicle center) cells; can have admixed larger cells (Figure 6-119)
- Translocation at t(14;18) causes overexpression of bcl-2
- Coexpression of CD10 and bcl-2 by immunohistochemistry (Figure 6-120)

MANTLE CELL LYMPHOMA
- Usually presents with widespread lymphadenopathy and frequent bone marrow involvement
- Gastrointestinal tract involved in 10% to 20% of patients; clinically occult involvement in up to 80% of patients

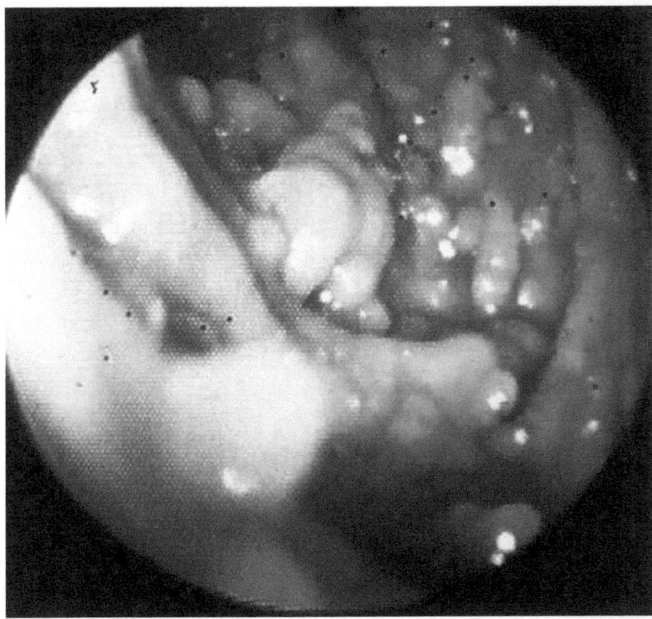

Figure 6-118. Endoscopic photograph of duodenum with follicular lymphoma. Notice the variably sized mucosal polyps (lymphomatous polyposis).

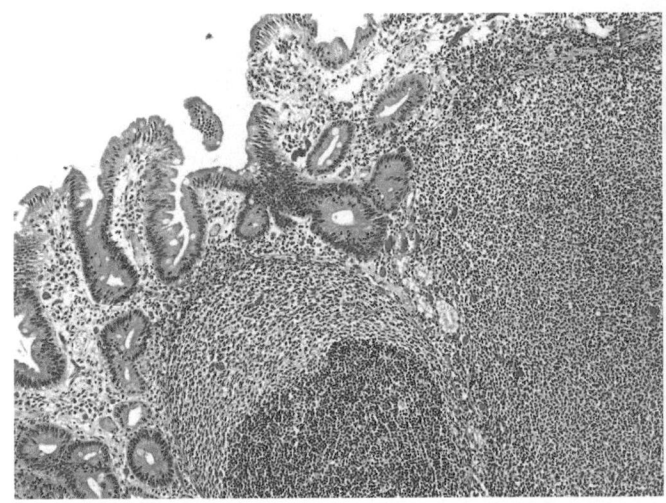

Figure 6-119. Follicular lymphoma involving duodenum showing small cleaved follicular center cells in a follicular arrangement.

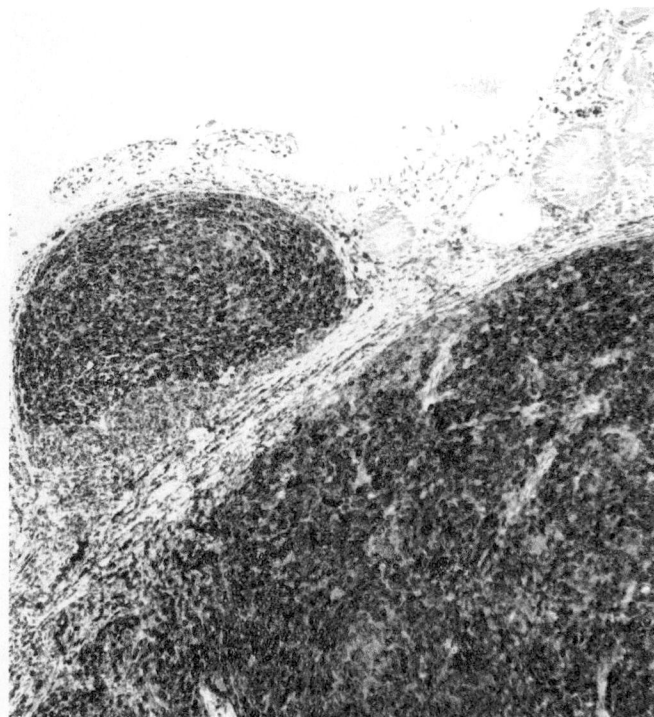

Figure 6-120. Follicular lymphoma showing prominent *bcl-2* immunostaining.

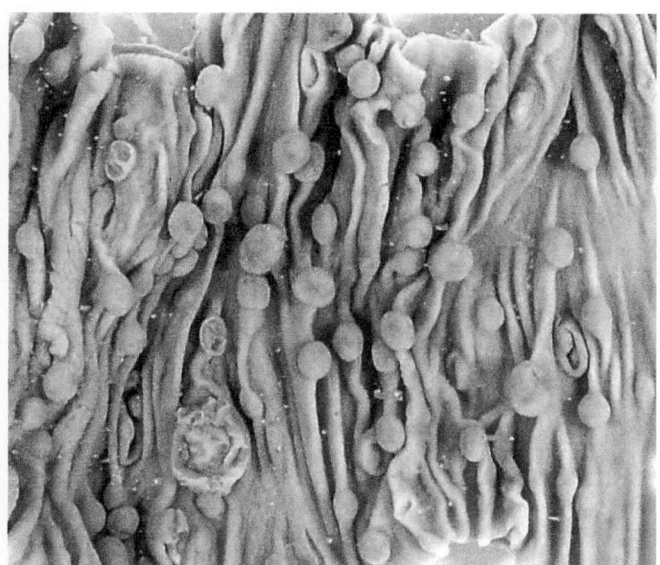

Figure 6-121. Colonic resection specimen demonstrating lymphomatous polyposis. The polyps themselves are spherical and attached to the mucosal folds by a small pedicle. Larger polyps show central ulceration.

- Can present with a mass, diffuse mucosal thickening, or lymphomatous polyposis (Figure 6-121)
- Composed of atypical small lymphocytes with irregular nuclear contours; may surround atrophic germinal centers (Figure 6-122)
- Coexpresses CD20 and CD5
- Translocation at t(11;14) causes overexpression of cyclin D1, which is considered definitional (Figure 6-123)

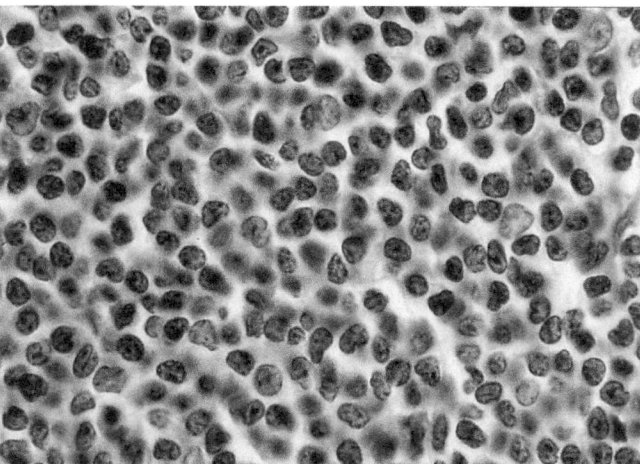

Figure 6-122. Mantle cell lymphoma involving the small intestine showing monotonous cells with a distinctive rim of cytoplasm. A small nucleolus is present in many of the cells.

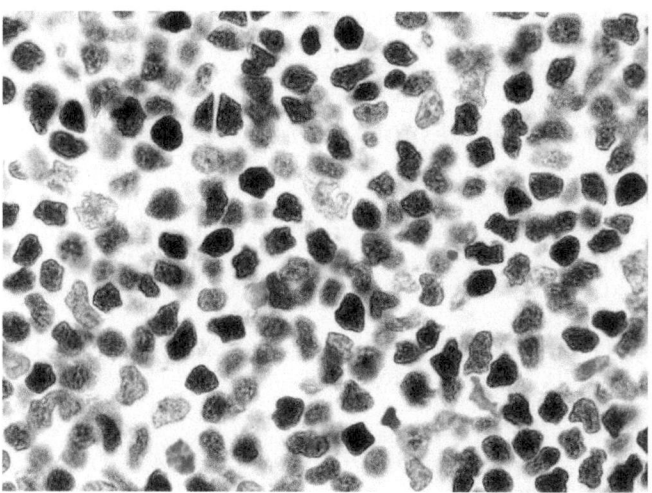

Figure 6-123. Mantle cell lymphoma. Cyclin D1 immunostain.

EXTRANODAL MARGINAL B-CELL LYMPHOMA OF MALT TYPE (ALSO SEE GASTRIC LYMPHOMA)
- Can present as lymphomatous polyposis
- Immunoproliferative small intestinal disease (IPSID, Mediterranean lymphoma) considered a variant
  - Can be associated with α heavy-chain disease

ENTEROPATHY-ASSOCIATED T-CELL LYMPHOMA
- Many cases associated with active or latent celiac sprue or refractory celiac sprue; typically affects patients in the sixth to seventh decades
- Causes small intestinal ulcers and strictures
- Poor prognosis
- Two histologic types
  - Pleomorphic lymphoma (80% of cases); cells are CD3 positive, CD56 negative, CD4 negative, CD5 negative, CD8 mostly negative (positive in 20% of cases); up to 70% of patients have had clinical Celiac sprue (Figure 6-124)

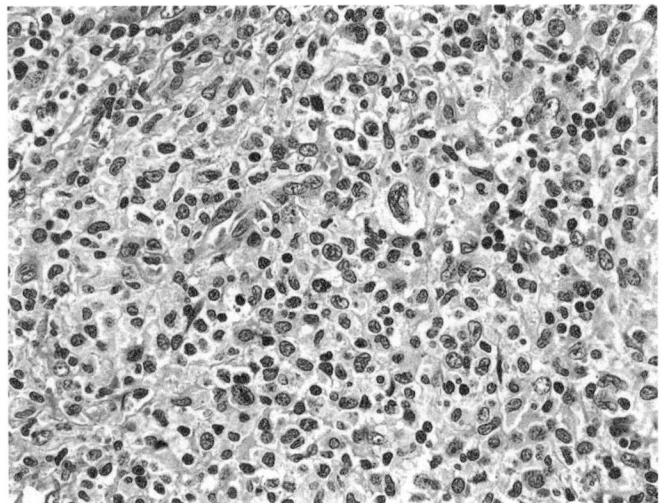

Figure 6-124. Pleomorphic enteropathy-associated T-cell lymphoma showing atypical lymphocytes of various sizes and shapes.

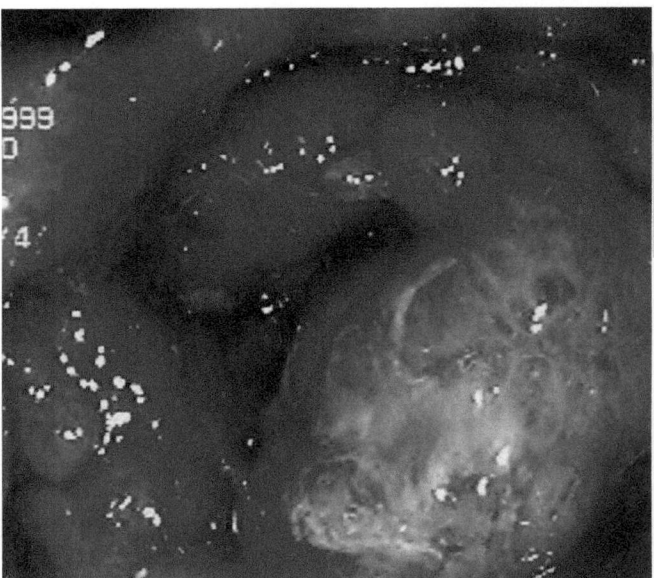

Figure 6-125. Endoscopic view of "rectal tonsil" demonstrating a large intraluminal polyp involving the rectum.

- Monomorphic small to medium cells; cells are CD56 positive (> 90%), CD8 positive (80%); much lower rate of clinical celiac sprue

Other Techniques for Diagnosis

- In addition to immunohistochemistry, flow cytometry, gene rearrangement studies, and fluorescence in situ hybridization (FISH) are crucial for the classification of lymphomas
- Extranodal marginal zone B-cell lymphoma of MALT type
  - Flow cytometry: CD19 and CD20 positive; CD5, CD10, and CD23 negative
  - FISH for t(11;18)
- Mantle cell lymphoma
  - Flow cytometry: CD20, CD5 positive; CD10 and CD23 negative
  - FISH for t(11;14)

Differential Diagnosis

- The main differential diagnosis is between benign reactive conditions and different variants of lymphoma
- Benign lymphoid hyperplasia in the gastrointestinal tract
  - Grossly or endoscopically present with multiple tan-white mucosal nodules 0.1 to 0.5 cm
  - May be anywhere in bowel but most common in ileum (Peyer patches), duodenum, and rectum (so-called rectal tonsil) (Figure 6-125)
  - Composed of variably sized lymphoid nodules with germinal centers; germinal centers have reactive changes, including tingible body macrophages, mitoses, nuclear debris, and phagocytosis (Figure 6-126)
  - Mixed inflammatory background consisting of small lymphocytes, plasma cells, and histiocytes
  - Remember that children often have marked lymphoid hyperplasia of the terminal ileum
  - No immunoglobulin light-chain restriction; no B-cell gene rearrangements

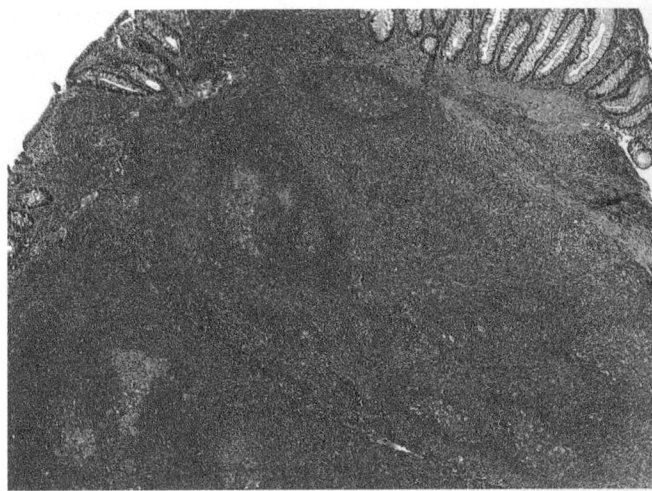

Figure 6-126. Lymphoid hyperplasia of the rectum shows follicular hyperplasia and scattered islands of pale-staining histiocytes.

PEARLS

- *Procure fresh tissue for flow cytometric analysis in suspected cases of lymphoma; gene rearrangement studies on paraffin blocks helpful*
- *Lymphoepithelial lesions suggest MALT lymphoma*
- *Ulcerated lesions in the jejunum (especially with a history of celiac sprue) suggest enteropathy-associated T-cell lymphoma*

SELECTED REFERENCES

Banks PM: Gastrointestinal lymphoproliferative disorders. Histopathology 50:42-54, 2007.

Freeman HJ, Chopra A, Clandinin MT, Thomson AB: Recent advances in celiac disease. World J Gastroenterol 17:2259-2272, 2011.

Kodama T, Ohshima K, Nomura K, et al: Lymphomatous polyposis of the gastrointestinal tract, including mantle cell lymphoma, follicular lymphoma and mucosa-associated lymphoid tissue lymphoma. Histopathology 47:467-478, 2005.

Riddell RH, Petras RE, Williams GT, Sobin LH: Tumors of the intestines. Atlas of Tumor Pathology Third Series, Fascicle 32. Washington, DC, Armed Forces Institute of Pathology, 2003.

ANAL CANAL

ANAL NEOPLASIA

- Proper classification requires careful clinical assessment
  - Classify lesions below the dentate line according to World Health Organization typing of skin tumors, and these should be treated accordingly

Clinical Features

CONDYLOMA ACUMINATUM

- More common in men, particularly men who have sex with men
- A form of squamous intraepithelial lesion associated with HPV infection
- Other risk factors include the following:
  - Cervical and vulvar condyloma
  - HIV infection
  - Pregnancy
  - Diabetes mellitus

SQUAMOUS INTRAEPITHELIAL LESIONS

- Can occur in anal canal (low-grade anal intraepithelial neoplasia [LGAIN] and high-grade anal intraepithelial neoplasia [HGAIN]) and perianal skin (low-grade squamous intraepithelial lesion [LSIL] and high-grade squamous intraepithelial lesion [HSIL])
- New terminology replaces anal canal intraepithelial neoplasia (AIN), bowenoid dysplasia, and squamous carcinoma in situ Bowen type (Bowen disease [BD])
- Squamous intraepithelial lesions are associated with HPV infection

ANAL CARCINOMA

- Arises from anal canal above dentate line
- About 95% are squamous cell carcinomas or variant squamous cell carcinomas
- Symptoms include rectal bleeding and pain
- Anal canal carcinomas occur at all ages (predominantly 40 to 60 years) and are more common in young men and older women
- Risk factors for anal canal carcinoma include the following:
  - Condyloma acuminatum
  - Squamous intraepithelial lesions
  - Crohn disease
  - Immunodeficient state

Gross and Endoscopic Pathology

CONDYLOMA ACUMINATUM

- Varies from single, small exophytic growths to cauliflower-like masses covering large areas (Figure 6-127)

SQUAMOUS INTRAEPITHELIAL LESIONS

- LGAIN/HGAIN: flat, generally single lesion in older patients
- LSIL/HSIL: slightly raised, scaly, reddish plaque on perianal skin

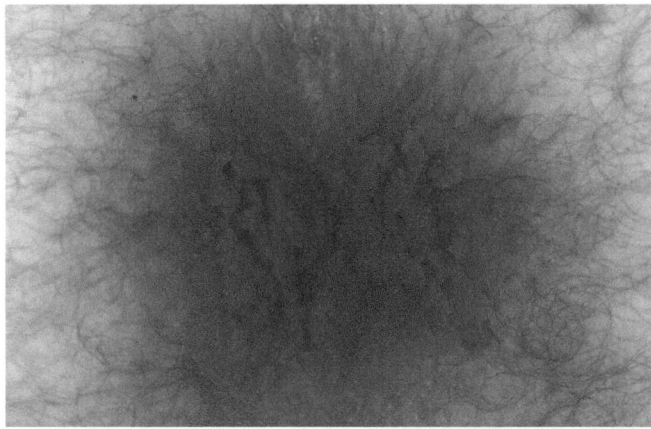

Figure 6-127. Condyloma acuminatum involving the anal canal and perianal skin (clinical photograph).

ANAL CARCINOMA

- Arises near dentate line
- May present as submucosal nodule or be diffusely infiltrative (Figure 6-128)
- May infiltrate prostate gland, vagina, or bladder

Histopathology

CONDYLOMA ACUMINATUM

- Acanthotic, papillomatous lesions with hyperkeratosis, koilocytotic atypia, and variable dysplasia; can be flat
- Discrete transition from adjacent normal squamous epithelium
- Variable chronic inflammation
- Typically associated with low-risk HPV types; HPV-16 and HPV-18 are associated with HGAIN, HSIL, and squamous carcinoma

SQUAMOUS INTRAEPITHELIAL LESIONS

- LGAIN and HGAIN
  - Thickened epithelium with variable degree of undifferentiated basal cell proliferation (analogous to cervical intraepithelial neoplasia) showing epithelial dysplasia
  - Variable chronic inflammatory response
  - Diffuse p16 immunostaining defines HGAIN and is associated with high-risk HPV types

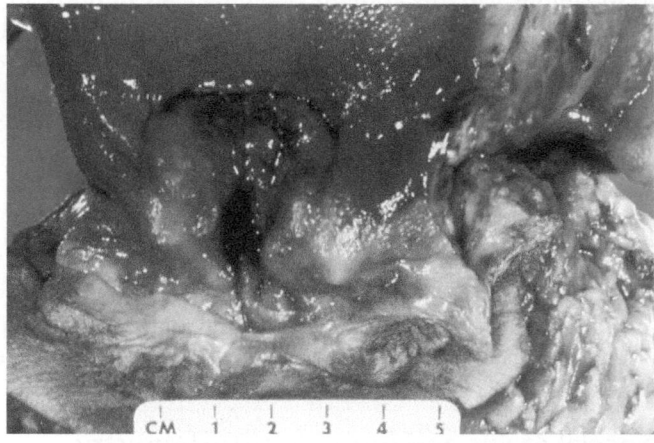

Figure 6-128. Resection specimen of anal squamous carcinoma. The focally ulcerated lesion undermines the rectal mucosa.

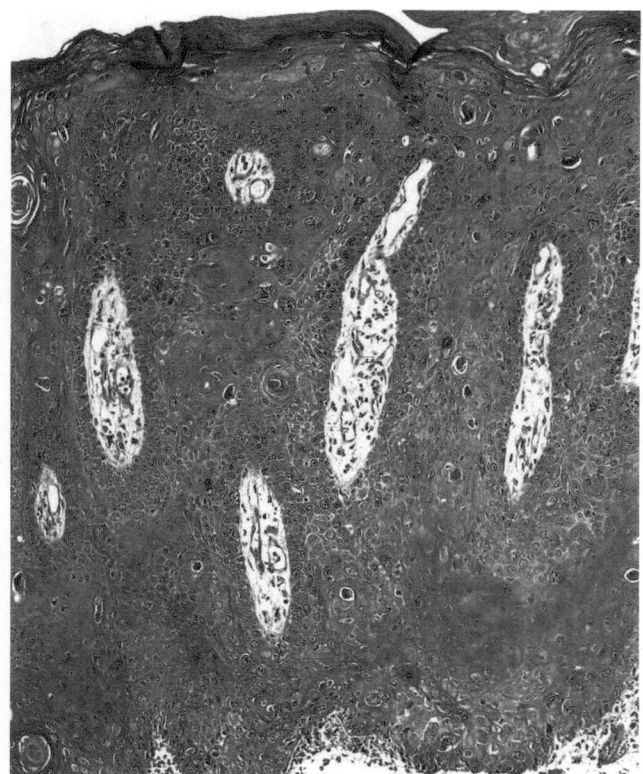

Figure 6-129. High-grade squamous intraepitheial lesion, showing full-thickness squamous epithelial atypia.

- LSIL and HSIL
  - Sharply demarcated area of acanthosis and hyperkeratosis with frequent parakeratosis and some degree of superficial maturation; epithelial dysplasia (Figure 6-129)
  - Koilocytotic atypia is usually present
  - Diffuse p16 immunostaining defines HSIL and is associated with high-risk HPV types

ANAL CARCINOMA

- Almost all are variants of squamous carcinomas
- About 50% of anal canal tumors are nonkeratinizing and are poorly differentiated
- Terms such as *basaloid, cloacogenic*, and *transitional carcinoma* are largely abandoned
- Squamous variants contain syncytial cells in nests and cords, often with central keratinization; a basaloid, transitional, and keratinizing squamous cell carcinoma pattern often coexists; sarcomatoid carcinoma and evidence of neuroendocrine or rhabdomyoblastic differentiation may be seen
- Basaloid pattern of squamous carcinoma
  - Characterized by peripheral palisading in tumor islands, although typically less than in basal cell carcinoma of skin (Figure 6-130)
- Other patterns of anal carcinoma include mucoepidermoid, adenoid cystic, colorectal-type adenocarcinoma, and undifferentiated carcinoma with neuroendocrine features, large cell and small cell type

Special Stains and Immunohistemistry

- Overexpression of p16 correlate with HGAIN/HSIL

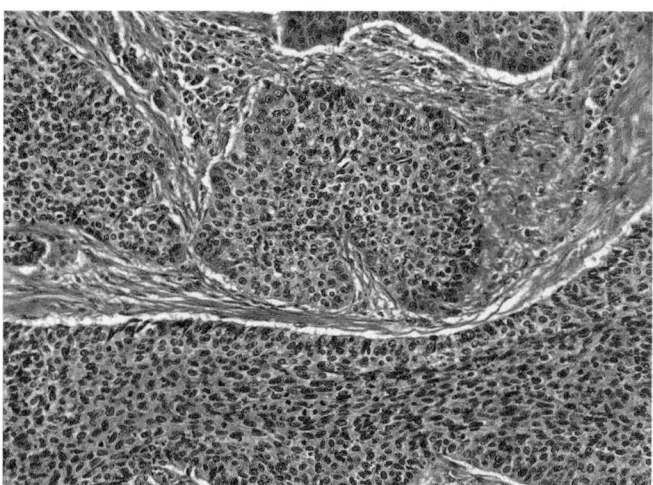

Figure 6-130. Squamous carcinoma of the anal canal showing insular-type infiltration, peripheral palisading of neoplastic cells, and retraction artifact.

- High-grade squamous carcinoma, especially the basaloid variant, can mimic high-grade neuroendocrine carcinoma and lymphoma; immunostaining for LCA, cytokeratin, and neuroendocrine markers (e.g., chromogranin and synaptophysin) can be helpful (Figure 6-131)

Other Techniques for Diagnosis

- Identification and typing of HPV in condyloma, dysplasia, and anal cancer by in situ hybridization or PCR can be done

Differential Diagnosis

VERRUCOUS CARCINOMA

- Differentiated from invasive well-differentiated carcinoma by its bulbous growth that pushes into the underlying stroma, compared with the infiltrative growth pattern of conventional squamous carcinoma
- Distinction from condyloma acuminatum is arbitrary; however, both require complete surgical excision

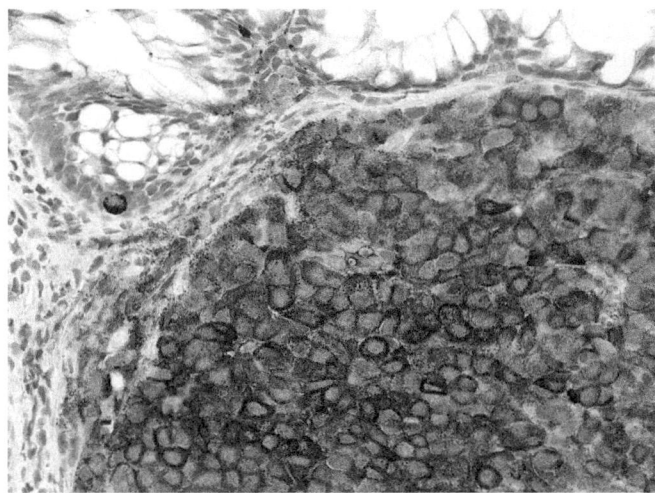

Figure 6-131. High-grade neuroendocrine carcinoma of the low rectum and anal canal, large cell type (chromogranin immunostain).

- Size greater than 2 cm and presence of fistulas and complex sinuses argue strongly for verrucous carcinoma over conventional squamous carcinoma or condyloma acuminatum

PAGET DISEASE

- Characterized by an intraepithelial proliferation of large, pale cells similar to those seen in melanoma; can mimic HGAIN and HSIL (Figure 6-132)
- Paget cells contain mucin and are PAS, mucicarmine, and Alcian blue stain positive; immunohistochemistry for CEA is often positive
- Can represent classic apocrine-type Paget disease but can also be seen in association with primary rectosigmoid adenocarcinoma (sometimes adenoma) and primary anal canal adenocarcinoma; although clinical assessment is paramount, immunostaining for CK7, CK20, and gross cystic disease protein can help differentiate these entities pathologically

ADENOCARCINOMA INVOLVING THE ANAL CANAL

- Adenocarcinoma involving the anal canal can represent downward extension of rectal adenocarcinoma, can arise primarily in the anal canal or perianal duct and glands, can arise primarily in Paget disease, or can complicate a chronic perianal fistula
  - Primary adenocarcinoma of the anal canal or perianal duct or glands shows no surface component and can have nonintestinal morphology
- Adenocarcinoma in chronic anorectal fistula usually occurs in men with a long history of perianal

disease; almost all cases reported have been mucinous adenocarcinoma

HIDRADENOMA PAPILLIFERUM

- Benign sweat gland tumor that can occur in the anus
- Shows a papillary pattern with two epithelial cell types
  - Columnar cell layer with apical blebs
  - Basal layer of cuboidal cells with eosinophilic PAS-positive cytoplasm

MALIGNANT MELANOMA

- Rare tumors; make up 1% of all primary melanomas and less than 1% of all anal tumors
- May contain large intraepithelial pale cells mimicking those of Paget and HGAIN/HSIL
- Adjacent squamous mucosa may demonstrate in situ melanoma with pagetoid melanocytes
- Positive immunostain for S-100 protein and HMB-45 and melan-A aid in diagnosis
- Tumor cells negative for mucin, cytokeratin, and CEA

PEARLS

- *If confronted with a tumor in the anal canal that is difficult to classify on routine H&E-stained sections, always remember the possibility of malignant melanoma*
  - *The anal canal is the third most common site for melanoma; frequently mimics a hemorrhoid clinically*
  - *Histologic appearance of anal melanoma can mimic solitary rectal ulcer syndrome, sarcoma (e.g., Kaposi sarcoma), lymphoma, basaloid carcinoma, and high-grade neuroendocrine carcinoma*
  - *Immunostains for S-100 protein, HMB-45, and melan-A should be considered*

SELECTED REFERENCES

Balachandra B, Marcus V, Jass JR: Poorly differentiated tumours of the anal canal: a diagnostic strategy for the surgical pathologist. Histopathology 50:163-174, 2007.

Bernick PE, Klimstra DS, Shia J, et al: Neuroendocrine carcinomas of the colon and rectum. Dis Colon Rectum 47:163-169, 2004.

Darragh TM, Colgan TJ, Cox JT, et al: The lower anogenital squamous terminology standardization project for HPV-associated lesions: background and consensus recommendations from the College of American Pathologists and the American Society for Colposcopy and Cervical Pathology. Arch Pathol Lab Med 136:1266-1297, 2012.

Riddell R, Petras RE, Williams G, Sobin L: Tumors of the small intestine, colon, and anus. Atlas of Tumor Pathology Third Series, Fascicle 32. Washington, DC, Armed Forces Institute of Pathology, 2003, pp 251-278.

Welton ML, Lambert R, Bosman FT: Tumours of the anal canal. In Bosman FT, Carneiro F, Hruban RH, Theise ND (eds): World Health Organization Classification of Tumours of the Digestive System. Lyon, IARC Press, 2010, pp 185-193.

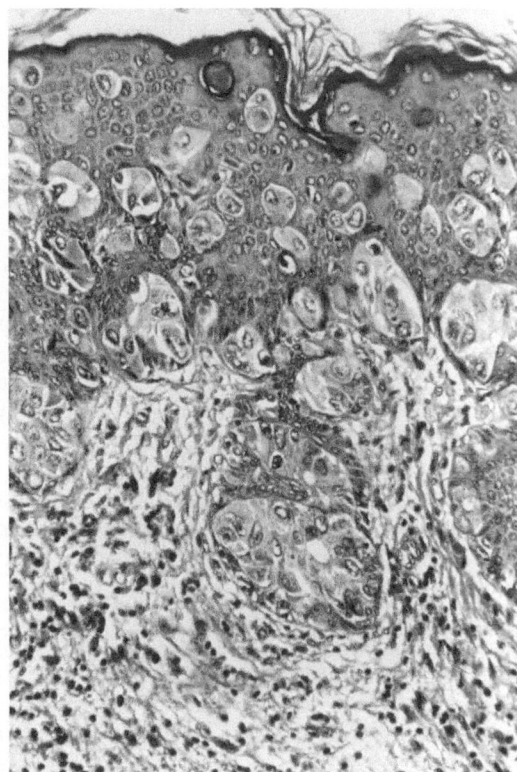

Figure 6-132. Paget disease of perianal skin. The epidermis contains individual and groupings of large pale vacuolated cells with some gland formation.

VERMIFORM APPENDIX

DEVELOPMENTAL ABNORMALITIES

- The appendix can be congenitally absent or hypoplastic
- Duplications can occur, usually in association with cecal duplication
- Diverticula are seen, but most are acquired from obstructive lesions of the appendix

APPENDICITIS

Clinical Features

- May occur at any age; peak age in teenage years and young adulthood
- About 10% of people in the United States are affected during their lifetime
- Elderly patients have higher mortality and complication rates
- Presentation includes periumbilical pain that radiates to the right lower abdominal quadrant, rebound tenderness, fever, and leukocytosis
- About 15% of appendices that are resected for a preoperative diagnosis of acute appendicitis are normal

Gross Pathology

- Typically the serosa is dull, hyperemic, and coated by fibrinous exudate and adhesion, and it may contain a discrete focus of perforation
- Cut surface may be frankly necrotic; lumen often contains blood-tinged pus
- When perforation is present, the mesoappendix is often congested and tense
- Appendiceal lumen may contain a fecalith

Histopathology

- Variable histologic features depend on the duration of inflammation
- Early lesions contain mild acute inflammation at the crypt bases with small mucosal erosions
- Advanced lesions contain submucosal and mural abscesses and extensive mucosal ulceration
- Gangrenous lesions show complete mural necrosis with acute periappendicitis

Special Stains and Immunohistochemistry

- Noncontributory

Other Techniques for Diagnosis

- Noncontributory

Differential Diagnosis

MUCOCELE

- Term should be used only as a gross description
- Characterized by cystic dilation of the appendix by mucus and is almost always associated with neoplastic process (mucinous cystadenoma or cystadenocarcinoma) (Figure 6-133)
- Existence of non-neoplastic cysts called *retention cysts* is debated; these are characterized by cystic appendices (< 1 cm) that are lined by atrophic or normal (nondysplastic) epithelium

ADENOCARCINOMA

- Mucinous adenocarcinoma is characterized by mucin-filled, neoplastic cysts lined by malignant, papillary mucinous epithelium with invasion
- Nonmucinous adenocarcinoma is identical to its colorectal adenocarcinoma counterpart

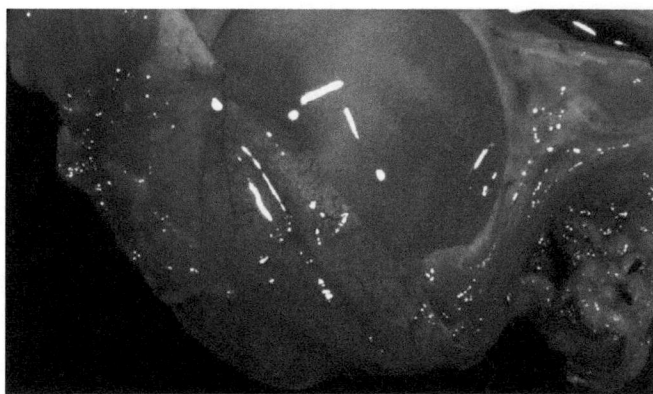

Figure 6-133. Mucocele of the vermiform appendix. The opened normal appendiceal lumen (*right*) is adjacent to a well-defined mucin-containing cyst.

PEARLS

- *Acute appendicitis is due to a combination of infection and luminal obstruction with ischemic damage, which in turn has many causes, including luminal fecalith (most common), lymphoid hyperplasia (often related to viral infection), foreign bodies, parasites (particularly* Enterobius vermicularis*), and fungi*
- *Always search for coexisting neoplasia, especially carcinoid tumor; the margin of excision should always be examined in appendectomy specimens*

SELECTED REFERENCES

Blair NP, Bugis SP, Turner LJ, MacLoed MM: Review of the pathologic diagnoses of 2,216 appendectomy specimens. Am J Surg 165:618-620, 1993.

Butler C: Surgical pathology of acute appendicitis. Hum Pathol 12:870-878, 1981.

APPENDICEAL NEOPLASMS

Clinical Features

MUCOCELE

- Gross term only
- Cystic dilation of the appendix by mucus caused by either a neoplastic or rarely an apparent non-neoplastic process; cysts larger than 1 cm should be considered neoplastic until proved otherwise
- Most are secondary to mucinous cystadenoma or cystadenocarcinoma; pseudomyxoma peritonei may occur if neoplastic process dissects through the wall of the appendix
- Non-neoplastic cysts, called retention cysts (*retention mucoceles*), are controversial, measure less than 1 cm, and are generally caused by sterile obstruction of the appendiceal lumen

MUCINOUS CYSTADENOMA

- Occurs in adults (mean age, 53 years; peak, seventh decade)
- Most present as mucoceles in asymptomatic patients
- About 20% to 25% are associated with separate primary colonic adenocarcinoma
- Often causes symptoms of appendicitis, palpable mass, or pseudomyxoma peritonei

ADENOCARCINOMA

- Uncommon in the appendix
- Typically found in adults 50 to 60 years old
- Often presents with symptoms of acute appendicitis; may cause pseudomyxoma peritonei
- Rarely recognized preoperatively

Gross and Endoscopic Pathology

MUCOCELE

- Cystic dilation of the appendix caused by accumulation of mucus
- Generally larger than 1 cm

MUCINOUS CYSTADENOMA

- Often sausage-like appendix
- Mucin-filled diverticula may be present

ADENOCARCINOMA

- Usually forms a mass at base of the appendix
- Can be a fungating mass with abundant mucus and necrosis
- May obliterate appendix, making exact site of origin difficult to determine

Histopathology

MUCINOUS CYSTADENOMA

- Lined by columnar cells showing epithelial dysplasia, most often low grade (Figure 6-134)
- Abundant mucus fills and dilates the appendiceal lumen
- Can extend into diverticula with rupture
- Hyalinization of appendiceal wall and dystrophic calcification are commonly seen
- Can be associated with pseudomyxoma peritonei

ADENOCARCINOMA

- Mucinous cystadenocarcinoma
  - Neoplastic glands infiltrate appendiceal wall with tumor desmoplasia (Figure 6-135)
  - Coexists with precursor mucinous cystadenoma
  - Can be associated with pseudomyxoma peritonei

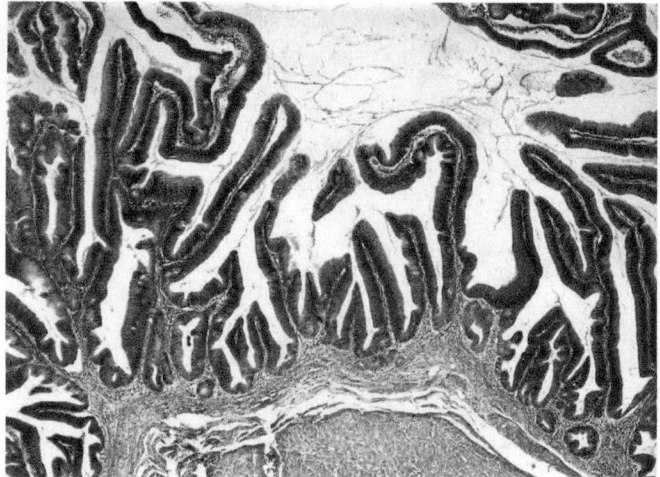

Figure 6-134. Mucinous cystadenoma of the appendix showing a villous adenoma similar to that seen in the colon.

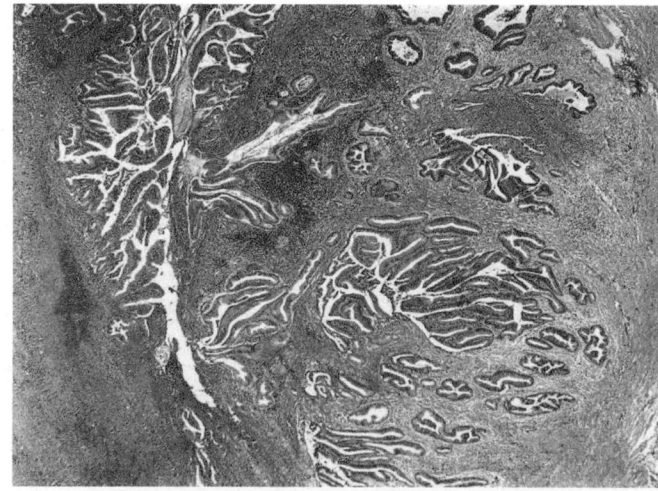

Figure 6-135. Invasive well-differentiated adenocarcinoma arising in association with a mucinous cystadenoma of the appendix (mucinous cystadenocarcinoma). There is an infiltrating pattern to the neoplastic glands, which are surrounded by a tumor desmoplasia.

- Nonmucinous adenocarcinoma
  - Identical to colorectal adenocarcinomas

PSEUDOMYXOMA PERITONEI

- Peritoneal accumulation of gelatinous ascites caused by benign or malignant neoplasms of the vermiform appendix
- Often composed of virtually acellular pools of mucus
- Prognosis varies depending on extent of pseudomyxoma (localized better than diffuse), status of primary tumor (benign better than malignant), cellularity within the mucus of the pseudomyxoma (no or few epithelial cells better than cellular mucus), and degree of dysplasia (low-grade dysplasia better than high-grade dysplasia and adenocarcinoma)
  - Even with diffuse intraperitoneal disease, patients with a benign primary tumor, low cellularity within the mucus, and low-grade dysplasia have a 70% 10-year survival rate
  - Patients usually die of sepsis and bowel obstruction and not cancer
  - In women, pseudomyxoma peritonei can occur with concomitant ovarian mucinous tumors; the vermiform appendix is the primary site in all cases

Special Stains and Immunohistochemistry

- PAS, mucicarmine, and Alcian blue stains are all positive in mucinous tumors (generally unnecessary)

Other Techniques for Diagnosis

- Cases of pseudomyxoma peritonei with a coexisting ovarian mucinous tumor have been studied with CK7, CK20, and *K-ras*; results usually support appendiceal origin of the tumors

Differential Diagnosis

RUPTURED ACUTE APPENDICITIS

- Characterized by acute inflammation, mural necrosis, and acute periappendicitis without dissecting mucus, neoplastic epithelium, or desmoplastic tissue reaction

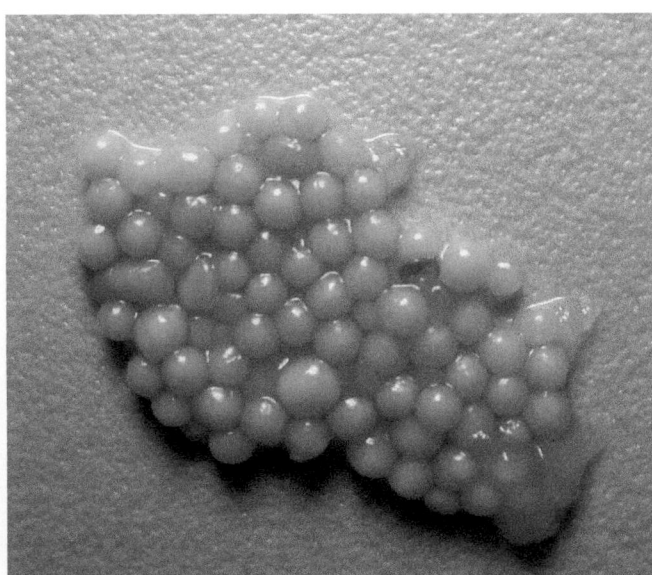

Figure 6-136. Myxoglobulosis of the vermiform appendix. The resected dilated appendix contained these intraluminal pearl-like globules along with a mucinous cystadenoma.

MYXOGLOBULOSIS

- May present with mucocele
- Term is applied to intraluminal tiny pearl-like globules that are often calcified (Figure 6-136)
- Histologically, eosinophilic laminations with external calcification are seen
- Can coexist with appendiceal mucinous neoplasia
- Lining of appendix can undergo pseudosynovial metaplasia

PEARLS

- *Because many appendiceal neoplasms present with acute appendicitis, all appendectomy specimens should be carefully examined grossly to detect subtle mural lesions or tumors; routine histologic examination of the appendiceal margin of excision is highly recommended*

SELECTED REFERENCES

Gonzalez JE, Hann SE, Trujillo YP: Myxoglobulosis of the appendix. Am J Surg Pathol 12:962-966, 1988.

Nitecki SS, Wolff BG, Schlinkert R, et al: The natural history of surgically treated primary adenocarcinoma of the appendix. Ann Surg 219:51-57, 1994.

Riddell RH, Petras RE, Williams GT, Sobin LH: Tumors of the intestines. Atlas of Tumor Pathology, Third Series, Fascicle 32. Washington, DC, Armed Forces Institute of Pathology, 2003.

Ronnett BM, Kurman RJ, Shmookler BM, et al: The morphologic spectrum of ovarian metastases of appendiceal adenocarcinomas: a clinicopathologic and immunohistochemical analysis of tumors often misinterpreted as primary ovarian tumors or metastatic tumors from other gastrointestinal sites. Am J Surg Pathol 21:1144-1155, 1997.

Ronnett BM, Kurman RJ, Zahn CM, et al: Pseudomyxoma peritonei in women: a clinicopathologic analysis of 30 cases with emphasis on site of origin, prognosis, and relationship to ovarian mucinous tumors of low malignant potential. Hum Pathol 26:509-524, 1995.

Ronnett BM, Zahn CM, Kurman RF, et al: Disseminated peritoneal adenomucinosis and peritoneal mucinous carcinomatosis: a clinicopathologic analysis of 109 cases with emphasis on distinguishing pathologic features, site of origin, prognosis, and relationship to "pseudomyxoma peritonei." Am J Surg Pathol 19:1390-1408, 1995.

Szych C, Staebler A, Connolly DC, et al: Molecular genetic evidence supporting the clonality and appendiceal origin of pseudomyxoma peritonei in women. Am J Pathol 154:1849-1855, 1999.

Young RH: Pseudomyxoma peritonei and selected other aspects of the spread of appendiceal neoplasms. Semin Diagn Pathol 21:134-150, 2004.

Young RH, Gilks CB, Sculy RE: Mucinous tumors of the appendix associated with mucinous tumors of the ovary and pseudomyxoma peritonei: a clinicopathologic analysis of 22 cases supporting an origin in the appendix. Am J Surg Pathol 15:415-429, 1991.

CARCINOIDS AND OTHER NONEPITHELIAL TUMORS OF THE VERMIFORM APPENDIX

Clinical Features

CARCINOID TUMORS

- Many are asymptomatic
- Can present with signs and symptoms of acute appendicitis

Gross and Endoscopic Pathology

- Present as a nodule or thickening of appendiceal wall

Histopathology

- Three variants described
  - Insular: typical midgut pattern of carcinoid tumor, well-demarcated variably sized islands composed of cells with uniform polygonal shape, little nuclear pleomorphism or mitotic activity with eosinophilic granular cytoplasm (Figure 6-137)
  - Tubular: dominant glandlike pattern sometimes with columns or ribbons and acinar arrangement of small neoplastic endocrine cells that lack pleomorphism, have little or no mitotic activity (Figure 6-138)
  - Goblet cell carcinoid
    - A misnomer; *crypt cell carcinoma* or *microglandular goblet cell adenocarcinoma* is the preferred name because these terms better reflect the true nature of the tumor
    - Small, well-defined clusters and strands and microglandular collections of mucus-secreting epithelial cells that resemble goblet cells infiltrate the appendiceal wall (Figure 6-139)

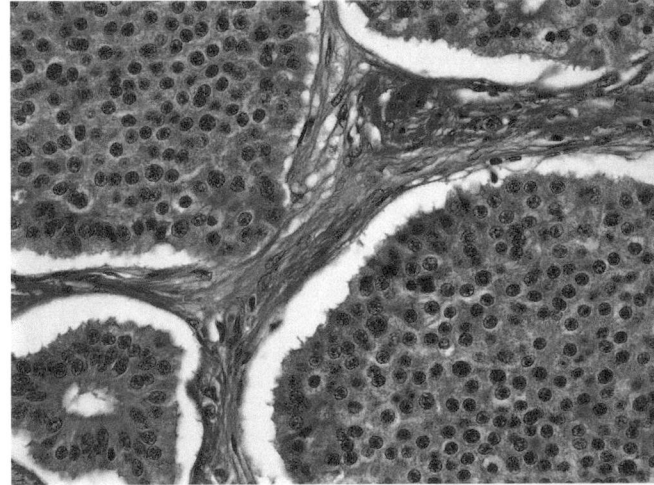

Figure 6-137. Carcinoid tumor of the appendix, midgut pattern with insular groupings of carcinoid tumor cells showing cytoplasmic granules, round nuclei, and a coarsely granular chromatin pattern.

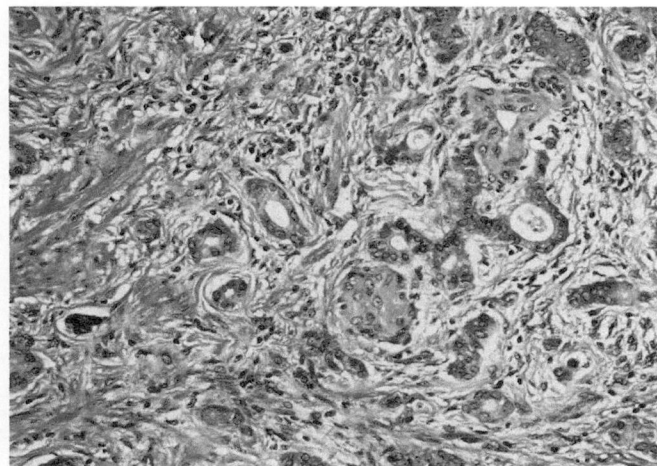

Figure 6-138. Tubular carcinoid of the appendix composed of ribbons and small tubular structures.

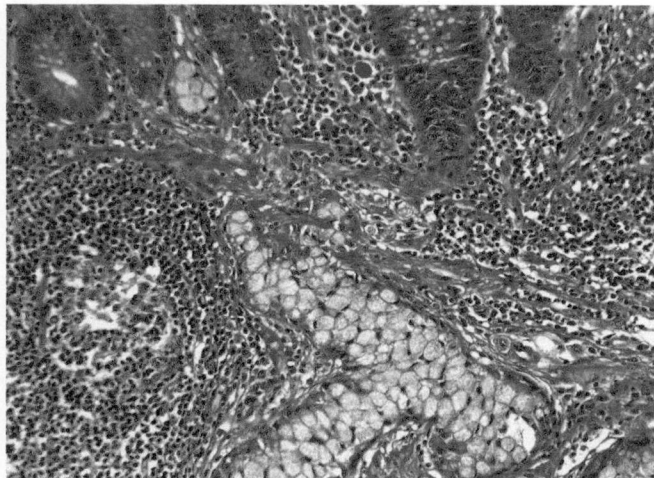

Figure 6-139. Appendiceal goblet cell carcinoid (microglandular goblet cell adenocarcinoma). Note the insular growth pattern of neoplastic cells showing prominent signet resembling mature goblet cells.

- Positive with pan-cytokeratin immunostains; usually negative for neuroendocrine markers such as chromogranin or synaptophysin, or can show scattered rare neuroendocrine cells
- Solid areas of growth, a complex infiltrative pattern, nuclear atypia with increased numbers of mitoses figures, and dissecting mucus usually signal dedifferentiation into a higher grade of adenocarcinoma

Special Stains and Immunohistochemistry

- Mucin stains can be done with goblet cell carcinoid but are usually not necessary
- Chromogranin and synaptophysin immunohistochemistry is helpful, especially in the differential diagnosis of tubular carcinoid versus carcinoma
- Tubular carcinoids are frequently positive for immunoreactive glucagon

Other Techniques for Diagnosis

- Noncontributory

Differential Diagnosis

- Fibrous obliteration of the lumen and appendiceal neuroma
  - These spindle cell proliferations can contain scattered neuroendocrine cells that represent hyperplasia
  - A definite insular or tubular growth pattern, extension of the cells into the muscularis propria or beyond, or the presence of a gross nodule indicates carcinoid tumor
- Tubular carcinoid versus well-differentiated adenocarcinoma
  - Immunohistochemistry for chromogranin and synaptophysin helpful
- Signet ring cell carcinoma versus goblet cell carcinoid
  - Signet ring cell carcinoma is more infiltrative, with increased pleomorphism and larger nuclei
- Neurofibroma, granular cell tumor, paraganglioma, ganglioneuroma, gastrointestinal stromal tumor, sarcoma, and lymphoma have been described primarily within the vermiform appendix but are extremely rare

PEARLS

- *Composite tumor with areas that look like conventional adenocarcinoma will act like conventional adenocarcinoma*
- *Discovery of carcinoid and variant tumors is usually a surprise in an appendectomy specimen removed either incidentally or for acute appendicitis; therefore, routine examination of the appendiceal margin or resection is recommended*
- *Indications for right hemicolectomy for appendiceal carcinoid tumor include size greater than 2 cm, invasion beyond muscularis propria, vascular invasion, incomplete excision (e.g., positive margin of resection), and coexisting adenocarcinoma*
- *CAP protocol should be used in reporting*

SELECTED REFERENCES

Burke AP, Sobin LH, Federspiel BH, et al: Goblet cell carcinoids and related tumors of the vermiform appendix. Am J Clin Pathol 94:27-35, 1990.

Modlin IM, Kidd M, Latich I, et al: Current status of gastrointestinal carcinoids. Gastroenterology 128:1717-1751, 2005.

Riddell RH, Petras RE, Williams GT, Sobin LH: Tumors of the intestines. In Atlas of Tumor Pathology, Third Series, Fascicle 32. Washington, DC, Armed Forces Institute of Pathology, 2003.

Washington MK, Tang LH, Berlin J, et al: Protocol for the examination of specimens from patients with neuroendocrine tumors (carcinoid tumors) of the appendix. Arch Pathol Lab Med 134:171-175, 2010.

Young RH: Pseudomyxoma peritonei and selected other aspects of the spread of appendiceal neoplasms. Semin Diag Pathol 21:134-150, 2004.

SECONDARY MALIGNANCIES IN THE GASTROINTESTINAL TRACT

GASTROINTESTINAL METASTATIC DISEASE

Clinical Features

ESOPHAGUS

- Primary tumors of the lungs, pharynx, thyroid, and stomach may invade the esophagus directly

- Breast, kidney, testicular, prostate, and pancreatic neoplasms can metastasize to the esophagus
- Breast cancer may produce strictures due to extensive lymphatic infiltration
- Melanoma metastasizes to the gastrointestinal tract in 43% of cases

STOMACH

- Stomach is a more common site of metastases than small or large bowel
- Most common gastric metastases are melanomas and carcinomas of the lung and breast
- Gastric metastases often have a targetoid endoscopic appearance due to extensive central necrosis (features particularly notable on radiologic examination)

SMALL INTESTINE

- Because primary small bowel tumors are so uncommon, metastases (carcinomas and sarcomas) are the most common tumors of the small bowel
- Larger tumors are often polypoid, causing obstruction, intussusception, or perforation
- Tumors near the ampulla may represent secondary involvement of the intestine by pancreaticobiliary adenocarcinoma; primary ampullary malignancies usually arise in a preexisting adenoma and have a better prognosis than pancreatitis biliary carcinoma
- Malignant melanoma is the most common small bowel metastasis and often produces obstruction
- About 5% of testicular tumors metastasize to the gastrointestinal tract
- Sarcomas only rarely metastasize to the small bowel
- Bronchogenic squamous carcinoma has a propensity to metastasize to the proximal jejunum

LARGE INTESTINE

- Most common spread of metastases to the colon is by peritoneal seeding, particularly at the pouch of Douglas (anterior wall of rectum)
- Prostatic carcinoma may directly invade the rectum, producing gastrointestinal rather than urinary symptoms
- Anal melanomas may extend into the rectum
- Most common colonic metastases in males are from noncolonic gastrointestinal tumors and lung carcinomas
- Most common colonic metastases in females are from ovarian, breast, and lung carcinomas
- Colonic metastases are often asymptomatic, but with large tumors, obstruction and bleeding may occur

APPENDIX

- Patients with mucinous tumors of the ovary may have a concurrent mucinous neoplasm in the appendix; all represent appendiceal primary tumors
- Other metastatic tumors reported include breast, stomach, cervix, and lung

Gross and Endoscopic Pathology

ESOPHAGUS

- Nonspecific

STOMACH

- Often have multiple tumors that commonly show extensive central necrosis

SMALL INTESTINE

- Intramural masses form submucosal nodules and eventually produce bulging polypoid masses
- Tumors may be circumferential
- Black tumors in the small intestine suggest melanoma; however, melanoma is often amelanotic
- Fleshy cut sections are typical for lymphoma (Figure 6-140)
- Ovarian metastases are most likely to present with carcinomatosis
- Ampullary tumors should be examined carefully to detect any residual adenoma (making the lesion more likely a primary small bowel neoplasm, rather than pancreatic)

LARGE INTESTINE

- Metastasis is suggested by a mural-centered mass not involving the overlying mucosa

Histopathology

ESOPHAGUS

- Metastatic carcinoma including breast carcinoma preferentially involves the submucosal lymphatics and leaves overlying mucosa intact

STOMACH

- Breast carcinoma may be diffusely infiltrative and difficult to distinguish from a primary poorly differentiated adenocarcinoma, diffuse type of Lauren

SMALL INTESTINE

- Ampullary tumors that are primary may have residual adenoma
- Pancreatic primary tumors with secondary involvement of the duodenum grow as an infiltrating, well-differentiated glandular proliferation or as highly anaplastic carcinoma with marked desmoplasia if high grade; often have non-neoplastic duodenal mucosa on the surface

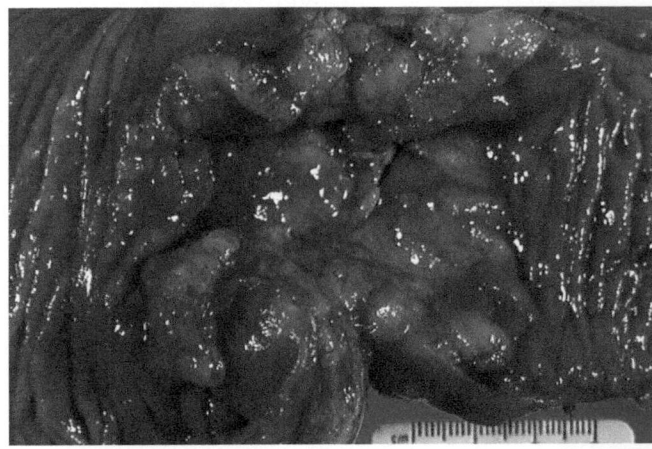

Figure 6-140. Resection specimen of large cell lymphoma involving the small intestine showing a stricturing and ulcerating mass lesion with a homogeneous, fleshy cut surface.

LARGE INTESTINE

- Primary colonic tumors may be distinguished from metastatic adenocarcinoma (such as lung) by the presence of extensive necrosis containing nuclear fragments (so-called dirty necrosis) along with lack of a surface component and predominant mural location

Special Stains and Immunohistochemistry

- In all cases, immunohistochemical markers unique to a specific site outside the gastrointestinal tract are helpful for diagnosing a metastasis (e.g., TTF-1 for lung primary)
- Estrogen receptor (ER) and progesterone receptor (PR) testing can be performed on a metastatic breast carcinoma, but these immunostains are not specific for breast cancer
- CEA and CA-125 immunostains may be used to determine whether a gastrointestinal tumor is primary (CEA positive) or ovarian (CA-125 positive)
- S-100 protein and HMB-45 are typically positive in metastatic malignant melanoma
- Primary colonic carcinoma
  - More likely to be positive for CEA and cytokeratin 20 and negative for cytokeratin 7
- Pulmonary adenocarcinoma
  - Tends to be positive for cytokeratin 7 and TTF-1 and negative for cytokeratin 20

Other Techniques for Diagnosis

- Noncontributory

Differential Diagnosis

- Clinical history is important
- Regardless of the site, tumors in the gastrointestinal tract that are not mucosal based or that predominantly involve the bowel wall and serosa should be considered potentially metastatic

PEARLS

- *Any small intestinal malignancy outside the ampullary region is more likely to be a metastatic tumor than a primary tumor*

SELECTED REFERENCES

Adair C, Ro JY, Sahin AA, et al: Malignant melanomas metastatic to gastrointestinal tract: a clinico-pathologic study. Int J Surg Pathol 2:3, 1994.

Berezauski K, Stastny J, Kornstein M, et al: Cytokeratin 7 and 20 and carcinoembryonic antigen in ovarian and colonic carcinoma. Mod Pathol 9:426, 1995.

Telerman A, Gerard B, van den Hevle B, et al: Gastrointestinal metastases from extra-abdominal tumors. Endoscopy 17:99-101, 1985.

Chapter 7
Hepatobiliary System

MATTHEW M. YEH • PAUL E. SWANSON

CHAPTER OUTLINE

VIRAL HEPATITIS

Clinical Features

HEPATITIS A VIRUS (HAV)
- Single-stranded RNA (ssRNA) virus (picornavirus)
- Transmission route: fecal-oral
- Incubation: 2 to 6 weeks
- Self-limited
- Not associated with chronic carrier state, chronic hepatitis, or hepatocellular carcinoma (HCC)

HEPATITIS B VIRUS (HBV)
- Partially circular double-stranded DNA virus (hepadnavirus)
- Transmission route: perinatal, sexual, and parenteral
- Incubation: 6 to 8 weeks
- Chronic infection (10%): persistent serum hepatitis B surface antigen (HBsAg) more than 6 months after diagnosis
- Associated with chronic hepatitis, fulminant hepatitis, cirrhosis, and HCC
- Anti-HBsAg confers long-term immunity

HEPATITIS C VIRUS (HCV)
- ssRNA virus (flavivirus like)
- Transmission route: parenteral

- Incubation: 6 to 12 weeks
- Highest rate of chronic hepatitis (60% to 80%) and persistent infection
- Associated with cirrhosis and HCC
- Anti-HCV does not confer immunity
- Serum transaminases: fluctuating

HEPATITIS D (DELTA AGENT) VIRUS
- Defective RNA virus requiring HBsAg (envelope protein) for infectivity
- Transmission route: parenteral
- Associated with cirrhosis and HCC

HEPATITIS E VIRUS
- ssRNA virus
- Water-borne infection
- Incubation: 6 weeks
- Virion shed in stools
- Usually self-limited
- High mortality rate among pregnant women

HEPATITIS G VIRUS
- Nonpathogenic

Gross Pathology
- Noncontributory

Histopathology

ACUTE VIRAL HEPATITIS

Injury is predominantly hepatocellular in the acini (zone 3)

- General features
  - Predominantly lymphocytic infiltrate, usually conspicuous in zone 3
  - Swollen hepatocytes with rarefied and granular cytoplasm
  - Apoptotic hepatocytes showing pyknotic nuclear remnants, shrunken and dense cytoplasm
  - Liver cell dropout with replacement by small groups of lymphocytes and macrophages
- Specific features
  - HAV: perivenular cholestasis; hepatitis with periportal inflammation (interface hepatitis) and dense portal infiltrate, including abundant plasma cells, or extensive microvesicular steatosis
  - HBV: ground-glass hepatocytes (indicating abundant HBsAg in the hepatocytes—evidence of viral infection) (Figure 7-1A)

CHRONIC VIRAL HEPATITIS

- Persistent liver injury with positive viral serology and abnormally high serum aminotransferase of >6 months' duration
- Injury is accentuated in the portal and periportal regions
- General features
  - Portal inflammatory infiltrate predominantly composed of lymphocytes with or without interface hepatitis of varying severity (Figure 7-1B)
  - Spotty or confluent necrosis with or without bridging necrosis
  - Portal fibrous expansion, periportal fibrosis, bridging fibrosis to cirrhosis (stages 1 to 4)
- Specific features
  - HBV: ground-glass hepatocytes
  - HCV: lymphoid aggregates or follicles with or without germinal centers, focal mild macrovesicular steatosis, damaged interlobular bile ducts

Special Stains and Immunohistochemistry

- Immunohistochemistry for hepatitis B core antigen (HBcAg), HBsAg, and hepatitis B e antigen (HBeAg)

Other Techniques for Diagnosis

- Electron microscopy: HBsAg in hepatocyte cytoplasm (22-nm spheres and rods)

Differential Diagnosis

- Serologic markers of viral infection are virtually essential to establish or exclude the diagnosis

ALCOHOLIC HEPATITIS

- Clinical history is important
- Fatty change is typical but not always present
- Many ballooned hepatocytes and Mallory-Denk bodies are usually seen
- Megamitochondria may be seen
- Lobular inflammatory foci (usually rich in neutrophils)
- Perivenular and pericellular fibrosis (chicken-wire pattern)

NONALCOHOLIC STEATOHEPATITIS (NASH)

- Significant steatosis is present, predominantly macrovesicular
- Zone 3 injury pattern with lobular inflammatory foci
- Ballooned hepatocytes and Mallory-Denk bodies are typical findings
- Megamitochondria may be seen
- Perivenular and pericellular fibrosis (chicken-wire pattern)

AUTOIMMUNE HEPATITIS

- Serologic markers important (positive antinuclear antibody [ANA], anti–smooth muscle antibody [ASMA], or liver-kidney microsomal antibody [LKM])
- Coexistent autoimmune diseases are common
- Prominent plasma cells in the portal and periportal region or deep within the parenchyma

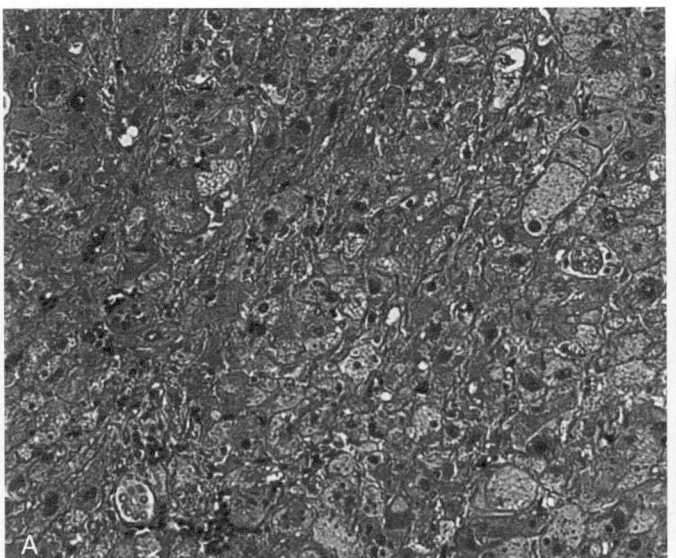
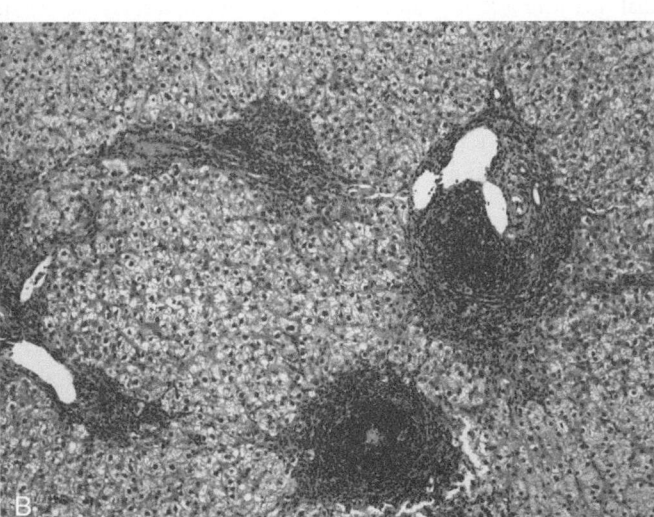

Figure 7-1. A, Ground-glass hepatocytes in hepatitis B. **B,** Chronic hepatitis C. Classic lymphoid aggregates with focal mild interface hepatitis.

- Marked interface hepatitis and parenchymal activity
- Bridging necrosis is common and may form hepatitis rosettes

EPSTEIN-BARR VIRUS (EBV) HEPATITIS
- Seen more often after transplantation
- Marked sinusoidal lymphoplasmacytic inflammatory infiltrate characteristically in single-file arrangement
- Marked hepatocellular regeneration

PRIMARY BILIARY CIRRHOSIS (PBC)
- Bile ductular reaction
- Florid duct lesion with granuloma
- Damage and loss of interlobular bile duct
- Positive antimitochondrial antibody (AMA)
- Cholestatic picture

PRIMARY SCLEROSING CIRRHOSIS
- Bile ductular reaction
- Periductal fibrosis and loss of interlobular bile duct
- Association with ulcerative colitis is common
- Characteristic beading on endoscopic retrograde cholangiopancreatography (ERCP)

DRUG HEPATITIS
- Clinical history is important (time course of drug use)
- Negative serologic markers of viral infection

PEARLS

- *Serologic markers of viral infection as well as the pattern of hepatic enzyme elevations are most important in distinguishing the many causes of hepatitis*

SELECTED REFERENCES

Batts KP, Ludwig J: Chronic hepatitis: an update on terminology and reporting. Am J Surg Pathol 19:1409-1417, 1995.

Gerber MA, Thung SN: The diagnostic value of immunohistochemical demonstration of hepatitis viral antigens in the liver. Hum Pathol 18:771-774, 1987.

Goodman ZD, Ishak KG: Histopathology of hepatitis C infection. Semin Liver Dis 15:70-81, 1995.

Ishak KG: Chronic hepatitis: morphology and nomenclature. Mod Pathol 7:690-713, 1994.

Sciot R, Van Damme B, Desmet VJ: Cholestatic features in hepatitis A. J Hepatol 3:172-181, 1986.

NONVIRAL INFECTIONS

Clinical Features
- High mortality rate
- Patients often have fever and right upper quadrant tenderness
- Surgical drainage is often required
- Bacterial abscesses are caused by portal spread of extrahepatic infection with *Staphylococcus aureus*, *Salmonella typhi*, and syphilis
- Parasitic abscesses are caused by *Entamoeba histolytica*, *Echinococcus* species, malaria, *Leishmania* species, *Ascaris lumbricoides*, and liver flukes (e.g., *Clonorchis sinensis*, *Fasciola hepatica*, and *Opisthorchis viverrini*)

Gross Pathology
- Bacteremic spread through arterial or portal system: multiple, soft, grossly necrotic lesions
- Bacteremic spread by direct extension or trauma: solitary, large, soft, grossly necrotic lesions

SYPHILIS
- Single or multiple soft well-circumscribed lesions (gummas) that eventually scar, resulting in hepar lobatum, which grossly resembles cirrhosis

ENTAMEBIASIS
- Well-circumscribed lesion containing thick, dark material

ECHINOCOCCAL (HYDATID) CYST
- Space-occupying cystic lesion with internal daughter cysts

ASCARIASIS
- Numerous foul-smelling cavities

MALARIA AND LEISHMANIASIS
- Hepatomegaly (secondary Kupffer cell hyperplasia)

Histopathology
BACTERIAL
- Marked neutrophilic infiltrate with hepatocyte destruction (Figure 7-2A)

SYPHILIS
- Congenital: neonatal hepatitis
- Tertiary: gummas (granulomatous abscesses), which heal as dense scars

ENTAMEBIASIS
- Necrotic debris with trophozoites at the periphery (Figure 7-2B)

ECHINOCOCCAL INFECTION
- Outer laminated non-nuclear layer, inner nucleated germinal layer with attached capsules containing numerous scolices that are released into the cyst cavity and give rise to daughter cysts
- Secondary cholangitis results from obstruction of intrahepatic bile ducts

ASCARIASIS
- Necrotic debris with granulomatous and eosinophilic response to degenerated parasites

LIVER FLUKES
- Biliary epithelial hyperplasia, cholangitis, and periductal fibrosis

MALARIA
- Kupffer cell hyperplasia and phagocytosis of ruptured erythrocytes

LEISHMANIASIS
- Kupffer cell hyperplasia and phagocytosis of organisms (Donovan bodies)

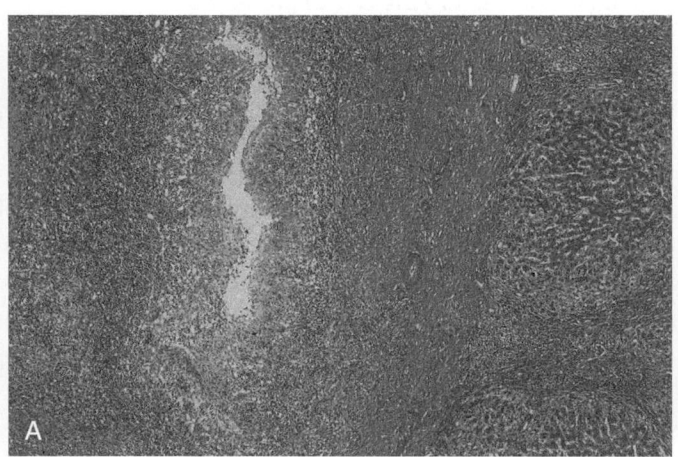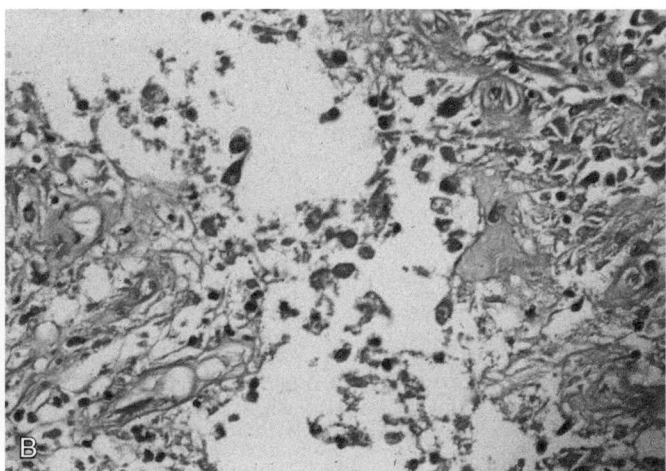

Figure 7-2. A, Bacterial abscess. Low-power view shows liver parenchyma with marked necrosis. **B,** Amebic abscess. Liver tissue showing necrotic debris with trophozoites at the center of the photomicrograph.

Special Stains and Immunohistochemistry

- Gram stain: helps highlight bacteria
- Warthin-Starry or Dieterle stain: syphilis
- Giemsa stain to identify amastigotes: leishmaniasis
- Direct examination for *Echinococcus* species scolices and liver flukes

Other Techniques for Diagnosis

- Culture may help identify organism

Differential Diagnosis

- See earlier discussion for specific infection characteristics

PEARLS

- *Amebic abscesses are more likely to spread into the thoracic cavity*
- *Echinococcal cysts should be removed intact*

SELECTED REFERENCES

Bissada AA, Bateman J: Pyogenic liver abscesses: a 7-year experience in a large community hospital. Hepatogastroenterology 38:17-20, 1991.

Koneman EW, Allen SD, Woods GL, et al (eds): Color Atlas and Textbook of Diagnostic Microbiology, 6th ed. Philadelphia, Lippincott Williams & Wilkins, 2005, pp 1244-1326.

DRUG-INDUCED LIVER DISEASE

Clinical Features

- Clinical history important (e.g., ingesting an agent known to cause liver disease)
- An appropriate time interval between exposure and onset of disease
- A histologic lesion known to be associated with the suspect drug
- Resolution of the lesion after withdrawal
- Can be acute or chronic

Histopathology

- Different agents may result in different liver injury patterns, such as the following:

- Zone 3 hepatocellular necrosis: acetaminophen
  - Mimicking acute viral hepatitis: antituberculous drugs, anesthetics, herbal medicine, nonsteroidal anti-inflammatory drugs
  - Cholestasis with duct damage and duct loss: amoxicillin and clavulanic acid (augmentin)
  - Vanishing bile duct: chlorpromazine, amoxicillin and flucloxacillin, haloperidol
  - Microvesicular steatosis: valproic acid, tetracycline, nucleoside analogues, salicylate (Reye syndrome)
  - Hypertrophic hepatic stellate cells and perivenular and pericellular fibrosis: hypervitaminosis A
  - Sinusoidal obstruction syndrome/veno-occlusive disease): pyrrolizidine alkaloids or chemotherapeutic agents associated with bone marrow transplantation
  - Steatohepatitis-like: amiodarone, tamoxifen
- Drug toxicity should always enter the differential diagnosis when abundant eosinophils or epithelioid granulomas are present or when hepatitis and cholestasis are both present

Special Stains and Immunohistochemistry

- Noncontributory

Other Techniques for Diagnosis

- Noncontributory

Differential Diagnosis

VIRAL HEPATITIS

- Positive serologic markers or viral nucleic acids
- Immunohistochemistry may help to detect viral antigens (e.g., HBV, cytomegalovirus [CMV], herpes simplex virus [HSV], EBV)

AUTOIMMUNE HEPATITIS

- Positive ANA, ASMA, and anti-LKM
- Prominent plasma cells
- Responds to corticosteroid

BILIARY OBSTRUCTION

- Image studies may help

PBC

- Positive AMA
- Florid duct lesion

PEARLS

- *Careful correlation of past and present history is essential, including use of herbal remedies and over-the-counter medications*
- *Rule out other liver diseases*

SELECTED REFERENCES

Geller SA, Petrovic LM: Effects of drugs and toxins on the liver. In Geller SA, Petrovic LM (eds): Biopsy Interpretation of the Liver. Philadelphia, Lippincott Williams & Wilkins, 2004, pp 111-124.

Scheuer PJ, Lefkowitch JH: Drugs and toxins. In Scheuer PJ, Lefkowitch JH (eds): Liver Biopsy Interpretation. London, WB Saunders, 2000, pp 134-150.

Zimmerman HJ: Hepatotoxicity: The Adverse Effects of Drugs and Other Chemicals on the Liver, 2nd ed. Philadelphia, Lippincott Williams & Wilkins, 1999.

Zimmerman HJ, Ishak KG: Hepatic injury due to drugs and toxins. In MacSween RNM, Burt AD, Portmann BC, et al (eds): Pathology of the Liver, 4th ed. Edinburgh, Churchill Livingstone, 2002, pp 621-709.

ALCOHOLIC LIVER DISEASE AND ALCOHOLIC STEATOHEPATITIS

Clinical Features

- Nonspecific symptoms including malaise, anorexia, weight loss, and tender hepatomegaly with mild elevation of serum bilirubin and alkaline phosphatase
- About 20% to 25% of heavy drinkers develop alcoholic steatohepatitis

Gross Pathology

- Early: large, soft, greasy, yellow liver
- Late: shrunken, mottled, red-brown liver with bile staining
- End-stage: cirrhosis

Histopathology

- Steatosis
- Zone 3 injury pattern
- Ballooning degeneration (Figure 7-3A)
- Lobular inflammatory infiltrates, especially rich in neutrophils
- Mallory-Denk bodies and megamitochondria (Figure 7-3B)

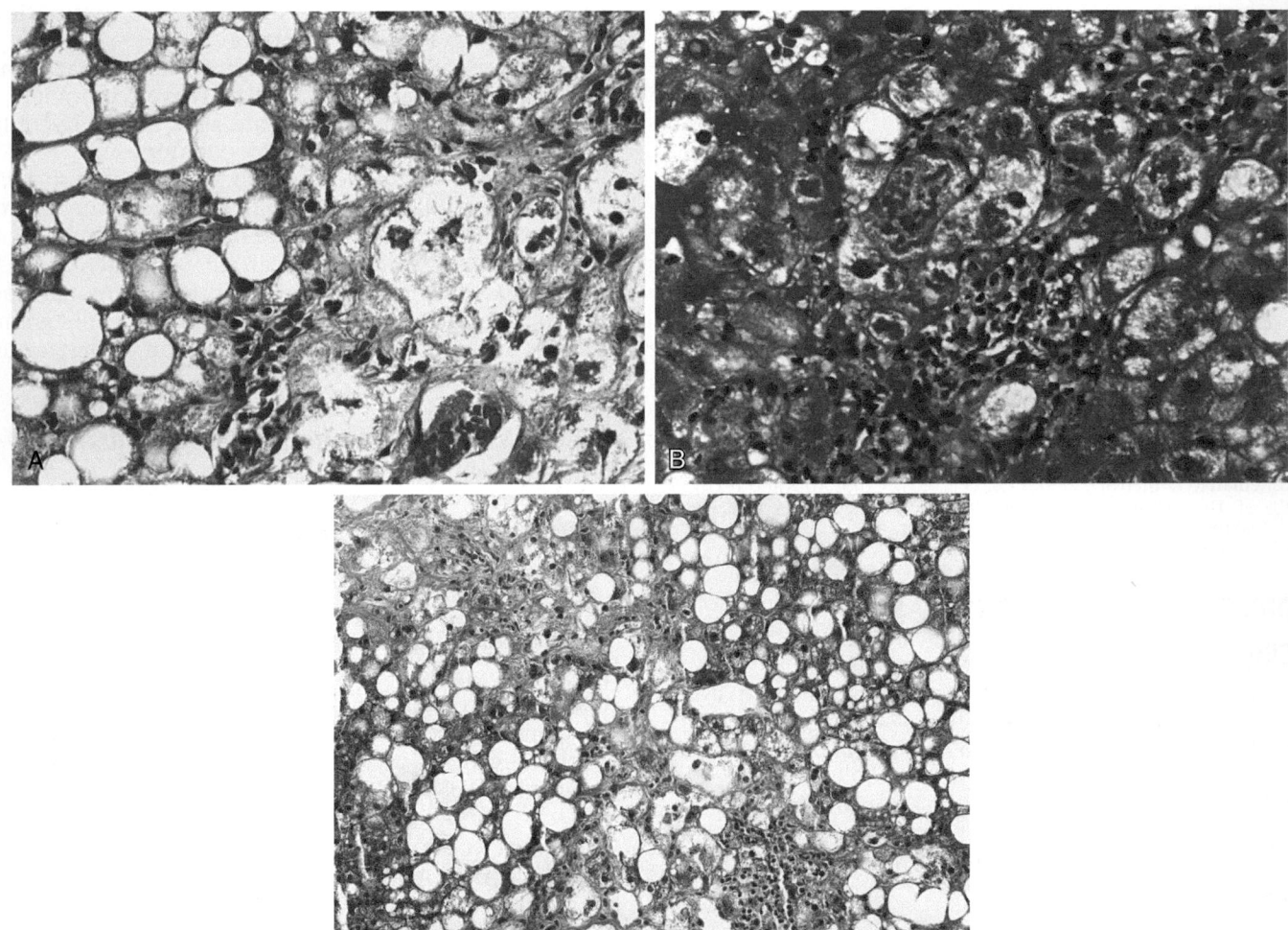

Figure 7-3. Steatohepatitis. **A,** Macrovesicular fat with ballooned hepatocyte and lobular inflammatory infiltrate. **B,** Mallory-Denk bodies are present in the ballooned hepatocytes with associated inflammatory foci. **C,** Pericellular and perisinusoidal fibrosis (chicken-wire pattern).

- Perivenular and pericellular fibrosis (Figure 7-3C)
- Bile ductular reaction
- Sclerosing hyaline necrosis

Special Stains and Immunohistochemistry

- Noncontributory

Other Techniques for Diagnosis

- Noncontributory

Differential Diagnosis

- Clinical history is essential
- Chronic viral hepatitis
- Positive serologic markers of viral infection
- Hepatocellular injury and initiation of fibrosis are more marked in the periportal areas, as opposed to steatohepatitis (perivenular and pericellular fibrosis and hepatocellular injury predominantly in zone 3 region)
- Mallory-Denk bodies are more common in steatohepatitis

FATTY LIVER OF PREGNANCY

- Typically occurs in third trimester of pregnancy
- Steatosis is microvesicular

NONALCOHOLIC STEATOHEPATITIS

- Steatosis is essential
- Glycogenated nuclei are more common
- Sclerosing hyaline necrosis or veno-occlusive lesion are not present

PEARLS

- *Major pathologic effects of alcohol are caused by interference with lipid metabolism, mitochondrial damage, and cytoskeletal injury*
- *Genetically determined susceptibility is thought to account for the fact that only 20% to 25% of heavy drinkers develop alcoholic steatohepatitis, whereas individuals with minimal to no alcohol intake may develop histologically identical nonalcoholic steatohepatitis*

SELECTED REFERENCES

Brunt EM: Alcoholic and nonalcoholic steatohepatitis. Clin Liver Dis 6:399-420, 2002.
Geller SA, Petrovic LM: Alcoholic liver disease. In Geller SA, Petrovic LM (eds): Biopsy Interpretation of the Liver. Philadelphia, Lippincott Williams & Wilkins, 2004, pp 134-149.
Scheuer PJ, Lefkowitch JH: Fatty liver and lesions in the alcoholic. In Scheuer PJ, Lefkowitch JH (eds): Liver Biopsy Interpretation. London, WB Saunders, 2000, pp 111-133.

NONALCOHOLIC FATTY LIVER DISEASE AND NONALCOHOLIC STEATOHEPATITIS

Clinical Features

- A manifestation of the metabolic (insulin resistance) syndrome
- Risk factors: central obesity, hyperglycemia, type II diabetes, arterial hypertension, and hypertriglyceridemia
- NASH is the progressive lesion of nonalcoholic fatty liver disease (NAFLD), which may progress to cirrhosis and liver failure

- Histologically, NASH is almost identical to alcoholic steatohepatitis but occurs in individuals who do not have significant alcohol history

Gross Pathology

- Early: large, soft, greasy, yellow liver
- Late: shrunken, mottled, red-brown liver with bile staining
- End-stage: cirrhosis

Histopathology

- Nonspecific steatosis in NAFLD
- Predominantly macrovesicular fatty change
- Typically starts in a zone 3 centrilobular pattern

NASH

- Begins as a zone 3 injury pattern consisting predominantly of macrovesicular steatosis, ballooned hepatocytes, and lobular inflammation
- Pigmented macrophages and acidophile bodies can be seen
- Cytoplasmic Mallory-Denk bodies (fibrillary eosinophilic material composed of intermediate cytokeratin filaments associated with ubiquitin, a protein from cytoskeletal injury)
- Zone 3 perivenular and pericellular fibrosis (chicken-wire pattern), which progresses to central-portal bridging
- Cirrhosis (end-stage disease)

Special Stains and Immunohistochemistry

- Immunohistochemical stains for ubiquitin and p62 have been developed to identify Mallory-Denk bodies
- Rearrangement of the intermediate filament cytoskeleton in ballooned hepatocytes can be demonstrated by the loss of cytoplasmic keratin 8/18 immunostaining and may be evaluated as a marker for the more objective detection of hepatocellular ballooning in NASH

Other Techniques for Diagnosis

- Noncontributory

Differential Diagnosis

- Clinical history is essential

CHRONIC VIRAL HEPATITIS

- Positive serologic markers of viral infection
- Inflammation is more accentuated in the portal and periportal areas
- Fibrosis initiates in portal regions
- Mallory-Denk bodies are more common in steatohepatitis

FATTY LIVER OF PREGNANCY

- Typically occurs in third trimester of pregnancy
- Steatosis is microvesicular

BILIARY OBSTRUCTION (ESPECIALLY PBC)

- Mallory-Denk bodies may be present and would most likely be seen in periportal as opposed to pericentral areas

WILSON DISEASE

- Mallory-Denk bodies may be present and would most likely be seen in periportal as opposed to pericentral areas
- Marked copper overload

INDIAN CHILDHOOD CIRRHOSIS

- Occurs almost exclusively in India
- Mallory-Denk bodies are often present
- Steatosis conspicuously absent
- Marked copper overload

PEARLS

- *Presence of Mallory-Denk bodies associated with lobular inflammatory infiltrates and steatosis (predominantly macrovesicular) in a zone 3 injury pattern suggests alcoholic or nonalcoholic steatohepatitis*
- *Mallory-Denk bodies may be present in other pathologic processes, including chronic cholestatic disease, Wilson disease, Indian childhood cirrhosis, and even HCCs (about 10%)*

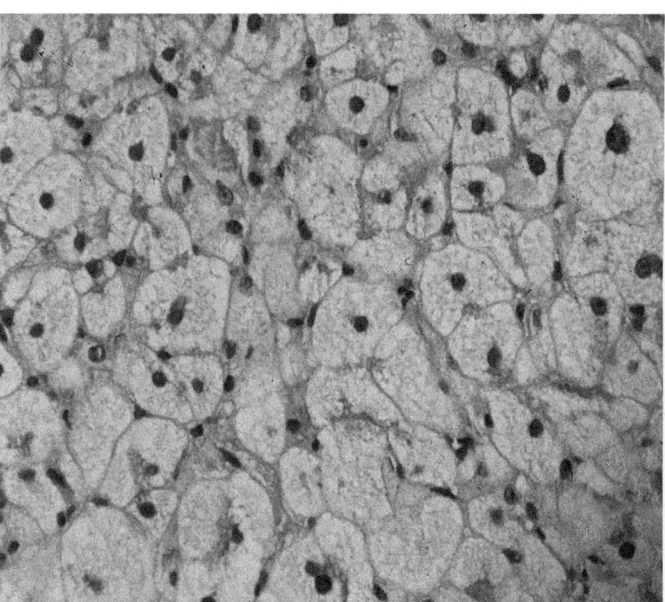

Figure 7-4. Acute fatty liver of pregnancy. Marked microvesicular transformation of hepatocytes.

SELECTED REFERENCES

Brunt EM: Nonalcoholic steatohepatitis: definition and pathology. Semin Liver Dis 21:3-16, 2001.

Brunt EM: Nonalcoholic steatohepatitis: pathologic features and differential diagnosis. Semin Diagn Pathol 22:330-338, 2005.

Guy CD, Suzuki A, Burchette JL, Brunt EM, et al: Nonalcoholic Steatohepatitis Clinical Research Network: costaining for keratins 8/18 plus ubiquitin improves detection of hepatocytes injury in nonalcoholic fatty liver disease. Hum Pathol 43:790-800, 2012.

Kleiner DE, Brunt EM, Van Natta M, et al: Design and validation of a histological scoring system for nonalcoholic fatty liver disease. Hepatology 41:1313-1321, 2005.

ACUTE FATTY LIVER OF PREGNANCY

Clinical Features

- Onset typically occurs during third trimester of pregnancy
- Bleeding, nausea and vomiting, jaundice, and occasionally coma
- Usually resolves after delivery

Gross Pathology

- Greasy, small, pale-yellow liver

Histopathology

- Microvesicular steatosis (Figure 7-4)
- Canalicular and intrahepatocytic cholestasis may occur
- Portal tract inflammation may be prominent

Special Stains and Immunohistochemistry

- Oil red O (on frozen-section slide) demonstrates microvesicular fat droplets

Other Techniques for Diagnosis

- Noncontributory

Differential Diagnosis

- Clinical history is essential

DRUG TOXICITY

- May show similar histologic features (e.g., tetracycline, valproic acid, nucleoside analogues), which are all associated with microvesicular fatty change
- Clinical history is required for definitive distinction

REYE SYNDROME

- Also shows microvesicular steatosis
- History of aspirin use
- Associated with encephalopathy

HCV

- Typically shows macrovesicular steatosis
- Shows lobular hepatitis and portal lymphoid aggregates

ALCOHOLIC STEATOHEPATITIS

- Mallory-Denk bodies are typically prominent and often associated with a neutrophilic infiltrate

PEARLS

- *Onset during pregnancy, usually third trimester*
- *Pathogenesis: defective intramitochondrial fatty acid oxidation*

SELECTED REFERENCES

Kaplan MM: Acute fatty liver of pregnancy. N Engl J Med 313:367-370, 1985.

Riely CA: Acute fatty liver of pregnancy. Semin Liver Dis 7:47-54, 1987.

Rolfes DB, Ishak KG: Acute fatty liver of pregnancy: a clinicopathologic study of 35 cases. Hepatology 5:1149-1158, 1985.

Rolfes DB, Ishak KG: Liver disease in pregnancy. Histopathology 10:555-570, 1986.

HEMOCHROMATOSIS

Clinical Features

- Abnormal accumulation of iron in liver, pancreas, myocardium, and other organs
- Hereditary: homozygous recessive
- Acquired: multiple transfusions, Bantu hemosiderosis (alcoholic beverages brewed in iron drums in sub-Saharan Africa)
- Most often presents in men older than 40 years
- Liver is the most severely affected organ
- Classic triad: cirrhosis, skin pigmentation, and diabetes mellitus (not as common now owing to early diagnosis and treatment)
- Patients may also have abdominal pain, cardiac dysfunction, and atypical arthritis
- Laboratory studies show increased serum iron and ferritin
- Increased risk for developing HCC

Gross Pathology

- Enlarged liver with dark-brown pigmentation
- Ultimately leads to cirrhosis with persistent dark-brown pigmentation

Histopathology

- Early: hemosiderin granules in cytoplasm of periportal hepatocytes
- Middle
  - Progressive involvement of lobule and eventually bile duct epithelium and Kupffer cells, resulting in hepatocyte necrosis, portal inflammation, and portal and bridging fibrosis (Figure 7-5A)
  - Lobular inflammation typically absent
- Late: fibrous septa develop over years with progression to cirrhosis with intense hemosiderin pigmentation

Special Stains and Immunohistochemistry

- Prussian blue stain for iron highlights increased iron deposition (Figure 7-5B)

Other Techniques for Diagnosis

- Hepatic iron index (HII): biochemical quantitation of hepatic iron in fresh tissue or paraffin block calculated as micromoles of iron per gram dry weight divided by patient's age
  - Homozygotes: HII greater than 2 (may be greater than 40)
  - Heterozygotes: less than 2
  - Normal individuals: less than 1
- Human leukocyte antigen (HLA) gene analysis: hemochromatosis gene is HLA-H located on the short arm of chromosome 6
  - Most common mutation is cysteine to tyrosine at amino acid 282

Differential Diagnosis

HEMOSIDEROSIS

- Patients typically have a cause for secondary iron overload (e.g., multiple transfusions, porphyria cutanea tarda, or chronic dietary iron overload as in Bantu siderosis)

CIRRHOSIS OF NONBILIARY ETIOLOGY

- Common to have iron overload in cirrhosis due to nonbiliary etiology (e.g., HCV, alcohol, NASH)

PEARLS

- *Iron is directly hepatotoxic; no inflammatory mediators released*
- *Women are less commonly affected and present later as a result of physiologic blood loss during menstruation and pregnancy*
- *Treatment is reduction of iron overload by phlebotomy*

SELECTED REFERENCES

Bacon BR, Britton RS: The pathology of hepatic iron overload: a free radical-mediated process. Hepatology 11:127-137, 1990.
Brunt EM: Pathology of hepatic iron overload. Semin Liver Dis 25:392-401, 2005.

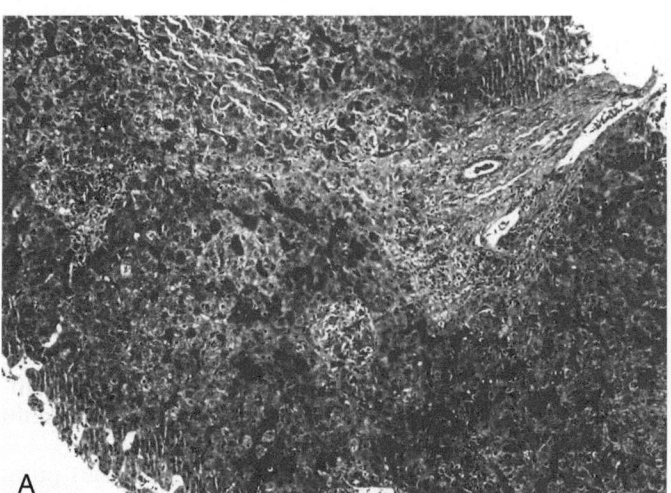
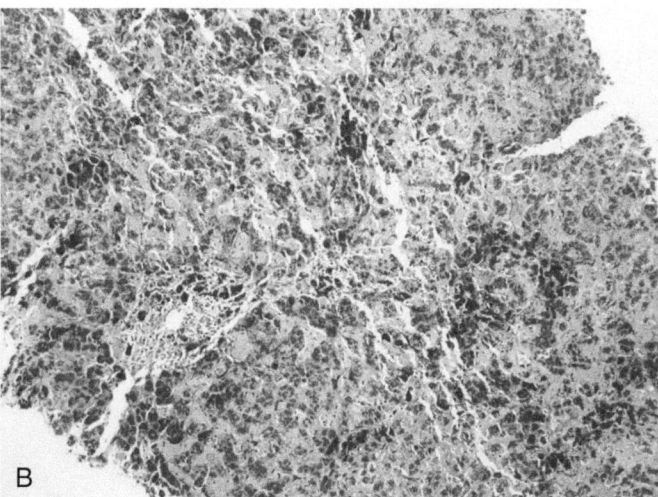

Figure 7-5. Hemochromatosis. A, Hepatocytes containing a large amount of iron. **B,** Prussian blue stain is strongly positive, highlighting the massive iron deposits.

Deugnier YM, Loreal O, Turlin B, et al: Liver pathology in genetic hemochromatosis: a review of 135 cases and their bioclinical correlations. Gastroenterology 104:228-234, 1992.

Deugnier YM, Turlin B, Powell LW, et al: Differentiation between heterozygotes and homozygotes in genetic hemochromatosis by means of a histologic hepatic iron index: a study of 192 cases. Hepatology 17:30-34, 1993.

WILSON DISEASE

Clinical Features

- Abnormal accumulation of copper in liver, brain, eyes, and other organs
- Variable age of onset
- Autosomal recessive
- Laboratory findings include decreased serum ceruloplasmin, increased hepatic copper, increased urinary excretion of copper
- Serum copper levels not helpful
- Most commonly presents with acute or chronic liver disease
- Neuropsychiatric symptoms are also frequent at presentation secondary to involvement of basal ganglia
- Kayser-Fleischer rings are diagnostic (green-brown deposits of copper in Descemet membrane in limbus of cornea)

Gross Pathology

- Liver eventually becomes cirrhotic

Histopathology

- Excessive copper granule in hepatocytes can only be seen with special stain (Figure 7-6)
- Mild to moderate fatty change
- Focal hepatocyte necrosis
- Glycogen vacuoles in hepatocyte nuclei
- Mallory-Denk bodies in periportal hepatocytes
- Acute and chronic hepatitis
- Cirrhosis following chronic hepatitis
- Rarely, massive liver necrosis

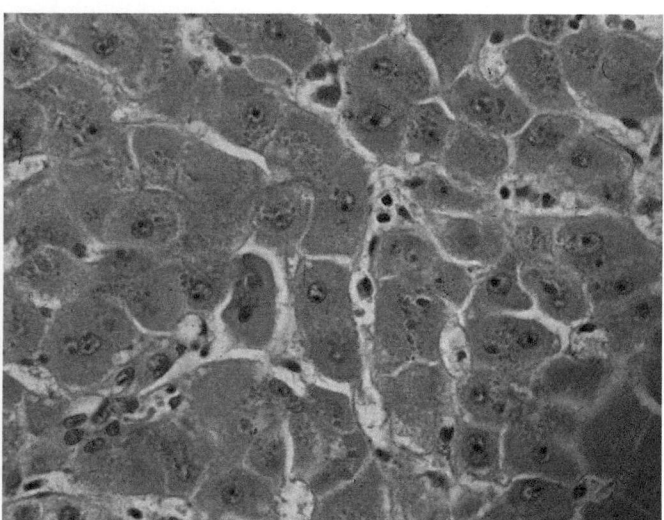

Figure 7-6. Wilson disease. High-power view shows liver cells containing cytoplasmic copper pigment.

Special Stains and Immunohistochemistry

- Rhodanine stain for copper positive
- Orcein stain for copper-associated protein positive

Other Techniques for Diagnosis

- Biochemical quantitation of hepatic copper in fresh tissue or paraffin block (more than 250 µg copper/1 g dry liver)

Differential Diagnosis

VIRAL HEPATITIS

- Serologic markers are positive
- No accumulation of copper

CHRONIC OBSTRUCTIVE CHOLESTASIS

- Lesser degree of copper accumulation

PEARLS

- *Normally free copper is absorbed in the stomach and duodenum, weakly bound to albumin, transferred to hepatocytes, and incorporated into α_2-globulin to form ceruloplasmin, which is re-secreted into plasma; senescent ceruloplasmin is taken up by hepatocytes, degraded by lysosomes, and excreted into bile*
- *Wilson disease gene is ATP7B on chromosome 13 and encodes a transmembrane copper-transporting adenosine triphosphatase (ATPase) located on canalicular membrane of hepatocytes*
- *Treatment is copper chelation with D-penicillamine*

SELECTED REFERENCES

Ludwig J, Moyer TP, Rakela J: The liver biopsy diagnosis of Wilson's disease: methods in pathology. Am J Clin Pathol 102:443-446, 1994.

Sternlieb I: Perspectives on Wilson's disease. Hepatology 12:1234-1239, 1990.

Stremmel W, Meyerrose KW, Niederau C, et al: Wilson disease: clinical presentation, treatment and survival. Ann Intern Med 115:720-726, 1991.

Stromeyer FW, Ishak KG: Histology of the liver in Wilson's disease: a study of 34 cases. Am J Clin Pathol 73:12-24, 1980.

α_1-ANTITRYPSIN DEFICIENCY

Clinical Features

- Variable age of onset
- Autosomal recessive disease caused by mutations of the polymorphic Pi (protease inhibitor) gene on chromosome 14
- Absent or decreased Pi activity results in unchecked activity of neutrophilic elastase leading to pulmonary emphysema (destruction of elastic fibers supporting alveolar spaces)
- The mutant polypeptide is abnormally folded, blocking its movements from the endoplasmic reticulum to Golgi and accumulating in the endoplasmic reticulum of hepatocytes
- In some patients, there is liver disease without pulmonary emphysema owing to functional mutant forms that inhibit neutrophil elastase but that are not appropriately degraded in hepatocytes

- Clinical hepatic presentations range from
  - Neonatal hepatitis with cholestatic jaundice
  - Young adults with recurrent attacks of hepatitis that either resolve or lead to chronic hepatitis and cirrhosis
  - Middle-aged to older adults with cirrhosis after a clinically silent course
- Increased risk for HCC, especially in homozygous patients
- Successful liver transplantation is curative

Gross Pathology

- Noncontributory

Histopathology

- Round to oval, variably sized eosinophilic globules most concentrated in periportal hepatocytes
- Otherwise variable histologic features
  - Neonatal hepatitis with or without cholestasis
  - Chronic hepatitic picture
  - Cirrhosis

Special Stains and Immunohistochemistry

- Eosinophilic globules are positive for periodic acid-Schiff (PAS) and resistant to diastase digestion (Figure 7-7)

Other Techniques for Diagnosis

- Identification of mutant protein by electrophoresis
- About 75 variants identified and named alphabetically according to migration on isoelectric gel
- Normal genotype is PiMM
- PiZZ is most clinically significant genotype (results from amino acid substitution of Glu to Lys) and shows the highest association with carcinoma
- Patients with PiMZ genotype have 50% normal α_1-antitrypsin and 50% mutant form
- Other mutant alleles include S (reduced levels of α_1-antitrypsin but no clinical disease) and null (no detectable protein)

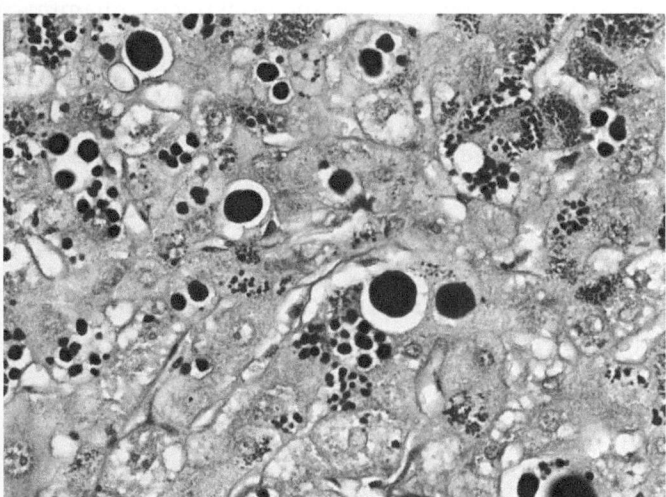

Figure 7-7. α_1-Antitrypsin deficiency. Hepatocytes containing intracytoplasmic eosinophilic globules (periodic acid–Schiff stain with diastase).

Differential Diagnosis

- Other types of chronic hepatitis and cirrhosis include viral, drug, and autoimmune hepatitis, but they do not demonstrate the PAS-positive and diastase-resistant globules that are characteristic of α_1-antitrypsin deficiency

PEARLS

- *α_1-Antitrypsin deficiency is one of the few liver diseases that can still be diagnosed in an end-stage liver explant because of the PAS-positive and diastase-resistant globules that remain in the hepatocyte cytoplasm*
- *This is a multifactorial disease in which there are heterogeneous genetic mutations, resulting in highly variable clinical presentations even among members of individual families*

SELECTED REFERENCES

Cohen C, Derose PB: Liver cell dysplasia in alpha 1-antitrypsin deficiency. Mod Pathol 7:31-36, 1994.
Deutsch J, Becker H, Aubock L: Histopathological features of liver disease in alpha-1-antitrypsin deficiency. Acta Paediatr 393(suppl):8-12, 1994.
Lomas DA, Evans DL, Finch JT, et al: The mechanism of Z alpha 1-antitrypsin accumulation in the liver. Nature 57:605-607, 1992.
Propst T, Propst A, Dietze O, et al: Alpha-1-antitrypsin deficiency and liver disease. Dig Dis 12:139-149, 1994.

AUTOIMMUNE HEPATITIS

Clinical Features

- Young and middle-aged women (female-to-male ratio of 7:3)
- Often associated with extrahepatic autoimmune disorders such as rheumatoid arthritis, thyroiditis, Sjögren syndrome
- Hyperglobulinemia
- Characterized by serum autoantibodies, classically ANA, ASMA, soluble liver antigen (SLA), and anti-LKM1
- Negative viral serologic markers
- Responsive to immunosuppressive therapy

Gross Pathology

- Noncontributory

Histopathology

- Significant portal and periportal inflammatory infiltrate with lymphocytes and plasma cells (prominent plasma cells are the hallmark) (Figure 7-8)
- Marked lobular inflammatory infiltrate with prominent plasma cells deep in the parenchyma
- Increased lobular apoptotic bodies
- Prominent interface hepatitis
- Bridging necrosis is common
- Severe hepatocellular injury with hepatitic rosette formation and syncytial giant hepatocytes

Special Stains and Immunohistochemistry

- Noncontributory

Other Techniques for Diagnosis

- Noncontributory

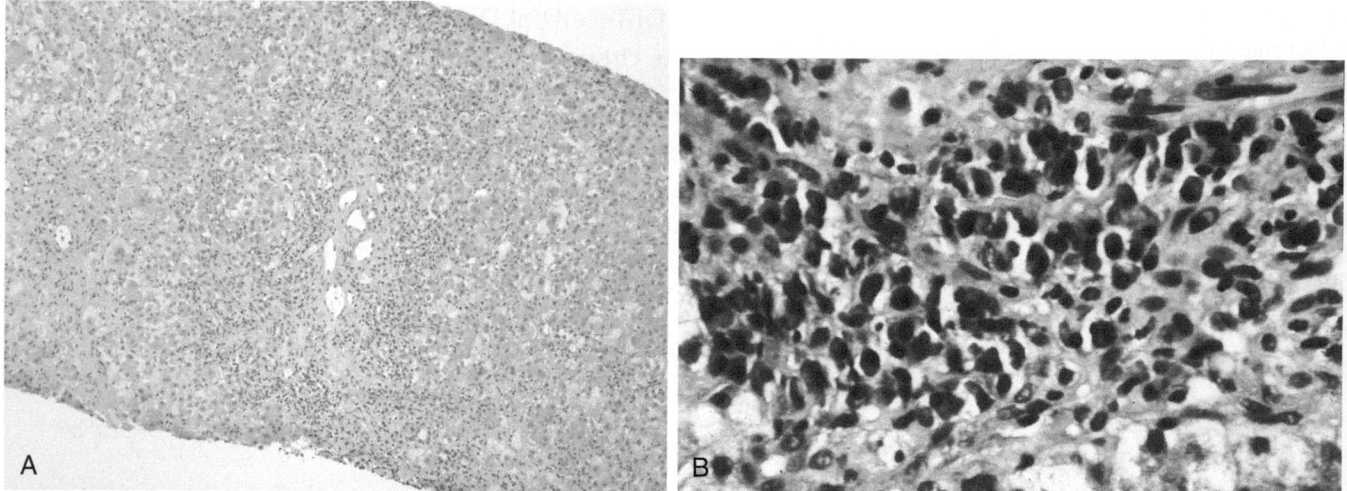

Figure 7-8. Autoimmune hepatitis. A, Low-power magnification shows marked interface hepatitis and lobular inflammation. **B,** Prominent portal and periportal infiltrate of plasma cells.

Differential Diagnosis

DRUG INJURY
- Clinical correlation and medication history including over-the-counter drugs is important in the differential diagnosis of this disease

CHRONIC VIRAL HEPATITIS
- Positive virologic and serologic markers
- Plasma cells less prominent
- Milder lobular hepatitis and interface hepatitis (especially in HCV)
- No association with autoimmune diseases

PEARLS

- *Most frequent in young women and associated with hyperglobulinemia and various serologic markers of autoimmune disease*
- *Rosette formation, although not specific, is highly suggestive of autoimmune hepatitis*
- *This is one of the few forms of chronic hepatitis that responds well to immunosuppressive therapy*

SELECTED REFERENCES

Bach N, Thung SN, Schaffner F: The histologic changes of chronic hepatitis C and autoimmune hepatitis: a comparative study. Hepatology 15:572-577, 1992.

Czaja AJ: Autoimmune hepatitis: evolving concepts and treatment strategies. Dig Dis Sci 40:435-456, 1995.

Johnson PJ, McFarlane IG: Meeting report. International Autoimmune Hepatitis Group. Hepatology 18:998-1005, 1993.

Washington MK: Autoimmune liver disease: overlap and outliers. Mod Pathol 20:S15-S30, 2007.

PRIMARY BILIARY CIRRHOSIS

Clinical Features
- Most commonly occurs in middle-aged women
- Serum AMAs in more than 90% of cases
- Insidious onset, with pruritus being the most common presenting symptom and jaundice developing later
- Elevated serum alkaline phosphatase, with hyperbilirubinemia developing later
- Chronic and progressive, with cirrhosis developing only after many years

Gross Pathology
- Early: unremarkable
- Late: finely granular capsule; bile-stained parenchyma
- Ultimately liver becomes cirrhotic (biliary type cirrhosis)

Histopathology
- Variability in stages of lesions (i.e., coexistence of different stages in single specimen)
- *Stage I (florid duct lesion)*: focal destruction of small and medium-sized bile ducts by granulomatous inflammation; bile duct epithelium irregular and hyperplastic; dense portal tract infiltrate of lymphocytes, macrophages, plasma cells, and eosinophils (Figure 7-9)
- *Stage II (ductular reaction)*: scarring; disappearance of small bile ducts; scarring of medium-sized bile ducts; proliferation of bile ductules in portal tracts; inflammation and interface hepatitis of adjacent periportal hepatic parenchyma
- *Stage III (scarring)*: small and medium-sized ducts scarce; little inflammation in fibrous septa or parenchyma; lymphoid aggregates with or without PAS-positive material representing residual basement membrane material in areas where ducts had been
- *Stage IV (cirrhosis)*: cirrhosis, often with a jigsaw pattern

Special Stains and Immunohistochemistry
- Noncontributory

Other Techniques for Diagnosis
- Noncontributory

Differential Diagnosis

PRIMARY SCLEROSING CHOLANGITIS (PSC)
- Characterized by periductal fibrosis and typical ERCP findings

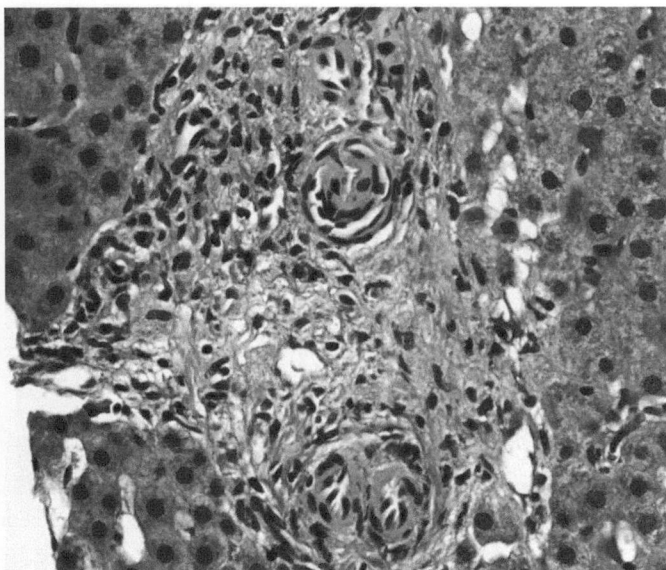

Figure 7-9. Primary biliary cirrhosis. A portal tract shows granulomatous inflammation, chronic inflammatory infiltrate, and paucity of bile ducts.

- Lacks the florid duct lesion seen in PBC
- Occurs in young men as opposed to middle-aged women
- Negative AMA
- Often associated with ulcerative colitis

AUTOIMMUNE HEPATITIS–PBC OVERLAP SYNDROME
- AMA and ANA positive with histologic features of both PBC and autoimmune hepatitis (more than the usual degree of lobular hepatitis, interface hepatitis, and plasma cell infiltrate)

AUTOIMMUNE CHOLANGITIS
- Histologically identical to PBC
- Patients are AMA negative and ANA positive

GRAFT-VERSUS-HOST DISEASE AND LIVER TRANSPLANT REJECTION
- Clinical history important
- Both can cause bile duct injury, lymphocytic cholangitis, and vanishing bile duct syndrome, which can resemble PBC

PEARLS
- *AMAs are against E2 subunit of pyruvate dehydrogenase complex on interlobular bile ducts in PBC*
- *Generally believed to be an autoimmune disease*
- *Liver transplantation is definitive treatment*

SELECTED REFERENCES

Berk PD: Primary biliary cirrhosis, Parts I and II. Semin Liver Dis 17:1-250, 1997.
Lacerda MA, Ludwig J, Dickson ER, et al: Antimitochondrial antibody-negative primary biliary cirrhosis. Am J Gastroenterol 90:247-249, 1995.
Mahl TC, Shockcor W, Boyer JL: Primary biliary cirrhosis: survival of a large cohort of symptomatic and asymptomatic patients followed for 24 years. J Hepatol 20:707-713, 1994.
Sherlock S: Primary biliary cirrhosis: clarifying the issues. Am J Med 96(suppl):27S-33S, 1994.

PRIMARY SCLEROSING CHOLANGITIS

Clinical Features
- More common in men in the third to fifth decades
- Characteristic beaded appearance of intrahepatic biliary tree by contrast radiography (ERCP) due to irregular strictures and secondary dilations of affected bile ducts
- About 70% of cases are associated with ulcerative colitis (conversely, only 4% of patients with ulcerative colitis have PSC)
- Elevated alkaline phosphatase and bilirubin
- Increased risk of cholangiocarcinoma (terminal event in about 10% of patients with PSC)

Gross Pathology
- Early: unremarkable
- Late: bile-stained, biliary-type cirrhosis

Histopathology
- Characterized by fibroinflammatory stricture of the bile ducts anywhere from the ampulla of Vater to the interlobular bile ducts
- *Stage I (portal)*: concentric periductal fibrosis and lymphocytic inflammation in portal tracts (Figure 7-10A and B)
- *Stage II (periportal)*: fibrosis extends into periportal parenchyma, interface hepatitis, and bile ductular reaction
- *Stage III (septal)*: obliteration of bile ducts and bridging fibrosis
- *Stage IV (cirrhotic)*: biliary-type cirrhosis (jigsaw pattern)
- Features of chronic cholestasis, especially pseudoxanthomatous changes, are commonly seen

Special Stains and Immunohistochemistry
- Noncontributory

Other Techniques for Diagnosis
- Noncontributory

Differential Diagnosis
WELL-DIFFERENTIATED CHOLANGIOCARCINOMA
- Heterogeneity of cells within individual glands
- Perineural invasion often seen
- Radiologic information is helpful

PBC
- Occurs more commonly in middle-aged women
- Typically positive for AMA
- Florid duct lesions followed by absence of bile duct as opposed to the fibroinflammatory obliteration of ducts seen in PSC

EXTRAHEPATIC OR LARGE DUCT INTRAHEPATIC BILIARY OBSTRUCTION
- Can give rise to a secondary sclerosing cholangitis similar to PSC

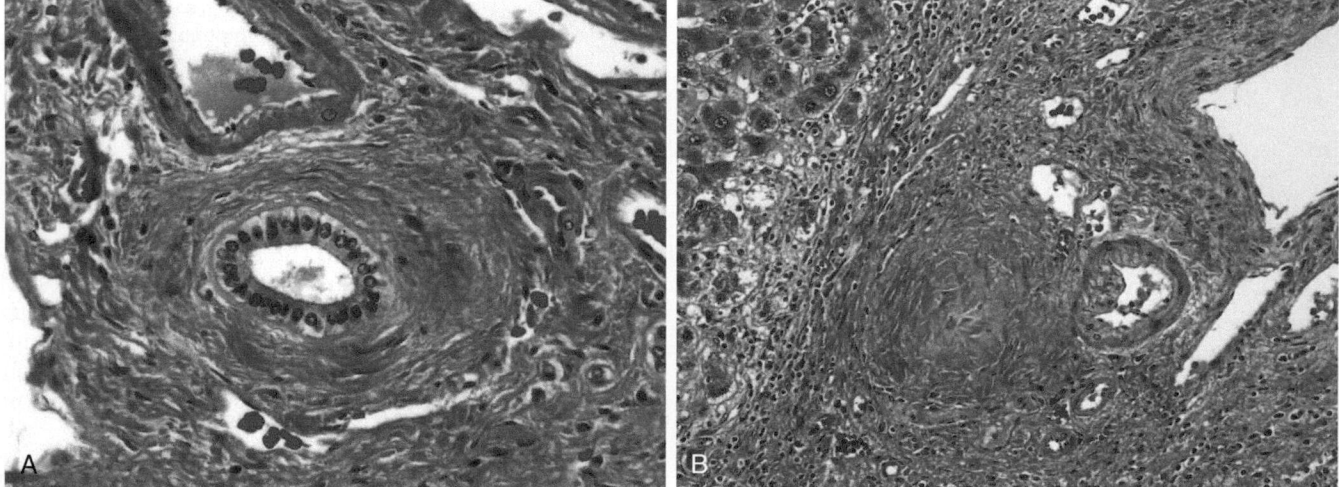

Figure 7-10. Primary sclerosing cholangitis. A, Histologic section of a portal field showing concentric periductal fibrosis. **B,** Histologic section of a portal field showing chronic inflammation and obliteration of the bile duct.

- Features suggestive of secondary cholangitis include marked ductular reaction and severe cholestasis with inspissated bile, which is often green and laminated
- Often see marked pseudoxanthomatous change and rapid onset (months) of biliary cirrhosis

PEARLS

- *Associated with chronic inflammatory bowel disease, particularly ulcerative colitis*
- *Increased risk for cholangiocarcinoma*
- *Characterized by fibroinflammatory obliteration of small and medium-sized bile ducts*
- *Liver transplantation is curative; however, disease may recur in transplanted liver*

SELECTED REFERENCES

Angulo P, Lindor KD: Primary sclerosing cholangitis. Hepatology 30:325-332, 1999.
Harnois DM, Lindor KD: Primary sclerosing cholangitis: evolving concepts in diagnosis and treatment. Dig Dis 15:23-41, 1997.
Lee YM, Kaplan MM: Primary sclerosing cholangitis. N Eng J Med 332:924-933, 1995.
Ueno Y, LaRusso NF: Primary sclerosing cholangitis. J Gastroenterol 29:531-543, 1994.

LIVER TRANSPLANTATION PATHOLOGY

Clinical Features

- Indications for liver transplantation include end-stage chronic liver disease, acute liver failure, and hepatic neoplasm
- The main complications of liver transplantation include surgical complications involving vascular or biliary structures, allograft rejection, recurrent diseases, acquired diseases, and complications of immunosuppressive therapy (opportunistic infections, posttransplantation lymphoproliferative diseases, and drug toxicities)

Gross Pathology

- Hyperacute and humoral allograft rejection: massive hemorrhagic necrosis
- Graft ischemia in early posttransplantation period: irregular geographic areas of infarction with a surrounding hemorrhagic border
- Ischemic bile duct necrosis: necrotic and bile-stained portal regions with surrounding centrilobular cholestasis

Histopathology

- Acute (cellular) rejection in allograft
  - Portal inflammation, bile duct damage, and endotheliitis are the characteristic histologic triad (Figure 7-11A)
  - Portal inflammatory infiltrate includes large lymphocytes, activated blast cells, plasmacytoid cells, macrophages, neutrophils, and eosinophils
  - The previous cell types are also involved in mediating bile duct damage and endotheliitis

Special Stains and Immunohistochemistry

- Noncontributory

Other Techniques for Diagnosis

- Noncontributory

Differential Diagnosis

RECURRENT HCV

- Typical portal infiltrate in recurrent chronic HCV rarely seen within first month after transplantation
- Endotheliitis usually milder
- Lymphocytic cholangitis usually milder and more localized

POST-TRANSPLANTATION LYMPHOPROLIFERATIVE DISEASE

- Immunohistochemistry of the lymphoid infiltrate demonstrates a clonal population that expresses EBV-associated proteins
- In situ hybridization demonstrates EBV nucleic acids

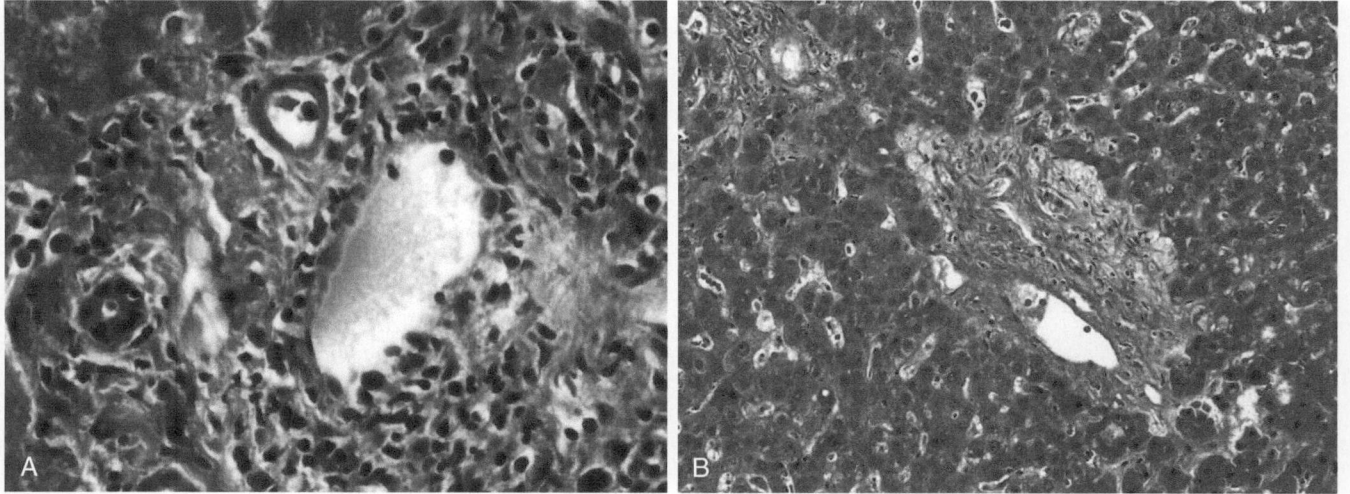

Figure 7-11. A, Acute cellular rejection. Portal inflammation, endotheliitis, and lymphocytic cholangitis. **B,** Chronic rejection. Loss of interlobular bile ducts in the portal tract.

CHRONIC (DUCTOPENIC) REJECTION IN ALLOGRAFT

- Loss of interlobular bile ducts (Figure 7-11B)
- Obliterative foam-cell arteriopathy with intimal aggregates of lipid-laden foamy macrophages in large and medium-sized arteries
- Centrilobular necrosis is a common finding

Special Stains and Immunohistochemistry

- CK7 for staining bile ductal epithelium
- PAS with diastase to stain basement membrane of the bile duct

Other Techniques for Diagnosis

- Noncontributory

Differential Diagnosis

RECURRENT PSC

- Periductal fibrosis present
- Typical ERCP finding
- Portal and periportal fibrosis

RECURRENT PBC

- Florid duct lesion
- Portal inflammation
- Portal and periportal fibrosis

PEARLS

- *A definitive diagnosis of ductopenic rejection is established with a formal count of at least 20 portal tracts showing loss of interlobular bile ducts from more than 50% of portal tracts (serial biopsies may be required to warrant adequate sampling and confident diagnosis)*
- *A diagnosis of rejection needs to be distinguished from other complications such as ischemia, biliary obstruction, infection, drug injury, and recurrent diseases*

SELECTED REFERENCES

Batts KP: Acute and chronic hepatic allograft rejection: pathology and classification. Liver Transpl Surg 5:S21-S29, 1999.

Demetris AJ, Batts KP, Dhillon AP, et al: Banff schema for grading liver allograft rejection: an international consensus document. Hepatology 25:658-663, 1997.

Hubscher SG, Portmann BC: Transplantation pathology. In Burt AD, Portmann BC, Ferrell LD (eds): MacSween's Pathology of the Liver, 5th ed. London, Churchill Livingstone, 2007, pp 815-880.

Jones KD, Ferrell LD: Interpretation of biopsy findings in the transplant liver. Semin Diagn Pathol 15:306-317, 1998.

CIRRHOSIS

Clinical Features

- Etiology: virtually all chronic liver diseases, including viral hepatitis, autoimmune hepatitis, alcoholic liver disease, nonalcoholic fatty liver disease, chronic biliary diseases, hemochromatosis, Wilson disease, α_1-antitrypsin deficiency, drugs, metabolic disorders, and cryptogenic disorders
- May be clinically silent
- Anorexia, weight loss, and weakness; ultimately debilitating
- Death due to progressive hepatic failure, complications of portal hypertension, or HCC

Gross Pathology

- Early: enlarged with or without greasy surface
- Late: shrunken with diffuse nodularity

Histopathology

- Diffuse nodules of regenerating hepatocytes surrounded by fibrous bands
- Arteries, bile ductules, and inflammatory infiltrate within fibrous septa
- Irregular ("jigsaw" pattern) nodules in biliary-type cirrhosis

Special Stains and Immunohistochemistry

- Trichrome: useful for determining the extent and pattern of fibrosis (Figure 7-12)
- Reticulin: useful for identifying thickened hepatic plates within regenerative nodules (two or three cell layers thick)

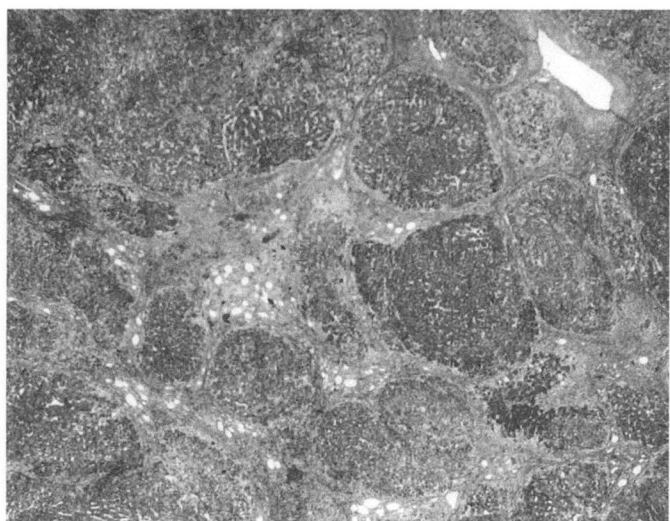

Figure 7-12. Cirrhosis. Nodular appearance of liver architecture surrounded by fibrous septa (trichrome stain).

Other Techniques for Diagnosis

- Noncontributory

Differential Diagnosis

- Distinguishing cirrhosis from other entities is important but may be sometimes challenging in a biopsy specimen because some histologic features may overlap

HIGH-GRADE DYSPLASTIC NODULES

- Plates more than two cells thick or areas of pseudoglandular formation may be seen
- Cytologic atypia with high nuclear-to-cytoplasmic ratio, hyperchromatic nuclei, irregular nuclear contour, and rare mitoses

HCC

- Nuclear atypia with increased nuclear-to-cytoplasmic ratio, hyperchromatic nuclei, and frequent mitotic activity
- Absence of portal tracts in the nodules
- Thick trabeculae or pseudoglandular formation and increased unpaired arteries may be seen

CONGENITAL HEPATIC FIBROSIS

- Large bands of collagen dividing liver into geographic areas
- Preservation of spatial relationships between vessels; therefore, not truly nodular
- Morphologically similar to biliary type cirrhosis
- Usually without inflammation or hepatocellular regeneration

NODULAR REGENERATIVE HYPERPLASIA

- Generalized or multiple hyperplastic parenchymal nodules without significant fibrosis
- Associated with myeloproliferative disorders, rheumatic diseases, chronic venous congestion, and drugs such as corticosteroids and chemotherapeutic agents

FOCAL NODULAR HYPERPLASIA

- Focal, distinct hypervascular lesion on image study
- Central scar
- Thickened arteries within fibrous septa

SUBCAPSULAR FIBROSIS

- Fibrosis does not extend down into the liver parenchyma

PEARLS

- *World Health Organization definition: cirrhosis is a diffuse process characterized by fibrosis and the conversion of normal liver architecture into structurally abnormal nodules*
- *Cirrhosis is the end stage of myriad different liver diseases, and the etiology is not always apparent from histopathologic examination*

SELECTED REFERENCES

Geller SA, Petrovic LM: Cirrhosis, hepatic fibrosis, and noncirrhotic portal hypertension. In Geller SA, Petrovic LM (eds): Biopsy Interpretation of the Liver. Philadelphia, Lippincott Williams & Wilkins, 2004, pp 228-238.
Scheuer PJ, Lefkowitch JH: Cirrhosis. In Scheuer PJ, Lefkowitch JH (eds): Liver Biopsy Interpretation. London, WB Saunders, 2000, pp 173-190.

FOCAL NODULAR HYPERPLASIA

Clinical Features

- Most common in women in third to fifth decades
- Can occur in both genders and any age group, including childhood
- Female-to-male ratio: adults, 2:1; children, 4:1
- Usually found incidentally at surgery or during image studies for unrelated symptoms
- Distinctive hypervascularity by arteriography
- Liver function tests usually normal
- Oral contraceptive use not an apparent etiologic factor

Gross Pathology

- Well-circumscribed but not encapsulated
- Lighter color than adjacent liver
- Often subcapsular
- Any size, but usually less than 5 cm in diameter
- Characteristic central stellate scar

Histopathology

- Nodules of hepatocytes with large central stellate scar (Figure 7-13A)
- Hepatocytes adjacent to the fibrous septa may show chronic cholestatic changes
- All components of normal liver lobule present (i.e., central veins and portal triads)
- Fibrous septa contain thickened vessels, numerous bile ductules, and varying degree of inflammatory cell infiltration
- Pseudoxanthomatous change (chronic cholestasis) adjacent to the fibrous septa

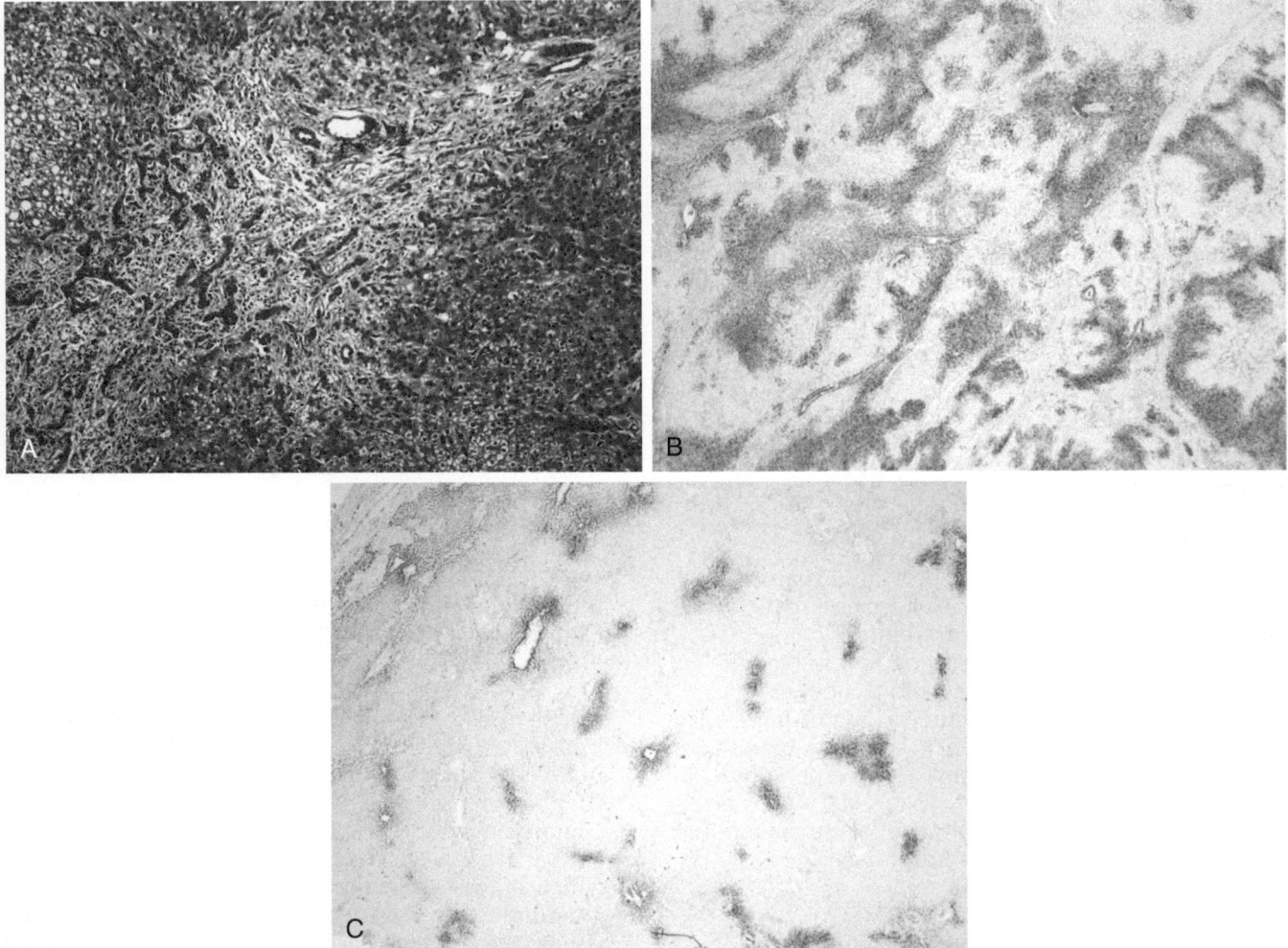

Figure 7-13. Focal nodular hyperplasia. A, Nodules of hepatocytes with large central stellate scar. Fibrous septa contain thickened vessels, numerous bile ductules, and a varying degree of inflammatory cell infiltration. **B,** Glutamine synthetase stain shows maplike pattern in focal nodular hyperplasia, **C,** Glutamine synthetase stain shows perivenular staining pattern in adjacent liver.

Special Stains and Immunohistochemistry

- Rhodanine stain to demonstrate accumulation of copper or Victoria blue stain to demonstrate copper-binding protein
- Glutamine synthetase immunohistochemical stain to demonstrate a maplike pattern of hepatocyte reactivity (Figure 7-13B and C)

Other Techniques for Diagnosis

- Noncontributory

Differential Diagnosis

HEPATIC ADENOMA

- No apparent fibrous septa
- Lack portal tracts
- No central scar
- Frequently see areas of infarction or hemorrhage
- Most occur in women; associated with oral contraceptive use
- Glutamine synthetase immunohistochemical stain to demonstrate perivenular hepatocyte staining without the maplike pattern

NODULAR REGENERATIVE HYPERPLASIA

- Diffuse process involving the entire liver
- No fibrous septa or central scar
- Clinically associated with a wide variety of extrahepatic disorders or medication

WELL-DIFFERENTIATED HCC

- Cells arranged in sheets or plates without portal tracts

CIRRHOSIS

- Generalized regenerative nodules surrounded by fibrous bands
- Arising in the background of underlying liver disease

PEARLS

- *Most characteristic features include central stellate scar, broad septa containing proliferating bile ducts, and the presence of all components of normal liver lobule*
- *Maplike immunostaining pattern of glutamine synthetase in hepatocytes*

SELECTED REFERENCES

Bioulac-Sage P, Cubel G, Taouji S, et al: Immunohistochemical markers on needle biopsies are helpful for the diagnosis of focal nodular hyperplasia and hepatocellular adenoma subtypes. Am J Surg Pathol 36:1691-1699, 2012.

Bioulac-Sage P, Laumonier H, Rullier A, et al: Over-expression of glutamine synthetase in focal nodular hyperplasia: a novel easy diagnostic tool in surgical pathology. Liver Int 29:459-465, 2009.

Ishak KG, Goodman ZD, Stocker JT: Benign hepatocellular tumors. In Atlas of Tumor Pathology, 3rd series, Fascicle 31. Washington, DC, Armed Forces Institute of Pathology, 2001, pp 9-48.

Makhlouf HR, Abdul-Al HM, Goodman ZD: Diagnosis of focal nodular hyperplasia of the liver by needle biopsy. Hum Pathol 36:1210-1216, 2005.

Nguyen BN, Flejou JF, Terris B, et al: Focal nodular hyperplasia of the liver: a comprehensive pathologic study of 305 lesions and recognitions of new histologic forms. Am J Surg Pathol 23:1441-1454, 1999.

HEPATIC ADENOMA

Clinical Features

- Characteristically affects women of child-bearing age
- Related to oral contraceptive use; decreasing incidence related to use of low-dose contraception
- Liver function tests usually within reference range
- Recognized risk factors: obesity and alcohol use
- Large tumors at risk for rupture or hemorrhage, may present as abdominal emergency
- Malignant transformation may occur, especially in β-catenin activated type
- Symptoms include epigastric and acute abdominal pain, the latter associated with rupture

Gross Pathology

- Any size; may measure up to 30 cm in diameter
- Usually solitary, well-defined, partially encapsulated, bulging mass
- Often subcapsular
- Multiple lesions may occur; > 10 adenomas indicates adenomatosis
- Different color from surrounding liver (yellow to tan or brown)
- Areas of necrosis or hemorrhage common

Histopathology

- Tightly packed, well-differentiated, glycogen-rich hepatocytes with abundant eosinophilic cytoplasm (Figure 7-14)
- No portal tracts
- Unpaired arteries
- Hepatocellular plates not thickened and pseudoglandular structures are rare

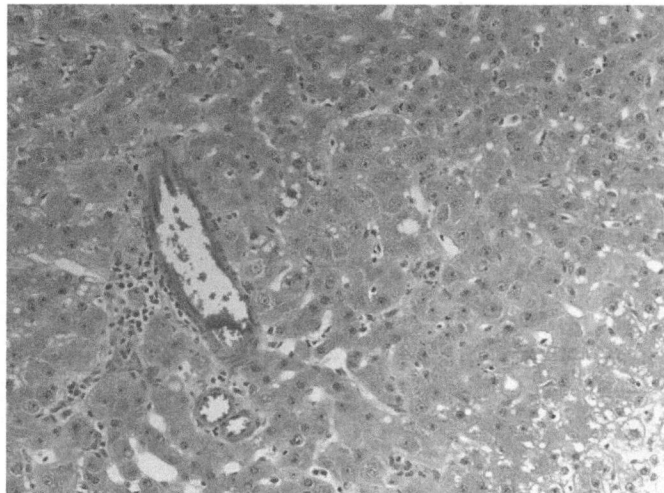

Figure 7-14. Hepatocytic adenoma. Proliferation of uniform liver cells characteristically lacking portal tracts.

- Intracellular and canalicular bile may be seen
- Fatty change often conspicuous
- Mitoses rare

Special Stains and Immunohistochemistry

- Hepatocyte antigen in paraffin (HepPar-1) and Arginase-1 positive
- Glypican-3 negative
- Glutamine synthetase stain shows perivenular staining pattern (except in the β-catenin activated subtype, which shows diffuse positivity; discussed later)
- β-catenin stain negative (membranous staining, unless in the β-catenin activated subtype, which shows nuclear staining)
- Current classification of hepatocytic adenoma (HCA) based on immunohistochemistry (Table 7-1)
- Occasional cases with "capillarization" of sinusoids (CD34 positivity similar to HCC)

Other Techniques for Diagnosis

- Noncontributory

Differential Diagnosis

FOCAL NODULAR HYPERPLASIA

- Central stellate scar
- Portal tracts and central veins present
- Bile ducts in fibrous septa; bile ductular reaction pattern often prominent
- Glutamine synthetase immunostain shows "maplike" staining pattern

TABLE 7-1	**CURRENT CLASSIFICATION OF HEPATIC ADENOMAS**			
	H-HCA	**B-HCA**	**I-HCA**	**Unclassified**
LFABP	− (loss of staining)	+	+	+
Glutamine synthetase	−	+ (diffuse staining)	−	−
β-catenin (nuclear expression)	−	+	−/+	−
SAA/CRP	−	−	+	−

H-HCA: HNF 1α-mutated HCA; B-HCA: β-Catenin activated HCA; I-HCA: Inflammatory HCA; LFABP: liver fatty acid binding protein; SAA: serum amyloid A; CRP: C reactive protein.

NODULAR REGENERATIVE HYPERPLASIA

- Diffuse process
- Portal tracts still present
- No gender predilection
- Clinically associated with a wide variety of extrahepatic disorders or medication history

WELL-DIFFERENTIATED HCC

- Underlying liver diseases and cirrhosis common
- Not female predominant

PEARLS

- *Focal process with absence of normal portal elements*
- *Composed of normal-appearing hepatocytes*
- *Difficult to separate from low-grade HCC in a needle biopsy*
- *Never occurs in cirrhosis (by convention); similar lesions in cirrhosis classified as low-grade dysplasia (macroregenerative nodule)*

SELECTED REFERENCES

Bioulac-Sage P, Cubel G, Taouji S, et al. Immunohistochemical markers on needle biopsies are helpful for the diagnosis of focal nodular hyperplasia and hepatocellular adenoma subtypes. Am J Surg Pathol 36:1691-1699, 2012.

DeCarlis L, Pirotta V, Rondinara GF, et al: Hepatic adenoma and focal nodular hyperplasia: diagnosis and criteria for treatment. Liver Transpl Surg 3:160-165, 1997.

Goodman ZD, Mikel W, Lubbers PR, et al: Kupffer cells in hepatocellular adenomas. Am J Surg Pathol 11:191-196, 1987.

Resnick MB, Kozakewich HP, Perez-Atayde AR: Hepatic adenoma in the pediatric age group: clinicopathological observations and assessment of cell proliferative activity. Am J Surg Pathol 19:1181-1190, 1995.

HEPATOCELLULAR CARCINOMA

Clinical Features

- Common carcinoma worldwide (eighth overall in women; fifth in men); strongly correlated with relative incidence of hepatitis B
- Most common primary hepatic malignancy in adults
- Most patients in Western countries are older than 50 years
- Fibrolamellar variant typically occurs in patients younger than 30 years
- Male-to-female ratio about 4:1
- Patients often present with abdominal pain, ascites, or hepatomegaly; early disease typically asymptomatic
- Elevated serum α-fetoprotein (AFP) in 60% to 80% of cases
- Serum AFP more than 100 times normal is diagnostic if malignant germ cell neoplasm is excluded
- Numerous associated risk factors, including cirrhosis, HBV (especially *Hbx* gene product) and HCV, fatty liver disease, alcohol, obesity, diabetes, hemochromatosis, progestational agents, anabolic steroids, aflatoxins, hepatocytic adenoma, ataxia-telangiectasia, α_1-antitrypsin deficiency, tyrosinemia, schistosomiasis
- DNA ploidy abnormalities (especially 8p loss of heterozygosity [LOH]); microsatellite instability, altered β-catenin expression, dysplasia, increases in transforming growth factor-α (TGF-α) and AFP expression, and increased proliferative activity often precede malignant transformation

Gross Pathology

- Soft, yellow-green or reddish nodules
- Highly variable in size
- Solitary, multinodular, and diffuse types
- Increasing numbers of small carcinomas (lesions < 3 cm) detected as a result of advances in diagnostic imaging techniques or examination of liver explants
- Advanced cases often associated with portal vein invasion or metastasis at diagnosis

Histopathology

- Three classic patterns: trabecular, acinar, and solid
  - Trabecular
    - Neoplastic hepatocytic cords greater than three cells thick lined by flat endothelial cells and lacking Kupffer cells
  - Acinar
    - Results from central degeneration of otherwise solid trabeculae eventually replaced by pseudoglandular spaces containing colloid-like material or bile
    - May also represent dilated canaliculi
  - Solid
    - Results from compression artifact or scarring; least common of three patterns
- Bile production by tumor cells is pathognomonic
- Neoplastic cells are variable in size, although typically large and polygonal, with central vesicular nuclei and prominent nucleoli (Figure 7-15A)
- Cytoplasmic and nuclear inclusions of different types are common; intranuclear inclusions are typically eosinophilic
- Highly pleomorphic cells with bizarre nuclei may occupy large areas
- Clear cells may predominate
- Carcinoma cell cords and clusters are surrounded by a network of sinusoidal vessels (Figure 7-15B)
- Bile canaliculi are present (grade dependent)
- Grading is based on degree of resemblance to normal liver
- Adjacent liver is commonly cirrhotic
- Fibrolamellar variant (distinctive histology)
  - Shows a prominent lamellar fibrous stroma (Figure 7-15C)
  - Composed of oncocytic-appearing malignant hepatocytes
  - Abundant and granular cytoplasm with prominent nucleoli
  - Pale bodies (fibrinogen materials) may be present in the cytoplasm
  - Calcification may be present within the tumor
  - Occurs in a noncirrhotic liver without underlying liver diseases
  - Almost always positive for CD68 in the cytoplasm
- Mixed HCC and cholangiocarcinoma (combined HCC-cholangiocarcinoma) are uncommon; requires elements of HCC and cholangiocarcinoma (see also "Special Stains and Immunohistochemistry")

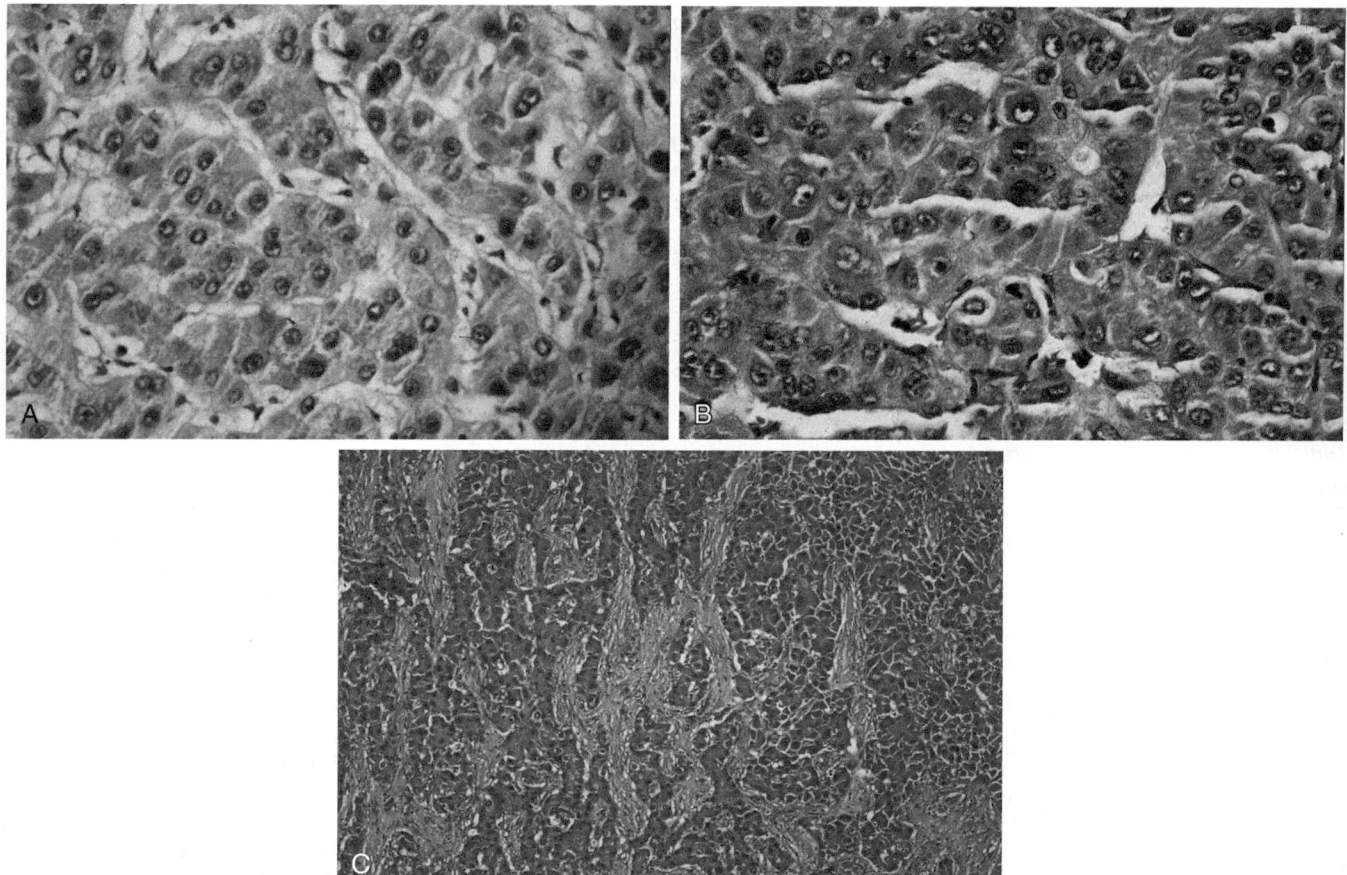

Figure 7-15. Hepatocellular carcinoma. A, Well-differentiated. Neoplastic liver cells with large nuclei, prominent nucleoli and fine granular cytoplasm arranged in a trabecular pattern. **B,** Poorly-differentiated. Note greater variation in cord size and nuclear size. **C,** Fibrolamellar type. Prominent fibrosis arranged in lamellar fashion around the neoplastic hepatocytes.

Special Stains and Immunohistochemistry

- AFP highly specific but insensitive (< 25% of cases positive)
- HepPar-1 (a urea cycle mitochondrial enzyme) highly sensitive for normal and neoplastic hepatocytes; specific in the proper histologic context, although metaplastic and neoplastic intestinal cells may also be positive
- Arginase (a manganese metalloenzyme active in the urea cycle): a recently developed immunohistochemical marker of hepatocytes and hepatocellular neoplasms, highly specific for hepatocyte differentiation, but cannot distinguish hepatocellular carcinoma from benign hepatocytic lesions
- Selected antithyroid transcription factor-1 (anti–TTF-1) antibodies label cytoplasm/mitochondria (not nucleus) of normal and neoplastic hepatocytes due to common epitope in TTF-1 on a novel mitochondrial peptide
- Glypican-3 may distinguish between non-neoplastic and neoplastic hepatocytes
- Low-molecular-weight keratins (keratins 8 and 18) positive, often with accentuation of subplasmalemmal cytoplasm
- Glutamine synthetase stain may show diffuse staining
- Keratin 7 occasionally positive
- Keratin 19, a biliary/hepatic progenitor cell marker, is expressed in a subset of HCC with poor prognosis

- Epithelial membrane antigen (EMA) typically negative, except in mixed HCC and cholangiocarcinoma; similar result with mucicarmine stains
- Polyclonal carcinoembryonic antigen (CEA) labels a non-CEA bile moiety; accentuates canaliculi; similar result with antibodies to CD10, multidrug-resistant p-glycoprotein, and occasionally villin
- Sinusoids often CD34 positive (so-called capillarization of sinusoids)
- Monoclonal CEA typically negative

Other Techniques for Diagnosis

- Electron microscopy: demonstration of bile canaliculi is pathognomonic of hepatocellular differentiation, but not HCC
  - Bile canaliculi show stubby microvilli and cell junctions of tight and intermediate types
  - Tumor cells resemble normal adult hepatocytes; typically numerous mitochondria, abundant electron-dense glycogen particles, and intracytoplasmic bile products
- Flow cytometry: aneuploidy correlates with higher grade but is also seen in dysplasia and is therefore not diagnostic of malignancy

Differential Diagnosis

- In general, HCC resembles normal liver in its platelike growth and cytology

Macroregenerative Nodule in Cirrhosis

- Presence of bile duct epithelial cells and chronic inflammation
- Absence of trabecular pattern
- Absence of significant cytologic atypia

High-Grade Dysplasia in Cirrhosis

- Disordered lobular architecture, but generally three or fewer cells in cords
- Focally prominent nuclear atypia
- Retention of portal elements
- Ki-67 proliferative index intermediate between cirrhosis and carcinoma
- TGF-α expression intermediate between cirrhosis and carcinoma

Cholangiocarcinoma

- Absence of bile production
- Glandular differentiation; positive for CEA and mucicarmine
- Positive for EMA; negative for HepPar-1 and glypican-3
- Keratin 19 typically present; keratins 8 and 18 (CAM 5.2) positive
- Villin in brush-border pattern
- Focal or variable CDX2 immunoreactivity

Focal Nodular Hyperplasia

- Liver cell plates less than three cells thick
- Cells have a normal nuclear-to-cytoplasmic ratio
- Absence of mitotic activity
- Central stellate scar
- Retention of portal elements; bile ductular reaction
- Glutamine synthetase stain shows maplike pattern

Hepatic Adenoma

- Liver cell plates less than three cells thick
- Slightly increased nuclear-to-cytoplasmic ratio, but no bizarre nuclei
- Absent or rare typical mitotic figures
- Glutamine synthetase stain shows the normal perivenular staining pattern

Hepatoblastoma

- Typically seen in young children
- Small polygonal or round cells; may resemble fetal liver
- Macrotrabecular pattern uncommon; closest resemblance to HCC
- Strong AFP immunoreactivity

Metastatic Endocrine Carcinoma

- Cords and ribbons mimic low-grade HCC
- Low-grade lesions have uniform round to oval nuclei
- Mitotic activity variable
- Granular cytoplasm typically positive for synaptophysin or CD56; may be chromogranin positive or positive for organ-specific endocrine peptides

Metastatic Nonendocrine Neoplasms

- Sharply demarcated from adjacent liver; often with hyperemic rim
- Uninvolved liver is typically normal (noncirrhotic)
- Selected immunoprofile compatible with specific lineage (remember melanoma); metastatic carcinoma often resembles primary cholangiocarcinoma

PEARLS

- *Extremely helpful features: platelike growth of tumor cells separated by vascular sinusoids and bile production*
- *Reactivity for HepPar-1 or arginase characteristic*
- *Stage is most important prognostic determinant*

Selected References

Brechot C: Pathogenesis of hepatitis B-virus-related hepatocellular carcinoma: old and new paradigms. Gastroenterology 127(suppl 1):556-561, 2004.

Durnez A, Verslype C, Nevens F, et al: The clinicopathological and prognostic relevance of cytokeratin 7 and 19 expression in hepatocellular carcinoma: a possible progenitor cell origin. Histopathology 49:138-151, 2006.

Govaere O, Komuta M, Berkers J, et al: Keratin 19: a key role player in the invasion of human hepatocellular carcinomas. Gut 2013, doi: 10.1136/gutjnl-2012-304351 [Epub ahead of print].

Pang Y, von Turkovich M, Wu H, et al: The binding of thyroid transcription factor 1 and hepatocyte paraffin 1 to mitochondrial proteins in hepatocytes: a molecular and immunoelectron microscopic study. Am J Clin Pathol 125:722-726, 2006.

Yan BC, Gong C, Song J, et al: Arginase-1: a new immunohistochemical marker of hepatocytes and hepatocellular neoplasms. Am J Surg Pathol 34:1147-1154, 2010.

Yeh MM, Larson AM, Campbell JS, et al: The expression of transforming growth factor-alpha in cirrhosis, dysplastic nodules, and hepatocellular carcinoma: an immunohistochemical study of 70 cases. Am J Surg Pathol 31:681-689, 2007.

HEPATOBLASTOMA

Clinical Features

- Most common liver neoplasm in children
- Occurs almost exclusively in infants
- About one third are associated with a variety of congenital anomalies, syndromes, or other childhood tumors: Beckwith-Wiedemann syndrome and familial adenomatous polyposis
- Serum AFP is often elevated
- Patients may present with virilization; result of ectopic sex hormone production
- Uncommon presentation: sexual precocity in boys with elevated serum and urine human chorionic gonadotropin (HCG)

Gross Pathology

- Solitary, unencapsulated, often large mass measuring up to 25 cm in diameter
- Variegated cut surface with areas of necrosis, cystic changes, and hemorrhage
- Normal surrounding liver

Histopathology

- Two types: epithelial (75%) and mixed epithelial and mesenchymal (25%)

Epithelial Type

- Components are *fetal* and *embryonal*, both invariably present in varying proportions and often intermingled
  - Fetal component
    - Fetal-type cells are polygonal and large with round to oval nuclei and with single nucleoli and clear or granular cytoplasm
    - Cells are organized into irregular plates with bile canaliculi and sinusoids
    - Commonly associated with extramedullary hematopoiesis

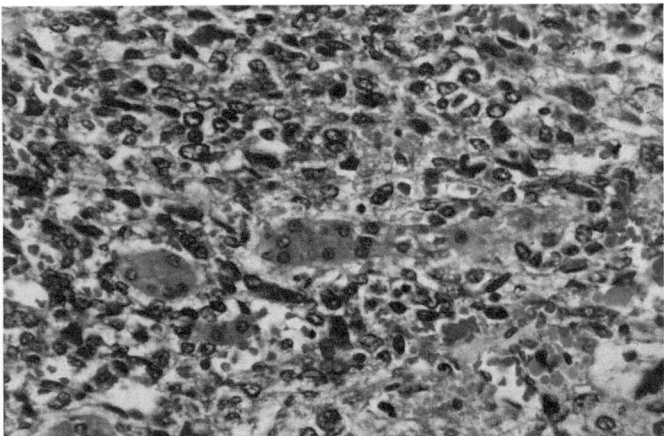

Figure 7-16. Hepatoblastoma. Tumor is composed of spindle cells with an embryonal appearance. Notice entrapped hepatocytes in the center of the photomicrograph.

- Embryonal component
  - Embryonal-type cells are smaller and elongated with hyperchromatic nuclei and scant cytoplasm (Figure 7-16)
  - Predominantly solid pattern with rosette-like clusters, cords, ribbons, and rarely tubules
- Variants of epithelial: anaplastic small cell and macrotrabecular
  - Anaplastic small cells arranged in sheets; histologically similar to neuroblastoma
  - Macrotrabecular component resembles HCC
- Intestinal-type glandular elements and areas of squamous metaplasia (often highly keratinized) uncommon
- Multinucleated giant cells may be associated with hormone production

MIXED EPITHELIAL AND MESENCHYMAL TYPE
- Fetal and embryonal epithelium component admixed with mesenchymal elements
- Mesenchymal component is usually osteoid, cartilage, or undifferentiated spindled cells
- Osteoid areas are typically keratin positive (metaplastic, not true mesenchyme)
- Other elements, such as striated muscle, and neural tissue, are rarely seen

Special Stains and Immunohistochemistry
- Keratin low molecular weight (keratins 8 and 18) and pan-keratin typically positive
- EMA typically positive
- HepPar-1 and glypican-3 positive
- AFP positive in fetal and embryonal cells
- Neuron-specific enolase (NSE), S-100 protein, and chromogranin often positive
- Bcl-2 variably positive

Other Techniques for Diagnosis
- Electron microscopy: immature hepatocytes in epithelial areas
- Flow cytometry: fetal type shows diploid DNA content; embryonal and anaplastic small cell are aneuploid in 50% of cases
- Cytogenetics
  - Complex karyotypes with gains of chromosomes 2 and X

- 11p15 LOH in Beckwith-Wiedemann syndrome
- Trisomy 2q and 20
- *Wnt* signaling pathway abnormalities (β-catenin and adenomatous polyposis coli [APC] mutations)
- Rarely *TP53* mutations

Differential Diagnosis

METASTATIC PRIMITIVE TUMOR OF INFANCY (NEPHROBLASTOMA AND NEUROBLASTOMA)
- Clinical history (i.e., evidence of primary) is essential
- Immunohistochemical stains may be of value in proper histologic context
  - WT-1 in nephroblastoma; keratin variable
  - Endocrine markers in the absence of keratin in neuroblastoma

HCC OF CHILDHOOD
- Generally resembles normal adult liver with platelike growth of tumor cells separated by CD34-positive vascular sinusoids
- Bile production by tumor cells

PEARLS

- *Hepatoblastoma is thought to arise from a multipotential blastema*
- *Poor prognostic indicators include age less than 1 year, large size, involvement of vital structures, predominance of anaplastic small cells or macrotrabeculae, and aneuploidy*

SELECTED REFERENCES

Chan ES, Pawel BR, Corao DA, et al: Immunohistochemical expression of glypican-3 in pediatric tumors: an analysis of 414 cases. Pediatr Dev Pathol 16:272-277, 2013.
Douglass EC: Hepatic malignancies in childhood and adolescence (hepatoblastoma, hepatocellular carcinoma, and embryonal sarcoma). Cancer Treat Res 92:201-212, 1997.
Raney B: Hepatoblastoma in children: a review. J Pediatr Hematol Oncol 19:418-422, 1997.
Schnater JM, Kohler SE, Lamers WH, et al: Where do we stand with hepatoblastoma? A review. Cancer 98:668-678, 2003.
Zynger DL, Gupta A, Luan C, et al: Expression of glypican 3 in hepatoblastoma: an immunohistochemical study of 65 cases. Hum Pathol 39:224-230, 2008.

BILE DUCT HAMARTOMA (Von MEYENBURG COMPLEX)

Clinical Features
- Usually incidental finding at surgery or autopsy
- Part of a spectrum of ductal plate malformations of the liver
- Often associated with polycystic liver or kidney disease

Gross Features
- Multiple white nodules up to several millimeters in diameter scattered throughout the liver
- Grossly mimics metastatic tumor

Histopathology
- Focal, well-demarcated lesions composed of a variable number of ductal structures embedded in a hyalinized stroma (Figure 7-17)

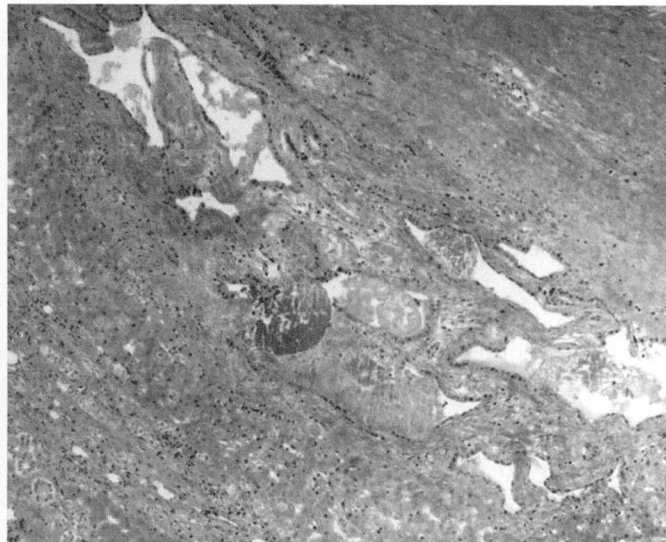

Figure 7-17. Bile duct hamartoma. Variable number of ductal structures embedded in a hyalinized stroma. The ductal structures are variably dilated and may have microcystic dilation with bile in the ductal lumens. The ductal lumens are lined by a flattened or cuboidal epithelium.

- Ductal structures are variably dilated and may have bile in the ductal lumens
- Ductal lumens are lined by a flattened or cuboidal epithelium
- No cytologic atypia

Special Stains and Immunohistochemistry

- Positive for CK7, CK19

Other Techniques for Diagnosis

- Noncontributory

Differential Diagnosis

PERIBILIARY GLAND HAMARTOMA (BILE DUCT ADENOMA)

- Usually single
- Composed of small tubular structures with no dilatation or bile

MESENCHYMAL HAMARTOMA

- Usually solitary
- Prominent myxoid stroma
- Contains hepatocyte islands
- Bile rarely present within the ducts

WELL-DIFFERENTIATED CARCINOMA (METASTATIC OR CHOLANGIOCARCINOMA)

- Histologically and cytologically malignant
- Clinical history important

PEARLS

- *A result of bile ductal plate malformation*
- *Often associated with polycystic liver or kidney disease*
- *Usually incidental finding*

SELECTED REFERENCES

Goodman ZD, Terracciano LM: Tumours and tumour-like lesions of the liver. In Burt AD, Portmann BC, Ferrel LD (eds): MacSween's Pathology of the Liver, 5th ed. London, Churchill Livingstone, 2007, pp 761-814.
Ishak KG, Goodman ZD, Stocker JT: Benign cholangiocellular tumors. In Atlas of Tumor Pathology, 3rd series, Fascicle 31. Washington, DC, Armed Forces Institute of Pathology, 2001, pp 49-70.

PERIBILIARY GLAND HAMARTOMA (BILE DUCT ADENOMA)

Clinical Features

- Usually asymptomatic and found incidentally at intra-abdominal surgery or autopsy
- Benign behavior

Gross Pathology

- Solitary, round or ovoid, well-demarcated but unencapsulated tumors, usually less than 1 cm in size
- Gray, white, yellow to tan in color, and firm in consistency

Histopathology

- Small tubules and acini with slight branching and tortuosity

PROLIFERATION OF PACKED UNIFORM TUBULAR STRUCTURE (FIGURE 7-18)

- Minimal luminal dilation and no cystic changes
- Tubules lined by single layer of cuboidal to columnar cells
- No bile in lumens
- May contain intracytoplasmic mucin
- No communication between tubular structures and interlobular bile ducts
- Fibrous stroma, which may be cellular or hyalinized
- Normally spaced portal tracts often present

Special Stains and Immunohistochemistry

- Positive for CK7, CK19

Other Techniques for Diagnosis

- Noncontributory

Differential Diagnosis

BILE DUCT HAMARTOMA

- Typically multiple

MESENCHYMAL HAMARTOMA

- Primarily found in infants
- Often cystic

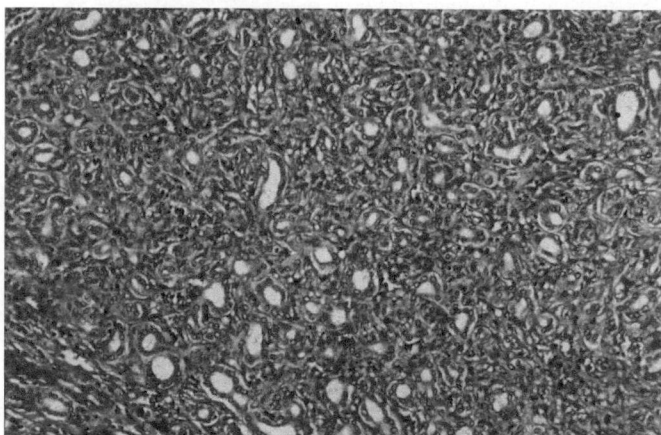

Figure 7-18. Peribiliary gland hamartoma (bile duct adenoma).

- Myxoid stroma
- Contains cords of hepatocytes

WELL-DIFFERENTIATED CARCINOMA (METASTATIC OR CHOLANGIOCARCINOMA)
- Variably pleomorphic cells within single gland
- Increased nuclear-to-cytoplasmic ratio

PEARLS

- *Hamartoma of peribiliary glands (small accessory glands of the major bile ducts)*
- *Not associated with dysplasia or malignancy*

SELECTED REFERENCES

Allaire GS, Rabin L, Ishak KG, et al: Bile duct adenoma: a study of 152 cases. Am J Surg Pathol 12:708-715, 1988.

Bhathal PS, Hughes NR, Goodman ZD: The so-called bile duct adenoma is a peribiliary gland hamartoma. Am J Surg Pathol 20:858-864, 1996.

Goodman ZD, Terracciano LM: Tumours and tumour-like lesions of the liver. In Burt AD, Portman BC, Ferrell LD (eds): MacSween's Pathology of the Liver, 5th ed. London, Churchill Livingstone, 2007, pp 761-814.

MUCINOUS CYSTIC NEOPLASM

Clinical Features
- Relatively rare neoplasm
- Almost exclusively a neoplasm of women
- Predominantly arises within the liver but may arise in the extrahepatic biliary tree, including the gallbladder

Gross Pathology
- Solitary and multilocular cystic neoplasm containing mucinous or clear fluid
- Multiple lobules of varying size
- Inner lining smooth, glistening, trabecular, or with papillary excrescences

Histopathology
- Lined by single layer of tall columnar cells that focally may become cuboidal, flattened, or even papillary (Figure 7-19A)
- Almost always mucinous
- Intestinal metaplasia with goblet cells can be present

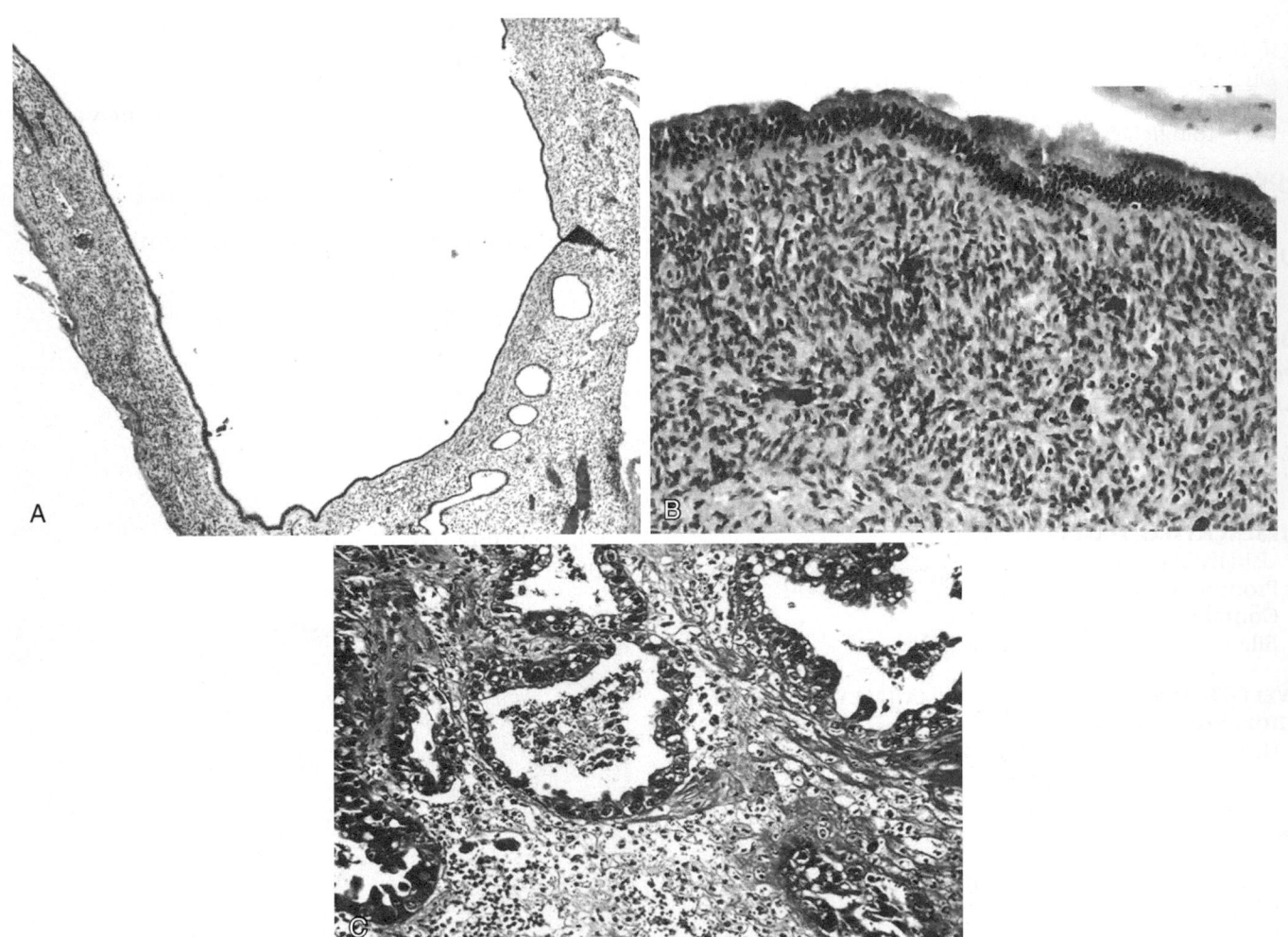

Figure 7-19. A, Biliary cystadenoma. The cyst is lined by a layer of tall columnar epithelium that focally may become cuboidal or flattened. **B,** Biliary cystadenoma. High-power photomicrograph showing the columnar epithelium resembling biliary epithelium with cytoplasmic mucin and an underlying ovarian-like stroma. **C,** Cystadenocarcinoma. Notice the stratification of the epithelium, and stromal invasion. *(Courtesy of Dr. Zachary Goodman, Armed Forces Institute of Pathology, Washington, DC.)*

- Ovarian-like stroma is a feature that mucinous cystic neoplasm in the liver shares with mucinous cystic neoplasm in the pancreas (Figure 7-19B)
- Ovarian-like stroma is exclusively present in women
- Varying degrees of dysplasia in the cystic epithelium may be seen
- Low-grade dysplasia (adenoma)
- Intermediate-grade dysplasia (borderline)
- High-grade dysplasia (carcinoma in situ), can develop into invasive cystadenocarcinoma

CYSTADENOCARCINOMA

- Most arise from preexisting mucinous cystic neoplasm
- Often show ovarian-type stroma in women
- Cytologic atypia, mitosis, and invasion of underlying stroma (Figure 7-19C)

Special Stains and Immunohistochemistry

- Keratin (7 and 19) and CEA: epithelial lining is positive
- Mucicarmine and Alcian blue: may demonstrate cytoplasmic mucin in epithelial cells
- Vimentin, smooth muscle actin (SMA), inhibin, estrogen receptor, and progesterone receptor: stromal component is positive

Other Techniques for Diagnosis

- Noncontributory

Differential Diagnosis

DEVELOPMENTAL CYSTS

- Unilocular
- No nuclear atypia

INTRADUCTAL PAPILLARY NEOPLASM OF THE BILE DUCT

- No ovarian-type stroma
- Also affects men
- Communicating with bile ducts

PEARLS

- *Characteristic underlying ovarian-like stroma*

SELECTED REFERENCES

Devaney K, Goodman ZD, Ishak KG: Hepatobiliary cystadenoma and cystadenocarcinoma: a light microscopic and immunohistochemical study of 70 patients. Am J Surg Pathol 18:1078-1091, 1994.
Weihing RR, Shintaku IP, Geller SA, Petrovic LM: Hepatobiliary and pancreatic mucinous cystadenocarcinomas with mesenchymal stroma: analysis of estrogen receptors/progesterone receptors and expression of tumor-associated antigens. Mod Pathol 10:372-379, 1997.
Wheeler DA, Edmondson HA: Cystadenoma with mesenchymal stroma (CMS) in the liver and bile ducts: a clinicopathologic study of 17 cases, 4 with malignant change. Cancer 56:1434-1445, 1985.

INTRADUCTAL PAPILLARY NEOPLASM OF THE BILE DUCT (IPNB)

Clinical Features

- Uncommon papillary neoplasm of the biliary tree
- May be solitary or may spread extensively along the biliary tree within or outside of the liver, including the gallbladder
- A biliary counterpart of intraductal papillary mucinous neoplasm (IPMN) in the pancreas
- Symptoms of biliary obstruction
- Curative resection difficult with frequent recurrence

Gross Pathology

- Dilated bile ducts with polypoid excrescences
- May contain inspissated mucus

Histopathology

- The involved bile ducts are dilated, containing papillary growth of columnar epithelial cells overlying fibrovascular stalks (Figure 7-20A)
- Lining epithelial cells may mimic biliary epithelium or show gastric or intestinal metaplasia (Figure 7-20B)
- Mucin production may be present
- Lining epithelial cells may show varying degrees of dysplasia and may progress to invasive carcinoma
- Low-grade intraepithelial neoplasia (adenoma)
- Intermediate grade intraepithelial neoplasia (borderline)

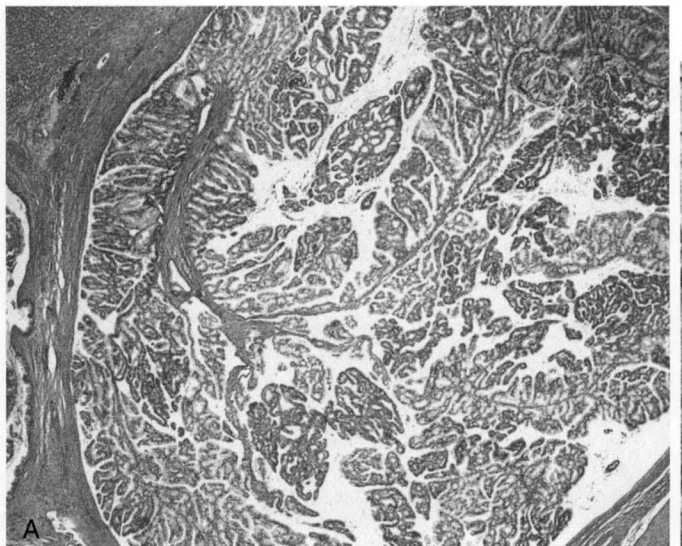
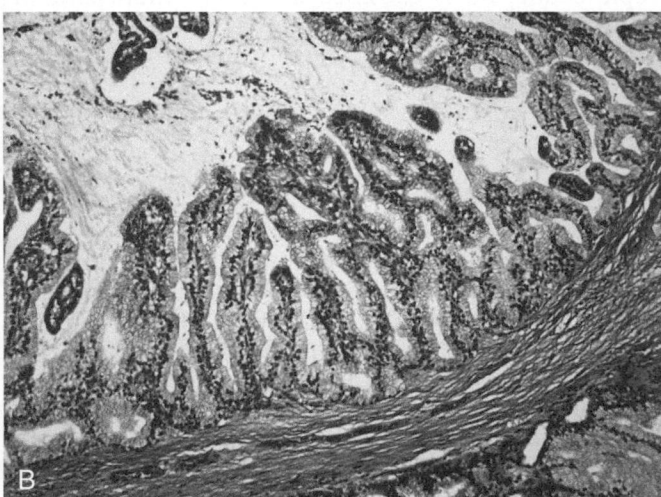

Figure 7-20. Biliary papillomatosis. A, The bile duct is dilated and filled with papillary outgrowth of epithelium. **B,** Higher power shows the lining epithelial cells with mucin production.

- High-grade intraepithelial neoplasia (carcinoma in situ)
- Malignant lesion: IPNB with an associated invasive carcinoma

Special Stains and Immunohistochemistry

- Lining cells positive for CK7, CK19

Other Techniques for Diagnosis

- Noncontributory

Differential Diagnosis

MUCINOUS CYSTIC NEOPLASM

- Ovarian-type stroma
- Almost exclusively occurs in women
- No communication with bile duct

PEARLS

- *Clinicopathologic features are similar to those of IPMN of the pancreas*
- *Geographic predilection; most large series reported in East Asia, where hepatolithiasis and clonorchiasis infestation are common*

SELECTED REFERENCES

Goodman ZD, Terracciano LM: Tumours and tumour-like lesions of the liver. In Burt AD, Portmann BC, Ferrell LD (eds): MacSween's Pathology of the Liver, 5th ed. London, Churchill Livingstone, 2007, pp 761-814.

Nakanuma Y, Sasaki M, Ishikawa A, et al: Biliary papillary neoplasm of the liver. Histol Histopathol 17:851-861, 2002.

Shibahara H, Tamada S, Goto M, et al: Pathologic features of mucin-producing bile duct tumors: two histopathologic categories as counterparts of pancreatic intraductal papillary-mucinous neoplasms. Am J Surg Pathol 28:327-338, 2004.

Zen Y, Fujii T, Itatsu K, et al: Biliary papillary tumors share pathological features with intraductal papillary mucinous neoplasm of the pancreas. Hepatology 44:1333-1343, 2006.

CHOLANGIOCARCINOMA: INTRAHEPATIC, EXTRAHEPATIC, AND HILAR (KLATSKIN TUMOR)

- This tumor arises from (or differentiates as) bile duct epithelium and is classified as either intrahepatic or extrahepatic
- Hilar (Klatskin) tumors are generally considered extrahepatic
- The main differences are in clinical presentation and gross appearance

Clinical Features

- Average age at presentation is 60 years
- Equal frequency in men and women
- More common in Southeast Asian countries, but incidence has increased since the 1990s in the United States
- Often preceded by biliary hyperplasia or dysplasia
- Can also arise in IPNB or mucinous cystic neoplasm
- Risk factors include ulcerative colitis, sclerosing cholangitis, cirrhosis, alcohol, viral hepatitis B and C, thorium dioxide (Thorotrast) exposure, *Clonorchis sinensis* infestation, intrahepatic bile duct lithiasis, and a variety of congenital anomalies of intrahepatic and extrahepatic bile ducts

- Most cases not associated with cirrhosis or hepatitis
- Normal serum AFP, elevated serum CEA
- Intrahepatic tumors present with abdominal pain and weight loss
- Hilar tumors often present as small lesions because their location results in early biliary obstruction
- Extrahepatic tumors also present with jaundice and ascites but tend to be larger than hilar lesions at presentation
- Frequently metastasizes to regional and peripancreatic lymph nodes
- Generally poor prognosis

Gross Pathology

- Intrahepatic
  - Gray-white, tough, scirrhous mass with finger-like extensions along major bile ducts and lymphatics
  - Can be large
  - Often multifocal
- Extrahepatic
  - Nodular or flat sclerotic lesions with deep penetration into the bile duct wall; less commonly polypoid superficial lesions
- Klatskin tumor (hilar)
  - Begins at hepatic duct junction and spreads along segments of biliary tree
  - Large green liver with collapse of gallbladder and extrahepatic ducts is characteristic

Histopathology

- Usually well-differentiated mucin-secreting adenocarcinomas with abundant fibrous stroma
- Typically do not show necrosis
- Heterogeneity of cells within same gland
- Increased nuclear-to-cytoplasmic ratio
- Prominent nucleoli
- Concentric layering of cellular stroma around neoplastic glands (Figure 7-21)
- Spreads between hepatic plates (sinusoidal growth) and along ducts and nerves
- Stromal and perineural invasion; vascular invasion less common than in HCC
- Metaplastic and dysplastic changes may be seen in adjacent biliary epithelium

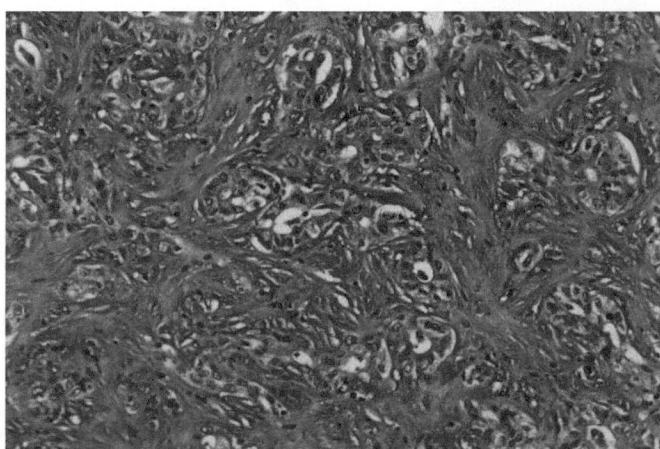

Figure 7-21. Cholangiocarcinoma. A characteristic feature of this lesion is the infiltrating nature of the glands surrounded by a marked desmoplastic stromal reaction.

- Sarcomatoid differentiation rare
- Occasionally admixed with trabeculae of neoplastic hepatocytes (mixed cholangiocarcinoma and HCC)

Special Stains and Immunohistochemistry

- Mucicarmine and PAS with diastase (PAS-D) positive
- EMA, MOC-31, keratins 7 and 19 positive
- Villin positive with brush-border accentuation; CD10 similar pattern
- CDX2 variable or weak reactivity
- CEA positive (will be positive with polyclonal anti-CEA but lacks the canalicular staining of HCC)
- Epidermal growth factor receptor protein (EGFR) positive (but so, too, HCC)

Other Techniques for Diagnosis

- Electron microscopy: nonspecific glandular characteristics
- Molecular studies
  - Expression of *C-myc, C-ras, c-erbB-2* oncogenes related to tumor differentiation (not diagnostically useful)
  - High incidence of *C-ras* oncogene mutation
  - Decreased β-catenin expression
  - Elevated *cox-2* expression

Differential Diagnosis

HCC

- Positive for low-molecular-weight keratin (with subplasmalemmal accentuation)
- Positive for HepPar-1, arginase, glypican-3
- Canalicular staining with polyclonal anti-CEA and CD10
- Sinusoidal endothelium CD34 positive
- Negative with monoclonal anti-CEA and MOC-31
- Absence of mucin
- Often resembles normal liver with thicker plates and cytologic pleomorphism; bile production

METASTATIC ADENOCARCINOMA

- More common in liver than cholangiocarcinoma
- Clinical history is important
- Virtually all colonic metastases show intraluminal necrosis

EPITHELIOID HEMANGIOENDOTHELIOMA

- Intracytoplasmic vacuoles; occasionally contain red blood cells
- Less often keratin positive
- Vascular markers positive

PEARLS

- *Perineural invasion is a helpful diagnostic feature, particularly on frozen section*
- *Clusters of small acini (periluminal sacculi of Beale) normally present in the extrahepatic duct wall should not be mistaken for invasive carcinoma*

SELECTED REFERENCES

Shaib YH, Davila JA, McGlynn K, El-Serag HB: Rising incidence of intrahepatic cholangiocarcinoma in the United States: a true increase? J Hepatol 40:472-477, 2004.
Tada M, Omata M, Ohto M: High incidence of ras gene mutation in intrahepatic cholangiocarcinoma. Cancer 69:1115-1118, 1992.
Thuluvath PJ, Rai R, Venbrux AC, et al: Cholangiocarcinoma: a review. Gastroenterologist 5:306-315, 1997.
Voravud N, Foster CS, Gilbertson JA, et al: Oncogene expression in cholangiocarcinoma and in normal hepatic development. Hum Pathol 20:1163-1168, 1989.

GALLBLADDER CARCINOMA

Clinical Features

- Marked female predominance
- Age peak in seventh decade; uncommon in patients younger than 50 years
- Higher incidence in Latin American countries
- Increased risk with cholelithiasis
- Other risk factors include porcelain gallbladder (end-stage calcifying cholecystitis), cholecystenteric fistula, anomalous pancreaticobiliary duct anastomosis, ulcerative colitis, adenomatous polyposis coli, and Gardner syndrome (APC mutations)
- Can present with right upper quadrant pain and anorexia
- More commonly found incidentally after cholecystectomy for cholelithiasis
- Increased serum alkaline phosphatase levels

Gross Pathology

- Two growth patterns
  - Diffuse growth (two thirds of cases)
  - Polypoid or papillary mass (one third of cases)
- Diffuse pattern can be mistaken for cholecystitis
- Carcinomatous gallbladders often contain calculi and exhibit marked mural fibrosis

Histopathology (Figure 7-22)

- Commonly associated with hyperplasia, gastric or intestinal metaplasia, dysplasia, or carcinoma in situ of adjacent mucosa
- Carcinoma in situ can extend into cystic duct and Aschoff-Rokitansky sinuses and *should not be mistaken for invasion*
- Most commonly invasive cancers are tubular adenocarcinomas that resemble cholangiocarcinoma
- Well-formed glands with wide lumens lined by one or more layers of highly atypical columnar or cuboidal cells surrounded by concentrically arranged cellular stroma
- Mucin production
- Characteristically better differentiated architecturally than cytologically
- Characteristically grows along nerves
- Regional lymph node metastases common
- Foci of intestinal differentiation common
- Choriocarcinoma-like elements rarely reported
- Other types: high-grade endocrine (small cell), adenosquamous, squamous (exceptionally rare), low-grade endocrine, and sarcomatoid

Special Stains and Immunohistochemistry

- Keratins 7 and 19 strongly positive; more likely than typical intrahepatic and extrahepatic cholangiocarcinoma to coexpress keratin 20
- CEA strongly positive
- Villin positive with brush-border accentuation
- CDX2 weak or variable

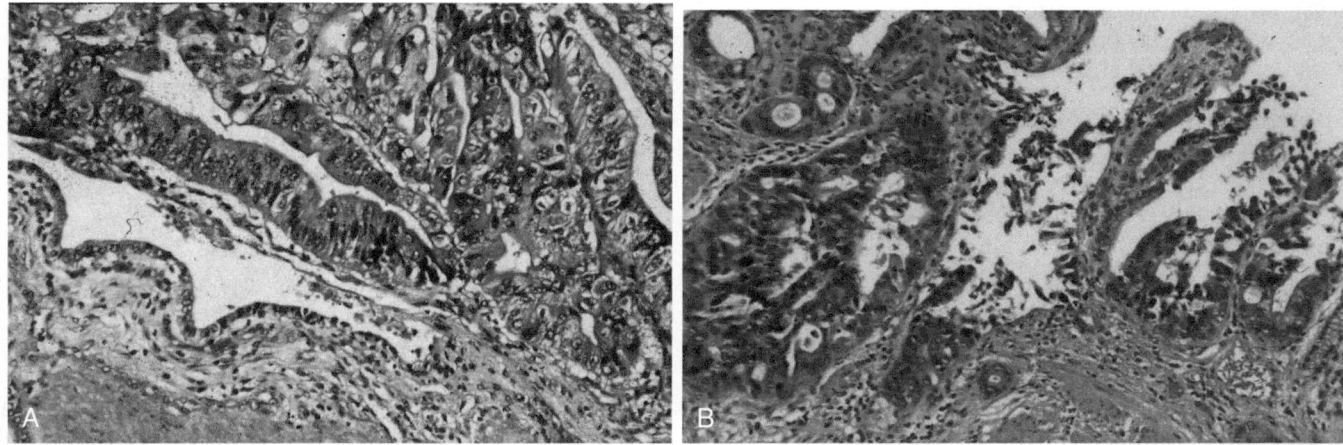

Figure 7-22. Adenocarcinoma of gallbladder. A, High-power view shows the transition between normal mucosa and malignant epithelium. **B,** Both in situ carcinoma and infiltrating carcinoma are evident in this photomicrograph.

- AFP occasionally positive

Other Techniques for Diagnosis

- Electron microscopy: adenocarcinoma cells show pleomorphic microvilli, mucin vacuoles, and abundant lysosomes (nonspecific features)
- Overexpression of *TP53* in most cases; more common in high-grade tumors; more common in gallbladder tumors than in extrahepatic cholangiocarcinomas

Differential Diagnosis

CHOLANGIOCARCINOMA

- Similar immunohistochemical staining pattern (although less often keratin 20 positive)
- Gross specimen and clinical information necessary to differentiate

HCC

- CEA negative except for bile canaliculi when using polyclonal antibodies, owing to cross-reactivity with non-CEA bile-associated glycoprotein
- Subplasmalemmal accentuation with low-molecular-weight keratin antibodies
- Absence of mucin

METASTATIC TUMORS

- Rare in gallbladder
- Most reported cases are melanoma, breast carcinoma, or renal cell carcinoma

PEARLS

- *Most important prognostic indicator is stage; low-stage lesions are effectively limited to those detected incidentally at cholecystectomy*
- *Thought to arise from a sequence of intestinal metaplasia, dysplasia, and in situ carcinoma*

SELECTED REFERENCES

Abi-Rached B, Neugut AI: Diagnostic and management issues in gallbladder carcinoma. Oncology 9:19-24, 1995.
Kamel D, Paakko P, Nuorva K, et al: P53 and c-erbB-2 protein expression in adenocarcinomas and epithelial dysplasias of the gallbladder. J Pathol 70:67-72, 1993.

Lee RG, Emond J: Prognostic factors and management of carcinomas of the gallbladder and extrahepatic bile ducts. Surg Oncol Clin N Am 6: 639-659, 1997.
Yamaguchi K, Enjoji M: Carcinoma of the gallbladder. Cancer 62:1425-1432, 1988.

HEPATIC METASTASES

Clinical Features

- Metastatic disease overall more common than primary hepatic malignancy in the Western world
- Liver is a common site for metastases from many primary sites, particularly the colon, breast, pancreas, lung, kidney, and stomach
- Sarcomas and malignant melanomas also metastasize to the liver
- Primary tumors of gallbladder, extrahepatic bile ducts, pancreas, and stomach frequently involve the liver by direct extension
- Resection with possibility of a cure may be indicated for single or multiple liver metastases from the colon and other primary sites
- Metastases are relatively rare in cirrhotic livers

Gross Pathology

- Hepatic metastases are usually discrete and well demarcated (grossly and histologically) from adjacent liver parenchyma; often with a hyperemic rim
- May be single or multiple, occasionally with infiltrative growth; may mimic either intrahepatic cholangiocarcinoma or HCC
- Diffusely infiltrative patterns may resemble primary liver tumors
- Occasionally metastases from the breast, prostate, or stomach can spread through the liver as small punctate lesions simulating cirrhosis
- Colonic metastases are usually multiple large nodules with marked central umbilication on the surface of the liver

Histopathology

- Depends on the primary malignancy
- Colon: prominent central necrosis in metastatic glandular lumens; mucin production can be abundant and may undergo calcification

- Squamous cell carcinoma: polygonal cells with abundant eosinophilic cytoplasm; may keratinize; if basaloid cells predominate, think upper aerodigestive or anal origin
- Lung and breast: often medium-sized nodules without extensive necrosis or hemorrhage and with early central umbilication; may be histologically indistinguishable if poorly differentiated
- Gallbladder: cluster around gallbladder bed and diminish in size with infiltration of hepatic parenchyma
- Malignant melanoma: large epithelioid or spindled cells with prominent nucleoli with or without pigment
- Prostate: epithelial cells with prominent nucleoli; acinar differentiation may not be conspicuous in some cases

Special Stains and Immunohistochemistry

- Immunohistochemical stains are relevant in both the clinical and histologic context; in selected cases, an immunohistochemical profile may confirm or augment the histologic and clinical impression; useful examples include (but are not limited to) the following:
  - Keratin 20 without keratin 7; villin (brush border); uniform CDX2: *lower intestinal tract*
  - Keratin 7 with variable or absent keratin 20; villin (brush border), keratin 17 or 19, weak or variable CDX2: *upper gastrointestinal tract and pancreaticobiliary* (additional markers, including mesothelin and MUC 1, 2, 4, 5 AC, and 6, may also be of value)
  - Keratin 7 without keratin 20; TTF-1, napsin, and surfactant A positive; CDX2 and villin negative: *pulmonary*
  - Keratin 7 and 20; CEA; high-molecular-weight keratin (including keratin 5/6); p63; GATA-3; absent CDX2: *urothelial*
  - Keratin 7 and 20 negative; CD10, EMA, PAX2/8 positive: *conventional type renal*
  - Keratin 7 and 20 negative; high-molecular-weight and p63 negative; prostate-specific antigen or prostatic acid phosphatase positive: *prostatic*
  - Thyroglobulin, TTF-1, PAX2/8 positive; surfactant negative: *thyroidal*
  - Gross cystic disease fluid protein-15, mammaglobin, S-100 protein positive; estrogen and progesterone receptor positive: *mammary*
  - Keratin 7, p53, CA-125, WT-1, PAX8, estrogen receptor protein positive; CEA negative: *nonmucinous mullerian* (serous more likely WT-1 positive; *mucinous mullerian* are CA-125, WT-1, PAX8 negative with an overall profile similar to intestinal carcinoma)
  - S-100 protein, GCDFP-15, androgen receptor protein positive; estrogen receptor protein negative: *salivary ductal* (other salivary gland lesions often coexpress S-100 protein and myoepithelial markers p63, SMA, and calponin)
  - S-100 protein, HM-B45, melan-A, tyrosinase, microphthalmia transcription factor (MiTF) positive; keratin negative: *melanocytic*
  - Synaptophysin, chromogranin A, NSE, CD56, CD57 positive; keratin variable; TTF-1 variable: *endocrine* (selected endocrine neoplasms have unique profiles, including calcitonin and TTF-1 in medullary thyroid and insulin, glucagon, somatostatin, and others in pancreatic endocrine neoplasms)
- Likelihood that immunohistochemistry will be helpful is inversely related to the grade of metastatic lesion

Other Techniques for Diagnosis

- Not likely to contribute

PEARLS

- *Metastasis more common than primary hepatic malignancy in the Western world*
- *Clinical history is most important, although some histologic patterns and selected immunohistochemical profiles may provide useful diagnostic information*
- *Number of metastases is important in the context of some cancers, especially colorectal adenocarcinoma, because some patients might be eligible for resection*
- *Gland formation with extensive central necrosis is characteristic of colonic metastases*

SELECTED REFERENCES

Kakar S, Gown AM, Goodman ZD, Ferrell LD: Best practices in diagnostic immunohistochemistry: hepatocellular carcinoma versus metastatic neoplasm. Arch Pathol Lab Med 131:1648-1654, 2007.

Ozcan A, Shen SS, Hamilton C, et al: PAX 8 expression in non-neoplastic tissues, primary tumors, and metastatic tumors: a comprehensive immunohistochemical study. Mod Pathol 24:751-764, 2011.

Sardi A, Akbarov A, Conaway G: Management of primary and metastatic tumors to the liver. Oncology 10:911-925, 1996.

PELIOSIS HEPATIS

Clinical Features

- Associated with use of anabolic steroids, oral contraceptives, thiopurines, and danazol
- Resolves after discontinuation of causative drugs
- Associated with hepatic infection by *Bartonella henselae* (causative organism of bacillary angiomatosis) in HIV-infected patients

Gross Pathology

- Liver parenchyma with focal blood lakes

Histopathology

- Large, intraparenchymal, blood-filled spaces and cysts surrounded by hepatocytes
- Blood-filled spaces without lining cells
- Disruption of sinusoids
- In *Bartonella*-associated cases: myxoid perisinusoidal stroma with clumps of granular material

Special Stains and Immunohistochemistry

- Reticulin stain demonstrates disruption of sinusoidal reticulin fibers
- Warthin-Starry stain positive in granular *Bartonella*-associated deposits

Other Techniques for Diagnosis

- Noncontributory

Differential Diagnosis

SINUSOIDAL DILATION
- Lacks cystic and cavernous change
- Sinusoidal reticulin intact

HEMANGIOMA
- Dilated vascular spaces lined by flattened endothelial cells
- Endothelial cells are CD31, CD34, factor VIII–related antigen (von Willebrand factor), D2-40 (podoplanin), and *Ulex europaeus I* positive

PEARLS

- *Most commonly related to use of androgenic anabolic steroids*
- *Associated with* Bartonella henselae, *especially in HIV-positive patients*

SELECTED REFERENCES

Cavalcanti R: Impact and evolution of peliosis hepatis in renal transplant recipients. Transplantation 58:315-316, 1994.
Koehler JE, Sanchez MA, Garrido CS: Molecular epidemiology of Bartonella infections in patients with bacillary angiomatosis-peliosis. N Engl J Med 337:1876-1883, 1997.
Perkocha LA: Clinical and pathological features of bacillary peliosis hepatis in association with human immunodeficiency virus infection. N Engl J Med 323:1581-1586, 1990.
Se KL: Liver pathology associated with the use of anabolic-androgenic steroids. Liver 12:73-79, 1992.

HEMANGIOMA

Clinical Features

- Most common hepatic neoplasm (in as many as 20% of autopsy cases)
- Typically asymptomatic
- Lesions larger than 4 cm may present with abdominal distention, mass, or pain
- Usually diagnosed in adulthood

Gross Pathology

- Usually solitary; most less than 4 cm
- Well-circumscribed, spongy, red-brown lesion
- Typically subcapsular

Histopathology

- Vascular spaces lined by single layer of bland endothelial cells (Figure 7-23)
  - Capillary: consists of small, thin-walled, anastomosing capillary-like vessels
  - Cavernous: consists of large irregular, dilated vascular spaces
- Intralesional thrombosis is common; Masson-like lesions may suggest a diagnosis of angiosarcoma
- Connective tissue stroma often shows areas of sclerosis and calcification

Special Stains and Immunohistochemistry

- Vascular markers (CD31, CD34, podoplanin, *Ulex europaeus I*, factor VIII–related antigen, and von Willebrand factor) positive
- Keratin negative

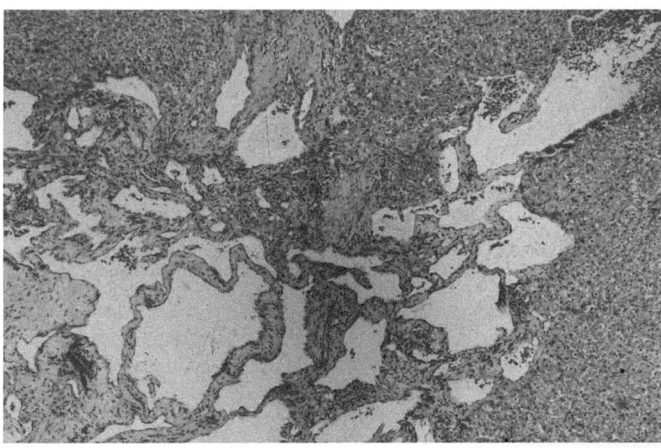

Figure 7-23. Liver hemangioma. Low-power photomicrograph of a liver section shows classic hemangioma composed of dilated vascular spaces.

Other Techniques for Diagnosis
- Noncontributory

Differential Diagnosis

PELIOSIS HEPATIS
- Consists of blood lakes without endothelial lining

ANGIOSARCOMA
- Multiple spongy hemorrhagic nodules with ill-defined borders
- Lining cells are large and show significant cytologic atypia
- Often has a high mitotic rate; occasional atypical mitotic figures

JUVENILE HEMANGIOENDOTHELIOMA
- Capillary-like vascular proliferation with plump endothelial cells
- Occasional mitotic figures
- Central fibrous scar
- Focal necrosis

EPITHELIOID HEMANGIOENDOTHELIOMA
- Multiple hepatic nodules with ill-defined borders
- Poorly defined vascular channels lined by atypical epithelioid cells

PEARLS

- *Usually incidental*
- *Most are the cavernous type*
- *Large or symptomatic lesions should be surgically excised*

SELECTED REFERENCES

Iqbal N, Saleem A: Hepatic hemangioma: a review. Tex Med 93:48-50, 1997.
Semelka RC, Sofka CM: Hepatic hemangiomas. Mag Reson Imaging Clin N Am 5:241-253, 1997.
Stanley P, Geer GD, Miller JH, et al: Infantile hepatic hemangiomas: clinical features, radiologic investigations, and treatment of 20 patients. Cancer 64:936-949, 1989.

INFANTILE HEMANGIOENDOTHELIOMA

Clinical Features

- Rare
- About 90% diagnosed in first year of life, male predominance
- Presents as abdominal mass or hepatomegaly
- Most symptomatic patients die from:
  - Arteriovenous shunt with risk for high-output congestive heart failure
  - Rupture
- Multicentricity precludes surgery; vascular ligation or embolization common means of treatment
- May involute or regress

Gross Pathology

- May be solitary or multicentric
- Marked variation in size (microscopic to greater than 15 cm)
- Central scar

Histopathology

- Capillary-like small vascular proliferation in periphery of lesion
- Lining endothelial cells plump, focally epithelioid
- Occasional mitotic figures identified
- Hypovascular stroma in center of lesion
- Central necrosis and calcification

Special Stains and Immunohistochemistry

- Vascular markers positive
- Keratin negative

Other Techniques for Diagnosis

- Noncontributory

Differential Diagnosis

CAPILLARY HEMANGIOMA
- Bland endothelial cells
- Lacks central scar

SO-CALLED INFANTILE ANGIOSARCOMA
- May be a variant of infantile hemangioendothelioma
- Endothelial cells more pleomorphic or kaposiform; may show intravascular budding
- Aggressive local infiltration, metastasis

ANGIOSARCOMA
- Increased nuclear atypia and mitotic activity
- Focal sinusoidal involvement

SELECTED REFERENCE

Dehner LP, Ishak KG: Vascular tumours of the liver in infants and children: a study of 30 cases and review of the literature. Arch Pathol 92:101-111, 1971.

EPITHELIOID HEMANGIOENDOTHELIOMA

Clinical Features

- Middle-aged patients, female predominance
- Slow growing
- Calcifications commonly seen by imaging studies
- Surgical excision often precluded by multifocal nature of lesion; liver transplantation is an effective means of treatment
- About 40% rate of recurrence
- About 30% may also involve spleen, lymph nodes, lung, or bone (metastasis versus metachronous primary disease)

Gross Pathology

- Hepatic nodules with ill-defined borders; 70% of cases multifocal
- Central scarlike areas with myxoid or calcified stroma

Histopathology

- Poorly defined vascular channels lined by atypical epithelioid tumor cells (Figure 7-24)
- Central scars contain dendritic tumor cells with vacuolated cytoplasm and only slight nuclear atypia
- Sparing of portal tracts
- Infiltrative borders
- Myxoid or sclerotic background

Special Stains and Immunohistochemistry

- Vascular markers (CD31, CD34, factor VIII-related antigen, podoplanin, *Ulex europaeus I*) positive
- Keratin (low molecular weight) occasionally positive
- Villin negative

Other Techniques for Diagnosis

- Electron microscopy: Weibel-Palade bodies

Differential Diagnosis

ANGIOSARCOMA
- Sinusoidal involvement
- Increased nuclear atypia and mitotic activity

CHOLANGIOCARCINOMA
- No blood-filled spaces
- True gland formation
- Keratin 7 and 19 and CEA positive
- Villin positive with brush-border pattern
- Vascular markers negative

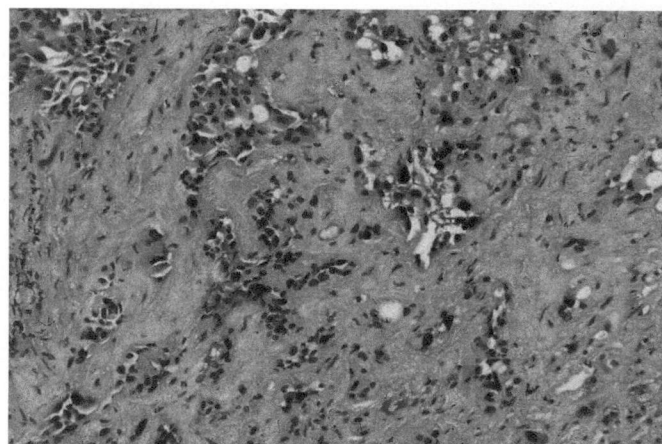

Figure 7-24. Epithelioid hemangioendothelioma. Proliferation of vascular channels lined by atypical epithelioid cells. Notice the sclerotic background.

METASTATIC CARCINOMA
- Keratin positive
- Vascular markers negative

MALIGNANT MELANOMA
- Nests and individual cells with prominent macronucleoli
- Melanin pigment occasionally seen
- S-100 protein, HMB-45, melan-A, tyrosinase, MiTF positive

PEARLS

- *Prognosis is more favorable than for angiosarcoma*
- *May involve several different organs at diagnosis (30% of cases)*

SELECTED REFERENCES

Fujii T, Zen Y, Sato Y, et al: Podoplanin is a useful marker for epithelioid hemangioendothelioma of the liver. Mod Pathol 21:125-130, 2008.
Ishak KG, Sesterhenn IA, Goodman MZD, et al: Epithelioid hemangioendothelioma of the liver: a clinicopathologic and follow-up study of 32 cases. Hum Pathol 15:839-852, 1984.
Kelleher MB, Iwatsuki S, Sheahan DG: Epithelioid hemangioendothelioma of liver: clinicopathological correlation of 10 cases treated by orthotopic liver transplantation. Am J Surg Pathol 13:999-1008, 1989.

ANGIOSARCOMA

Clinical Features

- Most common in men during the sixth and seventh decades
- Abdominal pain or hepatomegaly in most cases
- Associated with exposure to thorium dioxide (Thorotrast, a radiographic contrast material), vinyl chloride (plastics), arsenic, and anabolic steroids
- Latency period of many years
- Poor prognosis; metastasis at diagnosis not uncommon

Gross Pathology

- Multiple, spongy hemorrhagic nodules with ill-defined borders

Histopathology

- Variable patterns
- Growth of markedly atypical endothelial cells along existing sinusoids (often seen with other patterns)
- Predominantly cavernous with pseudopapillary projections of pleomorphic spindled to epithelioid mesenchymal cells and admixed hemorrhage (Figure 7-25)
- Occasional solid tumor cell nests without appreciable vascular spaces
- Individual malignant cells may be seen in adjacent hepatic parenchyma

Special Stains and Immunohistochemistry

- Vascular markers (CD31, CD34, podoplanin, factor VIII–related antigen, podoplanin, and *Ulex europaeus I*) positive, though often to a lesser degree than benign or low-grade vascular lesions

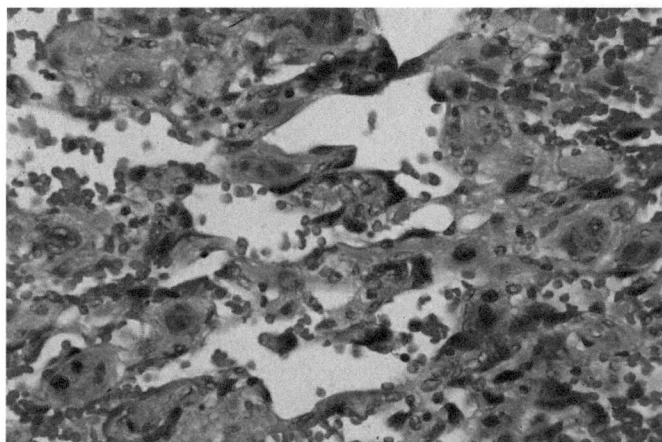

Figure 7-25. Angiosarcoma. Dilated vascular channels lined by pleomorphic, neoplastic, and endothelial cells.

- Keratin typically negative, but variable reactivity in some cases (especially epithelioid variants)
- Villin negative

Other Techniques for Diagnosis

- Electron microscopy: Weibel-Palade bodies
- Molecular studies: *K-ras-2* oncogene point mutations in vinyl chloride–associated cases

Differential Diagnosis

HCC
- Neoplastic cells positive for keratin and HepPar-1
- Negative for vascular markers (beware prominent CD34-positive sinusoidal endothelium)

CHOLANGIOCARCINOMA
- Neoplastic cells positive for keratin, villin (brush-border pattern), and CEA
- Negative for vascular markers

EPITHELIOID HEMANGIOENDOTHELIOMA
- Less prominent vascular differentiation
- Does not involve hepatic sinusoids
- Typically shows less cytologic atypia and a low mitotic rate
- Intracytoplasmic vacuoles may be present

METASTATIC CARCINOMA
- Neoplastic cells positive for keratins
- Negative for vascular markers

PEARLS

- *Increased risk associated with Thorotrast, vinyl chloride, and arsenic exposure*
- *Sinusoidal growth pattern characteristic*
- *Well-differentiated lesions may mimic benign vascular lesions; poorly differentiated lesions may be difficult to distinguish histologically from epithelial neoplasms*
- *Poor prognosis*

SELECTED REFERENCES

Lee FI, Smith PM, Bennett B, et al: Occupationally related angiosarcoma of the liver in the United Kingdom 1972-1994. Gut 39:312-318, 1996.

Ohsawa M, Kanno H, Aozasa K, et al: Use of immunohistochemical procedures in diagnosing angiosarcoma: evaluation of 98 cases. Cancer 75:2867-2874, 1995.

Selby DM, Stocker JT, Ishak KG: Angiosarcoma of the liver in childhood: a clinicopathologic and follow-up study of 10 cases. Pediatr Pathol 12:485-498, 1992.

Tamburro CH: Relationship of vinyl monomers and liver cancers: angiosarcoma and hepatocellular carcinoma. Semin Liver Dis 4: 158-169, 1984.

MESENCHYMAL HAMARTOMA

Clinical Features

- Rare benign lesion
- Presents during first 2 years of life
- Rare in adolescents and young adults
- Male-to-female ratio, 2:1
- Presents with abdominal swelling and palpable abdominal mass
- Related to polycystic disease, congenital hepatic fibrosis, and bile duct hamartoma
- Etiology uncertain (developmental anomaly versus ischemia versus neoplasm)

Gross Pathology

- Solitary spherical nodule
- Large (> 1 kg) soft fluctuant mass with a smooth surface
- Multiple cystic spaces filled with thin or viscous fluid
- Solid areas are variable: white and fibrous, yellow and myxoid, or brown and liver-like

Histopathology

- Low-power appearance resembles fibroadenoma
- Loose, edematous, myxoid connective tissue with dilated lymphatics, vessels, and fluid-filled spaces (Figure 7-26)
- Scattered disorganized and elongated branching bile ducts
- Scattered hepatocellular nodules
- Extramedullary hematopoiesis is common

Special Stains and Immunohistochemistry

- Noncontributory

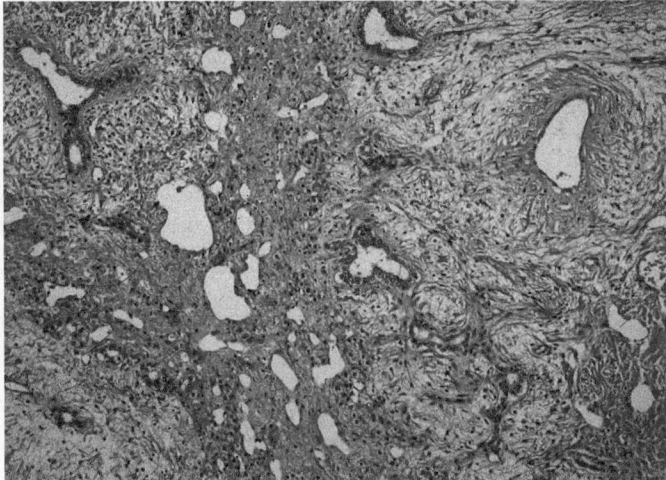

Figure 7-26. Mesenchymal hamartoma. Proliferation of loose connective tissue, dilated vessels, and scattered branching bile ducts.

Other Techniques for Diagnosis

- Electron microscopy: connective tissue component (myo)fibroblastic; admixed normal liver elements
- Flow cytometry: occasionally aneuploid

Differential Diagnosis

BILE DUCT ADENOMA

- Tubular structures with small or no lumens
- Lacks distinctive mesenchymal septa
- No liver cell islands
- May secrete mucin

BILE DUCT HAMARTOMA

- Characteristically multiple
- Composed of complex bile ducts in a fibrous stroma background

EMBRYONAL (UNDIFFERENTIATED) SARCOMA

- Found in prepubertal children
- Entirely mesenchymal tumor with few entrapped bile ducts
- Phenotypically diverse malignant cells
- Extensive necrosis

PEARLS

- *Mesenchymal hamartoma is a localized abnormality of ductal plates that is typically congenital*
- *Thought to arise in connective tissue of portal triads*

SELECTED REFERENCES

Craig JR: Mesenchymal tumors of the liver: diagnostic problems for the surgical pathologist. Pathology 3:141-160, 1994.

DeMaioribus CA, Lally KP, Sim K, et al: Mesenchymal hamartoma of the liver. Arch Surg 125:598-600, 1990.

Stocker JT, Ishak KG: Mesenchymal hamartoma of the liver. Pediatr Pathol 1: 245-267, 1983.

EMBRYONAL (UNDIFFERENTIATED) SARCOMA

Clinical Features

- Childhood neoplasm most common between ages 5 and 10 years; rare in adults
- No gender predilection
- No serum AFP elevation
- Presents with abdominal distention and weight loss
- Poor prognosis despite aggressive therapy

Gross Pathology

- Single, large, soft globular mass (10 to 30 cm)
- Variegated, solid, and cystic cut surface; pretreatment imaging studies often characteristic
- Fibrous pseudocapsule
- May show hemorrhage and necrosis

Histopathology

- Extensive necrosis; islands of viable neoplasm generally in periphery
- Loosely arranged pleomorphic spindled or stellate cells (Figure 7-27)

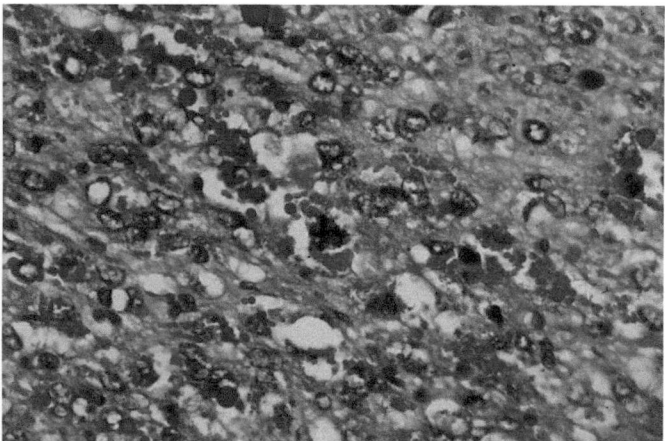

Figure 7-27. Embryonal (undifferentiated) sarcoma. Loosely arranged proliferation of spindle to oval cells with eosinophilic cytoplasm. Atypical mitosis is evident in the center portion of the photomicrograph.

- Scattered histiocytoid, fibrohistiocytoid, and myofibroblastic cells
- Fibroblast-like or smooth muscle–like fascicles or bundles of cells
- Minority population of cells resembling rhabdomyoblasts
- Scattered bizarre multinucleated giant cells
- Compact areas of more uniform round cells may be seen
- Variably sized eosinophilic globules in neoplastic cell cytoplasm and extracellular matrix
- Abundant acid mucopolysaccharide matrix
- Cystic, fluid-filled spaces secondary to degeneration are common
- Intermingled dilated benign bile ducts (entrapped), usually in periphery
- Extramedullary hematopoiesis in about 50% of cases

Special Stains and Immunohistochemistry

- PAS-D and α_1-antitrypsin: eosinophilic globules are positive
- Vimentin diffusely positive
- Keratin (pan-keratins and low-molecular-weight keratin) may be focally positive

Other Techniques for Diagnosis

- Electron microscopy: neoplastic cells show mesenchymal differentiation, including spindle-shaped cells with minimal cytoplasmic organelles and no desmosomal junctions
- Complex karyotype

Differential Diagnosis

PLEOMORPHIC SARCOMA (SO-CALLED MALIGNANT FIBROUS HISTIOCYTOMA)

- Typically occurs in elderly patients

- Positive for SMA (variable) and for histiocyte and lysosomal markers (CD68 and others)

PRIMARY AND METASTATIC HEPATIC SARCOMAS AND OTHER SPINDLE CELL NEOPLASMS

- Rarely encountered
- Monodirectional differentiation in an appropriate histologic context; examples include (but are not limited to) the following:
  - SMA and desmin: *leiomyosarcoma*
  - Muscle-specific actin, desmin, and caldesmon: *rhabdomyosarcoma* (spindled embryonal, solid alveolar, and pleomorphic variants)
  - SMA, HMB-45, and melan-A: *angiomyolipoma*
  - CD117, DOG-1, and CD34: *gastrointestinal stromal tumor*
  - S-100 protein, HMB-45, melan-A, tyrosinase, and MiTF: *melanoma*

ANAPLASTIC SMALL CELL HEPATOBLASTOMA

- Found in younger children
- Elevated serum AFP
- Monomorphic neoplastic cells

HCC WITH SARCOMATOID DIFFERENTIATION

- Elevated serum AFP
- Areas of typical HCC usually present (*beware limited sampling in biopsies*)
- Sarcomatoid areas more densely cellular than embryonal sarcoma
- Positive for keratin and HepPar-1

MESENCHYMAL HAMARTOMA

- Composed of benign elements
- Close association between mesenchymal and ductal components

PEARLS

- *Radiographic appearance of untreated lesion characteristic*
- *Must be considered in older prepubertal children with hepatic masses*
- *Purely mesenchymal neoplasm with phenotypic diversity*
- *Characteristic PAS-positive eosinophilic globules*

SELECTED REFERENCES

Aoyama C, Hachitanda Y, Sato JK, et al: Undifferentiated (embryonal) sarcoma of the liver: a tumor of uncertain histogenesis showing divergent differentiation. Am J Surg Pathol 15:615-624, 1991.

Craig JR: Mesenchymal tumors of the liver: diagnostic problems for the surgical pathologist. Pathology 3:141-160, 1994.

Stocker JT: An approach to handling pediatric liver tumors. Am J Clin Pathol 109(4 suppl 1):S67-S72, 1998.

Chapter 8
Pancreas

RALPH H. HRUBAN • MICHAEL CRUISE

CHAPTER OUTLINE

NONNEOPLASTIC ENTITIES

CHRONIC PANCREATITIS

Clinical Features

- Defined as irreversible loss of pancreatic parenchyma and function caused by inflammation
- Patients present with recurrent attacks of abdominal and back pain and evidence of loss of exocrine and endocrine pancreatic function including malabsorption, steatorrhea, and diabetes mellitus
- Alcohol abuse is the leading cause of chronic pancreatitis in Western countries
- Inherited genetic predispositions, such as hereditary pancreatitis caused by inherited mutations in the *PRSS1* or *SPINK1* genes and cystic fibrosis caused by inherited mutations in the *CFTR* gene, are increasingly being recognized as important predisposing factors; *PRSS1* and *SPINK1* mutations impair the inactivation of trypsin in the pancreas and thereby produce early onset of acute pancreatitis (often by age 10) and chronic pancreatitis (often by the age of 20); patients with mutations in *PRSS1* and *SPINK1* have approximately a 40% lifetime chance of developing pancreatic cancer
- Autoimmune (lymphoplasmacytic sclerosing) pancreatitis is associated with elevated serum IgG4 levels and other autoimmune diseases such as chronic sclerosing sialadenitis (Küttner tumor), primary sclerosing cholangitis, inflammatory bowel disease, retroperitoneal fibrosis (Ormond disease), and Riedel thyroiditis
- Chronic pancreatitis has a poor long-term prognosis with a 20-year mortality rate of 50%
- Chronic pancreatitis can clinically, radiologically, and pathologically mimic pancreatic cancer
- Pancreatic cancer can cause chronic pancreatitis, and longstanding chronic pancreatitis, particularly hereditary pancreatitis, can increase the risk of developing pancreatic cancer

Gross Pathology

- Diffuse atrophy of the gland with firm white fibrosis
- Early chronic pancreatitis may produce a localized ill-defined mass-like lesion that may mimic a pancreatic neoplasm
- Chronic pancreatitis secondary to alcohol abuse is characterized by pseudocyst formation and intraductal calculi

Histopathology

- Defined by inflammation with destruction of pancreatic parenchyma and replacement of the parenchyma by fibrous connective tissue and fat
- Lobular architecture of the parenchyma is retained (Figure 8-1)
- Remaining ductal epithelium can be atrophic or reactive
- Residual islets of Langerhans may aggregate producing enlarged islets that can mimic a neoplasm
- The islets may even abut nerves but the glands will not
- Autoimmune (lymphoplasmacytic sclerosing) pancreatitis is characterized by a duct-centric mixed plasma cell-rich inflammatory infiltrate, interstitial fibrosis, and venulitis (Figure 8-2A)

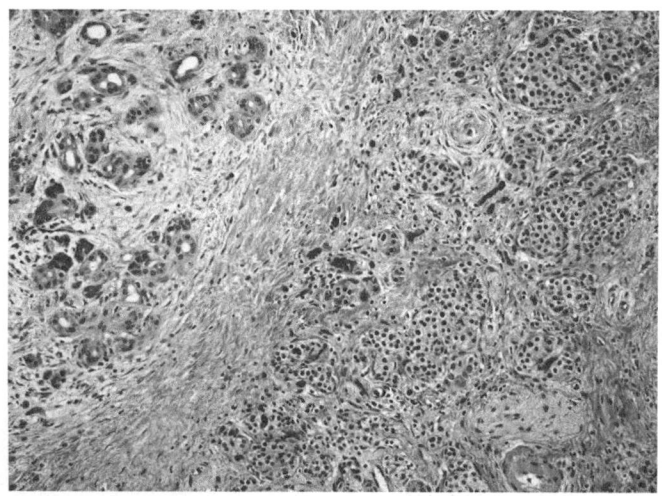

Figure 8-1. Chronic pancreatitis. Low-power view shows fibrosis and acinar dropout; however, the lobular architecture is maintained *(left)*. Note the aggregation of islets *(right)*.

Special Stains and Immunohistochemistry

- Immunolabeling for IgG4 may highlight increased numbers of IgG4 expressing plasma cells in autoimmune pancreatitis (Figure 8-2B)
- A Verhoeff-Van Gieson (VVG) elastin stain or Movat pentachrome stain can help highlight the venulitis typically seen in autoimmune pancreatitis (Figure 8-2C and D)

Other Techniques for Diagnosis

- Genetic testing for inherited mutations in the *PRSS1, SPINK1, and CFTR* genes is available for hereditary pancreatitis

Differential Diagnosis

INFILTRATING DUCTAL ADENOCARCINOMA

- Haphazard arrangement of glands with loss of lobular architecture at low power
- Glands immediately adjacent to muscular vessels
- Perineural invasion

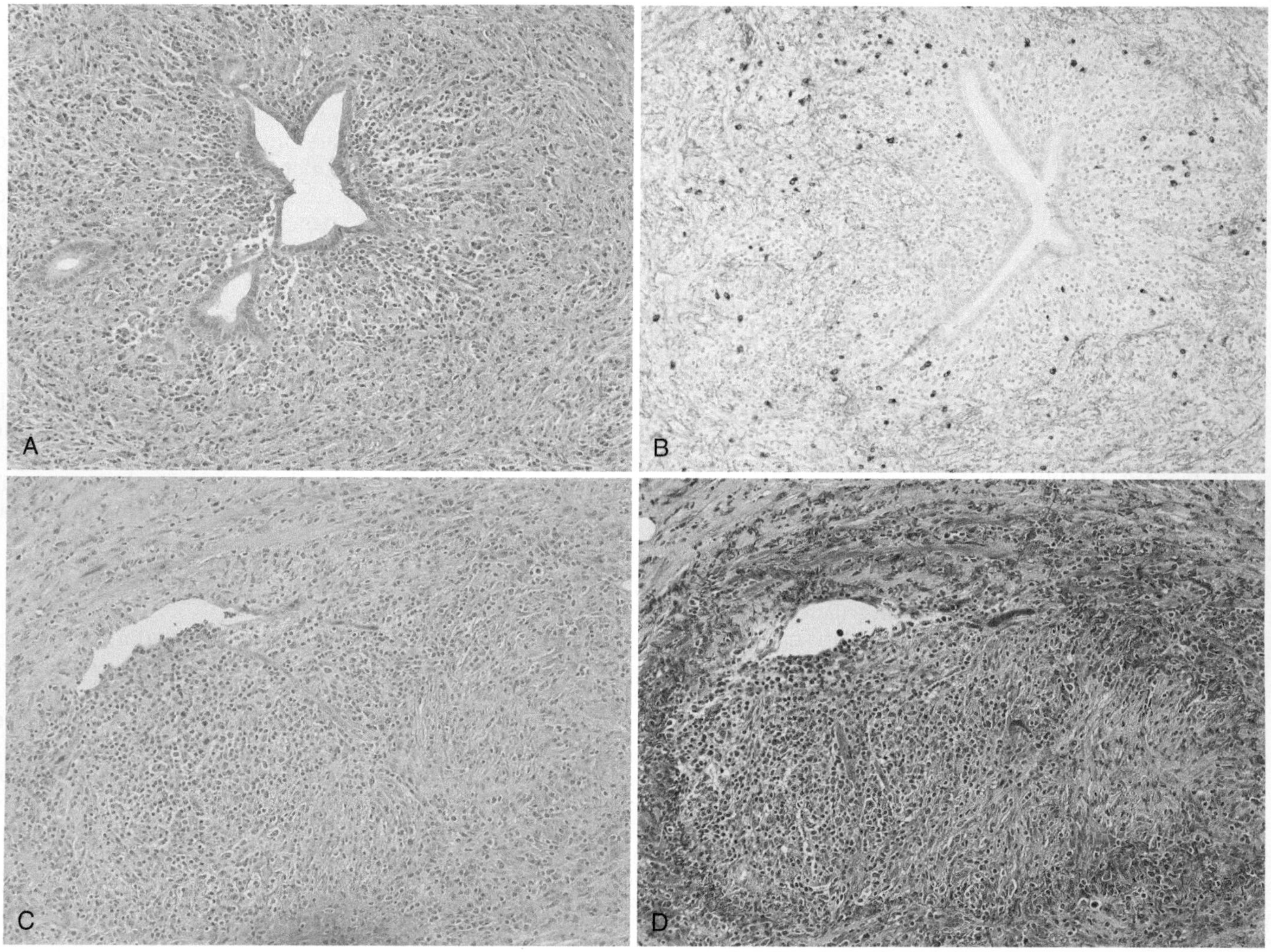

Figure 8-2. Autoimmune (lymphoplasmacytic sclerosing) pancreatitis. **A,** Characteristic mixed duct-centric inflammatory inflammation. **B,** IgG4 immunostain highlights the typical increase in IgG4 plasma cells. Venulitis, **C,** with partial involvement of the vein as highlighted by a Movat's stain, **D.**

- Vascular invasion
- Variation in the area of nuclei in a single gland by more than 4 to 1 ("4 to 1 rule")
- Incomplete lumina
- Luminal necrosis
- Loss of Smad4/Dpc4 expression

WELL-DIFFERENTIATED PANCREATIC NEUROENDOCRINE TUMOR

- Larger size and loss of the architecture of the normal islets
- Tendency to produce a single hormone (monoclonal)

PEARLS

- *Chronic pancreatitis can clinically and pathologically mimic pancreatic cancer, yet the two entities are treated vastly differently*
- *Growth pattern and location are the two most helpful features in distinguishing reactive from neoplastic glands*
- *Autoimmune pancreatitis is important to recognize because it may respond to treatment with steroids*
- *Avoid overdiagnosing the aggregated islets of Langerhans in chronic pancreatitis as a neuroendocrine tumor*

SELECTED REFERENCES

Applebaum-Shapiro SE, Finch R, Pfützer RH, et al: Hereditary pancreatitis in North America: the Pittsburgh-Midwest Multi-Center Pancreatic Study Group Study. Pancreatology 1:439-443, 2001.

Hruban RH, Pitman MB, Klimstra DS: Tumors of the Pancreas: Atlas of Tumor Pathology, Fourth Series, Fascicle 6 ed. Washington, DC, American Registry of Pathology and Armed Forces Institute of Pathology, 2007.

Klöppel G: Chronic pancreatitis, pseudotumors and other tumor-like lesions. Mod Pathol 20(suppl 1):S113-S131, 2007.

Klöppel G, Maillet B: Pathology of acute and chronic pancreatitis. Pancreas 8:659-670, 1993.

Whitcomb DC: Genetic risk factors for pancreatic disorders. Gastroenterology 14:1292-1302, 2013.

Zhang L, Notohara K, Levy MJ, et al: IgG4-positive plasma cell infiltration in the diagnosis of autoimmune pancreatitis. Mod Pathol 20:23-28, 2007.

PANCREATIC PSEUDOCYST

Clinical Features

- Accounts for 75% of cystic lesions of the pancreas
- The pathologic release of pancreatic enzymes causes the localized digestion of intra- and extrapancreatic tissues
- A complication of acute pancreatitis, often in the setting of chronic alcoholic pancreatitis
- May spontaneously resolve, may become infected, or may erode into adjacent organs

Gross Pathology

- Usually solitary
- Often involves peripancreatic tissues such as the lesser omental sac, the retroperitoneum between the stomach and transverse colon, and the space between the stomach and the liver
- Cysts filled with hemorrhagic necrotic debris rich in pancreatic enzymes
- Associated with peripancreatic hemorrhagic fat necrosis
- Ranges in size from 2 to 30 cm

Histopathology

- Locules contain necrotic and hemorrhagic debris with hemosiderin-laden macrophages
- Locules are lined by granulation and fibrous connective tissue and lack a true epithelial lining

Special Stains and Immunohistochemistry

- Noncontributory

Other Techniques for Diagnosis

- Elevated fluid amylase levels

Differential Diagnosis

CYSTIC NEOPLASMS OF THE PANCREAS

- Cystic neoplasms have a true epithelial lining and typically contain mucous or serous fluid
- Solid-pseudopapillary neoplasms can contain hemorrhagic and necrotic debris, but they will have poorly cohesive epithelial cells surrounding delicate branching blood vessels

PEARLS

- *Suspect a mimicker of a pseudocyst if the patient does not have a clinical history of acute or chronic pancreatitis, and when the pancreatic parenchyma is normal*
- *Extensive sampling may be necessary to demonstrate an epithelial lining in a cystic neoplasm*
- *Cyst fluid amylase levels should be high in pseudocysts*

SELECTED REFERENCES

Hruban RH, Pitman MB, Klimstra DS: Tumors of the pancreas. Atlas of Tumor Pathology, Fourth Series, Fascicle 6 ed. Washington, DC, American Registry of Pathology and Armed Forces Institute of Pathology, 2007.

Klöppel G: Pseudocysts and other non-neoplastic cysts of the pancreas. Semin Diagn Pathol 17:7-15, 2000.

Sanfey H, Aguilar M, Jones RS: Pseudocysts of the pancreas, a review of 97 cases. Am Surg 6:661-668, 1994.

LYMPHOEPITHELIAL CYST

Clinical Features

- Often an incidental finding
- Very rare
- Predominantly in men with a 4 to 1 male-to-female ratio
- Mean age ~55 years

Gross Pathology

- Can be unilocular or multilocular
- Mean size ~5 cm
- Well-demarcated, thin-walled cyst filled with keratinaceous (cheesy) debris (Figure 8-3A)

Histopathology

- Cyst lined by mature keratinizing squamous epithelium (Figure 8-3B)
- Subepithelial layer of lymphoid tissue often with germinal center formation
- Skin adnexal structures and cells with other directions of differentiation are, at most, focal

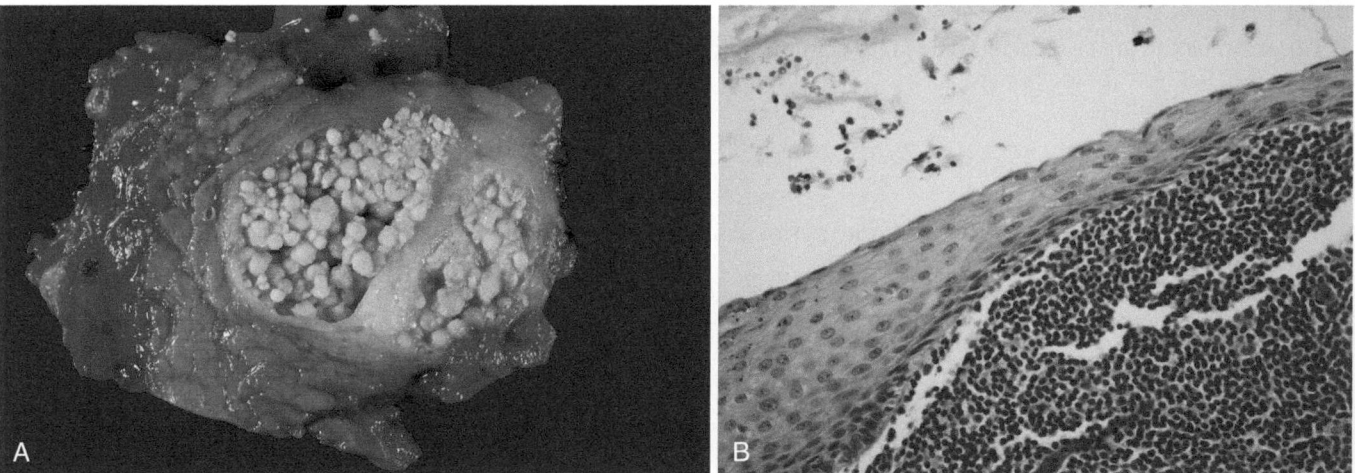

Figure 8-3. Lymphoepithelial cyst. A, Grossly the cyst is well-defined and filled with keratinaceous debris. **B,** Microscopically the cyst is lined by mature squamous epithelium with an underlying lymphoid infiltrate.

Special Stains and Immunohistochemistry

- Noncontributory

Other Techniques for Diagnosis

- Noncontributory

Differential Diagnosis

MATURE CYSTIC TERATOMA (DERMOID CYST)

- In addition to the squamous epithelium, these will have prominent skin adnexal structures and often mature mesenchymal elements such as cartilage

EPIDERMOID CYST IN HETEROTOPIC SPLEEN

- Distinctive cystic lesion that can also be lined by mature squamous epithelium, but, as the name suggests, these are present within splenic parenchyma

PEARLS

- *The keratinous debris can resemble the necrotic contents of a pseudocyst*
- *Unlike their counterparts in the head and neck, no relationship to immunosuppression (human immunodeficiency virus [HIV] infection), Sjögren disease, or Epstein-Barr Virus (EBV) infection has been found*
- *Although their pathogenesis is unknown, one proposal is squamous metaplasia of an obstructed, inflamed, and dilated duct*

SELECTED REFERENCES

Adsay NV, Hasteh F, Cheng JD, et al: Lymphoepithelial cysts of the pancreas: a report of 12 cases and a review of the literature. Mod Pathol 15:492-501, 2002.

Hruban RH, Pitman MB, Klimstra DS: Tumors of the pancreas. Atlas of Tumor Pathology, Fourth Series, Fascicle 6 ed. Washington, DC, American Registry of Pathology and Armed Forces Institute of Pathology, 2007.

Othman M, Basturk O, Groisman G, et al: Squamoid cyst of pancreatic ducts: a distinct type of cystic lesion in the pancreas. Am J Surg Pathol 31:291-297, 2007.

NEOPLASMS OF THE EXOCRINE PANCREAS

SEROUS CYSTIC NEOPLASMS

Clinical Features

- Slightly more common in women than in men with a female-to-male ratio of 7 to 3
- Mean age ~65 years
- Can be associated with the von Hippel-Lindau syndrome (VHL)
- Will present nonspecifically as large abdominal masses
- Majority are entirely benign with only a few case reports of aggressive behavior

Gross Pathology

- Can be cystic with innumerable small cysts (microcystic) or a few larger cysts (macrocystic), can be solid (solid serous adenoma), or can be combined with a well-differentiated pancreatic neuroendocrine tumor (especially in patients with VHL) (Figure 8-4A)
- Well-demarcated, often with a central stellate scar that may calcify
- Cysts are thin walled and contain watery straw-colored fluid

Histopathology

- Lined by a cuboidal epithelium with optically clear cytoplasm and round uniform nuclei (Figure 8-4B)
- Mitoses and nuclear pleomorphism are not seen
- Septa composed of relatively acellular fibrous connective tissue
- Solid variant is composed of sheets and nests of cells cytologically identical to the more common cystic variety

Special Stains and Immunohistochemistry

- Cells contain abundant glycogen and therefore stain with the periodic acid-Schiff (PAS) stain, and this staining is sensitive to diastase digestion

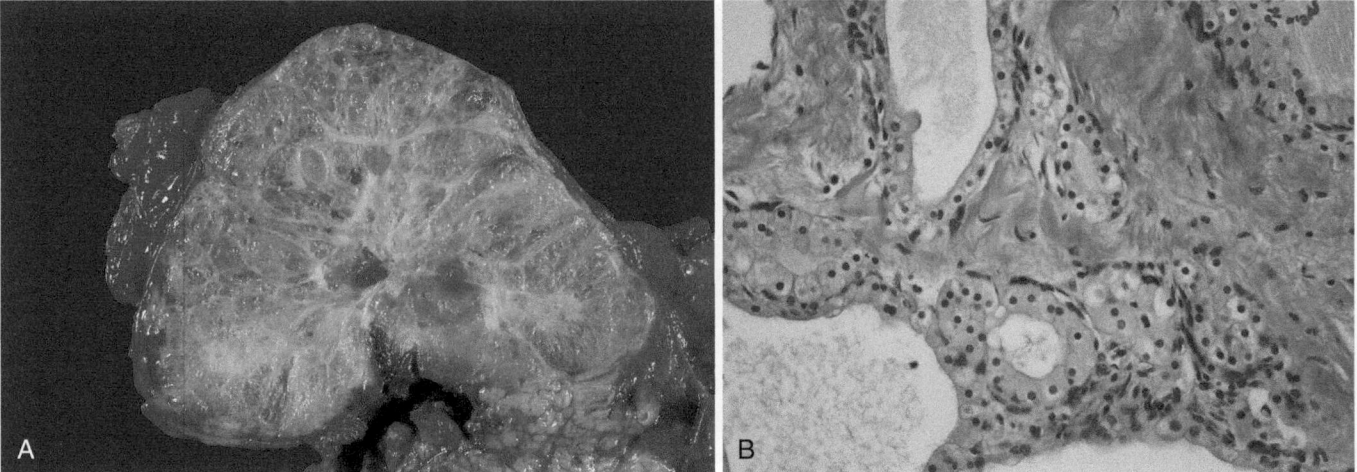

Figure 8-4. Serous cystadenoma. A, Grossly, the lesion has a central scar with innumerable thin-walled small cysts. **B,** The relatively small cysts are lined by a single layer of glycogen-rich cuboidal epithelial cells with round uniform nuclei.

- Epithelial cells label with antibodies to cytokeratin (AE1/AE3 and CAM5.2) and one third express epithelial membrane antigen (EMA)
- Immunolabeling for carcinoembryonic antigen (CEA), lipase, chromogranin, and amylase are negative

Other Techniques for Diagnosis

- Although rarely needed to establish the diagnosis, electron microscopy demonstrates abundant intracellular glycogen
- Some harbor mutations in the *VHL* gene or have loss of heterozygosity of the *VHL* locus on chromosome 3

Differential Diagnosis

MUCINOUS CYSTIC NEOPLASM
- Cyst has a thick wall and contains thick tenacious mucin
- Lined by tall columnar cells containing large quantities of mucin
- Distinctive ovarian-type stroma

INTRADUCTAL PAPILLARY MUCINOUS NEOPLASM
- Contains thick tenacious mucin
- Communicates with larger pancreatic ducts
- Lined by tall columnar cells containing mucin

METASTATIC RENAL CELL CARCINOMA
- Nuclear atypia and prominent nucleoli
- Immunolabels for vimentin, renal cell carcinoma marker (RCCma), PAX2, PAX8, and CD10

LYMPHANGIOMA
- Flat cells lining spaces
- Associated lymphoid aggregates in cyst walls
- Expresses CD31 and factor VIII-related antigen

PEARLS

- *The relationship of the cysts to the pancreatic ducts, the thickness of the cyst walls, and the cyst contents can all be used to support the diagnosis*
- *Radiologic feature of a central stellate scar can be characteristic*
- *Serous cystadenocarcinomas are extremely rare and can be distinguished from benign serous neoplasms only by their aggressive behavior (spread to other organs)*

SELECTED REFERENCES

Compton CC: Serous cystic tumors of the pancreas. Semin Diagn Pathol 17:43-55, 2000.
Galanis C, Zamani A, Cameron JL, et al: Resected serous cystic neoplasms of the pancreas: a review of 158 patients with recommendations for treatment. J Gastrointest Surg 11:820-826, 2007.
Hruban RH, Pitman MB, Klimstra DS: Tumors of the pancreas. Atlas of Tumor Pathology, Fourth Series, Fascicle 6 ed. Washington, DC, American Registry of Pathology and Armed Forces Institute of Pathology, 2007.

MUCINOUS CYSTIC NEOPLASMS

Clinical Features

- Much more common in women than in men with a female-to-male ratio of 20 to 1
- Mean age ~45 years
- Present nonspecifically as a large abdominal mass
- A third harbor an associated invasive adenocarcinoma
- The presence or absence of an associated invasive carcinoma drives prognosis

Gross Pathology

- The majority arise in the body or tail of the pancreas
- Usually solitary and multilocular
- Composed of large 1 to 3 cm thick-walled cysts containing tenacious mucin (Figure 8-5)
- The cysts do not communicate with the larger pancreatic ducts
- The lining of the cysts can be smooth or may have prominent papillary structures that project into the lumina

Histopathology

- Lined by tall columnar epithelium with varying degrees of cytologic and architectural atypia (Figure 8-6)
- Noninvasive tumors are classified into low-grade dysplasia, intermediate-grade dysplasia, or high-grade dysplasia (Figure 8-7)
- Dysplasia and even invasive cancer can be very focal
- The stroma is cellular and is histologically similar to ovarian stroma
- One third have an associated invasive ductal adenocarcinoma

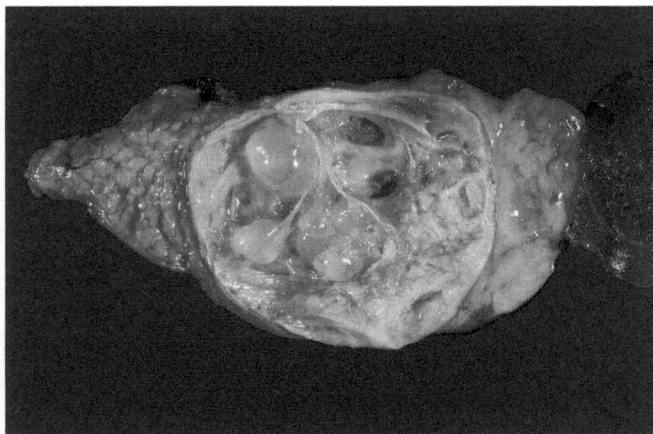

Figure 8-5. Mucinous cystic neoplasm. The neoplasm is composed of large well-demarcated mucin-containing cysts. As is typical, this tumor arose in the tail of the pancreas.

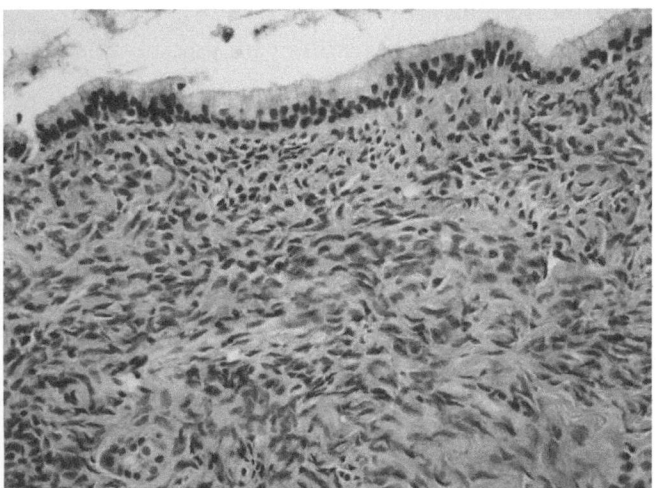

Figure 8-6. Mucinous cystic neoplasm with low-grade dysplasia. The cyst is lined by tall columnar cells with abundant intracellular mucin. Note the characteristic ovarian-type stroma.

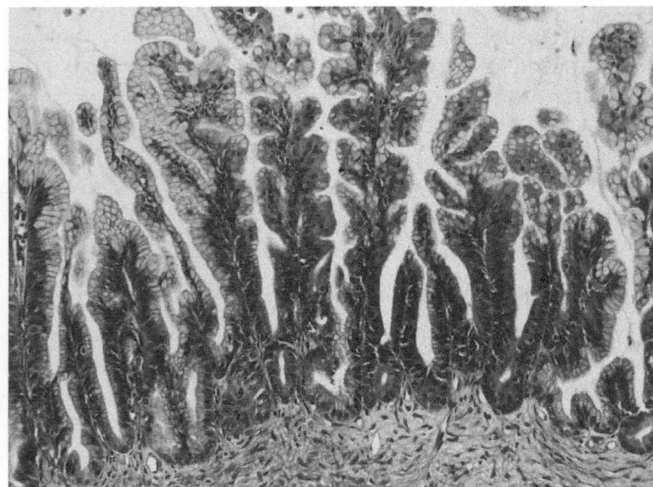

Figure 8-7. Mucinous cystic neoplasm with high-grade dysplasia. The mucin-producing epithelium is now architecturally complex and there is significant nuclear pleomorphism.

Special Stains and Immunohistochemistry

- Periodic acid-Schiff (PAS) with diastase treatment and mucicarmine positive
- The epithelium labels with antibodies to pan-cytokeratin and carcinoembryonic antigen (CEA); most will label with CK7, approximately two thirds will label with CK20, and two thirds will label with CDX2; up to 40% of cases have scattered chromogranin A expressing cells
- The stroma labels with antibodies to inhibin, and to progesterone and estrogen receptors

Other Techniques for Diagnosis

- May harbor *RNF43*, *KRAS2*, and *TP53* gene mutations
- Most noninvasive mucinous cystic neoplasms have intact Smad4/Dpc4 expression, whereas half of the invasive cancers associated with mucinous cystic neoplasms show loss of Smad4/Dpc4 expression

Differential Diagnosis

INTRADUCTAL PAPILLARY MUCINOUS NEOPLASM
- Located in the head more frequently than in the body/tail of the gland
- By definition, the cyst connects to the larger pancreatic ducts
- Has a paucicellular stroma, not the dense ovarian-type stroma

SEROUS CYSTIC NEOPLASM
- Contains thin, watery, straw-colored fluid
- Usually smaller (microcystic) and have thinner walls
- Central stellate scar
- Lined by cuboidal glycogen-rich cells

PSEUDOCYST
- Contains hemorrhagic and necrotic material
- Lacks an epithelial lining

PEARLS

- *The epithelium can be partially denuded. In these cases the diagnosis is suggested by the presence of ovarian-type stroma*
- *Because an invasive carcinoma can arise focally in these neoplasms, they should be entirely resected and thoroughly, if not completely, sampled for histologic examination*

SELECTED REFERENCES

Goh BK, Tan YM, Chung YF, et al: A review of mucinous cystic neoplasms of the pancreas defined by ovarian-type stroma: clinicopathological features of 344 patients. World J Surg 30:2236-2245, 2006.

Hruban RH, Pitman MB, Klimstra DS: Tumors of the pancreas. Atlas of Tumor Pathology, Fourth Series, Fascicle 6 ed. Washington, DC, American Registry of Pathology and Armed Forces Institute of Pathology, 2007.

Wilentz RE, Albores-Saavedra J, Hruban RH: Mucinous cystic neoplasms of the pancreas. Semin Diagn Pathol 17:31-42, 2000.

Zamboni G, Scarpa A, Bogina G, et al: Mucinous cystic tumors of the pancreas: clinicopathological features, prognosis, and relationship to other mucinous cystic tumors. Am J Surg Pathol 23:410-422, 1999.

INTRADUCTAL PAPILLARY MUCINOUS NEOPLASMS

Clinical Features

- Slightly more common in men than in women with a male-to-female ratio of 1.5 to 1
- Mean age ~65 years
- Arise in the head of the gland more commonly than in the body/tail
- Imaging may reveal a dilated main pancreatic duct
- May present with symptoms of chronic pancreatitis or symptoms of intermittent pancreatic duct obstruction
- A third have an associated invasive adenocarcinoma
- The presence or absence of an invasive component drives prognosis
- May be multifocal

Gross Pathology

- Most arise in the head of the gland
- Can be multifocal
- Cysts communicate with the larger pancreatic ducts (Figure 8-8A)
- Main duct-type involves the main pancreatic duct; branch duct-type involves a side-branch of the main duct
- Lining of the cysts can be relatively flat or may have large papillae

Histopathology

- Cysts lined by tall columnar epithelium with abundant intracellular and extracellular mucin (Figure 8-8B)
- The neoplastic epithelium involves the duct system of the pancreas
- Noninvasive neoplasms are classified into low-grade, intermediate-grade, and high-grade dysplasia
- The stroma is paucicellular
- One third have an associated invasive adenocarcinoma
- The invasive carcinoma can be a tubular (ductal) adenocarcinoma or a colloid (mucinous noncystic) adenocarcinoma; the designation colloid should be reserved for invasive adenocarcinomas with at least 80% colloid differentiation

Special Stains and Immunohistochemistry

- Periodic acid-Schiff with diastase treatment and mucicarmine positive
- The epithelium labels with antibodies to cytokeratin and CEA
- Intestinal type expresses the mucin MUC2, pancreatobiliary type expresses the mucin MUC1

Other Techniques for Diagnosis

- Can harbor *GNAS*, *RNF43*, *KRAS2*, or *TP53* gene mutations, and the prevalence of these mutations increases with increasing degrees of dysplasia
- Smad4/Dpc4 expression is usually intact in noninvasive lesions but may be lost in associated invasive carcinomas

Differential Diagnosis

MUCINOUS CYSTIC NEOPLASM

- Arises in women more often than in men
- Arises in the body/tail more often than in the head
- Cysts do not communicate with the larger pancreatic ducts
- Characteristic ovarian-type stroma

PANCREATIC INTRAEPITHELIAL NEOPLASIA (PanIN)

- Smaller (< 0.5 cm)
- Short stubby papillae relative to the long finger-like papillae of intraductal papillary mucinous neoplasms (Figure 8-8B)
- Expresses the mucin MUC1

PEARLS

- *Can be multifocal and are often associated with multifocal, smaller precursor lesions*
- *Be careful not to "overcall" small precursor lesions at surgical margins at the time of intraoperative consultation, as these lesions are common and are of no proven clinical significance; instead, reserve calling the parenchymal margins positive for instances in which the surgeon either has clearly grossly transected the neoplasm or has cut across a significant lesion with high-grade dysplasia*

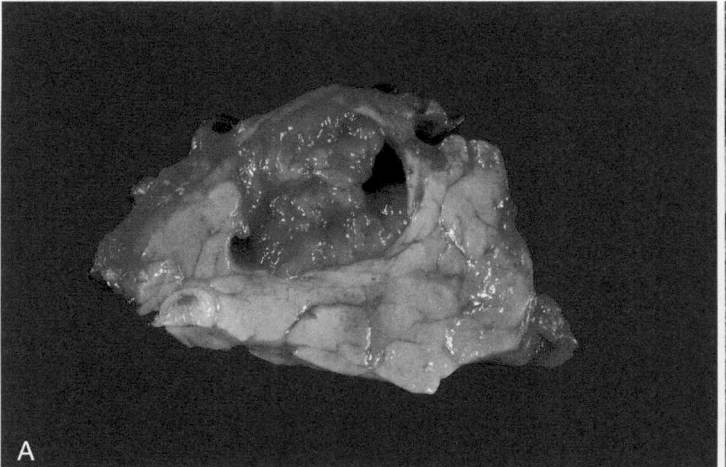
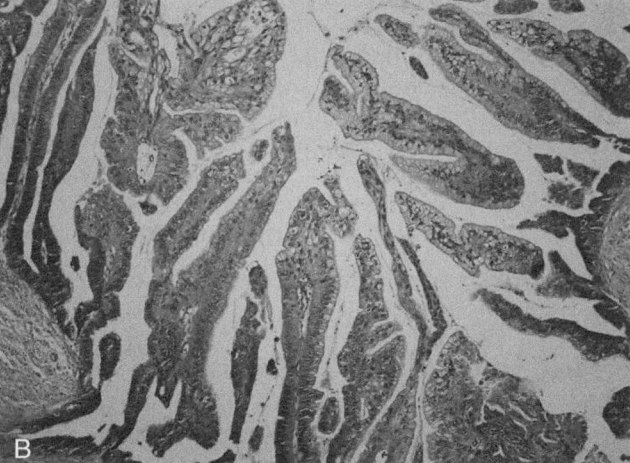

Figure 8-8. Intraductal papillary mucinous neoplasm. A, The lesion involves and expands the main pancreatic duct with an exuberant papillary proliferation. **B,** Low-power microscopic view shows a distended pancreatic duct filled with complex papillary structures lined by mucin-producing columnar cells.

- *Bivalving a resected specimen along a probe placed in the main pancreatic duct can help determine the relationship of the cysts to the duct system*
- *These neoplasms should be sampled extensively because the presence or absence of invasion is the most important prognosticator*
- *Colloid/mucinous differentiation in the invasive component portends a better prognosis*
- *Acellular mucin extruded into the stroma can mimic an associated invasive carcinoma*

SELECTED REFERENCES

Adsay NV, Merati K, Andea A, et al: The dichotomy in the preinvasive neoplasia to invasive carcinoma sequence in the pancreas: differential expression of MUC1 and MUC2 supports the existence of two separate pathways of carcinogenesis. Mod Pathol 15:1087-1095, 2012.

Chari ST, Yadav D, Smyrk TC, et al: Study of recurrence after surgical resection of intraductal papillary mucinous neoplasm of the pancreas. Gastroenterology 123:1500-1507, 2002.

Hruban RH, Pitman MB, Klimstra DS: Tumors of the pancreas. Atlas of Tumor Pathology, Fourth Series, Fascicle 6 ed. Washington, DC, American Registry of Pathology and Armed Forces Institute of Pathology, 2007.

Sohn TA, Yeo CJ, Cameron JL, et al: Intraductal papillary mucinous neoplasms of the pancreas: an updated experience. Ann Surg 239:788-797, 2004.

PANCREATIC INTRAEPITHELIAL NEOPLASIA (PanIN)

Clinical Features

- Too small (< 0.5 cm) to be detected reliably using currently available imaging techniques
- Believed to be a precursor to invasive ductal adenocarcinoma of the pancreas
- More common in the elderly
- More common in pancreata with an invasive carcinoma than in pancreata without a neoplasm

Gross Pathology

- Almost always too small to be appreciated grossly

Histopathology

- Epithelial proliferations within the smaller pancreatic ducts (Figure 8-9)
- May be flat or papillary
- The papillae are short and stubby
- Classified into PanIN-1, PanIN-2, and PanIN-3 based on the degree of architectural and cytologic dysplasia
- Lobular acinar units downstream of PanINs often show lobulocentric atrophy with scarring, presumably due to obstructive effects of exuberant duct epithelium

Special Stains and Immunohistochemistry

- Expresses the mucin MUC1

Other Techniques for Diagnosis

- Progressive accumulation of genetic alterations seen in invasive ductal adenocarcinoma; activating *KRAS2* gene mutations can be observed in low-grade PanINs (PanIN-1 lesions), inactivation of *p16/CDKN2A* in intermediate lesions (PanIN-2), and *TP53* and *SMAD4* loss in high-grade lesions (PanIN-3)

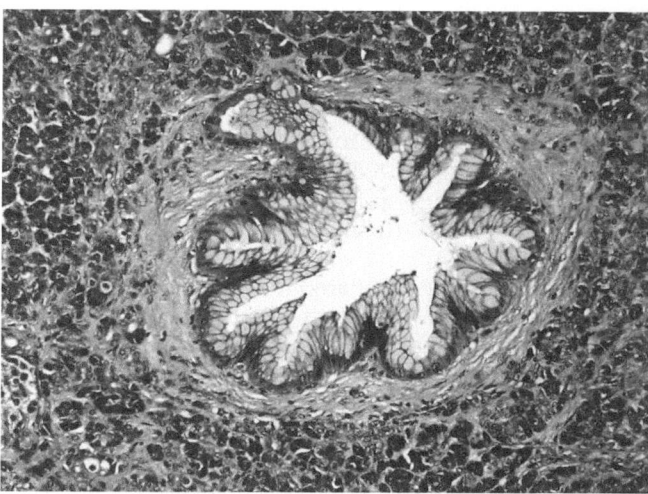

Figure 8-9. Pancreatic intraepithelial neoplasia. This papillary proliferation of epithelial cells projects into the lumen of a small duct. The papillae are shorter than those of intraductal papillary mucinous neoplasms.

Differential Diagnosis

INTRADUCTAL PAPILLARY MUCINOUS NEOPLASMS

- Grossly visible lesions (≥ 1 cm)
- Long finger-like papillae
- Abundant intracellular and extracellular mucin production
- Some express the mucin MUC2

INVASIVE DUCTAL ADENOCARCINOMA

- Haphazard growth pattern at low-power
- Glands immediately adjacent to muscular vessels
- Perineural invasion
- Vascular invasion
- Variation in the area of nuclei in a single gland by more than 4 to 1
- Incomplete lumina
- Luminal necrosis
- Loss of Smad4/Dpc4 expression

PEARLS

- *Avoid overstating the clinical significance of PanIN lesions, as PanINs, particularly low-grade PanINs are common in the population, particularly the elderly; thus, presence of a PanIN lesion at a margin in a resection for an invasive carcinoma has no clinical significance and in most cases should not prompt further surgery*
- *Avoid misdiagnosing the lobulocentric atrophy surrounding PanIN lesions as invasive carcinoma; the overall lobular pattern is intact in lobulocentric atrophy*

SELECTED REFERENCES

Hruban RH, Adsay NV, Albores-Saavedra J, et al: Pancreatic intraepithelial neoplasia: a new nomenclature and classification system for pancreatic duct lesions. Am J Surg Pathol 25:579-586, 2001.

Hruban RH, Takaori K, Klimstra DS, et al: An illustrated consensus on the classification of pancreatic intraepithelial neoplasia and intraductal papillary mucinous neoplasms. Am J Surg Pathol 28:977-987, 2004.

INVASIVE DUCTAL ADENOCARCINOMA AND ITS VARIANTS

Clinical Features

- Most patients are between 60 and 80 years old
- Strikes men slightly more than women
- Patients are usually not diagnosed until after the cancer has spread
- Most common symptoms include epigastric pain radiating to the back, weight loss, and painless jaundice
- The 5-year survival rate is only 5%

Gross Pathology

- Most arise in the head of the pancreas (65%)
- Firm, poorly defined sclerotic mass (Figure 8-10)
- Larger tumors sometimes undergo cystic degeneration
- They often obstruct the pancreatic and bile ducts resulting in upstream dilatation of these ducts (double duct sign)

Histopathology

- Ductal adenocarcinoma
  - Atypical gland-forming epithelial cells infiltrating into the stroma (Figure 8-11)
  - Loss of lobular architecture at low-power (haphazard growth pattern)
  - Glands immediately adjacent to muscular vessels (Figure 8-12)
  - Perineural invasion
  - Vascular invasion
  - Variation in the area of nuclei in a single gland by more than 4 to 1
  - Incomplete lumina
  - Luminal necrosis
- Adenosquamous carcinoma
  - Invasive carcinoma with both glandular and squamous differentiation
  - At least 30% of the neoplasm should have squamous differentiation

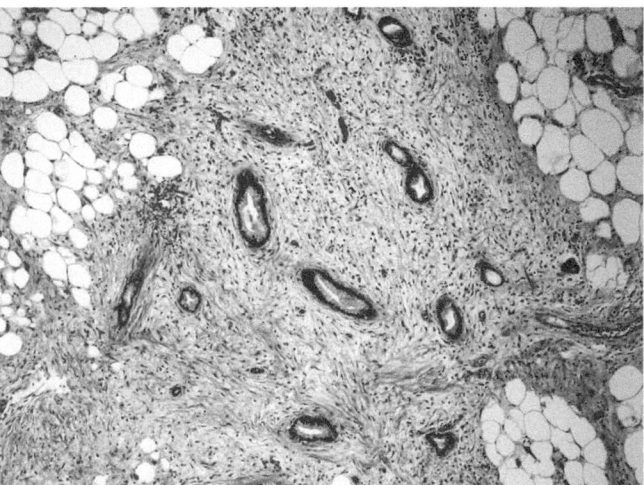

Figure 8-11. Well-differentiated infiltrating adenocarcinoma. Medium-power view shows a haphazard arrangement of the glands and the associated desmoplastic stroma.

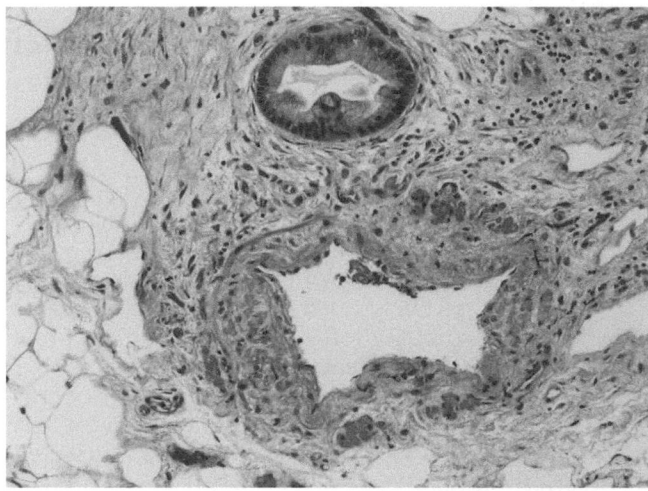

Figure 8-12. Well-differentiated infiltrating adenocarcinoma. This gland is immediately adjacent to a muscular vessel, a clue to the diagnosis of invasive carcinoma.

- Colloid carcinoma
  - Prominent extracellular mucin production with neoplastic cells "floating" in pools of extracellular stromal mucin (Figure 8-13)
  - By definition, at least 80% of the neoplasm has to have colloid differentiation
  - Almost always arises in association with an intraductal papillary mucinous neoplasm
- Hepatoid carcinoma
  - Large pink cell with prominent liver differentiation including the formation of trabeculae and sometimes even bile production
  - May express HepPar-1
  - Need to exclude a liver primary
- Medullary carcinoma
  - Poorly differentiated carcinoma with syncytial growth pattern, pushing boarders and an associated lymphocytic infiltrate
  - Usually microsatellite unstable

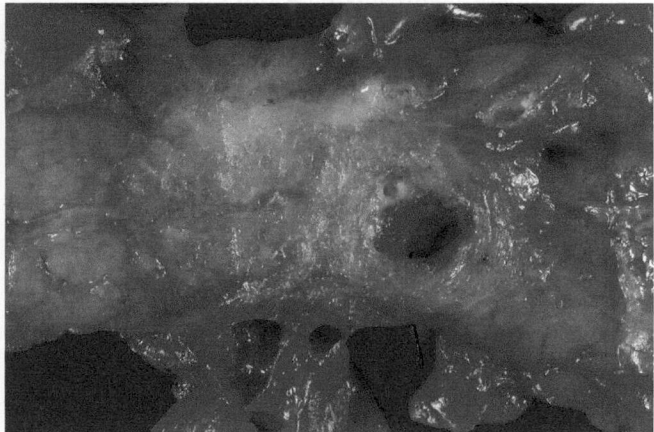

Figure 8-10. Infiltrating ductal adenocarcinoma. The lesion is a poorly defined infiltrating sclerotic mass arising in the body of the pancreas. Note the upstream dilatation of the pancreatic duct.

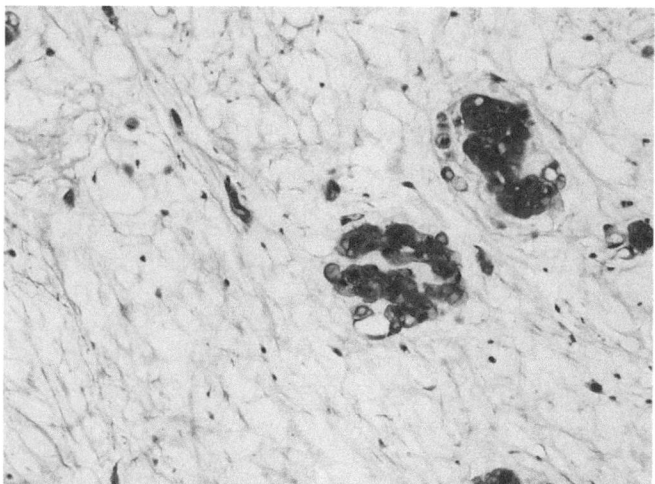

Figure 8-13. Colloid carcinoma. Neoplastic glands "float" in large pools of extracellular stromal mucin.

- Signet ring cell carcinoma
  - Infiltrating round noncohesive cells with prominent intracytoplasmic mucin vacuole
  - Loss of e-cadherin expression
  - Need to exclude gastric and breast primaries before making the diagnosis in the pancreas
- Undifferentiated carcinoma
  - Epithelial neoplasm without a definite direction of differentiation
  - Cells maybe large and bizarre in shape ("anaplastic"), they may be spindle shaped ("sarcomatoid"), or they may have a combination of glandular and spindle cell elements ("carcinosarcoma")
- Undifferentiated carcinoma with osteoclast-like giant cells
  - Neoplastic atypical mononuclear epithelial cells admixed with large nonneoplastic multinucleated osteoclast-like giant cells (Figure 8-14)

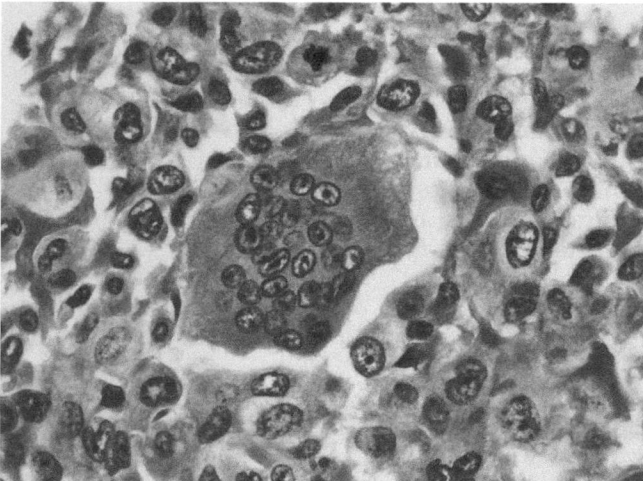

Figure 8-14. Undifferentiated carcinoma with osteoclast-like giant cells. High-power view shows a tumor composed of nonneoplastic large multinucleated osteoclast-like giant cells with uniform nuclei and admixed pleomorphic mononuclear neoplastic cells.

Special Stains and Immunohistochemistry

- Mucicarmine and periodic acid-Schiff (with and without diastase) stains highlight intracellular and extracellular mucin
- Immunolabeling for cytokeratin (7 and 19) will be positive, as is labeling for carcinoembryonic antigen, CA-19.9, and the mucin MUC1
- Loss of Smad4/Dpc4 expression observed in 55%

Other Techniques for Diagnosis

- Infiltrating ductal adenocarcinomas often harbor mutations in the *KRAS2, TP53, p16/CDKN2A* and *SMAD4/Dpc4* genes
- Medullary carcinomas frequently are microsatellite unstable
- Germline mutations in *BRCA2, STK11, PALB2, p16/CDKN2A, ATM,* and *PRSS1* genes are associated with increased risk for pancreatic cancer

Differential Diagnosis

CHRONIC PANCREATITIS
- Lobular arrangement maintained
- No perineural or vascular invasion
- No glands next to muscular vessels
- No luminal necrosis
- Complete lumina
- Only mild nuclear pleomorphism (< 4 to 1)
- Intact Smad4/Dpc4 expression, negative for CEA

ACINAR CELL CARCINOMA
- Cellular neoplasm with less desmoplastic stroma
- Acinar formations with basally placed nuclei and granular apical cytoplasm
- Single prominent nucleoli
- Expresses trypsin and chymotrypsin
- Immunolabel for bcl-10
- Negative for cytokeratin 7

PANCREATOBLASTOMA
- Squamoid nests
- Cellular neoplasm with less desmoplastic stroma
- Acinar formations with basally placed nuclei, granular apical cytoplasm, and single prominent nucleoli
- Expresses trypsin and chymotrypsin

SOLID-PSEUDOPAPILLARY NEOPLASM
- Predominantly in young women
- Neoplastic cells do not form true lumens
- Eosinophilic globules
- Cholesterol clefts
- Positive for CD10
- Nuclear labeling for beta-catenin

WELL-DIFFERENTIATED PANCREATIC NEUROENDOCRINE TUMOR
- Cellular neoplasm with less desmoplastic stroma
- Cells nest or form trabeculae
- Uniform nuclei with "salt and pepper" chromatin
- Positive for synaptophysin and chromogranin
- Negative for cytokeratin 7

METASTASES TO THE PANCREAS
- Clinical history of another primary
- Morphology unusual for a pancreatic primary including clear cells (renal primary) or signet ring cells (gastric or breast primary)
- Melanin pigment (melanoma)
- Absence of precursor lesions including IPMN and PanIN lesions

PEARLS

- *Despite their hugely different prognoses and treatment, adenocarcinomas of the pancreas can be difficult to distinguish from reactive glands of chronic pancreatitis; pattern of growth and location of the glands are the most helpful features*
- *Rule out metastases to the pancreas before diagnosing a primary signet ring cell carcinoma of the pancreas*
- *Pancreatic carcinoma has a very poor prognosis primarily because it is usually clinically detected at an advanced stage; early detection strategies would be expected to be very helpful in management and treatment*

SELECTED REFERENCES

Adsay NV, Bandyopadhyay S, Basturk O, et al: Chronic pancreatitis or pancreatic ductal adenocarcinoma? Semin Diagn Pathol 21:268-276, 2004.

Hruban RH, Pitman MB, Klimstra DS: Tumors of the pancreas. Atlas of Tumor Pathology, Fourth Series, Fascicle 6 ed. Washington, DC, American Registry of Pathology and Armed Forces Institute of Pathology, 2007.

Sharma S, Green KB: The pancreatic duct and its arteriovenous relationship: an underutilized aid in the diagnosis and distinction of pancreatic adenocarcinoma from pancreatic intraepithelial neoplasia. A study of 126 pancreatectomy specimens. Am J Surg Pathol 28:613-620, 2004.

ACINAR CELL CARCINOMA

Clinical Features
- Mostly in adults with a mean age of ~60 years
- Strikes males more than females, with a male-to-female ratio of 3.5 to 1
- Presenting signs and symptoms include weight loss, abdominal pain, nausea, and vomiting
- Fifteen percent present with metastatic fat necrosis, arthralgias, and peripheral eosinophilia caused by the release of lipase from the neoplasm

Gross Pathology
- Large well-circumscribed masses in head or tail of the pancreas (mean 10 cm)

Histopathology
- Most architecturally form acinar structures with basally oriented nuclei and granular apical cytoplasm
- Some form solid sheets of cells without well-formed acini
- Nuclei contain single prominent nucleoli (Figure 8-15)

Special Stains and Immunohistochemistry
- Immunolabel for trypsin, chymotrypsin, bd-10, and lipase

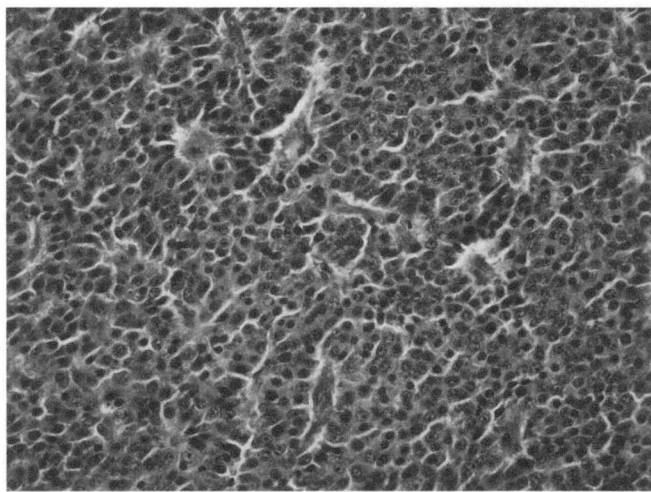

Figure 8-15. Acinar cell carcinoma. Although this particular example does not form well-defined acini, the single prominent nucleoli provide a clue to the diagnosis.

- Up to one third will have focal endocrine differentiation (if > 25%, then classify as mixed acinar-neuroendocrine)

Other Techniques for Diagnosis
- In contrast to ductal adenocarcinomas, acinar cell carcinomas rarely have *KRAS2* gene mutations

Differential Diagnosis

PANCREATOBLASTOMA
- The presence of squamoid nests distinguishes pancreatoblastomas from acinar cell carcinomas

WELL-DIFFERENTIATED PANCREATIC NEUROENDOCRINE TUMOR
- "Salt and pepper" nuclei
- Usually does not have single prominent nucleoli
- Diffusely expresses chromogranin and synaptophysin

SOLID-PSEUDOPAPILLARY NEOPLASM
- Predominantly in young women
- Does not form true lumens
- Eosinophilic globules
- Positive for CD10
- Nuclear labeling for beta-catenin

DUCTAL ADENOCARCINOMA
- Less cellular neoplasm with prominent desmoplastic stroma
- Gland formation with mucin production
- Nuclear pleomorphism
- Expresses cytokeratin 7, negative for trypsin, chymotrypsin, and lipase

PEARLS

- *Neoplastic cells with single prominent nucleoli should suggest the diagnosis of an acinar carcinoma*
- *Some grow as sheets of cells and do not form well-defined acini*
- *Mixed neuroendocrine-acinar carcinomas should be considered aggressive neoplasms similar to the pure acinar variety*

SELECTED REFERENCES

Hosoda W, Sasaki E, Murakami Y, et al: BCL10 as a useful marker for pancreatic acinar cell carcinoma, especially using endoscopic ultrasound cytology specimens. Pathol Int 63:176-182, 2013.

Hruban RH, Pitman MB, Klimstra DS: Tumors of the pancreas. Atlas of Tumor Pathology, Fourth Series, Fascicle 6 ed. Washington, DC, American Registry of Pathology and Armed Forces Institute of Pathology, 2007.

Klimstra DS, Heffess CS, Oertel JE, Rosai J: Acinar cell carcinoma of the pancreas: a clinicopathologic study of 28 cases. Am J Surg Pathol 16:815-837, 1992.

PANCREATOBLASTOMAS

Clinical Features

- Most, but not all, occur in children
- Associated with Beckwith-Wiedemann syndrome and familial adenomatous polyposis (FAP)
- Each presents clinically as a large abdominal mass
- Some patients have elevated alpha-fetoprotein levels

Gross Pathology

- Large well-circumscribed masses in head or tail of the pancreas (mean 10 cm)

Histopathology

- By definition, at least two components must be present: neoplastic cells with acinar differentiation and squamoid nests (Figure 8-16)
- Acinar formations have cells with basally placed nuclei and granular apical cytoplasm and single prominent nucleoli
- May also have cells with neuroendocrine and ductal differentiation
- Mesenchymal and primitive components may also be seen

Special Stains and Immunohistochemistry

- Acinar component expresses trypsin, chymotrypsin, and lipase
- Neuroendocrine component, if present, expresses chromogranin and synaptophysin

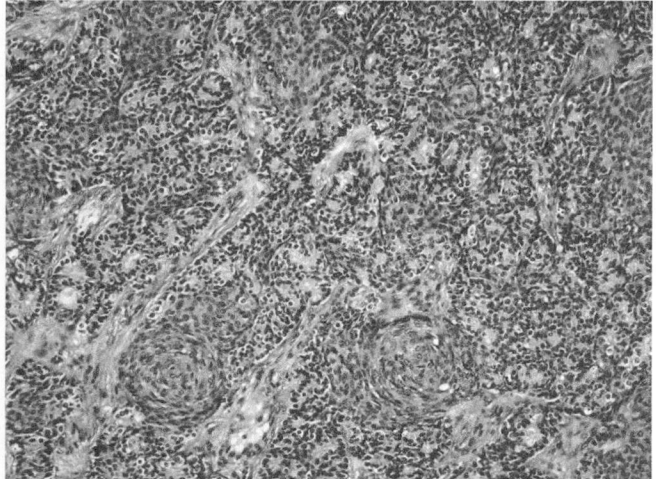

Figure 8-16. Pancreatoblastoma. Cells with acinar differentiation admixed with squamoid nests.

- Squamoid nests often not immunoreactive, but the nuclei of the cells in squamoid nests may contain biotin, which can cause a nonspecific labeling of these nuclei in immunostains

Other Techniques for Diagnosis

- Most have loss of heterozygosity of a highly imprinted region of chromosome 11p near the *WT-2* locus

Differential Diagnosis

ACINAR CELL CARCINOMA
- Usually, but not always, affects older patients
- Does not have squamoid nests
- Otherwise remarkably similar

WELL-DIFFERENTIATED PANCREATIC NEUROENDOCRINE TUMOR
- "Salt and pepper" nuclei
- Single prominent nucleoli are not typical
- Diffusely expresses chromogranin and synaptophysin

PEARLS

- *Should be thought of in children (but can occur in adults)*
- *Squamoid nests are key to the diagnosis*

SELECTED REFERENCES

Abraham SC, Wu TT, Klimstra DS, et al: Distinctive molecular genetic alterations in sporadic and familial adenomatous polyposis-associated pancreatoblastomas: frequent alterations in the APC/beta-catenin pathway and chromosome 11p. Am J Pathol 159:1619-1627, 2001.

Hruban RH, Pitman MB, Klimstra DS: Tumors of the pancreas. Atlas of Tumor Pathology, Fourth Series, Fascicle 6 ed. Washington, DC, American Registry of Pathology and Armed Forces Institute of Pathology, 2007.

Klimstra DS, Wenig BM, Adair CF, Heffess CS: Pancreatoblastoma: a clinicopathologic study and review of the literature. Am J Surg Pathol 19:1371-1389, 1995.

NEOPLASMS OF THE ENDOCRINE PANCREAS

WELL-DIFFERENTIATED PANCREATIC NEUROENDOCRINE TUMORS

Clinical Features

- Functional well-differentiated pancreatic neuroendocrine tumors (PanNETs) are associated with a clinical syndrome caused by the release of endocrine hormones by the neoplasm
- Functional PanNETs include insulinomas (hypoglycemia), glucagonomas (necrotizing migratory erythemia, stomatitis, and diabetes), gastrinomas (duodenal ulceration), and VIPomas (watery diarrhea, hypokalemia, and achlorhydria)
- Nonfunctional PanNETs may synthesize endocrine hormones, but do not produce a clinical syndrome
- Associated with multiple endocrine neoplasia type 1 (MEN1)
- Microadenomas are less than 0.5 cm
- Mitotic rate is an important prognosticator and should be well-documented

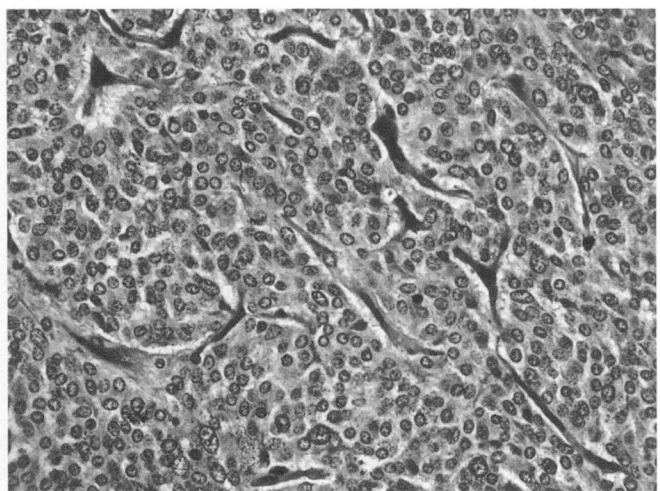

Figure 8-17. Well-differentiated pancreatic neuroendocrine tumor. Low-power view shows nests of uniform cells with "salt and pepper" chromatin.

Gross Pathology

- Arise in the head, body, and tail
- Well-demarcated
- Usually solid and soft, but some are cystic

Histopathology

- Cellular neoplasms with little stroma
- Nested or trabecular pattern of growth (Figure 8-17)
- Uniform nuclei with "salt and pepper" nuclei
- Amyloid deposition can be seen, especially in insulin-producing neoplasms
- Psammoma bodies are typically associated with somatostatin producing neoplasms

Special Stains and Immunohistochemistry

- Grimelius and Fontana-Masson stains positive
- Immunolabel with antibodies to chromogranin, synaptophysin, and CD56
- May immunolabel for specific hormones (insulin, glucagon, etc.)
- Immunolabel for cytokeratin (AE1/AE3 and CAM5.2), usually CK7 negative

Other Techniques for Diagnosis

- The MEN1 syndrome is caused by inherited (germline) mutations in the *MEN1* gene on chromosome 11q13
- May harbor mutations in *MEN1*, *DAXX*, *ATRX,* or the mTOR pathway genes

Differential Diagnosis

SOLID-PSEUDOPAPILLARY NEOPLASM

- Predominantly in young women
- Eosinophilic hyaline globules
- Poorly cohesive cells
- Cholesterol clefts
- Positive for CD10
- Nuclear labeling for beta-catenin

DUCTAL ADENOCARCINOMA

- Less cellular neoplasm with prominent desmoplastic stroma

- Gland formation with mucin production
- Nuclear pleomorphism
- Expresses cytokeratin 7, negative for chromogranin, synaptophysin, and CD56

ACINAR CELL CARCINOMA

- Acinar formation with basally placed nuclei and granular apical cytoplasm
- Single prominent nucleoli
- Expresses trypsin and chymotrypsin
- Acinar cell carcinoma can have a significant component with neuroendocrine differentiation (mixed acinar-neuroendocrine carcinomas), but the presence of histologic features of acinar cell carcinoma (acinar formation and large cells with prominent nucleoli) should distinguish these more aggressive neoplasms from the more indolent pure neuroendocrine neoplasms

PANCREATOBLASTOMA

- Squamoid nests
- Acinar formation with basally placed nuclei and granular apical cytoplasm and single prominent nucleoli
- Positive for trypsin and chymotrypsin

ISLET AGGREGATION IN CHRONIC PANCREATITIS

- Background of chronic pancreatitis
- Small focal lesion
- Polyclonal endocrine hormone production

PEARLS

- *Large PanNETs tend to be nonfunctioning as patients with functional neoplasms usually come to clinical attention early in the course of their disease*
- *All pancreatic neuroendocrine neoplasms > 0.5 cm should be considered malignant*
- *Mitotic rate is an important prognosticator and should be documented with immunolabeling for Ki-67*
- *Although functioning gastrinomas causing Zollinger-Elison syndrome can arise in the pancreas, they often arise in the duodenum in patients with the MEN1 syndrome*
- *When a hormone is expressed, insulinoma is the most common among neuroendocrine neoplasms arising in the pancreas*
- *Multiple synchronous or metachronous neoplasms may be observed in patients with MEN1*

SELECTED REFERENCES

Hruban RH, Pitman MB, Klimstra DS: Tumors of the pancreas. Atlas of Tumor Pathology, Fourth Series, Fascicle 6 ed. Washington, DC, American Registry of Pathology and Armed Forces Institute of Pathology, 2007.

Jiao Y, Shi C, Edil BH, et al: DAXX/ATRX, MEN1, and mTOR pathway genes are frequently altered in pancreatic neuroendocrine tumors. Science 331:1199-1203, 2011.

HIGH-GRADE NEUROENDOCRINE CARCINOMA (SMALL CELL CARCINOMA)

Clinical Features

- Rare neoplasm primarily in adults
- Affects males more often than females

- May be associated with a paraneoplastic syndrome such as Cushing syndrome
- Necessary to rule out a lung primary metastatic to the pancreas
- Extremely aggressive

Gross Pathology

- Solid white, poorly defined, often with necrosis

Histopathology

- Small round blue cell neoplasm
- Nuclear molding
- Minimal cytoplasm, inconspicuous nucleoli
- Extremely high mitotic rate (by definition, > 20 mitosis per 10 high-power fields, but usually much higher)

Special Stains and Immunohistochemistry

- Expresses cytokeratin, synaptophysin, and chromogranin
- Very high labeling index with Ki-67 (by definition >20%, but often exceeding 50%)

Other Techniques for Diagnosis

- In contrast to well-differentiated neuroendocrine tumors, *TP53* and *RB* are targeted in small cell carcinomas

Differential Diagnosis

PULMONARY SMALL CELL CARCINOMA METASTATIC TO THE PANCREAS

- Clinical history, imaging of the lungs

WELL-DIFFERENTIATED PANCREATIC NEUROENDOCRINE TUMOR

- Lower proliferative rate (<20 mitoses per 10 high-power fields)
- Uniform and more intense expression of synaptophysin and chromogranin

LYMPHOMA

- Uniform more dispersed sheets of round blue cells
- Lacks expression of neuroendocrine markers
- Expresses lymphoid markers (e.g., CD45)

PRIMITIVE NEUROECTODERMAL TUMORS (PNET) AND OTHER ROUND BLUE CELL TUMORS OF INFANCY AND CHILDHOOD

- Occur more commonly in pediatric patients
- Specific immunohistochemical and cytogenetic findings:
  - PNETs express CD99 and harbor the t(11:22)(q24;q12)) translocation
  - Intra-abdominal desmoplastic round cell tumors express desmin and harbor the t(11;22)(p13;q12) translocation
  - Rhabdomyosarcomas express MyoD

PEARLS

- *Small cell cancer of the lung must be excluded before establishing a pancreatic primary*

SELECTED REFERENCES

Manabe T, Miyashita T, Ohshio G, et al: Small carcinoma of the pancreas: clinical and pathologic evaluation of 17 patients. Cancer 62:135-141, 1988.
Yachida S, Vakiani E, White CM, et al: Small cell and large cell neuroendocrine carcinomas of the pancreas are genetically similar and distinct from well-differentiated pancreatic neuroendocrine tumors. Am J Surg Pathol 36:173-184, 2010.

NEOPLASMS OF UNCERTAIN DIRECTION OF DIFFERENTIATION

SOLID-PSEUDOPAPILLARY NEOPLASMS

Clinical Features

- Most occur in young women in their 20s and 30s, with a female-to-male ratio of 10 to 1 and a mean age of 30 years
- Present with nonspecific symptoms related to a large abdominal mass
- Rarely rupture producing hemoperitoneum
- Slow-growing, low-grade malignancy

Gross Pathology

- May arise in the head, body, or tail of the gland
- Solitary, often large (mean size 10 cm), well-demarcated masses
- Soft tan to yellow with areas of hemorrhage and cystic degeneration (Figure 8-18A)

Histopathology

- Uniform poorly cohesive cells (Figure 8-18B)
- Nuclear grooves
- Delicate branching blood vessels
- Hyaline globules (Figure 8-18C)
- Foam cells
- Cholesterol clefts

Special Stains and Immunohistochemistry

- Label with antibodies to CD10
- Nuclear labeling with antibodies to beta-catenin
- Hyaline globules label with antibodies to alpha-1 antitrypsin

Other Techniques for Diagnosis

- Beta-catenin gene mutations result in the nuclear accumulation of the beta-catenin protein

Differential Diagnosis

WELL-DIFFERENTIATED PANCREATIC NEUROENDOCRINE TUMOR

- Cells nest or form trabeculae
- "Salt and pepper" chromatin
- Expresses synaptophysin and chromogranin
- Membranous labeling with beta-catenin

DUCTAL ADENOCARCINOMA

- Less cellular neoplasm with prominent desmoplastic stroma
- Gland formation with mucin production
- Nuclear pleomorphism
- Expresses cytokeratin 7, negative for CD10
- Membranous labeling with beta-catenin

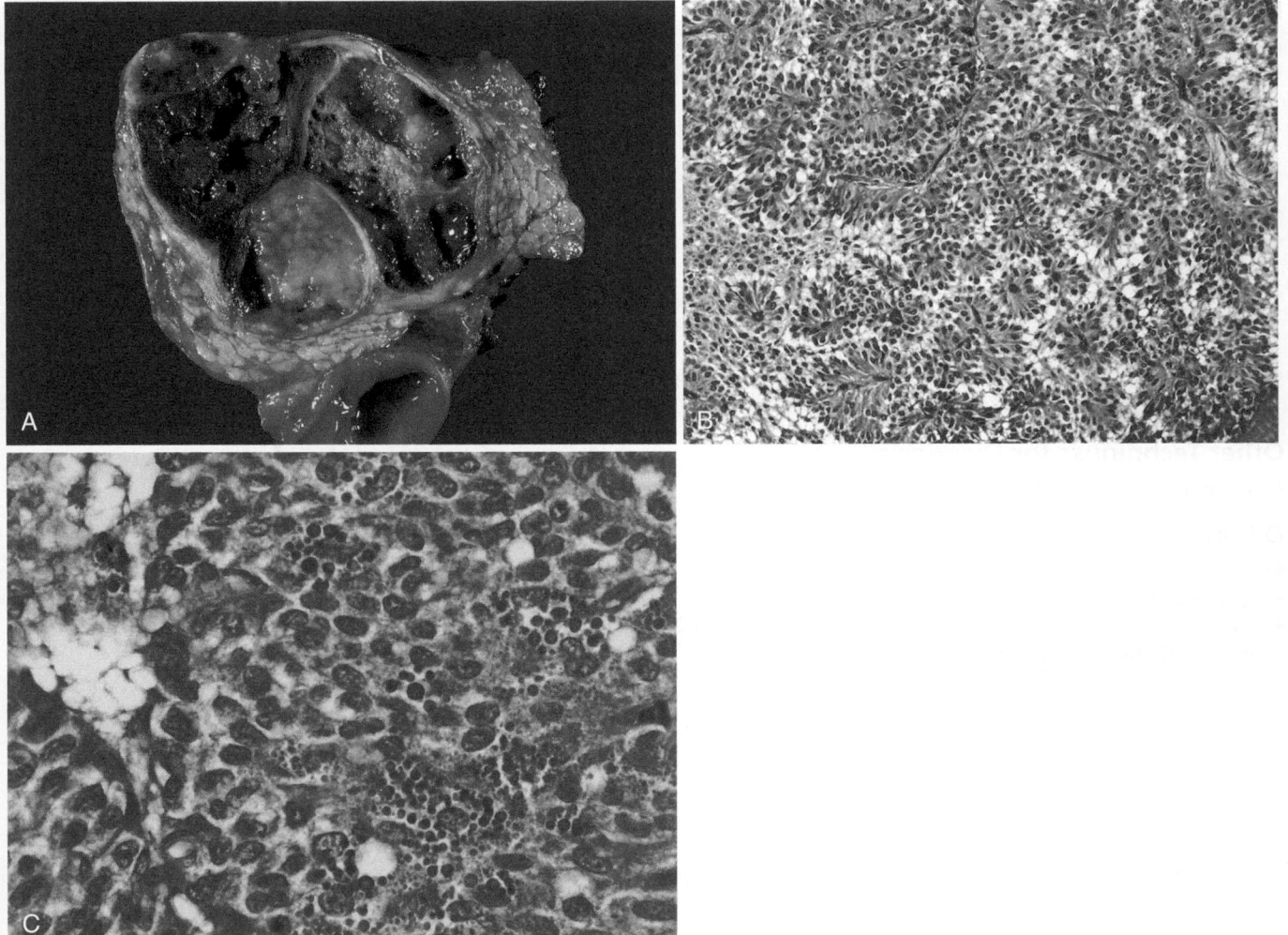

Figure 8-18. Solid-pseudopapillary neoplasm. A, Gross evaluation of the lesion demonstrates a predominantly solid lesion with areas of hemorrhage and cystic degeneration. **B,** Low-power view showing uniform poorly cohesive cells surrounding delicate blood vessels. **C,** Hyaline globules are a feature of these tumors.

ACINAR CELL CARCINOMA
- Acinar formation with basally placed nuclei and granular apical cytoplasm
- Single prominent nucleoli
- Label with antibodies to trypsin and chymotrypsin; most have a membranous pattern of labeling with antibodies to beta-catenin

PANCREATOBLASTOMA
- Squamoid nests
- Acinar formation with basally placed nuclei and granular apical cytoplasm
- Single prominent nucleoli
- Expresses trypsin and chymotrypsin

PEARLS

- *Should be at the top of the differential for a pancreatic neoplasm in a woman in her 20s and 30s*
- *Touch preparations can be extremely helpful in establishing the diagnosis, as they can highlight the delicate branching vasculature and poorly cohesive cells*
- *Hyaline globules are a clue to the diagnosis*

SELECTED REFERENCES

Abraham SC, Klimstra DS, Wilentz RE, et al: Solid-pseudopapillary tumors of the pancreas are genetically distinct from pancreatic ductal adenocarcinomas and almost always harbor beta-catenin mutations. Am J Pathol 160:1361-1369, 2002.

Hruban RH, Pitman MB, Klimstra DS: Tumors of the pancreas. Atlas of Tumor Pathology, Fourth Series, Fascicle 6 ed. Washington, DC, American Registry of Pathology and Armed Forces Institute of Pathology, 2007.

Klimstra DS, Wenig BM, Heffess CS: Solid-pseudopapillary tumor of the pancreas: a typically cystic carcinoma of low malignant potential. Semin Diagn Pathol 17:66-80, 2000.

METASTASES TO THE PANCREAS

Clinical Features

- History of a cancer in another organ

Gross Pathology

- Can be multiple
- Metastases from a renal primary are often yellow-orange in color
- Metastases from melanoma can be black/brown

Histopathology

- Clear cell neoplasm in metastatic renal cell carcinoma
- Signet ring cell neoplasm in metastatic gastric carcinoma and lobular carcinoma of the breast
- Melanin and single prominent nucleoli in metastatic melanoma

Special Stains and Immunohistochemistry

- PAX8, PAX2, CD10 and RCC mAb positive in metastatic renal cell carcinoma
- Gross cystic disease fluid protein (GCDFP), estrogen and progesterone receptor positive in metastatic mammary carcinoma
- S-100 protein, HMB-45, and melan-A positive in metastatic melanoma

Other Techniques for Diagnosis

- Noncontributory

Differential Diagnosis

DUCTAL ADENOCARCINOMA

- Prominent desmoplastic stroma
- Adjacent pancreatic intraepithelial neoplasia (PanIN) or intraductal papillary mucinous neoplasm
- Expresses cytokeratin 7
- About 55% have loss of Smad4/Dpc4

PEARLS

- *Know the patient's clinical history*
- *Radiology is crucial to the correct diagnosis*
- *Differentiation of pancreatic, biliary, and upper gastrointestinal tract neoplasms is difficult at best if one only relies on immunohistochemistry*

SELECTED REFERENCES

Adsay NV, Andea A, Basturk O, et al: Secondary tumors of the pancreas: an analysis of a surgical and autopsy database and review of the literature. Virchows Arch 444:527-535, 2004.

Chapter 9

Adrenal Gland

SYLVIA L. ASA • SANDRA E. FISCHER

CHAPTER OUTLINE

ADRENAL CORTICAL INSUFFICIENCY (ADDISON DISEASE)

Clinical Features

PRIMARY ADRENAL CORTICAL INSUFFICIENCY

- Etiology
  - Autoimmune etiology in 75% to 90% of cases, with circulating autoantibodies to endocrine antigens (21-OH, P-450scc, and 17-OH)
  - Other causes include infectious diseases such as tuberculosis, hemorrhage (sepsis), metastatic tumors, amyloidosis, adrenoleukodystrophy, and drugs
- Signs and symptoms: weakness, fatigue, salt craving, hypotension, anorexia and weight loss, hyperpigmentation (due to elevated adrenocorticotropic hormone [ACTH] and other pro-opiomelanocortin fragments)
- Biochemistry: decreased production of cortisol and aldosterone, elevated levels of ACTH and renin; hyponatremia and hyperkalemia may be seen as a result of decreased aldosterone
- Therapy: corticosteroid and mineralocorticoid replacement; fatal if not treated

SECONDARY ADRENAL CORTICAL INSUFFICIENCY

- Etiology: inadequate stimulation of the adrenal cortex as a result of low corticotropin-releasing hormone (CRH) or ACTH
  - May be seen after prolonged suppression of the hypothalamic-pituitary-adrenal axis by exogenous glucocorticoids or associated with destructive lesions of the hypothalamus or the pituitary gland
- Signs and symptoms: weakness, fatigue, anorexia, weight loss, hypopigmentation; hyperpigmentation does not occur
- Biochemistry: decreased cortisol and aldosterone as well as ACTH; renin and aldosterone levels are typically normal,

Gross Pathology

- Idiopathic form characterized by pale, shrunken adrenal gland, often weighing less than 2 to 3 g, with marked thinning of the cortical zone; severe atrophy may impair gross recognition of the adrenal glands
- Secondary forms often associated with adrenal enlargement and infiltration by inflammation or tumor (Figure 9-1A)

Histopathology

- Idiopathic form exhibits marked atrophy of the adrenal cortex, with intact medulla surrounded by fibrous tissue containing few small islands of atrophic cortical cells; lymphoid infiltrate is often present (Figure 9-1B, C, and D)
- Infiltrative forms due to inflammation or malignancy

Special Stains and Immunohistochemistry

- Special stains for microorganisms: may identify organisms in cases of infectious etiology

Other Techniques for Diagnosis

- Noncontributory

Differential Diagnosis

- One must distinguish between primary and secondary adrenal insufficiency
- If primary, one must attempt to determine etiology
  - Inflammatory; rule out infectious
  - Metastatic tumor
  - Amyloidosis (rare)

PEARLS

- *First described by Addison in 1855*
- *Must have destruction of more than 90% of adrenal gland before symptoms develop*
- *Immune form associated with autoimmune polyglandular syndromes (APS) type 1 and type 2 (Schmidt syndrome); APS type 1 is caused by mutations in the AIRE-1 gene*

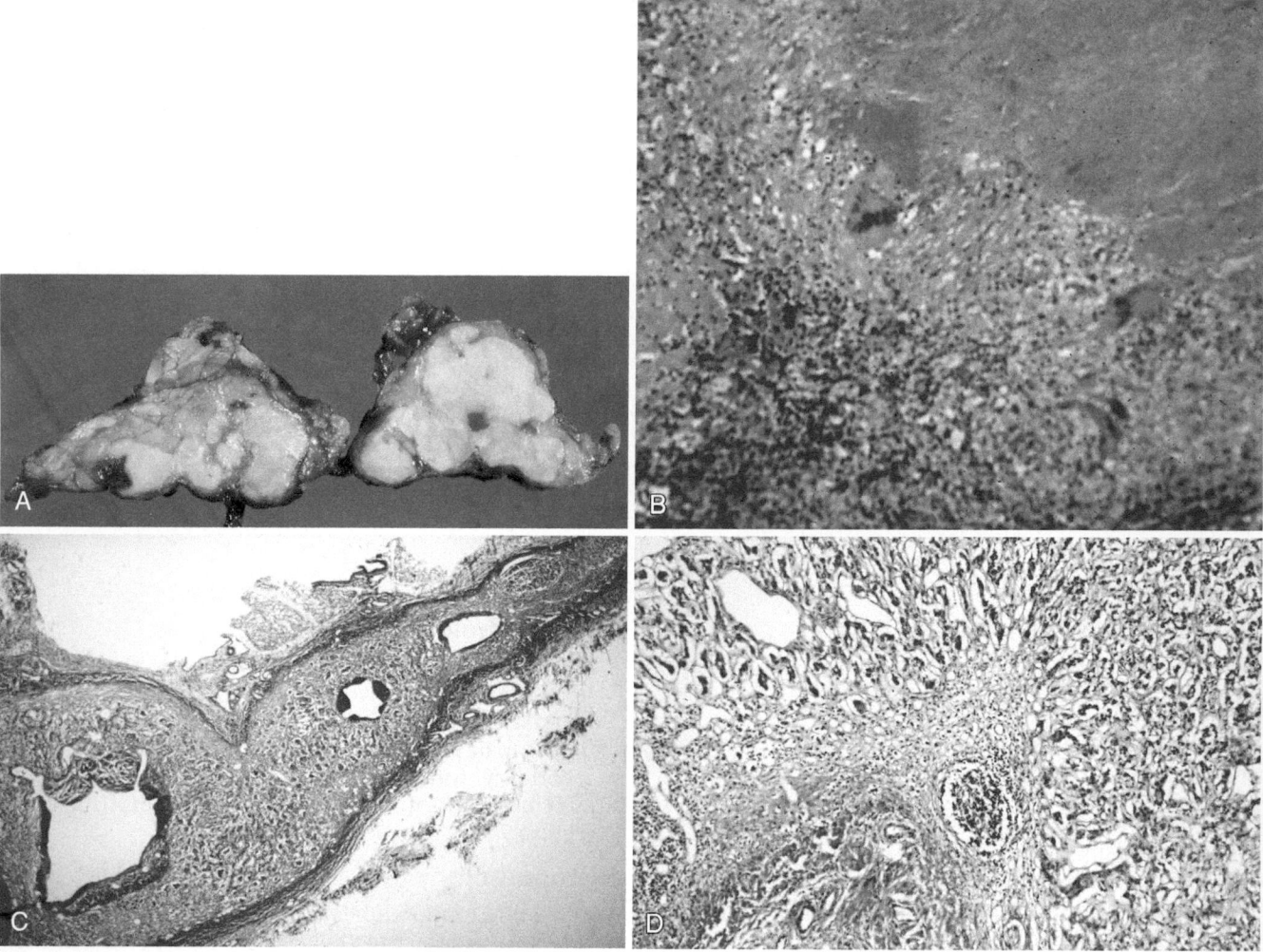

Figure 9-1. A, Addison disease due to tuberculosis infection. Tissue destruction due to tuberculosis infection results in adrenal enlargement, but the gland is replaced by necrotic yellow material. No normal tissue is identified. The surrounding fat is unremarkable. **B,** Addison disease due to tuberculosis infection. Caseating granuloma with giant cell reaction present in the adrenal cortex. **C,** Addison disease due to autoimmune inflammation. The adrenal is atrophic; the cortex is almost completely lost, and there is focal inflammation surrounding the residual medulla. **D,** Addison disease due to autoimmune inflammation. Inflammatory cells replace the cortex, and fibrosis is evident between the few residual cortical cells.

SELECTED REFERENCES

Fujieda K, Tajima T: Molecular basis of adrenal insufficiency. Pediatr Res 57:62R-69R, 2005.

Mitchell AL, Pearce SH: Autoimmune Addison disease: pathophysiology and genetic complexity. Nat Rev Endocrinol 8:306-316, 2012.

Shikama N, Nusspaumer G, Holländer GA: Clearing the AIRE: on the pathophysiological basis of the autoimmune polyendocrinopathy syndrome type-1. Endocrinol Metab Clin North Am 38:273-288, 2009.

Shulman DI, Palmert MR, Kemp SF: Adrenal insufficiency: still a cause of morbidity and death in childhood. Pediatrics 119:e484-e494, 2007.

Ten S, New M, Maclaren N: Clinical review 130: Addison's disease 2001. J Clin Endocrinol Metab 86:2909-2922, 2001.

CONGENITAL ADRENAL HYPERPLASIA (ADRENOGENITAL SYNDROME)

Clinical Features

- Etiology
  - Autosomal recessive disorder of cortisol biosynthesis resulting in impaired glucocorticoid feedback inhibition at the hypothalamic and pituitary levels, increased serum levels of CRH and ACTH, and adrenal hyperplasia
  - Results from a defect in one of the five enzymatic steps involved in steroid synthesis; 90% to 95% of cases are caused by deficiency of 21-hydroxylase, resulting in marked elevation of 17-hydroxyprogesterone, the main substrate for the enzyme
  - Unusual causes: 20,22-desmolase deficiency, 17α-hydroxylase deficiency, 3β-hydroxysteroid dehydrogenase deficiency, or 11 β-hydroxylase deficiency
  - Congenital lipoid adrenal hyperplasia
    - The most severe form of congenital adrenal hyperplasia (CAH), in which the synthesis of all gonadal and adrenal cortical steroids is markedly impaired
    - Lipoid CAH may be caused by a defect in either the steroidogenic acute regulatory (StAR) protein or P-450scc
- Epidemiology
  - Classic form occurs in 1 of 5000 to 15,000 live births
  - Nonclassic form occurs in 0.3% of the white population

- Signs and symptoms
  - Most common cause of ambiguous genitalia in newborn females; clinical presentation correlates with severity of 21-OH deficiency
  - Classic form
    - Can present as salt-wasting form or simple virilizing type
    - Newborn females typically show virilization at birth as a result of increased circulating androgens (clitoral hypertrophy and pseudohermaphroditism)
    - Postpubertal females have oligomenorrhea, hirsutism, and acne
    - Newborn males usually present with salt-losing crisis within days to weeks after delivery due to decreased synthesis of aldosterone (hypovolemia, hyperreninemia, and hyperkalemia can be life-threatening)
    - Males later show enlargement of external genitalia and precocious puberty
  - Nonclassic form
    - Affected individuals are normal at birth and do not have cortisol and aldosterone deficiency
    - Develop signs of androgen excess (virilization) in late childhood or puberty
    - May present as adrenal insufficiency during pregnancy
- Therapy
  - Pharmacologic treatment involves glucocorticoid and mineralocorticoid replacement and the use of androgen and estrogen antagonists
  - Bilateral adrenalectomy performed in selected cases
  - Gene therapy studies under way

Gross Pathology

- Bilateral adrenal gland enlargement with diffuse thickening of the cortex (Figure 9-2A)
- Adrenal glands may weigh up to 10 to 15 times normal weight
- Adrenals show a convoluted surface owing to numerous redundant folds

Histopathology

- Thickened adrenal cortex involving zona glomerulosa, zona fasciculata, and especially zona reticularis; poorly defined zonation (Figure 9-2B)

- Most cortical cells have lipid-depleted (compact) cytoplasm owing to sustained ACTH stimulation
- In lipoid CAH, the gland enlargement results from the accumulation of cholesterol esters in adrenal cortical cells; further damage with cell rupture and foreign-body granulomatous reaction to cholesterol clefts can be seen focally (Figure 9-2C)

Special Stains and Immunohistochemistry

- Noncontributory

Other Techniques for Diagnosis

- Genetic testing for 21-hydroxylase deficiency, or rarely 20,22-desmolase deficiency, 17α-hydroxylase deficiency, 3β-hydroxysteroid dehydrogenase deficiency, or 11 β-hydroxylase deficiency

Differential Diagnosis

ADRENAL CORTICAL HYPERPLASIA

- Primary hyperplasias are usually nodular unlike CAH; may be impossible to distinguish morphologically from ACTH-dependent hyperplasia

ADRENAL CORTICAL ADENOMA

- Discrete adrenal cortical nodule rather than diffuse hypertrophy, and usually unilateral

PEARLS

- *Defective adrenomedullary organogenesis owing to lack of glucocorticoids results in epinephrine deficiency and hypoglycemia*
- *Several reported cases of cortical adenomas and cortical carcinomas developing in children with congenital adrenal hyperplasia; may be related to persistent ACTH stimulation*
- *Adrenal cortical tumors may be seen developing in the testes/ovaries of patients with congenital cortical hyperplasia; believed to arise from ectopic adrenal cortical rests*

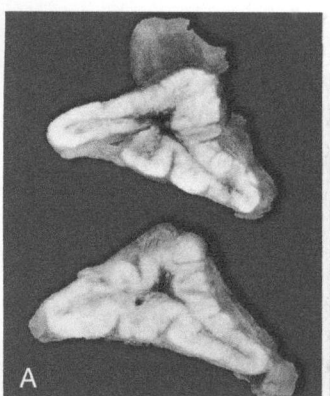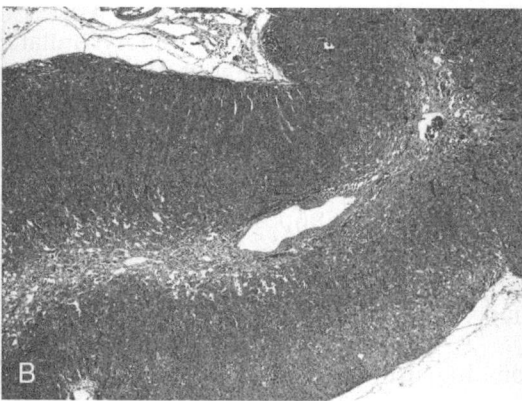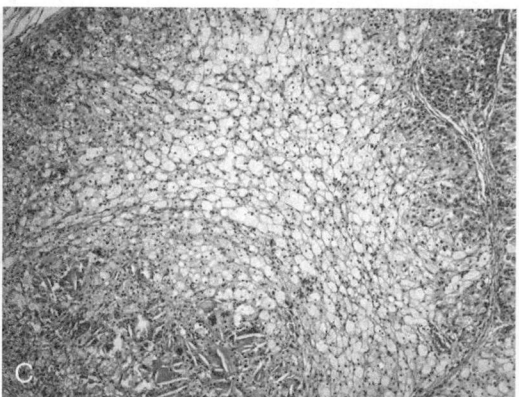

Figure 9-2. A, Congenital adrenal hyperplasia due to 21-hydroxylase deficiency. The adrenal glands are diffusely enlarged with lipid-depleted cortex. **B,** Congenital adrenal hyperplasia due to 21-hydroxylase deficiency. Microscopic examination of the diffusely enlarged gland shows a prominent cortex with poor zonation and predominantly compact cells. **C,** Lipoid congenital adrenal hyperplasia. The adrenal cortex is thickened by large clear adrenal cortical cells containing increased amount of lipid with focal cholesterol clefts and multinucleated giant histiocytes. (**A,** *Photo courtesy of Dr. Glenn P. Taylor, Hospital for Sick Children, Toronto.*)

SELECTED REFERENCES

Lekarev O, New MI: Adrenal disease in pregnancy. Best Pract Res Clin Endocrinol Metab 25:959-973, 2011.

Merke DP, Bornstein SR: Congenital adrenal hyperplasia. Lancet 365:2125-2136, 2005.

New MI, Abraham M, Yuen T, Lekarev O: An update on prenatal diagnosis and treatment of congenital adrenal hyperplasia. Semin Reprod Med. 30:396-399, 2012.

Ogilvie CM, Crouch NS, Rumsby G, et al: Congenital adrenal hyperplasia in adults: a review of medical, surgical and psychological issues. Clin Endocrinol 64:2-11, 2006.

Speiser PW, White PC: Congenital adrenal hyperplasia. N Engl J Med 349:776-788, 2003.

ADRENAL CORTICAL HYPERPLASIA

Clinical Features

- Two forms: primary (ACTH independent) and secondary (ACTH dependent)
- Etiology: depends on primary versus secondary
  - Primary adrenal cortical hyperplasia: due to germline mutations
    - Activating mutations of the ACTH receptor; illegitimate expression of membrane receptors (GIP receptor, β-adrenergic receptor, and LH receptor), and activating mutations of GNAS 1 in McCune-Albright syndrome result in ACTH-independent macronodular hyperplasia (AIMAH)
    - Inactivating germline mutations of the PRKAR1A and PDE11A genes are found in Carney complex and isolated primary pigmented nodular adrenal cortical disease (PPNAD)
    - Bilateral adrenal hyperplasia also seen in multiple endocrine neoplasia type 1 (MEN 1) syndrome and familial adenomatous polyposis
  - Secondary (ACTH-dependent) hyperplasia: due to ACTH excess from primary pituitary disease (corticotroph adenoma or hyperplasia) or ectopic ACTH production by tumors at other sites
- Signs and symptoms
  - Primary disorders may present with a variety of endocrine syndromes including Cushing syndrome, Conn syndrome, or virilization
  - Secondary disorder presents with severe Cushing syndrome, usually typical when pituitary dependent, and atypical (prominent wasting and pigmentation) when due to ectopic production by other malignancies
- Biochemistry
  - Variable, depending on clinical manifestations (Cushing, Conn, and virilization syndromes); ACTH levels usually low (suppressed) with primary forms and high in secondary conditions
- Therapy
  - Treatment of primary source of ACTH excess in secondary cases
  - Medical therapy to reduce glucocorticoid hypersecretion with ketoconazole, other drugs
  - Laparoscopic adrenalectomy for removal of adrenals followed by replacement therapies

Gross Pathology

- Non-neoplastic (polyclonal) condition consisting of nodular or diffuse hyperplasia of the adrenal cortex (Figure 9-3A and B)
- Degree of enlargement dependent on cause
  - Severe when due to ectopic ACTH or in ACTH-independent macronodular hyperplasia (AIMAH)
  - Mild to moderate with pituitary-dependent ACTH excess or PPNAD
  - Grossly undetectable when due to zona glomerulosa hyperplasia with Conn syndrome
- Almost always bilateral except for rare pigmented nodules showing prominent brown-black discoloration, which are more commonly unilateral
- Nodular form may show micronodules (< 1 cm) or macronodules (> 1 cm)
- Combination of nodular and diffuse types may be seen

Histopathology

- Adrenal cortex with diffuse hyperplasia or multinodular architecture, vague alveolar or trabecular pattern (Figure 9-3C)
- Cells are uniform in size with small, round nuclei
- Cells have vacuolated (clear) or eosinophilic (compact) granular cytoplasm
- Areas of lipomatous metaplasia may be seen
- Zona glomerulosa hyperplasia limited to periphery of gland, characterized by continuous layer of nests of cells with scant cytoplasm averaging five nests in thickness (Figure 9-3D)
- Mixture of large clear cells and small compact cells in AIMAH; pigmented nodules show enlarged, globular cortical cells with variable amounts of granular dark-brown pigment
- Cortical atrophy and disorganization of the normal zonation between nodules in PPNAD, as opposed to AIMAH, which shows characteristic interlobular hyperplasia

Special Stains and Immunohistochemistry

- PPNAD nodules stain for synaptophysin and 17α-hydroxylase cytochrome P-450; 3β-hydroxysteroid dehydrogenase staining is dominant in AIMAH nodules

Other Techniques for Diagnosis

- Noncontributory

Differential Diagnosis

ADRENAL CORTICAL ADENOMA

- Presence of solitary, unilateral lesions with evidence of autonomous growth favors adenoma
- Presence of small nodules adjacent to a larger nodule favors adrenal hyperplasia
- Definitive distinction between nodular hyperplasia and adrenal cortical adenoma can often be difficult or even impossible

PEARLS

- *Hyperplasia of the adrenal cortex (micronodular and diffuse) has been reported in cases of familial hyperaldosteronism type I (glucocorticoid-remediable aldosteronism), an autosomal dominant disorder caused by a hybrid gene formed by crossover between the ACTH-responsive regulatory portion of the 11 β-hydroxylase (CYP11B1) gene and the coding region of the aldosterone synthase (CYP11B2) gene; as a result, there is ACTH-responsive ectopic secretion of aldosterone in the zona fasciculata*

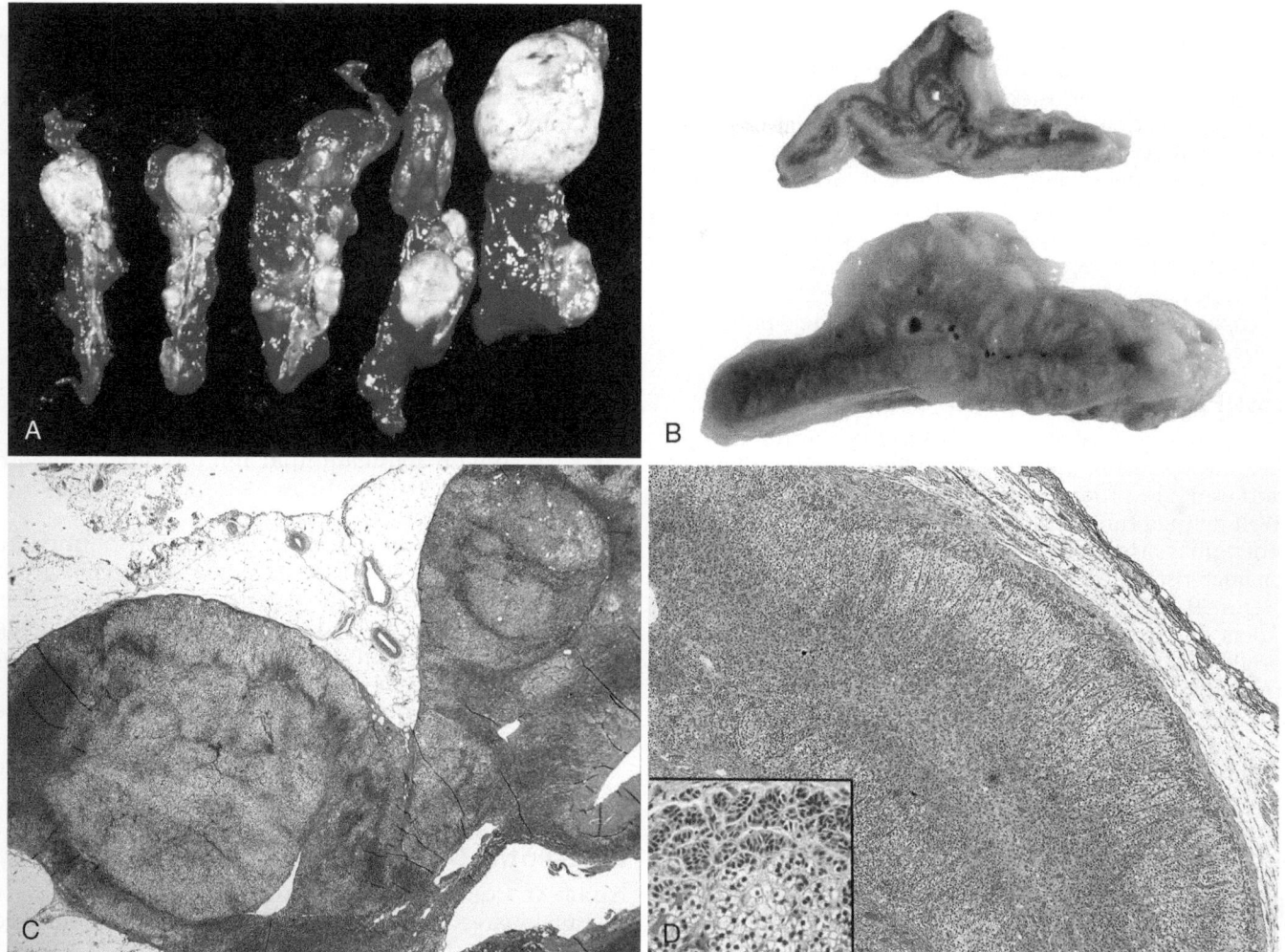

Figure 9-3. A, Macronodular adrenal cortical hyperplasia. Gross photograph showing multiple adrenal cortical nodules. **B,** Diffuse adrenal cortical hyperplasia. Gross photograph showing a normal adrenal gland (*top*) and a diffusely enlarged gland with a lipid-depleted cortex in a patient with ectopic adrenocorticotropic hormone syndrome (*bottom*). **C,** Macronodular adrenal cortical hyperplasia. Classic nodular adrenal cortical hyperplasia with multiple poorly defined cortical nodules composed of clear and compact cells. **D,** Zona glomerulosa hyperplasia. The adrenal gland is lined by a continuous layer of zona glomerulosa that is normally discontinuous. The cells are small and are on average five nests in thickness (*inset*).

SELECTED REFERENCES

Cazabat L, Ragazzon B, Groussin L, Bertherat J: PRKAR1A mutations in primary pigmented nodular adrenocortical disease. Pituitary 9:211-219, 2006.

Christopoulos S, Bourdeau I, Lacroix A: Clinical and subclinical ACTH-independent macronodular adrenal hyperplasia and aberrant hormone receptors. Horm Res 64:119-131, 2005.

Chui MH, Ozbey NC, Ezzat S, et al: Case report: adrenal LH/hCG receptor overexpression and gene amplification causing pregnancy-induced Cushing's syndrome. Endocrine Pathol 20:256-261, 2009.

Libe R, Bertherat J: Molecular genetics of adrenocortical tumors, from familial to sporadic diseases. Eur J Endocrinol 153:477-487, 2005.

Makras P, Toloumis G, Papadogias D, et al: The diagnosis and differential diagnosis of endogenous Cushing's syndrome. Hormones 5:231-250, 2006.

Mulatero P, Dluhy RG, Giacchetti G, et al: Diagnosis of primary aldosteronism: from screening to subtype differentiation. Trends Endocrinol Metab 16:114-119, 2005.

ADRENAL CORTICAL ADENOMA

Clinical Features

- Etiology
  - Most are sporadic with no known genetic basis
  - Association with familial disease (MEN 1, familial hyperaldosteronism, and congenital adrenal hyperplasia) can occur
  - Sporadic adenomas associated with Conn syndrome and hyperaldosteronism have mutations in the KCNJ5 potassium channel selectivity filter or in ATP1A1 and ATP2B3 encoding Na/K ATPases
  - Comparative genomic hybridization studies have demonstrated genetic alterations in 30% to 60% of adrenal adenomas; losses on chromosomes 2, 11q, and 17p, and gains on chromosomes 4 and 5 are the most common
  - *TP53* and *K-ras* mutations and loss of heterozygosity (LOH) of 11p15 and ACTH receptor are rare events in adenomas
- Signs and symptoms
  - Most adrenal cortical adenomas are asymptomatic (nonfunctional) and found incidentally
  - Patients may present with Cushing syndrome or hyperaldosteronism (Conn syndrome); virilization is rarely associated with adenomas, and feminization

in males is almost exclusively a sign of malignancy (see "Adrenal Cortical Carcinoma")
- Adenomas associated with Cushing syndrome and primary hyperaldosteronism are usually small and solitary; can rarely be multiple and bilateral
- Biochemistry
  - Variable, depending on clinical manifestations (Cushing, Conn, and virilization syndromes); ACTH levels usually low (suppressed), except in Conn syndrome
- Therapy
  - Laparoscopic tumor removal is the preferred treatment

Gross Pathology

- Adenomas associated with Cushing syndrome or hyperaldosteronism are usually solitary and unilateral and weigh less than 50 g (Figure 9-4B)
- Well-defined tumors appear encapsulated
- Adenomas associated with Conn syndrome have a characteristic bright-yellow or golden-yellow color (Figure 9-4A)
- Adenomas associated with Cushing syndrome may be bright yellow or tan and are associated with atrophy of the adjacent nontumorous gland
- All adenomas may show focal hemorrhage or necrosis (typically in larger lesions)
- Rarely, adenomas are diffusely pigmented black (pigmented adenoma) (Figure 9-4C)
- Oncocytic adrenal cortical adenomas have a dark-tan to mahogany-brown cut surface

Histopathology (Figure 9-4 D-H)

- Circumscribed tumor with pushing borders, lacks true capsule
- Typically has trabecular or alveolar (nesting) architecture
- Tumor cells are large and have round, regular nuclei with small, dotlike nucleoli; focal pleomorphism and large prominent nucleoli may be seen
- Absent or rare mitotic activity; never atypical mitoses
- Cytoplasm is abundant and "clear" or "compact"
  - In adenomas associated with Conn syndrome, cytoplasm is clear, lipid rich, and vacuolated; spironolactone bodies (small eosinophilic laminated intracytoplasmic inclusions) may develop in cells of the zona glomerulosa if patient is treated with spironolactone; these are best seen with the Luxol fast blue (LFB) stain
  - In adenomas associated with Cushing syndrome, cytoplasm may be clear or eosinophilic (compact), and in most tumors, both types may be seen
- Pigmented adenomas have cells with eosinophilic cytoplasm containing prominent granular yellow-brown pigment (lipofuscin)
- Oncocytic adenomas have cells with abundant granular eosinophilic cytoplasm; focal marked nuclear pleomorphism and nuclear pseudoinclusions may be seen
- Histologic appearance of the tumor cannot reliably predict accompanying clinical presentation; examination of the adjacent nontumorous gland is more helpful

- Atrophy of the normal cortex with loss of zona reticularis indicates Cushing syndrome with suppression of ACTH
- In patients with Conn syndrome, there may occasionally be hyperplasia of the zona glomerulosa (paradoxical hyperplasia)

Special Stains and Immunohistochemistry

- LFB for spironolactone bodies (Figure 9-4I)
- Immunohistochemistry for enzymes involved in steroidogenesis can distinguish function, but this is not used diagnostically
- MIB1 or Ki-67 labeling index usually below 2.5

Other Techniques for Diagnosis

- Electron microscopy
  - Cells contain abundant lipid and prominent smooth endoplasmic reticulum; mitochondria are also numerous (Figure 9-4J)
  - Mitochondrial morphology correlates with function: aldosterone-producing cells (zona glomerulosa differentiation) have flat, platelike, "lamellar" cristae, whereas glucocorticoid and sex steroid-producing cells (zona reticularis and fasciculata) have round or spherulated cristae (Figure 9-4K)
  - Pigmented adenomas contain many electron-dense granules consistent with lipofuscin (Figure 9-4L)
  - Spironolactone bodies are composed of concentric whorls of membranes

Differential Diagnosis

ADRENAL CORTICAL CARCINOMA

- Usually large mass with gross evidence of hemorrhage and necrosis
- Infiltrative borders typically invading into surrounding tissue
- Tumor cells show marked pleomorphism and frequent mitotic activity

EPITHELIOID ANGIOMYOLIPOMA

- An uncommon mesenchymal tumor with malignant potential, frequently associated with tuberous sclerosis complex
- Composed of sheets or nests of large polygonal epithelioid cells with abundant eosinophilic or occasionally clear cytoplasm, often with prominent nucleoli; may include multinucleated and markedly pleomorphic forms
- Exhibit immunoreactivity for both melanocytic and myoid markers
- Ultrastructural evidence of melanosomes and premelanosomes

PEARLS

- *Histologic appearance of adrenal cortical adenoma cannot be used to predict associated endocrine abnormality or syndrome, although the adjacent adrenal cortex may show atrophy (Cushing syndrome), or hyperplasia of the zona glomerulosa (Conn syndrome)*
- *Treatment is typically resection of the adrenal gland containing the adenoma*

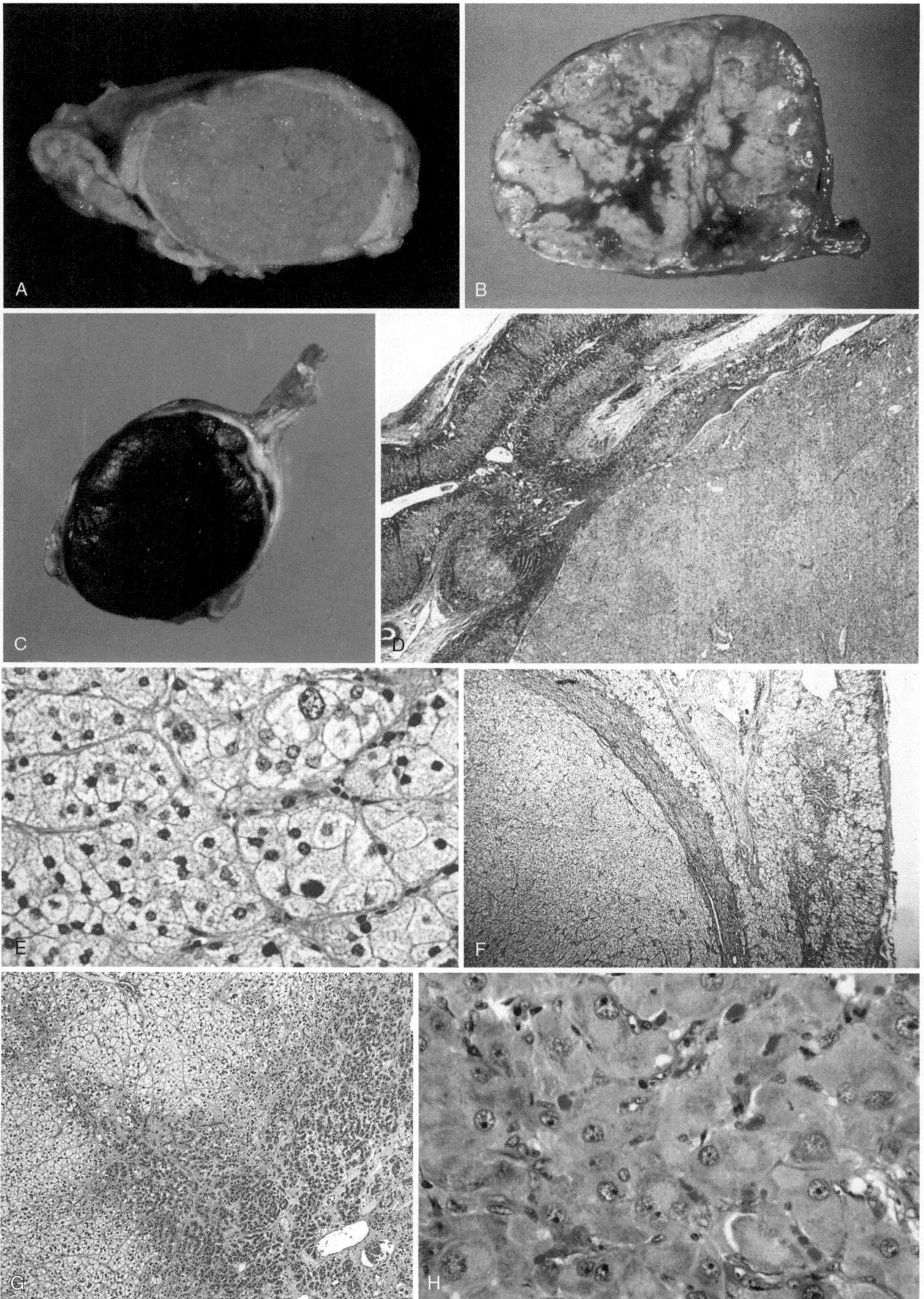

Continued

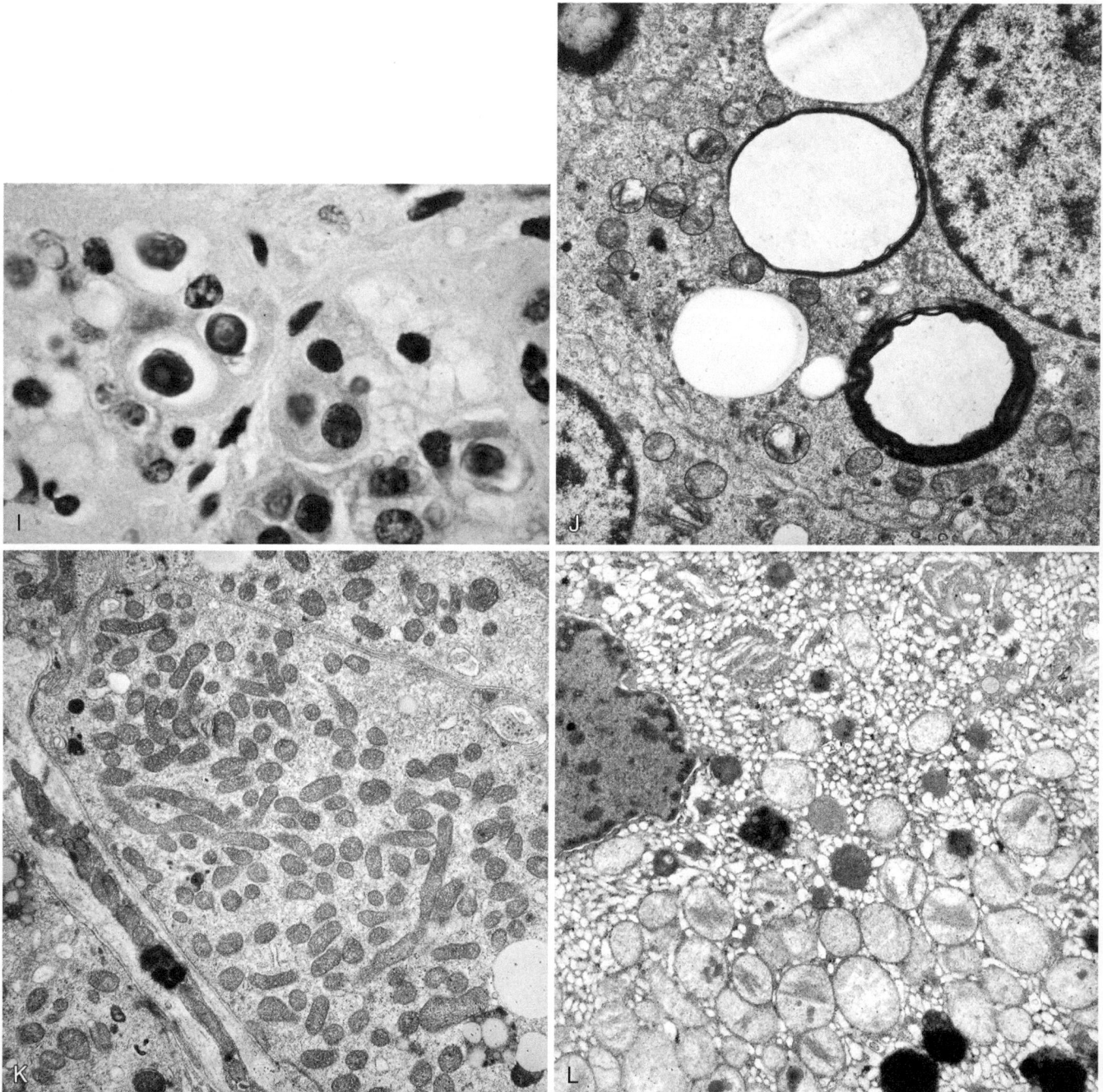

Figure 9-4. **A,** Adrenal cortical adenoma associated with Conn syndrome. Gross photograph shows that the tumor is well-delineated and bright golden-yellow. The adjacent adrenal is unremarkable. **B,** Adrenal cortical adenoma associated with Cushing syndrome. Gross photograph shows that the nodule is well-delineated and yellow with focal hemorrhage, and the adjacent gland shows marked atrophy. **C,** Adrenal cortical adenoma with pigmentation ("black adenoma"). Gross photograph shows that the nodule is well-delineated and dark black owing to pigment deposition. **D,** Adrenal cortical adenoma associated with Conn syndrome. On microscopy, there is a large, well-delineated but unencapsulated clear cell adenoma, and the adjacent gland has zona glomerulosa hyperplasia (see Figure 9-3D). **E,** Adrenal cortical adenoma associated with Conn syndrome. On microscopy, the tumor cells have abundant clear cytoplasm. **F,** Adrenal cortical adenoma associated with Cushing syndrome. On microscopy, there is a large, well-delineated but unencapsulated adenoma, and the adjacent gland exhibits marked atrophy with complete loss of the zona reticularis, indicating lack of adrenocorticotropic hormone stimulation. **G,** Adrenal cortical adenoma associated with Cushing syndrome. On microscopy, the adenoma has mixed clear and compact cell morphology with small round nuclei and abundant cytoplasm that varies from chromophobic to eosinophilic. **H,** Adrenal cortical adenoma, pigmented type. High-power view showing proliferation of a monomorphic population of adrenal cortical cells with large amounts of eosinophilic cytoplasm containing yellow-brown pigment. **I,** Adrenal cortical adenoma associated with Conn syndrome. The Luxol fast blue (LFB) stain highlights spironolactone bodies. **J,** Adrenal cortical adenoma associated with Conn syndrome. Electron microscopy shows that the tumor cells have abundant smooth endoplasmic reticulum; the mitochondria have flat platelike cristae, consistent with zona glomerulosa differentiation and mineralocorticoid production; and there are lamellated spironolactone bodies. **K,** Adrenal cortical adenoma associated with Cushing syndrome. Electron microscopy shows that the tumor cells have abundant smooth endoplasmic reticulum, and the mitochondria have tubulovesicular cristae, consistent with differentiation as steroid-producing cells. **L,** Adrenal cortical adenoma, pigmented type. Electron microscopy shows that the tumor cells have abundant smooth endoplasmic reticulum and numerous mitochondria, and there are large electron-dense granules consistent with complex lysosomes containing lipofuscin.

SELECTED REFERENCES

Beuschlein F, Boulkroun J, Osswald A, et al: Somatic mutations in ATP1A1 and ATP2B3 lead to aldosterone-producing adenomas and secondary hypertension. Nat Genet 45:440-444, 2013.

Funder JW: The genetic basis of primary aldosteronism. Curr Hypertens Rep 14:120-124, 2012.

Libe R, Bertherat J: Molecular genetics of adrenocortical tumors, from familial to sporadic diseases. Eur J Endocrinol 153:477-487, 2005.

Mete O, Asa SL: Morphologic distinction of cortisol-producing and aldosterone-producing adrenal cortical adenomas: not only possible but a critical clinical responsibility. Histopathology 60:1015-1016, 2012.

Mete O, van der Kwast TH: Epithelioid angiomyolipoma: a morphologically distinct variant that mimics a variety of intra-abdominal neoplasms. Arch Pathol Lab Med 135:665-670, 2011.

Mulatero P, Dluhy RG, Giacchetti G, et al: Diagnosis of primary aldosteronism: from screening to subtype differentiation. Trends Endocrinol Metab 16:114-119, 2005.

Ribeiro RC, Figueiredo B: Childhood adrenocortical tumours. Eur J Cancer 40:1117-1126, 2004.

Young WF Jr: The incidentally discovered adrenal mass. N Engl J Med 356:601-610, 2007.

ADRENAL CORTICAL CARCINOMA

Clinical Features

- Etiology
  - Sporadic adrenal cortical carcinoma is most common; however, it also occurs in hereditary syndromes: Li-Fraumeni, Beckwith-Wiedemann, MEN1, Carney complex, and hereditary isolated glucocorticoid deficiency syndrome
  - Sporadic carcinomas can harbor similar molecular defects, including germline and somatic mutations of *TP53*, *beta-catenin* and 17p13 LOH; rare *Menin* mutations, but frequent 11q13 LOH; 17q22-24 LOH (*PRKAR1A*); 11p15 LOH and *IGF-II* overexpression; 18p11 LOH (*MC2-R*)
- Epidemiology
  - Rare tumor; occurs in about 1 per 1 million population
  - Typically presents in fourth and fifth decades of life; less common in pediatric population
  - Equal incidence in males and females
- Signs and symptoms
  - Usually presents as incidental finding or associated with abdominal or flank pain; may present with a palpable abdominal mass or with evidence of distant metastasis
  - About 79% of carcinomas secrete hormones, and most functional tumors secrete cortisol with marked virilization owing to co-secretion of 17-ketosteroids and dehydroepiandrosterone (DHEA)
  - Less often, virilization in women and feminization in men can result from secretion of free testosterone and androstenedione, respectively
  - Mineralocorticoid excess is rare; however, combined secretion of cortisol and mineralocorticoid can occur
- Therapy
  - Tumor removal is the preferred treatment
  - Residual unresectable tumor or metastases treated with mitotane

Gross Pathology

- Usually large tumors weighing between 100 and 1000 g; may measure more than 20 cm (average, 14 to 15 cm) (Figure 9-5A)
- Irregular, variegated, tan-yellow mass with infiltrative borders
- Extension into adjacent soft tissue or surrounding organs is common
- Cut surface often shows extensive hemorrhage and necrosis

Histopathology

- Characteristic pattern is that of broad trabeculae with anastomosing architecture
- Other common patterns include solid or alveolar architecture
- Infiltrative growth pattern,
- Necrosis is common; often with calcification
- Tumor cells may resemble normal adrenal cortical cells; however, there is marked nuclear atypia, atypical and frequent mitoses (more than 5/50 high-power fields), vascular and extra-adrenal invasion, and necrosis (Figure 9-5B C and D)
- Although uncommon, intracytoplasmic eosinophilic hyaline globules may be seen and are better visualized with periodic acid–Schiff (PAS) staining
- Broad fibrous bands are a characteristic feature
- Diagnostic features of malignancy include size (weight, >100 g), vascular invasion, and metastasis

Special Stains and Immunohistochemistry

- Vimentin, inhibin-α, steroidogenic factor-1 (SF-1), and melan-A positive
- Cytokeratin may be negative or weakly positive
- Synaptophysin may be positive
- Chromogranin: negative
- Ki-67 labeling index may be helpful to separate adenomas from carcinomas and has prognostic relevance
- Beta-catenin nuclear translocation with loss of membrane staining
- P53 positivity may be diffuse and strong or negative when mutated
- Cyclin E: positive staining correlates with advanced stage

Other Techniques for Diagnosis

- Electron microscopy: prominent rough and smooth endoplasmic reticulum; mitochondria with spherulated cristae; intracellular lipid droplets may be seen; these features are useful to characterize metastatic lesions as derived from adrenal cortex (Figure 9-5E)
- Cytogenetic studies: 17p13 LOH, 11p15 uniparental disomy (UPD), and *IGF-II* overexpression are consistent findings

Differential Diagnosis

METASTASIS

- Separating adrenal cortical carcinoma from metastatic carcinomas from kidney and liver usually can be done using markers normally expressed in the adrenal cortex, including D11, SF-1, inhibin-α, and melan-A and markers of suspected primary site

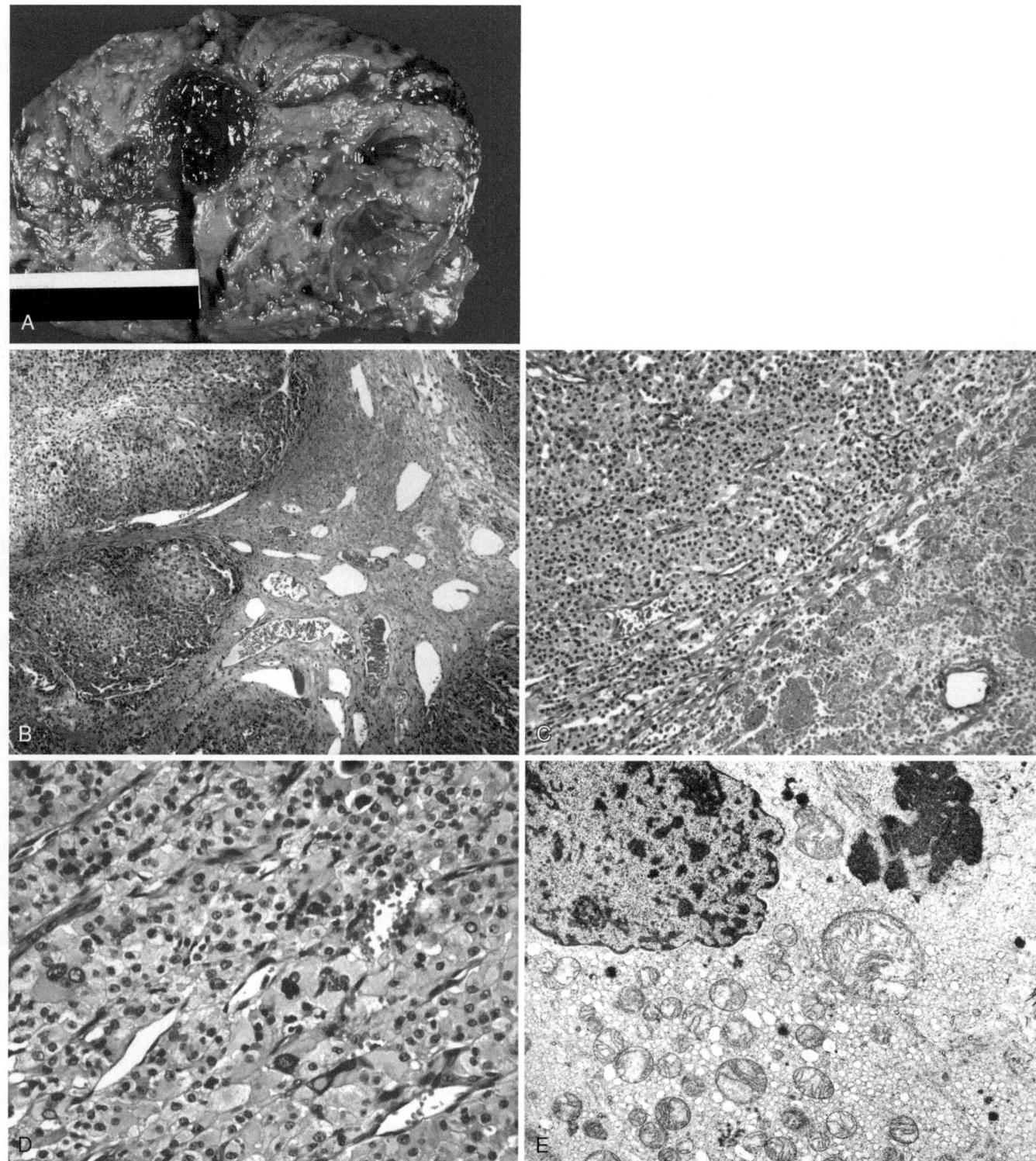

Figure 9-5. Adrenal cortical carcinoma. A, Gross photograph showing a large yellow tumor with areas of hemorrhage, necrosis, and cystic degeneration. **B** to **D,** On microscopy, the tumor is composed of a solid proliferation of neoplastic cells with moderately eosinophilic cytoplasm. There are areas of fibrosis **(B),** necrosis **(C),** and cytologic atypia **(D). E,** Electron microscopy characterizes the malignancy with prominent mitosis (*top right*) as derived from steroid-secreting cells by the prominence of smooth endoplasmic reticulum and the numerous large mitochondria with spherulated cristae.

ADRENAL CORTICAL ADENOMA

- Usually much smaller and lacks prominent hemorrhage or necrosis, pleomorphism, atypical mitotic figures, and vascular invasion

PHEOCHROMOCYTOMA

- Typically shows solid nesting architecture (Zellballen) with cells containing indiscreet cell borders, abundant intracytoplasmic hyaline globules, strong synaptophysin and chromogranin positivity, and S-100 protein highlighting sustentacular cells surrounding Zellballen

PEARLS

- *Adrenal cortical carcinoma has a high mortality rate, with death typically occurring within 2 to 3 years*
- *Large size, vascular invasion, and high mitotic rate are features of a more aggressive tumor*
- *Vascular invasion requires strict definition as in other endocrine glands: intravascular tumor cells with associated thrombus, but not tumor cells underlying intact endothelium*
- *Typical sites of metastasis include liver, lung, and lymph nodes*

SELECTED REFERENCES

Allolio B, Fassnacht M: Clinical review: adrenocortical carcinoma: clinical update. J Clin Endocrinol Metab 91:2027-2037, 2006.

Anselmo J, Medeiros S, Carneiro V, et al: A large family with Carney complex caused by the S147G PRKAR1A mutation shows a unique spectrum of disease including adrenocortical cancer. J Clin Endocrinol Metab 97:351-359, 2012.

Giordano TJ: Classification of adrenal cortical tumors: promise of the "molecular" approach. Best Pract Res Clin Endocrinol Metab 24:887-892, 2010.

Giordano TJ: The argument for mitotic rate-based grading for the prognostication of adrenocortical carcinoma. Am J Surg Pathol 35:471-473, 2011.

Libe R, Fratticci A, Bertherat J: Adrenocortical cancer: pathophysiology and clinical management. Endocr Relat Cancer 14:13-28, 2007.

Mete O, Asa SL: Pathological definition and clinical significance of vascular invasion in thyroid carcinomas of follicular epithelial derivation. Modern Pathol 24:1545-1552, 2011.

Morin E, Mete O, Wasserman J, et al: Carney's complex with adrenal cortical carcinoma. J Clin Endocrinol Metab 97:E202-E206, 2012.

Pan CC, Chen PC, Tsay SH, Ho DM: Differential immunoprofiles of hepatocellular carcinoma, renal cell carcinoma, and adrenocortical carcinoma. Appl Immunohistochem Mol Morphol 13:347-352, 2005.

Saeger W, Fassnacht M, Chita R, et al: High diagnostic accuracy of adrenal core biopsy: results of the German and Austrian adrenal network multicenter trial in 220 consecutive patients. Hum Pathol 34:180-186, 2003.

ADRENAL MEDULLARY HYPERPLASIA

Clinical Features

- Etiology: usually associated with MEN IIA and MEN IIB syndromes
  - MEN IIA (Sipple syndrome) autosomal dominant syndrome includes medullary carcinoma of thyroid, pheochromocytoma, and parathyroid hyperplasia
  - MEN IIB autosomal dominant syndrome but usually de novo sporadic germline mutations; includes medullary carcinoma of thyroid, pheochromocytoma, neuromas of the lip, mucous membranes, and gastrointestinal tract, and parathyroid hyperplasia
    - Occasionally associated with cystic fibrosis or Beckwith-Wiedemann syndrome
    - Not seen in other familial pheochromocytoma syndromes (SDHx mutation syndromes, von Hippel-Lindau disease, neurofibromatosis)
- Signs and symptoms
  - May resemble pheochromocytoma with paroxysmal hypertension, diaphoresis, and tachycardia
- Biochemistry
  - Elevated urinary catecholamine and metanephrine levels
- Therapy
  - Surgical resection of one or both adrenal glands is often indicated in both familial and sporadic forms

Gross Pathology

- Usually bilateral, with increased adrenal gland weight
- May be diffuse or have nodular architecture
- Nodules must be less than 1 cm to be considered hyperplasia (nodules greater than 1 cm are considered pheochromocytoma)
- Nodules are typically distinct and have a gray-tan cut surface

Histopathology

- Diffuse thickening of the medulla and expansion into the tail of the gland, with or without nodule formation, and with an increased medulla-to-cortex ratio (Figure 9-6)
- Enlarged cells with or without pleomorphism and increased mitotic activity may be seen
- Hyaline globules are commonly seen in patients with MEN II
- No reliable morphologic criteria distinguish hyperplasia from pheochromocytoma apart from size, which is the best indicator for distinguishing these two entities

Special Stains and Immunohistochemistry

- Noncontributory

Other Techniques for Diagnosis

- Flow cytometry: tumor cells are usually diploid
- Germline mutation of the *ret* proto-oncogene can be detected by molecular studies in MEN II patients

Differential Diagnosis

- Distinction between nodular adrenal medullary hyperplasia and pheochromocytoma is currently based on the size of the lesion

PEARLS

- *Armed Forces Institute of Pathology (AFIP) has designated adrenal medulla nodules less than 1 cm as medullary hyperplasia and nodules greater than 1 cm as pheochromocytoma*
- *Medullary hyperplasia is believed to be the initial pathologic change in the adrenal gland, leading subsequently to the development of pheochromocytoma*

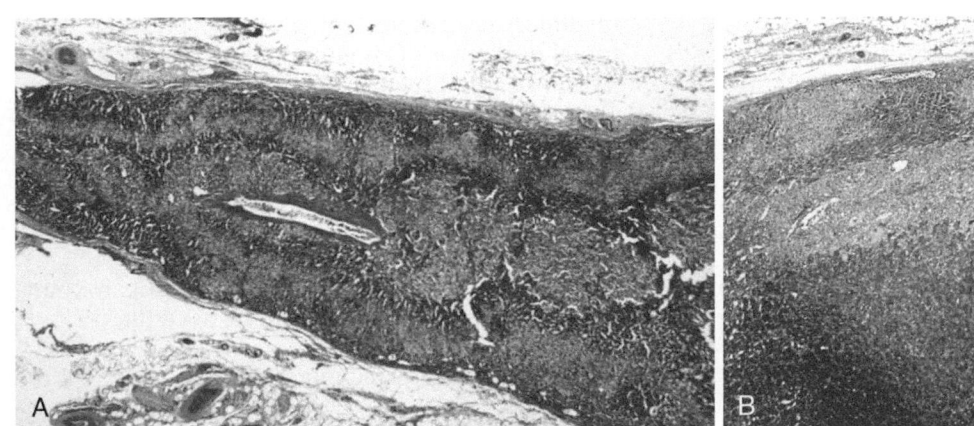

Figure 9-6. Adrenal medullary hyperplasia. A, Low-power view showing the adrenal gland with a diffusely hyperplastic medulla that extends all the way to the end of the wing. There is a suggestion of nodularity to the medulla. **B,** Low-power view showing the adrenal gland with nodules of hyperplastic medulla.

SELECTED REFERENCES

Carney JA, Sizemore GW, Sheps SG: Adrenal medullary disease in multiple endocrine neoplasia, type 2: pheochromocytoma and its precursors. Am J Pathol 66:279-290, 1976.

Carney JA: Familial multiple endocrine neoplasia: the first 100 years. Am J Surg Pathol 29:254-274, 2005.

DeLellis RA, Wolfe HJ, Gagel RF, et al: Adrenal medullary hyperplasia: a morphometric analysis in patients with familial medullary thyroid carcinoma. Am J Pathol 83:177-196, 1976.

Mete O, Asa SL: Precursor lesions of endocrine system neoplasms. Pathology 5:316-330, 2013.

Montgomery TB, Mandelstam P, Tachman ML, et al: Multiple endocrine neoplasia type IIb: a description of several patients and review of the literature. J Clin Hypertens 3:31-49, 1987.

Qupty G, Ishay A, Peretz H, et al: Pheochromocytoma due to unilateral adrenal medullary hyperplasia. Clin Endocrinol (Oxford) 47:613-617, 1997.

PHEOCHROMOCYTOMA

Clinical Features

- Etiology
  - Although classic teaching indicated that only 10% of pheochromocytomas were hereditary, more recent studies show that almost half of pheochromocytomas are hereditary; a small percentage of these are bilateral or multifocal, involving extra-adrenal paragangliomas
  - Germline mutations in *VHL* (3p26-25), resulting in von Hippel-Lindau disease; *RET* (10q11.2), resulting in MEN II; *NF1* (17q11.2), resulting in neurofibromatosis type 1 syndrome; or the succinate dehydrogenase genes *SDHA, SDHB, SDHC,* and *SDHD* (collectively "*SDH*x"), resulting in familial paraganglioma syndrome; other rare germline alterations implicated include mutations of *FP/TMEM127, KIF1Bbeta, PHD2/EGLN1,* and *MAX* (*MYC* associated factor *X* gene)
- Epidemiology
  - Sporadic tumors are usually diagnosed in patients aged 40 to 50 years, whereas hereditary forms are most often detected before age 40 years
- Signs and symptoms
  - Clinical presentation is paroxysmal and results from the direct actions of secreted catecholamines, including hypertension, tachycardia, pallor, headache, and anxiety; up to 25% of pheochromocytomas are asymptomatic
  - Anesthesia and tumor manipulation most often elicit a catecholamine crisis, but several drugs and food can also induce paroxysms
- Biochemistry
  - Diagnosis is made or confirmed based on measurements of urinary and plasma catecholamines, urinary metanephrines, and urinary vanillylmandelic acid (VMA)
- Imaging techniques
  - Computed tomography or magnetic resonance imaging and localization with functional ligands such as ^{123}I-MIBG
- Therapy
  - Laparoscopic tumor removal is the preferred treatment, after preoperative blocking of the effects of secreted catecholamines

Gross Pathology

- Variable size and weight (from few grams to > 2000 g)
- Round to oval, sharply circumscribed mass that is often encapsulated
- Cut surface shows a soft, variegated appearance with a dusky red-brown color (Figure 9-7A)
- Marked hemorrhage and necrosis may be seen; occasionally central cystic degeneration is seen
- Compression of the adjacent adrenal gland is common; tumor may cause marked attenuation of the adrenal gland around the tumor

Histopathology

- Tumor cells are arranged in well-defined nests, Zellballen appearance (Figure 9-7B and C)
- Distinct nests of tumor cells surrounded by thin strands of fibrovascular stroma that may (rarely) contain amyloid
- Rim of sustentacular cells may be seen at periphery of cell nests
- Tumor cells have varying size and shape with round nuclei, prominent nucleoli, and granular amphophilic to basophilic cytoplasm

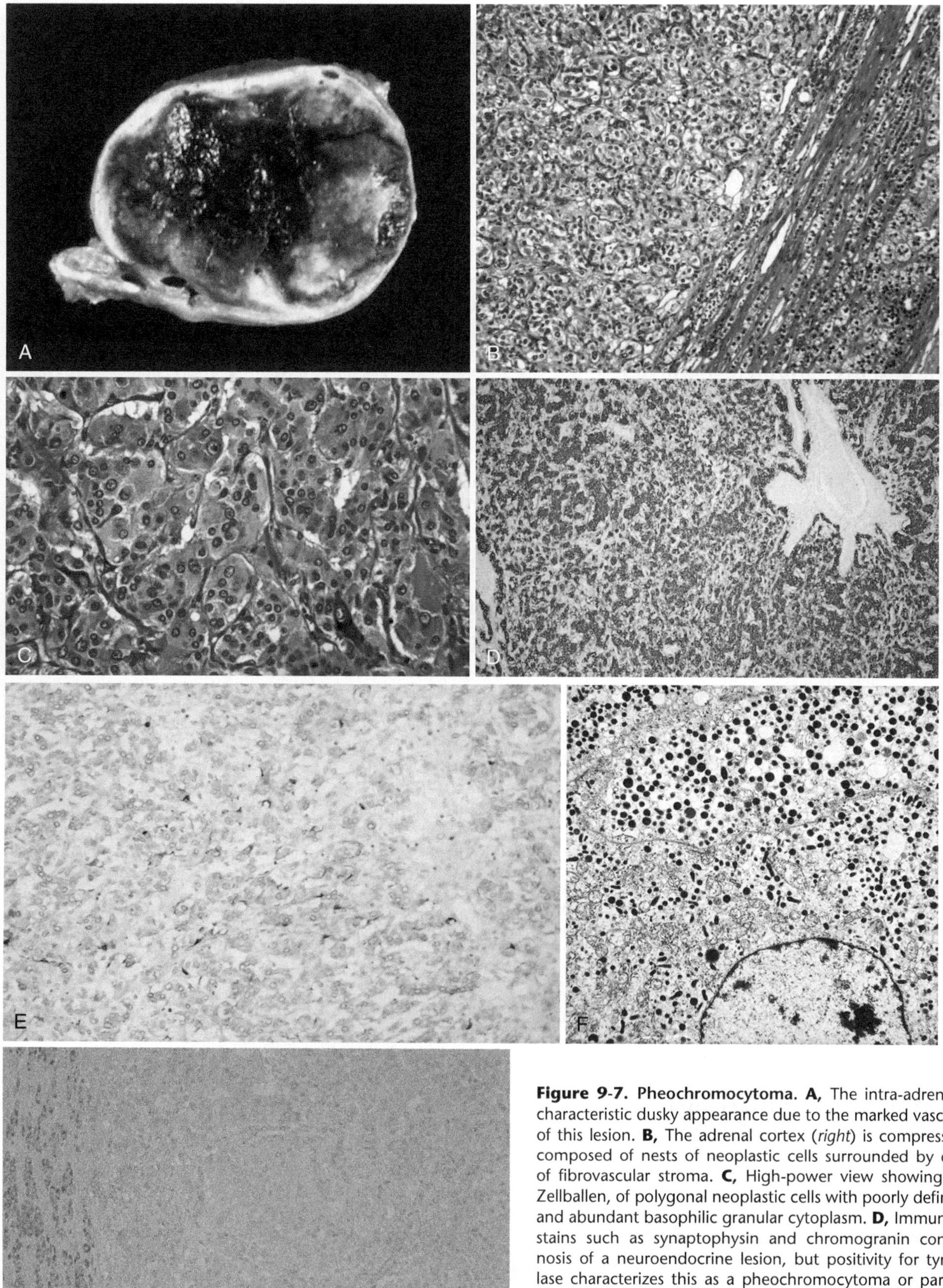

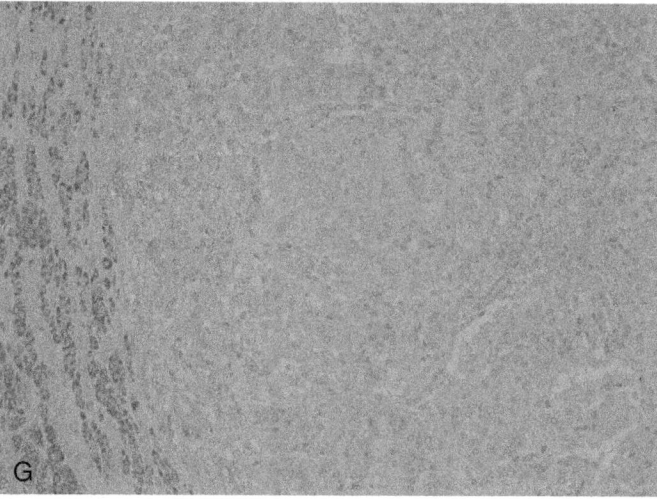

Figure 9-7. Pheochromocytoma. A, The intra-adrenal tumor has a characteristic dusky appearance due to the marked vascular congestion of this lesion. **B,** The adrenal cortex (*right*) is compressed by a tumor composed of nests of neoplastic cells surrounded by delicate strands of fibrovascular stroma. **C,** High-power view showing solid nests, or Zellballen, of polygonal neoplastic cells with poorly defined cell borders and abundant basophilic granular cytoplasm. **D,** Immunohistochemical stains such as synaptophysin and chromogranin confirm the diagnosis of a neuroendocrine lesion, but positivity for tyrosine hydroxylase characterizes this as a pheochromocytoma or paraganglioma. **E,** Immunohistochemical localization of S-100 protein decorates sustentacular cells that surround the nests of tumor cells. **F,** Electron microscopy identifies abundant electron-dense membrane-bound secretory granules of variable size and shape. **G,** Immunohistochemistry for SDHB is negative in this pheochromocytoma from a patient with a known SDHD mutation; the surrounding nontumorous gland retains positivity, consistent with no loss of heterozygosity in normal tissue.

- Nuclei often show inclusion-like structures due to intranuclear cytoplasmic invaginations
- Marked pleomorphism with bizarre tumor giant cells and numerous mitotic figures may be seen; *these features are not diagnostic of malignant behavior*
- Occasional tumors of patients with von Hippel-Lindau disease have marked stromal edema and lipid degeneration
- Tumors of patients with MEN II may be associated with adrenal medullary hyperplasia and may be multiple or bilateral
- Composite pheochromocytoma is a pheochromocytoma with areas resembling neuroblastoma, ganglioneuroblastoma (GNB), or typical ganglioneuroma

Special Stains and Immunohistochemistry

- Chromogranin, synaptophysin, tyrosine hydroxylase positive (Figure 9-7D)
- S-100 protein: immunoreactivity of sustentacular cells surrounding Zellballen; stain often decreases in malignant tumors (Figure 9-7E)
- Neurofilament and serotonin may show positivity
- HMB-45 may show focal or faint positivity
- Ki-67 may be helpful to assess proliferative activity
- SDHB immunohistochemistry is a valuable screen for genetic predisposition since loss of SDHB is identified with any SDHx mutation (Figure 9-7G)

Other Techniques for Diagnosis

- Electron microscopy: cells contain numerous neurosecretory granules (Figure 9-7F)
- Cytogenetic studies: allelic losses on chromosomes 1p, 3p, 3q, 17p, and 22q are common in hereditary and nonhereditary pheochromocytomas

Differential Diagnosis

ADRENAL CORTICAL ADENOMA

- Typically, adenomas appear golden-yellow on gross examination; pheochromocytomas with lipid degeneration can have a similar gross appearance, but stains for chromogranin and synaptophysin are diagnostic

NEUROBLASTOMA

- Typically found in children younger than 4 years; composed of small round blue cells often with pseudorosette formation

METASTATIC NEUROENDOCRINE CARCINOMA

- These lesions are usually positive for keratins and negative for tyrosine hydroxylase

PEARLS

- *Malignant behavior cannot be determined based on morphologic findings; only presence of distant metastases proves malignancy*
- *SDHB mutations, usually found in patients with extra-adrenal paragangliomas rather than adrenal pheochromocytomas, are correlated with malignancy*
- *Metastatic spread through lymphatic or hematogenous pathways most commonly involves lymph nodes, bones (particularly ribs and spine), lung, and liver*

- *Benign, surgically treated tumors have a 5-year survival rate of more than 95%; the 5-year survival rate of patients with malignant pheochromocytoma is about 44%*
- *Pheochromocytoma is rare in children and is most often extra-adrenal, multifocal, and associated with hereditary syndromes*
- *Tyrosine hydroxylase immunoreactivity in pheochromocytomas is helpful to rule out neuroendocrine carcinomas*

SELECTED REFERENCES

Eisenhofer G, Tischler AS, de Krijger RR: Diagnostic tests and biomarkers for pheochromocytoma and extra-adrenal paraganglioma: from routine laboratory methods to disease stratification. Endocr Pathol 23:4-14, 2012.

Mete O, Tischler AS, De Krijger R, et al: Protocol for the examination of specimens from patients with pheochromocytomas and extra-adrenal paragangliomas. Arch Pathol Lab Med 138:182-188, 2014.

Pacak K, Eisenhofer G, Ahlman H, et al: Pheochromocytoma: recommendations for clinical practice from the First International Symposium. October 2005. Nat Clin Pract Endocrinol Metab 3:92-102, 2007.

Tischler AS: Pheochromocytoma and extra-adrenal paraganglioma: updates. Arch Pathol Lab Med 132:1272-1284, 2008.

GANGLIONEUROMA

Clinical Features

- Etiology
  - Ganglioneuromas can present as de novo tumors or may arise from neuroblastomas and GNBs that underwent spontaneous maturation or after treatment with chemotherapy
- Epidemiology
  - Rare benign tumors found in older individuals; the median age at diagnosis ranges from 5.5 to 10 years; with a slight female predominance (1.5:1)
  - The most common locations are the posterior mediastinum (41%), retroperitoneum (37%), adrenal gland (21%), and neck (8%)
  - Most common tumor of sympathetic nervous system in adults
- Signs and symptoms
  - Most often manifests as an asymptomatic mass
  - May present with symptoms of catecholamine excess, rarely with diarrhea
- Biochemistry
  - Usually no abnormalities
  - May have elevated VMA and homovanillic acid (HVA) levels
  - Increased secretion of vasoactive intestinal peptide (VIP) or serotonin may cause diarrhea
- Therapy
  - Tumor removal is the preferred treatment

Gross Pathology

- Large, well circumscribed, although a true capsule is uncommon
- Measure from 1 cm to more than 15 cm; average about 8 cm
- Firm consistency with homogeneous, solid, tan-yellow to gray-white cut surface
- Occasionally multifocal

Histopathology

- Composed entirely of ganglion cells and stromal elements represented by Schwann cells and mature fibrous tissue (Figure 9-8)
- Ganglion cells have compact eosinophilic cytoplasm with distinct cell borders and a single eccentric nucleus with a prominent nucleolus; may contain granular golden-brown pigment (neuromelanin)
- Variable numbers of ganglion cells may be present; few may be seen, making distinction from neurofibroma difficult
- Mitotic activity and necrosis are absent
- Mast cells may be present, although tumor does not contain neuroblasts or intermediate cells

Special Stains and Immunohistochemistry

- S-100 protein positive
- Synaptophysin: ganglion cells positive
- Ganglion cells also stain for neurofilament, Neu-N

Other Techniques for Diagnosis

- Electron microscopy: ganglion cells have an eccentric nucleus with a prominent nucleolus; cytoplasm shows peripheral rough endoplasmic reticulum, and neurosecretory granules

Differential Diagnosis

NEUROFIBROMA

- Lacks ganglion cell differentiation

PEARLS

- *Ganglioneuroma is believed to be the fully differentiated counterpart of peripheral neuroblastic tumors*
- *Considered a benign tumor; however, malignant transformation to malignant peripheral nerve sheath tumor (MPNST) has been reported*
- *Thorough sampling needed to rule out less well-differentiated areas; all friable or hemorrhagic areas must be submitted for microscopic examination*

SELECTED REFERENCES

Khan AN, Solomon SS, Childress RD: Composite pheochromocytoma-ganglioneuroma: a rare experiment of nature. Endocr Pract 16:291-299, 2010.

Lonergan GJ, Schwab CM, Suarez ES, Carlson CL: Neuroblastoma, ganglioneuroblastoma, and ganglioneuroma: radiologic-pathologic correlation. Radiographics 22:91-134, 2002.

Mora J, Gerald WL: Origin of neuroblastic tumors: clues for future therapeutics. Exp Rev Mol Diagn 4:293-302, 2004.

Tischler AS: Divergent differentiation in neuroendocrine tumors of the adrenal gland. Semin Diagn Pathol 17:120-126, 2000.

GANGLIONEUROBLASTOMA

Clinical Features

- Epidemiology
  - Most often seen in patients 2 to 4 years old, and exceedingly rare after the age of 10 years; occurs with equal frequency in boys and girls
- Signs and symptoms
  - Patients often present with an abdominal mass or with abdominal tenderness
  - Most common tumor site is the abdomen, followed by the mediastinum, neck, and lower extremity
- Therapy
  - Prognosis and response to therapy is significantly more favorable than those of neuroblastoma

Gross Pathology

- Well-circumscribed mass with a variegated cut surface
- Tumor appearance varies depending on the amount of mature to immature elements, ranging from predominantly solid to cystic
- Firm tan-white areas (better differentiated component) and hemorrhagic areas (poorly differentiated component) may be seen
- Granular calcifications are often present

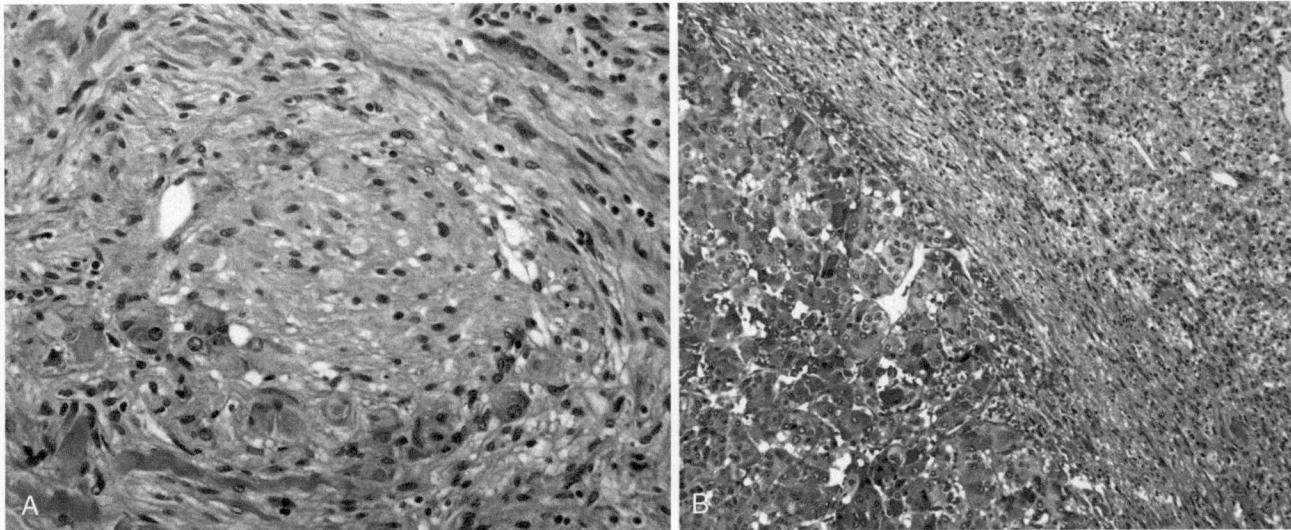

Figure 9-8. A, Ganglioneuroma. High-power view showing characteristic proliferation of spindle cells with wavy nuclei. Several classic ganglion cells are present in the center of the field. **B,** Composite pheochromocytoma and ganglioneuroma. The lesion consists of two components: a typical pheochromocytoma (*left*) and spindle cell ganglioneuroma (*right*).

Histopathology

- Shows histologic features similar to those of neuroblastoma, except that ganglion cell differentiation is present
- Variable amounts of neuroblastoma and ganglioneuroma are seen in the same tumor; typically the ganglioneuromatous component is in excess of 50% of the tumor
- Subtypes (International Neuroblastoma Pathology Committee)
  - *GNB: nodular classic* (abrupt transition between the neuroblastomatous nodule and the surrounding ganglioneuromatous component)
  - *GNB: nodular atypical* (no nodules are seen on gross or microscopic examination; ganglioneuromatous component is present as a thin rim; metastasis shows neuroblastomatous features)
  - *GNB: intermixed* (tumor is composed predominantly of gangliomatous component with well-delineated microscopic foci of neuroblastomatous component)
- These categories have prognostic significance: nodular has an unfavorable prognosis; intermixed has favorable prognosis

Special Stains and Immunohistochemistry

- Neuron-specific enolase (NSE), chromogranin, synaptophysin positive
- Neurofilament and Neu-N positive
- S-100 protein positive in spindle cell population

Other Techniques for Diagnosis

- Electron microscopy: cells with abundant filiform cell processes; cytoplasm showing distinct neurosecretory granules and neurotubules

Differential Diagnosis

Neuroblastoma

- Single population of small to medium-sized blue cells with no ganglion cells or evidence of differentiation

Ganglioneuroma

- Spindle cell population in a loose, myxoid background with distinct ganglion cells and no component of neuroblastoma

PEARLS

- *GNBs are transitional tumors of sympathetic cell origin that contain elements of both neuroblastoma and ganglioneuroma*
- *It has been suggested that nodular GNB evolves as a result of clonal proliferation of more aggressive malignant tumor cells in a neuroblastomatous component of what originally was a GNB of intermixed type maturing ganglioneuroma*
- *Nodules of nodular GNB may be identified by imaging studies and present with higher levels of urinary excretion of catecholamines compared with intermixed GNB and ganglioneuroma*

SELECTED REFERENCES

Guo YK, Yang ZG, Li Y, et al: Uncommon adrenal masses: CT and MRI features with histopathologic correlation. Eur J Radiol 62:359-370, 2007.

Joshi VV: Peripheral neuroblastic tumors: pathologic classification based on recommendations of International Neuroblastoma Pathology Committee (modification of Shimada classification). Pediatr Dev Pathol 3:184-199, 2000.

Koike K, Iihara M, Kanbe M, et al: Adult-type ganglioneuroblastoma in the adrenal gland treated by a laparoscopic resection: report of a case. Surg Today 33:785-790, 2003.

Rha SE, Byun JY, Jung SE, et al: Neurogenic tumors in the abdomen: tumor types and imaging characteristics. Radiographics 23:29-43, 2003.

Shimada H, Umehara S, Monobe Y, et al: International neuroblastoma pathology classification for prognostic evaluation of patients with peripheral neuroblastic tumors. Cancer 92:2451-2461, 2001.

NEUROBLASTOMA

Clinical Features

- Etiology
  - Malignant tumor of simpaticoadrenal lineage of the neural crest that can develop anywhere in the sympathetic nervous system
  - Genomic amplification of *MYCN* is common and consistently associated with poor outcome
  - Other biologic variables include deletions of 1p (25% to 35%), allelic loss of 11q (35% to 45%), and gain of 17q
- Epidemiology
  - Incidence of about 8 per 1×10^6 population; most common extracranial solid tumor of childhood
  - Accounts for more than 7% of malignancies in patients younger than 15 years; more than 85% occur in children younger than 4 years
  - Can occur in a variety of locations, with adrenal gland being most common site (50% to 80%)
  - Other common sites include posterior mediastinum (about 15%)
- Signs and symptoms
  - About 40% of patients present with localized disease ranging from an incidental adrenal mass discovered on prenatal ultrasound to large and invasive tumors
  - Classic signs of disseminated neuroblastoma include periorbital ecchymoses (raccoon eyes), proptosis, or both, due to metastasis to the bony orbit
  - Paraneoplastic syndromes include (1) intractable diarrhea and failure to thrive secondary to secretion of VIP and (2) opsoclonus-myoclonus syndrome (2% to 4%)
- Biochemistry
  - May produce catecholamines with increased levels of urinary VMA
- Therapy
  - Surgery, chemotherapy, radiotherapy, and biotherapy, as well as observation alone in selected cases, are used according to risk group based on the presence or absence of unfavorable biologic features

Gross Pathology

- Typically circumscribed, round to oval mass, often with a variegated, lobular cut surface; usually tan to gray-white (Figure 9-9A)

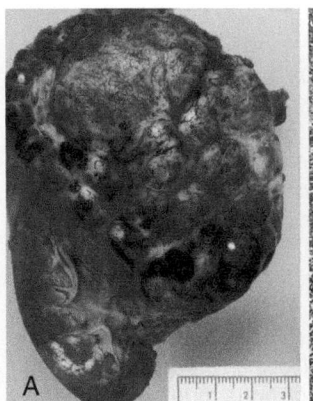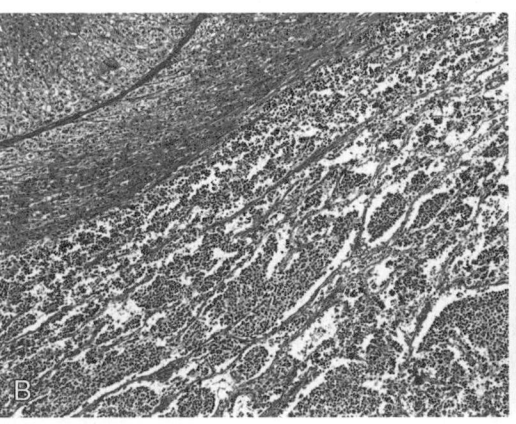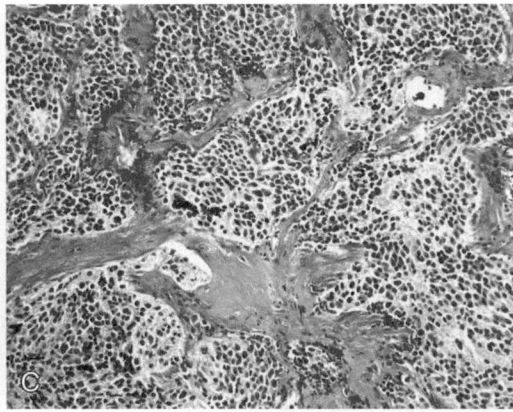

Figure 9-9. Neuroblastoma. A, The adrenal gland is replaced by a circumscribed, round to oval mass with a variegated, lobular appearance, invading into the kidney. **B,** Low-power view showing a monomorphic proliferation of small blue cells and adjacent residual adrenal cortex. **C,** High-power view showing a monomorphic proliferation of small blue cells with fine granular chromatin and indistinct cytoplasmic borders. Notice the fibrillary background. *(A, Photo courtesy of Dr. Glenn P. Taylor, Hospital for Sick Children, Toronto.)*

- May be variable in size ranging from less than 1 cm to greater than 10 cm
- Usually solitary and unicentric, but bilateral cases have been reported
- Typically solid but occasionally shows cystic degeneration
- Often shows marked hemorrhage, necrosis, or calcification
- Invasion into adjacent organs and soft tissue may be seen

Histopathology

- Cellular, small round blue cell tumor with vague lobular architecture (Figure 9-9B and C)
- Nodular aggregates of tumor cells separated by delicate fibrovascular septa
- Prominent Homer-Wright pseudorosettes (round spaces surrounded by palisading peripheral nuclei and filled with a faintly eosinophilic fibrillary matrix) may be seen
- Fibrillar matrix representing neuritic cell processes; resembles neuropil of the central nervous system
- Cells are medium sized and round to oval with high nuclear-to-cytoplasmic ratio and scant cytoplasm; hyperchromatic nuclei have stippled chromatin and inconspicuous nucleoli
- Hemorrhage and microcalcifications are common findings
- Variable mitotic activity
- Microscopic grading criteria (International Neuroblastoma Pathology Committee [INPC]): the criteria divide tumors into subtypes

- Neuroblastoma, undifferentiated: small, medium, or large round neuroblasts showing lack of differentiation or neuropil by routine light microscopy
- Neuroblastoma, undifferentiated, pleomorphic subtype: neuroblasts are large, with pleomorphic nuclei, prominent nucleoli, and moderate to abundant cytoplasm (some cells may have rhabdoid features); no neuropil
- Neuroblastoma, poorly differentiated: less than 5% neuroblasts show synchronous differentiation toward ganglion cells
- Neuroblastoma, differentiating: more than 5% neuroblasts show synchronous differentiation toward ganglion cells
- Mitosis karyorrhexis index (MKI) is based on percentage seen in 10 high-power fields (total of 5000 cells): less than 2% (low), 2% to 4% (intermediate), and more than 4% (high)
- Assessment of the MKI is crucial because it is used to determine prognostic categories (unfavorable versus favorable histology) in combination with the tumor differentiation and age of the patient (Table 9-1)

Special Stains and Immunohistochemistry

- NSE, chromogranin, synaptophysin positive
- Neurofilament and Neu-N positive
- S-100 protein: spindle cell population positive
- Cytokeratin positive
- Negative for desmin, myoglobin, vimentin, leukocyte common antigen (LCA), and CD99

TABLE 9-1	**PROGNOSIS FOR NEUROBLASTOMA**		
Age (Years)	**Differentiation**	**Mitosis Karyorrhexis Index**	**Prognostic Category**
<1.5	Undifferentiated	Any	Unfavorable histology
<1.5	Poorly differentiated or differentiating	Low or intermediate	Favorable histology
<1.5	Any	High	Unfavorable histology
1.5 to 5	Undifferentiated or poorly differentiated	Any	Unfavorable histology
1.5 to 5	Differentiating	Low	Favorable histology
1.5 to 5	Differentiating	Intermediate or high	Unfavorable histology
>5	Any	Any	Unfavorable histology

Other Techniques for Diagnosis

- Electron microscopy: characteristically shows cytoplasmic filaments, dense-core neurosecretory granules, and microtubules
- Cytogenetic studies: *MYCN* and 1p deletion by fluorescent in situ hybridization technique and DNA index by flow cytometry

Differential Diagnosis

GNB

- Shows evidence of differentiation in the form of ganglion cells, which may appear normal or abnormal

RHABDOMYOSARCOMA

- A rare tumor, usually arising in or around the kidney, composed of large tumor cells with eccentric nuclei and prominent nucleoli; large eosinophilic cytoplasmic inclusions are often seen
- Immunohistochemical stains: positive for desmin, negative for NSE, chromogranin, and synaptophysin

MALIGNANT LYMPHOMA

- Composed of diffuse sheets of atypical lymphoid cells without fibrovascular septa; lacks rosette formation and has no fibrillary matrix
- CD45 (LCA) positive; negative for NSE, chromogranin, and synaptophysin

EWING SARCOMA

- Typically found in long bones and occasionally in soft tissue
- Tumor cells frequently show intracytoplasmic glycogen (PAS positive) and are positive for CD99, negative for chromogranin and synaptophysin
- This tumor has a characteristic t(11;22) translocation

NEPHROBLASTOMA (WILMS TUMOR)

- Shows triphasic pattern consisting of blastema, stromal, and epithelial components
- Negative for synaptophysin, chromogranin, and NSE

PEARLS

- *DNA index is a prognostic marker for patients younger than 2 years with disseminated disease: near-diploid DNA content is associated with genomic instability and worse outcome, whereas hyperdiploidy (often near-triploidy) appears to be favorable*
- *May exhibit familial incidence (1% to 2%); may be associated with Hirschsprung disease, congenital central hypoventilation, pheochromocytoma, and neurofibromatosis type 1*
- *4S disease refers to stage 4S (S, special) that occurs in 5% of patients showing small localized primary tumors with metastasis in liver, skin, or bone marrow that almost always spontaneously regress (massive hepatomegaly can cause respiratory compromise in infants younger than 2 months) (Table 9-2)*

SELECTED REFERENCES

Fisher JP, Tweddle DA: Neonatal neuroblastoma. Semin Fetal Neonatal Med 17:207-215, 2012.

Maris JM, Hogarty MD, Bagatell R, Cohn SL: Neuroblastoma. Lancet 369:2106-2120, 2007.

Tan C, Sabai SM, Tin AS, et al: Neuroblastoma: experience from National University Health System, Singapore (1987-2008). Singapore Med J 53:19-25, 2012.

PRIMARY MALIGNANT MELANOMA

Clinical Features

- First observation in 1946; rare tumor with rigid diagnostic criteria
  - Only one adrenal gland involved
  - No medical history of melanoma or pigmented lesion
  - No evidence of endocrine disorders
  - Unequivocal histologic features of melanoma
- Epidemiology
  - Highly aggressive tumor that affects middle-aged adults; usually locally advanced with renal adhesions by the time of diagnosis

TABLE 9-2 NEUROBLASTOMA RISK GROUPS FOR PEDIATRIC ONCOLOGY GROUP AND CHILDREN'S GROUP CLINICAL PROTOCOLS

INS Stage	Age (Years)	MYCN Status	INPC Classification	DNA Ploidy	Risk Group
1	0-21	Any	Any	Any	Low
2A, 2B	<1	Any	Any	Any	Low
	>1-21	Not amplified	Any	—	Low
	>1-21	Amplified	FH	—	Low
	>1-21	Amplified	UH	—	High
3	<1	Not amplified	Any	Any	Intermediate
	<1	Amplified	Any	Any	High
	>1-21	Not amplified	FH	—	Intermediate
	>1-21	Not amplified	UH	—	High
	>1-21	Amplified	Any	—	High
4	<1	Not amplified	Any	Any	Intermediate
	<1	Amplified	Any	Any	High
	>1-21	Any	Any	—	High
4S	<1	Not amplified	FH	> 1	Low
	<1	Not amplified	Any	1	Intermediate
	<1	Not amplified	UH	Any	Intermediate
	<1	Amplified	Any	Any	High

FH, favorable histology; INPC, International Neuroblastoma Pathology Committee; INS, International Staging System; UH, unfavorable histology.

- Signs and symptoms
  - Presents as flank tenderness or palpable tumor; radiologic features are not specific
- Therapy
  - Surgical treatment (usually nephroadrenalectomy) is poorly effective, with a mortality rate near 100% in 2 years

Gross Pathology

- Unilateral brown to black tumor of variable size (8 to 17 cm)
- Cut surface often shows areas of hemorrhage and necrosis
- Gross appearance resembles pheochromocytoma

Histopathology

- Typical microscopic findings of malignant melanoma (Figure 9-10)
  - Large polygonal or spindle cells with marked nuclear polymorphism
  - Prominent nucleoli
  - Presence of abundant melanin pigment

Special Stains and Immunohistochemistry

- S-100 protein, Melan-A, HMB-45 positive
- Microphthalmia transcription factor positive
- Cytokeratin negative

Other Techniques for Diagnosis

- Electron microscopy: true melanin pigment seen in melanosomes or premelanosomes

Differential Diagnosis

PIGMENTED ADRENAL CORTICAL ADENOMA

- Usually associated with Cushing syndrome or primary hyperaldosteronism (Conn syndrome)
- Composed of cells with eosinophilic cytoplasm with a variable amount of golden-brown pigment (lipofuscin)
- S-100 protein and HMB-45 negative, but Melan-A positive

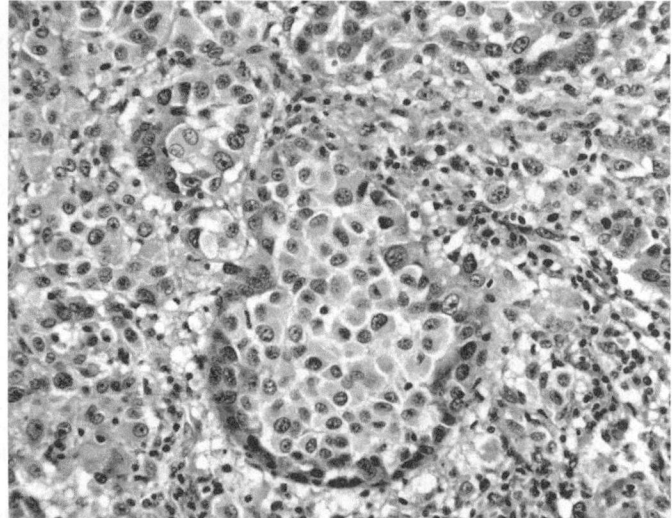

Figure 9-10. Malignant melanoma. High-power view showing large pleomorphic cells with abundant eosinophilic cytoplasm, large nuclei, and prominent nucleoli.

METASTATIC MELANOMA

- More common; it is often bilateral but otherwise similar to primary melanoma: a primary lesion can only be diagnosed if there is no current or history of malignant melanocytic lesion of skin

PIGMENTED PHEOCHROMOCYTOMA

- Exhibits immunoreactivity for neuroendocrine markers (chromogranin-A, synaptophysin), and on electron microscopy, cells contain numerous neurosecretory granules
- Also positive for HMB-45, and sustentacular cells show reactivity for S-100 protein

PEARLS

- *The histogenesis of primary adrenal melanoma is not fully elucidated; the pluripotent neural crest cells appear to link malignant melanoma and the adrenal medulla because they serve as precursors of melanocytes, neurons, glial cells of the peripheral nervous system, and adrenal chromaffin cells*
- *Both the argentaffin reaction and its disappearance after oxidative treatment are features shared by other nonmelanotic brown pigments, such as lipofuscin and neuromelanin*

SELECTED REFERENCES

Amerigo J, Roig J, Pulido F, et al: Primary malignant melanoma of the adrenal gland. Surgery 126:107-111, 1999.
Bastide C, Arroua F, Carcenac A, et al: Primary malignant melanoma of the adrenal gland. Int J Urol 13:608-610, 2006.
Bellezza G, Giasanti M, Cavaliere A, Sidoni A: Pigmented "black" pheochromocytoma of the adrenal gland: a case report and review of the literature. Arch Pathol Lab Med 128:e125-e128, 2004.
Granero LE, Al-Lawati T, Bobin JY: Primary melanoma of the adrenal gland, a continuous dilemma: report of a case. Surg Today 34:554-556, 2004.

MYELOLIPOMA

Clinical Features

- Etiology
  - A proliferation of hematopoietic elements
- Epidemiology
  - Usually found in older individuals (fifth to seventh decades); incidence in autopsy series is between 0.08% and 2%
  - Adrenal gland is the most common site
- Signs and symptoms
  - More than 50% of cases are asymptomatic and found incidentally; large tumors may present with flank or abdominal tenderness, constipation, vomiting, or as a palpable mass
  - Rarely may be associated with Cushing syndrome or Conn syndrome, usually associated with adrenal cortical adenoma

Gross Pathology

- Variable size and weight; range in size from few centimeters to greater than 30 cm
- Soft, fleshy, well-circumscribed tumor with pushing border

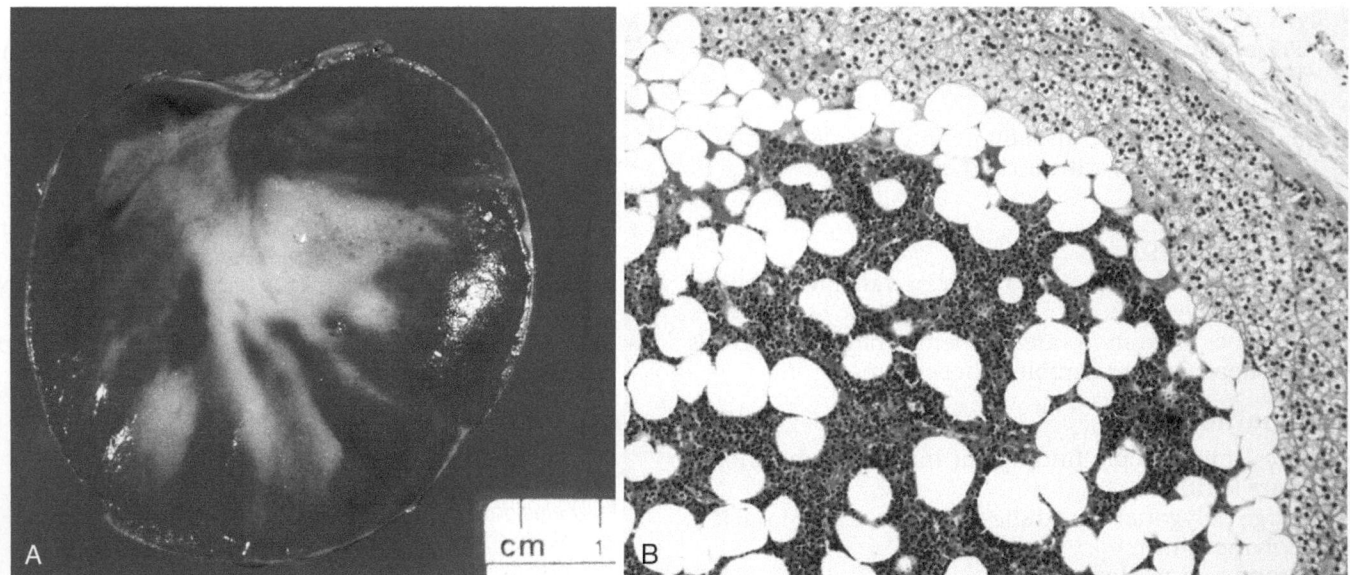

Figure 9-11. Myelolipoma. A, This large lesion has tan and red areas admixed with pale-yellow adipose tissue. The compressed adrenal is bright yellow (*top*). **B,** Classic features include the presence of bone marrow elements and adipose tissue.

- Variable color with tan-yellow and red-brown areas (Figure 9-11A)
- Large lesions may show areas of hemorrhage or necrosis; rarely, small cyst formation may be seen

Histopathology

- Composed of normal-appearing hematopoietic elements with all three cell lines typically represented (resembles normal bone marrow) (Figure 9-11B)
- Variable amount of mature adipose tissue is seen
- Compression of normal appearing adrenal cortex is seen at periphery

Special Stains and Immunohistochemistry

- Noncontributory

Other Techniques for Diagnosis

- Noncontributory

Differential Diagnosis

LIPOMA
- Rarely found in adrenal gland and is composed solely of mature adipose tissue; lacks bone marrow elements

ADENOLIPOMA
- Occasionally myelolipoma is associated with adrenal cortical adenoma

PEARLS

- *May be found in extra-adrenal sites, including liver, retroperitoneum, and stomach*
- *Occasionally associated with hypertension, similar to pheochromocytoma*
- *Etiology is controversial; the embolization of hematopoietic stem cells and ectopic myeloid hyperplasia has been implicated in the etiology; in addition, transformation of the zona reticularis into bone marrow tissue has been observed in mature rats after treatment with testosterone*

SELECTED REFERENCES

Al-Brahim N, Asa SL: Myelolipoma with adrenocortical adenoma: an unusual combination that can resemble carcinoma. Endocr Pathol 18:103-105, 2007.

Elsayes KM, Mukundam G, Narra VR, et al: Adrenal masses: MR imaging features with pathologic correlation. Radiographics 24(suppl 1): S73-S86, 2004.

Guo YK, Yang ZG, Li Y, et al: Uncommon adrenal masses: CT and MRI features with histopathological correlation. Eur J Radiol 62:359-370, 2007.

Lam KY, Lo CY: Adrenal lipomatous tumours: a 30 year clinicopathological experience at a single institution. J Clin Pathol 54:707-712, 2001.

Timonera ER, Paiva ME, Lopes JM, et al: Composite adenomatoid tumor and myelolipoma of adrenal gland: report of 2 cases. Arch Pathol Lab Med 132:265-267, 2008.

ADRENAL CYSTS AND PSEUDOCYSTS

Clinical Features

- Etiology
  - A heterogeneous group of lesions: true cysts versus pseudocysts
- Epidemiology
  - Rare (incidence between 0.06% and 0.18% in autopsy series, and about 5% of incidentally discovered adrenal lesions by computed tomography and magnetic resonance imaging)
  - Found at any age, with increased incidence in fourth to sixth decades; occur more frequently in women than men
  - Usually unilateral with no tendency to occur in either side
- Signs and symptoms
  - Mostly asymptomatic; when large they can present with gastrointestinal symptoms, lumbar or back pain, and palpable abdominal mass
  - Acute symptoms can occur due to rupture, cyst hemorrhage, or infection
  - May clinically and radiographically mimic retroperitoneal or adrenal neoplasms

- Therapy
  - Treatment depends on the underlying pathology, size of the cyst, associated symptoms, and occurrence of complications (small asymptomatic cysts with benign angiographic features can be managed by percutaneous aspiration and watch and follow)

Gross Pathology

- Typically of small size; can reach sizes of up to 30 cm
- Usually uniloculated; rarely multiloculated
- Cyst wall is composed of fibrotic tissue; areas of calcification may be seen
- Contains serous or serosanguineous fluid
- Cyst may contain clotted blood or degenerated thrombus (hemorrhagic cysts)
- Pushing border with compression of the adjacent adrenal gland parenchyma

Histopathology

- Four main groups: endothelial cysts (45%), pseudocysts (39%), epithelial cysts (9%), and parasitic cysts (7%)
  - Endothelial and epithelial cysts have true walls lined with endothelium and epithelium, respectively (true cysts)
  - Endothelial cysts include lymphangiomatous, angiomatous, and hamartomatous subtypes
  - Epithelial cysts are divided into cystic adenomas, glandular, or retention cysts, and cystic transformation of embryonal remnants
  - Pseudocysts usually arise after an episode of a prior adrenal hemorrhage and subsequent clot formation and are characterized by a fibrotic wall without a well-defined endothelial or epithelial lining (Figure 9-12)
  - Parasitic cysts are usually echinococcal in origin (hydatid cyst)
    - Mature adipose tissue or foci of myelolipomatous metaplasia are occasionally seen
    - Rim of compressed adrenal gland may be seen at the periphery

Special Stains and Immunohistochemistry

- Factor VIII, CD31: highlight endothelial cell lining
- Keratin stains can be used to identify an epithelial lining
- Elastic stain: may find elastic fibers within the fibrotic cyst wall

Other Techniques for Diagnosis

- Noncontributory

Differential Diagnosis

INFECTIONS

- Caseous necrosis of tuberculosis and other necrotizing infections

MYELOLIPOMA

- Typically forms a solid mass with a tan-yellow to red-brown cut surface and is composed entirely of mature adipose tissue and hematopoietic elements; cysts may rarely be seen but are typically small
- Adrenal cysts may show focal myelolipomatous differentiation but also have a fibrotic wall that is filled with proteinaceous debris, blood, or thrombus material

PEARLS

- *Hemorrhagic cysts may be associated with Beckwith-Wiedemann syndrome*
- *Cyst wall showing factor VIII and elastic positivity supports vascular and lymphatic nature of this lesion*
- *Pseudocysts tend to have mural, rimlike calcification more commonly than endothelial cysts, which tend to contain septal calcification*

SELECTED REFERENCES

Carvounis E, Marinis A, Arkadopoulos N, et al: Vascular adrenal cysts. Arch Pathol Lab Med 130:1722-1724, 2006.

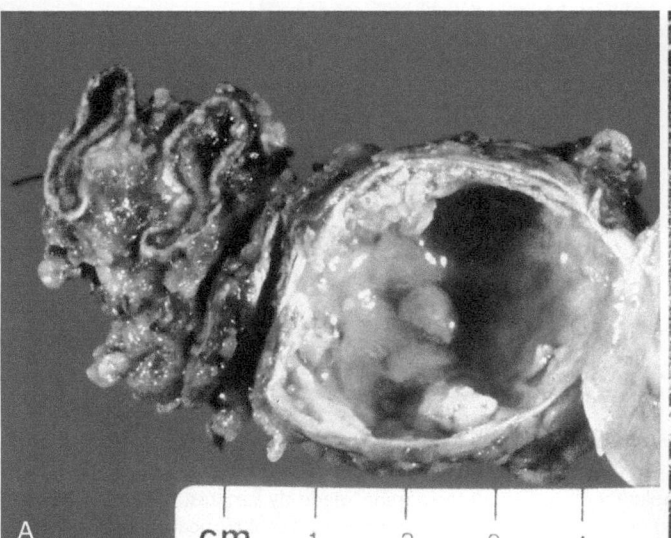
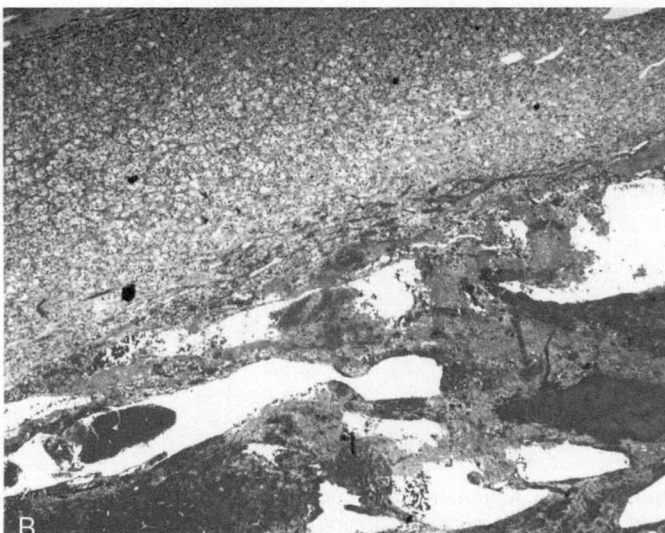

Figure 9-12. Pseudocyst of the adrenal gland. A, The adrenal cortex is intact, and there is a large cyst containing yellow necrotic material. **B,** Section showing adrenal cortex with an underlying hemorrhagic and cystic lesion containing necrotic material. Notice the lack of epithelial lining.

Elsayes KM, Mukundam G, Narra VR, et al: Adrenal masses: MR imaging features with pathologic correlation. Radiographics 24(suppl 1): S73-S86, 2004.

Guo YK, Yang ZG, Li Y, et al: Uncommon adrenal masses: CT and MRI features with histopathological correlation. Eur J Radiol 62:359-370, 2007.

Sanal HT, Kocaoglu M, Yildirim D, et al: Imaging features of benign adrenal cysts. Eur J Radiol 60:465-469, 2006.

Wedmid A, Palese M: Diagnosis and treatment of the adrenal cyst. Curr Urol Rep 11:44-50, 2010.

METASTATIC TUMORS

Clinical Features

- Epidemiology
  - Most common tumors of the adrenal gland
  - Bilateral adrenal gland involvement is found in about 50% of cases
  - Lung is most common primary tumor site, followed by stomach, esophagus, liver, bile ducts, pancreas, large intestine, kidney, and breast

- Signs and symptoms
  - About 90% are asymptomatic, affect elderly patients, and are diagnosed as part of multiorgan metastases
  - Patients may present with Addison disease (adrenal insufficiency) or peritoneal hemorrhage

Gross Pathology

- Often multifocal nodular disease
- Solitary lesions may mimic primary adrenal cortical carcinoma
- Typically involve adrenal cortex and often show extension into adjacent adipose tissue (Figure 9-13A)
- Tumors may occasionally show extension into vena cava
- Brown or black discoloration should raise suspicion of a metastatic melanoma

Histopathology

- Depends on primary site of malignancy (Figure 9-13B)
- Adenocarcinomas and squamous cell carcinomas are the most common subtypes

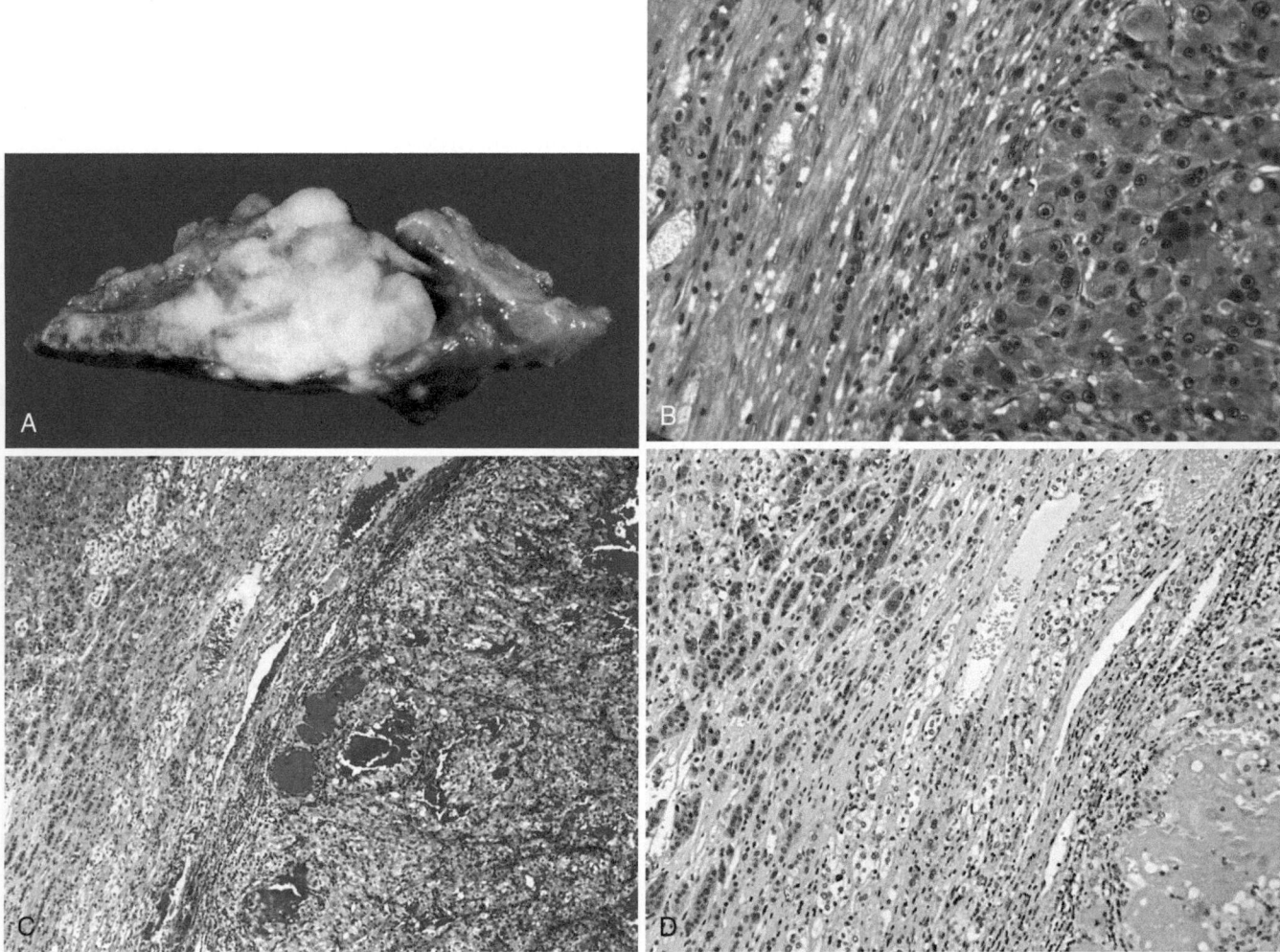

Figure 9-13. A, Metastatic adenocarcinoma. Gross photo showing complete replacement of the adrenal gland by a metastatic adenocarcinoma. **B,** Metastatic hepatocellular carcinoma. The adrenal cortex is compressed (*left*), and the tumor resembles an adrenal cortical adenoma; however, the presence of bile pigment is characteristic of hepatocellular carcinoma. **C,** Metastatic renal cell carcinoma. The adrenal cortex and medulla (*left*) are infiltrated by a clear cell tumor that forms tubules. **D,** Metastatic renal cell carcinoma. The adrenal cortex (*left*) stains for inhibin A, but the tumor (*right*) is negative for this marker.

- Lung and breast metastases typically show poorly differentiated carcinoma; squamous or glandular differentiation may be seen in metastatic lung carcinoma
- Renal cell carcinoma may be of clear cell morphology and mimic primary adrenal tumor (Figure 9-13C)
- Metastatic melanoma composed of large, polygonal cells with pleomorphic nuclei and prominent nucleoli; melanin pigment may be seen

Special Stains and Immunohistochemistry

- See "Differential Diagnosis"

Other Techniques for Diagnosis

- Noncontributory

Differential Diagnosis

- The use of markers normally expressed in the adrenal cortex, including D11, SF-1, inhibin-α, and melan-A, can be helpful in distinguishing primary from metastatic carcinomas; in contrast, markers of other lesions can be used to confirm metastasis
- Clinical history is important

METASTATIC MALIGNANT MELANOMA

- Distinction from primary malignant melanoma can be challenging (see "Primary Malignant Melanoma")

METASTATIC HEPATOCELLULAR CARCINOMA

- Can be difficult to distinguish from adrenal cortical cell carcinoma, especially when bile pigment is not present

within the tumor; well and moderately differentiated hepatocellular carcinoma is positive for HepPar-1, canalicular polyclonal carcinoembryonic antigen (pCEA), and canalicular CD10 by immunohistochemistry

METASTATIC RENAL CELL CARCINOMA (CLEAR CELL)

- Must be distinguished from adrenal cortical cell carcinoma
- Often there is adrenal gland involvement by direct extension of a renal cell carcinoma; renal cell carcinoma is immunoreactive for RCC, CD10, vimentin, and cytokeratin but not SF-1 or inhibin-α (Figure 9-13D)

PEARLS

- *Fine-needle aspiration is useful in diagnosing adrenal gland metastases*

SELECTED REFERENCES

Lack EE: AFIP Atlas of Tumor Pathology, fourth series, Fascicle 8: Tumors of the adrenal glands and extraadrenal paraganglia. Washington, DC, ARP Press, 2007.

Lam KY, Lo CY: Metastatic tumours of the adrenal glands: a 30-year experience in a teaching hospital. Clin Endocrinol 56:95-101, 2002.

Pan CC, Chen PC, Tsay SH, Ho DM: Differential immunoprofiles of hepatocellular carcinoma, renal cell carcinoma, and adrenocortical carcinoma. Appl Immunohistochem Mol Morphol 13:347-352, 2005.

Saeger W, Fassnacht M, Chita R, et al: High diagnostic accuracy of adrenal core biopsy: results of the German and Austrian Adrenal Network Multicenter Trial in 220 consecutive patients. Hum Pathol 34:180-186, 2003.

Chapter 10
Ureter, Urinary Bladder, and Kidney

CRISTINA MAGI-GALLUZZI • LAURA BARISONI • MING ZHOU

CHAPTER OUTLINE

URETER

URETERITIS CYSTICA et GLANDULARIS

Clinical Features

- One of the most common non-neoplastic urothelial proliferations
- Reactive urothelial proliferation that develops following an inflammatory stimulus
- Typically asymptomatic and found incidentally

Gross Pathology

- Nodular cobblestone appearance due to numerous small, superficial, fluid-filled cysts

Histopathology

URETERITIS CYSTICA
- Von Brunn nests (small nests of normal urothelial cells within lamina propria) with central lumens (cystic dilatation) lined by urothelial cells

URETERITIS GLANDULARIS
- Von Brunn nests with central lumens lined by columnar cells

Special Stains and Immunohistochemistry

- Noncontributory

Other Techniques for Diagnosis

- Noncontributory

Differential Diagnosis

UROTHELIAL HYPERPLASIA
- Increase in number of layers of urothelial cells
- Does not show nesting of urothelial cells

VON BRUNN NESTS
- Lacks formation of central cystic dilatation

PEARLS

- *Believed by some investigators to be a normal variant of the urothelial mucosa*
- *Most believe that an inflammatory stimulus is needed*
- *Must be considered in the differential diagnosis of ureteral and renal pelvic filling defects*

SELECTED REFERENCES

Duffin TK, Regan JB, Hernandez-Graulau JM: Ureteritis cystica with 17-year followup. J Urol 151:142-143, 1994.
Hochberg DA, Motta J, Brodherson MS: Cystitis glandularis. Urology 51:112-113, 1998.

UROTHELIAL CARCINOMA (TRANSITIONAL CELL CARCINOMA)

Clinical Features

- Relatively rare in the ureter; comprise 2% to 5% of urothelial neoplasms
- Similar etiologic and pathogenic agents as in bladder urothelial carcinoma: tobacco smoking is the most common risk factor; higher association with analgesic abuse; association with hereditary nonpolyposis colorectal cancer syndrome (HNPCC, Lynch syndrome)
- Clinical features are comparable to those lesions arising in the urinary bladder and include hematuria and flank pain
- More commonly results in urinary obstruction
- Can occur in any portion of the ureter; distal third is most common

Gross Pathology

- Low-grade tumors typically have a papillary architecture with delicate papillary fronds over the ureteral surface
- Higher-grade tumors often lack papillary architecture and show nodular, polypoid, or sessile pattern
- Ureteral wall is typically thickened and may show significant narrowing
- Ulceration and hemorrhage is often seen in high-grade tumors

Histopathology

GRADING OF UROTHELIAL CARCINOMAS
- To simplify the World Health Organization (WHO) (1973) system and avoid an intermediate cancer grade group (grade II), the WHO (2003)/International Society of Urological Pathology (ISUP) system classifies papillary urothelial carcinomas into only two grades:
  - Low-grade papillary urothelial carcinoma (LG-UC)
  - High-grade papillary urothelial carcinoma (HG-UC)

LOW-GRADE PAPILLARY UROTHELIAL CARCINOMA

- Exophytic growth pattern characterized by slender papillary fronds with obvious fibrovascular cores, frequent branching, and minimal fusion
- The papillae are lined by urothelium that shows an orderly appearance with easily recognizable variations in architectural and cytologic features
- Cells usually show minimal anaplasia; the nuclei are uniformly enlarged with mild differences in shape, contour, and chromatin distribution (Figure 10-1A)

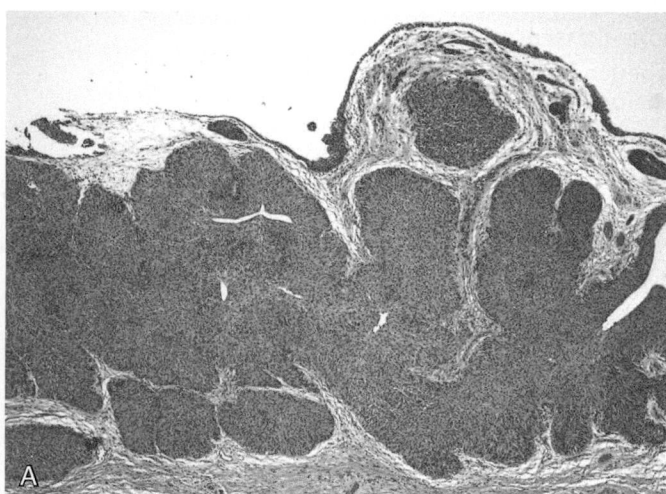

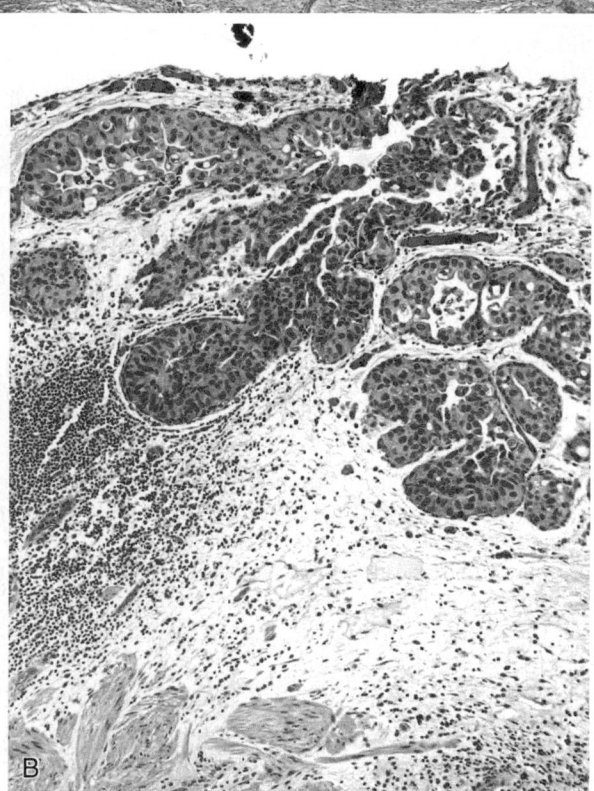

- Mitoses are infrequent

HIGH-GRADE PAPILLARY UROTHELIAL CARCINOMA

- May lack a distinct papillary architecture, although papillary remnants may persist
- The papillae are frequently fused and branching
- The pattern of disorder is predominant with easily recognizable variations in architectural and cytologic features
- Cells are large and irregular with a spectrum of nuclear pleomorphism ranging from moderate to marked; nucleoli may be prominent (Figure 10-1B)
- Bizarre or multinucleated tumor cells may be seen
- High mitotic activity; numerous atypical forms often seen
- Usually infiltrates the underlying subepithelial connective tissue or muscularis propria and grows in solid cords or nests
- Reactive desmoplastic stroma surrounds infiltrating nests of tumor cells
- Squamous differentiation is seen in more than 20% of cases

Special Stains and Immunohistochemistry

- Cytokeratin (high molecular weight and CK7) and p63: positive
- Carcinoembryonic antigen (CEA): positive (especially in high-grade tumors)

Other Techniques for Diagnosis

- Cytogenetic studies: similar findings as in urothelial carcinoma of the bladder

Differential Diagnosis

INVERTED PAPILLOMA

- Urothelial cords and trabeculae with uniform thickness, peripheral palisading, and central spindling and streaming
- Minimal cytologic atypia and low mitotic activity
- Lacks invasion into the muscularis propria

FIBROEPITHELIAL POLYP

- Typically solitary with a short, thin stalk
- Consists of a polyp of loose fibroconnective and fibrovascular tissue covered by normal-appearing urothelium

PEARLS

- *Urine cytology is helpful for evaluating ureteral lesions*
- *Prognosis is related to tumor stage (depth of invasion), grade (morphologic and cytologic features), and multifocality (presence of synchronous tumor in the renal pelvis)*

Figure 10-1. A, Low-grade papillary urothelial carcinoma of the ureter. The neoplasm shows a nodular and inverted pattern growth. Cells show minimal anaplasia; the nuclei are uniformly enlarged with mild differences in shape, contour, and chromatin distribution. **B,** High-grade urothelial carcinoma of the ureter. Ulceration and denudation of the urothelium are often seen in high-grade tumors of the ureter. Cells are large and irregular with moderate to marked nuclear pleomorphism. Infiltration of the underlying subepithelial connective tissue is common.

SELECTED REFERENCES

Eble JN, Sauter G, Epstein JI, et al (eds): Pathology and Genetics of Tumours of the Urinary System and Male Genitals Organs: World Health Classification of Tumours. Lyon, IARC Press, 2003.
Lehmann J, Suttmann H, Kovac I, et al: Transitional cell carcinoma of the ureter: prognostic factors influencing progression and survival. Eur Urol 51:1281-1288, 2007.

URINARY BLADDER

INFECTIOUS CYSTITIS

- Infectious cystitis can be caused by various microorganisms, including bacteria, fungi, viruses, and parasites
- Diagnosis relies primarily on urinalysis, urine culture, and empirical antimicrobial therapy

Malakoplakia
Clinical Features

- Most commonly found in the bladder; may be seen in the ureter, renal pelvis, testis, gynecologic tract, gastrointestinal tract, and lung
- Typically found in women; peak incidence in fifth decade
- Rarely seen in children
- Most patients present with typical symptoms of urinary tract infection
- Often culture *Escherichia coli* or other bacteria from the urine

Gross Pathology

- Multiple, soft, yellow-white, nodular plaques measuring less than 2 cm
- Involves mucosal surface

Histopathology

- Accumulation of histocytes with abundant eosinophilic granular cytoplasm (von Hansemann histiocytes) in the superficial lamina propria, typically underlying an intact urothelial layer (Figure 10-2)
- Michaelis-Gutmann bodies (small round basophilic intracytoplasmic or extracytoplasmic laminated structures with a bull's eye appearance) are found within histiocytes as well as within the interstitium
- Michaelis-Gutmann bodies are formed by precipitation of calcium or iron on bacteria or bacterial fragments
- Extensive fibrosis or marked acute and chronic inflammation may be seen

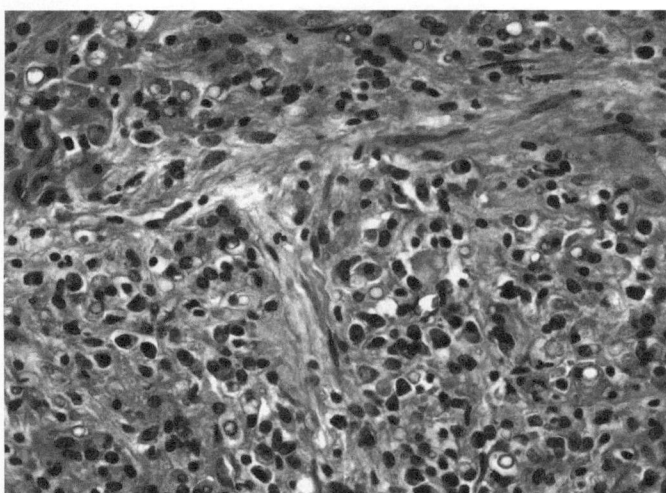

Figure 10-2. Malakoplakia. The lamina propria contains numerous histocytes with a large amount of eosinophilic granular cytoplasm and intracytoplasmic inclusions (Michaelis-Gutmann bodies).

Special Stains and Immunohistochemistry

- Von Kossa calcium and Perl's Prussian blue: Michaelis-Gutmann bodies are positive
- Periodic acid-Schiff (PAS): Von Hansemann and Michaelis-Gutmann bodies are positive

Other Techniques for Diagnosis

- Electron microscopy: Michaelis-Gutmann bodies consist of a dense core surrounded by a homogeneous zone composed of myelin figures; measure 5 to 10 μ in diameter

Differential Diagnosis

XANTHOGRANULOMATOUS CYSTITIS
- Lacks Michaelis-Gutmann bodies

LANGERHANS CELL HISTIOCYTOSIS
- Histiocytes are positive for CD1a and S-100

PEARLS

- *Terminology derived from the Greek words* plakos *(plaque) and* malakos *(soft)*
- *Believed to result from impairment of the ability of mononuclear cells to degrade phagocytosed bacteria*
- *Must identify Michaelis-Gutmann bodies in order to make the diagnosis*

SELECTED REFERENCES

Pusl T, Weiss M, Hartmann B, et al: Malacoplakia in a renal transplant recipient. Eur J Intern Med 17:133-135, 2006.
Tam VK, Kung WH, Li R, Chan KW: Renal parenchymal malacoplakia: a rare cause of ARF with a review of recent literature. Am J Kidney Dis 41:E13-E17, 2003.

NONINFECTIOUS CYSTITIS (POLYPOID CYSTITIS, FOLLICULAR CYSTITIS, GIANT CELL CYSTITIS)

Clinical Features

- Patients may present with urinary frequency, urgency, or dysuria
- Polypoid cystitis is often seen in patients with indwelling bladder catheters
- Follicular cystitis is frequently seen in patients with bladder carcinoma and urinary tract infection
- Giant cell cystitis is not a clinical entity; rather, it is a term used to describe the presence of atypical stromal cells in the lamina propria of the bladder
- Occasionally seen following radiation treatment

Gross Pathology

POLYPOID CYSTITIS
- Small polypoid mucosal lesions (may mimic bladder carcinoma)

FOLLICULAR CYSTITIS
- Mucosa showing erythematous gray-white nodules

GIANT CELL CYSTITIS
- Usually a subtle finding; erythematous bladder mucosa may be seen

Histopathology

POLYPOID CYSTITIS
- Broad fronds covered by benign-appearing urothelial cells
- Lamina propria is edematous with chronic inflammation and congested blood vessels

FOLLICULAR CYSTITIS
- Lamina propria contains scattered lymphoid follicles, usually with germinal centers

GIANT CELL CYSTITIS
- Atypical large stromal cells with bipolar or multipolar tapering eosinophilic processes and enlarged hyperchromatic nuclei (degenerative atypia); cells often contain multiple nuclei; mitoses are absent or rare (Figure 10-3)

Special Stains and Immunohistochemistry
- Noncontributory

Other Techniques for Diagnosis
- Noncontributory

Differential Diagnosis

BACTERIAL CYSTITIS
- Inflammatory component consists of acute inflammatory cells
- Bladder culture may yield positive results

LOW-GRADE PAPILLARY UROTHELIAL CARCINOMA
- May be confused with polypoid cystitis
- Typically shows branching delicate papillae rather than broad fronds
- Papillae are covered by atypical urothelial cells, which is much more pronounced than that seen in polypoid cystitis

MALIGNANT LYMPHOMA
- Must be distinguished from follicular cystitis
- Lymphomatous infiltrate typically shows a diffuse rather than follicular architecture

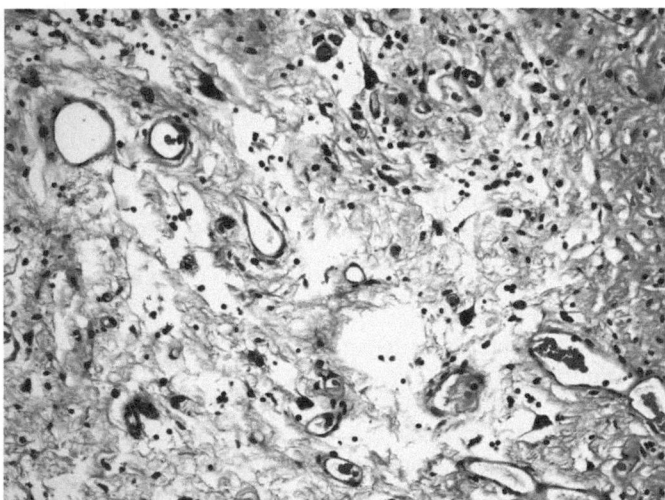

Figure 10-3. Giant cell cystitis. The lamina propria shows atypical large stromal cells with bipolar or multipolar tapering eosinophilic processes and multiple, enlarged hyperchromatic nuclei.

SARCOMA
- Must be distinguished from giant cell cystitis
- Sarcomatous stromal cells have a higher degree of nuclear atypia; mitoses are commonly found

PEARLS

- *Removal of the irritant (catheter, toxin) typically resolves the cystitis*
- *Often these conditions are asymptomatic and found incidentally*

SELECTED REFERENCES

Hansson S, Hanson E, Hjalmas K, et al: Follicular cystitis in girls with untreated asymptomatic or covert bacteriuria. J Urol 143:330-332, 1990.
Young RH: Papillary and polypoid cystitis: a report of eight cases. Am J Surg Pathol 12:542-546,1988.

TREATMENT-RELATED CYSTITIS

Clinical Features
- Bacillus Calmette-Guerin (BCG) cystitis is associated with intravesical instillation of Bacillus Calmette-Guerin used in the treatment of urothelial carcinoma in situ (CIS) and high-grade papillary urothelial carcinoma
- Radiation cystitis may be acute or chronic and can occur whenever the bladder is included in the treatment field
- Hemorrhagic cystitis is associated with radiation and chemotherapy; also seen with various chemical toxins (cyclophosphamide, busulfan) and viral infection (adenovirus in children), or may be idiopathic

Gross Pathology

GRANULOMATOUS CYSTITIS SECONDARY TO BACILLUS CALMETTE-GUERIN THERAPY (BCG CYSTITIS)
- Partially or entirely denuded bladder mucosa

RADIATION CYSTITIS
- Hyperemic and edematous bladder mucosa with thickened mucosal folds

HEMORRHAGIC CYSTITIS
- Hemorrhagic and edematous bladder mucosa

Histopathology

BCG CYSTITIS
- Superficial lamina propria shows discrete noncaseating granulomas containing epithelioid histiocytes and multinucleated giant cells
- Granulomas are associated with intense lymphocytic infiltrate
- Urothelium may show nonspecific reactive atypia or be denuded

RADIATION CYSTITIS (Figure 10-4)
- Lamina propria shows edema, hyperemia, and dilated blood vessels with fibrin
- Proliferation of urothelial nests within lamina propria "hugging" ectatic vessels

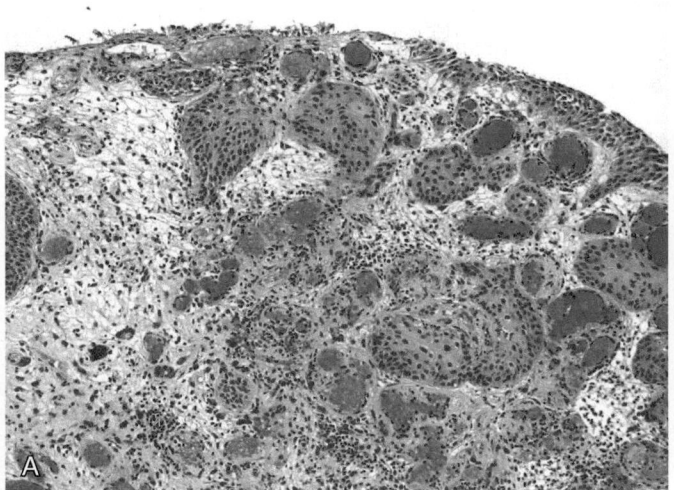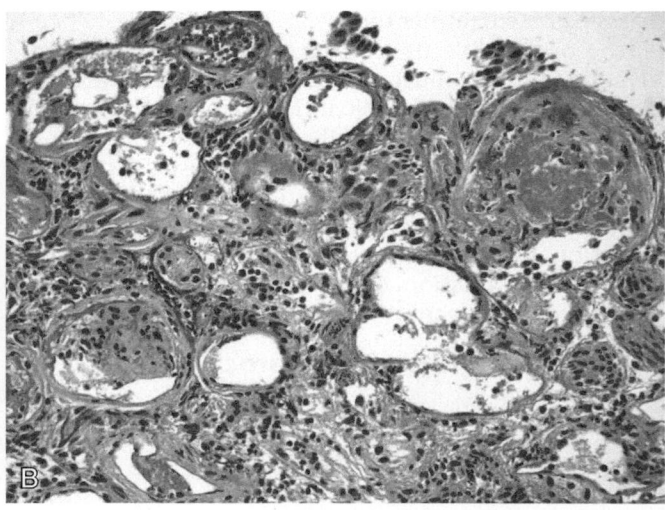

Figure 10-4. A, Radiation cystitis. Lamina propria shows edema, hyperemia, and thickened mucosal folds. The urothelium shows superficial ulceration and atypical cytologic features. The stroma contains extravasated erythrocytes, inflammation, and occasional bizarre multinucleated giant cells. **B,** Radiation cystitis. Late changes include superficial ulceration and dilated blood vessels with fibrinous exudate.

- Surface urothelium may shows desquamation, superficial ulceration, and atypical cytologic features mimicking CIS; however, atypia is degenerative and nuclear-cytoplasmic (N:C) ratio is low
- Bizarre giant cells and multinucleated cells are often present
- The stroma contains extravasated erythrocytes, inflammation, and hemosiderin deposition
- Late changes include collagenization of the lamina propria, myointimal proliferation or hyalinization of the arteriole's media, and often ulceration with fibrinous exudate

HEMORRHAGIC CYSTITIS
- Lamina propria shows hemorrhage and congested blood vessels
- Urothelium shows regenerative changes including nuclear pleomorphism
- Healing may result in hyperplastic urothelium with papillae formation
- Repeated bouts may result in a fibrotic, contracted bladder

Special Stains and Immunohistochemistry
- Acid-fast stain rarely reveals the presence of microorganisms in BCG cystitis

Other Techniques for Diagnosis
- Noncontributory

Differential Diagnosis
BACTERIAL CYSTITIS
- Inflammatory component consists of acute inflammatory cells
- Bladder culture may yield positive results

UROTHELIAL CARCINOMA IN SITU
- Cytologic atypia and architectural distortion are more pronounced and mitoses are frequently found

PEARLS
- *Acute symptoms of radiation cystitis may appear 4 to 6 weeks after the initiation of treatment; late symptoms appear as late as 10 years later*
- *Pathologist must be aware that these changes may be seen with a remote radiation or chemotherapy history*
- *Accurate clinical history is key to avoid misdiagnosis*

SELECTED REFERENCES
Chan TY, Epstein JI: Radiation or chemotherapy cystitis with "pseudo-carcinomatous" features. Am J Surg Pathol 28:909-913, 2004.
Wong-You-Cheong JJ, Woodward PJ, Manning MA, Davis CJ: From the archives of the AFIP: inflammatory and nonneoplastic bladder masses: radiologic-pathologic correlation. Radiographics 26:1847-1868, 2006.

INTERSTITIAL (HUNNER) CYSTITIS

Clinical Features
- Classically occurs in middle-aged and elderly women
- Interstitial cystitis is manifested by sensory hypersensitivity; patients present with urinary frequency, urgency, nocturia, suprapubic pressure, and pelvic and bladder pain
- Hematuria may be seen
- Urine is sterile and thus bladder culture is negative

Gross Pathology
- Cystoscopy may show petechial hemorrhage after inflation (glomerulation) and small linear ulcerations in the mucosa (Hunner ulcer)
- Scarring of bladder mucosa is often noted
- Longstanding cases may result in a fibrotic, contracted bladder with markedly diminished capacity
- Usually affects dome and posterolateral bladder walls

Histopathology
NONULCERATIVE OR EARLY DISEASE
- Multiple microhemorrhages are present within the lamina propria (glomerulations)

- Classic phase (Hunner ulcer)
- Single or multiple patches of reddened, ulcerated, or denuded bladder mucosa with fibrinous exudate often seen admixed with chronic inflammatory cells, including lymphocytes, plasma cells, and mast cells
- Characteristic feature is increase in mast cells within the mucosa, lamina propria, and muscularis propria
- Hemorrhage, edema, congestion, and fibrosis are also seen
- Occasionally there is no ulceration of the mucosa; only chronic inflammation, edema, hemorrhage, and granulation tissue are seen

Special Stains and Immunohistochemistry

- Noncontributory

Other Techniques for Diagnosis

- Noncontributory

Differential Diagnosis

Flat Urothelial Carcinoma in Situ (CIS)

- Denuding CIS exhibits ulceration, vascular congestion, and inflammation resembling interstitial cystitis
- Multiple tissue sections should be examined to search for atypical cells

Bacterial Cystitis

- Inflammatory component consists of acute inflammatory cells
- No increase in mast cells
- Bladder culture may yield positive results

Noninfectious Cystitis

- Features of polypoid cystitis, follicular cystitis, giant cell cystitis, or hemorrhagic cystitis
- No increase in mast cells

PEARLS

- *Only nonspecific features exist and must be correlated with clinical impression; no pathognomonic microscopic features currently exist*
- *Exclude CIS before a diagnosis of interstitial cystitis is rendered*

Selected References

Chai TC, Keay S: New theories in interstitial cystitis. Nat Clin Pract Urol 1:85-89, 2004.
Mayer R: Interstitial cystitis pathogenesis and treatment. Curr Opin Infect Dis 20:77-82, 2007.
Sant GR, Kempuraj D, Marchand JE, Theoharides TC: The mast cell in interstitial cystitis: role in pathophysiology and pathogenesis. Urology 69(4 Suppl):34-40, 2007.

CYSTITIS CYSTICA et GLANDULARIS

Clinical Features

- Common non-neoplastic lesion of the bladder
- Believed to be induced by chronic inflammatory stimulus
- Found most commonly in adults; occasionally seen in children
- Cystoscopically may occasionally mimic carcinoma

Gross Pathology

Cystitis Cystica

- Small submucosal cysts filled with clear yellow fluid

Cystitis Glandularis

- May not always be grossly visible
- Occasionally see irregular nodular mucosa

Histopathology

Cystitis Cystica

- Von Brunn nests within the lamina propria showing central cystic dilatation with spaces lined by urothelial or low cuboidal epithelium (Figure 10-5)
- Cysts are often filled with pale eosinophilic fluid

Cystitis Glandularis

- The epithelial lining of von Brunn nests undergoes glandular metaplasia
- Glands are lined by cuboidal to columnar cells without anaplasia
- Cells may contain mucin and occasionally goblet cells are present
- If the epithelium acquires intestinal-type goblet cells, this variant is called *cystitis glandularis with intestinal metaplasia* (if diffuse without urothelial cells: colonic metaplasia)

Special Stains and Immunohistochemistry

- Reactive urothelium shows CK20 immunoreactivity in only the umbrella cell layer
- p53 nuclear staining is predominantly negative with occasional weak positivity in the basal and parabasal intermediate cells
- CD44 can be overexpressed in the entire reactive urothelium or focally positive in intermediate cells

Other Techniques for Diagnosis

- Noncontributory

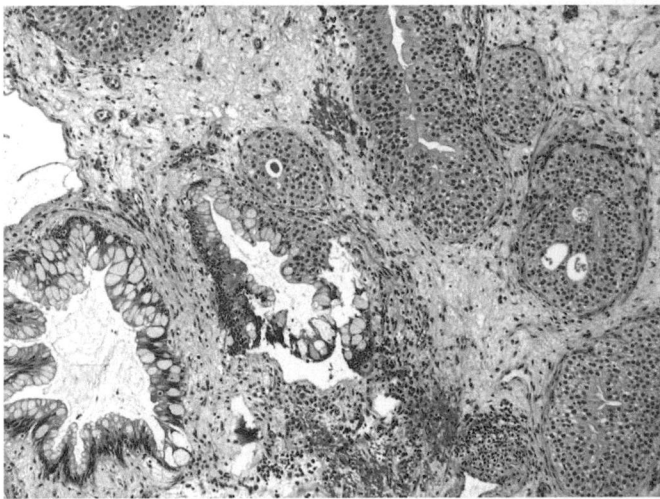

Figure 10-5. Cystitis cystica et glandularis. The lamina propria shows cystically dilated glands lined by urothelial cells *(right)*. In some cases the epithelial lining undergoes glandular metaplasia with intestinal-type goblet cells *(left)*. This variant is called *cystitis glandularis with intestinal metaplasia.*

Differential Diagnosis

UROTHELIAL CARCINOMA, NESTED VARIANT

- Florid von Brunn nest can be differentiated from nested variant of urothelial carcinoma by its lobular or linear array of the nests, flat noninfiltrative base, and lack of cytologic atypia

ADENOCARCINOMA

- Rare bladder neoplasm
- Atypical glands lined by stratified, pleomorphic cells with infiltration into the muscular layer
- Signet ring cells may be seen

PEARLS

- *Florid von Brunn nests, cystitis cystica, and cystitis glandularis are closely related reactive changes that may be seen in any portion of the urothelial tract*
- *Cystitis cystica et glandularis has no direct association with bladder cancer; coincidental coexistence may be seen*
- *Cystitis glandularis may be confused with adenocarcinoma, especially if extravasated mucin is present*
- *Believed to be associated with chronically irritated bladders; may resolve if source of inflammation is removed*

SELECTED REFERENCES

McKenney JK, Desai S, Cohen C, Amin MB: Discriminatory immunohistochemical staining of urothelial carcinoma in situ and nonneoplastic urothelium: an analysis of cytokeratin 20, p53, and CD44 antigens. Am J Surg Pathol 25:1074-1078, 2001.

Tamas EF, Epstein JI: Detection of residual tumor cells in bladder biopsy specimens: pitfalls in the interpretation of cytokeratin stains. Am J Surg Pathol 31:390-397, 2007.

Volmar KE, Chan TY, De Marzo AM, Epstein JI: Florid von Brunn nests mimicking urothelial carcinoma: a morphologic and immunohistochemical comparison to the nested variant of urothelial carcinoma. Am J Surg Pathol 27:1243-1252, 2003.

Young RH, Bostwick DG: Florid cystitis glandularis of intestinal type with mucin extravasation: a mimic of adenocarcinoma. Am J Surg Pathol 20:1462-1468, 1996.

NEPHROGENIC ADENOMA

Clinical Features

- Most cases involve the bladder; occasionally found in the urethra, ureter, or renal pelvis
- Found in young adults with a male predominance (2:1)
- Approximately half of the cases are found following genitourinary surgery, including renal transplantation
- Also associated with calculi, trauma, and cystitis
- Often asymptomatic, although patients frequently present with hematuria or dysuria

Gross Pathology

- Usually found over the posterior bladder wall
- May present as a papillary or polypoid exophytic mass or velvety lesion
- Sessile forms comprise approximately 25% to 30% of cases
- Papillary structures usually measure less than 1 cm; may rarely measure greater than 5 cm

Histopathology

- Classic histologic pattern is that of small tubules resembling renal tubules (Figure 10-6A)
- May also see papillary or flat architecture
- Tubules are lined by "hobnail" cells resembling endothelial-lined vascular spaces (Figure 10-6B)
- Tubules are often surrounded by a layer of hyalinized basement membrane
- Cells with oxyphilic or clear cytoplasm, or signet-ring-like cells, may also be seen
- Mitotic activity is rare
- Pale eosinophilic secretions are often found within the tubules
- A variable degree of acute and chronic inflammation and stromal edema are common in the background
- Typically confined to the lamina propria, it can on occasion focally involve the superficial lamina propria; rarely may have a deep infiltrative pattern into perinephric adipose tissue

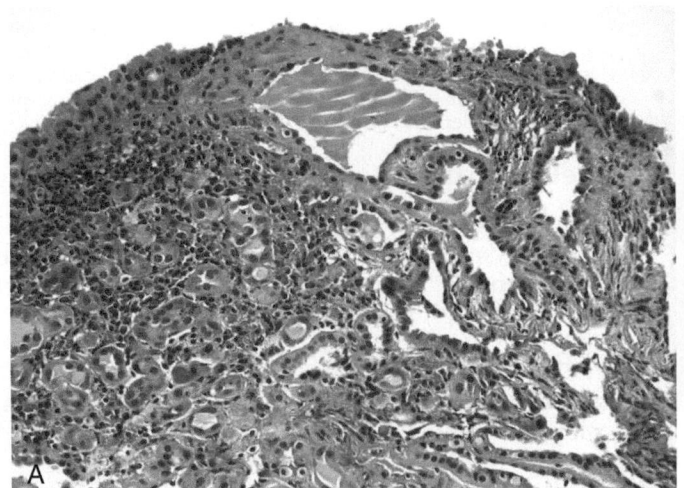
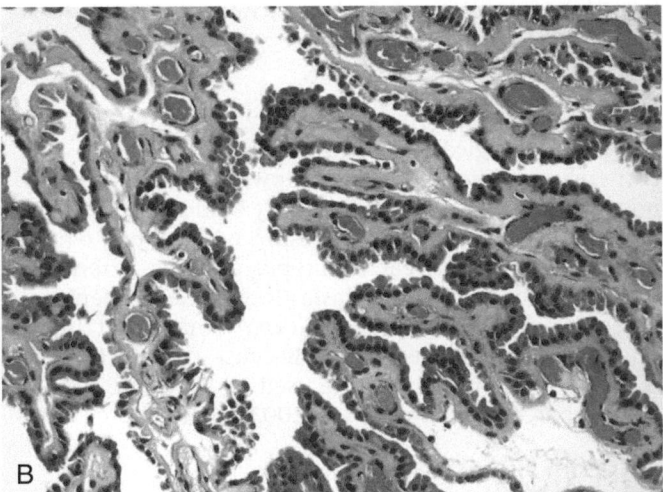

Figure 10-6. A, Nephrogenic adenoma. Proliferation of small tubules lined by cuboidal epithelium. No mitotic activity or nuclear pleomorphism are noted. Tubules are often surrounded by a layer of hyalinized basement membrane. Pale eosinophilic secretions are often found within the tubules. **B,** Nephrogenic adenoma. Papillary fronds lined by cuboidal eosinophilic cells with occasional "hobnail" features.

Special Stains and Immunohistochemistry

- Cytokeratin 7 (CK7), PAX2, and PAX8 are positive in the tubular lining cells
- Focal and weak PSA and PAP expression is detected in a subset of cases
- Most cases are positive for AMACR and negative for high molecular weight cytokeratin (34BE12)

Other Techniques for Diagnosis

- Noncontributory

Differential Diagnosis

PROSTATIC AND CLEAR CELL ADENOCARCINOMA

- Not typically associated with other clinical conditions
- Tubules with prominent nucleoli sometimes situated within muscle bundles
- Usually much larger
- Shows greater cytologic atypia and high mitotic rate

LOW-GRADE PAPILLARY UROTHELIAL CARCINOMA

- Papillae are covered by neoplastic urothelial cells rather than benign-appearing cuboidal cells
- Nested or microcystic variant of urothelial carcinoma exhibits greater atypia and increased mitoses at the deep invasive fronts

CAPILLARY HEMANGIOMA

- Negative for CK7 and positive for endothelial markers, such as CD31

PEARLS

- *Evidence in renal transplant patients suggests that nephrogenic adenoma is derived from tubular renal cells and is not a metaplastic proliferation of the urothelium*

SELECTED REFERENCES

Diolombi M, Ross HM, Mercalli F, et al: Nephrogenic adenoma: a report of 3 unusual cases infiltrating into perinephric adipose tissue. Am J Surg Pathol 37:532-538, 2013.
Piña-Oviedo S, Shen SS, Truong LD, et al: Flat pattern of nephrogenic adenoma: previously unrecognized pattern unveiled using PAX2 and PAX8 immunohistochemistry. Mod Pathol 26:792-798, 2013.

FLAT UROTHELIAL LESIONS

In 1998, the World Health Organization/International Society of Urological Pathology (WHO/ISUP) published a consensus classification. The following entities were included in the category for flat urinary bladder lesions: flat urothelial hyperplasia and flat lesion with atypia, which is further divided into reactive atypia, atypia of unknown significance, urothelial dysplasia (low-grade intraepithelial neoplasia), and flat urothelial carcinoma in situ (high-grade intraepithelial neoplasia). Because the 2003 WHO has accepted the nomenclature used in 1998, the system is currently referred to as WHO (2003)/ISUP.

Urothelial Hyperplasia
Clinical Features

- Rare benign urothelial lesion; it may be seen in the flat mucosa adjacent to a low-grade papillary urothelial lesion

Gross Pathology

- Noncontributory

Histopathology

- Markedly thickened urothelial mucosa without cytologic atypia
- Rather than requiring a specific number of cell layers, marked thickening compared with the adjacent normal urothelium is needed to diagnosis flat hyperplasia

Special Stains and Immunohistochemistry

- Noncontributory

Other Techniques for Diagnosis

- Frequent deletions of chromosome 9 detected by fluorescence in situ hybridization (FISH) have been reported in urothelial hyperplasias found in patients with papillary bladder cancer

Differential Diagnosis

UROTHELIAL DYSPLASIA

- Variable, often appreciable, loss of cell polarity with nuclear crowding and cytologic atypia that is not severe enough to merit a diagnosis of CIS

UROTHELIAL CARCINOMA IN SITU

- Pleomorphism, prominent nucleoli throughout the urothelium and upper-level mitoses

PEARLS

- *Regarded in the new WHO classification as a lesion without malignant potential*
- *Molecular analysis has shown that urothelial hyperplasia in bladder cancer patients may be chronologically related to papillary tumors*
- *In the absence of an associated papillary urothelial neoplasm, no treatment or follow-up is required*

SELECTED REFERENCES

Hartmann A, Moser K, Kriegmair M, et al: Frequent genetic alterations in simple urothelial hyperplasias of the bladder in patients with papillary urothelial carcinoma. Am J Pathol 154:721-727, 1999.
van Oers JM, Adam C, Denzinger S, et al: Chromosome 9 deletions are more frequent than FGFR3 mutations in flat urothelial hyperplasias of the bladder. Int J Cancer 119:1212-1215, 2006.

Urothelial Dysplasia
Clinical Features

- De novo dysplasia affects predominantly middle-aged men presenting occasionally with irritative bladder symptoms with or without hematuria

Gross Pathology

- Lesion may be inapparent or associated with erythema, erosion, or rarely ulceration

Histopathology

- Shows variable, often appreciable, loss of cell polarity, with nuclear crowding and cytologic atypia, that is not severe enough to merit a diagnosis of CIS (Figure 10-7)

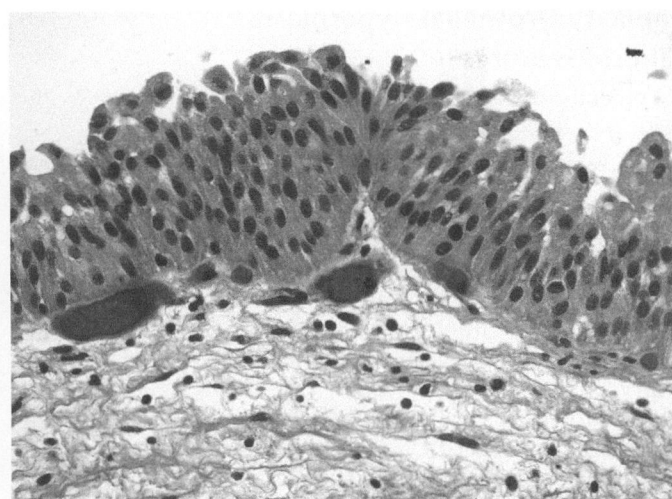

Figure 10-7. Urothelial dysplasia. The urothelium shows nuclear crowding and cytologic atypia. The cells have mildly altered chromatin distribution, slightly enlarged nuclei, inconspicuous nucleoli, and rare mitoses.

- Cells may have mildly altered chromatin distribution, slightly enlarged nuclei, inconspicuous nucleoli, and rare mitoses
- The thickness of the urothelium is usually normal; however, it may be increased or decreased
- Lamina propria may contain increased inflammation or neovascularity
- Urothelial dysplasia may involve von Brunn nests

Special Stains and Immunohistochemistry
- Aberrant CK20 expression
- p53 and Ki-67 overexpression

Other Techniques for Diagnosis
- Alteration of chromosome 9 and p53 allelic losses have been demonstrated

Differential Diagnosis

UROTHELIAL CARCINOMA IN SITU
- Typically shows pleomorphism, and prominent nucleoli throughout the urothelium
- Increased mitotic activity with upper-level mitosis
- Coarse chromatin pattern

REACTIVE INFLAMMATORY ATYPIA
- Presence of acute and chronic inflammation

UROTHELIAL ATYPIA OF UNKNOWN SIGNIFICANCE
- Presence of significant atypia and significant inflammation

PEARLS

- *Dysplasia in patients with noninvasive papillary neoplasms indicates urothelial instability and a marker for progression or recurrence*
- *De novo dysplasia progresses to urothelial neoplasia in 5% to 19% of patients*

SELECTED REFERENCES

Amin MB, McKenney JK: An approach to the diagnosis of flat intraepithelial lesions of the urinary bladder using the World Health Organization/International Society of Urological Pathology consensus classification system. Adv Anat Pathol 9:222-232, 2002.

Hodges KB, Lopez-Beltran A, Davidson DD, et al: Urothelial dysplasia and other flat lesions of the urinary bladder: clinicopathologic and molecular features. Hum Pathol 41:155-162, 2010.

Urothelial Carcinoma in Situ (CIS)

Clinical Features

- Patients are usually in their fifth to sixth decade
- Asymptomatic or symptomatic with dysuria, frequency, urgency, or even hematuria
- CIS is commonly multifocal and may be diffuse
- De novo (primary) CIS accounts for less than 1% to 3% of urothelial neoplasms but is seen in association with 45% to 65% of invasive urothelial carcinomas

Gross Pathology

- Bladder mucosa may be unremarkable or erythematous and edematous

Histopathology

- Urothelial carcinoma in situ (CIS) is a nonpapillary (i.e., flat) lesion in which the surface epithelium contains cells that are cytologically malignant (Figure 10-8)
- The term *CIS* is synonymous with "high-grade intraurothelial neoplasia"
- Nuclear anaplasia identical to high-grade papillary urothelial carcinoma
- The urothelium may be denuded, diminished in thickness, of normal thickness, or even hyperplastic
- There may be complete loss of polarity, marked crowding, and pleomorphism
- Nuclei are frequently hyperchromatic and have a coarse or condensed chromatin distribution

Special Stains and Immunohistochemistry

- CK20: diffuse strong cytoplasmic staining involving the full thickness of urothelium
- p53: nuclear staining may be diffuse throughout the full thickness

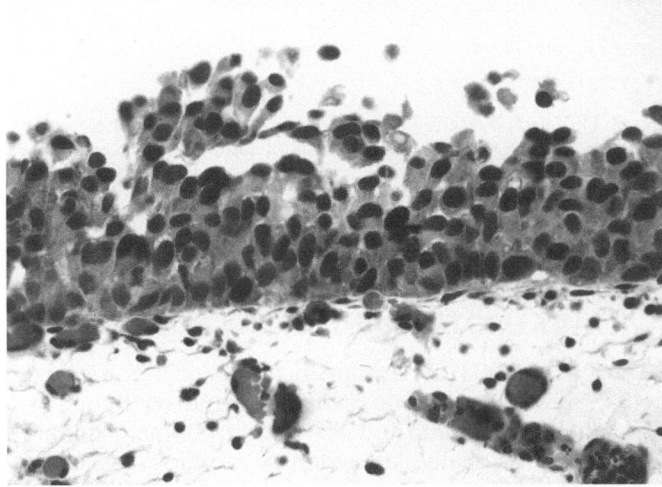

Figure 10-8. Urothelial carcinoma in situ. The entire thickness of the urinary bladder epithelium is replaced by neoplastic cells. There is complete loss of polarity, marked crowding, and pleomorphism. Nuclei are hyperchromatic and have a coarse or condensed chromatin distribution.

- CD44: expression limited to residual basal cell layer or negative

Other Techniques for Diagnosis

- Chromosome 9 deletions and p53 allelic losses have been frequently demonstrated

Differential Diagnosis

UROTHELIAL DYSPLASIA

- Cytologic atypia is not severe enough to merit a diagnosis of CIS
- Lacks pleomorphism comparable to high-grade papillary carcinoma, discohesion, or mitoses in the upper urothelium

REACTIVE ATYPIA

- Lacks nuclear pleomorphism
- Presence of acute and chronic inflammation

UROTHELIAL ATYPIA OF UNKNOWN SIGNIFICANCE

- Presence of significant atypia and significant inflammation

RADIATION-INDUCED ATYPIA

- Florid epithelial proliferation with cell enlargement, hyperchromasia, and prominent nucleoli
- Stromal fibrosis, subepithelial hemorrhage, and hyalinization of blood vessels

POLYOMA VIRUS INFECTION

- Nucleomegaly, high N:C ratio, and hyperchromasia
- Homogeneous, smudgy, basophilic, opaque nuclear inclusion
- Smooth nuclear membranes; nucleoli are absent

PEARLS

- *De novo CIS is less likely to progress to invasive disease than is secondary CIS*
- *BCG immunotherapy remains the most effective treatment and prophylaxis for CIS, reducing short-term tumor recurrence by about 20%, long-term recurrence by about 7%, disease progression, and mortality*

SELECTED REFERENCES

Oliva E, Pinheiro NF, Heney NM, et al: Immunohistochemistry as an adjunct in the differential diagnosis of radiation-induced atypia versus urothelial carcinoma in situ of the bladder: a study of 45 cases. Hum Pathol 44:860-866, 2013.
Yin H, He Q, Li T, Leong AS: Cytokeratin 20 and Ki-67 to distinguish carcinoma in situ from flat non-neoplastic urothelium. Appl Immunohistochem Mol Morphol 14:260-265, 2006.

PAPILLARY UROTHELIAL LESIONS

The WHO(2003)/ISUP classification of noninvasive papillary urothelial lesions comprises papillary hyperplasia, urothelial papilloma and inverted papilloma, papillary neoplasm of low malignant potential, and low-grade and high-grade papillary urothelial carcinoma. To avoid an intermediate cancer grade group (grade II), the WHO(2003)/ISUP system classifies papillary urothelial carcinoma into only two grades: low-grade papillary urothelial carcinoma and high-grade papillary urothelial carcinoma.

Papillary Urothelial Hyperplasia

Clinical Features

- Typically discovered on routine follow-up cystoscopy for papillary urothelial neoplasms

Gross Features

- Benign focally elevated lesion identified at cystoscopy, described as papillary, raised, sessile, or bleb like

Histopathology

- Undulating urothelium arranged into mucosal narrow papillary folds of varying heights; no detached papillary fronds
- The urothelium within papillary hyperplasia and the adjacent flat mucosa are often thicker than normal
- The cytologic findings are similar to that characteristic of normal urothelium

Special Stains and Immunohistochemistry

- Noncontributory

Other Techniques for Diagnosis

- Noncontributory

Differential Diagnosis

UROTHELIAL PAPILLOMA

- Well-developed, detached papillary fronds with branching fibrovascular cores of a papillary neoplasm are evident

PEARLS

- *Patients should be followed up, as papillary hyperplasia likely represents the precursor lesion to low-grade papillary urothelial neoplasms*

SELECTED REFERENCES

Swierczynski SL, Epstein JI: Prognostic significance of atypical papillary urothelial hyperplasia. Hum Pathol 33:512-517, 2002.
Taylor DC, Bhagavan BS, Larsen MP, et al: Papillary urothelial hyperplasia: a precursor to papillary neoplasms. Am J Surg Pathol 20:1481-1488, 1996.

Urothelial Papilloma

Clinical Features

- Benign papillary urothelial tumor lined by normal-appearing urothelium
- Slightly more common in men
- Tends to occur in younger patients and is seen in children
- Usually presents with gross hematuria

Gross Features

- Urothelial papillomas typically have a simple papillary architecture

Histopathology

- Papillary fronds are lined by normal-appearing urothelium, lacking atypia (Figure 10-9)
- Usually have a simple minimally branching arrangement and slender fibrovascular stalks with a predominantly exophytic pattern

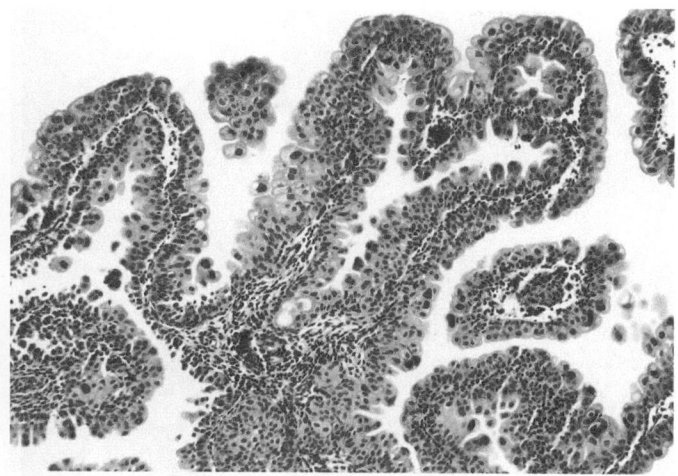

Figure 10-9. Urothelial papilloma. Papillary fronds are lined by normal-appearing urothelium. Superficial umbrella cells are often prominent, with abundant eosinophilic cytoplasm and vacuolization.

- Superficial umbrella cells are often prominent, with abundant eosinophilic cytoplasm, and vacuolization
- Mitoses are absent

Special Stains and Immunohistochemistry

- Cytokeratin 20: confined to the umbrella cells, similarly to normal urothelium

Other Techniques for Diagnosis

- Noncontributory

Differential Diagnosis

PAPILLARY NEOPLASM OF LOW MALIGNANT POTENTIAL (PUNLMP)

- Markedly thickened urothelium
- Mitoses may be present but are confined to the basal layers

PEARLS

- *Rarely recur; can progress to higher-grade disease*
- *Complete transurethral resection is the treatment of choice*

SELECTED REFERENCES

Magi-Galluzzi C, Epstein JI: Urothelial papilloma of the bladder: a review of 34 de novo cases. Am J Surg Pathol 28:1615-1620, 2004.

McKenney JK, Amin MB, Young RH: Urothelial (transitional cell) papilloma of the urinary bladder: a clinicopathologic study of 26 cases. Mod Pathol 16:623-629, 2003.

Inverted Papilloma

Clinical Features

- Rare benign urothelial tumor of unknown etiology
- More common in males and occurs at all ages; median age is 55 years
- Typically involves the bladder at the trigone, bladder neck, or prostatic urethra
- Frequently presents with hematuria

Gross Pathology

- Typically solitary flat or slightly raised polypoid mass with smooth contours
- Usually minimal exophytic component
- Most are smaller than 3 cm in diameter

Histopathology

- Characterized by anastomosing cords or islands of urothelium showing uniform width and minimal cytologic atypia; rare mitotic activity (Figure 10-10A)
- Tumor originates from the surface urothelium and extends down into the underlying lamina propria but not into the muscular bladder wall (Figure 10-10B)
- Small cystic spaces and true glandular differentiation with layer of mucin secreting cells may be seen
- The stromal component is mostly minimal and lacks inflammation

Special Stains and Immunohistochemistry

- Noncontributory

Other Techniques for Diagnosis

- Noncontributory

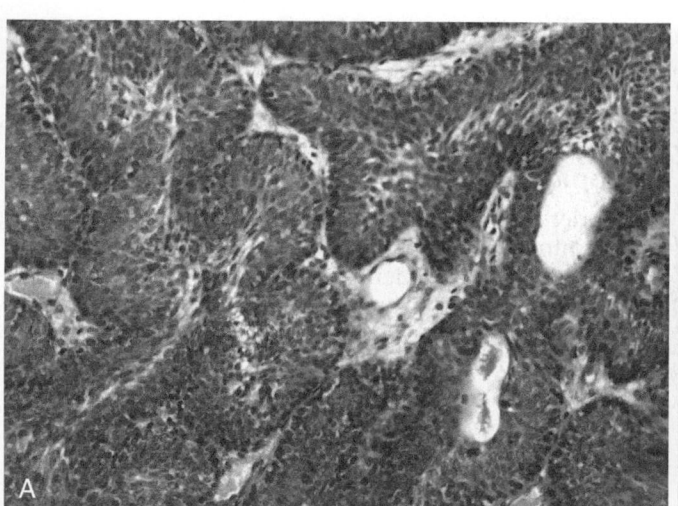
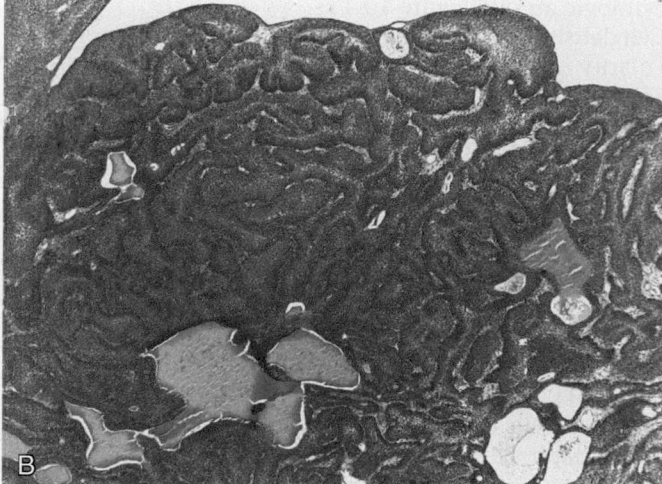

Figure 10-10. A, Inverted papilloma. The urothelial cells show minimal cytologic atypia. **B,** Inverted papilloma. Tumor originates from the surface urothelium and extends down into the underlying lamina propria. It forms anastomosing cords or islands of urothelium.

Differential Diagnosis

UROTHELIAL CARCINOMA
- Typically shows an exophytic papillary architecture
- Increased cytologic atypia and increased mitotic activity
- Invasive growth pattern is often noted

FLORID PROLIFERATION OF VON BRUNN NESTS
- Round nests without the anastomosing pattern

PEARLS

- *Relationship between inverted papilloma and low-grade papillary urothelial carcinoma is not fully understood*
- *Inverted papilloma is best treated by transurethral resection; occasional recurrences have been reported*
- *Occasionally coexistence with papillary urothelial carcinoma has been described, although it is unresolved whether there is an increased risk of this relationship*

SELECTED REFERENCES

Patel P, Reikie BA, Maxwell JP, et al: Long-term clinical outcome of inverted urothelial papilloma including cases with focal papillary pattern: is continuous surveillance necessary? Urology 82:857-860, 2013.

Sung MT, MacLennan GT, Lopez-Beltran A, et al: Natural history of urothelial inverted papilloma. Cancer 107:2622-2627, 2006.

Papillary Urothelial Neoplasm of Low Malignant Potential

Clinical Features

- Papillary urothelial neoplasm lined by urothelium with minimal atypia
- Slightly more common in men
- Mean age at diagnosis is 64.6 years (ranges from 29 to 94 years)
- Usually presents with gross or microscopic hematuria

Gross Features

- Small to 2-cm papillary tumor

Histopathology

- Discrete and slender papillary fronds lined by a thickened multilayered urothelium with minimal to absent cytologic atypia (Figure 10-11)
- Cell density appears to be increased compared to normal
- Polarity is preserved
- Mitoses are rare and have a basal location

Special Stains and Immunohistochemistry

- Cytokeratin 20: confined to the umbrella cells

Other Techniques for Diagnosis

- Noncontributory

Differential Diagnosis

NONINVASIVE LOW-GRADE PAPILLARY UROTHELIAL CARCINOMA
- Scattered cells with enlarged hyperchromatic nuclei
- More than rare mitotic figures

UROTHELIAL PAPILLOMA
- Lining urothelium is of normal thickness

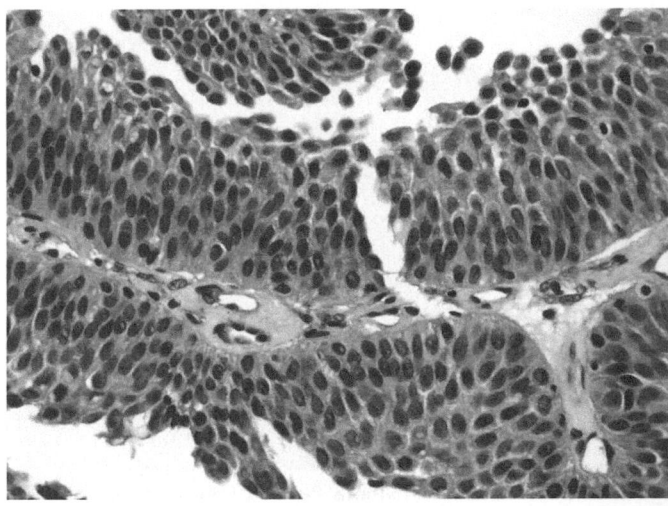

Figure 10-11. Papillary urothelial neoplasm of low malignant potential. Discrete and slender papillary frond lined by a thickened multilayered urothelium with minimal to absent cytologic atypia.

PEARLS

- *Recurrences occur but at a lower frequency than with papillary carcinoma*
- *Transurethral resection is the treatment of choice*

SELECTED REFERENCES

Jones TD, Cheng L: Papillary urothelial neoplasm of low malignant potential: evolving terminology and concepts. J Urol 175:1995-2003, 2006.

Lee TK, Chaux A, Karram S, et al: Papillary urothelial neoplasm of low malignant potential of the urinary bladder: clinicopathologic and outcome analysis from a single academic center. Hum Pathol 42:1799-1803, 2011.

Noninvasive Low-Grade Papillary Urothelial Carcinoma

Clinical Features

- Papillary neoplasm lined by urothelium with easily recognizable variation in architectural and cytologic features
- Slightly more common in men
- Mean age at diagnosis is 69.2 years (ranges from 28 to 90 years)
- Usually presents with gross or microscopic hematuria

Gross Features

- In the majority of the cases, the papillary tumor is single

Histopathology

- Slender papillary fronds showing frequent branching and minimal fusion (Figure 10-12)
- Lesion shows an orderly appearance with easily recognizable variations in architectural and cytologic features
- Nuclei are uniformly enlarged with mild variation in shape, contour, and chromatin distribution
- Mitoses are infrequent and may occur at any level

Special Stains and Immunohistochemistry

- p53 and Ki-67 expression is intermediate between papillary urothelial neoplasm of low malignant potential and high-grade urothelial carcinoma
- Negative or focal reactivity for CK20

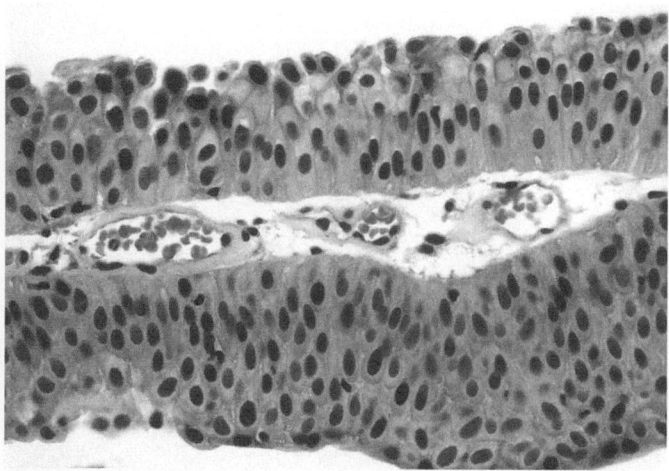

Figure 10-12. Noninvasive low-grade papillary urothelial carcinoma. Slender papillary frond lined by an orderly urothelium with easily recognizable variations in architectural and cytologic features. The nuclei are uniformly enlarged with mild differences in shape, contour, and chromatin distribution.

Other Techniques for Diagnosis

- Allelic loss of multiple chromosome loci has been reported

Differential Diagnosis

PAPILLARY UROTHELIAL NEOPLASM OF LOW MALIGNANT POTENTIAL

- Monotonous bland-appearing cells, lacking scattered cells with enlarged hyperchromatic nuclei

RARE MITOTIC FIGURES

- High-grade papillary urothelial carcinoma
- High degree of cytologic atypia with architectural distortion

PEARLS

- *Recurrence is common in approximately 48% to 71% of patients*
- *Progression to invasion and cancer deaths occurs in less than 5% of patients*
- *Transurethral resection is the treatment of choice; multifocal or recurrent disease is sometimes treated with intravesical immunotherapy*

SELECTED REFERENCES

Vardar E, Gunlusoy B, Minareci S, et al: Evaluation of p53 nuclear accumulation in low- and high-grade (WHO/ISUP classification) transitional papillary carcinomas of the bladder for tumor recurrence and progression. Urol Int 77:27-33, 2006.
Wu XR: Urothelial tumorigenesis: a tale of divergent pathways. Nat Rev Cancer 5:713-72, 2005.

Noninvasive High-Grade Papillary Urothelial Carcinoma

Clinical Features

- Usually presents with gross or microscopic hematuria

Gross Features

- Appearance varies from papillary to nodular/solid sessile lesion

Histopathology

- Papillary neoplasm characterized by a disorderly appearance of urothelium resulting from marked architectural and cytologic abnormalities, recognizable at low magnification
- Papillae are frequently fused and branching, although some may be delicate; extensive denudation may be present (Figure 10-13)
- Cytologically, there is a spectrum of pleomorphism ranging from moderate to marked
- There is marked variation in nuclear polarity, size, shape, and chromatin pattern; nucleoli may be prominent
- Mitotic figures, including atypical forms, are frequently seen at all levels of the urothelium

Special Stains and Immunohistochemistry

- Detection of p53 and ki67 is more frequent than in low-grade urothelial carcinoma
- Strong and diffuse reactivity for p16 and CK20

Other Techniques for Diagnosis

- Deletion of chromosome 9p seems to be an early event in the development of papillary urothelial carcinoma

Differential Diagnosis

LOW-GRADE PAPILLARY UROTHELIAL CARCINOMA

- Mild degree of cytologic atypia with minimum architectural distortion

PEARLS

- *Urothelial carcinoma with both low- and high-grade features is not uncommon*
- *Invasion both within the papillary cores and at the base of the lesions should be ruled out*

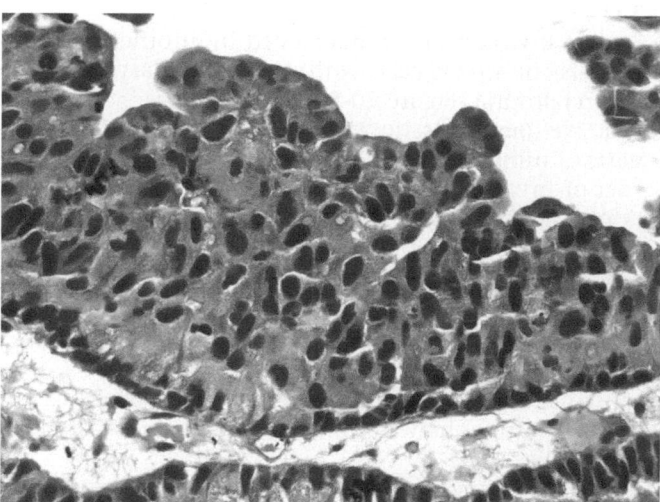

Figure 10-13. Noninvasive high-grade papillary urothelial carcinoma. Papillae are frequently fused and branching. Cytologically, there is moderate to marked pleomorphism with marked variation in nuclear polarity, size, shape, and chromatin pattern.

SELECTED REFERENCES

Chaux A, Karram S, Miller JS, et al: High-grade papillary urothelial carcinoma of the urinary tract: a clinicopathologic analysis of a post-World Health Organization/International Society of Urological Pathology classification cohort from a single academic center. Hum Pathol 43:115-120, 2012.

Mai KT, Flood TA, Williams P, et al: Mixed low- and high-grade papillary urothelial carcinoma: histopathogenetic and clinical significance. Virchows Arch 463:575-581, 2013.

Owens CL, Epstein JI: Significance of denuded urothelium in papillary urothelial lesions. Am J Surg Pathol 31:298-303, 2007.

Invasive Urothelial Carcinoma

Clinical Features

- Typically found in elderly individuals with a mean age greater than 65 years
- More frequently seen in men M:F=3:1
- Associated with tobacco smoking, many toxic chemicals (including nitrosamines), drugs (phenacetin, cyclophosphamide), infections (*Schistosoma hematobium*)
- Most common presenting symptom is painless hematuria
- Patients may have flank pain and obstructive symptoms

Gross Features

- Tumors usually involve the lateral or posterior bladder walls; occasionally involve the bladder dome
- Low-grade tumors typically have a papillary architecture appearing as multiple finger-like fronds over the bladder mucosa (see Noninvasive Low-Grade Papillary Urothelial Carcinoma)
- Higher-grade tumors often lack papillary architecture and show nodular, polypoid, or sessile pattern (see Noninvasive High-Grade Papillary Urothelial Carcinoma); focal remnants of papillary architecture may persist
- Bladder wall is typically thickened, firm, and gray-white
- Ulceration and hemorrhage is often seen in the high-grade tumors

Histopathology

UROTHELIAL CARCINOMA INVADING LAMINA PROPRIA (PT1)

- Foci of invasion are characterized by urothelial nests, clusters, or single cells within the papillary cores or lamina propria (Figure 10-14)
- Reactive desmoplastic stroma surrounds infiltrating nests of tumor cells
- Foci of invasive tumor may be associated with retraction artifact, mimicking vascular invasion

UROTHELIAL CARCINOMA INVADING MUSCULARIS PROPRIA (PT2)

- Usually nonpapillary tumors infiltrate the underlying muscularis propria
- Muscularis propria invasion is diagnosed when carcinoma infiltrates between thick distinct fascicles of muscle bundles
- Muscle invasion may or may not elicit a desmoplastic stromal response
- Even in cases of noninvasive disease, the pathologist should note whether muscularis propria is present in the biopsy specimen

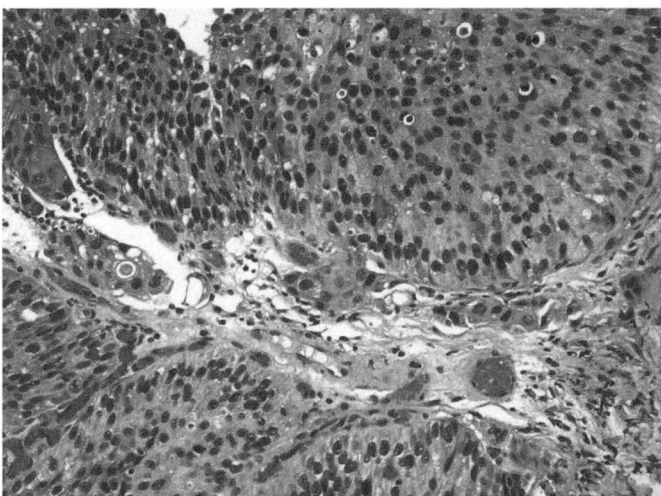

Figure 10-14. High-grade urothelial carcinoma invading lamina propria. Foci of invasion are characterized by urothelial nests within the lamina propria.

UROTHELIAL CARCINOMA INVADING ADIPOSE TISSUE AND SURROUNDING ORGANS (PT3 AND PT4)

- Adipose tissue is often present between detrusor muscle bundles, thus the presence of tumor in fat in a biopsy does not necessarily equate with involvement of perivesical fat

INVASIVE UROTHELIAL CARCINOMA: HISTOLOGIC VARIANTS

- Urothelial carcinoma has a propensity for divergent differentiation with the most common being squamous followed by glandular
- Presence of variant histology in general has no impact on clinical outcomes, although such tumors often have other adverse pathologic features such as higher stage

INFILTRATING UROTHELIAL CARCINOMA WITH SQUAMOUS DIFFERENTIATION

- Occurs in 21% of urothelial carcinomas of the bladder and 44% of tumors of the renal pelvis
- Clinical significance of squamous differentiation remains uncertain

INFILTRATING UROTHELIAL CARCINOMA WITH GLANDULAR DIFFERENTIATION

- Tubular or enteric glands with mucin secretions may be present in about 6% of urothelial carcinoma of the bladder

INFILTRATING UROTHELIAL CARCINOMA, NESTED VARIANT

- Aggressive neoplasm, with 70% of the patients dead 4 to 40 months after diagnosis, despite therapy
- This variant has a deceptively benign appearance that closely resembles von Brunn nests infiltrating the lamina propria (Figure 10-15)

INFILTRATING UROTHELIAL CARCINOMA, LARGE NESTED VARIANT

- Contains unevenly distributed medium to large cell nests with rounded to irregular contours, typically separated by abundant fibrous stromal tissue (Figure 10-16)

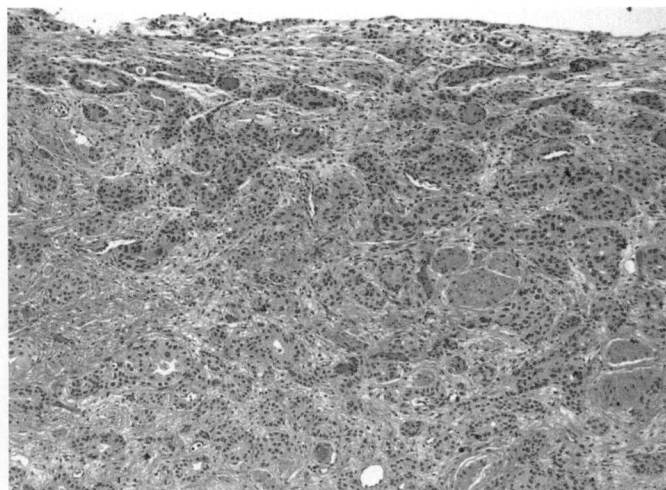

Figure 10-15. Infiltrating urothelial carcinoma, nested variant. This variant of urothelial carcinoma is characterized by closely packed, irregularly invading, crowded, or anastomosing nests of relatively bland neoplastic cells infiltrating the lamina propria.

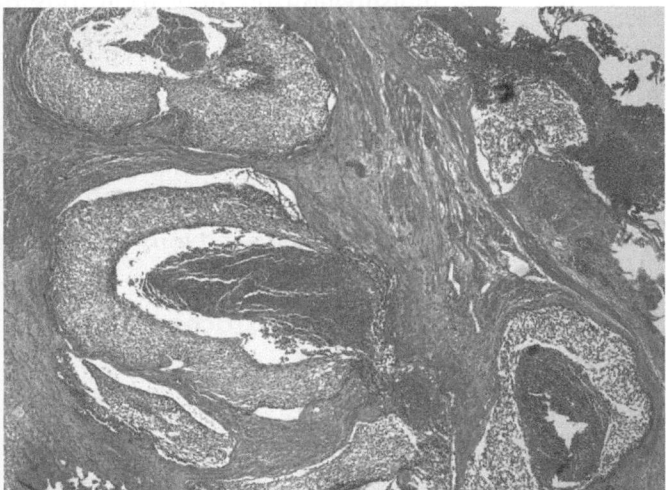

Figure 10-16. Infiltrating urothelial carcinoma, large nested variant. Tumor shows unevenly distributed large cell nests with rounded to irregular contours, separated by abundant fibrous stromal tissue.

- Displays deceptively bland cytologic features, often mimicking low-grade urothelial carcinoma
- Tumors frequently have a surface component often of low-grade papillary urothelial carcinoma, although in rare cases there may be an associated high-grade papillary component
- Invasion into the muscularis propria is commonly present with occasional cases displaying invasion into perivesical tissue

INFILTRATING UROTHELIAL CARCINOMA, MICROPAPILLARY VARIANT

- Resembles papillary serous carcinoma of the ovary
- Surface of the tumors shows slender, delicate papillary and villiform processes, often without a central vascular core
- Invasive portion is characterized by minute nests of cells or fine papillae contained within tissue retraction spaces, simulating lymphatic spaces
- Tumors are invariably muscle invasive, high grade

INFILTRATING UROTHELIAL CARCINOMA, LYMPHOEPITHELIOMA-LIKE

- Morphology is similar to lymphoepithelioma-like carcinoma in other organs with nests of tumor cells heavily infiltrated and masqueraded by lymphoplasmacytic cells
- Proportion of lymphoepithelioma-like carcinoma should be reported
- Behavior is uncertain as only few cases have been reported
- Pure form of lymphoepithelioma-like carcinoma is responsive to chemotherapy

Grading of Urothelial Carcinoma (see Noninvasive Low- and High-Grade Papillary Urothelial Carcinomas)

Special Stains and Immunohistochemistry

- Cytokeratin (high molecular weight, CK7, CK20), p63, and CD15: positive
- Carcinoembryonic antigen (CEA): positive (especially in high-grade tumors)
- GATA3: positive

Other Techniques for Diagnosis

- Cytogenetic studies: deletion of chromosome 9p is associated with superficial disease; abnormalities involving chromosome 17p are associated with disease progression; aneuploidy involving chromosomes 3, 7, and 17

Differential Diagnosis

POLYPOID CYSTITIS

- Must be distinguished from low-grade papillary transitional cell carcinoma
- Usually shows wider papillary structures and stromal edema
- Urothelium may show reactive atypia but usually less dysplasia than in transitional cell carcinoma

FLORID VON BRUNN NESTS

- Must be distinguished from nested and large nested variants of urothelial carcinoma
- Lobulated architecture with flat, noninvasive base
- Urothelial nests of relatively uniform size and shape and often associated with cystitis cystica et glandularis
- No significant cytologic atypia

NEPHROGENIC ADENOMA

- Must be distinguished from glandular component of urothelial carcinoma with glandular differentiation
- Classic histologic pattern is that of small tubules resembling renal tubules
- Papillary architecture can be confused with urothelial carcinoma
- Papillae and tubules are lined by benign cuboidal cells
- PAX2 and PAX8 positive, P63 and GATA3 negative

INVERTED PAPILLOMA

- Minimal cytologic atypia and low mitotic activity
- Lacks invasion into the muscularis propria

LOW-GRADE PAPILLARY UROTHELIAL CARCINOMA WITH INVERTED GROWTH PATTERN

- Must be distinguished from large nested variant of urothelial carcinoma

- Lacks invasive appearance and invasion into the muscularis propria
- Has rounded nests, which are fairly uniform in size and usually crowded

SQUAMOUS CELL CARCINOMA
- Pure squamous lesions lacking in situ and invasive urothelial component
- If an urothelial component is seen, the lesion should be classified as urothelial carcinoma with squamous differentiation

LYMPHOMA
- Must distinguish from lymphoepithelioma-like variant of urothelial carcinoma
- Islands of high-grade epithelial cells are not seen
- Cytokeratin is negative
- Leukocyte common antigen (LCA) is diffusely positive

PROSTATIC ADENOCARCINOMA
- Must distinguish from poorly differentiated bladder cancer
- Specimen is often obtained from the trigone or bladder neck
- p63, GATA3, and thrombomodulin are negative
- Prostate-specific antigen (PSA), prostate-specific acid phosphatase (PSAP), prostate specific membrane antigen (PSMA), p501s (prostein), and NKX3.1 are positive

PEARLS

- *Urine cytology is a valuable tool for managing patients with bladder cancer, especially high grade (best used as monitor for therapeutic response)*
- *Superficial urothelial tumors include those tumors that are confined to the lamina propria (stage T1); invasive cancer includes lesions that have invaded into the superficial muscularis propria (detrusor muscle) (stage T2a), deep muscularis propria (stage T2b), perivesical tissue (stage T3), and contiguous organs or tissues (stage T4)*
- *Low-grade urothelial carcinoma when completely excised virtually never metastasizes*
- *Despite the bland cytologic features, nested and large nested variants of urothelial carcinoma have well-documented metastatic potential*
- *Pathologist must comment on whether the biopsy material contains muscularis propria (detrusor muscle) and also whether or not there is muscularis propria invasion*
- *Superficial tumors have traditionally been treated with transurethral resection and intravesical chemotherapy or BCG, and muscle-invasive tumors have required radical cystectomy*

SELECTED REFERENCES

Chang A, Amin A, Gabrielson E, et al: Utility of GATA3 immunohistochemistry in differentiating urothelial carcinoma from prostate adenocarcinoma and squamous cell carcinomas of the uterine cervix, anus, and lung. Am J Surg Pathol 36:1472-1476, 2012.

Cox R, Epstein JI: Large nested variant of urothelial carcinoma: 23 cases mimicking von Brunn nests and inverted growth pattern of noninvasive papillary urothelial carcinoma. Am J Surg Pathol 35:1337-1342, 2011.

Magi-Galluzzi C, Zhou M, Epstein JI: Neoplasms of the urinary bladder. In Genitourinary Pathology: A Volume in Foundations in Diagnostic Pathology Series. Churchill Livingstone, Philadelphia, 2007, pp 176-189.

Samaratunga H, Delahunt B: Recently described and unusual variants of urothelial carcinoma of the urinary bladder. Pathology 44:407-418, 2012.

VILLOUS ADENOMA

Clinical Features

- Rare glandular neoplasm of the urinary bladder, which histologically mimics its enteric counterpart
- The lesion occurs in elderly patients (mean age 65 years)
- The most common locations are the urachus, dome, and trigone
- Patients often present with hematuria or irritative symptoms, occasionally with mucosuria
- Often coexists with in situ or invasive adenocarcinoma

Gross Features

- Papillary tumor indistinguishable from papillary urothelial carcinoma

Histopathology

- Blunt finger-like papillary architecture with central fibrovascular core, lined by pseudostratified columnar epithelium (Figure 10-17A)
- Epithelial cells display nuclear stratification, crowding, hyperchromasia, and occasional prominent nucleoli (Figure 10-17B)

Special Stains and Immunohistochemistry

- CK20, CK7 and CEA: positive
- EMA and acid mucin stains: frequently positive

Other Techniques for Diagnosis

- Noncontributory

Differential Diagnosis

WELL-DIFFERENTIATED ADENOCARCINOMA OF THE COLON OR BLADDER
- Degree of cytologic atypia similar to analogous colonic lesions
- Invasion into lamina propria

PEARLS

- *Presence of villous adenoma histology in a limited biopsy does not entirely exclude the possibility of adenocarcinoma, and complete excision is essential*

SELECTED REFERENCES

Chan TY, Epstein JI: In situ adenocarcinoma of the bladder. Am J Surg Pathol 25:892-899, 2001.

Cheng L, Montironi R, Bostwick DG: Villous adenoma of the urinary tract: a report of 23 cases, including 8 with coexistent adenocarcinoma. Am J Surg Pathol 23:764-771, 1999.

Seibel JL, Prasad S, Weiss RE, et al: Villous adenoma of the urinary tract: a lesion frequently associated with malignancy. Hum Pathol 33:236-241, 2002.

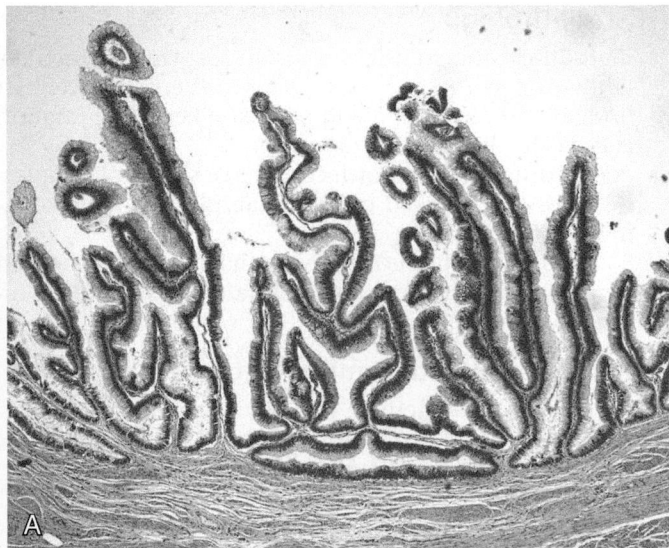

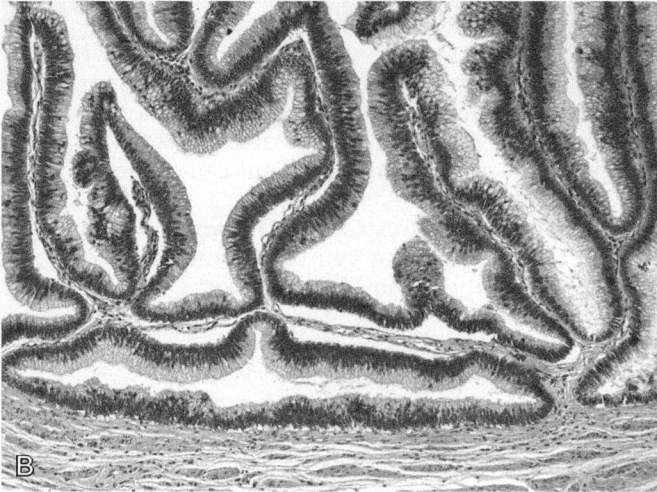

Figure 10-17. A, Villous adenoma. Neoplasm with blunt finger-like papillary architecture with central fibrovascular core, lined by pseudostratified columnar epithelium. **B,** Villous adenoma. Epithelial cells display nuclear stratification, crowding, hyperchromasia, and occasional prominent nucleoli.

ADENOCARCINOMA

Clinical Features

- Rare bladder neoplasm comprising approximately < 2% of all bladder tumors
- Divided into two groups:
  - Nonurachal adenocarcinoma
    - Accounts for two thirds of adenocarcinoma of the bladder
    - Found in adults with a mean age of 60 years
    - Most common presenting symptom is gross hematuria, followed by dysuria
    - Up to 40% of patients have metastatic disease at time of diagnosis
    - Occasionally associated with *Schistosoma hematobium* (less common association than with squamous cell carcinoma)
    - About 15% of tumors arise in patients with nonfunctioning bladder, and 85% are associated with exstrophy
  - Urachal adenocarcinoma
    - Primary carcinoma derived from the urachal remnants
    - Occurs in the fifth or sixth decade; the mean patient age is 50 years
    - Mucosuria occurs in approximately 25% of cases

Gross Features

NONURACHAL ADENOCARCINOMA

- Typically an exophytic, papillary, ulcerating mass arising from the bladder mucosa
- Usually involves the trigone or posterior bladder wall
- Often shows infiltrative margins
- May be sessile and cause a diffuse thickening of the bladder wall (resembles linitis plastica of the stomach); overlying bladder mucosa may be intact, leading to negative biopsies (signet ring cell variant)

URACHAL ADENOCARCINOMA

- Most form discrete masses over the dome of the bladder
- It may involve urachal remnants, forming a large mass in the anterior abdominal wall
- Overlying bladder mucosa may be intact or ulcerated
- Cut surface of the mass often shows abundant mucin

Histopathology

URACHAL AND NONURACHAL ADENOCARCINOMAS

- Mucinous carcinoma with pools of mucin containing single and groups of neoplastic cells (often resembles colonic adenocarcinoma)
- Neoplastic glands with an infiltrative growth pattern
- Glands are lined by large, pleomorphic cells with vesicular chromatin and prominent nucleoli; nuclear stratification is also common
- Signet ring cells may be seen
- Carcinoma in situ or intestinal metaplasia may be seen in nonurachal adenocarcinoma

URACHAL ADENOCARCINOMAS

- Criteria to classify a tumor as urachal adenocarcinoma
  - Location in the dome or anterior wall of the bladder
  - Sharp demarcation between tumor and normal surface epithelium
  - Lack of urothelial carcinoma
  - Typically adjacent mucosa lacks prominent cystitis glandularis
  - Bulk of tumor is in the bladder wall rather than luminal
  - Exclusion of primary adenocarcinoma located elsewhere that has spread secondarily to the bladder

Special Stains and Immunohistochemistry

- CK20, Leu M1 (CD15), and carcinoembryonic antigen (CEA): positive
- CK7: variably positive
- Villin: positive in the enteric type
- CDX-2: frequently positive; nuclear staining for β-catenin: negative

Other Techniques for Diagnosis

- Noncontributory

Differential Diagnosis

CYSTITIS CYSTICA ET GLANDULARIS
- Small submucosal cysts with benign cytologic features
- Typically small lesions without deep infiltration

NEPHROGENIC ADENOMA
- About 50% of cases found following genitourinary surgery
- Composed of small uniform tubules resembling proximal tubules of the kidney
- Usually much smaller than adenocarcinoma

ENDOMETRIOSIS
- Composed of endometrial glands and stroma
- Hemosiderin-laden macrophages often seen

METASTATIC ADENOCARCINOMA
- Presence of primary adenocarcinoma at distant site must be ruled out

PEARLS

- *Intestinal metaplasia is the precursor lesion in most nonurachal adenocarcinomas*
- *Treatment of urachal adenocarcinoma includes partial cystectomy with en bloc resection of the urachal ligament with the bladder dome and umbilicus*
- *Treatment of nonurachal adenocarcinoma includes cystectomy or cystoprostatectomy with pelvic lymph node dissection*
- *Overall prognosis is poor for both types*

SELECTED REFERENCES

Raspollini MR, Nesi G, Baroni G, et al: Immunohistochemistry in the differential diagnosis between primary and secondary intestinal adenocarcinoma of the urinary bladder. Appl Immunohistochem Mol Morphol 13:358-362, 2005.

Siefker-Radtke A: Urachal adenocarcinoma: a clinician's guide for treatment. Semin Oncol 39:619-624, 2012.

SQUAMOUS CELL CARCINOMA

Clinical Features
- Can involve the urinary bladder, renal pelvis, or occasionally the ureter
- Prevalence varies significantly depending on region of the world; it accounts for less than 5% of bladder carcinomas in areas where infection with *Schistosoma haematobium* is not endemic and 75% in areas where the infection is endemic
- Associated with *Schistosoma hematobium*
- Typically affects adults, with a slight male predominance
- Patients typically have a long duration of symptoms of cystitis and often have gross hematuria
- Bladder calculi and indwelling bladder catheters increase risk; tobacco is an important risk factor

Gross Pathology
- Typically large solid tumors often filling the bladder lumen and infiltrating the bladder wall
- Extensive necrosis is common

Histopathology

- Well-differentiated form consists of well-defined islands of squamous cells with prominent intercellular bridges and minimal pleomorphism; keratin formation is typically abundant
- Poorly differentiated form consists of sheets of neoplastic cells with marked cytologic atypia and focal squamous differentiation
- Squamous metaplasia often seen in adjacent epithelium
- Keratinizing squamous metaplasia or leukoplakia is often seen

Special Stains and Immunohistochemistry

- MAC387, Desmoglein-3, TRIM29: positive

Other Techniques for Diagnosis

- Noncontributory

Differential Diagnosis

UROTHELIAL CARCINOMA WITH SQUAMOUS DIFFERENTIATION
- If urothelial component is present, the tumor should not be classified as a squamous cell carcinoma
- Urothelial carcinoma in situ may be seen; it would never be seen in a pure squamous cell carcinoma

METASTATIC SQUAMOUS CELL CARCINOMA
- Presence of squamous cell carcinoma from local (cervix) or distant site must be ruled out

SQUAMOUS PAPILLOMA
- Lack of cytologic atypia and invasion

CONDYLOMA
- Presence of koilocytic cells

PEARLS

- *It comprises approximately 5% of all malignant bladder tumors*
- *The overall 5-year survival is 56%: 67% for patients with organ-confined tumor, and 19% for non-organ-confined tumor*
- *Treatment consists of radical cystectomy or cystoprostatectomy*
- *Overall poor prognosis*
- *Commonly develop local recurrence rather than distant metastases*
- *Metastases when present often involve bone*

SELECTED REFERENCES

Huang W, Williamson SR, Rao Q, et al: Novel markers of squamous differentiation in the urinary bladder. Hum Pathol 44:1989-1997, 2013.

Kassouf W, Spiess PE, Siefker-Radtke A, et al: Outcome and patterns of recurrence of nonbilharzial pure squamous cell carcinoma of the bladder: a contemporary review of The University of Texas M.D. Anderson Cancer Center experience. Cancer 110:764-769, 2007.

SMALL CELL CARCINOMA

Clinical Features
- Comprises less than 1% of primary bladder tumors

- Typically found in elderly men, with a 4:1 male-to-female ratio
- Most common presenting complaint is gross hematuria
- Patients often have extensive local involvement or distant metastases at the time of presentation

Gross Pathology

- Variable size, ranging from 2 cm to larger than 10 cm
- May have solid or papillary architecture
- Hemorrhage, necrosis, or mucosal ulceration are common

Histopathology

- Resembles small cell carcinoma of other sites
- Consists of uniform population of small to medium-sized cells with nuclear molding, scant cytoplasm, and nuclei with finely stippled chromatin and inconspicuous nucleoli
- Nuclei are hyperchromatic and show prominent folding
- Chromatin is dispersed, and nucleoli are inconspicuous
- Mitotic activity and apoptosis are prominent
- Diagnosis can be made on morphologic grounds alone, even if neuroendocrine differentiation cannot be demonstrated immunohistochemically
- Rarely see well-differentiated variant, which has features of carcinoid, including an organoid pattern

Special Stains and Immunohistochemistry

- Neuron-specific enolase (NSE), synaptophysin, and CD56: positive
- Chromogranin: positive in one third of cases
- Cytokeratin: typically positive; occasionally nonreactive

Other Techniques for Diagnosis

- Electron microscopy: tumor cells contain numerous dense core neurosecretory granules

Differential Diagnosis

METASTATIC SMALL CELL CARCINOMA
- Clinical correlation is needed to exclude presence of primary small cell carcinoma at distant site
- Identification of urothelial component, including urothelial carcinoma in situ, supports a bladder primary

MALIGNANT LYMPHOMA
- Consists of atypical lymphoid population
- Positive staining for LCA
- Negative staining for cytokeratin, synaptophysin, and chromogranin

PEARLS

- *Aggressive behavior with poor prognosis*
- *Overall 5-year survival rate for patients with local disease has been reported to be as low as 8%*
- *Treatment includes radical cystectomy or cystoprostatectomy in addition to multiagent chemotherapy*

SELECTED REFERENCES

Moretto P, Wood L, Emmenegger U, et al: Management of small cell carcinoma of the bladder: consensus guidelines from the Canadian Association of Genitourinary Medical Oncologists (CAGMO). Can Urol Assoc J 7: E44-E56, 2013.

Wang X, MacLennan GT, Lopez-Beltran A, Cheng L: Small cell carcinoma of the urinary bladder: histogenesis, genetics, diagnosis, biomarkers, treatment, and prognosis. Appl Immunohistochem Mol Morphol 15:8-18, 2007.
Zhao X, Flynn EA: Small cell carcinoma of the urinary bladder: a rare, aggressive neuroendocrine malignancy. Arch Pathol Lab Med 136:1451-1459, 2012.

INFLAMMATORY MYOFIBROBLASTIC TUMOR (IMT)/INFLAMMATORY PSEUDOTUMOR

Clinical Features

- Typically found in patients in second through fifth decades
- Slightly more common in women
- Usually presents with gross hematuria

Gross Pathology

- Typically pedunculated, nodular mass ranging in size from 2 to 5 cm
- May occasionally be sessile and extend into the underlying tissue

Histopathology

- Characterized by myofibroblastic cells resembling tissue-culture fibroblasts arranged in fascicles or more haphazardly (Figure 10-18)
- Background usually contains a sparse inflammatory component consisting of lymphocytes and plasma cells; eosinophils may also be numerous
- Prominent network of thin-walled blood vessels in an edematous or myxoid stroma with little-to-moderate collagen deposition is common
- Spindle cells may show focal pleomorphism
- Mitotic figures may be present and even frequent, but they are not atypical
- Infiltration into the muscularis propria may occur

Special Stains and Immunohistochemistry

- ALK protein: positive in two thirds of cases
- Cytokeratin: variable staining pattern

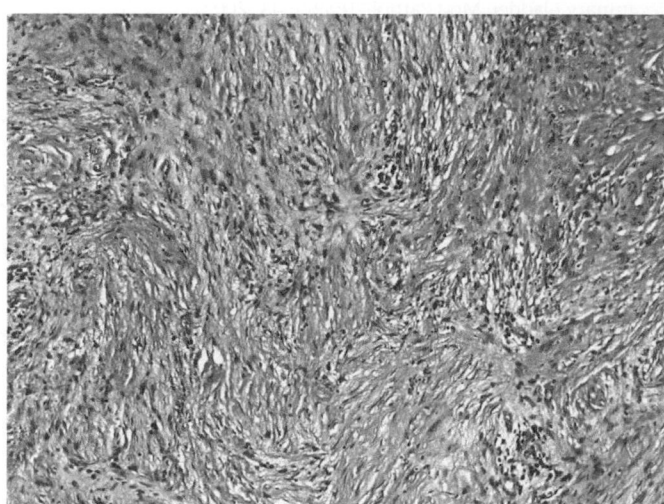

Figure 10-18. Inflammatory myofibroblastic tumor. The neoplasm is composed of a proliferation of spindle cells with a mixed inflammatory background.

- Smooth muscle actin (SMA): often positive
- Desmin: typically negative

Other Techniques for Diagnosis

- Translocation involving chromosome 2p23, site of the ALK gene

Differential Diagnosis

SARCOMATOID UROTHELIAL CARCINOMA/ CARCINOSARCOMA

- Consists of malignant epithelial and malignant mesenchymal components
- Numerous mitotic figures
- Lacks inflammatory background
- Lacks network of thin-walled blood vessels

LEIOMYOSARCOMA

- Overall, rare; however, it is the most common bladder sarcoma in older adults
- Usually shows infiltrative margins
- Typically shows cytologic atypia and increased mitotic activity with atypical mitotic figures
- More commonly shows immunohistochemical evidence of smooth muscle differentiation

PEARLS

- *Benign spindle cell neoplasm; complete surgical resection is the treatment of choice*
- *Most common misdiagnosis is that of malignant sarcoma or sarcomatoid carcinoma*
- *Most inflammatory pseudotumors are pedunculated and extend into the bladder lumen; occasionally they may be sessile and infiltrative*

SELECTED REFERENCES

Alquati S, Gira FA, Bartoli V, et al: Low-grade myofibroblastic proliferations of the urinary bladder. Arch Pathol Lab Med 137:1117-1128, 2013.
Shanks JH, Iczkowski KA: Spindle cell lesions of the bladder and urinary tract. Histopathology 55:491-504, 2009.
Sukov WR, Cheville JC, Carlson AW, et al: Utility of ALK-1 protein expression and ALK rearrangements in distinguishing inflammatory myofibroblastic tumor from malignant spindle cell lesions of the urinary bladder. Mod Pathol 20:592-603, 2007.
Young RH: Pseudotumors of the urinary bladder. Int J Surg Pathol 18(3 Suppl):101S-105S, 2010.

RHABDOMYOSARCOMA

Clinical Features

- Relatively common malignant neoplasm in children under the age of 15
- Most common bladder tumor of childhood
- Typically found before the age of 5
- Slightly more common in boys (male-to-female ratio of 3:2)
- Most tumors are of embryonal subtype and exophytic (polypoid), with or without a botryoid component
- Rare in adults, usually of the pleomorphic type
- Typically presents with hematuria or bladder outlet obstruction

Gross Pathology

- Grossly, embryonal rhabdomyosarcoma can be divided into two basic forms with prognostic impact: polypoid,

mostly intraluminal, associated with favorable prognosis (grapelike clusters, botryoid subtype), and deeply invasive tumors with a worse prognosis
- Typically occurs at the bladder trigone

Histopathology

- Tumor cells are small, round with scant cytoplasm, and hyperchromatic nuclei
- Typically a loose myxoid background is seen
- Large cells with abundant eosinophilic cytoplasm and cross striations (strap cells) may be seen

Special Stains and Immunohistochemistry

- Myogenin (myf4) and MyoD1: positive
- Desmin and pan-actin (HHF35): positive, but not specific
- Myosin and myoglobin: can be negative
- Cytokeratin: negative

Other Techniques for Diagnosis

- Electron microscopy: cells show thin actin and thick myosin filaments forming hexagonal pattern

Differential Diagnosis

SARCOMATOID CARCINOMA (CARCINOSARCOMA)

- Consists of malignant epithelial and malignant spindle cell components
- Islands of cells with epithelial differentiation are seen
- Cytokeratin positivity in the epithelial component

INFLAMMATORY MYOFIBROBLASTIC TUMOR (IMT)

- Background usually contains a sparse inflammatory component
- Prominent network of thin-walled blood vessels in an edematous or myxoid stroma
- Mitotic figures may be present and even frequent, but they are not atypical
- ALK-1 protein expression

PEARLS

- *Treatment includes surgery, radiation therapy, and chemotherapy; combination therapy has greatly improved survival in the pediatric age group*
- *Constitutes greater than 75% of bladder tumors in children*
- *Most common mesenchymal tumor of the urinary bladder*

SELECTED REFERENCES

Sukov WR, Cheville JC, Carlson AW, et al: Utility of ALK-1 protein expression and ALK rearrangements in distinguishing inflammatory myofibroblastic tumor from malignant spindle cell lesions of the urinary bladder. Mod Pathol 20:592-603, 2007.
Tavora F, Kryvenko ON, Epstein JI: Mesenchymal tumours of the bladder and prostate: an update. Pathology 45:104-115, 2013.

CARCINOSARCOMA/SARCOMATOID CARCINOMA WITH/WITHOUT HETEROLOGOUS ELEMENTS

Clinical Features

- Rare tumors of the urinary bladder
- Primarily affects elderly adults (seventh and eighth decades)

- Usually presents with hematuria or bladder outlet obstruction
- May rarely involve the ureter, renal pelvis, and bladder diverticulum
- Previous history of carcinoma treated by radiation or exposure to cyclophosphamide therapy is common

Gross Pathology

- Typically large polypoid mass measuring up to 10 to 12 cm in diameter with infiltrative margins

Histopathology

- Biphasic malignant neoplasm exhibiting morphologic or immunohistochemical evidence of epithelial and mesenchymal differentiation; presence or absence of heterologous elements should be mentioned in the diagnosis
- Malignant epithelial component is composed of urothelial, glandular, or small cell component showing variable degree of differentiation
- Mesenchymal component usually consists of pleomorphic, undifferentiated high-grade spindle cell neoplasm
- Most common heterologous element is osteosarcoma followed by chondrosarcoma, rhabdomyosarcoma, leiomyosarcoma, liposarcoma

Special Stains and Immunohistochemistry

- Cytokeratin (low molecular weight): epithelioid component is positive; some positivity in mesenchymal component may be seen
- Epithelial membrane antigen (EMA): may be positive but less frequently than cytokeratin
- Vimentin: mesenchymal component is positive
- Smooth muscle actin (SMA): may be positive in areas of smooth or striated muscle differentiation

Other Techniques for Diagnosis

- Noncontributory

Differential Diagnosis

Urothelial Carcinoma
- Malignant urothelial cells without malignant spindle cell component
- Vimentin negativity

Inflammatory Myofibroblastic Tumor/ Postoperative Spindle Cell Nodule
- Seen in association with recent therapeutic intervention, thus clinical history is important
- Most involve the genital tract of women or periprostatic tissue of men
- Reactive, highly cellular, spindle cell proliferation
- Often shows myxoid background with scattered small blood vessels and sparse neutrophilic infiltrate
- May have high mitotic rate; no abnormal mitoses

Malignant Spindle Cell Tumor, Including Leiomyosarcoma
- Primary sarcoma of the bladder is rare in adults
- Lacks epithelial component
- Negative for cytokeratin and EMA

PEARLS

- *Cytokeratin staining in both the epithelial and mesenchymal components supports a single cell line precursor theory*
- *Epithelial component may represent a minority of the tumor, thus extensive sectioning is required to identify an in situ or invasive epithelial component*
- *Aggressive tumor with poor prognosis*
- *Treatment consists of radical cystectomy or cystoprostatectomy; patients may also receive chemotherapy*

Selected References

Cheng L, Zhang S, Alexander R, et al: Sarcomatoid carcinoma of the urinary bladder: the final common pathway of urothelial carcinoma dedifferentiation. Am J Surg Pathol 35:e34-e46, 2011.
Gronau S, Menz CK, Melzner I, et al: Immunohistomorphologic and molecular cytogenetic analysis of a carcinosarcoma of the urinary bladder. Virchows Arch 440:436-440, 2002.

METASTATIC TUMORS AND SECONDARY EXTENSION

Clinical Features

- Metastases to the bladder or ureter are rare
- Majority of metastatic lesions are secondary to direct extension from tumors of the prostate, lower intestinal tract, and female genital tract
- Common primary tumors that metastasize to the bladder include breast, colon, or kidney carcinomas or malignant melanoma

Gross Pathology

- Often multiple tumors, typically located in the submucosa
- Focal ulceration of the urothelium overlying the mass may be seen

Histopathology

- Typically located within the bladder wall in a submucosal location
- Presence of a poorly differentiated tumor sparing the urothelial mucosa should raise suspicion of a possible metastasis
- Glandular differentiation is typically seen in metastatic colonic carcinoma; gland formation may also be seen in metastatic prostate carcinoma

Special Stains and Immunohistochemistry

- Prostate-specific antigen (PSA), prostate specific acid phosphatase (PSAP), p501s, NKX3.1: positive in metastatic prostate carcinoma
- S-100, Melan A, and HMB-45: positive in metastatic melanoma
- Villin, CDX-2: positive in metastatic colonic carcinoma

Other Techniques for Diagnosis

- Noncontributory

Differential Diagnosis

- Clinical history is important, especially the presence of a prostate carcinoma in men or a gynecologic tumor in women

PEARLS

- *Bladder metastases are most frequently a late event and are almost always associated with disseminated disease*
- *Patients typically have a poor prognosis*

SELECTED REFERENCES

Helpap B, Ayala AG, Grignon DJ, et al: Metastatic Tumors and Secondary Extension in Urinary Bladder: Tumors of the Urinary System and Male Genital Organs. WHO classification of tumors. Lyon, IARC Press, 2004, pp 148-149.

Suh N, Yang XJ, Tretiakova MS, et al: Value of CDX2, villin, and alpha-methylacyl coenzyme A racemase immunostain in the distinction between primary adenocarcinoma of the bladder and secondary colorectal adenocarcinoma. Mod Pathol 18:1217-1222, 2005.

KIDNEY

RENAL DYSPLASIA

Clinical Features

- Refers to presence of metanephric structure with aberrant nephronic differentiation
- Two main theories have been considered in its pathogenesis: a primary failure of ureteric bud activity and a disruption produced by fetal urinary flow impairment
- Most often *sporadic*, but may be syndromic and develop as part of a multiple malformation syndrome or chromosomal anomaly, some of which are *hereditary*
- Almost always accompanied by other urinary tract abnormalities
- Dysplastic kidneys are usually nonfunctional
- Large cystic dysplastic kidneys typically present as a palpable mass in a newborn; diagnosis confirmed by ultrasound
- Small dysplastic kidneys may remain asymptomatic for many years
- Bilateral disease results in oligohydramnios (Potter syndrome), and neonatal death from pulmonary hypoplasia

Gross Pathology

- Unilateral or bilateral involvement may be seen
- Distorted renal parenchyma with numerous variably sized cysts
- Dysplastic kidneys are usually enlarged; may occasionally be small

Histopathology

- Characteristic features include markedly disorganized kidney parenchyma with islands of cartilage and dysplastic ducts lined with columnar epithelium and surrounded by collars of spindle cells (Figure 10-19A)
- Cystic spaces lined by flattened epithelium (Figure 10-19B)
- Rudimentary glomeruli may be seen

Special Stains and Immunohistochemistry

- Noncontributory

Other Techniques for Diagnosis

- If multiple malformations are detected in a pediatric autopsy, it is important to obtain tissue for karyotype analysis

Differential Diagnosis

INFANTILE POLYCYSTIC KIDNEY DISEASE (AUTOSOMAL RECESSIVE)

- Often results in stillbirth or early neonatal death
- Cysts are in the cortex and medulla and do not congregate at the papillary tips
- Cartilaginous metaplasia or other dysplastic elements never seen

MEDULLARY CYSTIC DISEASE (AUTOSOMAL DOMINANT)

- Patients present with renal failure in first or second decade
- Cysts are located at the corticomedullary junction

MEDULLARY SPONGE KIDNEY

- Typically found in children or adolescents; not found at birth
- Ectasia of the papillary collecting ducts of one or more renal pyramids
- Renal function is normal
- Rare progression to end-stage renal disease

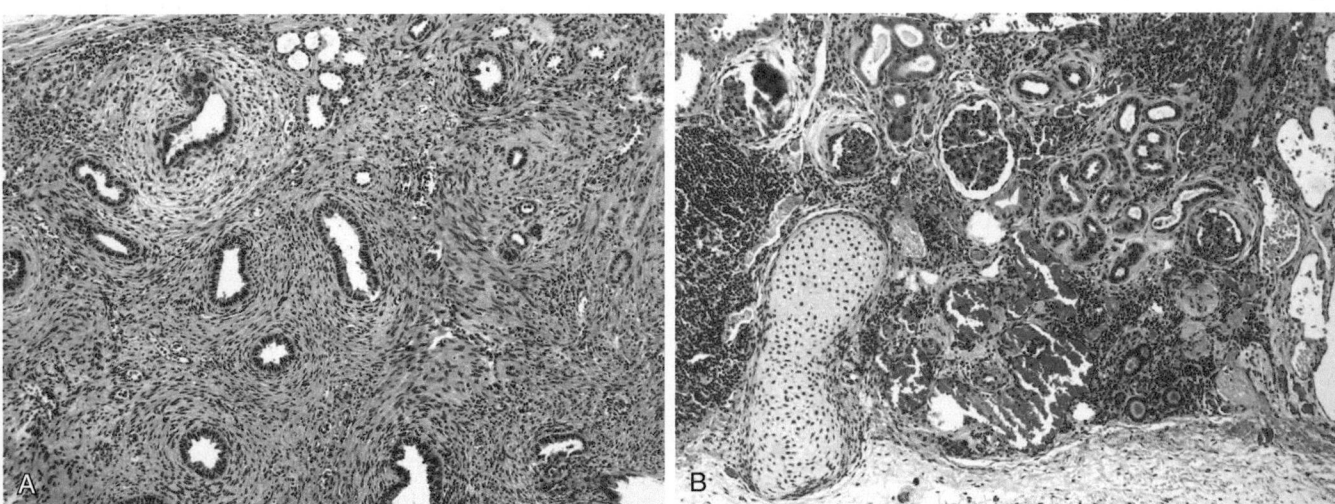

Figure 10-19. A, Renal dysplasia. Markedly disorganized kidney parenchyma with dysplastic ducts lined with columnar epithelium and surrounded by collars of spindle cells. **B,** Renal dysplasia. Island of cartilage and cystic spaces lined by flattened epithelium. Few glomeruli are seen.

PEARLS

- *Usually associated with congenital genitourinary abnormalities, including ureteral atresia*
- *Many investigators believe that renal dysplasia is associated with in utero urinary tract obstruction*
- *Unilateral disease is typically treated by nephrectomy*
- *Bilateral renal dysplasia ultimately results in renal failure*

SELECTED REFERENCES

Bisceglia M, Galliani CA, Senger C, et al: Renal cystic disease: a review. Adv Anat Pathol 13:256, 2006.
Woolf AS, Price KL, Scambler PJ, Winyard PJ: Evolving concepts in human renal dysplasia. J Am Soc Nephrol 15: 998-1007, 2004.

INFANTILE (AUTOSOMAL RECESSIVE) POLYCYSTIC KIDNEY DISEASE

Clinical Features

- Found in 1/10,000 to 1/50,000 live births
- Usually results in stillbirth or early neonatal death
- Abdominal distention due to massively enlarged kidneys
- Lungs may be poorly developed and hypoplastic owing to compression of the thoracic organs; fatal in 75% of cases
- Associated with congenital hepatic fibrosis in patients who survive infancy

Gross Pathology

- Always bilateral disease
- Massively enlarged kidneys with smooth external surface
- Renal parenchyma shows numerous small cysts involving the cortex and medulla
- Cysts are radially arranged and are oriented perpendicular to the renal capsule
- Calyceal system is normal

Histopathology

- Dilated collecting ducts lined by uniform cuboidal cells (Figure 10-20)
- Normal-appearing nephrons seen between cysts

Special Stains and Immunohistochemistry

- Noncontributory

Other Techniques for Diagnosis

- Cytogenetic studies: associated with single gene (PKHD1) mutation on chromosome 6p21-23: encodes for polyductin or fibrocystin

Differential Diagnosis

DYSPLASTIC KIDNEY

- Markedly disorganized kidney parenchyma with islands of cartilage and dysplastic ducts lined with columnar epithelium and surrounded by collars of spindle cells

MEDULLARY CYSTIC DISEASE

- Presents with renal failure in first or second decade
- Patients have polyuria and polydipsia as a result of salt wasting; develop uremia and growth retardation

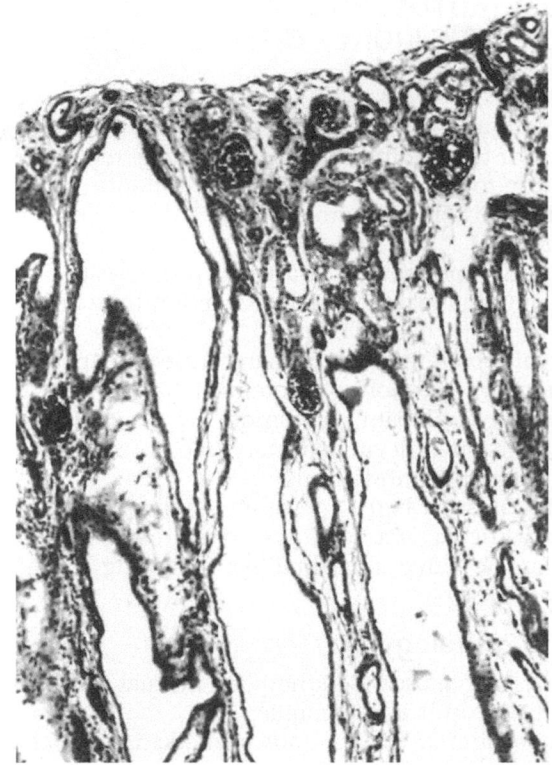

Figure 10-20. **Infantile polycystic kidney.** Characteristic dilated collecting ducts located perpendicular to the renal capsule.

- Kidneys are typically small; bilateral disease
- Cysts are numerous, less than 2 cm in diameter and located primarily at the corticomedullary junction
- Most patients develop end-stage renal disease within 5 years of diagnosis

MEDULLARY SPONGE KIDNEY

- Typically found in children or adolescents; not found at birth
- Kidneys are typically of normal size
- Multiple small cysts (< 0.5 cm) that involve the medullary pyramids and renal papillae and communicate with the collecting ducts
- Rare progression to end-stage kidney disease

PEARLS

- *Autosomal recessive disease*
- *Poor prognosis; often causes death in utero or shortly after birth*
- *Most cases are associated with multiple epithelium-lined cysts in the liver*

SELECTED REFERENCES

Dell KM: The spectrum of polycystic kidney disease in children. Adv Chronic Kidney Dis 18:339-347, 2011.
Garcia-Gonzalez MA, Menezes LF, Piontek KB, et al: Genetic interaction studies link autosomal dominant and recessive polycystic kidney disease in a common pathway. Hum Mol Genet 16:1940-1950, 2007.
Rossetti S, Harris PC: Genotype-phenotype correlations in autosomal dominant and autosomal recessive polycystic kidney disease. J Am Soc Nephrol 18:1374-1380, 2007.
Yoder BK: Role of primary cilia in the pathogenesis of polycystic kidney disease. J Am Soc Nephrol 18:1381-1388, 2007.

ADULT (AUTOSOMAL DOMINANT) POLYCYSTIC KIDNEY DISEASE

Clinical Features

- Found in 1/400 to 1/1000 live births
- One of the leading causes of end-stage renal disease in adults; found in 5% to 10% of all patients on dialysis
- Family history in approximately 70% to 75% of affected persons
- Typically presents in fourth to fifth decade after sufficient renal parenchyma destruction has occurred and renal failure has developed
- Usually presents with hematuria (secondary to stones, tumor, or infection) or proteinuria
- Chronic flank pain is common
- Patients often develop urinary tract infections
- Extrarenal manifestations
  - Intracranial berry aneurysms, hypertension, colonic diverticula, extrarenal cysts (pancreatic, hepatic), and cardiac valve abnormalities including mitral valve prolapse

Gross Pathology

- Early in the disease, kidneys are normal sized with few cysts in cortex and medulla
- Progression of disease leads to marked bilateral kidney enlargement with an increase in the size and number of cysts (may weigh up to 4 kg each) (Figure 10-21A)
- Kidneys have irregular contour due to numerous peripheral cysts
- Cysts range in size from few millimeters up to several centimeters; typically contain hemorrhagic or clear yellow fluid

Histopathology

- Cysts are lined by single layer of flat to cuboidal epithelium (Figure 10-21B)
- Small papillary projections may be seen
- Cysts contain proteinaceous material; calcified deposits are often seen
- Intervening kidney tissue typically shows interstitial fibrosis, lymphocytic infiltrate, tubular atrophy, and glomerular and vascular sclerosis
- Frequently associated with renal epithelial tumors (RCC)

Special Stains and Immunohistochemistry

- Noncontributory

Other Techniques for Diagnosis

- Cytogenetic studies:
  - Abnormality associated with chromosome 16 (16q13.3) in 85% of patients (involves PKD1 gene, which encodes a protein named polycystin 1)
  - Mutation involving chromosome 4 (4q21-23) in approximately 15% of cases (PKD2 gene, which encodes a protein named polycystin 2)

Differential Diagnosis

ACQUIRED CYSTIC DISEASE

- Patients typically have chronic renal failure and are on dialysis before cysts develop

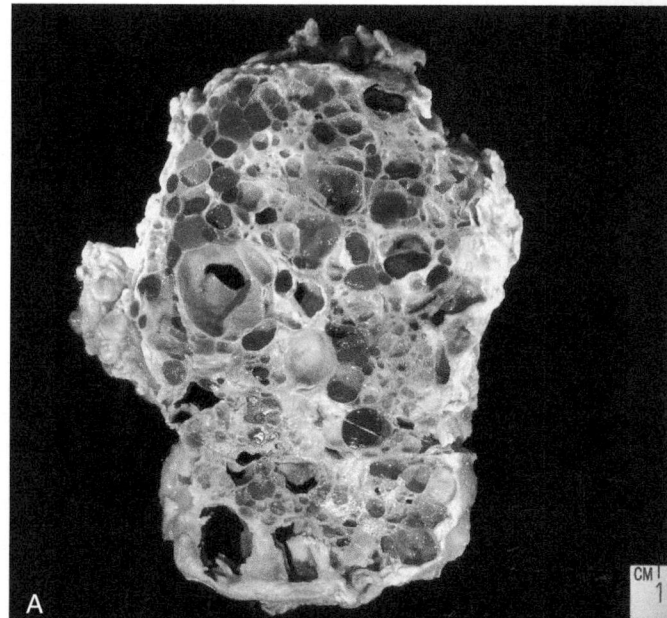

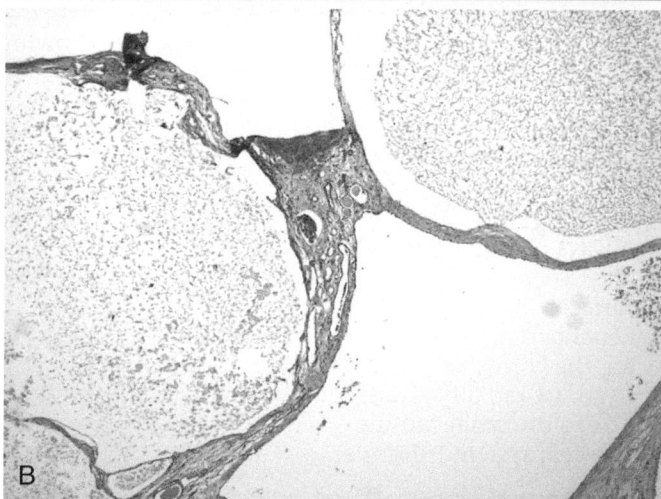

Figure 10-21. A, Adult polycystic kidney. Grossly the kidneys are markedly enlarged and show numerous cysts in the cortex and medulla. **B,** Adult polycystic kidney. Multiple cysts lined by flat cuboidal epithelium, some of which contain proteinaceous material.

- Kidney size reduced or only moderately enlarged
- Cysts are typically located in the cortex
- Lacks family history, which is typically present in polycystic kidney disease
- No associated extrarenal manifestations

PEARLS

- *Autosomal dominant disorder with high penetrance*
- *Almost 100% penetrance if patient lives to 80 years of age*
- *End-stage kidney disease is found in approximately 50% of patients by age 60*
- *The main and most effective therapy remains control of hypertension by renin-angiotensin-aldosterone system (RAAS) blockade*
- *Renal transplant is curative when patient develops end-stage kidney disease*

SELECTED REFERENCES

Czarnecki PG, Steinman TI: Polycystic kidney disease: new horizons and therapeutic frontiers. Minerva Urol Nefrol 65:61-68, 2013.

Helal I: Autosomal dominant polycystic kidney disease: new insights into treatment. Saudi J Kidney Dis Transpl 24:230-234, 2013.

Torres VE, Harris PC, Pirson Y: Autosomal dominant polycystic kidney disease. Lancet 369:1287-1301, 2007.

ACQUIRED CYSTIC DISEASE

Clinical Features

- Common finding in patients receiving hemodialysis or peritoneal dialysis
- Presence of cysts increases as time on dialysis increases
- Occasionally seen in patients with chronic renal insufficiency who are not on dialysis
- Pathogenesis of cyst formation remains largely unknown
- Often remains asymptomatic; may present with gross or microscopic hematuria
- Cyst formation is associated with increased risk of renal cell carcinoma

Gross Pathology

- Wide variation in size of cysts; from 1 mm up to several centimeters (Figure 10-22)
- Cysts are usually numerous; must be more than five to distinguish from incidental simple cysts
- Cysts are typically cortical
- Cysts usually contain clear, serous fluid; may contain hemorrhagic fluid
- Presence of solid areas suggests possible development of renal cell carcinoma

Histopathology

- Cysts are lined by single epithelial cell layer
- Epithelial lining may become hyperplastic and may occasionally develop into an adenoma or carcinoma

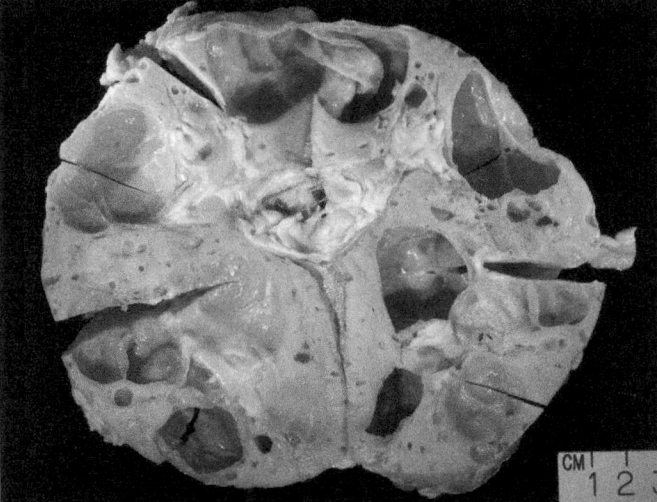

Figure 10-22. Acquired cystic disease. There is a wide variation in the size of cysts (from 1 mm up to several centimeters). Cysts are typically cortical and must be more than five to distinguish from incidental simple cysts.

- RCC in acquired cystic renal disease can be clear cell RCC, papillary RCC, chromophobe RCC, clear cell (tubulo)papillary RCC, and acquired cystic renal disease associated RCC
- Malignant tumors may develop in cystic areas or in adjacent kidney parenchyma
- Adjacent kidney parenchyma shows changes of end-stage kidney disease, including interstitial fibrosis, hyalinized glomeruli, and tubular atrophy

Special Stains and Immunohistochemistry

- Noncontributory

Other Techniques for Diagnosis

- Noncontributory

Differential Diagnosis

ADULT POLYCYSTIC KIDNEY DISEASE

- Kidneys are markedly enlarged and show numerous cysts in the cortex and medulla
- Family history is often present
- Found in third through fifth decades in patients without history of dialysis

PEARLS

- *Typically associated with hemodialysis or peritoneal dialysis*
- *Increased time on dialysis increases likelihood of cyst development*
- *Increased risk for subsequent development of renal cell carcinoma*
- *Patients are typically asymptomatic and do not require specific treatment*
- *CT scan is recommended to periodically evaluate cysts and look for development of suspicious masses*

SELECTED REFERENCES

Koljima Y, Takahara S, Miyake O, et al: Renal cell carcinoma in dialysis patients: a single center experience. Int J Urol 13:1045-1048, 2006.

Srigley JR, Delahunt B, Eble JN, et al: ISUP Renal Tumor Panel: The International Society of Urological Pathology (ISUP) Vancouver Classification of Renal Neoplasia. Am J Surg Pathol 37:1469-1489, 2013.

Tickoo SK, dePeralta-Venturina MN, Harik LR, et al: Spectrum of epithelial neoplasms in end-stage renal disease: an experience from 66 tumor-bearing kidneys with emphasis on histologic patterns distinct from those in sporadic adult renal neoplasia. Am J Surg Pathol 30:141-153, 2006.

XANTHOGRANULOMATOUS PYELONEPHRITIS

Clinical Features

- Subacute to chronic inflammatory lesion typically forming single or multiple mass lesions often mimicking a renal neoplasm
- Usually unilateral
- *Proteus* species and *E. coli* are the most common infective agents
- Most common presenting complaints are flank pain, fever, or a flank mass
- Nephrolithiasis is found in up to 70% of patients

Gross Pathology

- Kidney has dilated, thickened pelvis containing a staghorn calculus
- Yellow nodular tumor masses replace the renal pyramids
- Suppurative inflammation and edema begins within pelvic mucosa and sinus fat resulting in pelvicaliceal ulceration and fat necrosis
- Nodules may become confluent and eventually involve renal capsule, perinephric fat, and retroperitoneal tissue
- Diffuse form is most common; segmental form is polar and more common in children

Histopathology

- Xanthogranulomatous nodules have a zonal pattern
  - Central nidus of necrotic debris and neutrophils (microabscesses) with admixture of inflammatory cells, including lymphocytes, plasma cells
  - Surrounding sheets of lipid-laden macrophages with abundant clear cytoplasm (may resemble clear cell renal cell carcinoma) (Figure 10-23)
- Multinucleated giant cells and spindled fibroblasts surrounding macrophages (may resemble sarcomatoid carcinoma) may be seen

Special Stains and Immunohistochemistry

- CD68: macrophages are positive
- Cytokeratin: negative

Other Techniques for Diagnosis

- Noncontributory

Differential Diagnosis

CLEAR CELL RENAL CELL CARCINOMA
- Sheets of clear cells often with vague alveolar architecture
- Lacks inflammatory component
- Vimentin, cytokeratin, and CA9 (carbonic anhydrase IX) positive
- CD68 negative

SARCOMATOID CARCINOMA
- Polypoid mass often filling the bladder lumen
- Islands of cells with epithelial differentiation

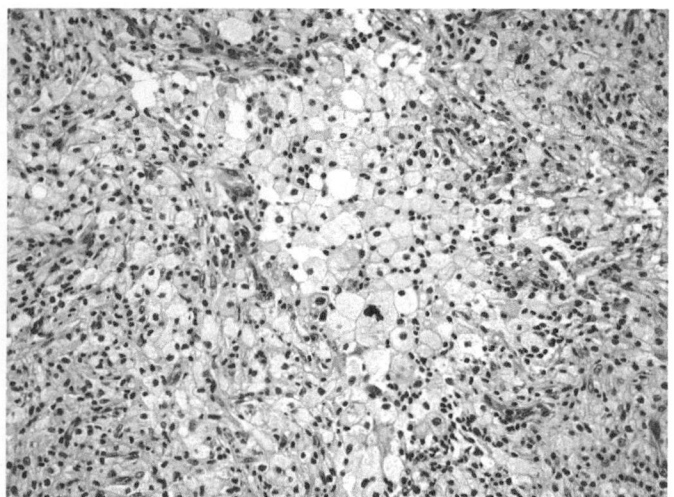

Figure 10-23. Xanthogranulomatous pyelonephritis. Collection of lipid-laden macrophages in a background of acute and chronic inflammatory cells.

- Cytokeratin positive
- CD68 negative

MALAKOPLAKIA
- Typically found in the urinary bladder
- Michaelis-Guttman bodies are characteristic

PEARLS

- *May clinically, radiologically, and pathologically mimic renal cell carcinoma*

SELECTED REFERENCES

Hendrickson RJ, Lutfiyya WL, Karrer FM, et al: Xanthogranulomatous pyelonephritis. J Pediatr Surg 41:e15-e17, 2006.
Li L, Parwani AV: Xanthogranulomatous pyelonephritis. Arch Pathol Lab Med 135:671-674, 2011.

ANGIOMYOLIPOMA

Clinical Features

- Majority are sporadic; 20% of cases are associated with tuberous sclerosis
- Majority of patients with tuberous sclerosis develop angiomyolipoma
- Tumors associated with tuberous sclerosis are usually asymptomatic; tumors are found earlier because these patients are all evaluated for kidney tumors
- Sporadic cases are larger and patients present with hematuria or flank or abdominal pain; rarely, retroperitoneal hemorrhage may occur

Gross Pathology

- Sporadic cases are typically single and unilateral
- Cases associated with tuberous sclerosis are typically multiple and bilateral
- Tumors are well circumscribed but unencapsulated
- Variegated appearance consisting of vascular and adipose tissue and gray-white solid areas corresponding to the smooth muscle component
- Necrosis is rarely seen but hemorrhage is common

Histopathology

- Triphasic tumor consisting of smooth muscle, mature adipose tissue, and thick-walled hyalinized blood vessels in varying proportion (Figure 10-24)
- One component may predominate
- Atypical features may occasionally be seen, including nuclear pleomorphism and mitosis
- Smooth muscle areas may show epithelioid differentiation with cells having abundant eosinophilic cytoplasm and large nuclei with prominent nucleoli

Special Stains and Immunohistochemistry

- Melanocytic markers: positive
- Smooth muscle markers: positive in smooth muscle component
- Epithelial markers: negative

Other Techniques for Diagnosis

- Noncontributory

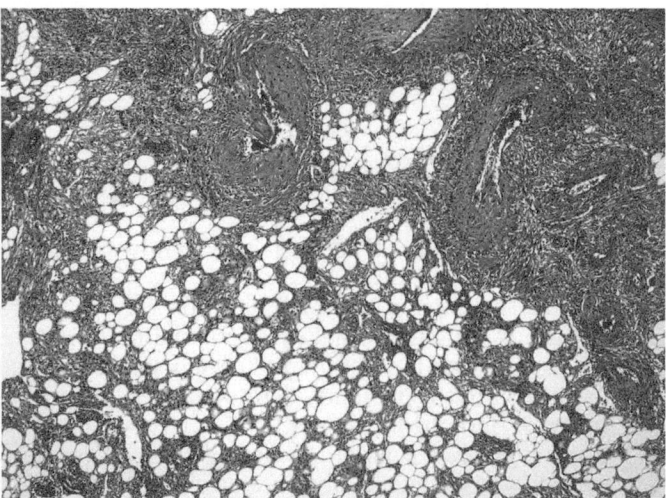

Figure 10-24. Angiomyolipoma. Classic angiomyolipoma of the kidney showing mature adipose tissue, smooth muscle, and blood vessels.

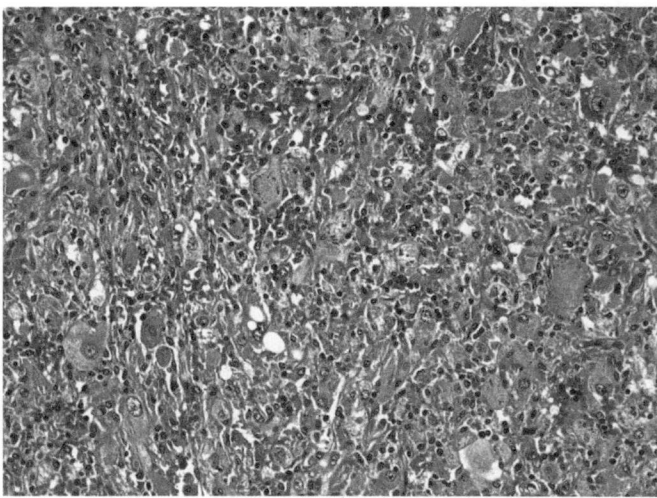

Figure 10-25. Epithelioid angiomyolipoma. Epithelioid angiomyolipoma is composed of stubby spindle cells and polygonal cells with eosinophilic cytoplasm. Occasional pleomorphic ganglion-like giant cells with amphophilic cytoplasm and eccentrically located nuclei are noted.

Differential Diagnosis

MALIGNANT SPINDLE CELL TUMORS, INCLUDING LEIOMYOSARCOMA

- Lack triphasic appearance
- Poorly circumscribed tumors with infiltrative borders
- Unequivocal high-grade, malignant cytologic features
- Negative for melanocytic markers

PEARLS

- *Tumor occasionally seen in the renal vein or in regional lymph nodes, but this is not a sign of malignant transformation*
- *Need to sample these tumors extensively to rule out the presence of coexisting renal cell carcinoma*
- *Must recognize that fatty tissue is part of lesion and not interpret it as an invasion into perirenal adipose tissue*

SELECTED REFERENCES

Rakowski SK, Winterkorn EB, Paul E, et al: Renal manifestations of tuberous sclerosis complex: incidence, prognosis, and predictive factors. Kidney Int 70:1777-1782, 2006.

Roma AA, Magi-Galluzzi C, Zhou M: Differential expression of melanocytic markers in myoid, lipomatous, and vascular components of renal angiomyolipomas. Arch Pathol Lab Med 131:122-125, 2007.

EPITHELIOID ANGIOMYOLIPOMA

Clinical Features

- Potentially malignant mesenchymal neoplasm with low metastatic potential
- Some patients are symptomatic and present with flank pain; in other the tumor is found incidentally in imaging studies
- Lack of fat makes their radiologic appearance resemble that of renal cell carcinoma
- Association with tuberous sclerosis

Gross Pathology

- Tumors are solid and extensively hemorrhagic
- Necrosis may be present

Histopathology

- Tumor consists entirely or predominantly (> 80%) of stubby spindle cells and polygonal cells with eosinophilic cytoplasm (Figure 10-25)
- A minor population of pleomorphic ganglion-like or multinucleated giant cells with amphophilic cytoplasm and eccentrically located nuclei and prominent nucleoli is present in 90% of cases
- Nuclear atypia and mitoses may be prominent
- Lymphovascular invasion, renal vein invasion, hilar and perinephric fat involvement may be present

Special Stains and Immunohistochemistry

- Melanocytic markers: positive
- Actins and desmin: frequently positive
- Epithelial markers: negative

Other Techniques for Diagnosis

- Noncontributory

Differential Diagnosis

HIGH-GRADE CARCINOMA

- Positive for epithelial markers
- Negative for melanocytic markers

PEARLS

- *Epithelioid angiomyolipomas constitute a small proportion of all angiomyolipomas (~5%)*
- *Minor epithelioid component in an otherwise classical angiomyolipoma does not impact its benign nature*
- *Rate of aggressive behavior among epithelioid angiomyolipomas, even when showing morphologic features previously reported to portend aggressive clinical behavior, is very low (~5%)*
- *Features more frequently observed in clinically malignant cases are older age, large tumor size, high percentage of epithelioid component, severe atypia, high percentage of atypical cells, high mitotic count, atypical mitotic figures, necrosis, lymphovascular invasion, and renal vein invasion*
- *Lymph nodes, liver, lung, and mesentery are the most common metastatic sites*

SELECTED REFERENCES

Aydin H, Magi-Galluzzi C, Lane BR, et al: Renal angiomyolipoma: clinicopathologic study of 194 cases with emphasis on the epithelioid histology and tuberous sclerosis association. Am J Surg Pathol 33:289-297, 2009.

Brimo F, Robinson B, Guo C, et al: Renal epithelioid angiomyolipoma with atypia: a series of 40 cases with emphasis on clinicopathologic prognostic indicators of malignancy. Am J Surg Pathol 34:715-722, 2010.

He W, Cheville JC, Sadow PM, et al: Epithelioid angiomyolipoma of the kidney: pathological features and clinical outcome in a series of consecutively resected tumors. Mod Pathol 26:1355-1364, 2013.

Nese N, Martignoni G, Fletcher CD, et al: Pure epithelioid PEComas (so-called epithelioid angiomyolipoma) of the kidney: a clinicopathologic study of 41 cases: detailed assessment of morphology and risk stratification. Am J Surg Pathol 35:161-176, 2011.

PAPILLARY ADENOMA

Clinical Features

- Usually incidental finding
- Often seen in patients receiving long-term hemodialysis and associated with acquired cystic disease; also more common in kidneys scarred from chronic pyelonephritis
- Occasionally associated with von Hippel-Lindau syndrome

Gross Pathology

- Small cortical tumors smaller than 5 mm
- Soft, well-circumscribed mass with yellow to gray cut surface
- Pushing borders occasionally compressing the adjacent kidney parenchyma

Histopathology

- Tubular, papillary, or tubulopapillary architecture; tubular pattern is most common (Figure 10-26)
- Lacks distinct capsule but does not have infiltrative border

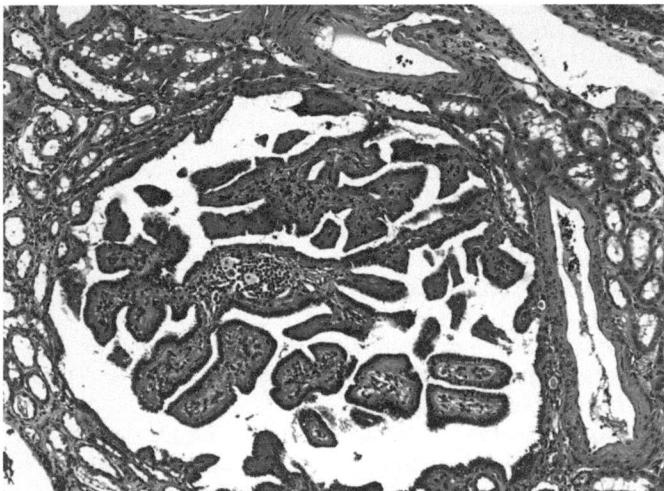

Figure 10-26. Papillary adenoma. Small tumor (< 5 mm) with papillary architecture. It lacks a distinct capsule but does not have an infiltrative border.

- Typically consists of densely packed tubules lined by small regular cuboidal cells with round to oval nuclei; low-grade nuclei similar to Fuhrman grades 1 and 2
- The nuclei show coarse chromatin and inconspicuous nucleoli
- Mitotic activity is rare
- Cells have high nuclear/cytoplasmic ratio with scant cytoplasm
- Psammomatous calcifications and foamy histiocytes may be present
- WHO 2004 classification of renal tumors regards any tumors as papillary adenomas in the following conditions:
  - Cortical tumor is composed of closely packed tubules with or without papillary architecture and ≤ 5 mm in greatest dimension
  - Cells are small, regular, and cuboidal with round to oval low-grade nuclei and rare or no mitotic activity
  - No areas of clear cell differentiation exist

Special Stains and Immunohistochemistry

- Positive for cytokeratin 7 and AMACR
- Negative for WT-1

Other Techniques for Diagnosis

- Cytogenetic studies: may be associated with trisomy 7 or 17, loss of Y chromosome in male patients

Differential Diagnosis

LOW-GRADE PAPILLARY RENAL CELL CARCINOMA (PRCC)

- May be histologically indistinguishable from papillary adenoma, so the size (5 mm) becomes the sole criterion that separates the two; however, one needs to be aware that the size may not perfectly correlate with the biologic behavior
- A papillary adenoma with nuclear grade ≥ 3 should be classified as papillary carcinoma

METANEPHRIC ADENOMA

- Usually larger
- Consists of tightly packed small acini
- Cells are small and have scant cytoplasm
- A panel of immunohistochemical stains (cytokeratin 7, WT-1, and AMACR) can aid the differential diagnosis, with metanephric adenoma positive for WT-1 and negative for cytokeratin 7 and AMACR, whereas papillary adenoma is positive for cytokeratin 7 and AMACR but negative for WT-1

PEARLS

- *Criteria to distinguish papillary adenoma from renal cell carcinoma are arbitrarily defined*
- *WHO 2004 criteria define cytologically benign tumor less than 5 cm and of low nuclear grade as adenoma and tumor more than 5 mm or of high nuclear grade as carcinoma*

SELECTED REFERENCES

Eble JN, Sauter G, Epstein JI, Sesterhenn IA (eds): Pathology and Genetics: Tumors of the Urinary System and Male Genital Organs. Lyon, IARC Press, 2004.

Wang KL, Weinrach DM, Luan C, et al: Renal papillary adenoma: a putative precursor of papillary renal cell carcinoma. Hum Pathol 38:239-246, 2007.

METANEPHRIC ADENOMA

Clinical Features

- Rare benign kidney tumor
- Female predominance with a female-to-male ratio of 2:1
- Found in childhood through adulthood, most commonly the fifth decade
- About 50% of cases symptomatic with hematuria and abdominal pain
- About 10% to 15% with polycythemia

Gross Pathology

- Unilateral, solitary, well-circumscribed but unencapsulated tumor
- Variable size ranging from smaller than 1 cm to 15 cm (mean, 5 cm)
- Cut surface shows soft, fleshy tan-yellow tissue
- Hemorrhage or necrosis may be seen

Histopathology

- Pushing border with no capsule or infiltration into surrounding kidney parenchyma
- Ordered array of small, tightly packed acini separated by acellular stroma (Figure 10-27)
- Papillary architecture may be seen
- Focal solid areas consisting of small round cells (blastema-like areas) infrequently seen
- Tumor cells are small and uniform with round to oval nuclei and scant cytoplasm
- Nuclei show delicate chromatin and inconspicuous nucleoli
- Rare to absent mitotic activity
- Microcalcifications may be seen

Special Stains and Immunohistochemistry

- Cytokeratin: AE1/3 positive in 50%, but cytokeratin 7 usually negative

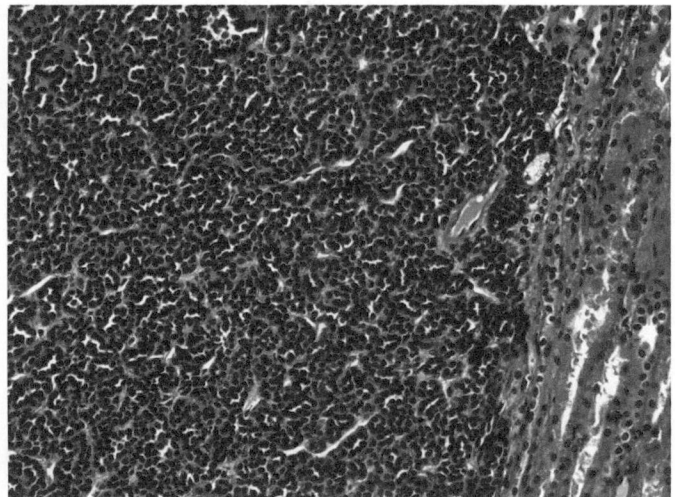

Figure 10-27. Metanephric adenoma. Proliferation of tubulopapillary structures within an acellular stroma background. Note the sharp border with the kidney.

- EMA, CD56: negative
- WT-1, CD57: positive
- AMACR: rarely positive in 5% to 10%

Other Techniques for Diagnosis

- Electron microscopy: cells have basal lamina and microvilli
- Flow cytometry: tumor cells almost always diploid
- BRAF V600E mutations are present in approximately 90% of cases

Differential Diagnosis

DIFFERENTIATED NEPHROBLASTOMA (EPITHELIAL PREDOMINANT WILMS TUMOR)

- Has a tumor capsule and may show a distinct triphasic pattern with blastema, stromal, and epithelial components after careful sampling
- Elongated or columnar nuclei with frequent mitotic activity
- Positive for CD56 and CD57

PAPILLARY RENAL CELL CARCINOMA, SOLID VARIANT

- Often has a tumor capsule or pseudocapsule
- Tumor cells have more abundant cytoplasm
- Foamy histiocytes and hemosiderin deposition common
- Cytokeratin 7, EMA, and AMACR positive, but WT-1 negative

PEARLS

- *Benign renal epithelial neoplasm probably representing the benign end of the metanephric tumors that also include Wilms tumor*
- *No reports of local recurrence or distant metastases*
- *May represent complete maturation of Wilms tumor; alternatively, metanephric adenoma may develop into Wilms tumor, as in the "neuroblastoma-ganglioneuroblastoma-ganglioneuroma" sequence*

SELECTED REFERENCES

Argani P: Metanephric neoplasms: the hyperdifferentiated, benign end of the Wilms tumor spectrum? Clin Lab Med 25:379-392, 2005.
Choueiri TK, Cheville J, Palescandolo E, et al: BRAF mutations in metanephric adenoma of the kidney. Eur Urol 62:917-922, 2012.
Mantoan Padilha M, Billis A, Allende D, et al: Metanephric adenoma and solid variant of papillary renal cell carcinoma: common and distinctive features. Histopathology 62:941-953, 2013.

RENAL ONCOCYTOMA

Clinical Features

- Accounts for approximately 5% to 10% of kidney tumors in adults
- Majority asymptomatic, although flank pain may be a presenting complaint; hematuria may be seen
- Computed tomography (CT) or magnetic resonance imaging (MRI) may identify central scar (spoke-wheel appearance)

Gross Pathology

- Well-circumscribed, homogeneous, cortical tumor
- Mahogany-brown cut surface

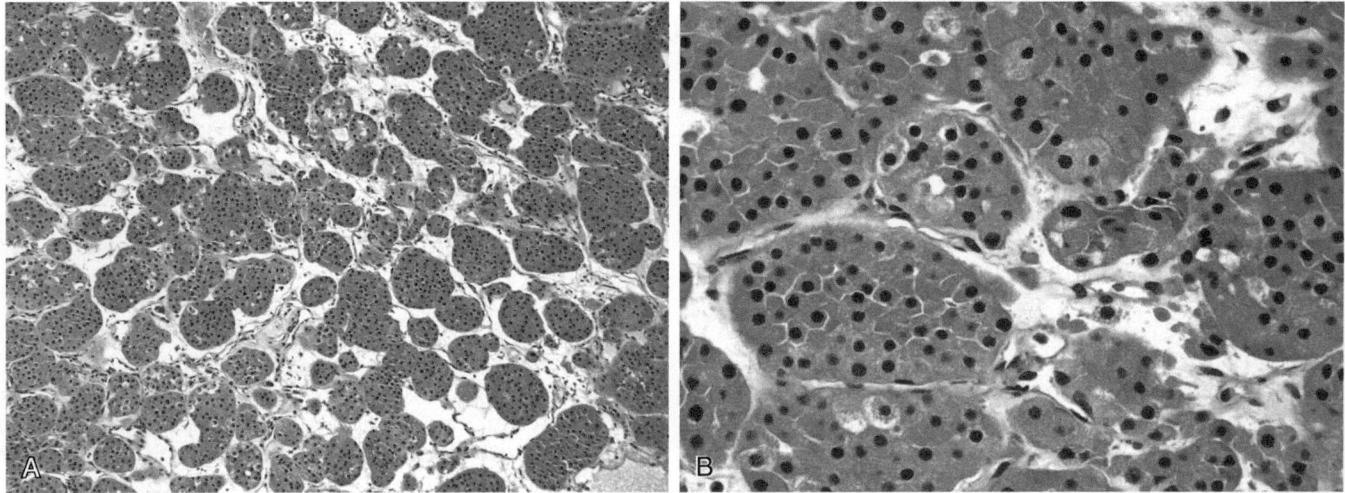

Figure 10-28. A, Oncocytoma. The tumor is composed of well-defined nests of tumor cells with abundant eosinophilic granular cytoplasm in an edematous stroma. **B,** Oncocytoma. High-power view shows the classical cytoplasmic and nuclear features of renal oncocytoma.

- Often shows a central, irregular, fibrous scar (approximately 40% of cases)
- Focal hemorrhage may be seen
- No grossly evident necrosis
- No renal vein invasion
- Bilateral or multicentric in 2% to 3% of cases

Histopathology

- Three histologic variants:
  - Classic (most common)
    - Organoid pattern with well-defined nests of tumor cells (Figure 10-28A and B)
    - Edematous, myxoid, or hyalinized stroma
    - Confluent nests of tumor cells can be seen at the periphery of the lesion; nests of tumor cells should be outlined by interlacing framework of thin fibrous septa
  - Tubulocystic
    - Variably sized tubular and cystic structures
    - Spaces often contain eosinophilic secretion
  - Mixed pattern
    - Composed of both organoid and tubular architecture
- Tumor cells have finely granular eosinophilic cytoplasm
- Round nuclei with smooth, regular contour and evenly distributed chromatin
- Presence of nucleoli is variable; may be absent or prominent
- Absence of mitotic figures
- Focally cells with hyperchromatic, smudged nuclei may be seen
- Other unusual features
  - Focal extension into perirenal fat, which has no adverse effect on the prognosis
  - Focal cytoplasmic clearing, especially in scarred area
- Histologic features that should never be seen include the following:
  - Gross extension into perirenal adipose tissue or gross vascular invasion
  - Papillary architecture
  - Sarcomatous or spindle cell areas

- Atypical mitotic figures
- Positive for colloidal iron stain

Special Stains and Immunohistochemistry

- Cytokeratin 7 stains single cells or clusters of cells
- Vimentin: negative
- S100A1: positive
- Hale's colloidal iron stain: negative or only stains luminal cytoplasm
- E-cadherin and kidney specific cadherin: positive
- Claudin 8: positive cytoplasmic staining

Other Techniques for Diagnosis

- Electron microscopy: cells have abundant, evenly distributed mitochondria and a paucity of other organelles
- Flow cytometry: usually diploid
- Cytogenetic studies: most oncocytomas are composed of a mixed population of cells with normal and abnormal karyotypes; some cases display loss of chromosomes 1 and 14; occasionally, t (5; 11) is observed

Differential Diagnosis

CLEAR CELL RENAL CELL CARCINOMA WITH EOSINOPHILIC CYTOPLASM

- Eosinophilic cytoplasm can be seen in high-grade clear cell RCC, but presence of clear cells or papillary structures precludes the diagnosis of oncocytoma
- Nuclear grade is usually high and mitosis readily identifiable
- Cytokeratin 7 negative, but vimentin positive
- E-cadherin: negative
- Chromophobe renal cell carcinoma, eosinophilic variant
- Sheetlike compact growth pattern
- "Raisinoid" nuclei and perinuclear halos
- Cytokeratin 7 diffusely positive; Hale's colloidal iron positive
- E-cadherin: positive
- S100A1: negative
- Claudin 8: positive membranous staining

RENAL ONCOCYTOSIS

- Renal parenchyma diffusely involved by numerous oncocytic nodules and oncocytic changes: infiltrative growth of oncocytic cells, cortical cysts with oncocytic features, oncocytic changes in non-neoplastic tubules
- Unilateral or bilateral
- May occur in a sporadic form or associated (1/2) with chronic renal failure/long-term hemodialysis

PEARLS

- *Believed to arise from the intercalated cells of collecting ducts*
- *Oncocytomas are benign tumors; previous reports of malignant oncocytomas are almost certain RCC misdiagnosed as oncocytomas*
- *Most common histologic features include well-defined nests of eosinophilic tumor cells separated by fine, delicate fibrous bands and a central fibrous scar*
- *Hybrid oncocytic tumors with features of both oncocytoma and chromophobe RCC (HOCT) can be seen in patients with Birt-Hogg-Dube syndrome*

SELECTED REFERENCES

Kim SS, Choi YD, Jin XM, et al: Immunohistochemical stain for cytokeratin 7, S100A1 and claudin 8 is valuable in differential diagnosis of chromophobe renal cell carcinoma from renal oncocytoma. Histopathology 54:633-635, 2009.

Kuroda N, Tanaka A, Ohe C, et al: Review of renal oncocytosis (multiple oncocytic lesions) with focus on clinical and pathobiological aspects. Histol Histopathol 27:1407-1412, 2012.

Petersson F, Gatalica Z, Grossmann P, et al: Sporadic hybrid oncocytic/chromophobe tumor of the kidney: a clinicopathologic, histomorphologic, immunohistochemical, ultrastructural, and molecular cytogenetic study of 14 cases. Virchows Arch 456: 355-365, 2010.

RENAL CELL CARCINOMA, CLEAR CELL TYPE

Clinical Features

- The most common variant of renal epithelial tumors, accounting for 2% of all malignancies and about 70% of renal cell carcinomas
- Primarily adults (sixth and seventh decades)
- Male predominance (male-to-female ratio of 2:1)
- Hematuria is single most common presenting sign
- Less than 10% present with classic triad of flank mass, pain, and hematuria

Gross Pathology

- Solitary renal cortical mass
- Bilaterality and multifocality more common in familial syndrome
- Well-circumscribed, lobulated with golden yellow cut surface
- Cystic change, hemorrhage, necrosis, and calcification often present

Histopathology

- Alveolar nests and sheets of clear cells interspersed by delicate vascular network (Figure 10-29)

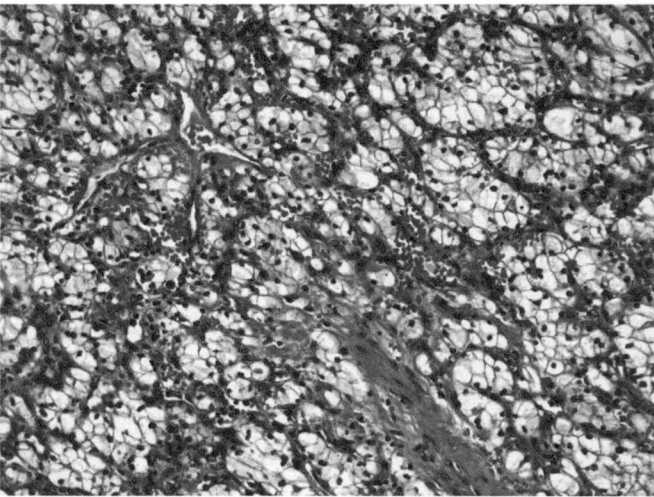

Figure 10-29. Renal cell carcinoma, clear cell type. Nests and sheets of clear cells interspersed by delicate vascular network.

- Other patterns are also seen, including trabecular, microcystic, and occasionally pseudopapillary, tubular
- Sarcomatoid differentiation is often in the form of spindle cells

Special Stains and Immunohistochemistry

- Cam 5.2, AE1/3, EMA, vimentin, CD10, CA9, and RCC antigen: positive
- Keratin 34BE12: negative
- S100 or CEA: only rarely positive
- PAX-2, PAX-8: positive

Other Techniques for Diagnosis

ELECTRON MICROSCOPY

- Abundant cytoplasmic lipid and glycogen
- Tubular differentiation: microlumens, microvilli, and brush border

MOLECULAR GENETICS

- Chromosome 3p deletion in the majority of sporadic clear cell RCC
- The four most commonly mutated genes are VHL, PBRM1, BAP1, and SETD2
- Mutation of the VHL gene in 34% to 56%, and promoter methylation in 20% of sporadic cases

Differential Diagnosis

CHROMOPHOBE RENAL CELL CARCINOMA

- Nonencapsulated mass with a homogenous, light brown cut surface
- Translucent and reticulated, not clear, cytoplasm
- Positive Hale's colloidal iron staining
- Diffuse positive cytokeratin 7

PAPILLARY RENAL CELL CARCINOMA

- Histiocytes and intracellular hemosiderin are usually present
- CK 7, AMACR positive
- CA9 negative
- Trisomy 7 and 17, loss of Y chromosome in male patients

CLEAR CELL (TUBULO) PAPILLARY RENAL CELL CARCINOMA

- Branched acini or ribbons lined with low-grade clear cells
- Nuclei polarized away from basement membrane toward the luminal surface of the acini and glands
- Cytokeratin 7, CA9, and keratin 34BE12: positive
- CD10 and AMACR: negative

ADRENOCORTICAL CARCINOMA

- Flocculated, not "water clear," cytoplasm
- EMA and cytokeratin: negative
- Inhibin and calretinin: positive

EPITHELIOID ANGIOMYOLIPOMA

- May have other components, such as fat or dysmorphic vessels
- Multinucleated epithelioid cells characteristic
- Negative for epithelial markers, but positive for melanocytic markers, such as HMB-45, Melan A, tyrosinase, MiTF

PEARLS

- *Most common histologic subtype of RCC*
- *Clear cytoplasm due to rich cytoplasmic glycogen and lipid contents*
- *Chromosome 3p alteration is the most common genetic change*
- *VHL gene and genes in hypoxia inducible pathway play critical role in the pathogenesis*

SELECTED REFERENCES

Amin MB, Amin MB, Tamboli P, et al: Prognostic impact of histologic subtyping of adult renal epithelial neoplasms: an experience of 405 cases. Am J Surg Pathol 26:281-291, 2002.

Fenner A: Genetics: a molecular atlas of clear cell renal cell carcinoma. Nat Rev Clin Oncol 10:485, 2013.

Jones TD, Eble JN, Cheng L: Application of molecular diagnostic techniques to renal epithelial neoplasms. Clin Lab Med 25:279-303, 2005.

Srigley JR, Delahunt B, Eble JN, et al; ISUP Renal Tumor Panel: The International Society of Urological Pathology (ISUP) Vancouver Classification of Renal Neoplasia. Am J Surg Pathol 37:1469-1489, 2013.

Zhou M, Roma A, Magi-Galluzzi C: The usefulness of immunohistochemical markers in the differential diagnosis of renal neoplasms. Clin Lab Med 25:247-257, 2005.

RENAL CELL CARCINOMA, PAPILLARY TYPE

Clinical Features

- Comprises approximately 10% to 15% of all renal cell carcinomas
- Majority sporadic, < 5% associated with hereditary papillary renal cell carcinoma syndrome that involves c-met gene on chromosome 7q31
- Signs and symptoms similar to clear cell RCC
- More likely to be bilateral or multiple than other renal cell carcinomas
- Significantly better outcome than that of the clear cell type

Gross Pathology

- Solitary, well-circumscribed cortical mass
- Fibrous pseudocapsule

- Necrosis and hemorrhage common
- More likely to be bilateral or multifocal than other renal cell carcinomas

Histopathology

- Papillae and tubulopapillary structures with true fibrovascular cores (Figure 10-30)
- Solid pattern due to tightly compact growth of papillae
- Foamy histiocytes expanding papillary core are characteristic
- Psammoma bodies common
- Subdivided into two types based on morphology
- Type I: papillae lined with single layer of cells, usually low-grade nuclear features and scant cytoplasm
- Type II: pseudostratified nuclei of higher nuclear grade and abundant eosinophilic cytoplasm
- Papillae may have abundant eosinophilic cytoplasm but low nuclear grade
- Sarcomatoid differentiation in 5% of cases

Special Stains and Immunohistochemistry

- Pan and low-molecular-weight cytokeratin: positive
- CK7 positive in 80% of type I and 20% type II
- EMA and vimentin positive in 50%
- CD10 and RCC antigen positive in majority of cases; PAX-8 positive

Other Techniques for Diagnosis

- Genetics: tri- or tetrasomy 7, 17, and loss of Y chromosome: the most common cytogenetic changes

Differential Diagnosis

PAPILLARY ADENOMA

- By WHO criteria, < 5 mm and low nuclear grade (Fuhrman grade 1 or 2)

CLEAR CELL (TUBULO) PAPILLARY RENAL CELL CARCINOMA

- Branched acini or ribbons lined with low-grade clear cells
- Nuclei polarized away from basement membrane toward the luminal surface of the acini and glands
- Cytokeratin 7, CA9, and keratin 34BE12: positive
- CD10 and AMACR: negative

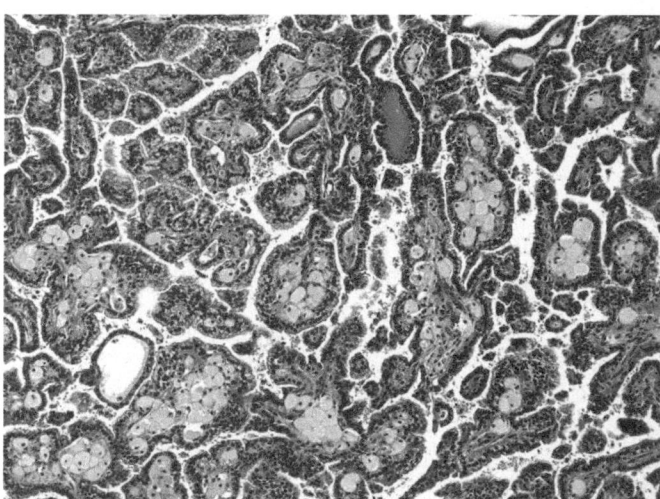

Figure 10-30. Renal cell carcinoma, papillary type. Papillae and tubulopapillary structures with true fibrovascular cores. Foamy histiocytes expanding papillary cores are characteristic.

METANEPHRIC ADENOMA

- Sharp circumscription from the kidney parenchyma without capsule
- Tightly packed tumor cells form small acini, tubulopapillary structures
- Tumor cells with scant cytoplasm, uniform nuclei without mitosis or nucleoli
- CK7 negative, but WT-1 positive

DIFFERENTIATED NEPHROBLASTOMA (EPITHELIAL PREDOMINANT WILMS TUMOR)

- Has a tumor capsule and may show a distinct triphasic pattern with blastema, stromal, and epithelial components after careful sampling
- Elongated or columnar nuclei with frequent mitotic activity
- CD56 positive

RCC ASSOCIATED WITH XP11.2/TFE3 TRANSLOCATION

- Often affects children and young adults
- Papillary structures lined by tumor cells with abundant clear to granular cytoplasm
- Psammomatous calcification and hyalinized fibrovascular cores are present
- Most epithelial markers, including cytokeratins and EMA, are negative
- Positive TFE3 stain is confirmatory

COLLECTING DUCT CARCINOMA

- Involving central region of the kidney
- Irregular, small glands and ducts in a loose collagenous chronically inflamed desmoplastic stroma
- Cells lining glands are high grade with pleomorphic nuclei; typically have hobnail appearance
- Associated tubular epithelial dysplasia

PEARLS

- *Second most common RCC subtypes*
- *Significantly better prognosis than clear cell RCC*
- *Trisomy 7 and 17 as well as the loss of Y chromosome are characteristic, but lacks VHL mutation*

SELECTED REFERENCES

Amin MB, Corless CL, Renshaw AA, et al: Papillary (chromophil) renal cell carcinoma: histomorphologic characteristics and evaluation of conventional pathologic prognostic parameters in 62 cases. Am J Surg Pathol 21:621-635, 1997.

Delahunt B, Eble JN: Papillary renal cell carcinoma: a clinicopathologic and immunohistochemical study of 105 tumors. Mod Pathol 10:537-544, 1997.

Eble JN, McCredie MR, Bethwaite PB, et al: Morphologic typing of papillary renal cell carcinoma: comparison of growth kinetics and patient survival in 66 cases. Hum Pathol 32:590-595, 2001.

RENAL CELL CARCINOMA, CHROMOPHOBE TYPE

Clinical Features

- About 5% of renal cell carcinoma
- Presents similarly to clear cell RCC
- Majority are sporadic; familial cases associated with Birt-Hogg-Dube syndrome
- Significantly better prognosis than clear cell RCC

Gross Pathology

- Solitary, spherical, well-circumscribed, pseudo-encapsulated mass
- Homogenous, tan or light brown cut surface

Histopathology

- Two histologic variants
  - Classic: finely reticulated pale cytoplasm with prominent cell membrane (Figure 10-31)
  - Eosinophilic: smaller cells with intense eosinophilic cytoplasm and prominent cell membrane
- "Koilocytic" nuclear atypia with wrinkled nuclear membrane and perinuclear halo
- Binucleation common
- Thick hyalinized blood vessels

Special Stains and Immunohistochemistry

- CK7 and EMA: diffusely positive
- RCC antigen: variably positive
- CD10 and S100A1: negative
- Hale's colloidal iron stain: positive-PAX-8 positive

Other Techniques for Diagnosis

- Electron microscopy
  - Abundant cytoplasmic microvesicles
  - Eosinophilic variant: abundant mitochondria, few microvesicles
- Molecular genetics:
  - Extensive chromosomal loss, most frequently involving chromosomes 1, 2, 6, 10, 13, 17, and 21

Differential Diagnosis

CLEAR CELL RENAL CELL CARCINOMA

- No "koilocytic nuclear atypia" or prominent cell membrane
- Hale's colloidal iron stain negative
- CK7 negative

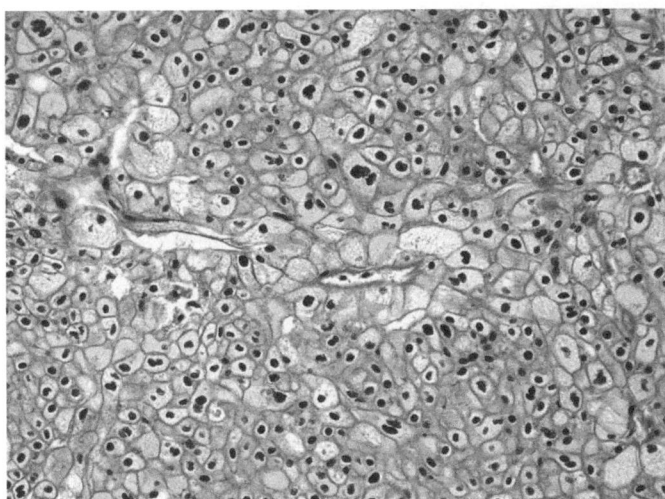

Figure 10-31. Renal cell carcinoma, chromophobe type. Proliferation of compact cells with finely reticulated pale cytoplasm and prominent cell membrane. "Koilocytic" nuclear atypia with wrinkled nuclear membrane and perinuclear halo, and binucleation are common.

ONCOCYTOMA

- Uniform nuclei without "koilocytic" nuclear atypia or prominent cell membranes
- Hale's colloidal iron stain highlights lumina, not the entire tumor cells
- CK7 stains single cells or small clusters of cells
- S100A1 positive

PEARLS

- *Third most common RCC subtype*
- *Significantly better prognosis than clear cell RCC; most patients are cured by nephrectomy*
- *Extensive chromosomal loss, distinct from clear cell and papillary RCC*

SELECTED REFERENCES

Abrahams NA, MacLennan GT, Khoury JD, et al: Chromophobe renal cell carcinoma: a comparative study of histological, immunohistochemical and ultrastructural features using high throughput tissue microarray. Histopathology 45:593-602, 2004.

Li G, Barthelemy A, Feng G, et al: S100A1: a powerful marker to differentiate chromophobe renal cell carcinoma from renal oncocytoma. Histopathology 50:642-647, 2007.

Tickoo SK, Amin MB, Zarbo RJ: Colloidal iron staining in renal epithelial neoplasms, including chromophobe renal cell carcinoma: emphasis on technique and patterns of staining. Am J Surg Pathol 22:419-424, 1998.

MULTILOCULAR CYSTIC RENAL CELL CARCINOMA

Clinical Features

- Rare variant (5%) of clear cell RCC
- Excellent prognosis; surgical resection is curative

Gross Pathology

- Well-circumscribed, entirely cystic mass of small and large cysts with serous or hemorrhagic content
- Occasionally calcified
- No solid expansile nodules of tumor cells

Histopathology

- Cysts lined by single layer of cells
- Small collections of clear epithelial cells within fibrous septa (Figure 10-32A and B)

Special Stains and Immunohistochemistry

- Identical to clear cell RCC

Other Techniques for Diagnosis

- Deletion of chromosome 3p identified in most tumors
- VHL gene mutation identified in 25% of cases

Differential Diagnosis

CYSTIC NEPHROMA

- Striking female predominant
- No clear cells within the fibrous septa
- Hyalinized or cellular stroma resembling ovarian stroma

RCC WITH EXTENSIVE CYSTIC CHANGE

- Presence of solid, expansile tumor nodules of any size excludes diagnosis of multilocular cystic renal cell carcinoma

PEARLS

- *A variant of clear cell RCC with excellent prognosis after surgical resection*
- *Strict diagnostic criteria should be applied to ensure the prognostic significance associated with the diagnosis; no solid expansile tumor nodule of any size is allowed*

SELECTED REFERENCES

Halat S, Eble JN, Grignon DJ, et al: Multilocular cystic renal cell carcinoma is a subtype of clear cell renal cell carcinoma. Mod Pathol 23:931-936, 2010.

Suzigan S, Lopez-Beltran A, Montironi R, et al: Multilocular cystic renal cell carcinoma: a report of 45 cases of a kidney tumor of low malignant potential. Am J Clin Pathol 125:217-222, 2006.

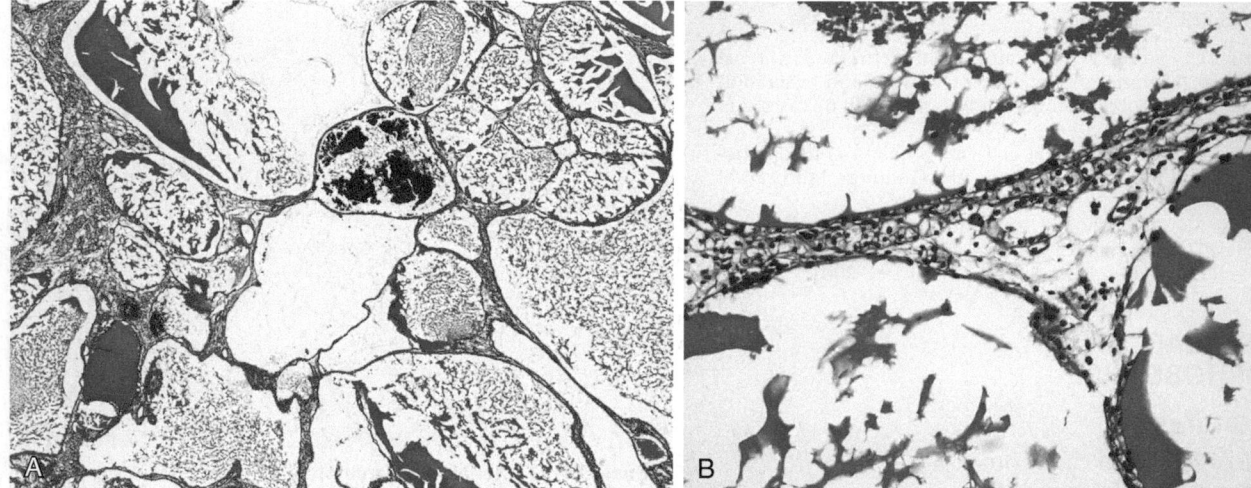

Figure 10-32. A, Multilocular cystic renal cell carcinoma. Cystic mass of small and large cysts with serous or hemorrhagic content. No solid expansile nodules of tumor cells are noted. **B,** Multilocular cystic renal cell carcinoma. Small collections of clear epithelial cells within fibrous septa.

COLLECTING DUCT CARCINOMA (CARCINOMA OF THE COLLECTING DUCTS OF BELLINI)

Clinical Features

- Rare, comprising approximately 0.1% of renal cell carcinomas
- Flank mass, pain and hematuria
- One third have metastasis at presentation

Gross Pathology

- Medullary location
- Light gray, white cut surface, with invasive borders
- Necrosis, hemorrhage, and cystic changes may be present

Histopathology

- Highly infiltrative border
- Tubular/tubulopapillary structure with tapered ends (Figure 10-33)
- Inflamed desmoplastic stroma
- High-grade nuclear features, brisk mitosis
- Intraluminal and intracytoplasmic mucin may be present
- Tubular epithelial dysplasia in adjacent kidney parenchyma

Special Stains and Immunohistochemistry
Histopathology

- Low- and high-molecular weight keratin (HMWCK), CK7, CEA, peanut agglutinin (PNA), and Ulex europaeus agglutinin (UEA): positive
- CD10: negative

Other Techniques for Diagnosis

- Electron microscopy
  - Well-formed cell junctions, short apical microvilli, and prominent basal lamina
- Molecular genetics
  - Not well characterized

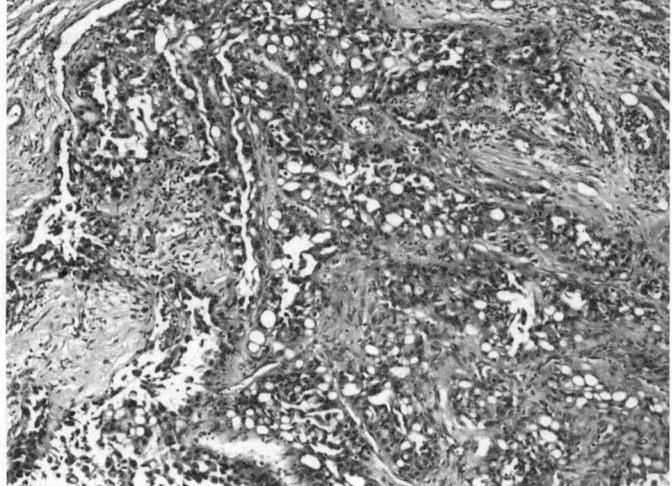

Figure 10-33. Collecting duct carcinoma. Tubular/tubulopapillary structures with tapered ends in an inflamed desmoplastic stroma.

Differential Diagnosis

PAPILLARY RENAL CELL CARCINOMA

- Typically located in the cortex
- Well circumscribed with a tumor capsule
- Histiocytes and hemosiderin deposition in papillary cores
- Lack inflamed desmoplastic stroma
- HMWCK and Ulex negative

UROTHELIAL CARCINOMA WITH GLANDULAR FEATURES

- Histology and immunoprofile similar to collecting duct carcinoma
- Urothelial carcinoma in renal calyces or pelvis favors the diagnosis of urothelial carcinoma

RENAL MEDULLARY CARCINOMA

- Affects exclusively patients with sickle trait or disease
- Sickle cells may be found within the tumor vessels
- INI-1 negative

METASTATIC CARCINOMA

- History of primary carcinoma
- Often multifocal with concentration at the corticomedullary junction
- Extensive involvement of perinephric fat and intravascular permeation

PEARLS

- *Rare, highly aggressive renal tumor*
- *Diagnosis is difficult and often is one of exclusion*
- *Consider this entity in the presence of a high-grade tumor with features reminiscent of papillary RCC, urothelial carcinoma, and clear cell RCC*

SELECTED REFERENCES

Peyromaure M, Thiounn N, Scotté F, et al: Collecting duct carcinoma of the kidney: a clinicopathological study of 9 cases. J Urol 170 (4 Pt 1):1138-1140, 2003.

Tokuda N, Naito S, Matsuzaki O, et al; Japanese Society of Renal Cancer: Collecting duct (Bellini duct) renal cell carcinoma: a nationwide survey in Japan. J Urol 176:40-43, 2006.

RENAL MEDULLARY CARCINOMA

Clinical Features

- Typically presents with gross hematuria; may present with abdominal or flank pain
- Almost always associated with sickle cell trait or sickle cell disease in a patient under 40 years old

Gross Pathology

- Ill-defined, poorly circumscribed mass predominantly located in the renal medulla, but often involving a majority of the renal parenchyma
- Typically extends into the calyces and pelvis and often invades into the perirenal adipose tissue
- Firm to rubbery lobulated tumor with tan-gray cut surface
- Typically shows extensive hemorrhage and necrosis

Histopathology

- Characteristically shows a reticular growth pattern; reminiscent of testicular yolk sac tumor on low-power examination

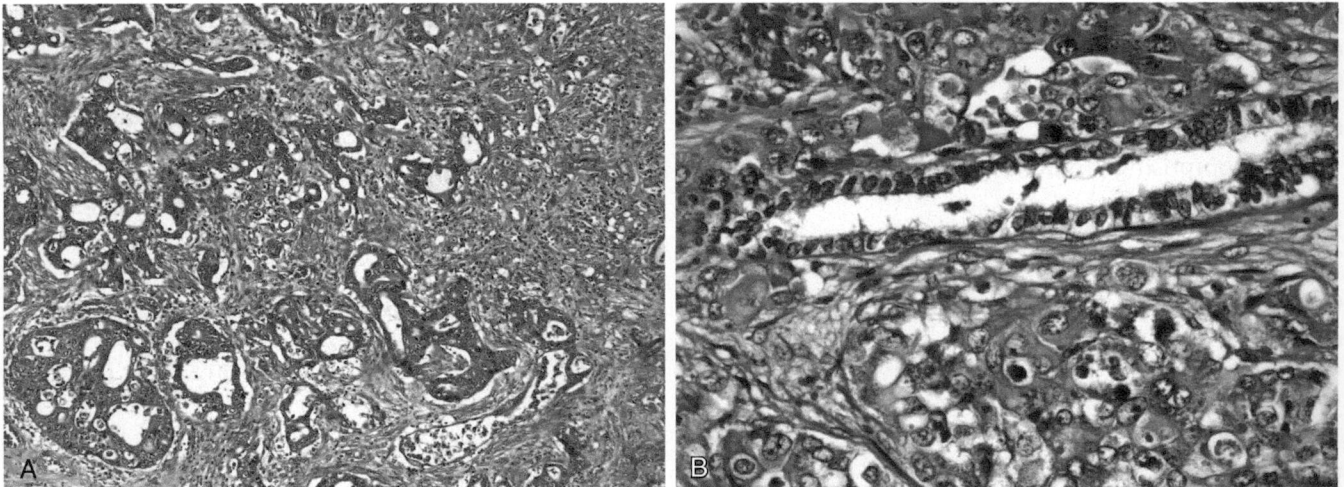

Figure 10-34. A, Renal medullary carcinoma. Proliferation of compact neoplastic ductlike structures resembling adenoid cystic carcinoma. **B,** Renal medullary carcinoma. High-power view shows neoplastic cells with large amount of eosinophilic cytoplasm, pleomorphic nuclei with a vesicular chromatin pattern, and prominent nucleoli. Sickled red cells are seen.

- Often shows areas with a more compact adenoid cystic appearance (Figure 10-34A)
- Solid sheets of poorly differentiated tumor cells are also commonly present
- Tumor cells have clear or vesicular nuclei with prominent nucleoli (Figure 10-34B)
- Desmoplastic stroma in the form of mucoid, myxoid, or edematous areas are typical findings
- Stroma typically shows variable degrees of inflammatory cells
- Most tumors show areas of hemorrhage and necrosis
- Lymphatic and vascular invasion is usually present
- Sickled red cells typically seen

Special Stains and Immunohistochemistry

- Cytokeratin: typically positive
- HMWCK: negative
- Negative INI-1 correlates with aggressive behavior

Other Techniques for Diagnosis

- Noncontributory

Differential Diagnosis

COLLECTING DUCT CARCINOMA

- Clinical history critical: patients have no sickle cell trait or disease
- Irregular, small glands and ducts in an inflamed desmoplastic stroma
- Cells lining glands are high grade with pleomorphic nuclei; typically have hobnail appearance

PEARLS

- *Previously referred to as collecting duct carcinoma, but now recognized as a unique entity*
- *Lymph node metastases are common at time of presentation; involvement of liver and lung is also common*
- *Radical nephrectomy is the treatment of choice; however, it is an aggressive tumor and most patients die within 1 year following diagnosis*

SELECTED REFERENCES

Figenshau RS, Easier JW, Ritter JH, et al: Renal medullary carcinoma. J Urol 159:711-713, 1998.

Swartz MA, Karth J, Schneider DT, et al: Renal medullary carcinoma: clinical, pathologic, immunohistochemical, and genetic analysis with pathogenetic implications. Urology 60:1083-1089, 2002.

MUCINOUS TUBULAR AND SPINDLE CELL CARCINOMA

Clinical Features

- Wide range of ages (17 to 82 years, mean 53)
- Female predominance
- Most tumors are asymptomatic and detected incidentally
- Prognosis favorable; best regarded as a low-grade carcinoma

Gross Pathology

- Well-circumscribed, homogeneous, tan-white-pinkish cut surfaces

Histopathology

- Comprising variable amounts of three components: elongated and compressed tubules, spindle-shaped epithelial cells, and a background extracellular mucinous material (Figure 10-35)
- Nuclei are bland, spherical or oval with inconspicuous nucleoli
- Necrosis, foamy histiocytes, and chronic inflammation may be present

Special Stains and Immunohistochemistry

- Cytokeratins CAM5.2, AE1/3, CK7, and CK19: positive
- AMACR: positive
- Markers of proximal tubules, including CD10 and villin: negative

Other Techniques for Diagnosis

- Molecular genetics: cytogenetic changes distinct from PRCC and clear cell RCC

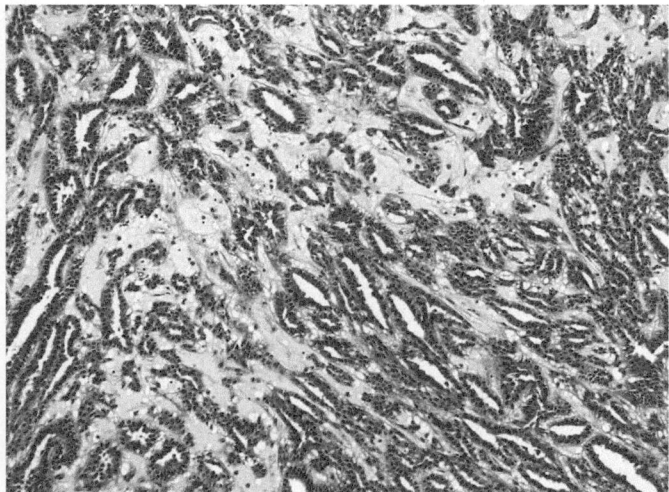

Figure 10-35. Mucinous tubular and spindle cell carcinoma. Elongated and compressed tubules are present in a background of extracellular mucinous material.

Differential Diagnosis

COLLECTING DUCT CARCINOMA
- Irregular, small glands and ducts in an inflamed desmoplastic stroma
- Cells lining glands are high grade with pleomorphic nuclei; typically have hobnail appearance

PAPILLARY RCC, SOLID VARIANT
- Compressed tubulopapillary structures forming solid or glomeruloid pattern
- Lacks spindle cell and mucinous components
- CK7, AMACR, CD10: positive

SARCOMATOID RCC
- Nondescript spindle cells, often with high nuclear grade
- Characteristic areas of preexisting RCC often seen after extensive sampling

PEARLS

- *Recently described low-grade carcinoma*
- *Classically comprising (1) mucinous stroma, (2) elongated and compressed tubules, and (3) bland spindle cells*
- *Immunohistochemically similar, but genetically distinct from PRCC*

SELECTED REFERENCES

Cossu-Rocca P, Eble JN, Delahunt B, et al: Renal mucinous tubular and spindle carcinoma lacks the gains of chromosomes 7 and 17 and losses of chromosome Y that are prevalent in papillary renal cell carcinoma. Mod Pathol 19:488-493, 2006.

Fine SW, Argani P, DeMarzo AM, et al: Expanding the histologic spectrum of mucinous tubular and spindle cell carcinoma of the kidney. Am J Surg Pathol. 30:1554-1560, 2006.

Shen SS, Ro JY, Tamboli P, et al: Mucinous tubular and spindle cell carcinoma of kidney is probably a variant of papillary renal cell carcinoma with spindle cell features. Ann Diagn Pathol 11:13-21, 2007.

RENAL CELL CARCINOMA ASSOCIATED WITH XP11.2/TFE3 TRANSLOCATION

Clinical Features

- Predominantly affects children and young adults
- Defined by several different translocation involving chromosome Xp11.2, all resulting in gene fusions involving the TFE3 gene
- The alveolar soft part locus (ASPL)-TFE3 carcinomas and those in adults characteristically present at advanced stage

Gross Pathology

- Similar to clear cell renal cell carcinoma
- Solitary cortical mass with tan-yellow cut surface, foci of hemorrhage and necrosis

Histopathology

- Papillary structures lined with abundant partially clear and partially eosinophilic cells are the most distinctive feature (Figure 10-36)
- Nested pattern made up of cells with abundant acidophilic cytoplasm is common
- Histology may vary with different chromosomal translocations
  - ASPL-TFE3: less compact, nested pattern; cells with voluminous clear to eosinophilic cytoplasm, discrete cell borders, vesicular chromatin, and prominent nucleoli; psammoma bodies and hyaline nodules frequent
  - PRCC-TFE3: compact, nested pattern; less abundant cytoplasm, fewer psammoma bodies, and hyaline nodules

Special Stains and Immunohistochemistry

- TFE3: confirmatory; cathepsin K positive
- EMA and other epithelial markers: usually negative or focally positive
- CD10 and RCC antigen consistently positive

Other Techniques for Diagnosis

- Cytogenetics: chromosomal translocation involving the TFE3 gene on Xp11.2, and several partner genes, including PRCC on 1q21, ASPL on 17q25, PSF on 1p34, and NonP on X chromosome

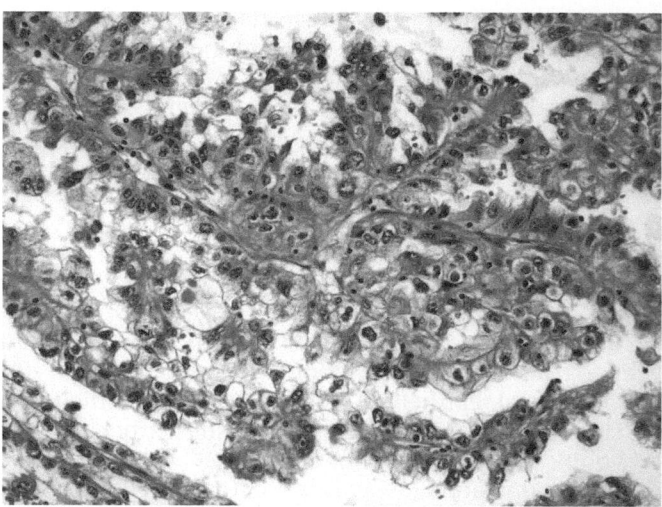

Figure 10-36. Renal cell carcinoma associated with Xp11.2/TFE3 translocation. The distinctive feature is the presence of papillary structures lined with cells with voluminous clear to eosinophilic cytoplasm, discrete cell borders, vesicular chromatin, and prominent nucleoli.

Differential Diagnosis

CLEAR CELL RCC

- Exceedingly rare in patients younger than 25 years old
- Nests of clear cells separated by delicate fibrovascular septa; papillary structures with clear cells rarely seen
- Epithelial markers positive, but TFE3 negative

PAPILLARY RCC

- RCC in children and young adults often has unusual morphology, including papillary architecture
- No alveolar or nested architecture, or clear cells
- TFE3 negative

PEARLS

- *Although RCC is rare in children and young adults, translocation-associated RCC accounts for 24% to 40% of RCC in this age group*
- *Most characteristic histologic feature is papillary structures lined with abundant partially clear and partially eosinophilic cells*
- *TFE3 immunostain is confirmatory*

SELECTED REFERENCES

Argani P, Olgac S, Tickoo SK, et al: Xp11 translocation renal cell carcinoma in adults: expanded clinical, pathologic, and genetic spectrum. Am J Surg Pathol 31:1149-1160, 2007.

Rao Q, Williamson SR, Zhang S, et al: TFE3 break-apart FISH has a higher sensitivity for Xp11.2 translocation-associated renal cell carcinoma compared with TFE3 or cathepsin K immunohistochemical staining alone: expanding the morphologic spectrum. Am J Surg Pathol 37:804-815, 2013.

RENAL CELL CARCINOMA ASSOCIATED WITH t(6;11)(p21;q12)/TFEB TRANSLOCATION

Clinical Features

- Predominantly affects children and young adults
- Defined by rearrangement between chromosome 6p21 and chromosome 11q12
- Patients presented with hematuria, abdominal pain, or asymptomatic renal mass detected incidentally on imaging studies
- Prognosis comparable with clear cell renal cell carcinoma

Gross Pathology

- Tumor generally forms a well circumscribed, homogeneous, tan-yellow-brown mass
- Satellite nodules may be observed

Histopathology

- Tumors feature a solid, nested pattern of growth, and demonstrated a biphasic population of neoplastic cells:
  - Polygonal epithelioid cells, with well-defined cell borders, and abundant cytoplasm, either eosinophilic and granular or clear
  - A subpopulation (5% to 30%) of smaller cells with dark nuclei clustering around hyaline material (basement membrane), sometimes with globular configuration
- Tubular structures may be seen together with micropapillary structures

- Neoplastic cells show clear cytoplasm with some elements characterized by granular and eosinophilic cytoplasm
- Mitoses are rare and necrosis is usually absent
- Some tumors demonstrate uncommon morphologic features, mimicking epithelioid angiomyolipoma, chromophobe cell RCC, clear cell RCC, and tubulocystic carcinoma

Special Stains and Immunohistochemistry

- TFEB (nuclear staining): confirmatory
- Cathepsin K, kidney-specific cadherin: positive
- TFE3: negative
- HMB45, Melan A, vimentin: always focally positive
- Epithelial markers (AE1/3, cytokeratin 7, cytokeratin 20, EMA): negative
- CD10: focally positive in a subset of cases

Other Techniques for Diagnosis

- Alpha-TFEB fusion can be detected by reverse transcriptase polymerase chain reaction or fluorescence in situ hybridization

Differential Diagnosis

CLEAR CELL RCC

- Exceedingly rare in patients younger than 25 years old
- Nests of clear cells separated by delicate fibrovascular septa
- Epithelial markers positive, but TFEB negative

PAPILLARY RCC

- RCC in children and young adults often has unusual morphology, including papillary architecture
- No alveolar or nested architecture, or clear cells
- TFEB negative

PEARLS

- *Most t(6;11) cases affecting children and young adults seem to be indolent*
- *TFEB immunostain is confirmatory*
- *Some have proposed grouping t(6;11) tumors and the Xp11 translocation carcinomas as members of the "MiTF/TFE translocation carcinoma family"*

SELECTED REFERENCES

Kuroda N, Tanaka A, Sasaki N, et al: Review of renal carcinoma with t(6;11)(p21;q12) with focus on clinical and pathobiological aspects. Histol Histopathol 28:685-690, 2013.

Rao Q, Liu B, Cheng L, et al: Renal cell carcinomas with t(6;11)(p21;q12): a clinicopathologic study emphasizing unusual morphology, novel alpha-TFEB gene fusion point, immunobiomarkers, and ultrastructural features, as well as detection of the gene fusion by fluorescence in situ hybridization. Am J Surg Pathol 36:1327-1338, 2012.

Srigley JR, Delahunt B, Eble JN, et al; ISUP Renal Tumor Panel: The International Society of Urological Pathology (ISUP) Vancouver Classification of Renal Neoplasia. Am J Surg Pathol 37:1469-1489, 2013.

RENAL CELL CARCINOMA ASSOCIATED WITH NEUROBLASTOMA

Clinical Features

- Rare, fewer than two dozens cases reported in the literature

- Occurs in long-term survivors of childhood neuroblastoma
- Diagnosis of neuroblastoma at 2 years of age; median age at diagnosis of renal cell carcinoma is 13.5 years

Gross Pathology

- Either kidney or both kidneys can be affected

Histopathology

- Morphologically heterogenous with some tumors showing solid and papillary architecture, cells with abundant eosinophilic cytoplasm
- Many tumors have typical clear cell appearance

Special Stains and Immunohistochemistry

- EMA, vimentin, CK8, CK18, and CK20: usually positive
- CK7, CK14, and CK19: negative

Other Techniques for Diagnosis

- Genetically different from other renal cell carcinoma types

Differential Diagnosis

- Renal cell carcinoma with eosinophilic cytoplasm
- Many renal cell carcinomas, including clear cell and papillary types, may have abundant eosinophilic cytoplasm, especially in high-grade tumors
- History of neuroblastoma is key to the diagnosis of postneuroblastoma RCC

PEARLS

- *Recently described renal cell carcinoma that affects survivors of childhood neuroblastoma*
- *Genetically different from other renal cell carcinoma types*

SELECTED REFERENCES

Dhall D, Al-Ahmadie HA, Dhall G, et al: Pediatric renal cell carcinoma with oncocytoid features occurring in a child after chemotherapy for cardiac leiomyosarcoma. Urology 70:178.e13-e15, 2007.
Koyle MA, Hatch DA, Furness PD III, et al: Long-term urological complications in survivors younger than 15 months of advanced stage abdominal neuroblastoma. J Urol 166:1455-1458, 2001.

RENAL CELL CARCINOMA, SARCOMATOID TYPE

Clinical Features

- Sarcomatoid differentiation can occur in all histologic subtypes of renal cell carcinoma and currently is not considered as a distinctive subtype
- Sarcomatoid differentiation is considered a poor prognostic sign

Gross Pathology

- Tumor is large with bulging, lobulated, soft and gray-white, fleshy cut surface
- Sarcomatoid component may appear firm and fibrous without hemorrhage and necrosis

Histopathology

- The sarcomatoid component is composed of nondescript malignant spindle cells

- Many resemble malignant fibrous histiocytoma
- Patterns reminiscent of leiomyosarcoma, fibrosarcoma, angiosarcoma, and rhabdomyosarcoma are rarely seen
- Carcinomatous component may be separated from the sarcomatous component, or the two components admixed together

Special Stains and Immunohistochemistry

- Immunohistochemistry: heterogenous staining patterns with variable cytokeratin and EMA staining in the spindle cells
- PAX8 has been reported to be positive; other RCC markers, including CD10 and RCC antigen, usually negative in sarcomatous areas

Other Techniques for Diagnosis

- Noncontributory

Differential Diagnosis

RENAL CELL CARCINOMA WITH SCAR AND GRANULATION TISSUE

- RCC, especially clear cell type, may have granulation tissue and scar within the tumor
- Fibroblastic reaction may be mistaken for sarcomatous differentiation
- Fibroblasts do not exhibit cytologic atypia

MUCINOUS TUBULAR AND SPINDLE CELL CARCINOMA

- Elongated compressed tubules and spindle cells in a mucinous, myxoid background
- Spindle cells have bland cytology and lack atypia

PRIMARY RENAL SARCOMA

- Rare
- Diagnosis can only be established after extensive sampling and immunohistochemical stains to rule out sarcomatoid RCC with a minor epithelial component

PEARLS

- *Sarcomatous differentiation can occur in all types of renal cell carcinoma*
- *Indicative of poor prognosis, regardless of the histologic subtypes of underlying RCC or the extent of sarcomatous component*
- *Graded as Fuhrman nuclear grade 4*

SELECTED REFERENCES

Delahunt B, Cheville JC, Martignoni G, et al; Members of the ISUP Renal Tumor Panel: The International Society of Urological Pathology (ISUP) grading system for renal cell carcinoma and other prognostic parameters. Am J Surg Pathol 37:1490-1504, 2013.
Kwak C, Park YH, Jeong CW, et al: Sarcomatoid differentiation as a prognostic factor for immunotherapy in metastatic renal cell carcinoma. J Surg Oncol 95:317-323, 2007.

RENAL CELL CARCINOMA, UNCLASSIFIED TYPE

Clinical Features

- Renal cell carcinoma that does not fit into any subtype of 2004 WHO classification

- Heterogeneous group of tumors with divergent clinical, morphologic, immunohistochemical, ultrastructural, or genetic characteristics

Gross Pathology

- Variable

Histopathology

- Histologic features that would fit into more than one category, including tumors with features of both oncocytoma and chromophobe RCC, clear cell RCC with papillary architecture, papillary RCC with clear cells
- High-grade carcinoma
- Sarcomatoid RCC with no recognizable or classifiable epithelial elements

Special Stains and Immunohistochemistry

- Noncontributory

Other Techniques for Diagnosis

- Noncontributory

Differential Diagnosis

Renal Cell carcinoma with Predominantly Sarcomatoid Differentiation

- Renal cell carcinoma with the epithelial component overrun by the sarcomatoid elements
- Extensive sampling of the tumor may reveal the coexisting epithelial component

Metastatic Carcinoma to the Kidney

- Patient often has a previous history of malignancy
- Metastatic tumor nodules are often multiple and concentrated along the corticomedullary junction
- Immunohistochemistry, especially lineage-specific markers (TTF-1 for lung and thyroid, thyroglobulin for thyroid, CDX-2 for gastrointestinal tract), may aid the differential diagnosis

PEARLS

- *"Wastebasket" for those cases of renal cell carcinoma that do not fit into any entities defined in the 2004 WHO classification*
- *The poorly differentiated and sarcomatoid carcinomas have aggressive behavior*

SELECTED REFERENCES

Amin MB, Amin MB, Tamboli P, et al: Prognostic impact of histologic subtyping of adult renal epithelial neoplasms: an experience of 405 cases. Am J Surg Pathol 26:281-291, 2002.

Zisman A, Chao DH, Pantuck AJ, et al: Unclassified renal cell carcinoma: clinical features and prognostic impact of a new histological subtype. J Urol 168:950-955, 2002.

CYSTIC NEPHROMA (MULTILOCULAR CYST)

Clinical Features

- Middle-aged adults
- Marked female predominance

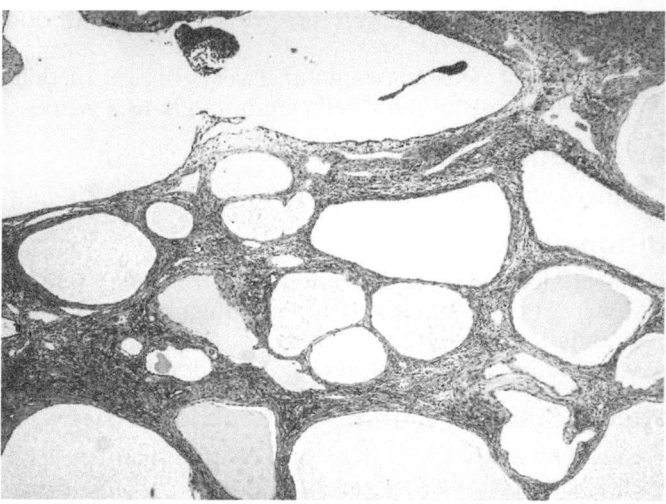

Figure 10-37. Cystic nephroma. Multiple cystic structures lined by a single layer of flattened or cuboidal cells.

- Usually asymptomatic
- Benign

Gross Pathology

- Solitary, encapsulated and well-circumscribed
- Thin-walled, multiloculated cystic
- Cystic spaces do not communicate with renal pelvis
- Focal hemorrhage is often seen

Histopathology

- Cysts are lined by single layer of flattened or cuboidal or low columnar cells with clear or eosinophilic cytoplasm (Figure 10-37)
- Stromal component is hyalinized or cellular which resembles ovarian stroma
- Renal nephron elements within stromal component should not be seen

Special Stains and Immunohistochemistry

- Cellular stroma positive for estrogen receptor (ER) and progesterone receptor (PR)

Other Techniques for Diagnosis

- Noncontributory

Differential Diagnosis

Mixed Epithelial and Stromal Tumor (MEST)

- MEST and cystic nephroma are considered to represent the morphologic continuum of the same entity
- MEST has solid component grossly and thick and solid septa (usually > 5 mm) microscopically

Cystic Renal Cell Carcinoma

- Shows focal areas of clear cells identical to those of clear cell renal cell carcinoma

Cystic Renal Dysplasia

- History of urinary obstruction or ureteral duplication
- Primitive renal tubules and fetal cartilage

Benign (Non-neoplastic) Renal Cysts

- Abnormal renal architecture
- Remnant nephrons in the septa

PEARLS

- *Pediatric cystic nephroma and cystic partially differentiated nephroblastoma are benign neoplasms currently considered to be a part of the spectrum of nephroblastoma*

SELECTED REFERENCES

Turbiner J, Amin MB, Humphrey PA, et al: Cystic nephroma and mixed epithelial and stromal tumor of kidney: a detailed clinicopathologic analysis of 34 cases and proposal for renal epithelial and stromal tumor (REST) as a unifying term. Am J Surg Pathol 31:489-500, 2007.

Zhou M, Kort E, Hoekstra P, et al: Adult cystic nephroma and mixed epithelial and stromal tumor of the kidney are the same disease entity: molecular and histologic evidence. Am J Surg Pathol 33: 72-80, 2009.

MIXED EPITHELIAL AND STROMAL TUMOR OF THE KIDNEY (MEST)

Clinical Features

- Rare benign tumor with striking female predominance
- Flank mass and pain, hematuria, or symptoms of urinary tract infection
- Estrogen imbalance is suspected etiologically

Gross Pathology

- Frequent central location in the kidney
- Well-circumscribed mass, frequently herniating into the renal pelvis
- Mixed solid and cystic cut surface

Histopathology (Figure 10-38)

- Biphasic: epithelial and stromal elements
  - Epithelial elements: cysts of variable sizes and tubules lined with flat, cuboidal, or low columnar cells; focal clear cells may be present
  - Stromal elements: variably cellular, from hypocellular collagen rich to hypercellular, ovarian stroma like, to smooth muscle bundles; fat may be present

Special Stains and Immunohistochemistry

- CK and vimentin: positive in epithelial elements
- Vimentin, actin, desmin, ER/PR: positive in stromal elements

Other Techniques for Diagnosis

- Noncontributory

Differential Diagnosis

CYSTIC NEPHROMA

- MEST and CN are currently considered to be the two diseases in the morphologic spectrum of the same entity (renal epithelial and stroma tumor)

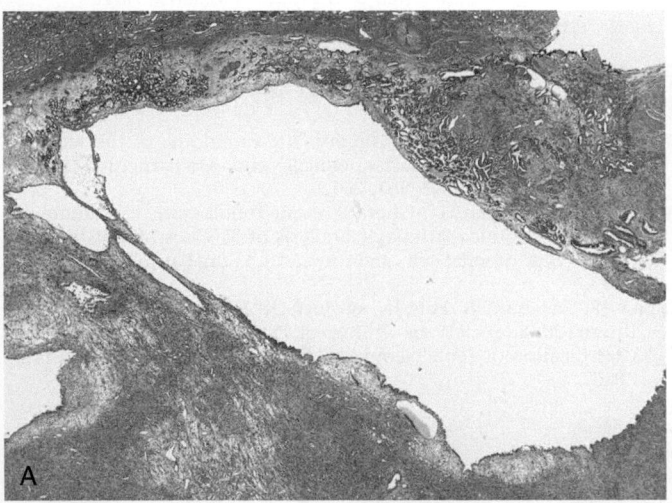
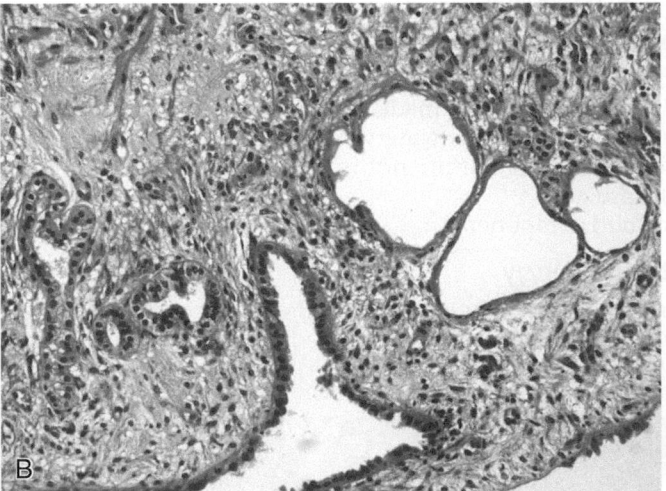
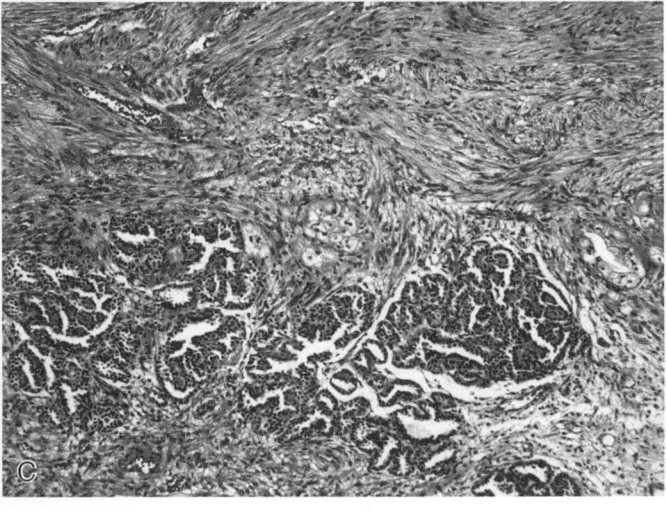

Figure 10-38. A, Mixed epithelial and stromal tumor of the kidney (MEST). Biphasic neoplasm with epithelial and stromal elements. **B,** Mixed epithelial and stromal tumor of the kidney (MEST). Epithelial elements consist of cysts of variable sizes and tubules lined with flat, cuboidal, or low columnar cells. **C,** Mixed epithelial and stromal tumor of the kidney (MEST). Stromal component is variably cellular, from hypocellular collagen-rich to hypercellular, ovarian stroma-like, to smooth muscle bundles.

- CN is morphologically much simpler without complex tubular and glandular structure or epithelial/stromal interaction

CYSTIC RENAL CELL CARCINOMA
- Shows focal areas of clear cells identical to those of clear cell renal cell carcinoma

PEARLS

- *Predominantly female patients with a history of estrogen imbalance*
- *Currently considered as renal epithelial and stromal tumor together with cystic nephroma*

SELECTED REFERENCES
Srigley JR, Delahunt B, Eble JN, et al; ISUP Renal Tumor Panel: The International Society of Urological Pathology (ISUP) Vancouver Classification of Renal Neoplasia. Am J Surg Pathol 37:1469-1489, 2013.

Zhou M, Kort E, Hoekstra P, et al: Adult cystic nephroma and mixed epithelial and stromal tumor of the kidney are the same disease entity: molecular and histologic evidence. Am J Surg Pathol 33: 72-80, 2009.

TUBULOCYSTIC CARCINOMA

Clinical Features
- Middle-aged adults
- Marked male predominance
- Usually unilateral

Gross Pathology
- Microcystic mass with a bubble-wrap appearance
- White spongy mass made of thin-walled translucent cysts filled with clear watery fluid
- Well demarcated from normal parenchyma, but not encapsulated
- No solid components

Histopathology
- Tumor with a tubulocystic architecture composed of cysts and small tubules, separated by delicate septa or by fibrotic stroma (Figure 10-39A)

- Tubules and cysts are lined by flat to columnar or hobnail eosinophilic cells (Figure 10-39B)
- Nuclei are regular, round to oval, with prominent nucleoli

Special Stains and Immunohistochemistry
- CD10, AMACR, CK19: positive
- CK7: weak

Other Techniques for Diagnosis
- Noncontributory

Differential Diagnosis

CYSTIC NEPHROMA
- Striking female predominance
- Cysts are usually larger and contain neither tubules nor epithelial cells in the septa

MULTILOCULAR CYSTIC RENAL CELL CARCINOMA
- Large cysts lined by clear cells, separated by fibrous septa containing nests of clear cells

PEARLS

- *Described as a variant of collecting duct carcinoma*
- *Should be considered as a new subtype of renal cell carcinoma, although not yet included in the WHO classification*
- *Seems to have an overall favorable prognosis, although cases with local recurrence or metastatic disease have been reported*

SELECTED REFERENCES
Alexiev BA, Drachenberg CB: Tubulocystic carcinoma of the kidney: a histologic, immunohistochemical, and ultrastructural study. Virchows Arch 462:575-581, 2013.

Amin MB, MacLennan GT, Gupta R, et al: Tubulocystic carcinoma of the kidney: clinicopathologic analysis of 31 cases of a distinctive rare subtype of renal cell carcinoma. Am J Surg Pathol 33:384-392, 2009.

Srigley JR, Delahunt B, Eble JN, et al; ISUP Renal Tumor Panel: The International Society of Urological Pathology (ISUP) Vancouver Classification of Renal Neoplasia. Am J Surg Pathol 37:1469-1489, 2013.

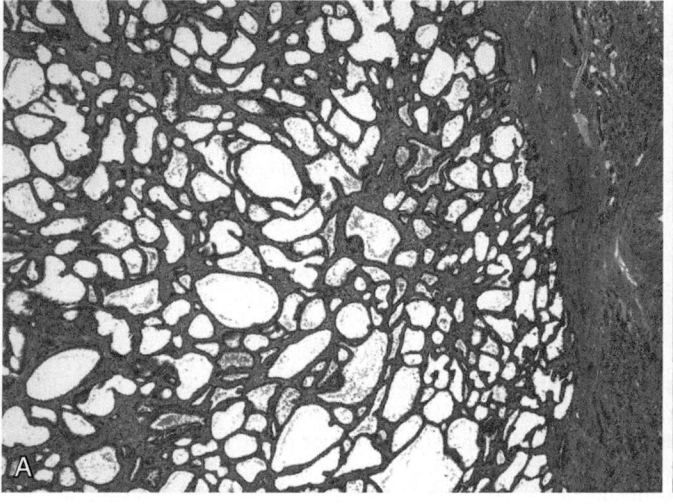
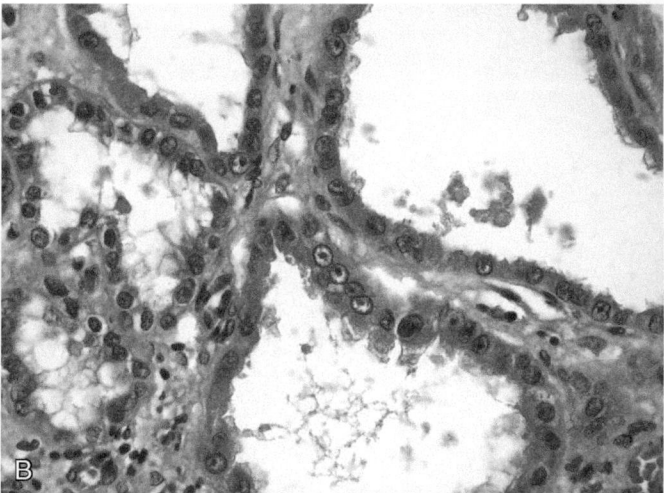

Figure 10-39. A, Tubulocystic carcinoma. Tumor with a tubulocystic architecture composed of cysts and small tubules, separated by delicate septa or by fibrotic stroma. **B,** Tubulocystic carcinoma. Tubules and cysts are lined by flat to cuboidal eosinophilic cells with round to oval nuclei and prominent nucleoli.

CLEAR CELL (TUBULO) PAPILLARY RENAL CELL CARCINOMA

Clinical Features

- Low-grade, low-stage renal cell tumor with cystic, tubuloacinar, or papillary architecture
- Comprises approximately 1% of all adult renal tumors
- Can arise in otherwise normal kidneys and in kidneys with end-stage renal disease
- Bilaterality has been reported

Gross Pathology

- Most tumors are cystic with a prominent fibrous capsule

Histopathology

- Composed mainly of cells with clear cytoplasm arranged in papillary patterns (Figure 10-40A)
- Cysts of different sizes often containing serosanguineous fluid or colloid-like secretion
- Branching tubules and acini and anastomosing clear cell ribbons with low-grade nuclei (Figure 10-40B)
- Nuclei are oriented away from the basement membrane and toward the apical surface of tubules

Special Stains and Immunohistochemistry

- CK7: diffuse membranous staining
- AMACR and FTE3: negative
- CAIX: positive in 90%
- CD10: negative in most cases
- PAX-8: positive

Other Techniques for Diagnosis

- Lack of gains of chromosomes 7 and 17
- Lack of losses of chromosome Y
- Lack of deletion of 3p

Differential Diagnosis

PAPILLARY RENAL CELL CARCINOMA

- AMACR and CK7 positive
- May display Fuhrman grade 3 and 4 nuclei

- Gains of chromosome 7 and 17
- Losses of chromosome Y

CLEAR CELL RENAL CELL CARCINOMA

- CAIX positive, but CK7 negative
- May display Fuhrman grade 3 and 4 nuclei
- Deletion of 3p

RCC ASSOCIATED WITH Xp11.2/TFE3 TRANSLOCATION

- Often affects children and young adults
- Papillary structures lined by tumor cells with abundant clear to granular cytoplasm
- Psammomatous calcification and hyalinized fibrovascular cores are present
- Cytokeratins and EMA: negative
- TFE3: positive
- Xp11.2/TFE3 translocation

PEARLS

- *Also reported as a renal angiomyoadenomatous tumor*
- *Most of the tumors reported are pT1 and Fuhrman nuclear grades 1 and 2*
- *No recurrence or metastasis reported to date*

SELECTED REFERENCES

Aydin H, Chen L, Cheng L, et al: Clear cell tubulopapillary renal cell carcinoma: a study of 36 distinctive low-grade epithelial tumors of the kidney. Am J Surg Pathol 34:1608-1621, 2010.

Pramick M, Ziober A, Bing Z: Useful immunohistochemical panel for differentiating clear cell papillary renal cell carcinoma from its mimics. Ann Diagn Pathol 17:437-440, 2013.

Rohan SM, Xiao Y, Liang Y, et al: Clear-cell papillary renal cell carcinoma: molecular and immunohistochemical analysis with emphasis on the von Hippel-Lindau gene and hypoxia-inducible factor pathway-related proteins. Mod Pathol 24:1207-1220, 2011.

Srigley JR, Delahunt B, Eble JN, et al; ISUP Renal Tumor Panel: The International Society of Urological Pathology (ISUP) Vancouver Classification of Renal Neoplasia. Am J Surg Pathol 37:1469-1489, 2013.

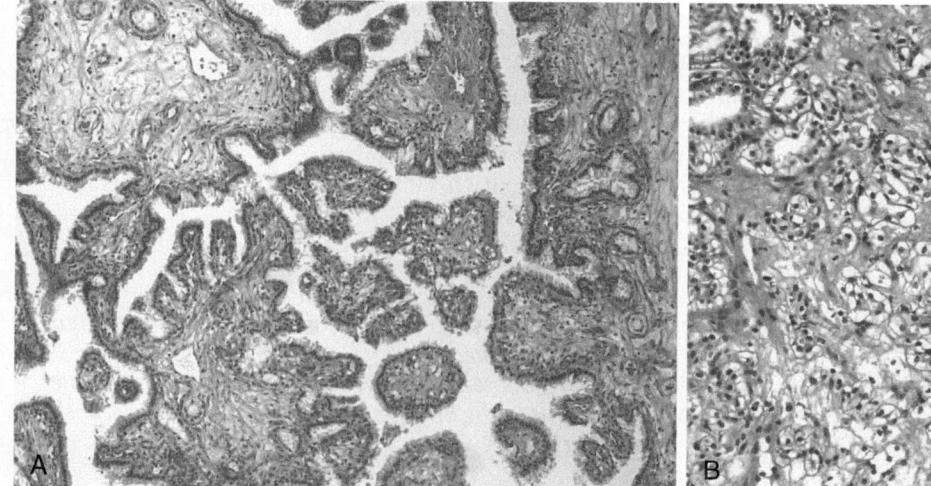
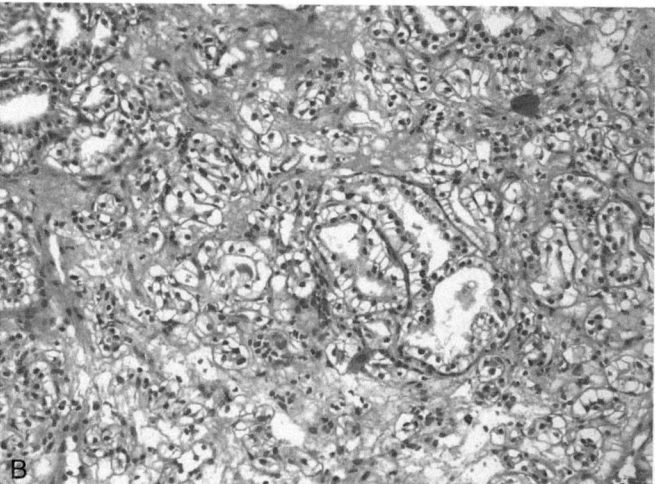

Figure 10-40. A, Clear cell (tubulo) papillary renal cell carcinoma. Tumor with predominantly papillary architecture. The papillae are lined by a single layer of cuboidal cells with a moderate amount of clear cytoplasm. **B,** Clear cell (tubulo) papillary renal cell carcinoma. Tumor with tubuloacinar architecture. The tubules and acini are lined with a single layer of cells with clear cytoplasm. The nuclei are oriented away from the basement membrane and toward the apical surface of tubules.

HEREDITARY LEIOMYOMATOSIS RENAL CELL CARCINOMA

Clinical Features

- Autosomal dominant tumor susceptibility syndrome characterized by predisposition to benign leiomyomas of skin and uterus and susceptibility to early-onset renal cell carcinoma and uterine leiomyosarcoma
- The predisposing gene is fumarate hydratase (FH) (1q42.3-q43)
- Low penetrance of RCC (20% to 30%)

Gross Pathology

- Typically unilateral and solitary tumors
- Frequently present at high stage with perinephric or venous invasion

Histopathology

- Architectural patterns include papillary, tubulopapillary, tubular, and solid
- Resembles type II papillary RCC due to tall neoplastic cells containing abundant eosinophilic cytoplasm lining the papillae
- Cysts, focal clear cell areas, and cribriforming may also be present
- Characteristic large nucleus with a very prominent inclusion-like orangeophilic or eosinophilic nucleolus, surrounded by a clear halo

Special Stains and Immunohistochemistry

- 2SC (2-succinyl cysteine); positive

Other Techniques for Diagnosis

- Loss of heterozygosity at 1q32 and 1q42-44

Differential Diagnosis

TUBULOCYSTIC CARCINOMA

- Tubules and cysts are lined by flat to columnar or hobnail eosinophilic cells
- Nuclei are regular, round to oval with prominent nucleoli

COLLECTING DUCT CARCINOMA

- Involving central region of the kidney
- Irregular, small glands and ducts in a loose collagenous chronically inflamed desmoplastic stroma
- Cells lining glands are high grade with pleomorphic nuclei; typically have hobnail appearance
- Associated tubular epithelial dysplasia

PEARLS

- *Associated with poor prognosis and frequent spread to regional lymph nodes*
- *Affected individuals harbor a germline heterozygous loss-of-function mutation of the FH gene*

SELECTED REFERENCES

Bardella C, El-Bahrawy M, Frizzell N, et al: Aberrant succination of proteins in fumarate hydratase-deficient mice and HLRCC patients is a robust biomarker of mutation status. J Pathol 225:4-11, 2011.

Merino MJ, Torres-Cabala C, Pinto P, Linehan WM: The morphologic spectrum of kidney tumors in hereditary leiomyomatosis and renal cell carcinoma (HLRCC) syndrome. Am J Surg Pathol 31:1578-1585, 2007.

Przybycin CG, Magi-Galluzzi C, McKenney JK: Hereditary syndromes with associated renal neoplasia: a practical guide to histologic recognition in renal tumor resection specimens. Adv Anat Pathol 20:245-263, 2013.

Srigley JR, Delahunt B, Eble JN, et al; ISUP Renal Tumor Panel: The International Society of Urological Pathology (ISUP) Vancouver Classification of Renal Neoplasia. Am J Surg Pathol 37:1469-1489, 2013.

BIRT-HOGG-DUBÉ–ASSOCIATED RENAL TUMOR

Clinical Features

- Familial occurrence of multiple skin lesions (fibrofolliculoma, trichodiscoma, and acrochordons)
- Association with multiple subtypes of renal neoplasia
- Birt-Hogg-Dubé gene locus is on 17p11.2; folliculin is the gene product

Gross Pathology

- Multiple bilateral renal tumors

Histopathology

- Three morphologic patterns, either in isolation or in combination
  - An admixture of areas typical of renal oncocytoma and chromophobe RCC
  - Scattered chromophobe cells in the background of a typical renal oncocytoma
  - Large eosinophilic cells with intracytoplasmic vacuoles
- Renal oncocytosis in the background renal parenchyma
- Tumor cells with cytoplasmic clearing but no prominent nuclear membrane irregularity

Special Stains and Immunohistochemistry

- CK7, CD117, parvalbumin: positive

Other Techniques for Diagnosis

- Noncontributory

Differential Diagnosis

CHROMOPHOBE RENAL CELL CARCINOMA

- Sheetlike compact growth pattern
- "Raisinoid" nuclei and perinuclear halos
- CK7 diffusely positive

RENAL ONCOCYTOMA

- Uniform nuclei without "koilocytic" nuclear atypia or prominent cell membranes
- CK7 stains single cells or small clusters of cells
- S100A1 positive

PEARLS

- *Indolent tumors; no evidence of aggressive behavior has been documented*
- *A subset (approximately 10%) of patients with germline mutations in the BHD gene does not have the typical skin findings*

SELECTED REFERENCES

Hes O, Petersson F, Kuroda N, et al: Renal hybrid oncocytic/chromophobe tumors: a review. Histol Histopathol 28:1257-1264, 2013.

Przybycin CG, Magi-Galluzzi C, McKenney JK: Hereditary syndromes with associated renal neoplasia: a practical guide to histologic recognition in renal tumor resection specimens. Adv Anat Pathol 20:245-263, 2013.

Schmidt LS, Warren MB, Nickerson ML, et al: Birt-Hogg-Dube syndrome, a genodermatosis associated with spontaneous pneumothorax and kidney neoplasia, maps to chromosome 17p11.2.Am J Hum Genet 69:876-882, 2001.

SDH-RELATED CARCINOMA

Clinical Features

- Syndrome linked to germline mutation of multiple subunits (SDHB/C/D) of the Krebs cycle enzyme, succinate dehydrogenase
- Presented with renal cell cancer at an early age (33 years, range 15 to 62)
- Family history of paraganglioma, pheochromocytoma, or gastrointestinal stromal tumor should raise awareness of possible SDH alterations
- Renal cancer can present as the only finding

Gross Pathology

- Typically unilateral and solitary tumor
- Well circumscribed or lobulated tumors frequently showing cystic change

Histopathology

- SDHB mutation associated tumors show oncocytic features
  - Composed of cuboidal cells with bubbly eosinophilic cytoplasm, indistinct cell borders, centrally placed nucleoli, and inconspicuous nucleoli (Figure 10-41)
  - Distinctive cytoplasmic inclusions, either vacuolated or containing eosinophilic fluid-like material
  - Cells are arranged in solid nests or in tubules surrounding central spaces
- SDHC/D mutation–associated tumors show features of clear cell RCC

Special Stains and Immunohistochemistry

- SDHB: negative

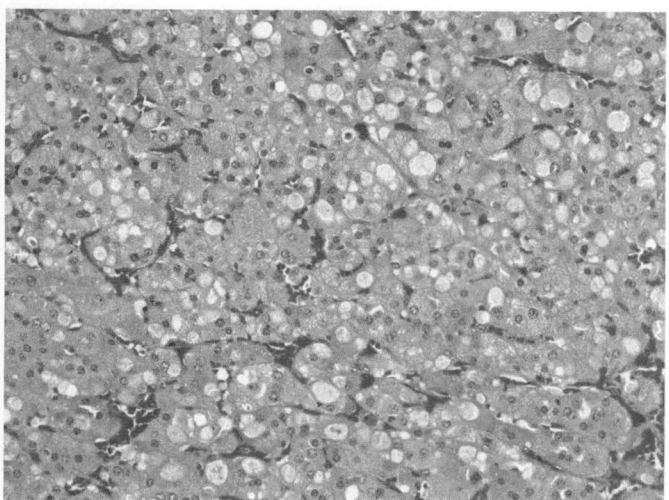

Figure 10-41. SDH related carcinoma. Tumor is composed of cuboidal cells with bubbly eosinophilic cytoplasm, indistinct cell borders, centrally placed nucleoli, and inconspicuous nucleoli.

Other Techniques for Diagnosis

- SDHB/C/D germline mutation testing in patients younger than 45

Differential Diagnosis

CLEAR CELL RENAL CELL CARCINOMA

- SDHB positive

RENAL ONCOCYTIC TUMORS

- SDHB positive

PEARLS

- *May have aggressive behavior, especially in younger individuals*
- *Two patients presented with widely metastatic disease*

SELECTED REFERENCES

Gill AJ, Pachter NS, Chou A, et al: Renal tumors associated with germline SDHB mutation show distinctive morphology. Am J Surg Pathol 35:1578, 2011.

Gill AJ, Pachter NS, Clarkson A, et al: Renal tumors and hereditary pheochromocytoma-paraganglioma syndrome type 4. N Engl J Med 364: 885, 2011.

Housley SL, Lindsay RS, Young B, et al: Renal carcinoma with giant mitochondria associated with germ-line mutation and somatic loss of the succinate dehydrogenase B gene. Histopathology 56:405-410, 2010.

Przybycin CG, Magi-Galluzzi C, McKenney JK: Hereditary syndromes with associated renal neoplasia: a practical guide to histologic recognition in renal tumor resection specimens. Adv Anat Pathol 20:245-263, 2013.

Ricketts CJ, Shuch B, Vocke CD, et al: Succinate dehydrogenase kidney cancer: an aggressive example of the Warburg effect in cancer. J Urol 188:2063-2071, 2012.

ACQUIRED CYSTIC DISEASE-ASSOCIATED RENAL CELL CARCINOMA

Clinical Features

- Subtype of RCC with unique morphologic features found exclusively in the background of end-stage renal disease (ESRD)
- Male predominance
- Patients on dialysis (4 to 12 years)

Gross Pathology

- Multiple and bilateral tumors have been reported
- Mostly well demarcated
- Predominantly solid with varying extent of cystic change

Histopathology

- Tumors show variegated architecture forming diffuse sheets, macro- and microcysts, tubulopapillary arrangements, and nests (Figure 10-42A)
- Characteristic inter- or intracellular microlumen formation and intratumoral deposition of oxalate crystals (Figure 10-42B)
- Large tumor cells with eosinophilic cytoplasm and mildly irregular nuclei (Fuhrman grade 3)
- Hemosiderin pigment frequently found in cytoplasm of tumor cells
- Proliferation and multilayering are occasionally present, creating papillary projections and small nests

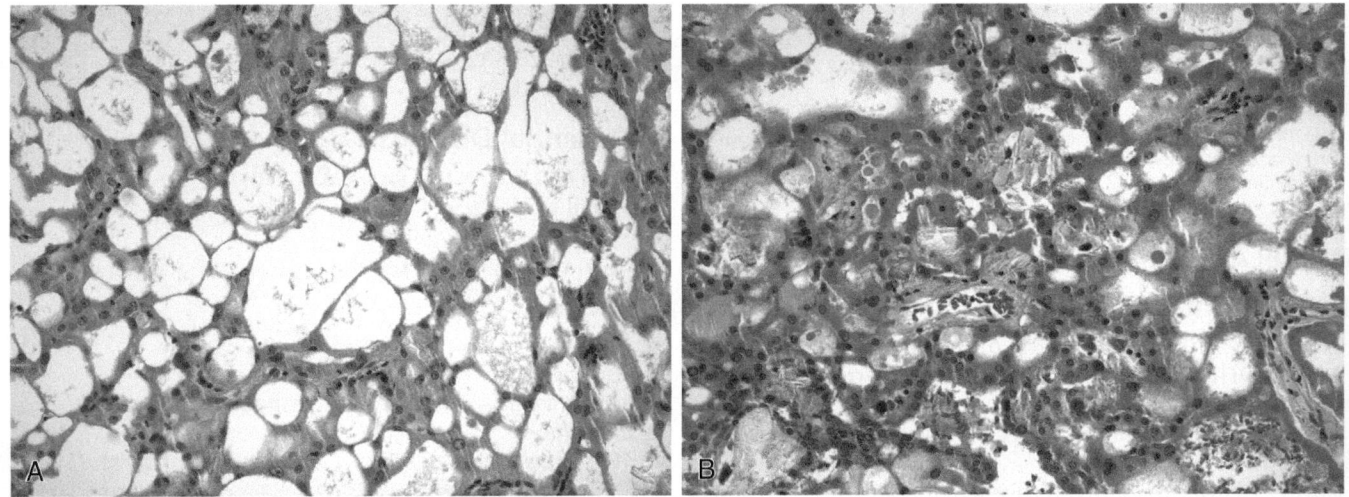

Figure 10-42. A, Acquired cystic disease-associated renal cell carcinoma. Tumor with typical microcystic pattern. Tumor cells are large with eosinophilic cytoplasm and mildly irregular nuclei. **B,** Acquired cystic disease-associated renal cell carcinoma. Tumor shows characteristic microlumen formation and intratumoral deposition of oxalate crystals.

Special Stains and Immunohistochemistry

- AMACR, CD10, pancytokeratin: positive
- CAIX, PAX-8: negative
- CK7: negative or variable

Other Techniques for Diagnosis

- Noncontributory

Differential Diagnosis

PAPILLARY RENAL CELL CARCINOMA
- AMACR, CD10, PAX-8, and CK7: positive

CLEAR CELL RENAL CELL CARCINOMA
- CAIX and PAX-8: positive
- CK7 and AMACR: negative

RENAL ONCOCYTOMA
- CD117 and E-cadherin positive

PEARLS

- *Incidence of RCC is increased 100-fold in the background of acquired cystic disease of the kidney compared to the general population*
- *Some have suggested relatively aggressive biologic behavior, whereas other authors have documented a generally indolent clinical course*

SELECTED REFERENCES

Ahn S, Kwon GY, Cho YM, et al: Acquired cystic disease-associated renal cell carcinoma: further characterization of the morphologic and immunopathologic features. Med Mol Morphol 46:225-232, 2013.

Kuroda N, Ohe C, Mikami S, et al: Review of acquired cystic disease-associated renal cell carcinoma with focus on pathobiological aspects. Histol Histopathol 26:1215-1218, 2011.

Srigley JR, Delahunt B, Eble JN, et al; ISUP Renal Tumor Panel: The International Society of Urological Pathology (ISUP) Vancouver Classification of Renal Neoplasia. Am J Surg Pathol 37:1469-1489, 2013.

RENOMEDULLARY INTERSTITIAL CELL TUMOR/MEDULLARY FIBROMA

Clinical Features

- Almost always asymptomatic lesions found incidentally in kidneys removed for other reasons or found at autopsy
- Found in up to 40% of autopsies

Gross Pathology

- Well-circumscribed, firm, gray-white nodule(s) in the kidney medulla
- Usually smaller than 0.5 cm in diameter
- Several nodules occasionally seen in same kidney

Histopathology

- Well-circumscribed nodule composed of haphazardly arranged, benign-appearing spindle cells (Figure 10-43)
- Typically paucicellular tumor with a loose collagenous or myxoid stroma

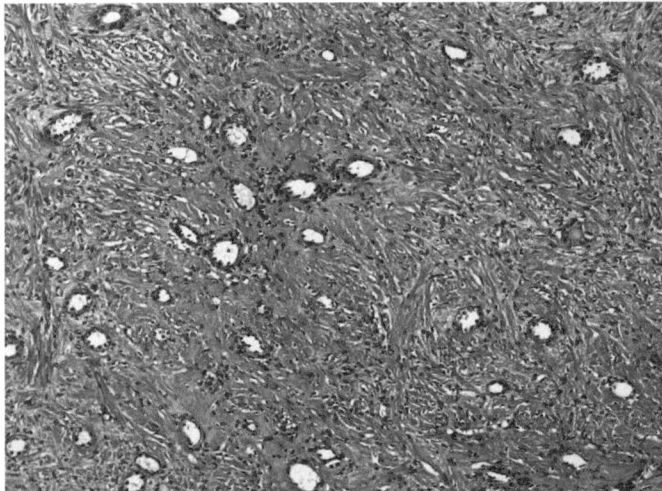

Figure 10-43. Renomedullary interstitial cell tumor/medullary fibroma. Well-circumscribed nodule composed of haphazardly arranged, benign-appearing spindle cells.

- Entrapped medullary tubules can be found at the periphery
- No mitotic activity or features of malignancy should be present

Special Stains and Immunohistochemistry

- Noncontributory

Other Techniques for Diagnosis

- Noncontributory

Differential Diagnosis

LEIOMYOMA

- Rare renal tumor
- Found in the cortex or capsule; not in the renal medulla
- Shows similar cytologic features as smooth muscle tumors at other sites

PEARLS

- *Cell of origin is the renomedullary interstitial cell, which functions in blood pressure control*
- *Lesions are almost always asymptomatic*

SELECTED REFERENCES

Dall'Era M, Das S: Benign medullary fibroma of the kidney. J Urol 164:2018, 2000.
Tamboli P, Ro JY, Amin MB, et al: Benign tumors and tumor-like lesions of the adult kidney. Part II: Benign mesenchymal and mixed neoplasms, and tumor-like lesions. Adv Anat Pathol 7:47-66, 2000.

JUXTAGLOMERULAR CELL TUMOR/RENIN-SECRETING TUMOR

Clinical Features

- Benign kidney tumor with differentiation toward the modified smooth muscle cells of the juxtaglomerular apparatus adjacent to the afferent arteriole at the hilus of the glomerulus
- Most commonly presents in patients younger than 30 years old
- Slight female predominance
- All patients have hypertension, which is corrected in majority of the cases by removal of the tumor
- Elevated renin level is characteristic; increased aldosterone levels with hypokalemia may occur

Gross Pathology

- Unilateral and solitary, well-circumscribed neoplasm in the cortex
- Cut surface shows a solid gray-white mass occasionally with small cystic spaces

Histopathology

- Classically has a diffuse architecture; trabecular or glomeruloid pattern may be seen
- Polygonal to spindle-shaped cells with oval bland nuclei
- Cells have moderate to abundant granular pink cytoplasm
- Loose myxoid stroma with scattered lymphocytic infiltrate

- Typically shows prominent vasculature with hemangiopericytoma-like pattern
- Mitotic activity is rare

Special Stains and Immunohistochemistry

- Smooth muscle actin, muscle-specific actin, and CD31: positive
- Renin: positive
- Cytokeratin, desmin, S-100, HMB-45: negative

Other Techniques for Diagnosis

- Electron microscopy: rhomboid, renin-specific crystalline structures

Differential Diagnosis

CLEAR CELL RENAL CELL CARCINOMA

- Lacks hypertension as presenting symptom
- Typically found in older patients
- Composed of sheets of clear cells with distinct cell borders

PEARLS

- *Small tumors can be localized by serum renin level in the renal vein*
- *Tumor is best treated surgically, typically with nephrectomy*
- *Blood pressure returns to normal levels following surgical resection*
- *No reports of local recurrence or metastases regardless of the type of surgical resection*

SELECTED REFERENCES

Lopez G-Asenjo JA, Blanco Gonzalez J, Ortega Medina L, Sanz Esponera J: Juxtaglomerular cell tumor of the kidney: morphological, immunohistochemical and ultrastructural studies of a new case. Pathol Res Pract 187:354-361, 1991.
Martin SA, Mynderse LA, Lager DJ, Cheville JC: Juxtaglomerular cell tumor: a clinicopathologic study of four cases and review of the literature. Am J Clin Pathol 116:854-863, 2001.

NEPHROBLASTOMA (WILMS TUMOR)

Clinical Features

- Common solid tumor of childhood; 90% found before age 6; peak ages are 2 to 5
- Rarely found in adults or neonates
- About 10% associated with dysmorphic syndromes
  - WAGR syndrome (Wilms tumor, aniridia, genital anomalies, and mental retardation deletion of chromosome 11p13 involving WT1 gene): 30% develop Wilms tumor
  - Denys-Drash syndrome (point mutation in WT-1 gene): 90% risk for Wilms tumor
  - Beckwith-Wiedemann syndrome (hemihypertrophy, macroglossia, omphalocele, visceromegaly, WT2 locus on 11p15)
  - Familial nephroblastoma (17q12-21 and 19q13.3-13.4)
- Patients usually present with an abdominal mass or abdominal tenderness; may present with hematuria, hypertension, or rarely with peritoneal symptoms if spontaneous rupture has occurred

- Treatment includes surgical resection, chemotherapy, and radiation
- Prognosis depends on tumor stage, histologic features, and patient age at time of diagnosis

Gross Pathology

- Typically single, well-circumscribed mass with lobulated appearance
- Variegated, bulging, pale-gray to tan-pink cut surface typically with extensive hemorrhage and necrosis; cyst formation may be seen
- Must carefully examine for evidence of spread into renal pelvis, renal vein, ureter, or perirenal adipose tissue
- Perirenal lymph node involvement may be found

Histopathology

- Classically shows triphasic pattern consisting of blastema, stromal, and epithelial components (Figure 10-44A)
- Biphasic or even monophasic tumors occasionally found
- Blastemal component is arranged in diffuse sheets or thin cords or as nodular aggregates; peripheral palisading of nuclei may be seen

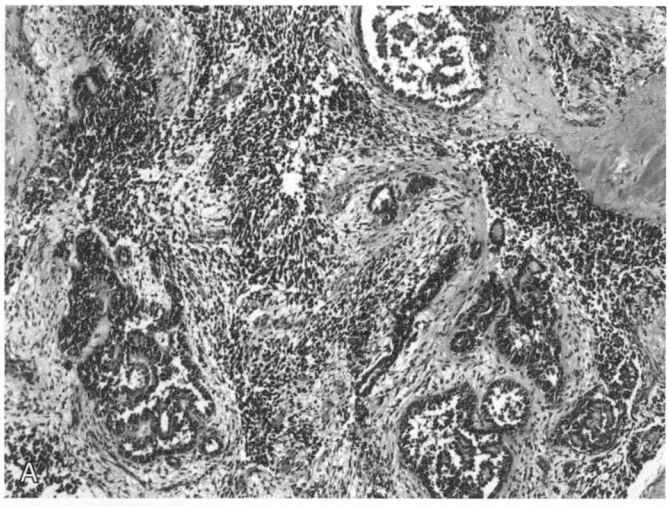

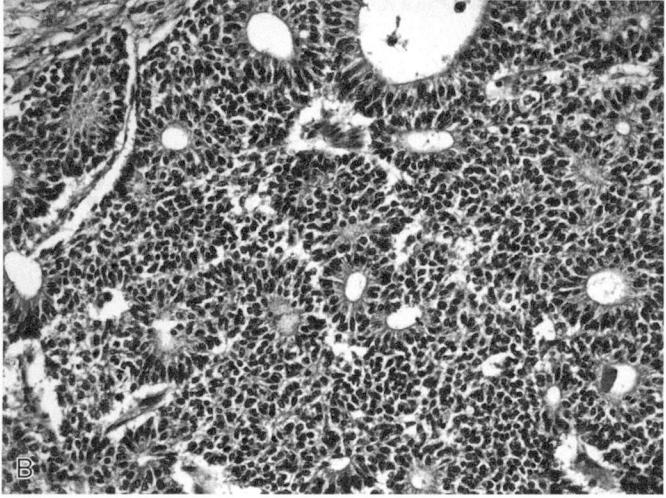

Figure 10-44. A, Nephroblastoma (Wilms tumor). Wilms tumor showing classical triphasic pattern consisting of blastema, stromal, and epithelial elements. **B,** Nephroblastoma (Wilms tumor). Wilms tumor showing classical epithelial component.

- Blastema consists of small, round cells with hyperchromatic nuclei showing coarse chromatin and scant cytoplasm
- Frequent mitotic activity is common
- Diffuse pattern shows poorly cohesive cells with infiltrative growth pattern
- Stroma is typically myxoid or fibromyxoid; differentiation toward skeletal muscle or less commonly cartilage, bone, fat, or neural tissue may be seen
- Epithelial component is in the form of poorly formed tubules to well-developed tubular or papillary structures (Figure 10-44B)
- Foci of squamous metaplasia or mucinous epithelium are not uncommon

Nuclear Anaplasia

- Presence of polyploidy multipolar mitotic figures, or nuclear enlargement with hyperchromasia (nuclei > 3× of adjacent non-neoplastic nuclei)
- Associated with responsiveness to therapy, rather than tumor aggressiveness

Special Stains and Immunohistochemistry

- Vimentin: highlights blastemal component
- WT-1: very low level or no expression in stromal area; diffuse expression in blastemal and early epithelial differentiation; patchy and variable expression in differentiated epithelium

Other Techniques for Diagnosis

- Electron microscopy
  - Can help distinguish between the tumors in the small round blue cell category (lymphoma, neuroblastoma) when only limited tissue is available
  - Shows cellular features resembling those of the developing metanephros
  - Blastemal cells have numerous organelles with many desmosomes, intermediate filaments, mitochondria, and cilia
- Cytogenetic studies
  - One third of sporadic Wilms tumors harbor WT-1 deletion and 10% harbor point mutation

Differential Diagnosis

NEUROBLASTOMA

- Most commonly found in the adrenal gland
- Homer-Wright pseudorosettes often seen
- Positive for chromogranin, synaptophysin, and NSE, negative for WT-1

SYNOVIAL SARCOMA

- Most cases are monophasic with short intersecting fascicles
- Cystic structures lined with hobnail cells
- WT-1 negative
- t(X; 18) translocation with SYT/SSX fusion transcripts

PRIMITIVE NEUROECTODERMAL TUMOR

- Grossly poorly circumscribed
- Primitive round cells with variable rosette formation
- CD99 positive and WT-1 negative

RHABDOID TUMOR
- Often presents with metastatic disease
- Tumor cells have large nucleoli and cytoplasmic inclusions
- Lacks triphasic pattern; no blastemal component

MESOBLASTIC NEPHROMA
- Typically found within first 3 months of life
- Composed of interlacing fascicles of bland spindle cells infiltrating among normal-appearing kidney structures

PEARLS

- *Embryonal neoplasm derived from nephrogenic blastemal cells*
- *Hereditary cases are more commonly bilateral*
- *All tumors must be generously sampled to determine the presence and extent of tumor anaplasia*
- *Anaplastic nephroblastoma is virtually never encountered in infants*
- *Common sites of metastasis include regional lymph nodes, lung, and liver*
- *Younger age at time of diagnosis is associated with a better prognosis*
- *Overall good prognosis; cure rate is approximately 90% following surgery, chemotherapy, and radiation*

SELECTED REFERENCES

Beckwith JB; Nephrogenic rests and the pathogenesis of Wilms' tumor: developmental and clinical considerations. Am J Med Genet 79:268-273, 1998.

Charles AK, Mall S, Watson J, Berry PJ: Expression of the Wilms' tumour gene WT1 in the developing human and in pediatric renal tumours: an immunohistochemical study. Mol Pathol 50:138-144, 1997.

Parham DM, Roloson GJ, Feely M, et al: Primary malignant neuroepithelial tumors of the kidney: a clinicopathologic analysis of 146 adult and pediatric cases from the National Wilms' Tumor Study Group Pathology Center. Am J Surg Pathol 25:133-146, 2001.

NEPHROGENIC RESTS AND NEPHROBLASTOMATOSIS

Clinical Features

- Nephrogenic rests are present in 25% to 40% of nephrectomy specimens with nephroblastoma
- Nephroblastomatosis refers to multifocal or diffuse nephrogenic rests
- Finding of nephrogenic rests increases the likelihood of subsequent development of nephroblastoma in the opposite kidney

Gross Pathology

- Hyperplastic nephrogenic rests form irregular subcortical or intraparenchymal yellow-tan lesions
- Nephroblastomatosis may cause diffuse cortical enlargement

Histopathology

- Nephrogenic rests are divided into perilobar and intralobar types

- Perilobar nephrogenic rests: composed of blastemal or tubular patterns and very little stroma at the periphery of the renal lobe
- Intralobar nephrogenic rests: ill-defined, stroma-rich lesions placed randomly within the renal lobe

Special Stains and Immunohistochemistry

- Noncontributory

Other Techniques for Diagnosis

- Noncontributory

Differential Diagnosis

- Nephroblastoma
- Presence of a fibrous tumor capsule
- Expansile and rounded contour

PEARLS

- *Finding of nephrogenic rests increases the likelihood of subsequent development of nephroblastoma in the opposite kidney*
- *The non-neoplastic kidney has to be sampled carefully*

SELECTED REFERENCES

Beckwith JB: Nephrogenic rests and the pathogenesis of Wilms' tumor: developmental and clinical considerations. Am J Med Genet 79:268-273, 1998.

Hennigar RA, O'Shea PA, Grattan-Smith JD: Clinicopathologic features of nephrogenic rests and nephroblastomatosis. Adv Anat Pathol 8:276-289, 2001.

CYSTIC PARTIALLY DIFFERENTIATED NEPHROBLASTOMA

Clinical Features

- Occurs with greater frequency in boys than in girls
- Almost all patients are younger than 24 months
- Palpable abdominal mass is the most common presentation

Gross Pathology

- Large, well-circumscribed mass with a fibrous pseudocapsule
- Cystic with variably sized cysts separated by thin septa
- No expansile solid component

Histopathology

- Cysts lined with flattened, cuboidal, or hobnail epithelium or lack lining epithelium undifferentiated and differentiated mesenchyme, blastema, and nephroblastomatous epithelial elements within the septa
- Termed *pediatric cystic nephroma* when no nephroblastomatous elements present

Special Stains and Immunohistochemistry

- Noncontributory

Other Techniques for Diagnosis

- Noncontributory

Differential Diagnosis

- Cystic nephroblastoma
- Presence of solid, expansile tumor nodule

PEARLS

- *Pediatric cystic nephroma is considered different from the adult cystic nephroma*

SELECTED REFERENCES

Eble JN, Bonsib SM: Extensively cystic renal neoplasms: cystic nephroma, cystic partially differentiated nephroblastoma, multilocular cystic renal cell carcinoma, and cystic hamartoma of renal pelvis. Semin Diagn Pathol 15:2-20, 1998.

Joshi VV, Beckwith JB: Multilocular cyst of the kidney (cystic nephroma) and cystic, partially differentiated nephroblastoma: terminology and criteria for diagnosis. Cancer 64:466-479, 1989.

MESOBLASTIC NEPHROMA

Clinical Features

- Most common congenital renal neoplasm; diagnosis typically made within first 3 months of life
- Uncommon in children older than 1 year; rarely found in adults
- Almost all infants present with an abdominal mass
- May occasionally recur; rare reports of metastases

Gross Pathology

- Centered in the renal sinus
- Classic mesoblastic nephroma: small with firm, whorled cut surface resembling leiomyoma
- Cellular mesoblastic nephroma: large, frequently soft, and cystic with foci of hemorrhage and necrosis

Histopathology

- "Classic" variant resembling benign fibromatosis; composed of interlacing fascicles of bland fibroblastic cells with infrequent mitoses; locally invasive, extending into adjacent renal parenchyma (Figure 10-45)
- "Cellular" variant, identical to infantile fibrosarcoma composed of sheets or ill-defined fascicles of densely packed plump cells with high mitotic activity; less invasive with pushing margins
- "Mixed" pattern is recognized when features of both are present in a single tumor

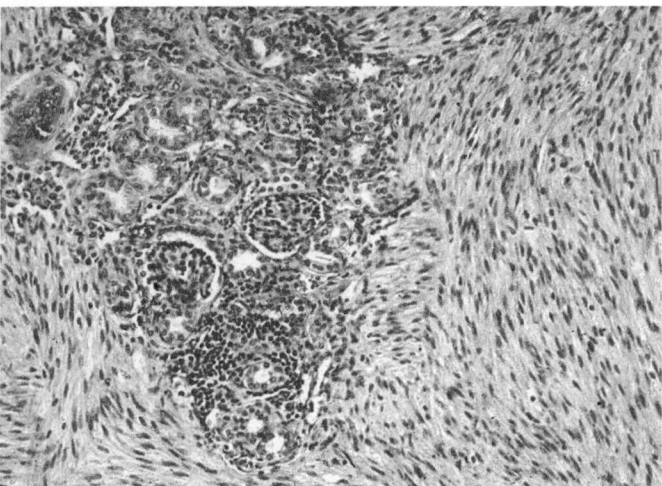

Figure 10-45. Mesoblastic nephroma. Proliferation of spindle cells infiltrating around renal structures.

Special Stains and Immunohistochemistry

- Vimentin: positive
- Smooth muscle actin (SMA): positive

Other Techniques for Diagnosis

- Electron microscopy: prominent network of endoplasmic reticulum
- Cytogenetics studies: cellular variant has trisomy 11 or t(12;15)(p13;q25)

Differential Diagnosis

NEPHROBLASTOMA (WILMS TUMOR)

- Blastemal component not present in mesoblastic nephroma
- Usually found in children older than 1 year of age
- Often bilateral

CLEAR CELL SARCOMA

- Typically found in older patients
- Classic histologic pattern consists of cords of uniform spindle-shaped cells with round to oval nuclei and a moderate amount of clear-pale cytoplasm in a collagenous background
- Often metastasizes to bone or other sites

RHABDOID TUMOR

- Often presents with metastatic disease
- Angiolymphatic invasion is often readily identified
- Tumor cells show nuclear pleomorphism and have large nucleoli and eosinophilic cytoplasmic inclusions

PEARLS

- *Treatment is surgical resection; complete resection renders excellent prognosis*
- *Tumor may recur; metastases are uncommon*
- *Risk for recurrence and metastasis includes cellular histology, stage III and above disease and involvement of intrarenal or sinus vessels*

SELECTED REFERENCES

Dal Cin P, Lipcsei G, Hermand G, et al: Congenital mesoblastic nephroma and trisomy 11. Cancer Genet Cytogenet 103:68-70, 1998.

Rubin BP, Chen CJ, Morgan TW, et al: Congenital mesoblastic nephroma t(12;15) is associated with ETV6-NTRK3 gene fusion: cytogenetic and molecular relationship to congenital (infantile) fibrosarcoma. Am J Pathol 153:1451-1458, 1998.

Truong LD, Williams R, Ngo T, et al: Adult mesoblastic nephroma: expansion of the morphologic spectrum and review of literature. Am J Surg Pathol 22:827-839, 1998.

CLEAR CELL SARCOMA

Clinical Features

- Rare renal tumor; approximately 5% of all pediatric kidney tumors
- Typically presents between ages 6 months and 5 years
- Presents with an abdominal mass; metastasis often evident at time of presentation
- Common sites of metastasis include bone, brain, lung, liver, soft tissue, and lymph nodes

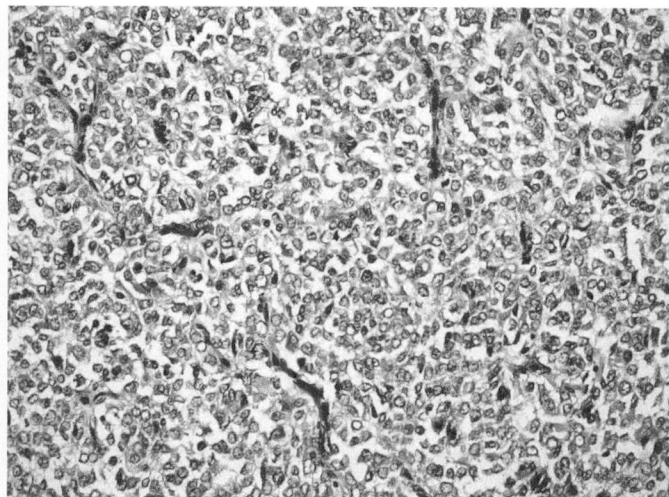

Figure 10-46. Clear cell sarcoma. Proliferation of cells with pale cytoplasm and pale, vesicular nuclei separated by delicate, regularly spaced fibrovascular arcade.

Gross Pathology

- Solitary tumor with variable size and weight; typically very large
- Appears well-circumscribed with compression of adjacent kidney parenchyma
- Uniform tan-white to gray color
- Often shows cystic areas
- Focal necrosis and hemorrhage may be seen but are rarely prominent

Histopathology

- Classic pattern: cords of cells with pale cytoplasm and pale, vesicular nuclei separated by delicate, regularly spaced fibrovascular arcades (Figure 10-46)
- Subtly infiltrating kidney-tumor interface with entrapment and separation of nephrons and tubules at the periphery
- Histologic variants: myxoid, sclerosing, cellular, epithelioid, spindle cell, and palisading patterns

Special Stains and Immunohistochemistry

- Vimentin, nerve growth factor receptor: positive
- Cytokeratin, Mic-2, S100, neural markers, desmin, and WT-1: negative

Other Techniques for Diagnosis

- Electron microscopy: primitive cells with abundant cytoplasmic processes and few poorly formed cell junctions; prominent collagen

Differential Diagnosis

NEPHROBLASTOMA (WILMS TUMOR)

- Shows heterologous cell types
- Blastemal component is not present in clear cell sarcoma

MESOBLASTIC NEPHROMA

- Typically discovered at birth; almost always before age 1
- Composed of bland spindle cells without significant clear cell differentiation
- Stroma often shows dilated staghorn vessels
- Rarely metastasizes

RHABDOID TUMOR

- Highly cellular tumor composed of large cells with prominent nucleoli and large eosinophilic cytoplasmic inclusions
- Cytokeratin positive

PEARLS

- *Highly aggressive tumor frequently associated with relapses and recurrences*
- *Metastases to bone and other extrapulmonary sites are common*
- *Treatment includes surgical resection and chemotherapy*

SELECTED REFERENCES

Furtwängler R, Gooskens SL, van Tinteren H, et al: Clear cell sarcomas of the kidney registered on International Society of Pediatric Oncology (SIOP) 93-01 and SIOP 2001 protocols: a report of the SIOP Renal Tumour Study Group. Eur J Cancer 49:3497-3506, 2013.

Gooskens SL, Furtwängler R, Vujanic GM, et al: Clear cell sarcoma of the kidney: a review. Eur J Cancer 48:2219-2226, 2012.

Schuster AE, Schneider DT, Fritsch MK, et al: Genetic and genetic expression analyses of clear cell sarcoma of the kidney. Lab Invest 83:1293-1299, 2003.

RHABDOID TUMOR

Clinical Features

- About 2% of all pediatric renal neoplasms
- Male-to-female ratio of 1.5:1
- Mean age of 13 months; usually < 24 months of age
- Hematuria, hypercalcemia, 15% associated with posterior fossa primitive neuroectodermal tumor (PNET)
- Highly lethal; 75% die within 1 year of diagnosis
- Widespread hematogenous and lymphatic metastases
- No effective therapy

Gross Pathology

- Moderately circumscribed, nonencapsulated mass
- Necrosis and hemorrhage common

Histopathology

- Sheets of uniform cells with the following:
  - Large vesicular nuclei
  - Prominent nuclei and cytoplasmic inclusions

Special Stains and Immunohistochemistry

- Epithelial markers: positive
- Characteristic pattern: focal but intense staining in a background of nonreactive cells
- INI-1 negative

Other Techniques for Diagnosis

- Electron microscopy: cytoplasmic inclusions consist of aggregates of intermediate filaments
- Cytogenetic studies: inactivation of *hSNF5/INI1* gene on chromosome 22 constitutes a molecular hallmark of rhabdoid tumor of the kidney

Differential Diagnosis

NEPHROBLASTOMA (WILMS TUMOR)

- Common solid tumor of childhood (typically in children ages 2 to 5)

- Typically shows a distinct triphasic pattern with blastema, stromal, and epithelial components

MESOBLASTIC NEPHROMA
- Composed of interlacing fascicles of bland spindle cells
- Cells lack intracytoplasmic inclusions

PEARLS
- *Common malignant tumor of childhood*
- *Cell of origin remains unknown*
- *Tumor cells resemble immature skeletal muscle but show no ultrastructural or immunohistochemical features of muscle differentiation*
- *Aggressive tumors; more than 50% of patients die within 1 year of diagnosis*
- *Infants have a dismal prognosis, whereas older children have a more favorable outcome*

SELECTED REFERENCES

Isaacs H Jr: Fetal and neonatal rhabdoid tumor. J Pediatr Surg 45:619-626, 2010.
Savla J, Chen TT, Schneider NR, et al: Mutations of the hSNF5/INI1 gene in renal rhabdoid tumors with second primary brain tumors. J Natl Cancer Inst 92:648-650, 2000.
Tomlinson GE, Breslow NE, Dome J, et al: Rhabdoid tumor of the kidney in the National Wilms' Tumor Study: age at diagnosis as a prognostic factor. J Clin Oncol 23:7641-7645, 2005.

METASTATIC TUMOR

Clinical Features
- Kidney is a common site for metastases from other malignant tumors
- Most common primary sites include lung, skin (malignant melanoma), gastrointestinal tract, ovary, testes, and contralateral kidney

Gross Pathology
- Metastatic tumors in the kidney are typically multiple and often bilateral
- May involve the cortex or medulla

Histopathology
- Depends on primary site
- Typically shows poorly differentiated carcinoma; glandular or squamous differentiation may be seen in metastatic carcinomas from the lung or gastrointestinal tract
- Malignant melanoma shows large, pleomorphic, polygonal cells with prominent nucleoli; melanin pigment may be seen

Special Stains and Immunohistochemistry
- S-100 protein and HMB-45: positive in metastatic melanoma

Other Techniques for Diagnosis
- Noncontributory

Differential Diagnosis
- Rarely have diagnostic difficulty with metastatic tumors involving the kidney, as primary tumor is typically well documented prior to development of kidney metastases

PEARLS
- *Primary tumor is usually known prior to the development of renal metastases*
- *Prognosis is poor*

SELECTED REFERENCES

Bracken RB, Chica G, Johnson DE, Luna M: Secondary renal neoplasms: an autopsy study. South Med J 72:806-807, 1979.
Murphy WM, Beckwith JB, Farrow GM: Tumors of the Kidney, Bladder and Related Urinary Structures: Atlas of Tumor Pathology, 3rd Series, Fascicle 11. Washington, DC, Armed Forces Institute of Pathology, 1994, pp 313-317.

KIDNEY: GLOMERULAR DISEASES

PODOCYTOPATHIES

Podocytopathies are a group of disorders where podocyte injury, often manifesting as foot process effacement, is considered the common denominator. Proteinuria is the clinical presentation.

Nonsclerosing Podocytopathies: Minimal Change Disease

Clinical Features
- Nephrotic syndrome, generally of sudden onset, with significant proteinuria
- Age of incidence varies from children to elderly patients, depending on etiology/pathogenesis, although most common in young children (boys more often than girls)
- Can present with acute renal failure in elderly or adults if secondary to use of certain nephrotoxic medications
- Hematuria in < 30% of cases

Histopathology
- Normal histology, by definition

Special Stains
- Periodic acid-Schiff (PAS) stain: normal cellularity and normal mesangial expansion
- Trichrome stain: no increase of mesangial matrix and a general absence of interstitial fibrosis and tubular atrophy
- Silver stain: normal thickness and contour of the glomerular basement membranes

Direct Immunofluorescence
- Generally negative

Electron Microscopy
- Extensive foot process effacement, although in partially treated forms focal effacement can be present (Figure 10-47)
- Extensive microvillus transformation with or without condensation of the actin-based cytoskeleton
- Generally normal glomerular basement membranes
- No deposits

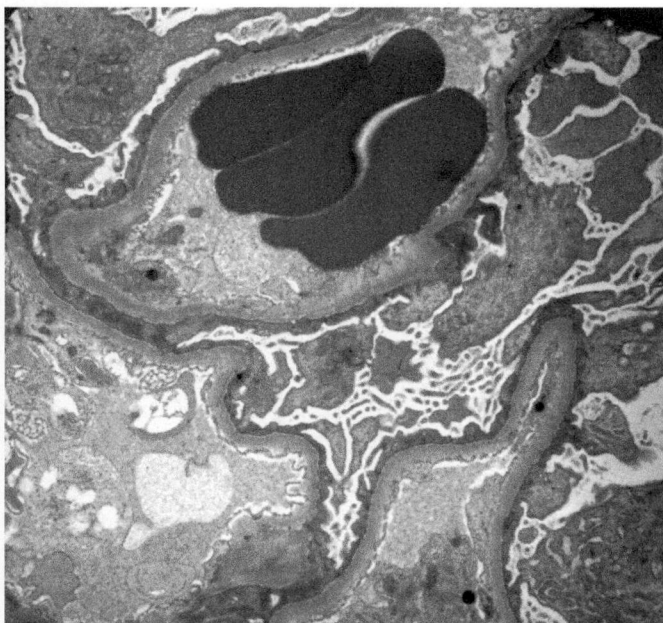

Figure 10-47. Minimal change disease. Podocytes foot processes are diffusely effaced. Microvillus transformation is also noted. The glomerular basement membranes are normal in thickness and contour (electron microscopy).

Differential Diagnosis

- Unsampled focal segmental glomerulosclerosis

PEARLS

- *Ultrastructural analysis is the key to demonstrate effacement*
- *Sectioning of the paraffin block is mandatory to avoid missing segmentally sclerotic lesions*
- *Foci of interstitial fibrosis and tubular atrophy are suspicious for an unsampled focal segmental glomerulosclerosis*
- *Once the diagnosis of minimal change disease is established, the differential diagnosis includes idiopathic versus other secondary causes and steroid sensitive versus steroid resistant forms*

SELECTED REFERENCES

Barisoni L, Schnaper HW, Kopp JB: Advances in the biology and genetics of the podocytopathies: implications for diagnosis and therapy. Arch Pathol Lab Med 133:201-216, 2009.

Oh J, Kemper MJ: Minimal change (steroid sensitive) nephrotic syndrome in children: new aspects on pathogenesis and treatment. Minerva Pediatr 64:197-204, 2012.

Sclerosing Lesions: Focal Segmental Glomerulosclerosis (FSGS) and Collapsing Glomerulopathy

Clinical Features

- Proteinuria, subnephrotic, nephrotic range or nephrotic syndrome, often sudden onset
- Most common cause of nephrotic syndrome in adults
- Azotemia

Etiology, Pathogenesis, and Classification

- Idiopathic
- Associated with monogenetic disorders (syndromic and nonsyndromic) or predisposing genetic background
- Secondary to immunologic and hematologic disorders, use of certain medications, environmental factors (i.e., viral infections [HIV]), circulating factors
- According to the Columbia classification, there are five variants: tip lesions, perihilar, not otherwise specified, cellular, and collapsing lesions

Histopathology

- FSGS with perihilar involvement (perihilar variant): segmental solidification of the tuft is at the hilum and may be accompanied by hyalinosis or foam cells
- FSGS with solidification of the tuft in nonspecified portion of the glomerulus (not otherwise specified variant): the segmental sclerosis may be accompanied by hyalinosis or foam cells
- FSGS with solidification of the tuft at the tip portion of the glomerulus (tip lesion variant): the segmental sclerosis may be accompanied by hyalinosis or foam cells and bridging of podocytes toward epithelial cells where the Bowman's capsule becomes proximal tubule (Figure 10-48A)
- Proliferative sclerosis lesions with podocytes, mesangial cells, and endothelial cell hypertrophy and hyperplasia (cellular variant); segmental or global collapse of the glomerular basement membranes accompanied by hypertrophy or hyperplasia of overlying podocytes (collapsing glomerulopathy or collapsing variant)
- Focal interstitial fibrosis and tubular atrophy may be present
- Interstitial inflammation can be present, generally more evident in cellular and collapsing forms

Special Stains

- PAS stain: shows segmental solidification of the tuft in sclerosing forms and reveals the location of the increased cellularity (cellular lesions: endocapillary and podocytes; collapsing glomerulopathy: podocytes) (Figure 10-48B)
- Trichrome stain: increase of mesangial matrix in the areas of sclerosis and in the areas of interstitial fibrosis
- Silver stain: normal thickness and contour of the glomerular basement membranes

Direct Immunofluorescence

- Generally negative

Electron Microscopy

- Variable amount of foot process effacement, with microvillous transformation and condensation of the actin-based cytoskeleton at the sole of podocytes
- Focal to extensive wrinkling of the glomerular basement membranes
- Tubuloreticular inclusions can be present in HIV-associated forms

Differential Diagnosis

- Glomerulonephritis with sclerosing lesions (i.e., IgA nephropathy with segmental sclerosis or healed/scarred necrotizing glomerulonephritis)

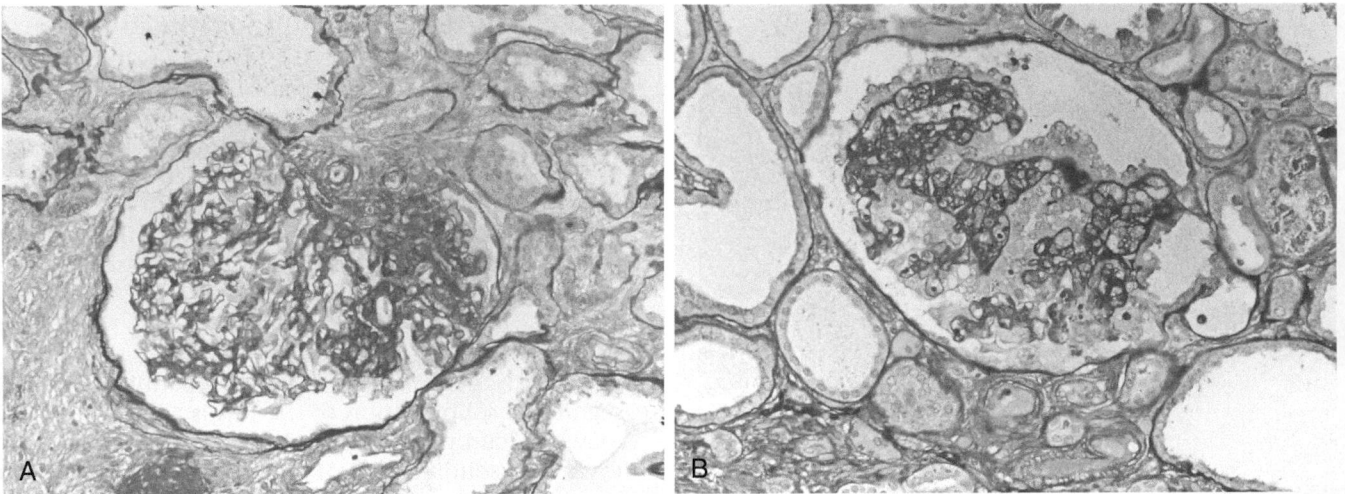

Figure 10-48. A, Focal segmental glomerulosclerosis. There is segmental solidification at the glomerular tuft with adhesion of the tuft to the Bowman's capsule (3 o'clock). Podocytes appear hypertrophic. The remaining portion of the glomerulus is unremarkable with glomerular membranes normal in thickness and contour and normally expanded mesangium (PAS × 40). **B,** Collapsing glomerulopathy. There is global wrinkling and folding of the glomerulus membrane with occlusion or subocclusion of the capillary lumina. Podocytes are markedly hypertrophic and hyperplastic, forming pseudocrescents, and containing protein reabsorption droplets (PAS positive). The urinary space appears enlarged (PAS × 40).

- Minimal change disease with incomplete effacement
- Focal global glomerulosclerosis where the segmental sclerosis is not sampled

PEARLS

- *Adequate sampling is essential*
- *Sectioning of the paraffin block is sometimes necessary to find the diagnostic lesion*

SELECTED REFERENCES

Barisoni L, Schnaper HW, Kopp JB: A proposed taxonomy for the podocytopathies: a reassessment of the primary nephrotic diseases. Clin J Am Soc Nephrol 2:529-542, 2007.

D'Agati VD, Alster JM, Jennette JC, et al: Association of histologic variants in FSGS clinical trial with presenting features and outcomes. Clin J Am Soc Nephrol 8:399-406, 2013.

COLLAGENOPATHIES

- Group of glomerulopathies characterized by altered morphology of the glomerular basement membranes, mesangium, or both
- A subset of collagenopathies represent genetically determined disorders that can affect collagen type IV (more commonly) or type III

Disorders of Collagen Type IV (Alport Disease, Thin Basement Membranes, and Benign Familiar Hematuria)

Clinical Features

- Hematuria, isolated (benign familiar hematuria and thin basement membranes disease)
- Hematuria is often followed by proteinuria and in some cases by increased serum creatinine (Alport disease and some cases of thin basement membranes disease)
- About 90% of X-liked males reach end-stage renal disease by the age of 40
- If Alport disease (X-linked) sensorineural deafness and ocular abnormalities are frequently detected
- Leiomyomatosis (rare)
- Age of incidence varies from children to elderly patients, depending on the type of mutations

Etiology, Pathogenesis, and Classification

- Mutations of the genes encoding for collagen type IV alpha 3, 4, or 5, leading to abnormal representation and configuration of the alpha chains in the basement membranes
- Three forms of collagen type disorders: benign familiar hematuria (never progresses and is characterized by hematuria alone), thin basement membranes disease (although generally with a benign course on occasion can mimic autosomal recessive Alport disease), and Alport disease
- About 85% of X-linked Alport disease cases are due to mutation of COL4A5
- About 15% of autosomal recessive or dominant Alport disease is due to mutations of COL4A3/4

Histopathology

- Normal histology in benign familiar hematuria, most of thin basement membranes disease and early phases of Alport disease
- Late phases of Alport disease: irregular thickness of the glomerular basement membranes and segmental solidification of the tuft (FSGS) with or without hyalinosis or foam cells
- Interstitial fibrosis and tubular atrophy
- Interstitial foam cells can be seen in Alport disease
- Arteriosclerosis and arteriolar hyalinosis can be present, especially in advanced forms

Special Stains

- PAS: normal cellularity
- Trichrome: increase of mesangial matrix in the areas of sclerosis and in the areas of interstitial fibrosis

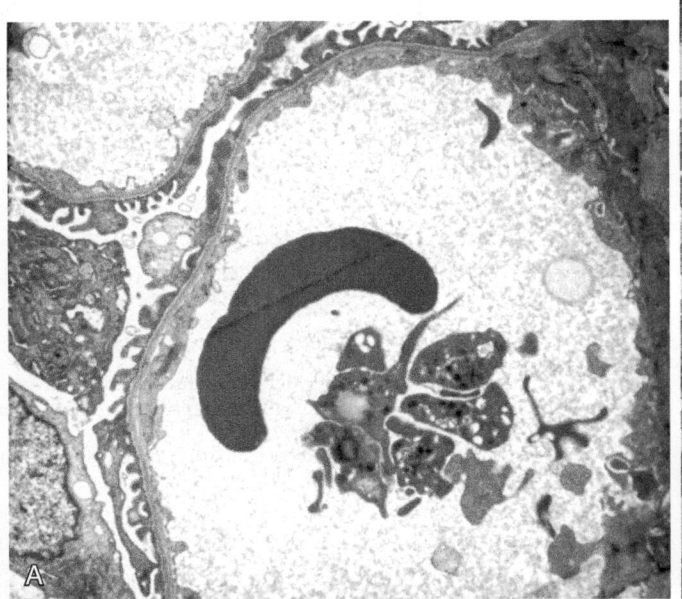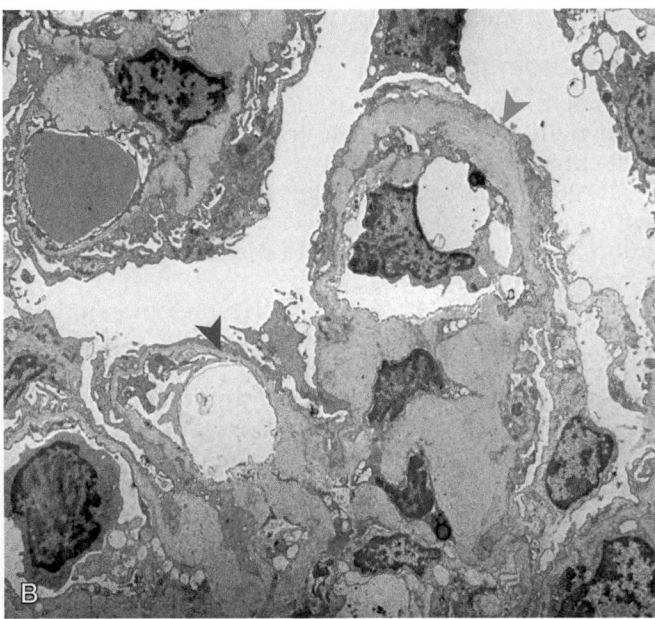

Figure 10-49. A, Thin base membrane disease. The glomerular membrane appears diffusely thinner than normal, measuring less than 200 nm (electron microscopy). **B,** Alport disease. The glomerular basement membranes are focally thin (red arrowhead) or markedly thickened (green arrowhead). The glomerular membranes are also irregular in texture, revealing extensive lamellation, with a basket-weave appearance. Podocytes are injured with extensive effacement (electron microscopy).

- Silver stain: irregular thickness of the glomerular basement membranes with diffuse thinning in benign familiar hematuria and thin basement membranes disease, to alternating thick and thin segments of the glomerular basement membranes in Alport disease

Direct Immunofluorescence

- Generally negative

Electron Microscopy

- Variable foot process effacement
- Glomerular basement membranes are thinner than normal (< 200 nm in thickness) in benign familiar hematuria and thin basement membranes disease (Figure 10-49A)
- In Alport disease, the glomerular basement membranes reveal irregular thickness with occasional breaks, and texture with electron-dense curvilinear particles alternating with electron lucent areas (basket-weave appearance); multilamellation and scalloping (Figure 10-49B)

Differential Diagnosis

- Other forms of focal segmental glomerulosclerosis
- Nail-Patella syndrome and type III collagen glomerulopathy
- Lamellation of the basement membranes can be seen in other diseases with remodeling of the glomerular basement membranes

PEARLS

- *Ultrastructural analysis is key to demonstrating abnormal glomerular basement membranes*
- *Interstitial foam cells are suspicious for Alport disease in a setting of hematuria and proteinuria*

SELECTED REFERENCES

Bekheirnia MR, Reed B, Gregory MC, et al: Genotype-phenotype correlation in X-linked Alport syndrome. J Am Soc Nephrol 21:876-883, 2010.

Heidet L, Gubler MC: The renal lesions of Alport syndrome. J Am Soc Nephrol 20:1210-1215, 2009.

ENDOTHELIOPATHIES

Thrombotic Microangiopathies (TMA)

Clinical Features

- Patients can present with nonspecific symptoms but also with fever, hypertension, mild proteinuria, microscopic hematuria, and renal failure
- Anemia, thrombocytopenia, peripheral smear schistocytes, and leukocytosis can also be detected in some of the thrombotic microangiopathic disorders
- Clinical and laboratory studies are necessary to determine etiology of the thrombotic microangiopathy changes

Etiology, Pathogenesis, and Classification

- *Thrombotic microangiopathy* is a descriptive term and indicates a variety of disorders characterized by endothelial cell injury and thrombosis, including the following:
  - Hemolytic uremic syndrome: typical (secondary to enterotoxin) and atypical (multifactorial)
  - Thrombotic thrombocytopenic purpura: secondary to deficiency of ADAMTS13, a zinc metalloprotease synthesized in the liver necessary for cleavage of vWF multimers; the deficiency is either due to genetic defect or acquired or due to the presence of autoantibodies against ADAMTS13
  - Malignant hypertension
  - Scleroderma renal crisis
  - Iatrogenic

• Autoimmune: antiphospholipid antibodies mediated

Histopathology

• Thrombotic microangiopathic changes can present with acute features, chronic features, or mixed acute and chronic
• Acute glomerular lesions include intracapillary thrombi with fragmented red blood cells, occasional margination of inflammatory cells, and thickening of the capillary walls (Figure 10-50)
• Chronic glomerular lesions have membranoproliferative features with double contours; mesangial and global sclerosis can be present
• Small arteries and arterioles show intima mucoid edema, intracapillary thrombi in the absence of significant inflammation, fragmented red blood cells in the vascular wall, and fibrinoid necrosis; chronic changes consist of onion skin appearance of vessels in malignant hypertension mediated forms, intimal fibrosis and hypertrophy with narrowing of vascular lumina, recanalization of thrombi
• The tubule-interstitium has features of acute injury in the acute phase or interstitial fibrosis and tubular atrophy in more chronic stages of the disease

Special Stains

• Silver stain: highlights the double contours (tram-track) in chronic TMA
• Elastin stain: highlights the extreme duplication of elastic lamina in malignant hypertension mediated forms
• Trichrome: highlights the intravascular thrombi and the fibrinoid necrosis

Direct Immunofluorescence

• Nonspecific positive stain for IgM, or sometimes IgG, and complement in the subendothelium
• Fibrinogen is positive in thrombi

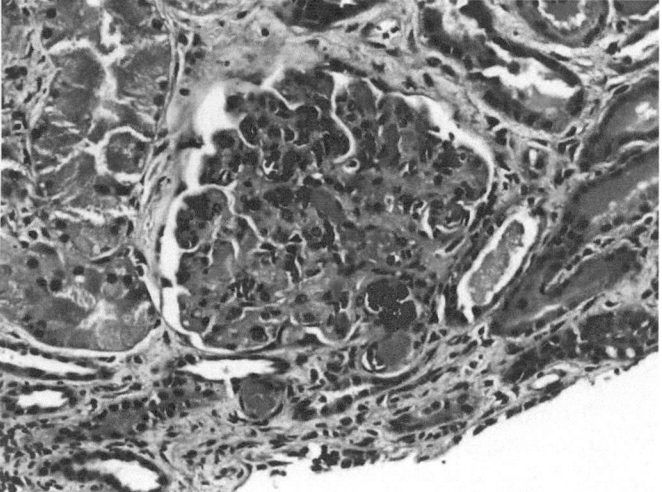

Figure 10-50. Thrombotic microangiopathy. The glomerulus appear mildly congested and containing numerous fibrin thrombi (pink on hematoxylin and eosin [H&E] stain). Marginating neutrophils are also seen. Thrombi can also be appreciated at the vascular pole of the glomerulus and in the afferent arteriolar lumen (H&E × 40).

Differential Diagnosis

• Membranoproliferative glomerulonephritis
• Once the presence of TMA has been determined, the differential diagnosis is between the various forms of TMA

PEARLS

• *TMA is a descriptive diagnosis; etiology needs to be clinically investigated*

SELECTED REFERENCES

Barbour T, Johnson S, Cohney S, Hughes P: Thrombotic microangiopathy and associated renal disorders. Nephrol Dial Transplant 27:2673-2685, 2012.
Benz K, Amann K: Thrombotic microangiopathy: new insights. Curr Opin Nephrol Hypertens 19:242-247, 2010.

ANTIBODY-MEDIATED DISEASES

Antibody-mediated disorders include a category of diseases manifesting as crescentic necrotizing glomerulonephritis. These diseases, also known in the past as rapidly progressive glomerulonephritis, have many histologic similarities and are mediated by circulating antibodies (against neutrophil components or the glomerular basement membranes collagen type IV alpha 3 chain).

Antineutrophil Cytoplasmic Antibody [ANCA]–Mediated Small Vessel Vasculitis

Clinical Features

• Rapid progressive renal failure with hematuria and proteinuria
• Sign of systemic vasculitis
• Skin involvement
• Serology positive for ANCA

Etiology, Pathogenesis, and Classification

• Auto-antibodies to neutrophil lysosomal components: MPO (p-ANCA) and PR3 (c-ANCA)
• ANCA activate neutrophils, which injure endothelium
• Granulomatosis with polyangiitis (75% PRs-ANCA+); microscopic polyangiitis (50% MPO-ANCA+); Churg Straus syndrome (60% MPO-ANCA+); renal limited crescentic glomerulonephritis (60% MPO-ANCA+)

Histopathology (Figure 10-51)

• Focal necrotizing glomerulonephritis with cellular crescents; cellular crescents contain proliferating of parietal epithelial cells, podocytes, inflammatory cells, and fibrin and occupy, obliterating, the urinary space, with a segmental or global distribution
• Segmental glomerular scars with fibrocellular and fibrous crescents in healed phases, containing progressively more fibroblasts and fibrosis compared to cellular crescents (chronic evolution of cellular crescents)
• Extraglomerular vascular involvement in the kidney in up to 35% of cases: leukocytoclastic vasculitis with endotheliitis to transmural arteritis and fibrinoid necrosis
• Often accompanied by interstitial inflammation

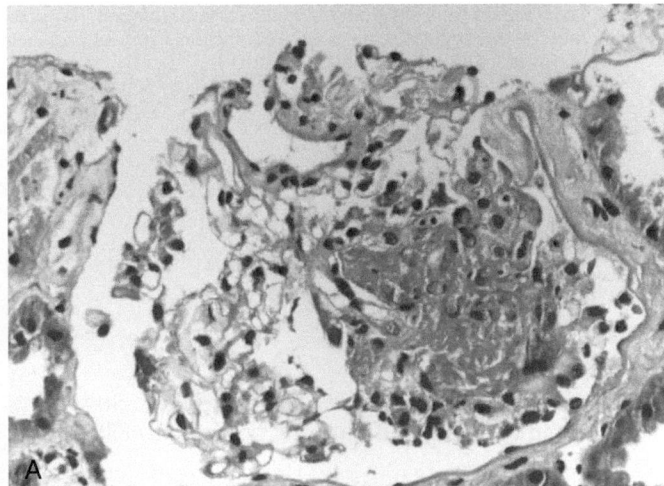

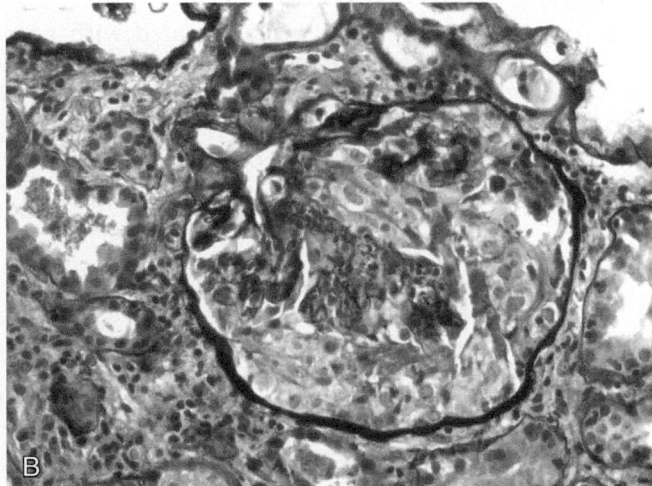

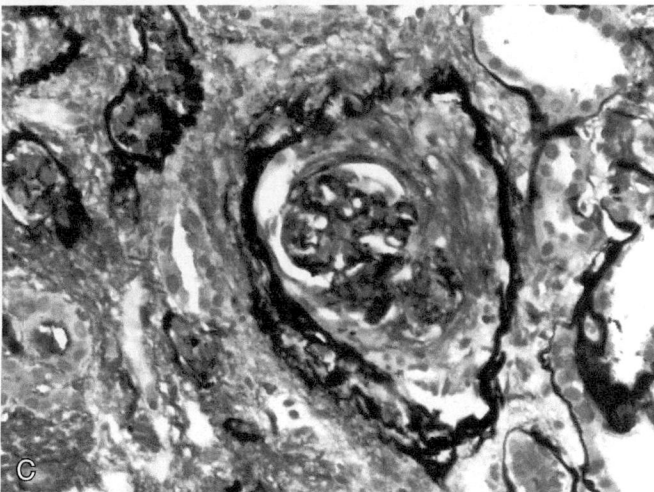

Figure 10-51. A, ANCA-mediated glomerulonephritis. Segmental area of fibrinoid necrosis of the tuft accompanied by marked podocytes hypertrophy and occasional marginating inflammatory cells (H&E × 60). **B,** ANCA-mediated glomerulonephritis. The urinary space is occupied by a cellular crescent containing epithelial cells, inflammatory cells, and fibrin. The glomerular tuft is compressed with occluded or sub-occluded capillaries. Marginating inflammatory cells are also noted (silver stain × 40). **C,** ANCA-mediated glomerulonephritis. Fibrocellular crescent. The glomerular tuft is compressed, and the urinary space is occupied by collagen and occasional fibroblasts and epithelial cells (H&E × 20).

- Interstitial granulomas are present in granulomatosis with polyangiitis form
- Acute tubular injury can be present in aggressive forms with red blood cells and fibrin in tubular lumina

Special Stains

- Trichrome stain highlights fibrin (red) in necrotizing lesions
- Elastin stain reveals rupture of the elastic lamina
- Silver shows rupture of Bowman's capsule in the areas of cellular crescents and disruption of the glomerular basement membranes in the areas of fibrinoid necrosis

Direct Immunofluorescence

- Negative

Other Techniques for Diagnosis

- Serology for ANCA

Differential Diagnosis

- Antiglomerular basement membrane disease
- IgA nephropathy with crescents: Henoch-Schönlein purpura
- Acute postinfectious glomerulonephritis

PEARLS

- *If suspected, multiple sections should be obtained to search for very focal lesions*
- *Nonaffected glomeruli are histologically unremarkable*

Selected References

Ford SL, Polkinghorne KR, Longano A, et al: Histopathologic and clinical predictors of kidney outcomes in ANCA-associated vasculitis. Am J Kidney Dis 63:227-235, 2014.
Jennette JC, Falk RJ, Bacon PA, et al: 2012 revised International Chapel Hill Consensus Conference nomenclature of vasculitides. Arthritis Rheum 65:1-11, 2013.

Anti-Glomerular Basement Membrane (GBM) Disease

Clinical Features

- About 1 in 1 million/year in the United States
- Peaks in second and sixth decades (young males and older females)
- Acute renal failure with hematuria and proteinuria
- Active sediment
- Pulmonary hemorrhage

Etiology, Pathogenesis, and Classification

- Autoantibodies against noncollagenous-1 domain of α-3 chain of collagen type IV (Goodpasture antigen)
- Strong association with HLA-DR and DQ antigens
- Anti-GBM disease can occur simultaneously with ANCA-mediated small vessel vasculitis
- Anti-GBM disease has been described to occur in some cases with membranous glomerulopathy

Histopathology

- Focal necrotizing glomerulonephritis with cellular crescents generally involving all glomeruli
- Segmental glomerular scars with fibrocellular and fibrous crescents in healed phases

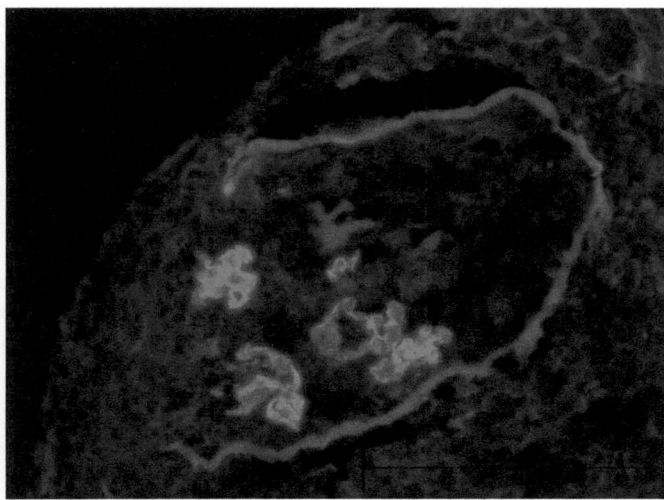

Figure 10-52. Anti-GBM disease. IgG is strongly positive with a linear pattern in the glomerular membrane and with less intensity in the Bowman's capsule (IgG × 40).

- Often accompanied by interstitial inflammation
- Acute tubular injury can be present in aggressive forms

Special Stains

- Trichrome stain highlights fibrin (red) in necrotizing lesions
- Silver shows rupture of Bowman's capsule in the areas of cellular crescents and disruption of the glomerular basement membranes in the areas of fibrinoid necrosis

Direct Immunofluorescence

- Linear positive stain in glomerular basement membranes for IgG (Figure 10-52)

Other Techniques for Diagnosis

- Indirect immunofluorescence on normal kidney incubated with the patient's serum

Differential Diagnosis

- ANCA-mediated crescentic and necrotizing glomerulonephritis
- IgA nephropathy with crescents: Henoch-Schönlein purpura
- Acute postinfectious glomerulonephritis
- Monoclonal immunoglobulin deposition disease

PEARLS

- *Most of the glomeruli are involved at the same time*
- *The rare nonaffected glomeruli are histologically unremarkable*
- *It can be superimposed on other diseases*

SELECTED REFERENCES

Srivastava A, Rao GK, Segal PE, et al: Characteristics and outcome of crescentic glomerulonephritis in patients with both antineutrophil cytoplasmic antibody and anti-glomerular basement membrane antibody. Clin Rheumatol 32:1317-1322, 2013.

Tang W, McDonald SP, Hawley CM, et al: Anti-glomerular basement membrane antibody disease is an uncommon cause of end-stage renal disease. Kidney Int 83:503-510, 2013.

IMMUNE-COMPLEX MEDIATED GLOMERULOPATHIES AND GLOMERULONEPHRITIS

Membranous Glomerulopathy

Clinical Features

- Nephrotic syndrome
- Affects generally adults with peak age 30 to 50 years
- Approximately 30% of patients progress to ESRD

Etiology, Pathogenesis, and Classification

- Primary: idiopathic forms are associated with autoantibodies to Phospholipase A2 receptors (in podocytes); congenital forms are associated with MMF antibodies
- Secondary: infections (hepatitis B, hepatitis C, syphilis)
- Autoimmune diseases (lupus, rheumatoid arthritis, thyroiditis), neoplastic processes, graph versus host disease

Histopathology

- Normal glomeruli (in early phases) to diffuse thickening of the glomerular basement membranes
- Mesangial expansion and proliferation may be present especially in secondary forms
- Glomerulitis associated with malignancy

Special Stains

- Silver stain shows spikes, holes or both according to the stage of the diseases (Figure 10-53A)
- Direct immunofluorescence
- IgG, C3, and kappa and lambda light chains are positive with a granular pattern in the glomerular basement membranes (Figure 10-53B)
- IgG4 (and to lesser degree IgG1) is positive in primary forms
- IgG1 and IgG2 are more frequently associated with secondary forms to neoplasia
- Tubular basement deposits can be present in secondary forms

Electron Microscopy

- Subepithelial electron-dense deposits (Figure 10-53C)
- The deposits may be situated between the extracellular matrix and the sole of podocytes (stage I); extracellular matrix can be present in between deposits (stage II); extracellular matrix can be in between and surrounding the deposits (stage III); electron lucent areas in areas previously containing electron-dense deposits (stage IV)
- Mesangial deposits can be present in secondary forms
- Extensive foot process effacement
- Tubular basement deposits can be present in secondary forms

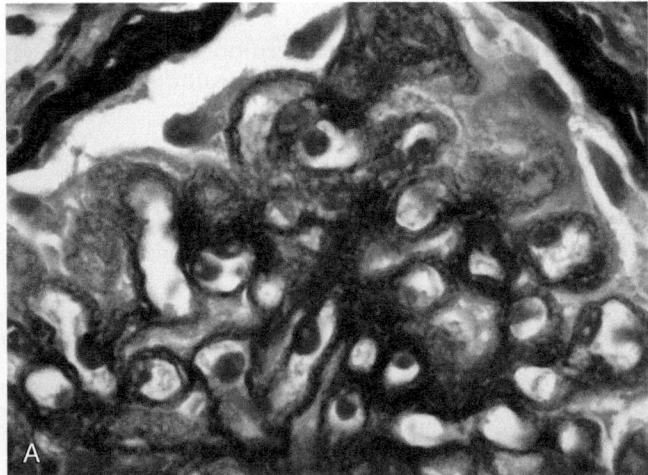

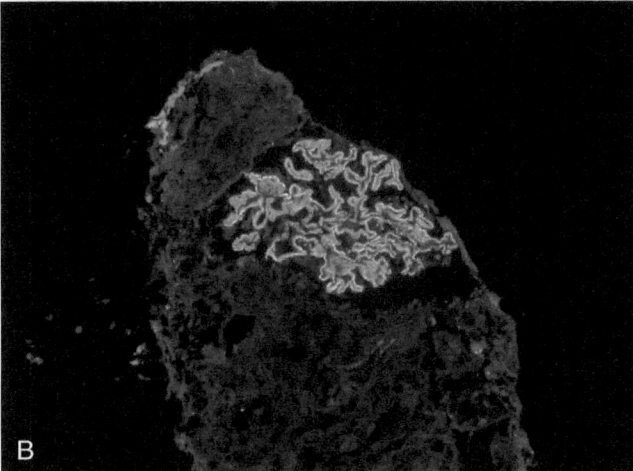

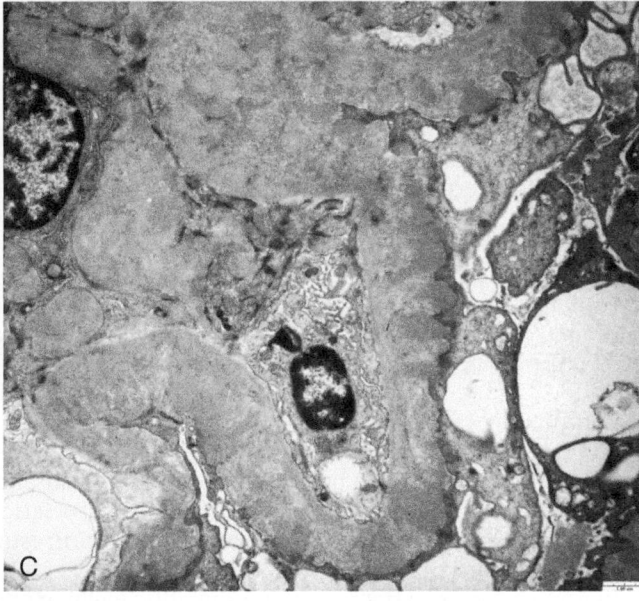

Figure 10-53. A, Membranous glomerulopathy. The glomerular membranes are diffusely thickened and irregular in texture and contour. Holes and pikes can be appreciated by silver stain. Podocytes are hypertrophic (silver stain × 100 oil). **B,** Membranous glomerulopathy. C3 is strongly positive in the glomerular basement membranes with a granular global pattern (C3 × 40). A similar pattern is seen with IgG, kappa, and lambda. **C,** Membranous glomerulopathy. Electron-dense deposits are present in the subepithelium. There is extracellular matrix interposition in between the deposits (spikes) (electron microscopy).

Other Techniques for Diagnosis

- Serology for phospholipase A2 receptors for primary forms
- Immunostaining for phospholipase A2 receptors is positive with a granular pattern in the glomerular basement membranes for primary forms associated with the autoantibodies

Differential Diagnosis

- Postinfectious glomerulonephritis
- Mediated membranoproliferative glomerulonephritis (MPGN) type III

PEARLS

- *Membranous glomerulopathy can occur with ANCA-mediated disease, anti-GBM disease, and other system disorders such as diabetes*

Selected References

Huang CC, Lehman A, Albawardi A, et al: Anti-neutral endopeptidase, natriuretic peptides disarrangement, and proteinuria onset in membranous nephropathy. Mod Pathol 26:799-805, 2013.
Larsen CP, Messias NC, Silva FG, et al: Determination of primary versus secondary membranous glomerulopathy utilizing phospholipase A2 receptor staining in renal biopsies. Mod Pathol 26:709-715, 2013.

Infection-Mediated Disease

Clinical Features

- Hypertension
- Oliguria, hematuria, proteinuria
- Hypocomplementemia
- Nephritis syndrome
- Can be associated with diabetes and neoplasia
- More frequent in males with bimodal peak (<6 and >40 years)

Etiology, Pathogenesis, and Classification

- Bacterial: poststreptococcal, nonstreptococcal, methicillin-resistant staphylococcus aureus
- Viral, rickettsia, fungi, parasites

Histopathology

- Mesangiopathic glomerulonephritis to membranoproliferative glomerulonephritis
- Crescents and necrosis can be occasionally seen
- Marginating neutrophils in glomerular capillaries (exudative glomerulonephritis)(Figure 10-54A)

Special Stains

- Humps, if large enough, can be seen by trichrome stain (red)

Direct Immunofluorescence

- IgG and C3 with a granular pattern in glomerular basement membranes and mesangium (Figure 10-54B)
- IgA and C3 in methicillin resistant staphylococcus aureus

Electron Microscopy

- Subepithelial humps (Figure 10-54C)
- Mesangial electron-dense deposits

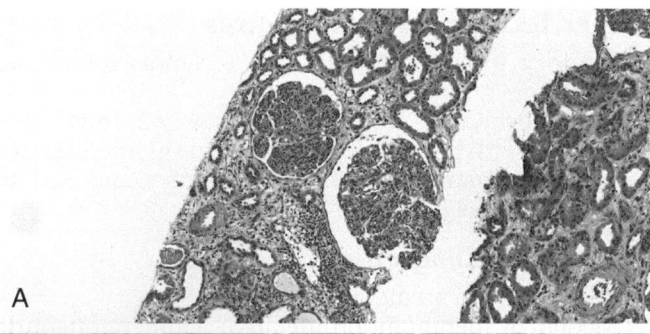
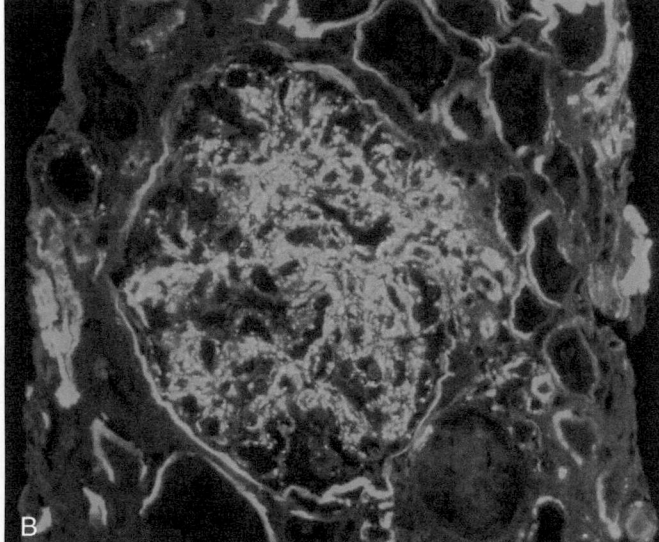
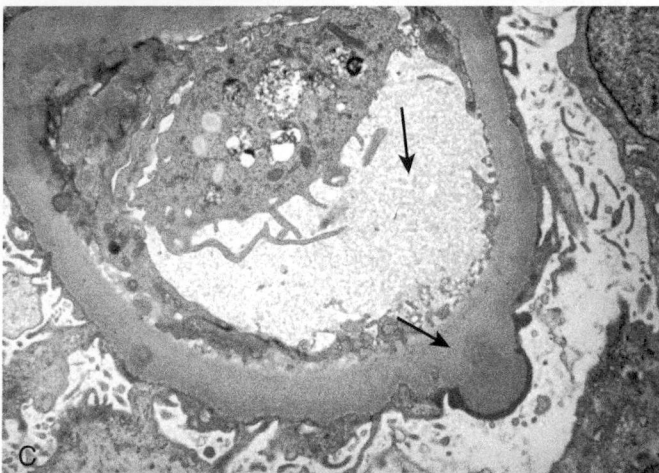

Figure 10-54. A, Postinfectious glomerulonephritis light microscopy. Two glomeruli with hypercellularity and lobulation of the tuft. Inflammatory cells are present (H&E × 20). **B,** Postinfectious glomerulonephritis (C3). Global granular staining in mesangium and glomerulus membrane (C3 × 40). **C,** Postinfectious glomerulonephritis. Typical subepithelial humps can be appreciated in postinfectious glomerulonephritis. Podocytes overlying humps reveal foot process effacement with condensation of the actin-based cytoskeleton (electron microscopy).

- Intramembranous and subendothelial electron-dense deposits
- Foot process effacement especially in areas over the humps
- Loss of fenestration and swelling of endothelial cells

Differential Diagnosis

- Membranoproliferative glomerulonephritis
- C3 glomerulopathy and C3 glomerulonephritis
- Cryoglobulinemic glomerulonephritis

PEARLS

- *Percentage of crescents increases the risk of ESRD*

SELECTED REFERENCES

Wen YK, Chen ML: The significance of atypical morphology in the changes of spectrum of postinfectious glomerulonephritis. Clin Nephrol 73:173-179, 2010.
Zeledon JI, McKelvey RL, Servilla KS, et al: Glomerulonephritis causing acute renal failure during the course of bacterial infections: histological varieties, potential pathogenetic pathways and treatment. Int Urol Nephrol 40:461-470, 2008.

IgA-Related Nephropathies
Clinical Features

- Most common glomerular disease worldwide
- Common in Asian population and rare in blacks
- It could be asymptomatic with hematuria or proteinuria; in > 80% of patients there is microhematuria with macrohematuria in approximately 40%; proteinuria varies from non-nephrotic to fully nephrotic in approximately 10% of patients
- Nephritic syndrome
- A small group of patients can also have acute renal failure or thrombotic microangiopathic changes
- Complement levels are normal
- Recurrence in transplant is approximately 30%

Etiology, Pathogenesis, and Classification

- Abnormal glycosylation of IgA1
- Increased activity of response with IgA production
- Genetic factors are involved in the pathogenesis (HLA-DQ); family history of nephritis can occur in approximately 10% of families and up to 50% in certain areas (Northern Italy and Eastern Kentucky)

Histopathology

- Highly variable from normal glomeruli by light microscopy to mesangial proliferation (if more than three mesangial cells per mesangial lobule), which could be focal or diffuse, and segmental or global (Figure 10-55A)
- Endocapillary proliferation with margination of inflammatory cells and endothelial cell swelling is also a feature in a portion of cases
- Segmental sclerosis can be present either in the absence of other features, resembling FSGS, or in association with endocapillary or extracapillary proliferation (suggesting a scar)
- In some patients, extracapillary proliferation (cellular crescents) and necrotizing lesions can be present; if in these cases there is positive stain for IgA in the mesangium in the absence of endocapillary features involving a large number of glomeruli, serology for ANCA is warranted to rule out a superimposed ANCA-mediated vasculitis
- Generally red blood cells can be appreciated in tubular lumina
- Variable interstitial fibrosis and tubular atrophy

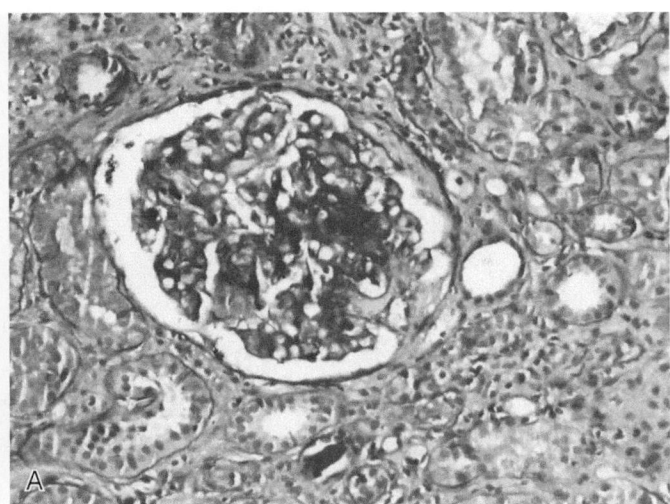
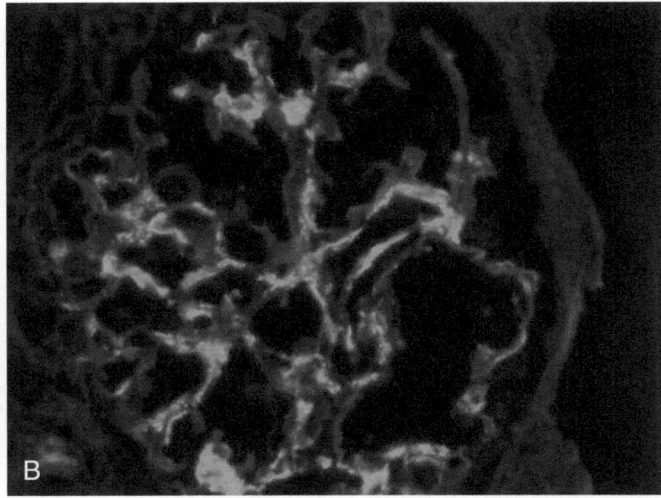

Figure 10-55. A, IgA nephropathy. Segmental mesangial expansion with mesangial cell hypercellularity. The glomerular basement membranes are normal in thickness and contour (PAS × 40). **B,** IgA nephropathy. Immunofluorescence stain for IgA is strongly positive in the mesangium (IgA × 40).

Special Stains

- PAS is helpful to evaluate mesangial hypercellularity

Direct Immunofluorescence

- Although other immunoglobulins can be weakly positive, IgA is always predominant with kappa and lambda light chains (lambda generally slightly stronger than kappa) and C3; C1q is positive in approximately 10% of cases (Figure 10-55B)
- The pattern of distribution is generally mesangial but a peripheral capillary positive stain can also be present, especially in the presence of endocapillary proliferation

Electron Microscopy

- Mesangial and paramesangial deposits are present in all cases, on occasion accompanied by subendothelial deposits, subepithelial deposits, intramembranous or resembling humps
- In approximately 40% of cases, diffuse or focal thinning of the glomerular basement membranes is present
- Foot process effacement generally correlates with the severity of proteinuria and is variable from case to case

Differential Diagnosis

- Henoch-Schönlein purpura, although some authors consider IgA nephropathy a renal limited form of HPS
- ANCA-associated vasculitis, in the absence of significant mesangial proliferation but if crescents and necrosis are present
- IgA-postinfectious glomerulonephritis, especially if humps are present on electron microscopy
- FSGS can resemble IgA nephropathy, but immunofluorescence and electron microscopy demonstrate mesangial deposits

PEARLS

- *Because of the high variability of morphologic glomerular damage, immunofluorescence is critical for the diagnosis*
- *According to the recent Oxford classification, the amount of interstitial fibrosis and tubular atrophy, as well as the presence of mesangial and endocapillary proliferation, determine the prognosis*

SELECTED REFERENCES

Bellur SS, Troyanov S, Cook HT, Roberts IS; Working Group of International IgA Nephropathy Network and Renal Pathology Society: Immunostaining findings in IgA nephropathy: correlation with histology and clinical outcome in the Oxford classification patient cohort. Nephrol Dial Transplant 26:2533-2536, 2011.

Wang H, Weening JJ, Yoshikawa N, Zhang H: The Oxford classification of IgA nephropathy: pathology definitions, correlations, and reproducibility. Kidney Int 76:546-556, 2009.

COMPLEMENT-MEDIATED GLOMERULONEPHRITIS AND IMMUNE-COMPLEX MEDIATED MEMBRANOPROLIFERATIVE GLOMERULONEPHRITIS (MPGN)

- The classification of MPGN has been revisited; a new classification system based on immunofluorescence findings divides the MPGN into immune-complex mediated forms (with Ig and C3 positive) and complement mediated forms (C3 only), independent of morphologic pattern by light microscopy

Immune-Complex Mediated MPGN (Type I and Type III)

Clinical Features

- More frequent in children, adolescents, and young adults
- The presentation is nephritic syndrome as well as nephrotic syndrome
- Hypocomplementemia
- May be triggered by an infection

Etiology, Pathogenesis, and Classification

- Idiopathic
- Secondary to hepatitis C

Histopathology

- Type I MPGN is characterized by lobulation of the tuft with endocapillary proliferation; double contours are always present and formed by interposition of mesangial cell cytoplasm and deposits; crescents, segmental or circumferential, can be present in approximately 20% of cases

- Type III MPGN—Burkholder—has features recapitulating both MPGN pattern as well as membranous pattern, with lobulation (mesangial proliferation and insudation); diffuse thickening of the capillary walls
- Type III MPGN—Anders and Strife—has features of both MPGN type I and C3 glomerulopathy, dense deposit disease; irregular thickening of capillary walls, less proliferation and lobulation of the tuft

Special Stains

- Silver and PAS show highlight the lobulation of the glomerular tuft and the double contours (tram track) (Figure 10-56A)
- In type III MPGN—Anders and Strife—silver stain shows negative areas in the glomerular basement membranes, with "moth-eaten" appearance and irregular thickening

Direct Immunofluorescence

- IgG and C3 are positive in the mesangium and in the capillary walls (lumpy-bumpy); IgM, IgA, and C1q can also be present
- The subendothelial deposits in type I often have a comma shape appearance, lining the inner surface of the glomerular basement membranes on one side and the endothelial cells or newly formed second layer of basement membrane on the other; MPGN type III has similar findings but often a more granular appearance in the basement membranes
- Focal positive staining can also be present in tubular basement membranes

Electron Microscopy

- Type I MPGN appearance is characterized by extensive proliferation and double contours formed by interposition of mesangial cell cytoplasm, electron-dense deposits, and inflammatory cells on occasion; electron-dense deposits can have a curvilinear, "sausage-string," appearance and be accompanied by occasional subepithelial as well as mesangial deposits
- Type III MPGN—Burkholder—shows an association with the previous findings, numerous subepithelial granular deposits
- Type III MPGN—Anders and Strife—has also numerous intramembranous and subepithelial deposits, or transmembrane deposits with disruption of the basement membranes (Figure 10-56B)

Differential Diagnosis

- Lupus nephritis class IV
- Postinfectious glomerulonephritis
- Mixed cryoglobulinemia
- Light chain deposition disease
- Chronic thrombotic microangiopathy

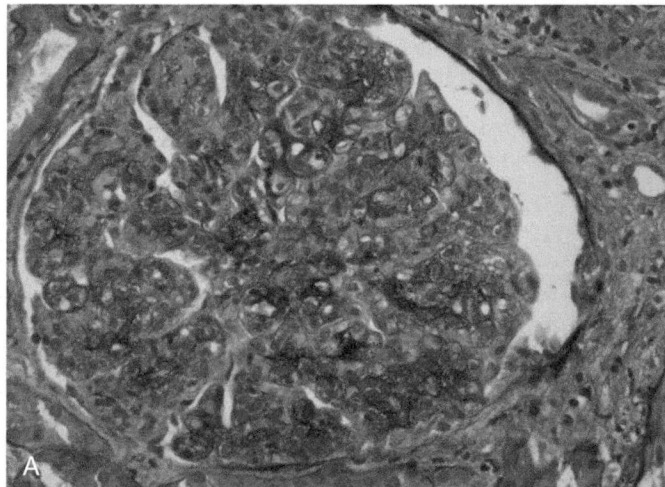

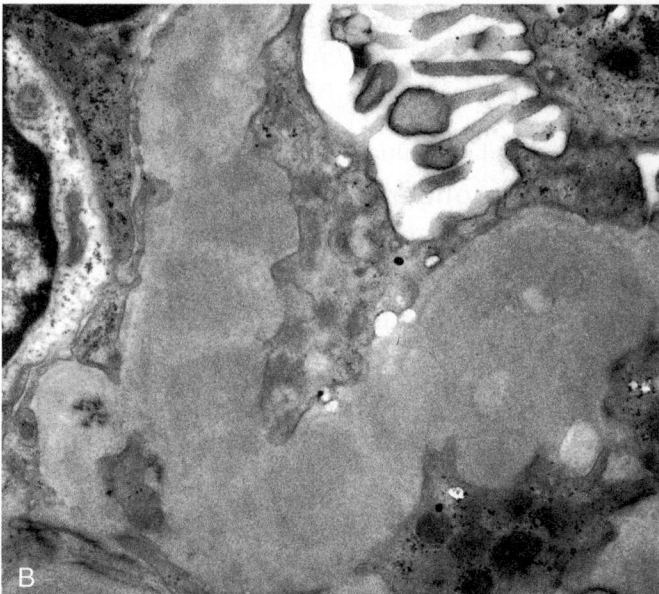

Figure 10-56. A, MPGN type I. There is mild enlargement of the glomerulus and significant hypercellularity due to the proliferation of mesangial and endothelial cells, and marginating inflammatory cells. The capillary lumina are partially occluded by the presence of extensive double contours in addition to the proliferation (silver stain × 60). **B,** MPGN type III. Electron-dense deposits are present throughout the glomerular membranes (electron microscopy).

PEARLS

- *If no immunoglobulins on immunofluorescence, consider diagnosis of C3 glomerulonephritis; whereas if immunoglobulins or evidence of classical pathway activation of complement, the diagnosis remains MPGN type I or III*
- *MPGN type III of Burkholder can mimic membranous glomerulopathy, mesangial deposits, and proliferation as well as intramembranous and subendothelial deposits help in the differential diagnosis*

SELECTED REFERENCES

Jain D, Green JA, Bastacky S, et al: Membranoproliferative glomerulonephritis: the role for laser microdissection and mass spectrometry. Am J Kidney Dis 63:324-328, 2014.

Sethi S, Fervenza FC: Membranoproliferative glomerulonephritis: pathogenetic heterogeneity and proposal for a new classification. Semin Nephrol 31:341-348, 2011.

C3 Glomerulopathies

Clinical Features

- More frequent in children, adolescents, and young adults
- The presentation is nephritic syndrome as well as nephrotic syndrome
- Hematuria, proteinuria, hypertension
- Hypocomplementemia

Etiology, Pathogenesis, and Classification

- Secondary to dysfunction of the alternative complement pathway with abnormalities in complement factor H, and complement factor HR1-5, C3bBb, factor I, C3 nephritic factor, and membrane cofactor protein
- The classification of C3 glomerulopathies includes the following:
  - C3 glomerulonephritis, when mimics morphologically MPGN type I and III but in the absence of immune-complex deposition (C3 only)
  - Dense deposit disease (DDD) previously known as MPGN type II

Histopathology

- Significant variability in morphologic presentation by light microscopy from no or minimal mesangiopathy to extensive double contours and full membranoproliferative pattern
- The DDD variant is characterized by irregular thickening of the basement membranes with mild mesangial proliferation

Special Stains

- Silver and PAS show highlight the lobulation of the glomerular tuft and the double contours (tram track) in proliferative C3 glomerulonephritis pattern
- In DDD, the silver stain shows negative areas in the glomerular basement membranes, with "moth-eaten" appearance and irregular thickening; periodic acid-Schiff is always positive

Direct Immunofluorescence

- C3 is strongly positive with a coarsely granular appearance to a "garland" pattern in dense deposits disease (Figure 10-57A)

Electron Microscopy

- C3 glomerulonephritis can mimic MPGN type I or type III with mesangial, subepithelial, intramembranous, and subendothelial deposits as described previously
- DDD has typical ribbon-like electron-dense ribbon material substitution in the basement membranes; deposits can be in the Bowman's capsule as well (Figure 10-57B)

Differential Diagnosis

- Immune complex–mediated MPGN type I and III
- Postinfectious glomerulonephritis
- Light chain deposition disease

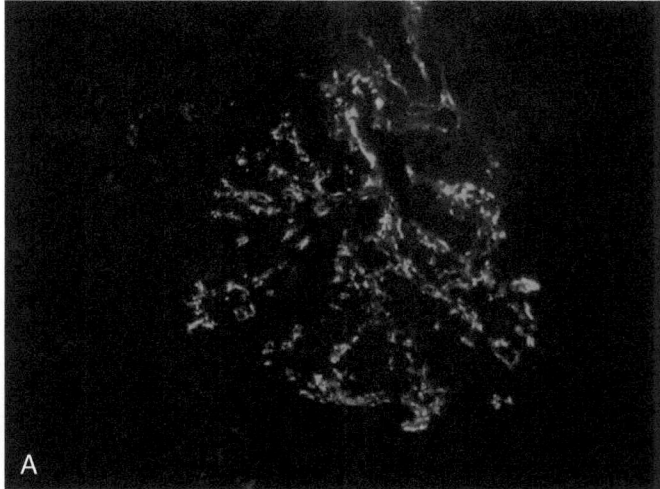
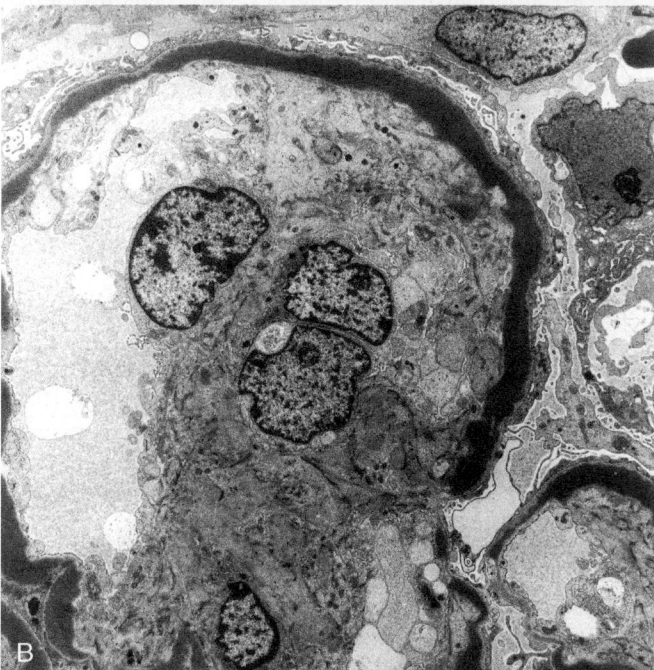

Figure 10-57. A, C3 glomerulonephritis. C3 is strongly positive in the mesangium (C3 × 40). **B,** Dense deposit disease. A ribbon-like deposition of strongly electron-dense material is seen in the glomerular basement membrane (electron microscopy).

PEARLS

- *Morphologic features with poor prognosis include older age, higher creatinine at presentation, and extracapillary proliferation*

Selected References

Pickering MC, D'Agati VD, Nester CM, et al: C3 glomerulopathy: consensus report. Kidney Int 84:1079-1089, 2013.
Sethi S, Fervenza FC, Zhang Y, et al: C3 glomerulonephritis: clinicopathological findings, complement abnormalities, glomerular proteomic profile, treatment, and follow-up. Kidney Int 82:4654-4673, 2012.

AUTOIMMUNE-MEDIATED DISEASE

- The most common autoimmune mediated renal disease is lupus nephritis, although other diseases such as rheumatoid arthritis and Sjögren syndrome can also manifest as glomerular or tubulointerstitial immune complex–mediated disorders

Lupus Nephritis
Clinical Features

- The clinical presentation of lupus nephritis varies according to the underlying lupus nephropathy class from subnephrotic proteinuria or hematuria, to nephrotic syndrome, nephritic syndrome with or without acute renal failure, and chronic renal failure
- The presentation may be gradual or with new onset
- Remitting and recurring course
- Approximately 80% of patients with lupus have lupus nephritis, of which 20% at presentation
- Relatively common disease, more frequent in females, African Americans, and Hispanics, with peak incidence between 15 and 40 years

Etiology, Pathogenesis, and Classification

- Autoimmune disease with autoantibody formation against various cellular component, although the most frequent and specific autoantibodies are those against double-strained DNA
- Environmental as well as genetic factors play a major role in the pathogenesis of lupus nephritis

Histopathology

- Six classes of lupus nephritis are part of the International Society of Nephrology/Renal Pathology Society (ISN/RPS) lupus classification system; although lupus nephritis affects all compartment of the kidney, the classification is based on glomerular lesions only; however, in the report, comments about all features need to be made and recapitulated in the activity and chronicity indices
  - Class I: normal glomerular histology but mesangial deposits by IF or EM
  - Class II: mesangial expansion and proliferation with mesangial deposits by IF or EM
  - Class III: segmental or global focal endocapillary proliferation involving < 50% of glomeruli; by electron microscopy, mesangial and subendothelial deposits are present
  - Class IV: segmental or global diffuse endocapillary proliferating involving 50% of glomeruli; by electron microscopy, mesangial, subendothelial, and occasionally subepithelial deposits are present
  - Class V: membranous pattern with thickening of the glomerular basement membranes and extensive granular deposits by IF and EM in the subepithelium
  - Class VI: sclerosing lupus nephritis, if globally sclerotic glomeruli are > 50%, but if there are also sclerosing class III and IV lesions, a combination of classes II and V and class III or IV and V is common
- Endocapillary proliferation defined by mesangial and endothelial cell proliferation, with occasional margination of inflammatory cells conferring a lobulated hypercellular appearance to the glomerulus; large subendothelial deposits can be appreciated (wire loops); the presence of endocapillary proliferation defines class III and IV (Figure 10-58A)

- Extracapillary proliferation: cellular crescents can be seen in all classes but are more commonly seen in class IV and then III; active and chronic lesions can be present at the same time: cellular crescents, fibrocellular crescents, and fibrous crescents
- Fibrinoid necrosis and karyorrhexis can also be present and are to be accounted for in the activity index of the biopsy; most common in class III and IV, rare in others
- The tubules and interstitium are also affected by chronic or active lesions; interstitial inflammation, often rich in plasma cells, and edema can be seen in acute phases; as the disease progresses, more interstitial fibrosis and tubular atrophy develop
- Vessels: various pattern of vascular involvement can be listed from normal to uncomplicated vascular deposition of Ig and complement, necrotizing vasculitis, thrombotic microangiopathy, and arterio-arteriolar sclerosis

Special Stains

- Silver stain shows double contours in classes III and IV and spikes and holes in class V
- Wire loops can be best appreciated with Masson trichrome stain

Direct Immunofluorescence

- The pattern of distribution of positive stain varies according to the class
  - Class I and II: mesangial only
  - Classes III and IV: granular mesangial, granular to semilinear, in the capillary walls involving only segments of the capillaries or the entire glomerulus
  - Class V: granular global in the basement membranes; mesangial deposits can be present
  - Class VI: the immunofluorescence stain may be weak in sclerosing forms
- Generally all immunoglobulins and complement are strongly positive, especially in proliferative forms (full-house positive stain) (Figure 10-58B)
- The presence of C1q is critical for the diagnosis (Figure 10-58C)
- Positive stain can also be seen in the tubular basement membranes and interstitium if active tubulointerstitial involvement

Electron Microscopy

- The distribution of electron-dense deposits reflects the lupus class, with purely mesangial deposits in classes I and II; mesangial, subendothelial, and occasionally subepithelial in classes III and IV; subepithelial in class V, although mesangial deposits can be seen as well
- The deposits can acquire a fingerprint substructural conformation in some of the cases (Figure 10-58D)
- Endothelial cells contain tubuloreticular inclusions, and especially in proliferative forms lose their typical fenestration (Figure 10-58E)
- Podocytes are generally injured with foot process effacement
- Electron-dense deposits can be present in tubular basement membranes and interstitium as well
- If immune-complex–mediated vasculopathy is present, electron-dense deposits can be detected in the subendothelium as well as in the media of small arteries and arterioles

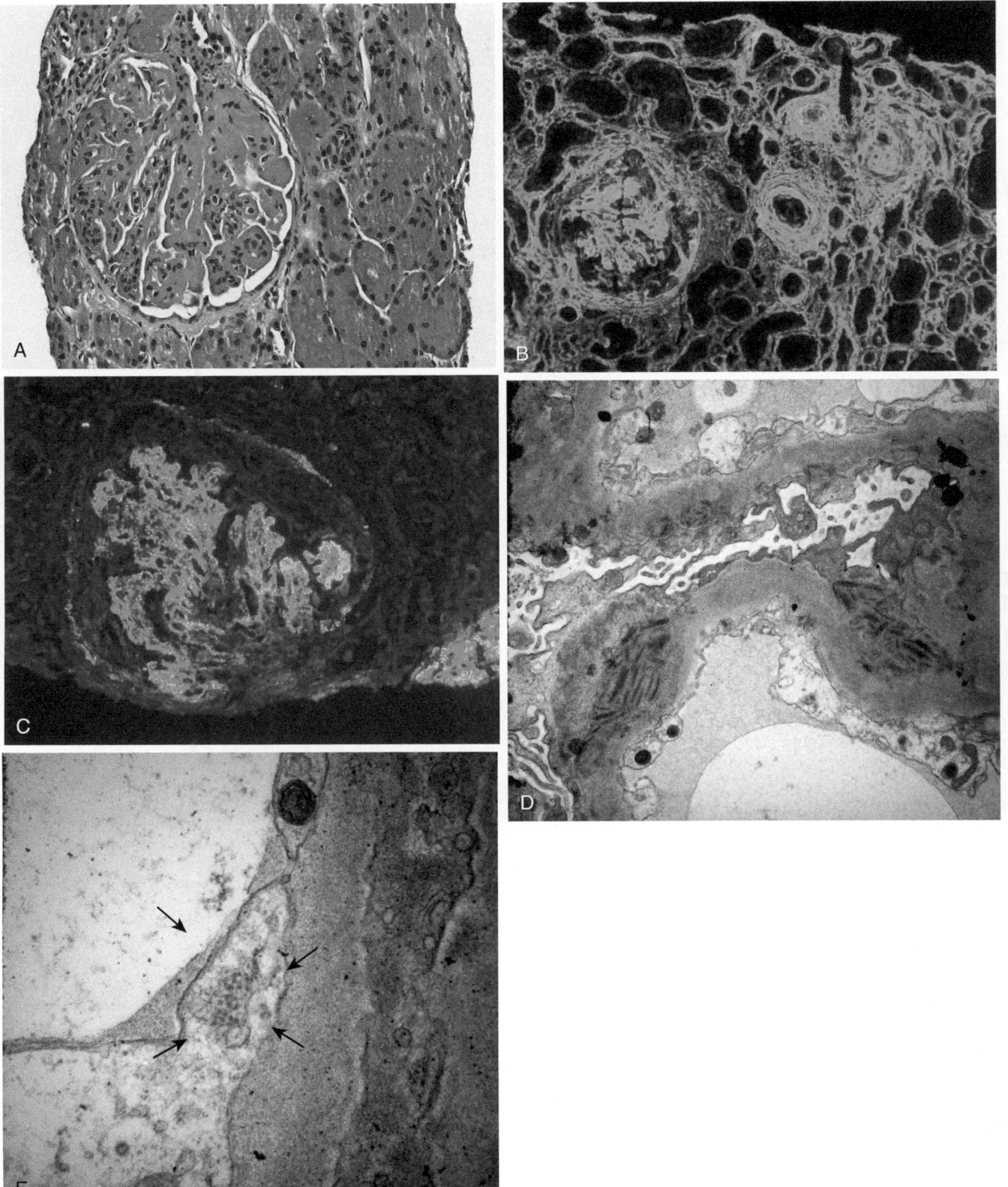

Figure 10-58. A, Proliferative lupus nephritis. Hypercellular glomerulus with large subendothelial eosinophilic deposits (wire loops). The capillary lumen is partially occluded (H&E × 40). **B,** Lupus nephritis–IgG. Strong positive granular stain in glomerular tuft, Bowman's capsule, tubular basement membranes, and interstitium and vascular walls (IgG × 40). **C,** Lupus nephritis–C1q. Strong positive granular stain in glomerular basement membranes and mesangium, and Bowman's capsule (C1Q × 60). **D,** Lupus nephritis. Subepithelial deposits with ultrastructural organization (fingerprints) (electron microscopy). **E,** Tubular reticular inclusions. Tubular reticular inclusions (arrows) in endothelial cells (electron microscopy).

Differential Diagnosis

- Membranoproliferative glomerulonephritis
- Postinfectious glomerulonephritis
- Idiopathic membranous glomerulopathy
- Drug-induced lupus nephritis
- ANCA and anti-GBM mediated disease
- Other autoimmune diseases with renal manifestations

PEARLS

- *Positive C1q is always helpful to suspect lupus*
- *Tubuloreticular inclusions are almost always present, although they can be detected in HIV-infected patients as well as in patients treated with interferon*
- *Activity and chronicity indices are important to guide the therapeutic approach*

Selected References

Furness PN, Taub N: Interobserver reproducibility and application of the ISN/RPS classification of lupus nephritis-a UK-wide study. Am J Surg Pathol 30:1030-1035, 2006.
Weening JJ, D'Agati VD, Schwartz MM, et al: The classification of glomerulonephritis in systemic lupus erythematosus revisited. J Am Soc Nephrol 15:241-250, 2004.

COMMON AND UNCOMMON METABOLIC DISORDERS

Diabetic Nephropathy

Clinical Features

- The early sign of diabetic nephropathy is microalbuminuria, which with time progressed to subnephrotic proteinuria and nephrotic range proteinuria
- Microalbuminuria occurs typically > 5 years from onset of diabetes
- Progressive loss of renal function, which is multifactorial: diabetes, associated hypertension, and probably use of multiple medications with potential nephrotoxicity, although the latter has not been demonstrated yet
- Microhematuria may occur, especially in the presence of papillary necrosis
- Hypertension and retinopathy

Etiology, Pathogenesis, and Classification

- Most common cause of ESRD in the United States
- Genetic predisposition: African Americans and Native Americans with type 2 diabetes are at higher risk

Histopathology

- Diabetic nephropathy is a progressive disease
  - Stage 1: normal glomeruli by light microscopy but thickening of the glomerular basement membranes by electron microscopy
  - Stage 2: diffuse mesangial expansion with or without increase in mesangial cellularity; by electron microscopy, glomerular basement membranes are thickened and mesangial areas contain increased collagen
  - Stage 3: diffuse nodular glomerulosclerosis (Kimmelstiel-Wilson lesions), with or without microaneurysms; abundant hyalinosis with occasional capsular drops

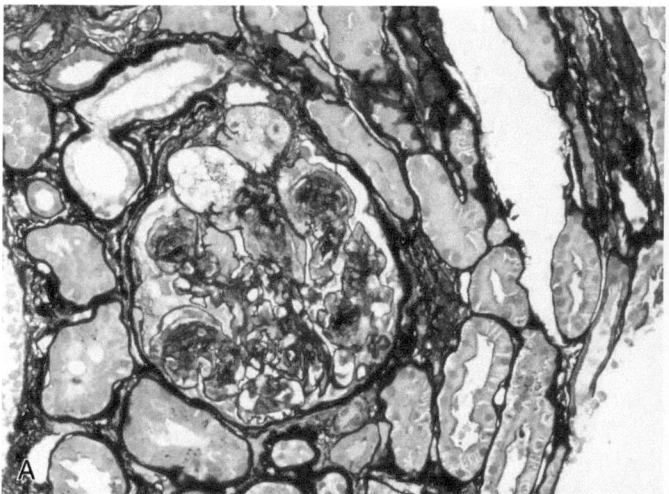

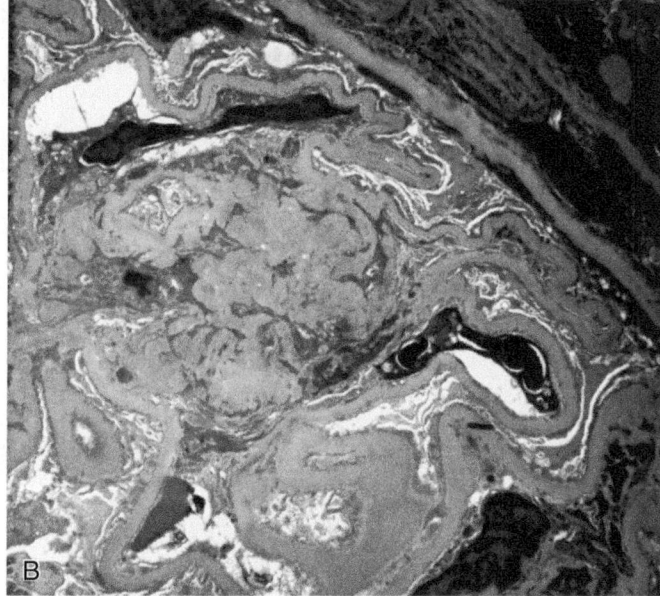

Figure 10-59. A, Diabetic nephropathy. Nodular glomerulosclerosis with microaneurysms and accumulation of abundant hyaline material (silver stain × 40). **B,** Diabetic nephropathy. By electron microscopy, the glomerulus membrane is diffusely thickened and mesangial areas are expanded. No electron-dense deposits are present (electron microscopy).

  - Stage 4: > 50% of glomeruli are globally sclerotic (Figure 10-59A)
- Glomerulomegaly
  - Fibrin caps: hyalinosis of capillaries
  - In a setting of diabetic nephropathy, globally sclerotic glomeruli generally maintain the normal size (if not larger) and contain abundant hyaline material
  - Increasing interstitial fibrosis and tubular atrophy with progression of the disease
  - Interstitial inflammation with occasional eosinophils, probably representing smoldering drug reaction
  - Proximal tubules may appear hypertrophic with numerous protein reabsorption droplets
- Arteriosclerosis
  - Significant arteriolar hyalinosis, which could be out of proportion compared to the severity of arteriosclerosis and involves both afferent and efferent arterioles

Special Stains

- Sclerotic nodules are strongly silver positive

Direct Immunofluorescence

- Linear positivity for IgG and albumin in glomerular and tubular basement membranes
- C3 and IgM are positive in the areas of glomerular and vascular hyalinosis
- Electron microscopy
- Diffuse thickening of the glomerular basement membranes, which can measure over 1000 nm (Figure 10-59B)
- Mesangial sclerosis with accumulation of collagen fibrils
- Electron-dense material, often with bubbly appearance, reflecting accumulation of hyaline insudates
- Podocytes reveal foot process effacement

Differential Diagnosis

- Idiopathic nodular glomerulosclerosis if there is no documented diabetes
- Chronic thrombotic microangiopathy: electron microscopy will reveal diffuse uniform thickening of the glomerular basement membranes and mesangial sclerosis
- Amyloidosis: sclerotic nodules are Congo red negative and silver positive

PEARLS

- *The hyaline lesions (capsular drops, fibrin caps, and significant arteriolar hyalinosis) are helpful for differential diagnosis*
- *Linear IgG may mimic anti GBM disease; however, in diabetic nephropathy, the presence of crescents is rare and albumin is always positive with a linear pattern as well*

SELECTED REFERENCES

Oh SW, Kim S, Na KY, et al: Clinical implications of pathologic diagnosis and classification for diabetic nephropathy. Diabetes Res Clin Pract 97:418-424, 2012.
Tervaert TW, Mooyaart AL, Amann K, et al; Renal Pathology Society: pathologic classification of diabetic nephropathy. J Am Soc Nephrol 21:556-563, 2010.

Fabry Disease
Clinical Features

- Genetic disorders that affect mostly males, although heterozygous females may be affected as well
- Multiorgan symptoms including skin (angiokeratomas), nervous system, kidney, and gastrointestinal system
- Mutations in AGAL occur in 1:40,000; the disease is often misdiagnosed or missed for long time
- Patients can present with renal dysfunction, strokes, cardiac dysfunction, skin manifestations, corneal opacities, and so on

Etiology, Pathogenesis, and Classification

- X-linked disease caused by mutation in AGAL gene encoding for α-galactosidase A, resulting in accumulation of lipids is many cell types and affecting multiple organs
- In kidney, α-galactosidase A accumulates in endothelial cells in glomeruli and interstitium, in podocytes, mesangial, smooth muscle, and tubular cells

Histopathology

- Glomeruli may appear normal at first; as the disease progresses, podocytes have a bubbly appearance and segmental sclerosis may develop; podocyte inclusions may be seen even on globally sclerotic glomeruli and are best visualized with toluidine blue stained thick sections
- Tubules show abundant vacuolizations representing the lysosomes filled with lipids
- Accumulation of lipids can also be seen in vascular walls (involving endothelium as well as myocytes) and interstitial capillary endothelial cells; again the best stain to visualize the inclusions by light microscopy is toluidine blue

Special Stains

- Toluidine blue

Direct Immunofluorescence

- Nonspecific

Electron Microscopy

- Diagnostic tool for Fabry disease demonstrating lysosomes filled with lipids with lamellated appearance (zebra bodies) in all cells of the kidney (Figure 10-60)
- Podocytes reveal foot process effacement

Other Techniques for Diagnosis

- Genetic testing

Differential Diagnosis

- Chloroquine toxicity may mimic Fabry disease inclusions
- FSGS, electron microscopy is critical for the diagnosis to visualize the lamellated bodies

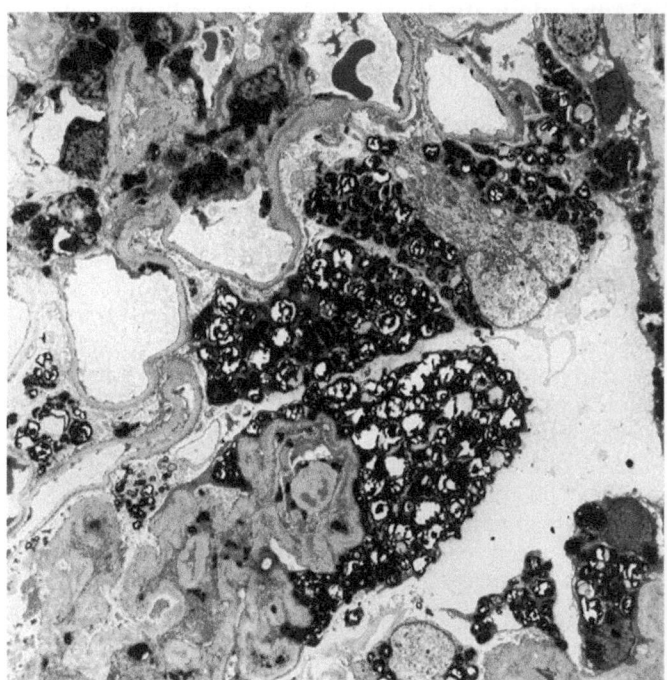

Figure 10-60. Fabry disease. Podocytes, endothelial cells, and mesangial cells contain numerous myelin figures (zebra bodies) (electron microscopy).

- Other metabolic disorders such as I-cell disease, for example, which rarely affect the kidney but characterized by accumulation of oligosaccharide

PEARLS

- *Electron microscopy is the key*
- *Heterozygous female may have few inclusions; the diagnosis still needs to be suspected and genetic counseling advised*
- *Exclude drug-induced forms*

SELECTED REFERENCES

Fogo AB, Bostad L, Svarstad E, et al: Scoring system for renal pathology in Fabry disease: report of the International Study Group of Fabry Nephropathy (ISGFN). Nephrol Dial Transplant 25:2168-2177, 2010.

Hirashio S, Taguchi T, Naito T, et al: Renal histology before and after effective enzyme replacement therapy in a patient with classical Fabry's disease. Nephrol 71:550-556, 2009.

ORGANIZED DEPOSITS

Organized deposits can be appreciated in a variety of diseases. The positive versus negative stain for Congo red is a critical step for the algorithmic approach to diagnosing these diseases, followed by immunofluorescence and electron microscopy contribution. Diseases with organized deposits include amyloidosis, monoclonal immunoglobulin deposition disease, monoclonal IgG glomerulonephritis, cryoglobulinemia, fibrillary glomerulopathy, immunotactoid glomerulopathy, type III collagen glomerulopathy, fibronectin glomerulopathy, and others.

Amyloidosis
Clinical Features

- Amyloidosis affecting the kidney generally presents with nephrotic range proteinuria and nephrotic syndrome
- It represents approximately 5% of nephrotic syndrome in adults
- Extrarenal manifestations are also frequent including heart failure, carpal tunnel syndrome, orthostatic hypotension, and liver, spleen, and tongue involvement

Etiology, Pathogenesis, and Classification

Although there are different forms of amyloidosis, those affecting the kidneys are AL amyloidosis, most frequently lambda light chain type over kappa; heavy chain type; AA amyloidosis, due to accumulation of serum amyloid A protein and associated with chronic inflammatory processes; transthyretin, although rarely affecting kidneys; α-fibrinogen, the most frequent genetic form affecting the kidney; β2 microglobulin, associated with dialysis; and leukocyte chemotactic factor 2.

Histopathology

- Deposition of amorphous, weakly eosinophilic acellular material in glomeruli, tubular basement membranes, interstitium, and vessels (Figure 10-61A)
- Glomeruli generally show progressively enlarged mesangium with nodules in more advanced stages, and irregular thickening of the glomerular basement membranes; pseudospikes pushing away the podocytes and made of

amyloid fibrils can be appreciated with special stains but also with hematoxylin and eosin stain (H&E stain)
- Tubules with basement membrane involvement may show irregular thickening of the basement membranes without atrophy
- Arteriolar intima contains nodules of pale material; arterioles and interlobular arteries are the most commonly involved

Special Stains

- Congo red is the diagnostic stain, showing apple green birefringence stain under polarized light in the areas where amyloidosis is present (Figure 10-61B)
- Thioflavin T and S is also an alternative stain
- Crystal violet stains violet the areas where amyloid is present, not commonly used
- AA amyloidosis has negative immunofluorescence with the standard panel but stains positive with antibodies against AA (by indirect immunofluorescence or immunohistochemistry)
- Antibodies against transthyretin, α-fibrinogen, β2 microglobulin, and leukocyte chemotactic factor 2 stain positive by indirect immunofluorescence or immunohistochemistry

Direct Immunofluorescence

- AL amyloidosis stains positive for one of the light chains, most commonly lambda over kappa (Figure 10-61C)
- Heavy chain amyloidosis stains positive for one Ig only
- Heavy/light chain amyloidosis stains positive for one Ig only and one light chain
- AA, transthyretin, α-fibrinogen, β2 microglobulin, and leukocyte chemotactic factor 2 amyloidosis are negative with the standard immunofluorescence panel

Electron Microscopy

- Confirmatory of the diagnosis by light microscopy with positive Congo red and shows deposition of randomly organized, nonbrunching fibrils, measuring generally from 9 to 11 nm in diameter in mesangium and glomerular basement membranes (Figure 10-61D)
- Transmural deposition of the fibrils in the basement membranes
- Podocyte foot process effacement

Other Techniques for Diagnosis

- Mass spectrometry

Differential Diagnosis

- Diabetic nephropathy: nodules are silver negative and Congo red positive in amyloidosis
- Light chain deposition disease: electron microscopy is key to demonstrate the presence of fibrils over powdery granular electron-dense material
- Fibrillary glomerulopathy: Congo red positive stain is key to make the diagnosis of amyloidosis over fibrillary glomerulopathy; amyloid fibrils are generally smaller
- If there is vascular involvement only, amyloidosis may mimic hyalinosis of the intima
- Collagenofibrotic glomerulopathy
- Nonamyloid monoclonal Ig deposition: lack of Congo red birefringence and structural organization on fibrils by electron microscopy

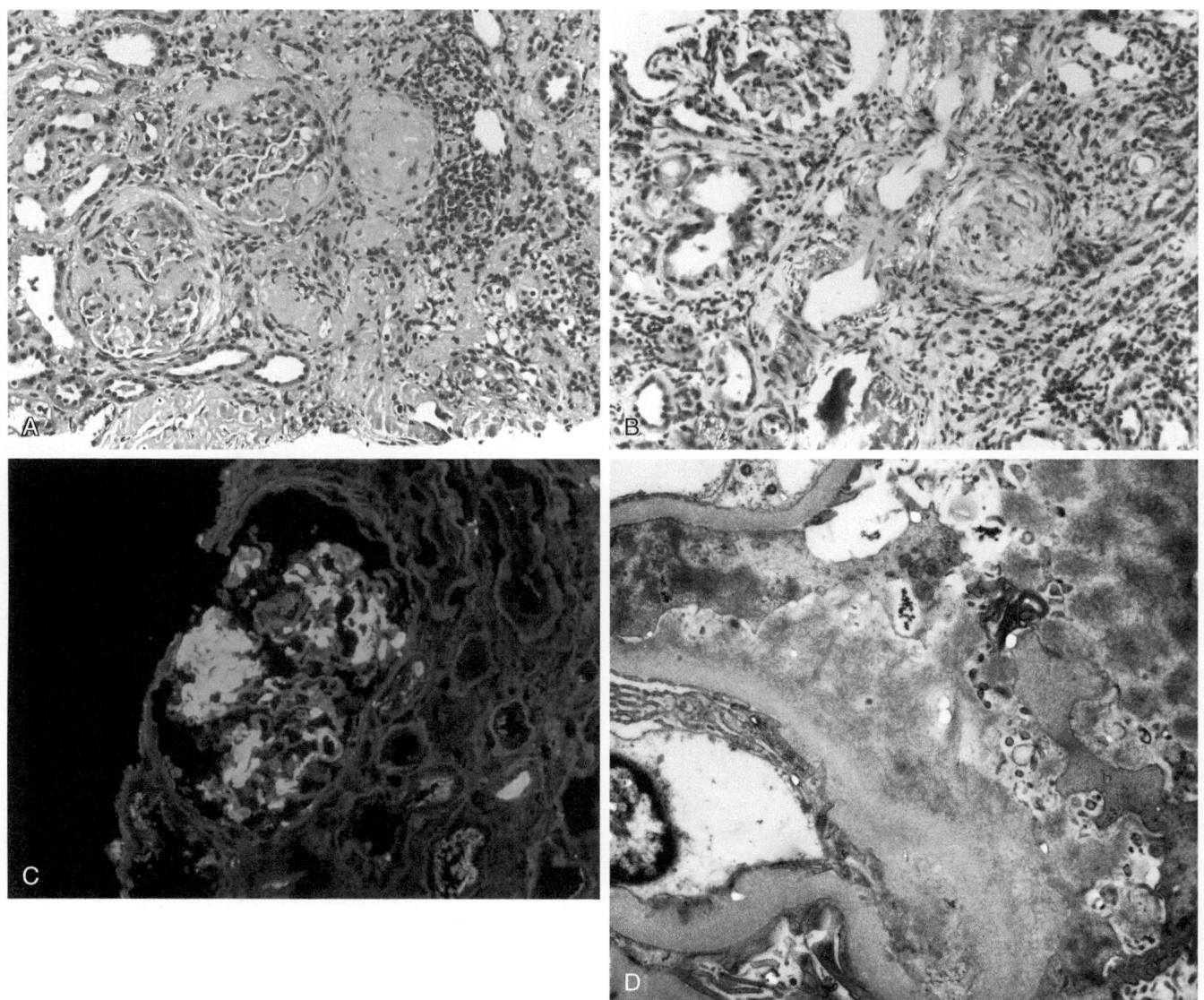

Figure 10-61. A, Amyloidosis. Globally sclerotic glomeruli as well as nonsclerotic glomeruli reveal extensive deposition of eosinophilic, amorphous, and acellular material. The same material is also present in the interstitium and vascular wall (6 o'clock) (H&E × 20). **B,** Amyloidosis. Apple green birefringence in the interlobular artery stained with Congo red and viewed under polarized light (Congo red × 40). **C,** Amyloidosis. Lambda light chain is positive in the mesangium and segmentally in the glomerular basement membranes (lambda × 40). **D,** Amyloidosis. Randomly organized nonbranching fibrils, measuring approximately 1 to 12 nm, are present in the glomerular basement membrane and subendothelium, pushing podocytes away (electron microscopy).

PEARLS

- *Evaluate Congo red birefringence with a good polarizing microscope and in the dark*

SELECTED REFERENCES

Herrera GA, Turbat-Herrera EA: Renal diseases with organized deposits: an algorithmic approach to classification and clinicopathologic diagnosis. Arch Pathol Lab Med 134:512-531, 2010.

Sethi S, Vrana JA, Theis JD, et al: Laser microdissection and mass spectrometry-based proteomics aids the diagnosis and typing of renal amyloidosis. Kidney Int 82:226-234, 2012.

KIDNEY: TUBULOINTERSTITIAL DISEASES

ISCHEMIA-INDUCED TUBULOINTERSTITIAL DAMAGE

The ischemic type of tubular injury may present as acute tubular injury from mild to frank tubular necrosis, renal cortical necrosis, or hepato-renal syndrome (due to elevated blood bilirubin causing direct toxicity to the tubules but also direct ischemia and decreased glomerular filtration rate). The most common form is acute tubular injury/necrosis.

Acute Tubular Injury/Necrosis
Clinical Features

- Acute renal failure is the typical presentation
- Oliguria to anuria
- Hypotension
- Urine sediment shows granular casts

Etiology, Pathogenesis, and Classification

- Ischemia (hypovolemia and decreased perfusion pressure) is the cause of 90% of acute tubular necrosis, with 10% only secondary to nephrotoxins

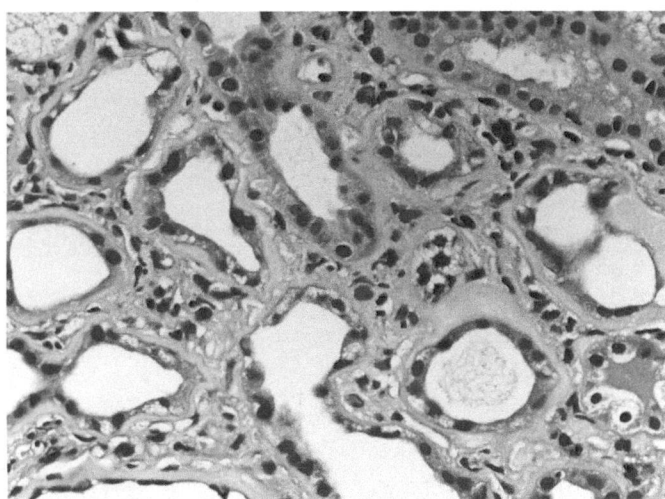

Figure 10-62. Acute tubular injury. Tubules reveal a flattened epithelium with occasional cytoplasmic vacuoles and loss of brush border. Interstitial edema and mild inflammation are also noted (H&E × 40).

Histopathology

- Necrosis and denudation of tubular epithelium in the early phase with cell loss, most prominent in distal nephrons
- Most cells have sublethal and non-necrotizing injury with loss of brush border and loss of apical portion of proximal tubular cells (Figure 10-62)
- Regeneration of tubular epithelium prominent in later phases, characterized by reepithelization of the tubules, with tubular cells with large nuclei and prominent nucleoli
- Interstitial edema with scant inflammatory cell infiltrate
- Glomeruli and blood vessels unremarkable

Special Stains

- PAS stain reveals reduced or absent brush borders

Electron Microscopy

- Loss of brush border and disruption of normal cellular architecture

Differential Diagnosis

- Acute interstitial nephritis, infectious type: prominent inflammation compared to ischemic forms
- Drug-induced interstitial nephritis: prominent inflammation compared to ischemic forms
- Autolysis

PEARLS

- *Most epithelial cells show sublethal injury with few necrotic tubular epithelial cells*
- *Prominent interstitial edema with scant inflammatory cell infiltrate*
- *Ischemic acute tubular necrosis (ATN) shows very little necrosis as opposed to toxin-related ATN*

SELECTED REFERENCES

Lameire N, Van Biesen W, Vanholder R: Acute renal failure. Lancet 365:417-430, 2005.

Solez K, et al: Difficulties in understanding human "acute tubular necrosis": analysis of 57 renal biopsies and a comparison with the glycerol model. Medicine (Baltimore) 58:362-376, 1979.

NEPHROTOXIC AGENT-INDUCED INTERSTITIAL NEPHRITIS

- Nephrotoxic agents can induce tubule-interstitial damage via various mechanisms including hypersensitivity reaction, direct damage of tubular cells' metabolism and cell production, and ischemic damage

DRUG-INDUCED INTERSTITIAL NEPHRITIS

Clinical Features

- Classic triad of fever, maculopapular rash, and eosinophilia in less than 50% of patients with acute renal failure about 2 weeks after drug exposure
- Eosinophils in urine
- Mild proteinuria and microscopic hematuria are usually present

Etiology, Pathogenesis, and Classification

- T-cell mediated hypersensitivity reaction is the usual mechanism
- Other mechanisms implicated: immune complex mediated, IgG mediated
- Drug classes implicated: antibiotics, nonsteroidal anti-inflammatory drugs (NSAIDs), diuretics, antiviral drugs, and others

Histopathology

- Interstitial inflammation with mixed inflammatory cell infiltrate and edema (Figure 10-63)
- Eosinophils are frequently found
- Tubulitis common during the active phase
- Granulomatous reaction can also occurs

Special Stains

- Bacterial and fungal stains do not reveal any organisms

Direct Immunofluorescence

- Immunofluorescence is usually nonreactive or nonspecific
- Electron microscopy
- Diffuse podocyte injury and foot process effacement seen in NSAID-induced disease

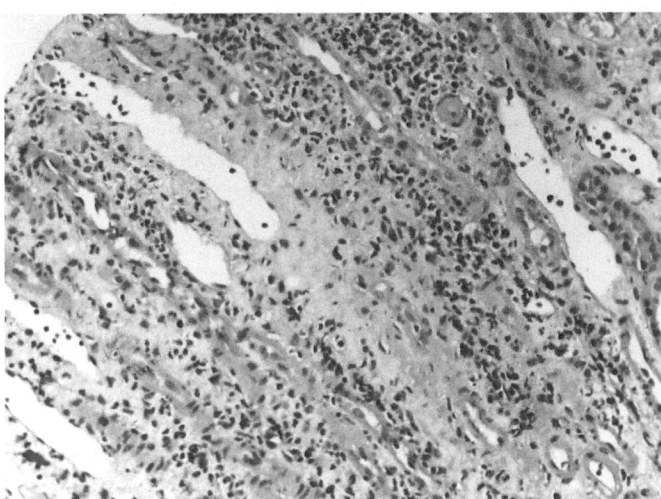

Figure 10-63. Drug-induced interstitial nephritis. Moderately to severe mononuclear inflammation with eosinophils in clusters in the medulla (H&E × 40).

Differential Diagnosis

- Acute tubular necrosis (ATN) with associated interstitial inflammation: inflammation is scant in ATN
- Autoimmune diseases: clinical history and serology will be helpful
- Infectious interstitial nephritis: special stains can reveal the infectious organisms and more neutrophilic and lymphocytic infiltrates and less of eosinophils
- If granulomas are present, sarcoidosis should be considered in the differential diagnosis as well as fungal or mycobacterial infection

PEARLS

- *If granulomas are present, GMS stain is mandatory*
- *Eosinophils are most commonly found at the corticomedullary junction*

SELECTED REFERENCES

Choudhury D, Ahmed Z: Drug-associated renal dysfunction and injury. Nat Clin Pract Nephrol 2:80, 2006.

Nasdasdy T, et al: Acute and chronic tubulointerstitial nephritis. In Jennette JC, et al: Herpinstall's Pathology of the Kidney, 6th ed. Philadelphia, Lippincott Williams & Wilkins, 2007, pp 1083-1109.

TUBULOINTERSTITIAL DAMAGE CAUSED BY TUBULAR OBSTRUCTION

Tubulointerstitial damage secondary to obstruction can be acute or chronic. Generally, intratubular casts are responsible for acute injury, presenting with sudden onset of acute renal failure. Those include myeloma cast nephropathy (most common), myoglobin cast nephropathy, and hemoglobin cast nephropathy. Chronic obstructive nephropathy is a more slowly progressive disease, secondary to structural abnormalities distal to the kidney.

Myeloma Cast Nephropathy

Clinical Features

- Constellation of signs and symptoms including anemia, bone pain, elevated creatinine levels, fatigue, and hypercalcemia
- Proteinuria with urine dipstick negative or only slightly positive for protein
- Diagnosis of myeloma can be confirmed by serum/urine electrophoresis

Etiology, Pathogenesis, and Classification

- Due to large amounts of free light chains produced
- Not all monoclonal light chains are toxic to kidney
- Renal toxicity is directly proportional to light chain concentration
- Mechanism of injury poorly understood but proposed mechanisms include direct toxicity and secondary to intratubular cast formation

Histopathology

- Casts can be diffuse or focal involving distal convoluted and collecting tubules (Figure 10-64A)

- Casts often have a fractured or crystalline appearance and are surrounded by multinucleated giant cells (Figure 10-64B)
- Tubular epithelial cells' surrounding casts appear reactive
- Interstitial fibrosis and interstitial lymphocytic infiltrate

Special Stains

- Myeloma casts are PAS negative versus Tamm-Horsfall casts (uromodulin) that are PAS positive

Direct Immunofluorescence

- Casts stain positive for monoclonal kappa or lambda light chains (Figure 10-64C and D)
- Often associated with light chain deposition disease features

Electron Microscopy

- Tubular casts have a distinctive composition of finely granular material of moderate electron density, often forming crystal-like structures

Differential Diagnosis

- Other forms of paraproteinemias, such as Waldenstrom macroglobulinemia
- Myoglobin or hemoglobin cast nephropathy: the casts do not have the typical hard fractured appearance of the myeloma casts
- Acute tubular injury with granular casts

PEARLS

- *Immunofluorescence is important for the diagnosis*
- *Clinical pathologic correlation is critical*

SELECTED REFERENCES

Herrera GA, Turbat-Herrera EA: Renal diseases with organized deposits: an algorithmic approach to classification and clinicopathologic diagnosis. Arch Pathol Lab Med 134:512-531, 2010.

Hutchison CA, Batuman V, Behrens J, et al; International Kidney and Monoclonal Gammopathy Research Group: The pathogenesis and diagnosis of acute kidney injury in multiple myeloma. Nat Rev Nephrol 8:43-51, 2011.

KIDNEY: VASCULAR DISEASES

Diseases affecting the renal vasculature can be classified based on their acute or chronic manifestations or by etiology. Acute vascular damage can be the result of malignant hypertension, acute thrombotic microangiopathic processes, vasculitis, cholesterol embolization, renal vein, or renal artery thrombosis. Chronic vascular damage can be the result of benign hypertension, renal artery stenosis, or fibromuscular dysplasia.

HYPERTENSIVE VASCULAR DISEASE

Clinical Features

- Lonstanding history of hypertension, in 95% of cases essential
- Often associated with obesity and diabetes
- African Americans are more frequently affected

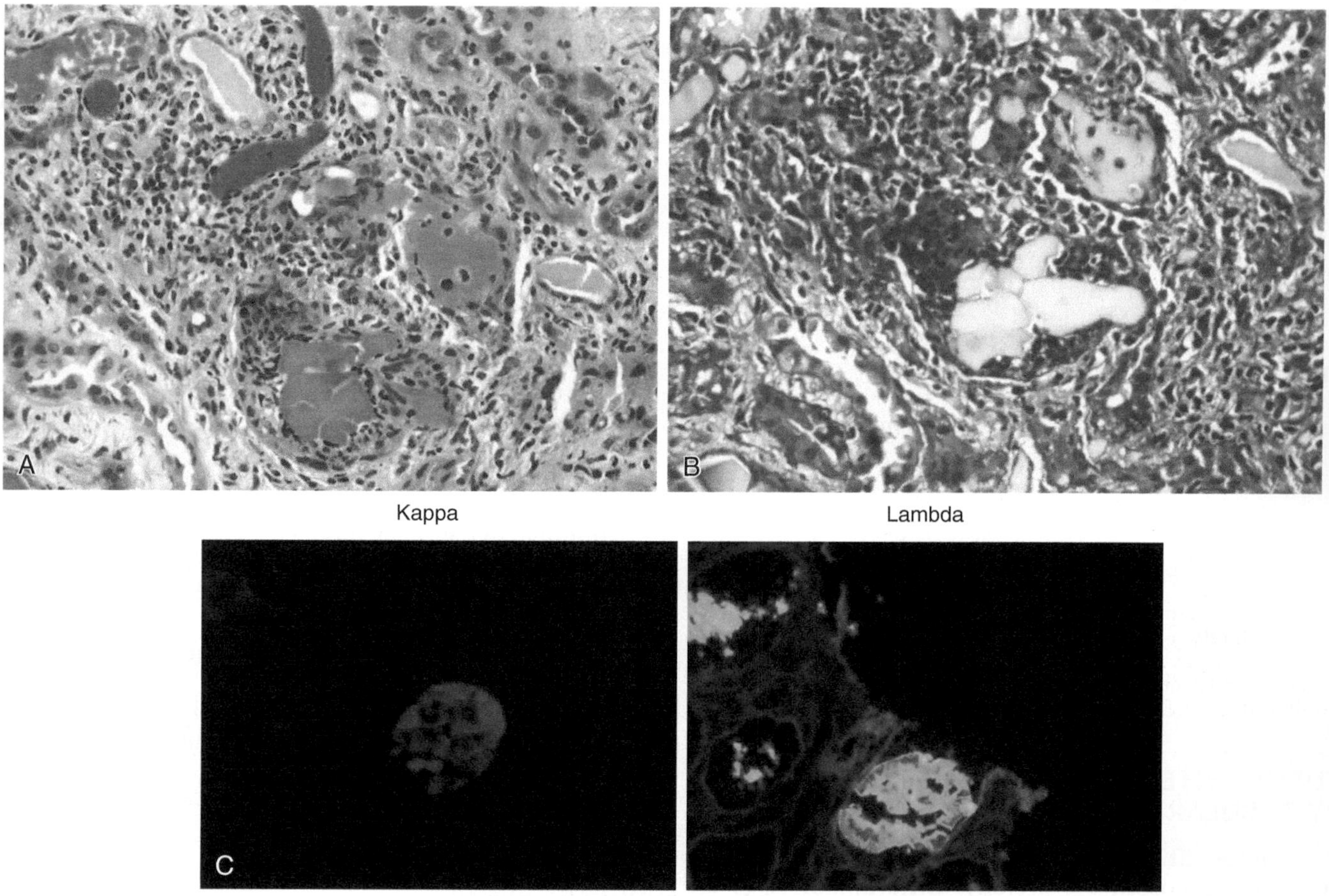

Kappa

Lambda

Figure 10-64. A, Myeloma cast nephropathy. Large hard eosinophilic and fractured intratubular casts with cellular reaction (H&E × 40). **B,** Myeloma cast nephropathy. The large hard, fractured intratubular casts with cellular reaction are PAS negative (PAS × 40). **C,** Myeloma cast nephropathy. Lambda is positive in intratubular casts, with kappa negative (kappa and lambda light chains × 60).

- Progressive loss of renal function
- Subnephrotic range proteinuria

Etiology, Pathogenesis, and Classification

- Predisposing genetic background
- Essential hypertension
- Secondary hypertension: renal artery stenosis, neoplastic processes, chronic glomerular disease

Histopathology

- Progressive global sclerosis, interstitial fibrosis, and tubular atrophy
- In some cases FSGS can develop as a secondary phenomenon to postadaptive mechanisms on a predisposing genetic background
- Ischemic type of retraction of the glomerular tuft not accompanied by podocyte hypertrophy
- Arteries show intimal fibrosis, duplication of the elastic lamina, and hypertrophy of the media (Figure 10-65)
- Arterioles have hyalinosis and hypertrophy of the media
- Endocrine type of tubular atrophy in renal artery stenosis

Special Stains

- Elastin highlights duplication of the elastic lamina
- Trichrome reveals the severity of interstitial fibrosis and tubular atrophy

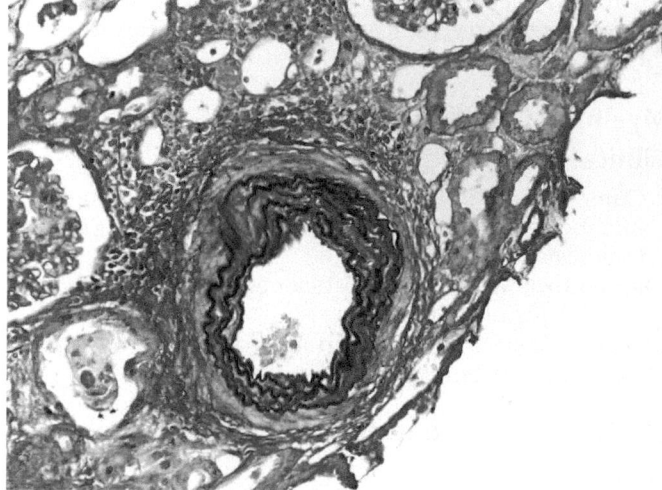

Figure 10-65. Arteriosclerosis. Duplication of elastic lamina with thickening of arterial wall and narrowing of the lumen (elastin × 40).

Direct Immunofluorescence

- Hyalin material stains with IgM and C3

Electron Microscopy

- Mild thickening or wrinkling of the glomerular basement membranes

- Variable amount of foot process effacement
- Accumulation of hyaline material that may mimic electron-dense deposits

Differential Diagnosis

- Primary focal segmental glomerulosclerosis

PEARLS

- *Clinical pathologic correlation is necessary to identify the underlying cause of the arterio- and arteriolosclerosis*

SELECTED REFERENCES

Hill GS: Hypertensive nephrosclerosis. Curr Opin Nephrol Hypertens 17:266-270, 2008.

Pirkle JL, Freedman BI: Hypertension and chronic kidney disease: controversies in pathogenesis and treatment. Minerva Urol Nefrol 65:37-50, 2013.

ATHEROMATOUS EMBOLI

Clinical Features

- Affect patients > 50 years, with Caucasian male predominance
- Presentation varies from acute renal failure to proteinuria or hematuria
- Fever and myalgia may be associated

Etiology, Pathogenesis, and Classification

- Atheroemboli occurs as acute events in patients with a recent history of invasive vascular procedures; however, they can also occur following trauma, cardiopulmonary resuscitation, or simply in a setting of diabetes, hypertension, and hypercholesterolemia

Histopathology

- Cholesterol clefts are present in vascular lumina and generally accompanied by cellular reaction with multinucleated giant cells (Figure 10-66)
- Glomeruli, arterioles, and arteries can be involved
- Morphologic evidence of hypertensive vascular disease is almost always present

Special Stains

- Not contributory

Direct Immunofluorescence

- Not contributory

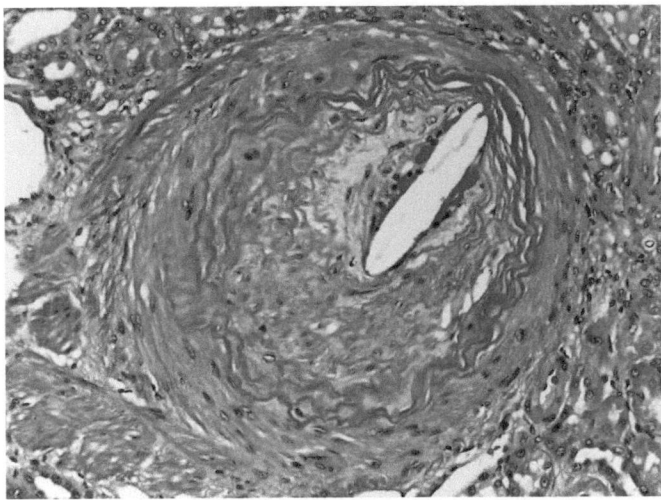

Figure 10-66. Atheroemboli. Intravascular cholesterol cleft, with cellular reaction, occluding an interlobular artery (H&E × 60).

Electron Microscopy

- In the presence of proteinuria, foot process effacement can be present, generally focal

Differential Diagnosis

- Handling artifacts

PEARLS

- *If suspected, extensive examination and deeper sections are necessary to demonstrate the presence of focal atheroemboli*

SELECTED REFERENCE

Mittal BV, Alexander MP, Rennke HG, Singh AK: Atheroembolic renal disease: a silent masquerader. Kidney Int 73:126-130, 2008.

The authors would like to acknowledge the following colleagues for their contribution:

David Brian Thomas, M.D.
Professor of Pathology
Renal Pathology Division
University of Miami, Miller School of Medicine
Miami, Florida

Bhavesh Papadi, M.D.
Genitourinary Pathology Fellow
University of Miami Hospital
Miami, Florida

Chapter 11
Male Genitourinary System

MICHAEL R. PINS

CHAPTER OUTLINE

PROSTATE GLAND

ACUTE AND CHRONIC PROSTATITIS

Clinical Features

- Clinical classification of acute and chronic prostatitis
  - Acute bacterial prostatitis
    - Prostate is swollen and tender on palpation
    - Often refractory to antibiotic therapy because the prostate is a "safe haven" for bacteria
    - Patients may present with recurrent urinary tract infections
    - Cultured organisms are the same as those seen in urinary tract infections (i.e., *Escherichia coli*, other gram-negative rods, and *Enterococcus* and *Staphylococcus* species)
  - Chronic bacterial prostatitis
    - Same as acute prostatitis, but symptoms are of longer duration
  - Chronic abacterial prostatitis
    - Most common form of clinical prostatitis
    - Presents similar to acute and chronic bacterial prostatitis
    - By definition, no organisms are cultured (idiopathic); however, infection by *Chlamydia*, *Ureaplasma*, or *Mycoplasma* species has been suggested
  - Granulomatous prostatitis
    - Nonspecific (idiopathic) granulomatous type
    - Patients are between 20 and 70 years of age (mean age, 60 years)
    - Patients present with obstructive symptoms, dysuria, fever, and chills; may have a history of urinary tract infection
    - Prostate on palpitation can be firm and indurated (may clinically mimic carcinoma)
    - After bacillus Calmette-Guérin (BCG) therapy: history of intracystic BCG therapy for transitional cell carcinoma (TCC) may be remote (Figure 11-1B)
    - Post-transurethral or postbiopsy granulomatous type: history of procedure up to 5 years ago
    - Infectious granulomatous type: history of infection by any one of the following
      - Bacteria (tuberculosis, syphilis, or brucella)
      - Fungi (cryptococcosis, blastomycosis, or coccidioidomycosis)
      - Viruses (herpes)
      - Parasites (schistosomiasis, echinococcosis)
  - Malakoplakia
    - Primarily affects men older than 50 years
    - Symptoms include fever, frequency, dysuria, and hematuria
    - Urine culture is often positive for *Escherichia coli*

Gross Pathology

- Acute and chronic bacterial and chronic abacterial prostatitis
  - Prostatic enlargement; may be soft and swollen
- Granulomatous prostatitis
  - Enlarged with firm, nodular parenchyma
  - Areas of infarction and necrosis with infectious granulomas are often seen

Histopathology

- Acute and chronic bacterial prostatitis
  - Prominent neutrophilic infiltrate with abscess formation
  - Neutrophils and necrotic debris may fill prostatic ducts and acini
  - Reactive glandular epithelium showing mild cytologic atypia; nuclei with prominent nucleoli may be seen (Figure 11-1A)
  - Glands may appear atrophic and have a pseudocribriform architecture owing to little glands budding off within lumen
  - Stroma is edematous and hyperemic
- Chronic abacterial prostatitis
  - Presence of neutrophils and lymphocytes in prostatic ducts and epithelium
  - Reactive glandular epithelium showing mild cytologic atypia; nuclei with prominent nucleoli may be seen
  - May be associated with glandular atrophy
- Granulomatous prostatitis
  - Nonspecific (idiopathic) granulomatous type
    - Admixture of histiocytes, plasma cells, eosinophils, neutrophils, lymphocytes, and giant cells
    - Cells arranged in sheets around ruptured ducts and acini
  - Post-BCG therapy
    - Mostly histiocytes and giant cells associated with ducts or acini (Figure 11-1B)
  - Posttransurethral or postbiopsy granulomatous type
    - Central zone of fibrinoid necrosis surrounded by palisading histiocytes and some multinucleated giant cells (Figure 11-1C)
    - Minimal chronic inflammatory infiltrate
    - Eosinophilic infiltrate typically present after recent prostate surgery (1 month after resection)
  - Infectious granulomatous type
    - Granulomatous inflammation, with or without necrosis
    - Eosinophils often present with parasitic infection
- Malakoplakia
  - Hansemann cells: histiocytes with clear or eosinophilic cytoplasm arranged in sheets with surrounding mixed chronic inflammatory infiltrate
  - Michaelis-Gutmann bodies: round, target-shaped structures found intracellularly and extracellularly

Special Stains and Immunohistochemistry

- Granulomatous prostatitis
  - Nonspecific granulomatous type
    - Stains positively for histiocytic markers, negative for epithelial markers
  - Infectious granulomatous type
    - May identify causative organism with special stains (Gomori methenamine silver [GMS], periodic acid-Schiff [PAS], acid-fast bacillus [AFB] stains)
  - Malakoplakia
    - Von Kossa calcium, iron, and PAS highlight Michaelis-Gutmann bodies

Other Techniques for Diagnosis

- Noncontributory

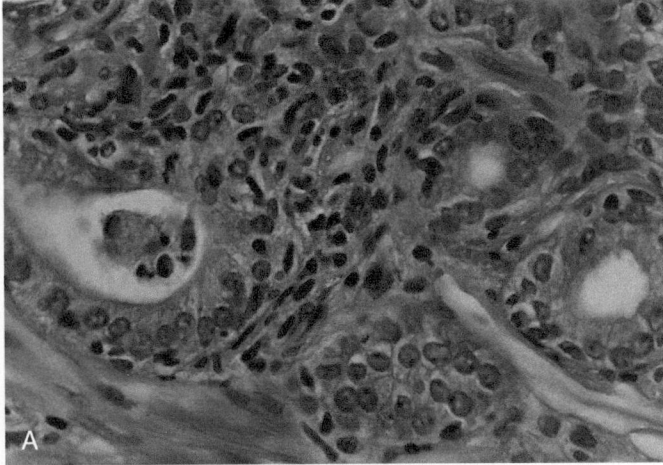

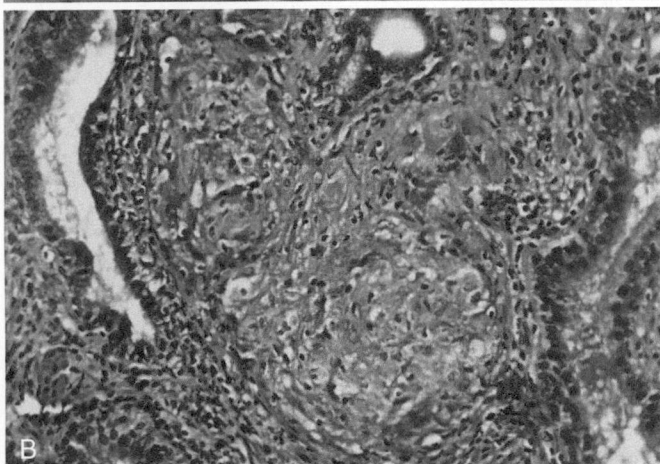

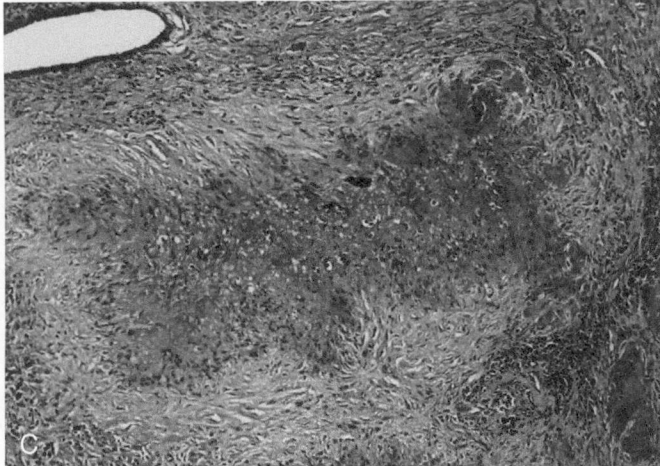

Figure 11-1. A, Chronic, focally acute prostatitis. Note the presence of reactive atypicality of the acinar epithelium in the form of conspicuous nucleoli. **B,** Iatrogenic granulomatous prostatitis. Noncaseating epithelioid granulomas and associated lymphocytic infiltrate in a patient receiving bacillus Calmette-Guérin therapy for urothelial cancer. **C,** Iatrogenic granulomatous prostatitis. Low-power view of palisading histiocytes after transurethral resection. Note the atrophic-appearing prostatic gland (*top left*).

Differential Diagnosis

NON-HODGKIN LYMPHOMA
- Rare in the prostate gland
- Proliferation of neoplastic lymphoid cells that typically infiltrate the prostatic stroma in diffuse sheets while sparing the ducts and acini

- Infiltration into surrounding periprostatic tissues is common
- Monoclonal lymphoid population seen with flow cytometry and immunohistochemistry
- Most common tumor subtype is diffuse large cell lymphoma, B-cell type

POORLY DIFFERENTIATED ADENOCARCINOMA (GLEASON GRADES 8 TO 10)
- Infiltrating tumor composed of a diffuse and focally glandular proliferation
- Malignant cells have pleomorphic nuclei and prominent nucleoli
- Neoplastic glands lack basal cell layer (negative high-molecular-weight cytokeratin [HMWCK] staining)
- Inflammatory cell infiltrate is unusual in adenocarcinoma

SARCOIDOSIS
- Patients typically have evidence of systemic disease; rare to have isolated prostate involvement
- Characterized by noncaseating granulomas composed of epithelioid histiocytes and giant cells
- Special stains for organisms are negative

PEARLS

- *Preferable to diagnose inflamed prostate specimens as having acute or chronic inflammation than as acute or chronic prostatitis (i.e., the latter are clinical diagnoses)*
- *Biopsy is not required because most prostatitis cases are effectively treated with antibiotics*
- *Patients with chronic prostatitis often have frequent recurrences, and histology correlates poorly with clinical findings (e.g., stromal and periglandular mononuclear cell infiltrates are normal in older men)*
- *All forms of prostatic disease may cause mild elevation of prostate-specific antigen (PSA)*

SELECTED REFERENCES

Nickel JC, True LD, Krieger JN, et al: Consensus development of a histopathological classification system for chronic prostatic inflammation. BJU Int 87:797-805, 2001.
Roberts RO, Lieber MM, Bostwick DG, Jacobsen SJ: A review of clinical and pathological prostatitis syndromes. Urology 49:809-821, 1997.

INFARCTION

Clinical Features

- Patients may be asymptomatic or present with urinary retention and hematuria
- Typically occurs in a background of nodular hyperplasia

Gross Pathology

- In general, the greater the degree of nodular hyperplasia, the greater the likelihood of infarction
- Central pale-yellow zone surrounded by hyperemic tissue

Histopathology

- Acute infarction
  - Central coagulative necrosis with surrounding hemorrhage (Figure 11-2)
  - Adjacent glands show reactive and metaplastic changes; typically squamous metaplasia

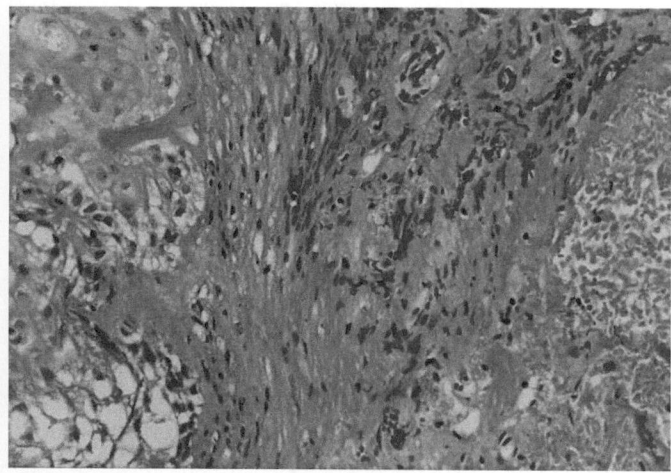

Figure 11-2. Prostatic infarct. Coagulative necrosis with hemorrhage (*right*) and early squamous metaplasia of prostatic glandular epithelium (*left*).

- Reactive glandular epithelium is characterized by cells with enlarged nuclei, prominent nucleoli, and mitotic figures
- Remote infarction
  - Central fibrous scar with hemosiderin admixed with small glands often showing squamous metaplasia

Special Stains and Immunohistochemistry
- Noncontributory

Other Techniques for Diagnosis
- Noncontributory

Differential Diagnosis
SQUAMOUS CELL CARCINOMA
- Rare in the prostate gland
- Infiltrative architecture composed of irregular nests or cords of malignant cells with squamous differentiation; areas of keratinization often seen
- Will typically have prominent desmoplastic changes in the surrounding stroma

PROSTATIC ADENOCARCINOMA, LOW GRADE
- Low-power magnification reveals uniform proliferation of small glands with irregular contours and irregular stromal spacing
- Neoplastic glands are lined by a single layer of epithelium (basal cell layer is absent)
- Higher-power magnification demonstrates cuboidal or columnar cells with abundant cytoplasm, enlarged nuclei, and prominent nucleoli
- Perineural infiltration is often present

PEARLS
- *Commonly seen at autopsy in men with marked hypotension who had had a urethral catheter in place*

SELECTED REFERENCE

Milord RA, Kahane H, Epstein JI: Infarct of the prostate gland: experience on needle biopsy specimens. Am J Surg Pathol 10:1378-1384, 2000.

HYPERPLASIA
Clinical Features
- Common in males after 60 years of age
- Patients may have symptoms of urinary obstruction (inability to initiate or terminate urinary flow) or may be asymptomatic

Gross Pathology
BENIGN (NODULAR) PROSTATIC HYPERPLASIA
- Multilobulated surface
- Variably sized nodules typically located around the prostatic urethra
- Peripheral zone appears compressed and atrophic
- Small foci of infarction may be seen

BASAL CELL AND CLEAR CELL CRIBRIFORM HYPERPLASIA
- Often incidental finding associated with benign (nodular) hyperplasia

ATYPICAL ADENOMATOUS HYPERPLASIA
- Nonspecific gross features

Histopathology
BENIGN (NODULAR) PROSTATIC HYPERPLASIA
- Well-circumscribed, nonencapsulated nodules
- Composed of hyperplastic epithelial and stromal components (Figure 11-3A)
  - Epithelial component
    - Large, irregularly shaped glands
    - Glands with a double cell layer and some with pseudostratification of secretory cells
    - Columnar cells with pale-staining granular cytoplasm
    - Papillae with fibrovascular cores
    - Chronic inflammatory infiltrate that surrounds glands
  - Stromal component
    - Composed of fibroblasts and smooth muscle cells

BASAL CELL PROLIFERATIONS
- Basal cell hyperplasia (BCH)
  - Typically an incidental finding
  - Forms well-defined, small solid nests of basal cells or glandular structures; may have an infiltrative architecture
  - Hyperplastic glands with proliferation of uniform basaloid cells that may occlude the glandular lumens (Figure 11-3B)
  - Glands showing peripheral nuclear palisading
  - Hypercellular, fibroblastic stroma
  - Often seen together with typical benign (nodular) prostatic hyperplasia
- BCH with nucleolomegaly (atypical BCH)
  - Architecture is similar to that of BCH
  - Differentiating feature is basaloid cells with prominent nucleoli

CLEAR CELL CRIBRIFORM HYPERPLASIA
- Almost always associated with benign (nodular) hyperplasia

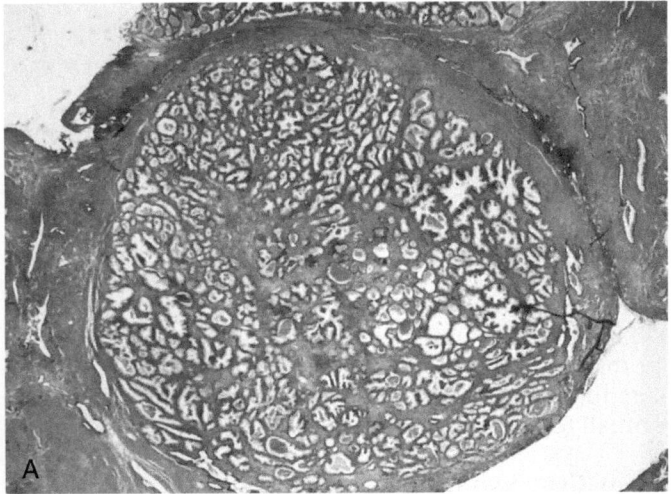

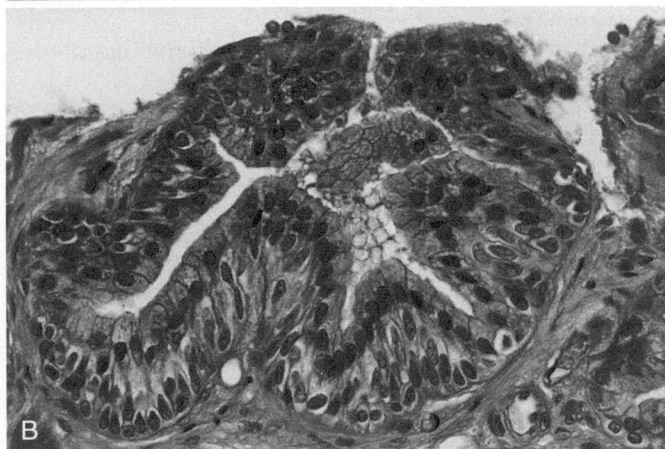

Figure 11-3. A, Benign (nodular) prostatic hyperplasia. Low-power view of a gland-rich hyperplastic nodule. Other nodules (not shown) may be stroma rich. **B,** Basal cell hyperplasia (BCH). Subluminal cell proliferation of basal cells characterized by elongated nuclei, longitudinal nuclear grooves, conspicuous nucleoli, and amphophilic cytoplasm. BCH showing enlarged nucleoli (atypical basal cell hyperplasia) should not be confused with high-grade prostatic intraepithelial neoplasia.

- Characterized by acini distended by a proliferation of cells with clear cytoplasm forming uniform round spaces
- Cells are cuboidal to columnar and have small hyperchromatic nuclei, indistinct nucleoli, and clear cytoplasm
- Basal cell layer is intact

SCLEROSING ADENOSIS
- Lobular or focally infiltrative glandular proliferation
- Glands may be round or compressed and have an angulated, slitlike appearance
- Glands have a double cell layer (may be difficult to appreciate) and a thickened basement membrane
- Cells contain medium-to-large nuclei with fine chromatin and typically indistinct nucleoli
- Stromal component contains plump spindle cells arranged randomly or in fascicles

ATYPICAL ADENOMATOUS HYPERPLASIA
- Architecturally similar to Gleason grade 1 or 2 adenocarcinoma

- Circumscribed proliferation of variably sized acini that may show focal infiltration at the periphery
- Tightly packed small glands intermixed with larger glands
- Basal cell layer may be discontinuous and indistinct but is usually focally present in at least some glands
- Glandular cells typically have pale to clear cytoplasm, small nuclei, and inconspicuous nucleoli; prominent nucleoli may occasionally be seen; however, macronucleoli (>3 μm) should not be present
- Corpora amylacea is often present (much less common in adenocarcinoma)

Special Stains and Immunohistochemistry
- HMWCK: highlights basal cell layer in benign (nodular) prostatic hyperplasia, BCH, clear cell cribriform hyperplasia, and sclerosing adenosis
- Muscle-specific actin (MSA) and S-100 protein positive for some basal and spindle cells in sclerosing adenosis (indicates myoepithelial differentiation)

Other Techniques for Diagnosis
- Noncontributory

Differential Diagnosis
PROSTATIC INTRAEPITHELIAL NEOPLASIA (PIN)
- Glands are large and branched with intraluminal papillary projections
- Nuclei are elongated, pseudostratified, and perpendicular to the basement membrane

PROSTATIC ADENOCARCINOMA, LOW GRADE
- Low-power microscopy reveals uniform proliferation of small glands with irregular contours and irregular stromal spacing
- Neoplastic glands are lined by a single layer of epithelium (basal cell layer is absent)
- Higher-power microscopy demonstrates cuboidal or columnar cells with abundant cytoplasm, enlarged nuclei, and prominent nucleoli
- Perineural infiltration is often present

CLEAR CELL CRIBRIFORM HYPERPLASIA VERSUS CRIBRIFORM ADENOCARCINOMA
- Cells in clear cell cribriform hyperplasia have distinct clear cytoplasm, small nuclei with indistinct nucleoli, and a prominent basal cell layer

PEARLS

- *Treatment for symptomatic hyperplasia is typically transurethral prostatectomy (TURP); occasionally treated with suprapubic prostatectomy*
- *May be treated with various drugs, including*
  - *Finasteride (androgen-converting enzyme inhibitor)*
  - *α₁-Adrenergic blockers*
- *Neoplastic nature of atypical adenomatous hyperplasia and its relationship to low-grade adenocarcinoma is an area of active investigation*
- *A diagnosis of carcinoma should not be made based on identification of a few malignant-appearing cells in a background clearly demonstrating atypical adenomatous hyperplasia*

SELECTED REFERENCES

Amin MB, Tamboli P, Verma M, Surgley JR: Postatrophic hyperplasia of the prostate gland: a detailed analysis of its morphology in needle biopsy specimens. Am J Surg Pathol 23:925-931, 1999.

Bostwick DG, Meiers I: Diagnosis of prostate carcinoma after therapy: review 2007. Arch Pathol Lab Med 131:360-371, 2007.

Bostwick DG, Svigley J, Grignon D, et al: Atypical adenomatous hyperplasia of the prostate: morphological criteria for its distinction from well-differentiated carcinoma. Hum Pathol 24:819-832, 1993.

Hameed O, Humphrey PA: Pseudoneoplastic mimics of prostate and bladder carcinomas. Arch Pathol Lab Med 134:427-443, 2010.

EPITHELIAL METAPLASIA

Clinical Features

UROTHELIAL AND TRANSITIONAL CELL METAPLASIA

- Describes a condition in which transitional epithelium is within the prostatic ducts and acini
- Often seen in infants and neonates
- Generally no clinical symptoms

SQUAMOUS METAPLASIA

- May be associated with infarction, estrogen therapy, androgen ablation, or radiation therapy
- Common in neonates
- Generally no clinical symptoms

Gross Pathology

- Nonspecific

Histopathology

UROTHELIAL AND TRANSITIONAL CELL METAPLASIA

- Localized to peripheral prostatic ducts and acini
- Urothelium admixed with alternating areas of cuboidal and columnar epithelium
- Cells are spindle to ovoid to polygonal and have ovoid nuclei overlapping in a streaming manner; nuclei are uniform and have prominent nuclear grooves
- May completely fill gland lumen forming a solid nest
- Differs from normal urothelium by lack of umbrella cells and presence of eosinophilic secretory lining cells

SQUAMOUS METAPLASIA

- Squamous differentiation (polygonal cells with eosinophilic cytoplasm) with variable keratin formation and intercellular bridging
- May be associated with infarcts and nodular prostatic hyperplasia; if associated with prostatic infarction, mild nuclear atypia may be seen

MUCINOUS METAPLASIA

- Haphazardly scattered or small groups of tall, mucin-filled goblet cells
- Cells have small, dark, basally oriented nuclei and abundant mucin-filled cytoplasm
- Can be found in association with normal and hyperplastic prostate glands, as well as in areas of urothelial metaplasia, BCH, or atrophy

Special Stains and Immunohistochemistry

- HMWCK positive in urothelial and transitional cells and squamous metaplasia
- Alcian blue and mucicarmine positive for intracytoplasmic acid mucin in mucinous metaplasia
- PAS positive for neutral mucin in mucinous metaplasia (diastase resistant)

Other Techniques for Diagnosis

- Noncontributory

Differential Diagnosis

TRANSITIONAL CELL CARCINOMA

- Carcinoma in situ (intraductal TCC) is typically present adjacent to the invasive component
- Infiltrative component consists of single or small groups of cells showing hyperchromatic, pleomorphic nuclei with chromatin clumping, multiple nucleoli, and angulated nuclear borders
- Mitotic figures and tumor necrosis are common
- Desmoplasia is typically associated with the invasive stromal component

SQUAMOUS AND ADENOSQUAMOUS CELL CARCINOMA

- Rare in prostate gland
- Infiltrative growth pattern composed of malignant cells with squamous features (keratin formation and intercellular bridging)
- Must exclude secondary involvement from extraprostatic sites (e.g., urinary bladder)
- Adenosquamous carcinoma composed of typical squamous cell carcinoma admixed with adenocarcinoma (patients usually have a history of radiation or hormonal therapy)

MUCINOUS ADENOCARCINOMA

- At least 25% of tumor consists of extracellular mucin lakes
- Neoplastic cells and glands float within lakes of extracellular mucin
- Cribriform pattern is most common, with mucin within the gland lumina and dissecting between the stroma
- Neoplastic cells have variable degree of cytologic atypia

PEARLS

- *None of the metaplastic cell types are associated with subsequent development of prostatic adenocarcinoma*

SELECTED REFERENCES

Leibovici D, Chiong E, Pisters LL, et al: Pathological characteristics of prostate cancer recurrence after radiation therapy: implications for focal salvage therapy. J Urol 188:98-102, 2012.

Rubin MA, Alloy Y, Molinie V, et al: Effects of long term finasteride treatment on prostate cancer morphology and clinical outcome. Urology 66:930-934, 2005.

PROSTATIC INTRAEPITHELIAL NEOPLASIA

Clinical Features

- High-grade prostatic intraepithelial neoplasia (PIN) is considered to be a premalignant condition based on morphologic, epidemiologic, and genetic features
- In autopsy series, high-grade PIN precedes carcinoma by 10 years and is common in the fourth decade of life

- Currently, high-grade PIN is associated with adenocarcinoma on rebiopsy in 25% of patients, significantly less than the 50% association reported in patients biopsied in the late 1980s (see "Pearls")
- Presence of high-grade PIN mandates rebiopsy; however, it is unclear that chasing PIN has any benefit (i.e., it simply results in the detection of clinically insignificant prostate cancers)
- Clinical significance of low-grade PIN is unclear; should not be diagnosed

Gross Pathology

- Nonspecific

Histopathology

- Low-grade PIN
  - Morphologic features not rigorously defined and subjective; should not be diagnosed
- High-grade PIN
  - Four patterns include tufted, cribriform, micropapillary, or flat
  - Cells have enlarged nuclei with prominent nucleoli (Figure 11-4)
  - Basal cells are present but may be attenuated

Special Stains and Immunohistochemistry

- HMWCK and p63: basal cell layer is immunopositive but may be thin and attenuated
- α-Methylacyl coenzyme A racemase (AMACR): high-grade PIN may be positive but more apical and granular and less intense than carcinoma

Other Techniques for Diagnosis

- Morphometric studies: high-grade PIN and adenocarcinoma have similar cytologic features (i.e., nuclear area, nuclear perimeter size, nuclear shape, amount and distribution of chromatin, and nucleolar changes)

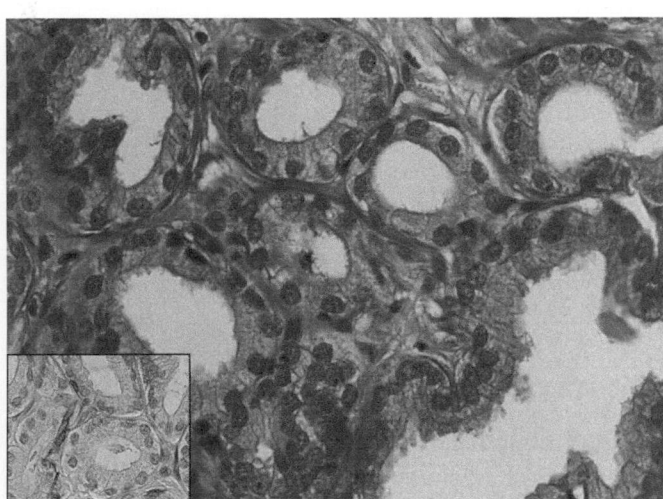

Figure 11-4. Prostatic intraepithelial neoplasia, high grade, flat type. Back-to-back glands lined by a single layer of epithelial cells with prominent nucleoli. Note the presence of attenuated basal cells (*inset*; high-molecular-weight cytokeratin immunohistochemical stain).

Differential Diagnosis

PROSTATIC ADENOCARCINOMA, LOW GRADE

- Low-power magnification reveals a uniform compact proliferation of small glands with irregular contours and irregular stromal spacing
- Neoplastic glands are lined by a single layer of epithelium (basal cell layer is absent)
- Higher magnification demonstrates cuboidal or columnar cells with abundant cytoplasm, enlarged nuclei, and prominent nucleoli
- Perineural infiltration is often present
- Negative staining for HMWCK (no basal cell layer)

PEARLS

- *The decreasing association between high-grade PIN and carcinoma is due to the following:*
  - *Increased number of cores performed per biopsy procedure with better targeting of peripheral zone*
  - *Changing patient population (younger, PSA screened) with lower prevalence or lower volume of adenocarcinoma; bayesian reasoning dictates that the positive predictive value of any test result (high-grade PIN on biopsy) is a function of the prevalence of disease (carcinoma) in the population being tested*
- *Diagnosis of high-grade PIN should be made conservatively (cells must show both nucleomegaly and nucleolomegaly)*

SELECTED REFERENCES

Dickinson SI: Premalignant and malignant prostate lesions: pathologic review. Cancer Control 17:214-222, 2010.

Iczkowski KA: Current prostate biopsy interpretation: criteria for cancer, atypical small acinar proliferation, high-grade prostatic intraepithelial neoplasia, and use of immunostains. Arch Pathol Lab Med 130:835-843, 2006.

Zynger DL, Yang X: High-grade prostatic intraepithelial neoplasia of the prostate: the precursor lesion of prostate cancer. Int J Clin Exp Pathol 2:327-338, 2009.

ADENOCARCINOMA: ACINAR (CONVENTIONAL) AND DISTINCT SUBTYPES (COLLOID [MUCINOUS], SIGNET RING CELL, DUCTAL TYPE, FOAMY GLAND, CARCINOSARCOMA [SARCOMATOID], ATROPHIC TYPE, PSEUDOHYPERPLASTIC)

Clinical Features

- Most common cause of cancer in men; second most common cause of cancer death after lung cancer
- One in five American men will be diagnosed with prostate cancer
- Occurs predominantly in men older than 50 years
- More prevalent in black men and rare in Asians
- Familial predisposition exists
- Because of the typical location of prostatic carcinoma (posterior aspects of the peripheral zone), urinary symptoms occur late; asymptomatic tumors are often detected by digital rectal examination or after routine examination that detects elevated PSA

- Advanced disease may cause obstructive symptoms (difficulty initiating or terminating urination, frequency, or dysuria)
- Metastases to bone may cause osteoblastic or osteolytic lesions; however, in men, the demonstration of osteoblastic bone metastases is virtually diagnostic of metastatic prostate carcinoma
- Back pain is a common finding in patients with metastatic disease
- Screening methods
  - Digital rectal examination: cancer focus may be nonpalpable or indurated
  - PSA levels greater than 4 ng/mL (some advocate 2 ng/mL) prompt biopsy
  - Random bilateral biopsies now standard of care in select patients with nonpalpable disease
  - Transrectal ultrasound with biopsy
- Elevated PSA is not sensitive or specific for prostatic cancer; other benign conditions, including inflammatory processes or nodular hyperplasia, may cause slight PSA elevation
- PSA levels do not distinguish between significant and insignificant cancers; identification of such biomarkers (e.g., EPCA-2, PCAs, TMPRSS2-ERG) is an active area of research
- Elevated PSA in patients after treatment for prostatic carcinoma is a useful indicator of recurrent or progressive disease

DUCTAL-TYPE ADENOCARCINOMA
- Cystoscopy often shows a polypoid lesion with extension into prostatic urethra
- Patients may present with urinary obstruction symptoms earlier than patients with typical prostatic adenocarcinoma

CARCINOSARCOMA (SARCOMATOID)
- Associated with a previous or current high-grade prostatic adenocarcinoma
- May have a history of radiation therapy for prior adenocarcinoma of prostate
- Serum PSA may be normal or only slightly elevated
- Carcinosarcoma and sarcomatoid carcinoma are often used interchangeably; however, by convention
  - *Carcinosarcoma* should be reserved for tumors that have distinct carcinomatous and sarcomatous elements by histology and immunohistochemistry
  - *Sarcomatoid carcinoma* should be used for tumors that show a transition between the two elements

Gross Pathology

ACINAR (CONVENTIONAL) ADENOCARCINOMA
- Often multifocal
- Preference for the posterior aspects of the peripheral zone (about 75% of tumors); this location renders tumor more likely to be palpable on digital rectal examination
- Small tumors typically show no gross abnormalities
- Neoplastic tissue is firm, gritty, and less spongy than the surrounding non-neoplastic prostate parenchyma; may show focal yellow discoloration

COLLOID (MUCINOUS) ADENOCARCINOMA
- Cut surface may be glistening or mucinous

DUCTAL-TYPE ADENOCARCINOMA
- May have papillary or polypoid mass extending into urethra

Histopathology (Figure 11-5)

ACINAR (CONVENTIONAL) ADENOCARCINOMA
- Constitutes more than 95% of prostate cancer
- Low-power magnification
  - Haphazard proliferation of crowded, but uniform, small acini with irregular contours; typically has an infiltrative pattern
  - Occasionally the neoplastic glands are larger and have a papillary or cribriform architecture
  - High-grade tumors tend to grow in cords, nests, or sheets
  - See Gleason grading system (Table 11-1)
- High-power magnification
  - Acini are lined by a single layer of epithelial cells; basal cell layer is absent
  - Epithelial cells are cuboidal or columnar and have abundant amphophilic cytoplasm and enlarged, variably pleomorphic nuclei with one or more prominent macronucleoli
  - Mitotic figures are a helpful feature of malignancy but are uncommon, especially in low-grade tumors
  - Features pathognomonic for carcinoma include glomeruloid structures, mucinous fibroplasias (collagenous micronodules), circumferential perineural invasion, and extraprostatic extension
  - Blue-tinged mucinous material, amorphous eosinophilic material, and crystalloid within lumina of neoplastic glands (less common in benign glands) may be seen
- Corpora amylacea is rare (much more common in benign conditions)

COLLOID (MUCINOUS) ADENOCARCINOMA
- Uncommon variant
- At least 25% of tumor consists of extracellular mucin lakes

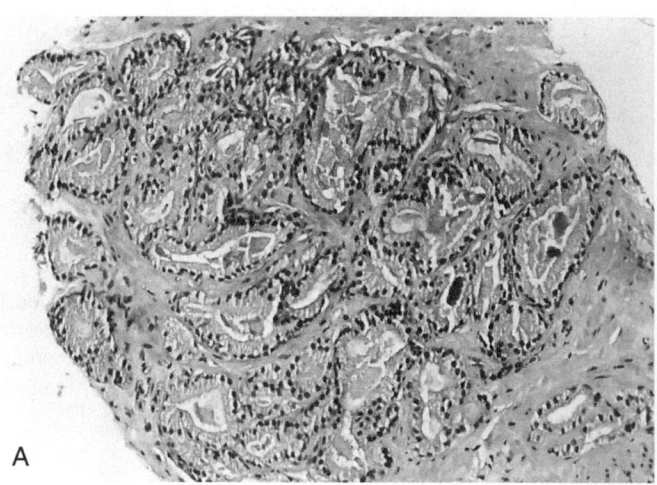

A

Figure 11-5. A, Prostatic adenocarcinoma on needle core. Gleason score 3 + 2: pattern 3 based on variability in the size of the acini, and pattern 2 based on good circumscription.

Continued

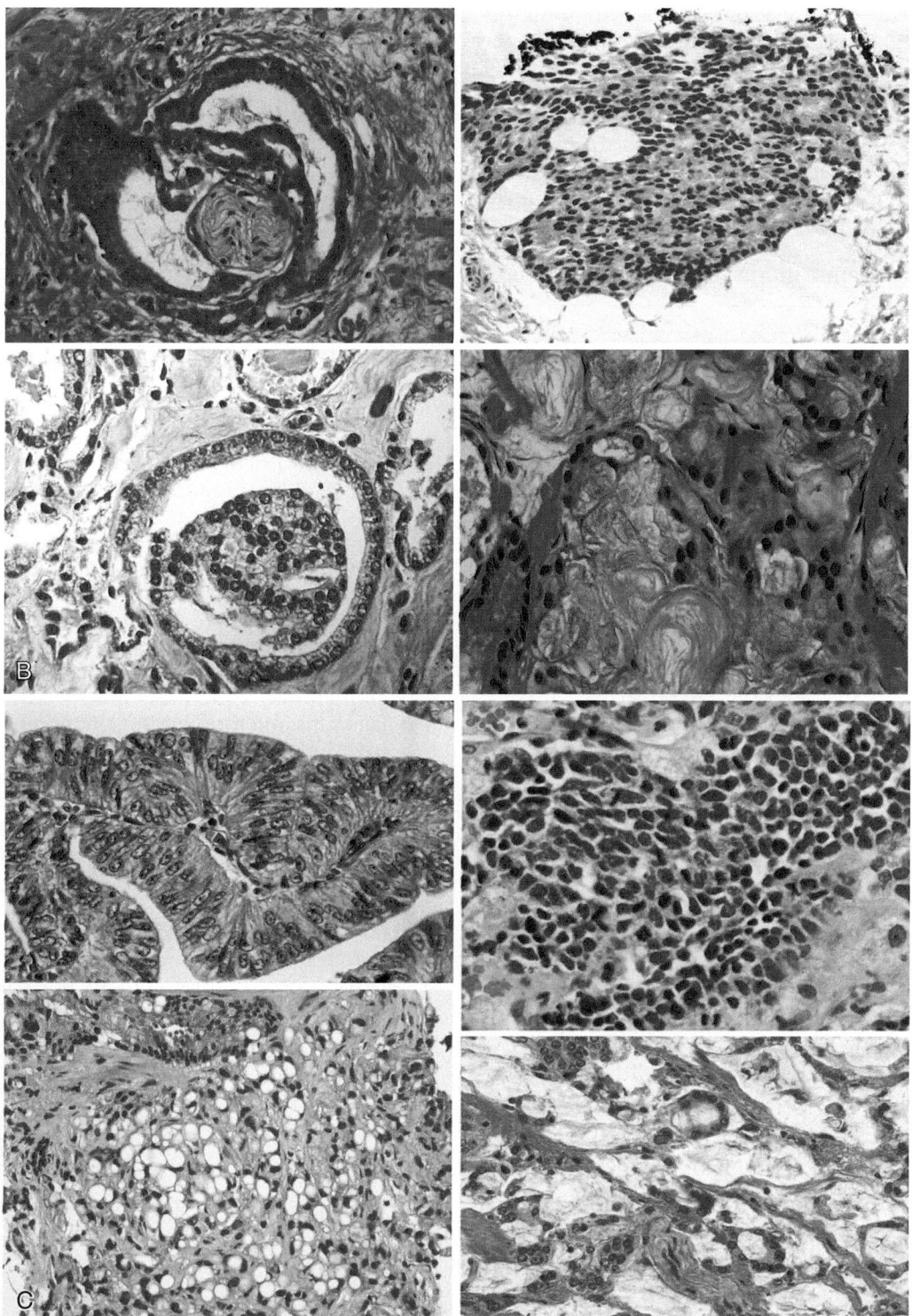

Figure 11-5—cont'd B, Histopathologic findings pathognomonic for prostatic adenocarcinoma. Circumferential perineural invasion (top left), extra-prostatic invasion (top *right*), glomeruloid bodies (*bottom left*), and mucinous fibroplasia and collagenolysis (*bottom right*). **C,** Variants of prostatic adeno-carcinoma. Ductal type showing tall columnar cells with marked nucleomegaly and nucleolomegaly (top left), neuroendocrine carcinoma in a patient with a history of treated acinar-type adenocarcinoma (*top right*), signet ring cell type with individual cells diffusely infiltrating (*bottom left*), and mucinous type with intraluminal and interstitial mucin (*bottom right*).

TABLE 11-1   **GLEASON GRADING SYSTEM**

Characteristics
- Based on a low-power view of architectural growth patterns of the tumor
- Patterns are grouped into five grades based upon ability to form glands (i.e., differentiation): Patterns range from1 through 5, with 1 being the most well differentiated
- Gleason score is the sum of the primary and secondary patterns
- If only one pattern is present, it is multiplied by 2 to get the Gleason score
- A threshold of at least 5% of the tumor no longer exists for the secondary pattern
- Grading aids in assessing malignant potential (stage and likelihood of PSA recurrence) and therapeutic decisions
- Higher scores represent poorly differentiated, highly aggressive adenocarcinomas and lower scores indicate a low malignant potential and are often of transition zone origin
- Good correlation between the prognosis and the degree of differentiation (i.e., Gleason grade)

2005 International Society of Urological Pathology Consensus Conference on Gleason Grading of Prostatic Carcinoma
- *Gleason pattern 1:* Circumscribed nodule of uniform, closely packed, medium-sized (larger than pattern 3) acini
- *Gleason pattern 2:* Like pattern 1 but less well circumscribed nodule and less uniform and more loosely arranged acini
- *Gleason pattern 3:* Infiltrative, variably sized acini -**or**- smoothly circumscribed, small cribriform glands
- *Gleason pattern 4:* Fused, irregular, infiltrative glands with poorly formed glandular lumina -**or**- smoothly circumscribed, large cribriform glands -**or**- poorly circumscribed (irregular) cribriform glands -**or**- hypernephromatoid (renal cell carcinoma-like)
- *Gleason pattern 5:* Sheets, cords or individual cells essentially lacking gland lumina -**or**- any pattern with comedo-type necrosis

Comments
- *Caveat:* Application of the 2005 consensus guidelines may result in upgrading in as many as one fourth of needle core biopsies; these changes lack rigorous clinical validation
- The primary pattern plus the highest grade pattern should be used to calculate the score on needle cores showing a tertiary pattern unless one of the patterns is less than 3; the primary pattern plus the secondary pattern should be used to calculate the score in radical prostatectomies showing a tertiary pattern with a comment on the tertiary pattern
- Grading of prostatic carcinoma variants/distinct patterns: Foamy gland, colloid (mucinous), and glomeruloid and mucinous fibroplasia (collagenous micronodule) patterns are grade 3 or 4 based upon their underlying architecture
  Signet ring cell, ductal-type, and pseudohyperplastic adenocarcinoma variants should be grade 5, 4, and 3, respectively
  Small cell, squamous, adenosquamous, and sarcomatoid carcinomas are not graded

---

- Neoplastic cells and glands float within lakes of extracellular mucin
- Cribriform pattern is most common, with mucin within the gland lumina and dissecting between stromal muscle fibers
- Neoplastic cells have variable degrees of cytologic atypia
- Typically associated with an acinar-type adenocarcinoma
- Considered Gleason grade 4 and is associated with aggressive biologic behavior

SIGNET RING CELL ADENOCARCINOMA
- At least 25% of tumor consists of cells with a cytoplasmic vacuole that displaces the nucleus to the side
- Cells diffusely infiltrate the stroma and invade perineural and vascular spaces as well as the prostatic capsule
- Other patterns of prostatic adenocarcinoma in the same tumor are typically seen

DUCTAL-TYPE ADENOCARCINOMA
- Located in the larger periurethral prostatic ducts and usually found in association with acinar-type adenocarcinoma
- Papillary and cribriform architecture composed of pseudostratified columnar cells; comedo necrosis may be seen
- Neoplastic cells have atypical large nuclei with coarse chromatin and large nucleoli
- Mitotic figures are common
- Considered Gleason grade 4 (or 5 if comedo necrosis is present); some consider this a subset of acinar adenocarcinoma, Gleason grade 4

FOAMY GLAND ADENOCARCINOMA
- Histologically characterized by cells with abundant foamy cytoplasm and bland nuclei
- May be underdiagnosed on needle core because of lack of nucleomegaly and nucleolomegaly
- Usually associated with higher-Gleason-score acinar-type adenocarcinoma; therefore, prognostic significance per se unclear

PSEUDOHYPERPLASTIC ADENOCARCINOMA
- Two patterns on low-power microscopy
  - Crowded glands lined by pseudostratified epithelium (truly pseudohyperplastic)
  - Large acini
- High-power microscopy shows nucleomegaly and nucleolomegaly
- May be underdiagnosed on needle core biopsy because the pseudostratified epithelium looks like hyperplasia or high-grade PIN on low-power microscopy and the large acinar pattern deviates from the more typical small acinar pattern

CARCINOSARCOMA (SARCOMATOID)
- Biphasic tumor: admixture of carcinoma and sarcoma components
- Sarcoma component consists of spindle cells with pleomorphic nuclei and high mitotic rate
- Common sarcoma patterns
  - Malignant fibrous histiocytoma-like
  - High-grade sarcoma-like, not otherwise specified
  - Fibrosarcoma-like
  - Leiomyosarcoma-like

- Elements resembling osteosarcoma, rhabdomyosarcoma, or chondrosarcoma may be present
- Carcinoma component is usually high grade

ATROPHIC-TYPE ADENOCARCINOMA
- Glandular proliferation with an infiltrative growth pattern
- Neoplastic cells have large nuclei with prominent nucleoli
- Glands lack a basal cell layer
- Generally associated with an adjacent acinar adenocarcinoma

TREATED ADENOCARCINOMA
- Androgen deprivation therapy
  - Smaller acini or single cells with loss of nucleolomegaly and cytoplasmic clearing (special stains may be required); residual carcinoma showing treatment effect should not be Gleason graded
  - Adjacent benign tissue shows stromal hyperplasia and gland involution with BCH and squamous metaplasia
- Radiation therapy
  - Smaller acini or single cells with cytoplasmic vacuolization (special stains may be required); residual carcinoma showing treatment effect should not be Gleason graded
  - Adjacent benign tissue shows glandular atrophy, nucleomegaly, nucleolomegaly, and BCH

Special Stains and Immunohistochemistry
- AMACR
  - Sensitive and specific marker for conventional (acinar) prostate cancer; positive in 82% to 100% of cases
  - Less sensitive in low-grade and hormone-treated conventional prostate cancer and prostate cancer variants, such as foamy gland, pseudohyperplastic, atrophic-type, and ductal-type prostate cancers
  - Positive but less intense, noncircumferential or only focal in high-grade PIN, atypical adenomatous hyperplasia, atrophy, nephrogenic adenoma, and benign glands adjacent to cancer
  - AMACR is less useful in evaluating metastases because many tumors in other organs are immunopositive
- HMWCK and p63
  - Stains basal cell cytoplasm (HMWCK) and nuclei (p63); therefore, negative in adenocarcinoma because basal cells are absent
- PSA and prostatic acid phosphatase (PAP) positive for tumor cells of mucinous, signet ring cell, and ductal-type variants of adenocarcinoma; also positive in epithelial component of carcinosarcoma
- Carcinoembryonic antigen (CEA) positive in some ductal-type variants of carcinoma
- Vimentin: spindle cell component of carcinosarcoma positive
- Desmin, smooth muscle actin (SMA), and S-100 protein: variable positivity in spindle cell component of carcinosarcoma

Other Techniques for Diagnosis
- Genetic studies: familial studies have demonstrated an 8q24 genetic variant that may be associated with prostate cancer risk; TMPRSS2-ERG fusion has been identified as an early molecular event in the development of prostate cancer
- Flow cytometry: diploid tumors have a more favorable outcome than tumors that are aneuploid

Differential Diagnosis

SCLEROSING ADENOSIS
- Lobular or focally infiltrative glandular proliferation composed of glands with a double cell layer (may be difficult to appreciate) and a thickened basement membrane
- Cells contain medium-sized to large nuclei with fine chromatin and indistinct nucleoli
- Stromal component contains plump spindle cells arranged randomly or in fascicles
- Cellular spindle cell component is positive for actin and S-100 protein (indicates myoepithelial differentiation)

ATYPICAL ADENOMATOUS HYPERPLASIA (ADENOSIS)
- Architecturally similar to Gleason grade 1 or 2 adenocarcinoma
- Circumscribed proliferation of variably sized acini that may show focal infiltration at the periphery
- Tightly packed small glands intermixed with larger glands
- Basal cell layer may be discontinuous and indistinct but is usually focally present in at least some glands (positive staining for HMWCK)
- Glandular cells typically have pale to clear cytoplasm, small nuclei, and inconspicuous nucleoli; distinct nucleoli may occasionally be seen; however, macronucleoli (> 3 μm) should not be present
- Corpora amylacea is often present (much less common in adenocarcinoma)
- Often seen adjacent to unequivocal adenocarcinoma

HIGH-GRADE PROSTATIC INTRAEPITHELIAL NEOPLASIA (PIN)
- Usually large acini lined by hyperplastic, pseudostratified epithelial cells with elongated, large nuclei with prominent nucleoli
- The "flat type" of PIN may show small acini with a single cell layer
- Basal cell markers (HMWCK or p63) often show attenuated basal cells
- AMACR often shows granular, apical cytoplasmic positivity in contrast to more diffuse staining seen in carcinoma

GLANDULAR ATROPHY AND PARTIAL ATROPHY/POSTATROPHIC HYPERPLASIA
- Atrophic glands may have a focally infiltrative architecture and thus may mimic atrophic-type adenocarcinoma
- Atrophic glands have open lumens and are lined by cells with an increased nuclear-to-cytoplasmic ratio and inconspicuous nucleoli
- Atrophic-type adenocarcinoma is associated with an adjacent acinar adenocarcinoma

CLEAR CELL CRIBRIFORM HYPERPLASIA VERSUS CRIBRIFORM ADENOCARCINOMA
- Cells in clear cell cribriform hyperplasia have distinct clear cytoplasm, small nuclei with indistinct nucleoli, and a prominent basal cell layer

TRANSITIONAL CELL CARCINOMA

- Typically, TCC involves the urethra or prostatic ducts in patients with a history of carcinoma in situ of the urinary bladder who have been treated conservatively
- Carcinoma in situ (intraductal TCC) is typically present adjacent to the invasive component
- Lacks glandular differentiation
- Mitotic figures and tumor necrosis are common
- Stains negative for PSA and PAP

ADDITIONAL MICROSCOPIC MIMICS OF PROSTATIC ADENOCARCINOMA:

- Basal cell hyperplasia, Cowper's glands, mesonephric remnant hyperplasia, mucous gland metaplasia, nephrogenic adenoma, paraganglion tissue, radiation changes, seminal vesicles/ejaculatory duct, squamous metaplasia, urothelial metaplasia, verumontanum mucosal hyperplasia, and xanthoma cells

PEARLS

- *Prostatic carcinoma is typically multifocal, and gross examination usually underestimates the extent of disease*
- *Tumors of the transitional zone are less aggressive than tumors of the peripheral zone*
- *Metastases typically involve the pelvic or para-aortic lymph nodes and axial skeleton (most commonly lumbar vertebrae)*
- *Only in recent years has a survival advantage been demonstrated with the onset of widespread PSA screening; however, this same advantage has also been observed in Europe, where PSA screening is less common*
- *AMACR staining quality may be affected by technologist expertise, run-to-run variability, and the use of monoclonal (P504S) versus polyclonal antibodies, with the latter showing more background staining*
- *Total androgen blockade therapy is commonly used as an adjunct to postradiation therapy for treatment of adenocarcinoma metastases*
  - *Luteinizing hormone–releasing hormone agonists (e.g., leuprolide)*
  - *Direct antiandrogens (e.g., flutamide)*
- *Endocrine therapy is used to deprive tumor cells of testosterone and is typically used in patients with widespread metastatic disease (orchiectomy or estrogen administration decreases or eliminates testicular production of testosterone)*
- *Cryotherapy and radiation implants are being used more frequently as alternatives to radical prostatectomy*
- *In general, the presence of lymph node metastases precludes radical prostatectomy*
- *Small prostatectomies should be completely submitted for histopathologic examination, but larger prostatectomies may be partially submitted as long as all of the posterior aspect, apex, and base are submitted (see Iremashvili et al., 2013); the 2010 TNM guidelines require documentation of the following:*
  - *Volume and laterality of tumor*
  - *Status of the prostate pseudocapsule (intact or disrupted)*
  - *Extent of involvement of the pseudocapsule ("not involved," "penetration without perforation," or "extracapsular extension" [T3a])*
  - *Presence or absence of seminal vesicle invasion (T3b)*
  - *Presence or absence of invasion of adjacent structures including external sphincter, rectum, bladder, levator muscles, or pelvic wall (T4)*
  - *Gleason score, which is now the preferred grading system*
- *Ten-year survival rate for all stages of adenocarcinoma is about 50%*
  - *Localized tumor: 10-year survival rate is 95%*
  - *Adenocarcinoma with metastases to regional lymph nodes: 40% survival at 10 years*
  - *Adenocarcinoma with metastases to distant organs: 10% survival at 10 years*

SELECTED REFERENCES

Berney DM, Fisher G, Kattan MW, et al: Pitfalls in the diagnosis of prostate cancer: retrospective review of 1791 cases with clinical outcome. Histopathology 51:452-457, 2007.

Bostwick DG, Meiers I: Atypical small acinar proliferation in the prostate: clinical significance in 2006. Arch Pathol Lab Med 130:952-957, 2006.

Clyne M: Prostate cancer: TMPRSS2: ERG—the root of the problem? Nature Rev Urol 10:248, 2013.

Edge SB, Byrd DR, Compton CC, et al (eds): AJCC Cancer Staging Manual, 7th ed. New York, Springer, 2010, pp 457-468.

Egevad L, Mazzucchelli R, Montironi R: Implications of the International Society of Urological Pathology Modified Gleason Grading System. Arch Pathol Lab Med 136:426-434, 2012.

Epstein JI, Allsbrook WC, Amin MB, et al: The 2005 International Society of Urological Pathology (ISUP) consensus conference on Gleason grading of prostatic carcinoma. Am J Surg Pathol 29:1228-1242, 2005.

Iczkowski KA: Current prostate biopsy interpretation: criteria for cancer, atypical small acinar proliferation, high-grade prostatic intraepithelial neoplasia, and use of immunostains. Arch Pathol Lab Med 130:835-843, 2006.

Iremashvili V, Lokeshwar SD, Soloway MS, et al: Partial sampling of radical prostatectomy specimens: detection of positive margins and extraprostatic extension. Am J Surg Pathol 37:219-225, 2013.

Kristiansen G: Diagnostic and prognostic molecular markers for prostate cancer. Histopathol 60:125-141, 2012.

Prensner JR, Rubin MA, Wei JT, et al: Beyond PSA: the next generation of prostate cancer biomarkers. Sci Transl Med 4:127rv3, 2012.

Srigley JR and Members of the Cancer Committee, College of American Pathologists: Updated protocol for the examination of specimens from patients with carcinomas of the prostate gland. Arch Pathol Lab Med 130:936-946, 2006.

ADENOID CYSTIC/BASAL CELL CARCINOMA

Clinical Features

- Serum PSA and PAP levels are typically not elevated
- Benign and malignant basal cell lesions are relatively uncommon (reported in less than 6% to 9% of cases); benign basal cell proliferations make up most of them

Gross Pathology

- Nonspecific

Histopathology

- Basal cell tumors consist of a spectrum of disease ranging from BCH to atypical BCH to basal cell adenoma to basal cell carcinoma (BCC); historically a, basal cell tumor with a cribriform architecture has been referred to as an adenoid basal cell tumor or adenoid cystic carcinoma (ACC); BCC and ACC are now considered parts of a morphologic continuum

BASAL CELL CARCINOMA

- Infiltrative clusters of basaloid cells
- Often have prominent desmoplastic stromal response
- Must demonstrate one or more of the following features: necrosis, perineural invasion, or infiltration outside prostatic capsule

BASAL CELL CARCINOMA WITH CRIBRIFORM SPACES (ADENOID CYSTIC CARCINOMA)

- Histologic features similar to those of adenoid cystic carcinoma of the salivary glands
- Cells form poorly circumscribed, infiltrative nodules surrounded by a loose or myxoid stroma
- Nests show peripheral nuclear palisading around adenoid cystlike spaces that contain mucinous, eosinophilic, or hyaline material
- Focal squamous differentiation with keratin production may be seen
- Basaloid cells are uniform and have round hyperchromatic nuclei
- Perineural invasion is rare
- Low malignant potential; no reports of metastasis (believed by some authors to be part of BCH and adenoma)

Special Stains and Immunohistochemistry

- PSA and PAP typically positive
- HMWK: focal weak positivity in basaloid cells

Other Techniques for Diagnosis

- Noncontributory

Differential Diagnosis

BASAL CELL HYPERPLASIA

- Often see other findings of androgen blockade including stromal and glandular involution and squamous metaplasia
- Lacks cytologic atypicality, infiltrative growth and desmoplasia seen in adenoid cystic/basal cell carcinoma

SCLEROSING ADENOSIS

- Lobular or focally infiltrative proliferation composed of glands with a double cell layer (may be difficult to appreciate) and a thickened basement membrane
- Cells contain medium-sized to large nuclei with fine chromatin and indistinct nucleoli
- Cellular spindle cell stroma with evidence of myoepithelial differentiation demonstrated by positive staining for S-100 protein and MSA

ATYPICAL ADENOMATOUS HYPERPLASIA

- Circumscribed proliferation of variably sized acini that may show focal infiltration at the periphery
- Tightly packed small glands intermixed with larger glands
- Some glands may show a basal cell layer (positive for HMWCK)

- Glandular cells typically have pale to clear cytoplasm, small nuclei, and inconspicuous nucleoli; prominent nucleoli may occasionally be seen; however, macronucleoli (> 3 μm) should not be present

ADENOCARCINOMA, CRIBRIFORM TYPE

- Typical cytologic features of malignancy, including cuboidal or columnar cells with abundant amphophilic cytoplasm, enlarged nuclei, and one or more prominent macronucleoli
- Absence of basal cell layer (negative for HMWCK)

PEARLS

- *Typically treated with transurethral resection; controversy still exists regarding treatment for basal cell carcinoma*
- *Basal cell lesions in the prostate form a spectrum of disease behavior that is typically benign*
- *Malignant behavior in adenoid basal cell tumor has not been demonstrated*

SELECTED REFERENCES

Ali TZ, Epstein JI: Basal cell carcinoma of the prostate: a clinicopathologic study of 29 cases. Am J Surg Pathol 31:697-705, 2007.
Begnami MD, Quezado M, Pinto P, et al: Adenoid cystic / basal cell carcinoma of the prostate: review and update. Arch Pathol Lab Med 131:637-640, 2007.
Fine SW: Variants and unusual patterns of prostate cancer: clinicopathologic and differential diagnostic considerations. Adv Anat Pathol 19:204-216, 2012.
Humphry PA: Histological variants of prostatic carcinoma and their significance. Histopathol 60:59-74, 2012.
Tan PH, Billis A: Basal cell carcinoma. In Eble JN, Sauter G, Epstein JI, Sesterhenn IA (eds): World Health Organization Classification of Tumours: Pathology and Genetics: Tumours of the Urinary System and Male Genital Organs. Lyon, IARC Press, 2004, p 206.

NEUROENDOCRINE (SMALL CELL) CARCINOMA

Clinical Features

- Rarely occurs de novo; patients usually have a history of treated prostate cancer
- Most show no evidence of hormonal secretion; however, paraneoplastic syndromes can occur
  - Cushing syndrome (most common)
  - Malignant hypercalcemia
  - Syndrome of inappropriate antidiuretic hormone (SIADH)
  - Eaton-Lambert syndrome
- May have minor elevations of serum PSA
- Metastasizes through hematogenous (liver, brain) rather than lymphatic channels

Gross Pathology

- Nonspecific

Histopathology

- Histologic features similar to those of small cell carcinoma of the lung
- Necrosis is commonly seen in small cell carcinoma
- Typical acinar pattern of adenocarcinoma is present in more than 50% of cases; the neuroendocrine component should not be assigned a Gleason score

Special Stains and Immunohistochemistry

- Neuron-specific enolase (NSE), chromogranin, and cytokeratin typically positive
- PSA and PAP: often negative or only focally positive
- AMACR: 50% positive
- Secretory products may be present within neoplastic cells
  - Adrenocorticotropic hormone (ACTH), serotonin, calcitonin, human chorionic gonadotropin (HCG), thyroid-stimulating hormone (TSH), and bombesin

Other Techniques for Diagnosis

- Electron microscopy: neuroendocrine cells contain round, regular membrane-bound neurosecretory granules, measuring 100 to 400 nm

Differential Diagnosis

METASTATIC SMALL CELL CARCINOMA FROM BLADDER OR LUNG

- Clinical history is important
- Lacks associated acinar adenocarcinoma that is usually seen in primary neuroendocrine carcinoma of the prostate gland
- Thyroid transcription factor-1 (TTF-1) immunostain not useful

NON-HODGKIN LYMPHOMA

- Primary prostatic lymphoma is rare
- Neoplastic lymphoid population infiltrating around ducts and acini (typically spares prostatic glands)
- Infiltration into surrounding periprostatic tissue is common
- Positive for leukocyte common antigen (LCA)
- Negative for cytokeratin, NSE, chromogranin, and other neuroendocrine markers

PEARLS

- *Many acinar-type prostatic adenocarcinomas show immunohistochemical evidence of neuroendocrine differentiation, the significance of which is unknown*
- *Neuroendocrine carcinoma of the prostate may respond to small cell carcinoma–directed chemotherapy but is clinically aggressive*
- *Neuroendocrine carcinoma is more aggressive when androgen receptors are expressed (10 months' survival time versus more than 30 months' survival time)*

SELECTED REFERENCES

di Sant'Agnese PA, Egevad L, Epstein JI, et al: Neuroendocrine tumors. In Eble JN, Sauter G, Epstein JI, Sesterhenn IA (eds): World Health Organization Classification of Tumours: Pathology and Genetics: Tumours of the Urinary System and Male Genital Organs. Lyon, IARC Press, 2004, pp 207-208.

Fine SW: Variants and unusual patterns of prostate cancer: clinicopathologic and differential diagnostic considerations. Adv Anat Pathol 19:204-216, 2012.

Furtado P, Lima MVA, Nogueira C, et al: Review of small cell carcinomas of the prostate. Prostate Cancer, 2011:543272, 2011.

Humphry PA: Histological variants of prostatic carcinoma and their significance. Histopathol 60:59-74, 2012.

TRANSITIONAL CELL CARCINOMA

Clinical Features

- Rare primary prostate gland tumor (represents 1% to 3% of primary prostatic gland malignancies)
- Common symptoms include hematuria or urinary obstruction
- PSA not elevated
- Three modes of prostatic involvement
  - Primary tumor of prostatic urethra, ducts, or acini
  - Secondary mucosal involvement from a prior or currently active bladder cancer
  - Direct invasion from bladder cancer infiltrating through the bladder wall

Gross Pathology

- Nodular proliferation in prostatic urethra
- Nonspecific nodular architecture with involvement of prostatic ducts and acini

Histopathology

- Carcinoma in situ (intraductal TCC) is typically present adjacent to the invasive component; may involve the urethra, the prostatic ducts and acini, and occasionally the ejaculatory ducts and seminal vesicles
- Infiltrative component consists of small groups or single cells with hyperchromatic, pleomorphic nuclei with chromatin clumping, multiple nucleoli, and angulated nuclear borders
- Mitotic figures and tumor necrosis are common
- Elicits a desmoplastic stromal reaction
- Pagetoid spread and squamous metaplasia may be seen

Special Stains and Immunohistochemistry

- HMWCK, CK7, and CK20 variably positive
- PSA and PAP negative

Other Techniques for Diagnosis

- Noncontributory

Differential Diagnosis

PROSTATIC ADENOCARCINOMA

- Gleason grade 5 adenocarcinoma with comedo necrosis may be difficult to distinguish from TCC
- Focal gland formation can typically be found after careful evaluation of multiple sections
- Not associated with TCC in situ
- Positive for PSA, PAP, or AMACR

PEARLS

- *Typically TCC involves the urethra or prostatic ducts in patients with a history of carcinoma in situ of the bladder who have been treated*
- *Prostatic urethra urothelial carcinoma involving the prostate can rarely be mucinous (urothelial mucinous adenocarcinoma of the prostate)*
- *Prostatic stromal involvement by TCC is by definition stage T4 disease and carries a poor prognosis*
- *Radical cystoprostatectomy is the typical treatment*

SELECTED REFERENCES

Fine SW: Variants and unusual patterns of prostate cancer: clinicopathologic and differential diagnostic considerations. Adv Anat Pathol 19:204-216, 2012.

Grignon DJ: Urothelial carcinoma. In Eble JN, Sauter G, Epstein JI, Sesterhenn IA (eds): World Health Organization Classification of Tumours: Pathology and Genetics: Tumours of the Urinary System and Male Genital Organs. Lyon, IARC Press, 2004, pp 202-204.

Humphry PA: Histological variants of prostatic carcinoma and their significance. Histopathol 60:59-74, 2012.

Srinivasan M, Parwani AV: Diagnostic utility of p63/P501S double sequential immunohistochemical staining in differentiating urothelial carcinoma from prostate carcinoma. Diagn Pathol 6:67-73, 2011.

SQUAMOUS CELL CARCINOMA AND ADENOSQUAMOUS CARCINOMA

Clinical Features

- Rare in the prostate gland
- Typically found in older age group (mean age of about 70 years)
- Two clinical scenarios
  - Primary, de novo squamous cell carcinoma
  - Associated with treated (radiation or hormone ablation) adenocarcinoma
- Serum PSA and PAP are usually normal
- Metastatic bone lesions osteolytic, in contrast to adenocarcinoma, which causes osteoblastic bone lesions
- Most commonly associated with squamous cell carcinoma of the urinary bladder

- May be associated with *Schistosoma haematobium* infection

Gross Pathology (Figure 11-6A)

- Nonspecific

Histopathology

- Similar histologic features to squamous cell carcinoma of other sites
- Malignant squamous cells arranged in cords and nests with an infiltrative architecture
- Two forms of carcinoma
  - Pure squamous carcinoma
    - Rare
    - Infiltrative growth pattern composed of malignant cells with squamous features (keratin formation and intercellular bridging) (Figure 11-6B,C)
    - No gland formation
    - No patient history of radiation or hormonal therapy
    - Must exclude secondary involvement from extraprostatic sites (e.g., bladder)
  - Adenosquamous carcinoma
    - Admixture of adenocarcinoma and squamous cell carcinoma
    - Typically associated with a history of radiation or hormonal therapy

Special Stains and Immunohistochemistry

- PSA and PAP are positive in glandular component of adenosquamous carcinoma; pure squamous cell carcinoma is typically negative

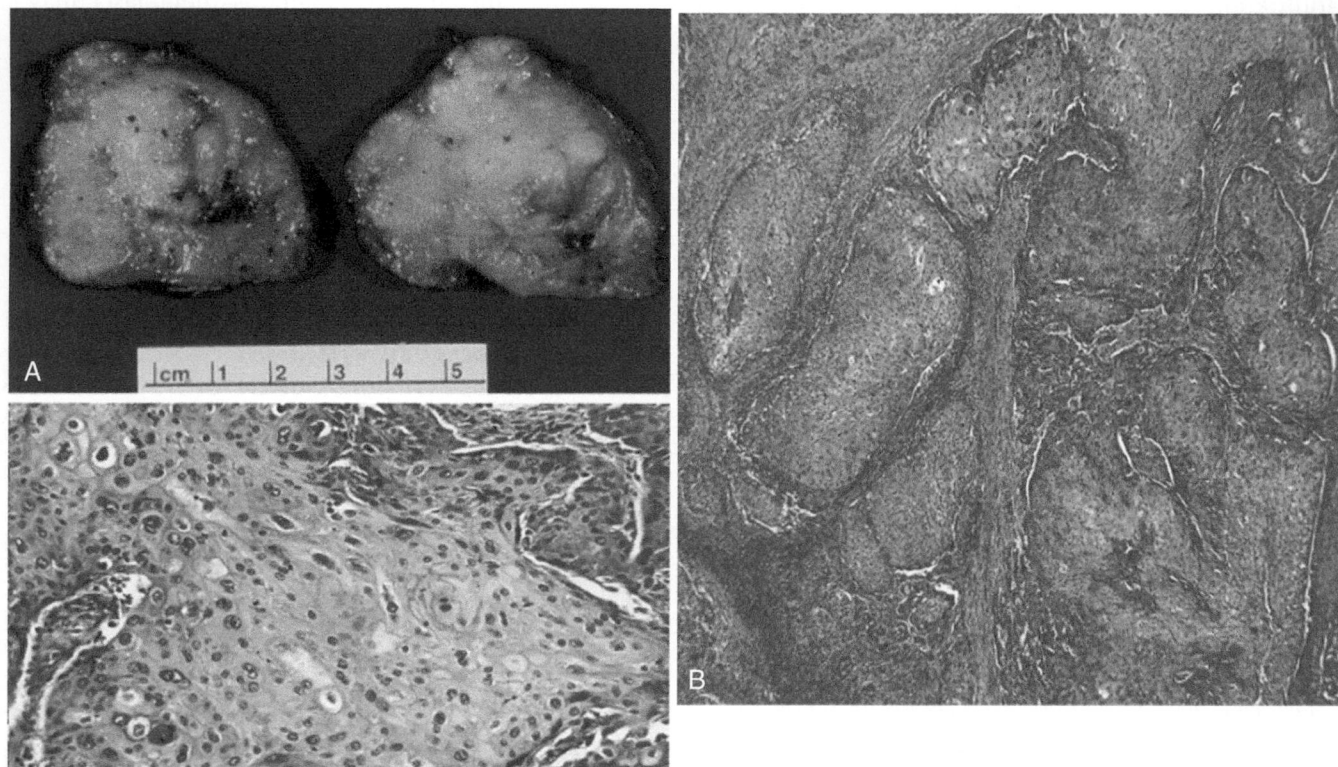

Figure 11-6. Primary squamous cell carcinoma of the prostate. A, Cross sections showing nodular growth replacing the gland. Low-power **(B)** and high-power **(C)** photomicrographs showing infiltrative squamous cell carcinoma with keratinization.

Other Techniques for Diagnosis

- Noncontributory

Differential Diagnosis

SQUAMOUS METAPLASIA

- Commonly associated with prostatic infarction
- Lacks significant cytologic atypia and tumor necrosis

PROSTATIC PRIMARY

- Much more common to have a squamous cell carcinoma in the prostate gland as metastatic disease or direct extension from adjacent organs (i.e., urinary bladder) than as a prostatic primary

PEARLS

- *Behaves in an aggressive manner (mean survival of 14 months, regardless of therapy)*
- *Unresponsive to androgen-deprivation therapy*

SELECTED REFERENCES

Arva NC, Das K: Diagnostic dilemmas of squamous differentiation in prostate carcinoma: case report and review of the literature. Diagn Pathol 6:46-54, 2011.

Fine SW: Variants and unusual patterns of prostate cancer: clinicopathologic and differential diagnostic considerations. Adv Anat Pathol 19:204-216, 2012.

Humphry PA: Histological variants of prostatic carcinoma and their significance. Histopathol 60:59-74, 2012.

Van der Kwast TH: Squamous neoplasms. In Eble JN, Sauter G, Epstein JI, Sesterhenn IA (eds): World Health Organization Classification of Tumours: Pathology and Genetics: Tumours of the Urinary System and Male Genital Organs. Lyon, IARC Press, 2004, pp 205-206.

PHYLLODES TUMOR

Clinical Features

- Rare neoplasm
- Wide age range
- Patients present with symptoms associated with prostatic enlargement, which include urinary obstruction, hematuria, and dysuria

Gross Pathology

- Multinodular solid, gray-white mass
- Cut surface may be spongy or cystic
- Variable size; may be larger than 25 cm in diameter

Histopathology

- Biphasic tumor composed of epithelial and stromal components
  - Epithelial cells are cuboidal to columnar, arranged in a double-layer lining glands, cysts, or slitlike spaces
  - Stellate to spindle stromal cells arranged in a loose, myxoid background
- Glandular or cystic spaces compressed by cellular stroma into a leaflike configuration (Figure 11-7)
- Likelihood of recurrence and malignant behavior is associated with a high stromal to epithelial ratio (stromal hypercellularity), cellular atypia, and high mitotic rate

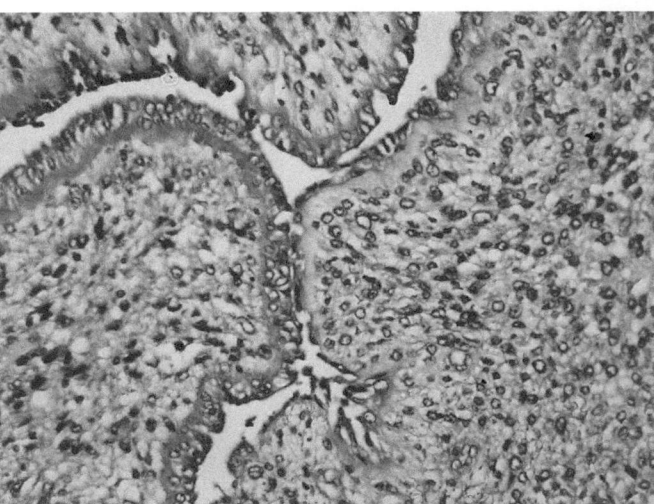

Figure 11-7. Prostatic phyllodes tumor. Proliferation of specialized prostatic stroma bulging into prostatic glands and creating clefted spaces.

Special Stains and Immunohistochemistry

- Vimentin: stromal component is typically positive
- PSA and PAP: epithelial cells may be positive
- SMA negative

Other Techniques for Diagnosis

- Noncontributory

Differential Diagnosis

STROMAL HYPERPLASIA

- Benign prostatic hyperplasia nodule with stromal overgrowth may be large
- Lacks epithelial component and leaflike configuration

GIANT MULTILOCULAR PROSTATIC CYSTADENOMA

- Solitary cystic tumor with a surrounding dense fibrous stroma
- Numerous, variably sized cystic spaces lined by a benign-appearing prostatic epithelium
- Lacks leaflike configuration

POSTOPERATIVE SPINDLE CELL PROLIFERATION

- Rare reactive spindle cell proliferation that may occur after transurethral prostate resection (previously resected prostate tissue must show no evidence of a mesenchymal or spindle cell tumor)
- Benign cytologic features and variable mitotic rate (uniform cells with no nuclear pleomorphism and no atypical mitotic figures)
- Lacks epithelial component

SOLITARY FIBROUS TUMOR OF THE PROSTATE

- Low-power view has variable cellularity and lacks leaflike configuration
- High-power view has spindled cells insinuating themselves into bands of collagen

LEIOMYOMA OR LEIOMYOSARCOMA

- Monophasic hypercellular spindle cell neoplasm without epithelial component
- Positive for SMA and desmin

SARCOMATOID CARCINOMA

- Malignant spindle cell proliferation admixed with a malignant epithelial component
- Spindle cell component may predominate; cytokeratin positivity, the distinguishing feature, may be weak and focal

PEARLS

- *Most are cured by surgical resection and follow a benign clinical course; however, biologic behavior is difficult to predict based on histologic features*
- *Tumors with overtly malignant stromal component have given rise to distant metastases (most commonly lung and bone)*
- *Diagnosis on needle biopsy may be difficult*

SELECTED REFERENCES

Cheville J, Algaba F, Boccon-Gibod L, et al: Mesenchymal tumors. In Eble JN, Sauter G, Epstein JI, Sesterhenn IA (eds): World Health Organization Classification of Tumours: Pathology and Genetics: Tumours of the Urinary System and Male Genital Organs. Lyon, IARC Press, 2004, pp 209-211.

Paner GP, Aron M, Hansel DE, et al: Non-epithelial neoplasms of the prostate. Histopathol 60:166-186, 2012.

Tavora F, Kryvenko ON, Epstein JI: Mesenchymal tumors of the bladder and prostate: an update. Pathol 45:104-115, 2013.

RHABDOMYOSARCOMA

Clinical Features

- Most common sarcoma of the prostate
- Occurs primarily between birth and 6 years of age
- Most common in the head and neck, followed by the genitourinary tract
- About 20% of childhood cases occur in the genitourinary tract
- Rare cases reported in older men
- Presents with pelvic mass and urethral obstruction
- Pelvic mass may cause bladder displacement and rectal compression

Gross Pathology

- Large, gray-white mass typically measuring 5 to 10 cm
- Appears grossly circumscribed but is typically infiltrative microscopically

Histopathology

EMBRYONAL RHABDOMYOSARCOMA

- Most common subtype
- Mixture of sheets of primitive, undifferentiated, round to spindle cells admixed with haphazardly arranged rhabdomyoblasts in a myxoid stroma
- Primitive cells are small and round with dark nuclei and minimal cytoplasm
- Variable numbers of strap cells, with or without cross-striations
- Variable mitotic activity

ALVEOLAR, BOTRYOID, AND PLEOMORPHIC PATTERNS

- These patterns are rare
- Botryoid pattern consists of polypoid fragments covered with urothelium that often extends into the urethra or bladder

Special Stains and Immunohistochemistry

- Vimentin, MSA, desmin, and myoglobin positive
- Stains negatively for cytokeratin, LCA, NSE, PSA, and PAP

Other Techniques for Diagnosis

- Electron microscopy: rhabdomyoblasts have cytoplasmic myofilaments and Z bands
- Flow cytometry: tumor cells are typically aneuploid

Differential Diagnosis

- Must rule out metastasis from other primitive childhood small round blue cell tumors
- Non-Hodgkin lymphoma
  - Typically found in older age groups
  - Neoplastic lymphoid cells infiltrating stroma in diffuse sheets or patches; ducts and acini are typically spared
  - Positive for LCA
  - Composed of a monoclonal lymphoid population

PEARLS

- *Presence of strap cells or rhabdomyoblasts is diagnostic*
- *Treatment typically consists of surgery, chemotherapy, and radiotherapy*
- *The prostate and urinary bladder are considered "unfavorable prognosis" sites*

SELECTED REFERENCES

Ferrer FA, Isakoff M, Koyle MA: Bladder/prostate rhabdomyosarcoma: past, present and future. J Urol 176:1283-1291, 2006.

Janet NL, May AW, Akins RS: Sarcoma of the prostate: a single institution review. Am J Clin Pathol 32:27-29, 2009.

LYMPHOMA

Clinical Features

- Most common in older men (mean age, 60 years)
- Presents with urinary obstruction symptoms
- Primary lymphoma involves the prostate gland without extraglandular involvement (i.e., liver, spleen, lymph nodes, peripheral blood)
- Secondary involvement of the prostate gland by a systemic lymphoma is more common than primary prostate lymphoma
- Systemic symptoms (fever, chills, night sweats, and weight loss) are infrequent and typically seen only in patients with disseminated disease

Gross Pathology

- Diffuse enlargement of the prostate gland
- Tan, homogeneous, rubbery parenchyma

Histopathology

- Proliferation of neoplastic lymphoid cells that typically infiltrate the prostatic stroma in diffuse sheets while sparing the ducts and acini
- Infiltration into surrounding periprostatic tissues is common
- Most common subtype is diffuse large cell lymphoma, B-cell type; small cleaved cell lymphoma is also relatively common
- Hodgkin disease is rare

Special Stains and Immunohistochemistry

- LCA positive (non-Hodgkin lymphoma)
- Refer to Chapter 14 for specific immunohistochemistry profiles

Other Techniques for Diagnosis

- Flow cytometric immunophenotyping using fresh tissue is useful in documenting clonality and for subtyping lymphomas (refer to Chapter 14)

Differential Diagnosis

CHRONIC PROSTATITIS WITH FOLLICULAR HYPERPLASIA

- Mixed inflammatory infiltrate with germinal center formation
- Inflammation is typically within duct lumina and in the glandular epithelium
- Nonclonal lymphocytic population

GRANULOMATOUS PROSTATITIS

- Admixture of histiocytes, plasma cells, eosinophils, neutrophils, lymphocytes, and giant cells
- Inflammatory cells cause destruction of the prostatic ducts and acini

NEUROENDOCRINE CARCINOMA

- Characteristic prostatic adenocarcinoma associated with a neuroendocrine carcinoma, which may range from a low-grade neuroendocrine carcinoma (carcinoid) to a small cell undifferentiated carcinoma (oat cell carcinoma)
- Areas of necrosis are typical in small cell carcinoma
- Positive for cytokeratin, NSE, chromogranin, and other neuroendocrine markers
- Negative for LCA

RHABDOMYOSARCOMA

- Typically found in younger age group
- Mixture of sheets of primitive, undifferentiated, round to spindle cells admixed with haphazardly arranged rhabdomyoblasts in a myxoid stroma
- Positive for MSA, desmin, and myoglobin
- Negative for LCA

PEARLS

- *Surgery is used mainly for relief of urinary obstruction symptoms*
- *Poor prognosis; death typically results within 2 years of diagnosis*

SELECTED REFERENCES

Bostwick DG, Mann RB: Malignant lymphomas involving the prostate: a study of 13 cases. Cancer 56:2932-2938, 1985.

Chu PG, Huang Q, Weiss LM: Incidental and concurrent malignant lymphomas discovered at the time of prostatectomy and prostate biopsy: a study of 29 cases. Am J Surg Pathol 29:693-699, 2005.

TESTIS

CRYPTORCHIDISM

Clinical Features

- Usually unilateral (75%)
- Occurs in 3% to 4% of term infants and in up to 20% of premature infants
- Undescended testicles typically descend by 3 months of age (< 1% remain undescended at 1 year of age)
- Associated with an inguinal hernia in 10% to 20% of cases
- Most cryptorchid testes are found in the inguinal canal
- Right testicle is more commonly involved
- Patients with undescended and surgically descended cryptorchid testes have decreased fertility and increased risk for certain germ cell and non–germ cell tumors
- Normal descent of testes is under hormonal control

Gross Pathology

- Cryptorchid testes are smaller and softer than normal testes

Histopathology

- Histologic changes in cryptorchid testis occur by age 2 years
- Seminiferous tubules may be small or ring shaped and have areas of tubular sclerosis or atrophy (Figure 11-8)
- Spermatogonia may be decreased in number and irregularly distributed or totally absent
- Sertoli cells are increased in number; Leydig cell hyperplasia may be prominent
- Interstitium is typically widened and edematous
- Normally descended testis contralateral to the cryptorchid testis often shows many of the same histologic features

Special Stains and Immunohistochemistry

- Noncontributory

OTHER TECHNIQUES FOR DIAGNOSIS

- Noncontributory

Differential Diagnosis

- Causes of testicular maldescent include anatomic abnormalities of the gubernaculum, hormonal dysfunction, mechanical impairment, and gonadal dysgenesis

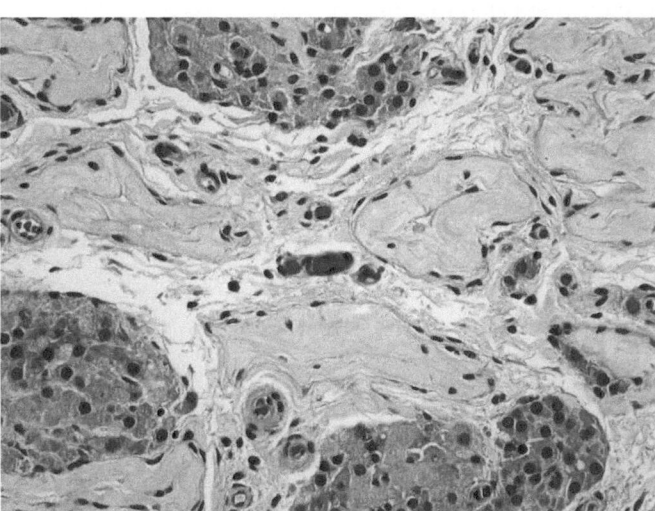

Figure 11-8. Cryptorchidism. Complete tubular sclerosis and mild Leydig cell hyperplasia.

PEARLS

- *Testicles normally descend from their intra-abdominal location to the scrotum in two phases, both of which are under hormonal control; defects in the transabdominal phase are much less common than defects in the inguinal or scrotal phase*
- *Patients with cryptorchidism have a 5 to 10 times higher risk for testicular malignancy than the general population; orchiopexy does not reduce the risk for cancer but does make detection easier*
- *Most common consequence is infertility*
- *Early orchiopexy (surgical placement of the testis in the scrotum) may have a positive effect on fertility; orchiopexy after 4 years of age does not increase fertility*

SELECTED REFERENCES

Fan R, Zhang J, Cheng L, et al: Testicular and paratesticular pathology in the pediatric population: a 20 year experience at Riley hospital for children. Pathol Res Pract 209:404-408, 2013.
Ferguson L, Agoulnik AI: Testicular cancer and cryptorchidism. Front Endocrinol 4:32-50, 2013.

TESTICULAR CYSTS

Clinical Features

- Usually unilateral
- May be difficult to distinguish from cysts of testicular adnexa by ultrasound
- May be difficult to distinguish from neoplastic cysts by ultrasound

Gross Pathology

- Albugineal cysts are usually uniloculated, centered in the visceral tunica albuginea, and contain clear fluid
- Epidermoid cysts are usually uniloculated, abut the visceral tunica albuginea; and contain laminated, granular, friable material (Figure 11-9)
- Rete testes cysts (cystic dysplasia of the rete testes) are usually multiloculated, retiform, centered in the testicular hilum, and contain clear fluid

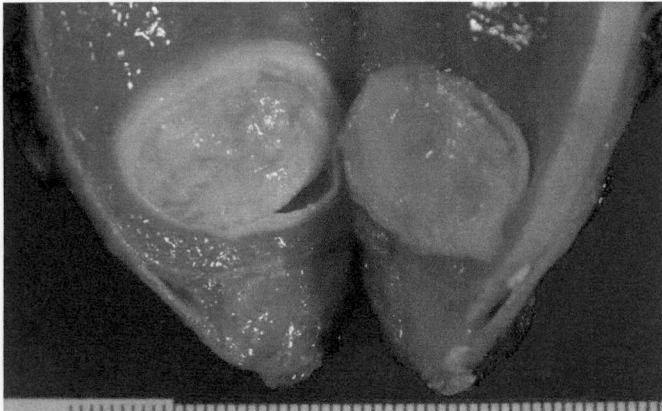

Figure 11-9. Epidermoid cyst. Hemisected testis showing sharply circumscribed cyst in testicular parenchyma, abutting tunica albuginea and containing laminated material.

Histopathology

- Albugineal cysts are at least partially lined by low cuboidal serosal epithelium
- Epidermoid cysts are lined by attenuated squamous epithelium, contain keratinaceous material, and, by definition, lack adnexal structures and germinal elements
- Rete testes cysts (cystic dysplasia of the rete testes) are lined by attenuated, low cuboidal epithelium

Special Stains and Immunohistochemistry

- Noncontributory

Other Techniques for Diagnosis

- Noncontributory

Differential Diagnosis

- Dermoid cysts are lined by keratinizing squamous epithelium but also have adnexal structures
- Teratomas may be mostly cystic lined by keratinizing squamous epithelium but also have teratomatous elements

PEARLS

- *Complete submission of epidermoid cysts is required to rule out dermoid cysts and teratoma*

SELECTED REFERENCE

Algaba F, Mikuz G, Boccon-Gibod L, et al: Pseudoneoplastic lesions of the testis and paratesticular structures. Virchows Arch 451:987-997, 2007.

HYDROCELE

Clinical Features

- Most are idiopathic; may be associated with inguinal hernia, scrotal trauma, orchitis, or testicular tumors
- May be secondary to congenital lack of closure of the processus vaginalis, resulting in a communication with the peritoneal cavity
- Characterized by accumulation of serous fluid between the parietal and visceral tunica vaginalis
- Patients present with a testicular mass that transilluminates
- Occasionally patients present with acute testicular enlargement secondary to hemorrhage; lack of transillumination may necessitate orchiectomy

Gross Pathology

- Clear serous fluid-filled cavity compresses adjacent testis
- Hemorrhage or infection may cause fluid to become opaque
- Tunica may be thickened in long-standing lesions

Histopathology

- Fluid-filled cavity lined by flattened or cuboidal mesothelial cells
- Mesothelium may be hyperplastic or cytologically atypical

Special Stains and Immunohistochemistry

- Noncontributory

Other Techniques for Diagnosis

- Noncontributory

Differential Diagnosis

SPERMATOCELE

- Usually located near rete testis or caput epididymis
- Contains spermatozoa

MESOTHELIAL CYST

- Usually located anterior or lateral to testis
- May arise within the tunica vaginalis, tunica albuginea, epididymis, or rarely the spermatic cord
- May be multiloculated

SELECTED REFERENCE

Haynes JH: Inguinal and scrotal disorders. Surg Clin North Am 86:371-381, 2006.

ORCHITIS

Clinical Features

VIRAL ORCHITIS

- Mumps is most common; coxsackievirus B is also relatively common
- Although the mumps viral syndrome occurs primarily in adolescent children, mumps orchitis is seen in postpubertal individuals
- Manifests with testicular pain
- Usually appears shortly after or during the viral syndrome, which includes parotitis
- Testicular involvement is seen in 15% to 30% of mumps infections
- May be bilateral
- Infrequent in childhood

BACTERIAL ORCHITIS

- *Escherichia coli* is the most common causative agent
- May be acute or chronic
- Usually associated with infection elsewhere in the genitourinary tract

GRANULOMATOUS ORCHITIS

- Usually a chronic process
- Associated with a variety of organisms; often associated with systemic or extratesticular infection
- May be idiopathic

Gross Pathology

- Acute: testicle is swollen and edematous
- Chronic: testicle is firm and often has a thickened tunica

Histopathology

VIRAL ORCHITIS

- Acute inflammation seen during acute infection
- Long-term infection results in patchy interstitial fibrosis and atrophy of seminiferous tubules; often involves both testes

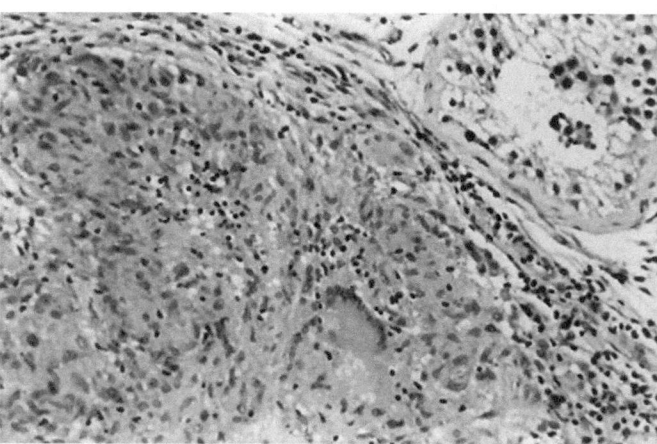

Figure 11-10. Idiopathic granulomatous orchitis. Intratubular, non-necrotizing granulomas.

BACTERIAL ORCHITIS

- Often associated with bacterial epididymitis
- Prominent neutrophilic infiltrate with abscess formation
- Chronic bacterial orchitis may show granulomatous inflammation; lacks intratubular giant cells

SYPHILITIC ORCHITIS

- Characterized by edema and diffuse lymphoplasmacytic inflammation
- Defining features include obliterative endarteritis with perivascular lymphocytes and plasma cells
- Gumma formation may be seen

Special Stains and Immunohistochemistry

- Stains for microorganisms can be useful to identify bacteria and fungi

Other Techniques for Diagnosis

- Noncontributory

Differential Diagnosis

INFECTIOUS GRANULOMATOUS ORCHITIS

- Specific agents (e.g., mycobacteria, brucellosis, fungi) must be demonstrated by special stains, culture, or serology

NONINFECTIOUS GRANULOMATOUS ORCHITIS

(Figure 11-10)
- Sarcoidosis
  - Isolated (i.e., nonsystemic) testicular involvement is extremely rare
  - Characterized by noncaseating granulomas composed of epithelioid histiocytes and giant cells
- Idiopathic granulomatous orchitis
  - No organisms are identified

SEMINOMA

- May be associated with a florid granulomatous reaction, but diagnostic foci of seminoma are at least focally present
- Intratubular germ cell neoplasia seen in residual seminiferous tubules
- Placental alkaline phosphatase (PLAP), OCT 3/4, and CD117 immunopositivity seen in seminoma cells

Malakoplakia

- Diagnostic Michaelis-Gutmann bodies readily demonstrated by iron or calcium stain
- Often associated with chronic *Escherichia coli* infection

PEARLS

- *Healing infection typically shows prominent granulation tissue and fibrosis*
- *Tuberculosis may involve the testes; more common in underdeveloped countries or immunocompromised patients*

SELECTED REFERENCES

Roy S, Hooda S, Parwani AV: Idiopathic granulomatous orchitis. Pathol Res Pract 207:275-278, 2011.

Yap RL, Jang TL, Gupta R, et al: Xanthogranulomatous orchitis. Urology 63:176-177, 2006.

MALAKOPLAKIA

Clinical Features

- Typically presents with testicular enlargement with or without tenderness
- Often associated with chronic bacterial infections, particularly *Escherichia coli*
- Rarely seen in children

Gross Pathology

- Testicular enlargement with focal areas of firm, tan-yellow tissue (Figure 11-11A)

Histopathology

- Normal testicular architecture is obscured by a mixed inflammatory infiltrate including abundant macrophages with abundant eosinophilic cytoplasm (von Hansemann histiocytes) (Figure 11-11B)
- Destruction of the seminiferous tubules
- Intracytoplasmic and extracellular laminated concretions represent Michaelis-Gutmann bodies

Special Stains and Immunohistochemistry

- Von Kossa calcium and Prussian blue stains highlight Michaelis-Gutmann bodies (Figure 11-11C)
- PAS stains eosinophilic, undigested, bacterial debris in macrophage cytoplasm

Other Techniques for Diagnosis

- Electron microscopy may demonstrate bacilli in core of Michaelis-Gutmann bodies

Differential Diagnosis

IDIOPATHIC GRANULOMATOUS ORCHITIS

- Usually has significant giant cell component
- Lacks Michaelis-Gutmann bodies

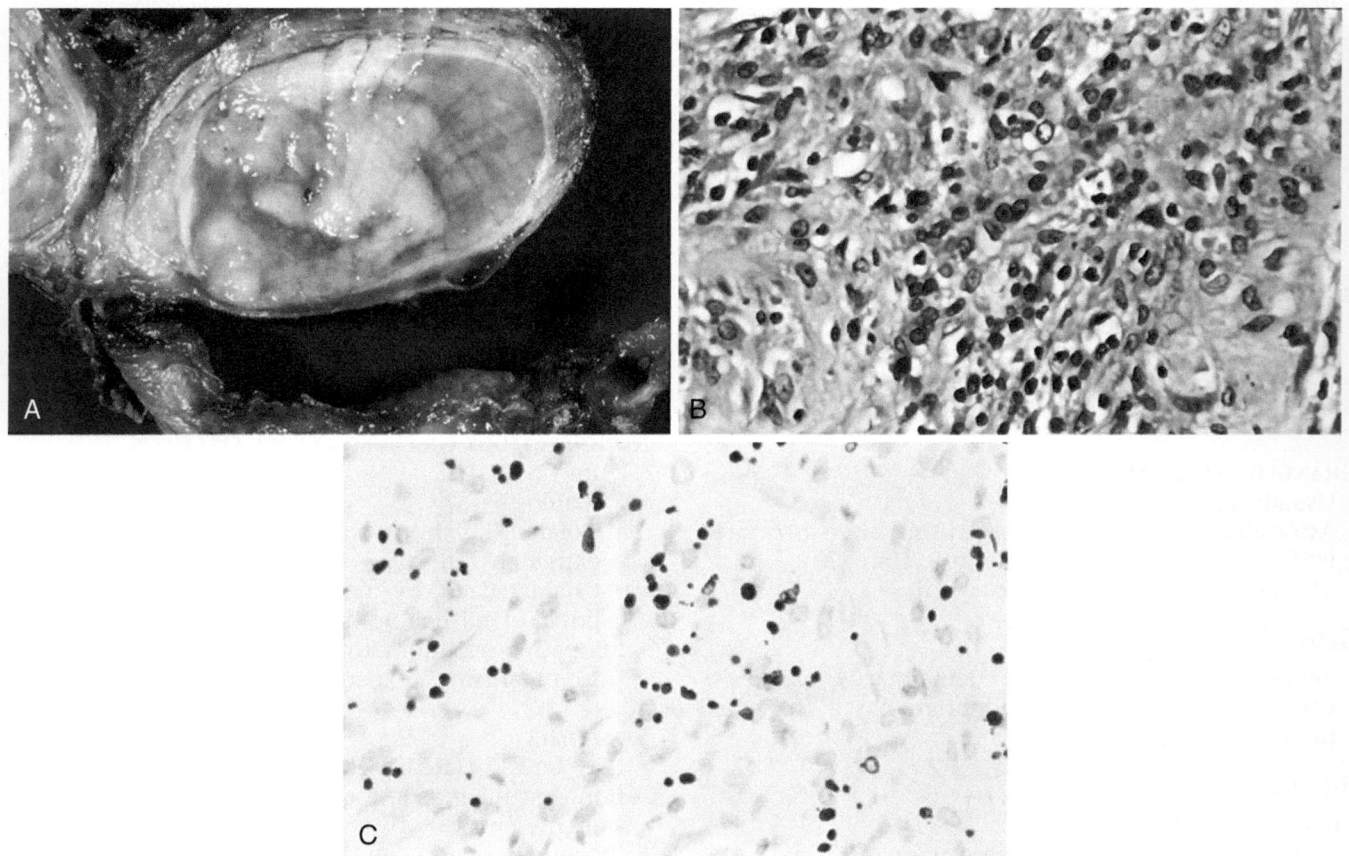

Figure 11-11. Testicular malakoplakia. A, Hemisected testis showing nodular, tan tissue replacing testicular parenchyma with marked peritesticular fibrosis. **B,** High-power photomicrograph showing a mixed inflammatory infiltrate composed mainly of macrophages with abundant eosinophilic cytoplasm. **C,** A von Kossa histochemical stain for calcium nicely highlights Michaelis-Gutmann bodies.

LYMPHOMA

- Clonal lymphocytic proliferation, usually large cell lymphoma, B-cell type
- Characteristic interstitial growth pattern with sparing of the seminiferous tubules
- Lacks Michaelis-Gutmann bodies

SEMINOMA WITH GRANULOMATOUS RESPONSE

- Diagnostic seminoma is at least focally present
- PLAP-immunopositive seminoma cells
- Lacks Michaelis-Gutmann bodies

PEARLS

- *Chronic inflammatory disorder*
- *Many organs may be involved; urinary bladder is most commonly affected*

SELECTED REFERENCES

Kostakopoulos A, Giannakopoulos S, Demonakou M, Deliveliotos C: Malakoplakia of the testis. Int Urol Nephrol 29:461-463, 1997.
Waisman J: Malakoplakia outside the urinary tract. Arch Pathol Lab Med 131:1512, 2007.

TORSION

Clinical Features

- Torsion of the spermatic cord is the most common cause of testicular infarction
- Trauma and lesions of the spermatic cord vessels may also cause infarction
- Compression of the spermatic cord veins with continued arterial inflow can lead to venous infarction
- Patients typically present with acute onset of testicular pain

Gross Pathology

- Early vascular compromise is manifested by testicular congestion and swelling
- Infarcted testes are enlarged and consist of soft, necrotic, hemorrhagic tissue (Figure 11-12)

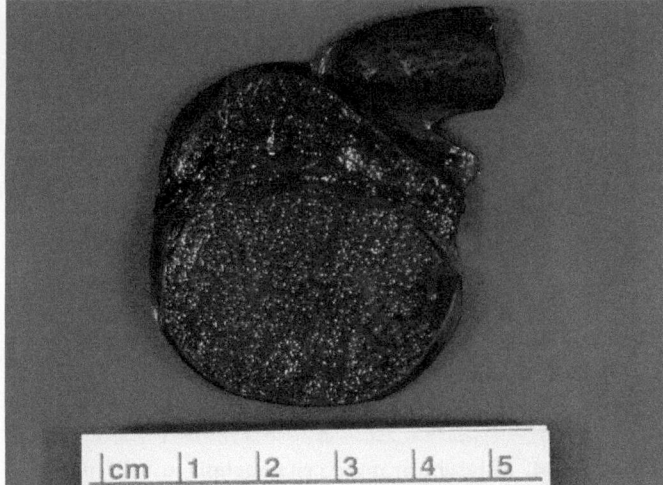

Figure 11-12. Testicular torsion. Hemisected orchiectomy specimen showing a venous-type hemorrhagic infarct involving testis and epididymis *(bottom)* and spermatic cord *(top)*.

Histopathology

- Changes range from intense congestion to extravasation of blood into the testicular interstitium and epididymis
- Eventually the entire testis becomes necrotic and hemorrhagic

Special Stains and Immunohistochemistry

- Noncontributory

Other Techniques for Diagnosis

- Noncontributory

Differential Diagnosis

GERM CELL TUMOR WITH EXTENSIVE NECROSIS AND HEMORRHAGE

- Foci of typical germ cell tumor is almost invariably present somewhere in the testis; identification may require several histologic sections

PEARLS

- *If surgical intervention is delayed for more than 8 hours, the testis is usually not viable*

SELECTED REFERENCES

Hadziselimovic F, Snyder H, Duckett J, Howards S: Testicular histology in children with unilateral testicular torsion. J Urol 136:208-210, 1986.
Rosenstein D, McAninch JW: Urologic emergencies. Med Clin North Am 688:495-518, 2004.

MALE INFERTILITY

Clinical Features

- In general, infertility is defined as lack of conception after 1 year of unprotected coitus
- Male factors are responsible for 40% to 50% of infertile couples
- In general, male infertility is broken down into pretesticular (hormonal), testicular (75% of cases), and posttesticular (obstruction of outflow) causes

Gross Pathology

- Testicular atrophy

Histopathology

- Seminiferous tubules
  - Show similar changes regardless of underlying cause
  - Tubular hyalinization
- Germinal epithelium
  - May show arrest at any stage (spermatogonia → primary spermatocytes → secondary spermatocytes → spermatids → spermatozoa)
  - May be completely attenuated with only Sertoli cells remaining (Sertoli-only syndrome) (Figure 11-13)
- Interstitium
  - May show varying degrees of fibrosis
  - Leydig cell hypoplasia or hyperplasia may be present
- Blood vessels
  - Atherosclerosis is a common cause of low sperm count, particularly in older individuals

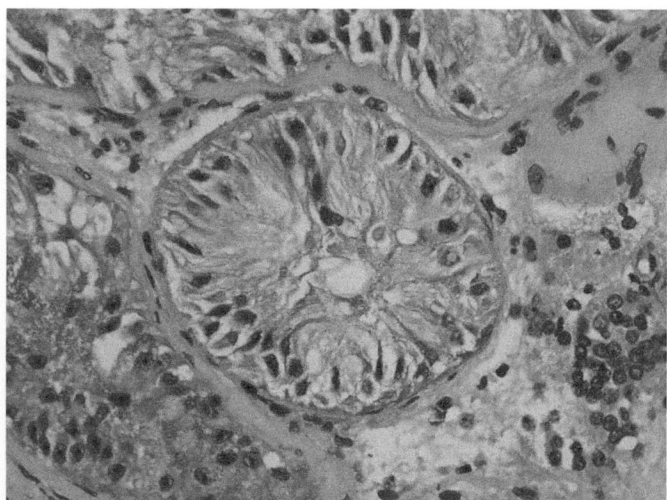

Figure 11-13. Sertoli-only tubule. Loss of germinal epithelium and persistence of Sertoli cells characterized by elongated cytoplasmic processes and pyramidal nuclei with prominent nucleoli.

Special Stains and Immunohistochemistry

- PLAP may be necessary to identify intratubular germ cells

Other Techniques for Diagnosis

- Noncontributory

Differential Diagnosis

- Causes of male infertility are numerous and include inflammatory, reactive or reparative, iatrogenic, infectious, and vascular-related processes
- Pathologic findings, which are often nonspecific, must be viewed in the context of the clinical evaluation

PEARLS

- *Many genetic syndromes are associated with infertility, including Klinefelter syndrome, Down syndrome, and Prader-Willi syndrome; also, structural abnormalities of the Y chromosome are associated*
- *Endocrine dysfunction, including Cushing syndrome, diabetes mellitus, and hyperprolactinemia, may result in infertility*
- *Prostate cancer treated with chemotherapy, radiation, or surgery may render the patient infertile*
- *Treatment of infertility is variable and depends on the patient's underlying condition*

SELECTED REFERENCES

McLachlan RI, Raipert-De Meyts E, Hoei-Hansen CE, et al: Histologic evaluation of the human testis—approaches to optimising the clinical value of the assessment: mini review. Hum Reprod 22:2-16, 2007.

Nistal M, Paniaqua R: Non-neoplastic diseases of the testis. In Bostwick DG, Eble JN (eds): Urologic Surgical Pathology. Philadelphia, Mosby–Year Book, 1997, pp 496-535.

INTRATUBULAR GERM CELL NEOPLASIA

Clinical Features

- Originally called carcinoma in situ

- May be found in testicular biopsies performed on patients at high risk for germ cell tumors (high-risk conditions include cryptorchidism, prior testicular germ cell tumor, family history, gonadal dysgenesis, and androgen insensitivity syndrome)
- Considered a precursor lesion to germ cell neoplasia
- Almost invariably seen in orchiectomy specimens removed for germ cell neoplasia

Gross Pathology

- Typically has an unremarkable gross appearance; features associated with cryptorchidism, such as atrophy or fibrosis, may be seen

Histopathology

- Neoplastic intratubular germ cells typically form a single layer along the seminiferous tubules and may involve the rete testis (Figure 11-14)
- Malignant germ cells are pleomorphic and have abundant vacuolated cytoplasm, large nuclei with coarse chromatin, and two or more nucleoli
- Spermatogenesis is severely diminished or absent in the affected tubule

Special Stains and Immunohistochemistry

- PLAP positive
- PAS positive, diastase sensitive (tumor cell cytoplasm contains glycogen)

Other Techniques for Diagnosis

- Noncontributory

Differential Diagnosis

GERMINAL EPITHELIUM WITH MATURATION ARREST

- May show some PAS positivity but is almost invariably PLAP negative
- Cells lack significant nuclear pleomorphism

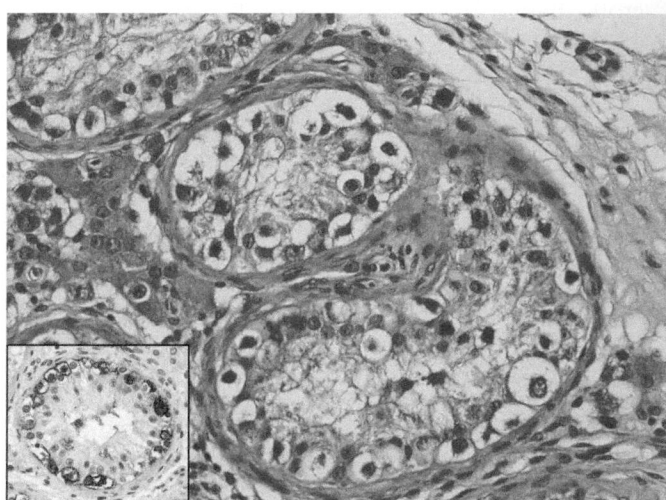

Figure 11-14. Intratubular germ cell neoplasia, usual type. Large malignant cells with vacuolated cytoplasm scattered along the basement membrane of the seminiferous tubules. Note the absence of spermatogenesis. Placental alkaline phosphatase immunohistochemical stain highlights the malignant germ cells (*inset*).

SELECTED REFERENCES

Emerson RE, Cheng L: Premalignancy of the testis and paratestis. Pathology 45:264-272, 2013.
Ulbright TM: Germ cell tumors of the gonads: a selective review emphasizing problems in differential diagnosis, newly appreciated, and controversial issues. Mod Pathol 18 (suppl 2):S61-S79, 2005.

SEMINOMA

Clinical Features

- Most common pure testicular germ cell neoplasm
- Typically occurs between 30 and 40 years of age (10 years older than nonseminomatous germ cell tumors); rare before puberty
- Presents as a painless testicular mass; may cause dull aching sensation
- Elevated HCG in 7% to 25% of cases (due to presence of syncytiotrophoblastic cells); α-fetoprotein (AFP) levels are usually normal

Gross Pathology

- Multinodular with bulging, cream to tan, fleshy cut surface
- Tumor typically replaces entire testis
- Yellow foci of necrosis may be seen in large tumors
- Extension into paratesticular structures occurs in 10% of cases
- Foci of punctate hemorrhage may indicate admixed syncytiotrophoblastic elements

Histopathology

- Composed of diffuse sheets of tumor cells with intervening branching fibrous septa; cells may be loosely cohesive, giving an appearance of cystlike or tubular spaces
- Interstitial growth pattern with preservation of seminiferous tubules may be seen at the periphery of the tumor
- Tumor cells are round to polyhedral and have pale to clear cytoplasm with well-defined cell borders; uniform, round to oval nuclei with finely granular chromatin; and one or two prominent nucleoli (Figure 11-15)
- Infrequent mitotic activity
- Nearly all tumors contain a lymphocytic infiltrate composed predominantly of T cells; lymphoid infiltrate is most dense in the perivascular areas and in the fibrous septa
- Granulomas consisting of small clusters of epithelioid histiocytes and multinucleated giant cells are seen in about 50% of cases
- Pagetoid spread may be seen within seminiferous tubules or rete testis

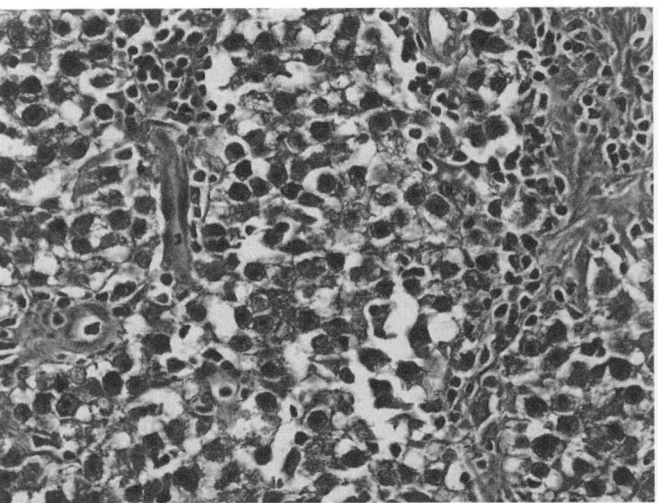

Figure 11-15. Seminoma. Monotonous population of cells with clear to eosinophilic cytoplasm and prominent, centrally placed nucleoli associated with a mild lymphocytic infiltrate in the thin, fibrous septa.

- Many tumors show scarring with hyalinized deposits of collagen; ossification of the fibrous septa can occur
- Single cells or small groups of syncytiotrophoblasts may be seen in 10% to 20% of cases and are often associated with foci of hemorrhage
- Anaplastic seminoma
  - Higher cellularity with increased nuclear pleomorphism
  - Three or more mitoses per high-power field (hpf)
- Prominent giant cells

Special Stains and Immunohistochemistry

- PLAP strongly positive and CD117 positive
- Cytokeratin: only patchy immunopositivity
- PAS: cytoplasmic positivity due to intracytoplasmic glycogen
- HCG: isolated syncytiotrophoblastic cells are positive
- Epithelial membrane antigen (EMA) uniformly negative

Other Techniques for Diagnosis

- Cytogenetic studies: isochromosome 12p is almost always present
- DNA content is usually aneuploid in the range of triploid to hypotetraploid

Differential Diagnosis

EMBRYONAL CARCINOMA

- Solid architecture (which may resemble seminoma) is usually mixed with tubular or papillary architecture
- Tumor cells have poorly defined borders and pleomorphic nuclei with prominent macronucleoli
- Lacks regular fibrous septa and prominent lymphocytic infiltrate
- Is CD30 positive, shows greater positivity for cytokeratin and weaker PLAP staining

YOLK SAC TUMOR

- Solid architecture (which may resemble seminoma) is usually mixed with many other patterns
- Usually shows hyaline globules and extracellular basement membrane material

- Lacks fibrous septa and dense lymphoid infiltrate
- Is AFP and glypican 3 positive, OCT 3/4 negative, and shows greater positivity for cytokeratin and weaker PLAP staining

LYMPHOMA
- Typically occurs in older population
- More frequently bilateral
- Interstitial growth pattern with lymphomatous infiltrate surrounding seminiferous tubules
- Not associated with intratubular germ cell neoplasia
- Negative for PLAP

SERTOLI CELL TUMOR
- Solid architecture with clear cytoplasm (which is rarely seen in malignancy and may resemble seminoma) is often at least focally associated with a more conventional tubular pattern
- Cells have clear cytoplasm, which is due to the presence of lipid rather than glycogen
- Not associated with intratubular germ cell neoplasia
- Is negative for PLAP and OCT 3/4 and often at least focally inhibin positive

CHORIOCARCINOMA
- Unlike choriocarcinoma, the syncytiotrophoblastic cells of seminoma are not associated with cytotrophoblasts (non-bilaminar) and are not arranged in nodular aggregates

PEARLS

- *Identical tumor in the ovary is called dysgerminoma*
- *Seminomas that have a greater lymphocytic infiltrate may be associated with a better prognosis*
- *Combined orchiectomy plus radiation leads to a 95% cure rate in low-stage patients*

SELECTED REFERENCES

Beyer J, Albers P, Altena R, et al: Maintaining success, reducing treatment burden, focusing on survivorship: highlights from the third European Consensus Conference on diagnosis and treatment of germ cell cancer. Ann Oncol 24:878-888, 2011.

Edge SB, Byrd DR, Compton CC, et al (eds): AJCC Cancer Staging Manual, 7th ed. New York: Springer, 2010, pp 469-478.

Ulbright TM: The most common, clinically significant misdiagnoses in testicular tumor pathology and how to avoid them. Adv Anat Pathol 15:18-27, 2008.

Woodward PJ, Heidenreich A, Looijenga LHJ, et al: Germ cell tumors. In Eble JN, Sauter G, Epstein JI, Sesterhenn IA (eds): World Health Organization Classification of Tumours: Pathology and Genetics: Tumours of the Urinary System and Male Genital Organs. Lyon, IARC Press, 2004, pp 221-249.

SPERMATOCYTIC SEMINOMA

Clinical Features
- Rare germ cell tumor that occurs only in the testis
- Typically affects patients aged 50 to 60 years
- Patients present with painless, often longstanding testicular enlargement
- Not associated with cryptorchidism or other forms of germ cell neoplasia
- Serum tumor markers are not elevated
- Excellent prognosis

Gross Pathology
- Typically multinodular
- May measure up to 15 cm; typically 2 to 5 cm
- Variable cut surface with areas of fleshy, white tissue, mucoid material, hemorrhage, and cystic degeneration (Figure 11-16A)

Histopathology
- Polymorphous population of cells arranged in sheets, cords, or small nests (Figure 11-16B)
  - Small cells: 6 to 8 µm, smudged chromatin, and scant cytoplasm
  - Intermediate cells: 15 to 20 µm, scant cytoplasm, and round nuclei with granular or filamentous chromatin
  - Giant cells: 50 to 100 µm, uninucleate or multinucleate, and may show filamentous chromatin
- Lacks a lymphoid infiltrate, granulomas are not seen and not associated with intratubular germ cell neoplasia

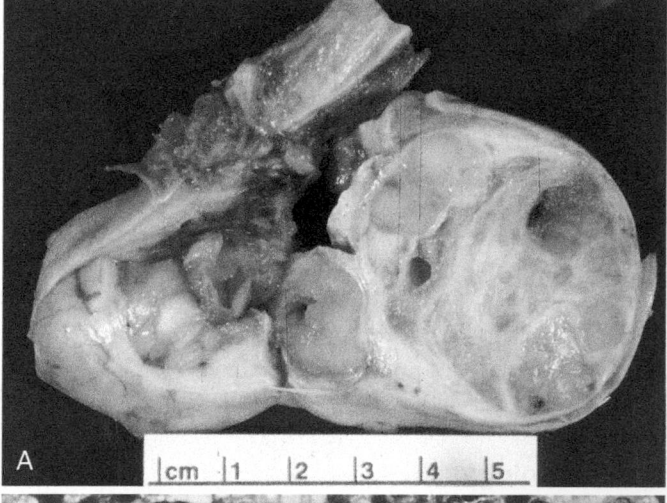

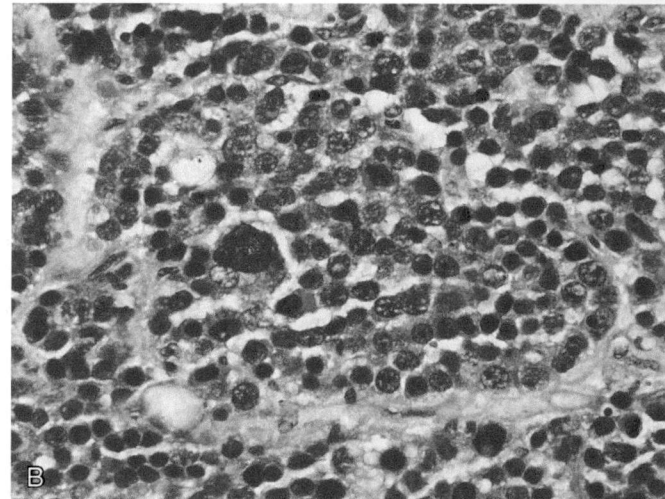

Figure 11-16. Spermatocytic seminoma. A, Hemisected orchiectomy specimen showing nodules with a glistening cut surface and cystic spaces separated by fibrous septa. **B,** Characteristic small, intermediate, and large cell types. Note the absence of lymphocytes in the fibrous septa.

Special Stains and Immunohistochemistry

- Cytokeratin: positivity may be seen in a perinuclear, dotlike pattern
- PAS negative (cells do not contain glycogen)
- PLAP may be focally positive
- Cells are negative for vimentin, SMA, desmin, AFP, HCG, CEA, and LCA

Other Techniques for Diagnosis

- Electron microscopy: tumor cells have intercellular bridges, macula adherens-type junctions, and filamentous chromosomes with lateral fibrils
- Characteristically lacks isochromosome 12p

Differential Diagnosis

CLASSIC SEMINOMA
- Affects younger patients
- May be associated with other germ cell tumor types
- Composed of a single cell type and cells contain abundant cytoplasmic glycogen
- Fibrous septa with prominent lymphoid infiltrate
- Strong PLAP positivity

PEARLS

- *Not associated with intratubular germ cell neoplasia*
- *Orchiectomy alone is curative; essentially no metastatic potential*

SELECTED REFERENCES

Edge SB, Byrd DR, Compton CC, et al (eds): AJCC Cancer Staging Manual. 7th ed. New York: Springer, 2010, pp 469-478.
Woodward PJ, Heidenreich A, Looijenga LHJ, et al: Germ cell tumors. In Eble JN, Sauter G, Epstein JI, Sesterhenn IA (eds): World Health Organization Classification of Tumours: Pathology and Genetics: Tumours of the Urinary System and Male Genital Organs. Lyon, IARC Press, 2004, pp 221-249.

EMBRYONAL CARCINOMA

Clinical Features

- Common component of mixed germ cell tumors (present in 85% of cases)
- Pure embryonal carcinoma is rare, accounting for less than 5% of testicular germ cell neoplasms
- Presents as a testicular mass; gynecomastia or clinically evident metastasis is seen in 40% of patients at presentation
- Serum AFP and HCG may be slightly elevated (related to yolk sac tumor and choriocarcinoma components in mixed tumors); pure embryonal carcinoma is negative

Gross Pathology

- Poorly circumscribed, variegated, gray-white mass with areas of hemorrhage and necrosis
- Tumor typically does not replace entire testis

Histopathology

- Cohesive clusters of primitive, anaplastic epithelial cells are seen in three major patterns: solid, tubular-glandular, and papillary
- Tumor cells have abundant cytoplasm and large, vesicular, pleomorphic nuclei with prominent macronucleoli;

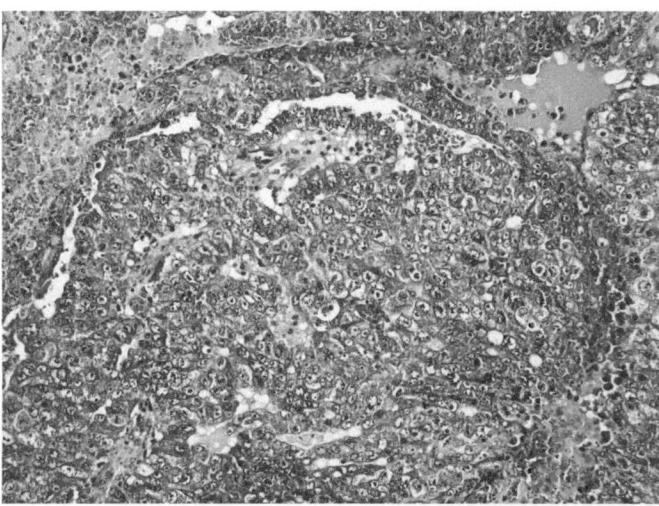

Figure 11-17. Embryonal carcinoma. Glandular and diffuse growth of cells with marked pleomorphism and associated hemorrhage.

cell borders are ill-defined, and the nuclei appear crowded or overlapping (Figure 11-17)
- Foci of coagulative necrosis are common
- Mitotic rate is high, and karyorrhectic fragments are frequently seen
- Teratocarcinoma
  - Used to describe a mixed germ cell tumor composed of embryonal carcinoma and teratoma

Special Stains and Immunohistochemistry

- Cytokeratin strongly positive
- PLAP: patchy positivity is seen in more than 85% of cases
- CD30 (Ki-1) typically positive
- EMA negative

Other Techniques for Diagnosis

- Cytogenetic studies
  - Isochromosome 12p is often found
  - Interstitial deletion 12(p13;q22) is found in nonseminomatous germ cell neoplasms
- DNA index ranges from 1.4 to 1.6 (significantly lower than in seminoma)

Differential Diagnosis

SEMINOMA
- Typically arranged in solid sheets; lacks glands, tubules, or papillae
- Tumor cells have well-defined borders with more uniform, evenly spaced nuclei
- Weaker cytokeratin immunopositivity, CD30 negative and stronger reactivity for PLAP and CD117

YOLK SAC TUMOR
- Variable tumor architecture, which commonly is microcystic or solid
- Usually shows hyaline globules and extracellular basement membrane material
- Lacks fibrous septa and dense lymphoid infiltrate
- Positive for cytokeratin and AFP
- Commonly seen together as part of a mixed germ cell tumor (distinction between the two components may be difficult)

CHORIOCARCINOMA
- Predominantly hemorrhagic background
- Strongly immunopositive for HCG

PEARLS

- *Embryonal carcinoma is a frequent component of mixed germ cell tumors and is rarely seen as a pure tumor*
- *Intratubular germ cell neoplasia is frequently seen in association with embryonal carcinoma*
- *Poor prognostic factors include older age, high elevations of serum tumor markers (lactate dehydrogenase), and higher tumor stage*
- *Overall, more aggressive than seminomas*

SELECTED REFERENCES

Beyer J, Albers P, Altena R, et al: Maintaining success, reducing treatment burden, focusing on survivorship: highlights from the third European Consensus Conference on diagnosis and treatment of germ cell cancer. Ann Oncol 24:878-888, 2011.

Edge SB, Byrd DR, Compton CC, et al (eds): AJCC Cancer Staging Manual, 7th ed. New York: Springer, 2010, pp 469-478.

Woodward PJ, Heidenreich A, Looijenga LHJ, et al: Germ cell tumors. In Eble JN, Sauter G, Epstein JI, Sesterhenn IA (eds): World Health Organization Classification of Tumours: Pathology and Genetics: Tumours of the Urinary System and Male Genital Organs. Lyon, IARC Press, 2004, pp 221-249.

YOLK SAC TUMOR

Clinical Features

- Most common testicular tumor in children younger than 3 years
- Pure yolk sac tumor occurs in children from birth to 9 years, with a median age of 18 months; rare in adults
- In adults, yolk sac tumor usually occurs as a component of mixed germ cell tumor
- Patients typically present with a painless testicular mass
- Almost all patients have an elevated AFP level

Gross Pathology

- Nonencapsulated, solid, gray-white to tan, homogeneous mass with a myxoid or gelatinous cut surface; cystic change may be seen
- In adults, because yolk sac tumor is usually only one component of a mixed germ cell tumor, the appearance is variable and may include areas of hemorrhage or necrosis

Histopathology (Figure 11-18)

- Numerous patterns are recognized in yolk sac tumor and include mixed and transitional forms of the following
  - Microcystic (most common pattern)
    - Microcystic appearance results from the presence of intracellular vacuoles, which gives the tumor a lacelike or reticular pattern
    - Extracellular spaces surrounded by cords of tumor cells may be seen
    - Vacuolated cells have compressed nuclei, which resemble lipoblasts
    - Surrounding stroma is often myxoid
    - Solid and myxomatous patterns are often combined with the microcystic subtype
  - Solid (common pattern)
    - Composed of sheets of uniform cells with pale to clear cytoplasm and well-defined borders

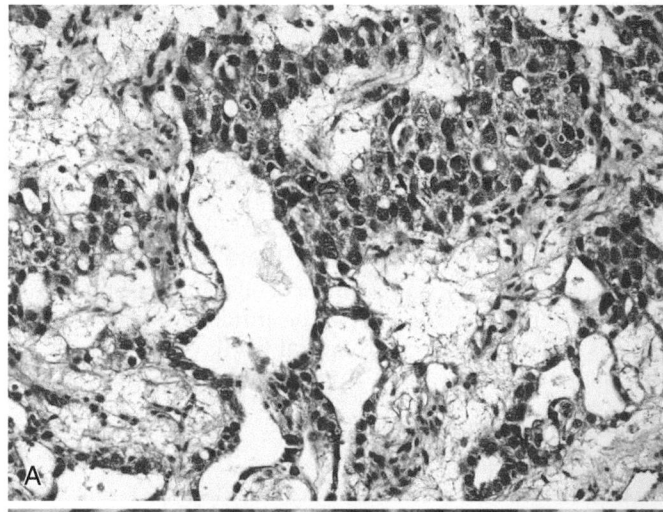

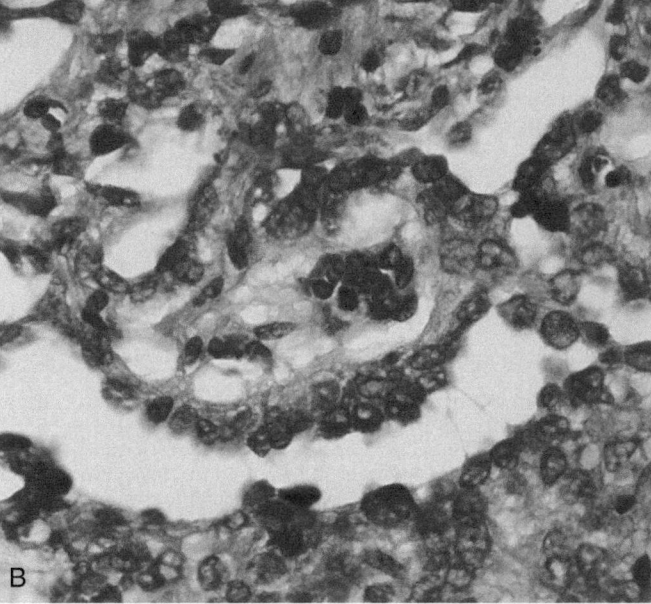

Figure 11-18. Yolk sac tumor. A, Tubuloalveolar and diffuse architectural patterns shown here represent just two of many described for yolk sac tumor. Note the brightly eosinophilic, intracytoplasmic, hyaline globules. **B,** A Schiller-Duval body with characteristic fibrovascular core.

- Prominent thin-walled blood vessels may be present
- May have a focal microcystic pattern
- No lymphoid component or fibrous septa
  - Myxomatous (common pattern)
    - Consists of cytokeratin-positive epithelioid to spindle cells in a myxoid stroma
    - Prominent vascular network
    - Typically intermixed with the microcystic pattern
  - Endodermal sinus
    - Characteristic Schiller-Duval or glomeruloid bodies (formed by a central blood vessel and rim of fibrous tissue surrounded by malignant epithelium); seen in about half of cases
    - May be a component in any of the other patterns
  - Papillary
    - Papillae are lined by cuboidal, low columnar, or hobnail cells and project into cystic spaces

- Papillae may have well-formed or inconspicuous fibrovascular cores
- Frequently intermixed with the endodermal sinus pattern
- Glandular and alveolar
  - Focally present in up to 30% of cases
  - Composed of round or tubular glands that may show a simple or complex pattern
  - May show areas of polyvesicular vitelline, myxomatous, solid, or microcystic patterns
- Macrovesicular
  - Coalescence of microcystic spaces forms large, round to irregular cystic spaces
  - Frequently has an adjacent microcystic pattern
- Polyvesicular vitelline
  - Round, irregular, or dumbbell-shaped vesicular structures lined by flat, bland epithelium
  - Abundant myxoid and loose fibrous stroma
- Hepatoid
  - Present in up to 20% of cases; often only small, scattered foci
  - Composed of polygonal, eosinophilic cells with vesicular nuclei and prominent nucleoli, arranged in sheets or trabeculae (resembles hepatocellular carcinoma)
  - Contains abundant AFP
  - Hyaline globules are common
- Sarcomatoid (uncommon pattern)
  - Composed of a cellular proliferation of cytokeratin-positive spindle cells
  - Often intermixed with the microcystic pattern but may be associated with any of the other subtypes
  - Tumor cells in all patterns may have intracellular, round, hyaline globules, ranging from 1 μm to more than 50 μm in diameter

Special Stains and Immunohistochemistry

- Cytokeratin: strong diffuse positivity
- PLAP: variable positivity in 40% to 85% of cases
- Vimentin: immunopositivity is seen in the spindle cells of the myxomatous and sarcomatoid patterns
- AFP: patchy, cytoplasmic immunopositivity in 50% to 100% of cases; intense staining is seen in areas with a hepatoid pattern
- α1-Antitrypsin: 50% of cases are positive
- Intracellular hyaline globules are PAS positive, diastase resistant, and usually negative for AFP

Other Techniques for Diagnosis

- Electron microscopy: epithelial cells with junctional complexes, occasional apical microvilli, flocculent material in dilated endoplasmic reticulum, and cytoplasmic glycogen; electron-dense, non–membrane-bound bodies correspond to the hyaline globules
- Adult cases are almost all aneuploid and may show isochromosome 12p
- Childhood cases lack the isochromosome 12p, and about 30% are diploid

Differential Diagnosis

SEMINOMA

- Unlike in seminoma, the solid pattern of yolk sac tumor lacks the prominent lymphoid component and the fibrous septa

EMBRYONAL CARCINOMA

- May show transitional patterns that are similar to those of yolk sac tumor but is typically composed of more pleomorphic, atypical cells
- Commonly seen together as part of a mixed germ cell tumor (distinction between the two components may be difficult)
- Positive for CD30 (Ki-1); negative for AFP

JUVENILE GRANULOSA CELL TUMOR

- Typically found in infants younger than 5 months
- May show architectural pattern similar to that of yolk sac tumor
- Tumor cells lack intracellular hyaline globules
- No Schiller-Duval bodies
- Negative for AFP

PEARLS

- *Also called endodermal sinus tumor*
- *Pediatric yolk sac tumor is the most common testicular neoplasm in prepubertal children; constitutes about 80% of testicular tumors in children*
- *Not associated with cryptorchidism*
- *Five-year survival rate is about 90%*
- *In adults, up to 45% of nonseminomatous germ cell tumors have yolk sac tumor elements*

SELECTED REFERENCES

Beyer J, Albers P, Altena R, et al: Maintaining success, reducing treatment burden, focusing on survivorship: highlights from the third European Consensus Conference on diagnosis and treatment of germ cell cancer. Ann Oncol 24:878-888, 2011.

Edge SB, Byrd DR, Compton CC, et al (eds): AJCC Cancer Staging Manual, 7th ed. New York: Springer, 2010, pp 469-478.

Woodward PJ, Heidenreich A, Looijenga LHJ, et al: Germ cell tumors. In Eble JN, Sauter G, Epstein JI, Sesterhenn IA (eds): World Health Organization Classification of Tumours: Pathology and Genetics: Tumours of the Urinary System and Male Genital Organs. Lyon, IARC Press, 2004, pp 221-249.

TERATOMA

Clinical Features

- Pure teratoma occurs in children with a mean age of 20 months; unusual in children older than 4 years
- Childhood tumors are frequently found by parent or during routine physical examination
- Teratomatous elements are found in 50% of mixed germ cell tumors in adults
- Pure mature teratomas in prepubertal children do not metastasize

Gross Pathology

- Typically 5 to 10 cm
- Variable appearance with solid areas and multiple cysts (<1 cm in diameter) containing watery to mucoid fluid
- Semitranslucent nodules of gray-white cartilage may be seen
- Immature areas are typically composed of fleshy or hemorrhagic tissue

Histopathology

- Consists of any combination of mature or immature ectodermal, endodermal, and mesodermal elements including cartilage, smooth and skeletal muscle, neuroglia, enteric-type glands, squamous epithelial islands, respiratory or transitional epithelium, fetal neuroepithelium, undifferentiated blastema, or embryonic tubules (Figure 11-19)
- Somatic-type malignancies (carcinoma or sarcoma) may occur and show expansile or infiltrative overgrowth of the teratomatous elements

Special Stains and Immunohistochemistry

- Immunohistochemical reactivity is as expected for the various tissue types present
- AFP: positivity may be seen in enteric or respiratory glands or liver-like tissue
- CEA and α_1-antitrypsin: epithelial areas may show positivity

Other Techniques for Diagnosis

- Tumors usually have an aneuploid DNA content in the hypotriploid range
- Cytogenetic studies: isochromosome 12p may be seen

Differential Diagnosis

DERMOID CYST

- Very rare, benign, predominantly cystic tumor composed of epidermis and adnexal structures such as hair follicles and sebaceous glands
- Term should not be used when nonectodermal or immature elements are present
- No intratubular germ cell neoplasia in the residual seminiferous tubules

NONDERMOID BENIGN TERATOMA

- Extremely rare, benign tumor composed of mature ectodermal (without adnexal structures) and mesodermal elements

- Can be distinguished from potentially malignant postpubertal teratomas by <u>absence</u> of cytologic atypia, intratubular germ cell neoplasia, tubular sclerosis, impaired spermatogenesis, and evidence of chromosome 12p abnormalities

EPIDERMOID CYST

- Uncommon benign cyst with a lining of keratinizing squamous epithelium without associated adnexal structures

MIXED GERM CELL TUMOR

- Much more common in postpubertal patients
- Adequate sampling is needed to determine the presence of other germ cell tumor components

SOMATIC-TYPE MALIGNANCY (CARCINOMA OR SARCOMA)

- Somatic-type malignancy arising in a teratoma (i.e., immature elements in a teratoma can look like a carcinoma or a sarcoma)
- Must show infiltrative or expansile overgrowth of the teratoma
- Amount of overgrowth required has not been rigorously defined

PEARLS

- *Second most common testicular germ cell tumor in children*
- *Some cases have associated congenital anomalies, including spina bifida, retrocaval ureters, hemihypertrophy, and inguinal hernia*
- *Prepubertal patients with pure mature teratoma are cured by orchiectomy*
- *Postpubertal patients rarely, if ever, have pure mature teratoma (metastases may resemble the original tumor or be composed of other germ cell elements)*
- *Except for nondermoid benign teratoma, all teratomas in postpubertal males are potentially malignant*

SELECTED REFERENCES

Beyer J, Albers P, Altena R, et al: Maintaining success, reducing treatment burden, focusing on survivorship: highlights from the third European Consensus Conference on diagnosis and treatment of germ cell cancer. Ann Oncol 24:878-888, 2011.

Edge SB, Byrd DR, Compton CC, et al (eds): AJCC Cancer Staging Manual, 7th ed. New York: Springer, 2010, pp 469-478.

Semjen D, Kalman E, Tornoczky T, et al: Further evidence of the existence of benign teratomas of the postpubertal testis. Am J Surg Pathol 38:580-581, 2014.

Woodward PJ, Heidenreich A, Looijenga LHJ, et al: Germ cell tumors. In Eble JN, Sauter G, Epstein JI, Sesterhenn IA (eds): World Health Organization Classification of Tumours: Pathology and Genetics: Tumours of the Urinary System and Male Genital Organs. Lyon, IARC Press, 2004, pp 221-249.

Zhang C, Berney DM, Hirsch MS, et al: Evidence supporting the existence of benign teratomas of the postpubertal testis. A clinical, histopathologic, and molecular genetic analysis of 25 cases. Am J Surg Pathol 37:827-835, 2013.

CHORIOCARCINOMA

Clinical Features

- Typically a component of mixed germ cell tumors; pure choriocarcinoma is extremely rare

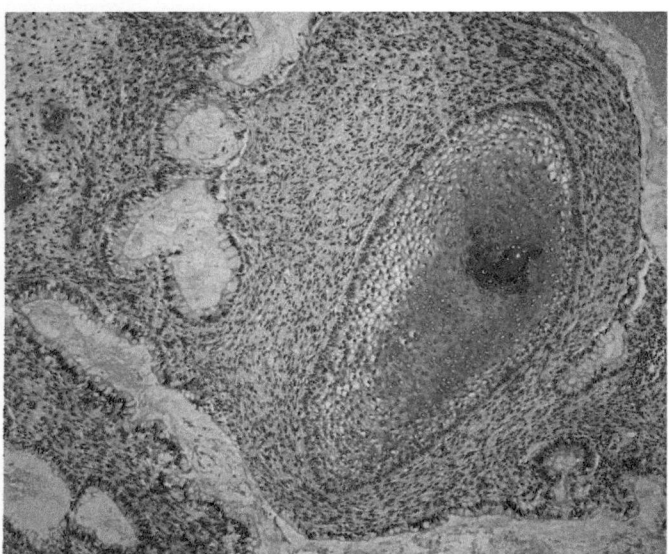

Figure 11-19. Teratoma. Low-power view showing mixed epithelial and stromal elements. Immature elements should not be confused with a somatic malignancy such as a carcinoma or sarcoma.

- Patients present between the second and third decades; not reported before puberty
- Patients often present with symptoms secondary to metastases to lung, brain, or gastrointestinal tract; testicular tumor may be occult
- Serum HCG is usually highly elevated

Gross Pathology

- Testis may appear normal externally
- Often forms a small tumor with focal hemorrhage and necrosis (Figure 11-20B)
- Tumor regression may leave only a fibrous scar

Histopathology

- Characterized by an intimate mixture of cytotrophoblasts and syncytiotrophoblasts (Figure 11-20A)
  - Cytotrophoblasts: mononucleated cells with pale to clear cytoplasm and well-defined cell borders
  - Syncytiotrophoblasts: large, multinucleated cells with smudged chromatin and vacuolated, eosinophilic cytoplasm
- Hemorrhage and necrosis are typically prominent
- Angioinvasion is commonly seen

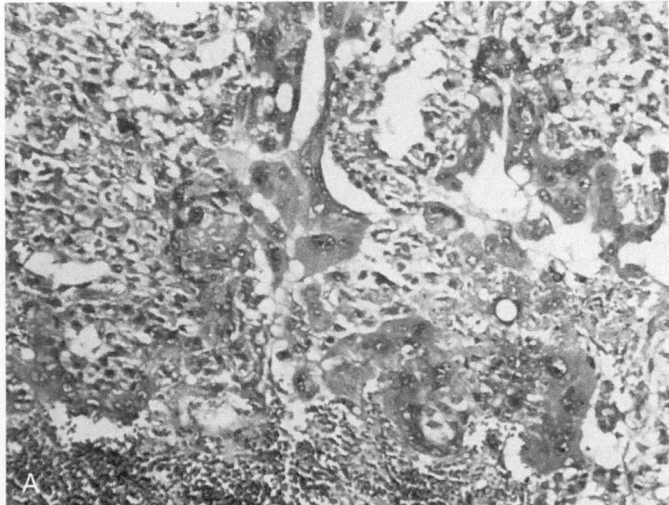

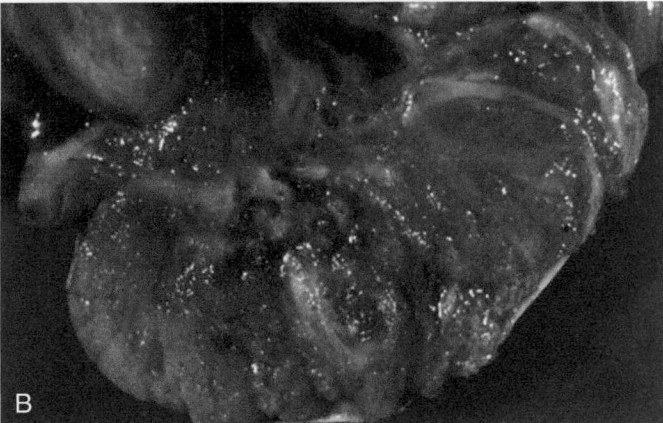

Figure 11-20. A, Choriocarcinoma. Bilaminar distribution of syncytiotrophoblasts and cytotrophoblasts with associated hemorrhage. **B,** Mixed germ cell tumor. Hemisected orchiectomy specimen showing characteristically heterogeneous cut surface with solid, hemorrhagic, and necrotic areas.

- Typically seen as a component of a mixed germ cell tumor; pure tumors are rare
- Teratocarcinoma: used to describe a mixed germ cell tumor composed of embryonal carcinoma and teratoma

Special Stains and Immunohistochemistry

- HCG: immunopositivity is strongest in syncytiotrophoblasts and weak or absent in cytotrophoblasts
- Cytokeratin and EMA typically positive
- CEA and PLAP may be positive

Other Techniques for Diagnosis

- Electron microscopy: syncytiotrophoblasts have prominent rough endoplasmic reticulum and interdigitating microvilli on the cell surface; desmosomes are seen in both cytotrophoblasts and syncytiotrophoblasts

Differential Diagnosis

MIXED GERM CELL TUMOR CONTAINING FOCI OF CHORIOCARCINOMA

- Adequate sampling is needed to differentiate pure choriocarcinoma from the much more common mixed germ cell tumor containing foci of choriocarcinoma

SEMINOMA

- Syncytiotrophoblasts occurring in a seminoma are scattered as single cells or small clusters without any associated cytotrophoblastic cells
- Degenerated cells in other germ cell tumors, particularly embryonal carcinoma, may resemble syncytiotrophoblasts but are HCG negative

PEARLS

- *Choriocarcinoma has almost always metastasized by the time of presentation*
- *Pure choriocarcinoma carries a worse prognosis than other germ cell tumors; mixed germ cell tumors with choriocarcinoma components have a worse prognosis than those without choriocarcinoma elements*
- *Radiation therapy is ineffective, but choriocarcinoma is chemosensitive*

SELECTED REFERENCES

Beyer J, Albers P, Altena R, et al: Maintaining success, reducing treatment burden, focusing on survivorship: highlights from the third European Consensus Conference on diagnosis and treatment of germ cell cancer. Ann Oncol 24:878-888, 2011.

Edge SB, Byrd DR, Compton CC, et al (eds): AJCC Cancer Staging Manual, 7th ed. New York: Springer, 2010, pp 469-478.

Woodward PJ, Heidenreich A, Looijenga LHJ, et al: Germ cell tumors. In Eble JN, Sauter G, Epstein JI, Sesterhenn IA (eds): World Health Organization Classification of Tumours: Pathology and Genetics: Tumours of the Urinary System and Male Genital Organs. Lyon, IARC Press, 2004, pp 221-249.

LEYDIG CELL TUMOR

Clinical Features

- Classified as a sex cord–stromal tumor
- Makes up about 3% of all testicular tumors
- Two peaks of incidence: children between 5 and 10 years of age (not seen before 2 years of age) and adults between ages 20 and 60 years

- Children present with isosexual pseudoprecocious puberty, and 10% have gynecomastia
- Adults present with testicular swelling; 30% have gynecomastia
- Associated with cryptorchidism and testicular atrophy
- Malignant behavior is seen in 10% of cases; benign behavior in prepubertal patients

Gross Pathology

- Well-circumscribed, solid or lobulated intratesticular nodule 2 to 5 cm in diameter (Figure 11-21A)
- Variably yellow, brown, or tan cut surface
- Hemorrhage and necrosis are uncommon

Histopathology

- Tumor cells are typically arranged in solid sheets; less commonly, nests or pseudoglandular pattern (Figure 11-21B)
- Cells are polygonal and have round nuclei with prominent central nucleoli and abundant eosinophilic cytoplasm
- Intracytoplasmic lipofuscin pigment can be seen, particularly in postpubertal patients
- Rod-shaped intracytoplasmic crystals of Reinke are seen in about 40% of cases
- Accumulated lipid may produce cells with clear, finely vacuolated cytoplasm
- Mitotic activity is typically low; ≥ 3 mitoses/10 hpf has been correlated with malignant behavior

Special Stains and Immunohistochemistry

- Vimentin and androgenic hormones: variable positivity

Other Techniques for Diagnosis

- Electron microscopy: cells have features of steroid synthesis, including lipid droplets, prominent smooth endoplasmic reticulum, and mitochondria with tubular cristae; crystals of Reinke appear as sharp geometric shapes, such as hexagons or rhomboid structures
- DNA aneuploidy can be seen in clinically benign tumors but has been associated with malignant behavior

Differential Diagnosis

LEYDIG CELL HYPERPLASIA

- May form nodules but has an interstitial pattern with preservation of the seminiferous tubules
- May be multifocal
- Lacks crystals of Reinke

LARGE CELL CALCIFYING SERTOLI CELL TUMOR

- Often bilateral and multifocal
- Cells have abundant eosinophilic cytoplasm and are arranged in a myxoid or collagenous stroma that is frequently calcified or ossified
- Lacks crystals of Reinke

SEMINOMA

- Must be differentiated from Leydig cell tumor with clear cells
- Tumor cells are round to polyhedral and have pale to clear cytoplasm with well-defined cell borders; uniform, round to oval nuclei with finely granular chromatin and one or two prominent nucleoli

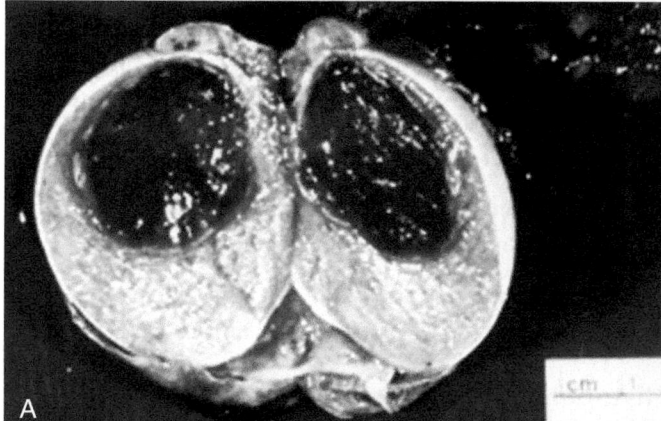

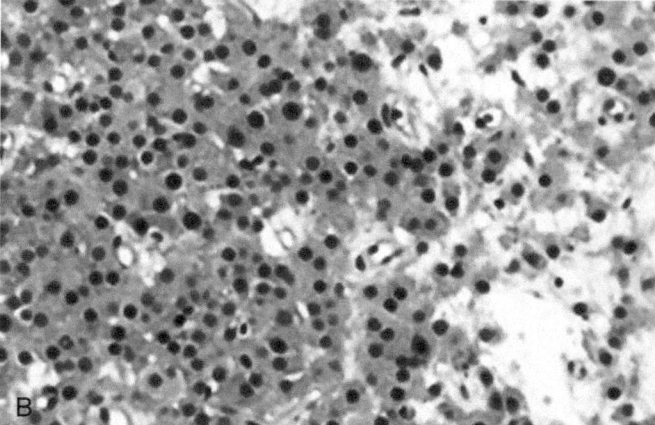

Figure 11-21. Leydig cell tumor. A, Hemisected orchiectomy specimen showing small, well-circumscribed, brown parenchymal nodule. **B,** Sheets of bland cells with a large amount of eosinophilic cytoplasm, rounded nuclei, and prominent nucleoli.

- Tumor cells have abundant intracytoplasmic glycogen
- Fibrous septa with lymphoid component surrounding tumor cells
- PLAP positive

PEARLS

- *Sex cord–stromal tumor composed of androgen-producing cells*
- *Tumor may elaborate androgens or estrogens*
- *Prepubescent children present with pseudoprecocious puberty and have a uniformly benign course*
- *Most tumors (90%) behave in a benign fashion; 10% are invasive and produce metastases*
- *Tumor size, mitotic index, cytologic atypia, necrosis, angiolymphatic invasion, and infiltration into paratesticular structures have all been associated with malignant behavior*

SELECTED REFERENCES

Hofmann M, Schlegel PG, Hippert F, et al: Testicular sex cord stromal tumors: analysis of patients from the MAKEI study. Pediatr Blood Cancer 60:1651-1655, 2013.

Sesterhenn IA, Jacobsen GK, Cheville J, et al: Sex cord gonadal stromal tumours. In Eble JN, Sauter G, Epstein JI, Sesterhenn IA (eds): World Health Organization Classification of Tumours: Pathology and Genetics: Tumours of the Urinary System and Male Genital Organs. Lyon, IARC Press, 2004, pp 250-258.

SERTOLI CELL TUMOR

Clinical Features

- Rare sex cord–stromal tumor constituting about 1% of testicular neoplasms
- Can occur at any age but most common in middle age
- Patients typically present with a testicular mass; gynecomastia or impotence due to estrogen production may be presenting complaint
- Children may develop gynecomastia but usually do not have isosexual pseudoprecocious puberty
- About 10% are malignant; malignancy can occur in prepubescent children
- Sclerosing variant presents without hormonal symptoms and is uniformly benign
- Large cell calcifying variant occurs in patients younger than 20 years and is a component of Carney syndrome in 40% of cases
- Intratubular large cell-hyalinizing Sertoli cell neoplasia may be associated with Peutz-Jeghers syndrome

Gross Pathology

- Solid, gray-white nodule typically smaller than 3 cm (Figure 11-22A)

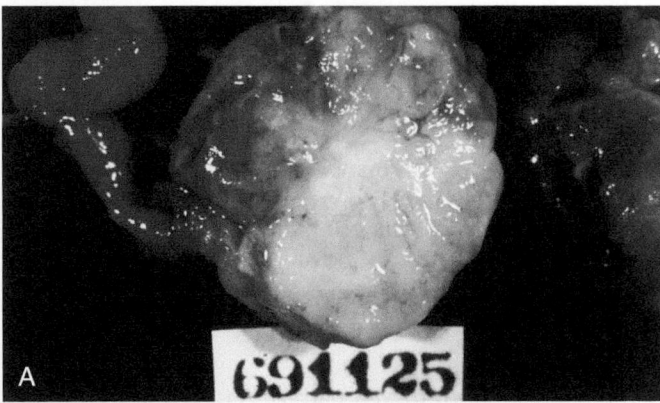
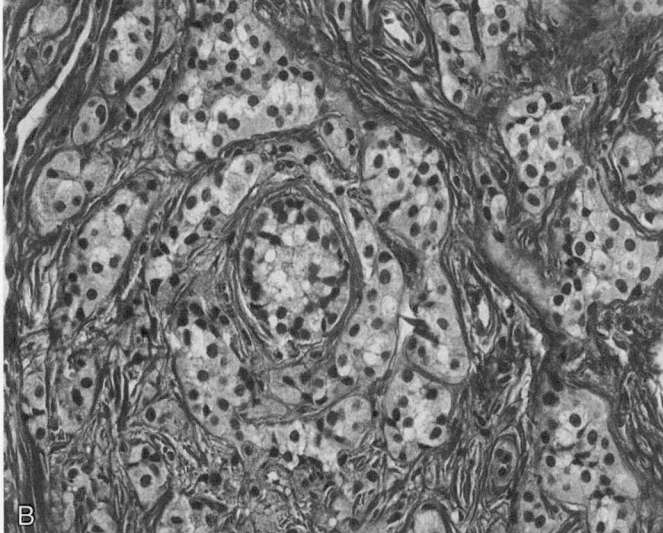

Figure 11-22. Sertoli cell tumor. A, Hemisected orchiectomy specimen showing a homogeneous, rubbery cut surface. **B,** Tubular arrangement of cells with vacuolated cytoplasm in a collagenous background.

- Large cell calcifying variant, usually tan-yellow with gritty calcifications; multifocal and bilateral in 40% of cases

Histopathology

- Tumor cells are typically arranged in a trabecular pattern and form cordlike structures resembling immature seminiferous tubules (Figure 11-22B)
- Tumor cells usually have clear or vacuolated cytoplasm owing to lipid accumulation and oval nuclei with moderate-sized nucleoli
- Sclerosing variant
  - Has dense collagenous stroma
- Large cell calcifying variant
  - Composed of cells with abundant eosinophilic cytoplasm in a myxoid or collagenous stroma that is frequently calcified or ossified (Figure 11-23A and B)
  - May have an intratubular component

Special Stains and Immunohistochemistry

- Immunostaining variable but tend to be S-100, inhibin, cytokeratin, vimentin, and calretinin (focal) positive and EMA negative

Other Techniques for Diagnosis

- Electron microscopy: cells have features of steroid synthesis, including lipid droplets, prominent smooth endoplasmic reticulum, and mitochondria with tubular cristae; adjacent cells are connected by desmosomes; perinuclear arrays of filaments (Charcot-Böttcher filaments) are pathognomonic for Sertoli cell differentiation and are present in all variants

Differential Diagnosis

SEMINOMA

- Typically arranged in solid sheets rather than tubules
- Tumor cells have abundant intracytoplasmic glycogen instead of lipid
- Fibrous septa with prominent lymphoid infiltrate
- Typically shows adjacent intratubular germ cell neoplasia

ADENOMATOID TUMOR (VERSUS SCLEROSING VARIANT OF SERTOLI CELL TUMOR)

- Centered in paratesticular tissue with only occasional extension into testicular parenchyma
- Inhibin immunonegative and usually EMA immunopositive

TESTICULAR WELL-DIFFERENTIATED NEUROENDOCRINE (CARCINOID) TUMOR

- Insular (nontrabecular) growth pattern at least focally
- May be associated with teratoma
- Neuroendocrine immunomarkers (chromogranin, synaptophysin, or NSE) uniformly positive

LEYDIG CELL TUMOR (VERSUS LARGE CELL CALCIFYING VARIANT OF SERTOLI CELL TUMOR)

- Typically grows in sheets, nests, and rarely cords
- Lacks tubular architecture, intratubular growth, and calcifications
- Cytoplasmic lipofuscin pigment and Reinke crystals

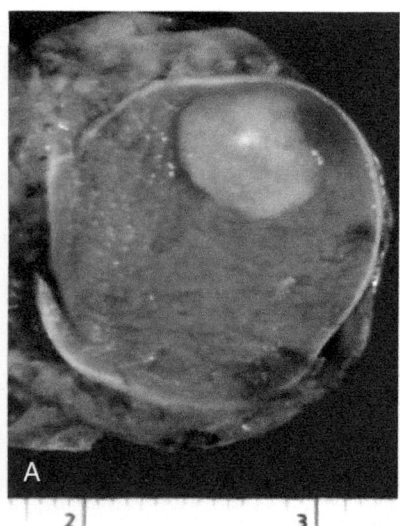
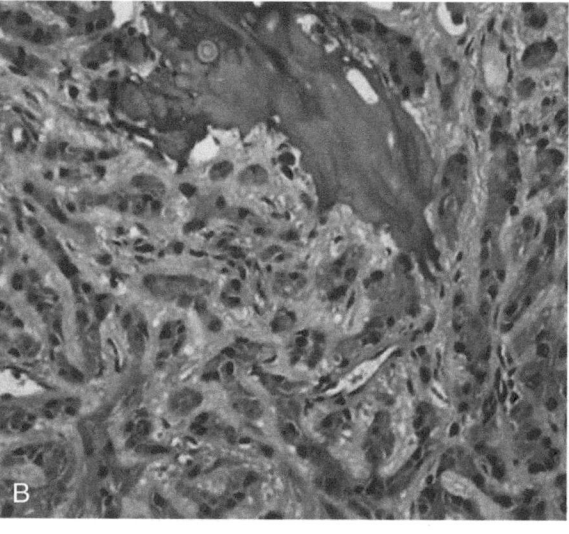

Figure 11-23. Sertoli cell tumor, large cell calcifying variant. A, Sharply circumscribed, intraparenchymal tumor bulging from the surface of the hemisected testis with central, yellow-white calcification. **B,** Cords of polygonal cells with abundant eosinophilic cytoplasm in a myxofibromatous stroma with calcification.

ANDROGEN INSENSITIVITY SYNDROME OR TESTICULAR FEMINIZATION
- Patients may develop a nodular lesion of closely packed tubules lined by Sertoli cells, but these nodules also contain intervening Leydig cells

PEARLS

- *Rare sex cord–stromal tumor*
- *Malignant behavior in up to 10% of cases*
- *Charcot-Böttcher filaments on EM are pathognomonic for Sertoli cell differentiation*
- *Diagnosis of large cell calcifying Sertoli cell tumor should prompt an investigation for other components of Carney syndrome*

SELECTED REFERENCES

Hofmann M, Schlegel PG, Hippert F, et al: Testicular sex cord stromal tumors: analysis of patients from the MAKEI study. Pediatr Blood Cancer 60:1651-1655, 2013.

Sesterhenn IA, Jacobsen GK, Cheville J, et al: Sex cord gonadal stromal tumours. In Eble JN, Sauter G, Epstein JI, Sesterhenn IA (eds): World Health Organization Classification of Tumours: Pathology and Genetics: Tumours of the Urinary System and Male Genital Organs. Lyon, IARC Press, 2004, pp 250-258.

GRANULOSA CELL TUMOR

Clinical Features
- Rare sex cord–stromal tumor with adult and juvenile subtypes
- Adult type
  - Least common sex cord–stromal tumor
  - Occurs in patients 15 to 75 years old
  - Presents with a testicular mass and is frequently associated with gynecomastia
  - Benign behavior; essentially no metastatic potential
- Juvenile type
  - Most common non–germ cell tumor of neonates
  - Restricted to infants younger than 5 months
  - Presents with a testicular mass without hormonal symptoms

- May be associated with gonadal dysgenesis or sex chromosome anomalies
- Malignant behavior has not been reported

Gross Pathology
- Solitary gray, yellow to tan nodule with solid and cystic areas
- May be up to 10 cm in diameter

Histopathology

ADULT TYPE
- Microfollicular or solid pattern
- Characterized by Call-Exner bodies (small follicles containing eosinophilic material and nuclear debris)
- Tumor cells have round to oval nuclei, often with characteristic nuclear grooves and scant, pale cytoplasm
- Mitotic figures are uncommon

JUVENILE TYPE
- Follicular, solid, or mixed pattern (Figure 11-24)
- Basophilic material within follicles is mucicarmine positive

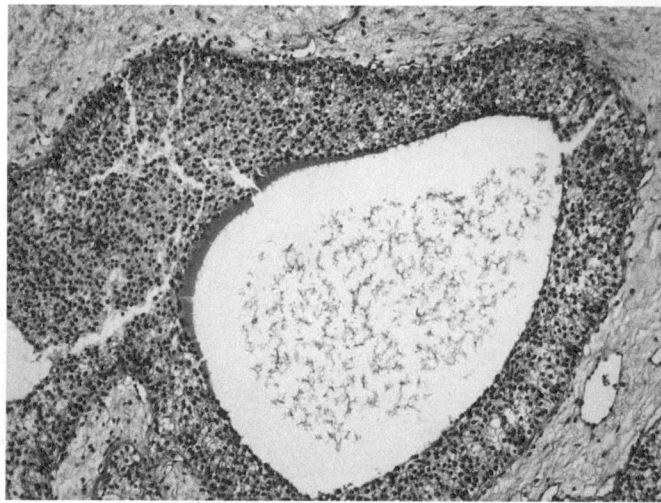

Figure 11-24. Granulosa cell tumor, juvenile type. Follicle-like structure consisting of uniformly bland cells and partially lined by eosinophilic material.

- Solid areas may have a hyalinized, collagenous stroma
- Tumor cells are round to polyhedral and have hyperchromatic nuclei with identifiable nucleoli and abundant pale to eosinophilic cytoplasm
- Mitoses may be frequent

Special Stains and Immunohistochemistry

- Cytokeratin (predominantly 8 and 18) positive
- Vimentin positive mucicarmine
  - Intrafollicular material in juvenile granulosa cell tumors is positive
  - Adult granulosa cell tumors are mucicarmine negative

Other Techniques for Diagnosis

- Noncontributory

Differential Diagnosis

CARCINOID TUMOR

- May resemble adult granulosa cell tumors, but the tumor cells lack nuclear grooves and have characteristic granular chromatin
- Positive for neuroendocrine immunohistochemical markers

YOLK SAC TUMOR

- May have a cystic or solid pattern and thus resemble juvenile granulosa cell tumors
- Tumor cells typically have characteristic intracellular hyaline globules
- May show characteristic Schiller-Duval bodies
- Positive for AFP

PEARLS

- *Juvenile-type granulosa cell tumor in adults is rare*
- *Juvenile-type granulosa cell tumor is the most common non–germ cell tumor in infants*
- *Malignant behavior is not seen in the juvenile type of testicular granulosa cell tumor*

SELECTED REFERENCES

Hofmann M, Schlegel PG, Hippert F, et al: Testicular sex cord stromal tumors: analysis of patients from the MAKEI study. Pediatr Blood Cancer 60:1651-1655, 2013.
Sesterhenn IA, Jacobsen GK, Cheville J, et al: Sex cord gonadal stromal tumours. In Eble JN, Sauter G, Epstein JI, Sesterhenn IA (eds): World Health Organization Classification of Tumours: Pathology and Genetics: Tumours of the Urinary System and Male Genital Organs. Lyon, IARC Press, 2004, pp 250-258.

GONADOBLASTOMA

Clinical Features

- Occurs in the abnormal, dysgenetic gonads of patients with an intersex syndrome or in undescended testes
- Phenotypically, male patients present in childhood or early adolescence
- Usually an incidental finding in gonads removed for other indications
- Bilateral involvement is seen in one third of cases
- Typically has a benign clinical course; however, in 10% to 50% of cases, there is an associated germ cell neoplasm

Gross Pathology

- Solid, gray to yellow-brown tumor, ranging in size from less than 1 mm up to several centimeters
- Cut surface may be soft, fleshy, or firm, or may appear chondroid
- May have scattered, gritty calcification or be almost totally calcified

Histopathology

- Germ cells and cells of sex cord–stromal differentiation arranged in well-defined nests with surrounding connective tissue stroma
- Cells surround amorphous eosinophilic material (hyaline)
- Germ cells resemble seminoma, immature testicular germ cells, or spermatogonia (large cells have vesicular nuclei with finely granular chromatin and prominent nucleoli); mitotically active (Figure 11-25)
- Epithelial cells of sex cord–stromal origin resemble immature Sertoli or granulosa cells (small, uniform, round or elongated cells with scanty cytoplasm and pale nuclei); mitotically inactive
- May have foci of calcification or hyalinization
- An associated germ cell tumor may be seen

Special Stains and Immunohistochemistry

- PAS: seminoma-like cells are positive owing to abundant glycogen

Other Techniques for Diagnosis

- Electron microscopy: Sertoli-like sex cord cells may contain Charcot-Böttcher filaments

Differential Diagnosis

SERTOLI CELL NODULE WITH INTRATUBULAR GERM CELL NEOPLASIA

- Usually a microscopic lesion in a nondysgenetic gonad with foci of neoplastic germ cells variably distributed among the Sertoli cells

PEARLS

- *Although pure gonadoblastoma is a benign lesion, prognosis depends on the presence and behavior of any associated germ cell neoplasm*
- *Bilateral orchiectomy is recommended because of the high incidence of bilaterality of gonadoblastoma and risk for associated germ cell neoplasm*

SELECTED REFERENCE

Ulbright TM: Tumours containing both sex cord/gonadal stromal elements. Gonadoblastoma. In Eble JN, Sauter G, Epstein JI, Sesterhenn IA (eds): World Health Organization Classification of Tumours: Pathology and Genetics: Tumours of the Urinary System and Male Genital Organs. Lyon, IARC Press, 2004, pp 259-262.

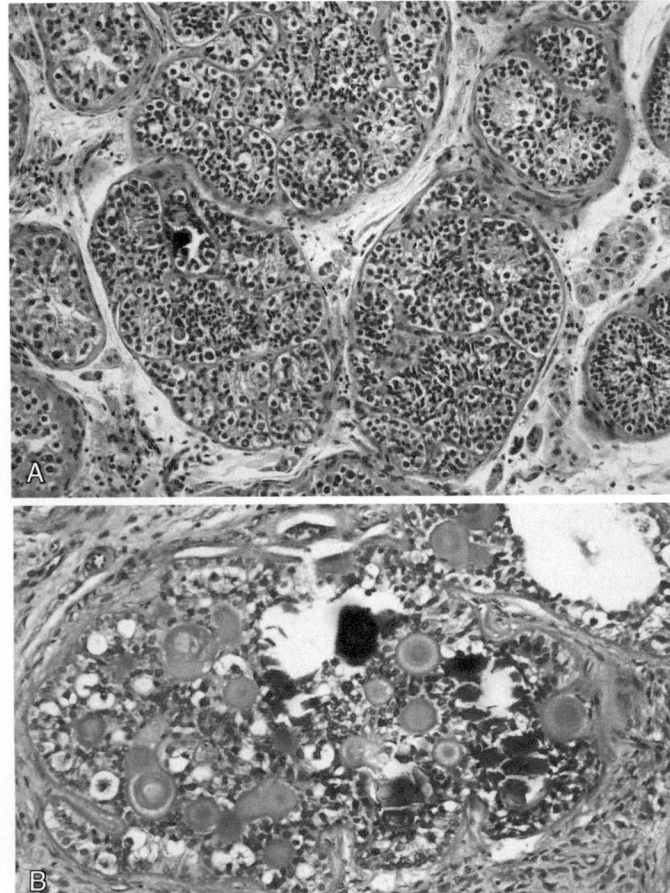

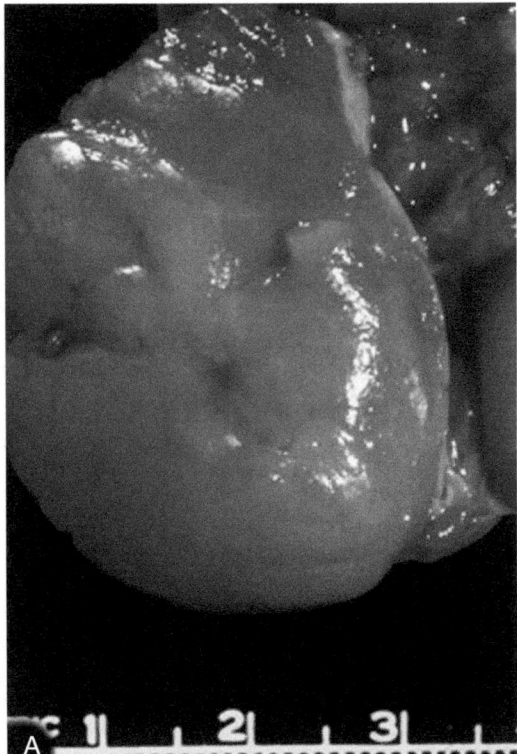

Figure 11-25. A, Gonadoblastic congeries. Germ cells in a patient with intratubular germ cell neoplasia (usual type) incidentally involving a Sertoli cell nodule or congeries. This should not be confused with gonadoblastoma. **B,** Gonadoblastoma. Mixed population of Sertoli cells and neoplastic germ cells associated with hyalinization and microcalcifications.

LYMPHOMA

Clinical Features

- Primary testicular lymphoma is rare; subclinical testicular involvement in the late stages of disseminated disease is more common
- Lymphoma makes up about 5% of all testicular tumors
- Most common malignant testicular tumor in patients older than 50 years

Gross Pathology

- Part or the entire testis is replaced by a single mass or multiple nodules
- Cut surface is cream to tan, soft, fleshy, and homogeneous (Figure 11-26A)
- Spread to the epididymis or spermatic cord is seen in up to 50% of cases

Histopathology

- Lymphoid infiltrate shows a characteristic interstitial growth pattern typically sparing the seminiferous tubules (Figure 11-26B)

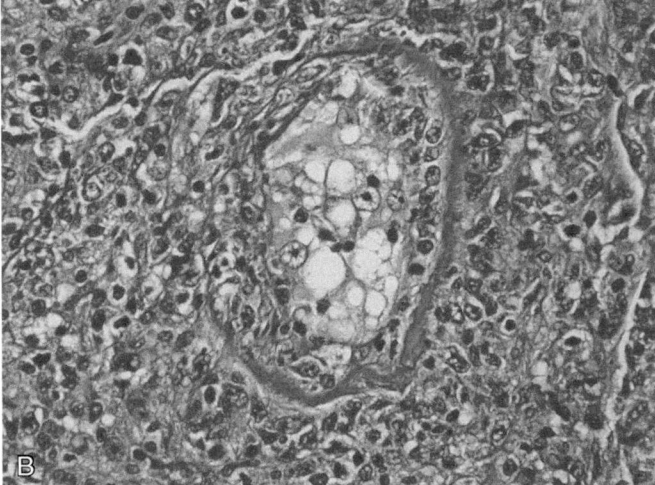

Figure 11-26. Non-Hodgkin lymphoma, large cell type. A, Hemisected orchiectomy specimen with characteristic homogeneous tan-yellow cut surface in a 60+-year-old patient. **B,** Interstitial growth of malignant lymphoid cells surrounding and partially involving a hyalinized seminiferous tubule.

- Most common histologic type is diffuse large cell lymphoma, B-cell type
- Follicular lymphoma and Hodgkin disease are rare in the testis

Special Stains and Immunohistochemistry

- B-cell lymphomas make up about 90% of testicular lymphomas
- Immunohistochemical markers are as expected for the various types of lymphoma

Other Techniques for Diagnosis

- As with other lymphomas, flow cytometry, molecular diagnostic techniques, and cytogenetics may be crucial (refer to Chapter 14)

Differential Diagnosis

SEMINOMA

- Composed of glycogen-rich cells with well-defined borders and prominent lymphocytic infiltrate
- Positive for PLAP

CHRONIC ORCHITIS

- Contains a heterogeneous population of inflammatory cells consisting of lymphocytes, plasma cells, and neutrophils that typically involve the seminiferous tubules
- Long-term infection results in patchy interstitial fibrosis and atrophy of seminiferous tubules; often involves both testes

PEARLS

- *Lymphoma accounts for more than 50% of testicular tumors in men older than 60 years*
- *Primary lymphoma limited to the testis is rare*

SELECTED REFERENCES

Ahmad SS, Idris SF, Follows GA, et al: Primary testicular lymphoma. Clin Oncol 24:358-365, 2012.
Horne MJ, Adeniran AJ: Primary diffuse large B-cell lymphoma of the testis. Arch Pathol Lab Med 135:1363-1367, 2011.

PARATESTICULAR ADNEXA AND SPERMATIC CORD

EPIDIDYMITIS

Clinical Features

- May be acute or chronic depending on inciting agent and duration of disease
- Acute cases present with unilateral painful swelling of the epididymis and scrotum
- Acute epididymitis may be caused by bacteria (enteric gram-negative rods, *Neisseria gonorrhoeae*, *Chlamydia trachomatis*), viruses (mumps, cytomegalovirus), or trauma
- Chronic epididymitis is associated with tuberculosis, leprosy, sarcoidosis, fungi, and sperm granulomas
- Usually occurs in conjunction with orchitis or after trauma
- Most cases are due to retrograde spread by urine reflux
- Rarely seen as a surgical specimen

Gross Pathology

- Acute infection: epididymis is thickened, congested, and edematous and has a variable fibrinopurulent exudate
- Chronic infection: epididymis is indurated and scarred; calcification or calculi may be seen

Histopathology

- Microscopic features vary depending on the causative agent
- Bacterial infection is associated with neutrophilic microabscesses, edema, and tubular destruction; xanthogranulomas may be seen
- Cases of *C. trachomatis* infection show minimally destructive periductal and intraepithelial inflammation
- Viral infection leads to vascular congestion, edema, and interstitial lymphocytic infiltrates
- Tuberculous epididymitis has prominent caseating granulomas
- Lepromatous epididymitis leprosy shows perivascular and perineural lymphocytic infiltrates with sheets of macrophages containing acid-fast organisms
- Typical noncaseating granulomas may be seen in sarcoidosis
- Fungi usually cause necrotizing granulomas and abscesses
- Traumatic epididymitis shows vascular congestion and patchy blood extravasation
- Sperm granulomas cause foreign body–type reactions due to extravasated sperm

Special Stains and Immunohistochemistry

- Special stains for bacteria or fungi may be helpful
- Immunohistochemistry for *C. trachomatis* or viral agents may be performed

Other Techniques for Diagnosis

- Noncontributory

Differential Diagnosis

- Differential diagnosis depends on clinical features and identification of the specific inciting agent

PEARLS

- *Presentation and microscopic features depend on the inciting agent*
- *Urethral or epididymal aspirate smears and cultures are useful in identifying the causative agent*
- *Diagnosis is generally based on clinical symptoms and culture results*
- *Treatment is typically medical; rarely seen as a surgical specimen*

SELECTED REFERENCE

Hedger MP: Immunophysiology and pathology of inflammation in the testis and epididymis. J Androl 32:625-640, 2011.

CYSTS OF TESTICULAR ADNEXA

Clinical Features

- Often discovered as part of the clinical workup for infertility
- May be difficult to distinguish from cysts of testicular cysts by ultrasound
- May be difficult to distinguish from neoplastic cysts by ultrasound

Gross Pathology

- Spermatocele is usually unilocular, may be located anywhere along the flow of spermatozoa, contains clear or milky fluid, and has a floppy cyst wall
- Epididymal cyst may involve head, body, or tail, usually unilocular, contains clear or milky fluid, and has a rubbery cyst wall
- Cystic ductus efferentia are multiloculated and, by definition, lie between the rete testis and head of epididymis (Figure 11-27)

Histopathology

- Spermatocele is lined by attenuated epithelium and associated with spermatozoa
- Epididymal cyst lined by epididymal epithelium that may be hyperplastic or attenuated
- Cystic ductus efferentia is lined low cuboidal epithelium and not associated with epididymal smooth muscle

Special Stains and Immunohistochemistry

- Noncontributory

Other Techniques for Diagnosis

- Noncontributory

Differential Diagnosis

- Dermoid cysts are lined by keratinizing squamous epithelium but also have adnexal structures
- Teratomas may be mostly cystic lined by keratinizing squamous epithelium but also have teratomatous elements

PEARLS

- *Complete submission of epidermoid cysts is required to rule out dermoid cysts and teratoma*

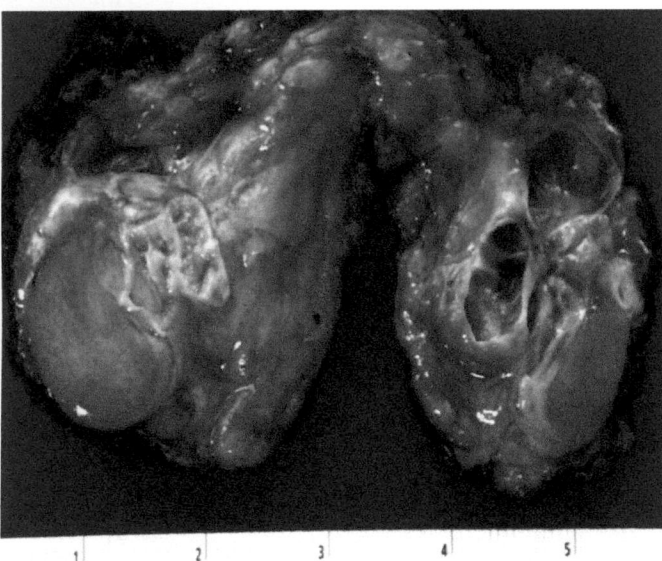

Figure 11-27. Cystic ductus efferentia. Hemisected orchiectomy specimen showing paratesticular, multiloculated cyst abutting testicular hilum.

SELECTED REFERENCE

Algaba F, Mikuz G, Boccon-Gibod L, et al: Pseudoneoplastic lesions of the testis and paratesticular structures. Virchows Arch 451:987-997, 2007.

LIPOMA

Clinical Features

- Accounts for up to 90% of spermatic cord tumors
- Usually occurs in adults but can be seen at all ages

Gross Pathology

- Well-circumscribed, lobulated mass of mature, yellow adipose tissue

Histopathology

- Composed of mature, variably sized adipocytes with no nuclear pleomorphism or mitotic activity; similar to that of lipoma at other sites
- Variants include angiolipoma and combinations of fibrous or myxoid types
- Hibernoma may rarely be seen

Special Stains and Immunohistochemistry

- Noncontributory

Other Techniques for Diagnosis

- Noncontributory

Differential Diagnosis

WELL-DIFFERENTIATED LIPOSARCOMA

- Rare in this location
- Greater nuclear pleomorphism and higher mitotic rate
- Distinction between true (i.e., neoplastic) lipoma and so-called lipoma of the cord associated with inguinal hernias (prolapsed portions of preperitoneal adipose tissue) is somewhat arbitrary

PEARLS

- *Most common paratesticular tumor*

SELECTED REFERENCE

Lioe TF, Biggart JD: Tumours of the spermatic cord and paratesticular tissue: a clinicopathological study. Br J Urol 71:600-606, 1993.

ADENOMATOID TUMOR

Clinical Features

- Most common neoplasm of the paratesticular tissues
- Seen at all ages; peak incidence between 20 and 40 years of age
- Typically located in lower pole of epididymis; may be found in tunica albuginea or spermatic cord (Figure 11-28A)
- Presents as a painless, unilateral, solitary, solid mass that does not transilluminate
- May extend into testis, but behavior is uniformly benign

Gross Pathology

- Usually smaller than 5 cm; solitary, gray-white, well-demarcated, firm nodule
- Cut surface is homogeneous and fibrous with a whorled appearance; occasional yellow areas may be seen

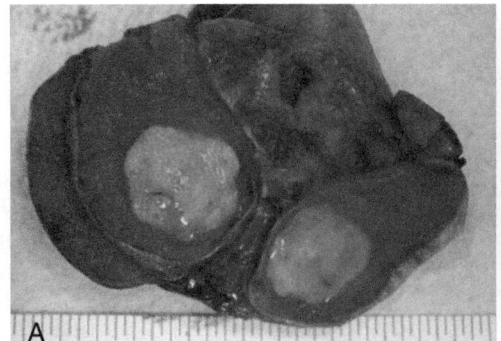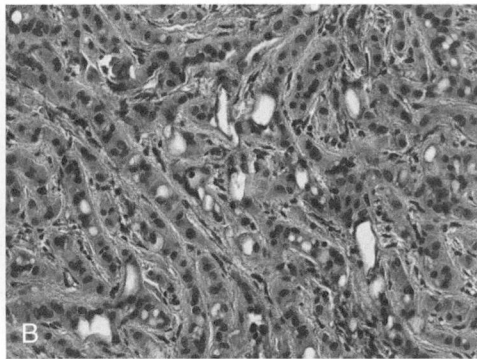

Figure 11-28. Adenomatoid tumor. A. Hemisected testis showing a rare example of a parenchymal tumor that was only focally abutting the tunica albuginea. **B.** Characteristic variably sized tubular structures with a pseudoinfiltrative growth pattern lined by bland, low cuboidal epithelial cells.

Histopathology

- Composed of two major components: epithelial-like cells and fibrous stroma
  - Epithelial-like cells
    - Form networks of round, oval, or slitlike tubules, irregular cysts, or small cords
    - Cells lining the tubules may be flat, cuboidal, or low columnar and have round to oval nuclei and abundant dense cytoplasm (Figure 11-28B)
    - Cytoplasm may contain intracytoplasmic vacuoles, giving the appearance of signet ring cells
  - Fibrous stroma
    - May be hyalinized or contain smooth muscle
    - Stroma often contains lymphoid aggregates or patchy lymphocytic infiltrate
    - Infiltrative border with extension into the testicular parenchyma may be present
    - Lymphoid aggregates may be seen within the tumor or at the periphery

Special Stains and Immunohistochemistry

- Mesothelial markers (thrombomodulin, HBME-1, CK5/6, OC125, calretinin, and cytokeratin) positive
- Alcian blue: may be positive (hyaluronidase sensitive)
- CEA, Leu-M1, inhibin, and factor VIII negative

Other Techniques for Diagnosis

- Electron microscopy: numerous microvilli on the luminal surface of the epithelial-like cells with well-developed desmosomes on the lateral surfaces

Differential Diagnosis

METASTATIC CARCINOMA
- Typically occurs in an older age group
- Usually bilateral
- Demonstrates frankly malignant cells that may show hyaluronidase-resistant positive mucin staining

SCLEROSING SERTOLI CELL TUMOR
- Centered in testicular parenchyma with occasional extension into paratesticular tissues
- Usually inhibin immunopositive and EMA immuno-negative

ADENOCARCINOMA OF THE RETE TESTIS
- Rare tumor
- Typically forms an ill-defined mass at the testicular hilum

- May have a solid or tubulopapillary growth pattern
- Composed of pleomorphic cells with large nuclei and prominent nucleoli
- Poor prognosis

MALIGNANT MESOTHELIOMA
- Highly cellular tumor composed of pleomorphic cells with high mitotic rate
- Characteristic immunohistochemical profile

PEARLS

- *Firm, well-demarcated paratesticular mass with epithelial-like elements in a fibrous stroma*
- *Uniformly benign behavior*

SELECTED REFERENCE

Amin MB: Selected other problematic testicular and paratesticular lesions: rete testis neoplasms and pseudotumors, mesothelial lesions, and secondary tumors. Mod Pathol 18(suppl 2):S131-S145, 2005.

PAPILLARY CYSTADENOMA OF THE EPIDIDYMIS

Clinical Features

- Accounts for one third of primary epididymal tumors
- Age range is from 15 to 70 years, with a slight peak in the second and third decades of life
- May present as a small nodule in the head of the epididymis
- About 40% are bilateral
- May be seen in patients with von Hippel-Lindau disease

Gross Pathology

- Well-circumscribed, often encapsulated nodule, typically 1 to 5 cm in diameter
- Multicystic mass with a mottled gray-tan, yellow, and brown cut surface
- Fluid within the cysts may be clear, yellow, or hemorrhagic

Histopathology

- Composed of dilated ducts and cystic spaces with papillary projections
- Cystic spaces and papillae are lined by a single or double layer of cuboidal to tall columnar cells with clear or vacuolated cytoplasm

- Tumor cells are filled with glycogen and secretory droplets and have cilia at the luminal surface
- Stroma is densely fibrous with focal areas of hyalinization and patchy chronic inflammation
- Small foci of lipogranulomatous inflammation may be seen

Special Stains and Immunohistochemistry

- PAS: tumor cells are PAS positive, diastase sensitive because of their high glycogen content

Other Techniques for Diagnosis

- Noncontributory

Differential Diagnosis

PAPILLARY CARCINOMA

- Tumors with extensive papillary projections may appear solid and must be differentiated from papillary carcinoma, which tends to be more cellular and shows a greater degree of pleomorphism

PEARLS

- *Almost two thirds of the cases of cystadenoma occur in patients with von Hippel-Lindau disease*
- *Clinical behavior is uniformly benign*

SELECTED REFERENCE

Kuhn MT, Maclennan GT: Benign neoplasms of the epididymis. J Urol 174:723, 2005.

FIBROUS PSEUDOTUMOR

Clinical Features

- Second most common mass-forming lesion of the testicular adnexa (most common is adenomatoid tumor)
- Diffuse or localized proliferation involving the tunicae, epididymis, or spermatic cord
- Reported in patients ranging from 7 to 95 years of age; peak incidence in the third decade
- About 30% of patients report a history of trauma or epididymo-orchitis

Gross Pathology

- Firm, white cut surface
- In the localized form, there may be single or multiple nodules ranging from less than 0.5 cm up to almost 10 cm in diameter
- Diffuse form is characterized by a diffuse thickening of the involved tissues

Histopathology

- Characteristically shows a spindle cell proliferation with a whorled appearance and areas of hyalinized collagen
- Focal hypercellularity may be seen
- Stroma contains a variable inflammatory cell infiltrate consisting of lymphocytes, plasma cells, histiocytes, and scattered eosinophils
- Calcification and ossification may be present
- About half of the lesions may show features of fibroxanthoma, sclerosing lipogranuloma, or sclerosing hemangioma

Special Stains and Immunohistochemistry

- Cytokeratin, SMA, and S-100 protein negative

Other Techniques for Diagnosis

- Noncontributory

Differential Diagnosis

SPINDLE CELL MESOTHELIOMA

- Consists of cells with eosinophilic cytoplasm in a background of cytokeratin-positive cells
- Features of mesothelial cell origin seen on electron microscopy

IDIOPATHIC FIBROMATOSIS

- Typically a more diffuse process with less inflammatory infiltrate
- May be seen in association with fibromatosis of the retroperitoneum

SARCOMA

- Generally hypercellular neoplasm composed of malignant cells with pleomorphic nuclei
- High mitotic rate often with atypical forms
- Less inflammatory cell infiltrate

LEIOMYOMA AND NEUROFIBROMA

- Best differentiated with immunohistochemistry

PEARLS

- *Fibrous pseudotumor is a reactive, non-neoplastic fibrous proliferation that may clinically mimic a testicular neoplasm*

SELECTED REFERENCES

Frias-Kletecka MC, MacLennan GT: Benign soft tissue tumors of the testis. J Urol 182:312-313, 2009.
Polsky EG, Ray C, Dubilier LD: Diffuse fibrous pseudotumor of the tunica vaginalis testis, epididymis, and spermatic cord. J Urol 171:1625-1626, 2004.

LEIOMYOMA AND LEIOMYOSARCOMA

Clinical Features

LEIOMYOMA

- Relatively common tumor of the epididymis
- Variable age range; rare in children
- Associated with a hernia sac or hydrocele in up to 20% of cases
- Bilateral in up to 40% of cases

LEIOMYOSARCOMA

- More common in the spermatic cord than in the epididymis
- Peak incidence in the sixth and seventh decades

Gross Pathology

LEIOMYOMA

- Well-defined, variably sized, round, firm, gray-white mass
- Whorled, bulging, homogeneous cut surface

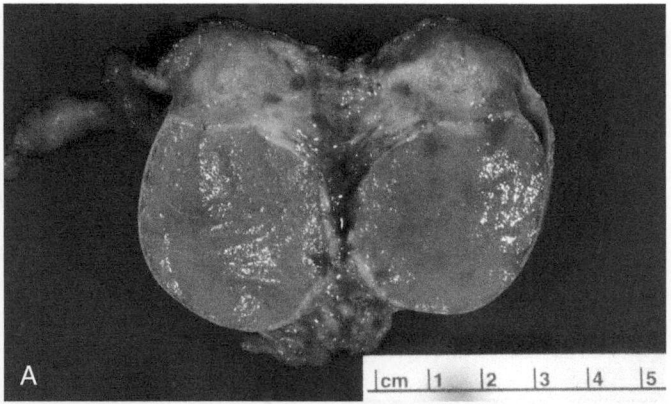

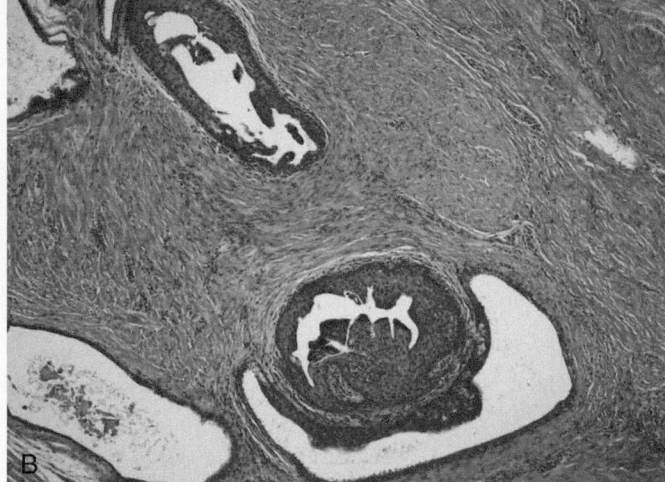

Figure 11-29. Smooth muscle hyperplasia of testicular adnexa. A, Hemisected orchiectomy specimen showing normal testicular parenchyma and an adjacent rubbery white mass involving the epididymis. **B,** Smooth muscle intimately associated with epididymal tissue with secondary dilation and squamous metaplasia.

LEIOMYOSARCOMA
- Similar to leiomyoma; more commonly has areas of necrosis and hemorrhage (Figure 11-30)

Histopathology
LEIOMYOMA
- Spindle cell proliferation composed of interlacing bundles of uniform, spindled smooth muscle cells
- Rare or absent mitotic activity

LEIOMYOSARCOMA
- Cellular spindle cell proliferation that typically shows greater nuclear pleomorphism
- High mitotic rate (≥ 1 to 2 mitoses/hpf)
- Hemorrhage and necrosis are common, especially in high-grade tumors
- Definitive features to distinguish leiomyoma from low-grade leiomyosarcoma are lacking

Special Stains and Immunohistochemistry
- Vimentin, SMA, and desmin positive

Other Techniques for Diagnosis
- Electron microscopy: cells have features of smooth muscle differentiation with bundles of thin filaments and pinocytotic vesicles

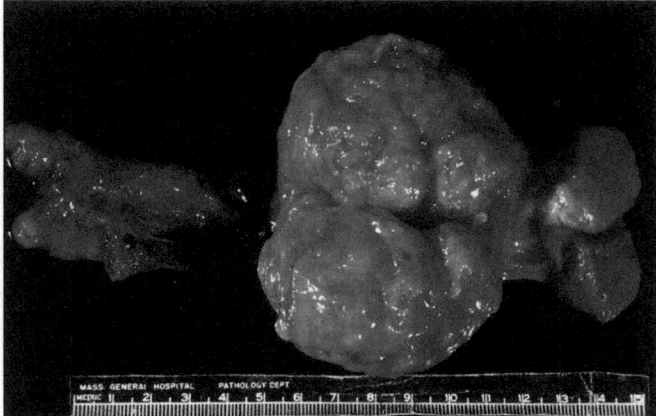

Figure 11-30. Leiomyosarcoma. Radical orchiectomy specimen showing a rubbery, tan, lobulated mass in the midportion of the spermatic cord.

Differential Diagnosis
LOW-GRADE LEIOMYOSARCOMA VERSUS LEIOMYOMA
- See "Histopathology"

FIBROUS MESOTHELIOMA
- Negative for SMA

LIPOSARCOMA WITH SMOOTH MUSCLE DEDIFFERENTIATION
- Increased MDM2 nuclear immunopositivity
- MDM2 amplification by fluorescent in situ hybridization

EMBRYONAL RHABDOMYOSARCOMA, SPINDLE CELL TYPE
- Rhabdomyoblasts at least focally present
- Immunopositive for myogenin and myoglobin and immunonegative for H-caldesmon

SMOOTH MUSCLE HYPERPLASIA OF TESTICULAR ADNEXA
- Fascicles of bland smooth muscle cells insinuating themselves between dilated epididymal (Figure 11-29)

PEARLS
- *Mitotic rate appears to be the most reliable criterion to distinguish between leiomyoma and low-grade leiomyosarcoma; necrosis, high mitotic activity, hypercellularity, and marked nuclear pleomorphism suggest malignancy*
- *Treatment of both leiomyoma and leiomyosarcoma is typically orchiectomy; role of retroperitoneal dissection for leiomyosarcoma is controversial*
- *Leiomyosarcoma frequently recurs locally and often metastasizes; about one third of patients die from metastatic disease*

SELECTED REFERENCE
Fisher C, Goldblum JR, Epstein JI, et al: Leiomyosarcoma of the paratesticular region: a clinicopathological study. Am J Surg Pathol 25:1143-1149, 2001.

LIPOSARCOMA

Clinical Features
- Most common paratesticular sarcoma in adults (overall, rare in this location)

- Typically found in adults between the ages of 40 and 90 years
- Presents as large, firm, slowly growing mass within the scrotum or inguinal canal

Gross Pathology

- Resembles lipoma; more often multinodular; cut surface is yellow and may be soft or firm (Figure 11-31A)
- Focal mucinous areas or necrosis may be seen

Histopathology

- Well-differentiated liposarcoma
  - Most common subtype
  - Composed of enlarged, mature adipocytes that typically have atypical, hyperchromatic nuclei
  - Varying numbers of vacuolated lipoblasts
  - Often have prominent areas of sclerosis
- Dedifferentiated liposarcoma
  - Dedifferentiated (i.e., nonlipogenic) areas usually high-grade (pleomorphic) but may show low-grade, smooth muscle differentiation
  - The well-differentiated component may be difficult to document
- Myxoid and pleomorphic liposarcomas may be seen but are less common in the paratesticular tissues

Special Stains and Immunohistochemistry

- Oil red O and Sudan black: lipoblasts contain intracellular lipid vacuoles that are positive with fat stains

Other Techniques for Diagnosis

- Cytogenetic studies: well-differentiated liposarcoma is associated with ring chromosome 12; myxoid liposarcoma is associated with t(12;16)
- Increased MDM2 nuclear immunopositivity and MDM2 amplification by fluorescent in situ hybridization (Figure 11-31B)

Differential Diagnosis

LIPOMA

- Much more common in this location

- Composed of benign-appearing, mature adipocytes with small, eccentric, compressed nuclei
- No lipoblasts

SCLEROSING LIPOGRANULOMA

- Generally occurs in younger patients
- May involve the penis, scrotum, spermatic cord, or perineum
- Granulomatous and mixed inflammatory infiltrate in a sclerotic background
- Scattered foreign-body giant cells

PEARLS

- *Most tumors are well-differentiated; may recur after local excision*
- *Typically more indolent behavior compared to other sarcomas*
- *Poorly differentiated liposarcoma is rare in this location but may produce distant metastases*
- *Treatment is typically radical orchiectomy, usually without lymph node dissection; may rarely need to perform hemiscrotectomy to obtain negative margins*

SELECTED REFERENCES

Dotan ZA, Tal R, Golijanin D, et al: Adult genitourinary sarcoma: the 25-year Memorial Sloan-Kettering experience. J Urol 176:2033-2038, 2006.
Montgomery E, Fisher C: Paratesticular liposarcoma: a clinicopathologic study. Am J Surg Pathol 27:40-47, 2003.

RHABDOMYOSARCOMA

Clinical Features

- Second most common tumor of the paratesticular tissues, behind only adenomatoid tumor
- About 60% of cases occur in the first two decades of life; peak incidence at 10 years of age
- About 95% of patients present with a mass in the scrotum, with only rare involvement of the testicular parenchyma

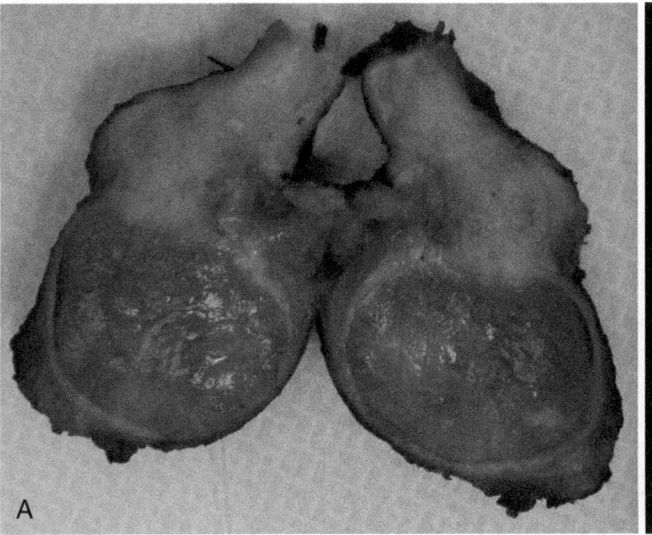
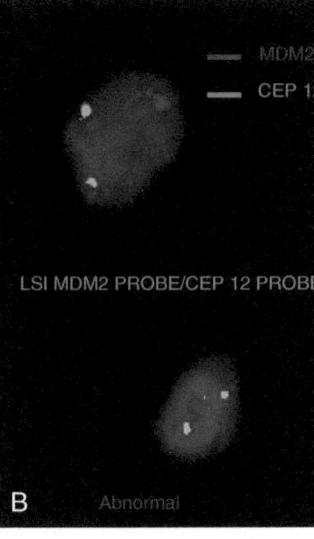

Figure 11-31. Spermatic cord dedifferentiated liposarcoma. A, Hemisected testis showing a rubbery mass in the distal aspect of the spermatic cord. **B,** Fluorescent in situ hybridization shows amplification of the MDM2 gene.

- Frequent local recurrences and pelvic lymph node metastases are seen necessitating radical orchiectomy and retroperitoneal lymph node dissection
- Prognosis for stage I or II disease is excellent after surgery, radiation therapy, and chemotherapy

Gross Pathology

- Encapsulated, lobulated, smooth, gray-white, glistening mass that displaces and does not typically involve the testicular parenchyma (typically does not invade testicular tissue) (Figure 11-32A)
- Tumor size ranges from 1 to 20 cm
- Focal hemorrhage and cystic degeneration may be seen

Histopathology

- Embryonal rhabdomyosarcoma
  - Most common subtype (makes up 90% of rhabdomyosarcomas in the paratesticular tissues)
  - The spindle cell type (which is more common in this site) shows interlacing fascicles of spindle cells with eosinophilic cytoplasm; the "not otherwise specified" type shows alternating myxoid and cellular areas, the latter consisting of a mix of primitive-appearing, polygonal cells and spindle cells with variable amounts of eosinophilic cytoplasm (Figure 11-32B)
  - Variable numbers of strap cells, with or without cross-striations, and bizarre "tadpole" cells
  - Alveolar, botryoid, and pleomorphic types are rare at this site

Special Stains and Immunohistochemistry

- MSA, desmin, and myosin: rhabdomyoblasts are typically positive
- Cytokeratin negative

Other Techniques for Diagnosis

- Electron microscopy: rhabdomyoblasts have cytoplasmic myofilaments and Z bands

Differential Diagnosis

- Metastasis from other primitive childhood tumors (small round blue cell tumors)
- Leiomyosarcoma (versus embryonal rhabdomyosarcoma, spindle cell type)
  - Lacks rhabdomyoblasts
  - H-caldesmon immunopositive and myogenin and myoglobin immunonegative

SELECTED REFERENCES

Fan R, Zhang J, Cheng L, et al: Testicular and paratesticular pathology in the pediatric population: a 20 year experience at Riley hospital for children. Pathol Res Pract 209:404-408, 2013.

Keskin S, Ekenel M, Basaran M, et al: Clinicopathological characteristics and treatment outcomes of adult patients with paratesticular rhabdomyosarcoma (PRMS): a 10-year single-centre experience. Can Urol Assoc J 6:42-45, 2012.

MALIGNANT MESOTHELIOMA OF THE TUNICA VAGINALIS

Clinical Features

- Rare tumor but second most common paratesticular malignancy
- Often associated with a hydrocele
- Bimodal age distribution with peaks in the third to fourth and sixth to eighth decades
- History of asbestos exposure may be present

Gross Pathology

- Solid or partially cystic tumor
- Multiple shaggy, friable nodules or diffuse thickening of the tunica vaginalis

Histopathology

- Similar histology to malignant mesothelioma of the lung
- Variable histologic features, including epithelial, spindle cell, or biphasic patterns
- Epithelial pattern is most common (70% to 80% of cases)
  - Complex structures have papillary projections, tubuloalveolar structures, and solid sheets of cells (Figure 11-33)
  - Cells lining the papillary structures and tubuloalveolar spaces are usually rounded and cuboidal but may be flattened

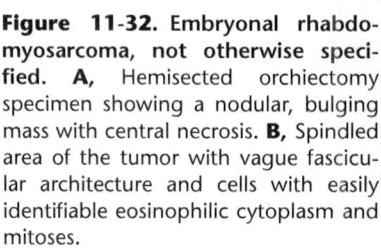

Figure 11-32. Embryonal rhabdomyosarcoma, not otherwise specified. **A,** Hemisected orchiectomy specimen showing a nodular, bulging mass with central necrosis. **B,** Spindled area of the tumor with vague fascicular architecture and cells with easily identifiable eosinophilic cytoplasm and mitoses.

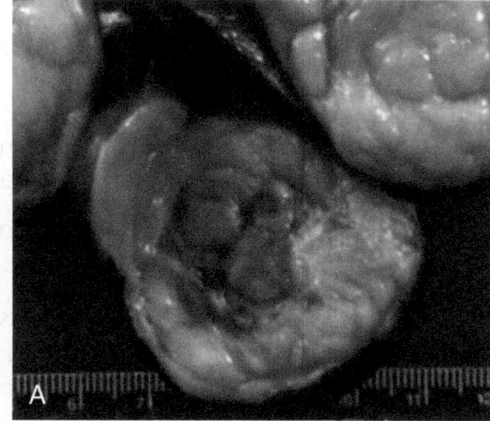
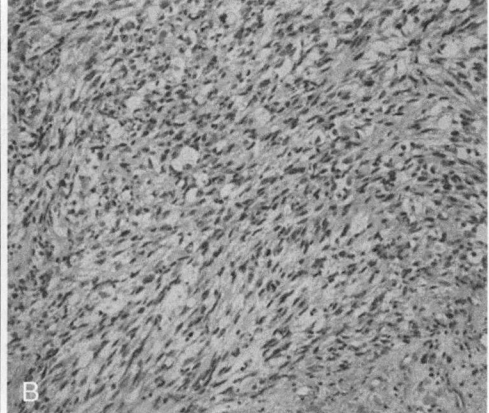

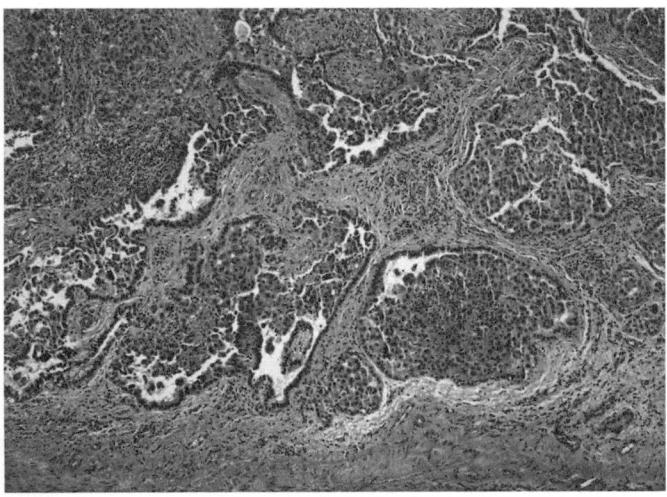

Figure 11-33. Malignant mesothelioma of tunica. Neoplasm composed of complex tubuloalveolar structures lined by low cuboidal epithelium extending from the tunica (*bottom*).

- Cells arranged in solid sheets often have an epithelioid appearance, with eosinophilic cytoplasm and large round central, vesicular nuclei with prominent nucleoli
- Variable mitotic rate
- Marked pleomorphism and bizarre cells are rare
- Psammoma bodies may be seen in the papillary areas

Special Stains and Immunohistochemistry

- Cytokeratin 5 and 6, EMA, calretinin (nuclear more than cytoplasmic), GLUT1, telomerase, p53, vimentin positive
- CEA, Leu-M1 negative
- Alcian blue positive; PAS and mucicarmine negative

Other Techniques for Diagnosis

- Electron microscopy: tumor cells have long, slender microvilli; tonofilaments; desmosomes; and perinuclear mitochondria

Differential Diagnosis

BENIGN REACTIVE MESOTHELIAL PROLIFERATION
- Commonly seen in hernia sacs
- Usually small and solitary with simple papillary processes
- Minimal cytologic atypia

FLORID ATYPICAL MESOTHELIAL HYPERPLASIA
- May show some features of malignancy: cytologic atypia, numerous mitoses, and tubulopapillary architecture
- No true invasion of stroma other than superficial entrapment; cytokeratin stains may be helpful
- Tends to be p53 and EMA immunonegative and desmin immunopositive

ADENOCARCINOMA, METASTATIC OR PRIMARY
- Best differentiated with immunohistochemistry (CEA, Leu-M1, and mucin positivity) or electron microscopy (tumor cells have short microvilli)

SELECTED REFERENCES

Chen X, Sheng W, Wang J: Well-differentiated papillary mesothelioma: a clinicopathological and immunohistochemical study of 18 cases with additional observation. Histopathology 62:805-813, 2013.

Churg A, Colby TV, Cagle P, et al: The separation of benign and malignant mesothelial proliferations. Am J Surg Pathol 24:1183-1200, 2000.

SEMINAL VESICLE

CARCINOMA OF THE SEMINAL VESICLE

Clinical Features
- Rare tumor occurring in patients older than 50 years
- Symptoms include urinary retention, dysuria, and hematuria
- Only a few cases diagnosed early enough for cure

Gross Pathology
- Infiltrative tumor that replaces the seminal vesicle and may extend into the prostate gland or contralateral seminal vesicle
- Obstruction of the urethra and one or both ureters is common
- Tumors may grow to 10 to 15 cm in diameter

Histopathology
- Most tumors are papillary adenocarcinomas; some may be undifferentiated or mucinous and elicit a desmoplastic stromal response
- Tumor cells are columnar or polygonal and have vesicular nuclei, clear cytoplasm, and variably prominent nucleoli
- In situ adenocarcinoma may be present in adjacent seminal vesicle epithelium

Special Stains and Immunohistochemistry
- Consistently CA-125 and CEA positive; PSA and PAP negative
- Usually CK7 and HMWCK positive; CK20 negative
- AMACR staining unknown

Other Techniques for Diagnosis
- Noncontributory

Differential Diagnosis
PROSTATIC ADENOCARCINOMA
- More commonly involves both seminal vesicles
- PSA and PAP positive; CA-125 negative

URINARY BLADDER ADENOCARCINOMA

- Best distinguished clinically depending on site of primary tumor
- CA-125 negative

TRANSITIONAL CELL CARCINOMA

- Best distinguished clinically depending on site of primary tumor
- CK20 positive; CA-125 negative

PEARLS

- *Carcinoma of the seminal vesicle should only be diagnosed if it can be demonstrated that the tumor arises in the seminal vesicle (may invade the prostate gland or bladder from outside)*
- *Prostate, colon, and bladder must be ruled out as primary site of malignancy before diagnosis of primary seminal vesicle is made*
- *Overall, tumors involving both the prostate gland and the seminal vesicle are much more likely to be of prostatic origin*
- *May be impossible to determine site of primary tumor in infiltrative high-grade tumors that involve multiple organs*
- *Disease has aggressive clinical course with poor prognosis*

SELECTED REFERENCES

Ormsby AH, Haskell R, Jones D, Goldblum JR: Primary seminal vesicle carcinoma: an immunohistochemical analysis of four cases. Mod Pathol 13:46-51, 2000.

Thiel R, Effert P: Primary adenocarcinoma of the seminal vesicles. J Urol 186:1891-1896, 2002.

URETHRA

URETHRAL POLYPS

FIBROEPITHELIAL POLYP

Clinical Features

- Rare lesion
- Occurs only in males
- Usually congenital
- Patients usually present between 3 and 9 years of age with hematuria, urinary retention, and infection

Gross Pathology

- Polypoid mass arising in the prostatic urethra adjacent to the verumontanum

Histopathology

- Polyp lined by urothelium with variable stromal inflammation
- Surface ulceration may be seen
- Squamous metaplasia may be present

CARUNCLE

Clinical Features

- Found exclusively in women; usually in later life

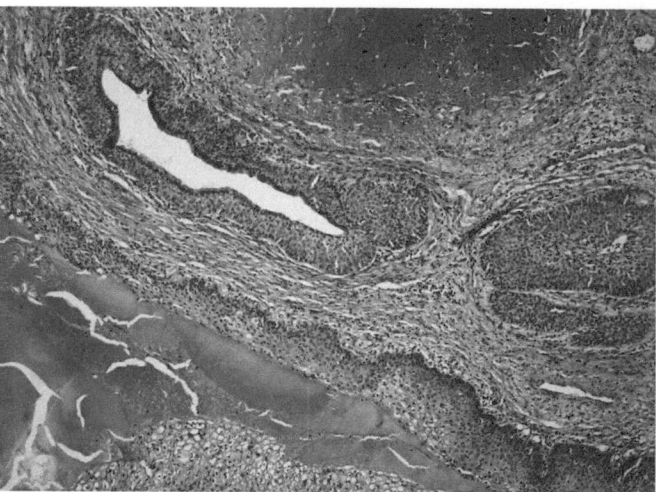

Figure 11-34. Urethral caruncle. Seen only in women but illustrated in this chapter for completeness. Inflamed urothelium and stroma associated with hemorrhage and vascular ectasia.

- Patients present with a red, painful mass at the external urethral meatus and frequently have dysuria, urinary frequency, or obstruction

Gross Pathology

- Small (1 to 2 cm), pedunculated or sessile polypoid lesion in the distal urethra
- Fleshy, hemorrhagic appearance

Histopathology

- Polypoid mass lined by urothelial (transitional) or squamous epithelium that is often hyperplastic (Figure 11-34)
- Lamina propria consists of loose fibroblastic connective tissue that is richly vascular and has extravasated red blood cells and mixed inflammation

NEPHROGENIC ADENOMA

Clinical Features

- Arises in response to chronic irritation or trauma
- Most common in young adult males
- Usually incidental finding at endoscopy; may cause hematuria
- Benign condition with no increased risk for malignancy; coexistent adenocarcinoma occasionally seen

Gross Pathology

- Flattened erythematous plaque or discrete papillary lesion

Histopathology

- May show papillary or flat configuration
  - Flat lesions have a loose stroma with scattered mixed inflammatory cells and numerous small tubules lined by uniform cuboidal cells with hyperchromatic, round to oval nuclei (Figure 11-35)
  - Papillae have similar lining cells with associated small stromal tubules and mixed inflammation
  - Pale eosinophilic secretions are often found within the tubules

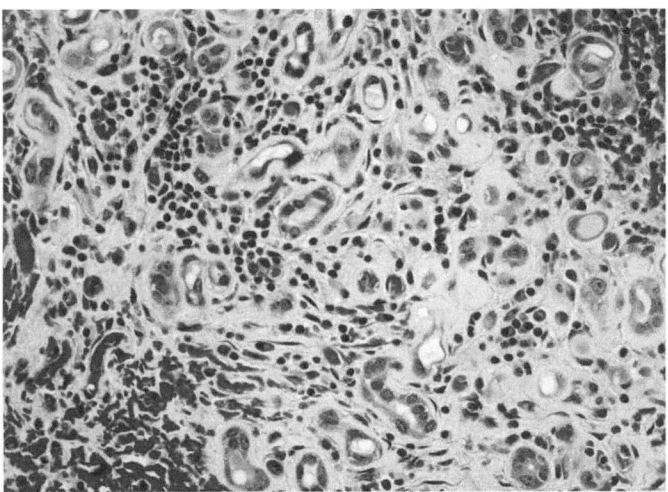

Figure 11-35. Nephrogenic adenoma arising in a urethral diverticulum. Variably sized glandular spaces lined by uniformly bland, low cuboidal epithelial cells in an edematous background.

Special Stains and Immunohistochemistry

- Tubular secretion may be PAS positive, diastase resistant, or mucicarmine positive
- Epithelial cells are negative for PSA and PAP

Other Techniques for Diagnosis

- Noncontributory

Differential Diagnosis

ADENOCARCINOMA

- Usually much larger and more commonly causes clinical symptoms, including dysuria and hematuria
- Glandular structures are composed of pleomorphic cells with a high mitotic rate

PROSTATIC URETHRAL POLYP

Clinical Features

- Usually asymptomatic; may cause hematuria
- More commonly seen in adults but may present at earlier ages

Gross Pathology

- Small, discrete, velvet-like papillary growths

Histopathology

- Papillary fronds with thin fibrovascular cores
- Lined by prostatic acinar epithelium with abundant clear to eosinophilic cytoplasm
- Small basally oriented nuclei without conspicuous nucleoli

Special Stains and Immunohistochemistry

- PSA: epithelial cells are positive

Other Techniques for Diagnosis

- Noncontributory

Differential Diagnosis

- Cytologic features need to be carefully examined to distinguish prostatic urethral polyp from intraluminal extension of prostatic adenocarcinoma

SELECTED REFERENCE

Demirican M, Ceran C, Karaman A, et al: Urethral polyps in children: a review of the literature and report of two cases. Int J Urol 13:841-843, 2006.

CARCINOMA OF THE URETHRA

Clinical Features

- Rare tumor
- Most common in older women
- Usually located in the prostatic or membranous portion of the urethra
- Patients usually present with symptoms associated with urinary obstruction
- May have purulent or bloody discharge
- Tumors of the anterior urethra may be palpable

Gross Pathology

- On endoscopy, the tumor may have an exophytic growth pattern or an area of ulceration

Histopathology

- Usually squamous cell carcinomas; tumors with transitional cell differentiation may be seen
- Tumors of transitional cell type may be papillary or flat and may be of any histologic grade
- Squamous cell carcinomas are usually well to moderately differentiated with little keratinization; however, verrucous carcinomas may be seen in the distal urethra
- Spindle cell variants of both transitional cell and squamous cell carcinomas may occur

Special Stains and Immunohistochemistry

- Cytokeratin: positivity may aid in differentiating the spindle cell variant from sarcoma

Other Techniques for Diagnosis

- Noncontributory

Differential Diagnosis

- Secondary involvement of the urethra by TCC of the bladder is much more common than primary urethral carcinoma
- Intramucosal pagetoid spread of TCC may be seen in the urethra in association with TCC of the bladder but is rare in primary urethral carcinoma

PEARLS

- *Spread of a TCC of the bladder into the urethra is much more common than primary urethral carcinoma*
- *Overall these tumors are aggressive primarily, resulting in local destruction; they occasionally metastasize*

SELECTED REFERENCE

Mostofi FK, Davis CJ Jr, Sesterhenn IA: Carcinoma of the male and female urethra. Urol Clin North Am 19:347-358, 1992.

ADENOCARCINOMA OF THE PERIURETHRAL GLANDS

Clinical Features

- Rare tumor (only few reported cases)
- Appears to be more common in women
- May present with symptoms of urinary obstruction, hematuria, or dysuria
- Advanced tumors may present as a perineal mass with skin ulceration

Gross Pathology

- Tumors arising in Cowper glands involve the posterior urethra or perineum
- Tumors arising in the periurethral glands of Littre involve the anterior urethra

Histopathology

- Variety of growth patterns and cell types described
  - Tubular or papillary growth pattern with or without intracytoplasmic mucin
  - Cuboidal or columnar cells with eosinophilic to clear cytoplasm and large, hyperchromatic nuclei (Figure 11-36)
  - Clear cell variant is composed of large clear cells with abundant cytoplasmic glycogen

Special Stains and Immunohistochemistry

MUCINOUS TUMORS
- Positive for cytokeratin
- Negative for PSA and PAP

CLEAR CELL CARCINOMA
- May show PAS positivity with diastase sensitivity

Other Techniques for Diagnosis

- Noncontributory

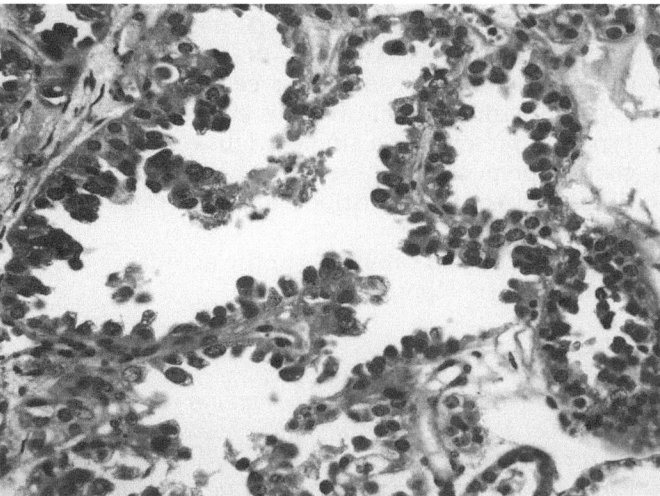

Figure 11-36. Clear cell adenocarcinoma arising in a urethral diverticulum in a female. Hobnail cells with eosinophilic cytoplasm (eosinophilic variant of clear cell carcinoma).

Differential Diagnosis

PROSTATIC OR UROTHELIAL ADENOCARCINOMA
- Periurethral involvement by prostatic or urothelial adenocarcinoma can often be ruled out based on clinical history

PEARLS

- *These tumors are rare in men*
- *Urethral adenocarcinomas are more prevalent in women and may arise in a background of chronic irritation (i.e., diverticulum) and mucinous metaplasia or may arise from Skene glands or the periurethral glands of Littre*

SELECTED REFERENCES

Murphy DP, Pantuck AJ, Amenta PS, et al: Female urethral adenocarcinoma: immunohistochemical evidence of more than one tissue of origin. J Urol 161:11881-11884, 1999.
Ullmann AS, Ross OA: Hyperplasia, atypia and carcinoma in-situ in prostatic periurethral glands. Am J Clin Pathol 47:497-504, 1967.

PENIS

PENILE FIBROMATOSIS (PEYRONIE DISEASE)

Clinical Features

- Patients present with painful erection and bending or constriction of the erect penis
- Commonly affects middle-aged or older men; rare before the age of 40 years
- Associated with other superficial fibromatoses, including palmar or plantar sites (Dupuytren and Ledderhose disease, respectively) in 10% to 25% of patients
- Clinical course is variable; spontaneous resolution is seen in one third of patients

Gross Pathology

- Circumscribed, firm plaque or nodule on the dorsal surface of the penile shaft
- Inelasticity of the plaques causes penile curvature and pain with erection; may cause urethral constriction

Histopathology

- Proliferative (early) phase shows increased cellularity and less collagen compared with advanced lesions
- Tumor cells are bland with fibroblastic and myofibroblastic features; rarely have focal mitotic activity, associated inflammation, and giant cells (Figure 11-37)
- Advanced lesions may show hyalinization with foci of bone or cartilage formation

Special Stains and Immunohistochemistry

- SMA: variable positivity (indicative of myofibroblastic differentiation)

Other Techniques for Diagnosis

- Cytogenetic studies: various nonrandom karyotypic abnormalities may be seen (commonly trisomy 3 or 8)

Differential Diagnosis

- Diagnosis is made based on characteristic clinical history and presentation

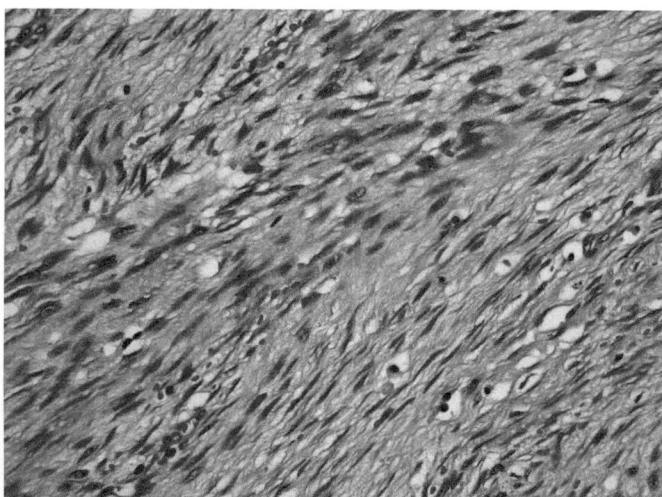

Figure 11-37. Penile fibromatosis (Peyronie disease). Fascicles of mature fibroblasts with elongated, tapered nuclei.

PEARLS

- *Histologic features are often less dramatic than clinical presentation*
- *May resolve spontaneously, remain stable for many years, or progress*
- *Treatment options include resection of the penile plaques, radiotherapy, or steroid injections*
- *May be related to scarring secondary to urethritis, coital trauma, or urethral instrumentation; often idiopathic*

SELECTED REFERENCES

Gonzalez-Cadavid NF, Rajfer J: Mechanisms of disease: new insights into the cellular and molecular pathology of Peyronie's disease. Nat Clin Pract Urol 2:291-297, 2005.
Greenfield JM, Levine LA: Peyronie's disease: etiology, epidemiology and medical treatment. Urol Clin North Am 32:469-478, 2005.

BALANITIS XEROTICA OBLITERANS

Clinical Features

- Penile equivalent of vulvar lichen sclerosus
- Atrophy of the epidermis and dermal connective tissue of the genital skin
- Asymptomatic white patch on glans or prepuce; may involve the urethral meatus

Gross Pathology

- Clinically, affected skin is white and fibrotic

Histopathology

- Orthokeratotic hyperkeratosis, epidermal atrophy, upper dermal collagenization, and patchy lymphoplasmacytic infiltrate in the upper dermis (Figure 11-38)

Special Stains and Immunohistochemistry

- Noncontributory

Other Techniques for Diagnosis

- Noncontributory

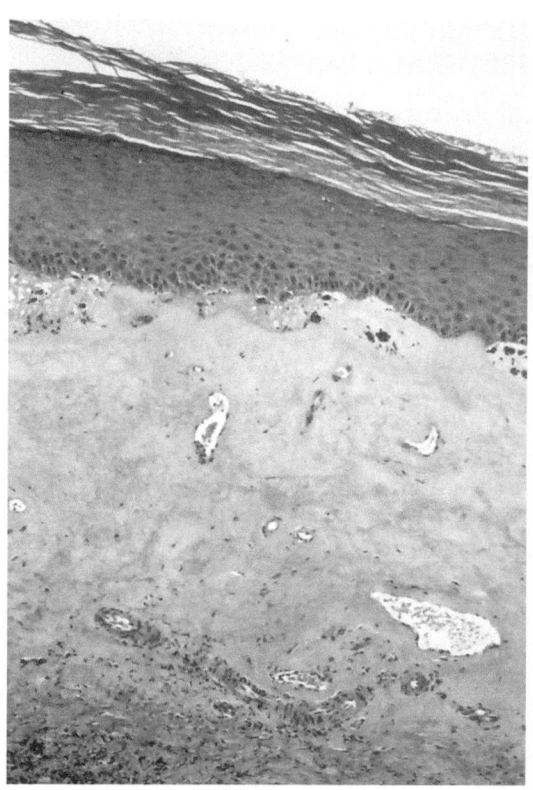

Figure 11-38. Balanitis xerotica obliterans. Characteristic subepithelial acellular collagenization with linear lymphocytic infiltrate. Epidermis may be normal or atrophic.

Differential Diagnosis

LICHEN SIMPLEX CHRONICUS

- Can show orthokeratotic hyperkeratosis, but unlike balanitis xerotica obliterans, it usually shows epidermal hyperplasia and no dermal collagenization

LICHEN PLANUS

- Prominent band of chronic inflammatory cells that can obscure the dermoepidermal junction
- Balanitis xerotica obliterans has a less dense lymphocytic infiltrate

PLASMA CELL (ZOON) BALANITIS (BALANITIS CIRCUMSCRIPTA PLASMACELLULARIS)

- Clinically looks like squamous cell carcinoma in situ and occurs almost exclusively in uncircumcised men
- Typically presents as a single bright-red patch on the glans or prepuce
- Characterized by a distinct upper dermal band of plasma cells
- Prominent dilated capillaries in the dermis
- Lacks collagen deposition

PEARLS

- *Many of the same histopathologic features useful in the differential diagnosis of inflammatory lesions of the vulva are useful in the penis*
- *Variable treatment options include circumcision, laser ablation, steroid treatments, and antifungal agents*
- *May rarely progress to squamous cell carcinoma, particularly if persistent or not treated*

SELECTED REFERENCES

Philippou P, Shabbir M, Ralph DJ, et al: Genital lichen sclerosis/balanitis xerotica obliterans in men with penile carcinoma: a critical analysis. BJU Int 111:970-976, 2013.

Velazquez EF, Cubilla AL: Lichen sclerosis in 68 patients with squamous cell carcinoma of the penis: frequent atypias and correlation with special carcinoma variants suggest a precancerous role. Am J Surg Pathol 27:1448-1453, 2003.

CONDYLOMA ACUMINATUM (GENITAL WART)

Clinical Features

- Most common tumor-like lesion of the penis
- Caused by human papillomavirus (HPV)
- Incidence of 5% among men aged 20 to 40 years

Gross Pathology

- Lesions are located on corona of glans, fossa navicularis, or penile meatus
- Involvement of penile shaft, scrotal skin, and perineum may be seen
- Lesions appear as pink to tan, flat, or papillary cauliflower-like nodules
- Can be large with pushing growth (giant condyloma of Buschke-Löwenstein)

Histopathology

- Exophytic growth with branching, papillary structures covered by hyperplastic squamous epithelium showing orderly maturation (Figure 11-39)
- Koilocytes: cells with raisinoid, hyperchromatic, binucleated nuclei with perinuclear halos
- Hyperkeratosis and parakeratosis
- Minimal cytologic atypia with mitoses confined to the basal layer

Special Stains and Immunohistochemistry

- HPV can be demonstrated with immunohistochemistry
- HPV types 6 and 11 are associated with nondysplastic genital warts

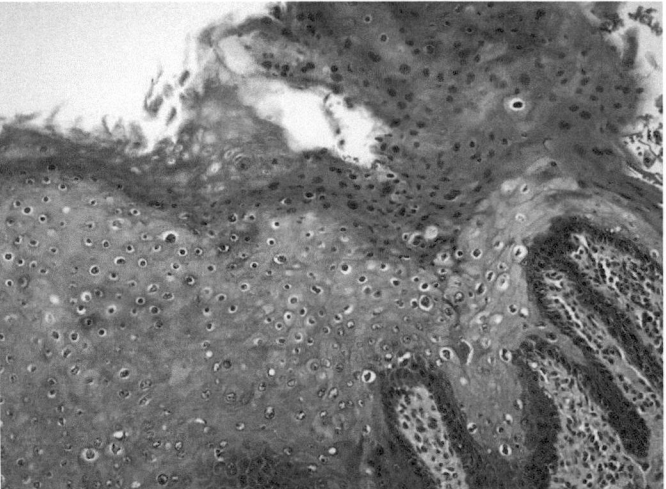

Figure 11-39. Condyloma acuminatum. Foreskin showing epidermal hyperplasia, hyperkeratosis, and parakeratosis with characteristic human papillomavirus cytopathic effect.

Other Techniques for Diagnosis

- In situ hybridization can demonstrate viral HPV DNA

Differential Diagnosis

VERRUCOUS CARCINOMA

- Shows acanthosis, hyperkeratosis, parakeratosis, and sometimes koilocyte-like cells similar to condyloma
- Typically has a broad invasive growth pattern at the deep margin
- Not associated with HPV

PEARLS

- *Previous treatment with podophyllin or laser therapy may cause bizarre cytologic changes suggestive of malignancy*
- *Variable treatment consisting of podophyllin, laser therapy, radiation, or conservative surgical resection*
- *Patients with condyloma are at increased risk for developing penile squamous cell carcinoma*

SELECTED REFERENCES

Hartwig S, Syrjanen S, Dominiak-Felden G, et al: Estimation of the epidemiological burden of human papillomavirus-related cancers and non-malignant diseases in men in Europe: a review. BMC Cancer 20:12-30, 2012.

Rubin MA, Kleter B, Zhou M, et al: Detection and typing of human papillomavirus DNA in penile carcinoma: evidence for multiple independent pathways of penile carcinogenesis. Am J Pathol 159:1211-1218, 2001.

PENILE CARCINOMA IN SITU: ERYTHROPLASIA OF QUEYRAT

Clinical Features

- Usually occurs in men between the ages of 50 and 70 years
- Patients typically present with a plaque on the glans penis or prepuce
- Circumcision protects against the development of erythroplasia
- About 10% of cases progress to invasive squamous cell carcinoma

Gross Pathology

- Shiny, elevated, red, velvety erythematous plaque on the glans or prepuce
- Solitary lesion in more than 50% of cases

Histopathology

- Squamous epithelium shows full-thickness dysplasia without invasion of the basement membrane (Figure 11-40)
- Dysplastic cells demonstrate loss of polarity and lack normal maturation; cells have large, irregular hyperchromatic nuclei, multinucleation, and numerous typical and atypical mitotic figures
- Scattered dyskeratotic cells are seen throughout the epithelium
- Underlying lichenoid inflammation and vascular proliferation are common

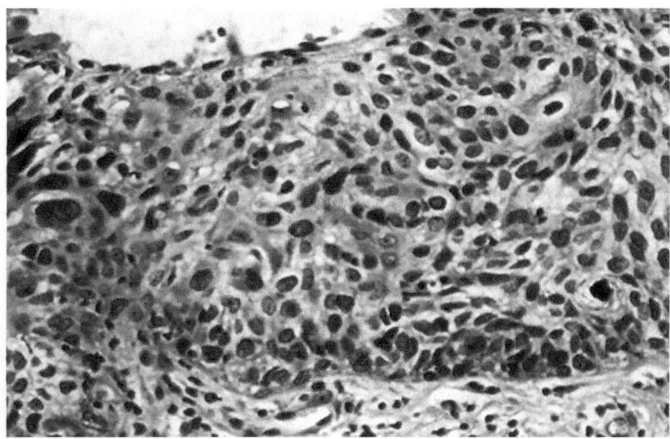

Figure 11-40. Erythroplasia of Queyrat or Bowen disease. Both show epithelium with full-thickness dysplasia.

Special Stains and Immunohistochemistry

- HPV demonstrable in up to 80% of lesions

Other Techniques for Diagnosis

- HPV DNA can be demonstrated with in situ hybridization techniques; HPV types 16 and 18 are most common

Differential Diagnosis

BOWEN DISEASE

- Histologic features of erythroplasia of Queyrat and Bowen disease are almost identical; differentiation is based on clinical presentation and biologic behavior

BOWENOID PAPULOSIS

- Affects younger men
- Often multifocal
- Typically shows slightly less dysplasia
- Does not progress to invasive squamous cell carcinoma

PEARLS

- *Unlike Bowen disease, erythroplasia is limited to the glans and prepuce and occurs in somewhat older patients*
- *About 10% incidence of progression to invasive squamous cell carcinoma*

PENILE CARCINOMA IN SITU: BOWEN DISEASE

Clinical Features

- Usually occurs in men 40 to 60 years old
- Typically presents as a scaly plaque
- About 5% to 10% of cases progress to invasive squamous cell carcinoma
- Reported association with visceral (lung, gastrointestinal tract, and genitourinary tract) malignancies in up to 33% is debatable

Gross Pathology

- Crusted, sharply demarcated scaly plaque on the shaft of the penis

Histopathology

- Squamous epithelium has full-thickness dysplasia without invasion of basement membrane
- Dysplastic cells demonstrate loss of polarity and lack normal maturation; cells have large, irregular hyperchromatic nuclei, multinucleation, and numerous typical and atypical mitotic figures
- Scattered dyskeratotic cells are seen throughout the epithelium
- Underlying lichenoid inflammation and vascular proliferation are common
- Often has prominent hyperkeratosis and parakeratosis
- Commonly involves the pilosebaceous units

Special Stains and Immunohistochemistry

- HPV demonstrable in up to 80% of lesions

Other Techniques for Diagnosis

- HPV DNA can be demonstrated with in situ hybridization techniques; HPV types 16 and 18 are most common

Differential Diagnosis

ERYTHROPLASIA OF QUEYRAT

- Histologic features of erythroplasia of Queyrat and Bowen disease are almost identical; differentiation is based on clinical presentation and biologic behavior

BOWENOID PAPULOSIS

- Affects younger men
- Often multifocal
- Typically shows slightly less dysplasia
- Does not progress to invasive squamous cell carcinoma

PEARLS

- *Unlike erythroplasia of Queyrat, Bowen disease arises on the skin of the penile shaft and occurs in somewhat younger patients*
- *About 5% to 10% incidence of progression to invasive squamous cell carcinoma*
- *Many authors use the term* Bowen disease *for carcinoma in situ of the skin and* erythroplasia of Queyrat *for carcinoma in situ of the glans penis*

SELECTED REFERENCE

Cubilla AL, Velazquez EF, Young RH: Epithelial lesions associated with invasive penile squamous cell carcinoma: a pathologic study of 288 cases. Int J Surg Pathol 12:351-364, 2004.

BOWENOID PAPULOSIS

Clinical Features

- Usually seen in young adults (typically 20 to 40 years of age)
- Multiple papules or coalescent papules seen on the penile shaft or perineum
- Responds to topical therapy or local excision; may regress spontaneously
- Does not progress to invasive squamous cell carcinoma

Gross Pathology

- Multiple papules, 2 to 10 mm in diameter
- Papules may coalesce to form plaques resembling condyloma acuminatum

Histopathology

- Squamous epithelium showing variable degrees of acanthosis, papillomatosis, hyperkeratosis, and parakeratosis
- Scattered atypical keratinocytes and mitotic figures
- Shows more maturation than carcinoma in situ

Special Stains and Immunohistochemistry

- HPV: present in some cases (especially types 16 and 18)

Other Techniques for Diagnosis

- In situ hybridization techniques may demonstrate HPV DNA

Differential Diagnosis

- Bowen disease and erythroplasia of Queyrat
- Histologically, bowenoid papulosis is essentially identical to Bowen disease
- Unlike erythroplasia of Queyrat and Bowen disease, bowenoid papulosis affects younger men, is more often multifocal, shows somewhat less dysplasia, and does not progress to invasive squamous cell carcinoma

PEARLS

- *Does not progress to invasive squamous cell carcinoma*
- *Responds to local or topical therapy; may regress spontaneously*

SELECTED REFERENCES

Bhojwani A, Biyani CS, Nicol A, Powell CS: Bowenoid papulosis of the penis. Br J Urol 80:508, 1997.
Su CK, Shipley WU: Bowenoid papulosis: a benign lesion of the shaft of the penis misdiagnosed as squamous carcinoma. J Urol 157:1361-1362, 1997.

SQUAMOUS CELL CARCINOMA

Clinical Features

- Accounts for less than 1% of malignancy in males, but accounts for up to 95% of penile malignancies
- Wide geographic variation; high rates in Uganda, Brazil, Jamaica, Mexico, and Haiti (areas where circumcision is not routinely practiced)
- Usually occurs in older men; rare before the age of 40 years
- Patients typically present with a slow-growing, exophytic or ulcerating penile mass; may have pain or difficulty voiding
- Risk factors include lack of circumcision, poor hygiene, phimosis, and HPV
- Extremely rare in men circumcised in infancy
- Retention of smegma or its derivatives may have an irritating effect
- Almost 50% of the patients have phimosis
- HPV type 11, 16, 18, or 30 can be demonstrated in about 50% of cases
- Often clinically neglected and may metastasize to bilateral inguinal and iliac lymph nodes

Gross Pathology

- Exophytic or ulcerating mass arising on the glans or prepuce

Histopathology

- Well-differentiated invasive squamous cell carcinoma
  - Composed of atypical squamous cells that extend down from a thickened hyperkeratotic, papillomatous surface and infiltrate through the underlying basement membrane (Figure 11-41A)
  - Limited nuclear atypia and pleomorphism
  - Keratin pearls may be numerous
  - Intercellular bridges are prominent
- Higher-grade invasive squamous cell carcinoma
  - Composed of large cells with hyperchromatic nuclei and moderate to marked pleomorphism depending on grade
  - Ulcerated surface and invasive architecture with infiltration of the tumor through the basement membrane
  - Increased mitotic rate; atypical mitoses are common in poorly differentiated tumors

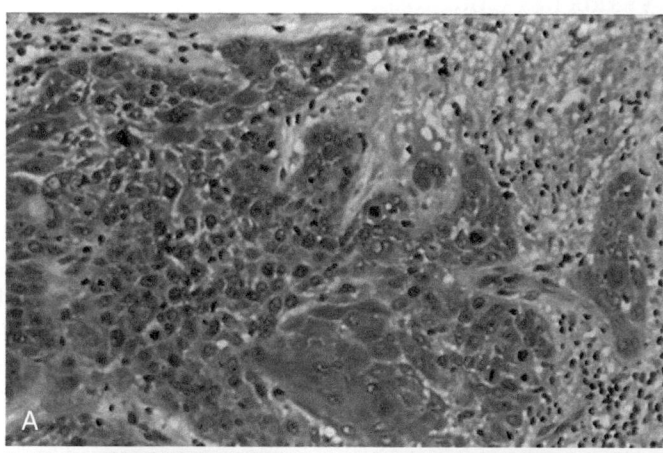

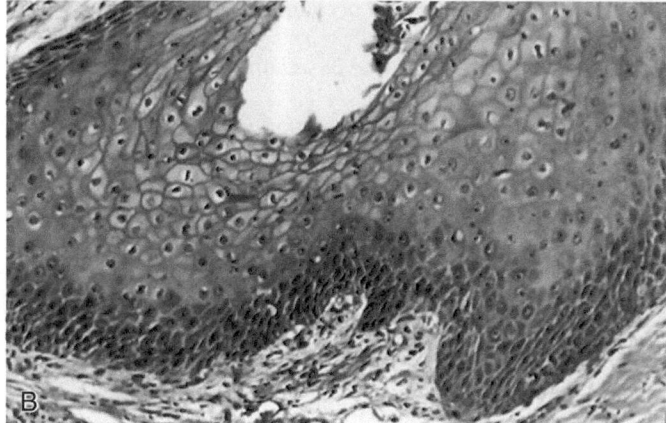

Figure 11-41. A, Typical penile squamous cell carcinoma. Superficially invasive squamous cell carcinoma with keratinization. **B,** Well-differentiated squamous cell carcinoma. Tumor cells invade in a bulbous, pushing manner similar to that seen in a verrucous carcinoma; however, the degree of cytologic atypicality is too great for that diagnosis.

- Poorly differentiated tumors typically have focal areas of necrosis
  - Fewer keratin pearls
- Two main growth patterns are seen: fungating-exophytic and ulcerating-infiltrative
- Exophytic tumors are usually well-differentiated and have extensive keratinization
- Ulcerating tumors tend to be on the glans and are moderately or poorly differentiated
- Rare squamous cell carcinomas have a predominantly spindle cell pattern with marked nuclear pleomorphism and high mitotic rates with only focal areas of identifiable squamous differentiation

Special Stains and Immunohistochemistry

- Cytokeratin positive

Other Techniques for Diagnosis

- Electron microscopy: tumor cells have bundles of tonofilaments and desmosomes
- HPV DNA can be demonstrated by in situ hybridization
- Flow cytometric analysis of DNA ploidy and S-phase fractions may have prognostic significance

Differential Diagnosis

VERRUCOUS CARCINOMA

- Histologic characteristics similar to those for well-differentiated squamous cell carcinoma (Figure 11-41B)
- Typically has a broad pushing pattern of infiltration
- Low mitotic rate
- Much better prognosis with essentially no metastatic potential

PENILE SARCOMAS

- Various penile sarcomas enter into the differential diagnosis of poorly differentiated and spindle cell types of squamous cell carcinoma
- Sarcoma is typically cytokeratin negative

PEARLS

- *Squamous cell carcinoma accounts for most penile malignancies*
- *Wide variation in incidence based on geography and cultural practices*
- *Stage, specifically depth of invasion (epithelium, lamina propria, corpus spongiosum, corpus cavernosum), and lymph node status are prognostically important*
- *Almost 40% of patients have inguinal lymph node metastases at presentation; widespread metastases typically occur late in the course of the disease*

SELECTED REFERENCES

Chaux A, Cubilla AL, Haffner MC, et al: Combining routine morphology, p16INK4a immunohistochemistry and in situ hybridization for the detection of human papillomavirus infection in penile carcinomas: a tissue microarray study using classifier performance analyses. Urol Oncol 2013 Mar 13. doi:pii: S1078-1439(12)00158-5. http://dx.doi.org/10.1016/j.urolonc.2012.04.017 [Epub ahead of print.]

Edge SB, Byrd DR, Compton CC, et al (eds): AJCC Cancer Staging Manual, 7th ed. New York: Springer, 2010, pp 447-455.

VERRUCOUS CARCINOMA

Clinical Features

- Most commonly seen in middle-aged men
- Most arise in the coronal sulcus
- Behaves as a locally aggressive neoplasm; essentially no metastatic potential
- Not associated with HPV

Gross Pathology

- Large, fungating, warty tumor
- Surface of tumor is frequently ulcerated

Histopathology

- Endophytic and exophytic papillary growth consisting of acanthotic, hyperkeratotic, and parakeratotic squamous mucosa
- Minimal cytologic atypia and rare mitotic activity
- Deep margin of the tumor shows a pushing, broad area of infiltration
- True koilocytosis with large, wrinkled nuclei and perinuclear halos are not seen

Special Stains and Immunohistochemistry

- Consistent absence of HPV

Other Techniques for Diagnosis

- In situ hybridization fails to demonstrate HPV DNA

Differential Diagnosis

CONDYLOMA ACUMINATUM AND GIANT CONDYLOMA OF BUSCHKE-LÖWENSTEIN

- True koilocytic atypia
- Positive for HPV

INVASIVE SQUAMOUS CELL CARCINOMA

- Greater cytologic atypia, higher mitotic rate, and a more diffusely infiltrative growth pattern

HYBRID TUMORS

- Hybrid tumors with features of both well-differentiated squamous cell carcinoma and verrucous carcinoma may occur

PEARLS

- *True verrucous carcinomas with no metastatic potential are relatively rare*
- *May recur frequently and be locally destructive*
- *Tumors with features of both verrucous carcinoma and squamous cell carcinoma (so-called hybrid squamous-verrucous carcinoma) are relatively common*

SELECTED REFERENCE

Cubilla AL, Dillner J, Schellhammer PF, et al: Tumours of the penis: verrucous carcinoma. In Eble JN, Sauter G, Epstein JI, Sesterhenn IA (eds): World Health Organization Classification of Tumours: Pathology and Genetics: Tumours of the Urinary System and Male Genital Organs. Lyon, IARC Press, 2004, p 286.

PENILE SARCOMA

General Features

- Rare tumor composing less than 5% of penile malignancies
- As a group, penile sarcomas are the second most common penile malignancy
- Peak incidence is between 40 and 60 years of age; rhabdomyosarcoma may be seen in children
- Most present as nodules or masses on the penile shaft
- Most common histologic types include Kaposi sarcoma, epithelioid hemangioendothelioma, leiomyosarcoma, fibrosarcoma, and epithelioid sarcoma

KAPOSI SARCOMA

Clinical Features

- About 20% of male patients with AIDS-related Kaposi sarcoma have penile lesions
- Tumors usually involve the glans or penile shaft
- Involvement of the glans or corpus spongiosum may cause urethral obstruction

Gross Pathology

- Red to purple patches, plaques, or nodules

Histopathology

- Patch stage
  - Dilated irregular vascular spaces, interspersed mononuclear cell infiltrate, extravasated red blood cells, and hemosiderin-laden macrophages
- Plaque stage
  - Vascular spaces become lined by plump spindle cells and there are variable perivascular spindle cell aggregates
- Nodular stage
  - Small and slitlike vascular spaces are scattered among sheets of plump spindle cells
  - Frequent mitotic activity, hemorrhage, and hemosiderin-laden macrophages

PEARLS

- *Usually associated with other systemic lesions seen in patients with HIV infection*

EPITHELIOID HEMANGIOENDOTHELIOMA

Clinical Features

- Rare vascular tumor that arises in the corpora cavernosum

Gross Pathology

- Red to purple, vaguely circumscribed, spongy nodule

Histopathology

- Anastomosing vascular spaces lined by plump to cuboidal cells with an epithelioid appearance
- Most are low grade, but some tumors may show marked pleomorphism, hemorrhage, and necrosis

Special Stains and Immunohistochemistry

- Immunohistochemical markers for vascular differentiation such as factor VIII, CD31, and CD34 may be useful

Other Techniques for Diagnosis

- Electron microscopy: Weibel-Palade bodies are characteristic of endothelial cell differentiation

Differential Diagnosis

POORLY DIFFERENTIATED OR METASTATIC CARCINOMA

- Positive for cytokeratin and negative for vascular markers

PEARLS

- *Low-grade tumors usually follow an indolent course*
- *High-grade tumors have been reported to metastasize to lymph nodes, lung, liver, and bone*

LEIOMYOSARCOMA

Clinical Features

- Usually occurs in men between 40 and 70 years of age

Gross Pathology

- Well-circumscribed, superficial or deep-seated, tan-gray nodule
- Firm and whorled to myxoid cut surface

Histopathology

- Composed of interwoven fascicles of spindle cells
- Cigar-shaped nuclei with variable nuclear pleomorphism and hyperplasia
- At least 1 to 2 mitoses/hpf

Special Stains and Immunohistochemistry

- Tumor cells are positive for vimentin, desmin, and SMA

Other Techniques for Diagnosis

- Electron microscopy: cell cytoplasm contains bundles of thin filaments and pinocytotic vesicles with surrounding basal lamina

PEARLS

- *Superficial tumors arising from dermal smooth muscle respond well to local excision but may recur*
- *Deep tumors arising from the smooth muscle of the corpora tend to invade the urethra and metastasize early, leading to a poor prognosis despite radical surgery*

FIBROSARCOMA

Clinical Features

- Slowly growing, nontender mass on the dorsum of the shaft or glans

Gross Pathology

- Soft to firm mass with infiltrative borders and fleshy cut surface

Histopathology

- Spindle cell neoplasm with infiltrative borders

- Differentiation ranges from spindle cells growing in a well-ordered herringbone pattern to high-grade tumors with marked nuclear pleomorphism, frequent mitoses, and necrosis

Special Stains and Immunohistochemistry

- Vimentin positive
- Cytokeratin, desmin, and SMA negative

Other Techniques for Diagnosis

- Electron microscopy: bipolar spindle cells without intercellular junctions; organelles consist of rough endoplasmic reticulum and mitochondria

Differential Diagnosis

LEIOMYOSARCOMA

- Positive for SMA

SPINDLE CELL VARIANT OF SQUAMOUS CELL CARCINOMA

- At least focally cytokeratin positive

PROLIFERATIVE (EARLY) PHASE OF FIBROMATOSIS (PEYRONIE DISEASE)

- Only focal cytologic atypia

EPITHELIOID SARCOMA

Clinical Features

- Age range typically 20 to 40 years
- Patients present with a slow-growing, painless subcutaneous mass that may ulcerate the overlying skin
- May cause erectile pain or dysuria

Gross Pathology

- Gray to tan, firm nodules
- Central areas of necrosis and degeneration may be seen

Histopathology

- Cellular neoplasm with an infiltrative growth pattern and nodular architecture
- Tumor cells are arranged in nodules surrounded by hyalinized stroma and may have central necrosis and cystic degeneration
- Large, polygonal cells with abundant eosinophilic cytoplasm and vesicular nuclei with prominent nucleoli (Figure 11-42)
- Frequent mitotic activity

Special Stains and Immunohistochemistry

- Vimentin positive
- Cytokeratin typically positive
- EMA: greater than 50% of cases are positive

Other Techniques for Diagnosis

- Noncontributory

Differential Diagnosis

ULCERATING INFILTRATING SQUAMOUS CELL CARCINOMA

- Positive for cytokeratin but negative for vimentin

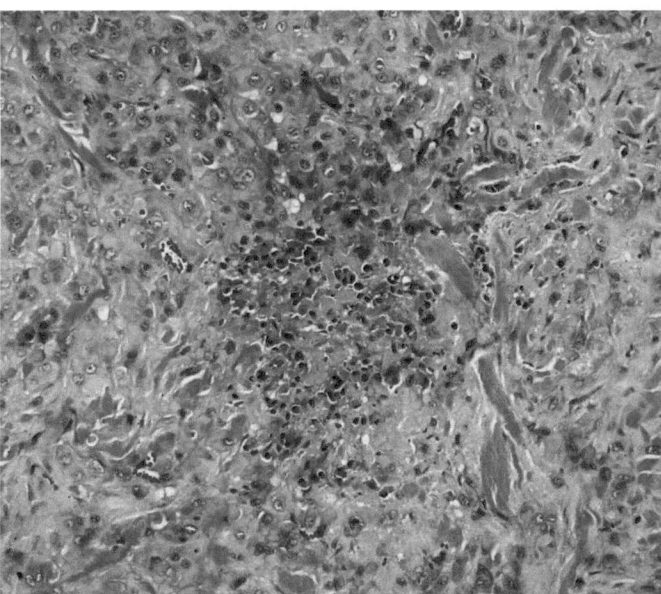

Figure 11-42. Epithelioid sarcoma involving penile dermal tissue. Proliferation of polygonal cells with eosinophilic cytoplasm and associated with hyalinized bands of collagen and central necrosis.

ULCERATING GRANULOMATOUS REACTIONS

- Cells are positive for histiocytic markers
- Other spindle cell sarcomas
- Negative for cytokeratin and EMA

SELECTED REFERENCE

Katona TM, Lopez-Beltran A, MacLennan GT, et al: Soft tissue tumors of the penis: a review. Anal Quant Cytol Histol 28:193-206, 2006.

SCROTUM

IDIOPATHIC SCROTAL CALCINOSIS

Clinical Features

- Idiopathic deposition of calcified nodules in the scrotal skin
- Calcification of dermal connective tissue may arise from eccrine duct cysts; however, residual cyst epithelium is often not apparent (Figure 11-43A)
- Typically found in young adults
- Multiple long-standing painless nodules up to 3 cm in diameter

Gross Pathology

- Hard, chalky, gray to white nodules
- Overlying skin is usually intact but may be ulcerated

Histopathology

- Dermal lesions consisting of granules and globules of calcific material (Figure 11-43B)
- Variable giant cell and granulomatous reaction

Special Stains and Immunohistochemistry

- Noncontributory

Other Techniques for Diagnosis

- Noncontributory

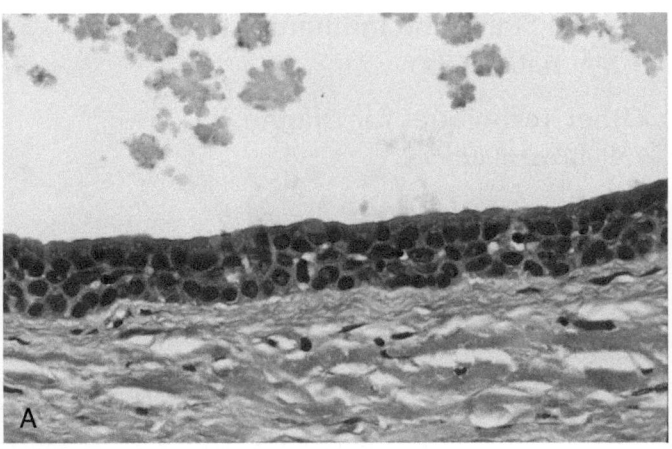
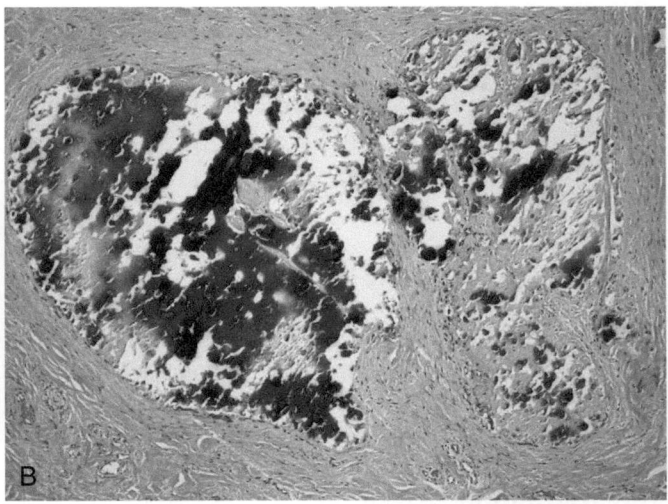

Figure 11-43. A, Scrotal cyst. Dilated eccrine duct with intraluminal calcifications. **B,** Scrotal calcinosis. Calcified nodules embedded in a dense connective tissue matrix.

Differential Diagnosis

CALCIFICATION OF PREEXISTING EPIDERMAL OR PILAR CYST
- Presence of keratinaceous debris

PEARLS

- *Treatment may be unnecessary for asymptomatic lesions*
- *Excision may be necessary for infected, recurrent, or extensive lesions*

SELECTED REFERENCE

Pompeo A, Molina WR, Pohlman GD, et al: Idiopathic scrotal calcinosis: a rare entity and a review of the literature Can Urol Assoc J 7:E439-E441, 2013.

PAGET DISEASE

Clinical Features
- Rare in this location
- Penile and scrotal Paget disease is usually associated with a primary visceral (bladder, prostate, urethra, or rectum) or perineal (skin adnexal) malignancy
- Typically occurs in the sixth and seventh decades of life
- Patients present with a scaly, eczematous lesion on the scrotum or penis

Gross Pathology
- Scaly, indurated, eczematous plaque

Histopathology
- Low power shows single cells or clusters of atypical cells with radial and some degree of vertical intraepidermal spread (Figure 11-44)
- Tumor cells have variable nuclear pleomorphism and vacuolated cytoplasm

Special Stains and Immunohistochemistry
- CEA positive
- S-100 protein negative

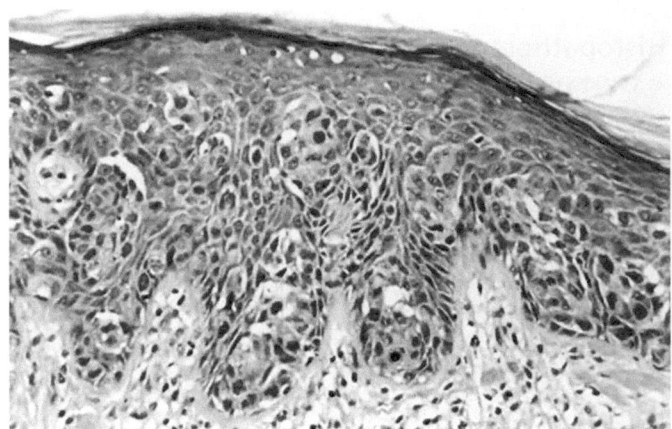

Figure 11-44. Penile Paget disease. Large atypical cells with clear cytoplasm showing intraepidermal spread.

- PAS, mucicarmine, and Alcian blue stain positive (tumor cells contain intracytoplasmic neutral and acid mucopolysaccharides)

Other Techniques for Diagnosis
- Noncontributory

Differential Diagnosis

MALIGNANT MELANOMA
- Similar pattern of intraepidermal spread, but S-100 protein positive and CEA negative
- Lacks intracytoplasmic mucin

SQUAMOUS CELL CARCINOMA
- Can show a similar low-power pattern of spread
- Typically has greater degree of invasion with infiltration into underlying tissue

PEARLS

- *Visceral malignancy must be ruled out with any case of penile or scrotal Paget disease*

SELECTED REFERENCES

Bagby CM, MacLennan GT: Extramammary Paget's disease of the penis and scrotum. J Urol 182:2908-2909, 2009.

Wang Z, Lu M, Dong GQ, et al: Penile and scrotal Paget's disease: 130 Chinese patients with long-term follow-up. BJU Int 102:485-488, 2008.

SQUAMOUS CELL CARCINOMA

Clinical Features

- First cancer linked to occupational exposure of 3'4'-benzpyrene
- Originally described in chimney sweeps; also seen in workers in other occupations with coal or petroleum exposure
- Typically occurs in sixth or seventh decade of life
- Ipsilateral inguinal lymphadenopathy is found at presentation in 50% of cases

Gross Pathology

- Early lesions are slow-growing, solitary papules or nodules
- Later lesions are ulcerated and have raised, rolled edges and a seropurulent discharge

Histopathology

- Well to moderately differentiated squamous cell carcinoma
- Keratinization is common
- Surrounding skin shows acanthosis, hyperkeratosis, and dysplasia

Special Stains and Immunohistochemistry

- Noncontributory

Other Techniques for Diagnosis

- Noncontributory

Differential Diagnosis

- Includes a wide variety of inflammatory and neoplastic skin lesions

PEARLS

- *Most common malignant tumor of the scrotum; much less frequent than penile squamous cell carcinoma*
- *First cancer linked by occupational exposure to a carcinogen*
- *Prognosis depends on stage; overall prognosis is poor (typically, 30% to 40% 5-year survival rate)*

SELECTED REFERENCES

Johnson TV, Hsiao W, Delman KA, et al: Scrotal cancer survival is influenced by histology: a SEER study. World J Urol 31:585-590, 2013.

Peng W, Feng G, Lu H, et al: A case report of scrotal carcinoma and review of the literature. Case Rep Oncol 5:434-438, 2012.

Chapter 12
Female Reproductive System

PINCAS BITTERMAN • VIJAYA B. REDDY

CHAPTER OUTLINE

VULVA

Inflammatory dermatologic diseases that affect hair-bearing skin elsewhere on the body may also occur on the vulva (see Chapter 2). A selected group of disorders are addressed here primarily because of the frequency with which they are seen on the vulva.

LICHEN SCLEROSUS (CHRONIC ATROPHIC VULVITIS)

Clinical Features
- Most common in postmenopausal white women
- Tends to develop slowly but is insidious and progressive
- Stenosis of introitus may occur

Gross Pathology
- Flat, often symmetrical white plaques involving labia majora, labia minora, clitoris, and often the perineum

Histopathology
- Hyperkeratosis, thinned epidermis with blunting of rete ridges (Figure 12-1A)

- Hydropic degeneration of basal cells
- Papillary dermal edema and homogenization of collagen
- Patchy bandlike lymphocytic infiltrate underlying the abnormal dermis
- Loss of melanocytes in affected area

Special Stains and Immunohistochemistry
- Noncontributory

Other Techniques for Diagnosis
- Noncontributory

Differential Diagnosis
LICHEN PLANUS
- Dense bandlike lymphoid infiltrate that obscures the dermoepidermal junction (Figure 12-1B)
- Other sites (mucosal and nonmucosal) often involved
- Colloid bodies (degenerated keratinocytes and basement membrane material) may be present
- Lichen simplex chronicus
- Hyperkeratosis associated with epidermal hyperplasia rather than atrophy
- No papillary dermal edema or homogenization

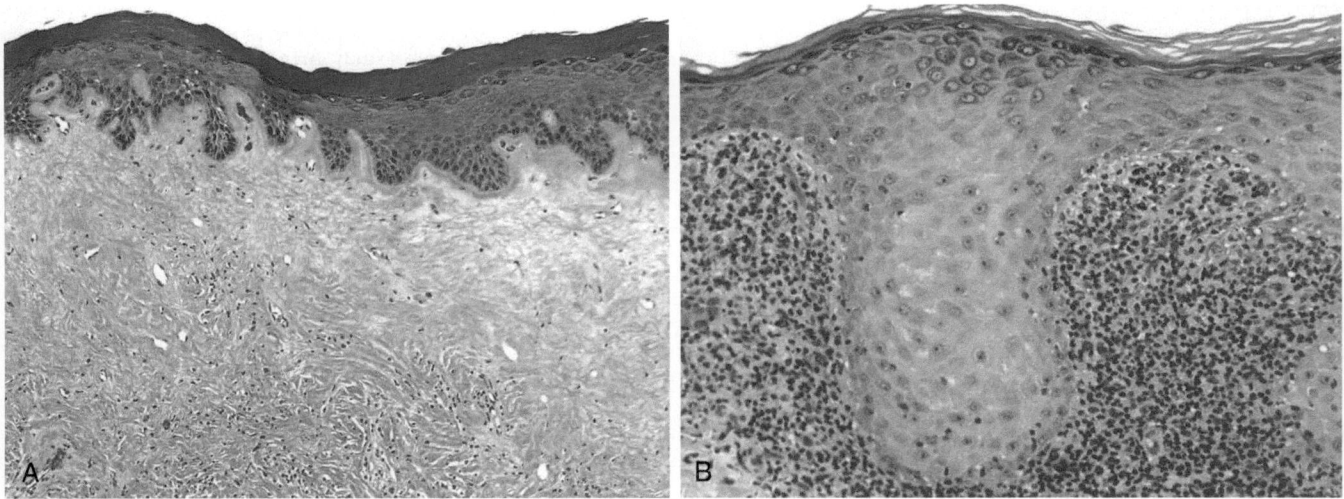

Figure 12-1. A, Lichen sclerosus. Hyperkeratosis and collagenization of the superficial dermis is evident. A patchy inflammatory cell infiltrate is present below the zone of dermal changes. **B,** Lichen planus. Hyperkeratosis, wedge-shaped hypergranulosis, irregular epidermal hyperplasia, and a bandlike inflammatory cell infiltrate that obscures the dermoepidermal junction.

PEARLS

- *Lichen sclerosus may be present adjacent to squamous cell carcinoma; however, it is not regarded as a precancerous condition*
- *Associated with a small but significant risk of squamous cell carcinoma in postmenopausal women (up to 5% of cases)*
- *Topical corticosteroids are the mainstay of treatment*

SELECTED REFERENCES

Chiesa-Vottero A, Dvoretsky PM, Hart WR: Histopathologic study of thin vulvar squamous cell carcinomas and associated cutaneous lesions: a correlative study of 48 tumors in 44 patients with analysis of adjacent vulvar intraepithelial neoplasia types and lichen sclerosus. Am J Surg Pathol 30:310-318, 2006.

Fistarol SK, Itin PH: Diagnosis and treatment of lichen sclerosus: an update. Am J Clin Dermatol 14:27-47, 2013.

Raspollini MR, Asirelli G, Moncini D, Taddei GL: A comparative analysis of lichen sclerosus of the vulva and lichen sclerosus that evolves to vulvar squamous cell carcinoma. Am J Obstet Gynecol 197:592-595, 2007.

LICHEN SIMPLEX CHRONICUS (SQUAMOUS CELL HYPERPLASIA, HYPERPLASTIC DYSTROPHY)

Clinical Features

- Adult women
- Commonly presents with vulvar pruritus
- Treated with topical corticosteroids and antipruritics

Gross Pathology

- Gray-white plaques, often edematous and excoriated

Histopathology

- Hyperkeratosis, hypergranulosis, and epithelial thickening (Figure 12-2)
- Normal maturation of epidermal keratinocytes
- In squamous cell hyperplasia, there are no significant dermal changes

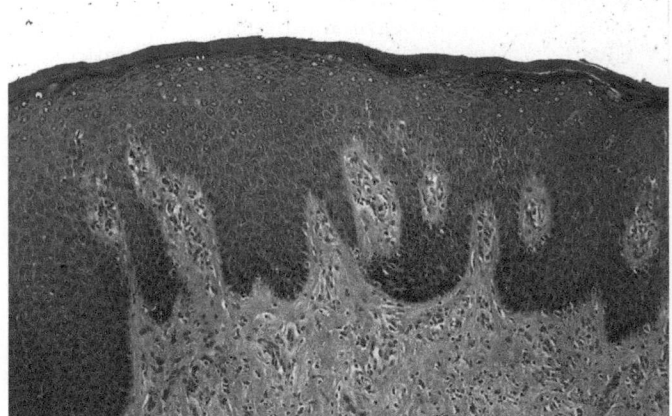

Figure 12-2. Squamous cell hyperplasia (ex-hyperplastic dystrophy). Hyperkeratosis, acanthosis, and mild chronic inflammation within the dermis.

- In lichen simplex chronicus, there is dermal fibrosis with vertically oriented collagen bundles and a chronic inflammatory cell infiltrate

Special Stains and Immunohistochemistry

- Noncontributory

Other Techniques for Diagnosis

- Noncontributory

Differential Diagnosis

- Diagnosis of lichen simplex chronicus is one of exclusion because the changes may be superimposed on practically any dermatosis; a careful evaluation to exclude a primary dermatosis is necessary

PEARLS

- *Lichen simplex chronicus and squamous cell hyperplasia are not known to be associated with an increased risk of squamous cell carcinoma*

SELECTED REFERENCES

Fox H, Wells M: Recent advances in the pathology of the vulva. Histopathology 42:209-216, 2003.

Stewart KM: Clinical care of vulvar pruritus, with emphasis on one common cause, lichen simplex chronicus. Dermatol Clin 28:669-680, 2010.

LICHEN PLANUS

Clinical Features

- Most common in women over 40 years old
- Symptoms include vulvar pruritus, burning or asymptomatic
- Vulvo-gingival syndrome: involvement of the vulva, vagina, and oral mucosa by white lacelike plaques

Gross Pathology

- Variable appearance: white, lacelike plaques, papules, erosive desquamative lesions

Histopathology

- Hyperkeratosis, hypergranulosis and epithelial hyperplasia
- Bandlike predominantly lymphoid infiltrate that obscures the dermoepidermal junction
- Civatte (cytoid) bodies (degenerated keratinocytes forming eosinophilic bodies)
- Parakeratosis is generally absent

Special Stains and Immunohistochemistry

- Noncontributory

Other Techniques for Diagnosis

- Noncontributory

Differential Diagnosis

LICHEN SCLEROSUS

- Absence of wedge-shaped hypergranulosis, cytoid bodies and bandlike lymphocytic infiltrate obscuring the dermoepidermal junction
- There is epidermal atrophy in lichen sclerosus rather than hyperplasia
- Presence of papillary dermal edema and homogenized collagen

LICHEN SIMPLEX CHRONICUS

- Epidermal hyperplasia and hyperkeratosis similar to lichen planus
- Bandlike lymphoid infiltrate at the dermoepidermal junction is not characteristic of lichen simplex chronicus

PEARLS

- *Thinned epithelium and postinflammatory hypopigmentation in advanced disease may make it difficult to differentiate from lichen sclerosus*
- *Involvement of vaginal and oral mucosa (vulvo-vaginal-gingival syndrome), regarded as an erosive form of lichen planus, is characteristic*

SELECTED REFERENCES

Ball SB, Wojnarowska F: Vulvar dermatoses: lichen sclerosus, lichen planus, and vulval dermatitis/lichen simplex chronicus. Semin Cutan Med Surg 17:182, 1998.

Cooper SM, Ali I, Baldo M, Wojnarowska F: The association of lichen sclerosus and erosive lichen planus of the vulva with autoimmune disease: a case-control study. Arch Dermatol. 144:1432, 2008.

Simpson RC, Thomas KS, Leighton P, Murphy R: Diagnostic criteria for erosive lichen planus affecting the vulva: an international electronic-Delphi consensus exercise. Br J Dermatol 169:337-343, 2013.

VULVAR CYSTS

Clinical Features

- Generally asymptomatic
- Occur at any age
- Incidental finding on clinical examination

Gross Pathology

- Single or multiple thin-walled cysts several millimeters in diameter

Histopathology

- None of the cysts show atypia of the lining epithelium

EPIDERMAL INCLUSION CYST

- Similar to those seen in skin
- Lined by stratified squamous epithelium with a preserved granular layer
- Laminated keratin material in the lumen

BARTHOLIN DUCT CYST

- Dilated segment of obstructed Bartholin gland duct
- Noncornified squamous, transitional, or cuboidal lining
- Accumulation of secretions in the lumen but no laminated keratin

MUCINOUS CYST

- Lined by a single layer of columnar mucinous epithelium (Figure 12-3)
- Focal squamous metaplasia may be present

MESONEPHRIC-LIKE CYST

- Lined by a single layer of cuboidal to columnar epithelium
- May be attenuated by pressure from cyst contents (clear fluid)
- Smooth muscle layer around basement membrane

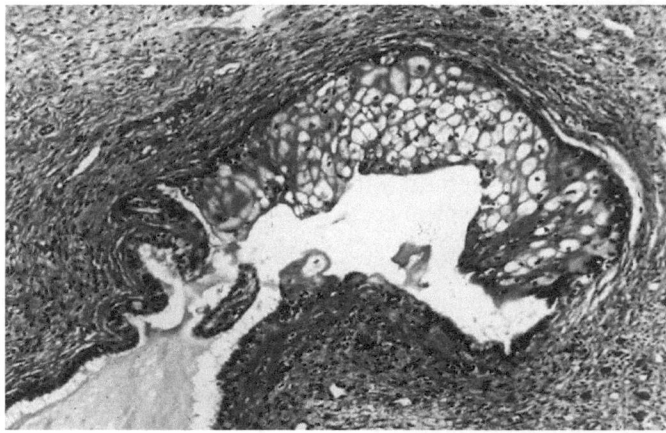

Figure 12-3. Mucous cyst. Cystic space lined by simple mucus-secreting cells. Squamous metaplasia of the epithelium lining the cyst wall is evident.

CILIATED CYST

- Rare
- Ciliated and secretory columnar epithelial cell lining
- May show pseudostratification
- No muscle layer
- Absent cellularity of surrounding stroma

MESOTHELIAL CYST

- Thin-walled cyst lined by a single layer of flattened mesothelial cells

PERIURETHRAL CYST

- Cyst lined by transitional epithelium

Special Stains and Immunohistochemistry

- Noncontributory

Other Techniques for Diagnosis

- Noncontributory

Differential Diagnosis

CILIATED CYST VERSUS ENDOMETRIOSIS

- In endometriosis, the glands may be ciliated; however, endometrial-type stroma is necessary for diagnosis

PEARLS

- *None of the previously listed cysts are associated with malignancy*
- *Surgical excision is curative*

SELECTED REFERENCES

Hamada M, Kiryu H, Ohta T, Furue M: Ciliated cyst of the vulva. Eur J Dermatol 14:347-349, 2004.

Patil S, Sultan AH, Thakar R: Bartholin's cysts and abscesses. J Obstet Gynecol 27:241-245, 2007.

Peters WA III: Bartholinitis after vulvovaginal surgery. Am J Obstet Gynecol 178:1143-1144, 1998.

PAPILLARY HIDRADENOMA (HIDRADENOMA PAPILLIFERUM)

Clinical Features

- Occurs mainly in middle-aged women in the labia majora, labia minora, and perineum
- Cutaneous adnexal origin (i.e., apocrine sweat glands)
- Some may arise from the mammary-like glands that occur in the vulva (ectopic breast tissue)
- Identical appearance to intraductal papillomas of the breast

Gross Pathology

- Round, firm, dome-shaped nodule that is 1 to 2 cm in diameter
- On occasion, slightly tender and ulcerated if neglected

Histopathology

- Complex papillary structures with fine fibrovascular cores lined by two cell layers (Figure 12-4)
- Inner layer of columnar or cuboidal cells, sometimes with apocrine appearance
- Basal layer of flattened myoepithelial cells

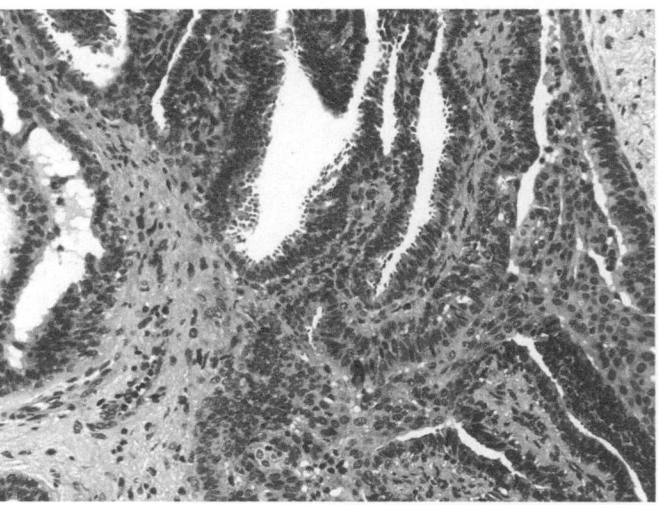

Figure 12-4. Papillary hidradenoma. Papillary structures with fibrovascular cores covered by two layers of cells: a basal layer of flattened myoepithelial cells and a luminal layer of tall columnar cells with decapitation secretions.

Special Stains and Immunohistochemistry

- S-100 protein, SMMS and P63 are positive in the myoepithelial cells
- Periodic acid-Schiff (PAS) focally positive in the epithelial cells

Other Techniques for Diagnosis

- Noncontributory

Differential Diagnosis

ADENOCARCINOMA

- Nuclear pleomorphism and mitotic figures
- Absence of myoepithelial layer

OTHER SKIN AND SKIN ADNEXAL TUMORS

- The vulva and its adnexal structures may be rarely affected by other skin tumors that occur in other sites (refer to Chapter 2 for a detailed discussion)

PEARLS

- *Papillary hidradenoma is the only cutaneous adnexal tumor that is seen in the vulva with any frequency*

SELECTED REFERENCES

Baker GM, Selim MA, Hoang MP: Vulvar adnexal lesions: a 32-year, single-institution review from Massachusetts General Hospital. Arch Pathol Lab Med 137:1237-1246, 2013.

Kazakov DV, Mikyskova I, Kutzner H, et al: Hidradenoma papilliferum with oxyphilic metaplasia: a clinicopathological study of 18 cases, including detection of human papillomavirus. Am J Dermatopathol 27:102-110, 2005.

HERPES VIRUS INFECTION

Clinical Features

- Genital herpes virus infection (HSV) is a highly contagious sexually transmitted infection typically caused by HSV type II and occasionally by HSV type I

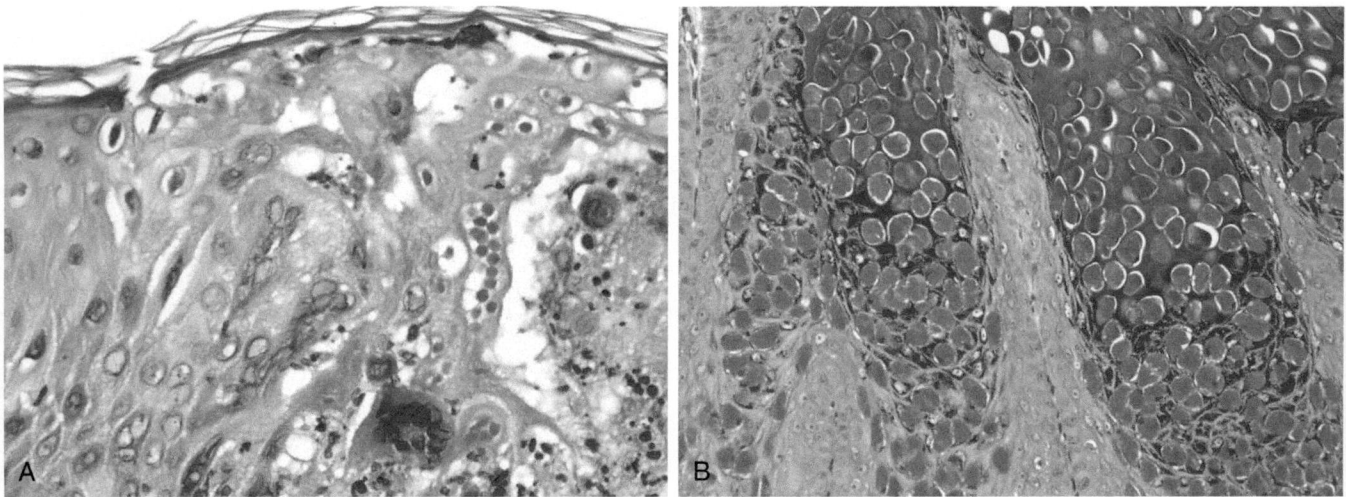

Figure 12-5. A, Herpes virus infection. Epidermal necrosis and multinucleated giant cells with nuclear clearing and margination of chromatin. **B,** Molluscum contagiosum. Epidermal hyperplasia and invaginations filled with classic eosinophilic intracytoplasmic inclusions.

- Typically presents with asymptomatic vesicles that may ulcerate and become painful or become infected secondarily by bacteria
- Recurrences are common

Gross Pathology

- Small, smooth vesicles, 3 to 6 mm
- Often arranged in clusters

Histopathology

- Balloon degeneration of epithelial cells
- Epidermal necrosis and vesiculation (Figure 12-5A)
- Multinucleated keratinocytes with ground-glass nuclear inclusions and margination of chromatin

Special Stains and Immunohistochemistry

- In situ hybridization or immunostain for HSV may be useful for confirmation

Other Techniques for Diagnosis

- Polymerase chain reaction (PCR) and viral cultures

Differential Diagnosis

- None, when the classic cytopathic effects of herpes virus are present
- Identical histologic changes are seen in HSV and varicella-zoster virus infections

PEARLS

- *Diagnosis can be made from a cytology preparation of the scraping of the base of a vesicle or ulcer (Tzanck smear)*

SELECTED REFERENCES

Bernstein DI, Bellamy AR, Hook EW 3rd, et al: Epidemiology, clinical presentation, and antibody response to primary infection with herpes simplex virus type 1 and type 2 in young women. Clin Infect Dis 56:344-345, 2013.

Yeung-Yue KA, Brentjens MH, Lee PC, Tyring SK: Herpes simplex viruses 1 and 2. Dermatol Clin 20:249-266, 2002.

MOLLUSCUM CONTAGIOSUM

Clinical Features

- Contagious DNA viral disease
- Spreads by close contact
- Most lesions regress spontaneously

Gross Pathology

- Small, smooth papules that measure 0.3 mm to 1 cm
- Central umbilication
- Usually multiple and discrete

Histopathology

- Marked epidermal hyperplasia surrounding a central crateriform invagination that may extend deep into the dermis (Figure 12-5B)
- Brightly eosinophilic intracytoplasmic inclusions within the hyperplastic squamous epithelium that are discharged into the crater as the epithelium matures with cornification
- In older lesions, the inclusions may appear more basophilic
- The crateriform invagination may rupture and invoke a marked inflammatory response in the dermis; the inclusions may be difficult to identify in the inflammatory background

Special Stains and Immunohistochemistry

- Noncontributory

Other Techniques for Diagnosis

- PCR

Differential Diagnosis

- None when the characteristic inclusions are identified

PEARLS

- *Most lesions regress spontaneously*
- *Central umbilication of papule is a helpful finding for clinical diagnosis*
- *Diagnosis may be made by cytologic examination of scrapings from a papule*

SELECTED REFERENCES

Epstein WL: Molluscum contagiosum. Semin Dermatol 11:184-189, 1992.
Trama JP, Adelson ME, Mordechai E: Identification and genotyping of molluscum contagiosum virus from genital swab samples by real-time PCR and pyrosequencing. J Clin Virol 40:325-329, 2007.

CONDYLOMA ACUMINATUM

Clinical Features

- Spread by sexual contact
- Human papilloma virus (HPV) types 6 and 11 are the most common associated types
- Lesions turn white upon application of 3% to 5% acetic acid under colposcopic examination
- Usually asymptomatic

Gross Pathology

- Exophytic lesions of variable size
- Usually multiple and often confluent

Histopathology

- Papillomatous epidermal hyperplasia
- Hyperkeratosis and parakeratosis (Figure 12-6A)
- Prominent granular cell layer
- Koilocytes in superficial epithelial layer (pathognomic feature) (Figure 12-6B)
  - Enlarged cells with perinuclear cytoplasmic clearing (halos)
  - Enlarged or pyknotic nuclei with irregular membranes (raisinoid)
  - Binucleate and multinucleate forms are common
- Mitotic figures and cytologic atypia when present are confined to the lower third of the epithelium; if mitotic figures and atypia are present in the middle one third, the lesion is regarded as condyloma with VIN 2

Special Stains and Immunohistochemistry

- A p16 immunohistochemical stain is helpful in excluding aggressive HPV types (e.g., 16, 18, 31, 45)

Other Techniques for Diagnosis

- Polymerase chain reaction (PCR) or in situ hybridization (ISH): identification of specific HPV type, usually 6 or 11

Differential Diagnosis

HIGH-GRADE SQUAMOUS INTRAEPITHELIAL NEOPLASIA (VULVAR INTRAEPITHELIAL NEOPLASIA [VIN] 2-3)

- Usually flat lesions with or without koilocytic changes
- Nuclear pleomorphism and hyperchromasia and abnormal mitoses
- Cytologic atypia is present above the lower third of the epithelium

SQUAMOUS CELL HYPERPLASIA AND LICHEN SIMPLEX CHRONICUS

- No koilocytes are present
- Lacks HPV by PCR and DNA analysis

SQUAMOUS PAPILLOMA

- Lacks hyperkeratosis
- Lacks koilocytosis

PEARLS

- *HPV-6 is most commonly associated with condyloma acuminatum*
- *HPV-11 is not uncommon*
- *Most lesions regress spontaneously*
- *Progression to a high-grade squamous intraepithelial lesion and even to a squamous cell carcinoma has been reported*

SELECTED REFERENCES

Srodon M, Stoler MH, Baber GB, Kurman RJ: The distribution of low and high-risk HPV types in vulvar and vaginal intraepithelial neoplasia (VIN and VAIN). Am J Surg Pathol 30:1513-1518, 2006.
Vinokurova S, Wentzensen N, Einenkel J, et al: Clonal history of papillomavirus-induced dysplasia in the female lower genital tract. J Natl Cancer Inst 97:1816-1821, 2005.

VULVAR INTRAEPITHELIAL NEOPLASIA (VIN)

Clinical Features

- Most common in premenopausal women
- Discolored, raised plaques, often white after application of (5%) acetic acid at colposcopic examination

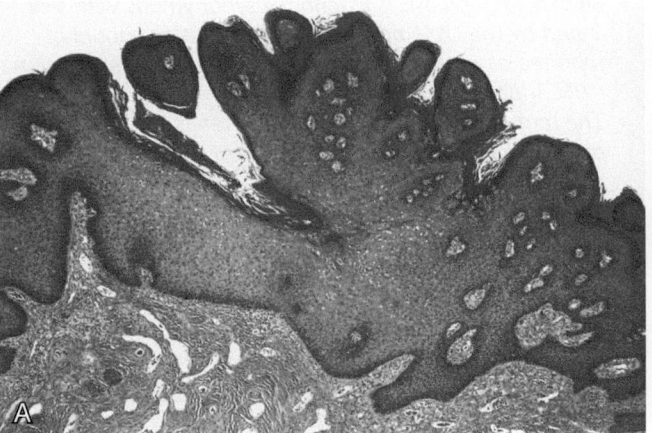
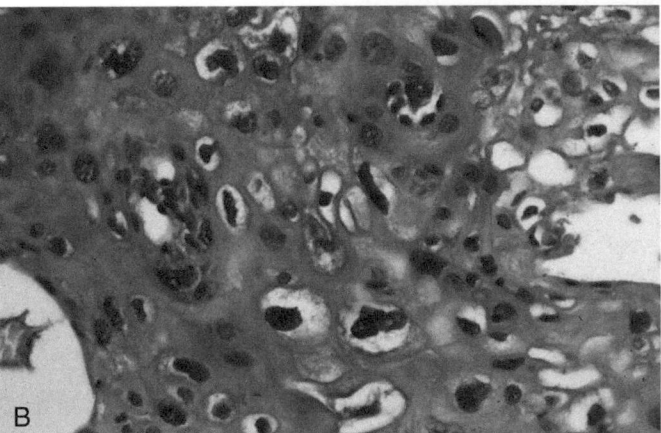

Figure 12-6. Condyloma acuminatum. A, Low-power view demonstrates an exophytic lesion associated with acanthosis and hyperkeratosis. **B,** High-power view shows classic koilocytotic cells with prominent perinuclear halos.

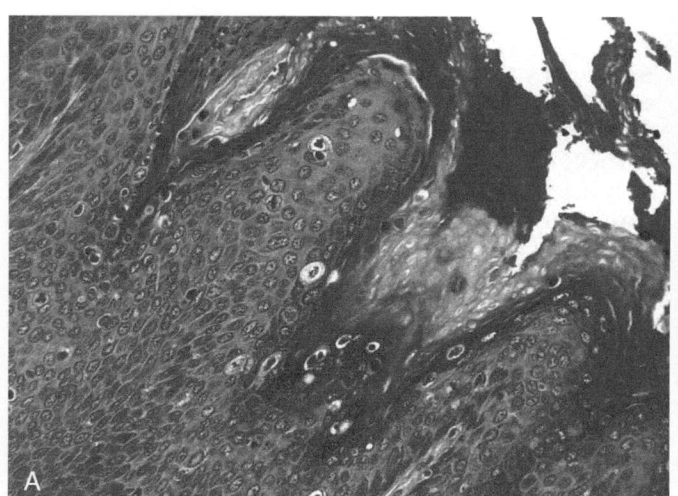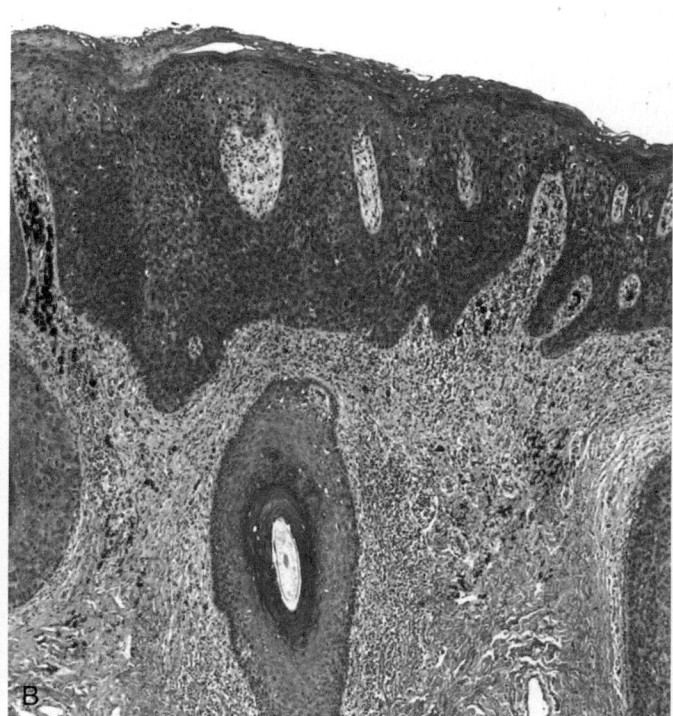

Figure 12-7. Vulvar intraepithelial neoplasia (VIN)3. A, Vulvar skin with hyperkeratosis and finger-like projections showing severe nuclear atypia and lack of maturation. **B,** Full-thickness dysplasia of the epithelium with overlying parakeratosis. Notice the uniformity of the lesion.

Gross Pathology

- Flat or papular discolored lesions, often white but may be red, gray, brown, or black

Histopathology

VIN 1 (LOW-GRADE SQUAMOUS INTRAEPITHELIAL LESION)

- Nuclear pleomorphism and hyperchromasia involving the lower third of the epithelium
- Increased mitotic activity in the lower third

VIN 2 AND 3 (HIGH-GRADE SQUAMOUS INTRAEPITHELIAL LESION)

- Nuclear pleomorphism and hyperchromasia involving the lower two thirds (VIN 2) or full thickness of the epithelium (VIN 3) (Figures 12-7A and B)
- Binucleate and multinucleate cells are often present
- Atypical mitotic figures are readily identifiable
- Koilocytosis may be seen within or adjacent to the lesion

Special Stains and Immunohistochemistry

- Positive for p16
- MIB-1 index high

Other Techniques for Diagnosis

- PCR, ISH: HPV-16 is commonly identified
- Ploidy: High-grade VIN lesions usually contain an aneuploid population of cells

Differential Diagnosis

PAGET DISEASE

- Epidermis with scattered, highly atypical single cells with pale cytoplasm (adenocarcinoma cells)

- Atypical cells positive for mucin, HER-2-neu, and carcinoembryonic antigen (CEA)

PEARLS

- *The Lower Anogenital Squamous Terminology (LAST) standardization project for HPV-related lesions recommended a two-tiered nomenclature for noninvasive HPV-associated squamous proliferations of the lower anogenital tract, low-grade and high-grade squamous intraepithelial lesions (LSIL and HSIL), which may be further qualified with the appropriate IN terminology that includes the site designation (VAIN for vaginal, VIN for vulvar and CIN for cervical)*
- *Condyloma acuminatum including flat condyloma is regarded as a low-grade squamous intraepithelial lesion in the LAST terminology*
- *Bowenoid papulosis is essentially synonymous with VIN 3 and by the LAST project recommendation should be reported as a high-grade squamous intraepithelial lesion (VIN 3, Bowenoid papulosis)*
- *The term* erythroplasia of Queyrat *refers to a high-grade squamous intraepithelial lesion (VIN 3) in mucous membranes of the vulvar vestibule that are often red*
- *Squamous intraepithelial lesions, particularly the low-grade lesions, may spontaneously regress, especially in young or pregnant women*
- *Local excision is the current recommended therapy*

SELECTED REFERENCES

Darragh TM, Colgan TJ, Cox JT, et al: The lower anogenital squamous terminology standardization project for HPV-associated lesions: background and consensus recommendations from the College of American Pathologists and the American Society for Colposcopy and Cervical Pathology. Arch Pathol Lab Med 136:1266-1297, 2012.

Goffin F, Mayrand MH, Gauthier P, et al: High-risk human papillomavirus infection of the genital tract of women with a previous history or current high-grade vulvar intraepithelial neoplasia. J Med Virol 78:814-819, 2006.

Hart WR: Vulvar intraepithelial neoplasia: historical aspects and current status. Int J Gynecol Pathol 20:16-30, 2001.

Rodolakis A, Diakomanolis E, Vlachos G, et al: Vulvar intraepithelial neoplasia (VIN): diagnostic and therapeutic challenges. Eur J Gynaecol Oncol 24:317-322, 2003.

SQUAMOUS CELL CARCINOMA

Clinical Features

- Generally two patient populations
  - Young women with history of smoking and concomitant HPV-associated lesions
  - Postmenopausal women with well-differentiated squamous cell carcinoma and no evidence of HPV infection

Gross Pathology

- Superficially invasive: red papule, white plaque, or irregular ulcerated lesion, smaller than 2 cm
- Invasive: exophytic papillary mass or endophytic ulcer, usually solitary

Histopathology

- Full-thickness involvement of epithelium by pleomorphic cells with high nuclear-to-cytoplasmic ratio and mitotic activity (carcinoma in situ/HSIL)
- Atypical mitotic figures are often readily identifiable
- Superficially invasive squamous cell carcinoma
  - Depth of invasion ≤ 1 mm as measured from the basement membrane of the nearest dermal papilla to the point of deepest point of invasion
  - Less than 2 cm in diameter
- Invasive squamous cell carcinoma (Figures 12-8A and B)
  - Greater than 1 mm in depth of invasion
  - Variable degree of squamous differentiation (i.e., keratin pearl formation)
    - Gynecologic Oncology Group (GOG) grade 1: no undifferentiated cells; keratin pearls are present
    - GOG grade 2: less than 50% undifferentiated cells
    - GOG grade 3: greater than 50% undifferentiated cells

SPINDLE CELL SQUAMOUS CARCINOMA

- Pleomorphic spindle cells that are keratin positive
  - Acantholytic squamous cell carcinoma
- Pseudogland formation caused by acantholysis
- Variants of squamous cell carcinoma

BASALOID CARCINOMA

- Endophytic growth with dense hyalinized stroma
- Nests and cords of basaloid cells with minimum cytoplasm
- Overlying squamous epithelium often shows high-grade VIN
- Associated with synchronous or metachronous tumors of the vagina and cervix

VERRUCOUS CARCINOMA

- Synonymous with giant condyloma of Buschke-Löwenstein
- Exophytic growth resembling papilloma
- No fibrovascular cores or cytologic atypia
- Invasion is defined by large, cytologically bland cells in bulbous nests with pushing borders

WARTY (CONDYLOMATOUS) CARCINOMA

- Squamous carcinoma with papillary exophytic growth
- Fibrovascular fronds
- Numerous koilocytes
- Irregularly outlined nests of invasive tumor at base
  - Squamous cell carcinoma with tumor giant cells
    - Nonkeratinizing with pleomorphic multinucleate tumor giant cells

Special Stains and Immunohistochemistry

- Cytokeratin positive
- Strongly positive p16 in basaloid and warty squamous cell carcinoma

Other Techniques for Diagnosis

- PCR, ISH: HPV-16 detected in about 75% of tumors, especially in younger women with history of VIN

Differential Diagnosis

BASAL CELL CARCINOMA: AS PER BASAL CELL CARCINOMA OF SKIN

- Adenoid pattern: in addition has tubular and glandlike differentiation
- Basosquamous: includes foci of squamous cell carcinoma

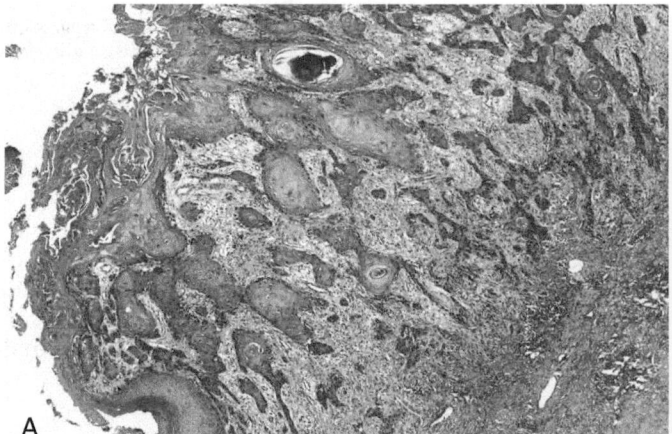
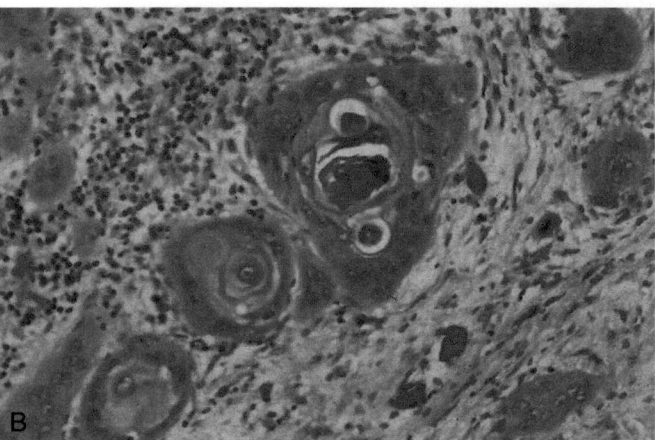

Figure 12-8. Infiltrating squamous cell carcinoma. A, Well-differentiated infiltrating squamous cell carcinoma. **B,** High-power view shows infiltrating sheets of squamous cells with keratinization and prominent stromal reaction (desmoplasia).

Amelanotic Malignant Melanoma
- Negative for cytokeratin
- Positive for S-100 protein, melan-A, and HMB-45
- No keratinization or squamous pearl formation

Epithelioid Sarcoma
- Absent intraepithelial component
- Aggregates of atypical epithelioid cells resembling granulomas
- Deeper location in the mucosa (near fascia)

Pseudoepitheliomatous Hyperplasia
- Bland cytology
- Normally maturing squamous epithelium
- Usually a reactive process

Metastatic Squamous Cell Carcinoma
- Clinical history is important
- Generally metastatic tumor will be present deep in the dermis
- No connection to the overlying epidermis

PEARLS

- *According to the consensus recommendations of the LAST project, the term* superficially invasive squamous cell carcinoma (SISCCA) *is recommended for minimally invasive squamous cell carcinoma of the lower anogenital tract that has been completely excised and is potentially amenable to conservative therapy*
- *Important prognostic factors are tumor thickness, depth of invasion, tumor diameter, and vascular and lymphatic space invasion*
- *The risk for inguinal node involvement increases significantly in tumors with a depth of invasion greater than 1 mm*
- *The invasive component is often better differentiated than the intraepithelial component*
- *Tumors with a depth of invasion > 1 to 2 mm have relatively low but unpredictable rates of inguinal node involvement*
- *Wide local excision appears to be the preferred treatment for superficially invasive carcinoma*
- *Tumors greater than 1 mm in depth could also be treated by partial or total vulvectomy with inguinal node dissection*

SELECTED REFERENCES

Chiesa-Vottero A, Dvoretsky PM, Hart WR: Histopathologic study of thin vulvar squamous cell carcinomas and associated cutaneous lesions: a correlative study of 48 tumors in 44 patients with analysis of adjacent vulvar intraepithelial neoplasia types and lichen sclerosus. Am J Surg Pathol 30:310-318, 2006.
Darragh TM, Colgan TJ, Cox JT, et al: The lower anogenital squamous terminology standardization project for HPV-associated lesions: background and consensus recommendations from the College of American Pathologists and the American Society for Colposcopy and Cervical Pathology. Arch Pathol Lab Med 136:1266-1297, 2012.
Hauspy J, Beiner M, Harley I, et al: Sentinel lymph node in vulvar cancer. Cancer 110:1015-1023, 2007.

MALIGNANT MELANOMA

Clinical Features

- Most common in the labia and in older women
- High mortality rate even when localized
- Most often diagnosed when deeply invasive
- Local recurrences are frequent
- Overall 5-year survival between 40% and 50%

Gross Pathology

- Pigmented macule, papule, or plaque

Histopathology

- Similar to melanoma in cutaneous sites (see Chapter 2)

Special Stains and Immunohistochemistry

- S-100 protein, melan-A, and HMB-45 positive
- Cytokeratin and CEA negative

Other Techniques for Diagnosis

- Noncontributory

Differential Diagnosis

Paget Disease
- More common in skin from the breast
- Immunohistochemical profile (mucin and CEA positive; melan-A and HMB-45 negative) is the opposite of the profile for malignant melanoma

High-Grade Squamous Intraepithelial Lesions (VIN 3)
- Dysplastic cells lack prominent nucleoli
- Positive for p16 and negative for mucin, CEA, HMB-45, melan-A, and S-100 protein

PEARLS

- *Clinically pigmented appearance of the lesion is characteristic, but up to 35% of vulvar melanomas can be amelanotic*
- *Vulvar melanoma is a disease of older women often associated with a worse prognosis than cutaneous melanomas and high rates of local recurrences and satellite lesions*

SELECTED REFERENCES

Mert I, Semaan A, Winer I, et al: Vulvar/vaginal melanoma: an updated surveillance epidemiology and end results database review, comparison with cutaneous melanoma and significance of racial disparities. Int J Gynecol Cancer 23:1118-1125, 2013.
Ragnarsson-Olding BK, Kanter-Lewensohn LR, Lagerlof B, et al: Malignant melanoma of the vulva in a nationwide, 25-year study of 219 Swedish females: clinical observations and histopathologic features. Cancer 86:1273-1284, 1999.

BARTHOLIN GLAND CARCINOMA

Clinical Features

- Presents in older women
- Clinically may be mistaken for a cyst or abscess
- About 20% present with inguinal lymph node metastasis
- Treated by wide excision or vulvectomy with inguinal-femoral lymph node dissection

Gross Pathology

- Solid infiltrative tumor that occupies the anatomic site of the Bartholin gland (Figure 12-9)

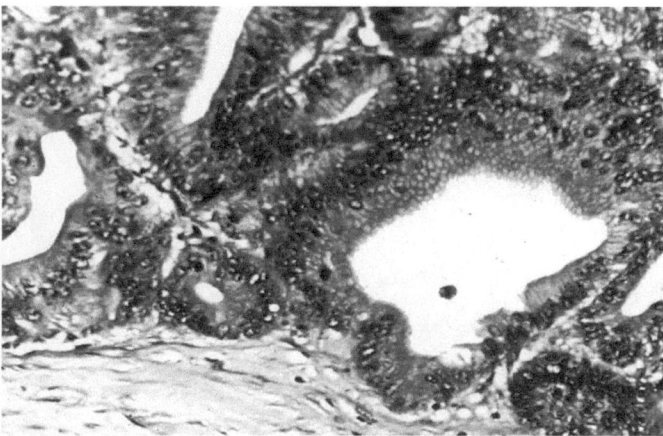

Figure 12-9. Bartholin gland adenocarcinoma. High-power view shows back-to-back neoplastic glands demonstrating nuclear stratification and hyperchromasia.

Histopathology

- Squamous cell carcinoma (about 40%)
  - Usual appearance of squamous cell carcinoma (SCC)
- Adenocarcinoma (40%)
  - Generally typical features of adenocarcinoma: malignant glands
  - Intracytoplasmic mucin
  - CEA-positive cells
- Adenoid cystic carcinoma (about 10%)
- Transitional cell carcinoma (about 5%)
- Adenosquamous carcinoma (about 5%)

Special Stains and Immunohistochemistry

- Cytokeratin positive
- CEA positive
- S-100 protein positive in adenoid cystic carcinoma

Other Techniques for Diagnosis

- None

Differential Diagnosis

METASTATIC ADENOCARCINOMA VERSUS PRIMARY BARTHOLIN GLAND TUMOR

- Metastases are rare in this location
- May resemble organ of origin
- Clinical history is most important

SKIN ADNEXAL ADENOCARCINOMA VERSUS BARTHOLIN GLAND ADENOCARCINOMA

- Usually well differentiated
- Morphologically the tumor resembles adnexal structure of origin

METASTATIC SQUAMOUS CELL CARCINOMA VERSUS BARTHOLIN GLAND SQUAMOUS CELL CARCINOMA

- Usually only weakly positive for CEA
- Clinical history is most important

PEARLS

- *Nodal metastasis is seen in up to 40% of patients, and distant metastasis (lungs, bone) may also occur*

- *Adenoid cystic type of Bartholin gland carcinoma generally has a better prognosis than other types*
- *Adenosquamous type generally has a worse prognosis than squamous cell carcinoma of the vulva*
- *Adenocarcinoma has the highest rate of lymph node metastasis*

SELECTED REFERENCES

Finnan MA, Barre G: Bartholin's gland carcinoma, malignant melanoma and other rare tumours of the vulva. Best Pract Res Clin Obstet Gynaecol 17:609-633, 2003.

Khanna G, Rajni, Azad K: Bartholin gland carcinoma. Indian J Pathol Microbiol 53:171-172, 2010.

Woida FM, Ribeiro-Silva A: Adenoid cystic carcinoma of the Bartholin gland: an overview. Arch Pathol Lab Med 131:796-798, 2007.

EXTRAMAMMARY PAGET DISEASE

Clinical Features

- Most common in postmenopausal white women
- Fluorescein is useful to visualize the lesion before excision
- Often presents with pruritus
- Most develop de novo in epidermis and probably represent adenocarcinoma in situ of the cutaneous sweat ducts
- Slowly progressive disease
- Not necessarily associated with underlying vulvar invasive cancer in contrast to mammary Paget disease
- Therapy is wide local excision

Gross Pathology

- Pink to red eczematous patches with white foci due to hyperkeratosis

Histopathology

- Irregularly defined lesion often larger than clinical impression
- Abnormal cells in the epidermis concentrated in the basal layer but may also be present superficially and in skin appendages
- Intraepithelial tumor cells singly or in small groups
- Large cells with round nuclei often containing large nucleoli
- Pale cytoplasm or vacuolated signet ring cells (Figure 12-10)
- Adenocarcinoma may be seen in underlying dermis in about 10% to 20% of cases

Special Stains and Immunohistochemistry

- Cytokeratin 7 and CEA positive
- PAS with diastase, mucin, and Alcian blue positive
- May be HER-2-neu positive

Other Techniques for Diagnosis

- Noncontributory

Differential Diagnosis

VIN

- Usually associated with HPV infection
- More regular involvement of basal layer

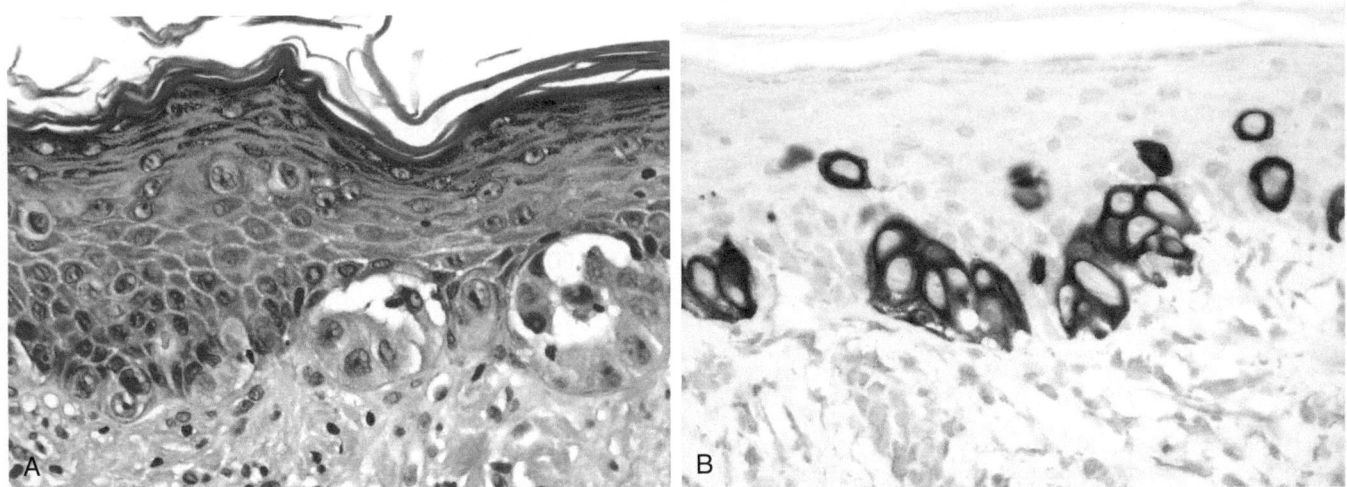

Figure 12-10. Paget disease. A, Neoplastic cells in small groups near the basal cell layer and above it. The cells have pale cytoplasm, round nuclei, and prominent nucleoli. **B,** Paget cells are strongly immunoreactive for cytokeratin 7.

- Smaller cells with less prominent nucleoli
- Negative for mucin, CEA, low-molecular-weight cytokeratin (LMWCK), and HER-2-neu

SUPERFICIAL SPREADING MALIGNANT MELANOMA
- Positive for S-100 protein, melan-A, and HMB-45
- Negative for mucin, cytokeratin, and HER-2-neu
- Cells may contain melanin pigment

PEARLS

- *Generally not associated with HPV*
- *Occasionally associated with underlying adenocarcinoma or primary breast carcinoma including Paget disease*
- *Mucin positivity is a helpful diagnostic feature*
- *Recurrences are frequent because lesions are often more extensive than can be appreciated clinically*

SELECTED REFERENCES

Baker GM, Selim MA, Hoang MP: Vulvar adnexal lesions: a 32-year, single-institution review from Massachusetts General Hospital. Arch Pathol Lab Med 137:1237-1246, 2013.
Petković S, Jeremić K, Vidaković S, et al: Paget's disease of the vulva: a review of our experience. Eur J Gynaecol Oncol 27:611-612, 2006.

GRANULAR CELL TUMOR

Clinical Features

- Peripheral nerve sheath tumor seen uncommonly in the vulva
- Presents as a painless, slow-growing, subcutaneous mass
- Generally occurs in the labia majora, clitoris, or mons pubis
- Local recurrences are common
- Malignant tumors are extremely rare

Gross Pathology

- Well-demarcated, firm mass

Histopathology

- Nonencapsulated with pushing or infiltrative borders
- Composed of irregular nests and sheets of polyhedral cells with indistinct borders, abundant eosinophilic granular cytoplasm, and relatively small nuclei
- The overlying epithelium may show pseudoepitheliomatous hyperplasia

Special Stains and Immunohistochemistry

- S-100 protein positive
- PAS positive

Other Techniques for Diagnosis

- Noncontributory

Differential Diagnosis

LEIOMYOMA, NEUROFIBROMA, AND DERMATOFIBROMA
- Generally lack the classic granular cytoplasm seen in granular cell tumors
- Pseudocarcinomatous hyperplasia on the surface of granular cell tumor may be misdiagnosed as squamous cell carcinoma in superficial biopsies

PEARLS

- *Much more common in other locations (i.e., tongue)*
- *May enlarge rapidly during pregnancy*
- *Examination of the margins of resection is most important*

SELECTED REFERENCES

Kondi-Pafiti A, Kairi-Vassilatou E, Liapis A, et al: Granular cell tumor of the female genital system: clinical and pathologic characteristics of five cases and literature review. Eur J Gynaecol Oncol 31:222-224, 2010.
Wolber R, Wilkinson E, Talerman A, et al: Granular cell tumors of the vulva with pseudocarcinomatous hyperplasia: a comparative morphologic analysis with squamous cell carcinoma. Int J Gynecol Pathol 10:59-66, 1991.

ANGIOMYOFIBROBLASTOMA

Clinical Features

- Benign tumor, rare

- Presents as a painless mass, typically <5 cm, occasionally pedunculated
- Clinical impression is often a Bartholin gland cyst

Gross Pathology

- Well circumscribed, nonencapsulated
- Tan-white cut surface

Histopathology

- Alternating zones of hyper and hypocellularity with irregularly distributed abundant thin-walled blood vessels
- Bland spindled, oval, plasmacytoid and epithelioid stromal cells with eosinophilic cytoplasm that tend to aggregate around the blood vessels (Figure 12-11)
- Variably edematous to collagenous matrix
- Occasional multinucleated cells and rare to absent mitotic activity
- Adipose tissue may be present within the tumor
- Scattered lymphocytes and mast cells are usually present

Special Stains and Immunohistochemistry

- Vimentin and desmin positive
- Smooth muscle actin (SMA) negative
- S-100 protein, ER, PR, and CD34 variably positive

Other Techniques for Diagnosis

- Noncontributory

Differential Diagnosis

AGGRESSIVE ANGIOMYXOMA

- Less cellular, homogeneous, and characterized by infiltrative borders
- Medium to large muscular vessels in clusters

PEARLS

- *Treated by local excision*

SELECTED REFERENCES

Nasu K, Fujisawa K, Takai N, Miyakawa I: Angiomyofibroblastoma of the vulva. Int J Gynecol Cancer 12:228-231, 2002.

Sims SM, Stinson K, McLean FW, et al: Angiomyofibroblastoma of the vulva: a case report of a pedunculated variant and review of the literature. J Low Genit Tract Dis 16:149-154, 2012.

AGGRESSIVE ANGIOMYXOMA

Clinical Features

- Usually seen in premenopausal women
- Presents as a poorly demarcated mass in the vulva, perineum, and pelvis
- Locally aggressive, deeply invasive tumor, often larger than clinically appreciated
- Wide local excision is the treatment of choice

Gross Pathology

- Soft gelatinous mass with ill-defined margins
- Clusters of vessels are visible on cut surface

Histopathology

- Myxoid stroma with benign spindled fibroblasts and myofibroblasts (Figure 12-12)
- Numerous haphazardly arranged medium-large sized, often hyalinized blood vessels
- Perivascular cuffs of collagen and bundles of smooth muscle cells
- Entrapped fat, neural elements, or glandular elements may be present

Special Stains and Immunohistochemistry

- Spindle cells positive for SMA, ER, and PR
- S-100 protein and CD34 may be positive

Other Techniques for Diagnosis

- Noncontributory

Differential Diagnosis

SUPERFICIAL ANGIOMYXOMA (CUTANEOUS MYXOMA)

- Superficial location, small size and good circumscription
- Neutrophils are often present
- Lack thick-walled muscular vessels
- Negative for desmin, ER and PR

ANGIOMYOFIBROBLASTOMA

- Superficial location and well-defined margins
- Cellular areas, thin-walled blood vessels, and perivascular condensation of cells

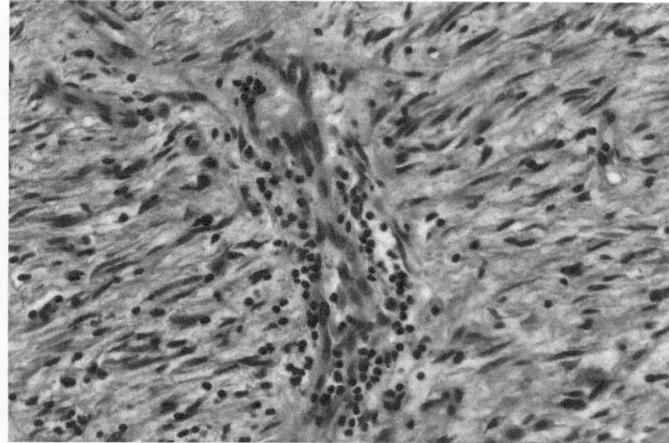

Figure 12-11. Angiomyofibroblastoma. Spindle-shaped tumor cells with perivascular distribution. A prominent perivascular chronic inflammatory infiltrate is noted.

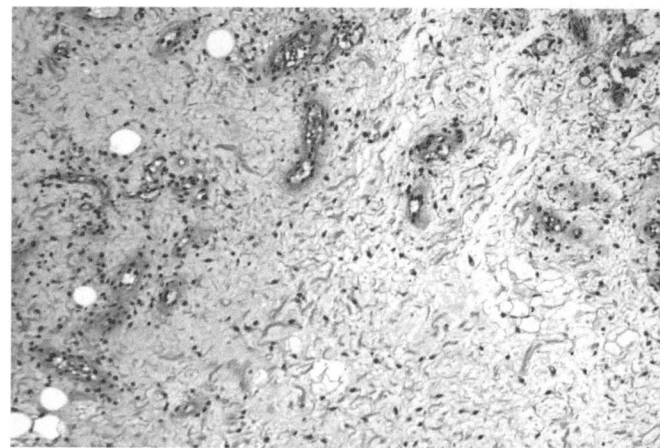

Figure 12-12. Aggressive angiomyxoma. Prominent myxoid stroma with small blood vessels.

PEARLS

- *Locally aggressive with significant rate of local recurrence*

SELECTED REFERENCES

Abu JI, Bamford WM, Malin G, et al: Aggressive angiomyxoma of the perineum. Int J Gynecol Cancer 15:1097-1100, 2005.
Dierickx I, Deraedt K, Poppe W, Verguts J: Aggressive angiomyxoma of the vulva: a case report and review of literature. Arch Gynecol Obstet 277:483-487, 2008.
Ribaldone R, Piantanida P, Surico D, et al: Aggressive angiomyxoma of the vulva. Gynecol Oncol 95:724-728, 2004.
Sutton BJ, Laudadio J: Aggressive angiomyxoma. Arch Pathol Lab Med. 136:217-221, 2012.

LEIOMYOSARCOMA

Clinical Features

- Most common vulvar sarcoma but overall quite rare
- Occurs in women of any age
- Usually arises in labia majora
- Often presents with pain
- Treatment is wide excision
- Metastasis to lung and liver have been reported

Gross Pathology

- Well-defined firm mass with infiltrative edges
- Focal hemorrhage, necrosis, and cystic degeneration

Histopathology

- Interlacing bundles of spindle cells with perinuclear clearing and nuclear atypia
- A prominent epithelioid cell component is seen rarely
- The background may be myxoid and or hyalinized
- Coagulative necrosis and areas of hemorrhage
- Greater than 5 mitotic figures/10 high-power fields (hpf)

Special Stains and Immunohistochemistry

- Cytokeratin: occasional positive cells
- Vimentin, desmin, and SMA positive

Other Techniques for Diagnosis

- Noncontributory

Differential Diagnosis

DERMATOFIBROSARCOMA PROTUBERANS

- Storiform pattern
- Rare cytologic atypia and mitotic figures
- Negative for SMA and desmin but positive for CD34

AGGRESSIVE ANGIOMYXOMA

- Multiple clusters of muscular blood vessels
- Generally lacks cytologic atypia and mitotic activity

PEARLS

- *Tumors > 5 cm in diameter have a higher rate of recurrence*
- *Some tumors may have minimal cytologic atypia, but infiltrative margins, coagulative necrosis, and a mitotic count > 5 mitotic figures/10 hpf help distinguish them from leiomyomas*

SELECTED REFERENCES

Nielsen GP, Rosenberg AE, Koerner FC, et al: Smooth-muscle tumors of the vulva: a clinicopathological study of 25 cases and review of the literature. Am J Surg Pathol 20:779-793, 1996.
Shankar S, Todd PM, Rytina E, Crawford RA: Leiomyosarcoma of the vulva. J Eur Acad Dermatol Venereol 20:116-117, 2006.

OTHER SARCOMAS

- The following mesenchymal tumors rarely arise in the vulvar subcutaneous tissue:
  - Embryonal rhabdomyosarcoma, generally in children
  - Dermatofibrosarcoma protuberans
  - Malignant fibrous histiocytoma
  - Epithelioid sarcoma
  - Malignant rhabdoid tumor
  - Angiosarcoma
  - Hemangiopericytoma
  - Kaposi sarcoma
  - Alveolar soft part sarcoma
  - Malignant schwannoma (neural)
  - Liposarcoma
- In the vulva, these sarcomas are identical to their counterparts in soft tissue
- Refer to Chapters 2 and 17 for detailed discussions

SELECTED REFERENCES

Nucci MR, Fletcher CDM: Vulvovaginal soft tissue tumors: update and review. Histopathology 36:97-108, 2000.
Ulutin HC, Zellars RC, Frassica D: Soft tissue sarcoma of the vulva: a clinical study. Int J Gynecol Cancer 13:528-531, 2003.

VAGINA

Both atresia and total absence of the vagina are extremely uncommon.

VAGINAL POLYP (FIBROEPITHELIAL POLYP, MESODERMAL STROMAL POLYP)

Clinical Features

- Occurs in women of childbearing age
- Usually discovered incidentally during pelvic examination

Gross Pathology

- Soft polypoid or papillary mass usually in the lower third of the vagina, typically < 4 cm in size (Figure 12-13)

Histopathology

- Squamous epithelium with underlying fibrovascular stroma
- Plump, cytologically atypical myofibroblasts may be present in the stroma
- Bizarre multinucleate giant cells may also be present
- Mitotic activity is generally low

Special Stains and Immunohistochemistry

- Stromal cells positive for vimentin, desmin, ER, PR

Other Techniques for Diagnosis

- Noncontributory

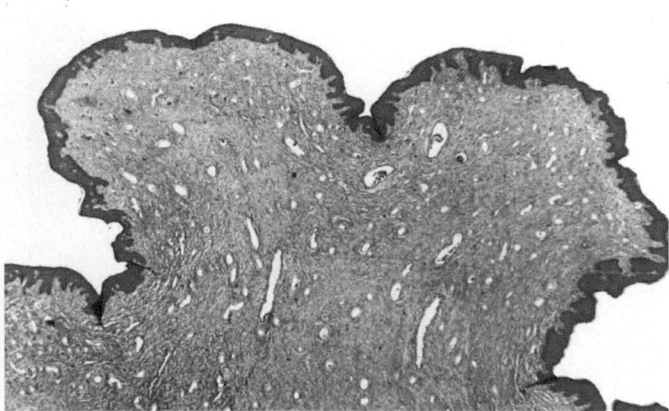

Figure 12-13. Vaginal (fibroepithelial) polyp. Polypoid lesion composed of fibrous connective tissue covered by mature squamous epithelium.

Differential Diagnosis

SARCOMA BOTRYOIDES
- Patients are generally younger than 5 years
- Population of small round blue undifferentiated cells
- Cellular cambium layer
- Rhabdomyoblasts

PEARLS

- *Clinically benign; important to recognize to avoid misdiagnosing as condyloma or sarcoma*

SELECTED REFERENCES

Kurman R, Norris H, Wilkinson E: Atlas of Tumor Pathology: Tumors of the Cervix, Vagina, and Vulva, 3rd Series, Fascicle 4. Washington DC, Armed Forces Institute of Pathology, 1992, pp 170-172.
Nucci MR, Young RH, Fletcher CDM: Cellular pseudosarcomatous fibroepithelial stromal polyps of the lower female genital tract: an underrecognized lesion often misdiagnosed as sarcoma. Am J Surg Pathol. 24; 231-240, 2000.

SQUAMOUS PAPILLOMA

Clinical Features
- May be seen in vagina, vulvar vestibule, or cervix
- Usually asymptomatic

Gross Pathology
- Several millimeters or larger in diameter
- Clustered papillary lesions

Histopathology
- Fibrovascular core with papillary fronds
- Mature, squamous epithelial lining (Figure 12-14)
- No koilocytes

Special Stains and Immunohistochemistry
- Noncontributory

Other Techniques for Diagnosis
- Noncontributory

Differential Diagnosis

CONDYLOMA ACUMINATUM
- Arborizing architecture

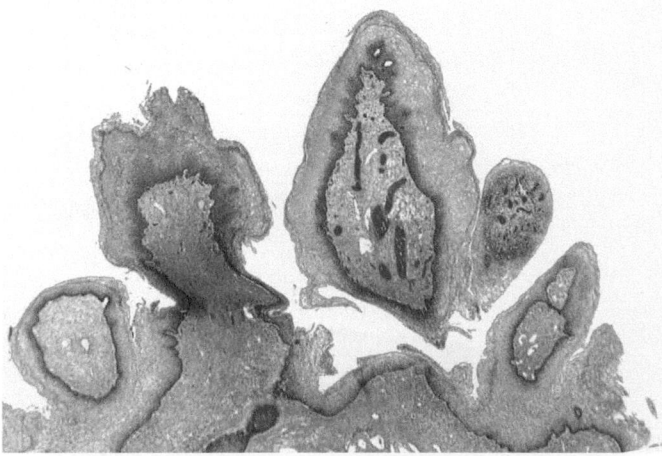

Figure 12-14. Squamous papilloma. Papillary lesion lined by mature nonkeratinizing squamous epithelium.

- Koilocytosis
- HPV-6 or HPV-11 associated

VAGINAL (FIBROEPITHELIAL) POLYP
- Thinner squamous lining
- Polypoid rather than papillary
- Cellular stroma with occasional large pleomorphic cells

PEARLS

- *Clinically benign; important to recognize to avoid misdiagnosing as condyloma or squamous cell carcinoma*

SELECTED REFERENCE

Kurman R, Norris H, Wilkinson E: Atlas of Tumor Pathology: Tumors of the Cervix, Vagina, and Vulva, 3rd Series, Fascicle 4. Washington DC, Armed Forces Institute of Pathology, 1992, p 141.

VAGINAL INTRAEPITHELIAL NEOPLASIA (VAIN)

Clinical Features
- Relatively rare compared with the incidence of cervical squamous intraepithelial lesions
- Usually occurs in postmenopausal women
- Frequently associated with squamous cell carcinomas of cervix or vulva
- HPV infection and cervical or vulvar intraepithelial neoplasia are risk factors
- Usually asymptomatic

Gross Pathology
- Roughened pink or white discolored epithelium
- Occasional gross abnormality

Histopathology

VAIN 1 (LOW-GRADE SQUAMOUS INTRAEPITHELIAL LESION)
- Nuclear pleomorphism and hyperchromasia involving the lower third of the epithelium
- Increased mitotic activity in the lower third
- Flat condylomata acuminata are best classified as VAIN 1

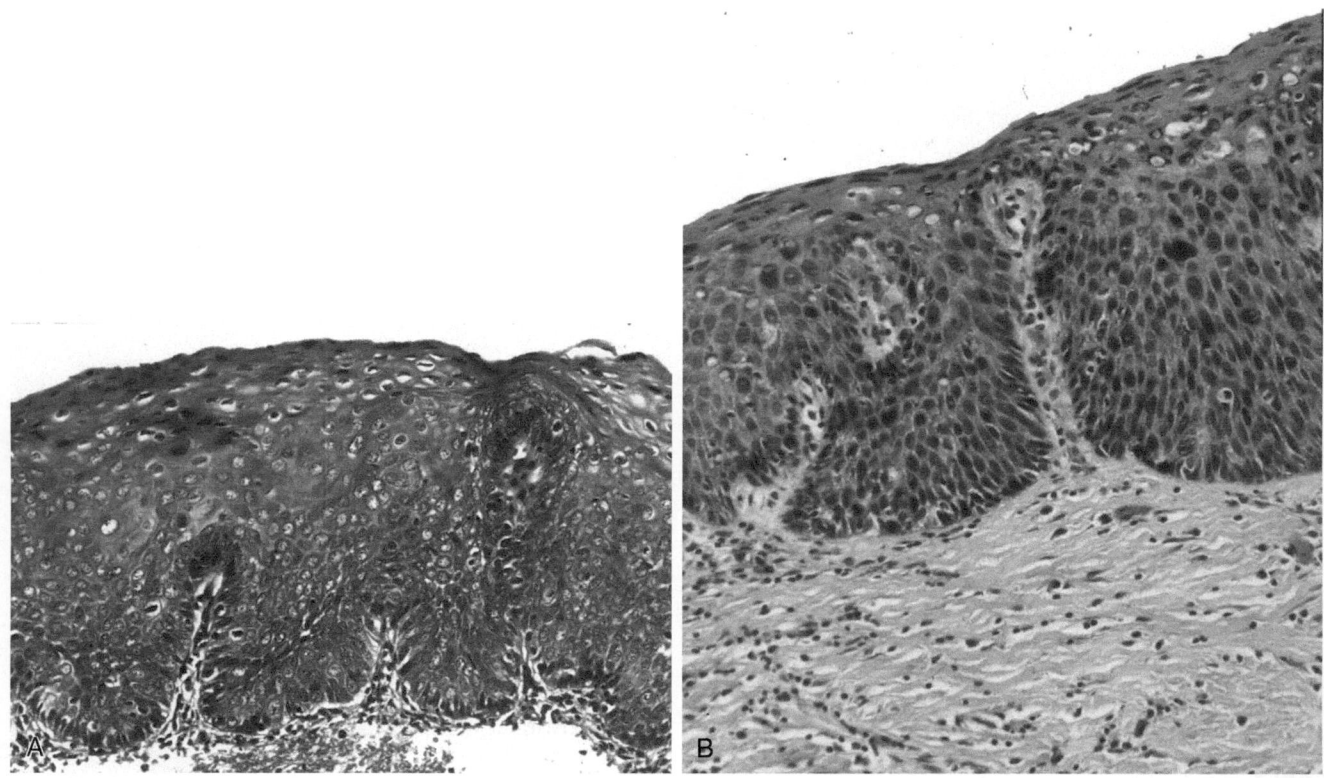

Figure 12-15. A, Vaginal intraepithelial neoplasia (VAIN) 2. Dysplastic cells occupy the lower two thirds of the epithelium. **B,** Vaginal intraepithelial neoplasia (VAIN) 3. The dysplastic cells are present throughout the full thickness of the epithelium.

VAIN 2 AND VAIN 3 (HIGH-GRADE SQUAMOUS INTRAEPITHELIAL LESION)

- Nuclear pleomorphism and hyperchromasia involving the lower two thirds (VAIN 2) or full thickness (VAIN 3) of the epithelium (Figure 12-15)
- Binucleate and multinucleate cells are often present
- Atypical mitotic figures are readily identifiable
- Koilocytosis may be seen within or adjacent to the lesion

Special Stains and Immunohistochemistry

- p16 positivity in HSIL

Other Techniques for Diagnosis

- HPV subtypes may be identified by PCR or ISH

Differential Diagnosis

ATROPHY

- Thinned epithelium without squamous atypia or koilocytosis
- No mitotic activity

IMMATURE SQUAMOUS METAPLASIA

- Nuclear pleomorphism is not dramatic
- Minimal if any mitosis

RADIATION CHANGE

- Preserved nuclear-to-cytoplasmic ratio
- Vacuolated cytoplasm
- Smudged chromatin
- Multinucleation
- Lack of mitotic activity

REACTIVE ATYPIA

- Prominent nucleoli
- Lack of nuclear membrane irregularities

PEARLS

- *Less than 10% progress to invasive carcinoma*
- *Laser ablation and topical 5-fluorouracil are alternative treatments*

SELECTED REFERENCES

Darragh TM, Colgan TJ, Thomas Cox J, et al: The lower anogenital squamous terminology standardization project for HPV-associated lesions: background and consensus recommendations from the College of American Pathologists and the American Society for Colposcopy and Cervical Pathology. Arch Pathol Lab Med 136:1266-1297, 2012.

Drodon M, Stoler MH, Baber GB, Kurman RJ: The distribution of low and high-risk HPV types in vulvar and vaginal intraepithelial neoplasia (VIN and VAIN). Am J Surg Pathol 30:1513-1518, 2006.

Jones RW, Rowan DM: Spontaneous regression of vulvar intraepithelial neoplasia 2-3. Obstet Gynecol 96:470-472, 2000.

SQUAMOUS CELL CARCINOMA

Clinical Features

- Most common malignant vaginal neoplasm, but rare
- One fiftieth of the incidence of cervical squamous cell carcinoma
- Most common in postmenopausal women
- Treatment is radiation therapy

Gross Pathology

- Superficially invasive: red papule, white plaque, or irregular ulcerated lesion
- Invasive: exophytic papillary mass or endophytic ulcer, usually solitary

Histopathology

- Keratinizing with squamous pearl formation or nonkeratinizing
- Syncytial sheets of cells with variable amounts of eosinophilic cytoplasm
- Distinct cell borders and intercellular bridges
- Variants
  - Verrucous carcinoma
    - Rare variant
    - Bulbous solid masses composed of bland squamous cells that push into the stroma (Figure 12-16)
    - Generally koilocytes are not evident
    - Lymph node metastasis is rare
  - Warty (condylomatous) carcinoma
    - Squamous cell carcinoma with numerous koilocytes
    - Exophytic growth

Special Stains and Immunohistochemistry

- Noncontributory

Other Techniques for Diagnosis

- Noncontributory

Differential Diagnosis

AMELANOTIC MALIGNANT MELANOMA

- Negative for cytokeratin
- Positive for S-100 protein and HMB-45
- Absent keratinization and squamous pearl formation

PSEUDOEPITHELIOMATOUS HYPERPLASIA

- Bland cytology
- Normally maturing squamous epithelium
- Absent stromal nests dissociated from basal layer
- Commonly a reactive process

METASTATIC SQUAMOUS CELL CARCINOMA

- Clinical history is fundamental
- Generally metastatic tumor will be present deep in the submucosa
- Absent overlying intraepithelial component

PEARLS

- *Tumors with less than 3 mm depth of stromal invasion and also verrucous carcinomas have low rates of lymph node metastasis*
- *Verrucous carcinomas should not be treated with radiation therapy because they are radioresistant and may transform to higher-grade squamous carcinomas*

SELECTED REFERENCES

Medeiros F, Nascimento AF, Crum CP: Early vulvar squamous neoplasia: advances in classification, diagnosis, and differential diagnosis (review). Adv Anat Pathol 12:20-26, 2005.

Roma AA, Hart WR: Progression of simplex (differentiated) vulvar intraepithelial neoplasia to invasive squamous cell carcinoma: a prospective case study confirming its precursor role in the pathogenesis of vulvar cancer. Int J Gynecol Pathol 26:248-253, 2007.

VAGINAL ADENOSIS

Clinical Features

- Associated with diethylstilbestrol (DES) exposure, most frequently in utero
- Occurs in about one third of women exposed to DES
- Young women aged 30 to 50 are most commonly affected
- Red granular spots that do not stain with iodine
- Excessive mucoid vaginal discharge is a common symptom
- Glandular epithelium may be observed colposcopically (Figure 12-17)
- May also occur with 5-fluorouracil and carbon dioxide laser therapy

Gross Pathology

- Red granular patches
- Upper third of anterior wall is the most common location

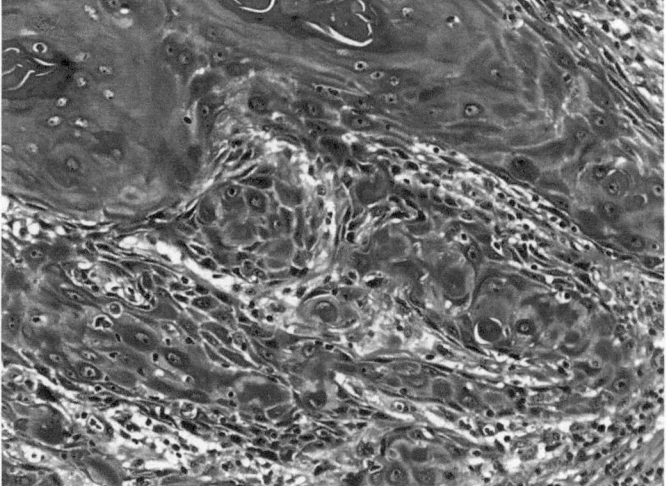

Figure 12-16. Infiltrating squamous cell carcinoma. Nests and clusters of neoplastic cells invade the stroma.

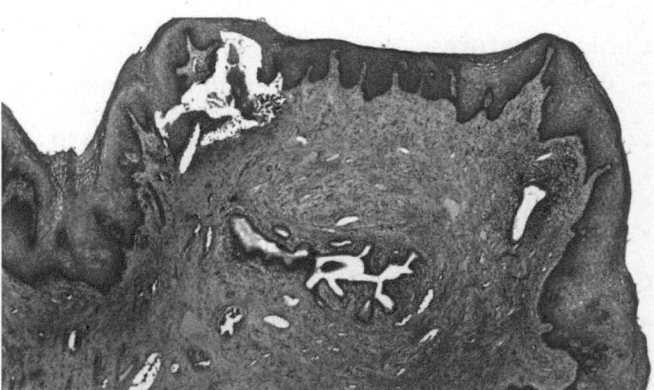

Figure 12-17. Vaginal adenosis. Low-power view demonstrates glandular epithelium at the junction of the mucosa and submucosa/lamina propria in the vagina.

Histopathology

- Endocervical type mucosa replaces squamous lining of vagina
- Mucinous glands are present in the lamina propria
- On occasion, ciliated epithelium or endometrial-type glands are present, particularly in lower third of vagina
- In longstanding lesions, the glands undergo replacement by metaplastic squamous epithelium; obliterated glands or mucin droplets may still be identified in these lesions

Special Stains and Immunohistochemistry

- Noncontributory

Other Techniques for Diagnosis

- Noncontributory

Differential Diagnosis

METASTATIC ADENOCARCINOMA

- Cytologic atypia
- Clinical history

PEARLS

- *DES was prescribed to women in the 1940s and 1950s to prevent miscarriages*
- *History of exposure to DES is important*
- *Vaginal adenosis usually regresses spontaneously*
- *Rarely associated with clear cell carcinoma of vagina and cervix*
- *No treatment is required*

SELECTED REFERENCES

Kurman R, Norris H, Wilkinson E: Atlas of Tumor Pathology: Tumors of the Cervix, Vagina, and Vulva, 3rd Series, Fascicle 4. Washington DC, Armed Forces Institute of Pathology, 1992, pp 146-152.

McCluggage WG: Recent developments in vulvovaginal pathology. Histopathology 54:156-173, 2009.

Robboy SJ, Hill EC, Sandberg EC, Czernobilsky B: Vaginal adenosis in women born prior to the diethylstilbestrol era. Hum Pathol 17:488-492, 1986.

Robboy SJ, Szyfelbein WM, Goellner JR, et al: Dysplasia and cytologic findings in 4,589 young women enrolled in diethylstilbestrol-adenosis (DESAD) project. Am J Obstet Gynecol 140:579-586, 1981.

CLEAR CELL ADENOCARCINOMA

Clinical Features

- Often but not always associated with in utero exposure to DES
- Occurs in less than 0.2% of women exposed to DES
- Generally occurs in women about 20 years of age
- Often presents with vaginal bleeding and discharge
- May be asymptomatic

Gross Pathology

- Occurs anywhere in the vagina
- Polypoid or nodular mass
- Less commonly flat or ulcerated

Histopathology

- Tubulocystic and solid are the most common patterns

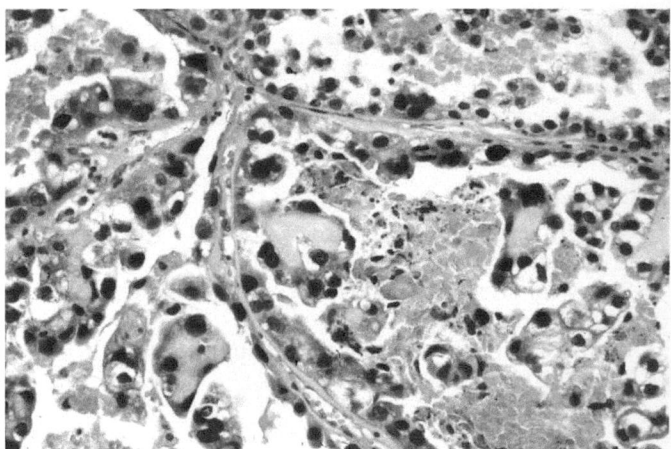

Figure 12-18. Clear cell adenocarcinoma, papillary pattern. The papillae are lined by large pleomorphic cells showing clear cytoplasm. Focal necrosis is present.

- Papillary, tubular, and trabecular patterns may also be seen
- Tumor cells are polyhedral with round, atypical nuclei and clear cytoplasm containing glycogen (Figure 12-18)
- Hobnail cell is a characteristic finding (cell with a nucleus that protrudes beyond the boundaries of the cell into a luminal, tubular, or cystic space)
- Less commonly, the epithelial cells are flattened, cuboidal, oxyphilic, or signet ring
- Adenosis is usually identified adjacent to tumor
- Intracellular hyaline structures and psammoma bodies are common

Special Stains and Immunohistochemistry

- Cytokeratin positive
- PAS positive (intracytoplasmic glycogen)
- PAS with diastase and mucin negative (mucin may be positive in glandular lumina)

Other Techniques for Diagnosis

- Noncontributory

Differential Diagnosis

METASTATIC CLEAR CELL CARCINOMA FROM THE OVARY

- Clinical history is essential

METASTATIC RENAL CELL OR ADRENAL CARCINOMA

- Clinical history is fundamental
- Centrally located nuclei with prominent nucleoli
- Absent gland formation and hobnail cells
- Prominent vascularity

PEARLS

- *Associated with in utero exposure to DES*
- *Adenosis believed to be a precursor lesion*
- *High risk for nodal metastasis if depth of invasion is greater than 3 mm*
- *More aggressive than squamous cell carcinoma*
- *Treatment of early-stage disease: vaginectomy with radical hysterectomy and lymphadenectomy to prevent recurrence*
- *Radiation therapy indicated for advanced disease*

SELECTED REFERENCES

Herbst AL, Anderson S, Hubby MM, et al: Risk factors for the development of diethylstilbestrol associated clear cell adenocarcinoma: a case-control study. Am J Obstet Gynecol 154:814-822, 1986.

Robboy SJ, Anderson MC, Russell P: Pathology of the Female Reproductive Tract. London, Churchill Livingstone, 2002, pp 92-97.

Sander R, Nuss RC, Rhatigan RM: Diethylstilbestrol-associated vaginal adenosis followed by clear cell adenocarcinoma. Int J Gynecol Pathol 5:362-370, 1986.

RHABDOMYOMA

Clinical Features

- Rare; occurs in middle-aged women
- Presents with vaginal bleeding and dyspareunia

Gross Pathology

- Polypoid mass, less commonly flat or ulcerated

Histopathology

- Bland skeletal muscle cells with fetal or adult-type appearance
- Cells are spindle to oval with abundant eosinophilic cytoplasm with cross striations and plump oval nuclei without atypia or mitosis
- Cells are surrounded by a fibrous stroma

Special Stains and Immunohistochemistry

- Positive for actin, desmin, caldesmon, myoglobin, and myosin

Other Techniques for Diagnosis

- Noncontributory

Differential Diagnosis

EMBRYONAL RHABDOMYOSARCOMA (SARCOMA BOTRYOIDES)

- Occurs at a younger age as a rapidly growing infiltrative mass
- Presence of cambium layer
- Pleomorphic strap cells with mitosis

PEARLS

- *Fewer than 25 cases reported*
- *Unremarkable overlying squamous mucosa*
- *Benign behavior*

SELECTED REFERENCES

López JI, Brouard I, Eizaguirre B: Rhabdomyoma of the vagina. Eur J Obstet Gynecol Reprod Biol 45:147-148, 1992.

López Varela C, López de la Riva M, La Cruz Pelea C: Vaginal rhabdomyomas. Int J Gynaecol Obstet 47:169-170, 1994.

EMBRYONAL RHABDOMYOSARCOMA (SARCOMA BOTRYOIDES)

Clinical Features

- Most common vaginal sarcoma
- Occurs in infants and girls younger than 5 years
- Aggressive tumor
- Classically presents as a mass of small translucent nodules protruding from the vagina
- May present with bleeding and discharge and extension to bladder and rectum
- Metastasis to lung or bone usually occurs later in the course of the disease

Gross Pathology

- Classic appearance is a sessile or pedunculated tumor of numerous translucent gray, grapelike, polypoid masses
- Hemorrhagic areas
- Most common location is anterior vaginal wall

Histopathology

- Tumor is organized histologically in layers
  - Superficial attenuated layer of squamous epithelium (Figure 12-19A)
  - Underlying cambium layer composed of small, round to spindled, primitive blue cells with dense hyperchromatic nuclei and minimal cytoplasm (Figure 12-19B)
    - Cells may invade the overlying epithelium
  - Underlying sparsely cellular region with scattered small round blue cells as noted previously in an edematous or myxoid stroma
    - Rhabdomyoblasts are found in this region
      - Large irregular, elongated, or "strap" cells with prominent eosinophilic cytoplasm
      - Cross-striations may be seen but are not required to make the diagnosis
      - Cells may appear to condense around blood vessels

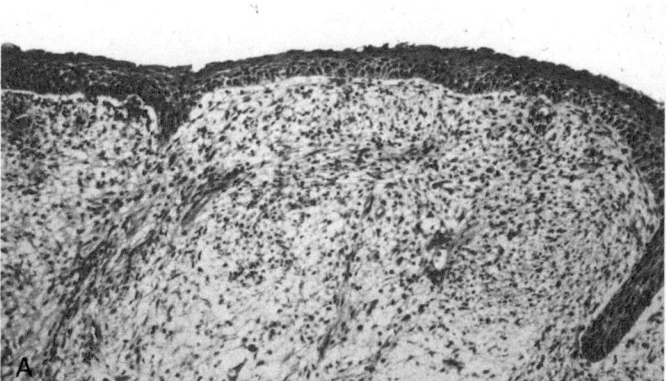
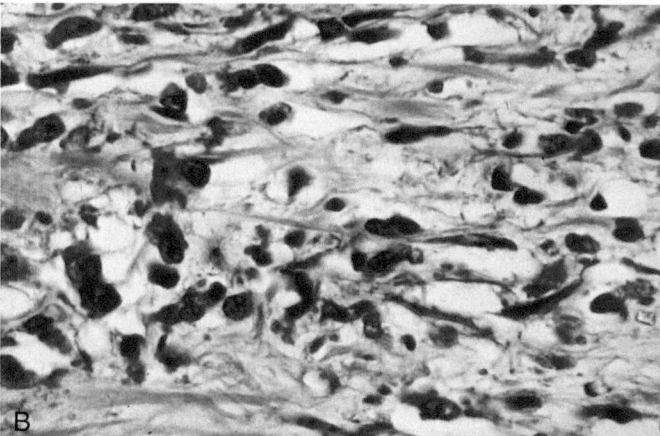

Figure 12-19. Embryonal rhabdomyosarcoma (sarcoma botryoides). **A,** Low-power view demonstrates a proliferation of pleomorphic tumor cells beneath the squamous epithelium. **B,** High-power view demonstrates myxoid stroma containing round to spindled neoplastic cells with eosinophilic cytoplasm.

- Brisk mitotic activity
- Small islands of hyaline cartilage may be present

Special Stains and Immunohistochemistry

- Vimentin, desmin, myogenin, and myo-D1 positive

Other Techniques for Diagnosis

- Noncontributory

Differential Diagnosis

Müllerian Papilloma

- In the differential not because of histologic similarity, but rather because of its similar clinical presentation in infants and young girls
- Papillary tumor with broad fibrovascular cores lined by cuboidal or mucinous epithelium
- Absence of cytologic atypia and mitotic activity

Vaginal Polyp (Mesodermal Stromal Polyp)

- Usually seen in adult women
- Essentially a fibroepithelial polyp as seen histologically in other sites
- Polypoid (as opposed to grapelike) mass
- Edematous fibrous tissue covered by squamous epithelium
- Lymphocytes may be present in the fibrous stroma
- No cambium layer
- Absent small round undifferentiated blue cells and rhabdomyoblasts
- Negative for desmin, myogenin, and myo-D1

Rhabdomyoma

- Usually occurs in middle-aged women
- Numerous well-developed rhabdomyoblasts
- No nuclear atypia or mitotic figures
- Absence of cambium layer
- Absent small round undifferentiated blue cells

PEARLS

- *Aggressive tumor with rapid local invasion and high rate of local recurrence*
- *Survival has significantly improved by combination of surgery, radiation, and new multiagent chemotherapeutic regimens*

Selected References

Fernandez-Pineda I, Spunt SL, Parida L, Krasin MJ, et al: Vaginal tumors in childhood: the experience of St. Jude Children's Research Hospital. J Pediatr Surg 46:2071-2075, 2011.

Hemida R, Goda H, Abdel-Hady el-S, El-Ashry R: Embryonal rhabdomyosarcoma of the female genital tract: 5 years' experience. J Exp Ther Oncol 10:135-137, 2013.

Nucci MR, Fletcher CD: Vulvovaginal soft tissue tumours: update and review. Histopathology 36:97-99, 2000.

OTHER SARCOMAS

- Leiomyosarcoma, epithelioid sarcoma, and malignant fibrous histiocytoma may also present as primary sarcomas of the vagina
- Refer to Chapter 17 for a detailed discussion

CERVIX

ENDOCERVICAL POLYP

Clinical Features

- Most common new growth of the cervix
- Multigravidas during the fourth to sixth decades are the typical patients with polyps
- Majority are discovered as incidental finding; most common symptom is abnormal vaginal bleeding

Gross Pathology

- Rounded or elongated with a smooth or lobulated surface
- Most commonly single
- May measure from millimeters to a few centimeters

Histopathology

- Variety of patterns
- Varying amounts of squamous or endocervical epithelium depending on proximity to cervical os (Figure 12-20)
- Stroma consists of dense fibroconnective tissue with thin and thick-walled vessels

Special Stains and Immunohistochemistry

- Noncontributory

Other Techniques for Diagnosis

- Noncontributory

Differential Diagnosis

Microglandular Adenosis (Hyperplasia)

- Tightly packed glands in a relatively ordered distribution
- Neutrophils are commonly present in the glandular lumina
- Acute and chronic inflammation in the stroma

Papillary Adenofibroma

- Extremely rare and benign
- Leaflike pattern of glandular epithelium compressed by a dense fibrous stroma

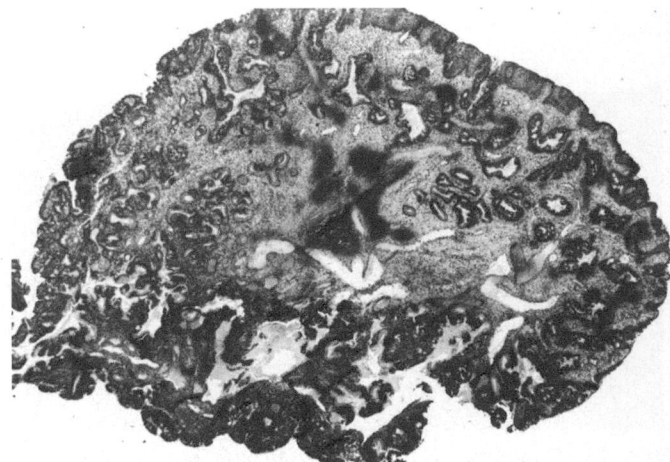

Figure 12-20. Endocervical polyp. Polypoid lesion composed of endocervical mucous glands.

SELECTED REFERENCES

Kurman R, Norris H, Wilkinson E: Atlas of Tumor Pathology: Tumors of the Cervix, Vagina, and Vulva, 3rd Series, Fascicle 4. Washington DC, Armed Forces Institute of Pathology, 1992, pp 77-78.
Wright TC, Ronnett BM, Ferenczy A: Benign diseases of the cervix. In Kurman R (ed): Blaustein's Pathology of the Female Genital Tract, 6th ed. New York, Springer, 2011, pp 155-191.

MICROGLANDULAR HYPERPLASIA

Clinical Features

- Incidental finding in cervical specimens mostly in women of reproductive age
- May present with postcoital spotting or bleeding
- Associated with history of oral contraceptive use, pregnancy, or postpartum condition

Gross Pathology

- Single or multiple polypoid lesions resembling small cervical polyps

Histopathology

- Single or multiple foci of crowded glands have variable amounts of mucin (Figure 12-21)
- Variably sized glands include rare mitotic figures (1 mitotic figure/10 hpf)
- Uniform small round nuclei have even chromatin
- Focal squamous metaplasia and some signet ring cells may be present
- Neutrophils are commonly present in the glandular lumina
- Stroma separating the glands shows acute and chronic inflammatory cells

Special Stains and Immunohistochemistry

- CEA generally negative
- Mucin positive

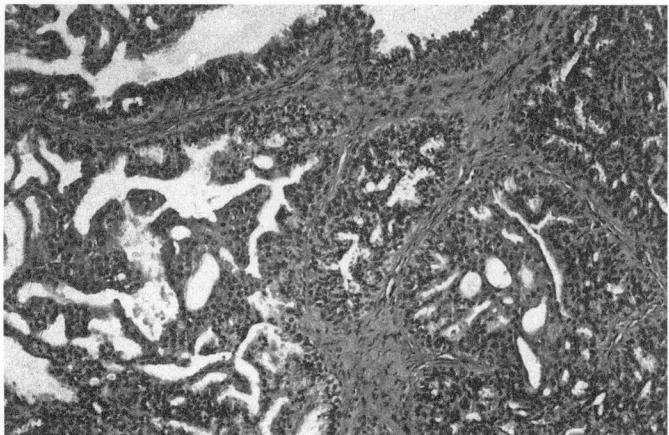

Figure 12-21. Microglandular hyperplasia. Tightly packed variously sized glands lined by flattened to cuboidal cells.

Other Techniques for Diagnosis

- Noncontributory

Differential Diagnosis

CLEAR CELL AND CLASSIC CERVICAL ADENOCARCINOMA

- Papillary and glandular patterns
- Irregular infiltration of cervical stroma by markedly atypical cells with nuclear pleomorphism
- Brisk mitotic rate
- Clear cytoplasm contains mostly glycogen rather than mucin

SELECTED REFERENCES

Greeley C, Schroeder S, Silverberg SG: Microglandular hyperplasia of the cervix: a true "pill" lesion? Int J Gynecol Pathol 14:50-54, 1995.
Witkiewicz AK, Hecht JL, Cviko A, et al: Microglandular hyperplasia: a model for the de novo emergence and evolution of endocervical reserve cells. Hum Pathol 36:154-161, 2005.
Young RH, Scully RE: Atypical forms of microglandular hyperplasia of the cervix simulating carcinoma. Am J Surg Pathol 13:50-56, 1989.

SQUAMOUS INTRAEPITHELIAL LESION (SIL) OR CERVICAL INTRAEPITHELIAL NEOPLASIA (CIN) AND CARCINOMA IN SITU

Clinical Features

- Most common in premenopausal women
- Discolored raised plaques, often white after application of acetic acid (3% to 5%), at colposcopy
- High-grade lesions (high-grade squamous intraepithelial lesions and carcinoma in situ [CIS]) may have a mosaic or cobblestone appearance
- Variety of risk factors, including high number of sexual partners, early age at initiation of sexual activity, and unprotected sex
- Smoking is a cofactor
- Greater than 95% of cervical dysplasias are related to HPV infection

Gross Pathology

- Flat or papular discolored lesions, often white or red

Histopathology

LOW-GRADE SQUAMOUS INTRAEPITHELIAL LESION (LGSIL; CERVICAL INTRAEPITHELIAL NEOPLASIA [CIN] 1) (Figures 12-22 and 12-23A)

- Nuclear pleomorphism and hyperchromasia involving the lower third of the epithelium
- Irregular chromatin with inconspicuous nucleoli
- Increased mitotic activity in the lower third
- Most display HPV effect
- Condylomata acuminata are considered LSIL

HIGH-GRADE SQUAMOUS INTRAEPITHELIAL LESION (HGSIL; CIN 2 OR 3 AND CIS) (Figures 12-23B,C,D)

- Nuclear pleomorphism and hyperchromasia involving the lower two thirds (HGSIL; CIN 2) or the entire thickness of the epithelium (HGSIL; CIN 3; CIS)

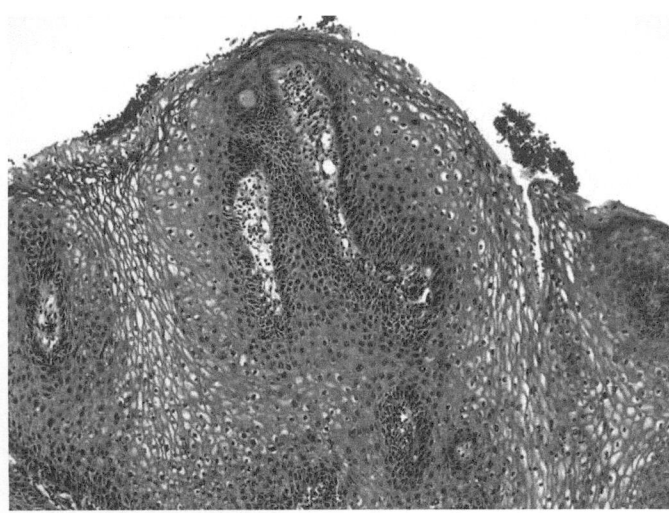

Figure 12-22. Cervical condyloma (cervical intraepithelial neoplasia 1 with human papillomavirus). Hyperplastic epithelium with cells containing irregular cytoplasmic halos and enlarged, binucleate, pyknotic nuclei.

- Irregular chromatin with inconspicuous nucleoli
- High nuclear-to-cytoplasmic ratio and atypical mitotic figures are identifiable
- Binucleate and multinucleate cells are often present but less than in LGSIL
- HPV is occasionally present within the lesion, more commonly adjacent to the lesion
- Involvement of underlying endocervical glands may be seen and should not be confused with microinvasive carcinoma

Special Stains and Immunohistochemistry

- Strong and diffuse nuclear and cytoplasmic positivity for p16 in the full thickness or at least two thirds of the thickness helps confirm a diagnosis of HGSIL (Figure 12-23E)
- MIB-1/Ki-67 positivity in the lower two thirds to full thickness of the epithelium in HGSIL

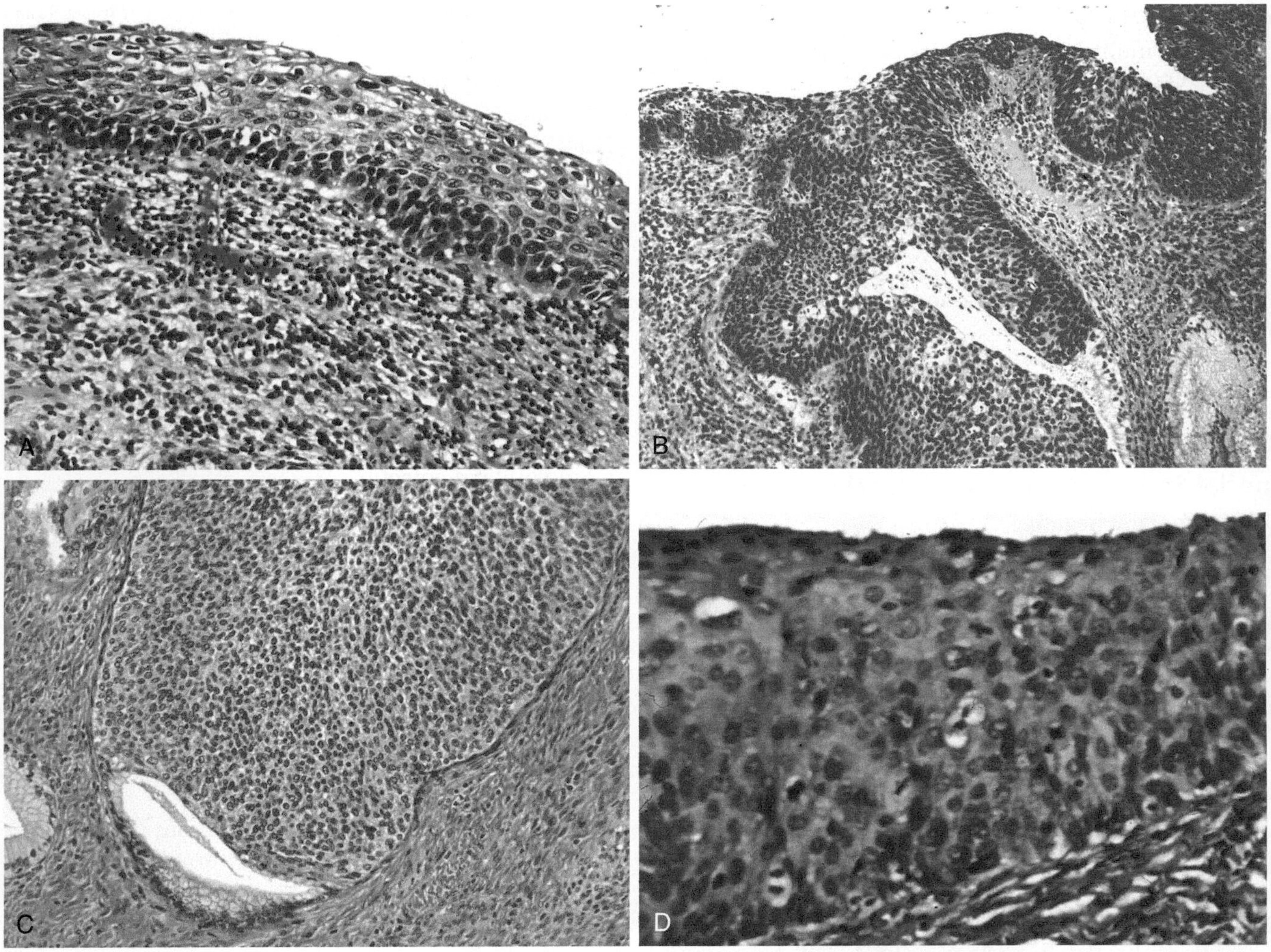

Figure 12-23. A, Low-grade squamous intraepithelial lesion (cervical intraepithelial neoplasia grade 1 [CIN 1]). Dysplastic cells occupy the lower third of the epithelium. The upper two thirds shows koilocytosis. **B,** High-grade squamous intraepithelial lesion (CIN 2). Squamous mucosa featuring dysplastic cells that involve the endocervical gland. **C,** High-grade squamous intraepithelial lesion (carcinoma in situ) with gland involvement. Atypical squamous cells involving endocervical gland. **D,** High-grade squamous intraepithelial lesion (CIN 3). Squamous mucosa with atypical cells and mitotic figures involving the full thickness of the epithelium.

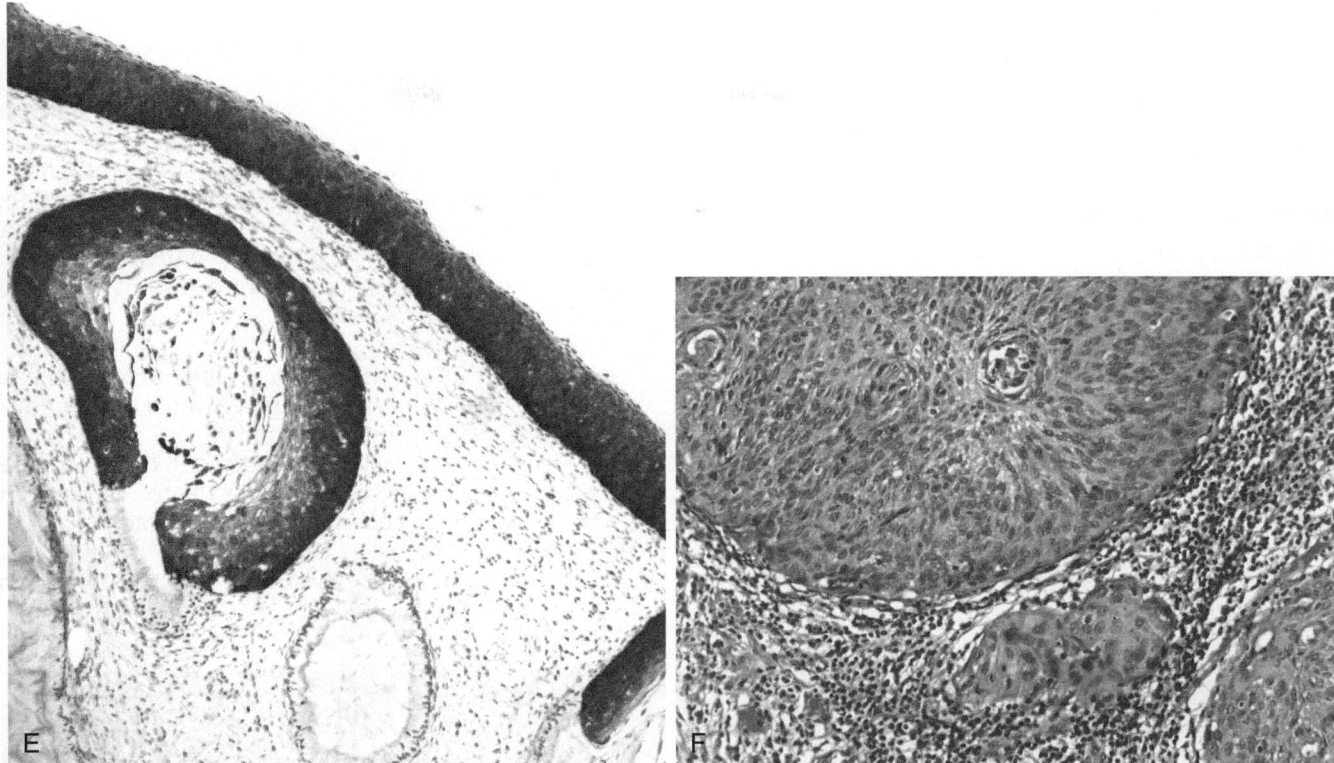

Figure 12-23—cont'd E, High-grade squamous intraepithelial lesion (carcinoma in situ) with gland involvement. A p16 stain showing strong and diffuse positivity. **F,** Microinvasive squamous cell carcinoma. Irregular nests of squamous cell carcinoma surrounded by stromal reaction.

Other Techniques for Diagnosis

- PCR and ISH: High-risk HPV types 16 and less commonly 18 are present in HGSIL, whereas a spectrum of types rarely including 6,11 can be found in LGSIL
- Ploidy: dysplastic lesions usually contain an aneuploid population of cells

Differential Diagnosis

ATROPHY
- Preserved polarity
- Basal cells in the full thickness of the epithelium
- No nuclear pleomorphism or mitotic figures
- Resolves after a 2-week course of locally applied estrogen therapy

IMMATURE SQUAMOUS METAPLASIA
- Retains cellular polarity
- Clearly defined cell membranes
- Absent nuclear atypia and atypical mitoses
- Residual mucin may be seen

REACTIVE ATYPIA
- Associated with inflammation
- Prominent nucleoli
- Retained polarity and nuclear-to-cytoplasmic ratio
- No atypical mitoses
- Changes more pronounced at the base
- Halos mimicking koilocytosis may be present

MICROINVASIVE CARCINOMA VERSUS HGSIL (CIN 3/CIS) WITH GLAND INVOLVEMENT
- No basement membrane around invasive foci

- Irregular infiltration of stroma instead of rounded nests (Figure 12-23 F)
- Stromal reaction, either desmoplastic or inflammatory

PEARLS

- *SIL is usually multifocal*
- *SIL, particularly low-grade lesions (CIN 1), may spontaneously regress, especially in young or pregnant women*
- *LGSIL may be followed clinically, whereas HGSIL CIN (2 or 3) and CIS are generally followed by loop electrocautery excision procedure (LEEP) or cold knife cone and endocervical curetting to determine the extent of dysplasia*
- *Because of the preceding statement, it is essential to distinguish between LGSIL (CIN 1) and HGSIL (CIN 2-3); if both low- and high-grade lesions are present, a diagnosis of HGSIL is appropriate*
- *Vaccination for HPV is effective in about 60% to 70% of patients*

SELECTED REFERENCES

Bosch FX, de Sanjose S: The epidemiology of human papillomavirus infection and cervical cancer. Dis Markers 23:213-227, 2007.

Castle PE, Schiffman M, Wheeler CM, et al: Evidence for frequent regression of cervical intraepithelial neoplasm-grade 2. Obstet Gynecol 113:18-25, 2009.

Fadare O, Rodriguez R: Squamous dysplasia of the uterine cervix: tissue sampling-related diagnostic considerations in 600 consecutive biopsies. Int J Gynecol Pathol 26:469-474, 2007.

Focchi GR, Silva ID, Nogueira-de-Souza NC, et al: Immunohistochemical expression of p16(INK4A) in normal uterine cervix, nonneoplastic epithelial lesions, and low-grade squamous intraepithelial lesions. J Low Genit Tract Dis 11:98-104, 2007.

McCluggage WG: Immunohistochemistry as a diagnostic aid in cervical pathology. Pathology 39:97-111, 2007.

Song SH, Lee JK, Oh MJ, et al: Risk factors for the progression or persistence of untreated mild dysplasia of the uterine cervix. Int J Gynecol Cancer 16:1608-1613, 2006.

Waxman AG, Zsemlye MM: Preventing cervical cancer: the Pap test and the HPV vaccine. Med Clin North Am 92:1059-1082, 2008.

INVASIVE SQUAMOUS CELL CARCINOMA
(Figure 12-24A-H)

Clinical Features

- Young women with history of smoking and concomitant HPV-associated lesions
- Microinvasive or invasive
- Microinvasive tumors rarely metastasize

Gross Pathology

- Microinvasive: red papule, white plaque, or irregular ulcerated lesion
- Invasive: exophytic papillary mass or endophytic ulcer, usually solitary

Histopathology

- Usually associated with high-grade dysplasia or CIS
  - Full-thickness involvement of epithelium or cervical glands by pleomorphic cells with high nuclear-to-cytoplasmic ratio and mitotic activity
- Atypical mitotic figures are often readily identifiable
- Variable degree of squamous differentiation, including keratin pearl formation
  - GOG grading as described under "Vulva"
- Desmoplastic reaction is a helpful finding associated with invasion
- Microinvasive
  - Tumor depth less than 3 mm as measured from basal layer of overlying surface epithelium to the point of deepest invasion by the tumor
  - If invasion is present only adjacent to an involved gland, the measurement is from the top of the gland to the point of deepest invasion by tumor
  - Tumor diameter is less than 7 mm
- Vascular space invasion is not present in microinvasive carcinoma

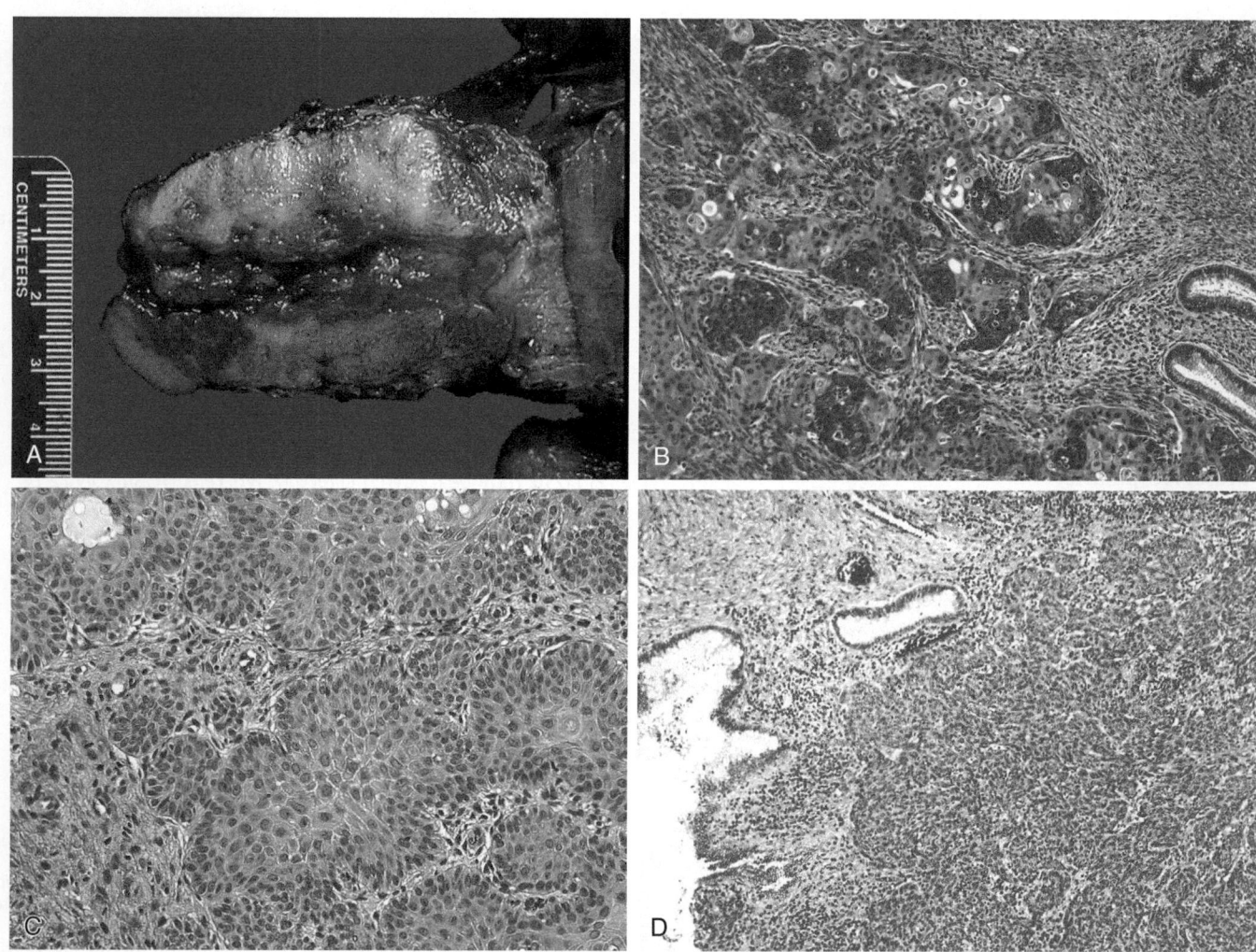

Figure 12-24. A, Invasive squamous cell carcinoma of the cervix (gross photograph). Endocervix with endophytic, deeply invasive white to tan ill-defined tumor involving the cervical wall. **B,** Invasive squamous cell carcinoma, keratinizing type. Irregular nests of pleomorphic squamous cells with dyskeratosis infiltrating reactive stroma with inflammatory cells. **C,** Squamous metaplasia. In contrast to invasive squamous cell carcinoma, the sheets of metaplastic cells show rounded borders as they involve endocervical glands. The nuclear-to-cytoplasmic ratio is not altered, and desmosomes are obvious. **D,** Nonkeratinizing squamous cell carcinoma (invasive). Continuous sheets of malignant cells with no discernible intercellular bridges adjacent to an unremarkable endocervical gland (grade 3).

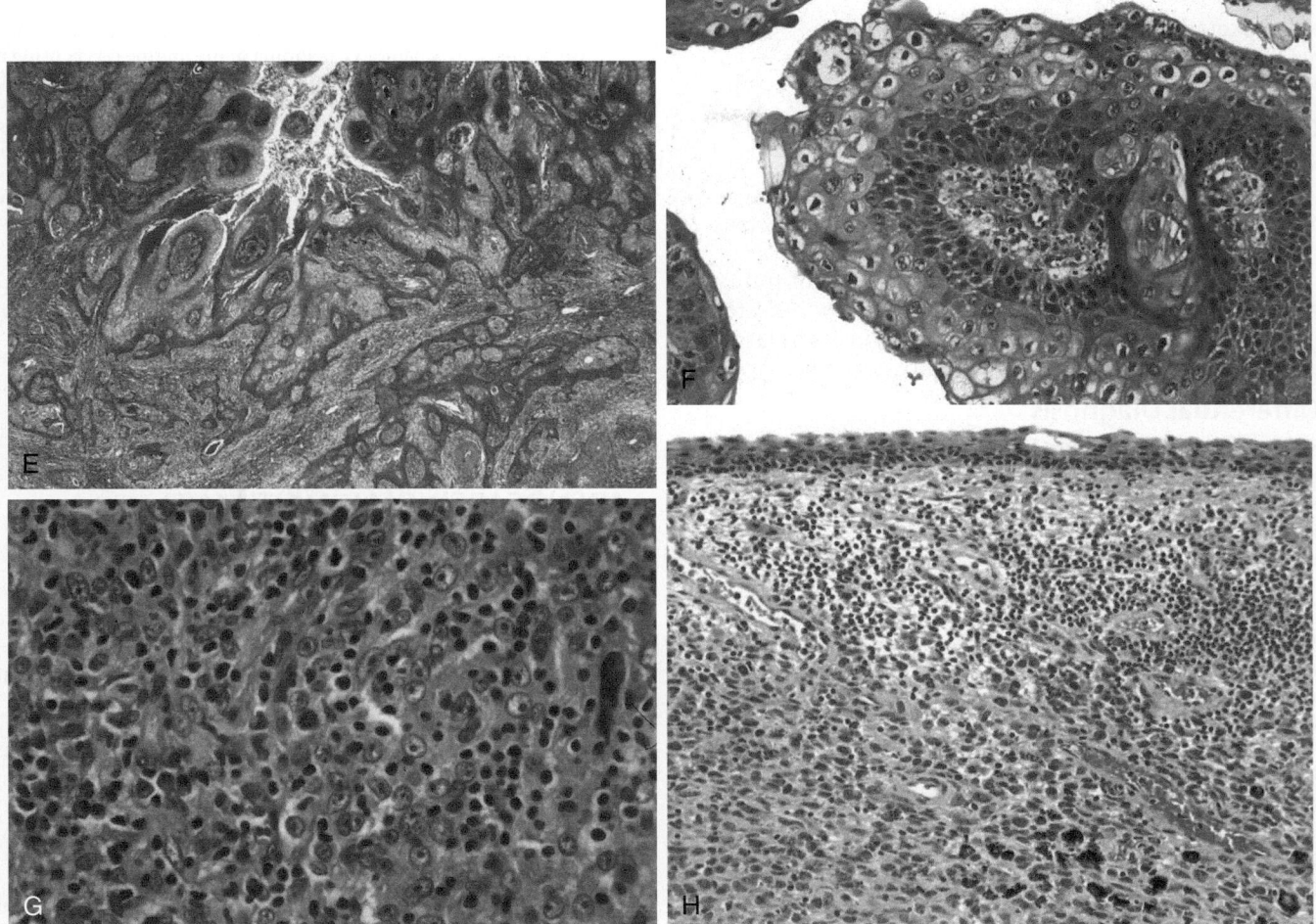

Figure 12-24—cont'd E, Warty (condylomatous) squamous cell carcinoma. Low-power view demonstrates frondlike papillae with marked keratinization. Stromal invasion is present. **F,** Warty (condylomatous) squamous cell carcinoma. High-power view demonstrates classic epithelial papillae with condylomatous changes. **G,** Lymphoepithelioma-like carcinoma. Large pleomorphic neoplastic cells with abundant eosinophilic cytoplasm, irregular nuclei, and prominent nucleoli. Notice the marked lymphoplasmacytic infiltrate in the background. **H,** Malignant melanoma. Melanoma cells infiltrate the submucosa. Melanin pigment is present focally.

- Invasive
  - Greater than 3 mm in depth of invasion
  - Generally greater than 7 mm in diameter
- Types of squamous cell carcinoma of cervix
  - Keratinizing
    - Nests, cords, or single malignant polygonal epithelial cells with high nuclear-to-cytoplasmic ratio, nuclear pleomorphism with irregular chromatin, and eosinophilic cytoplasm
    - Atypical mitoses
    - Variable degree of necrosis
    - Keratin pearl formation or individual cell keratinization
  - Nonkeratinizing
    - Usually rounded nests, as above
    - Absent keratin pearl formation
  - Verrucous
    - Well-differentiated squamous cell carcinoma with minimal cytologic atypia
    - Exophytic, often bulky tumor
    - Hyperkeratosis on the surface
    - Characterized by a bulbous pushing border rather than a truly invasive border

  - Rarely metastasizes
  - Associated with HPV-6 and its subtypes
  - Warty (condylomatous)
    - Papillary exophytic growth
    - Fibrovascular fronds
    - Squamous differentiation
    - Numerous koilocytes
    - Irregularly outlined nests of invasive tumor at base
  - Papillary (transitional)
    - Rare variant with papillary architecture
    - Papillae are lined by several layers of cytologically atypical spindled cells with frequent mitotic activity
    - Squamous differentiation may be focally present
    - Resembles transitional cell carcinoma of the genitourinary tract histologically
  - Lymphoepithelioma-like carcinoma
    - Well-circumscribed tumor
    - Discrete nests of nonkeratinizing epithelial cells with vesicular nuclei and abundant cytoplasm
    - Prominent lymphoplasmacytic inflammatory infiltrate between and around nests
    - Negative for Epstein-Barr virus (EBV)

Special Stains and Immunohistochemistry

- Cytokeratin and p63 positive
- CEA focally positive
- Mucin negative

Other Techniques for Diagnosis

- PCR and ISH
  - HPV-16, -18, -31, -35, and other types have been detected in greater than 95% of tumors, especially in younger women with history of CIN
  - HPV-16 has been detected in about 75% of tumors
- *Ras* oncogene product p21 overexpression: detected by PCR or ISH; associated with poor prognosis in large cell keratinizing and nonkeratinizing carcinomas

Differential Diagnosis

SQUAMOUS METAPLASIA WITH GLAND INVOLVEMENT
- Nuclear atypia absent
- Rare mitotic figures
- Metaplastic glands rounded
- No stromal reaction

GLASSY CELL CARCINOMA
- High mitotic activity
- Distinct cell borders
- Prominent nucleoli
- Ground-glass cytoplasm

SMALL CELL CARCINOMA
- Neuroendocrine patterns (e.g., round nests, trabeculae, ribbons, and rosettes)
- Hyperchromatic smudged chromatin
- No nucleoli
- Neuroendocrine differentiation by immunohistochemistry (chromogranin, synaptophysin positive) or electron microscopy (dense neurosecretory granules)

MALIGNANT MELANOMA
- Although rare, both primary and metastatic melanomas can occur in the cervix
- Melanin pigment when present is helpful in differentiating melanoma from poorly differentiated carcinoma; however, melanoma can be amelanotic
- Negative for cytokeratin
- Positive for S-100 protein, melan-A, and HMB-45

METASTATIC SQUAMOUS CELL CARCINOMA
- Clinical history is important
- Generally, metastatic tumor is present deep in the mucosa

PEARLS

- *Important prognostic indicators are tumor thickness, depth of invasion, tumor diameter, and vascular space invasion*
- *The invasive component is often better differentiated than the intraepithelial component*
- *Microinvasive carcinoma may be treated with cervical cone (cold knife) and endocervical curettage if the cone shows focal microinvasion and free margins*
- *If curettage is positive, hysterectomy may be indicated*
- *Invasive carcinomas are treated by radical hysterectomy with or without adjuvant therapy depending on stage of the tumor*

SELECTED REFERENCES

Chao A, Wang TH, Lee YS, et al: Molecular characterization of adenocarcinoma and squamous carcinoma of the uterine cervix using microarray analysis of gene expression. Int J Cancer 119:91-98, 2006.

Horn LC, Hentschel B, Braumann UD: Malignancy grading, pattern of invasion, and juxtatumoral stromal response (desmoplastic change) in squamous cell carcinoma of the uterine cervix. Int J Gynecol Pathol 27:606-607, 2008.

Hsu KF, Huang SC, Shiau AL, et al: Increased expression level of squamous cell carcinoma antigen 2 and 1 ratio is associated with poor prognosis in early-stage uterine cervical cancer. Int J Gynecol Cancer 17:174-181, 2007.

Kokka F, Verma M, Singh N, et al: Papillary squamotransitional cell carcinoma of the uterine cervix: report of three cases and review of the literature. Pathology 38:584-586, 2006.

Papanikolaou A, Kalogiannidis I, Misailidou D, et al: Results on the treatment of uterine cervix cancer: ten years experience. Eur J Gynaecol Oncol 27:607-610, 2006.

Pecorelli S: Revised FIGO staging for carcinoma of the vulva, cervix, and endometrium. Int J Gynaecol Obstet 105:103-104, 2009.

ADENOCARCINOMA IN SITU (AIS)

Clinical Features

- Occurs in women in third and fourth decades
- Significantly less common than squamous cell carcinoma in situ
- Precursor lesion to invasive adenocarcinoma, but not in all cases
- Usually asymptomatic
- Often diagnosed incidentally during workup of abnormal Papanicolaou (Pap) test or cervical dysplasia
- Most common symptom is vaginal bleeding (60% of patients)
- Increasing incidence (related to improved detection in Pap smears collected with the current endocervical brush)
- Associated with HPV 18 infection more often than squamous lesions
- Risk factors include obesity, hypertension, and oral contraceptives with progesterone content
- Thirty to 50% of cases are associated with CIN and invasive squamous cell carcinoma of the cervix

Gross Pathology

- Usually above the squamocolumnar junction
- Unifocal lesion but can be multifocal occasionally
- Rarely visible colposcopically

Histopathology

- Replacement of the normal glandular epithelium by malignant epithelium
- High nuclear-to-cytoplasmic ratio
- Irregular chromatin and inconspicuous nucleoli (Figure 12-25A)
- Cellular stratification
- Mitotic activity and apoptotic bodies are characteristic
- Endocervical (most common), intestinal, and endometrioid types
- Absent stromal desmoplasia
- Morphologic types include endocervical, intestinal, endometrioid, villoglandular, and adenosquamous variants

Special Stains and Immunohistochemistry

- A p16, usually positive (Figure 12-25B)
- Vimentin generally negative
- CEA and Mucin positive

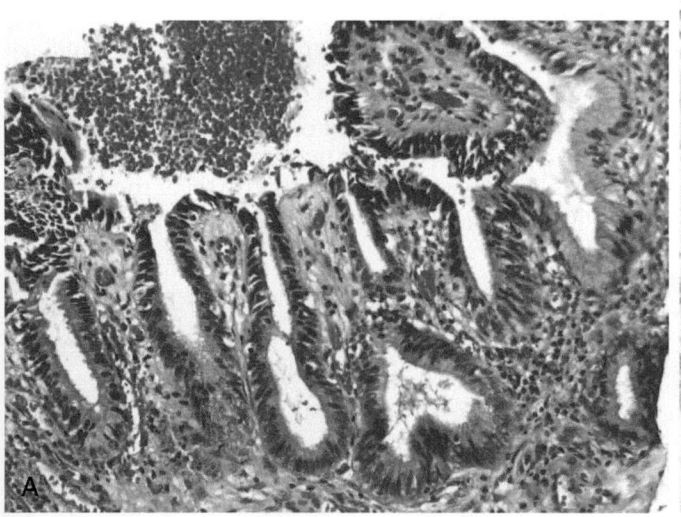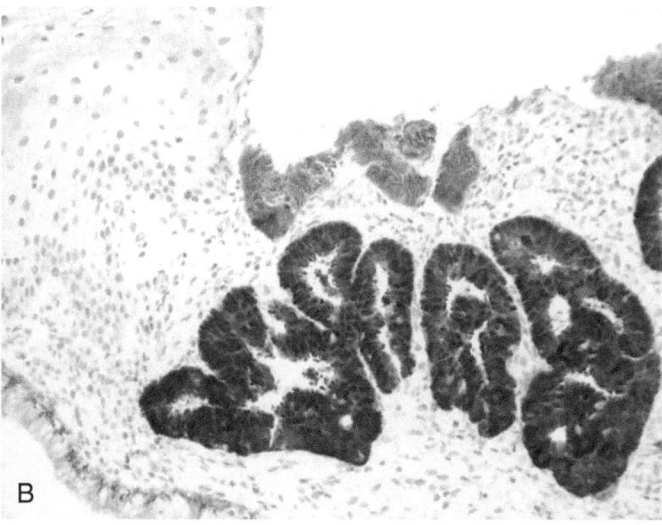

Figure 12-25. Adenocarcinoma in situ of the cervix. A, Endocervical glands lined by cells with hyperchromatic nuclei and mitosis. **B,** Immunohistochemical stain for p16 is strongly positive.

Other Techniques for Diagnosis
- PCR or ISH often positive for HPV

Differential Diagnosis
REACTIVE GLANDULAR ATYPIA
- Prominent nucleoli
- No stratification
- Associated with inflammation

MICROINVASIVE ADENOCARCINOMA
- Adenocarcinoma infiltrates less than 5 mm of the cervical stroma and is less than 7 mm wide
- Reactive stroma, glands extending deeper than normal glands, and glands adjacent to thick-walled blood vessels are features that distinguish AIS from microinvasive adenocarcinoma

INVASIVE ADENOCARCINOMA
- Infiltration of the stroma by malignant glands
- Glands present deep in the wall of the cervix
- Glands may show budding, papillary growth, or cribriforming
- Stromal response includes inflammatory cells and desmoplasia

MICROGLANDULAR HYPERPLASIA
- Small polypoid lesion
- Lobular arrangement
- Dense concentration of benign glands with luminal neutrophils

TUBAL METAPLASIA
- Few glands involved
- Nuclear atypia absent
- Ciliated epithelium

ENDOMETRIOSIS
- Endometrial glands and stroma are present in cervical tissue
- Hemosiderin-laden macrophages may also be present

PEARLS

- *Associated with HPV infection*
- *Increasingly detected in Pap smears as a result of the use of the endocervical brush, which reaches higher into the endocervical canal than does the spatula*
- *Treatment is cervical cone with free surgical margins or hysterectomy*
- *Recurrence may follow second conization because of residual adenocarcinoma in situ at the endocervical canal or lower uterine segment or hysterectomy*
- *30-50% of cases coexist with CIN*
- *Glandular dysplasia is suggested as the precursor lesion; however, the coexistence of glandular dysplasia and AIS is uncommon*

SELECTED REFERENCES

Ceballos KM, Shaw D, Daya D: Microinvasive cervical adenocarcinoma (FIGO stage 1A tumors): results of surgical staging and outcome analysis. Am J Surg Pathol 30:370-374, 2006.

Colgan TJ, Lickrish GM: The topography and invasive potential of cervical adenocarcinoma in situ, with and without associated squamous dysplasia. Gynecol Oncol 36:246-249, 1990.

McCluggage WG. Immunohistochemistry as a diagnostic aid in cervical pathology. Pathology 39:97-111, 2007.

Park JJ, Sun D, Quade BJ, et al. Stratified mucin-producing intraepithelial lesions of the cervix: adenosquamous or columnar cell neoplasia? Am J Surg Pathol 24:1414-1419, 2000.

Tase T, Okagaki T, Clark BA, et al: Human papillomavirus DNA in adenocarcinoma in situ, microinvasive adenocarcinoma of the uterine cervix, and coexisting cervical squamous intraepithelial neoplasia. Int J Gynecol Pathol 8:8-17, 1989.

Yap OW, Hendrickson MR, Teng NN, Kapp DS: Mesonephric adenocarcinoma of the cervix: a case report and review of the literature. Gynecol Oncol 103:1155-1158, 2006.

Zaino RJ: Glandular lesions of the uterine cervix. Mod Pathol 13:261-274, 2000.

INVASIVE ADENOCARCINOMA
(Figure 12-26A-F)

Clinical Features
- Increased incidence

- Affected patients are slightly older (fourth and fifth decades) than patients with squamous cell carcinoma
- Associated with HPV infection
- Risk factors include obesity, hypertension, and oral contraceptives with progesterone content
- More than 40% of cases are associated with SIL and on occasion invasive squamous cell carcinoma of the cervix
- May present with a watery discharge

Gross Pathology

- Generally exophytic, polypoid, nodular, or papillary

Histopathology

- Variable combinations of cell types
- Mixed cell type if any two or more of the following types listed represent more than 10% of the total tumor volume

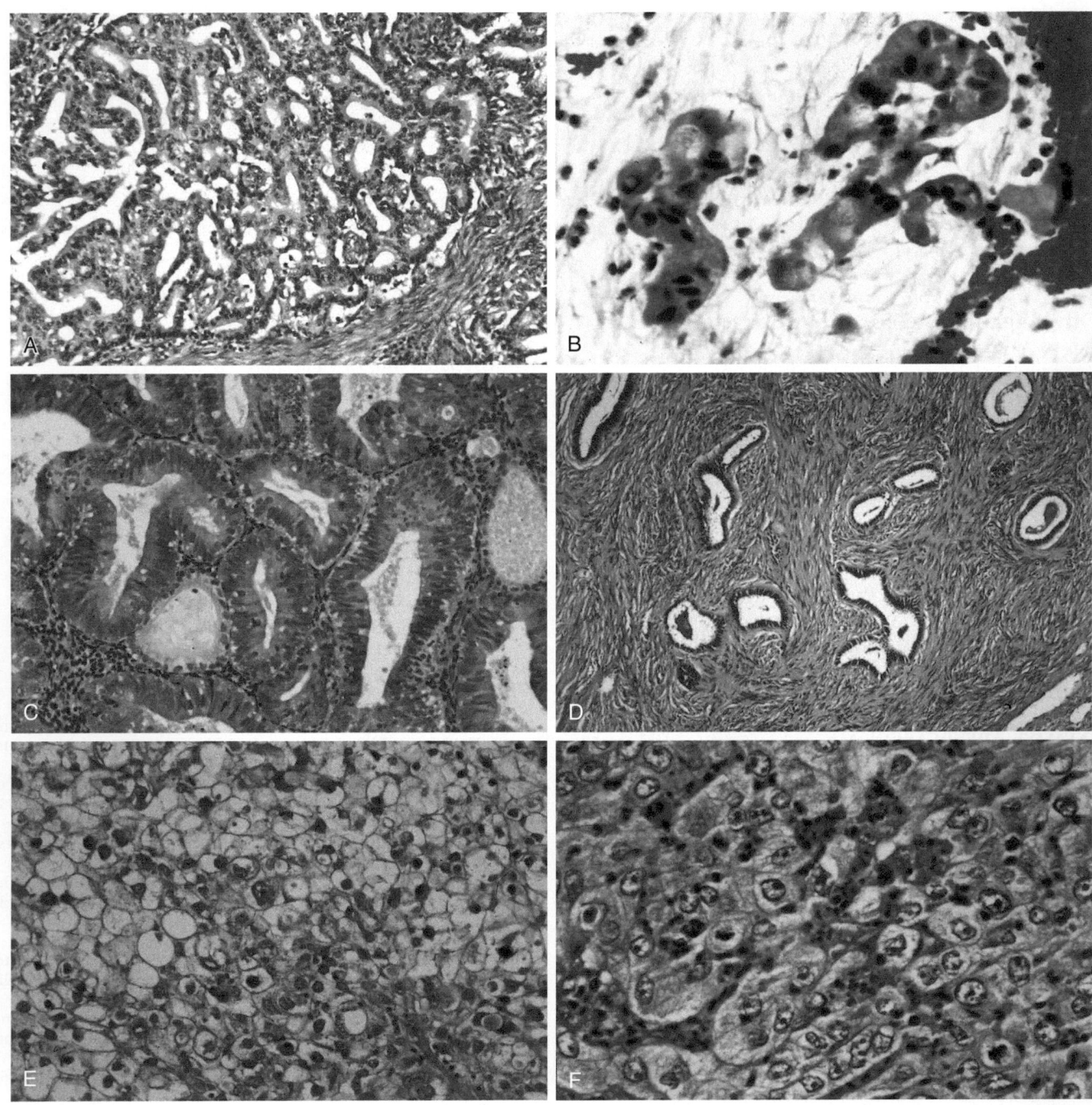

Figure 12-26. A, Moderately differentiated invasive adenocarcinoma of the cervix. Crowded glands and nuclear pleomorphism. **B,** Mucinous adenocarcinoma of the cervix. Clusters of neoplastic mucinous epithelium in lakes of extracellular mucin. **C,** Well-differentiated endometrioid adenocarcinoma of the cervix. Confluent glandular pattern with minimal desmoplastic stroma identical to uterine corpus endometrioid adenocarcinoma. **D,** Minimal deviation adenocarcinoma (adenoma malignum). Low-power view demonstrates irregular neoplastic endocervical glands associated with desplasia. **E,** Clear cell carcinoma of the cervix. Solid proliferation of neoplastic cells with clear cytoplasm. **F,** Glassy cell carcinoma of the cervix. Large neoplastic cells with finely granular ground-glass cytoplasm, prominent nuclei, and nucleoli. The stroma contains inflammatory cells, including eosinophils.

- Mucinous endocervical
  - Resembles normal endocervical epithelium
  - Occasionally papillary
- Mucinous intestinal
  - Pseudostratified columnar epithelium with goblet cells
- Mucinous signet ring cell
  - Compressed nucleus with abundant intracytoplasmic mucin
  - Usually not a prominent component
- Endometrioid
  - Stratified epithelial cells with minimal granular cytoplasm resembling malignant endometrial glands
  - Intracytoplasmic mucin absent
- Minimal deviation adenocarcinoma (adenoma malignum)
  - Cytologically bland glands, usually mucinous endocervical type
  - Irregular, branching glands of variable sizes
  - Increased numbers of glands at surface and extending deep into the wall of the cervix (> 5 mm)
  - Stromal desmoplasia may be present
  - Cervical biopsy may not be deep enough to permit the diagnosis
- Well-differentiated papillary villoglandular
  - Patients generally in third or fourth decade
  - May be deeply invasive
  - Complex branching papillary architecture
  - Stratified columnar lining: endocervical, endometrioid, or intestinal type
  - Minimal cytologic atypia
  - Scant mucin
- Clear cell
  - Often associated with DES exposure
  - Tubulocystic and solid are the most common patterns
  - Papillary, tubular, and trabecular patterns may also be seen
  - Tumor cells are polyhedral with round, atypical nuclei and clear cytoplasm containing glycogen
  - The hobnail cell is a common and characteristic finding: cell in which the nucleus protrudes beyond the boundaries of the cell into the luminal, tubular, or cystic space
  - Less commonly, the epithelial cells are flattened, cuboidal, oxyphilic, or signet ring
  - Psammoma bodies or intracellular hyaline bodies may be seen
- Adenocarcinoma with features of carcinoid tumor
  - Occasionally an adenocarcinoma may contain areas of neuroendocrine carcinoma positive for neuroendocrine markers
  - Paraendocrine syndromes are rare
  - Not responsive to the usual treatment modalities
- Grading (not as definitive as corpus cancer)
  - Well-differentiated: more than 50% glands
  - Moderately differentiated: 10% to 50% glands
  - Poorly differentiated: less than 10% glands
- Depth of invasion is measured from the surface
  - Microinvasive adenocarcinoma
    - Adenocarcinoma infiltrates less than 5 mm of the cervical stroma and is less than 7 mm wide

- The measurement is from the basement membrane of the overlying endocervical or ectocervical surface
- Most are associated with synchronous and often extensive adenocarcinoma in situ
- Reactive stroma, glands extending deeper than normal glands, and glands adjacent to thick-walled blood vessels are features that distinguish AIS from microinvasive adenocarcinoma
- Excellent prognosis with conservative surgical therapy

Special Stains and Immunohistochemistry

- CEA usually positive in mucinous adenocarcinomas and negative in normal endocervical glands

Other Techniques for Diagnosis

- HPV often detected by PCR or ISH

Differential Diagnosis

MICROGLANDULAR HYPERPLASIA
- Polypoid lesion
- Lobular arrangement
- Dense concentration of benign glands
- CEA negative

ADENOCARCINOMA IN SITU
- Glands are not present deep in the wall of cervix
- Minimal glandular budding, papillary growth, or cribriforming
- Absence of stromal response (or desmoplasia)

METASTATIC ADENOCARCINOMA
- Clinical history essential
- Surface involvement is generally absent
- Extensive lymphatic invasion

DIRECT EXTENSION OF ENDOMETRIAL ADENOCARCINOMA
- Clinical history of endometrial carcinoma
- Absence of endocervical glandular or in situ adenocarcinoma
- Negative for HPV infection
- The distinction may be difficult
- Mucinous endometrial adenocarcinoma is also positive for CEA and negative for vimentin

PEARLS

- *Associated with HPV infection*
- *Increasingly detected in Pap smears as a result of the use of the endocervical brush, which reaches higher into the endocervix than does the spatula*
- *Standard treatment is radical hysterectomy with pelvic lymphadenectomy*
- *Radiation therapy is preferred for tumors that are larger than 5 cm at the time of diagnosis*
- *Generally tumors smaller than 1 cm do not metastasize to lymph nodes*
- *Prognosis correlates with stage and grade (of the tumor)*

SELECTED REFERENCES

Ceballos KM, Shaw D, Daya D: Microinvasive cervical adenocarcinoma (FIGO stage 1A tumors): results of surgical staging and outcome analysis. Am J Surg Pathol 30:370-374, 2006.

Gilks CB, Young RH, Aguirre P, et al: Adenoma malignum (minimal deviation adenocarcinoma) of the uterine cervix: a clinicopathological and immunohistochemical analysis of 26 cases. Am J Surg Pathol 13:717-729, 1989.

Kurman RJ, Ronnett BM, Sherman ME, et al: Tumors of the cervix, vagina and vulva. American Registry of Pathology in conjunction with Armed Forces Institute of Pathology, Washington, DC, 2009.

Wang SS, Sherman ME, Silverberg SG, et al: Pathological characteristics of cervical adenocarcinoma in a multi-center US-based study. Gynecol Oncol 103:541-546, 2006.

Young RH, Clement PB: Endocervical adenocarcinoma and its variants: their morphology and differential diagnosis. Histopathology 41:185-207, 2002.

Zaino RJ: Symposium part I: Adenocarcinoma in situ, glandular dysplasia, and early invasive adenocarcinoma of the uterine cervix. Int J Gynecol Pathol 21:314-326, 2002.

ADENOSQUAMOUS CARCINOMA

Clinical Features

- Occurs in women of all ages
- Risk factors as in squamous cell carcinoma: smoking, multiple sexual partners, and low socioeconomic status
- Less common than adenocarcinoma

Gross Pathology

- Polypoid endocervical mass

Histopathology

- Poorly differentiated squamous cell carcinoma intermingled with high-grade adenocarcinoma
- Intracytoplasmic and luminal mucin usually present in the glandular component

Special Stains and Immunohistochemistry

- CEA may be positive in adenocarcinoma
- Mucin positive if mucin is present

Other Techniques for Diagnosis

- Noncontributory

Differential Diagnosis

DIRECT EXTENSION OF ADENOCARCINOMA OF ENDOMETRIUM

- Bulky tumor in the endometrium
- Usually less squamous differentiation
- More likely endometrioid than mucinous adenocarcinoma
- Precursor lesion in the uterine corpus (i.e., endometrial hyperplasia) is helpful

ENDOCERVICAL CARCINOMA WITH SYNCHRONOUS SQUAMOUS CELL CARCINOMA

- Separate tumors with no intermingling
- Endometrial or endocervical precursor lesions (i.e., hyperplasia or dysplasia [CIN], respectively) are helpful

PEARLS

- *Mixed carcinoma*
- *Occurs in women of any age*
- *Treatment and prognosis as for other invasive cervical carcinomas*

SELECTED REFERENCE

Bethwaite P, Yeong ML, Holloway L: The prognosis of adenosquamous carcinoma of the uterine cervix. Br J Obstet Gynecol 99:745-750, 1992.

NEUROENDOCRINE TUMORS

Clinical Features

- Uncommon
- Occurs in women in third and fourth decades
- Aggressive tumor
- Paraendocrine syndromes may manifest

Gross Pathology

- Often ulcerating tumors

Histopathology

- Highly cellular
- Sheets of tightly packed small cells with minimal cytoplasm and round to spindled nuclei (Figure 12-27)
- Smudged chromatin with inconspicuous nucleoli
- Few scattered larger pleomorphic cells
- Brisk mitotic rate is often present
- Vascular space invasion is frequently identified
- Squamous or glandular differentiation makes up less than 10% of tumor volume
- Similar to pulmonary small cell carcinoma

Special Stains and Immunohistochemistry

- Cytokeratin positive
- Chromogranin positive in about 50% of tumors
- Synaptophysin and neuron-specific enolase (NSE) positive in a significant number of tumors
- Serotonin and somatostatin rarely positive

Other Techniques for Diagnosis

- PCR, ISH: HPV-18 has been detected; less commonly HPV-16

Differential Diagnosis

POORLY DIFFERENTIATED, NONKERATINIZING SQUAMOUS CELL CARCINOMA

- May be difficult to distinguish if cells are small
- No neuroendocrine differentiation

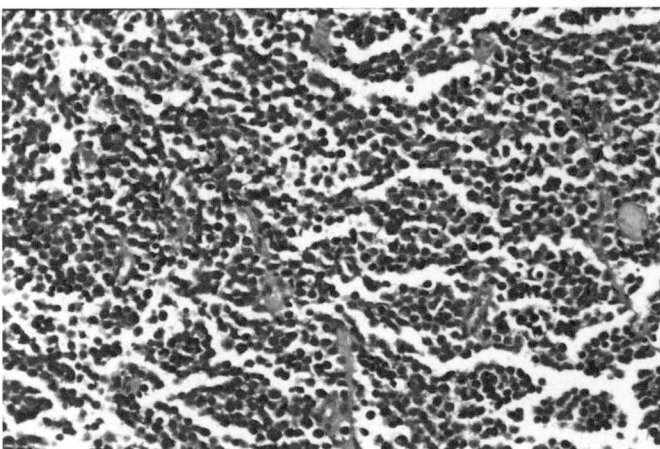

Figure 12-27. Small cell carcinoma of the cervix. Low-power view demonstrates a solid proliferation of small uniform neoplastic cells mimicking a malignant lymphoma.

POORLY DIFFERENTIATED ADENOCARCINOMA
- Gland formation makes up less than 10% of tumor volume
- Neuroendocrine differentiation is absent

LYMPHOMA
- Cells less tightly packed
- Positive for CD45 (leukocyte common antigen)
- No neuroendocrine differentiation

PEARLS
- *Treatment is radical hysterectomy with bilateral pelvic and periaortic lymph node dissection*
- *Adjuvant radiation therapy if lymph node metastases are present*
- *Aggressive tumor with frequent recurrence and poor survival*
- *Distant metastases common*

SELECTED REFERENCES
Ambros RA, Park JS, Shah KV, Kurman RJ: Evaluation of histologic, morphometric, and immunohistochemical criteria in the differential diagnosis of small cell carcinomas of the cervix with particular reference to human papillomavirus types 16 and 18. Mod Pathol 4:586-593, 1991.

Gersell DJ, Mazoujian G, Mutch DG, Rudloff MA: Small-cell undifferentiated carcinoma of the cervix: a clinicopathologic, ultrastructural, and immunocytochemical study of 15 cases. Am J Surg Pathol 12:684-698, 1988.

Stoler MH, Mills SE, Gersell DJ, Walker AN: Small-cell neuroendocrine carcinoma of the cervix: a human papillomavirus type-18 associated tumor. Am J Surg Pathol 15:28-32, 1991.

Werness BA, Levine AJ, Howley PM: Association of human papillomavirus types 16 and 18 E6 proteins with p53. Science 248:76-79, 1990.

Zivanovic O, Leitao MM Jr, Park KJ, et al: Small cell neuroendocrine carcinoma of the cervix: analysis of outcome, recurrence pattern and the impact of platinum-based combination chemotherapy. Gynecol Oncol 112:590-593, 2009.

METASTATIC ADENOCARCINOMA

Clinical Features
- Ovarian carcinoma is the most common tumor metastatic to the cervix
- Breast is the most common extragenital source of tumor metastatic to the cervix
- Endometrial carcinomas may spread by direct extension to the cervical stroma; this occurrence increases the stage of the corpus cancer (II versus I)
- Metastases may present with vaginal bleeding

Gross Pathology
- Generally tumors metastasize to the outer surface
- Direct extension from the endometrium may be detected within the endocervical canal

Histopathology
- As per the primary tumor
- Tumors from the endometrium may be difficult to distinguish from primary cervical tumors, which may arise simultaneously
- The absence of CIN in the presence of subepithelial infiltrates or prominent lymphatic permeation suggests metastatic disease

Special Stains and Immunohistochemistry
- As per the primary tumor

Other Techniques for Diagnosis
- CEA is generally positive in cervical adenocarcinoma but negative in endometrial tumors, whereas vimentin is positive in endometrial tumors but not cervical adenocarcinoma
- CDX2 is commonly positive in cervical adenocarcinoma (mucinous type) but negative in endometrial carcinoma
- Generally, p16 is positive in cervical adenocarcinomas

Differential Diagnosis

METASTATIC CARCINOMA VERSUS PRIMARY CERVICAL CARCINOMA
- The absence of CIN and adenocarcinoma in situ in the presence of subepithelial infiltrates or prominent lymphatic permeation suggests metastatic disease
- Endometrial and cervical adenocarcinomas may be synchronous and indistinguishable
- Clinical history is essential

PEARLS
- *The absence of CIN in the overlying epithelium suggests metastatic disease*
- *Clinical history is essential*

SELECTED REFERENCES
Kurman R (ed): Blaustein's Pathology of the Female Genital Tract, 6th ed. New York, Springer, 2011, p 295.

Lemoine NR, Hall PA: Epithelial tumors metastatic to the uterine cervix: a study of 33 cases and review of the literature. Cancer 57:2002-2005, 1986.

UTERUS

ENDOMETRIUM

ACUTE ENDOMETRITIS

Clinical Features
- Most often associated with pelvic inflammatory disease (PID)
- May be associated with pregnancy
- Elevated temperature, leukocytosis, discomfort, and pain

Gross Pathology
- When secondary to PID, presents with a tubo-ovarian complex with fibrous adhesions, fibrinous exudate, congestion, and edema
- Associated with intrauterine device (IUD) use and may be seen in compressed endometrium overlying large leiomyomas

Histopathology
- Numerous neutrophils in the stroma and several glands
- Ectatic blood vessels
- Fibrin exudate
- Hemorrhage

Special Stains and Immunohistochemistry
- Tissue Gram stain to identify microorganisms

Other Techniques for Diagnosis

- Noncontributory

Differential Diagnosis

MENSTRUATION

- Vacuoles in the distended glands
- Decidual change in the stroma and stromal neutrophils

PEARLS

- *Clinical history is important, particularly as it relates to the menstrual cycle*
- *Aseptic abortion is a possibility in some areas of USA and worldwide*
- *Patient may present with acute abdomen*

SELECTED REFERENCES

Crum CP, Hornstein MD, Nucci MR: Hertig and beyond: a systematic and practical approach to the endometrial biopsy. Adv Anat Pathol 10:301-318, 2003.

Silverberg SG: The endometrium. Arch Pathol Lab Med 131:372-382, 2007.

CHRONIC ENDOMETRITIS

Clinical Features

- Common condition
- May be asymptomatic, although may present with pelvic pain when associated with menstrual irregularities
- Associated with IUD use and may be identified in compressed endometrium overlying large leiomyomas

Gross Pathology

- Generally the findings are nonspecific

Histopathology

- Plasma cells must be identified in the endometrial stroma (Figure 12-28)
- Endometrium is difficult to date (i.e., glands appear variable in terms of phase [early, mid, and late secretory endometrium or proliferative])

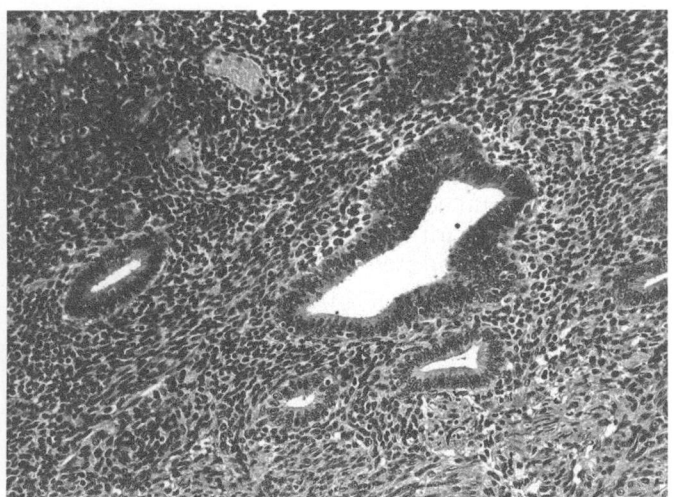

Figure 12-28. Chronic endometritis. Endometrial glands and stroma in which plasma cells are present.

- Focal crowding mimicking hyperplasia
- Glandular epithelium may show mild cytologic atypia and focal or diffuse spindled stroma

Special Stains and Immunohistochemistry

- Noncontributory

Other Techniques for Diagnosis

- Noncontributory

Differential Diagnosis

ENDOMETRIAL HYPERPLASIA

- Stromal plasma cells are unusual
- Diffuse process

ENDOMETRIAL ADENOCARCINOMA

- Confluent or cribriform glandular architecture with cytologic atypia
- Stromal desmoplasia or necrosis may be present

PEARLS

- *Lymphocytes are normally present in the endometrium, as are neutrophils in the late secretory and early proliferative phases; therefore, the diagnosis of chronic endometritis requires plasma cells*
- *In the presence of chronic endometritis, the diagnosis of hyperplasia should be made with caution*

SELECTED REFERENCES

Kiviat NB, Eschenbach DA, Paavonen JA, et al: Endometrial histopathology in patients with culture-proved upper genital tract infection and laparoscopically diagnosed acute salpingitis. Am J Surg Pathol 14:167-175, 1990.

Rotterdam H: Chronic endometritis: a clinicopathologic study. Pathol Annu 13:209-231, 1978.

ENDOMETRIAL POLYP (Figure 12-29A-D)

Clinical Features

- Common
- Most often seen in middle-aged and postmenopausal women
- Often presents with abnormal bleeding
- Tamoxifen effect

Gross Pathology

- Usually solitary and highly variable in size
- Most commonly arises in the fundus
- Broad based and sessile, pedunculated or slender stalk

Histopathology

- Irregularly outlined glands that may be out of phase with the endometrium
- Fibrovascular stalk or fibrous stroma with several thick-walled vessels
- Metaplastic epithelium, particularly squamous, may be present
- Polyps in the lower uterine segment may contain endocervical as well as endometrial glands
- If the stroma contains abundant muscle, the polyp may be referred to as *adenomyomatous polyp*

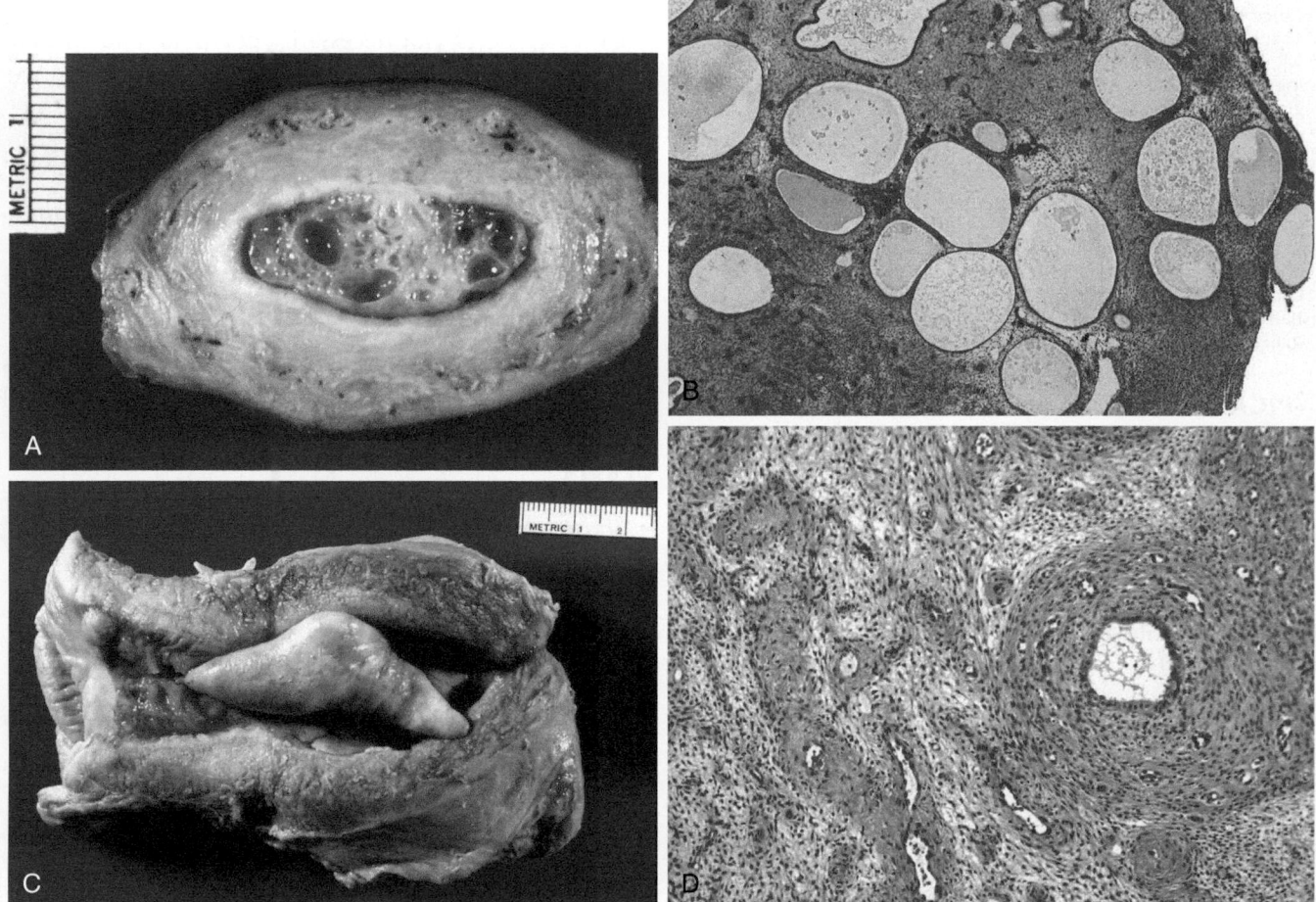

Figure 12-29. Endometrial polyp. A, Cross section of the uterus shows an endometrial polyp filling the endometrial cavity. **B,** Atrophic glandular epithelium is visible. The cystic dilated glands are lined by low columnar to cuboidal epithelium. **C,** The endometrial cavity shows a broad-based polypoid lesion. The external surface is smooth, tan, and glistening. **D,** Endometrial glands surrounded by thick-walled blood vessels.

- Absence of cytologic atypia, usually with epithelial lining on three sides
- Hyperplasia might be present and confined to the polyp

Special Stains and Immunohistochemistry
- Noncontributory

Other Techniques for Diagnosis
- Noncontributory

Differential Diagnosis

ENDOMETRIAL HYPERPLASIA
- Diffuse process involving the entire endometrium or, if curetted, most of the fragments
- Crowded glands with or without cytologic atypia
- Generally thick-walled vessels absent in hyperplasia

POLYPOID ADENOCARCINOMA
- Malignant epithelial cells lining back-to-back glands
- Absence of fibrous stroma and thick-walled vessels

ADENOFIBROMA
- Extremely rare and benign
- Lobulated polypoid mass with small cystic spaces and fibrous stroma

- Spaces lined by müllerian epithelium

ADENOSARCOMA
- Stromal cells are cytologically atypical with mitosis
- Cells are generally packed tightly around nonmalignant glands
- Characteristic leaflike pattern reminiscent of phyllodes tumor of breast

PEARLS

- *Less than 0.5% of otherwise benign polyps show focal adenocarcinoma confined to the polyp; excision of the polyp might be curative in these cases if the adjacent endometrium is normal*
- *Polyps arise from the basalis layer of the endometrium*
- *Inversion of chromosome 6 has been identified as a nonrandom mutation in endometrial polyp*

SELECTED REFERENCES

Deligdisch L, Kalir T, Cohen CJ, et al: Endometrial histopathology in 700 patients treated with tamoxifen for breast cancer. Gynecol Oncol 78:181-186, 2000.

Kelly P, Dobbs SP, McCluggage WG: Endometrial hyperplasia involving endometrial polyps: report of a series and discussion of the significance in an endometrial biopsy specimen. Br J Obstet Gynaecol 114:944-950, 2007.

Kim KR, Peng R, Ro JY, Robboy SJ: A diagnostically useful histopathologic feature of endometrial polyp: the long axis of endometrial glands arranged parallel to surface epithelium. Am J Surg Pathol 28:1057-1062, 2004.

Le Donne M, Lentini M, De Meo L, et al: Uterine pathologies in patients undergoing tamoxifen therapy for breast cancer: ultrasonographic, hysteroscopic and histological findings. Eur J Gynaecol Oncol 26:623-626, 2005.

Mittal K, Da Costa D: Endometrial hyperplasia and carcinoma in endometrial polyps: clinicopathologic and follow-up findings. Int J Gynecol Pathol 27:45-48, 2008.

Shushan A, Revel A, Rojansky N: How often are endometrial polyps malignant? Gynecol Obstet Invest 58:212-215, 2004.

ATYPICAL POLYPOID ADENOMYOMA

Clinical Features

- Most common in women in the late reproductive years
- Usually presents with abnormal bleeding
- Benign clinical course; curettage alone may be curative

Gross Pathology

- Solitary polypoid mass that often involves the lower uterine segment

Histopathology

- Random arrangement of numerous glands with irregular outlines in a smooth muscle stroma consisting of small fascicles generally with few mitoses if any (Figure 12-30)
- Epithelial cells are atypical with loss of polarity but no outright pleomorphism
- Squamous metaplasia and morules with occasional central necrosis are common

Special Stains and Immunohistochemistry

- Noncontributory

Other Techniques for Diagnosis

- Noncontributory

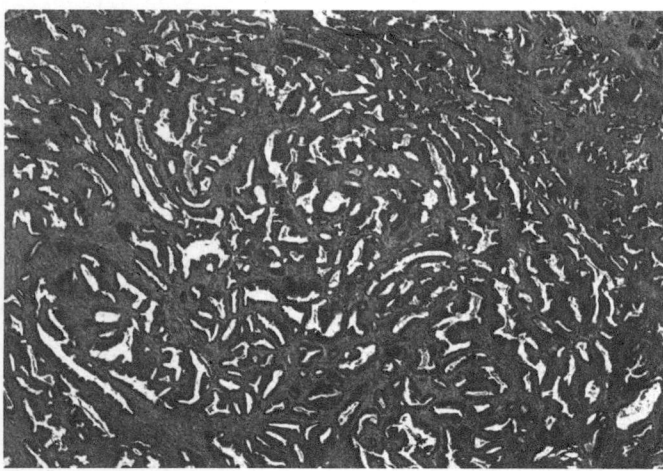

Figure 12-30. Atypical polypoid adenomyoma. Low-power view demonstrates a polypoid lesion composed of a proliferation of compact irregular glands without invasion of the stroma or desmoplasia.

Differential Diagnosis

ENDOMETRIAL HYPERPLASIA

- Diffuse process, not necessarily polypoid, and without smooth muscle stroma

INFILTRATING CARCINOMA

- Reactive fibrous stroma and absence of short bundles of smooth muscle stroma
- Marked architectural and cytologic atypia including cribriforming of glands

METAPLASTIC CARCINOMA (CARCINOSARCOMA)

- Epithelial component as endometrial adenocarcinoma
- Malignant spindle component of highly atypical cells with dense cellularity and cytologic pleomorphism plus a high mitotic rate with atypical forms

PEARLS

- *This lesion is distinguished by short smooth muscle bundles*
- *Location of the lesion and age of the patient are helpful for differential diagnosis*

SELECTED REFERENCES

Heatley MK: Atypical polypoid adenomyoma: a systematic review of the English literature. Histopathology 48:609-610, 2006.

Mazur MT: Atypical polypoid adenomyomas of the endometrium. Am J Surg Pathol 5:473-482, 1981.

ENDOMETRIAL HYPERPLASIA
(Figure 12-31A-D)

Clinical Features

- Can arise at any age, but most common in middle-aged to postmenopausal women
- Usually presents with abnormal bleeding
- Risk factors include obesity, nulliparity, increased endogenous estrogen (i.e., estrogen-producing ovarian tumors and exogenous estrogen; common denominator is continuous exposure to unopposed estrogen)
- Endometrium may be thickened on ultrasound, and uterus may be enlarged on clinical examination
- Inactivation of *PTEN* tumor suppressor gene is associated with the development of hyperplasia and related cancers

Gross Pathology

- Endometrium appears thickened and increased in volume
- May appear diffusely polypoid; more commonly appears normal and has a soft, velvety surface

Histopathology

- Glands are increased in number and crowded with an increased amount of stroma
- Ratio of glands to stroma is elevated
- Most often the diagnosis is made in proliferative-phase endometrium and rarely in secretory phase, as the glands normally appear crowded
- In simple hyperplasia, the glands are crowded but generally round

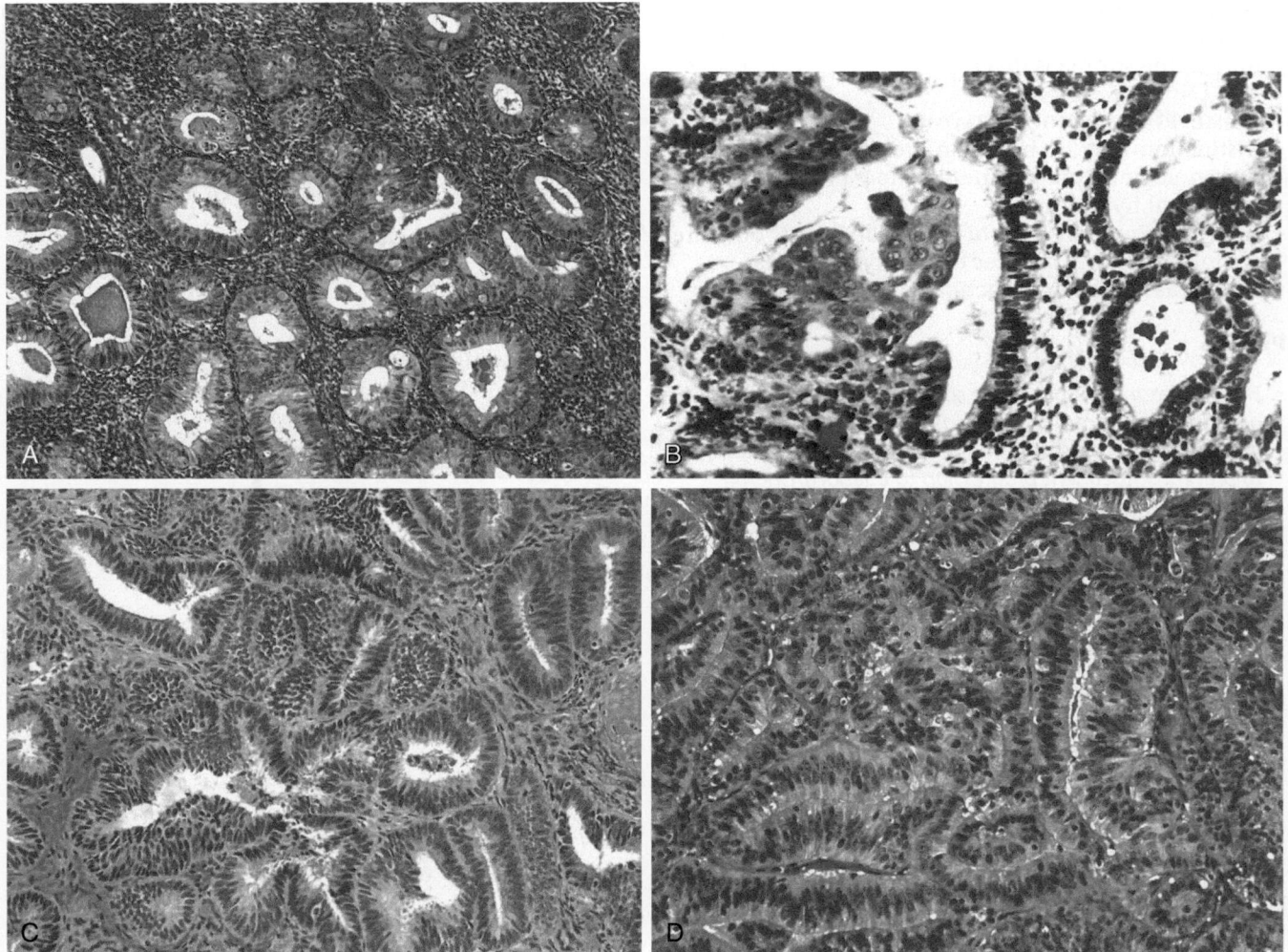

Figure 12-31. A, Simple endometrial hyperplasia without atypia. Crowded endometrial glands lacking cytologic atypia and surrounded by abundant endometrial stroma. **B,** Simple endometrial hyperplasia with squamous metaplasia. The squamous and glandular components lack cytologic atypia. **C,** Complex endometrial hyperplasia without atypia. Marked glandular crowding is present, whereas only minimal endometrial stroma is identified. **D,** Complex endometrial hyperplasia with atypia. Endometrial curettage displaying haphazardly arranged glands lined by cells with atypical nuclei surrounded by minimal stroma.

- In complex hyperplasia, the glands show irregular branching but no cribriforming pattern
- In both simple and complex patterns, stromal tissue is present between all glands
- Both simple and complex hyperplasia may show normal or atypical cytology
- Atypia may be focal and is characterized by cells featuring increased nuclear-to-cytoplasmic ratios, large hyperchromatic, pleomorphic, rounded nuclei with hyperchromasia, and prominent nucleoli
- Both architecture and cytology are taken into consideration, but normal versus atypical cytology is more clinically relevant than simple versus complex architecture
- Various types of metaplasia, particularly squamous, may be present

Special Stains and Immunohistochemistry

- Noncontributory

Other Techniques for Diagnosis

- Cytogenetics: atypical hyperplasias are more likely to be aneuploid and more commonly have mutations shared with carcinomas of the endometrium

Differential Diagnosis

PROLIFERATIVE ENDOMETRIUM

- Even distribution of glands without irregular outpouchings or cellular atypia
- Glands are generally similarly oriented from the base to the surface

ENDOMETRIAL POLYP

- Focal process
- Fibrotic stroma, numerous thick-walled vessels, and epithelial lining on three sides

CYSTIC ATROPHY

- Atrophic glands lined by a single layer of often flattened epithelium
- Number of glands is generally less, and stroma is atrophic

CHRONIC ENDOMETRITIS
- May resemble hyperplasia; however, plasma cell infiltrate in the stroma is diagnostic

ENDOMETRIAL ADENOCARCINOMA
- Distinction may be based on architectural pattern, as the cytologic atypia may not be more pronounced than in atypical hyperplasia
- Cribriforming and back-to-back glands without intervening stroma are features of adenocarcinoma
- Desmoplastic stromal reaction to infiltrating glands

PEARLS

- *Hyperplasia may respond to a course of progestin therapy; adenocarcinoma (grade I) may as well but much less often*
- *If hyperplasia is persistent the treatment is hysterectomy to prevent subsequent progression to adenocarcinoma*
- *Endometrial adenocarcinoma has been identified in up to 25% of uteri removed for atypical hyperplasia when using the criteria described by Kurman et al. in 1982*
- *The term* endometrial intraepithelial neoplasia *(EIN) is occasionally used to refer to precursor lesions of endometrial carcinoma; however, this terminology is not commonly used*

SELECTED REFERENCES

Kurman RJ, Kaminski PF, Norris HJ: The behavior of endometrial hyperplasia: a long-term study of "untreated" hyperplasia in 170 patients. Cancer 56:403-412, 1985.
Kurman RJ, Norris HJ: Evaluation of criteria for distinguishing atypical endometrial hyperplasia from well-differentiated carcinoma. Cancer 49:2457-2549, 1982.
Marchesoni D, Driul L, Fabiani G, et al: Endometrial histologic changes in post-menopausal breast cancer patients using tamoxifen. Int J Gynaecol Obstet 75:257-262, 2001.
Mutter GL: Endometrial intraepithelial neoplasia (EIN): will it bring order to chaos? The Endometrial Collaborative Group. Gynecol Oncol 76:287-290, 2000.
Silverberg SG: Hyperplasia and carcinoma of the endometrium. Semin Diagn Pathol 5:135-153, 1988.
Silverberg SG: Problems in the differential diagnosis of endometrial hyperplasia and carcinoma. Mod Pathol 13:309-327, 2000.
Zaino RJ, Kauderer J, Trimble CL, et al: Reproducibility of the diagnosis of atypical endometrial hyperplasia: a Gynecologic Oncology Group study. Cancer 106:804-811, 2006.
Zaino RJ, Kurman R, Herbold D, et al: The significance of squamous differentiation in endometrial carcinoma: data from a Gynecologic Oncology Group study. Cancer 68:2293-2302, 1991.

ENDOMETRIAL INTRAEPITHELIAL CARCINOMA (EIC)

Clinical Features
- Likely precursor lesion of uterine serous carcinoma
- Presents in postmenopausal age women with a median age of 60
- Also known as "carcinoma in situ" and uterine surface carcinoma

Gross Pathology
- None

Histopathology
- Markedly atypical nuclei with prominent nucleoli identical to those of invasive serous carcinoma
- Lines the surface endometrium, surface of polyps and glands
- The cells may show a papillary contour
- The adjacent endometrium is atrophic in most cases

Special Stains and Immunohistochemistry
- P53 is positive
- Ki-67 shows a high proliferative index

Other Techniques for Diagnosis
- Noncontributory

Differential Diagnosis

SEROUS CARCINOMA
- Stromal desmoplasia
- Confluent papilloglandular pattern
- Larger than 10 mm in dimension

EOSINOPHILIC AND HOBNAIL METAPLASIA
- Enlarged smudged nuclei with a degenerated appearance
- Absence of prominent nucleoli

TUBAL METAPLASIA
- A mixture of enlarged hyperchromatic nuclei without prominent nucleoli admixed with other cells (i.e., ciliated and intercalated cells)

PEARLS

- *Most commonly present in association with serous carcinoma*
- *Lacks desmoplasia or a confluent pattern*
- *Not associated with uterine endometrioid carcinoma*

SELECTED REFERENCES

Ambros RA, Sherman ME, Zahn CM, et al: Endometrial intraepithelial carcinoma: a distinctive lesion specifically associated with tumors displaying serous differentiation. Hum Pathol 26:1260-1267, 1995.
Jarboe EA1, Pizer ES, Miron A, et al: Evidence for a latent precursor (p53 signature) that may precede serous endometrial intraepithelial carcinoma. Mod Pathol 22:345-350, 2009.
Wheeler DT, Bell KA, Kurman RJ, Sherman ME: Minimal uterine serous carcinoma: diagnosis and clinicopathologic correlation. Am J Surg Pathol 24:797-806, 2000.

ENDOMETRIAL CARCINOMA
(Figure 12-32A-J)

Two generally accepted types are endometrial adenocarcinoma preceded by hyperplasia (type I) and endometrial adenocarcinoma preceded by endometrial intraepithelial carcinoma (EIC) with or without atrophy (type II).

Clinical Features
- Risk factors include obesity, nulliparity, late menopause, estrogen-producing ovarian tumors (generally stomal), and exogenous estrogen (generally type I)
- Common denominator is continuous exposure to unopposed estrogen (type I)
- Commonly preceded by hyperplasia (type I)
- Usually presents with abnormal vaginal bleeding (types I and II)
- Ultrasound or computed tomography scan findings range from thickened endometrium to extensive tumor (types I and II)

Gross Pathology

- Uterus may be grossly enlarged
- Tumor usually arises in the corpus
- Often single dominant mass; mostly soft, tan to white, and friable
- Endometrium may be diffusely thickened
- Cut surface through endomyometrium is compulsory to show depth of invasion

Histopathology

ENDOMETRIOID

- Most common type
- Crowded, complex branching glands with cribriform architecture and back-to-back glands without intervening stroma
- Loss of polarity and cytologic atypia: large, round nuclei with prominent nucleoli, nuclear membrane condensation

- Glands may infiltrate into the myometrium, inducing a desmoplastic response
- Grading is based on the degree of glandular differentiation versus solid areas
  - Grade 1: less than 5% of the tumor is composed of solid areas
  - Grade 2: 5% to 50% of the tumor is composed of solid areas
  - Grade 3: greater than 50% of the tumor is composed of solid areas
- Prominent nuclear atypia and mitotic figures increase the grade by one (i.e., grade 1 tumors with marked atypia should be classified as grade 2)

ADENOCARCINOMA WITH SQUAMOUS DIFFERENTIATION

- Malignant glands with benign or malignant squamous foci (squamous differentiation)
- Areas of squamous differentiation are not regarded as solid areas in the grading

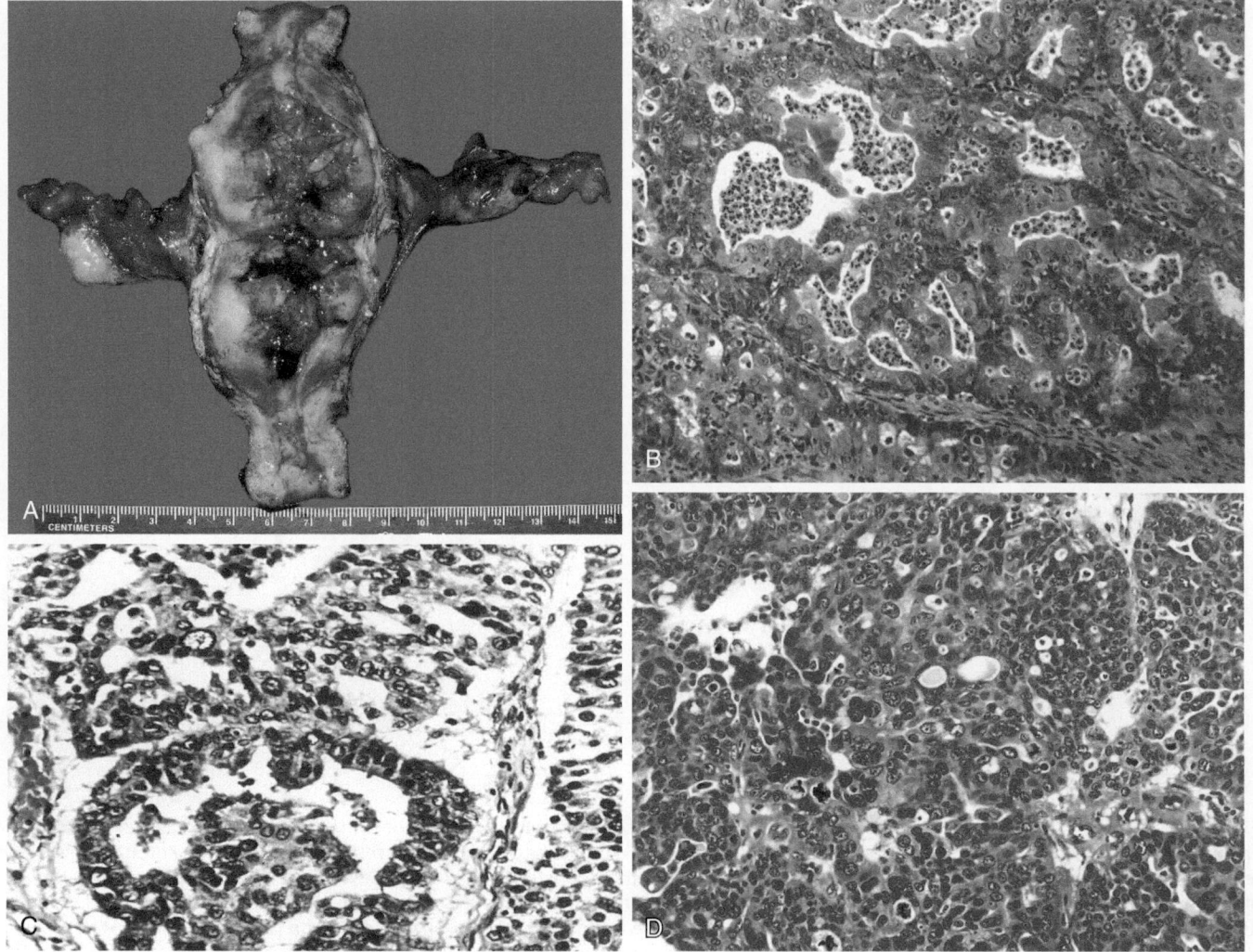

Figure 12-32. A, Endometrial adenocarcinoma. An ill-defined tan to yellow mass with hemorrhage fills the entire endometrial cavity and extends to the endocervix. **B,** Well-differentiated endometrial adenocarcinoma, endometrioid type (grade 1). Back-to-back glands and no solid component. **C,** Moderately differentiated endometrial adenocarcinoma, endometrioid type (grade 2), with nuclear pleomorphism. Cribriform glands and solid foci represent 25% of the tumor volume. **D,** Poorly differentiated endometrial adenocarcinoma, endometrioid type. Minimal gland formation and marked nuclear pleomorphism are seen.

Continued

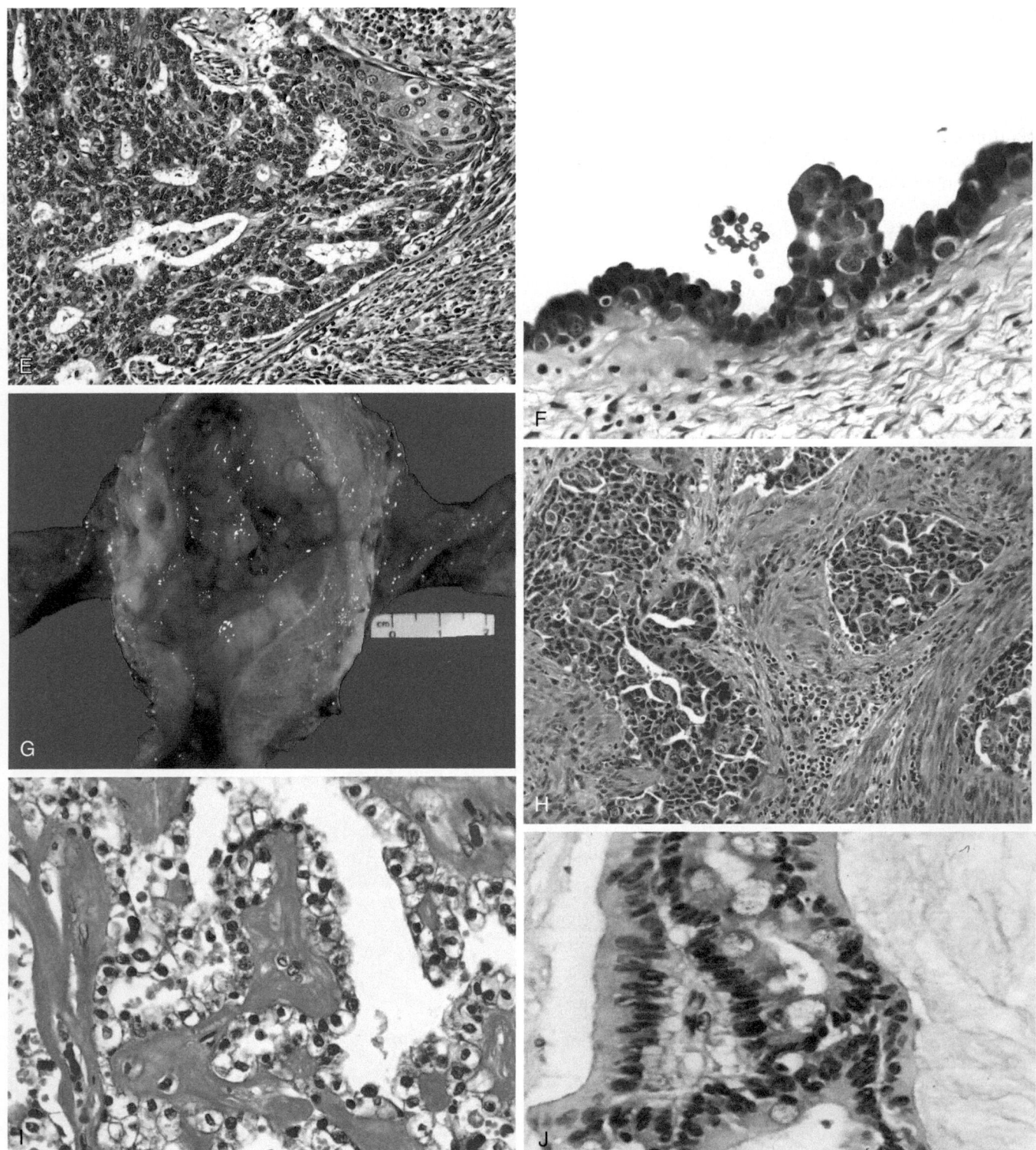

Figure 12-32—cont'd E, Endometrioid adenocarcinoma with squamous differentiation. **F,** Endometrial intraepithelial carcinoma. Section of endomyometrium lined by a single layer of endometrium showing marked nuclear pleomorphism and stratification. The morphology is characteristic of serous differentiation. **G,** Serous carcinoma of the endometrium. Exophytic tan to pink tumor with focal necrosis and superficial invasion of the myometrium. **H,** Serous carcinoma of the endometrium. Papillary structures lined by pleomorphic cells and infiltrating the surrounding desmoplastic stroma. **I,** Clear cell carcinoma of the endometrium. The tumor is composed of sheets of large pleomorphic cells with abundant clear cytoplasm. **J,** Mucinous carcinoma of the endometrium. Neoplastic glands with a papillary configuration. The glands are lined by uniform columnar mucinous cells with minimal stratification. Lakes of extracellular mucinous material are evident.

- Grade of the tumor is based on the morphologic features of the glandular component exclusively
- Squamous differentiation is characterized by intercellular bridges, sharp cell borders, opaque eosinophilic cytoplasm, and squamous pearl formation or keratinization

VILLOGLANDULAR ADENOCARCINOMA
- Common variant of endometrioid adenocarcinoma
- Short blunt papillae lined by cells, as described under "Invasive Adenocarcinoma"
- Generally, the cytologic atypia is low grade
- Papillary carcinoma showing high-grade cytology should be classified as serous

SECRETORY ADENOCARCINOMA
- Commonly associated with hormonal therapy and generally low grade
- Well-differentiated glands that resemble secretory endometrium; generally grade 1
- Malignant clear cells with glycogen-filled cytoplasm and secretions in the glandular lumens

CILIATED CARCINOMA
- Endometrioid adenocarcinoma with ciliated cells
- This variant is usually low grade (grade 1)

SEROUS CARCINOMA
- Generally presents in women in their 60s or older
- Usually preceded by atrophic endometrium or EIC type II
- Thick and thin papillae with marked nuclear pleomorphism
- Cellular stratification, apoptotic bodies, and tumor necrosis
- Psammoma bodies may be present (30% of cases)
- By definition, a high-grade tumor with poor prognosis (grade 3)

CLEAR CELL CARCINOMA
- Usually preceded by atrophic endometrium type II
- By definition, a high-grade tumor (grade 3)
- Architecture may be papillary, glandular, solid, or mixed
- Cells are those of a high-grade endometrioid adenocarcinoma but contain abundant clear cytoplasm filled with glycogen
- Clear cells feature pleomorphic nuclei and hobnail cells (nuclei of atypical cells protrude into the glandular lumens)

OTHER RARE VARIANTS, INCLUDING MUCINOUS ADENOCARCINOMA AND SQUAMOUS CELL CARCINOMA
- Mucinous adenocarcinoma is diagnosed when more than 50% of the tumor cells demonstrate mucinous differentiation
- Squamous cell carcinoma is a rare primary tumor of the endometrium and should be diagnosed only in the absence of a cervical squamous cell carcinoma
- Associated with ichthyosis uteri (squamous metaplasia of endometrial lining)

MIXED CARCINOMA
- Two or more of the above cell types with a minimum volume of 10% per type

UNDIFFERENTIATED CARCINOMAS
- Several variable phenotypes, which include small cell (neuroendocrine differentiation), giant cell, and spindle cell types

Special Stains and Immunohistochemistry
- Cytokeratin positive in all types
- Vimentin often positive; useful in distinguishing primary endometrial carcinomas from endocervical adenocarcinomas
- CEA often negative
- Mucicarmine positive in mucinous type; may be positive in endometrioid, essentially negative in clear cell
- PAS positive in clear cell, negative with diastase digestion

Other Techniques for Diagnosis
- Endometrial carcinomas, particularly endometrioid type, express estrogen and progesterone receptors
- Clear cell and serous carcinomas are mostly negative for estrogen and progesterone receptors, p53 positive, and often aneuploid with *c-myc* gene amplification

Differential Diagnosis
ENDOMETRIAL HYPERPLASIA
- Stroma between glands, lacks cribriforming and a back-to-back glandular pattern
- Absence of complex papilloglandular areas with cellular atypia, and desmoplasia

METASTATIC ADENOCARCINOMA
- Usually infiltrates from the serosal surface into the myometrium
- Rarely present in the endometrium
- Clinical history important

ATYPICAL POLYPOID ADENOMYOMA
- Randomly arranged glands in smooth muscle stroma without desmoplasia
- Slightly atypical cells with loss of polarity but not outright malignant pattern: lack cribriforming or back-to-back arrangement
- Squamous morulas usually present

PEARLS
- *Depth of myometrial invasion is an important prognostic parameter; therefore, a well-oriented section (or sections if necessary) from endomyometrium to serosa is imperative*
- *Endometrioid pattern is the most common*
- *Presence of squamous differentiation is not prognostically significant*
- *Villoglandular type is generally low grade*
- *Serous and clear cell carcinomas (type II) are by definition high grade (grade 3)*

SELECTED REFERENCES
Blanco LZ, Heagley DE, Lee JC, et al: Immunohistochemical characterization of squamous differentiation and morular metaplasia in uterine endometriod adenocarcinoma. Int J Gynecol Pathol. 32(3):283-292, 2013.

Clement PB, Young RH: Endometrioid carcinoma of the uterine corpus: a review of its pathology with emphasis on recent advances and problematic aspects. Adv Anat Pathol 9:145-184, 2002.

Kapucuoglu N, Bulbul D, Tulunay G, Temel MA: Reproducibility of grading systems for endometrial endometrioid carcinoma and their relation with pathologic prognostic parameters. Int J Gynecol Cancer 18:790-796, 2008.

Lax SF, Kurman RJ, Pizer ES, et al: A binary architectural grading system for uterine endometrial endometrioid carcinoma has superior reproducibility compared with FIGO grading and identifies subsets of advance-stage tumors with favorable and unfavorable prognosis. Am J Surg Pathol 24:1202-1208, 2000.

Modica I, Soslow RA, Black D, et al: Utility of immunohistochemistry in predicting microsatellite instability in endometrial carcinoma. Am J Surg Pathol 31:744-751, 2007.

Sagae S, Saito T, Satoh M, et al: The reproducibility of a binary tumor grading system for uterine endometrial endometrioid carcinoma, compared with FIGO system and nuclear grading. Oncology 67:344-350, 2004.

Sherman ME: Theories of endometrial carcinogenesis: a multidisciplinary approach. Mod Pathol 13:295-308, 2000.

Sherman ME, Bitterman P, Rosenshein NB, et al: Uterine serous carcinoma: a morphologically diverse neoplasm with unifying clinicopathologic features. Am J Surg Pathol 16:600-610, 1992.

Silverberg SG: The endometrium. Arch Pathol Lab Med 131:372-382, 2007.

Silverberg SG, Kurman RJ, Nogales F, et al: Tumours of the uterine corpus: epithelial tumours and related lesions. In Travassoli FA, Devilee P (eds): World Health Organization Classification of Tumours: Pathology and Genetics: Tumours of the Breast and Female Genital Organs. Lyon, IARC Press, 2003, pp 221-232.

Soslow RA, Bissonnette JP, Wilton A, et al: Clinicopathologic analysis of 187 high-grade endometrial carcinomas of different histologic subtypes: similar outcomes belie distinctive biologic differences. Am J Surg Pathol 31:979-987, 2007.

Yemelyanova A, Ji H, Shih IeM, et al: Utility of p16 expression for distinction of uterine serous carcinomas from endometrial endometrioid and endocervical adenocarcinomas: immunohistochemical analysis of 201 cases. Am J Surg Pathol 33:1504-1514, 2009.

ADENOFIBROMA

Clinical Features

- Extremely rare and benign
- Arises in perimenopausal and postmenopausal women
- Commonly presents with abnormal vaginal bleeding

Gross Pathology

- Lobulated polyploid neoplasm of variable size confined to endometrium
- Tan-brown, focally hemorrhagic cut surface
- Commonly, cut surface shows numerous small cysts

Histopathology

- Benign stroma and glands (< 4 mitotic figures/10 hpf)
- Often contains numerous cystic spaces and papillary projections lined by unremarkable cuboidal, columnar, tubal, or other epithelial cells (Figure 12-33)

Special Stains and Immunohistochemistry

- Noncontributory

Other Techniques for Diagnosis

- Noncontributory

Differential Diagnosis

ADENOSARCOMA
- Markedly atypical stromal cells and a mitotic index of more than 5 mitotic figures/10 hpf
- Benign endometrial glands

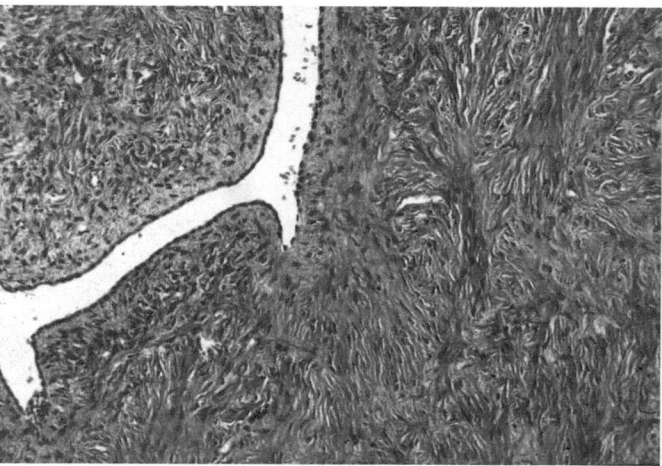

Figure 12-33. Adenofibroma. Cleftlike space lined by cuboidal cells surrounded by hypocellular collagenous stroma.

PEARLS

- *Hysterectomy is the treatment of choice to prevent local recurrence and to exclude more aggressive lesions, such as adenosarcoma*

SELECTED REFERENCES

Bettaieb I, Mekni A, Bellil K, et al: Endometrial adenofibroma: a rare entity. Arch Gynecol Obstet 275:191-193, 2007.

Clement PB, Scully RE: Müllerian adenofibroma of the uterus with invasion of myometrium and pelvic veins. Int J Gynecol Pathol 9:363-371, 1990.

Gallardo A, Prat J: Mullerian adenosarcomas: a clinicopathologic and immunohistochemical study of 55 cases challenging the existence of adenofibroma. Am J Surg Pathol 33:278-288, 2009.

Vellios F, Ng AB, Reagen JW: Papillary adenofibroma of the uterus: a benign mesodermal mixed tumor of müllerian origin. Am J Clin Pathol 60:543-551, 1973.

ADENOSARCOMA

Clinical Features

- May occur at any age and usually presents with abnormal bleeding
- Arises in the endometrium and rarely in the cervix

Gross Pathology

- Solitary sessile polypoid mass that often fills the entire endometrial cavity
- Cut surface is tan-gray with small cysts and focal hemorrhage and necrosis

Histopathology

- Leaflike glandular pattern featuring epithelial-lined broad papillary fronds with a cellular mesenchymal stroma cuffing cystlike spaces and clefts (reminiscent of phyllodes tumor of breast)
- Stroma is atypical, particularly dense in periglandular regions, with mitosis ranging from 4 or 5 to 20 mitotic figures/10 hpf (Figure 12-34)
- Epithelial lining is most often endometrioid but may also be mucinous, serous, squamous, or clear cell
- Sex cord–like elements: plump epithelioid cells with foamy cytoplasm arranged in a trabecular, insular, or tubular pattern are present in about 5% of tumors

- Mesenchymal stroma is usually homologous (e.g., fibrous sarcoma); heterologous elements include rhabdomyosarcoma more commonly than chondrosarcoma

Special Stains and Immunohistochemistry

- Cytokeratin positive in the epithelial component
- Vimentin positive in stromal component
- Desmin, MSA may be positive in heterologous rhabdomyosarcomatous component
- MIB-1 index: high proliferative index around glands and cysts

Other Techniques for Diagnosis

- Noncontributory

Differential Diagnosis

ADENOFIBROMA
- Bland fibrotic stroma with cystic spaces, glands, and papillary projections without cytologic atypia
- Fibrous stroma is cellular, but cells are not atypical
- Stromal mitotic activity is fewer than four mitotic figures/10 hpf

CARCINOSARCOMA (METAPLASTIC CARCINOMA)
- Presence of malignant epithelial and spindle cell components

HOMOLOGOUS SARCOMA
- Absence of leaflike pattern and absence of epithelial structures

PEARLS

- *Benign epithelial component and malignant mesenchymal component*
- *Periepithelial stromal cellularity is highly characteristic of adenosarcoma*
- *Myometrial invasion in about 20% of cases*
- *Sarcomatous overgrowth, deep myometrial invasion, and extrauterine involvement at time of diagnosis are associated with increased risk for recurrence and metastasis*
- *About 25% to 40% recur, and 5% metastasize (typically sarcomatous component only)*

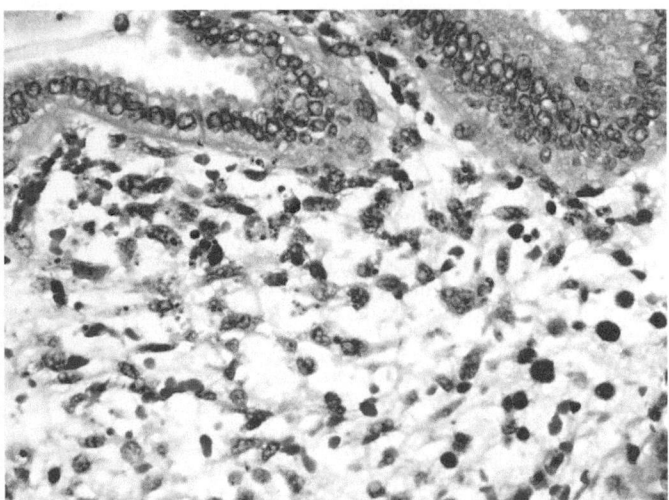

Figure 12-34. Adenosarcoma. Pleomorphic spindle cells with mitotic figures and nonmalignant but atypical epithelium.

SELECTED REFERENCES

Clement PB, Scully RE: Müllerian adenosarcoma of the uterus: a clinicopathologic analysis of 100 cases with a review of the literature. Hum Pathol 21:363-381, 1990.
Clement PB, Scully RE: Müllerian adenosarcomas of the uterus with sex cord-like elements: a clinicopathologic analysis of eight cases. Am J Clin Pathol 91:664-672, 1989.
Gallardo A, Prat J: Müllerian adenosarcomas: a clinicopathologic and immunohistochemical study of 55 cases challenging the existence of adenofibroma. Am J Surg Pathol 33:278-288, 2009.
Lyle P, Evans R, Jarboe E, et al: Biphasic tumors of the female genital tract. Oncology 19:1178-1190, 2005.
Soslow RA, Ali A, Oliva E: Müllerian adenosarcomas: an immunophenotypic analysis of 35 cases. Am J Surg Pathol 32:1013-1021, 2008.

CARCINOSARCOMA (METAPLASTIC CARCINOMA MALIGNANT MIXED MESODERMAL TUMOR)

Clinical Features

- Often associated with history of pelvic radiation therapy
- Usually arises in postmenopausal women
- Presents with abnormal bleeding and abdominal or pelvic pain
- Bulky tumors that are often visible protruding through cervical os

Gross Pathology

- Large friable polypoid mass
- Often the tumor fills the entire endometrial cavity, invading deeply into the myometrium and extending out through the cervical os (Figure 12-35A)
- Variegated cut surface with hemorrhage and necrosis
- Hard foci may be present owing to heterologous elements such as bone or cartilage

Histopathology

- Intimate admixture of malignant glands (endometrial adenocarcinoma) and malignant spindle cells (sarcoma) (Figure 12-35B)
- Adenocarcinoma may be any type of endometrial adenocarcinoma
- Malignant spindle cell component may be either of the following:
  - Homologous: often high-grade, spindled, round, or giant cells sometimes resembling fibrosarcoma, leiomyosarcoma, or stromal sarcoma
  - Heterologous: rhabdomyosarcoma (most common), chondrosarcoma, osteosarcoma, or mixture; less common are liposarcoma or neuroectodermal differentiation (Figure 12-35C and D)
- Scattered cells in each tumor display hybrid features, mixture of spindle and epithelial

Special Stains and Immunohistochemistry

- Vimentin: both epithelial and spindle cell components positive
- Cytokeratin 8/18: epithelial component diffusely positive; spindle cell components focally positive
- Desmin, Myoglobin: rhabdomyomatous component positive
- S-100 protein: chondrosarcoma or liposarcoma positive
- CD10: positive in stromal sarcoma component

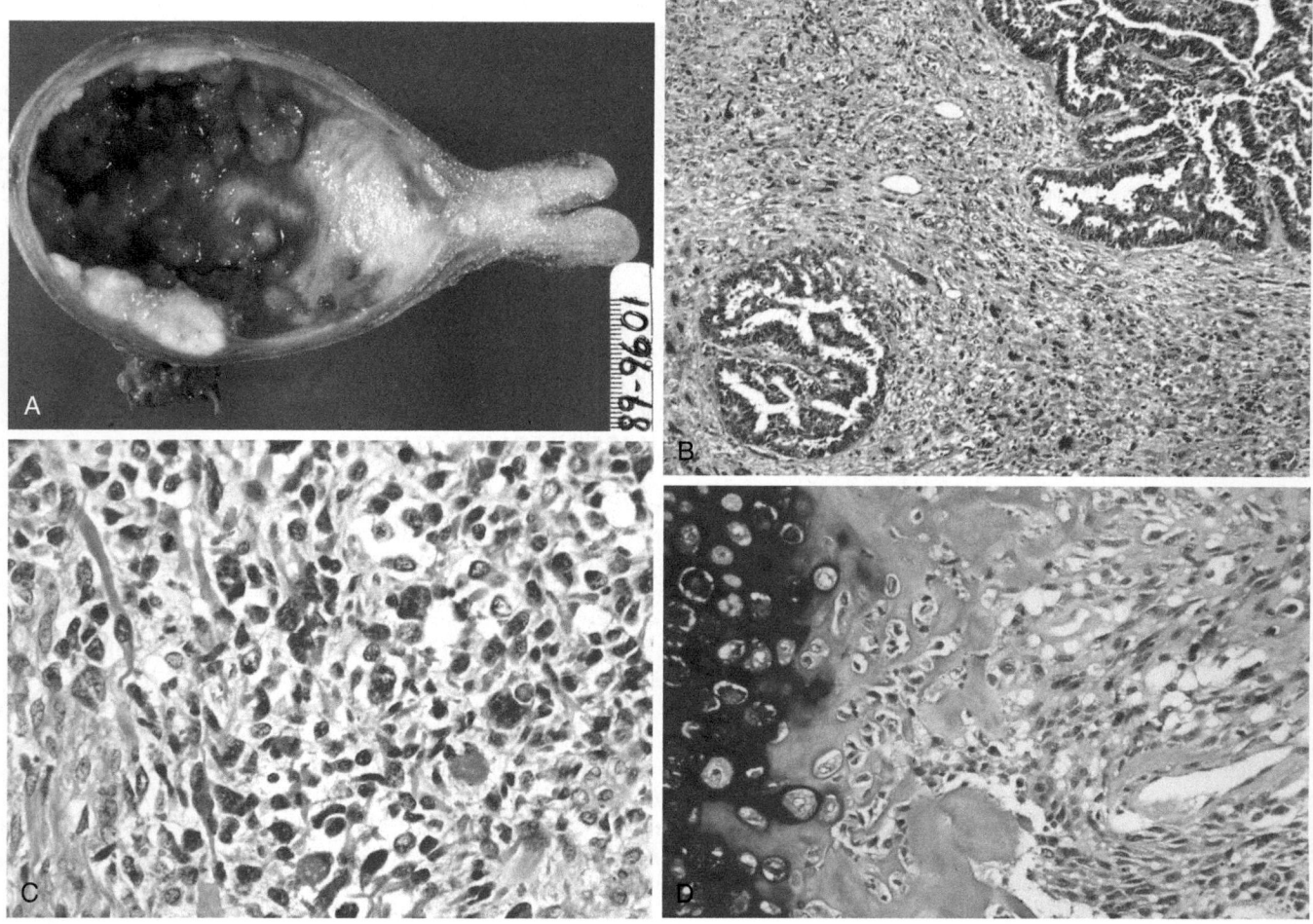

Figure 12-35. Carcinosarcoma (metaplastic carcinoma). A, Large nodular exophytic tumor mass filling the entire endometrial cavity. **B,** Biphasic morphology displaying malignant glands and markedly pleomorphic spindle cells with mitotic figures. **C,** Heterologous metaplastic carcinoma. Numerous rhabdomyoblasts are evident. **D,** Heterologous metaplastic carcinoma. The neoplasm shows chondroid and osseous differentiation.

Other Techniques for Diagnosis

- Electron microscopy is rarely used

Differential Diagnosis

POORLY DIFFERENTIATED ENDOMETRIAL CARCINOMA

- Lacks biphasic population of cells
- Diffusely positive for cytokeratin

ADENOSARCOMA

- Lacks malignant epithelial component

PEARLS

- *Malignant epithelial and spindle cell components*
- *In endometrial curettage, often only the carcinomatous component is identified*
- *Early metastases are epithelial*
- *Late metastases are both epithelial and spindle cell or exclusively spindle cell (sarcomatous overgrowth)*
- *Lungs are a common site of metastasis*
- *Prognosis is poor*

SELECTED REFERENCES

Bitterman P, Chun B, Kurman RJ: The significance of epithelial differentiation in mixed mesodermal tumors of the uterus: a clinicopathologic and immunohistochemical study. Am J Surg Pathol 14:317-328, 1990.

Cimbaluk D, Rotmensch J, Scudiere J, et al: Uterine carcinosarcoma: immunohistochemical studies on tissue microarrays with focus on potential therapeutic targets. Gynecol Oncol 105:138-144, 2007.

McCluggage WG: Uterine carcinosarcomas (malignant mixed müllerian tumors) are metaplastic carcinomas. Int J Gynecol Cancer 12:687-690, 2002.

Silverberg SG, Major FJ, Blessing JA, et al: Carcinosarcoma (malignant mixed mesodermal tumor) of the uterus: a Gynecologic Oncology Group pathologic study of 203 cases. Int J Gynecol Pathol 9:1-19, 1990.

MYOMETRIUM

ADENOMYOSIS

Clinical Features

- Non-neoplastic and most common in adult women

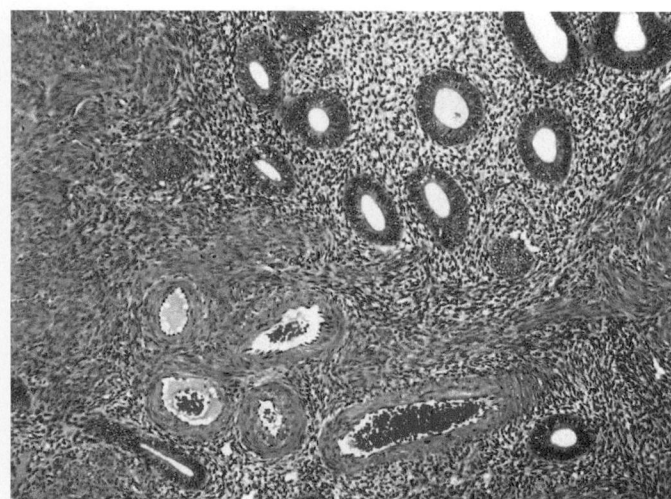

Figure 12-36. Adenomyosis. Endometrial glands deep in the myometrial smooth muscle surrounded by endometrial stroma and adjacent blood vessels.

- Presents with a palpably enlarged uterus and abnormal bleeding or dysmenorrhea; often associated with leiomyomas
- Commonly an incidental finding in hysterectomy specimen

Gross Pathology

- Thickened myometrium with focal soft, discolored areas or small cysts

Histopathology

- Islands of endometrial glands surrounded by endometrial stroma within the myometrium or endometrial stroma exclusively (Figure 12-36)
- Often the glands appear inactive, and hemosiderin is generally absent
- Endometrial glands in the myometrium that are more than 2 to 2.5 mm away from the basalis in a properly oriented section are required for diagnosis

Special Stains and Immunohistochemistry

- CD10 positive, confirming endometrial stroma rather than smooth muscle around the glands

Other Techniques for Diagnosis

- Noncontributory

Differential Diagnosis

NORMAL ENDOMETRIUM THAT IS CUT TANGENTIALLY

- Deeper levels may demonstrate that the glands in question are actually continuous with the endometrium

ENDOMETRIAL CARCINOMA INVOLVING ADENOMYOSIS

- Malignant glands, perhaps with cribriforming surrounded by endometrial stroma; not regarded as myometrial invasion

INVASIVE ADENOCARCINOMA

- Malignant glands and desmoplastic or inflammatory stromal response

STROMAL TUMOR

- Tumor mass composed of stromal cells with or without lymphatic or vascular space invasion and no glands

ADENOMATOID TUMOR

- Flat cuboidal epithelial lining glandular spaces as opposed to endometrial glands
- Mesothelial origin
- No endometrial stroma
- Uncommon

PEARLS

- *It is important to have a properly oriented histologic section because tangential sections may mimic adenomyosis*

SELECTED REFERENCE

Parrott E, Butterworth M, Green A, et al: Adenomyosis: a result of disordered stromal differentiation. Am J Pathol 159:623-630, 2001.

LEIOMYOMA

Clinical Features

- Benign neoplasm, more commonly referred to as *"fibroid"* by gynecologists
- Most common tumor in women as well as in the uterus
- Rare in women younger than 20 years of age and increasingly common in women older than 30 years
- Small tumors may be asymptomatic
- Larger tumors may cause pain, dysmenorrhea, urinary difficulties, changes in bowel habits, and, in extreme cases, infertility; often diagnosed on pelvic examination
- Tumors may be more specifically localized by ultrasound

Gross Pathology

- Often multiple
- Discrete, well-circumscribed masses with firm, whorled, tan-white cut surfaces (Figure 12-37A)
- Cystic degeneration is often present in larger tumors
- Hyalinization and calcification may be extensive
- Hemorrhage and degenerative necrosis are not prominent findings; no coagulative necrosis present
- Three types
  - Subserosal: located immediately beneath the serosa; may be pedunculated
  - Intramural: within myometrium
  - Submucosal: located immediately beneath the endometrium

Histopathology

- Interlacing fascicles of bland monomorphic spindle (smooth muscle) cells
- Well-circumscribed borders with mitotic activity of fewer than five mitotic figures/10 hpf
- Pseudocapsuled; hyalinized areas and calcifications may be present
- Occasionally, the entire leiomyoma may be hyalinized, suggesting an infarcted neoplasm
- Endometritis may be present in the overlying endometrium if compressed by leiomyoma
- Variants
  - Cellular leiomyoma
    - Densely cellular (Figure 12-37B)
    - Mitotic activity is fewer than five mitotic figures/10 hpf
    - No coagulative necrosis or cellular pleomorphism
  - Epithelioid leiomyoma

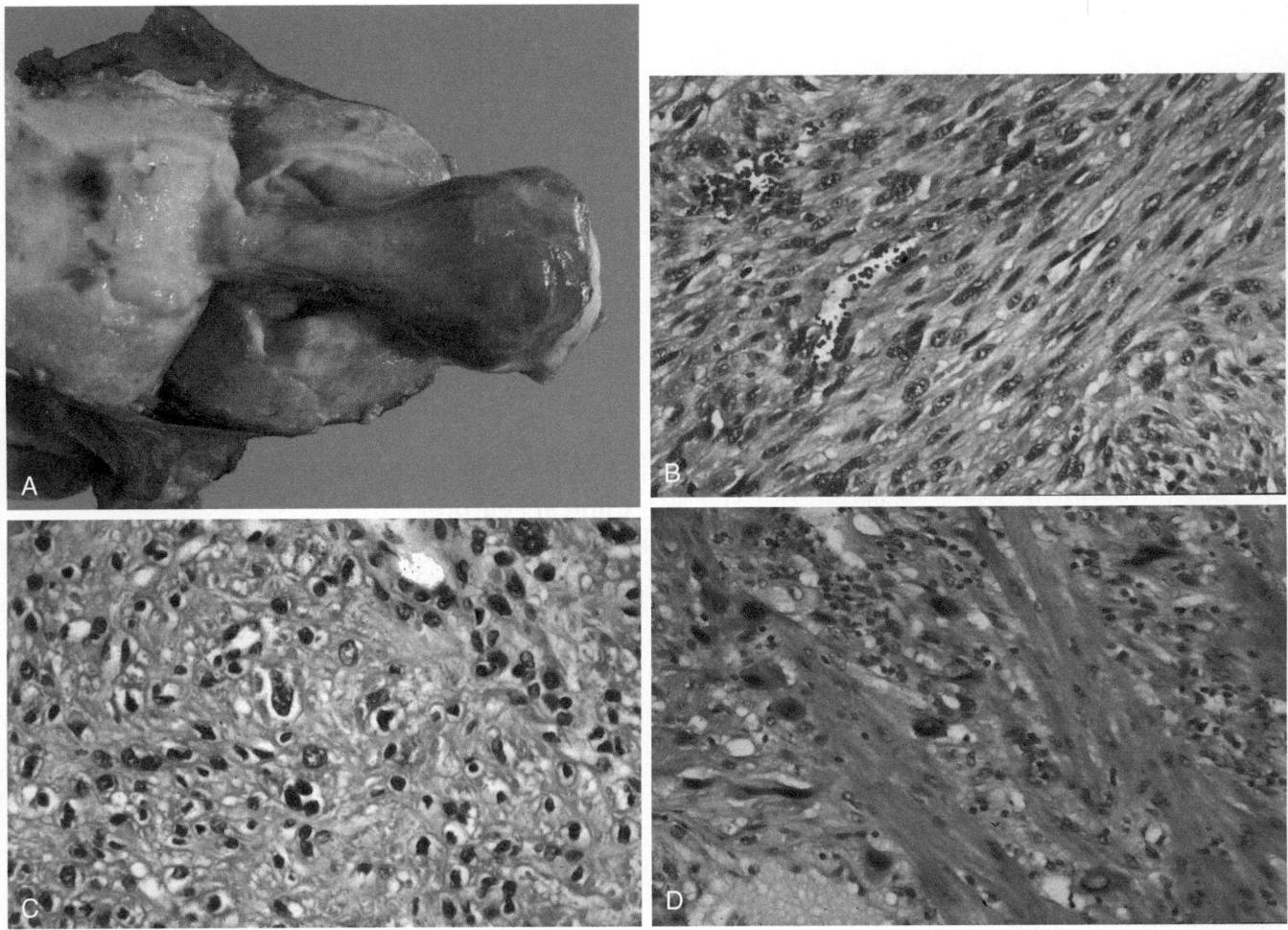

Figure 12-37. A, Pedunculated leiomyoma. Solid tan mass protruding into the cervical canal. **B,** Cellular leiomyoma. The tumor is composed of densely cellular fascicles of smooth muscle cells with minimal intervening collagen. **C,** Epithelioid leiomyoma. The tumor is composed of round to polygonal cells. Focally the tumor cells show clear cytoplasm. **D,** Bizarre (symplastic) leiomyoma. Large atypical cells show hyperchromatic nuclei with chromatin smudging.

- Round polygonal (epithelioid) cells
- Leiomyoblastoma: cells with eccentric nuclei and granular eosinophilic cytoplasm, hyalinization
- Clear cell: round polygonal cells with abundant clear cytoplasm (Figure 12-37C)
- Plexiform: rows and columns of round polygonal cells separated by fibrous stroma
- Mitotic activity of fewer than five mitotic figures/10 hpf in all variants
- Bizarre leiomyoma (also referred to as *symplastic, pleomorphic,* or *atypical*)
  - Bizarre giant cells grouped focally or scattered in an otherwise typical leiomyoma (Figure 12-37D)
  - Mitotic activity of fewer than five mitotic figures/10 hpf and no coagulative necrosis
- Lipoleiomyoma
  - Mostly composed of benign adipocytes with occasional smooth muscle cells
- Mitotically active leiomyoma
  - Occurs in women younger than 35 years of age
  - Cytologic atypia and necrosis are absent
  - Mitotic activity more than 5 mitotic figures/10 hpf, perhaps up to 20 mitotic figures/10 hpf

- Intravenous leiomyomatosis (IVL)
  - Rare condition characterized by leiomyomas that extend into myometrial veins and continue beyond the uterus
  - Intravenous leiomyomatosis shows no tendency to metastasize
- Benign metastasizing leiomyoma
  - Rare condition characterized by leiomyoma in distant sites such as lungs
  - Metastasis may occur years after the diagnosis of typical uterine leiomyoma

Special Stains and Immunohistochemistry

- Vimentin positive
- Desmin, caldesmon, SMA positive
- Cytokeratin negative (rare positive cells)
- Estrogen and progesterone receptors often positive

Other Techniques for Diagnosis

- Electron microscopy demonstrates actin filaments with associated dense bodies as well as incomplete basal lamina (features characteristic of smooth muscle cells)

Differential Diagnosis

LEIOMYOSARCOMA

- Cellular neoplasm with moderate to severe cytologic pleomorphism
- Hemorrhage and coagulative necrosis
- Generally more than 10 mitotic figures/hpf
- Infiltrating borders, and perhaps metastatic at time of presentation

STROMAL NODULE

- Smaller bland round and spindled cells resembling endometrial stroma
- Positive for CD10 with occasional cells positive for SMA

LOW-GRADE STROMAL SARCOMA

- Wormlike masses representing lymphatic invasion may be seen grossly within the myometrium
- Smaller, bland round and spindled cells with minimal cytoplasm resembling endometrial stroma
- May find admixture of stromal and epithelioid glandular or sex cord–like components
- CD10 is positive

PEARLS

- *Leiomyomas are hormonally responsive; that is, most shrink after menopause*
- *The following variants are regarded as atypical or of uncertain malignant potential:*
  - *Epithelioid, bizarre, and intravenous leiomyomatosis*
  - *Tumors in women older than 35 years that show mild cytologic atypia and more than five mitotic figures/10 hpf*

SELECTED REFERENCES

Clement PB, Young RH, Scully RE: Intravenous leiomyomatosis of the uterus: a clinicopathological analysis of 16 cases with unusual histologic features. Am J Surg Pathol 12:932-934, 1988.

Lee HJ, Choi J, Kim KR: Pulmonary benign metastasizing leiomyoma associated with intravenous leiomyomatosis of the uterus: clinical behavior and genomic changes supporting a transportation theory. Int J Gynecol Pathol 27:340-345, 2008.

Leitao MM, Soslow RA, Nonaka D, et al: Tissue microarray immunohistochemical expression of estrogen, progesterone, and androgen receptors in uterine leiomyomata and leiomyosarcoma. Cancer 101:1455-1462, 2004.

O'Connor DM, Norris HJ: Mitotically active leiomyomas of the uterus. Hum Pathol 21:223-227, 1990.

Toledo G, Oliva E: Smooth muscle tumors of the uterus: a practical approach. Arch Pathol Lab Med 132:595-605, 2008.

LEIOMYOSARCOMA

Clinical Features

- Rapidly growing tumor that usually arises in postmenopausal women
- Large tumor that may cause pain, dysmenorrhea, urinary difficulties, changes in bowel habits, and, in extreme cases, infertility
- Often diagnosed on pelvic examination and specifically localized by ultrasound
- May have spread into the pelvic cavity by the time of presentation
- Often detected as an incidental finding in hysterectomy specimens
- Distant metastases may occur months or years later, often in the lungs
- Treatment is total abdominal hysterectomy with salpingo-oophorectomy and tumor debulking, and radiation; chemotherapeutic agents have not proved effective
- Prognosis is variable depending on stage and grade

Gross Pathology

- Usually solitary
- Large, poorly circumscribed mass, often extending beyond the uterine serosa (Figure 12-38A)
- Soft, fleshy, variegated cut surface showing hemorrhage and necrosis

Histopathology

- Densely cellular tumor composed of interlacing fascicles of pleomorphic spindled cells (Figure 12-38B)
- Coagulative necrosis is often present

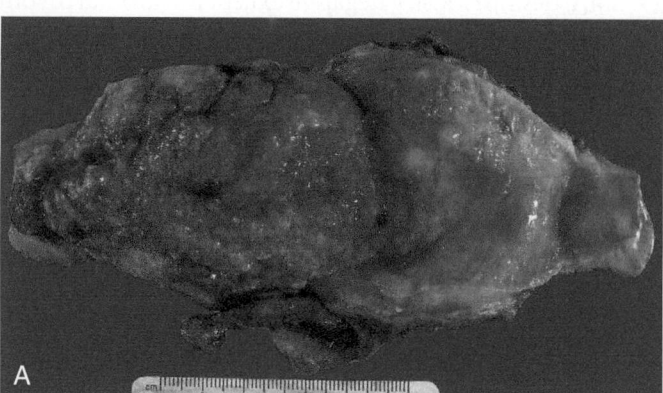
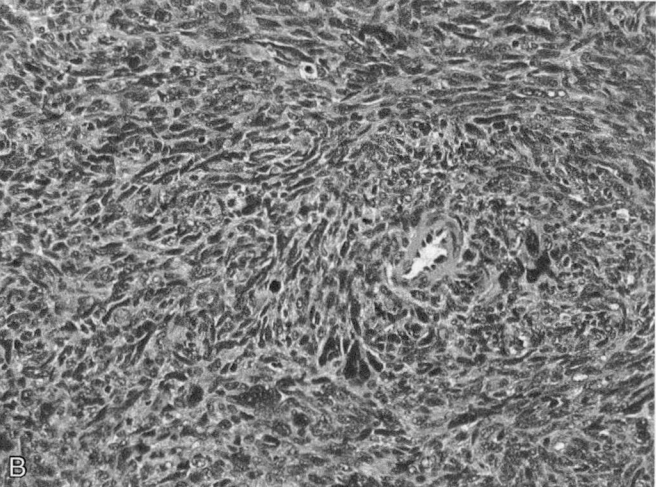

Figure 12-38. A, Leiomyosarcoma. Uterine cavity displaying a soft, ill-defined tan mass with necrosis and hemorrhage filling the endometrial cavity and infiltrating the myometrium. **B,** Leiomyosarcoma. Interlacing bundles of pleomorphic spindle cells with large nuclei, prominent nucleoli, and mitotic figures.

- Mitoses are generally greater than 10 to 20/10 hpf in areas with highest mitotic activity (viewed with a 40× objective)
- Infiltrative margins with occasional vascular invasion
- Variants
  - Epithelioid
    - Rounded, highly atypical polygonal cells with necrosis and increased mitosis
  - Myxoid
    - Myxoid matrix that makes tumor appear less cellular and mitotically active
    - Infiltrates myometrium and vessels

Special Stains and Immunohistochemistry

- Vimentin positive
- SMA, desmin, caldesmon, and other muscle markers positive
- Estrogen and progesterone receptors positive in better differentiated areas
- Cytokeratin negative

Other Techniques for Diagnosis

- Noncontributory

Differential Diagnosis

MITOTICALLY ACTIVE LEIOMYOMA

- Women younger than 35 years
- Smaller and well circumscribed
- Absence of coagulative necrosis, cytologic atypia, and vascular invasion

HIGH-GRADE STROMAL SARCOMA (UNDIFFERENTIATED SARCOMA)

- Numerous evenly distributed small blood vessels
- Absence of interlacing fascicular pattern
- Originates in endometrium and extends down into myometrium
- Negative or only focally positive for SMA and other muscle markers; may show CD10 positivity

METAPLASTIC CARCINOMA (CARCINOSARCOMA)

- Malignant glands admixed with malignant spindle cell component

PEARLS

- *Much less common than leiomyomas*
- *Characterized by hypercellularity, cytologic atypia, and mitotic activity generally more than 10 mitotic figures/10 hpf*
- *Large tumors (>10cm) with coagulative necrosis and >10 mitotic figures/hpf have a dismal prognosis (<5 years survival)*
- *Tumors with high mitotic activity (> 5 to 10 mitotic figures/hpf) but lacking significant cytologic atypia and necrosis should be classified as smooth muscle tumors of uncertain malignant potential (STUMP), or atypical leiomyomas*
- *Myxoid leiomyosarcoma: mitotic count should be performed in more cellular areas*

SELECTED REFERENCES

Berchuck A, Rubin SC, Hoskins WJ, et al: Treatment of uterine leiomyosarcoma. Obstet Gynecol 71:845-850, 1988.
Giuntoli RL 2nd, Metzinger DS, DiMarco CS, et al: Retrospective review of 208 patients with leiomyosarcoma of the uterus: prognostic indicators, surgical management, and adjuvant therapy. Gynecol Oncol 89:460-469, 2003.
Ip PP, Cheung AN, Clement PB: Uterine smooth muscle tumors of uncertain malignant potential (STUMP): a clinicopathologic analysis of 16 cases. Am J Surg Pathol 33:992-1005, 2009.
King ME, Dickersin GR, Scully RE: Myxoid leiomyosarcoma of the uterus: a report of six cases. Am J Surg Pathol 6:589-598, 1982.
O'Neill CJ, McBride HA, Connolly LE, McCluggage WG: Uterine leiomyosarcomas are characterized by high p16, p53 and M1B1 expression in comparison with usual leiomyomas, leiomyoma variants and smooth muscle tumors of uncertain malignant potential. Histopathology 50:851-858, 2007.
Prayson RA, Goldblum JR, Hart WR: Epithelioid smooth-muscle tumors of the uterus: a clinicopathologic study of 18 patients. Am J Surg Pathol 21:383-391, 1997.
Toledo G, Oliva E: Smooth muscle tumors of the uterus: a practical approach. Arch Pathol Lab Med 132:595-605, 2008.

STROMAL NODULE

Clinical Features

- Rare, benign tumor
- Occurs at any age, but generally in older, postmenopausal women
- Usually presents with abnormal bleeding
- Uterus may be palpably enlarged

Gross Pathology

- Well-circumscribed, solid, soft, tan-gray mass
- Unencapsulated with pushing margins

Histopathology

- Small uniform oval to spindled cells resembling endometrial stromal cells (Figure 12-39A)
- Minimal cytologic atypia and generally fewer than 10 mitotic figures/10 hpf
- Numerous thin-walled vessels evenly spaced among stromal cells and resembling spiral arterioles
- Rare small foci of necrosis, cystic degeneration, foam cells, calcification, decidualization, and sex cord–like structures

Special Stains and Immunohistochemistry

- CD10 positive
- Vimentin positive
- Reticulin positive surrounding individual cells
- Cytokeratin only focally positive, except in sex cord elements
- SMA, desmin mostly negative except for stromal myoma
- Epithelial membrane antigen (EMA) negative

Other Techniques for Diagnosis

- Noncontributory

Differential Diagnosis

LEIOMYOMA

- Unevenly spaced, thick-walled vessels
- Spindled cells and interlacing fascicles
- Positive for SMA, desmin, smooth muscle myosin (SMMS), only focally positive for CD10

LOW-GRADE STROMAL SARCOMA

- Infiltrative margins
- Prominent lymphovascular invasion

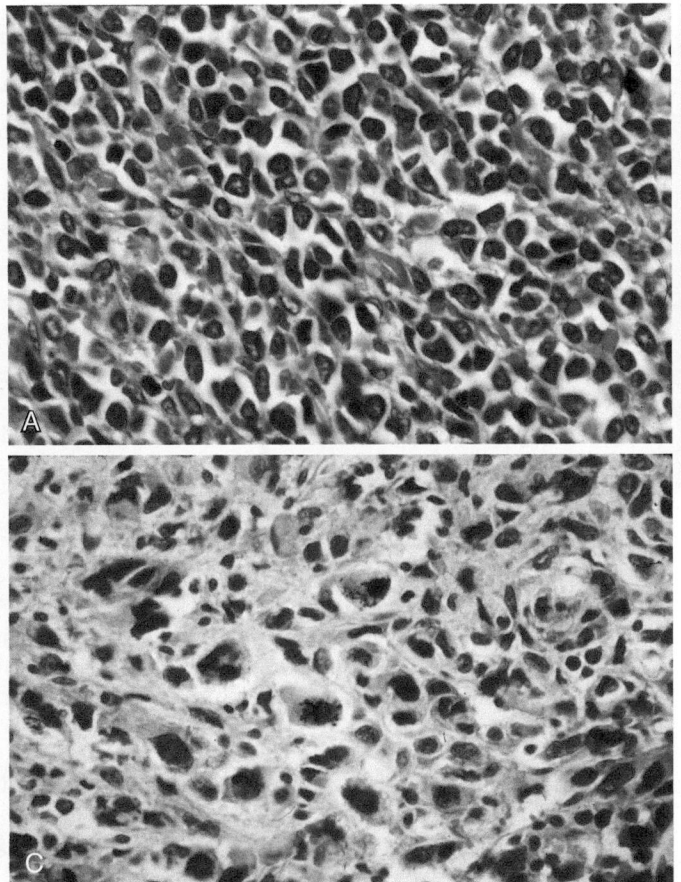

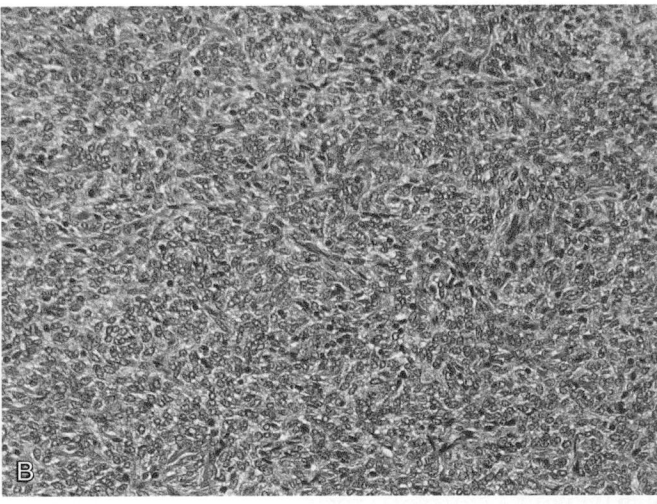

Figure 12-39. A, Endometrial stromal nodule. The neoplastic cells are uniform in size and shape, and they have minimal cytologic atypia and no mitotic figures. **B,** Low-grade endometrial stromal sarcoma. Round to spindled cells with bland nuclei, no mitotic figures, and small plexiform blood vessels. **C,** High-grade endometrial stromal sarcoma (undifferentiated sarcoma). High mitotic activity and nuclear pleomorphism are evident.

HEMANGIOPERICYTOMA

- Extremely rare in the uterus
- Large branching staghorn vessels
- Definitively diagnosed by immunohistochemistry demonstrating neoplastic cells with pericytic differentiation

PEARLS

- *Benign without recurrence even if excised without hysterectomy*
- *Usually expresses estrogen and progesterone receptors*

SELECTED REFERENCES

Baker P, Oliva E: Endometrial stromal tumours of the uterus: a practical approach using conventional morphology and ancillary techniques. J Clin Pathol 60:235-243, 2007.

Chang KL, Crabtree GS, Lim-Tan SK, et al: Primary uterine endometrial stromal neoplasms: a clinicopathologic study of 117 cases. Am J Surg Pathol 14:415-438, 1990.

Kempson RL, Hendrickson MR: Pure mesenchymal neoplasms of the uterine corpus: selected problems. Semin Diagn Pathol 5:172-198, 1988.

LOW-GRADE ENDOMETRIAL STROMAL SARCOMA

Clinical Features

- Rare tumor that usually presents with abnormal vaginal bleeding
- Occurs at any age, but most common in older premenopausal or postmenopausal women
- Uterus is often palpably enlarged

Gross Pathology

- Well-circumscribed mass, diffusely infiltrative mass, or multiple confluent masses
- Wormlike masses within myometrium (gross manifestation of lymphovascular invasion)
- Foci of hemorrhage, necrosis, or cystic degeneration
- Gross extrauterine extension in about 30% of cases at time of diagnosis

Histopathology

- Extensively infiltrative margins
- Plugs of tumor within lymphovascular spaces and myometrium (hence, former name *endolymphatic stromal myosis*)
- Variable numbers of mitotic figures, generally 10 to 20 mitotic figures/10 hpf
- Cells with minimal atypia resembling endometrial stromal cells (Figure 12-39B)
- Foci of epithelioid differentiation appearing as glandular or sex cord–like elements
- Foci of hemorrhage and necrosis are occasionally present
- Calcification, decidualization, cystic degeneration, and foam cells may be identified

Special Stains and Immunohistochemistry

- CD10, vimentin positive
- Cytokeratin occasionally focally positive
- EMA negative
- SMA, desmin: mostly negative (useful in distinguishing from smooth muscle tumors)

Other Techniques for Diagnosis

- Noncontributory

Differential Diagnosis

STROMAL NODULE

- Lack of lymphovascular invasion
- Noninfiltrating (pushing) margins

HIGH-GRADE STROMAL SARCOMA

- Marked cytologic atypia
- Atypical mitotic figures and necrosis

HEMANGIOPERICYTOMA

- Rare in uterus
- Large, branching staghorn vessels

INTRAVENOUS LEIOMYOMATOSIS

- Purely smooth muscle with irregularly spaced, thick-walled vessels
- Uncommon admixture of stromal cells or, rarely, epithelial components
- More abundant cytoplasm
- Intracytoplasmic myofibrils demonstrated by trichrome or electron microscopy
- Positive for SMA, MSA, desmin

METAPLASTIC CARCINOMA VERSUS LOW-GRADE ENDOMETRIAL STROMAL SARCOMA WITH PROMINENT EPITHELIOID ELEMENTS

- Metaplastic carcinoma has glands that are outright malignant
- Generally does not show plugging of lymphovascular spaces

ADENOSARCOMA

- Papillary folds with slitlike or dilated glands composed of cells with nuclei that are epithelial, not stromal
- Generally demarcated from surrounding atypical stroma with some mitotic figures

PEARLS

- *Mitotic activity is not predictive of aggressive behavior*
- *Distinction from high-grade stromal sarcoma is based on the absence of marked cytologic atypia, only minimal necrosis, and atypical mitotic figures*
- *Treatment is usually total abdominal hysterectomy with bilateral salpingo-oophorectomy with debulking of extrauterine tumor*
- *Recurrence is common even after several years*

SELECTED REFERENCES

Baker P, Oliva E: Endometrial stromal tumors of the uterus: a practical approach using conventional morphology and ancillary techniques. J Clin Pathol 60:235-243, 2007

Chang KL, Crabtree GS, Lim-Tan SK, et al: Primary uterine endometrial stromal neoplasms: a clinicopathologic study of 117 cases. Am J Surg Pathol 14:415-438, 1990.

Czernobilsky B: Uterine tumors resembling ovarian sex cord tumors: an update. Int J Gynecol Pathol 27:229-235, 2008.

Fekete PS, Vellios F: The clinical and histologic spectrum of endometrial stromal neoplasms: a report of 41 cases. Int J Gynecol Pathol 3:198-212, 1984.

Leath CA III, Huh WK, Hyde J Jr, et al: A multi-institutional review of outcomes of endometrial stromal sarcoma. Gynecol Oncol 105:630-634, 2007.

McCluggage WG, Sumathi VP, Maxwell P: CD10 is a sensitive and diagnostically useful immunohistochemical marker of normal endometrial stroma and of endometrial stromal neoplasms. Histopathology 39:273-278, 2001.

HIGH-GRADE ENDOMETRIAL STROMAL SARCOMA (UNDIFFERENTIATED SARCOMA)

Clinical Features

- Rare tumor that generally occurs in postmenopausal women
- Usually presents with abnormal bleeding or pelvic pain
- Aggressive tumor, with less than 50% 5-year survival rate

Gross Pathology

- Grossly infiltrative masses, confluent mass, or diffuse infiltration of myometrium
- Endometrial involvement, hemorrhage, and necrosis are common
- Wormlike infiltration of myometrium is usually absent

Histopathology

- Pronounced cytologic atypia; however, cells may still resemble endometrial stromal cells
- Mitotic activity is generally more than 10 mitotic figures/10 hpf with atypical forms (Figure 12-39C)
- Uneven distribution of thin-walled vascular spaces
- Coagulative necrosis
- There may be areas composed of undifferentiated bizarre or giant sarcoma cells
- Heterologous elements, including rhabdomyosarcoma or chondrosarcoma
- Epithelioid foci and wormlike plugs are generally absent
- Frequent lymphovascular invasion
- May be morphologically indistinguishable from other uterine sarcomas leiomyosarcoma in particular

Special Stains and Immunohistochemistry

- Vimentin positive
- Cytokeratin and CD10 focally positive
- EMA negative
- SMA generally negative (useful in distinguishing from leiomyosarcoma)
- S-100 protein positive if chondrosarcomatous component present

Other Techniques for Diagnosis

- Noncontributory

Differential Diagnosis

LOW-GRADE STROMAL SARCOMA

- Minimal cytologic atypia
- Evenly spaced vessels
- Wormlike projections of tumor
- May have epithelioid elements

UNDIFFERENTIATED ENDOMETRIAL SARCOMA

- Lacks endometrial stromal differentiation

METAPLASTIC CARCINOMA
- Malignant epithelial and spindle cell components are present

LEIOMYOSARCOMA
- Evidence of smooth muscle differentiation by hematoxylin and eosin (H&E) and immunohistochemistry
- Whorling pattern of plump, atypical spindle cells as opposed to more random streaming distribution of cells in stromal sarcoma

ADENOSARCOMA
- Benign glandular epithelium

OTHER SARCOMAS (E.G., MALIGNANT FIBROUS HISTIOCYTOMA, RHABDOMYOSARCOMA, OSTEOSARCOMA)
- All of these are rare as primary tumors in the uterine corpus
- These lack cell populations that resemble endometrial stromal cells

POORLY DIFFERENTIATED ENDOMETRIAL CARCINOMA
- Positive for cytokeratin

PEARLS

- *Cytologic atypia has proved more accurate than mitotic count in distinguishing low-grade from high-grade stromal sarcomas as well as in predicting behavior*
- *Necrosis is generally present, and epithelioid elements and wormlike endolymphatic stromal projections are generally absent*
- *Treatment is usually total abdominal hysterectomy with bilateral salpingo-oophorectomy and tumor debulking*
- *Distinction from leiomyosarcoma has no clinical significance*

SELECTED REFERENCES

Chang KL, Crabtree GS, Lim-Tan SK, et al: Primary uterine endometrial stromal neoplasms: a clinicopathologic study of 117 cases. Am J Surg Pathol 14:415-438, 1990.

Farhood AI, Abrams J: Immunohistochemistry of endometrial stromal sarcoma. Hum Pathol 22:224-230, 1991.

Feng W, Malpica A, Robboy SJ et al: Prognostic value of the diagnostic criteria distinguishing endometrial stromal sarcoma, low grade from undifferentiated endometrial sarcoma, 2 entities within the invasive endometrial stromal neoplasia family. Int J Gynecol Pathol. 32(3):299-306, 2013.

Nucci MR, O'Connell JT, Huettner PC, et al: H-caldesmon expression effectively distinguishes endometrial stromal tumors from uterine smooth muscle tumors. Am J Surg Pathol 24:455-463, 2001.

Oliva E, Clement PB, Young RH: Endometrial stromal tumors: an update on a group of tumors with a protean phenotype. Adv Anat Pathol 7:257-281, 2000.

Oliva E, Clement PB, Young RH, Scully RE: Mixed endometrial stromal and smooth muscle tumors of the uterus: a clinicopathologic study of 15 cases. Am J Surg Pathol 22:997-1005, 1998.

ENDOSALPINGIOSIS

Clinical Features

- Benign glands with fallopian tube–like epithelium, sometimes with calcifications
- Present often in the pelvic peritoneum: covering the uterus, fallopian tubes, omentum, laparotomy scars, and so on; rarely in retroperitoneal lymph nodes
- Affects women of reproductive age with a mean age of 30 years, rarely occurs in postmenopausal women

- Generally an incidental finding
- Originates in the secondary müllerian system
- Associated with atypical proliferative serous tumors

Gross Pathology

- Multiple small fluid filled cysts measuring < 5 mm may be seen on the peritoneum covering the uterus, fallopian tubes, and ovaries

Histopathology

- Glands of varying size and shapes and occasionally cystic lined by a single layer of benign tubal type epithelium
- Loose or dense connective tissue stroma
- Psammoma bodies in the gland lumina and stroma

Special Stains and Immunohistochemistry

- Noncontributory

Other Techniques for Diagnosis

- Noncontributory

Differential Diagnosis

EXTRAOVARIAN SEROUS CYSTADENOMA
- Solitary mass of significant size or fibromatous stroma
- Implants of borderline serous tumors

PEARLS

- *Atypical endosalpingiosis refers to cellular endosalpingiosis with cellular stratification and atypia and is to be considered in the differential diagnosis of peritoneal serous borderline tumors*
- *May represent the precursor lesion of ovarian serous tumors*

SELECTED REFERENCE

Zinser KR, Wheeler JE: Endosalpingiosis in the omentum: a study of autopsy and surgical material. Am J Surg Pathol 6:109-117, 1982.

OVARY

Inflammatory conditions of the ovary are uncommon and generally associated with PID or systemic infections such as tuberculosis. Immune oophoritis is a rare condition and most commonly a diagnosis of exclusion. Neoplasms of the ovary represent most of the pathology.

MISCELLANEOUS CONDITIONS

FOLLICULAR CYST AND CORPUS LUTEUM CYST

Clinical Features

FOLLICULAR CYSTS
- Common; they occur at any age, but often in the reproductive years
- Occasionally associated with McCune-Albright syndrome
  - Polyostotic fibrous dysplasia, irregular patches of pigmented skin, and endocrine dysfunction, especially precocious puberty in girls

CORPUS LUTEUM CYSTS
- Occur frequently during the reproductive years
- Usually an incidental finding

- May present as a palpable mass with endocrine manifestations like increased estrogen production and menstrual irregularities
- Rupture and bleeding into the peritoneum is relatively common

Gross Pathology

- Follicular cysts are typically unilocular with a thin wall and smooth inner surface, usually smaller than 10 cm in diameter, and filled with serous fluid (Figure 12-40A)
- Corpus luteum cysts are larger than 2 cm, have a smooth yellow lining, and have bloody fluid

Histopathology

FOLLICULAR CYST

- Inner layer of granulosa cells separated by the basement membrane from outer layer of theca interna cells; both are often luteinized (Figure 12-40B)
- Granulosa cells
  - Small and round with scanty cytoplasm
  - Hyperchromatic nuclei with occasional grooves
- Theca interna cells
  - Larger with abundant cytoplasm and mixed with vessels

CORPUS LUTEUM CYST

- Thin inner layer of connective tissue

- Outer layer of luteinized, large vacuolated granulosa cells and smaller theca interna cells

Special Stains and Immunohistochemistry

- Reticulin stain: highlights reticular network around theca interna cell layer in a follicular cyst

Other Techniques for Diagnosis

- Noncontributory

Differential Diagnosis

- Serous cystadenoma versus follicular cyst
  - Presence of a theca interna layer points toward follicular cyst
  - May be diagnosed as a simple cyst if unclear
- Corpus luteum versus corpus luteum cyst
  - Corpus luteum contains a cavity that is usually filled with blood (Figure 12-40C)
  - It displays luteinization effect of the cells
  - Cyst is greater than 2 cm in diameter and has a smooth rather than a folded contour (Figure 12-40D)
- Endometriosis versus hemorrhagic corpus luteum cyst
  - Peripheral theca interna cells are present, and organized blood clot is more typical of cysts

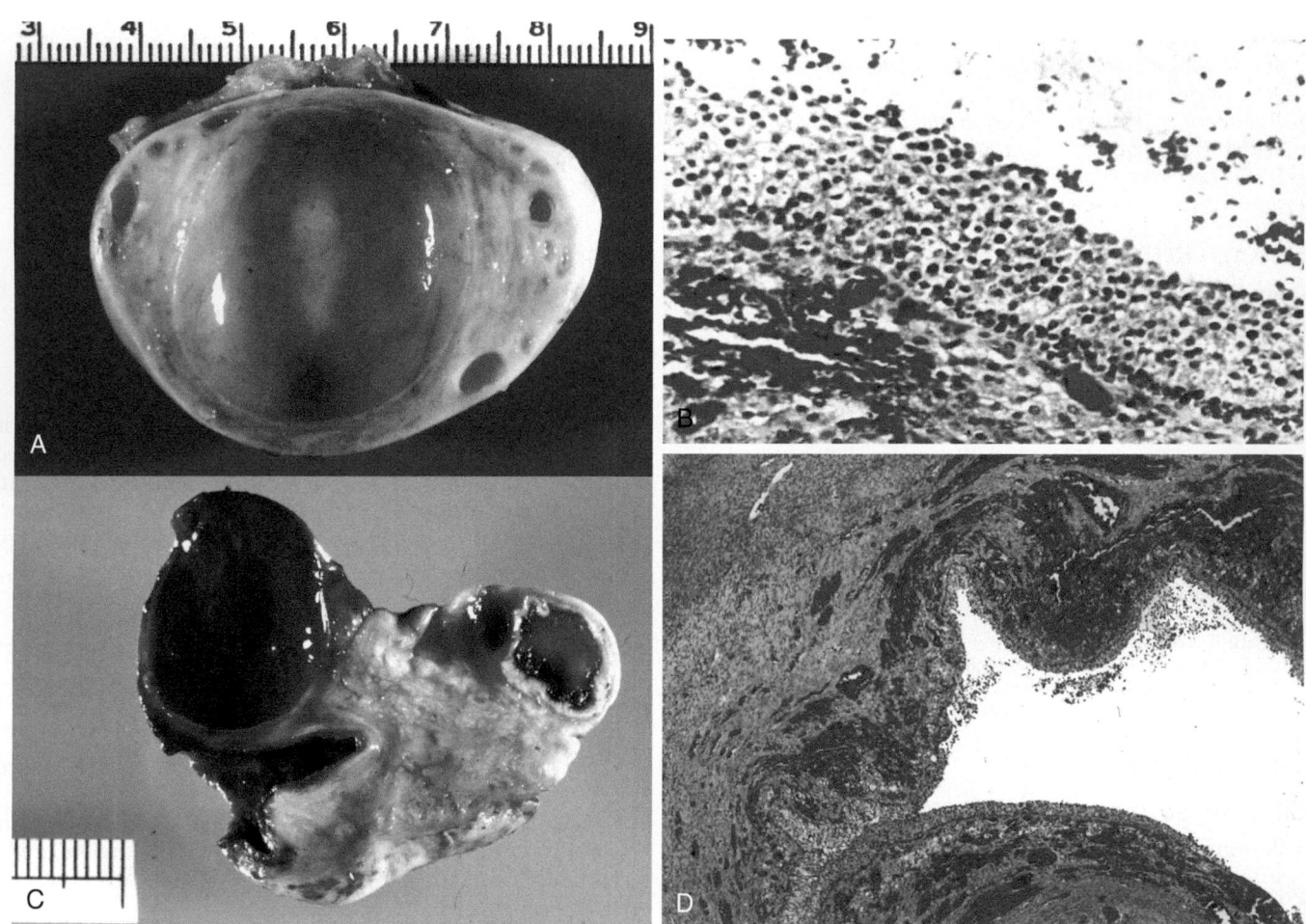

Figure 12-40. A, Follicular cyst. Cross section shows a thin-walled unilocular cyst. **B,** Follicular cyst. The cyst wall is lined by an inner layer of granulosa cells and an outer layer of theca interna cells. **C,** Hemorrhagic corpus luteum. Multiple well-demarcated cysts displaying a yellow rim and intraluminal blood. **D,** Corpus luteum. Low-power view shows a classic convoluted cyst wall surrounded by hemorrhagic stroma.

- Endometriosis must show endometrial glands, stroma, or hemosiderin pigment; the presence of two of the three is diagnostic

PEARLS

- *Most regress spontaneously within 2 months*
- *The large, solitary, luteinized follicular cyst of pregnancy and puerperium is usually an incidental finding during cesarean section or physical examination, with a median diameter of 25 cm; it consists of a lining of luteinized cells with hyperchromatic, pleomorphic nuclei*

SELECTED REFERENCES

Adashi EY, Hennebold JD, Higgins RV, et al: Comparison of fine-needle aspiration cytologic findings of ovarian cysts with ovarian histologic findings. Am J Obstet Gynecol 180:550-553, 1999.
Irving JA, Clement PB: Nonneoplastic lesions of the ovary. In Kurman R, Ellenson LH, Ronnett BM (eds): Blaustein's Pathology of the Female Genital Tract, 6th ed. New York, Springer, 2011, pp 591-594.
Scully RE, Young RH, Clement PB: Atlas of Tumor Pathology: Tumors of the Ovary, Maldeveloped Gonads, Fallopian Tube, and Broad Ligament, 3rd Series, Fascicle 23. Washington, DC, Armed Forces Institute of Pathology, 1998, pp 409-410.

HYPERREACTIO LUTEINALIS

Clinical Features

- Associated with conditions in which high levels of human chorionic gonadotropin (HCG) are secreted, such as pregnancy and gestational trophoblastic disease (GTD)
- Usually asymptomatic, but may present as a palpable mass or abdominal pain related to hemorrhage, torsion, or rupture

Gross Pathology

- Large ovary with multiple bilateral, thin-walled cysts filled with serous or bloody fluid resulting in massive ovarian enlargement

Histopathology

- Large cysts lined by enlarged, luteinized theca interna cells, and sometimes luteinized granulosa and stromal cells
- Ovarian stroma and the theca interna layer may be noticeably edematous

Special Stains and Immunohistochemistry

- Noncontributory

Other Techniques for Diagnosis

- Noncontributory

Differential Diagnosis

LARGE, SOLITARY LUTEINIZED FOLLICLE CYST OF PREGNANCY AND PUERPERIUM

- Ovaries in hyperreactio luteinalis contain multiple cysts

PEARLS

- *Present in about 10% to 45% of women with GTD; the cysts regress after removal of the trophoblastic elements*
- *Rarely coexists with a pregnancy luteoma*

SELECTED REFERENCES

Irving JA, Clement PB: Nonneoplastic lesions of the ovary. In Kurman R, Ellenson LH, Ronnett BM (eds): Blaustein's Pathology of the Female Genital Tract, 6th ed. New York, Springer, 2011, pp 594-596.
Schenker JG: Clinical aspects of ovarian hyperstimulation syndrome. Eur J Obstet Gynecol Reprod Biol 85:13-20, 1999.
Scully RE, Young RH, Clement PB: Atlas of Tumor Pathology: Tumors of the Ovary, Maldeveloped Gonads, Fallopian Tube, and Broad Ligament, 3rd Series, Fascicle 23. Washington, DC, Armed Forces Institute of Pathology, 1998, pp 424-426.

POLYCYSTIC OVARIAN SYNDROME
(Figure 12-41A,B)

Clinical Features

- Characterized by numerous subcortical in particular follicular cysts, in both ovaries, anovulation, infertility, hirsutism, oligomenorrhea, and obesity
- Also known as Stein-Leventhal syndrome; affects 3.5% to 7% of females, usually in the third decade
- Most cases show an increased luteinizing hormone (LH): follicle-stimulating hormone (FSH) ratio, whereas occasional cases show hyperprolactinemia

Gross Pathology

- Both ovaries are round and usually two to five times the normal size
- Many small, superficial cysts visible under a smooth, thick, gray-white outer cortex
- Central homogeneous stroma lacking corpora lutea or albicantia

Histopathology

- Superficial cortex is thickened, hypocellular, and collagenous, frequently with thick-walled blood vessels
- Multiple follicular cysts lined by an inner nonluteinized granulosa and an outer hyperplastic luteinized theca interna (follicular hyperthecosis)
- Corpora lutea are usually absent

Special Stains and Immunohistochemistry

- Noncontributory

Other Techniques for Diagnosis

- Noncontributory

Differential Diagnosis

PREGNANCY

- Luteinization of both granulosa and theca interna

STROMAL HYPERTHECOSIS

- Polycystic ovaries show stromal hyperthecosis, but stromal hyperthecosis, as an entity, is idiopathic

PEARLS

- *Pelvic ultrasound may help in diagnosis*
- *Hyperandrogenemia, with increased conversion of androstenedione to estrone*
- *Endometrium may show hyperplasia or adenocarcinoma in some cases*
- *Virilism is rarely present*

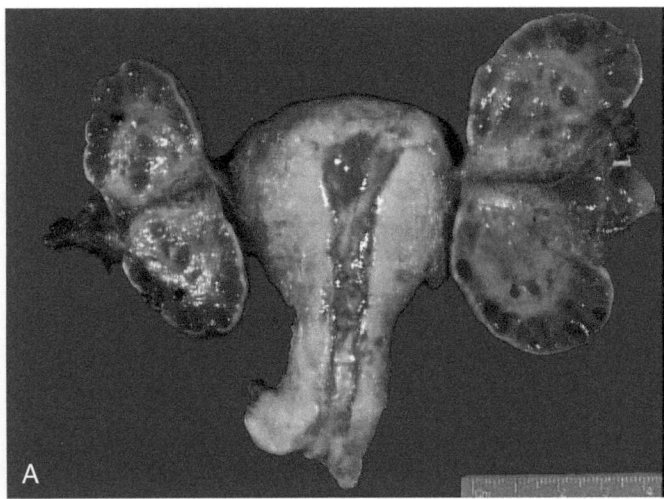
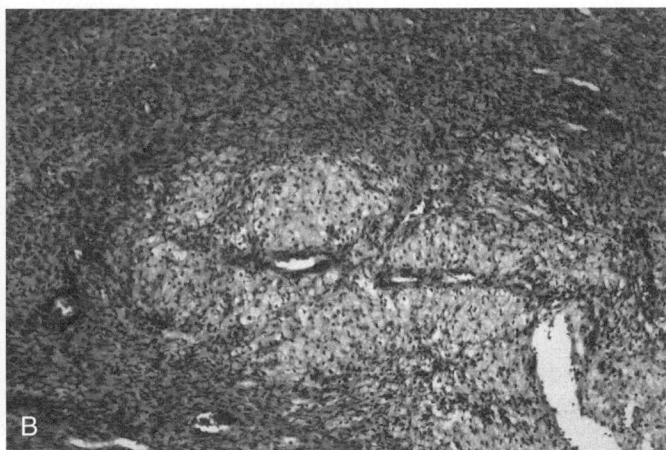

Figure 12-41. Polycystic ovary. A, Cross section of both ovaries show cortical fibrosis and multiple cystic follicles. **B,** Expanded ovarian cortex exhibits focal nodular luteinization.

• *Hyperandrogenism, insulin resistance, and acanthosis nigricans (HAIR-AN) syndrome may be associated and includes insulin resistance, acanthosis nigricans, and hyperandrogenism*

SELECTED REFERENCES

Gordon CM: Menstrual disorders in adolescents: excess androgens and the polycystic ovary syndrome. Pediatr Clin N Am 46:519-543, 1999.

Guzick D: Polycystic ovary syndrome: symptomatology, pathophysiology, and epidemiology. Am J Obstet Gynecol 179:S89-S93, 1998.

Norman RJ, Dewailly D, Legro RS, et al: Polycystic ovary syndrome. Lancet 370:685-697, 2007.

Scully RE, Young RH, Clement PB: Atlas of Tumor Pathology: Tumors of the Ovary, Maldeveloped Gonads, Fallopian Tube, and Broad Ligament, 3rd Series, Fascicle 23. Washington, DC, Armed Forces Institute of Pathology, 1998, pp 410-413.

Taylor AE: Understanding the underlying metabolic abnormalities of polycystic ovary syndrome and their implications. Am J Obstet Gynecol 179: S94-S100, 1998.

STROMAL HYPERPLASIA AND HYPERTHECOSIS

Clinical Features

• Patients with stromal hyperthecosis are usually in their sixth to ninth decades; occasional familial cases
• Stromal hyperthecosis in the premenopausal patient may present as virilization, obesity, hypertension, and glucose intolerance; less often it may resemble polycystic ovarian syndrome; some cases show endometrial hyperplasia or adenocarcinoma
• Stromal hyperplasia typically presents in the sixth or seventh decade and may be associated with androgen hypersecretion, endometrial adenocarcinoma, obesity, hypertension, and decreased glucose tolerance

Gross Pathology

• Bilateral involvement with or without ovarian enlargement
• White or yellow tissue occupies a variable percentage of each ovary
• Nodular hyperthecosis may appear as multiple yellow nodules

Histopathology

• Stromal hyperthecosis exhibits luteinization of stromal cells not attached to the follicles, arranged singly and in clusters; rarely as nodules, with a typical background of stromal hyperplasia (Figure 12-42)
  • Luteinized stromal cells are oval or round with eosinophilic or vacuolated cytoplasm and round, plump nuclei
• Stromal hyperplasia displays minimal collagen production and a diffuse or vaguely nodular proliferation of small stromal cells; the nodules commonly coalesce

Special Stains and Immunohistochemistry

• Oil red O stain: may highlight lipid in vacuolated luteinized cells in stromal hyperthecosis

Other Techniques for Diagnosis

• Noncontributory

Differential Diagnosis

LUTEINIZED THECOMA VERSUS STROMAL HYPERTHECOSIS

• Most thecomas are unilateral and form a distinct nodule or tumor

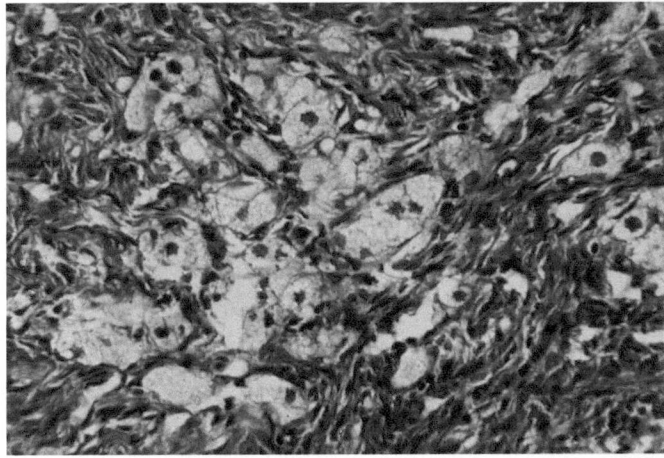

Figure 12-42. Stromal hyperthecosis. Foci of luteinized stromal cells are present within the ovarian stroma.

- The pockets or collections of lutein cells in stromal hyperthecosis are surrounded by small hyperplastic stromal cells with minimal collagen production

FIBROMA VERSUS STROMAL HYPERPLASIA
- Fibroma is composed of cells with larger nuclei and characteristic production of large amounts of collagen; typically measures greater than 3 cm in diameter

LOW-GRADE ENDOMETRIAL STROMAL SARCOMA VERSUS STROMAL HYPERPLASIA
- Endometrial stromal sarcoma of the ovary, which is rare, shows significant ovarian enlargement, marked cellularity, mitotic activity, and regularly distributed arterioles

PEARLS

- *Stromal hyperthecosis, with additional edema and fibrosis, may accompany the HAIR-AN syndrome, which is characterized by hyperandrogenism, insulin resistance, and acanthosis nigricans*

SELECTED REFERENCES

Scully RE, Young RH, Clement PB: Atlas of Tumor Pathology: Tumors of the Ovary, Maldeveloped Gonads, Fallopian Tube, and Broad Ligament, 3rd Series, Fascicle 23. Washington, DC, Armed Forces Institute of Pathology, 1998, pp 413-416.
Sluijmer AV, Heineman MJ, Koudstaal J, et al: Relationship between ovarian production of estrone, estradiol, testosterone, and androstenedione and the ovarian degree of stromal hyperplasia in postmenopausal women. Menopause 5:207-210, 1998.

MASSIVE EDEMA AND FIBROMATOSIS

Clinical Features

- Enlargement of one or both ovaries with peak incidence in the second decade
- Presents with abdominal pain
- Abnormal menstruation and androgenic manifestations may be present

Gross Pathology

- Usually unilateral, sometimes with torsion of the ovarian pedicle
- Massive edema
  - Pearly white ovarian surface with seeping fluid
  - Cut section reveals watery or gelatinous tissue with numerous cystic follicles under the capsule
  - Averages 12 cm in diameter, often with hemorrhage
- Fibromatosis
  - Smooth or lobulated ovarian surface, sometimes with cysts; averages about 11 cm in diameter

Histopathology

MASSIVE EDEMA
- Pale, edematous, hypocellular stroma; spared outer cortex
- Follicles widely separated with venous congestion and lymphatic dilation
- Clusters of lutein cells and foci of fibromatosis may be present

FIBROMATOSIS
- Proliferating spindle cells and collagen production enveloping occasional follicles
- Clusters of lutein cells and foci of edema may be present

Special Stains and Immunohistochemistry
- Noncontributory

Other Techniques for Diagnosis
- Noncontributory

Differential Diagnosis

EDEMATOUS FIBROMA VERSUS MASSIVE EDEMA
- Follicles and their derivatives are present in massive edema

FIBROMA VERSUS FIBROMATOSIS
- Follicles and their derivatives are present in fibromatosis

PEARLS

- *Cortical stromal hyperplasia and hyperthecosis are often associated*

SELECTED REFERENCES

Nielsen GP, Young RH: Fibromatosis of soft tissue type involving the female genital tract: a report of two cases. Int J Gynecol Pathol 16:383-386, 1997.
Scully RE, Young RH, Clement PB: Atlas of Tumor Pathology: Tumors of the Ovary, Maldeveloped Gonads, Fallopian Tube, and Broad Ligament, 3rd Series, Fascicle 23. Washington, DC, Armed Forces Institute of Pathology, 1998, pp 416-420.

PREGNANCY LUTEOMA

Clinical Features
- Ovarian enlargement during pregnancy related to HCG stimulation
- Most patients are black and multiparous; peak incidence in third and fourth decades
- May present with hirsutism or virilization; infants born to such mothers frequently show virilism

Gross Pathology
- Multiple in one half of cases, and bilateral in one third
- Small to large nodules ranging from a few millimeters to 20 cm in diameter
- Soft, well-circumscribed, yellow-brown, or gray on cut surface with areas of hemorrhage

Histopathology
- Well-circumscribed nodules composed of solid proliferations of uniform polygonal cells with abundant eosinophilic, granular cytoplasm (Figure 12-43)
- Nuclei are round and relatively large; may be hyperchromatic with moderate mitotic activity, in a sparse intercellular stroma divided by reticulin fibers into clusters

Special Stains and Immunohistochemistry
- Noncontributory

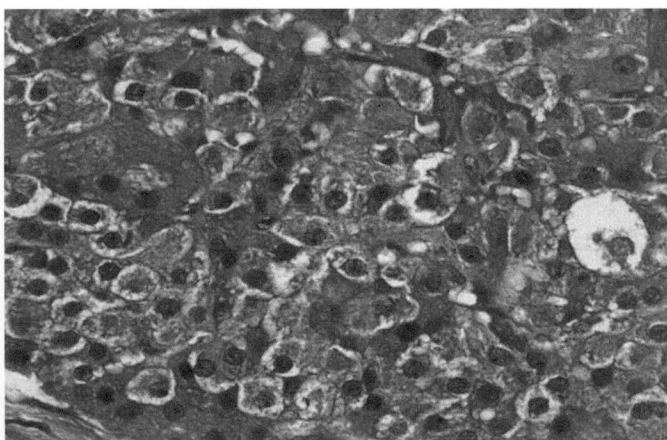

Figure 12-43. Pregnancy luteoma. Solid proliferation of polygonal luteinized cells with abundant eosinophilic granular cytoplasm.

Other Techniques for Diagnosis

- Noncontributory

Differential Diagnosis

LUTEINIZED THECOMA
- Unilateral and unrelated to pregnancy in most cases
- Contains moderate to large amounts of lipid, as opposed to little or no lipid in pregnancy luteoma
- Background of fibroma or typical thecoma with thin reticulin-positive fibers surrounding individual cells rather than clusters

LIPID-POOR STEROID CELL TUMOR
- Both may be virilizing
- Rarely bilateral; if mitotic activity is brisk, more likely to show nuclear atypia

PEARLS

- *Usually an incidental finding*
- *After delivery, the ovaries regress and return to normal size within a few weeks*

SELECTED REFERENCES

Cronje HS, Niemand I, Bam RH, Woodruff JD: Review of the granulosa-theca cell tumors from the Emil Novak ovarian tumor registry. Am J Obstet Gynecol 180:323-327, 1999.

Rodriguez M, Harrison TA, Nowacki MR, Saltzman AK: Luteoma of pregnancy presenting with massive ascites and markedly elevated CA 125. Obstet Gynecol 94:854, 1999.

Scully RE, Young RH, Clement PB: Atlas of Tumor Pathology: Tumors of the Ovary, Maldeveloped Gonads, Fallopian Tube, and Broad Ligament, 3rd Series, Fascicle 23. Washington, DC, Armed Forces Institute of Pathology, 1998, pp 422-424.

ENDOMETRIOSIS

Clinical Features

- Common in women of childbearing age
- Defined as the presence of endometrial tissue outside the uterine corpus
- Complications include rupture or hemorrhage
- May occur in any organ system and mimic neoplasia

Gross Pathology

- Red, blue, or dark-brown nodules or cysts with a raised or puckered appearance, often with fibrous adhesions on involved serosal surfaces
- "Powder burns" refer to ecchymotic or brown areas
- Endometriotic cysts frequently involve the ovaries, are often bilateral, and are usually less than 10 cm in diameter
- Cyst lining is ragged and dark-brown to yellow and contains thick chocolate-colored material (chocolate cyst) (Figure 12-44A)

Histopathology

- Characterized by epithelium and stroma reminiscent of endometrium (Figure 12-44B)
- Hemosiderin-laden macrophages are also usually present
- Appearance varies with hormonal fluctuations of the menstrual cycle
- Menstruation may cause hemorrhage into the glands and stroma with a consequent inflammatory reaction consisting predominantly of histiocytes
- Pseudoxanthoma cells are histiocytes that have transformed the red blood cells into glycolipid, hemofuscin, and hemosiderin pigment
- Postmenopausal women show atrophic glands similar to the endometrium
- Extensive fibrosis may be present

Special Stains and Immunohistochemistry

- CD10 highlights the endometrial stroma

Other Techniques for Diagnosis

- Noncontributory

Differential Diagnosis

ENDOMETRIOID CYSTADENOMA
- Extremely rare and lined by stratified endometrial type epithelium
- Does not contain endometrial-like stroma or pseudoxanthoma cells

HEMORRHAGIC CORPUS LUTEUM CYST VERSUS ENDOMETRIOSIS
- Presence of peripheral theca interna cells and organized blood clot are more typical of a corpus luteum cyst
- Endometriosis requires the presence of endometrial glands, stroma, or hemosiderin pigment (Figure 12-44C)

PEARLS

- *Hyperplastic and atypically proliferating changes similar to those seen in the endometrium may be present (i.e., hyperplasia, metaplasia)*
- *About 0.5% of cases have a malignant neoplasm arising from the endometriotic lesion; associated with a hyperestrogenic state*
- *Endometrioid and clear cell adenocarcinoma are the most frequent associations*

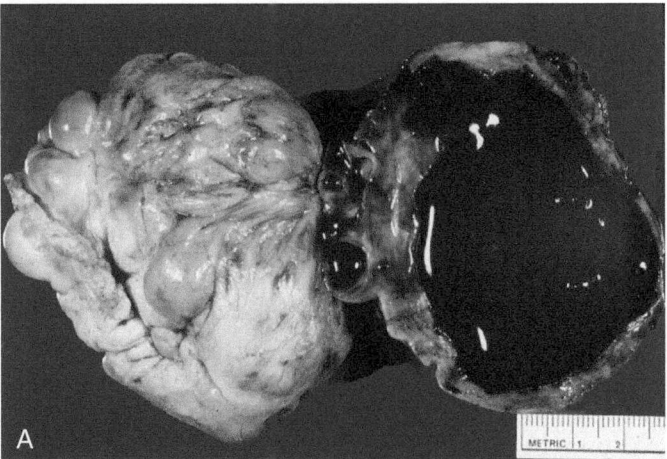

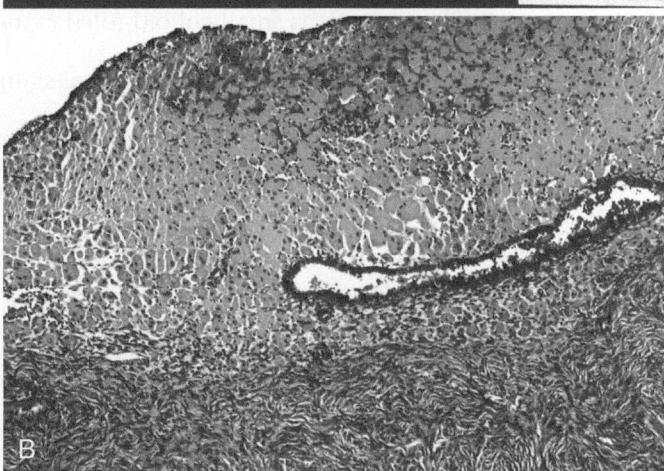

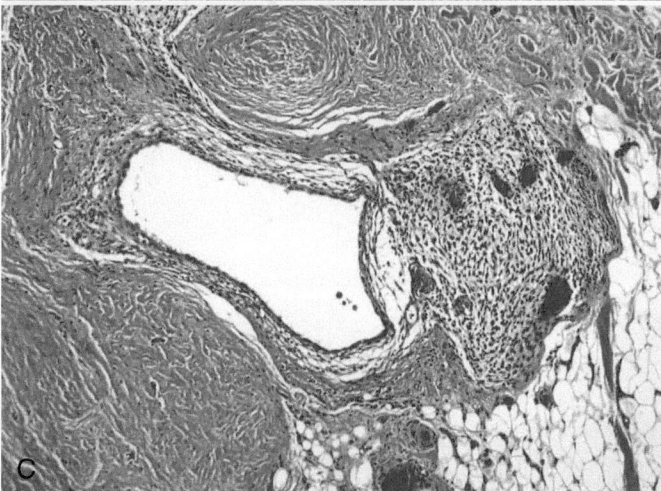

Figure 12-44. Endometrioma. A, Cystic ovary filled with blood and with a glistening external surface. **B,** Cyst lined by cuboidal epithelium associated with endometrial stroma and hemosiderin-laden macrophages. Adjacent ovarian stroma can be seen. **C,** Endometriosis, presenting as an abdominal mass. Endometrial glands, stroma, and adjacent adipose tissue can be seen.

SELECTED REFERENCES

Clement PB: The pathology of endometriosis: a survey of the many faces of a common disease emphasizing diagnostic pitfalls and unusual and newly appreciated aspects. Adv Anat Pathol 14:241-260, 2007.

Miyakoshi K, Tanaka M, Gabionza D, et al: Decidualized ovarian endometriosis mimicking malignancy. AJR Am J Roentgenol 171:1625-1626, 1998.

Scully RE, Young RH, Clement PB: Atlas of Tumor Pathology: Tumors of the Ovary, Maldeveloped Gonads, Fallopian Tube, and Broad Ligament, 3rd Series, Fascicle 23. Washington, DC, Armed Forces Institute of Pathology, 1998, pp 430-434.

Wells M: Recent advances in endometriosis with emphasis on pathogenesis, molecular pathology, and neoplastic transformation. Int Gynecol Pathol 23:316-320, 2004.

SURFACE EPITHELIAL-STROMAL TUMORS

These are the most common tumors of the ovary. Table 12-1 shows the pathogenesis of ovarian cancer.

SEROUS TUMORS

BENIGN SEROUS TUMORS
(Figure 12-45A-C)

Clinical Features

- Common ovarian neoplasms with a peak incidence in the fifth decade
- Makes up about 70% of all serous tumors
- One of the two most common ovarian neoplasms seen in pregnancy

Gross Pathology

- Bilateral in about 10% of cases
- Cystadenomas: usually one (sometimes more) smooth, glistening, thin-walled cyst filled with clear, watery, serous (occasionally mucinous or hemorrhagic) fluid
- Papillary cystadenomas: inner lining with small polypoid excrescences and an underlying cystic component
- Surface papillomas: coarse papillary projections on the outer surface of the ovary without a cystic cavity
- Adenofibromas and cystadenofibromas are predominantly solid fibrous tumors with a variable number of fluid-filled glands or cysts and firm papillary excrescences

TABLE 12-1	**PATHOGENESIS OF OVARIAN CANCER**

Type I
Low grade with a precursor lesion in a stepwise fashion
—Represented by cystadenomas and borderline tumors
—Most often presents at stage 1; slow growing, indolent
—Generally remains low grade but can progress to high grade
—*K-ras/BRAF* mutations in 65%, and *TP53* mutation in 8%
Includes
—Serous carcinoma (grade 1)
—Mucinous, endometrioid, and clear cell carcinomas and transitional cell carcinoma (Brenner and non-Brenner)
Type II
High grade, arises de novo, and most often presents at a high stage
Rapidly growing, aggressive
About 70% have *p53* mutation, whereas *K-ras/BRAF* mutation is rare (1%)
Includes
—Serous carcinoma (grade 2 or 3)
—Malignant mixed müllerian tumor (carcinosarcoma)

Histopathology

- In general, serous neoplasms mimic the epithelium of the fallopian tube
- Cysts, papillae, and glands are lined mainly by a single layer of cuboidal to low-columnar ciliated cells without significant nuclear atypia; they may also be lined by nonciliated cuboidal to columnar secretory cells (Figure 12-45E-G)
- Epithelium may be flattened by accumulated serous fluid in the lumen
- Stroma varies from dense and fibrous to distinctly edematous (Figure 12-45H)
- Psammoma bodies may be rarely present
- Variants include cystadenoma and papillary cystadenoma, surface papilloma, and adenofibroma and cystadenofibroma
- Cystadenofibromas are characterized by broad fibrous papillary structures lined by epithelium, which is generally serous; other epithelia (i.e., mucinous, etc.) are less common

Special Stains and Immunohistochemistry

- Noncontributory

Other Techniques for Diagnosis

- Noncontributory

Differential Diagnosis

EPITHELIAL INCLUSION CYST VERSUS SMALL SEROUS CYSTADENOMA

- Epithelial inclusion cyst is less than 1 cm in diameter

FOLLICLE CYST VERSUS SEROUS CYSTADENOMA

- Both may have an atrophic lining, but the presence of a theca interna layer and inner granulosa cells points toward follicle cyst
- May be diagnosed as simple cyst if the morphology of the lining is unclear

STRUMA OVARII VERSUS SEROUS CYSTADENOMA

- Struma ovarii always contains small colloid-filled cysts
- Histologically identical to thyroid tissue
- Positive for thyroglobulin immunohistochemical stain (Figure 12-45I)

RETE CYSTADENOMA VERSUS SEROUS CYSTADENOMA

- Rete cystadenomas are rare tumors arising in the rete ovarii (ovarian hilus)

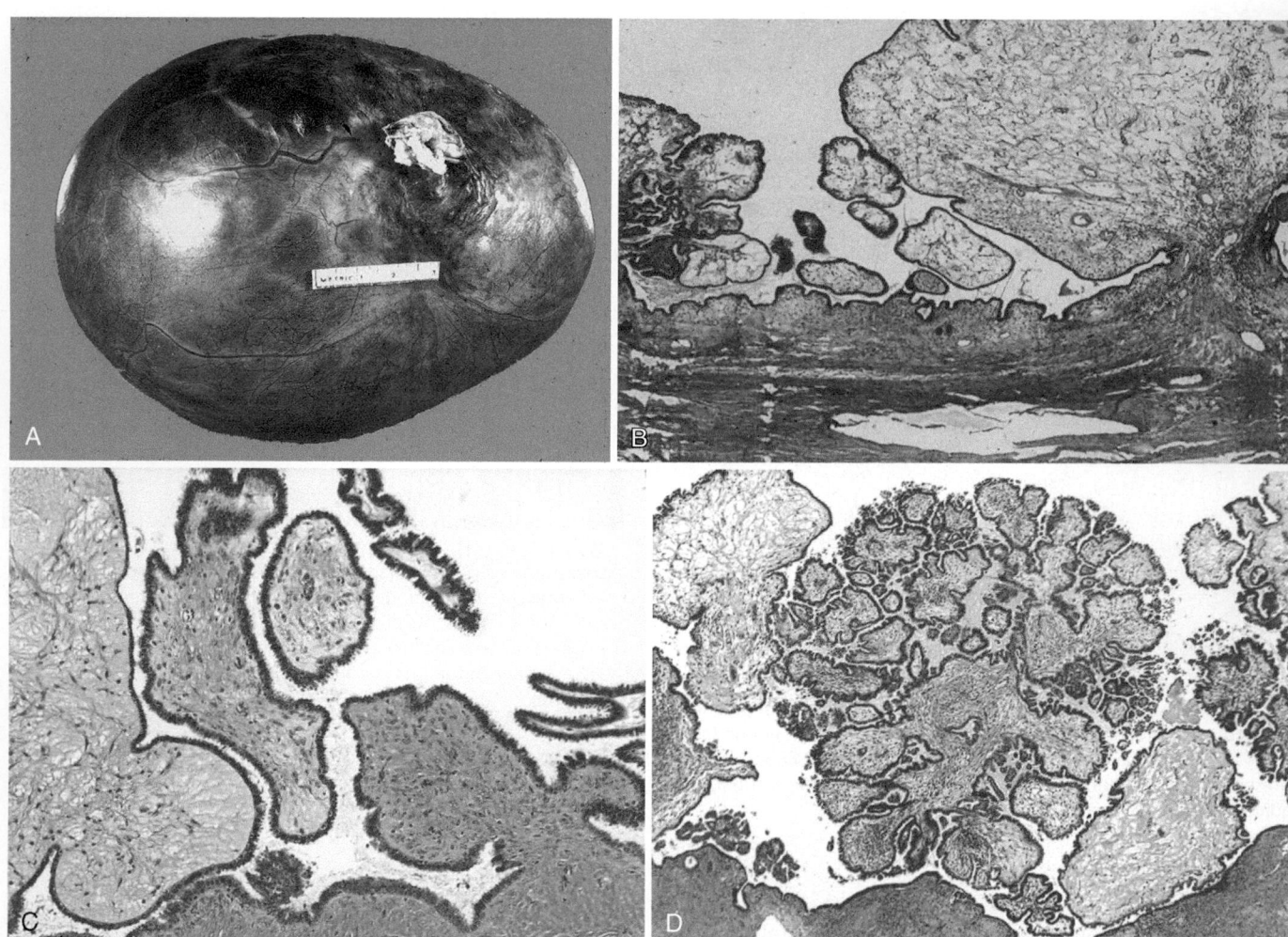

Figure 12-45. A, Benign serous tumor. The external surface of the cyst is smooth and glistening with a marked vascular pattern. **B,** Benign serous tumor. Papillary structures lined by a single layer of cuboidal epithelium. **C,** Serous cystadenofibroma. Papillary structures with a prominent stromal component. **D,** Borderline serous tumor. Cystic ovary showing tan to yellow papillary excrescences.

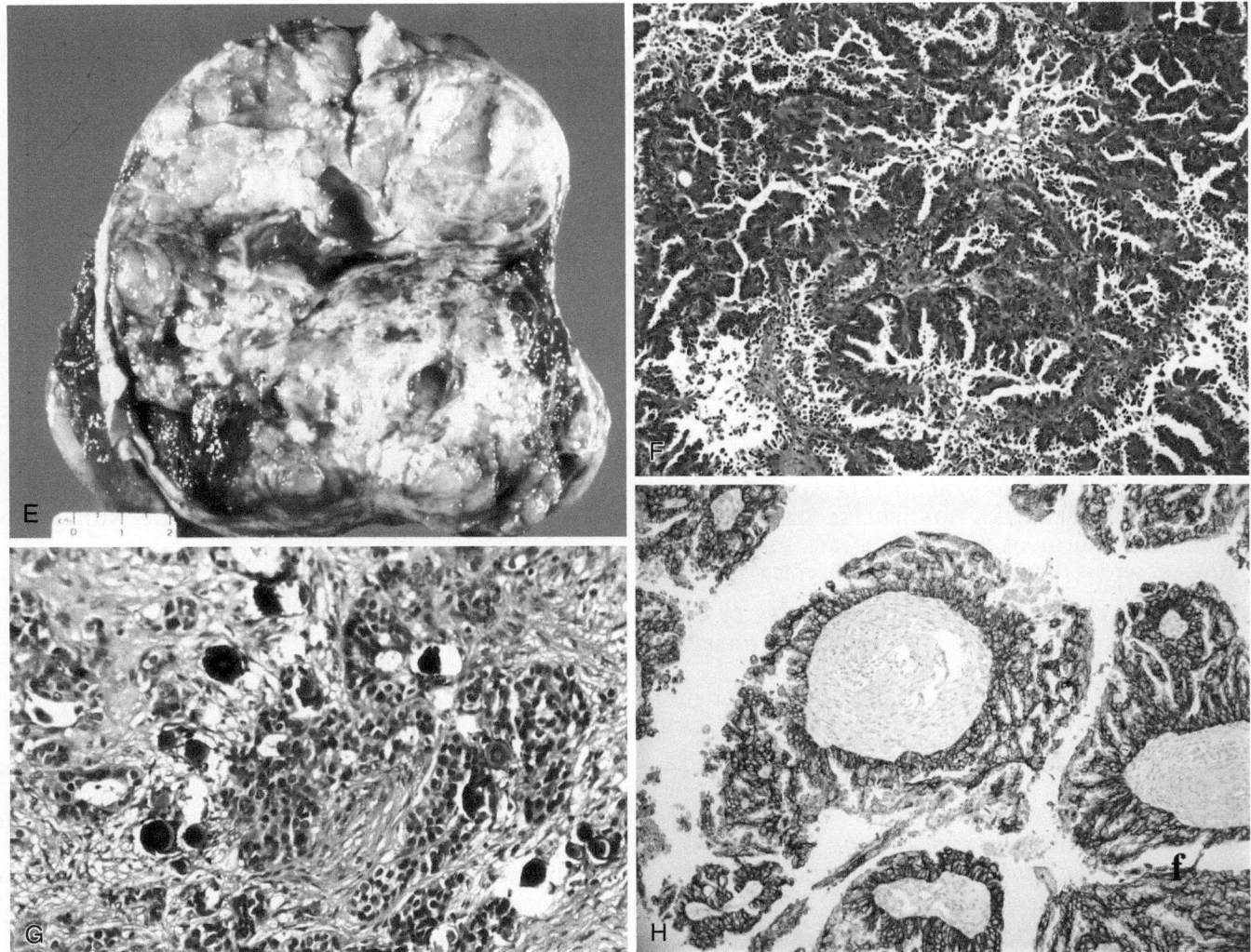

Figure 12-45—cont'd E, Serous borderline tumor. Complex branching papillae lined by stratified epithelial cells with formation of cellular buds. **F,** Papillary serous carcinoma. Cut surface shows a solid tumor with focal cystic changes. **G,** Papillary serous carcinoma. Moderately differentiated tumor composed of crowded papillae lined by pleomorphic cells. **H,** Papillary serous carcinoma. Poorly differentiated tumor invading into the surrounding stroma. Several psammoma bodies are evident. **I,** Serous carcinoma of the ovary. WT-1 stain is strongly positive, confirming the serous differentiation. Coexpression of *p53* is also characteristic of high grade ovarian serous carcinoma.

- Lined by nonciliated epithelium, showing crevices along their inner surfaces
- Smooth muscle and hilus cells commonly present in their walls

PEARLS

- *Cystectomy, or oophorectomy is curative*

SELECTED REFERENCE

Scully RE, Young RH, Clement PB: Atlas of Tumor Pathology: Tumors of the Ovary, Maldeveloped Gonads, Fallopian Tube, and Broad Ligament, 3rd Series, Fascicle 23. Washington, DC, Armed Forces Institute of Pathology, 1998, pp 51-79.

ATYPICAL PROLIFERATIVE SEROUS TUMOR (SEROUS BORDERLINE TUMOR) (Figure 12-45D-E)

Clinical Features

- Peak incidence between 30 and 60 years of age
- Makes up 5% to 10% of all serous tumors

Gross Pathology

- Bilateral in 25% to 30% of cases
- Gross is similar to that of benign tumors or with excrescences on the surface
- Cysts lined by abundant, fine, somewhat firm papillary projections

Histopathology

- Complex, hierarchical branching papillae with small papillary projections on the surface lined by epithelium showing cellular buds and nuclear stratification
- No destructive stromal invasion
- Cells generally have scant cytoplasm and bland nuclei but may have moderate to abundant eosinophilic cytoplasm with round hyperchromatic nuclei and obvious nucleoli
- Psammoma bodies may be present
- Micropapillary serous carcinoma (MPSC) with no stromal invasion is regarded as variant of atypical proliferative serous tumor and is regarded as low-grade carcinoma

- Tumor is characterized by long, thin, nonhierarchical papillae without fibrovascular support arising from edematous large papillae without invasion of the stroma
- Variants are similar to those listed in benign serous tumors
- Peritoneal implants: proliferating epithelium with complex glands with or without psammoma bodies resembling the ovarian tumor, which are not regarded as metastasis
  - Implants may also be identified in lymph nodes

Special Stains and Immunohistochemistry

- Weak or negative *p53* essentially excludes high-grade serous carcinoma
- WT-1 positive

Other Techniques for Diagnosis

- Noncontributory

Differential Diagnosis

ENDOCERVICAL-LIKE BORDERLINE MUCINOUS TUMOR VERSUS MUCIN-SECRETING BORDERLINE SEROUS TUMOR
- Borderline mucinous tumor cells are mucin filled, whereas serous tumors contain merely apical mucin

RETIFORM SERTOLI-LEYDIG CELL TUMOR (SLCT)
- Peak incidence in first decade, sometimes presenting with androgenic manifestations
- Tubular and cystic structures lined by one or more layers of cells with round, regular nuclei and scanty cytoplasm

PEARLS

- *Surgical excision of tumors confined to the ovaries results in survival without recurrence in the majority (> 95%) of patients*
- *Postoperative recurrences can occur many years later*

SELECTED REFERENCES

Burks RT, Kurman RJ, Seidman JD, Shih IM: Serous borderline tumours of the ovary. Histopathology 47:310-315, 2005.
Gershenson DM, Silva EG, Tortolero-Luna G, et al: Serous borderline tumors of the ovary with noninvasive peritoneal implants. Cancer 83:2157-2163, 1998.
Hart WR: Borderline epithelial tumors of the ovary. Mod Pathol 18(suppl 2):S33-S50, 2005.
Kurman RJ, Shih IM: Pathogenesis of ovarian cancer: lessons from morphology and molecular biology and their clinical implications. Int J Gynecol Pathol 27:151-160, 2008.
Seidman JD, Kurman RJ: Subclassification of serous borderline tumors of the ovary into benign and malignant types: a clinicopathologic study of 65 advanced stage cases. Am J Surg Pathol 20:1331-1345, 1996.
Yemelyanova A, Mao TL, Nakayama N, et al: Low-grade serous carcinoma of the ovary displaying a macropapillary pattern of invasion. Am J Surg Pathol 32:1800-1806, 2008.

SEROUS CARCINOMA LOW GRADE (MICROPAPILLARY OR PSAMMOMATOUS)

Clinical Features

- Mean age of patients is 45 for micropapillary (Figure 12-45F-I); psammocarcinomas have a mean age of 54
- Asymptomatic pelvic mass in low stage
- Abdominal pain, fullness, or distention are common in advanced stage
- Well-differentiated low-grade tumor micropapillary is the most common pattern and cribriform is less frequent

Gross Pathology

- Bilaterality in 80% to 90%, and greater than 90% are advanced stage tumors
- Tumors with an exophytic component are more often associated with advance-stage cancer
- Tumors are generally cystic with papillary, tan to yellow excrescences
- Psammocarcinoma is most often of peritoneal origin

Histopathology

- Large, edematous bulbous papillae from which emanate smaller papillae with nonhierarchical branching of fine lacelike pattern with low-grade nuclei infiltrating the ovarian stroma
- Glands and tubules arranged in a cribriform fashion lined by mild to moderately atypical cuboidal cells
- Psammoma bodies are present in most well-differentiated papillary tumors
  - The tumor cells show low-grade nuclei with only occasional mitotic figures
  - Psammocarcinoma features numerous psammoma bodies with a scarce epithelial component

HIGH GRADE

Clinical Features

- Most common malignant ovarian neoplasm, with a peak incidence between 40 and 70 years of age and constituting about 20% to 25% of all serous tumors
- Serum shows elevated level of CA-125 (not specific for serous tumors or malignancy)
- The great majority originate in the fimbria of either fallopian tubes

Gross Pathology

- Bilateral in about 65% of cases
- Well-differentiated forms are partly solid, but mostly cystic, papillary tumors
- Surface serous carcinomas include large hemorrhagic papillary excrescences on the surface of the ovary
- Poorly differentiated tumors show solid areas of friable, necrotic, and hemorrhagic tissue with few recognizable papillae
- Tumor adhesion to adjacent structures is common

Histopathology

- Cellular tumor with obvious invasion of the connective tissue stroma (desmoplasia)
- May contain few papillae, which are generally thick, but the tumors are mostly composed of solid sheets of cells with pleomorphic nuclei
- Hyperchromatic nuclei and atypical mitoses are characteristic of high-grade tumors along with cellular budding and stratification
- Variants include cystadenocarcinoma, surface carcinoma, and carcinoma arising in adenofibroma
- In the majority of cases the fallopian tube shows serous tubal intraepithelial carcinoma (STIC)

Special Stains and Immunohistochemistry

- Vimentin positive
- CA-125 positive

- More than 60% of high-grade tumors and less than 10% of low-grade tumors positive for p53
- Cytokeratin, WT-1, and EMA positive

Other Techniques for Diagnosis
- Noncontributory

Differential Diagnosis
PAPILLARY CLEAR CELL CARCINOMA VERSUS PAPILLARY SEROUS CARCINOMA
- Clear cell carcinoma displays plump hobnail cells with large nuclei, cells with clear cytoplasm, or oxyphilic cells
- Papillae are more regular and may have hyalinized cores

ENDOMETRIOID CARCINOMA VERSUS POORLY DIFFERENTIATED SEROUS CARCINOMA
- Papillae and glands in endometrioid carcinoma are larger and more regular (villoglandular), without cellular budding
- Squamous differentiation is commonly associated with endometrioid carcinoma and rarely with serous carcinoma
- Psammoma bodies are rare in endometrioid carcinomas

ADULT GRANULOSA CELL TUMOR (AGCT) VERSUS SOLID SEROUS CARCINOMA
- Cell necrosis in serous carcinoma may be confused for Call-Exner bodies
- Serous carcinomas are positive for EMA and diffusely positive for keratin 8/18, whereas EMA is negative in AGCT, and keratin 8/18 shows focal positivity only
- Inhibin is positive in AGCT and generally negative in serous carcinoma; likewise with calretinin

RETIFORM SLCT
- Rare tumor with a peak incidence in first decade, sometimes presenting with androgenic manifestations
- Tubular and cystic structures; tubules lined by one or more layers of cells with round, regular nuclei and scanty cytoplasm; most retiform tumors are seen with other SLCT subtypes

PEARLS
- *Most high-grade tumors show extensive intraperitoneal dissemination at diagnosis*

SELECTED REFERENCES
Burks RT, Sherman ME, Kurman RJ: Micropapillary serous carcinoma of the ovary: a distinctive low-grade carcinoma related to serous borderline tumors. Am J Surg Pathol 20:1319-1330, 1996.

Dehari R, Kurman RJ, Logani S, Shih IM: The development of high-grade serous carcinoma from atypical proliferative (borderline) serous tumors and low-grade micropapillary serous carcinoma: a morphologic and molecular genetic analysis. Am J Surg Pathol 31:1007-1012, 2007.

Kobel M, Kalloger SE, Baker PM, et al: Diagnosis of ovarian carcinoma cell type is highly reproducible: a transcanadian study. Am J Surg Pathol 34:984-993, 2010.

Kurman RJ, Shih IM: Pathogenesis of ovarian cancer: lessons from morphology and molecular biology and their clinical implications. Int J Gynecol Pathol 27:151-160, 2008.

Kurman RJ, Shih I-M: The origin and pathogenesis of epithelial ovarian cancer: a proposed unifying theory. Am J Surg Pathol 34:433-443, 2010.

Seidman JD, Yemelyanova A, Zaino RJ, Kurman RJ: The fallopian tube-peritoneal junction: a potential site of carcinogenesis. Int J Gynecol Pathol 30:4-11, 2011.

MUCINOUS TUMORS
BENIGN MUCINOUS TUMOR
Clinical Features
- Make up about 75% to 85% of all mucinous tumors
- Peak incidence in fourth and fifth decades
- Most common epithelial tumor in pregnancy
- Signs and symptoms may be related to acute torsion

Gross Pathology
- Bilateral in 2% to 4% of cases
- Large, mucin-filled, multiloculated tumor with a smooth inner lining (Figure 12-46A)
- Stromal component of adenofibroma is firm and fibrous

Histopathology
- In general, mucinous tumors mimic endocervical and intestinal epithelium
- Cysts, papillary structures, and cryptlike structures are lined by a single layer of columnar cells with clear, apical mucin and small basally located nuclei (picket fence–like) or intestinal-type epithelium with goblet cells (Figure 12-46B)
- Fibrocollagenous walls and stroma
- Mucinous tumors may have argyrophil and Paneth cells
- Variants include cystadenoma and adenofibroma or cystadenofibroma

Special Stains and Immunohistochemistry
- PAS highlights mucinous material
- Cytokeratin 7 is generally positive

Other Techniques for Diagnosis
- Noncontributory

Differential Diagnosis
SEROUS CYSTADENOMA
- Mucinous cystadenomas may have a cuboidal epithelium similar to serous cystadenoma, but with intracytoplasmic mucin and without ciliated cells

HETEROLOGOUS SLCT
- Contains glands and cysts lined by mucinous epithelium that may be similar to the lining in benign mucinous tumors
- Foci of SLCT of intermediate differentiation are characterized by cords of darkly staining Sertoli cells separated by a stroma containing Leydig cells with abundant eosinophilic cytoplasm
- Areas of immature skeletal muscle, cartilage, or both may be seen

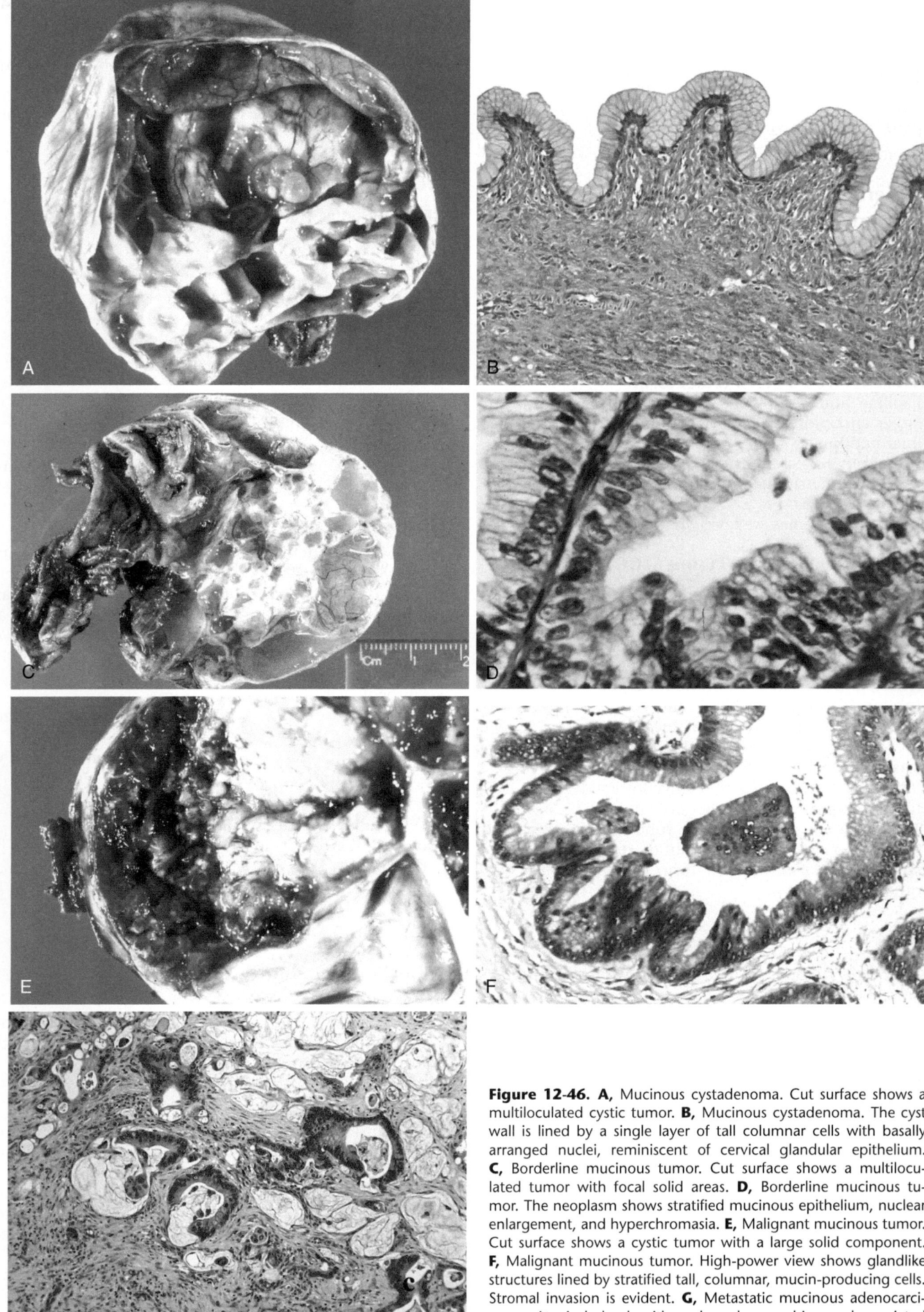

Figure 12-46. A, Mucinous cystadenoma. Cut surface shows a multiloculated cystic tumor. **B,** Mucinous cystadenoma. The cyst wall is lined by a single layer of tall columnar cells with basally arranged nuclei, reminiscent of cervical glandular epithelium. **C,** Borderline mucinous tumor. Cut surface shows a multiloculated tumor with focal solid areas. **D,** Borderline mucinous tumor. The neoplasm shows stratified mucinous epithelium, nuclear enlargement, and hyperchromasia. **E,** Malignant mucinous tumor. Cut surface shows a cystic tumor with a large solid component. **F,** Malignant mucinous tumor. High-power view shows glandlike structures lined by stratified tall, columnar, mucin-producing cells. Stromal invasion is evident. **G,** Metastatic mucinous adenocarcinoma. Atypical glands with nuclear pleomorphism and associated mucin infiltrate the omentum. An ovarian primary is unlikely.

Mucinous Carcinoid Tumor versus Epithelial Mucinous Tumor

- Mucinous carcinoid tumors are mostly solid and only rarely predominantly cystic on gross examination
- Argyrophil and argentaffin cells may be present in mucinous carcinoid tumors but are less abundant
- Generally positive for chromogranin and synaptophysic immunostains

PEARLS

- *Mucinous tumors are associated with dermoid cysts in 3% to 5% of cases, along with appendiceal mucoceles and pseudomyxoma peritonei*
- *Mucinous cystadenomas are associated with benign transitional cell tumors (Brenner)*
- *Pseudomyxoma peritonei: condition featuring extensive mucinous ascites, cystic and bland epithelial implants on the peritoneal surfaces, and adhesions most commonly in association with an appendiceal lesion (e.g., mucocele) or, less likely, mucinous ovarian tumor*
- *Treatment consists of surgical excision of the tumor*
- *Important to thoroughly sample tumor to exclude areas of borderline or malignancy*

SELECTED REFERENCES

Hart WR: Mucinous tumors of the ovary: a review. Int J Gynecol Pathol 24:4-25, 2005.

Hristov AC, Young RH, Vang R, et al: Ovarian metastases of appendiceal tumors with goblet cell carcinoidlike and signet ring cell patterns: a report of 30 cases. Am J Surg Pathol 31:1502-1511, 2007.

Raab SS, Robinson RA, Jensen CS, et al: Mucinous tumors of the ovary: interobserver diagnostic variability and utility of sectioning protocols. Arch Pathol Lab Med 121:1192-1198, 1997.

Scully RE, Young RH, Clement PB: Atlas of Tumor Pathology: Tumors of the Ovary, Maldeveloped Gonads, Fallopian Tube, and Broad Ligament, 3rd Series, Fascicle 23. Washington, DC, Armed Forces Institute of Pathology, 1998, pp 81-105.

Shiohara S, Shiozawa T, Shimizu M, et al: Histochemical analysis of estrogen and progesterone receptors and gastric-type mucin in mucinous ovarian tumors with reference to their pathogenesis. Cancer 80:908-916, 1997.

Yemelyanova AV, Vang R, Judson K, et al: Distinction of primary and metastatic mucinous tumors involving the ovary: analysis of size and laterality data by primary site with reevaluation of an algorithm for tumor classification. Am J Surg Pathol 32:128-138, 2008.

ATYPICAL PROLIFERATIVE MUCINOUS TUMOR (MUCINOUS BORDERLINE TUMOR)

Clinical Features

- Makes up about 10% to 15% of all mucinous tumors
- Peak incidence in third to fifth decades; intestinal-type tumors present later than endocervical-like tumors
- Tumors consisting of mostly intestinal-type cells are more common
- Occasional cases show elevation in serum inhibin

Gross Pathology

- Bilateral in about 7% of intestinal-type tumors and 40% of endocervical-like tumors; both types are the largest ovarian epithelial tumors
- Averages 15 to 20 cm in diameter
- Similar to benign mucinous tumor in gross appearance, but the cyst lining shows bulging masses and papillary projections more often (Figure 12-46C)
- Intestinal-type tumors are usually larger and more loculated

Histopathology

- Increased crowding of cysts, glands, and papillae, with areas of glandular budding, nuclear atypia, and stratification, but lacking destructive stromal invasion (Figure 12-46D)
- Tumor cells are usually mucin filled and have irregular nuclei, large nucleoli, and increased mitotic activity
- Most show mixed mucinous differentiation (intestinal and/or endocervical)
- Tumors made up of predominantly endocervical-like cells are less common and are often associated with infiltration by acute inflammatory cells
- Foreign-body giant cells may be seen in association with mucin from ruptured cysts
- Variants include mucinous adenofibroma

Special Stains and Immunohistochemistry

- CK7 and mucin positive

Other Techniques for Diagnosis

- Noncontributory

Differential Diagnosis

HETEROLOGOUS SLCT

- Contains glands and cysts lined by areas of mucinous epithelium, which may be similar to a borderline mucinous tumor
- Foci of SLCT of intermediate differentiation also seen, with cords of darkly staining Sertoli cells separated by a stroma containing Leydig cells with abundant eosinophilic cytoplasm
- Areas of immature skeletal muscle, cartilage, or both may be seen

PEARLS

- *More than 95% of mucinous carcinomas are of gastrointestinal origin, appendiceal in particular*
- *Intestinal-type tumors may be associated with pseudomyxoma peritonei but are less likely to have associated endometriosis than endocervical-like tumors*
- *Surgical excision of tumors confined to the ovaries may occasionally be associated with recurrence, spread, and rarely death*
- *Important to thoroughly sample tumor to exclude areas of invasive malignant tumor*

SELECTED REFERENCES

Bradley RF, Stewart JH, Russell GB, et al: Pseudomyxoma peritonei of appendiceal origin: a clinicopathologic analysis of 101 patients uniformly treated at a single institution, with literature review. Am J Surg Pathol 30:551-559, 2006.

Ronnett BM, Kurman RJ, Zahn CM, et al: Pseudomyxoma peritonei in women: a clinicopathologic study of 30 cases with emphasis on site of origin, prognosis and relationship to ovarian mucinous tumors of low malignant potential. Hum Pathol 56:509-524, 1995.

Ronnett BM, Shmookler BM, Sugarbaker PH, Kurman RJ: Pseudomyxoma peritonei: new concepts in diagnosis, origin, nomenclature, and relationship to mucinous borderline (low malignant potential) tumors of the ovary. Anat Pathol 2:197-226, 1997.

Seidman JD, Elsayed AM, Sobin LH, Tavassoli FA: Association of mucinous tumors of the ovary and appendix: a clinicopathologic study of 25 cases. Am J Surg Pathol 17:22-34, 1993.

Szych C, Staebler A, Connolly DC, et al: Molecular genetic evidence supporting the clonality and appendiceal origin of pseudomyxoma peritonei in women. Am J Pathol 154:1849-1855, 1999.

MUCINOUS CARCINOMA (MALIGNANT MUCINOUS TUMOR) (Figure 12-46E-G)

Clinical Features

- Makes up about <5% of all mucinous tumors
- Peak incidence in fourth to seventh decades
- Some patients show elevated levels of CEA, CA-19-9, inhibin, and CA-125

Gross Pathology

- Bilateral in <20% of cases
- Cystic spaces with papillae mixed with solid masses; sometimes the tumor is completely solid
- Hemorrhage and necrosis have been reported

Histopathology

- Cellular tumor containing crowded glands, cysts, papillae, or solid sheets of stratified mucinous cells, with stromal invasion by single or small groups of cells or glands, displaying a desmoplastic stromal response
- Cells with hyperchromatic nuclei, atypical mitoses with eosinophilic cytoplasm, and abundant mucin, sometimes with signet ring forms
- Large pools of extracellular mucin with associated histiocytes and less often a foreign-body giant cell reaction
- Variants include mucinous carcinoma arising in mucinous adenofibroma

Special Stains and Immunohistochemistry

- Vimentin negative
- Cytokeratin 7 and 20 positive
- CEA: positive cytoplasmic staining

Other Techniques for Diagnosis

- Noncontributory

Differential Diagnosis

SEROUS AND ENDOMETRIOID ADENOCARCINOMAS

- May contain abundant luminal mucin but minimal intracytoplasmic mucin
- WT-1 positive in serous, negative in endometrioid and mucinous
- CEA positive in mucinous, negative in serous and endometrioid

HETEROLOGOUS SLCT

- Contains glands and cysts lined by areas of mucinous epithelium, which may be similar to a malignant mucinous tumor
- Foci of SLCT of intermediate differentiation showing cords of darkly staining Sertoli cells separated by

stroma containing Leydig cells with abundant eosinophilic cytoplasm
- Areas of immature skeletal muscle, cartilage, or both may be seen

KRUKENBERG TUMOR

- Metastatic mucin-secreting adenocarcinoma with signet ring cells originating from an extragenital source
- Breast and gastrointestinal tract are the most common primary sites
- Contains goblet cells in the stroma and is usually bilateral

PEARLS

- *Treatment consists of surgery, sometimes with chemotherapy depending on the stage and grade of the tumor*
- *About 40% 5-year survival rate, with recurrences often occurring in the lungs*

SELECTED REFERENCES

Raab SS, Robinson RA, Jensen CS, et al: Mucinous tumors of the ovary: interobserver diagnostic variability and utility of sectioning protocols. Arch Pathol Lab Med 121:1192-1198, 1997.

Scully RE, Young RH, Clement PB: Atlas of Tumor Pathology: Tumors of the Ovary, Maldeveloped Gonads, Fallopian Tube, and Broad Ligament, 3rd Series, Fascicle 23. Washington, DC, Armed Forces Institute of Pathology, 1998, pp 81-105.

Seidman JD, Kurman RJ, Ronnett BM: Primary and metastatic mucinous adenocarcinomas in the ovaries: incidence in routine practice with a new approach to improve intraoperative diagnosis. Am J Surg Pathol 27:985-993, 2003.

Tabrizi AD, Kalloger SE, Kobel M: Primary ovarian mucinous carcinoma of intestinal type: significance of pattern of invasion and immunohistochemical expression profile in a series of 31 cases. Int J Gynecol Pathol 29:99-107, 2010.

ENDOMETRIOID TUMORS

Clinical Features

- Most are malignant; benign and borderline variants are rare
- Peak incidence in fifth decade; women with endometrioid carcinoma and endometriosis in the same ovary are 5 to 10 years younger on average
- May be associated with ovarian or pelvic endometriosis and endometrial carcinoma; serum CA-125 is elevated in most cases

Gross Pathology

- Most tumors are unilateral; about 30% of malignant tumors are bilateral
- Similar in gross appearance to previously mentioned tumors but may contain obvious foci of endometriosis
- Carcinomas measure up to 20 cm in diameter, are predominantly solid, but may contain papillae; some contain cysts are filled with bloody or mucinous fluid

Histopathology

- In general, endometrioid tumors mimic the epithelium of the endometrium, containing cells with basophilic cytoplasm, elongated nuclei, and obvious nucleoli (Figure 12-47)

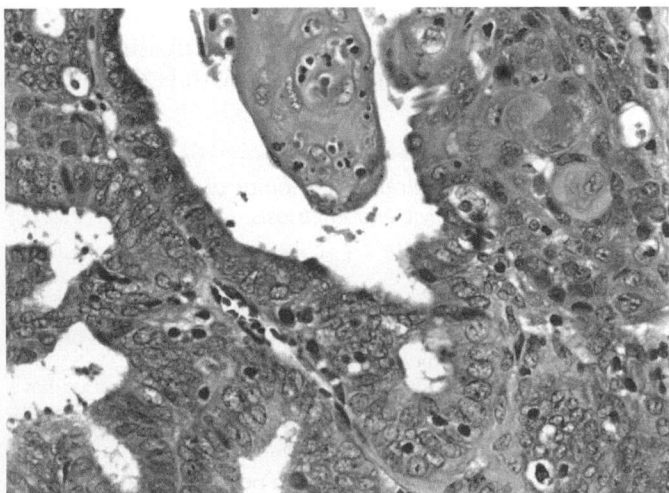

Figure 12-47. Endometrioid carcinoma of ovary. Endometrial-like glands and areas of squamous differentiation.

- Benign endometrioid tumor (rare)
  - Usually have an adenofibromatous pattern with mature glands in a fibrous stroma

ATYPICAL PROLIFERATIVE ENDOMETRIOID TUMOR (ENDOMETRIOID BORDERLINE TUMOR)
- No stromal invasion
- Usually has an adenofibromatous pattern with fibrous stroma and squamous morulas

MALIGNANT ENDOMETRIOID TUMOR (ENDOMETRIOID CARCINOMA)
- Characterized by stromal invasion and cribriforming of glands
- Often displays squamous differentiation
- Graded as other epithelial tumors

Special Stains and Immunohistochemistry

- Vimentin positive in malignant tumors

Other Techniques for Diagnosis

- Noncontributory

Differential Diagnosis

POORLY DIFFERENTIATED SEROUS CARCINOMA VERSUS ENDOMETRIOID CARCINOMA
- Serous carcinoma contains irregular, slitlike glands, with smaller, complex papillae, cellular budding, and frequent psammoma bodies
- Squamous differentiation points toward endometrioid carcinoma

MUCINOUS CARCINOMA VERSUS ENDOMETRIOID CARCINOMA
- Mucinous carcinoma contains abundant luminal mucin and goblet cells with mucin-rich cytoplasm
- Vimentin negative and CEA positive

SLCT VERSUS ENDOMETRIOID CARCINOMA
- SLCT has a well-differentiated epithelium that is more abundant, has smaller tubules, and has only small amounts of intraluminal mucin

- SLCT does not contain an adenofibromatous component or squamous differentiation

MALIGNANT MIXED MÜLLERIAN TUMOR VERSUS ENDOMETRIOID ADENOCARCINOMA
- Endometrioid adenocarcinoma may contain prominent foci of spindled epithelial cells, but they are less atypical than both the epithelial and spindle cell components of a malignant mixed mullerian tumor

PEARLS

- *Borderline tumors typically have a relatively benign course, if low stage*
- *Endometrioid carcinomas are associated with the same risk factors as endometrial carcinomas*
- *Endometrioid and clear cell carcinomas are the most common tumors arising adjacent to or within endometriosis*

SELECTED REFERENCES

Acs G, Pasha T, Zhang PJ: WT1 is differentially expressed in serous, endometrioid, clear cell, and mucinous carcinomas of the peritoneum, fallopian tube, ovary, and endometrium. Int J Gynecol Pathol 23:110-118, 2004.
Cho KR, Shih IM: Ovarian cancer. Annu Rev Pathol Mech Dis 4:287-313, 2009.
Garg PP, Kerlikowske K, Subak L, Grady D: Hormone replacement therapy and the risk of epithelial ovarian carcinoma: a meta-analysis. Obstet Gynecol 92:472-479, 1998.
Heaps JM, Nieberg RK, Berek JS: Malignant neoplasms arising in endometriosis. Obstet Gynecol 75:1023-1028, 1990.
Scully RE, Young RH, Clement PB: Atlas of Tumor Pathology: Tumors of the Ovary, Maldeveloped Gonads, Fallopian Tube, and Broad Ligament, 3rd Series, Fascicle 23. Washington, DC, Armed Forces Institute of Pathology, 1998, pp 107-128.

CLEAR CELL TUMORS

Clinical Features

- Most are malignant, with rare benign and borderline variants
- Malignant tumors often occur in nulliparous women; peak incidence in fifth decade
- Associated with endometriosis

Gross Pathology

- Most tumors are cystic with solid areas, but some are predominantly solid; often bilateral
- Focal hemorrhage and necrosis may be present
- Clear cell carcinomas average 15 cm in diameter, often have surface adhesions; typically consist of thick-walled unilocular, sometimes multilocular, cysts with white or yellow-tan solid papillary or nodular protrusions into the lumen

Histopathology

BENIGN CLEAR CELL TUMOR
- Usually have an adenofibromatous pattern with mature glands in a fibrous stroma

ATYPICAL PROLIFERATIVE CLEAR CELL TUMOR (CLEAR CELL BORDERLINE TUMOR)
- Usually an adenofibromatous pattern with atypical glands in a fibrous stroma

CLEAR CELL CARCINOMA (MALIGNANT CLEAR CELL TUMOR)

- May show papillary, tubulocystic, solid, or mixed patterns with stromal invasion
- Polyhedral, glycogen-rich clear cells containing round or angular atypical nuclei with frequent abnormal mitoses
- Clear cells line papillae (which usually have hyalinized cores), tubules, and cysts or may be arranged in nests
- Nucleoli are generally not present, and hyaline globules are common
- Hobnail cells have plump hyperchromatic nuclei and line papillae, tubules, and cysts (Figure 12-48)
- Less often cells are cuboidal, flat, oxyphilic, or mucin-containing signet ring cells

Special Stains and Immunohistochemistry

- PAS highlights abundant glycogen in clear cells
- Mucin negative
- α-Fetoprotein (AFP) rarely positive
- Cytokeratin positive

Other Techniques for Diagnosis

- Noncontributory

Differential Diagnosis

DYSGERMINOMA

- Peak incidence in second and third decades
- Dysgerminoma cell is large and round with smooth edges; it contains a central nucleus with one or more prominent nucleoli
- Dysgerminoma has thin fibrous bands within an almost pure lymphocytic infiltrate

YOLK SAC TUMOR (YST)

- Peak incidence in first and second decades
- YSTs and clear cell tumors may have a loose edematous pattern
- YST displays primitive nuclei and may demonstrate simple papillae arranged around a single central vessel (Schiller-Duval bodies) typical of the endodermal sinus tumor
- YST may show several other patterns or may be admixed with other forms of germ cell tumor (mixed germ cell tumor)

- YSTs are AFP positive
- Clear cell carcinoma may be admixed with other types of carcinoma, often endometrioid, or with endometriosis

PEARLS

- *Clear cell and endometrioid carcinomas are associated with ovarian and pelvic endometriosis*

SELECTED REFERENCES

Cathro HP, Stoler MH: The utility of calretinin, inhibin, and WT1 immunohistochemical staining in the differential diagnosis of ovarian tumors. Hum Pathol 36:195-201, 2005.

Chan JK, Teo D, Hu JM, et al: Do clear cell ovarian carcinomas have poorer prognosis compared to other epithelial cell types? A study of 1411 clear cell ovarian cancers. Gynecol Oncol 109:370-376, 2008.

Heaps JM, Nieberg RK, Berek JS: Malignant neoplasms arising in endometriosis. Obstet Gynecol 75:1023-1028, 1990.

Matias-Guiu X, Lerma E, Prat J: Clear cell tumors of the female genital tract. Semin Diagn Pathol 14:233-239, 1997.

Scully RE, Young RH, Clement PB: Atlas of Tumor Pathology: Tumors of the Ovary, Maldeveloped Gonads, Fallopian Tube, and Broad Ligament, 3rd Series, Fascicle 23. Washington, DC, Armed Forces Institute of Pathology, 1998, pp 141-151.

Shimizu M, Nikaido T, Toki T, et al: Clear cell carcinoma has an expression pattern of cell cycle regulatory molecules that is unique among ovarian adenocarcinomas. Cancer 85:669-677, 1999.

TRANSITIONAL CELL TUMORS (BRENNER TUMORS) (Figure 12-49A-C)

Clinical Features

- Most are benign transitional (Brenner) tumors; peak incidence in fifth decade
- Borderline tumors and transitional cell carcinomas usually occur in seventh decade
- May be associated with estrogenic or, less often, androgenic manifestations

Gross Pathology

- Most benign transitional cell tumors (Brenner) are small (< 2 cm in diameter), lobulated, white to yellow, and sharply circumscribed
- Small to large cystic spaces are not uncommon
- Borderline: rare, may be solid or cystic with papillae or nodular projections
- Transitional cell carcinomas are more often bilateral (15%) and appear both solid and cystic
- If a benign component is present, the tumors may be classified as *ex-Brenner*

Histopathology

- In general, transitional cell tumors mimic the urothelium

BENIGN TRANSITIONAL CELL TUMOR (BENIGN BRENNER TUMOR)

- Well-defined solid or partially cystic nests and trabeculae of transitional cells with pale cytoplasm and oval, often grooved nuclei
- Cysts are lined by mucinous or other glandular epithelium and filled with eosinophilic material
- Stroma is dense and fibrotic, sometimes with calcifications

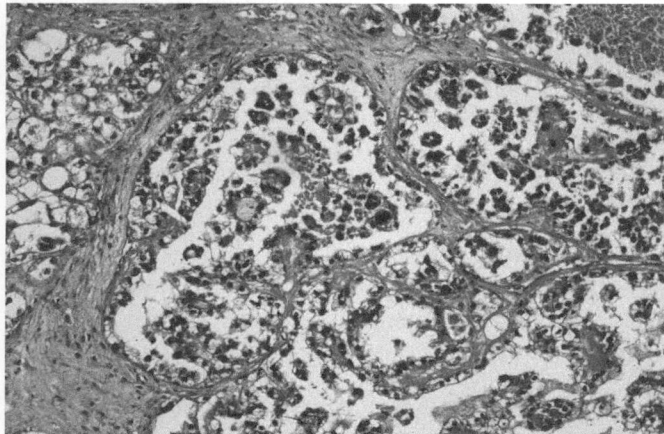

Figure 12-48. Clear cell carcinoma. Low-power view demonstrates a papillary pattern with hobnail-shaped and pleomorphic clear cells.

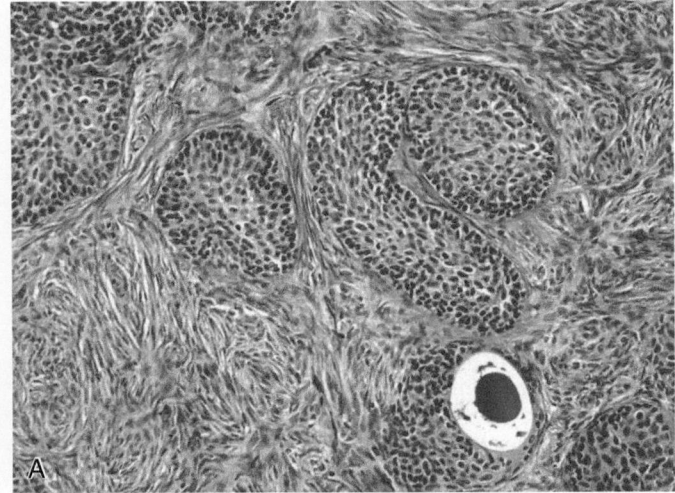

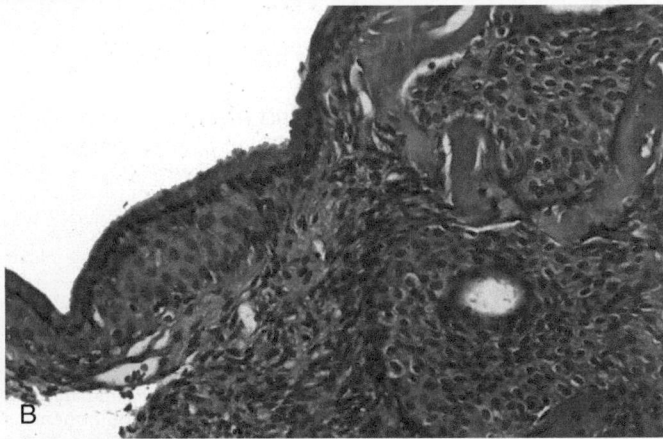

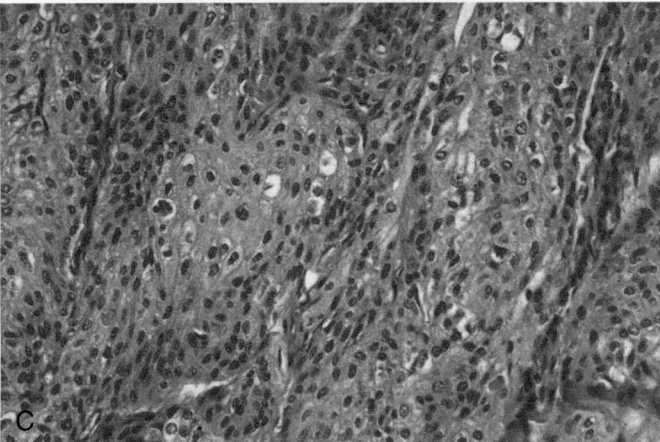

Figure 12-49. A, Brenner tumor. Solid nests of epithelial cells with grooved nuclei surrounded by a stroma composed of tightly packed, spindle-shaped cells. **B,** Brenner tumor associated with mucinous cystadenoma. Low-power view demonstrates both components. **C,** Borderline transitional cell tumor featuring solid proliferation of epithelial cells with nuclear atypia. There is no invasion of the stroma.

ATYPICAL PROLIFERATIVE TRANSITIONAL CELL TUMOR (BORDERLINE)

- Atypical urothelial-like cells in poorly defined nests with no stromal invasion
- Focal necrosis and mitotic figures are occasionally present

TRANSITIONAL CELL CARCINOMA

- Destructive stromal invasion with desmoplasia and occasional necrosis
- Pleomorphic urothelial single and nests of cells with mitotic figures and an intracystic papillary pattern, sometimes with small pools of mucin

Special Stains and Immunohistochemistry

- Cytokeratin 8/18 positive
- Cytokeratin 20 negative

Other Techniques for Diagnosis

- Noncontributory

Differential Diagnosis

MUCINOUS CYSTADENOMA

- Benign Brenner tumors may contain large mucinous cysts but have foci of transitional cells at the periphery of the mucinous cells

POORLY DIFFERENTIATED AND UNDIFFERENTIATED SURFACE EPITHELIAL CARCINOMA

- Surface epithelial carcinomas usually grow in diffuse masses; may have a pattern simulating papillary transitional cell carcinoma, but this is usually due to pseudopapillae resulting from central necrosis with dropout of necrotic cellular debris

PEARLS

- *Occasionally Brenner tumors are associated with a dermoid cyst, or less often with struma ovarii, carcinoid tumor, or mucinous cystadenomas*
- *Transitional cell carcinoma has a poor prognosis, unless confined to one ovary, with an overall 5-year survival rate of 35%*

SELECTED REFERENCES

Cho KR, Shih IM: Ovarian cancer. Annu Rev Pathol Mech Dis 4:287-313, 2009.
Costa MJ, Hansen C, Dickerman A, Scudder SA: Clinicopathologic significance of transitional cell carcinoma pattern in nonlocalized ovarian epithelial tumors (stages 2-4). Am J Clin Pathol 109:173-180, 1998.
Gersell DJ: Primary ovarian transitional cell carcinoma: diagnostic and prognostic considerations. Am J Clin Pathol 93:586-588, 1990.
Ogawa K, Johansson SL, Cohen SM: Immunohistochemical analysis of uroplakins, urothelial specific proteins, in ovarian Brenner tumors, normal tissues, and benign and neoplastic lesions of the female genital tract. Am J Surg Pathol 155:1047-1050, 1999.
Scully RE, Young RH, Clement PB: Atlas of Tumor Pathology: Tumors of the Ovary, Maldeveloped Gonads, Fallopian Tube, and Broad Ligament, 3rd Series, Fascicle 23. Washington, DC, Armed Forces Institute of Pathology, 1998, pp 153-162.

MALIGNANT MIXED MÜLLERIAN TUMOR

Clinical Features

- Classified in the endometrioid category
- Rare tumor occurring in postmenopausal women; peak incidence in sixth decade
- Poor prognosis

Gross Pathology

- Typically large, averaging 15 to 20 cm in diameter
- Most are unilateral
- Solid, or partly cystic, with areas of necrosis and hemorrhage
- Yellow to brown cut surface
- Bone or cartilage may be palpated on occasion

Histopathology

- Epithelial-stromal variant of endometrioid tumor containing malignant epithelial elements (carcinoma) and mesenchymal elements (sarcoma) (Figure 12-50)
- Epithelial elements
  - These include serous or endometrioid carcinoma
  - Squamous cell, clear cell, or mucinous differentiation may be seen
  - Bizarre cells with hyperchromatic nuclei and cells with intracytoplasmic hyaline bodies may be present
- Mesenchymal elements are homologous (native to the female genital tract), such as stromal sarcoma, fibrosarcoma, or leiomyosarcoma; or heterologous (foreign tissue), including chondrosarcoma (most common), rhabdomyosarcoma, or osteosarcoma

Special Stains and Immunohistochemistry

- Reticulin stain highlights areas of undifferentiated carcinoma
- Cytokeratin and EMA highlight areas of undifferentiated carcinoma
- Vimentin highlights areas of sarcoma, although carcinoma may be focally positive

Other Techniques for Diagnosis

- Noncontributory

Differential Diagnosis

IMMATURE TERATOMA

- Occurs in younger women, peak incidence in first and second decades; rare in women older than 50 years of age
- Contains elements of all three germ cell layers, particularly immature neuroectodermal tissue

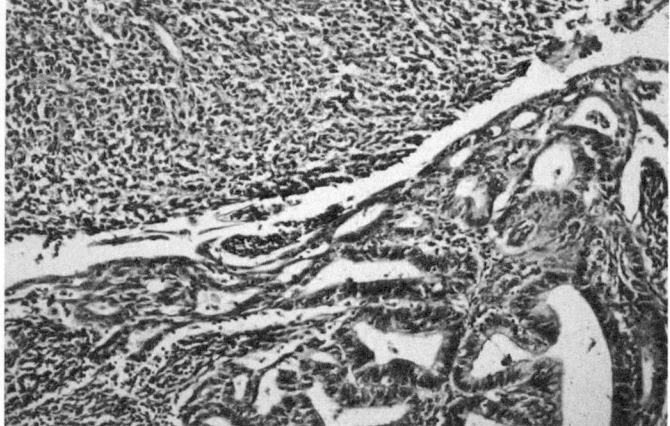

Figure 12-50. Malignant mixed mesodermal tumor (carcinosarcoma). Malignant epithelial and mesenchymal components are evident.

- Lacks a malignant component of müllerian type
- Cartilage has an embryonic or fetal appearance, rather than that of chondrosarcoma

SLCT

- May contain islands of cartilage or rhabdomyoblasts but also shows characteristic Leydig cells, sex cord formations, tubules, or endodermal tissues
- May lead to virilization
- Inhibin positive; rarely EMA positive

ADENOSARCOMA

- Rare tumors showing nonmalignant endometrioid epithelium, sometimes with pseudostratification, and a malignant hypercellular stroma with nuclear atypia
- Peak incidence in fifth decade

PEARLS

- *Spreads beyond the ovary in more than half of cases at surgery*
- *Epithelial or sarcomatous components metastasize early to the omentum, pelvic organs, and liver; poor prognosis with rapid progression*

SELECTED REFERENCES

Abeln EC, Smit VT, Wessels JW, et al: Molecular genetic evidence for the conversion hypothesis of the origin of malignant mixed müllerian tumours. J Pathol 183:424-431, 1997.

Kounelis S, Jones MW, Papadaki H, et al: Carcinosarcomas (malignant mixed müllerian tumors) of the female genital tract: comparative molecular analysis of epithelial and mesenchymal components. Hum Pathol 29:82-87, 1998.

Scully RE, Young RH, Clement PB: Atlas of Tumor Pathology: Tumors of the Ovary, Maldeveloped Gonads, Fallopian Tube, and Broad Ligament, 3rd Series, Fascicle 23. Washington, DC, Armed Forces Institute of Pathology, 1998, pp 128-131.

Wang P, Lee R, Lin G, et al: Malignant mixed mesodermal tumors of the ovary: preoperative diagnosis. Gynecol Obstet Invest 47:69-72, 1999.

SEX CORD–STROMAL TUMORS

FIBROMA

Clinical Features

- Most common sex cord–stromal tumor
- Nonfunctioning tumor with peak incidence in fourth decade
- Occasionally occurs as a component of Meigs syndrome: ascites, hydrothorax (usually right sided), and ovarian fibroma; Meigs syndrome has been reported with other solid ovarian tumors
- May be associated with basal cell nevus syndrome (Gorlin syndrome), an autosomal dominant disorder consisting of numerous basal cell carcinomas beginning in early life, odontogenic keratocysts, erythematous pitting of the palms and soles, calcification of the cerebral falx, frequent skeletal anomalies, and other abnormalities, including bilateral ovarian fibromas

Gross Pathology

- Greater than 90% bilateral and larger than 3 cm in diameter (averages 5 to 6 cm)

- If less than 1 cm, classified as fibromatous nodule
- Hard, chalky white, whorled appearance on cut section, often with areas of edema; occasionally hemorrhagic with sporadic calcifications (Figure 12-51A)

Histopathology

- Intersecting bundles of spindle cells, often in a storiform pattern (Figure 12-51B)
- Moderately cellular without nuclear atypia and infrequent mitotic figures (fewer than four mitotic figures/10 hpf)
- Diffuse intercellular edema is common
- Minor sex cord elements (tubules) may occasionally be identified

Special Stains and Immunohistochemistry

- Inhibin may be focally positive
- Vimentin positive

Other Techniques for Diagnosis

- Noncontributory

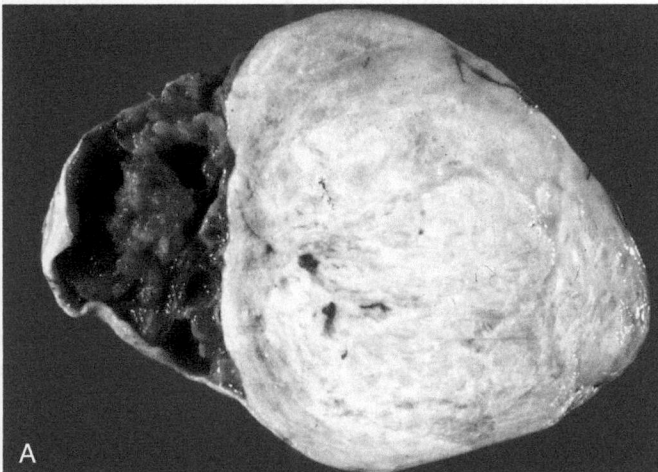

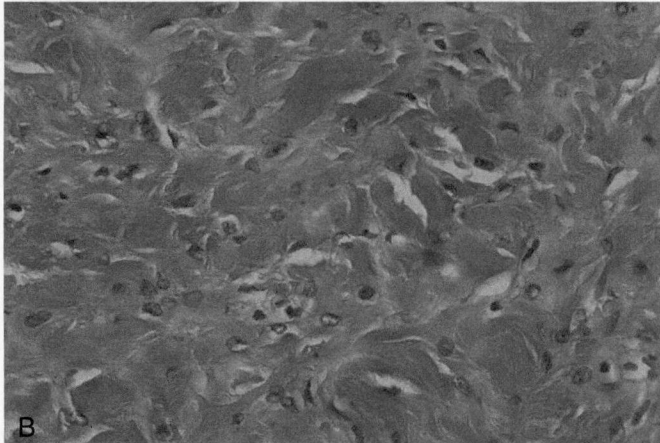

Figure 12-51. Ovarian fibroma. A, Cross section shows a well-circumscribed, chalky-white, solid tumor mass. **B,** This particular lesion shows a prominent hyalinized fibrous stroma with a scanty spindle cell component.

Differential Diagnosis

THECOMA

- Spectrum between fibroma and thecoma (fibrothecoma)
- Thecoma displays large cells with abundant pale cytoplasm
- Typically estrogenic, contains intracytoplasmic lipids, and is inhibin positive

MASSIVE EDEMA AND FIBROMATOSIS

- Edema: usually unilateral with marked intercellular edema, which is characteristic
- Fibromatosis shows stromal cell proliferation with abundant dense collagen
- Envelops rather than displaces follicles, corpora lutea, and corpora albicantia

PEARLS

- *Considered benign unless nuclear pleomorphism and mitotic figures are present (i.e., fibrosarcoma)*

SELECTED REFERENCES

Abad A, Cazorla E, Ruiz F, et al: Meigs' syndrome with elevated CA125: case report and review of the literature. Eur J Obstet Gynecol Reprod Biol 82:97-99, 1999.

Irving JA, Alkushi A, Young RH, Clement PB: Cellular fibromas of the ovary: a study of 75 cases including 40 mitotically active tumors emphasizing their distinction from fibrosarcoma. Am J Surg Pathol 30:929-938, 2006.

Scully RE, Young RH, Clement PB: Atlas of Tumor Pathology: Tumors of the Ovary, Maldeveloped Gonads, Fallopian Tube, and Broad Ligament, 3rd Series, Fascicle 23. Washington, DC, Armed Forces Institute of Pathology, 1998, 194-197.

THECOMA

Clinical Features

- Usually occurs in postmenopausal women; peak incidence in sixth decade
- In younger patients, luteinized thecomas are much more common than the classic type; they are typically estrogenic and often present with uterine bleeding
- This causes an increased incidence of endometrial hyperplasia and carcinoma

Gross Pathology

- Most are unilateral and measure up to 10 cm in diameter
- Lobulated, solid, yellow tumor sometimes with cystic change, hemorrhage, and necrosis (Figure 12-52A)
- Foci of calcification may be seen

Histopathology

- Typical and luteinized variants
- Typical thecoma is composed of sheets and bundles of swollen, lipid-laden, theca-like cells and a variable fibrous component with less than 10% granulosa cells (Figure 12-52B)
- Nuclei are round to spindled and have mild atypia and infrequent mitoses
- Stroma may show obvious hyaline plaques and focal calcification

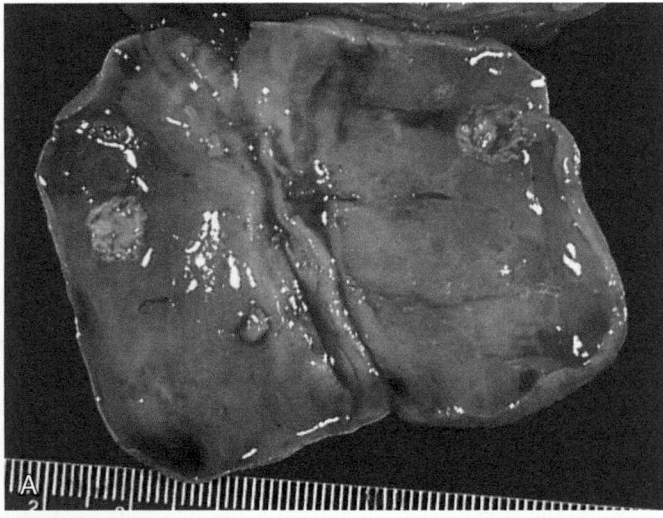

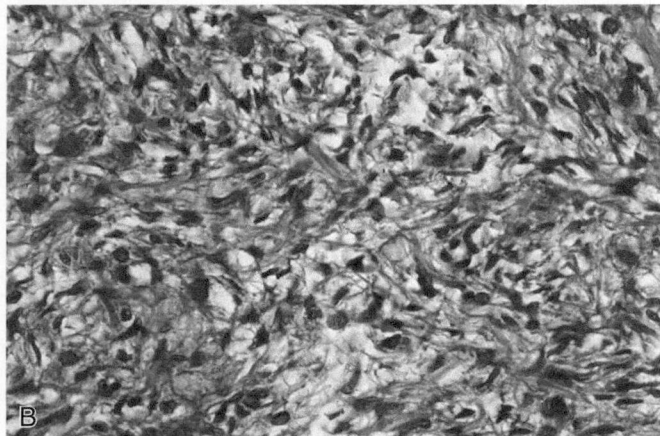

Figure 12-52. Thecoma. A, Cut surface shows a well-circumscribed, tan-yellow, solid tumor mass replacing the ovary. **B,** The tumor is composed predominantly of plump spindle cells with pale cytoplasm. Focally, the tumor cells have vacuolated cytoplasm.

- Luteinized thecomas show luteinized stromal cells and luteinized theca-like cells, with abundant clear or eosinophilic cytoplasm and central, round nuclei

Special Stains and Immunohistochemistry

- Reticulin highlights reticulin fibers surrounding individual tumor cells
- Inhibin positive
- Oil red O positive on fresh tissue (frozen section)

Other Techniques for Diagnosis

- Noncontributory

Differential Diagnosis

FIBROMA

- Spectrum exists between fibroma and thecoma (fibrothecoma)
- Large cells with abundant pale cytoplasm; lipid-laden cells are absent
- Fibromas are not associated with steroid hormone production

STEROID CELL TUMOR

- Steroid cell tumors may show extensive luteinization and a fibromatous component

- Fibromatous component accounts for less than 10% of the tumor
- Typically androgenic, does not show hyaline plaques, and is often malignant

STROMAL HYPERTHECOSIS

- Almost always bilateral
- Lutein cells are mixed with small hyperplastic stromal cells with minimal collagen production

PREGNANCY LUTEOMA

- Multiple in about 50% of cases
- Contain little or no lipid
- Lacks intersecting bundles of spindle cells

PEARLS

- *Most tumors are benign and treated with surgical resection*

SELECTED REFERENCES

Nocito AL, Sarancone S, Bacchi C, Tellez T: Ovarian thecoma: clinicopathological analysis of 50 cases. Ann Diagn Pathol 12:12-16, 2008.
Staats PN, McCluggage WG, Clement PB, Young RH: Luteinized thecomas (thecomatosis) of the type typically associated with sclerosing peritonitis: a clinical, histopathologic, and immunohistochemical analysis of 27 cases. Am J Surg Pathol 32:1273-1299, 2008.

ADULT GRANULOSA CELL TUMOR

Clinical Features

- Represents 1% to 2% of ovarian tumors
- Occurs in middle-aged and older women
- Most women are postmenopausal, with a peak incidence in the fifth decade
- May secrete estrogen, resulting in endometrial hyperplasia and, in less than 5% of cases, endometrial carcinoma
- Endocrine manifestations include irregular excessive uterine bleeding sometimes preceded by amenorrhea in reproductive-age women and uterine bleeding in postmenopausal women
- May present with a palpable mass, abdominal pain, or swelling; occasionally acute abdominal symptoms due to rupture and bleeding into the peritoneum

Gross Pathology

- Usually unilateral and averages 12 cm in diameter
- Solid, soft, yellow-tan or gray tumor with cystic areas and hemorrhage (Figure 12-53A)
- Sometimes blood-filled cysts predominate, mixed with solid areas

Histopathology

- The amount of granulosa cells varies; they are mixed with stromal theca cells and fibroblasts
- Microfollicular pattern
  - Groups of granulosa cells forming Call-Exner bodies: small, round cystic spaces containing eosinophilic material or pyknotic nuclei (Figure 12-53B)

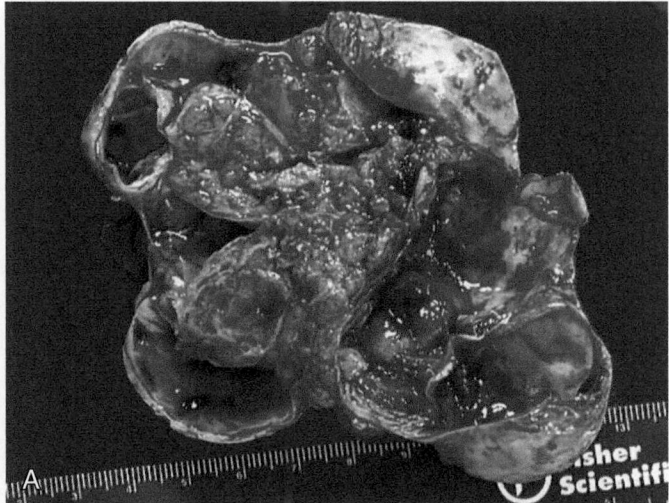

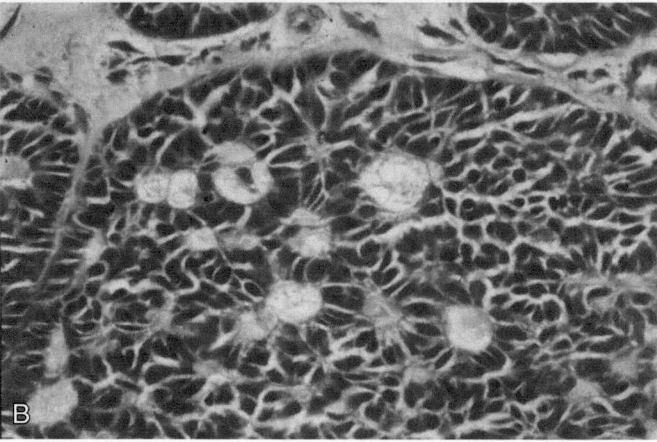

Figure 12-53. Adult granulosa cell tumor. A, Cut surface of the tumor showing a variegated tan appearance with hemorrhage and yellow foci. **B,** Characteristic round to oval nuclei with grooves, inconspicuous nucleoli, and Call-Exner body.

- Cells are round to oval and contain scanty cytoplasm with pale, angular to round, often grooved nuclei, with variable mitotic activity
- AGCT occasionally contains a component of luteinized granulosa cells, with abundant eosinophilic cytoplasm or cells with enlarged, hyperchromatic nuclei, including multinucleate forms
- Trabecular pattern consists of cords of cells
- Insular pattern
  - Sheets of tumor cell in a geographic arrangement
- Macrofollicular pattern
  - Displays large cysts lined by granulosa cells
- Water silk pattern
  - Cells arranged in undulated rows
- Gyriform pattern is characterized by zigzag cords of cells
- Diffuse and sarcomatoid patterns are less differentiated; shows increased nuclear pleomorphism, spindle cells, mitotic activity, and prominent nucleoli
- Call-Exner bodies are rare

Special Stains and Immunohistochemistry

- Reticulin stain: highlights sparse reticulin surrounding aggregates of granulosa cells
- Vimentin, inhibin, and calretinin positive and CD56 often positive
- EMA, cytokeratin 7, desmin negative

Other Techniques for Diagnosis

- Noncontributory

Differential Diagnosis

UNDIFFERENTIATED CARCINOMA AND ADENOCARCINOMA

- Carcinomas with serous differentiation in particular are bilateral in more than 25% of cases; often spread beyond the ovary and may be necrotic
- Cells are large and hyperchromatic, with pleomorphic nuclei, many mitosis, and psammoma bodies if serous; stroma is fibrous and often desmoplastic

THECOMA, CELLULAR FIBROMA, AND FIBROSARCOMA

- Classic AGCT cellular patterns are absent; reticulin stain is diffuse
- AGCT is rarely composed exclusively of spindle cells ("sarcomatous") variant

CARCINOID TUMOR

- Glands with regular margins and eosinophilic secretions; nuclei are round, uniform, and coarsely stippled with rare mitotic figures
- Abundant eosinophilic cytoplasm separates the nuclei from the lumen of glands
- Neuroendocrine and several keratin immunohistochemical markers are positive

HYPERCALCEMIC SMALL CELL CARCINOMA

- Hypercalcemia and a higher rate of extraovarian spread favor the diagnosis
- Hyperchromatic, somewhat pleomorphic, nongrooved nuclei with frequent mitoses reminiscent of small cell carcinoma of the lung
- No evidence of estrogen excess and occasional mucinous epithelium

ENDOMETRIAL STROMAL SARCOMA

- Extremely rare
- Large, yellow to tan tumor, often with foci of hemorrhage and necrosis; solid, partially cystic, or rarely predominantly cystic
- Diffuse arrangement of small, oval to spindle-shaped cells with scanty cytoplasm; small arteries distributed throughout tumor
- May have areas of sex cord–like patterns, and endometriosis is not unusual
- High-grade tumor: mitotic rate is brisk; tumor is at an advanced stage and frequently bilateral
- Reticulin stain highlights individual cells surrounded by fibrils

PEARLS

- *Spread is largely within the pelvis and lower abdomen*
- *May recur decades later: 10-year survival rate ranges from 80% to 90% if stage I*

SELECTED REFERENCES

Fontanelli R, Stefanon B, Raspagliesi F, et al: Adult granulosa cell tumor of the ovary: a clinicopathologic study of 35 cases. Tumori 84:60-64, 1998.

Leuverink EM, Brennan BA, Crook ML, et al: Prognostic value of mitotic counts and Ki-67 immunoreactivity in adult-type granulosa cell tumour of the ovary. J Clin Pathol 61:914-919, 2008.

Ranganath R, Sridevi V, Shirley SS, Shantha V: Clinical and pathologic prognostic factors in adult granulosa cell tumors of the ovary. Int J Gynecol Cancer 18:929-933, 2008.

Roth LM: Recent advances in the pathology and classification of ovarian sex cord-stromal tumors. Int J Gynecol Pathol 25:199-215, 2006.

Schneider DT, Calaminus G, Harms D, et al: Ovarian sex cord-stromal tumors in children and adolescents. J Reprod Med 50:439-446, 2005.

Scully RE, Young RH, Clement PB: Atlas of Tumor Pathology: Tumors of the Ovary, Maldeveloped Gonads, Fallopian Tube, and Broad Ligament, 3rd Series, Fascicle 23. Washington, DC, Armed Forces Institute of Pathology, 1998, pp 169-180.

JUVENILE GRANULOSA CELL TUMOR

Clinical Features

- Juvenile granulosa cell tumor (JGCT) occurs in children and young adults in first three decades
- Most prepubertal children present with a palpable mass and estrogenic effects, including isosexual pseudoprecocity, and irregular uterine bleeding
- Postpubertal patients present with a mass, abdominal pain or swelling, menstrual irregularities, and occasionally rupture and ascites

Gross Pathology

- Similar to adult granulose cell tumor, with an average diameter of 12.5 cm
- Most are unilateral, yellow-tan, or gray solid tumors
- Cysts, sometimes with bloody fluid, are common, as are necrosis and hemorrhage

Histopathology

- Features solid sheets of cells mixed with small immature follicles of varying sizes and shapes containing secretions; nuclear atypia and many mitoses may be present
- The cells line the follicles, blending into diffusely cellular areas, commonly mixed with theca interna cells in the stroma
- Granulosa cells have round, hyperchromatic, ungrooved nuclei with abundant eosinophilic or clear, vacuolated cytoplasm; luteinization is frequent

Special Stains and Immunohistochemistry

- Reticulin highlights sparse reticulin fibrils surrounding aggregates of granulosa cells
- Mucicarmine usually highlights follicular secretions
- Inhibin and vimentin positive
- EMA negative

Other Techniques for Diagnosis

- Noncontributory

Differential Diagnosis

ADULT GRANULOSA CELL TUMOR

- Follicles are more regular in size and shape and contain eosinophilic basement membrane material with degenerating nuclei
- Cells have scanty cytoplasm, and extensive luteinization is absent

- Nuclei are pale, angular to round, and often grooved, with variable mitotic activity

YST, EMBRYONAL CARCINOMA

- Affects children and young adults; peak incidence in first decade
- Associated with endocrine manifestations, such as isosexual precocious puberty (elevated HCG) in embryonal carcinoma; YST is positive for AFP
- Follicular pattern is absent, and nuclei appear primitive

THECOMA

- Infrequent before 30 years of age, shows rare mitotic activity
- JGCT may contain areas lacking follicles and occasionally shows a predominance of theca cells, causing confusion with thecoma
- Thorough sampling of JGCT to demonstrate follicles, along with reticulin stain, helps to establish the diagnosis JGCT

HYPERCALCEMIC SMALL CELL CARCINOMA

- Hypercalcemia and a higher rate of extraovarian spread favor the diagnosis
- Small cell carcinoma displays numerous mitotic figures and necrosis
- Evidence of estrogen excess and mucinous epithelium favors AGCT
- Follicles typically contain eosinophilic, rather than mucicarminophilic, fluid

PEARLS

- *Most patients do well after surgical resection; some completely cured*
- *Most recurrences are within 3 postoperative years*

SELECTED REFERENCES

Cronjé HS, Niemand I, Bam RH, Woodruff JD: Granulosa and theca cell tumors in children: a report of 17 cases and literature review. Obstet Gynecol Surv 53:240-247, 1998.

Hildebrandt RH, Rouse RV, Longacre TA: Value of inhibin in the identification of granulosa cell tumors of the ovary. Hum Pathol 28:1387-1395, 1997.

Ligtenberg MJ, Siers M, Themmen AP, et al: Analysis of mutations in genes of the follicle-stimulating hormone receptor signaling pathway in ovarian granulosa cell tumors. J Clin Endocrinol Metab 84:2233-2234, 1999.

McCluggage WG: Immunoreactivity of ovarian juvenile granulosa cell tumours with epithelial membrane antigen. Histopathology 46:235-236, 2005.

Schneider DT, Calaminus G, Harms D, et al: Ovarian sex cord-stromal tumors in children and adolescents. J Reprod Med 50:439-446, 2005.

Scully RE, Young RH, Clement PB: Atlas of Tumor Pathology: Tumors of the Ovary, Maldeveloped Gonads, Fallopian Tube, and Broad Ligament, 3rd Series, Fascicle 23. Washington, DC, Armed Forces Institute of Pathology, 1998, pp 180-186.

SCLEROSING STROMAL TUMOR

Clinical Features

- Rare, benign, occurring mostly in first three decades, with a peak incidence in the second decade

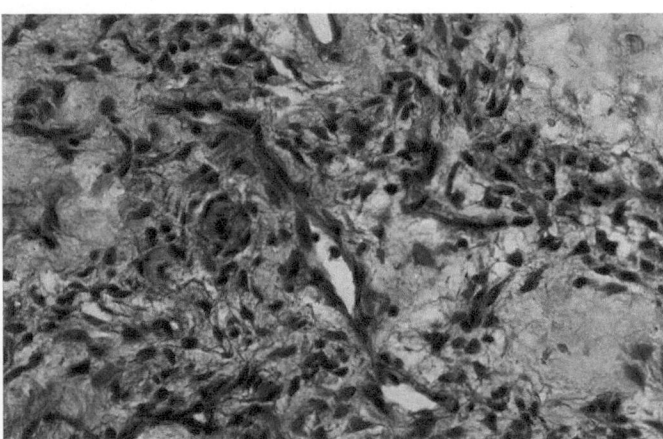

Figure 12-54. Sclerosing stromal tumor. Pseudolobular pattern with edematous connective tissue and prominent thin-walled vessels.

Gross Pathology

- Unilateral, solid, discrete, white tumor that is sharply demarcated
- Frequently with foci of edema, cyst formation, and yellow discoloration

Histopathology

- Moderately cellular pseudolobules with numerous thin-walled vessels (Figure 12-54)
- Pseudotubules are composed of fibroblasts and lipid-laden, vacuolated cells separated by edematous connective tissue or dense collagenous stroma
- Sclerosis is present within the nodules, but mitoses are identified only rarely

Special Stains and Immunohistochemistry

- Inhibin positive
- CD34, CD31 positive

Other Techniques for Diagnosis

- Noncontributory

Differential Diagnosis

THECOMA VERSUS FIBROMA

- Thecoma is typically an estrogenic tumor with peak incidence in sixth decade; shows characteristic and distinct lutein cells
- Fibroma is a nonfunctioning tumor with peak incidence in fourth decade; may have diffuse edema
- Hyaline plaques may be a noticeable feature, especially with thecoma

PEARLS

- *Rarely forms a unilocular cyst*
- *Scarce association with estrogen secretion*

SELECTED REFERENCES

Kawauchi S, Tsuji T, Kaku T, et al: Sclerosing stromal tumor of the ovary: a clinicopathologic, immunohistochemical, ultrastructural, and cytogenetic analysis with special reference to its vasculature. Am J Surg Pathol 22:83-92, 1998.

Kostopoulou E, Moulla A, Giakoustidis D, Leontsini M: Sclerosing stromal tumors of the ovary: a clinicopathologic, immunohistochemical and cytogenetic analysis of three cases. Eur J Gynaecol Oncol 25:257-260, 2004.

Scully RE, Young RH, Clement PB: Atlas of Tumor Pathology: Tumors of the Ovary, Maldeveloped Gonads, Fallopian Tube, and Broad Ligament, 3rd Series, Fascicle 23. Washington, DC, Armed Forces Institute of Pathology, 1998, pp 197-200.

Tiltman AJ, Haffajee Z: Sclerosing stromal tumors, thecomas, and fibromas of the ovary: an immunohistochemical profile. Int J Gynecol Pathol 18:254-258, 1999.

SERTOLI CELL TUMOR

Clinical Features

- Rare tumor best regarded as low-grade malignancy
- Mostly affects women of childbearing age; peak incidence in the second decade
- Usually nonfunctioning but may be estrogenic or occasionally androgenic

Gross Pathology

- Unilateral, solid, lobulated tumor averaging 9 cm in diameter
- Variegated, yellow or brown cut surface

Histopathology

- Well-differentiated Sertoli cell tumor contains round or elongated hollow or solid tubules separated by fibrous stroma devoid of Leydig cells
- Hollow tubules are lined by cuboidal, columnar cells with moderate to abundant pale, occasionally eosinophilic, cytoplasm, and rare to absent nuclear atypia and mitoses (Figure 12-55)
- Solid tubules may be closely packed with small nuclei and scanty cytoplasm or large cells with abundant cytoplasmic lipid (lipid-rich Sertoli cell tumor)
- Stroma may be hyalinized and focally replace the tubules

Special Stains and Immunohistochemistry

- Cytokeratin and inhibin positive
- EMA negative
- Calretinin, focal

Other Techniques for Diagnosis

- Noncontributory

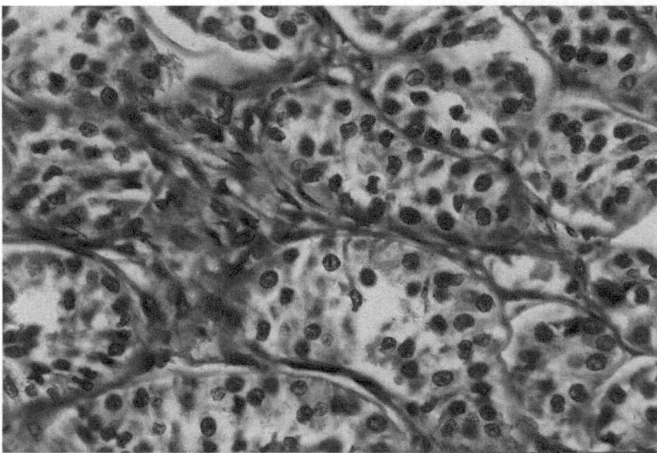

Figure 12-55. Sertoli cell tumor. The tumor is composed of closely packed tubules lined by cuboidal to columnar epithelial cells. Notice the lack of nuclear atypia.

Differential Diagnosis

SERTOLI-LEYDIG CELL TUMOR
- Presence of several clusters of Leydig cells or their spindle cell precursors

CARCINOID TUMOR
- May rarely have a solid tubular pattern
- Distinguished with immunohistochemical stains for neuroendocrine markers (chromogranin, synaptophysin) and by diffuse cytokeratin positivity

PEARLS

- *Excellent prognosis when well differentiated ("tubular adenoma")*

SELECTED REFERENCES

Costa MJ, Ames PF, Walls J, Roth LM: Inhibin immunohistochemistry applied to ovarian neoplasms: a novel, effective, diagnostic tool. Hum Pathol 28:1247-1254, 1997.

Oliva E, Alvarez T, Young RH: Sertoli cell tumors of the ovary: a clinicopathologic and immunohistochemical study of 54 cases. Am J Surg Pathol 29:143-156, 2005.

Rishi M, Howard LN, Bratthauer GL, Tavassoli FA: Use of monoclonal antibody against human inhibin as a marker for sex cord-stromal tumors of the ovary. Am J Surg Pathol 21:583-589, 1997.

Scully RE, Young RH, Clement PB: Atlas of Tumor Pathology: Tumors of the Ovary, Maldeveloped Gonads, Fallopian Tube, and Broad Ligament, 3rd Series, Fascicle 23. Washington, DC, Armed Forces Institute of Pathology, 1998, pp 203-204.

Zhao C, Bratthauer GL, Barner R, et al: Comparative analysis of alternative and traditional immunohistochemical markers for the distinction of ovarian Sertoli cell tumor from endometrioid tumors and carcinoid tumor: a study of 160 cases. Am J Surg Pathol 31:255, 2007.

SERTOLI-LEYDIG CELL TUMOR

Clinical Features

- Androgen-secreting tumor that may occur at any age; peak incidence in the second decade; patients with the retiform subtype are 10 years younger on average
- Plasma testosterone, androstenedione, and other androgen levels may be high; androgenic manifestations may occur with virilization or hirsutism
- Half of patients have no endocrine symptoms, but rather abdominal swelling or pain

Gross Pathology

- Most are unilateral, confined to the ovary, and average 10 cm in diameter
- Solid, lobulated, yellow-tan to reddish brown masses, but may have a cystic component, especially with heterologous or retiform tumors
- Poorly differentiated tumors are larger and show more hemorrhage and necrosis

Histopathology

- Differentiation
  - Well differentiated
    - Hollow or solid tubular pattern with round, oval, elongated, or irregular tubules in a fibrous stroma mixed with clusters of Leydig cells
  - Intermediate differentiation
    - Nodular appearance with dense cellular areas showing occasional mitoses separated by hypocellular fibrous or edematous stroma
    - Cellular areas contain less-differentiated tubules, clusters, and cords of immature Sertoli cells that have small hyperchromatic nuclei and sparse cytoplasm
    - Sertoli cells separated by stromal cells and Leydig cells with abundant pale cytoplasm and round nuclei with prominent nucleoli with or without heterologous elements (Figure 12-56)
  - Poorly differentiated
    - Diffuse pattern of densely packed pleomorphic spindle-shaped cells (sarcoma-like) with frequent mitotic figures
- Heterologous elements
  - Benign mucinous epithelium of gastrointestinal type, with goblet, argentaffin, and argyrophil cells often present is the most common component, seen in about 15% to 20% of SLCTs, except in the well-differentiated subtype
  - Immature skeletal muscle, cartilage, or both may be identified
- Retiform
  - Significant proportion of cells akin to rete epithelial cells with patterns similar to rete testis, including tubular and cystic structures
  - Morphology of the tubules is identical to tubules in a well-differentiated SLCT
  - Most retiform tumors exhibit other SLCT patterns

Special Stains and Immunohistochemistry

- Inhibin positive

Other Techniques for Diagnosis

- Noncontributory

Differential Diagnosis

MUCINOUS TUMORS
- Cysts and glands lined by benign, proliferating, or malignant mucinous cells resembling intestinal or endometrioid epithelium without SLCT elements

ENDOMETRIOID CARCINOMA
- Endometrioid glands, squamous differentiation, occasional adenofibromatous component; may show intraluminal mucin in the glands

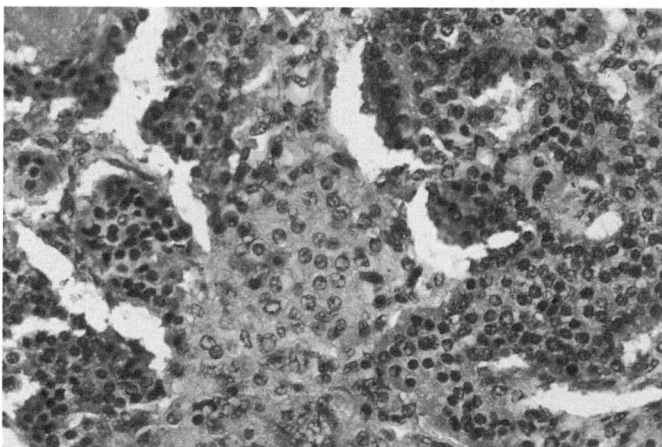

Figure 12-56. Sertoli–Leydig cell tumor of intermediate differentiation. Sheets of immature Sertoli cells and clusters of Leydig cells with abundant eosinophilic cytoplasm are present at the center of the photomicrograph.

MALIGNANT MIXED MÜLLERIAN TUMOR

- May contain heterologous elements, including cartilage or rhabdomyoblasts, but lacks Sertoli and/or Leydig cells and other components
- High-grade malignant epithelial cells with müllerian (e.g., serous, clear) differentiation, but no androgenic secretions
- Cytokeratin and EMA highlight carcinoma, whereas inhibin is negative

PEARLS

- *Occasional association with androgenic manifestations*
- *Androgen secretion may result in erythrocytosis*
- *Rarely associated with sarcoma botryoides of the cervix, thyroid disease, and rare familial occurrence*

SELECTED REFERENCES

Lantzsch T, Stoerer S, Lawrenz K, et al: Sertoli-Leydig cell tumors. Arch Gynecol Obstet 264:206-208, 2001.

Mooney EE, Man YG, Bratthauer GL, Tavassoli FA: Evidence that Leydig cells in Sertoli-Leydig cell tumors have a reactive rather than a neoplastic profile. Cancer 86:2312-2317, 1999.

Roth LM: Recent advances in the pathology and classification of ovarian sex cord-stromal tumors. Int J Gynecol Pathol 25:199-215, 2006.

Scully RE, Young RH, Clement PB: Atlas of Tumor Pathology: Tumors of the Ovary, Maldeveloped Gonads, Fallopian Tube, and Broad Ligament, 3rd Series, Fascicle 23. Washington, DC, Armed Forces Institute of Pathology, 1998, pp 205-219.

SEX CORD TUMOR WITH ANNULAR TUBULES

Clinical Features

- Sex cord tumor with annular tubulus (SCTAT) is a relatively rare tumor; most patients are of childbearing age
- One third of cases are associated with Peutz-Jeghers syndrome (PJS)
- Estrogenic manifestations may be present, including menstrual irregularities and isosexual precocious puberty

Gross Pathology

- Tumors associated with PJS are usually small, multifocal, bilateral, and focally calcified; tumors not associated with PJS are relatively large, solid, and yellow
- Cysts may be seen in both types

Histopathology

- SCTAT is characterized by simple and complex annular tubules encircling hyaline material; simple tubules are shaped like a ring
- Complex tubules are more numerous and form intercommunicating rings; if associated with PJS, calcification of the tubules may be present
- Rings are lined by epithelial cells that have abundant pale cytoplasm oriented toward the center of the ring and a peripheral nucleus

Special Stains and Immunohistochemistry

- Inhibin is positive focally

Other Techniques for Diagnosis

- Noncontributory

Differential Diagnosis

GONADOBLASTOMA

- Stromal and germ cell tumor components must be present; not associated with PJS
- Almost always occurs in phenotypic women with underlying gonadal disorders

PEARLS

- *Benign, incidental finding at autopsy or surgery when seen in patients with PJS*
- *Malignant in one fourth of cases; characteristically spreads through lymphatics*
- *Considered a specific sex cord–stromal tumor with a potential for bidirectional differentiation toward granulosa cell or Sertoli cell tumors*

SELECTED REFERENCES

Connolly DC, Katabuchi H, Cliby WA, Cho KR: Somatic mutations in the STK11/LKB1 gene are uncommon in rare gynecological tumor types associated with Peutz-Jeghers syndrome. Am J Pathol 156:339-345, 2000.

Scully RE, Young RH, Clement PB: Atlas of Tumor Pathology: Tumors of the Ovary, Maldeveloped Gonads, Fallopian Tube, and Broad Ligament, 3rd Series, Fascicle 23. Washington, DC, Armed Forces Institute of Pathology, 1998, pp 219-223.

GYNANDROBLASTOMA

Clinical Features

- Extremely rare tumor that usually presents in young adults but may occur at any age
- May have androgenic or estrogenic manifestations

Gross Pathology

- Solid, pale tumor less than 6 cm in diameter

Histopathology

- Well-differentiated with granulosa and Sertoli cell components
- Tumors should contain more than 10% of the minor component to warrant the diagnosis

Special Stains and Immunohistochemistry

- Noncontributory

Other Techniques for Diagnosis

- Noncontributory

Differential Diagnosis

GRANULOSA CELL TUMOR

- If Sertoli cells are present, they represent less than 10% of the total tumor volume

SERTOLI TUMOR OR SERTOLI-LEYDIG TUMOR

- If granulosa cells are present, they represent less than 10% of the total tumor volume

SEX CORD TUMOR WITH ANNULAR TUBULES

- Simple and complex tubules forming intercommunicating rings and encircling hyaline material often associated with PJS

PEARLS

- *Extremely rare tumor*
- *Almost always benign*

SELECTED REFERENCES

Jaworski RC, Fryatt JJ, Turner TB, Osborn RA: Gynandroblastoma of the ovary. Pathology 18:348-351, 1986.
Kalir T, Friedman F Jr: Gynandroblastoma in pregnancy: case report and review of literature. Mt Sinai J Med 65:292-295, 1998.
Scully RE, Young RH, Clement PB: Atlas of Tumor Pathology: Tumors of the Ovary, Maldeveloped Gonads, Fallopian Tube, and Broad Ligament, 3rd Series, Fascicle 23. Washington, DC, Armed Forces Institute of Pathology, 1998, pp 219-222.

STROMAL LUTEOMA

Clinical Features

- Small benign steroid cell tumor
- Usually develops in postmenopausal women; peak incidence in fifth decade
- Frequently estrogenic with abnormal vaginal bleeding; occasionally androgenic

Gross Pathology

- Solitary, unilateral, well-circumscribed solid tumor, at least 5 mm in diameter, but almost always less than 3 cm
- Gray-white or yellow in most cases with occasional brown-red foci

Histopathology

- Round nodules of lutein cells that, by definition, are confined within ovarian stroma
- Stroma is usually sparse and sometimes focally fibrotic
- Luteinized cells arranged diffusely or in nests and cords, containing eosinophilic cytoplasm with little lipid; nuclei are small and round with one prominent nucleolus and rare mitoses
- Sometimes degeneration produces irregular spaces that may simulate glands or vessels

Special Stains and Immunohistochemistry

- Noncontributory

Other Techniques for Diagnosis

- Noncontributory

Differential Diagnosis

STROMAL HYPERTHECOSIS

- Microscopic nests of lutein cells may develop (nodular hyperthecosis) but are less than 5 mm in diameter; the nodules are typically multiple

PEARLS

- *Presumably arises from the ovarian stroma*
- *Stromal hyperthecosis is present in the ipsilateral or contralateral ovary in most cases*

SELECTED REFERENCES

Outwater EK, Wagner BJ, Mannion C, et al: Sex cord-stromal and steroid cell tumors of the ovary. Radiographics 18:1523-1546, 1998.
Rao BR, Slotman BJ: Ovarian tumors with endocrine manifestations. Curr Therapy Endocrinol Metab 6:260-262, 1997.
Scully RE, Young RH, Clement PB: Atlas of Tumor Pathology: Tumors of the Ovary, Maldeveloped Gonads, Fallopian Tube, and Broad Ligament, 3rd Series, Fascicle 23. Washington, DC, Armed Forces Institute of Pathology, 1998, pp 227-228.

LEYDIG CELL TUMOR

Clinical Features

- Rare, benign steroid cell, known as a *hilus cell tumor*; peak incidence in fifth decade
- Androgenic manifestations are classic, including hirsutism and virilization
- Occasionally, estrogenic manifestations are present

Gross Pathology

- Unilateral, well-circumscribed, solid, usually less than 5 cm in diameter, located near the hilum, and hemorrhage frequently present
- Usually red-brown to yellow, or dark brown to black (Figure 12-57A)

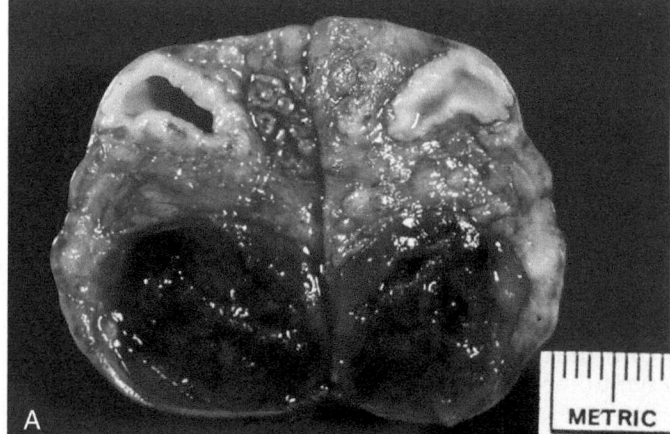

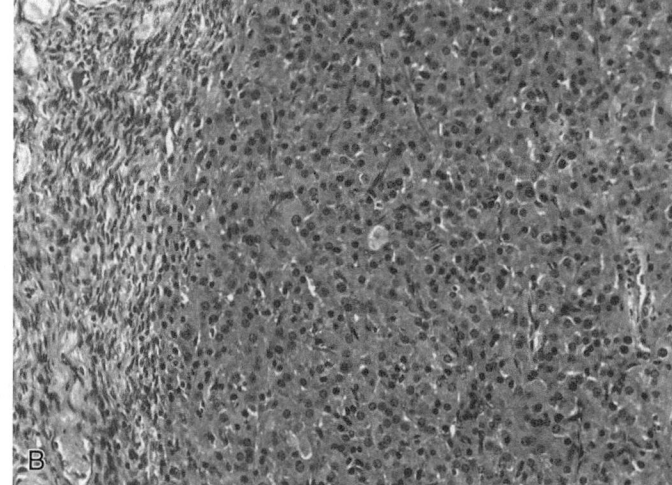

Figure 12-57. Leydig cell tumor. A, Cross section shows a well-circumscribed, reddish brown tumor. **B,** Well-circumscribed proliferation of a homogeneous population of eosinophilic cells with a low nuclear-to-cytoplasmic ratio, nuclei with noticeable chromatin, and discrete nucleoli.

Histopathology

- Sheets, cords, or clusters of polyhedral cells with abundant eosinophilic, finely granular cytoplasm, which may contain small lipid vacuoles (Figure 12-57B)
- By definition, elongated eosinophilic crystalloids of Reinke are present in the cytoplasm; however, these may not be obvious
- Large, centrally located hyperchromatic nuclei often with one or more prominent nucleoli and rare mitoses; fibrinoid degeneration of vessels walls is common
- Anuclear eosinophilic zones separate cellular areas and surround blood vessels

Special Stains and Immunohistochemistry

- Inhibin positive

Other Techniques for Diagnosis

- Electron microscopy highlights rod-shaped crystals of Reinke, which are hexagonal in cross section

Differential Diagnosis

SLCT

- Tubular pattern, Sertoli cells plus Leydig cells characterize the tumor
- Mixed population of different types of cells

PEARLS

- *Originate most often in the hilus but may arise from the ovarian stroma (nonhilar type)*

SELECTED REFERENCES

Baiocchi G, Manci N, Angeletti G, et al: Pure Leydig cell tumour (hilus cell) of the ovary: a rare cause of virilization after menopause. Gynecol Obstet Invest 44:141-144, 1997.
Scully RE, Young RH, Clement PB: Atlas of Tumor Pathology: Tumors of the Ovary, Maldeveloped Gonads, Fallopian Tube, and Broad Ligament, 3rd Series, Fascicle 23. Washington, DC, Armed Forces Institute of Pathology, 1998, pp 228-232.

GERM CELL TUMORS

MATURE CYSTIC TERATOMA (DERMOID CYST)

Clinical Features

- Dermoid cyst is one of the most common ovarian tumors
- Occurs most commonly in adult women during the reproductive years
- Often asymptomatic, but patients may present with pain, swelling, or uterine bleeding

Gross Pathology

- Bilateral in about 15% of cases, smaller than 15 cm, and may be multiple in one ovary
- Combination solid and cystic mass with white to gray external surface
- Opened cysts may contain visible hair, cheeselike sebaceous material, skin, bone, cartilage, fat, thyroid tissue, brain tissue, and teeth (Figure 12-58A)

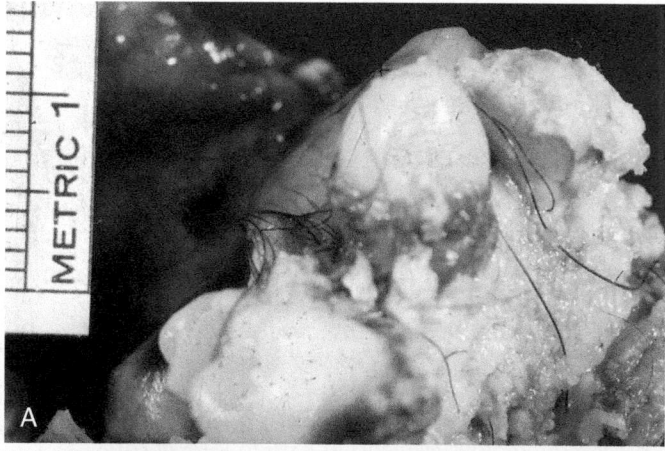

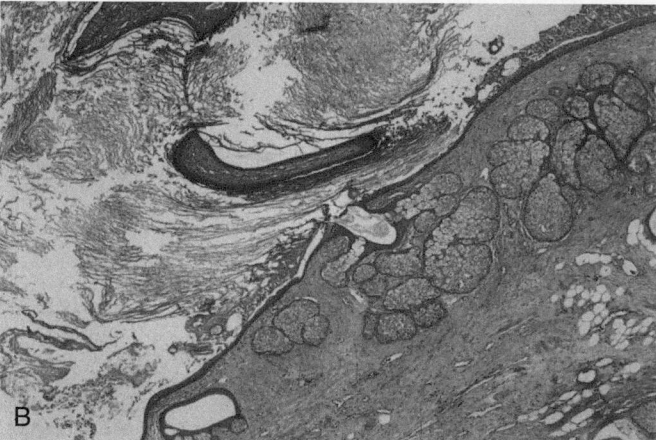

Figure 12-58. Mature cystic teratoma (dermoid cyst). A, Cut surface shows a cystic lesion containing sebaceous material and teeth. **B,** The cavity of the cyst is lined by keratinized squamous epithelium with underlying cutaneous structures.

Histopathology

- Mature (adult-type) tissues, typically representing all three germ layers
- Often consists of ectodermal tissues with a cyst lined by mature epidermis and its appendages and rare (if any) mitoses (Figure 12-58B)
- Neuroectodermal elements: glial, peripheral nervous tissue, cerebrum, and cerebellum are common
- Mesodermal elements like smooth muscle, bone, teeth, cartilage, and fat may be present
- Endodermal elements include respiratory and gastrointestinal epithelium, thyroid tissue and others

Special Stains and Immunohistochemistry

- Stains correspond to tissues present

Other Techniques for Diagnosis

- Noncontributory

Differential Diagnosis

IMMATURE TERATOMA

- Contains immature elements, most commonly glial; on occasion, cartilage and others

PEARLS

- *Dermoid cysts are lined by keratinizing squamous epithelium with skin appendages*
- *Skin may be admixed with struma ovarii, carcinoid tumor, or solid teratoma; a foreign-body giant cell reaction may occur with rupture*
- *Dermoid cysts may be present in the contralateral ovary in patients with yolk sac tumor or immature teratoma about 5% to 10% of the time*
- *Treatment: cystectomy*
- *Malignant transformation—usually to squamous cell carcinoma—is rare (<3%) and presents in postmenopausal women or older*
- *Primary carcinoid tumors of the ovary are associated with other teratomatous elements in 85% to 90% of cases*

SELECTED REFERENCES

Hurwitz JL, Fenton A, McCluggage WG, McKenna S: Squamous cell carcinoma arising in a dermoid cyst of the ovary: a case series. BJOG 114:1283-1287, 2007.

Iwasa A, Oda Y, Kaneki E, et al: Squamous cell carcinoma arising in mature cystic teratoma of the ovary: an immunohistochemical analysis of its tumorigenesis. Histopathology 1:98-104, 2007.

Park JY, Kim DY, Kim JH, et al: Malignant transformation of mature cystic teratoma of the ovary: experience at a single institution. Eur J Obstet Gynecol Reprod Biol 141:173, 2008

Vang R, Gown AM, Zhao C, et al: Ovarian mucinous tumors associated with mature cystic teratomas: morphologic and immunohistochemical analysis identifies a subset of potential teratomatous origin that shares features of lower gastrointestinal tract mucinous tumors more commonly encountered as secondary tumors in the ovary. Am J Surg Pathol 31:854-869, 2007.

MATURE SOLID TERATOMA

Clinical Features

- Slow-growing, benign tumor with peak incidence in first and second decades
- Uncommon and asymptomatic until large

Gross Pathology

- Unilateral large, mostly solid tumor with minimal hemorrhage or necrosis

Histopathology

- Solid tumor with morphologic features resembling mature cystic teratoma
- Composed exclusively of mature elements: endoderm, mesoderm, and ectoderm (Figure 12-59)
- Neural tissue sometimes predominates; only rare mitoses are identified
- Important to thoroughly sample the tumor to exclude immature elements

Special Stains and Immunohistochemistry

- Noncontributory

Other Techniques for Diagnosis

- Noncontributory

Differential Diagnosis

IMMATURE TERATOMA

- Characterized by the presence of immature elements, most commonly glial

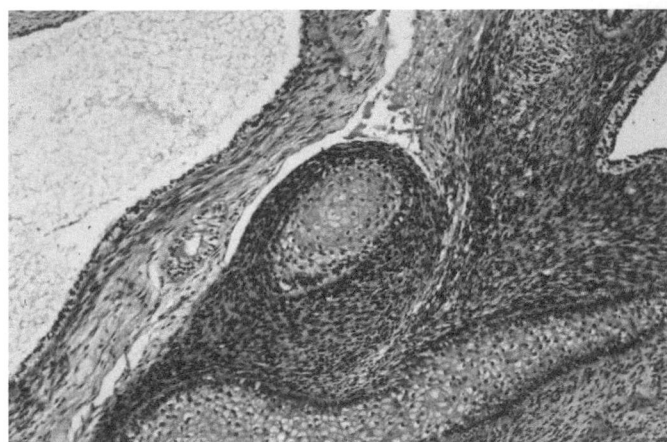

Figure 12-59. Mature solid teratoma. The lesion is composed of cartilage, glandular epithelium, and fibrous tissue.

PEARLS

- *Surgical resection is curative if immature teratoma has been ruled out*
- *Rarely associated with mature glial peritoneal implants, but prognosis is still excellent*

SELECTED REFERENCES

Calame JJ, Schaberg A: Solid teratomas and mixed müllerian tumors of the ovary: a clinical, histological, and immunocytochemical comparative study. Gynecol Oncol 33:212-221, 1989.

Scully RE, Young RH, Clement PB: Atlas of Tumor Pathology: Tumors of the Ovary, Maldeveloped Gonads, Fallopian Tube, and Broad Ligament, 3rd Series, Fascicle 23. Washington, DC, Armed Forces Institute of Pathology, 1998, pp 272-273.

DYSGERMINOMA

Clinical Features

- Most common malignant germ cell tumor; more frequent in women with ovarian dysgenesis; one of the two most common ovarian neoplasms seen in pregnancy
- Pure or mixed with other malignant germ cell components
- Primarily affects young women; peak incidence in second and third decades
- Most patients have elevated serum lactic dehydrogenase and isoenzyme-1, which can be used as tumor markers
- Occasionally produces HCG, manifesting with isosexual precocious puberty and menstrual irregularities
- One of the two most common ovarian neoplasms seen in pregnancy

Gross Pathology

- Mostly a unilateral solid, soft tumor with a median diameter of 15 cm
- More often bilateral in patients with gonadal dysgenesis
- External surface is smooth and gray-white; cut surface is lobulated, gray-white, with hemorrhage or necrotic areas giving it a yellow, pink, or tan color (Figure 12-60A)

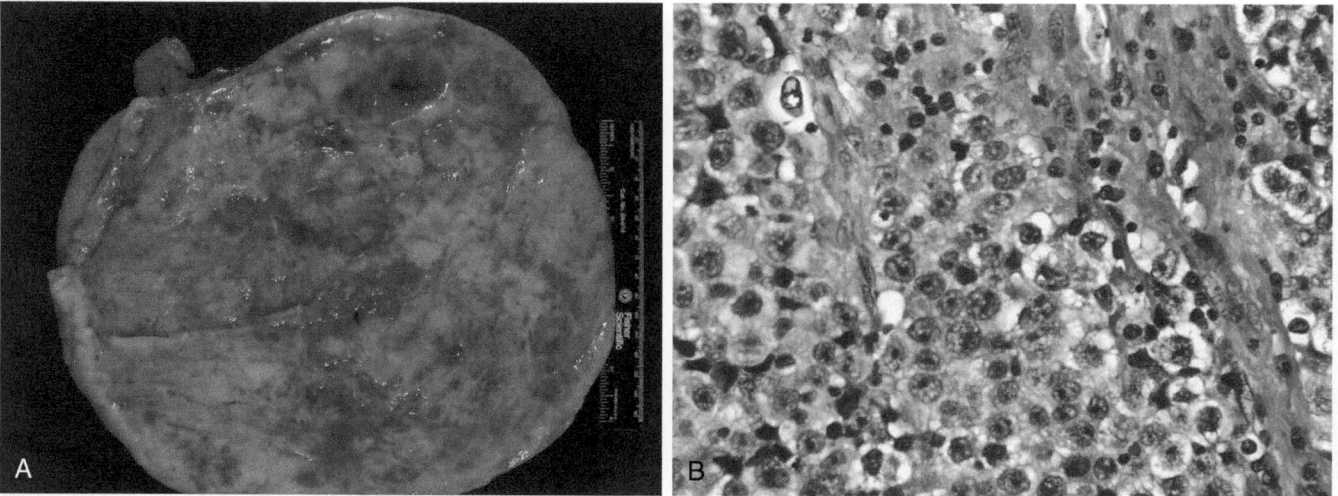

Figure 12-60. Dysgerminoma. A, Twenty-centimeter ovary with a solid tan lobulated appearance on the cut surface. **B,** Sheets of large germ cells with prominent nucleoli and fibrous bands with plasma cells and lymphocytes.

- Important to sample tumor extensively to exclude other germ cell elements (especially variegated and cystic areas)

Histopathology

- Uniform clusters, nests, and cords of large, round cells with abundant, clear, glycogen-rich cytoplasm, separated by lymphocyte-infiltrated fibrous stroma (Figure 12-60B)
- Nuclei are centrally located, large, round, and vesicular, with clumped chromatin and one to several prominent nucleoli; frequent mitoses, necrosis, and hemorrhage
- Noncaseating granulomas and multinucleate syncytiotrophoblastic giant cells may be seen; not regarded as choriocarcinomatous component, although HCG might be elevated
- Frequently dysgerminomas are combined with other germ cell neoplasms, forming mixed tumors; calcifications suggests the presence of a gonadoblastoma

Special Stains and Immunohistochemistry

- Placental alkaline phosphatase (PLAP) and vimentin positive
- Cytokeratin is usually negative and EMA is negative
- PAS highlights glycogen-rich cytoplasm of tumor cells

Other Techniques for Diagnosis

- Noncontributory

Differential Diagnosis

SOLID YOLK SAC TUMOR

- Solid tumor with increased nuclear variation, hyaline bodies, and rare stromal lymphocytes
- AFP positive

EMBRYONAL CARCINOMA

- Composed of focal tubuloglandular structures and larger cells with larger markedly hyperchromatic nuclei without lymphocytic infiltration of the stroma
- Most contain syncytiotrophoblastic giant cells and stain positively for cytokeratin

DIFFUSE CLEAR CELL CARCINOMA

- Polygonal cells with eccentric, hyperchromatic nuclei, usually without prominent nucleoli and glycogen-filled cytoplasm; plasma cells may be prominent
- Less often positive for PLAP, but almost always positive for cytokeratin and EMA

LYMPHOMA

- Often bilateral
- Cells lack cytoplasmic glycogen; stain positively for CD45 and negatively for PLAP

PEARLS

- *Most patients do not have menstrual abnormalities and are capable of bearing children*
- *Treated with surgery and radiation; recurrences are treated with chemotherapy*
- *Metastatic spread late in the course of the disease, first through lymphatics and later hematogenously to the liver, lungs, and bones*
- *Five-year survival rate for a pure tumor in stage 1 ranges from 90% to 95%*
- *Sampling is of utmost importance to exclude a mixed germ cell tumor*

SELECTED REFERENCES

Guillem V, Poveda A: Germ cell tumours of the ovary. Clin Transl Oncol 9:237-243, 2007.

Merino MJ, Jaffe G: Age contrast in ovarian pathology. Cancer 71(2 suppl):537-544, 1993.

Reddy KB, Ahuja VK, Kannan V, et al: Dysgerminoma of the ovary: a retrospective study. Australas Radiol 41:262-265, 1997.

Roth LM, Talerman A: Recent advances in the pathology and classification of ovarian germ cell tumors. Int J Gynecol Pathol 25:305, 2006.

Scully RE, Young RH, Clement PB: Atlas of Tumor Pathology: Tumors of the Ovary, Maldeveloped Gonads, Fallopian Tube, and Broad Ligament, 3rd Series, Fascicle 23. Washington, DC, Armed Forces Institute of Pathology, 1998, pp 239-245.

Sever M, Jones TD, Roth LM, et al: Expression of CD117 (c-kit) receptor in dysgerminoma of the ovary: diagnostic and therapeutic implications. Mod Pathol 18:1411-1416, 2005.

YOLK SAC TUMOR

Clinical Features

- Malignant tumor also referred to as *endodermal sinus tumor* (EST), which is a common subtype
- Peak incidence in second and third decades; rare after age 40 years
- Presents with abdominal pain associated with a mass
- Elevated serum AFP; levels may be useful in monitoring the effectiveness of therapy

Gross Pathology

- Unilateral, large tumor averaging 15 cm in diameter with a smooth external surface
- Soft, solid, gray-yellow mass on cut section, often containing cysts (Figure 12-61A)
- Frequent areas of hemorrhage and necrosis
- Several morphologic variants

Histopathology

- Reticular pattern of small cystic spaces lined by cells with clear cytoplasm containing glycogen or lipid (Figure 12-61B)
- Hyperchromatic, irregular, and large nuclei with prominent nucleoli; frequent mitoses and loose connective tissue stroma
- Schiller-Duval bodies are characteristic, particularly in EST (Figure 12-61C)
  - Glomeruloid, epithelial-lined space containing a polypoid projection covered by cuboidal to columnar cells with a single central vessel
- Frequent hyaline globules
- Other structural variants include polyvesicular, hepatoid, glandular, papillary, myxomatous, macrocystic, and solid
  - Polyvesicular-vitelline shows many small cysts, giving a honeycomb appearance; background of dense cellular stroma lined by columnar, cuboidal, or flat epithelium
  - Hepatoid (usually a minor component); mimics hepatocellular carcinoma
    - Composed of groups of polygonal cells with abundant eosinophilic cytoplasm and a central nucleus with single nucleolus
    - Abundant hyaline bodies are present
  - Glandular (mostly a minor component); may mimic endometrioid adenocarcinoma
    - Intestinal variant contains nests of cells in a cribriform pattern
    - Endometrioid-like variant contains glandular or villoglandular pattern
    - Simple or pseudostratified columnar epithelium may show subnuclear or supranuclear vacuoles
    - Hepatoid cells within gland lumens mimic squamous morulas

Special Stains and Immunohistochemistry

- AFP positive cytoplasmic staining, may be focal or diffuse
- α₁-Antitrypsin positive cytoplasmic staining, may be focal
- Creatine kinase positive cytoplasmic staining

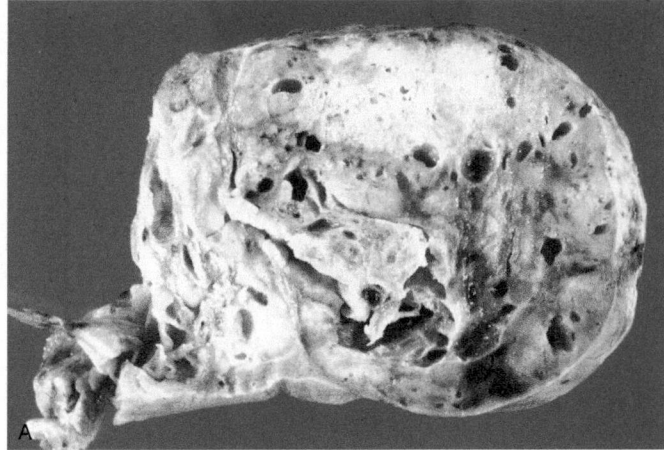
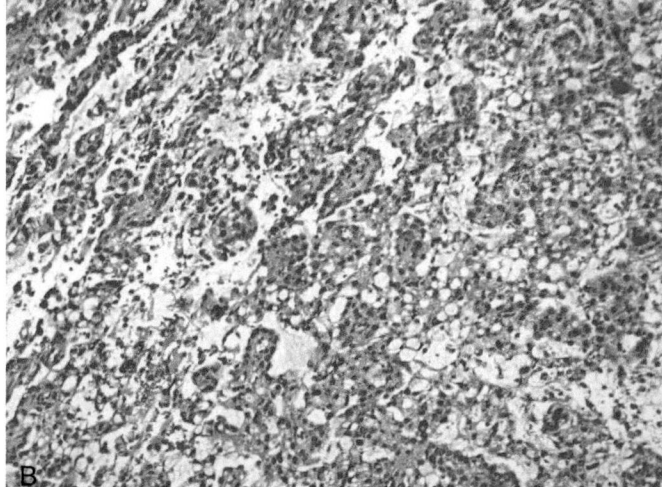
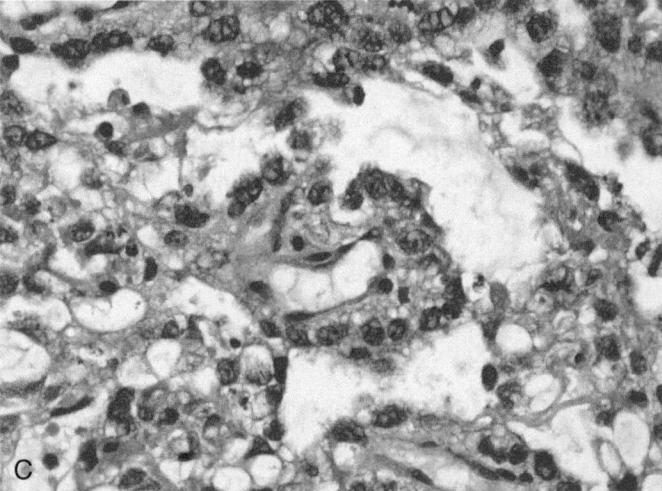

Figure 12-61. Yolk sac tumor (endodermal sinus tumor). **A,** Formalin-fixed firm, smooth, gray-yellow tumor mass with occasional cysts. **B,** Low-power view shows the classic microcystic pattern. **C,** This image shows the typical perivascular distribution of the neoplastic cells (Schiller-Duval bodies).

- EMA negative
- PAS highlights hyaline globules and basement membrane material in tumors with parietal differentiation; present in most YSTs

Other Techniques for Diagnosis

- Noncontributory

Differential Diagnosis

CLEAR CELL CARCINOMA

- Peak incidence in fifth decade
- Can have loose reticular pattern similar to YST
- May show other müllerian differentiation (i.e., endometrioid, serous) or a background of endometriosis
- Polyhedral glycogen-rich clear cells with atypical nuclei and frequent mitoses with occasional nucleoli
- Hyaline globules are common
- Epidermal growth factor receptor (EGFR) is positive in 25% of cases
- Cytokeratins positive
- AFP rarely positive

ENDOMETRIOID ADENOCARCINOMA

- Peak incidence in fifth decade; may be associated with ovarian or pelvic endometriosis
- AFP negative
- Endometrioid-like YST will show foci of more common YST variants

HEPATOID CARCINOMA

- Rare tumor, usually in postmenopausal women
- AFP positive
- More nuclear atypia than YST
- Hepatoid YST shows foci of more common YST variants

DYSGERMINOMA

- Uniform round cells with abundant, clear, glycogen-rich cytoplasm, separated by lymphocyte-infiltrated fibrous stroma
- Cytokeratin is usually negative; AFP negative

PEARLS

- *Rapidly growing, highly malignant tumor*
- *Often spreads outside of the ovary to the peritoneum or retroperitoneal lymph nodes*
- *May be seen in association with endometrioid or mucinous tumors, pregnancy, or gonadal dysgenesis; may be mixed with other germ cell tumors*
- *Treatment with combination chemotherapy*
- *Dermoid cyst present in either ovary in about 5% to 15% of cases*

SELECTED REFERENCES

Dällenbach P, Bonnefoi H, Pelte MF, Vlastos G: Yolk sac tumours of the ovary: an update. Eur J Surg Oncol 32:1063-1075, 2006.
Nawa A, Obata N, Kikkawa F, et al: Prognostic factors of patients with yolk sac tumors of the ovary. Am J Obstet Gynecol 184:1182-1188, 2001.
Scully RE, Young RH, Clement PB: Atlas of Tumor Pathology: Tumors of the Ovary, Maldeveloped Gonads, Fallopian Tube, and Broad Ligament, 3rd Series, Fascicle 23. Washington, DC, Armed Forces Institute of Pathology, 1998, pp 245-255.
Tewari K, Cappuccini F, Disaia PJ, et al: Malignant germ cell tumors of the ovary. Obstet Gynecol 95:128-133, 2000.

EMBRYONAL CARCINOMA

Clinical Features

- Rare tumor affecting children and young adults; peak incidence in first decade
- HCG often elevated and may be used as a tumor marker
- Signs and symptoms related to an adnexal mass and sometimes associated with endocrine manifestations, including isosexual precocious puberty and irregular bleeding

Gross Pathology

- Unilateral, smooth-surfaced, solid tumor with a median diameter of 17 cm
- Gray-white or yellow with foci of hemorrhage or necrosis (Figure 12-62A)
- Variegated pattern may be seen depending on other germ cell elements present

Histopathology

- Solid, papillary, or glandular pattern with sheets and nests of malignant large ovoid or polygonal cells forming syncytiotrophoblastic giant cells in a fibrotic stroma (Figure 12-62B)
- Cells display abundant granular, eosinophilic cytoplasm
- Pleomorphic nuclei are centrally located, round, and vesicular with irregular membranes and often contain prominent nucleoli; cleftlike spaces are often present
- Frequent, sometimes abnormal, mitoses with foci of necrosis and hemorrhage
- Usually combined with other germ cell elements, most commonly YST

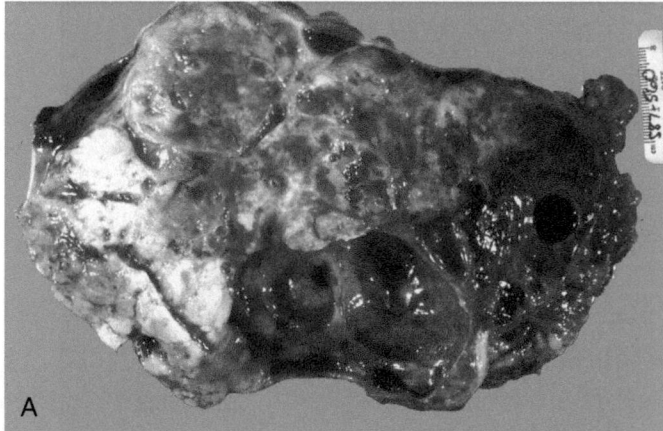

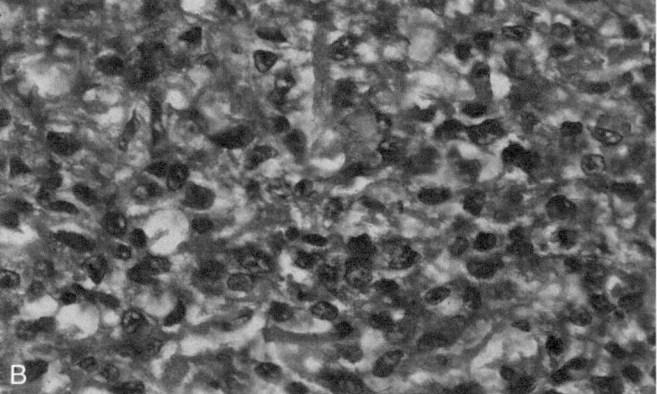

Figure 12-62. Embryonal carcinoma. **A,** Cross section shows a lobulated gray-white tumor that is partially cystic and hemorrhagic. **B,** Solid pattern composed of large polygonal cells with poorly defined cytoplasmic borders.

Special Stains and Immunohistochemistry

- Cytokeratin positive
- PLAP positive in syncytiotrophoblasts
- EMA negative

Other Techniques for Diagnosis

- Noncontributory

Differential Diagnosis

DYSGERMINOMA

- Consists of relatively smaller, more uniform cells, arranged in clumps and cords, in a fibrous stroma infiltrated with lymphocytes and rare syncytiotrophoblasts

YST

- Smaller cells with clear, glycogen-rich cytoplasm arranged in a reticular pattern mixed with solid areas
- Schiller-Duval bodies are classic; rare syncytiotrophoblasts

JUVENILE GRANULOSA CELL TUMOR

- Focal follicle formation with relatively less nuclear atypia; positive inhibin

PEARLS

- *Treatment: surgery and postoperative chemotherapy*

SELECTED REFERENCES

Chang MC, Vargas SO, Hornick JL, et al: Embryonic stem cell transcription factors and D2-40 (podoplanin) as diagnostic immunohistochemical markers in ovarian germ cell tumors. Int J Gynecol Pathol 28:347, 2009.

Oliver RT: Germ cell cancer. Curr Opin Oncol 11:236-241, 1999.

Scully RE, Young RH, Clement PB: Atlas of Tumor Pathology: Tumors of the Ovary, Maldeveloped Gonads, Fallopian Tube, and Broad Ligament, 3rd Series, Fascicle 23. Washington, DC, Armed Forces Institute of Pathology, 1998, pp 255-257.

Talerman A: Germ cell tumors of the ovary. Curr Opin Obstet Gynecol 9:44-47, 1997.

POLYEMBRYOMA

Clinical Features

- Rare malignant tumor typically occurring in children and young adults
- May have elevation of serum AFP and HCG

Gross Pathology

- Typically, a unilateral, solid tumor with areas of hemorrhage and necrosis

Histopathology

- Numerous embryoid bodies, resembling early embryos in different stages of development, scattered in a fibrous or edematous stroma
- More differentiated embryoid body contains an embryonic disk, amniotic cavity, yolk sac, and extraembryonic mesenchyme
- Embryonic disk elements consist of an ectodermal layer of tall columnar cells and an endodermal layer of cuboidal cells
- Occasionally chorionic elements, including syncytiotrophoblastic giant cells, are present

- Embryoid bodies may appear as a normal early embryo or may appear malformed
- Seen in association with other neoplastic germ cell elements, usually mature or immature teratoma

Special Stains and Immunohistochemistry

- AFP highlights yolk sac component and hepatic elements
- α_1-Antitrypsin may highlight yolk sac component of embryoid bodies and hepatic elements
- HCG highlights syncytiotrophoblastic elements

Other Techniques for Diagnosis

- Noncontributory

Differential Diagnosis

RETIFORM SLCT

- Peak incidence in first decade, sometimes presenting with androgenic manifestations
- Tubular and cystic structures; tubules lined by one or more layers of cells with round, regular nuclei and scanty cytoplasm; most retiform tumors are seen with other SLCT subtypes

PEARLS

- *Embryoid bodies probably arise from multipotential malignant embryonal cells and never appear to develop beyond the 18-day stage*
- *Invasion of adjacent structures and distant metastases usually seen*
- *Treatment consists of surgical excision and chemotherapy*

SELECTED REFERENCES

Chapman DC, Grover R, Schwartz PE: Conservative management of an ovarian polyembryoma. Obstet Gynecol 83:879-882, 1994.

Scully RE, Young RH, Clement PB: Atlas of Tumor Pathology: Tumors of the Ovary, Maldeveloped Gonads, Fallopian Tube, and Broad Ligament, 3rd Series, Fascicle 23. Washington, DC, Armed Forces Institute of Pathology, 1998, pp 257-258.

Williams SD: Ovarian germ cell tumors: an update. Semin Oncol 25:407-413, 1998.

CHORIOCARCINOMA

Clinical Features

- Pure choriocarcinoma is rare; occurs in children and young adults
- Presents with an adnexal mass, pain, and sometimes hemoperitoneum
- Serum levels of HCG are elevated, manifesting as isosexual precocious puberty in children and as signs of ectopic pregnancy in adults

Gross Pathology

- Unilateral solid, gray-white hemorrhagic tumor, sometimes with necrosis
- Depends on other germ cell components

Histopathology

- Most are a component of a mixed germ cell tumor and characterized by a mixture of cytotrophoblast and syncytiotrophoblast (Figure 12-63)

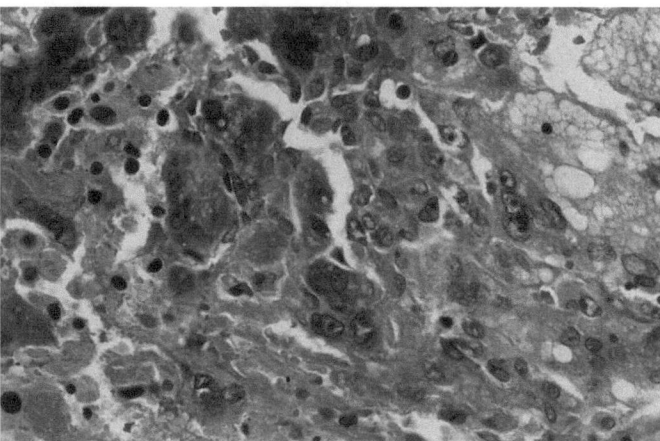

Figure 12-63. Primary ovarian choriocarcinoma. Both components are present: cytotrophoblast and syncytiotrophoblast.

- Cytotrophoblastic cells placed centrally within the tumor surrounded by syncytiotrophoblastic cells, frequently with associated hemorrhage
- Mononucleate cytotrophoblasts show clear cytoplasm and obvious cell borders; small, centrally located, round, hyperchromatic vesicular nuclei with prominent nucleoli
- Multinucleate syncytiotrophoblastic cells are large and basophilic with vacuolated cytoplasm and many hyperchromatic nuclei

Special Stains and Immunohistochemistry

- HCG, PLAP highlight syncytiotrophoblastic cells
- Cytokeratin highlights cytotrophoblastic and syncytiotrophoblastic cells
- Human placental lactogen (HPL) highlights syncytiotrophoblastic cells
- HCG highlights cytotrophoblasts

Other Techniques for Diagnosis

- Noncontributory

Differential Diagnosis

EMBRYONAL CARCINOMA
- Isolated syncytiotrophoblastic cells may be present
- Pleomorphic cells of embryonal carcinoma have large nuclei with irregular chromatin; these cells are positive only for cytokeratin

DYSGERMINOMA
- Isolated syncytiotrophoblastic cells may be present
- Uniform round cells with abundant clear cytoplasm negative for cytokeratin

YST
- Isolated syncytiotrophoblastic cells may be present
- Small cystic spaces formed by mononuclear cells
- YST cells are positive for AFP
- Hyaline globules and Schiller-Duval bodies may be seen

POORLY DIFFERENTIATED SURFACE EPITHELIAL TUMORS
- Solid carcinomas occurring in older women may show apparent trophoblastic differentiation, with isolated giant cells which are HCG negative

- Immunohistochemically, this tumor may be positive for WT-1, EGFR, and cyclooxygenase-2

PEARLS

- *Highly malignant, spreading locally, intra-abdominally, and through lymphatics and blood vessels*
- *Treatment consists of surgery with chemotherapy*

SELECTED REFERENCES

Chang MC, Vargas SO, Hornick JL, et al: Embryonic stem cell transcription factors and D2-40 (podoplanin) as diagnostic immunohistochemical markers in ovarian germ cell tumors. Int J Gynecol Pathol 28:347, 2009.

Ezzat A, Raja M, Bakri Y, et al: Malignant ovarian germ cell tumours: a survival and prognostic analysis. Acta Oncol 38:455-460, 1999.

Scully RE, Young RH, Clement PB: Atlas of Tumor Pathology: Tumors of the Ovary, Maldeveloped Gonads, Fallopian Tube, and Broad Ligament, 3rd Series, Fascicle 23. Washington, DC, Armed Forces Institute of Pathology, 1998, pp 258-260.

IMMATURE TERATOMA

Clinical Features

- Rare, rapidly growing, malignant tumor presenting in childhood; peak incidence in first and second decades
- Asymptomatic until large, then symptoms are related to an abdominal or pelvic mass

Gross Pathology

- Typically a unilateral tumor with a median diameter of 18 cm, showing capsular perforation in half of cases and adhesions to neighboring structures
- Predominantly solid, but frequently mixed with small fluid-filled cysts
- Sometimes composed of one or more large cysts with solid areas in the wall
- Soft, variegated cut surface often with areas of hemorrhage and necrosis
- Areas of bone, cartilage, or hair may be present

Histopathology

- Made up of haphazardly arranged immature tissues derived from ectoderm, mesoderm, and endoderm; typically mixed with mature elements
- Ectodermal elements are mostly composed of neural tissue, including neuroepithelial rosettes and tubules, glia, and neuroblastic tissue (Figure 12-64)
- Mesodermal elements include cartilage, muscle, and immature mesenchyme
- Endodermal elements usually consist of tubules lined by columnar epithelium
- Important to sample all teratomas extensively for histologic grading, with neuroectodermal tissue being by far the most common immature tissue identified
  - Grade 0: all tissues mature; no mitotic activity
  - Grade 1: minor foci of abnormally cellular or immature tissue mixed with mature elements; slight mitotic activity
  - Grade 2: moderate quantities of immature tissue mixed with mature elements; moderate mitotic activity

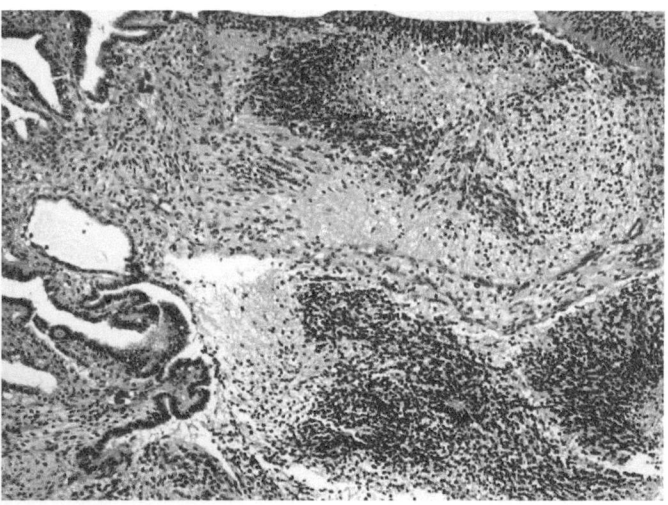

Figure 12-64. Immature teratoma. Small round blue and immature neural cells with rosettes associated with neuropil and mucinous glands.

SELECTED REFERENCES

Bezuidenhout J, Schneider JW, Hugo F, Wessels G: Teratomas in infancy and childhood at Tygerberg Hospital, South Africa, 1973 to 1992. Arch Pathol Lab Med 121:499-502, 1997.

Cushing B, Giller R, Ablin A, et al: Surgical resection alone is effective treatment for ovarian immature teratoma in children and adolescents: a report of the pediatric oncology group and the children's cancer group. Am J Obstet Gynecol 181:353-358, 1999.

Heifetz SA, Cushing B, Giller R, et al: Immature teratomas in children. Pathologic considerations: a report from the combined Pediatric Oncology Group/Children's Cancer Group. Am J Surg Pathol 22:1115-1124, 1998.

Kojs Z, Urbanski K, Reinfuss M, et al: Pure immature teratoma of the ovary: analysis of 22 cases. Eur J Gynaecol Oncol 18:534-536, 1997.

McCluggage WG: Ovarian neoplasms composed of small round cells: a review. Adv Anat Pathol 11:288-296, 2004.

O'Connor DM, Norris HJ: The influence of grade on the outcome of stage I ovarian immature (malignant) teratomas: the reproducibility of grading. Int J Gynecol Pathol 13:283, 1994.

Ulbright TM: Gonadal teratomas: a review and speculation. Adv Anat Pathol 11:10-23, 2004.

- Grade 3: large quantities of immature tissue; high mitotic activity
- A two-tier grading system is also used (low versus high)

Stains and Immunohistochemistry

- Neural markers, including chromogranin and synaptophysin; GAFP and S-100 protein highlight neuroectodermal tissue

Other Techniques for Diagnosis

- Noncontributory

Differential Diagnosis

MATURE SOLID TERATOMA

- Thorough sampling should be performed to exclude immature elements

MALIGNANT MIXED MULLERIAN TUMOR

- Occurs in postmenopausal women; peak incidence between the ages of 50 and 70 years
- Composed of typical carcinomatous and sarcomatous cells

PRIMITIVE NEUROECTODERMAL TUMOR (PNET)

- Resemble PNETs seen in the central nervous system
- Peak incidence in second to fourth decades; hormonal manifestations
- Average diameter 14 cm

PEARLS

- *Mature cystic teratoma (dermoid cyst) may exist simultaneously in the contralateral ovary*
- *Spreads most commonly through peritoneal implantation, less commonly through lymphatics to retroperitoneal, para-aortic, and distant lymph nodes, and only rarely hematogenously to lungs, liver, and other organs*
- *Histologic grading is helpful in determining treatment and prognosis*
- *Poor prognosis for higher-grade tumors (grade 2 or 3), with treatment consisting of surgery and chemotherapy*

MONODERMAL TERATOMAS: STRUMA OVARII

Clinical Features

- Occurs most commonly during the reproductive years and is usually asymptomatic
- Some patients may present with a painful mass, swelling, or ascites; uterine bleeding has been reported
- Occasionally associated with thyrotoxicosis and thyroid enlargement

Gross Pathology

- Typically unilateral, less than 10 cm in diameter, and smooth surfaced
- Solid, brown or green-brown, glistening tissue separated by fibrous septa, with or without an associated mature cystic teratoma
- Fluid-filled cysts containing brown to green gelatinous fluid
- Hemorrhage, necrosis, and fibrosis reported

Histopathology

- Composed solely or predominantly of mature thyroid tissue or adenoma with small and large follicles lined by a layer of columnar, cuboidal, or flattened epithelium (Figure 12-65A)
- Follicles with colloid mixed with solid, cellular areas and sometimes cysts
- Can include oxyphilic, clear cell, and solid tubular forms
- May show changes similar to that of the thyroid gland, including hyperplasia, or thyroiditis
- Carcinoma is rare

Special Stains and Immunohistochemistry

- PAS highlights colloid
- Thyroglobulin highlights thyroglobulin in the struma component

Other Techniques for Diagnosis

- Noncontributory

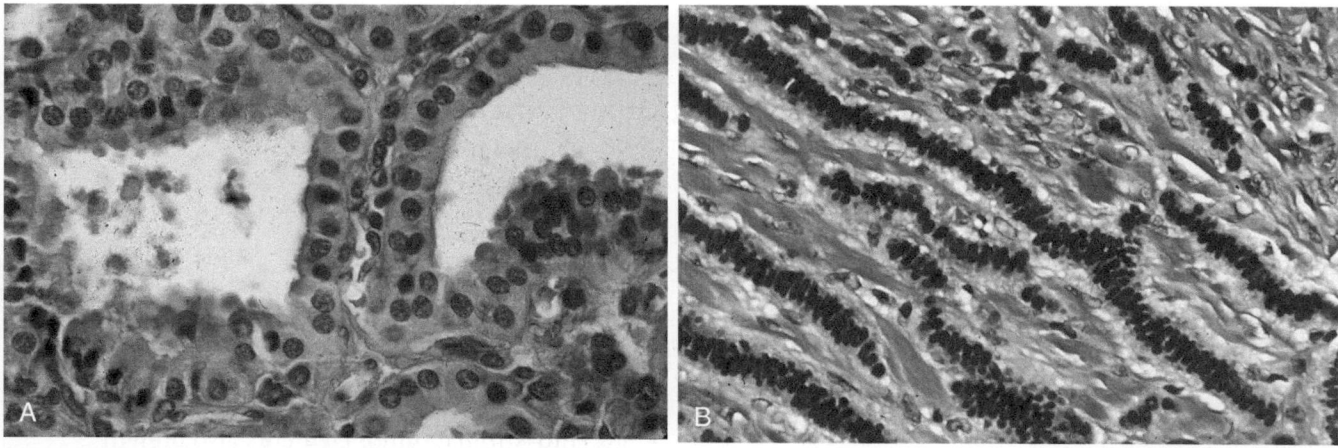

Figure 12-65. A, Struma ovarii. The neoplasm shows small papillary projections similar to those in hyperactive thyroid tissue. **B,** Carcinoid tumor. Trabecular pattern composed of long cords of neuroendocrine tumor cells surrounded by dense collagenous stroma.

Differential Diagnosis

MUCINOUS CYSTIC TUMOR
- Cyst content is usually colorless gelatinous material; cystic struma ovarii may contain green-brown gelatinous fluid
- Cyst is lined by mucinous epithelium with abundant intracytoplasmic mucin

SEROUS CYSTADENOMA
- Struma ovarii may rarely take the form of a unilocular, thin-walled cyst containing watery fluid; always shows at least one recognizable thyroid follicle

STEROID CELL TUMORS
- May be confused with an oxyphilic thyroid adenoma, but no thyroid follicles are present
- Struma ovarii shows calcium oxalate crystals and immunoreactivity for thyroglobulin

SERTOLI CELL TUMOR
- May be mistaken for a solid tubular adenoma
- Struma ovarii shows true thyroid follicles and calcium oxalate crystals and immunoreactivity for thyroglobulin

PEARLS

- *Thyroid tissue is commonly found as a component of mature cystic teratoma*
- *Regarded as a teratoma with an exclusively or mainly thyroid tissue component*
- *Generally benign and treated with surgical excision*
- *Infrequently complicated by ascites, adhesions, or malignant change with metastases*

SELECTED REFERENCES

Papadias K, Kairi-Vassilatou E, Kontogiani-Katsaros K, et al: Teratomas of the ovary: a clinicopathological evaluation of 87 patients from one institution during a 10-year period. Eur J Gynaecol Oncol 26:446-448, 2005.

Robboy SJ, Shaco-Levy R, Peng RY, et al. Malignant struma ovarii: an analysis of 88 cases, including 27 with extraovarian spread. Int J Gynecol Pathol 28:405, 2009.

Roth LM, Miller AW 3rd, Talerman A: Typical thyroid-type carcinoma arising in struma ovarii: a report of 4 cases and review of the literature. Int J Gynecol Pathol 27:496-506, 2008.

Roth LM, Talerman A: The enigma of struma ovarii. Pathology 39:139-146, 2007.

MONODERMAL TERATOMAS: CARCINOID TUMOR

Clinical Features

- Primary carcinoid tumors of the ovary are associated with other teratomatous elements in 85% to 90% of cases
- Most commonly an insular carcinoid; age range from 30 to 80 years
- Occasional presentation with carcinoid syndrome; more often with older patients
- Carcinoid syndrome consists of flushing, diarrhea, abdominal cramping, and, often, cardiac involvement
- Elevated urinary 5-hydroxyindole acetic acid (5-HIAA)

Gross Pathology

- Unilateral yellow-tan, small nodular neoplasm projecting into a dermoid cyst
- Less often found in a mucinous cystic tumor or mature solid teratoma
- Can predominate as a large, firm, homogeneous mass

Histopathology

- Insular carcinoid resembles a midgut carcinoid with discrete groups of small uniform cells separated by fibrous stroma (Figure 12-65B)
- Cells are uniform with abundant cytoplasm, nuclei with coarse chromatin, and rare mitoses; most are associated with other teratomatous components
- Variants also include trabecular, strumal, and goblet cell

Special Stains and Immunohistochemistry

- Chromogranin, synaptophysin, and NSE positive

Other Techniques for Diagnosis

- Noncontributory

Differential Diagnosis

GRANULOSA CELL TUMOR (MICROFOLLICULAR PATTERN)

- Mimics insular carcinoid showing round to oval cells with pale cytoplasm and round, often grooved nuclei; neuroendocrine markers are negative
- Mitotic activity is generally higher in carcinoid tumors

PEARLS

- *Tumor usually confined to the ovary*
- *Strumal carcinoid consists of a combination of thyroid and carcinoid components*

SELECTED REFERENCES

Athavale RD, Davies-Humphreys JD, Cruickshank DJ: Primary carcinoid tumours of the ovary. J Obstet Gynaecol 24:99-101, 2004.

Scully RE, Young RH, Clement PB: Atlas of Tumor Pathology: Tumors of the Ovary, Maldeveloped Gonads, Fallopian Tube, and Broad Ligament, 3rd Series, Fascicle 23. Washington, DC, Armed Forces Institute of Pathology, 1998, pp 291-300.

Soga J, Osaka M, Yakuwa Y: Carcinoids of the ovary: an analysis of 329 reported cases. J Exp Clin Cancer Res 19:271-280, 2000.

MIXED MALIGNANT GERM CELL TUMORS

Clinical Features

- Mixture of two or more germ cell tumors with their characteristic morphologies

Gross Pathology

- Tumor needs to be sampled extensively, especially in hemorrhagic, necrotic areas and distinct-appearing foci, to identify all the components

Histopathology

- Patterns described for each separate germ cell tumor may be combined in different variations and amounts in one tumor
- Usually two components: most often dysgerminoma and YST, or dysgerminoma combined with other germ cell neoplasms (Figure 12-66)
- Other tumors typically have between three and five types

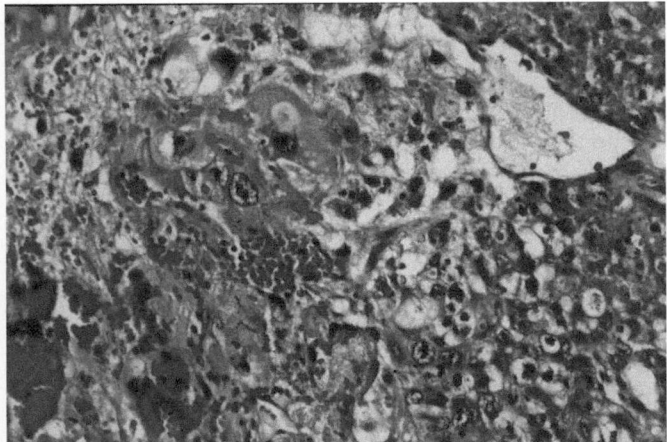

Figure 12-66. Malignant mixed germ cell tumor. A mixture of choriocarcinoma and embryonal carcinoma components is evident.

Special Stains and Immunohistochemistry

- See specific tumor types

Other Techniques for Diagnosis

- Noncontributory

Differential Diagnosis

GYNANDROBLASTOMA

- Extremely rare
- Granulosa cell tumor component present, representing more than 10% of tumor volume

GONADOBLASTOMA

- Occurs in phenotypic women with gonadal dysgenesis
- Sex cord–stromal tumor elements also present

METASTATIC CARCINOMA

- Clinical history is of extreme importance
- Lacks histologic features of germ cell tumors and is characterized by glands and sheets of malignant epithelial cells
- Negative for AFP, PLAP, HPL, and HCG

PEARLS

- *Tumor must be sampled extensively; each component and its quantity needs to be mentioned in the diagnosis in descending order of prevalence*
- *Prognosis may depend on the quantity of most aggressive component*

SELECTED REFERENCES

Akahira J, Ito K, Kosuge S, et al: Ovarian mixed germ cell tumor composed of dysgerminoma, endodermal sinus tumor, choriocarcinoma and mature teratoma in a 44-year-old woman: case report and literature review. Pathol Int 48:471-474, 1998.

Scully RE, Young RH, Clement PB: Atlas of Tumor Pathology: Tumors of the Ovary, Maldeveloped Gonads, Fallopian Tube, and Broad Ligament, 3rd Series, Fascicle 23. Washington, DC, Armed Forces Institute of Pathology, 1998, pp 260-262.

Tewari K, Cappuccini F, Disaia PJ, et al: Malignant germ cell tumors of the ovary. Obstet Gynecol 95:128-133, 2000.

OTHER TUMORS

GONADOBLASTOMA

Clinical Features

- Mixed germ cell and sex cord–stromal tumor affect children and young adults
- Almost always found in phenotypic women with an underlying gonadal disorder
  - Usually 46XY pure gonadal dysgenesis or mixed gonadal dysgenesis
  - Often associated with 45X or 46XY karyotype
- Presentation may include signs of virilization
- Can occur in phenotypic male or normal women with a history of pregnancy

Gross Pathology

- Solid, slightly lobulated, and often speckled with calcifications or totally calcified

- Brown, yellow, or gray ranging from a microscopic lesion to 8 cm in diameter, and frequently bilateral
- Large tumors usually show dysgerminoma overgrowth
- Gonad may be of uncertain nature: abdominal or inguinal testis, or a gonadal streak

Histopathology

- Germ cell or cells of sex cord–stromal differentiation arranged in nests; cells surround amorphous eosinophilic material (hyaline) (Figure 12-67)
- Large germ cells resembling dysgerminoma and seminoma, immature testicular germ cells, or spermatogonia
- Malignant cells contain vesicular nuclei with finely granular chromatin and prominent nucleoli and mitotic activity
- Epithelial cells of sex cord–stromal origin resemble immature Sertoli or granulosa cells: small, uniform, round or elongated cells, with scanty cytoplasm and pale nuclei; mitotically inactive
- Cells resembling lutein or Leydig cells are identified in the stroma between nests
- May show foci of calcification, hyalinization, or overgrowth by a malignant germ cell neoplasm (usually dysgerminoma)

Special Stains and Immunohistochemistry

- Noncontributory

Other Techniques for Diagnosis

- Noncontributory

Differential Diagnosis

Dysgerminoma

- In patients with gonadal dysgenesis and a Y chromosome, gonadoblastoma is always a possibility
- Gonadoblastoma within dysgerminoma may appear as a small focus of calcification or a nest of typical gonadoblastoma

Sex Cord Tumor with Annular Tubules

- Steroid cell tumor characterized by simple and complex annular tubules encircling hyaline material with few mitotic figures; lacks a germ cell component

- Tumors associated with PJS may show focal calcification of the tubules

PEARLS

- *Patient may have a malignant germ cell neoplasm in the contralateral ovary*

Selected References

Gibbons B, Tan SY, Yu CC, et al: Risk of gonadoblastoma in female patients with Y chromosome abnormalities and dysgenetic gonads. J Paediatr Child Health 35:210-213, 1999.
Iezzoni JC, Von Kap-Herr C, Golden WL, Gaffey MJ: Gonadoblastomas in 45,X/46,XY mosaicism: analysis of Y chromosome distribution by fluorescence in situ hybridization. Am J Clin Pathol 108:197-201, 1997.
Pauls K, Franke FE, Büttner R, Zhou H: Gonadoblastoma: evidence for a stepwise progression to dysgerminoma in a dysgenetic ovary. Virchows Arch 447:603-609, 2005.
Scully RE, Young RH, Clement PB: Atlas of Tumor Pathology: Tumors of the Ovary, Maldeveloped Gonads, Fallopian Tube, and Broad Ligament, 3rd Series, Fascicle 23. Washington, DC, Armed Forces Institute of Pathology, 1998, pp 307-310.

HYPERCALCEMIC SMALL CELL CARCINOMA

Clinical Features

- Hypercalcemic small cell carcinoma (HSCC) is most associated with paraendocrine hypercalcemia
- Occurs predominantly in young patients; peak incidence in second decade

Gross Pathology

- Unilateral, fleshy, solid, cream-colored to pale yellow–gray tumor
- Frequent hemorrhage and necrosis, cystic degeneration, and focal softening

Histopathology

- Sheets, nests, and cords of small round cells with sparse cytoplasm (Figure 12-68)
- Large cells are often present displaying hyperchromatic nuclei with one or two small nucleoli and abundant eosinophilic cytoplasm

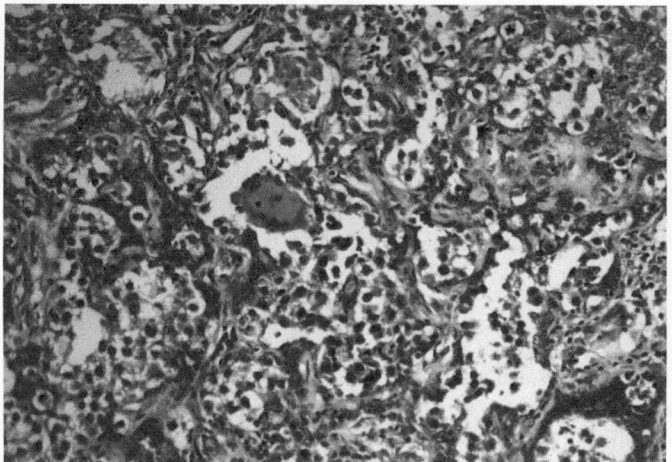

Figure 12-67. Gonadoblastoma. Low-power view shows solid nests of tumor cells surrounded by thin connective tissue stroma.

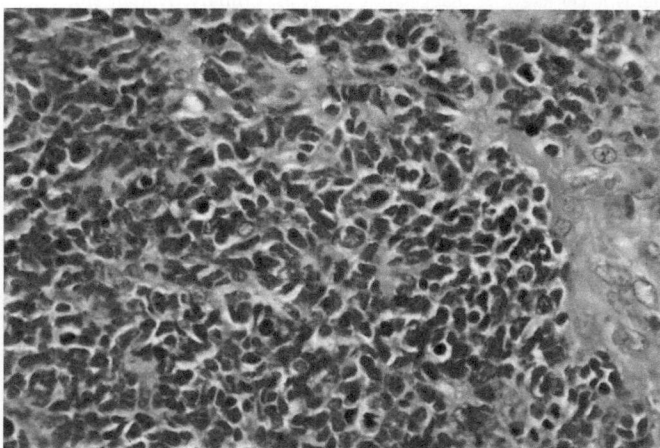

Figure 12-68. Hypercalcemic small cell carcinoma. Solid proliferation of neoplastic cells with a fine chromatin pattern and scanty cytoplasm.

- Brisk mitotic rate, necrosis, and occasional intracytoplasmic eosinophilic globules
- Small follicle-like structures containing eosinophilic material may be present
- Some tumors contain mucinous epithelium or focal mucin production

Special Stains and Immunohistochemistry

- Generally noncontributory
- Undifferentiated tumor negative for neuroendocrine markers, inhibin, and CEA

Other Techniques for Diagnosis

- Noncontributory

Differential Diagnosis

GRANULOSA CELL TUMOR (ADULT)

- Older age group (AGCT); functional, and not hypercalcemic
- Uniform cells forming Call-Exner bodies with much lower mitotic rate
- Less hyperchromatic cells sometimes with grooved nuclei (AGCT)
- Much lower rate of extraovarian spread

LYMPHOMA

- Lymphoma with an unusual insular or follicular pattern may mimic
- Diffuse HSCC may resemble malignant lymphoma
- Different immunohistochemical profile (CD45, B-cell markers, or T-cell markers positive)

PEARLS

- *Rarely familial*
- *Extraovarian spread often present and poor prognosis*

SELECTED REFERENCES

Hamilton S, Beattie GJ, Williams AR: Small cell carcinoma of the ovary: a report of three cases and review of the literature. J Obstet Gynaecol 24:169-172, 2004.

Lindboe CF: Large cell neuroendocrine carcinoma of the ovary. APMIS 115:169-176, 2007.

Mebis J, De Raeve H, Baekelandt M, et al: Primary ovarian small cell carcinoma of the pulmonary type: a case report and review of the literature. Eur J Gynaecol Oncol 25:239-241, 2004.

Seidman JD: Small cell carcinoma of the ovary of the hypercalcemic type: *p53* protein accumulation and clinicopathologic features. Gynecol Oncol 59:283-287, 1995.

Young RH, Oliva E, Scully RE: Small cell carcinoma of the ovary, hypercalcemic type: a clinicopathological analysis of 150 cases. Am J Surg Pathol 18:1102-1116, 1994.

METASTATIC TUMORS

Clinical Features

- Ovarian masses are metastatic tumors in less than 10% of cases
- Most common primary sites is the gynecologic tract. Other sites include intestine, stomach, and breast
- *Krukenberg tumor* originally referred to gastric carcinomas metastatic to the ovaries; currently it refers to cancers with signet ring cells of any origin

Gross Pathology

- Ill-defined, occasionally mucinous masses that are bilateral in about 70% of cases
- Hematogenous spread is an important factor, but transcoelomic dissemination, direct extension, and lymphatics also play a role
- Solitary or multiple discrete nodules and surface tumor deposits
- Predominantly solid, but may form one or more cysts (Figure 12-69A)

Histopathology

- Tumor on the surface, often with a desmoplastic stroma, multiple nodules, and blood or lymph vessel invasion and morphology different from that of primary ovarian tumors
- Usually adenocarcinoma
- Krukenberg tumors may completely replace the ovarian parenchyma with signet ring cells and glandular structures (Figure 12-69B)

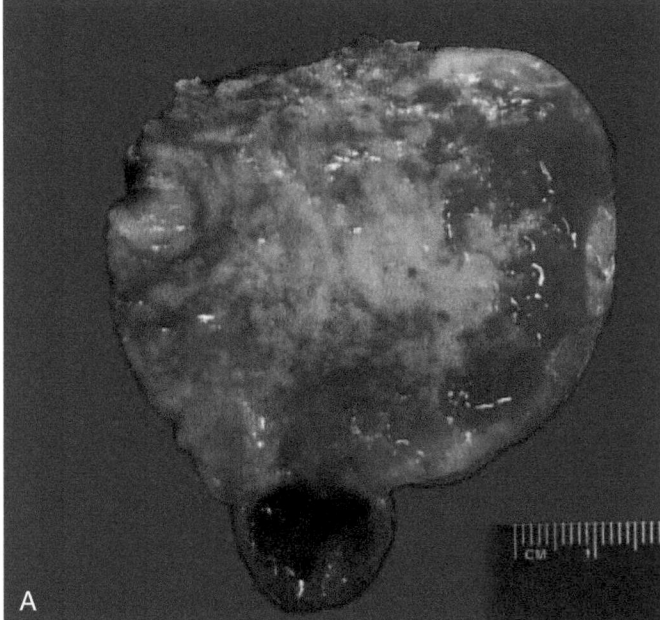

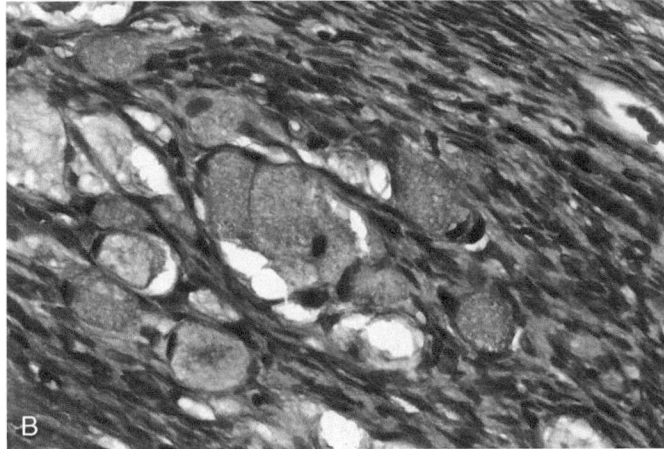

Figure 12-69. A, Metastatic gastric carcinoma, signet ring cell type. Cut surface shows the tumor replacing almost the entire ovarian stroma. A multinodular gelatinous tumor with cystic change is evident. **B,** Krukenberg tumor. Tumor cells are infiltrating the ovarian stroma. Notice the signet ring nature of the cells.

Special Stains and Immunohistochemistry

- See specific tumors
- Mucin positive in Krukenberg tumors and other types of mucin-producing carcinomas (e.g., intestinal, pancreatic, and occasionally breast)

Other Techniques for Diagnosis

- See specific tumors

Differential Diagnosis

- Clinical history is most important
- Metastatic tumors usually involve the cortex and the hilum of the ovary
- Histochemical and immunohistochemical stains as per suspected site of origin

PRIMARY MUCINOUS ADENOCARCINOMA VERSUS KRUKENBERG TUMOR

- Primary mucinous adenocarcinomas are typically unilateral with rare signet ring cells in the stroma, as opposed to Krukenberg tumors, which are bilateral in more than 70% of patients and essentially composed of signet ring cells
- Primary mucinous carcinoma is <5% of epithelial tumors
- This differential is often challenging in the absence of clinical history

PEARLS

- *May also include appendiceal carcinoid and pancreatic tumors as well as small cell carcinoma, malignant melanoma, malignant lymphoma, and leukemia*
- *Relevant clinical history, search for primary tumor elsewhere, and careful gross and histologic examination are important in the diagnosis of metastatic tumors*

SELECTED REFERENCES

Hart WR: Diagnostic challenge of secondary (metastatic) ovarian tumors simulating primary endometrioid and mucinous neoplasms. Pathol Int 55:231-243, 2005.

Khunamornpong S, Lerwill MF, Siriaunkgul S, et al: Carcinoma of extrahepatic bile ducts and gallbladder metastatic to the ovary: a report of 16 cases. Int J Gynecol Pathol 27:366-379, 2008.

Scully RE, Young RH, Clement PB: Atlas of Tumor Pathology: Tumors of the Ovary, Maldeveloped Gonads, Fallopian Tube, and Broad Ligament, 3rd Series, Fascicle 23. Washington, DC, Armed Forces Institute of Pathology, 1998, pp 335-372.

Yemelyanova AV, Vang R, Judson K, et al: Distinction of primary and metastatic mucinous tumors involving the ovary: analysis of size and laterality data by primary site with reevaluation of an algorithm for tumor classification. Am J Surg Pathol 32:128-138, 2008.

Young RH: From Krukenberg to today: the ever present problems posed by metastatic tumors in the ovary. Part I. Historical perspective, general principles, mucinous tumors including the Krukenberg tumor. Adv Anat Pathol 13:205-227, 2006.

FALLOPIAN TUBE

ACUTE AND CHRONIC SALPINGITIS

Clinical Features

- Young and middle-aged women who may present with acute abdomen
- Considered an ascending infection that may result in infertility
- Culprits: *Chlamydia* species or *Neisseria gonorrhoeae* followed by polymicrobial infection
- Less commonly associated with curettage or IUD placement
- Granulomatous salpingitis may be caused by tuberculosis, parasitosis, actinomycosis, or even systemic diseases such as Crohn disease and sarcoidosis

Gross Pathology

- Acute: tubal lumen distended by pus and secretions (Figure 12-70A)

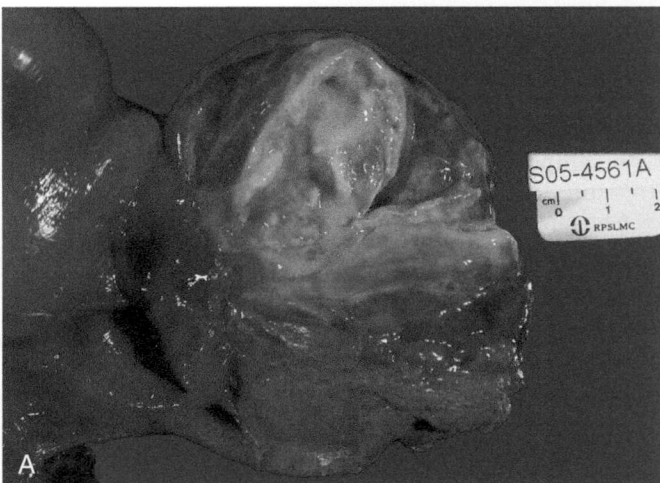

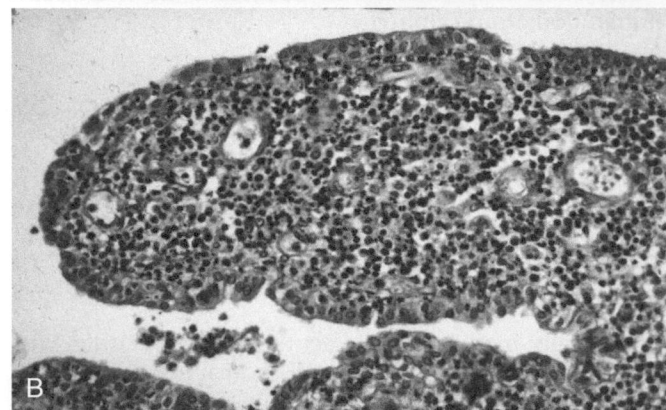

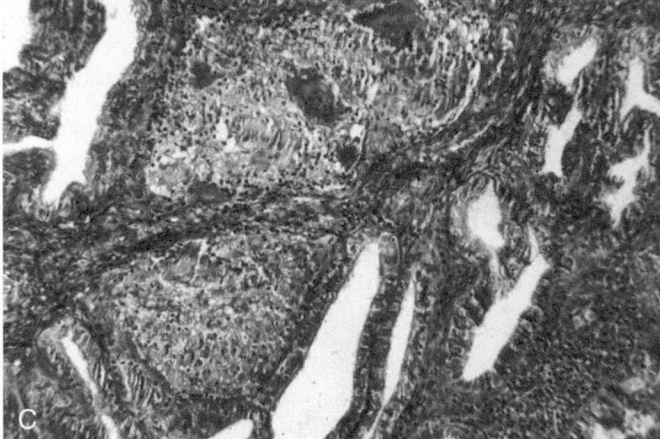

Figure 12-70. A, Acute salpingitis. Cross section shows a dilated fallopian tube containing purulent material. **B,** Acute salpingitis. Marked neutrophilic exudate in the tubal mucosa. The lumen also contains inflammatory exudate material. **C,** Granulomatous salpingitis (tuberculous salpingitis). Multiple granulomas and multinucleate giant cells are present (*center*).

- Massive hemorrhage may result in hemosalpinx
- Chronic: fibrotic tubal wall with adhesions

Histopathology

- Acute
  - Marked acute inflammation in plicae and tubal wall, fibrinous adhesions with congestion and edema (Figure 12-70B)
  - Pyosalpinx: mucosal ulceration with purulent exudate within lumen
  - Hematosalpinx: blood-filled lumen resulting from massive hemorrhage
- Chronic
  - Lymphoplasmacytic infiltrate in plicae and paratubal fibrous adhesions
  - Lymphofollicular hyperplasia suggests chlamydial infection
- Granulomatous
  - Caseating granulomas (tuberculosis) or noncaseating granulomas, such as in sarcoidosis (Figure 12-70C)
- End stage
  - Hydrosalpinx: thinned wall with clear hypocellular fluid in the lumen

Special Stains and Immunohistochemistry

- Gram stain may identify bacterial organisms
- Fite stain may identify mycobacteria in necrotizing granulomatous salpingitis

Other Techniques for Diagnosis

- Noncontributory

Differential Diagnosis

ECTOPIC PREGNANCY

- Particularly when hemosalpinx is present and serum HCG is elevated
- Immature villi or trophoblasts in clotted blood or tubal lumen
- Clinically may present as acute abdomen; clinical differential diagnosis includes PID and acute appendicitis
- May result in infertility

SELECTED REFERENCES

Fortier KJ, Haney AF: The pathologic spectrum of uterotubal junction obstruction. Obstet Gynecol 65:93-98, 1985.

Lareau SM, Beigi RH: Pelvic inflammatory disease and tubo-ovarian abscess. Infect Dis Clin North Am 22:693-708, 2008.

TUMOR-LIKE LESIONS

ENDOMETRIOSIS

Clinical Features

- Tube is frequently involved; other organs may also be affected
- Generally occurs in women of reproductive age and is associated with infertility
- May also occur after tubal ligation (*postsalpingectomy endometriosis*)

Gross Pathology

- Serosal nodules or dark areas of discoloration

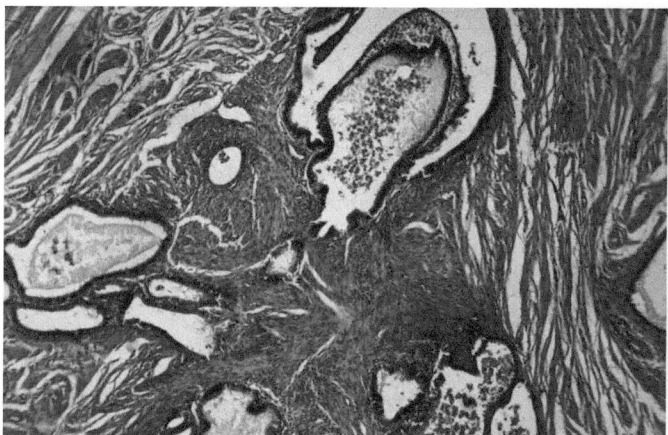

Figure 12-71. Endometriosis of the fallopian tube. The tubal wall contains endometrial glands and stroma.

Histopathology

- Identical to the morphology previously described in the ovary (Figure 12-71)
- In postsalpingectomy endometriosis, the endometrial glands with stroma extend from the mucosal surface into the wall at the site of the proximal stump

Special Stains and Immunohistochemistry

- CD10 highlights endometrial stroma

Other Techniques for Diagnosis

- Noncontributory

Differential Diagnosis

PHYSIOLOGIC EXTENSION OF ENDOMETRIAL TISSUE INTO THE FALLOPIAN TUBE

- Endometrial glands with stroma replace mucosa of isthmic portion of tube
- May fill lumen, resulting in occlusion of tube (endometrial colonization)

SALPINGITIS ISTHMICA NODOSA

- Dilated spaces lined by ciliated tubal epithelium (nonendometrial) within the thickened wall of the fallopian tube (similar to colonic diverticula)

METASTATIC ADENOCARCINOMA

- Glands are malignant
- Absent endometrial stroma around glands

PEARLS

- *Fallopian tube is a common site of endometriosis*
- *Serosal and subserosal process, which also involves other pelvic organs*
- *Must be differentiated from physiologic extension of endometrium (mucosal replacement)*

SELECTED REFERENCE

Scully RE, Young RH, Clement PB: Atlas of Tumor Pathology: Tumors of the Ovary, Maldeveloped Gonads, Fallopian Tube, and Broad Ligament, 3rd Series, Fascicle 23. Washington, DC, Armed Forces Institute of Pathology, 1998, pp 477-498.

SALPINGITIS ISTHMICA NODOSA

Clinical Features

- Most common in young women in the third or fourth decade
- Predisposes to ectopic pregnancy and is associated with infertility
- Pathogenesis is unclear

Gross Pathology

- Often bilateral
- Fallopian tubes display an intact serosal surface
- Isthmic nodules (1 to 2 cm) in the wall of the fallopian tube

Histopathology

- Outpouchings of tubal epithelium in the thickened muscle wall of the fallopian tube
- Small nests or cysts with tubal epithelium lining spaces surrounded by a muscle coat

Special Stains and Immunohistochemistry

- Noncontributory

Other Techniques for Diagnosis

- Noncontributory

Differential Diagnosis

ENDOMETRIOSIS

- Classic microscopic features as previously described in the ovary
- Glands tightly cuffed by endometrial stroma (not muscle coat)
- Generally present over serosal surface; no connection of glands to tubular lumen

METASTATIC ADENOCARCINOMA

- Glands are malignant
- No ciliated epithelial lining
- Desmoplastic or inflammatory stromal response dissecting muscle fibers

PEARLS

- *Salpingitis isthmica nodosa is analogous to adenomyosis in the uterus*
- *Unclear pathogenesis but associated with infertility and ectopic pregnancy*
- *Glands have been shown to connect to tubal lumen*

SELECTED REFERENCES

Majmudar B, Henderson PH, Semple E: Salpingitis isthmica nodosa: a high-risk factor for tubal pregnancy. Obstet Gynecol 62:73-78, 1983.
Scully RE, Young RH, Clement PB: Atlas of Tumor Pathology: Tumors of the Ovary, Maldeveloped Gonads, Fallopian Tube, and Broad Ligament, 3rd Series, Fascicle 23. Washington, DC, Armed Forces Institute of Pathology, 1998, pp 477-498.

TUBAL ECTOPIC PREGNANCY

Clinical Features

- From 1% to 2% of all conceptions are ectopic; fallopian tube is the most common site
- Number one risk factor is chronic salpingitis (35% to 45% have a history of PID)
- Other risk factors include congenital tubal anomalies, salpingitis isthmica nodosa, and endometriosis
- Often patients present emergently with tubal rupture and hemorrhagic shock
- Elevated serum HCG
- Ultrasound examination may identify the gestational sac

Gross Pathology

- Most commonly ampullary, although it may occur in isthmus or fimbriated end
- Blood-filled dilated lumen with chorionic villi that may be identified grossly
- Most cases contain at least one embryo (Figure 12-72A)

Histopathology

- Intermediate trophoblasts in tubal wall and vessels
- Syncytiotrophoblasts are present
- Lamina propria often shows decidual change (Figure 12-72B)
- Chorionic villi may invade muscularis and then serosa
- Microscopically identifiable embryo in most cases (Figure 12-72C)
- Atherosclerotic changes in tubal vessels
- Uterine curettage shows gestational change, including Arias-Stella reaction and decidualization, but no chorionic villi or trophoblasts
  - Arias-Stella reaction: due to gestational-hormonal effect on the endometrium featuring hypersecretory endometrial glands with complex architecture, hobnail cells, and nuclear atypia

Special Stains and Immunohistochemistry

- Cytokeratin positive in trophoblasts
- HPL positive in intermediate trophoblasts
- HCG positive in syncytiotrophoblasts

Other Techniques for Diagnosis

- Noncontributory

Differential Diagnosis

MISSED ABORTION OF INTRAUTERINE PREGNANCY

- Absent chorionic villi, trophoblasts, or embryonic tissue

PLACENTAL SITE TROPHOBLASTIC TUMOR (PST; PSTT)

- Absent chorionic villi or embryonic tissue

PEARLS

- *Commonly associated with PID*
- *Patients often present emergently with hemorrhagic shock after tubal rupture*
- *Hematosalpinx results from rupture of maternal vessels*
- *An embryo is often present; the most common outcome is abortion*

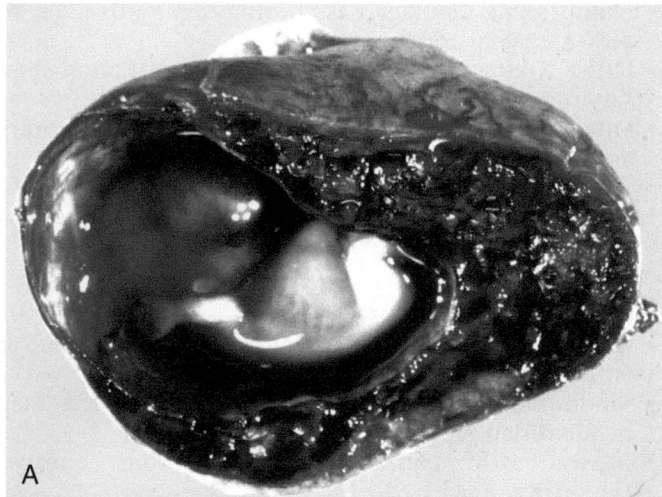

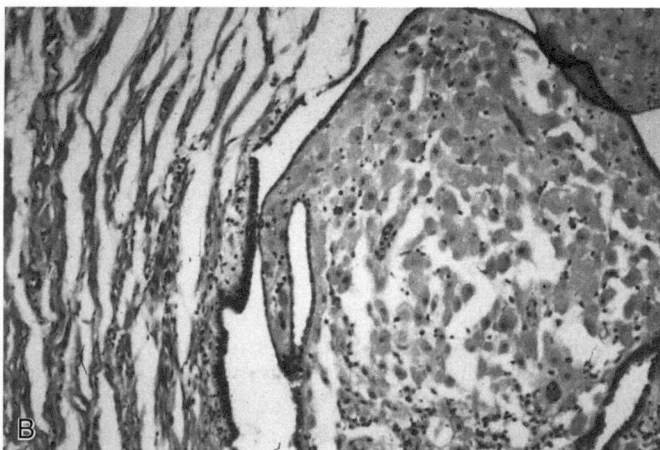

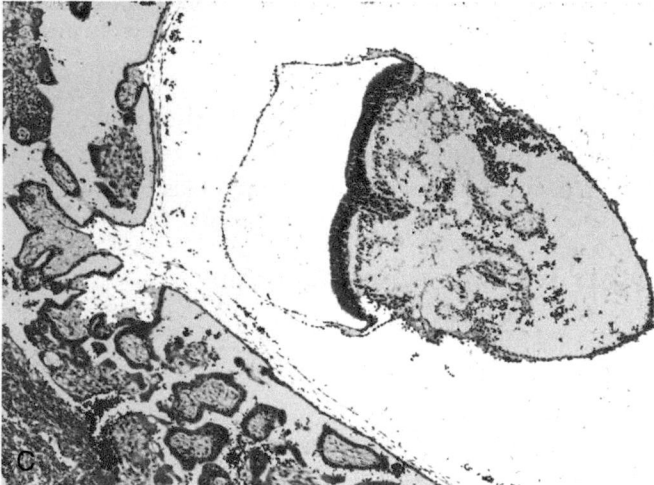

Figure 12-72. Tubal pregnancy. A, Cut surface shows a well-formed embryo. **B,** The lamina propria shows decidual changes. **C,** Histologic section of a tubal pregnancy shows a 7- to 10-day-old embryo (*right side*).

SELECTED REFERENCES

Jacques SM, Qureshi F, Ramirez NC, Lawrence WD: Retained trophoblastic tissue in fallopian tubes: a consequence of unsuspected ectopic pregnancies. Int J Gynecol Pathol 16:219-224, 1997.

Scully RE, Young RH, Clement PB: Atlas of Tumor Pathology: Tumors of the Ovary, Maldeveloped Gonads, Fallopian Tube, and Broad Ligament, 3rd Series, Fascicle 23. Washington, DC, Armed Forces Institute of Pathology, 1998, pp 493-498.

BENIGN TUMORS

ADENOMATOID TUMOR

Clinical Features

- Most common benign neoplasm of the fallopian tube
- Usually occurs in adult women and often asymptomatic

Gross Pathology

- Mesothelial origin
- Well-circumscribed, 1- to 2-cm, firm, yellow-gray nodule within the muscle wall
- Most often unilateral

Histopathology

- Adenomatoid and glandular patterns are most common
- Solid and cystic patterns are less common (Figure 12-73)
- Luminal spaces may contain acid mucin
- Hyperplasia of surrounding smooth muscle

Special Stains and Immunohistochemistry

- Cytokeratin, vimentin, EMA, calretinin and WT-1 positive
- Mucicarmine, CD31, CEA negative
- SMA positive in the surrounding smooth muscle

Other Techniques for Diagnosis

- Electron microscopy: features of mesothelial cells, including long slender microvilli, intracellular lumina, and intracytoplasmic filaments in bundles

Differential Diagnosis

LYMPHANGIOMA

- Positive for D2-40, CD31, and factor VIII; negative for cytokeratin

LEIOMYOMA

- As described in the uterus

MALIGNANT MESOTHELIOMA

- Poorly circumscribed tumor with cytologic atypia and mitosis; rare

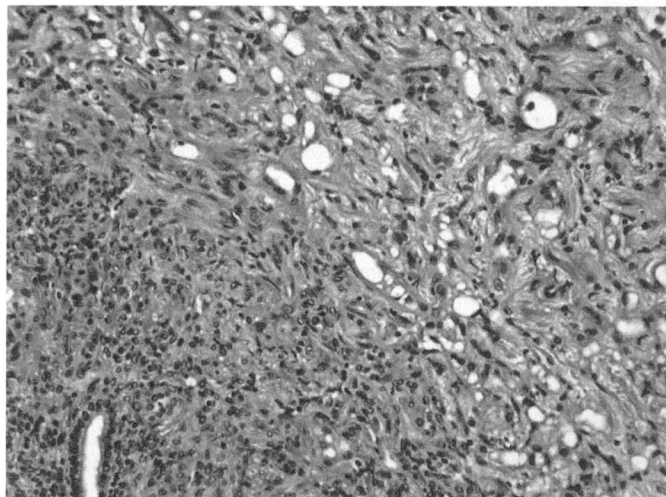

Figure 12-73. Adenomatoid tumor. Tumor composed of small slit-like spaces lined by cuboidal epithelium.

METASTATIC ADENOCARCINOMA
- Most likely from a gynecologic primary; extremely rare from extrapelvic organs

INVASIVE PRIMARY ADENOCARCINOMA
- Rare; tumor originates in the mucosa and extends through the wall

PEARLS

- *Arises from the peritoneal mesothelium and is essentially a benign mesothelioma*
- *May represent a nodular reactive mesothelial hyperplasia*

SELECTED REFERENCE

Scully RE, Young RH, Clement PB: Atlas of Tumor Pathology: Tumors of the Ovary, Maldeveloped Gonads, Fallopian Tube, and Broad Ligament, 3rd Series, Fascicle 23. Washington, DC, Armed Forces Institute of Pathology, 1998, pp 477-480.

OTHER BENIGN TUMORS

Clinical Features

- Mostly incidental findings; the most common is epithelial papilloma
- Most common benign mesenchymal tumor is leiomyoma
- Other epithelial, stromal, or neural tumors are extremely rare

Gross Pathology

- Epithelial tumors: small papillary or cystic mucosal lesions
- Mesenchymal tumors: small, well-circumscribed intramural nodules

Histopathology

- Epithelial papilloma: branching fibrovascular stalk lined by a single layer of benign nonciliated columnar or oncocytic epithelial cells (Figure 12-74)
- Other tumors show identical morphology to their counterparts in other sites

Special Stains and Immunohistochemistry

- Noncontributory

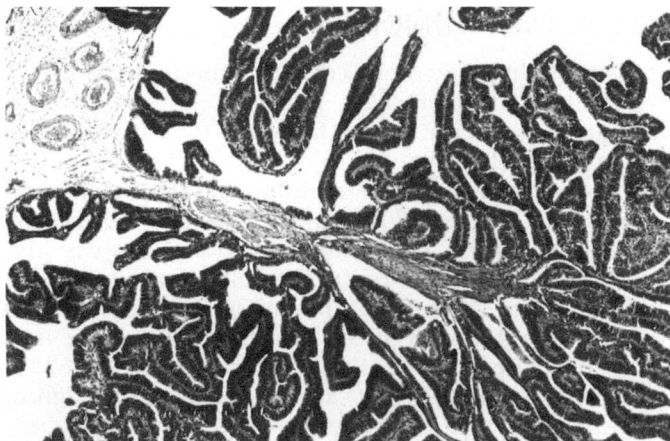

Figure 12-74. Epithelial papilloma. Papillary lesion lined by a single layer of uniform, nonciliated columnar cells.

Other Techniques for Diagnosis

- Noncontributory

Differential Diagnosis

ADENOMATOUS HYPERPLASIA
- Rare preneoplastic process showing epithelial cell stratification and crowding with loss of polarity, cytologic atypia, and occasional mitoses

METASTATIC ADENOCARCINOMA
- Patients have history of a primary malignant tumor elsewhere

PEARLS

- *Generally benign tumors are incidental findings of no clinical significance*

SELECTED REFERENCES

Bartnik J, Powell WS, Moriber-Katz S, Amenta PS: Metaplastic papillary tumor of the fallopian tube: case report, immunohistochemical features, and review of the literature. Arch Pathol Lab Med 113:545-547, 1989.
Doleris A, Macrez F: Endosalpingeal papillomas. Gynecology 3:289-308, 1988.
Gisser SD: Obstructing fallopian tube papilloma. Int J Gynecol Pathol 5:179-182, 1986.
Keeney GL, Thrasher TV: Metaplastic papillary tumor of the fallopian tube: a case report with ultrastructure. Int J Gynecol Pathol 7:86-92, 1988.

MALIGNANT TUMORS

CARCINOMA

Clinical Features

- Rare, occurring in the sixth and seventh decades, and frequently bilateral
- May present with vaginal bleeding, clear discharge, pelvic pain, or pelvic mass (Figure 12-75A)
- Almost always invasive at time of diagnosis
- Serum CA-125 may be elevated

Gross Pathology

- Swollen tube filled and distended by solid and papillary tumor
- Bulk of the tumor is within the tube

Histopathology

- Serous Tubal Intra-epithelial Carcinoma (STIC)
- Carcinoma in situ (CIS)
  - Flat or papillary proliferation of atypical cuboidal tubal epithelial cells with large, stratified, pleomorphic nuclei, clumped chromatin, irregular nuclear membranes with loss of polarity, and high mitotic activity (Figure 12-75B)
  - Serous intraepithelial carcinoma (STIC) is perhaps the most common precursor of ovarian serous carcinoma
  - A transitional area between benign and malignant epithelium may be identified
- Invasive adenocarcinoma
  - Most common type is serous carcinoma histologically identical to ovarian counterpart
  - Less common types include mucinous, endometrioid, and clear cell

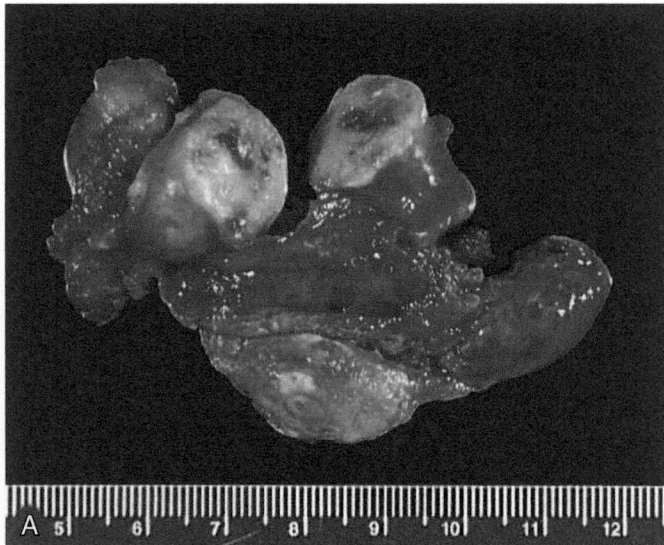

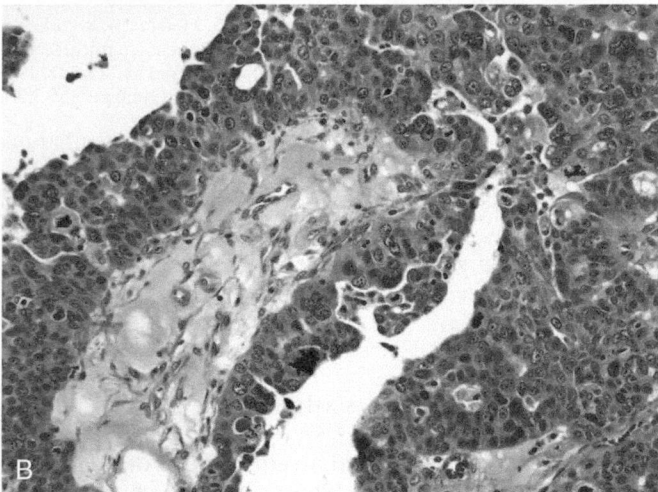

Figure 12-75. A, Serous carcinoma of the fallopian tube. Cut surface of an engorged fallopian tube filled with tan to yellow tumor with central hemorrhage and necrosis. Adjacent paratubal cyst and atrophic ovary. **B,** Papillary serous carcinoma. The papillary tumor shows cellular pleomorphism and marked nuclear stratification. Invasion of the lamina propria is present in other areas of the lesion.

Special Stains and Immunohistochemistry

- As per ovarian counterparts

Other Techniques for Diagnosis

- Noncontributory

Differential Diagnosis

METASTATIC CARCINOMA

- Overwhelmingly more common than primary fallopian tube malignancies
- Presence of tubal CIS supports the diagnosis of primary tubal malignancy
- Clinical history is most helpful

BENIGN TUBAL EPITHELIAL TUMORS

- Absence of cytologic atypia and mitotic activity

PEARLS

- *Primary cancers of the fallopian tube are rare and have a poor prognosis*
- *Morphologically, they resemble their ovarian counterparts*
- *Serous cancer is the most common*
- *Dysplastic epithelium adjacent to areas of outright malignancy is helpful*

SELECTED REFERENCES

Acs G, Pasha T, Zhang PJ: WT1 is differentially expressed in serous, endometrioid, clear cell, and mucinous carcinomas of the peritoneum, fallopian tube, ovary, and endometrium. Int J Gynecol Pathol 23:110-118, 2004.

Alvarado-Cabrero I, Young R, Vamvakas E, Scully R: Carcinoma of the fallopian tube: a clinicopathological study of 105 cases with observations on staging and prognostic factors. Gynecol Oncol 72:367-379, 1999.

Callahan MJ, Crum CP, Medeiros F, et al: Primary fallopian tube malignancies in BRCA-positive women undergoing surgery for ovarian cancer risk reduction. J Clin Oncol 1:3985-3990, 2007.

Jarboe E, Folkins A, Nucci MR, et al: Serous carcinogenesis in the fallopian tube: a descriptive classification. Int J Gynecol Pathol 27:1-9, 2008.

Medeiros F, Muto MG, Lee Y, et al: The tubal fimbria is a preferred site for early adenocarcinoma in women with familial ovarian cancer syndrome. Am J Surg Pathol 30:230-236, 2006.

Moore KN, Moxley KM, Fader AN, et al: Serous fallopian tube carcinoma: a retrospective, multi-institutional case-control comparison to serous adenocarcinoma of the ovary. Gynecol Oncol 107:398-403, 2007.

Roh MH, Kindelberg D, Crum CP: Serous tubal intraepithelial carcinoma and the dominant ovarian mass: clues to serous tumor origin? Am J Surg Pathol 33:376-383, 2009.

Visvanathan K, Vang R, Shaw P, et al: Diagnosis of serous tubal intraepithelial carcinoma based on morphologic and immunohistochemical features: a reproducibility study. Am J Surg Pathol. 35(12):1766-1775, 2011.

SARCOMAS AND MIXED TUMORS

- Leiomyosarcoma, although rare, is the most common sarcoma of the fallopian tube
- Carcinosarcoma, which is extremely rare, may arise in the fallopian tube

SELECTED REFERENCES

Buchwalter CL, Jenison EL, Fromm M, et al: Pure embryonal rhabdomyosarcoma of the fallopian tube. Gynecol Oncol 67:95-101, 1997.

Carlson JA, Ackerman BL, Wheeler JE: Malignant mixed müllerian tumor of the fallopian tube. Cancer 71:187-192, 1993.

Hellstrom A, Auer G, Silversward C, Pettersson F: Malignant mixed müllerian tumor of the fallopian tube: the Radiumhemmet series, 1923-1993. Int J Gynecol 5 (suppl):68-73, 1995.

METASTATIC TUMORS

- Overwhelmingly more common than primary fallopian tube malignancies
- Tumor metastatic to the fallopian tube usually originates within the pelvis
- Tubal involvement by lymphoma has been reported
- May extend from endometrium to mucosal surface of tube
- May invade the serosal surface by vascular space invasion or direct extension from a pelvic mass
- Presence of squamous differentiation implies metastasis; primary squamous cell carcinoma of the tube is extremely rare
- Presence of tubal in situ carcinoma suggests a diagnosis of primary tubal malignancy
- Synchronous tubal and other gynecologic organ tumors may occur
- Clinical history is essential

SELECTED REFERENCE

Scully RE, Young RH, Clement PB: Atlas of Tumor Pathology: Tumors of the Ovary, Maldeveloped Gonads, Fallopian Tube, and Broad Ligament, 3rd Series, Fascicle 23. Washington, DC, Armed Forces Institute of Pathology, 1998, pp 482-484.

GESTATIONAL TROPHOBLASTIC DISEASE

EXAGGERATED PLACENTAL SITE (EXAGGERATED IMPLANTATION SITE)

Clinical Features

- Occurs during normal pregnancy or in association with abortion or hydatidiform mole

Gross Pathology

- Gestational endometrium

Histopathology

- Extensive infiltration of myometrium by intermediate trophoblast (IT) which show single hyperchromatic nuclei) and some syncytiotrophoblast (ST) which are multinucleated
- Invasion of spiral arterioles by IT may be noted at implantation site; however, mitoses are rare, and chorionic villi may be present

Special Stains and Immunohistochemistry

- Cytokeratin positive
- HPL positive in intermediate trophoblasts
- HCG positive in syncytiotrophoblasts

Other Techniques for Diagnosis

- Noncontributory

Differential Diagnosis

PLACENTAL SITE NODULE

- Well-circumscribed and extensively hyalinized

PLACENTAL SITE TROPHOBLASTIC TUMOR (PST; PSTT)

- Deeply invades the myometrium
- Composed predominantly of sheets of intermediate trophoblasts with mitotic figures

CHORIOCARCINOMA

- Alternating areas of cytotrophoblasts, IT, and ST
- Vascular invasion may be prominent, and chorionic villi are absent
- May be extensively necrotic or hemorrhagic

EPITHELIOID TROPHOBLASTIC TUMOR

- Extremely rare
- Features markedly atypical mononucleated trophoblastic cells with a striking epithelioid appearance

PEARLS

- *Formerly referred to as* syncytial endometritis *or benign chorionic invasion*
- *Shows rare mitosis*
- *Preservation of normal uterine architecture*

SELECTED REFERENCES

Castrillon DH, Sun D, Weremowicz S, et al: Discrimination of complete hydatidiform mole from its mimics by immunohistochemistry of the paternally imprinted gene product p57KIP2. Am J Surg Pathol 25:1225, 2001.

Li J, Shi Y, Wan X, et al: Epthelioid trophoblastic tumor: a clinicopathological and immunohistochemical study of seven cases. Med Oncol 28:294-299, 2011.

Papadopoulos AJ, Foskett M, Seckl MJ, et al: Twenty-five years' clinical experience with placental site trophoblastic tumors. J Reprod Med 47:460-464, 2002.

PLACENTAL SITE NODULE (PLACENTAL SITE PLAQUE; INVOLUTING IMPLANTATION SITE)

Clinical Features

- Occurs in women of reproductive age
- Often presents with abnormal bleeding or is asymptomatic
- Generally without elevation in serum HCG

Gross Pathology

- Often not grossly visible
- Single or multiple tan-yellow excrescences or nodules may be identified in the endometrium

Histopathology

- Nodules and plaques of IT and rare ST
- Round cells with hyperchromatic nuclei, irregular membranes, and rare mitotic figures
- Abundant amphophilic, eosinophilic, or vacuolated cytoplasm and extensive hyalinization
- Central collapsed vascular lumina (thought to represent hyalinized spiral arterioles)

Special Stains and Immunohistochemistry

- Cytokeratin positive
- HPL focally positive in IT
- HCG rarely positive

Other Techniques for Diagnosis

- Noncontributory

Differential Diagnosis

PSTT (PST)

- Larger, poorly circumscribed, minimal hyalinization
- More cellular with brisk mitotic rate and atypical nuclei
- Deeply invades myometrium with necrosis
- Composed predominantly of IT; elevated HCG

PEARLS

- *Believed to represent unresorbed involuted placental site*
- *Benign; no treatment required even if diagnosed in curettage specimen*

SELECTED REFERENCE

Silverberg S, Kurman R: Atlas of Tumor Pathology: Tumors of the Uterine Corpus and Gestational Trophoblastic Disease, 3rd Series, Fascicle 3. Washington, DC, Armed Forces Institute of Pathology, 1992, pp 274-277.

HYDATIDIFORM MOLE: COMPLETE MOLE

Clinical Features

- Complete mole (CM) is the most common form of GTD; presents in second trimester
- Serum HCG continues to rise after 14 weeks of gestation instead of normal drop
- Uterus is disproportionately enlarged
- Vaginal bleeding suggests spontaneous abortion of mole
- Past history of mole increases the risk for future molar pregnancy
- Increased incidence of choriocarcinoma in patients with history of CM
- More common in Asia, Africa, and Latin America

Gross Pathology

- Grapelike clusters of vesicles corresponding to swollen villi microscopically (Figure 12-76A)
- Entire specimen appears involved

Histopathology

- All villi are abnormal; most are enlarged and rounded with cystic swelling
- Central cisternae, or empty spaces without vessels in the center of the villi, are readily identified (Figure 12-76B)
- Irregular diffuse circumferential proliferation of trophoblasts instead of normal, even, perivillous distribution
- Absence of fetal parts, including nucleated red blood cells

Special Stains and Immunohistochemistry

- HCG diffusely positive
- PLAP positive in syncytiotrophoblast
- HPL positive in intermediate trophoblast
- Positive for p53 in complete moles (owing to proliferation of cytotrophoblast)
- Focally positive for p57

Other Techniques for Diagnosis

- Cytogenetics: usually diploid 46XX
  - All chromosomes derived from sperm (androgenesis), hence absence of fetal parts
  - Less commonly 46XY and rarely triploid

Differential Diagnosis

PARTIAL MOLE

- Biphasic populations of normal and hydropic villi

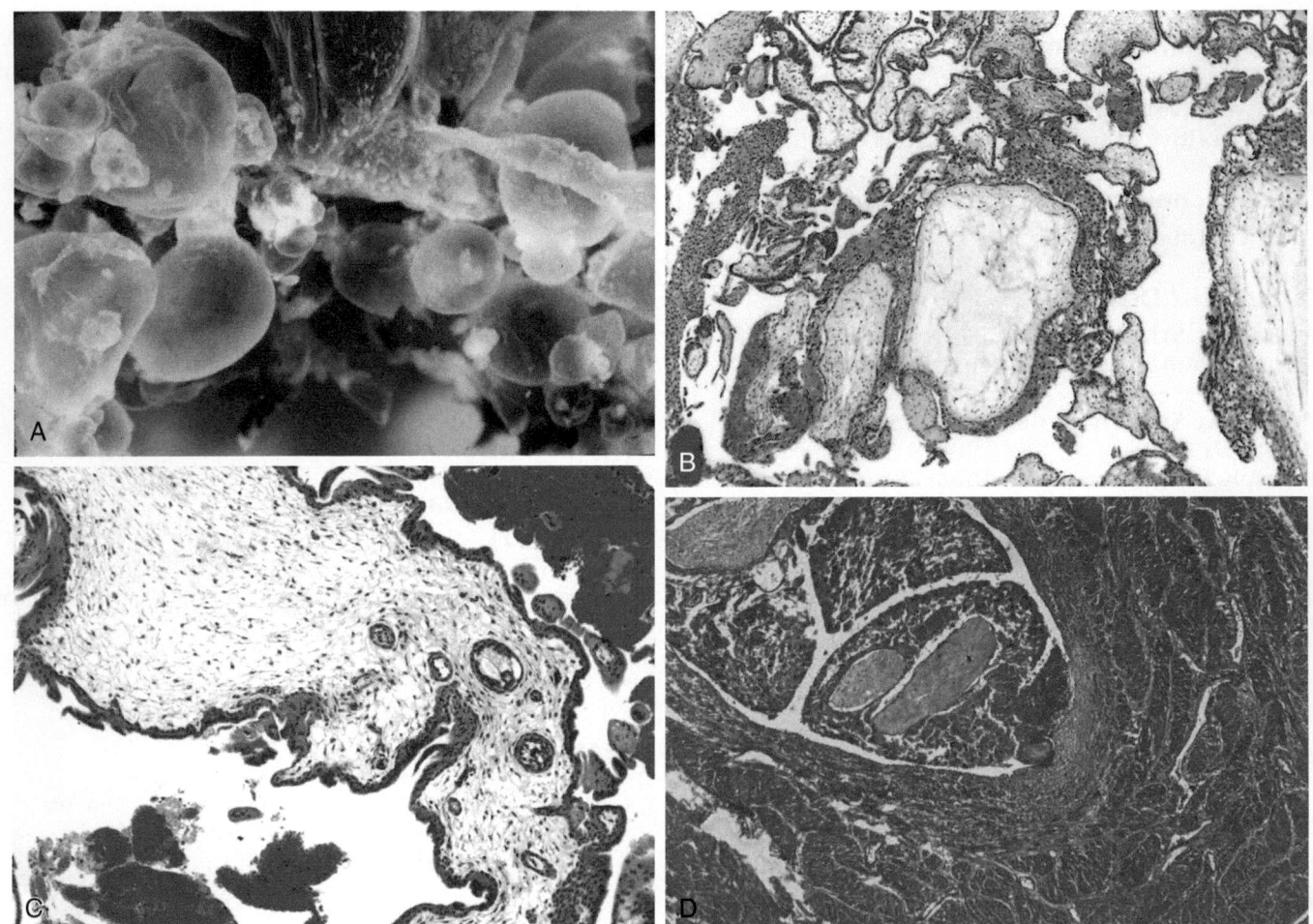

Figure 12-76. A, Complete mole. Gross appearance of the villi showing marked hydropic change reminiscent of bunches of grapes. **B,** Complete mole. Hydropic villi with cisterns and trophoblastic proliferation. **C,** Partial mole. Enlarged hydropic villus with scalloped borders and trophoblastic pseudoinclusions within the stroma. **D,** Invasive mole. Within the myometrial wall, there are several enlarged molar villi surrounded by concentric trophoblastic proliferation.

- Chorionic villi with irregular, scalloped borders with few if any central cisternae
- Fetal parts (e.g., nucleated red blood cells) may be seen
- Less pronounced, more focal trophoblastic proliferation
- Triploid by cytogenetics

EARLY NONMOLAR PREGNANCY
- Edematous villi are not apparent grossly
- Villous edema on microscopic examination is focal and mild
- Polar as opposed to circumferential trophoblastic proliferation, which lacks atypia, and rare to absent cisternae

CHORIOCARCINOMA
- Absent chorionic villi
- Myometrial and vascular invasion with necrosis

PSTT (PST)
- Absence of chorionic villi in greater than 98% of cases
- Proliferation of atypical IT rather than cytotrophoblast and syncytiotrophoblast

PEARLS

- *About 2% of complete molar gestations are followed by choriocarcinoma*
- *About 10% to 20% develop persistent GTD*
- *CM should be distinguished from partial moles because of the higher incidence of persistent GTD and choriocarcinoma in the former*
- *Therapy is complete evacuation by curettage with follow-up monitoring of serum HCG*
  - *Levels should be down to normal by day 60*
  - *If levels continue to rise, chemotherapy may be indicated*

SELECTED REFERENCES

Fisher RA, Lawler SD, Ormerod MG, et al: Flow cytometry used to distinguish between complete and partial hydatidiform moles. Placenta 8:249-256, 1987.
Shih I-M: Gestational trophoblastic lesions. In Nucci MR, Oliva E (eds): Gynecologic Pathology. Churchill Livingstone Elsevier, London, 2009, pp 645-665.
Silverberg S, Kurman R: Atlas of Tumor Pathology: Tumors of the Uterine Corpus and Gestational Trophoblastic Disease, 3rd Series, Fascicle 3. Washington, DC, Armed Forces Institute of Pathology, 1992, pp 233-238.
Szulman A: Complete hydatidiform mole: clinico-pathologic features. In Szulman A, Buchsbaum H (eds): Gestational Trophoblastic Disease, vol 7. New York, Springer-Verlag, 1987, pp 27-36.
Yap KL, Hafez MJ, Mao TL, et al: Lack of a y-chromosomal complement in the majority of gestational trophoblastic neoplasms. J Oncol 2010:364508, 2010.

HYDATIDIFORM MOLE: PARTIAL MOLE

Clinical Features

- Partial mole (PM) revealed by abnormal uterine bleeding
- Uterus is often small for gestational age
- Slightly elevated serum HCG level

Gross Pathology

- Few grapelike vesicular villi admixed with normal-appearing villi

Histopathology

- Edematous villi with irregular, scalloped borders admixed with normal-appearing villi (Figure 12-76C)
- Trophoblast proliferation is focal, as opposed to circumferential in CM
- Fetal vessels often contain nucleated red blood cells

Special Stains and Immunohistochemistry

- HCG strongly positive
- PLAP weakly positive (less cytotrophoblast proliferation, therefore fewer syncytiotrophoblasts)
- Weaker p53 than in complete mole (less cytotrophoblast proliferation)
- Diffuse p57 positivity

Other Techniques for Diagnosis

- Cytogenetics: most are triploid 69XXX or 69XXY (fertilization of one ovum by two sperm)

Differential Diagnosis

COMPLETE MOLE
- All villi are abnormal; many are hydropic
- Villi have more rounded borders with frequent central cisternae and more pronounced circumferential trophoblastic proliferation
- Absence of fetal parts
- Diploid by cytogenetics

EARLY NONMOLAR PREGNANCY
- Villous edema is not grossly visible and is microscopically focal and mild
- Focal polar trophoblast proliferation without atypia
- Absence of scalloping of villous borders
- Generally diploid by cytogenetics

PEARLS

- *Fetal parts, such as nucleated red blood cells, may be identified in villous capillaries*
- *Less common than complete moles*
- *Risk for persistent GTD is 5% to 10%*
- *Lower to negligible risk for subsequent choriocarcinoma (<1%) than for complete mole*

SELECTED REFERENCES

Fisher RA, Lawler SD, Ormerod MG, et al: Flow cytometry used to distinguish between complete and partial hydatidiform moles. Placenta 8:249-256, 1987.
Genest DR: Partial hydatidiform mole: clinicopathological features, differential diagnosis, ploidy and molecular studies, and gold standards for diagnosis. Int J Gynecol Pathol 20:315-332, 2001.
McConnell TG, Murphy KM, Hafez M, et al: Diagnosis and subclassification of hydatidiform moles using p57 immunohistochemistry and molecular genotyping: validation and prospective analysis in routine and consultation practice settings with development of an algorithmic approach. Am J Surg Pathol 33:805-817, 2009.
Paradinas FJ: The diagnosis and prognosis of molar pregnancy: the experience of the National Referral Centre in London. Int J Gynaecol Obstet 6(suppl 1):S57-S64, 1998.
Shih I-M: Gestational trophoblastic lesions. In Nucci MR, Oliva E (eds): Gynecologic Pathology. Churchill Livingstone Elsevier, London, 2009, pp 645-665.
Smith EB, Szulman AE, Hinshaw W, et al: Human chorionic gonadotropin levels in complete and partial hydatidiform moles and in nonmolar abortuses. Am J Obstet Gynecol 149:129-132, 1984.

INVASIVE HYDATIDIFORM MOLE

Clinical Features

- Extremely rare occurrence
- Presents with vaginal bleeding
- Uterine enlargement
- Persistently elevated HCG
- Most follow complete rather than partial molar pregnancy

Gross Pathology

- Invades the myometrium and shows irregular borders and hemorrhage
- May extend through the serosa and beyond to adnexa

Histopathology

- Abnormal chorionic villi with features of PM or CM penetrate myometrium or myometrial vascular spaces (Figure 12-76D)
- Proliferation of cytotrophoblastic and syncytiotrophoblastic cells
- Fetal parts are rarely identified (most arise from complete moles)

Special Stains and Immunohistochemistry

- Generally as per CM
- HCG diffusely positive
- PLAP positive in ST
- HPL positive in IT
- Positive for p53 as in CM (owing to proliferation of cytotrophoblasts)

Other Techniques for Diagnosis

- Cytogenetics: usually diploid 46XX as per complete moles; triploid if invasive partial mole (rare)

Differential Diagnosis

NONINVASIVE HYDATIDIFORM MOLE

- Absence of hydropic villi in myometrium or vascular spaces (trophoblast may be present in myometrium as a normal occurrence)

PLACENTA ACCRETA, INCRETA, OR PERCRETA

- Normal villi without molar change
- Absence of chorionic villi in blood vessels

CHORIOCARCINOMA

- Absence of chorionic villi
- Dimorphic population of cytotrophoblast and ST

PEARLS

- *Sequelae of complete moles*
- *Significant morbidity may result from uterine rupture and hemorrhage*
- *Responsive to chemotherapy*
- *Hydropic villi may embolize to lungs and brain but do not grow and usually regress spontaneously*
- *Differential diagnosis of persistent elevation of serum HCG following curettage of molar pregnancy is invasive mole versus choriocarcinoma, both of which respond to chemotherapy; tissue diagnosis is not often clinically indicated in this situation*

SELECTED REFERENCES

Castrillon DH, Sun D, Weremowicz S, et al: Discrimination of complete hydatidiform mole from its mimics by immunohistochemistry of the paternally imprinted gene product p57KIP2. Am J Surg Pathol 25:1225-1230, 2001.

Genest DR, Dorfman DM, Castrillon DH: Ploidy and imprinting in hydatidiform moles: complementary use of flow cytometry and immunohistochemistry of the imprinted gene product p57KIP2 to assist molar classification. J Reprod Med 47:342-346, 2002.

Kalhor N, Ramirez PT, Deavers MT, et al: Immunohistochemical studies of trophoblastic tumors. Am J Surg Pathol 33:633-638, 2009.

Shih I-M. Gestational trophoblastic lesions. In Nucci MR, Oliva E (eds): Gynecologic Pathology. Churchill Livingstone Elsevier, London, 2009, pp 645-665.

GESTATIONAL CHORIOCARCINOMA

Clinical Features

- Often presents with irregular bleeding and discharge of bloody, brown fluid
- High levels of serum HCG (tens of thousands)
- Complete mole is a risk factor (5% to 6% of cases)
- Older age (> 40 years) is also a risk factor
- Rapidly invasive and widely metastatic: most commonly to vagina and lungs, followed by brain, bone marrow, and liver
- Highly responsive to chemotherapy (in contrast to nongestational or extrauterine choriocarcinoma)

Gross Pathology

- Usually present within uterine cavity but may also arise in sites of ectopic pregnancy (uncommon)
- Soft, fleshy, tan-white tumor
- Variegated cut surface with large areas of necrosis, cystic degeneration, and hemorrhage

Histopathology (Figure 12-77A,B)

- Purely trophoblastic proliferation: chorionic villi are absent
- Alternating areas of cytotrophoblast and ST or IT
  - Cytotrophoblasts
    - Small mononuclear cells with pale granular or clear cytoplasm and distinct cell borders
    - May be mitotically active
  - Syncytiotrophoblasts
    - Larger multinucleate cells
    - Opaque cytoplasm with vacuoles
  - Intermediate trophoblasts
    - Medium-sized cells with single nucleus
    - Opaque cytoplasm without vacuoles
    - Irregular cell borders
- Marked nuclear pleomorphism and brisk mitotic rate
- Central necrosis and hemorrhage (owing to rapid growth) and prominent vascular invasion

Special Stains and Immunohistochemistry

- HCG positive in syncytiotrophoblast
- HPL positive in intermediate trophoblast
- Cytokeratin positive in all forms of trophoblast
- CEA may be positive

Other Techniques for Diagnosis

- Noncontributory

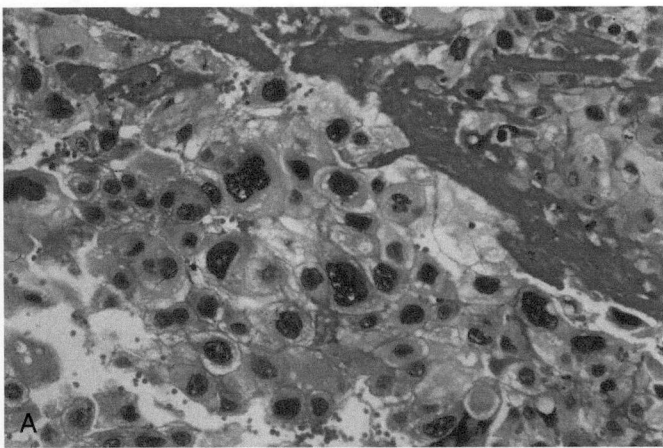

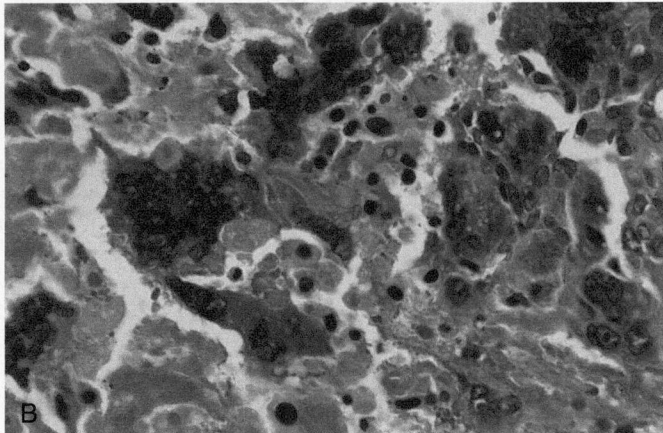

Figure 12-77. Choriocarcinoma. A, Mixed population of neoplastic cells featuring intermediate trophoblast and binucleate and multinucleate neoplastic cells. Cytotrophoblast cells are not readily identified in this picture. **B,** A mixture of cytotrophoblast and syncytiotrophoblast cells is present in this lesion.

Differential Diagnosis

EARLY NONMOLAR PREGNANCY
- Smaller numbers of randomly arranged trophoblastic cells with or without villi
- Serum HCG levels will return to normal following curettage or spontaneous abortion

HYDATIDIFORM MOLE
- Hydropic villi present grossly and microscopically

INVASIVE MOLE
- Hydropic villi present grossly and microscopically within the myometrium

PSTT (PST)
- Lower serum HCG levels (around 1000)
- Predominance of IT (HPL much higher than HCG immunohistochemically)
- Fibrin within and around vessel walls
- Less hemorrhage and necrosis

POORLY DIFFERENTIATED CARCINOMA
- Usually not biphasic
- Negative HCG and HPL immunohistochemically
- Negative serum HCG level (unless in pregnant patient)

EPITHELIOID TROPHOBLASTIC TUMOR
- Pleomorphic mononucleate trophoblastic cells predominate
- Remarkable epithelioid appearance
- Less necrosis and hemorrhage than choriocarcinoma

PEARLS

- *Characteristic biphasic pattern of cytotrophoblast and ST (less commonly, IT and ST)*
- *There is a variant that is composed of highly atypical intermediate cells in a rich fibrovascular network*
- *Primary tumor may be so extensively necrotic that in patients with metastatic disease the primary may not be found*
- *Gestational choriocarcinoma is highly responsive to chemotherapy (cure rate approaches 100%), whereas nongestational and extrauterine choriocarcinomas are significantly more resistant*

SELECTED REFERENCES

Brewer JI, Mazur MT: Gestational choriocarcinoma: its origin in the placenta during seemingly normal pregnancy. Am J Surg Pathol 5:267-277, 1981.

Duncan DA, Mazur MT: Trophoblastic tumors: ultrastructural comparison of choriocarcinoma and placental-site trophoblastic tumor. Hum Pathol 20:370-381, 1989.

Mazur MT: Metastatic gestational choriocarcinoma: unusual pathologic variant following therapy. Cancer 63:1370-1377, 1989.

Seckl MJ, Fisher RA, Slerno G, et al: Choriocarcinoma and partial hydatidiform moles. Lancet 356:36-39, 2000.

PLACENTAL SITE TROPHOBLASTIC TUMOR (PSTT; PST)

Clinical Features

- Presents with amenorrhea or abnormal bleeding
- Most follow a normal pregnancy or missed abortion (rather than molar pregnancy)
- Uterus is often enlarged, and uterine perforation may occur
- Low but persistently elevated serum HCG level
- Most are considered benign (75% to 85%)

Gross Pathology

- Variable gross pathology: circumscribed or ill-defined borders
- Confined to myometrium, extension into endometrial cavity, or invasion to serosa
- Soft with a tan cut surface with small foci of tumor necrosis

Histopathology

- Predominance of intermediate trophoblast
  - Medium-sized cells with single nucleus, opaque bluish cytoplasm, and no vacuoles
  - Cells may be atypical and mitotically active with irregular cell borders
- Trophoblast infiltrates and splits the myometrial smooth muscle fibers (Figure 12-78)
- There is vascular invasion from the periphery of the vessel to the lumen with eventual replacement of the entire vessel wall
- Fibrinoid material is deposited in the vessel wall

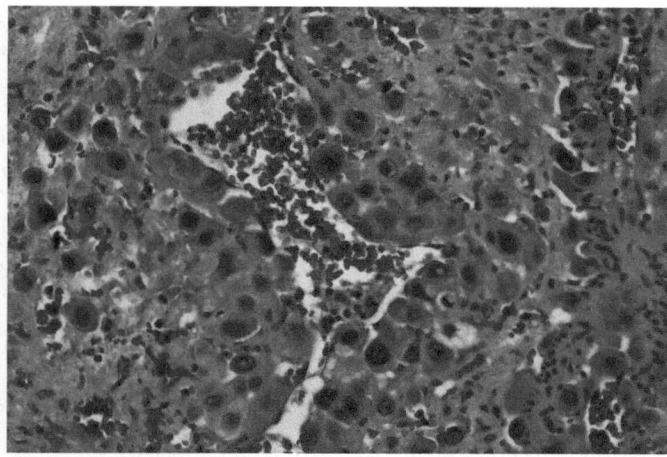

Figure 12-78. Placental site trophoblastic tumor. Intermediate trophoblast surrounds and invades the blood vessel wall.

- Poor prognostic indicators include high cellularity, high mitotic index, marked necrosis, local spread, and distant metastasis (lungs, liver, peritoneal cavity, brain)

Special Stains and Immunohistochemistry

- Cytokeratin positive
- HPL positive diffusely (predominance of intermediate trophoblast)
- HCG positive focally

Other Techniques for Diagnosis

- Cytogenetics: diploid by flow cytometry

Differential Diagnosis

EXAGGERATED PLACENTAL SITE

- Microscopic focus
- Serum HCG level returns to normal following curettage

PLACENTAL SITE NODULES AND PLAQUES

- Small and well circumscribed
- Extensive hyalinization
- Absence of cytologic atypia and mitoses
- Serum HCG level returns to normal following curettage

CHORIOCARCINOMA

- High elevation of serum HCG: tens of thousands (mIU/mL)
- Biphasic trophoblastic population with marked hemorrhage and necrosis
- Absence of fibrinoid material in and around vessels

Epithelioid Leiomyosarcoma

- Normal serum HCG level
- Lack of fibrinoid material in and around vessels
- Cytokeratin HCG and HPL are negative

POORLY DIFFERENTIATED CARCINOMA

- No fibrinoid deposits in vessel walls
- Negative HCG and HPL immunohistochemically
- Negative serum HCG level (except in pregnant patients)

PEARLS

- *These tumors are believed to result from dysregulation of extravillous IT as evidenced by myometrial infiltration and vascular invasion recapitulating implantation site*
- *Most are benign (10% to 15% are malignant)*
- *Malignant tumors do not respond to chemotherapy*
- *May be associated with a renal syndrome of hematuria and proteinuria with eosinophilic deposits in glomerular capillaries*
- *Treated with hysterectomy*

SELECTED REFERENCES

Baergen RN, Rutgers JL, Young RH, et al: Placental site trophoblastic tumor: a study of 55 cases and review of the literature emphasizing factors of prognostic significance. Gynecol Oncol 100:511-520, 2006.

Duncan DA, Mazur MT: Placental site trophoblastic tumor: a study of 55 cases and review of the literature emphasizing factors of prognostic significance. Gynecol Oncol 100:511-520, 2006.

Papadopoulos AJ, Foskett M, Seckl MJ, et al: Twenty-five years' clinical experience with placental site trophoblastic tumors. J Reprod Med 47:460-464, 2002.

Chapter 13

Breast

MARIA J. MERINO-NEUMANN

CHAPTER OUTLINE

SUBAREOLAR ABSCESS

Clinical Features

- Develops in lactating and nonlactating breasts, usually in nonlactating breasts
- Found in women of any age, typically during reproductive years
- Can be seen after reduction mammoplasty
- May resemble inflammatory carcinoma clinically
- May present as a painful, erythematous, and edematous breast
- Organisms associated with abscess formation include bacteria such as *Staphylococcus, Proteus, Bacteroides*, and *Streptococcus* species
- Tuberculosis may be the cause in endemic areas
- May have a tendency to recur and to form extended fistulas

Gross Pathology

- Incision and drainage of acute lesion yields purulent drainage
- Chronic lesion may show development of a fistula from the abscess cavity to the overlying skin

Histopathology

- Extensive neutrophilic inflammatory infiltrate associated with surrounding breast ducts (Figure 13-1)
- Involved ducts show extensive squamous metaplasia, with cell debris and keratin plugs in lactiferous ducts
- Foreign-body giant cell reaction may be seen

Special Stains and Immunohistochemistry

- Special stains for microorganisms (Gomori methenamine silver [GMS], periodic acid–Schiff [PAS], and acid-fast bacillus [AFB]) are negative

Other Techniques for Diagnosis

- Noncontributory

Differential Diagnosis

PLASMA CELL MASTITIS

- Inflammation consists primarily of plasma cells with admixed lymphocytes rather than neutrophils

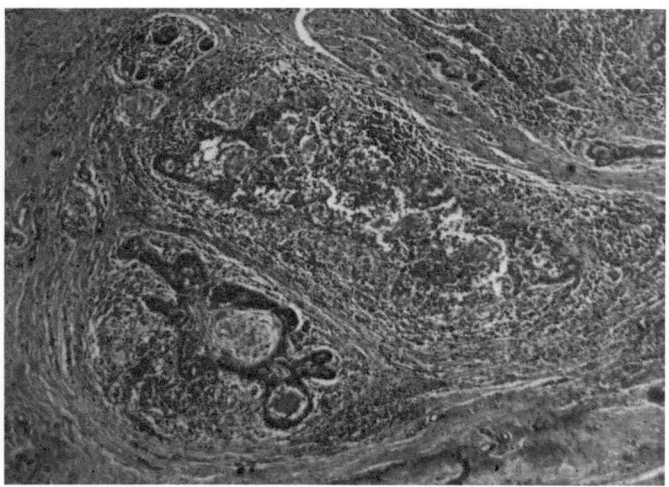

Figure 13-1. Subareolar abscess. Dilated ductal structures lined by metaplastic squamous epithelium are noted. The lumens contain keratinous and cellular debris. Mixed inflammatory cells are seen in the background.

GRANULOMATOUS LOBAR MASTITIS

- Granulomatous inflammation in and around breast lobules

PEARLS

- *Incision, drainage, and course of antibiotics is first-line treatment*
- *May require surgical resection of nipple and major duct system if sinus tract develops or in cases that repeatedly recur*

SELECTED REFERENCES

Ergin AB, Cristofanilli M, Daw H: Recurrent granulomatous mastitis mimicking inflammatory breast cancer. BMJ Case Rep Jan 25;2011.

Li S, Grant CS, Degnim A, Donohue J: Surgical management of recurrent subareolar breast abscesses: Mayo Clinic experience. Am J Surg 192:528-529, 2006.

Versluijs-Ossewaarde FN, Roumen RM, Goris RJ: Subareolar breast abscesses: characteristics and results of surgical treatment. Breast J 11:179-182, 2005.

PLASMA CELL MASTITIS

Clinical Features

- Typically found in women in second to fourth decades
- Usually found several years (average interval, 4 years) after cessation of lactation
- Presents with acute onset of breast tenderness, redness, and nipple discharge
- Following acute episode, a hard, palpable mass often remains mimicking carcinoma
- May be associated with axillary lymphadenopathy

Gross Pathology

- Large, dilated ducts containing thick, tan-yellow secretion

Histopathology

- Extensive lymphoplasmacytic infiltrate in and around ducts and lobules (Figure 13-2)

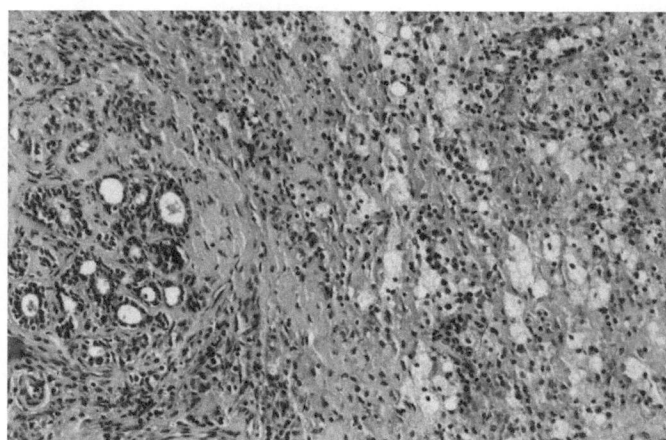

Figure 13-2. Plasma cell mastitis. Dense lymphoplasmacytic infiltrate is noted around a lobular unit. Xanthomatous reaction is also evident.

- Hyperplasia of ductal epithelium often seen
- Areas of necrosis may be present
- Scattered granulomas and histiocytes (xanthomatous reaction) are common

Special Stains and Immunohistochemistry

- Special stains for microorganisms (GMS, PAS, AFB) are negative

Other Techniques for Diagnosis

- Noncontributory

Differential Diagnosis

GRANULOMATOUS LOBAR MASTITIS

- Consists primarily of granulomatous inflammation with a minor component of plasma cells

TUBERCULOUS MASTITIS

- Granulomatous inflammation with caseating necrosis
- May occasionally be positive for AFB

PEARLS

- *Clinically mimics carcinoma*
- *May be diagnosed by fine-needle aspiration, but hyperplastic ductal epithelium should not be mistaken for carcinoma*
- *Excisional biopsy is curative and avoids possible skin ulceration or fistula formation*

SELECTED REFERENCES

Baslaim MM, Khayat HA, Al-Amoudi SA: Idiopathic granulomatous mastitis: a heterogeneous disease with variable clinical presentation. World J Surg 31:1677-1681, 2007.

Ming J, Meng G, Yuan Q, et al: Clinical characteristics and surgical modality of plasma cell mastitis: analysis of 91 cases. Am Surg 79:54-60, 2013.

Tavassoli FA: Plasma cell mastitis. In Pathology of the Breast, 2nd ed. Stamford, CT, Appleton & Lange, 1999, pp 792-793.

GRANULOMATOUS LOBAR MASTITIS (GRANULOMATOUS MASTITIS)

Clinical Features

- Etiology unknown, but has been linked to pregnancy, hormonal therapy, infection with corynebacterium, and autoimmune disorders
- Appears after pregnancy
- Usually presents about 2 years postpartum; may be seen many years later
- Typically presents as a distinct, hard breast mass
- Clinically mimics carcinoma

Gross Pathology

- Firm to hard breast mass, usually located peripherally
- Mass often has a nodular architecture
- Measures up to 8 cm; usually 4 to 6 cm

Histopathology

- Granulomatous inflammation in and around breast lobules (granulomatous lobulitis)
- Inflammatory reaction in lobules consisting of granulomas, multinucleated giant cells, plasma cells, and eosinophils (Figure 13-3)
- Fat necrosis and small abscess formation occasionally present

Special Stains and Immunohistochemistry

- Special stains for microorganisms (GMS, PAS, AFB) are negative
- Cytokeratin or other epithelial markers can help identify or rule out carcinoma obscured by florid granulomatous reaction

Other Techniques for Diagnosis

- Noncontributory

Differential Diagnosis

PLASMA CELL MASTITIS
- Marked plasma cell infiltrate in and around lobules
- Associated ductal epithelial hyperplasia is often seen

TUBERCULOUS MASTITIS
- Granulomatous inflammation with caseating necrosis, possibly AFB positive

BREAST ABSCESS
- Well-defined aggregates of acute inflammatory cells (abscess formation)

SARCOIDOSIS
- Primary sarcoid of the breast is uncommon
- Noncaseating, sarcoid-type granulomas typically are diffuse and found between breast lobules

CAT SCRATCH DISEASE
- Granulomatous reaction in lymph nodes that may involve intramammary lymph nodes

PEARLS

- *Appears after pregnancy*
- *Clinically mimics carcinoma*
- *Classic histologic picture is an inflammatory reaction in and around lobules with numerous multinucleated giant cells*
- *May recur and require many surgical treatments*

SELECTED REFERENCES

Gautier N, Lalonde L, Tran-Thanh D, et al: Chronic granulomatous mastitis: imaging, pathology and management. Eur J Radiol 82:e165-e175, 2013.

Lacambra M, Thai TA, Lam CC, et al: Granulomatous mastitis: the histological differentials. J Clin Pathol 64:405-411, 2011.

Marriott DA, Russell J, Grebosky J, et al: Idiopathic granulomatous lobular mastitis masquerading as a breast abscess and breast carcinoma. Am J Clin Oncol 30:564-565, 2007.

Yau FM, Macadam SA, Kuusk U, et al: The surgical management of granulomatous mastitis. Ann Plast Surg 64:9-16, 2010.

FAT NECROSIS

Clinical Features

- May present with a painless palpable breast mass or with breast tenderness
- May clinically and mammographically mimic carcinoma
- Believed to be related to trauma, most commonly previous breast surgery; other possibly related etiologic factors include cyst aspiration, radiotherapy, warfarin use, breast infection

Gross Pathology

- Typically of small size (< 2 cm)
- Single or multiple firm, round or irregular masses
- Tan-yellow streaks and often areas of dense fibrosis
- Areas of hemorrhage may be seen
- Cystic degeneration and calcification may develop

Histopathology

- Abundant lipid-laden and foamy macrophages surrounding small cystic spaces
- Foreign-body giant cells and chronic inflammation (lymphoplasmacytic infiltrate) are typical (Figure 13-4)

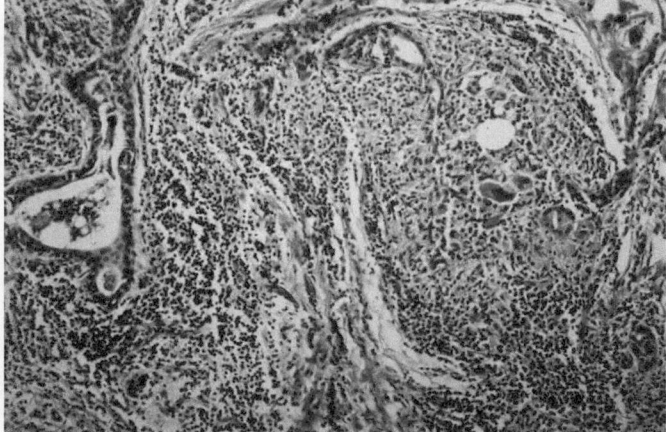

Figure 13-3. Granulomatous mastitis. The granulomatous inflammation distorts the lobular unit and shows giant cells.

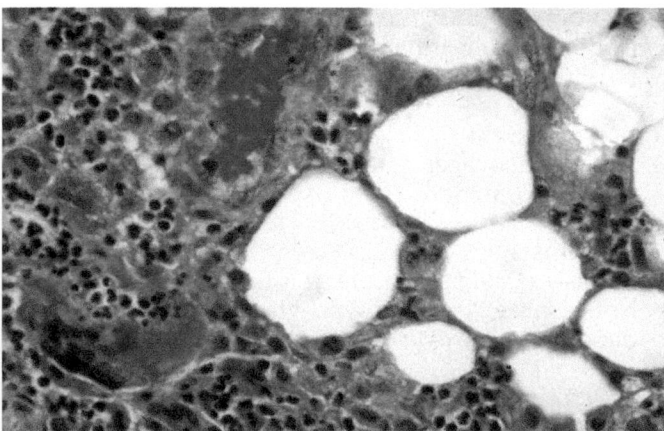

Figure 13-4. Fat necrosis. Fat vacuoles surrounded by chronic inflammatory cells and giant cells.

- Fibroblastic proliferation and collagen deposition seen in older lesions
- Scar formation and peripheral calcification are late manifestations

Special Stains and Immunohistochemistry

- CD68: histiocytes are positive
- S-100 protein negative, although it can stain the fat
- Cytokeratin negative

Other Techniques for Diagnosis

- Noncontributory

Differential Diagnosis

INFILTRATING DUCTAL CARCINOMA

- Neoplastic cells show cytologic atypia and increased mitotic activity and lack vacuolated cytoplasm seen in cells of fat necrosis
- Tumor cells are cytokeratin positive and CD68 negative

GRANULAR CELL TUMOR

- Nests or sheets of polygonal cells with abundant eosinophilic granular cytoplasm
- Lacks associated giant cells and lymphoplasmacytic infiltrate
- Granular cells are S-100 protein positive

PEARLS

- *History of trauma found in greater than 50% of cases*
- *Fat necrosis is almost always found surrounding previous biopsy cavity*
- *Skin changes that mimic carcinoma may be seen*
- *Mammographically, peripheral calcification, described as eggshell calcifications, may be seen*

SELECTED REFERENCES

Miller JA, Festa S, Goldstein M: Benign fat necrosis simulating bilateral breast malignancy after reduction mammoplasty. South Med J 91:765-767, 1998.
Tan PH, Lai LM, Carrington EV, et al: Fat necrosis of the breast: a review. Breast 15:313-318, 2006.
Trombetta M, Valakh V, Julian TB, et al: Mammary fat necrosis following radiotherapy in the conservative management of localized breast cancer: does it matter? Radiother Oncol 97:92-94, 2010.

DIABETIC MASTOPATHY

Clinical Features

- Most cases found in females with type 1 diabetes mellitus, with exogenous insulin use
- Widely reported in premenopausal women, with broad age distribution (teenage years up to fifth or sixth decade)
- Bilateral in about 50% of cases
- Presenting complaint is usually a hard, nontender, freely mobile breast mass
- Mammographic findings are nonspecific

Gross Pathology

- Hard, homogeneous, white-gray breast tissue
- Typically no distinct tumor is identified

Histopathology

- Dense, collagenous stroma (keloid-like) with proliferation of benign-appearing fibroblasts (Figure 13-5)
- No cytologic atypia
- Lymphocytic infiltrate around small blood vessels, in and around lobules and ducts
- Vascular calcifications may be present

Special Stains and Immunohistochemistry

- Lymphocytes are typically CD20 positive (B-cell lineage)

Other Techniques for Diagnosis

- Noncontributory

Differential Diagnosis

GRANULOMATOUS LOBAR MASTITIS

- Granulomatous inflammation in and around breast lobules

BREAST ABSCESS

- Prominent neutrophilic inflammatory infiltrate

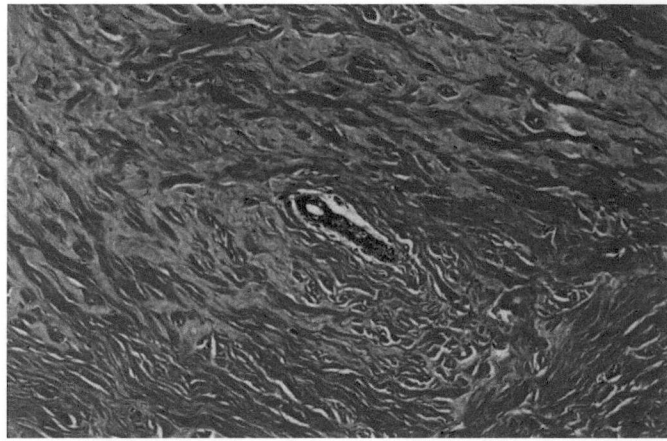

Figure 13-5. Diabetic mastopathy. Atrophic duct surrounded by dense collagenous stroma.

FIBROCYSTIC CHANGE

- Shows heterogeneous histologic features that may include cyst formation, apocrine metaplasia, adenosis, and ductal epithelial hyperplasia

PEARLS

- *Contributory factor may be alterations in collagen metabolism that exist in diabetic patients*
- *Self-limited condition primarily affecting premenopausal women*
- *Excisional biopsy is adequate treatment; rare cases have recurred*

SELECTED REFERENCES

Chan CL, Ho RS, Shek TW, Kwong A: Diabetic mastopathy. Breast J 19:533-538, 2013.

Dorokhova O, Fineberg S, Koenigsberg T, Wang Y: Diabetic mastopathy, a clinicopathological correlation of 34 cases. Pathol Int 62:660-664, 2012.

Fong D, Lann MA, Finlayson C, et al: Diabetic (lymphocytic) mastopathy with exuberant lymphohistiocytic and granulomatous response: a case report and review of the literature. Am J Surg Pathol 30:1330-1336, 2006.

Hunfeld KP, Bassler R: Lymphocytic mastitis and fibrosis of the breast in long-standing insulin-dependent diabetics: a histopathologic study on diabetic mastopathy and report of ten cases. Gen Diagn Pathol 143:49-58, 1997.

JUVENILE OR VIRGINAL HYPERTROPHY

Clinical Features

- Typically occurs in young girls (< 16 years)
- History of rapid growth of one or both breasts to massive, persistent proportions; overlying skin hyperemia and necrosis can occur
- Benign findings on mammography

Gross Pathology

- Diffuse process involving one or both breasts
- Discrete masses are not seen

Histopathology

- Characterized by proliferation of connective tissue and ductal structures (Figure 13-6)

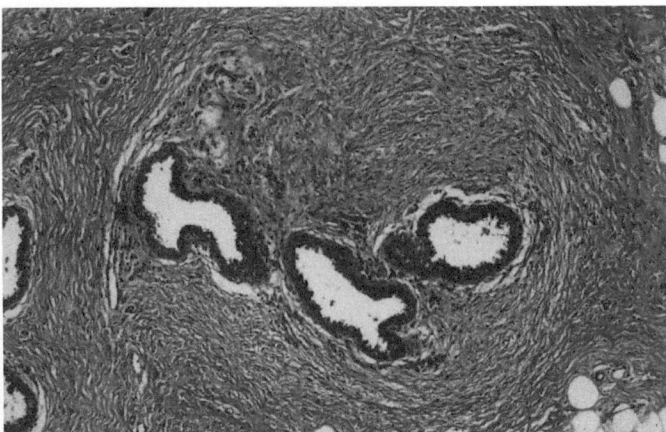

Figure 13-6. Juvenile hypertrophy. Ductal structures surrounded by loose proliferating connective tissue.

- Lacks normal lobular development
- May be histologically identical to gynecomastia

Special Stains and Immunohistochemistry

- Noncontributory

Other Techniques for Diagnosis

- Noncontributory

Differential Diagnosis

JUVENILE FIBROADENOMA

- Discrete nodules measuring an average of 2 to 3 cm in diameter that are able to be "shelled out" from surrounding breast tissue
- Hypercellular collagenous stroma with proliferation of slitlike, branching ducts

PEARLS

- *Cases in which each breast weighed more than 17 pounds have been reported*
- *Histologically resembles gynecomastia of the male breast*
- *May be related to hypersensitivity of mammary tissue to estrogen stimulation that occurs during puberty*
- *Usually sporadic, but familial cases have been described;* PTEN *gene mutation has been linked to virginal hypertrophy with increased risk for malignant transformation*

SELECTED REFERENCES

Govrin-Yehudain J, Kogan L, Cohen HI, Falik-Zaccai F: Familial juvenile hypertrophy of the breast. J Adolesc Health 35:151-155, 2004.

Koves IH, Zacharin M: Virginal breast hypertrophy of an 11 year old girl. J Pediatr Child Health 43:315-317, 2007.

Netscher D, Mosharrafa AM, Laucirica R: Massive asymmetric virginal breast hypertrophy. South Med J 89:434-437, 1996.

GRANULAR CELL TUMOR

Clinical Features

- Typically found in premenopausal women
- Presents as a firm, painless, solitary mass more frequently in the upper inner quadrant
- Mimics carcinoma on mammography

Gross Pathology

- Firm, hard mass with well-circumscribed or occasionally infiltrative borders
- Typically measures less than 5 cm
- Gray-white or tan cut surface
- May grossly mimic infiltrating carcinoma

Histopathology

- Composed of nests or sheets of polygonal cells with abundant eosinophilic cytoplasmic granules
- Cells have uniform, round nuclei with open chromatin and prominent nucleoli
- Occasional mitotic figures may be seen
- Infiltrative growth pattern; often surrounds nerves and infiltrates adipose tissue (Figure 13-7)
- Surface epithelium may show pseudoepitheliomatous hyperplasia

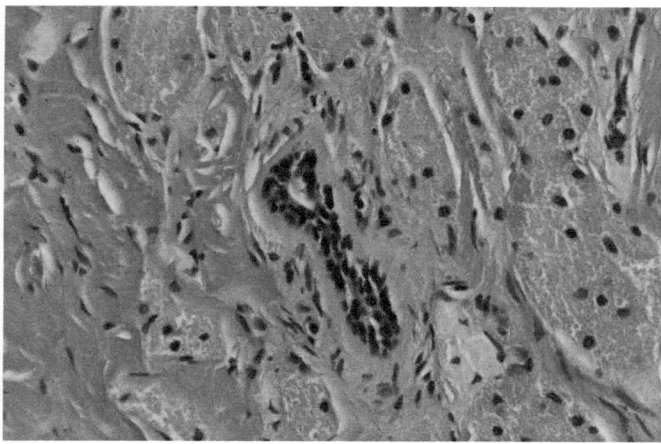

Figure 13-7. Granular cell tumor. Microscopically, the tumor cells infiltrate the breast parenchyma in small nests separated by delicate fibrous bands.

Special Stains and Immunohistochemistry

- S-100 protein: highlights cytoplasmic granularity with strong cytoplasmic and nuclear staining
- CD68 can be positive
- Carcinoembryonic antigen (CEA): diffuse immunoreactivity
- Cytokeratin and epithelial membrane antigen (EMA) negative
- Actin, myoglobin, desmin negative

Other Techniques for Diagnosis

- Electron microscopy demonstrates myelin figures and numerous lysosomes

Differential Diagnosis

HISTIOCYTIC LESIONS, INCLUDING FAT NECROSIS AND MAMMARY DUCT ECTASIA

- Granular cell tumor is usually not immunoreactive with histiocyte-associated antigens, such as α_1-antitrypsin and α_1-antichymotrypsin, but reactivity for CD68 is seen

APOCRINE CARCINOMA

- Tumor cells are large, with pleomorphic nuclei and prominent nucleoli
- Typically shows an associated intraductal component
- Positive for cytokeratin

METASTATIC NEOPLASMS, INCLUDING ONCOCYTIC RENAL CELL CARCINOMA, MELANOMA, AND ALVEOLAR SOFT PART SARCOMA

- Malignant histologic features, along with panel of immunohistochemical stains, including cytokeratin, EMA (positive in renal cancer), MART-1, HMB-45 (positive in melanoma), and myoglobin (positive in alveolar sarcoma), help in the differential diagnosis

PEARLS

- *Virtually always benign; only rare reports of metastasis*
- *Eosinophilic cytoplasmic granules are due to abundant lysosomes*
- *Treated by wide local excision; may recur if not completely resected*

SELECTED REFERENCES

Gavriilidis P, Michalopoulou I, Baliaka A, Nikolaidou A: Granular cell breast tumour mimicking infiltrating carcinoma. BMJ Case Rep, 2013.
Mátrai Z, Langmár Z, Szabó E, et al: Granular cell tumour of the breast: case series and review of the literature. Eur J Gynaecol Oncol 31:636-640, 2010.

FIBROCYSTIC CHANGES

Clinical Features

- Most common condition involving the female breast
- Affects primarily premenopausal women (third to fifth decades)
- Bilateral and multifocal
- Irregular, firm, and nodular breast tissue with discrete lumps
- Breasts often tender
- Breast nodularity typically fluctuates with the menstrual cycle

Gross Pathology

- Irregular, rubbery, fibrotic breast tissue
- Macroscopic cysts containing clear or turbid fluid often seen
- Blue-domed cysts may be present

Histopathology (Figures 13-8, 13-9 and 13-10)

CYST FORMATION

- Variably sized cysts lined by flattened or cuboidal epithelial cells

STROMAL FIBROSIS

- Dense periductal and perilobular fibrosis

APOCRINE METAPLASIA

- Cysts lined by large, polygonal cells with abundant granular, eosinophilic cytoplasm and small, hyperchromatic nuclei

SCLEROSING ADENOSIS

- Multiple well-defined foci are usually present
- Proliferation of attenuated ductules with preservation of the lobular configuration

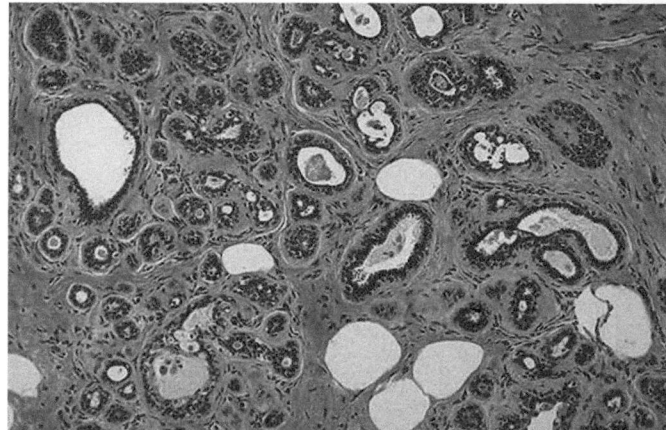

Figure 13-8. Fibrocystic changes characterized by cyst formation, stromal fibrosis, and sclerosing adenosis.

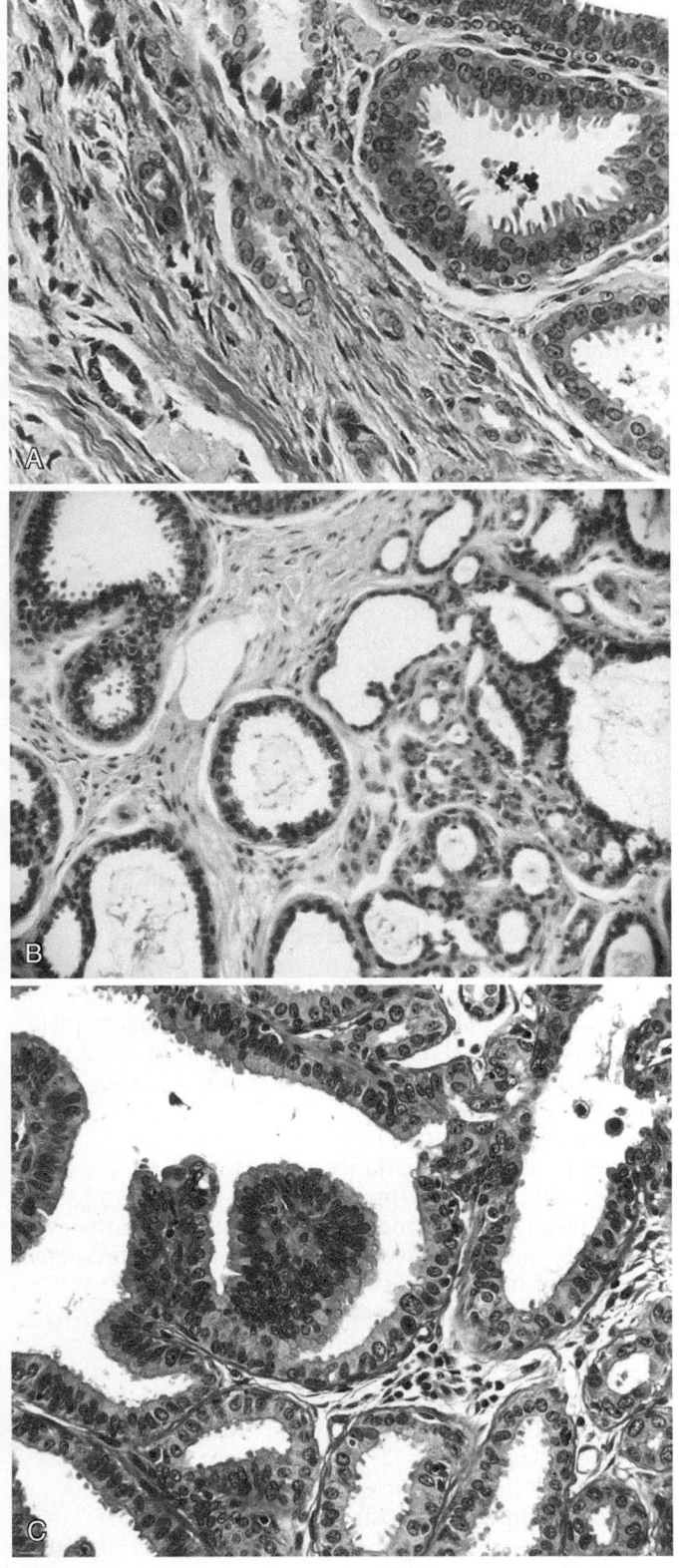

Figure 13-9. Fibrocystic changes with columnar cell lesions. A, Dilated acini showing columnar cell change are lined by two cell layers with occasional apical snouts, luminal secretions, and no atypia. Distended acini showing (**B**) columnar cell change and (**C**) columnar cell hyperplasia with cytologic atypia (flat epithelial atypia) are lined by more than two layers, with occasional papillary formation and cell atypia.

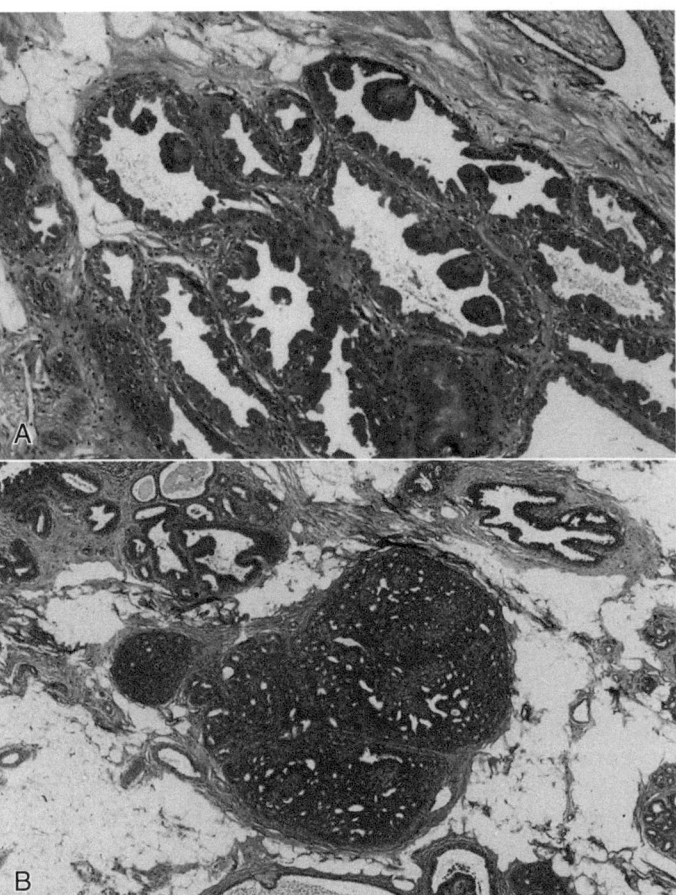

Figure 13-10. A, Apocrine metaplasia. Dilated ducts lined by metaplastic apocrine cells. The cells are columnar and have granular pink cytoplasm. **B,** Ductal hyperplasia without atypia. The ductal spaces are distended by a solid proliferation of hyperplastic ductal cells. Notice prominent fenestrations with variable size of the secondary lumens.

- Increased stromal and myoepithelial cells
- Microcalcifications are often seen in ducts or stroma

EPITHELIAL HYPERPLASIA WITHOUT ATYPIA (USUAL DUCTAL HYPERPLASIA)
- Proliferation of ductal cells forming duct lumens filled with a heterogeneous population of round to oval cells
- The nuclei of these cells grow, creating a streaming pattern
- Irregular, slitlike fenestrations are often seen at the periphery of the ducts
- Cells can grow as bands that cross the lumen of the duct

COLUMNAR CELL LESIONS (CCLs)
- Enlarged acini of terminal ductal lobular units (TDLUs) lined by columnar cells with occasional luminal secretions and calcification
  - Columnar cell change (CCC)
    - Distended acini with undulating borders; up to two epithelial layers; ovoid nuclei oriented perpendicular to basement membrane and inconspicuous nucleoli; infrequent mitosis; apical snouts may

be seen with occasional luminal secretions and calcification
  • No nuclear atypia is seen
• Columnar cell hyperplasia (CCH)
  • More than two cell layers with papillary formation; apical snouts, secretions, and calcifications are common
• Flat epithelial atypia (CCC and CCH with cytologic atypia)
  • Acini with rigid contours, round nuclei with nucleoli not oriented perpendicular to basement membrane, occasional mitosis; epithelial cells in three to five layers with cytologic atypia

Special Stains and Immunohistochemistry

• ER, PR, BCL-2, low molecular weight keratin (CK8, 18, 19 positive in CCL)
• Negative for p53, C-erb-B2 (HER-2-neu) and high molecular weight keratin (CK5/6, CK14, 34beta E12)

Other Techniques for Diagnosis

• Noncontributory

Differential Diagnosis

FIBROMATOSIS

• Greater cellularity composed of elongated spindle cells
• Lacks cyst formation and other features that characterize fibrocystic changes

ATYPICAL DUCTAL HYPERPLASIA (ADH) OR DUCTAL CARCINOMA IN SITU (DCIS)

• Shows greater cytologic atypia and complex architectural changes than CCLs with atypia (flat epithelial atypia)

PEARLS

• *May clinically mimic carcinoma*
• *Most common diagnosis made after lumpectomy (> 50% of all surgical procedures involving the breast)*
• *Typically displays several features, including cyst formation, apocrine metaplasia, fibrosis, chronic inflammation, and epithelial hyperplasia without atypia*
• *CCLs show 16q loss; may represent early lesion of low-grade DCIS*
• *Believed to be related to hormonal imbalance involving estrogen and progesterone; oral contraceptives decrease risk for fibrocystic changes*
• *Sclerosing adenosis is associated with a slight (1.5 to 2 times) increased risk for carcinoma*
• *No increased risk for carcinoma associated with apocrine metaplasia, stromal fibrosis, or mild ductal epithelial hyperplasia without atypia; florid ductal hyperplasia without atypia increases risk for carcinoma slightly (1.5 to 2 times)*

SELECTED REFERENCES

Aulmann S, Braun L, Mietzsch F, et al: Transitions between flat epithelial atypia and low-grade ductal carcinoma in situ of the breast. Am J Surg Pathol 36:1247-1252, 2012.

Biggar MA, Kerr KM, Erzetich LM, Bennett IC: Columnar cell change with atypia (flat epithelial atypia) on breast core biopsy-outcomes following open excision. Breast J 18:578-581, 2012.
Ellis IO: Intraductal proliferative lesions of the breast: morphology, associated risk and molecular biology. Mod Pathol 23(suppl 2):S1-S7, 2010.
Sudarshan M, Meguerditchian AN, Mesurolle B, Meterissian S: Flat epithelial atypia of the breast: characteristics and behaviors. Am J Surg 201:245-250, 2011.

ADENOSIS

Clinical Features

• Primarily affects premenopausal women (third and fourth decades)
• Typically found in association with fibrocystic changes but may form solitary firm masses mimicking cancer
• May be found in biopsy material removed for suspicious or indeterminate microcalcifications

Gross Pathology

• Findings are often those of fibrocystic changes with areas of fibrosis and cyst formation
• Florid adenosis tumors are well circumscribed; sclerotic tumors tend to be less well defined at borders
• Lesions with abundant microcalcifications have a gritty cut surface

Histopathology (Figure 13-11)

• Usually consists of a circumscribed, benign proliferation of ductal structures
• Ducts have an oval or elongated contour
• Well-defined epithelial and myoepithelial layers
• Microcalcifications are often seen
• Increase in cell size, but no evidence of nuclear pleomorphism, normal mitoses, focal necrosis, or infarction can be seen in florid adenosis, especially during pregnancy and lactation
• Sclerosing adenosis can involve nerves
• Several patterns and variants of adenosis exist
  • Sclerosing adenosis (most common variant)
    • Multiple well-defined foci are usually present
    • Proliferation of attenuated ductules with preservation of the lobular configuration
    • Increased stromal and myoepithelial cells
    • Dense stroma surrounding ducts
    • Microcalcifications are often seen
  • Apocrine adenosis
    • Ductule proliferation with extensive apocrine metaplasia
    • Cells with large nucleolus
  • Microglandular adenosis (rare variant)
    • Haphazard arrangement of small, round ductules lacking lobular architecture that simulate an infiltrative pattern
    • Background shows hypocellular, collagenous stroma
    • Proliferating ducts often extend around normal breast ducts and lobules and may extend into adjacent adipose tissue

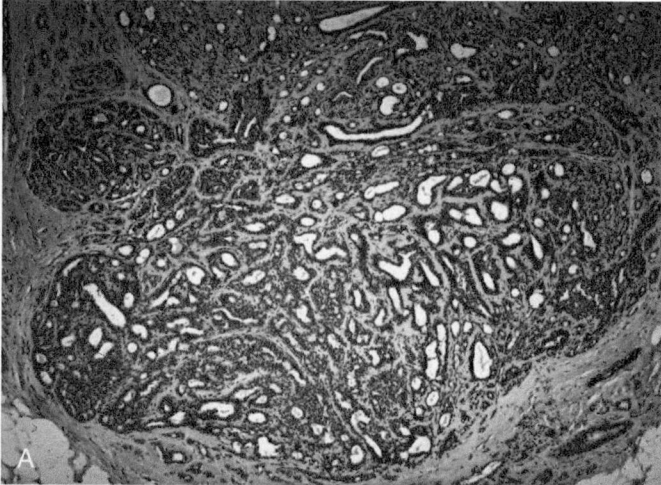
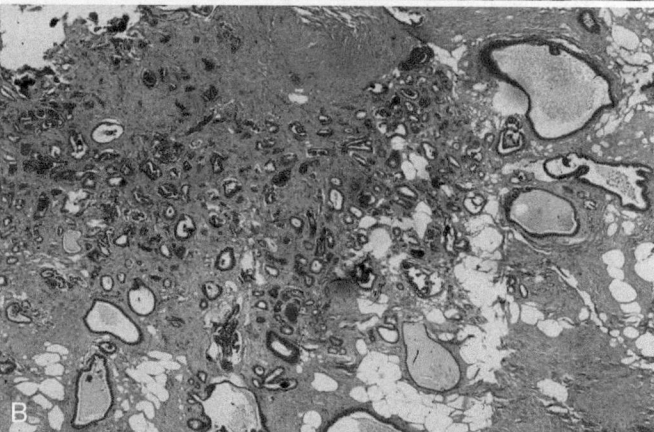
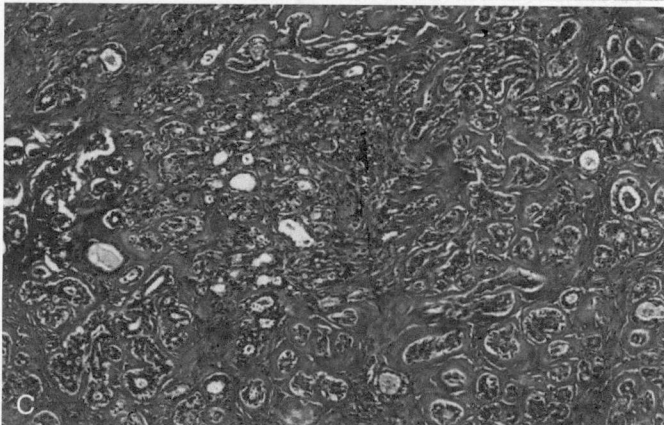

- Atypical microglandular adenosis has foci of both typical adenosis and areas of more complex structure and cytologic atypia
- Myoepithelial layer is absent (negative for S-100 protein, smooth muscle actin [SMA], smooth muscle myosin heavy-chain, and p63)
- Positive for collagen IV
- Usually negative for EMA and ER
- Adenosis tumor: grossly recognized mass formed by numerous adjacent foci of adenosis

Special Stains and Immunohistochemistry

- Cytokeratin, S-100, and cathepsin D highlight epithelial cells of microglandular adenosis
- SMA, S-100, smooth muscle myosin heavy chain, and p63 highlight myoepithelial cell layer
- PAS, laminin, and collagen IV highlight basement membrane of sclerosing adenosis

Other Techniques for Diagnosis

- Noncontributory

Differential Diagnosis

INFILTRATING TUBULAR CARCINOMA

- Haphazardly arranged ducts with angulated, open lumens and bridges of epithelial cells
- Absent myoepithelial layer (also absent in microglandular adenosis)
- Lumens lack eosinophilic secretions
- Lining cells have eosinophilic cytoplasm and often show apical snouts
- Reactive, fibroblastic stroma with desmoplasia often seen
- Often associated with an intraductal carcinoma component
- Usually positive for EMA and ER

INFILTRATING LOBULAR CARCINOMA

- Classically shows small, uniform, rounded cells infiltrating in single-file lines or alveolar pattern
- Lacks lobular configuration and myoepithelial cell layer (similar to microglandular adenosis)

PEARLS

- *Classically sclerosing adenosis is a ductule proliferation that maintains a lobular architecture*
- *Myoepithelial cell proliferation in sclerosing adenosis is helpful to distinguish from carcinoma*
- *Microglandular adenosis is often difficult to distinguish from tubular carcinoma; best distinguishing features include the shape of the ductules and the stromal characteristics*
- *Adenosis has been shown to be associated with a slight increased risk for carcinoma (1.5 to 2 times)*

Figure 13-11. A, Sclerosing adenosis. Well-circumscribed area of closely packed ducts retaining a lobular configuration. **B,** Sclerosing adenosis showing dense collagenous stroma between the proliferating tubules. Notice multiple microcalcifications in the tubules. **C,** Microglandular adenosis. Proliferation of tubules lacking lobular architecture in a dense collagenous background.

- Duct lumens contain a colloid-like eosinophilic, secretory material (PAS positive)
- Bland cytologic features with cells typically showing clear or vacuolated cytoplasm and rare mitotic figures

SELECTED REFERENCES

Salarieh A, Sneige N: Breast carcinoma arising in microglandular adenosis: a review of the literature. Arch Pathol Lab Med 131:1397-1399, 2007.

Seidman JD, Ashton M, Lefkowitz M: Atypical apocrine adenosis of the breast: a clinicopathologic study of 37 patients with 8.7 year follow up. Cancer 77:2529-2537, 1996.

Shin SJ, Simpson PT, Da Silva L, Jayanthan J, et al: Molecular evidence for progression of microglandular adenosis (MGA) to invasive carcinoma. Am J Surg Pathol 33:496-504, 2009.

Wen YH, Weigelt B, Reis-Filho JS: Microglandular adenosis: a nonobligate precursor of triple-negative breast cancer? Histol Histopathol 28:1099-1108, 2013.

RADIAL SCLEROSING LESION AND RADIAL SCAR

Clinical Features

- Uncommon before 30 years of age
- Typically small and therefore usually nonpalpable but may form palpable masses
- Usually an incidental finding; associated with adenosis and fibrocystic changes
- Mammographically shows a dense central radiolucent zone with thin, linear densities radiating outward; microcalcifications may be seen
- Can mimic carcinoma on mammography
- In many patients, this lesion is multifocal or bilateral; clustering of scars may occur

Gross Pathology

- Typically of small size, rarely larger than 1 cm (*radial scar* refers to lesions < 1 cm; *complex sclerosing lesion* describes lesions > 1 cm)
- Shows irregular, stellate, dense fibrotic tissue; may grossly mimic carcinoma

Histopathology

- Pseudoinfiltrative lesions
- Central collagenous scar showing fibrosis and elastosis, with entrapped ducts showing dual epithelial and myoepithelial layer; basement membrane intact (Figure 13-12)
- Epithelial proliferation with stellate or radial arrangement of ductules resembling sclerosing adenosis
- Commonly seen fibrocystic changes, including ductal hyperplasia, duct ectasia, adenosis, and papillomatosis surrounding fibrotic zone
- Ducts may show squamous metaplasia
- Perineural infiltration by benign ducts may be seen

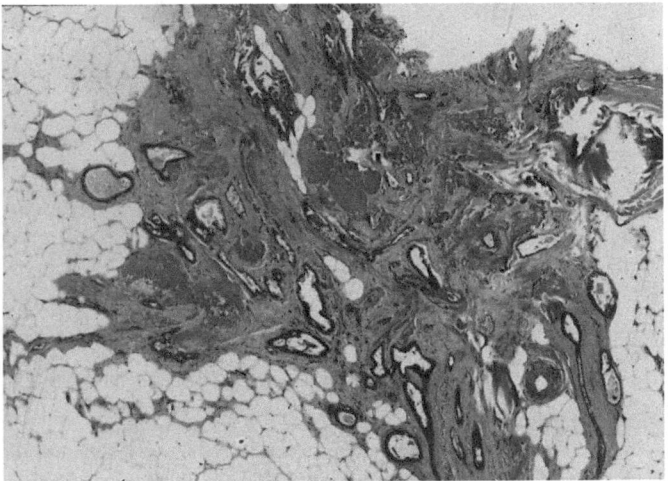

Figure 13-12. Radial scar. Central collagenous scar surrounded by proliferating ducts in a radial pattern resembling sclerosing adenosis.

- Necrosis is rare, but small areas can be present
- Ducts should not infiltrate into adjacent adipose tissue

Special Stains and Immunohistochemistry

- p63, CD10, SMA, and S100 highlight myoepithelial layer

Other Techniques for Diagnosis

- Noncontributory

Differential Diagnosis

TUBULAR CARCINOMA
- Ducts do not have a myoepithelial cell layer
- Often infiltrates into surrounding fatty tissue

PEARLS

- *Most commonly seen in association with adenosis*
- *Can grossly and histologically mimic carcinoma*
- *Presence of a myoepithelial layer and lack of infiltration are the best distinguishing characteristics*
- *Carcinoma has been seen to arise in a background of a radial scar*
- *Believed to be benign but associated with atypia and malignancy; radial scar may be an independent risk factor for the development of carcinoma*

SELECTED REFERENCES

Andacoglu O, Kanbour-Shakir A, Teh YC, et al: Rationale of excisional biopsy after the diagnosis of benign radial scar on core biopsy: a single institutional outcome analysis. Am J Clin Oncol 36:7-11, 2013.

Eusebi V, Millis RR: Epitheliosis, infiltrating epitheliosis, and radial scar. Semin Diagn Pathol 27:5-12, 2010.

Sanders ME, Page Dl, Simpson JF, et al: Interdependence of radial scar and proliferative disease with respect to invasive breast carcinoma risk in patients with benign breast biopsies. Cancer 1:1453-1461, 2006.

Tóth D, Sebő É, Sarkadi L, et al: Role of core needle biopsy in the treatment of radial scar. Breast 21:761-763, 2012.

INTRADUCTAL PAPILLOMA (SOLITARY AND MULTIPLE)

Clinical Features

SOLITARY PAPILLOMA
- Typically arises from lactiferous ducts in central breast tissue (beneath the areola) and often presents with serous or bloody nipple discharge
- Usually found in women in their fifth or sixth decade

MULTIPLE PAPILLOMAS
- Multiple papillary masses typically located in peripheral breast tissue in contiguous branches of the ductal system
- Occurs in younger women (40s and early 50s)
- Occurs far less frequently than solitary papillomas

Gross Pathology

- Large papillomas may be visible in the lumen of a dilated or cystic duct
- Palpable lesions typically measure 2 to 3 cm, but cystic lesions can be larger than 10 cm

Histopathology

- Organized papillary proliferation of ductal epithelium on a frond-forming fibrovascular core or stroma (Figure 13-13A and B)
- Any degree of epithelial hyperplasia of the usual type may be seen
- Fusion of papillae often results in glandlike spaces or solid areas

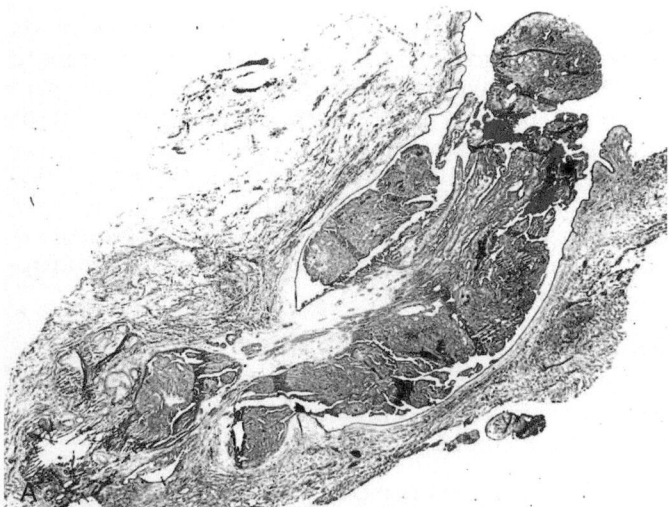

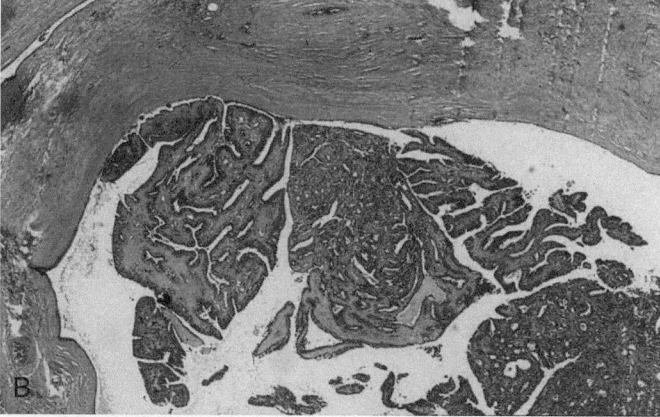

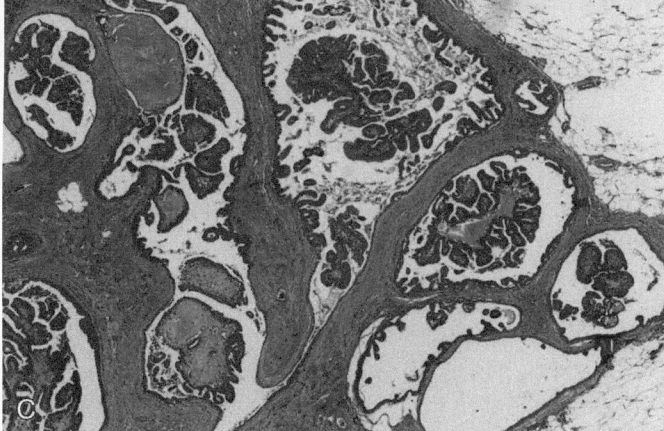

Figure 13-13. Intraductal papilloma. A, Dilated duct showing papillary proliferation on a sclerotic fibrovascular core. **B,** Distended duct showing a papillary lesion with a delicate fibrovascular core. **C,** Multiple intraductal papillomas. Distended ducts showing multiple papillary lesions.

- Presence of a myoepithelial cell layer in papillae and around glandular spaces, although it can be focally absent
- Papillomas may show apocrine, squamous, mucinous, clear cell, or sebaceous metaplasia
- Sclerosis of the cores with entrapment of ductal epithelium may occur and may be mistaken for invasive carcinoma
- Infarction associated with torsion of the cores may happen, hindering evaluation of atypia and malignancy
  - Solitary papilloma
    - Papillae with single layer of cuboidal to columnar epithelium; focal epithelial hyperplasia may be seen
    - Typically shows minimal cellular atypia and rare mitotic activity
    - May show extreme distortion and fusion of papillary fronds (solid intraductal papilloma) or marked sclerosis (sclerosing papilloma)
  - Multiple papillomas
    - Multiple papillomas with involvement of more than one duct system or multiple foci within a single duct system (Figure 13-13C)
    - Arise in terminal duct lobular units and may extend into terminal
    - May show prominent epithelial hyperplasia
    - Atypia may develop with papillae lined by pseudostratified, elongated epithelial cells
  - Atypical papilloma (papilloma with atypia, papilloma with ADH) and papilloma with DCIS
    - Papillomas with foci of epithelial proliferation with full architectural and cytologic criteria for the diagnosis of ADH or DCIS
    - Papillomas with non-high-grade DCIS when lesion is larger than 3 mm
    - Papillomas with ADH (atypical papillomas) when lesion is smaller than or equal to 3 mm
    - DCIS most often of low or intermediate nuclear grade with solid, cribriform, or micropapillary patterns; small necrotic foci may be present
    - Focal loss or reduction of myoepithelial cells in the ADH and DCIS foci
    - Presence of large atypical or higher-grade lesion foci or necrosis should prompt designation of *carcinoma in situ arising within a papilloma*

Special Stains and Immunohistochemistry

- SMA, calponin, S-100 protein, smooth muscle myosin heavy chain, and p63 highlight myoepithelial cells
- ER stains a variable minority of epithelial cells in papillomas without atypia, with diffuse positivity in ADH and low-grade DCIS foci
- High-molecular-weight cytokeratins (HMWCKs), such as 5/6, 14, and 34βE12, stain epithelial cells in papillomas without atypia, whereas ADH and low-grade DCIS foci are negative
- Combination of ER positivity and HMWCK negativity is a useful indicator of neoplastic population in an intraductal papillary proliferation
- CD34/factor VIII demonstrate vascular endothelial cells within fibrovascular cores (helps distinguish between endothelial and myoepithelial cells)

Other Techniques for Diagnosis

- Noncontributory

Differential Diagnosis

PAPILLARY DCIS

- Prominent neoplastic proliferation of epithelial cells showing papillary architecture and features of intraductal carcinoma characterized by unequivocal comedo, cribriform, solid, or micropapillary architecture; no apocrine metaplasia; necrosis often seen

ENCAPSULATED (INTRACYSTIC) PAPILLARY CARCINOMA AND NONINVASIVE PAPILLARY CARCINOMA

- Papillary proliferation growing within dilated ducts and consisting entirely of papillae lacking a myoepithelial cell layer; studies failed to demonstrate myoepithelial cells at the periphery of tumor nodules

PEARLS

- *Papillomas, solitary and multiple, without atypia have been shown to be associated with an increased risk for malignancy, the risk being greater with multiple lesions*
- *Women with multiple papillomas with atypia have a particularly high breast cancer risk*
- *Clinical significance of atypical papillary lesions is uncertain, and complete excision is recommended with careful follow-up*
- *Deferring the diagnosis of carcinoma to paraffin sections is recommended when diagnosis of an intraductal papilloma is made on frozen section*
- *Loss of heterozygosity (LOH) at loci 16p13 is identified in papillomas with florid hyperplasia*
- *Frozen sections are not recommended on papillary lesions*
- *Most important feature for distinguishing between a benign papilloma and a papillary carcinoma is the presence of a uniform myoepithelial layer in the proliferating papillary intraluminal component*
- *Presence of apocrine metaplasia within the lesion favors a benign diagnosis*

SELECTED REFERENCES

Collins LC, Schnitt SJ: Papillary lesions of the breast: Selected diagnostic and management issues. Histopathology 52:20-29, 2008.

Jakate K, De Brot M, Goldberg F, et al: Papillary lesions of the breast: impact of breast pathology subspecialization on core biopsy and excision diagnoses. Am J Surg Pathol 36:544-551, 2012.

Richter-Ehrenstein C, Tombokan F, Fallenberg EM, et al: Intraductal papillomas of the breast: diagnosis and management of 151 patients. Breast 20:501-504, 2011.

Shamonki J, Chung A, Huynh KT, et al: Management of papillary lesions of the breast: can larger core needle biopsy samples identify patients who may avoid surgical excision? Ann Surg Oncol 20:4137-4144, 2013.

FLORID PAPILLOMATOSIS OF THE NIPPLE

Clinical Features

- May be seen at any age, typically in middle-aged women (fourth and fifth decades)
- Rarely reported in men
- Frequently presents with serous or bloody nipple discharge
- Pain or itching may be experienced
- Palpable mass is present in most cases
- May resemble Paget disease clinically

Gross Pathology

- Generally forms a discrete mass
- Nipple frequently shows ulceration, erythema, and scaling

Histopathology

- Characteristic feature is florid ductal hyperplasia with lesions grouped into four subtypes according to their growth pattern: sclerosing papillomatosis, papilloma, adenosis, and mixed proliferative patterns (Figure 13-14A and B)
- Myoepithelial cell hyperplasia is common, but in sclerosing lesions may be inconspicuous or absent
- Foci of necrosis and normal mitosis may be present
- Areas of ADH, DCIS, or invasive carcinoma within papillomatosis may be seen

Special Stains and Immunohistochemistry

- SMA, calponin, S-100 protein, smooth muscle myosin heavy chain, and p63 highlight myoepithelial cells
- Keratin 34betaE12 highlights epithelial cells

Other Techniques for Diagnosis

- Noncontributory

Differential Diagnosis

PAGET DISEASE

- Identification of neoplastic tumor cells within epidermis of nipple that stain for Her-2 neu

DCIS OR INVASIVE CARCINOMA

- Often present when florid papillomatosis is found
- May be associated with or be present away from area of papillomatosis
- Intraductal carcinoma should show a cribriform, comedo, solid, or micropapillary architecture and may show necrosis

PEARLS

- *Benign epithelial tumor arising in the large ducts of the nipple*
- *Treatment involves complete excision, usually with removal of the nipple*
- *Associated with concomitant or subsequent carcinoma in 10% of cases; carcinoma may be found anywhere in the breast*

SELECTED REFERENCES

Brownstein MH, Phelps RG, Magnin PH: Papillary adenoma of the nipple: analysis of fifteen new cases. J Am Acad Dermatol 12:707-715, 1985.

Rosen PP, Caicco JA: Florid papillomatosis of the nipple: a study of 51 patients, including nine with mammary carcinoma. Am J Surg Pathol 10:87-101, 1986.

Rosen PP, Oberman HA: Atlas of Tumor Pathology: Tumors of the Mammary Gland, 3rd Series, Fascicle 7. Washington, DC, Armed Forces Institute of Pathology, 1993.

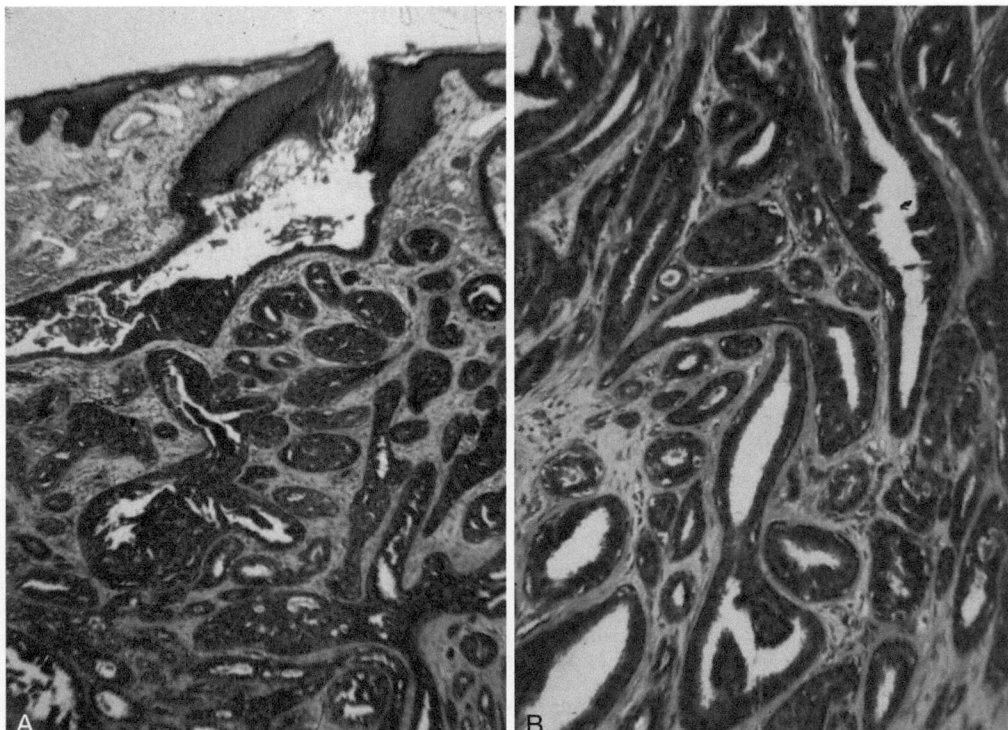

Figure 13-14. Florid papillomatosis. A, Distended ducts filled with hyperplastic ductal cells are extending into the upper dermis. **B,** Tubular arrangement with focal ductal hyperplasia and fibrous stroma.

PSEUDOANGIOMATOUS STROMAL HYPERPLASIA

Clinical Features

- Found in women of childbearing age but can also affect men with gynecomastia
- Presents as a firm, palpable, nontender, solitary breast mass or area of thickening
- Can be found as an incidental finding in patients undergoing biopsies for other reasons

Gross Pathology

- Well-circumscribed and typically encapsulated
- Variable size (typically 3 to 4 cm)
- Cut section demonstrates a fibrous, tan-white, homogeneous tumor

Histopathology

- Characterized by complex, anastomosing, empty slitlike spaces (pseudoangiomas) in a dense collagenous stroma (Figure 13-15)
- Empty spaces lined by monomorphic myofibroblastic spindle cells resembling endothelial cells
- Can form solid foci of prominent spindle cells

Special Stains and Immunohistochemistry

- Vimentin positive in spindle cells lining pseudoangiomatous spaces
- CD34 positive in most lesions
- CD31 mostly negative
- SMA variably reactive
- Cytokeratin, factor VIII negative

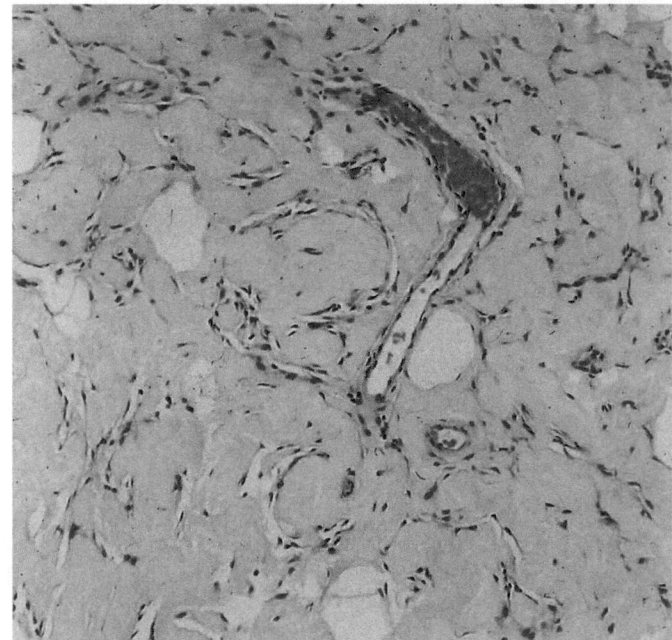

Figure 13-15. Pseudoangiomatous stromal hyperplasia. Complex anastomosing slitlike spaces in a dense collagenous background.

Other Techniques for Diagnosis

- Electron microscopy: pseudoangiomatous spaces lined by cells showing fibroblastic differentiation

Differential Diagnosis

HEMANGIOMA

- Slitlike spaces are vascular channels and often contain blood

- Lining cells are endothelial and show cytokeratin, CD31, factor VIII, and *U. europaeus* positivity

LOW-GRADE ANGIOSARCOMA
- Intercommunicating vascular spaces lined by atypical endothelial cells with hyperchromatic nuclei
- Infiltrative architecture typically extending into adjacent breast tissue

PEARLS

- *Pseudoangiomatous stromal hyperplasia is a benign lesion that must be distinguished from low-grade angiosarcoma*
- *Treatment is wide local excision; clear margins are necessary to avoid recurrences*
- *Development may be related to hormonal factors*
- *Positivity for CD34 supports the diagnosis*

SELECTED REFERENCES

Bowman E, Oprea G, Okoli J, et al: Pseudoangiomatous stromal hyperplasia (PASH) of the breast: a series of 24 patients. Breast J 18:242-247, 2012.

Drinka EK, Bargaje A, Erşahin ÇH, et al: Pseudoangiomatous stromal hyperplasia (PASH) of the breast: a clinicopathological study of 79 cases. Int J Surg Pathol 20:54-58, 2012.

Ferreira M, Albarracin CT, Resetkova E: Pseudoangiomatous stromal hyperplasia tumor: a clinical, radiologic and pathologic study of 26 cases. Mod Pathol 21:201-207, 2008.

Gresik CM, Godellas C, Aranha GV, et al: Pseudoangiomatous stromal hyperplasia of the breast: a contemporary approach to its clinical and radiologic features and ideal management. Surgery 148:752-757, 2010.

ADENOMA

Clinical Features
- Some may represent unusual types of fibroadenomas
- All present as breast masses
- Lactating adenoma is often recognized during pregnancy or while lactating

Gross Pathology
- Well-defined, circumscribed, tan-yellow tumors
- Typically less than 5 cm in greatest diameter
- Lactating adenomas may be multiple

Histopathology

TUBULAR ADENOMA
- Proliferation of benign glands of uniform size and shape (Figure 13-16A)
- Lined by a single layer of epithelial cells showing bland nuclear features
- Myoepithelial cells surround each gland

LACTATING ADENOMA
- Proliferation of benign ducts with preservation of a lobular architecture; typically sharply delineated from the surrounding breast tissue
- Ducts lined by benign-appearing epithelial cells with vacuolated cytoplasm; may show hobnail appearance (Figure 13-16B)
- Duct lumens contain eosinophilic secretions

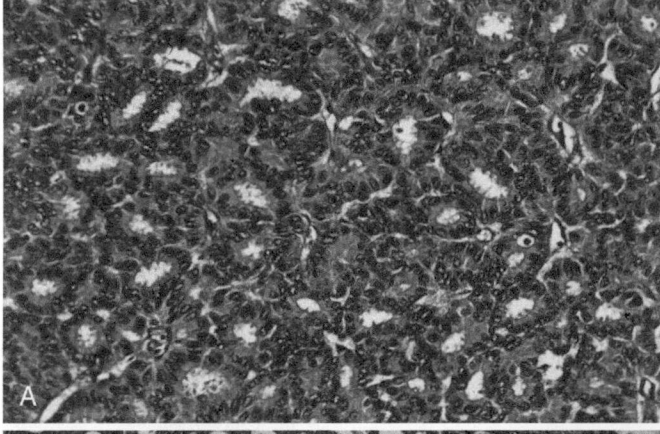

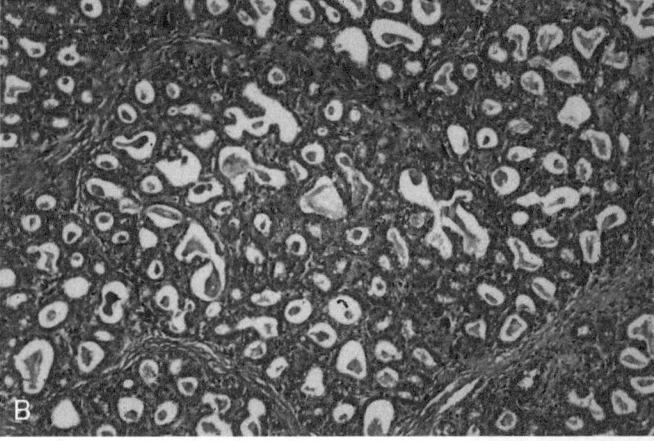

Figure 13-16. A, Tubular adenoma. Densely packed ductal structures lined by epithelial and myoepithelial cells. **B,** Lactating adenoma. The ducts are lined by vacuolated secretory cells. The lumens contain secretory material.

- Typically shows increased secretion if removed postpartum, less secretion if removed during pregnancy
- Prone to infarction during pregnancy

APOCRINE ADENOMA
- Extremely rare lesions
- Discrete mass, homogeneous throughout, sharply demarcated from surrounding breast tissue and composed of benign breast ducts with apocrine epithelium and minimal supportive stromal component
- Often shows papillary and cystic architecture

Special Stains and Immunohistochemistry
- SMA, S-100, and p63 highlight myoepithelial cell layer
- PAS highlights luminal secretion in lactating adenoma

Other Techniques for Diagnosis
- Noncontributory

Differential Diagnosis

TUBULAR CARCINOMA
- Composed of small angulated ducts with infiltrative growth pattern
- Lacks myoepithelial cell layer
- Shows reactive, desmoplastic stroma surrounding proliferating ducts

- *Tubular adenomas do not recur after excision and show no increased risk for subsequent carcinoma*
- *Lactating adenomas may infarct, causing significant pain*
- *Apocrine adenoma is a discrete mass composed of benign breast ducts all showing apocrine epithelium*
- *Carcinoma can develop in adenomas*

SELECTED REFERENCES

Maiorano E, Albrizio M: Tubular adenoma of the breast: an immuno-histochemical study of ten cases. Pathol Res Pract 191:1222-1230, 1995.

O'Hara MF, Page DL: Adenomas of the breast and ectopic breast under lactational influences. Hum Pathol 16:707-712, 1985.

Sumkin JH, Perrone AM, Harris KM, et al: Lactating adenoma: US features and literature review. Radiology 206:271-274, 1998.

FIBROADENOMA

Clinical Features

- Most common breast tumor in adolescents and young women
- Hormonally sensitive, usually involutes during menopause
- Often develops in transplant recipients receiving cyclosporine
- Presents as discrete, nontender, palpable breast mass
- Typically solitary but can be multifocal or bilateral
- Giant fibroadenomas are larger than 5 cm or weigh more than 500 g

Gross Pathology

- Tan-white to gray, firm to rubbery, round to oval mass
- Well-circumscribed and typically encapsulated
- No infiltration into surrounding fatty breast tissue
- Most fibroadenomas measure up to 3 cm

Histopathology

- Benign tumor that arises from lobules and stroma of the terminal duct–lobular unit
- Typically shows a well-defined capsule (Figure 13-17)

- Characteristic features include a collagenous stroma and distorted, slitlike, elongated ducts
- Variable degree of stromal cellularity
- Fibrocystic changes (apocrine metaplasia, adenosis, ductal epithelial hyperplasia) are common associated findings
- Benign multinucleated giant cells may be seen

Special Stains and Immunohistochemistry

- Noncontributory

Other Techniques for Diagnosis

- Noncontributory

Differential Diagnosis

TUBULAR CARCINOMA

- Composed of small, angulated ducts with infiltrative growth pattern
- Desmoplastic stromal response surrounding ducts

PHYLLODES TUMOR

- Fibroadenomas are 50 times more common than phyllodes tumor
- Shows an exaggerated intracanalicular growth pattern (leaflike structure) exceeding that which is typical for a fibroadenoma
- Often shows increased cytologic atypia and mitotic activity
- Unequivocal malignant areas may be seen

TUBULAR ADENOMA

- Composed of regular benign breast ducts of similar size and shape
- Distinction between these two benign entities is of little importance; they are believed to be related to each other and may occasionally show overlapping histologic features, but neither shows an increased risk for carcinoma

- *Some use the term* juvenile fibroadenoma *when the tumor is found in young girls; often larger with greater degree of stromal cellularity when compared with typical fibroadenoma*
- *Most common breast tumor in young women*
- *Karyotypic abnormalities are detected in about 20% to 30% of fibroadenomas*
- *No increased risk for malignant transformation or subsequent carcinoma in the setting of noncomplex fibroadenomas and negative family history of breast cancer*
- *Lobular carcinoma in situ (LCIS) is the most common malignancy found in fibroadenoma*
- *Rare cases of invasive lobular and ductal carcinoma arising in fibroadenomas have been reported*
- *Excision biopsy with narrow margins is adequate treatment; rare recurrence if incompletely excised*

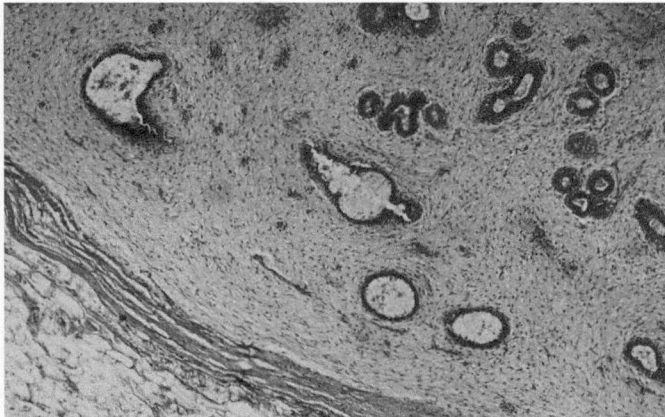

Figure 13-17. Fibroadenoma. Delicate capsule surrounds this fibroadenoma. The glandular and stromal components are evident.

SELECTED REFERENCES

Abe M, Miyata S, Nishimura S, et al: Malignant transformation of breast fibroadenoma to malignant phyllodes tumor: long-term outcome of 36 malignant phyllodes tumors. Breast Cancer 18:268-272, 2011.

Lerwill MF: Biphasic lesions of the breast. Semin Diagn Pathol 21: 48-56, 2004.

Limite G, Esposito E, Sollazzo V, et al: Lobular intraepithelial neoplasia arising within breast fibroadenoma. BMC Res Notes 12;6:267, 2013.

PHYLLODES TUMOR

Clinical Features

- Rare tumor; about 1% of all breast tumors
- Usually affects adults (fifth and sixth decades); rarely found in pediatric age group
- History of a rapidly growing, discrete, palpable breast mass
- Aggressive with high rate of recurrence

Gross Pathology

- Variably sized, discrete, gray-tan mass with firm consistency (Figure 13-18A)
- Variegated, lobulated cut surface; cleft formation may be seen
- Areas of necrosis and hemorrhage (more common in malignant lesions) (Figure 13-18B)

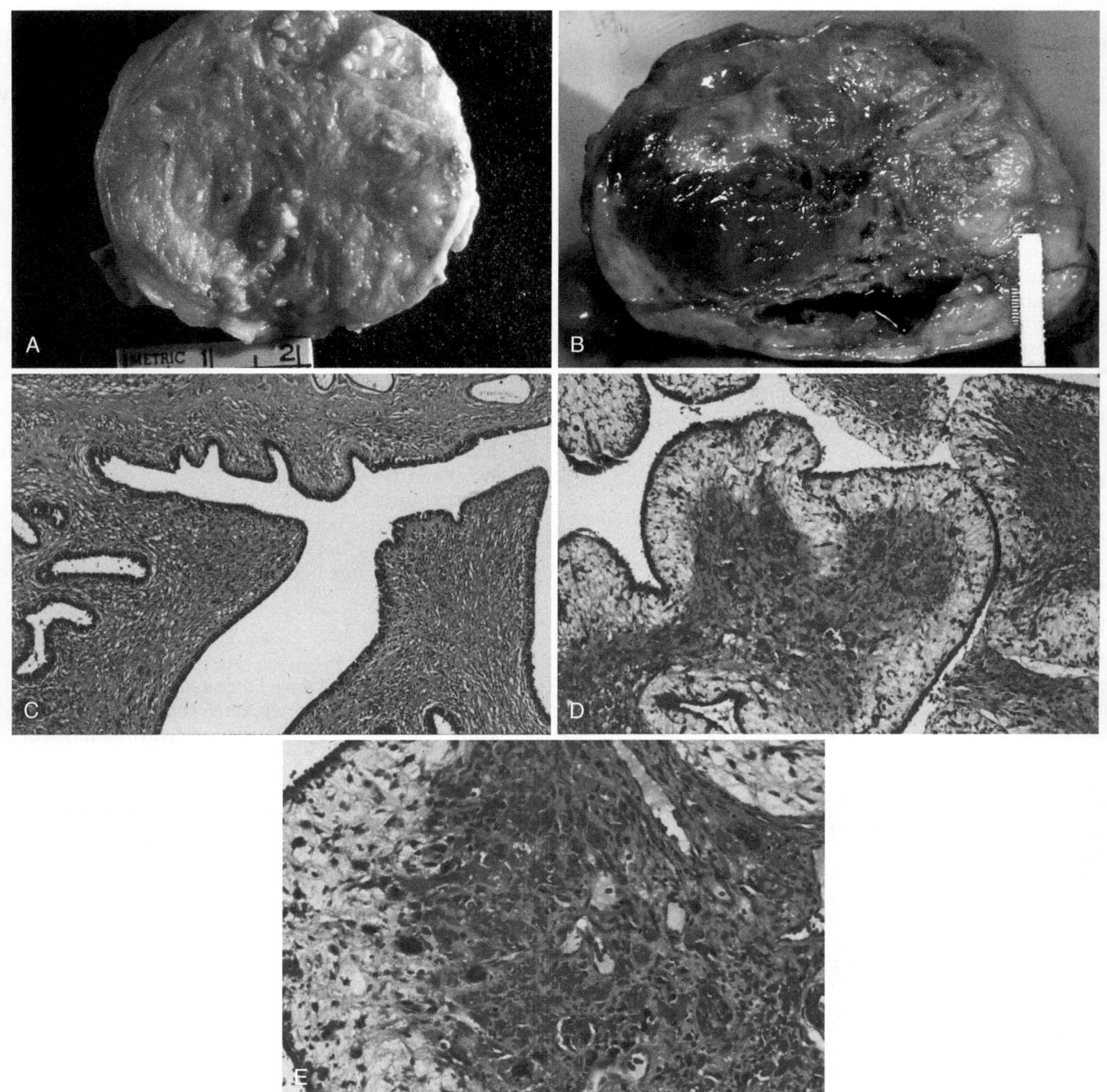

Figure 13-18. Phyllodes tumor. A, Benign phyllodes tumors are variably sized, discrete masses of firm consistency. **B,** Malignant phyllodes tumors frequently show areas of necrosis and hemorrhage. **C,** The benign neoplasm shows leaflike pattern with mild cellular stroma. **D,** The malignant tumor displays a leaflike pattern with highly cellular stroma and cytologic pleomorphism. **E,** This malignant phyllodes tumor shows marked nuclear pleomorphism and mitotic activity of the stromal component.

Histopathology

- Composed of both mesenchymal and epithelial elements
- May be well-circumscribed or microscopically invasive
- Adipose tissue within stroma is seen in about one third of phyllodes tumors (in biopsies)
- Epithelial component
  - Elongated, leaflike epithelial proliferation (similar to that seen in fibroadenoma) (Figure 13-18C)
  - Squamous metaplasia of ductal epithelium
- Mesenchymal component
  - Increased stromal cellularity typically in periductal regions (greater than seen in fibroadenoma)
  - Cellular atypia or increased mitotic activity may be seen
- Metaplastic change is common in both epithelial and stromal elements
  - Metaplastic bone, cartilage, fat, or muscle can be present in mesenchymal component (more frequent in malignant tumors)
- Classified as benign, borderline, or malignant based on histologic features
  - Malignant phyllodes tumor
    - In general show cellular stroma with nuclear pleomorphism and overgrowth (10 fields with no epithelium), increased mitotic activity, and infiltrative margins (Figure 13-18 D and E)
    - Sarcomatous appearance with increased cellularity and atypia; heterologous mesenchymal differentiation may be seen
    - High mitotic rate (more than five mitotic figures/10 high-power fields [hpf])
    - Stromal overgrowth with loss of epithelial component
    - Areas of necrosis
    - Infiltrative tumor margin
  - Benign phyllodes tumor
    - In general, stromal cells are not markedly pleomorphic; mitoses are few (> 4) and show well-circumscribed edges
  - Variable cellularity
    - Minimal pleomorphism
    - Low mitotic activity
    - No necrosis
    - Well-defined tumor margin
  - Low-grade malignant or borderline phyllodes tumor
    - Tumors with some but not all of the above features, two to five mitoses/10 hpf, and moderate stromal cellularity)

Special Stains and Immunohistochemistry

- Cytokeratin highlights epithelial component
- Vimentin stromal cells positive
- Actin, desmin variably positive
- CD34 and β-Catenin frequently expressed in stromal cell

Other Techniques for Diagnosis

- Electron microscopy: most tumor cells show fibroblastic and myofibroblastic differentiation
- Flow cytometry: most malignant tumors are aneuploid and have a high proliferative index

Differential Diagnosis

JUVENILE FIBROADENOMA

- Lacks the exaggerated intracanalicular growth pattern (leaflike architecture) characteristic of phyllodes tumor
- Shows uniform stromal cellularity
- No pleomorphism or mitotic activity

CARCINOSARCOMA

- Rarely found in the breast
- Characterized by malignant epithelial and stromal components that are distinct and separate from each other

PEARLS

- *Benign phyllodes tumors closely resemble fibroadenomas but are typically more cellular and show an exaggerated intracanalicular growth pattern*
- *In young girls, the surgical approach may be different for fibroadenoma and benign phyllodes tumor; a narrow margin is reasonable with fibroadenoma, but because of the possibility of recurrence, a phyllodes tumor should be excised with wider margins*
- *Lymph node dissection is not indicated because malignant tumors spread hematogenously (to lungs, pleura, and bones)*
- *May recur locally, and malignant variants may metastasize*
- *Metastases usually contain only sarcomatous component*
- *ER and PR are not useful to determine prognosis*
- *Gain of chromosome 1q is common in phyllodes tumors; stromal p53 gene expression and complex karyotypic abnormalities are more commonly observed in malignant tumors*

SELECTED REFERENCES

Ho SK, Thike AA, Cheok PY, et al: Phyllodes tumours of the breast: the role of CD34, vascular endothelial growth factor and β-catenin in histological grading and clinical outcome. Histopathology 63:393-406, 2013.

Jang JH, Choi MY, Lee SK, et al: Clinicopathologic risk factors for the local recurrence of phyllodes tumors of the breast. Ann Surg Oncol 19:2612-617, 2012.

Kim S, Kim JY, Kim do H, et al: Analysis of phyllodes tumor recurrence according to the histologic grade. Breast Cancer Res Treat 141:353-363, 2013.

Lee AHS: Recent developments in the histological diagnosis of spindle cell carcinoma, fibromatosis and phyllodes tumor of the breast. Histopathology 52:45-57, 2008.

ATYPICAL DUCTAL HYPERPLASIA AND DUCTAL CARCINOMA IN SITU

Clinical Features

- Age distribution similar to that of invasive mammary carcinomas
- Usually not associated with a palpable breast mass
- Mammogram may show suspicious calcifications
- May be an incidental finding in breast biopsy performed for other reasons

Gross Pathology

- Comedo DCIS may show small areas of necrosis within dense fibrotic breast tissue
- ADH and noncomedo-type DCIS usually show no distinct gross pathologic changes

Histopathology

ADH

- Lesion that measures less than 2 to 3 mm or involves only two duct spaces
- Epithelial cell proliferation within breast ducts (Figure 13-19A)
- Consists of a monotonous cell population similar to that seen in DCIS
- Typically shows more nuclear overlapping and indistinct cell membranes when compared with DCIS (Figure 13-19B)
- Secondary lumens show irregular borders with variable size and shape; lack the rounded, punched-out appearance of DCIS
- No necrosis
- Criteria for diagnosis of ADH
  - Diagnosis of ADH is made when cytologic features are typical of DCIS, but the characteristic architecture of DCIS is lacking, or
  - Characteristic cytologic features and architecture of DCIS are seen but only focally present within one or two ducts

DCIS (SEVERAL WELL-RECOGNIZED VARIANTS EXIST)

- Comedocarcinoma
  - Ducts showing extensive epithelial cell proliferation with marked pleomorphism and central necrosis; mitosis can be present (Figure 13-19C)
  - Must have high-grade (grade III) nuclei and central necrosis
  - Periductal fibrosis and inflammation
  - May extend into adjacent lobules
  - Retrograde cancerization of lobules is often present
  - May be multifocal; large lesions can be palpable
- Cribriform type
  - Epithelial cell proliferation with formation of secondary lumens (Figure 13-19D)
  - Secondary lumens are round and have a clean, punched-out appearance (Figure 13-19E)
  - Areas of necrosis may be seen
  - Cells have round nuclei and distinct cell membranes; no or minimal nuclear overlapping
  - Uniform population of monotonous cells; may show mild to moderate atypia (Figure 13-19F)

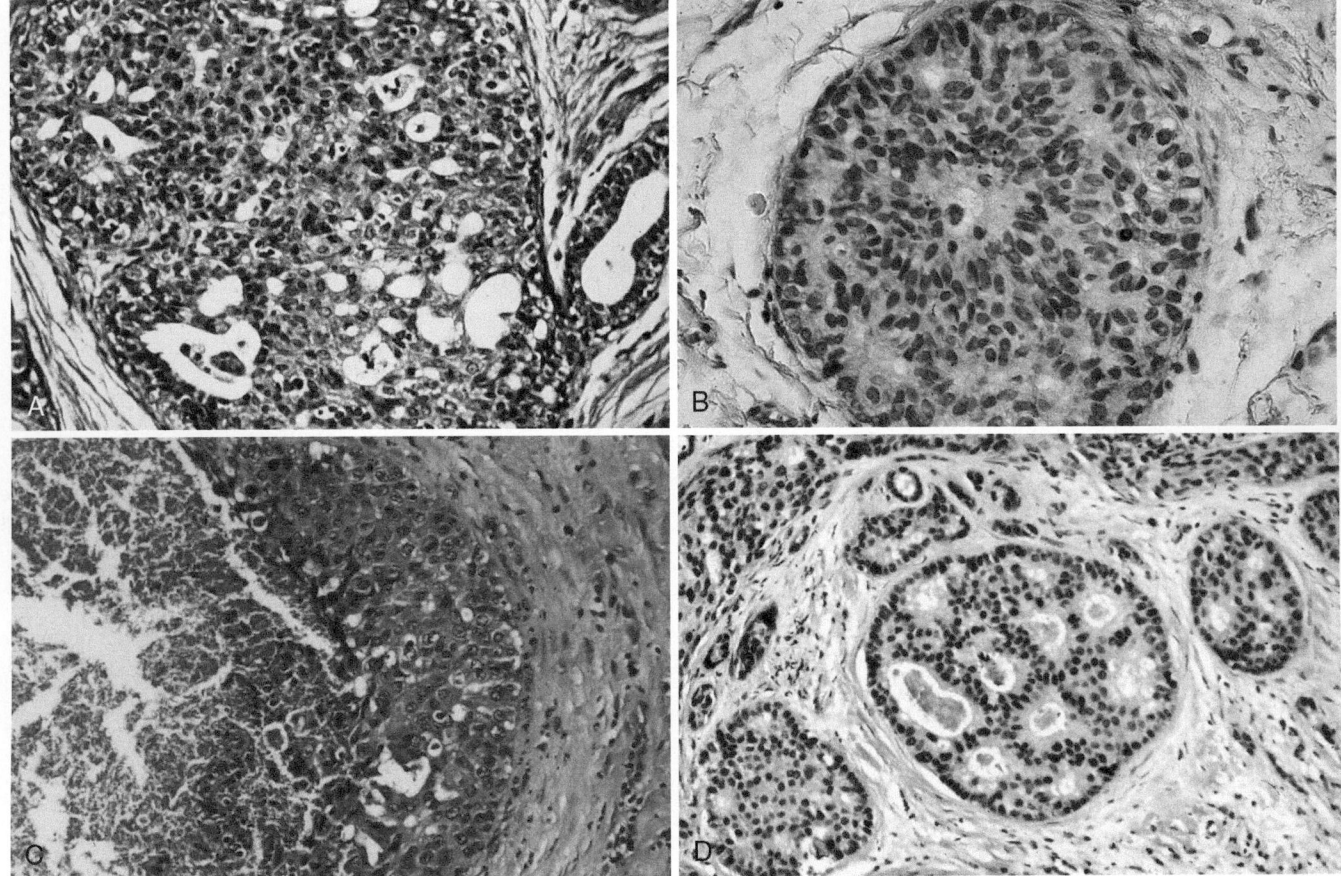

Figure 13-19. A, Atypical ductal hyperplasia. Duct involved by a complex proliferation of epithelial cells. Notice the irregularity of the luminal spaces. Scattered small myoepithelial cells can also be seen. **B,** Atypical ductal hyperplasia, uniform cell proliferation. Notice some cellular overlap and irregularity of secondary lumens. **C,** Ductal carcinoma in situ, comedo type. High-grade ductal carcinoma in situ with central necrosis, large pleomorphic nuclei, and prominent nucleoli. **D,** Ductal carcinoma in situ, cribriform type. Several ducts displaying proliferation of epithelial cells with formation of secondary lumens. Notice that the secondary lumens are round and have clean, punched-out borders. Central necrosis is also noted.

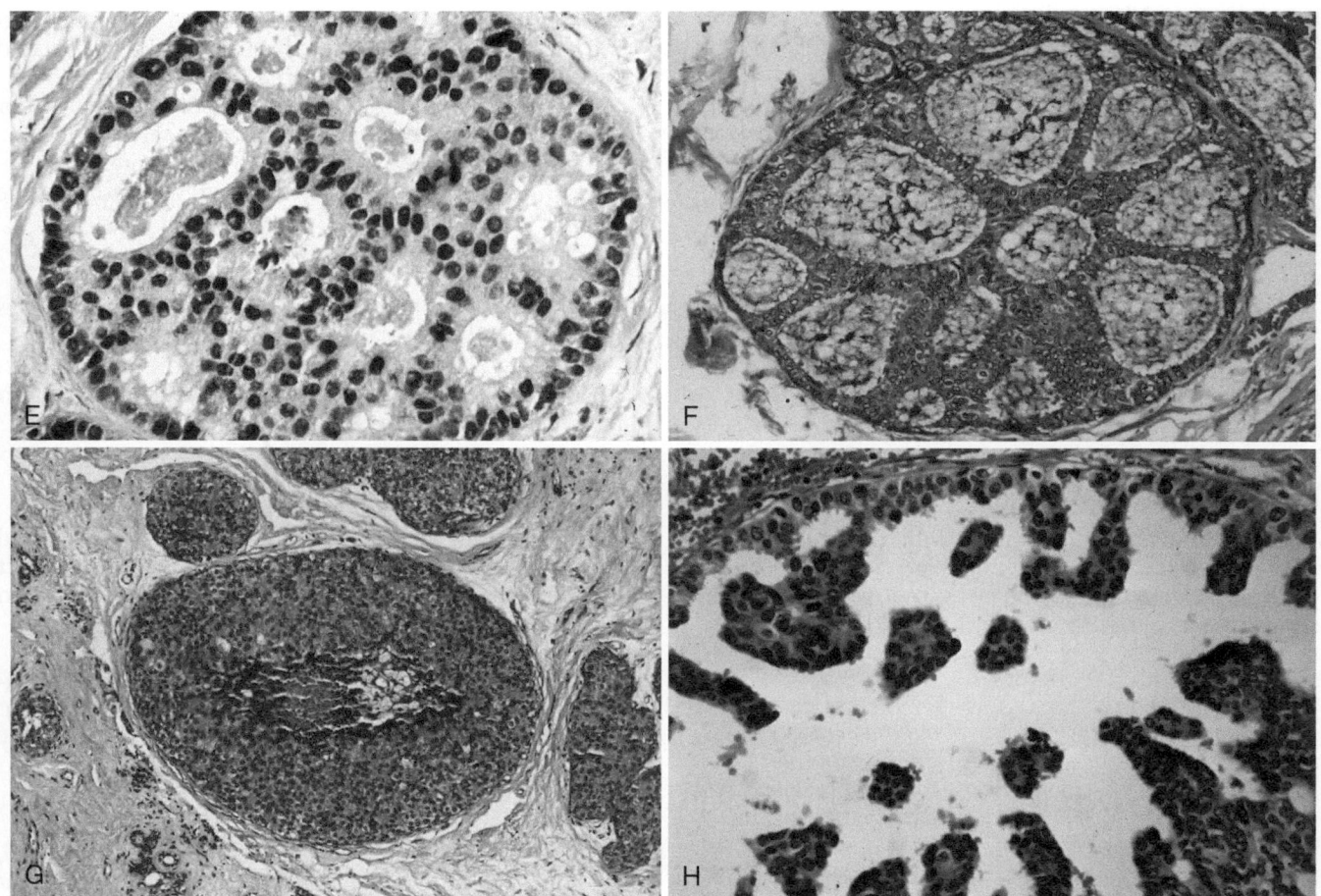

Figure 13-19, cont'd E, Ductal carcinoma in situ, cribriform type. The tumor shows sharp, well-demarcated, punched-out lumens. Central necrosis is also noted. **F,** Ductal carcinoma in situ, cribriform type. Distended duct displaying classic cribriform pattern. **G,** Ductal carcinoma in situ, solid type. Several distended ducts demonstrating a solid proliferation of uniform epithelial cells. Central necrosis is seen. **H,** Ductal carcinoma in situ, micropapillary type. Dilated duct containing a proliferation of a monomorphic cell population forming epithelial tufts around the duct.

- Low mitotic activity
- Solid type
  - Ducts are completely filled and distended with proliferating epithelial cells (Figure 13-19G)
  - Round to polygonal cells with distinct cell membranes and no or minimal nuclear overlapping
  - Central necrosis may be seen; high-grade nuclear features seen in comedo variant are not seen
  - Uniform population of monotonous cells; may show mild to moderate atypia
  - Usually intermediate grade
- Micropapillary type
  - Uniform epithelial cells forming small papillary tufts extending into the lumen of the duct
  - Papillary projections are regularly spaced around the duct (Figure 13-19H)
  - Lining cells usually show minimal cytologic atypia
  - Combination of micropapillary and cribriform types occasionally seen
  - Involves the breast extensively

Special Stains and Immunohistochemistry

- C-erb-B2 (HER-2-neu): more commonly positive in high-grade tumors

- Mib-1 (Ki-67): higher percentage (>20%) of tumor cells positive in high-grade tumors
- ER and PR: lower-grade tumors more frequently positive

Other Techniques for Diagnosis

- Chromosomal losses have been seen in low grade DCIS at 16q and 17p, whereas high-grade DCIS shows losses at 8p, 11q, 13q, and others

Differential Diagnosis

ADH Versus Intraductal Carcinoma

- Diagnosis of ADH is made when cytologic features are typical of DCIS but the characteristic architecture of DCIS is lacking, or
- Characteristic cytologic features and architecture of DCIS are seen but are only focally present within one or two ducts or the lesion measures 2 to 3 mm

Invasive Ductal Carcinoma

- Shows infiltration of the neoplastic cells outside the basement membrane of the duct
- Immunohistochemical staining for basement membrane proteins, including laminin or type IV collagen, may help identify areas of invasion by showing loss of continuity of the basement membrane

TABLE 13-1	**GRADING OF INTRADUCTAL CARCINOMA**
Grade	**Characteristics**
High	Marked cytologic atypia and necrosis; high mitotic rate
	All comedocarcinomas are high grade by definition
Intermediate	Cribriform, solid, or micropapillary types with minimal nuclear pleomorphism and necrosis or moderate nuclear pleomorphism without necrosis
Low	Cribriform, solid, or micropapillary types with minimal nuclear pleomorphism and no necrosis

LCIS

- Typically shows small, uniform cells that fill and distend the lobular unit
- Intraductal carcinoma (Table 13-1) involving lobules shows larger cells with greater nuclear pleomorphism

PEARLS

- *Occasionally multicentric or bilateral but much less frequently than lobular carcinomas*
- *Typically treated by excisional biopsy following radiologic needle localization with or without radiation therapy*
- *Occasionally occult microinvasive carcinoma is found*
- *Lymph node metastases may be seen in about 3% of comedocarcinomas (these cases are believed to actually have microinvasion that is not identified)*
- *Aneuploid tumors have been shown to be more likely to recur after excisional biopsy*
- *Carcinoma risk*
  - *ADH is associated with a 400% to 500% increased risk for carcinoma*
  - *ADH is a marker for subsequent invasive carcinoma, which usually develops at the site of disease*
  - *DCIS (especially comedocarcinoma) shows high likelihood of progression to invasive carcinoma*

SELECTED REFERENCES

Han K, Nofech-Mozes S, Narod S: Expression of HER2neu in ductal carcinoma in situ is associated with local recurrence. Clin Oncol (R Coll Radiol) 24:183-189, 2012.

Kerlikowske K, Molinaro AM, Gauthier ML, et al: Biomarker expression and risk of subsequent tumors after initial ductal carcinoma in situ diagnosis. J Natl Cancer Inst 102:627-637, 2010.

Vandenbussche CJ, Khouri N, Sbaity E, et al: Borderline atypical ductal hyperplasia/low-grade ductal carcinoma in situ on breast needle core biopsy should be managed conservatively. Am J Surg Pathol 3:913-923, 2013.

Zhou W, Jirström K, Amini RM, et al: Molecular subtypes in ductal carcinoma in situ of the breast and their relation to prognosis: a population-based cohort study. BMC Cancer 13:512, 2013.

ATYPICAL LOBULAR HYPERPLASIA AND LOBULAR CARCINOMA IN SITU

Clinical Features

- No palpable lesion is present
- Typically found as an incidental lesion in biopsy performed for a different indication or may be associated with invasive lobular carcinoma
- Mammography is not useful in detecting either ALH or LCIS; nonspecific calcifications may be seen
- Multicentric and bilateral disease is often present
- LCIS shows high probability of progressing to invasive lobular carcinoma (about 25% to 35% of cases)

Gross Pathology

- LCIS by itself usually causes no gross pathologic changes
- Extensive LCIS may cause a firm granular cut surface
- Proliferative lesions (fibrocystic changes) are often associated with both ALH and LCIS and are what often prompts biopsy

Histopathology

ATYPICAL LOBULAR HYPERPLASIA (ALH)

- Neoplastic cells are evenly spaced, round to polygonal cells with bland nuclei, scant cytoplasm, and indistinct cell borders; cells usually lack intracytoplasmic mucin droplets and show minimal or no loss of cohesion
- Involved lobules show residual ductule lumens
- Lobules are filled with neoplastic cells, but there is no significant distention of involved lobular units (Figure 13-20A)
- Involvement of only a single lobular unit and usually less than 50% of the acini

LCIS

- Proliferation of evenly spaced, round to polygonal, monotonous cells with small, bland nuclei, clear or eosinophilic cytoplasm, and indistinct cell borders (Figure 13-20B and C)
- Signet ring cells (cells with intracytoplasmic vacuoles containing mucin, which compresses the nucleus to the periphery of the cell) are often seen
- Neoplastic cells causing expansion and distention of lobular unit (more than 50% of the acini)
- Intervening stroma between involved ductules are typically seen; confluent ductules may be seen when massively distended
- Pagetoid spread of neoplastic cells into adjacent ducts may be seen
- Necrosis is rare
- Pleomorphic LCIS (PLCIS) shows pleomorphic nuclei grade III, with more obvious nucleoli, and is more likely associated with comedo-type necrosis and microcalcifications

Special Stains and Immunohistochemistry

- Mucicarmine or Alcian blue and PAS highlight signet ring cells (intracytoplasmic mucin)
- ER and PR show variable reactivity
- HER-2 and p53, E-cadherin negative
- PLCIS immunohistochemistry profile is often ER, PR negative, and C-erb-B2 (HER-2-neu) positive; glycoprotein of cystic breast disease (GCDFP-15) and p53 show increased immunoreactivity

Other Techniques for Diagnosis

- Genetic alterations common to both processes include loss at 19q13.2, 11q13, and 16q21 and gains at 20q13

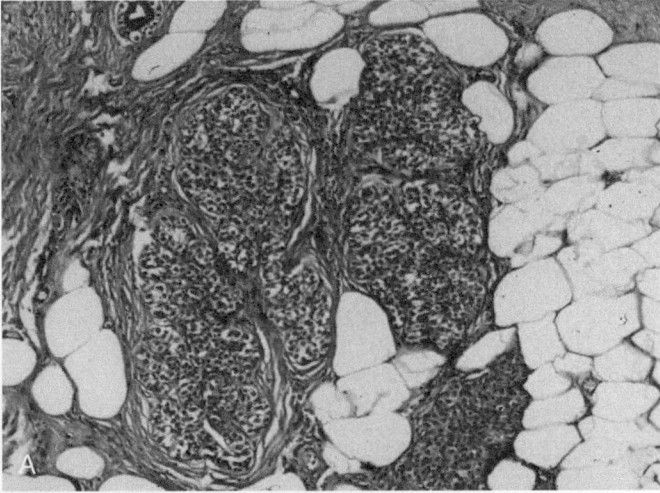

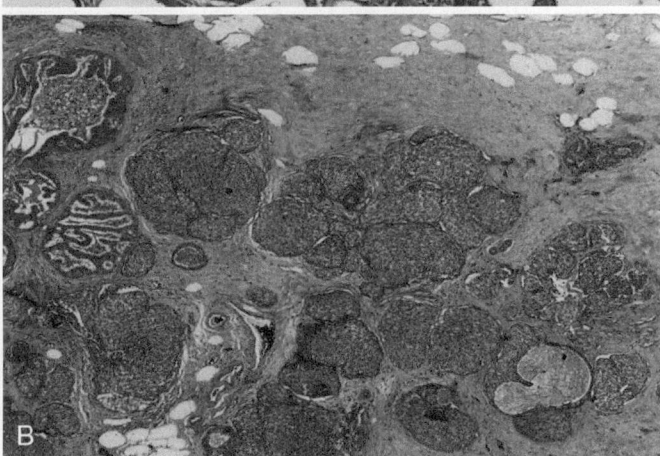

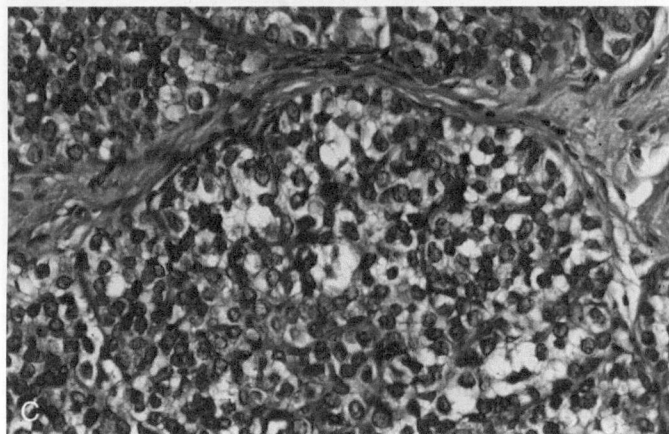

Figure 13-20. A, Atypical lobular hyperplasia. Mildly distended lobular unit filled with a small round monomorphic population of epithelial cells. **B,** Lobular carcinoma in situ. Several distended lobular units filled with a monotonous population of small round neoplastic cells. **C,** Lobular carcinoma in situ. Classic histologic features of lobular carcinoma in situ. Notice the small size and uniformity of the neoplastic cells.

Differential Diagnosis

DCIS INVOLVING LOBULES

- Typically shows larger cells with greater pleomorphism
- Neoplastic cells show distinct cell borders
- Small ductule formation with rosette-like pattern

- Presence of intracytoplasmic mucin (mucicarmine positivity) favors LCIS
- Mitosis and necrosis may be present

PEARLS

- *Many investigators believe that no prognostic information is gained by distinguishing between ALH and LCIS; some use the term* lobular neoplasia *(or more recently,* in situ lobular neoplasia*) to encompass both ALH and LCIS*
- *High probability of multicentricity and bilaterality (up to 50% of cases)*
- *Follow-up surgical excision is recommended when the diagnosis of AHL or LCIS is made on core needle biopsy*
- *Loss or down-regulation of E-cadherin (CDH1) gene is the most important molecular feature of lobular neoplasias*
- *Carcinoma risk*
  - *Eight- to 10-fold risk and four- to fivefold risk for developing invasive carcinoma after a diagnosis of LCIS*
  - *ALH and LCIS are markers for subsequent invasive carcinoma, which may develop at any location within the breast or in the contralateral breast, with greater risk in the ipsilateral breast*
  - *Recommended treatment includes close follow-up and hormonal therapy*
  - *Treated LCIS progresses to invasive carcinoma at a rate similar to that for untreated DCIS*
  - *May develop invasive carcinoma of any type, although invasive lobular carcinoma is most common after a diagnosis of ALH or LCIS*

SELECTED REFERENCES

Dabbs DJ, Schnitt SJ, Geyer FC, et al: Lobular neoplasia of the breast revisited with emphasis on the role of E-cadherin immunohistochemistry. Am J Surg Pathol 37:e1-e11, 2013.

Karabakhtsian RG, Johnson R, Sumkin J, Dabbs DJ: The clinical significance of lobular neoplasia on core biopsy. Am J Surg Pathol 31 (suppl):717-723, 2007.

Page DL, Schuyler PA, Dupont WD, et al: Atypical lobular hyperplasia as a unilateral predictor of breast cancer risk: a retrospective cohort study. Lancet 361:125-129, 2003.

Rendi MH, Dintzis SM, Lehman CD, et al: Lobular in-situ neoplasia on breast core needle biopsy: imaging indication and pathologic extent can identify which patients require excisional biopsy. Ann Surg Oncol 19:914-921, 2012.

INFILTRATING DUCTAL CARCINOMA

Clinical Features

- Most frequently diagnosed mammary carcinoma
- Wide age distribution; most commonly occurs in those 40 to 60 years of age
- Risk factors include positive family history of breast carcinoma, early menstruation, late menopause, and nulliparity
- Often presents as palpable or mammographically suspicious calcifications
- Skin ulceration, dimpling (peau d'orange), or nipple discharge and retraction may be seen
- Prognosis depends on numerous factors; most important is lymph node status

Gross Pathology

- Hard, fibrotic mass typically with stellate, infiltrative borders
- Rare tumors appear circumscribed with pushing borders
- Gray-white color with gritty, yellow-white streaks
- Gross evidence of necrosis may be seen
- Wide variation in size depending on duration of growth before treatment

Histopathology

- Infiltrating tumor composed of clusters or sheets of tumor cells together with single or cords of neoplastic cells
- Neoplastic cells often form tubules or glands
- Prominent lymphoplasmacytic response seen in 15% to 20% of cases
- Angiolymphatic or perineural invasion often seen, especially in high-grade lesions
- Most cases show intraductal carcinoma involving adjacent ducts; LCIS involving adjacent lobules may be seen
- Grading determined by cytologic and architectural features (Table 13-2), (Figure 13-21A-C)

Special Stains and Immunohistochemistry

- ER and PR
  - Positive in most grade I and grade II lesions
  - Higher-grade (grade III) tumors are typically ER and PR negative
  - Occasionally ER positive and PR negative (about 10% to 15% of cases)
- C-erb-B2 (HER-2-neu): more commonly positive in high-grade tumors
- CK8/18, CK19, CK7, EMA, and E-cadherin positive
- Mib-1 (Ki-67): higher percentage of tumor cells positive in high-grade tumors

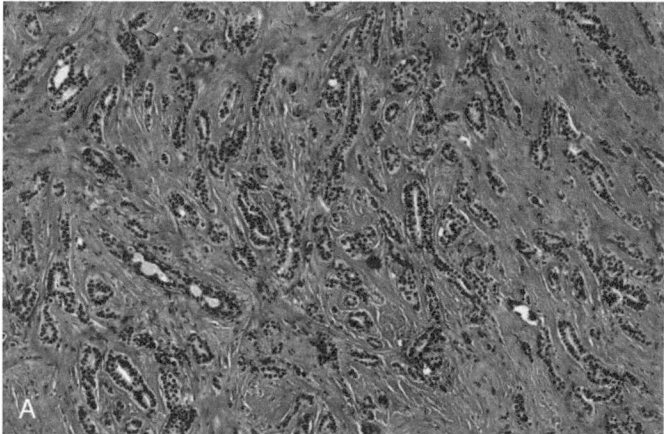
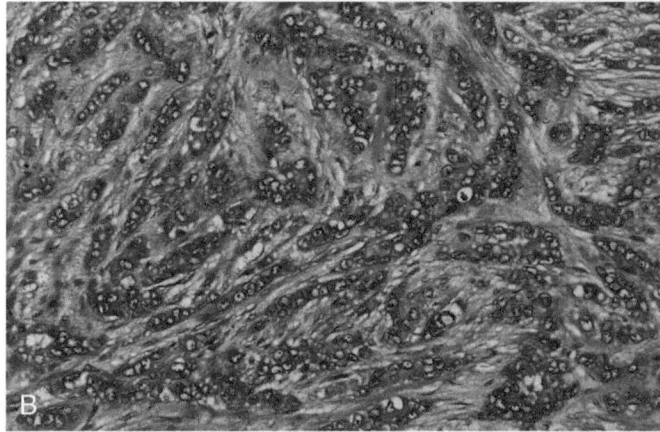
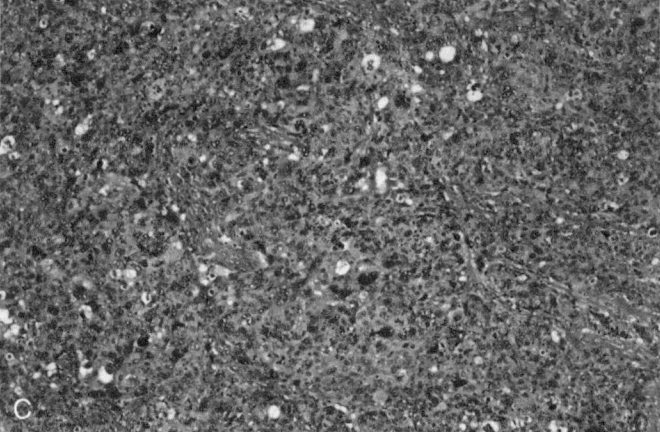

Figure 13-21. Infiltrating ductal carcinoma. A, Well differentiated (grade I). **B,** Moderately differentiated (grade II). **C,** Poorly differentiated (grade III).

TABLE 13-2	**GRADING OF INVASIVE DUCTAL CARCINOMA**
Grade	**Characteristics**
I	Distinct duct formation composing 75% of overall architecture
	Minimal variation in cell size
	Minimal pleomorphism with nuclear size equal to that of a normal duct epithelial cell nucleus; inconspicuous nucleoli
	Rare mitotic activity
II	Less than 75% tubule formation
	Increased variation in cell size (twofold to threefold variation)
	Tumor cells with larger nuclei, coarse chromatin, and distinct nucleoli
	Increased mitotic activity
III	Lacks distinct tubule formation
	Marked variation in cell size (greater than threefold variation)
	Marked nuclear pleomorphism with hyperchromatic nuclei showing coarse chromatin and prominent, often multiple nucleoli
	Numerous mitotic figures; atypical mitoses often seen

Other Techniques for Diagnosis

- Molecular studies
  - Mutation of *ras* proto-oncogene found in about 10% to 30% of breast carcinomas
  - Two to threefold amplification of *C-erb-B2* (*HER-2-neu*) reported in up to 30% of breast carcinomas

Differential Diagnosis

INFILTRATING TUBULAR CARCINOMA

- Composed of small, well-formed, angulated glands with open lumens and minimal pleomorphism

INFILTRATING LOBULAR CARCINOMA

- Neoplastic cells are small and uniform; typically infiltrates in single-file (linear) or alveolar pattern

RADIAL SCAR

- Shows central zone of fibrosis and elastosis with stellate or radial arrangement of ductules
- No infiltration into adjacent adipose tissue
- Proliferating ducts show myoepithelial cells

SCLEROSING ADENOSIS

- Benign ductule proliferation that retains lobular architecture
- Lacks infiltration into surrounding adipose tissue
- Ductules show a myoepithelial cell layer

PEARLS

- *Often difficult to distinguish between well-differentiated infiltrating ductal carcinoma (grade I) and tubular carcinoma*
- *Invasive ductal carcinomas that are associated with a high percentage (>25%) of DCIS show a higher likelihood of recurrence and treatment failure*
- *Overall survival is significantly lower in patients with C-erb-B2 (Her-2-neu)-positive tumors*
- *Tumors with increased S-phase fraction (SPF) or abnormal ploidy show decreased disease-free survival*
- *Presence of p53 mutation is associated with a worse prognosis*
- *Lymph node status appears to be the most predictive prognostic factor*
- *Sentinel lymph node biopsy is an alternative to axillary lymph node dissection*
- *Factors associated with increased risk for invasive breast carcinoma include the following:*
  - *Family history of breast cancer, especially in first-degree relatives*
  - *Patients positive for tumor suppressor genes BRCA1 (chromosome 17) and BRCA2 (chromosome 13) show up to an 85% lifetime risk for breast carcinoma*
  - *Early menarche, late menopause*
  - *Obesity*
  - *Delivery of first child after age 30 years*
  - *Li-Fraumeni syndrome (associated with presence of p53 tumor suppressor gene)*
  - *Heterologous carriers of the ataxia-telangiectasia (ATM) gene*
  - *Cowden disease (gastrointestinal polyps, multiple trichilemmomas, and increased risk for thyroid and breast carcinomas); associated with abnormal gene on chromosome 10*

SELECTED REFERENCES

Ahmed SS, Thike AA, Iqbal J, et al: Sentinel lymph nodes with isolated tumour cells and micrometastases in breast cancer: clinical relevance and prognostic significance. J Clin Pathol 67:243-250, 2014.

Feeley LP, Mulligan AM, Pinnaduwage D, et al: Distinguishing luminal breast cancer subtypes by Ki67, progesterone receptor or TP53 status provides prognostic information. Mod Pathol 2013 Sep 20 (Epub ahead of print).

Sanpaolo P, Barbieri V, Genovesi D: Prognostic value of breast cancer subtypes on breast cancer specific survival, distant metastases and local relapse rates in conservatively managed early stage breast cancer: a retrospective clinical study. Eur J Surg Oncol 37:876-882, 2011.

Santarpia L, Iwamoto T, Di Leo A, et al: DNA repair gene patterns as prognostic and predictive factors in molecular breast cancer subtypes. Oncologist 18:1063-1073, 2013.

INFILTRATING LOBULAR CARCINOMA

Clinical Features

- Similar age distribution and risk factors as infiltrating ductal carcinoma
- Accounts for 5% to 14% of all invasive breast carcinomas
- Presents as a mass with poorly defined margins
- High incidence of multifocal or bilateral disease (up to 20%)
- May not be identified on mammograms

Gross Pathology

- Variable size (may be of microscopic size to well-defined, large masses to large tumors that are diffusely present throughout the breast)
- Typically forms a hard mass with irregular, infiltrative borders

Histopathology

- Classic growth pattern shows tumor cells in a linear or single-file (Indian filing) pattern in a sclerotic background; cells may show mucin-filled vacuoles sometimes resulting in signet ring cells (Figure 13-22A and B)
- Other common growth patterns and subtypes include the following:
  - Solid: irregular solid nests of tumor cells
  - Tubulolobular: small tubule formation with linear infiltration
  - Alveolar: numerous small round aggregates of tumor cells separated by fibrous tissue
  - Apocrine and histiocytoid subtypes: tumor cells resemble macrophages with copious cytoplasm and prominent nucleoli
  - Pleomorphic subtype: tumors with high-grade nuclei and high mitotic index (Figure 13-22C and D)
- Tumor cells concentrically arranged around ducts (targetoid or bull's-eye pattern)
- Uniform, small bland cells with round nuclei and inconspicuous nucleoli
- Often associated with LCIS

Special Stains and Immunohistochemistry

- Mucicarmine, Alcian blue, and PAS positive in signet ring cells containing intracytoplasmic sialomucin
- Mib-1 (Ki-67): variable proliferative activity
- ER and PR: variable reactivity
- C-erb-B2 (HER-2-neu): about 30% of tumors show 2+ or 3+ positivity
- E-cadherin: negative
- GCDFP 15: positive

Other Techniques for Diagnosis

- Noncontributory

Differential Diagnosis

SCLEROSING ADENOSIS

- Ductule proliferation that retains lobular architecture
- Lacks infiltration into surrounding adipose tissue
- Myoepithelial cells present

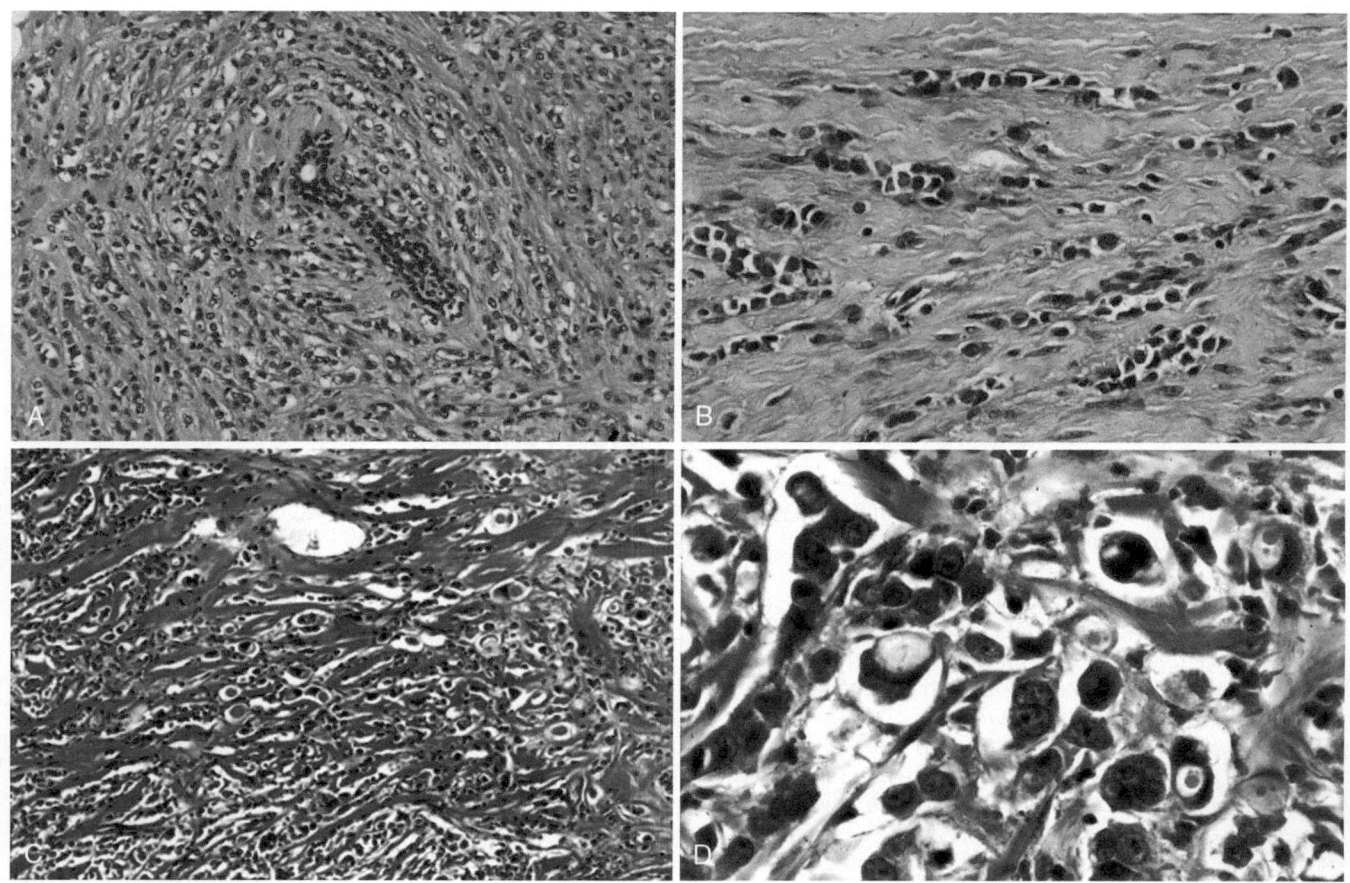

Figure 13-22. Infiltrating lobular carcinoma. A, Classic targetoid pattern. **B,** Classic growth pattern of linear or "single-file" infiltration. **C,** Pleomorphic cell variant. **D,** Pleomorphic cell variant. Tumor cells infiltrating stroma are highly pleomorphic, some with signet ring cell morphology.

INFILTRATING DUCTAL CARCINOMA
- Neoplastic cells often form distinct ducts
- Typically composed of large, pleomorphic cells with prominent nucleoli and numerous mitotic figures

MALIGNANT LYMPHOMA
- Small, noncohesive cells
- Immunohistochemistry negative for cytokeratin and EMA and positive for lymphoid markers

PEARLS

- *Loss or down-regulation of E-cadherin (CDH1) gene is the most important molecular feature of lobular neoplasias*
- *Most frequent breast carcinoma to be multifocal or bilateral*
- *Tubulolobular variant may be better categorized with ductal-type carcinomas*
- *Classic cytogenetic changes of the classic variant are loss of 16q and 1p gain resembling grade I ductal carcinomas*
- *Cytogenetic profile of pleomorphic variant resembles more grade III ductal carcinoma with overexpression of HER-2-neu (with gene amplification), p53 positivity, and loss of ER and PR expression*
- *Classic form of invasive lobular carcinoma has better prognosis than other subtypes*

- *Higher likelihood of metastases to the ovary, bone marrow, serosal surfaces, and cerebrospinal fluid when compared with invasive ductal carcinomas*

SELECTED REFERENCES

Hariby AM, Hughes TA: In situ and invasive lobular neoplasia of the breast. Histopathology 52:58-66, 2008.

Karabakhtsian RG, Johnson R, Sumkin J, Dabbs DJ: The clinical significance of lobular neoplasia on breast core biopsy. Am J Surg Pathol 31:717-723, 2007.

Pai K, Baliga P, Shrestha BL: E-cadherin expression: a diagnostic utility for differentiating breast carcinomas with ductal and lobular morphologies. J Clin Diagn Res 7:840-844, 2013.

Rakha EA, van Deurzen CH, Paish EC, et al: Pleomorphic lobular carcinoma of the breast: is it a prognostically significant pathological subtype independent of histological grade? Mod Pathol 26:496-501, 2013.

TRIPLE NEGATIVE CARCINOMAS

Clinical Features

- Account for 10% to 17% of all breast carcinomas
- Found more frequently in women younger than 50 years
- More common in premenopausal women

- Behave as biologically aggressive cancers, with most deaths occurring in the first 5 years
- Heterogeneous group of tumors defined by the absent expression of ER, PR, and Her-2

Gross Pathology

- Tumors are of relatively large size
- Tumors have pushing borders

Histopathology

- Most triple negative breast cancers are of a basal-like phenotype (tumors with basal cytokeratin, myoepithelial, and epidermal growth factor receptor [EGFR] expression) and are high-grade ductal carcinomas of no specific type; many high-grade metaplastic carcinomas and medullary carcinomas exhibit a basal-like immunophenotype
- Triple negative breast cancers have high-grade nuclear features, high mitotic rate, and geographic tumor necrosis (Figure 13-23A)
- Areas of squamous metaplasia and differentiation are seen, and spindled and sarcomatoid foci may be present
- Variable lymphocytic inflammatory infiltrate may be seen

Special Stains and Immunohistochemistry

- ER, PR, and HER-2-neu negative
- Cytokeratins 5/6, 14, 17 positive in most basal-like phenotype tumors (Figure 19-23B)
- EGFR positive in most basal-like phenotype tumors
- SMA and p63 positive in most basal-like phenotype tumors

Other Techniques for Diagnosis

- Tissue microarray gene expression profiling identified triple negative breast cancers as tumors that have negativity for hormone receptors and HER-2-neu

Differential Diagnosis

- Some tumors may mimic large cell lymphomas

PEARLS

- BRCA1 *gene-related breast cancers, triple negative breast cancers, and basal-like breast cancers are a closely related group of carcinomas with significant morphologic, phenotypic, and genetic overlap*
- *Triple negative breast cancers of basal-like morphology favor a hematogenous spread with metastatic deposits to lungs and brain and less to axillary nodes and bones*
- *Tumors may show objective response to neoadjuvant chemotherapeutic regimens, but lack of complete pathologic response implies a poor prognosis*

SELECTED REFERENCES

Hudis CA, Gianni L: Triple-negative breast cancer: an unmet medical need. Oncologist 16(suppl 1):1-11, 2011.

Kim JE, Ahn HJ, Ahn JH, et al: Impact of triple-negative breast cancer phenotype on prognosis in patients with stage I breast cancer. J Breast Cancer 15:197-202, 2012.

Pai K, Baliga P, Shrestha BL: E-cadherin expression: a diagnostic utility for differentiating breast carcinomas with ductal and lobular morphologies. J Clin Diagn Res 7:840-844, 2013.

Rakha EA, van Deurzen CH, Paish EC, et al: Pleomorphic lobular carcinoma of the breast: is it a prognostically significant pathological subtype independent of histological grade? Mod Pathol 26:496-501, 2013.

Reis-Filho JS, Tutt ANJ: Triple negative tumours: a critical review. Histopathology 52:108-118, 2008.

MEDULLARY CARCINOMA

Clinical Features

- Rare, about 3% of all mammary carcinomas
- Similar age distribution as infiltrating ductal carcinoma, although some reports suggest a younger age (35 years)
- Mammography shows well-circumscribed mass; may mimic fibroadenoma
- Good prognosis

Gross Pathology

- Firm, discrete mass (typically 2 to 3 cm)

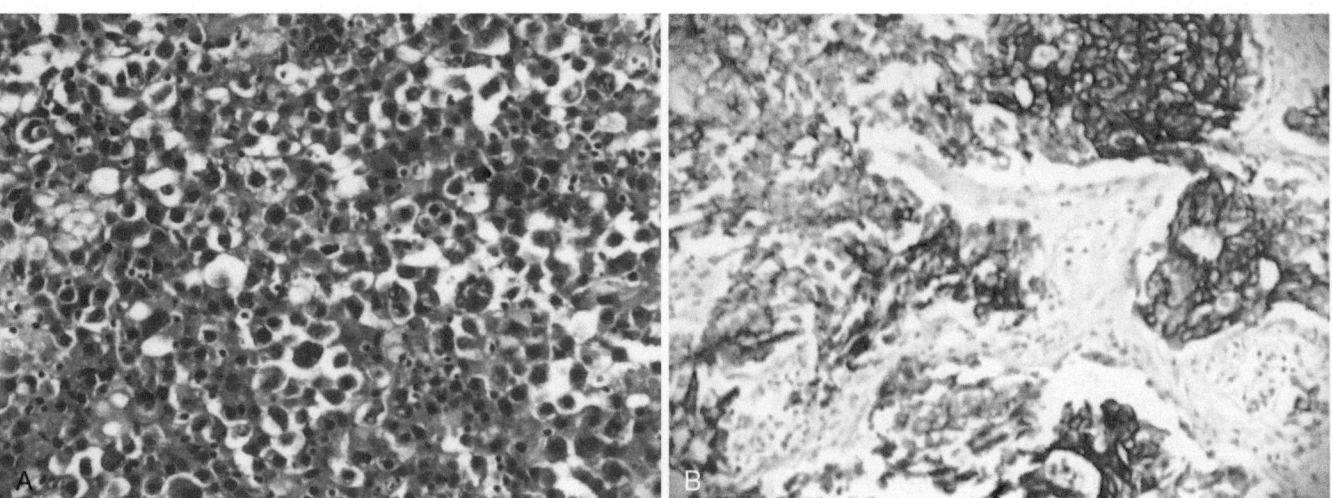

Figure 13-23. Triple negative breast carcinomas. A, Triple negative breast carcinomas are high-grade neoplasms with high-grade nuclear features. **B,** Cytokeratin 5/6 is positive in most, but these tumors are estrogen receptor, progesterone receptor, and C-erb-B2 negative.

- Noninvasive tumors that are typically well circumscribed; often show distinct capsule
- Faintly nodular, soft, tan-brown or gray tumor

Histopathology

- Poorly differentiated tumor with syncytial pattern (> 75% of tumor) (Figure 13-24)
- Pleomorphic cells with high nuclear grade and numerous mitoses
- Must show a prominent lymphoplasmacytic response around tumor cells
- No invasion into surrounding adipose tissue
- Well-defined margins with pushing borders
- Glandular or ductal structures should not be seen

Special Stains and Immunohistochemistry

- Cytokeratin 5/6, p53, and Mib-1 positive
- ER and PR negative in more than 90% of cases
- C-erb-B2 (HER-2-neu) negative
- EGFR frequently expressed
- Frequently associated with BRCA1 mutations

Other Techniques for Diagnosis

- Flow cytometry: tumor cells typically aneuploid or polypoid

Differential Diagnosis

INFILTRATING DUCTAL CARCINOMA

- Typically does not show extensive syncytial pattern
- Less prominent lymphocytic infiltrate
- Infiltrative borders

PEARLS

- *Relatively better prognosis than infiltrating ductal carcinoma*
- *Patients have decreased likelihood of axillary lymph node metastases*
- *Designation of atypical medullary carcinoma should be avoided because these lesions have been shown to behave similarly to infiltrating ductal carcinomas*

SELECTED REFERENCES

Khomsi F, Ben Bachouche W, Bouzaiene H, et al: Typical medullary carcinoma of the breast: a retrospective study of about 33 cases. Gynecol Obstet Fertil 35:1117-1122, 2007.

Kostianets O, Antoniuk S, Filonenko V, Kiyamova R: Immunohistochemical analysis of medullary breast carcinoma autoantigens in different histological types of breast carcinomas. Diagn Pathol 7:161, 2012.

Marginean F, Rakha EA, Ho BC, et al: Histological features of medullary carcinoma and prognosis in triple-negative basal-like carcinomas of the breast. Mod Pathol 23:1357-1363, 2010.

Vincent-Salomon A, Gruel N, Lucchesi C, et al: Identification of typical medullary breast carcinoma as a genomic sub-group of basal-like carcinomas, a heterogeneous new molecular entity. Breast Cancer Res 9:R24, 2007.

MUCINOUS (COLLOID) CARCINOMA

Clinical Features

- Constitutes less than 2% of all breast carcinomas
- Typically presents as a discrete mass
- Older women are more commonly affected
- Mammogram shows a well-defined tumor

Gross Pathology

- Well-circumscribed, gelatinous mass

Histopathology

- Clusters of infiltrating tumor cells surrounded by lakes of extracellular mucin (Figure 13-25)
- Extracellular mucin must make up greater than 50% of the tumor
- May have alveolar, cribriform, or papillary configuration or infiltrate as diffuse sheets of cells
- Gland formation is not typically seen
- Classified as type A, which does not have neuroendocrine differentiation and is paucicellular, and type B, with neuroendocrine differentiation and increased cellularity
- Intraductal carcinoma often involves peripheral ducts

Special Stains and Immunohistochemistry

- Cytokeratin 7 positive
- Cytokeratin 20 typically negative

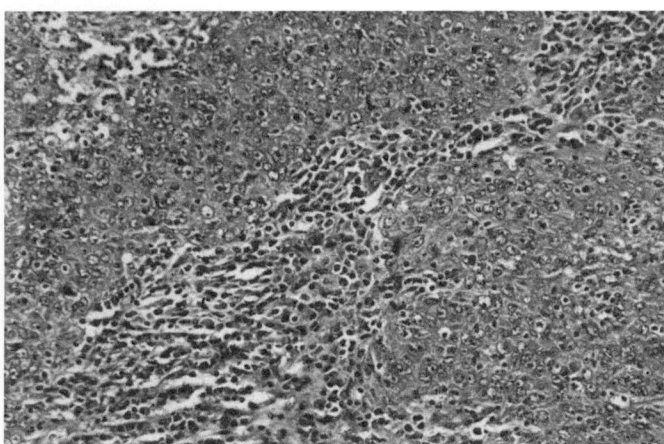

Figure 13-24. Medullary carcinoma. Composed of a proliferation of large neoplastic cells with vesicular nuclear chromatin and prominent nucleoli. Syncytial growth pattern is visible. Characteristic lymphoplasmacytic infiltrate is also evident.

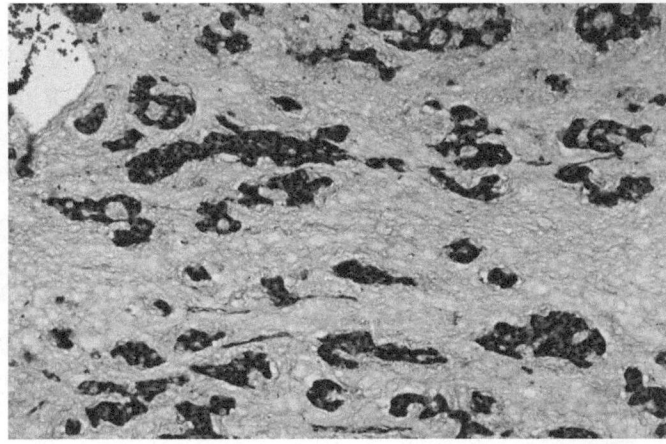

Figure 13-25. Mucinous (colloid) carcinoma. Numerous clusters of neoplastic ductal cells surrounded by pools of extracellular mucin material.

- PAS highlights intracellular mucin
- ER and PR: variable reactivity, usually positive
- Her-2 negative in most cases
- Neuroendocrine markers positive in type B

Other Techniques for Diagnosis

- Electron microscopy: demonstrates intracellular mucin (mucigen granules)
- Flow cytometry: pure mucinous carcinomas are almost always diploid; mixed tumors with areas of invasive ductal carcinoma are more commonly aneuploid

Differential Diagnosis

MUCOCELE-LIKE TUMOR

- Benign epithelial-lined cysts containing mucin
- No tumor cells floating in the extracellular mucin
- Extracellular mucin dissecting through fibrous stroma

MIXED MUCINOUS CARCINOMA

- Lesions with minimal mucin (<50% of tumor) relative to epithelial component

METASTATIC MUCINOUS OVARIAN OR PANCREATIC CARCINOMA

- Exceedingly rare
- Malignant epithelial cells are positive for cytokeratin 20

PEARLS

- *Mucinous carcinoma is a variant of invasive ductal carcinoma*
- *Lymph node metastases are found in fewer than 20% of patients*
- *Mucinous carcinoma is associated with an excellent prognosis with increased survival compared with infiltrating ductal carcinoma*

SELECTED REFERENCES

Kryvenko ON, Chitale DA, Yoon J, et al: Precursor lesions of mucinous carcinoma of the breast: analysis of 130 cases. Am J Surg Pathol 37:1076-1084, 2013.

Molavi D, Argani P: Distinguishing benign dissecting mucin (stromal mucin pools) from invasive mucinous carcinoma. Adv Anat Pathol 15:1-17, 2008.

Tan PH, Tse GM, Bay BH: Mucinous breast lesions: diagnostic challenges. J Clin Pathol 61:11-19, 2008.

TUBULAR CARCINOMA

Clinical Features

- Wide age distribution (second to eighth decades), usually fourth decade
- Pure tubular carcinoma makes up about 2% of all invasive mammary carcinomas
- Presents as a palpable breast mass
- May not show a mass in mammography (20%)
- May show skin changes if superficially located

Gross Pathology

- Most lesions are less than 2cm in diameter
- Firm, stellate, sclerotic appearance

Histopathology

- Infiltrative margins often extending into adjacent adipose tissue
- May be multifocal
- Composed of small, angulated tubules with open lumens (Figure 13-26A and B)
- Tubules are haphazardly arranged in dense collagenous stroma showing a desmoplastic response surrounding the neoplastic ducts
- Bland cytologic features, including cells with small nuclei and eosinophilic cytoplasm; rare mitotic activity; apical snouts present
- Tubules lack myoepithelial cells
- Pure tubular carcinoma must show virtually 100% tubular architecture
- DCIS is an associated finding in up to 40% of cases; 10% are associated with LCIS
- May have mixed forms; tubulolobular type or ductal carcinoma with tubular features

Special Stains and Immunohistochemistry

- ER positive in most cases
- SMA and S-100 protein negative (lack of myoepithelial cells)
- Her-2 and EGFR negative

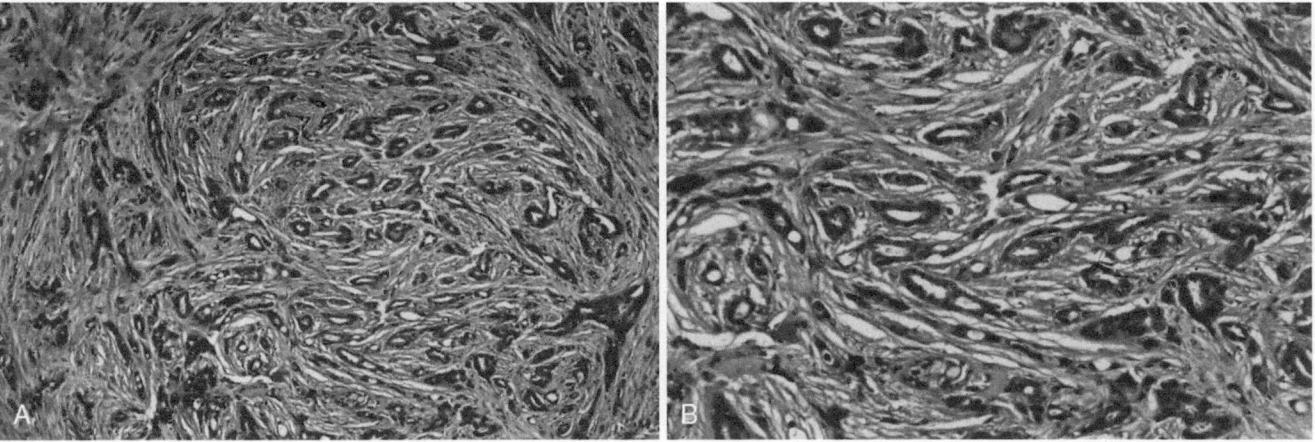

Figure 13-26. Tubular carcinoma. A, Characterized by a proliferation of tubular structures in a background of loose desmoplastic stroma. **B,** The neoplastic tubules have open lumens and are lined by a single layer of epithelial cells.

Other Techniques for Diagnosis

- Noncontributory

Differential Diagnosis

SCLEROSING ADENOSIS

- Lobular architecture is maintained
- Tubules are lined by myoepithelial cells

MICROGLANDULAR ADENOSIS

- Haphazard arrangement of round ductules lacking lobular architecture and stellate configuration (similar to tubular carcinoma)
- Background shows hypocellular, collagenous stroma
- Ductal cells typically show clear or vacuolated cytoplasm
- Usually negative for EMA and ER
- Lumens often contain eosinophilic, PAS-positive secretions

MIXED TUMORS (TUBULOLOBULAR OR DUCTAL CARCINOMA WITH TUBULAR FEATURES)

- Tumor is not completely composed of well-formed tubules
- Invasive ductal or lobular carcinoma makes up more than 5% to 25% of tumor

PEARLS

- *Highly differentiated form of invasive ductal carcinoma*
- *Rare perineural, vascular, or lymphatic invasion*
- *Axillary lymph node involvement is seen in less than 10% of cases*
- *Associated microcalcifications are present in more than 50% of cases*
- *Relatively good prognosis compared with infiltrating ductal carcinoma*

SELECTED REFERENCES

Abdel-Fatah TM, Powe DG, Hodi Z, et al: High frequency of coexistence of columnar cell lesions, lobular neoplasia, and low grade ductal carcinoma in situ with invasive tubular carcinoma and invasive lobular carcinoma. Am J Surg Pathol 31:417-426, 2007.

Dejode M, Sagan C, Campion L, et al: Pure tubular carcinoma of the breast and sentinel lymph node biopsy: a retrospective multi-institutional study of 234 cases. Eur J Surg Oncol 39:248-254, 2013.

Fernández-Aguilar S, Simon P, Buxant F, et al: Tubular carcinoma of the breast and associated intra-epithelial lesions: a comparative study with invasive low-grade ductal carcinomas. Virchows Arch 447:683-687, 2005.

Marchiò C, Sapino A, Arisio R, Bussolati G: A new vision of tubular and tubulo-lobular carcinomas of the breast, as revealed by 3-D modelling. Histopathology 48:556-562, 2006.

PAPILLARY CARCINOMA (INTRADUCTAL, INTRACYSTIC, ENCAPSULATED, AND INVASIVE)

Clinical Features

- Rare breast tumor; makes up 1% to 2% of mammary carcinomas
- Age distribution is similar to that of other mammary carcinomas; patients are older than those with solitary intraductal papillomas
- Most patients have a palpable mass
- Associated with higher likelihood of nipple discharge (often hemorrhagic) and nipple retraction
- Rounded, circumscribed mass with rare microcalcifications on mammography

Gross Pathology

- Usually well-circumscribed mass with pushing borders
- Tan-gray tumor; may be focally hemorrhagic
- Typically cystic with obvious papilla formation

Histopathology

- Papillary lesions composed of numerous complex epithelial fronds proliferating into a distended duct lumen (Figure 13-27A,B)

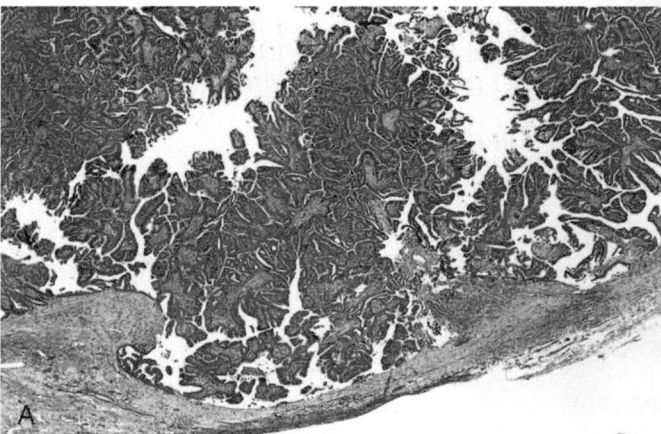

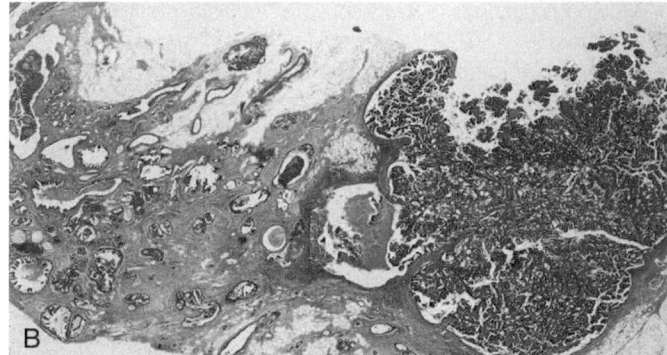

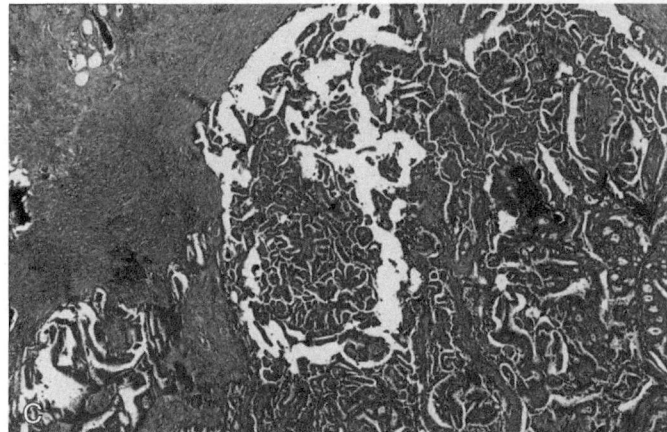

Figure 13-27. A, Intracystic papillary carcinoma. Distended duct with highly complex proliferating epithelial fronds with absence of a myoepithelial cell layer are the hallmark of encapsulated, intracystic, and intraductal papillary carcinoma. **B,** Intracystic papillary carcinoma with non–high-grade ductal carcinoma in situ. **C,** Infiltrating papillary carcinoma. Stromal invasion is evident in the left lower corner.

- Must demonstrate papillae with absence of myoepithelial cell layer; in addition, studies have failed to demonstrate myoepithelial cells at the periphery of tumor nodules
- Apocrine metaplasia is not a feature
- Diagnosis of invasive papillary carcinoma should be made only with identification of unequivocal stromal invasion (tumor should be clearly present beyond the capsule of the lesion) (Figure 13-27C)

Special Stains and Immunohistochemistry

- SMA, calponin, S-100 protein, smooth muscle myosin heavy chain, and p63 demonstrate focal or complete lack of myoepithelial cell layer
- ER and PR stains typically positive C-erb-B2 (HER-2-neu) negative
- HMWCK (5/6, 14, 34βE12) stains are negative in neoplastic cells
- CEA positive in 85% of papillary carcinomas and negative in benign papillary lesions

Other Techniques for Diagnosis

- LOH on chromosome 16q23 appears to be limited to papillary carcinomas
- LOH at *TP53* locus significantly associated with malignant papillary lesions
- Flow cytometry: tumor cells may be diploid or occasionally aneuploid (of little help in distinguishing benign papillomas from papillary carcinoma)

Differential Diagnosis

Benign Papilloma Versus Intraductal Papillary Carcinoma

- Myoepithelial cell layer must be demonstrated in benign lesions and is absent in papillary carcinoma
- Degree of cytologic atypia and complexity is typically not helpful in distinguishing benign papillomas from intraductal papillary carcinoma
- Apocrine metaplasia is present in benign lesions
- Papillary carcinoma is typically CEA positive, diffusely ER/PR positive, and lacks HMWCK expression

Invasive Papillary Carcinoma

- Complex papillary proliferation with unequivocal stromal invasion

PEARLS

- *Intraductal (intracystic, encapsulated) papillary carcinoma, long considered a variant of intraductal carcinoma, may represent a form of low-grade carcinoma, being part of a spectrum of progression from in situ to invasive disease*
- *Patients with intraductal papillary carcinoma are typically good candidates for breast-conserving surgery*
- *Invasive papillary carcinoma rarely shows nodal metastases*

Selected References

Carder PJ, Garvican J, Haigh I, Liston JC: Needle core biopsy can reliably distinguish between benign and malignant papillary lesions of the breast. Histopathology 46:320-327, 2005.

Collins LC, Schnitt SJ: Papillary lesions of the breast: selected diagnostic and management issues. Histopathology 52:20-29, 2008.
Khoury T, Hu Q, Liu S, Wang J: Intracystic papillary carcinoma of breast: interrelationship with in situ and invasive carcinoma and a proposal of pathogenesis: array comparative genomic hybridization study of 14 cases. Mod Pathol 27:194-203, 2014.
Rakha EA, Gandhi N, Climent F, et al: Encapsulated papillary carcinoma of the breast: an invasive tumor with excellent prognosis. Am J Surg Pathol 35:1093-1103, 2011.
Wynveen CA, Nehhozina T, Akram M, et al: Intracystic papillary carcinoma of the breast: an in situ or invasive tumor? Results of immunohistochemical analysis and clinical follow-up. Am J Surg Pathol 35:1-14, 2011.

METAPLASTIC CARCINOMA

Clinical Features

- Uncommon, occurring in less than 3% of breast cancer patients
- Typically presents as palpable breast mass
- Rapid growth is common
- Mammogram shows a well-defined tumor

Gross Pathology

- Distinct, firm mass with circumscribed margins
- Nodular or cystic areas can be seen

Histopathology

- Heterogenous group of lesions, simply designated as biphasic (mixed carcinomatous and sarcomatoid components) or monophasic (sarcomatoid elements only)
- Carcinomatous component is usually of a high grade and typically a poorly differentiated ductal carcinoma with glandular and tubular formation or the presence of intracellular or extracellular mucin production; additional subtypes include squamous component with intercellular bridges with or without keratin pearl formation
- Spindle cell proliferation or sarcomatous component is usually of a high grade with occasional heterologous elements, including bone or cartilage; fibromatosis-like metaplastic carcinoma appears to be a low-grade variant (Figure 13-28)

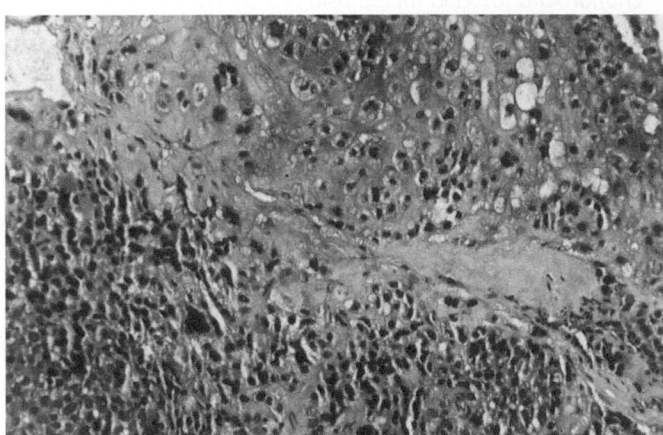

Figure 13-28. Metaplastic carcinoma. High-grade ductal carcinoma is seen in the lower portion of the photomicrograph. Notice metaplastic cartilaginous tissue in the upper area.

- Metaplastic changes include squamous metaplasia with or without keratin formation, chondroid metaplasia, or metaplastic bone
- Spindle cell proliferation or sarcomatous appearance may be seen
- Metastases from metaplastic carcinoma may consist of metaplastic elements, adenocarcinoma, or both
- Focal metaplastic changes in other invasive tumor subtypes (tubular, medullary, and lobular) may be seen

Special Stains and Immunohistochemistry

- Cytokeratin (AE1/AE3, 5/6, and 14): epithelial component positive; spindle cell component focally positive
- EMA: epithelial component positive; may be focally positive in mesenchymal areas
- Vimentin: typically positive in both epithelial and mesenchymal components
- ER, PR, and Her-2 usually negative
- Positive for p63 in the spindle and sarcomatous component
- EGFR overexpressed and amplified

Other Techniques for Diagnosis

- Noncontributory

Differential Diagnosis

INFILTRATING DUCTAL CARCINOMA
- Lacks metaplastic elements

ADENOSQUAMOUS CARCINOMA
- Rare variant of metaplastic carcinoma
- Mixture of malignant glandular and epidermoid elements in dense fibrous stroma

SQUAMOUS CELL CARCINOMA
- Composed entirely of neoplastic, typically keratinizing squamous cells

PEARLS

- *Most common metaplastic change is squamous metaplasia*
- *Squamous metaplasia has little impact on prognosis; chondroid or osteoid metaplasia has a negative impact on prognosis*

SELECTED REFERENCES

Abd El Hafez A, Shawky Ael-A: Analysis of metaplastic breast carcinoma: FNAC; histopathology and immunohistochemistry are complementary for diagnosis. Breast Dis 34:67-75, 2013.

Cooper CL, Karim RZ, Selinger C, et al: Molecular alterations in metaplastic breast carcinoma. J Clin Pathol 66:522-528, 2013.

Luini A, Aguilar M, Gatti G, et al: Metaplastic carcinoma of the breast, an unusual disease with worse prognosis: the experience of the European Institute of Oncology and review of the literature. Breast Cancer Res Treat 101:349-353, 2007.

Rungta S, Kleer CG: Metaplastic carcinomas of the breast: diagnostic challenges and new translational insights. Arch Pathol Lab Med 136:896-900, 2012.

Song Y, Liu X, Zhang G, et al: Unique clinicopathological features of metaplastic breast carcinoma compared with invasive ductal carcinoma and poor prognostic indicators. World J Surg Oncol 11:129, 2013.

SECRETORY CARCINOMA (JUVENILE CARCINOMA)

Clinical Features

- Rare, less than 1% of all breast cancers
- Affects women of any age; increased incidence in children and young adults (mean age, 25 years)
- Patients present with distinct painless breast mass; can be located near the areola

Gross Pathology

- Well-defined, circumscribed, nodular mass
- Cut surface shows gray-white or tan tumor
- Variable size (0.6 to 12 cm); larger lesions typically found in older women

Histopathology

- Proliferation of variably sized ducts with loss of the normal lobular architecture
- Tumor forms cystic spaces filled with abundant pale-pink secretion (Figure 13-29)
- Both intracellular and extracellular secretory material
- Neoplastic ductal epithelial cells are small with bland nuclei and abundant pale, eosinophilic, granular, and vacuolated cytoplasm; rare mitotic activity
- Ducts lack a myoepithelial layer
- Often shows an intraductal component, which may be papillary, cribriform, solid, or comedo type

Special Stains and Immunohistochemistry

- Mucicarmine- and diastase-resistant PAS: luminal secretion positive
- CEA (polyclonal), EMA, S-100, and α-lactalbumin positive
- ER and PR show variable reactivity but are frequently negative

Other Techniques for Diagnosis

- Electron microscopy: cytoplasm shows numerous membrane-bound secretory vacuoles lined by microvilli
- Genetics: ETV6-NTRK3 fusion gene, the product of t(12:1 5)(p13;q25) translocation, is expressed

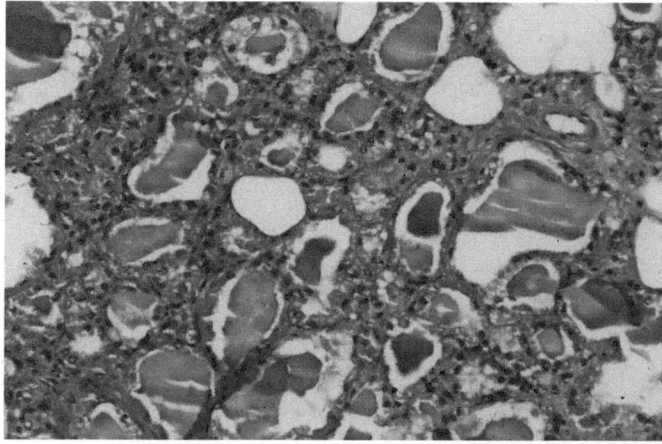

Figure 13-29. Secretory carcinoma. Secretory material in the neoplastic lumens. Notice the uniformity of the nuclei.

Differential Diagnosis

LACTATING ADENOMA

- Typically presents during pregnancy or while lactating
- Sharply circumscribed mass
- Myoepithelial cell layer is present (SMA and S-100 protein positive)

SECRETORY CHANGES

- Lobulocentric hypersecretory changes
- Occur in nonparous breast
- Associated with hormonal and other drug intake

PEARLS

- *Good prognosis compared with other invasive carcinomas (age related), especially in patients younger than 20 years*
- *Axillary lymph node metastasis can rarely be seen; increased incidence of axillary node metastases in patients older than 20 years; distant metastases are extremely rare*
- *Radiation and chemotherapy are not usually part of treatment*

SELECTED REFERENCES

Diallo R, Schaefer K-L, Bankfalvi A, et al: Secretory carcinoma of the breast: a distinct variant of invasive ductal carcinoma assessed by comparative genomic hybridization and immunohistochemistry. Hum Pathol 34:1299-1305, 2003.

Laé M, Fréneaux P, Sastre-Garau X, et al: Secretory breast carcinomas with ETV6-NTRK3 fusion gene belong to the basal-like carcinoma spectrum. Mod Pathol 22:291-298, 2009.

Li D, Xiao X, Yang W, et al: Secretory breast carcinoma: a clinicopathological and immunophenotypic study of 15 cases with a review of the literature. Mod Pathol 25:567-575, 2012.

Osako T, Takeuchi K, Horii R, et al: Secretory carcinoma of the breast and its histopathological mimics: value of markers for differential diagnosis. Histopathology 63:509-519, 2013.

Tognon C, Knezevich SR, Huntsman D, et al: Expression of the ETV6-NTRK3 gene fusion as a primary event in human secretory breast carcinoma. Cancer Cell 2:367-376, 2002.

APOCRINE CARCINOMA

Clinical Features

- Uncommon breast tumor; incidence of pure apocrine carcinoma varies from less than 1% to 4%
- Presents as a firm, distinct breast mass (similar to other breast carcinomas)
- Age distribution similar to that of other breast carcinomas
- Mammographic findings similar to those of typical infiltrating ductal carcinoma

Gross Pathology

- Firm, tan-brown tumor with infiltrative or well-defined margins
- Focal cyst formation may be seen

Histopathology

- Tumor composed of nests or sheets of neoplastic apocrine cells showing large pleomorphic nuclei with prominent and often multiple nucleoli (Figure 13-30A)
- Cells show abundant eosinophilic cytoplasm; may be granular and vacuolated (Figure 13-30B)
- Gland formation often with apocrine snouts may be seen
- Intraductal apocrine carcinoma may have solid, cribriform, micropapillary, or comedo architecture
- Apocrine carcinoma must be composed almost completely of apocrine cells

Special Stains and Immunohistochemistry

- Diastase-resistant PAS: cytoplasmic granules positive
- CEA positive in most cases
- Cytokeratin and GCDFP-15 positive
- Androgen receptor (AR) positive in many cases
- ER and PR show variable positivity
- S-100 protein negative

Other Techniques for Diagnosis

- Molecular studies suggest that apocrine carcinomas are characterized by overexpression of the AR and metabolism-related genes

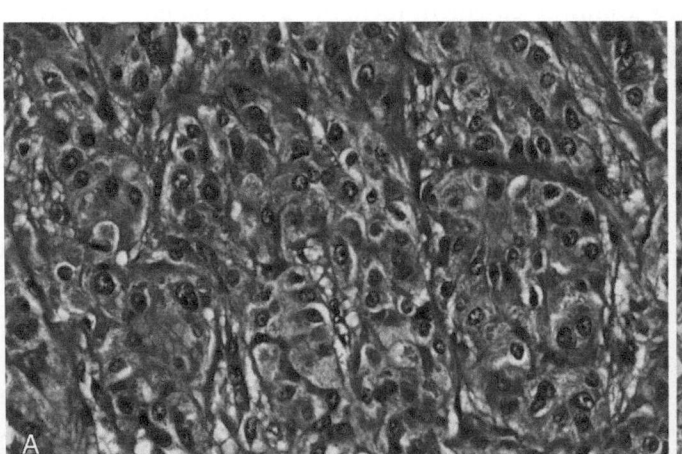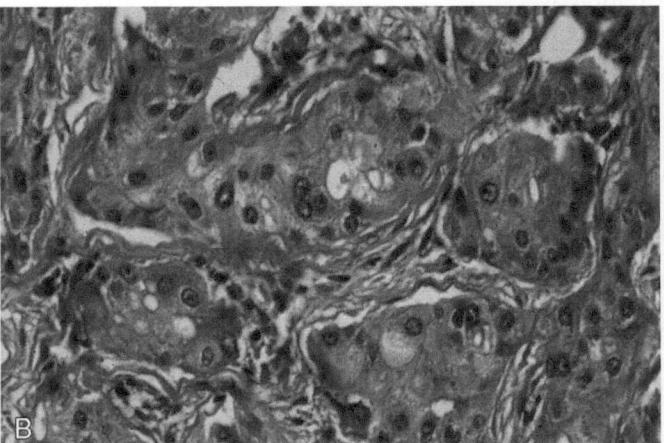

Figure 13-30. Infiltrating apocrine carcinoma. A, Classic histologic features include a large amount of pink granular cytoplasm and prominent nucleoli. **B,** Notice the pink granular cytoplasm and the prominent nucleoli.

- Electron microscopy: apocrine cells contain numerous mitochondria, empty vesicles, and osmiophilic membrane-bound secretory granules

Differential Diagnosis

SCLEROSING ADENOSIS WITH APOCRINE METAPLASIA

- Typically has lobular arrangement without infiltrative pattern
- Benign-appearing apocrine cells without pleomorphic nuclei and prominent nucleoli

PEARLS

- *Apocrine metaplasia is a common finding and is associated with benign proliferative conditions (fibrocystic changes)*
- *Malignant tumors with focal apocrine differentiation should not be called apocrine carcinoma; must be nearly completely composed of apocrine cells*
- *Apocrine differentiation within invasive or in situ tumors plays little role in determining prognosis or treatment*
- *Similar natural history to that of nonapocrine-infiltrating ductal carcinoma*

SELECTED REFERENCES

Dellapasqua S, Maisonneuve P, Viale G, et al: Immunohistochemically defined subtypes and outcome of apocrine breast cancer. Clin Breast Cancer 1:95-102, 2013.

Farmer P, Bonnefoi H, Becette V, et al: Identification of molecular apocrine breast tumours by microarray analysis. Oncogene 24:4660-4671, 2005.

Honma, N, Takubo K, Akiyama F: Expression of GCDFP-15 and AR decreases in larger or node-positive apocrine carcinomas of the breast. Histopathology 47:195-201, 2005.

Japaze H, Emina J, Diaz C: "Pure" invasive apocrine carcinoma of the breast: a new clinicopathologic entity? Breast 14:3-10, 2005.

Tavassoli FA, Norris HJ: Intraductal apocrine carcinoma: a clinicopathologic study of 37 cases. Mod Pathol 7:813-818, 1994.

Vranic S, Schmitt F, Sapino A, et al: Apocrine carcinoma of the breast: a comprehensive review. Histol Histopathol 28:1393-1409, 2013.

ADENOID CYSTIC CARCINOMA

Clinical Features

- Rare lesion accounting for less than 0.5% of all breast carcinomas
- Found in the same age distribution as other mammary carcinomas
- Presents as a palpable breast mass, typically periareolar or subareolar
- Patients may have nipple discharge
- Mammographic findings are often nonspecific

Gross Pathology

- Variable size (0.7 to 12 cm); most measure less than 3 cm
- Firm, well-circumscribed, pale, tan-gray tumor
- Nodular architecture is common
- Small cyst formation occasionally seen

Histopathology

- Tumor composed of epithelial and myoepithelial cells

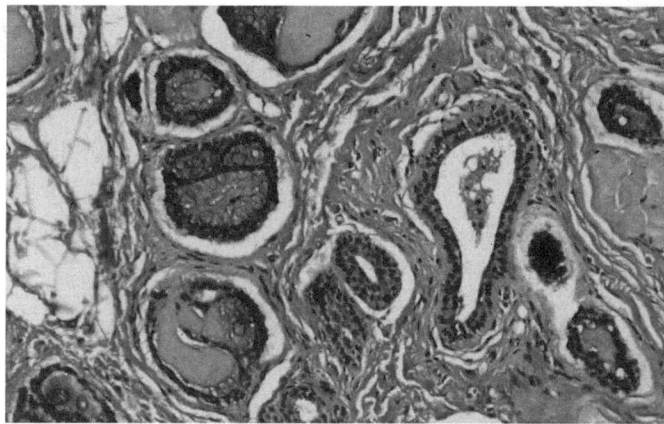

Figure 13-31. Adenoid cystic carcinoma. Classic cribriform pattern of adenoid cystic carcinoma. Notice the eosinophilic basement membrane-like material.

- Invasive tumor forming distinct islands and cords of neoplastic cells
- Characteristically shows proliferating glands (adenoid component) and abundant eosinophilic basement membrane–like material or hyaline globules (Figure 13-31)
- Solid, cribriform, tubular, or trabecular architecture may be seen
- Tumor composed of two distinct cell types: basal cell population (believed to be related to myoepithelial cells) and cells with bright eosinophilic cytoplasm
- Areas of squamous differentiation and sebaceous features may be seen
- Divided into grades I, II, and III
  - Grade I: composed of glandular and cystic areas; no solid zones
  - Grade II: solid areas make up less than 30% of the tumor
  - Grade III: solid areas make up more than 30% of the tumor

Special Stains and Immunohistochemistry

- S-100 protein, cytokeratin 14, calponin, p63: basaloid cells positive
- SMA: basaloid cells positive
- Cytokeratin 7: highlight eosinophilic cell population
- Laminin: basement membrane–like material positive
- ER and PR typically negative

Other Techniques for Diagnosis

- Electron microscopy
  - Basaloid cells show few organelles with cytoplasmic projections and well-developed desmosomes
  - Eosinophilic cells are spindled or cuboid with microvilli at the luminal border and abundant tonofilaments

Differential Diagnosis

INVASIVE CRIBRIFORM CARCINOMA

- Rare breast tumor, composed entirely of cribriform pattern
- Lacks dual cell population
- Lacks eosinophilic basement membrane–like material
- Negative for S-100 protein and SMA

CYLINDROMA
- Benign skin tumor overlying the breast

PEARLS

- *Much less aggressive than other mammary carcinomas*
- *Salivary gland adenoid cystic is much more aggressive than its breast counterpart*
- *No evidence of perineural invasion*
- *Rarely metastasizes to axillary lymph nodes*
- *May occasionally recur or metastasize (usually to lungs) many years after treatment*
- *Alterations of chromosome 6q present (similar to related salivary gland tumors)*

SELECTED REFERENCES

Bhosale SJ, Kshirsagar AY, Patil RK, et al: Adenoid cystic carcinoma of female breast: a case report. Int J Surg Case Rep 4:480-482, 2013.

Fargahi S, Gu M: Adenoid cystic carcinoma of the breast diagnosed by fine needle aspiration. Cytopathology 23:205-207, 2012.

Page DL: Adenoid cystic carcinoma of breast, a special histopathologic type with excellent prognosis. Breast Cancer Res Treat 93:189-190, 2005.

Pia-Foschini M, Reis-Filho JS, Eusebi V, Lakhani SR: Salivary glandlike tumours of the breast: surgical and molecular pathology. J Clin Pathol 56:497-506, 2003.

Vranic S, Bender R, Palazzo J, Gatalica Z: A review of adenoid cystic carcinoma of the breast with emphasis on its molecular and genetic characteristics. Hum Pathol 44:301-309, 2013.

Wetterskog D, Lopez-Garcia MA, Lambros MB, et al: Adenoid cystic carcinomas constitute a genomically distinct subgroup of triple-negative and basal-like breast cancers. J Pathol 226:84-96, 2012.

INFLAMMATORY CARCINOMA

Clinical Features

- Represents about 1% to 8% of all breast cancers and is the most aggressive form
- Typically presents as swelling and diffuse induration of the mammary skin along with rapid enlargement of the breast
- Often associated with skin retraction and dimpling (peau d'orange)
- Palpable mass often not present
- May present with enlarged axillary lymph nodes

Gross Pathology

- Mammary skin is erythematous and thickened
- Must be associated with an invasive mammary carcinoma

Histopathology

- Usually associated with an infiltrating ductal carcinoma (typically high grade or poorly differentiated)
- Must have tumor present in dilated dermal lymphatic channels (Figure 13-32)
- Lymphoplasmacytic infiltrate seen around involved lymphatic spaces
- Tumor emboli usually seen throughout breast tissue

Special Stains and Immunohistochemistry

- ER and PR usually negative
- Usually positive for p53

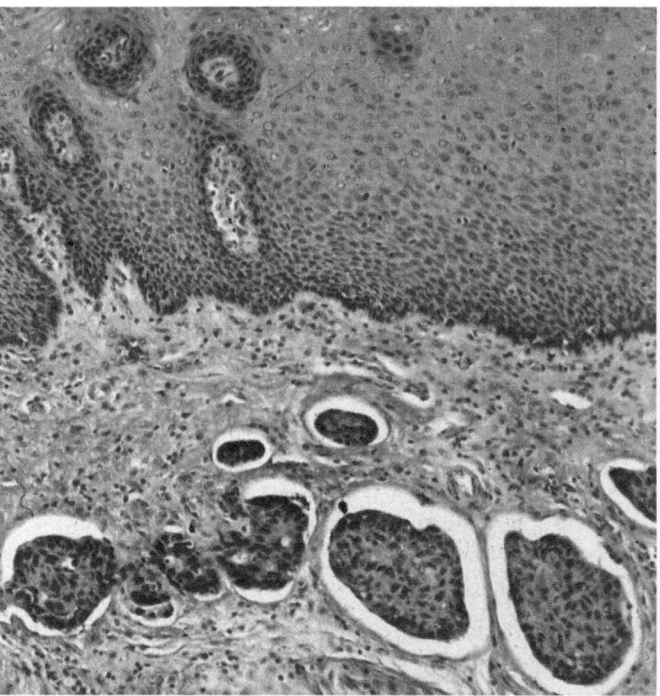

Figure 13-32. Inflammatory carcinoma. Dermal and lymphatic spread of tumor cells, which is characteristic of inflammatory carcinoma.

- C-erb-B2 (HER-2-neu) usually positive
- E-cadherin usually positive

Other Techniques for Diagnosis

- Noncontributory

Differential Diagnosis

METASTATIC CARCINOMA
- Lacks underlying invasive mammary carcinoma, which is needed for diagnosis of inflammatory carcinoma

PEARLS

- *Must have an invasive breast cancer and tumor in dermal lymphatics to make the diagnosis*
- *Associated with amplified expression of C-erb-B2 (HER-2-neu) proto-oncogene*
- *Treatment combination of neoadjuvant chemotherapy, mastectomy, and radiotherapy results in local control in about 80% of patients; axillary dissection is not typically performed; recurrence is seen in about 20% of patients*
- *Poor prognosis; less than 40% 5-year survival rate*
- *Overexpression of RhoC oncoprotein and loss of the LIBC/WISP3 gene has been associated with inflammatory breast cancer, highly invasive phenotype*

SELECTED REFERENCES

Crane K: Elucidating an uncommon disease: inflammatory breast cancer. J Natl Cancer Inst 103:1358-1360, 2011.

Dawood S, Merajver SD, Viens P, et al: International expert panel on inflammatory breast cancer: consensus statement for standardized diagnosis and treatment. Ann Oncol 22:515-523, 2011.

Wu M, Merajver SD: Molecular biology of inflammatory breast cancer: applications to diagnosis, prognosis, and therapy. Breast Dis 22:25-34, 2005/2006.

Robertson FM, Bondy M, Yang W, et al: Inflammatory breast cancer: the disease, the biology, the treatment. CA Cancer J Clin 60:351-375, 2010.

Schairer C, Li Y, Frawley P, Graubard BI, et al: Risk factors for inflammatory breast cancer and other invasive breast cancers. J Natl Cancer Inst 105:1373-1384, 2013.

PAGET DISEASE OF THE NIPPLE

Clinical Features

- More frequent in postmenopausal women (sixth decade); can affect males
- Usually unilateral lesion with nipple pain or irritation
- Nipple erythema, ulceration, or discharge may be present
- About 50% of patients have a palpable, hard, underlying breast mass
- May have no clinical abnormality; found on routine histologic section of nipple
- Overall found in 1% to 4% of women with breast carcinoma

Gross Pathology

- Dilated ducts in subareolar breast tissue may be seen
- Many patients have an obvious invasive mammary carcinoma
- Rarely, no carcinoma is found in mastectomy specimen

Histopathology

- Characteristic finding is Paget cell in the epidermis of the nipple
- Paget cells are large and round with large nuclei, prominent nucleoli, and abundant pale vacuolated cytoplasm (Figure 13-33)

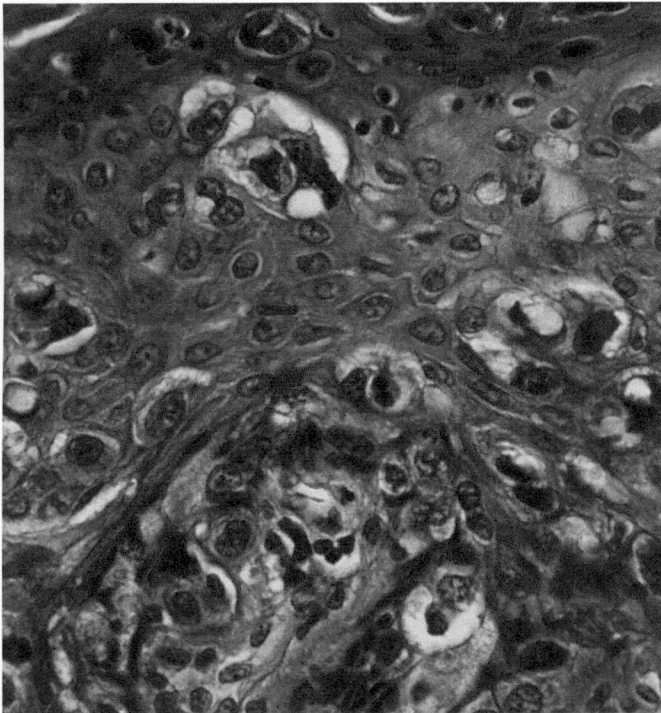

Figure 13-33. Paget disease. Classic histologic features of this entity, including large pleomorphic cells with vacuolated cytoplasm involving the epidermis.

- Cytoplasm may contain mucin (about 50% to 60% of cases) and occasionally melanin
- Paget cells may occur in small clusters, with occasional glandlike structures with a lumen, or singly within the epidermis
- Associated carcinoma is almost always seen with Paget disease
- Associated lesion is usually intraductal carcinoma (solid and comedo form), often with an infiltrating component
- Paget disease rarely occurs without associated mammary carcinoma (<5% of cases)

Special Stains and Immunohistochemistry

- Mucicarmine and PAS positive in about 50% to 60% of cases
- Cytokeratin 7, EMA, CEA, GCDFP-15 positive
- HMWCK negative
- HER-2-neu and p53 positive in more than 90% of cases
- AR positive, ER often positive
- S-100 protein typically negative

Other Techniques for Diagnosis

- Noncontributory

Differential Diagnosis

MALIGNANT MELANOMA

- Not associated with intraductal or invasive mammary carcinoma
- Immunohistochemical staining pattern is characteristic
  - Positive for S-100 and HMB-45
  - Typically negative for CEA, EMA, and C-erb-B2 (HER-2-neu)

BOWEN DISEASE (SQUAMOUS CELL CARCINOMA IN SITU)

- Not associated with intraductal or invasive mammary carcinoma

CLEAR CELL CHANGE OF KERATINOCYTES

- Large cells with small nuclei
- Vacuolated, empty cytoplasm; no cytoplasmic mucin

PEARLS

- *Immunohistochemical stains are helpful in confirming the diagnosis of Paget disease*
- *Typically results from superficial spread of underlying intraductal or invasive carcinoma*
- *Prognosis is based on extent of underlying carcinoma*
- *Treatment is usually mastectomy with lymph node excision regardless of whether obvious breast mass is identified*
- *Adjuvant chemotherapy (tamoxifen) may be an option for premenopausal women with positive nodes*

SELECTED REFERENCES

Bianco MK, Vasef MA: HER-2 gene amplification in Paget disease of the nipple and extramammary site: a chromogenic in situ hybridization study. Diagn Mol Pathol 15:131-135, 2006.

Chen CY, Sun LM, Anderson BO: Paget disease of the breast: changing patterns of incidence, clinical presentation, and treatment in the U.S. Cancer 107:1448-1458, 2006.

Hanna M, Jaffer S, Bleiweiss IJ, Nayak A: Minimally invasive mammary Paget's disease without an underlying breast carcinoma. Virchows Arch 463:471-473, 2013.

Sanders M, Lester S: Paget disease of the breast with invasion from nipple skin into the dermis. Arch Pathol Lab Med 137:307, 2013.

Sandoval-Leon AC, Drews-Elger K, Gomez-Fernandez CR, et al: Paget's disease of the nipple. Breast Cancer Res Treat 141:1-12, 2013.

Yim JH, Wick MR, Philpott GW, et al: Underlying pathology in mammary Paget's disease. Ann Surg Oncol 4:287-292, 1997.

HEMANGIOMA

Clinical Features

- Often presents as a palpable breast lesion or as a suspicious lesion on mammogram
- May be an incidental finding in mastectomy performed for carcinoma

Gross Pathology

- Typically less than 2 cm
- Firm, well-defined hemorrhagic mass within breast parenchyma

Histopathology

- Typically found in perilobular region
- Tumor composed of dilated, congested vascular channels
- Vascular spaces lined by benign-appearing endothelial cells (Figure 13-34)
- Vessels surrounded by fibrous stroma
- Cavernous hemangiomas are the most common form
- No evidence of mitosis or necrosis

Special Stains and Immunohistochemistry

- CD31, factor VIII, CD34: endothelial cells positive
- Mib-1 shows low values

Other Techniques for Diagnosis

- Noncontributory

Differential Diagnosis

LOW-GRADE ANGIOSARCOMA

- Typically several centimeters larger than hemangiomas
- Poorly defined with infiltrative margins
- Composed of complex anastomosing vascular spaces

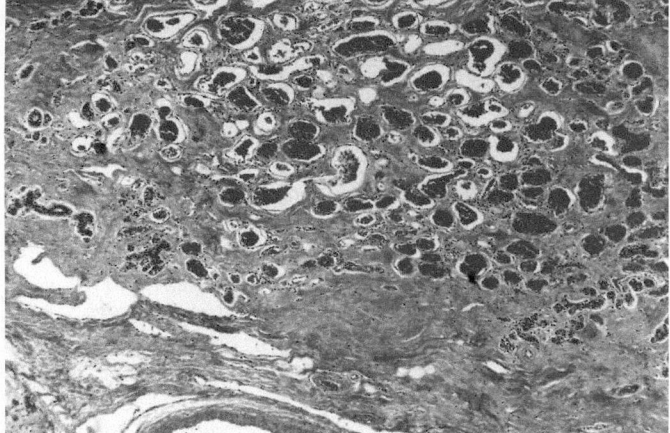

Figure 13-34. Hemangioma. The neoplasm is composed of well-spaced vascular channels lined by flat endothelial cells.

- Endothelial cells show atypical features with hyperchromatic nuclei; occasional mitotic activity may be seen
- Often shows thrombi, necrosis, and hemorrhage

PSEUDOANGIOMATOUS STROMAL HYPERPLASIA (PASH)

- Composed of anastomosing, empty, slitlike spaces, lined by myofibroblasts with endothelial-like nuclei
- Lining cells (myofibroblasts) are variably reactive for CD34 and SMA, negative for factor VIII, and rarely positive for CD31

PEARLS

- *Complete excision is recommended to render an accurate diagnosis*
- *No recurrences or malignant transformations have been documented*
- *Infantile hemangiomas have been associated with decreased Hox-A5 gene expression and immunopositivity for GLUT1*
- *Immunohistochemistry for Ki-67 may assist in the differentiation between hemangioma and low-grade angiosarcoma*

SELECTED REFERENCES

Brodie C, Provenzano E: Vascular proliferations of the breast. Histopathology 52:30-44, 2008.

Hoda SA, Cranor ML, Rosen PP: Hemangiomas of the breast with atypical histological features: further analysis of histological subtypes confirming their benign character. Am J Surg Pathol 16:553-560, 1992.

Tilve A, Mallo R, Pérez A, Santiago P: Breast hemangiomas: correlation between imaging and pathologic findings. J Clin Ultrasound 40:512-517, 2012.

ANGIOSARCOMA

Clinical Features

- Overall rare breast tumor
- May be found in women of all ages; mean age, between 30 and 40 years
- Presents as a rapidly growing typically painless mass; often causes red-blue discoloration of the overlying skin
- More commonly found in irradiated breasts
- Cases of primary angiosarcoma arising in pregnant women are well documented

Gross Pathology

- Variably sized mass ranging from 1 to 20 cm, average size of 4 to 5.5 cm
- Typically have infiltrative margins
- Cut surface shows an ill-defined, friable, spongy, and hemorrhagic mass (Figure 13-35A)
- Cystic degeneration and necrosis often seen in higher-grade lesions

Histopathology

- Divided into three grades depending on histologic findings (low grade, intermediate grade, and high grade)
  - Low grade (grade I)
    - Tumor consists of open, irregular vascular channels (Figure 13-35B)
    - Tumor characteristically infiltrates into adjacent breast lobules

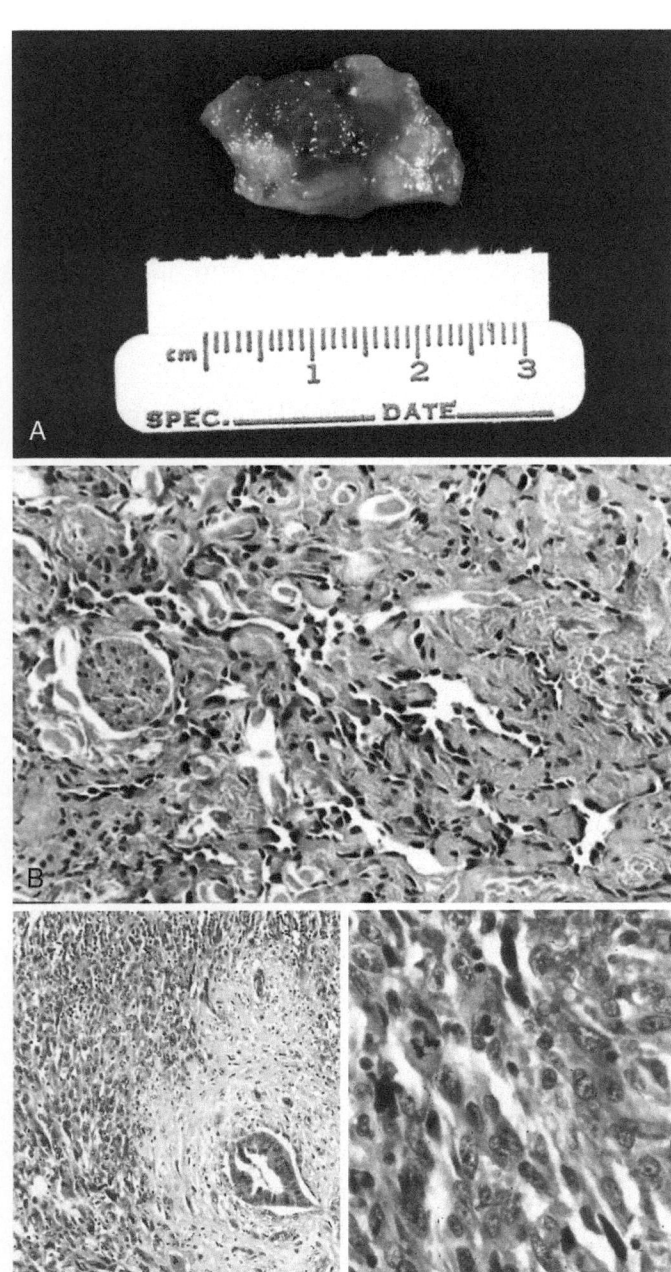

Figure 13-35. Angiosarcoma. A, Grossly, angiosarcomas are friable, spongy hemorrhagic masses. **B,** Under light microscopy, they can be low grade with minimal atypia. **C,** Section shows frankly malignant spindle cell neoplasm with marked cytologic pleomorphism. **D,** Frequent mitotic figures including atypical ones can be seen.

- Hyperchromatic nuclei may be seen, but nuclei lack significant pleomorphism
- Mitotic activity is rare to absent
- Endothelial tufting is minimal
- Papillary formations, solid and spindle cell areas, blood lakes, and necrosis are absent
- May appear deceptively benign
- Intermediate grade (grade II)
  - Shows irregular vascular channels with focal areas of increased cellularity due to endothelial tufting

and papillary fronds that project into the vascular lumens
- Degree of cellularity is used to distinguish low-grade from intermediate-grade tumors
- Tumor cells are hyperchromatic and show a moderate degree of pleomorphism
- Show infiltration into adjacent breast lobules
- Mitotic activity and solid and spindle cell areas are infrequent
- Blood lakes and necrosis are absent
- High grade (grade III)
  - Highly cellular lesion with endothelial tufting and increased degree of papillary formation
  - Tumor cells show marked pleomorphism (Figure 13-35C)
  - High mitotic rate often with atypical mitotic figures (Figure 13-35D)
  - Typically extensive hemorrhage with blood lake formation
  - Necrosis is typically present
  - Solid or spindle cell areas resembling fibrosarcoma or malignant fibrous histiocytoma may be seen

Special Stains and Immunohistochemistry

- Factor VIII, CD31, and CD34: endothelial cells positive (> 90% of cases)
- Cytokeratin negative in most cases, but epithelioid areas may be positive in up to 35% of cases

Other Techniques for Diagnosis

- Electron microscopy: features associated with endothelial cells are seen, including Weibel-Palade bodies, intermediate filaments, and pinocytotic vesicles

Differential Diagnosis

HEMANGIOMA
- Typically smaller and better defined than angiosarcoma
- Lacks malignant cytologic features
- Does not infiltrate breast lobules
- Usually located in perilobular region

PASH
- Well-circumscribed lesions with a tan-white, homogeneous cut surface
- Composed of anastomosing, slitlike spaces in a dense collagenous stroma
- Lining cells are negative for CD31 and factor VIII

PEARLS

- *Correlation between patient age and clinical outcome is significant; high-grade lesions are more common in younger patients and have a worse prognosis*
- *Tumor grade is the most important prognostic factor*
- *High-grade (grade III) lesions have a poor prognosis*
- *Low- and intermediate-grade tumors (grades I and II) have increased disease-free and overall survival rates*
- *Treatment includes total mastectomy; axillary dissection is not indicated because these tumors rarely metastasize to axillary lymph nodes*
- *The role of adjuvant chemotherapy remains unclear, but chemotherapy for patients with high-grade lesions should be considered*

SELECTED REFERENCES

Billings SD, McKenney JK, Folpe AL, et al: Cutaneous angiosarcoma following breast-conserving surgery and radiation: an analysis of 27 cases. Am J Clin Pathol 28:781-788, 2004.

Colwick S, Gonzalez A, Ngo N, et al: Bilateral radiation-induced angiosarcoma of the breast. Breast J 19:547-549, 2013.

Hui A, Henderson M, Speakman D, Skandarajah A: Angiosarcoma of the breast: a difficult surgical challenge. Breast 21:584-589, 2012.

Mentzel T, Schildhaus HU, Palmedo G, et al: Postradiation cutaneous angiosarcoma after treatment of breast carcinoma is characterized by MYC amplification in contrast to atypical vascular lesions after radiotherapy and control cases: clinicopathological, immunohistochemical and molecular analysis of 66 cases. Mod Pathol 25: 75-85, 2012.

POSTMASTECTOMY ANGIOSARCOMA (STEWART-TREVES SYNDROME)

Clinical Features

- Arises in a lymphedematous upper extremity after mastectomy, with or without radiotherapy; in irradiated patients, it arises outside of the treated field
- Associated with chronic lymphedema, but pathogenesis is unknown
- Occurs in less than 0.45% of postmastectomy patients
- Typically presents about 10 years after mastectomy
- Presents as subtle, blue-purple discoloration of skin and can progress into large nodules and superficial vesicles that contain hemorrhagic fluid

Gross Pathology

- Early lesions appear as hemorrhagic foci on the skin surface and are confined to the superficial soft tissue (Figure 13-36A)
- Advanced disease presents as multiple hemorrhagic tumor nodules involving deeper soft tissue and muscle

Histopathology

- Proliferation of irregular, variably sized interconnecting vascular spaces lined by large endothelial cells with hyperchromatic, atypical nuclei (Figure 13-36B)
- Highly atypical endothelial cells with large pleomorphic nuclei showing prominent nucleoli and numerous mitotic figures
- Papillary structures may be seen within neoplastic vessels
- Dense collagenous background

- Infiltrative borders with involvement of surrounding fibroadipose tissue
- Typically, changes of chronic lymphedema are seen, including hyperplasia of the epidermis, subcutaneous edema, fibrosis, mild chronic inflammation, and small-vessel proliferation with reactive endothelial cells

Special Stains and Immunohistochemistry

- CD34, CD31, and factor VIII: endothelial cells are positive
- Cytokeratin negative

Other Techniques for Diagnosis

- Electron microscopy: features associated with endothelial cells are seen, including Weibel-Palade bodies, intermediate filaments, and pinocytotic vesicles

Differential Diagnosis

POSTIRRADIATION ANGIOSARCOMA
- Develops in field of radiation, not in area of chronic lymphedema
- Typically develops within 5 years after irradiation

KAPOSI SARCOMA
- May be difficult to differentiate from early findings in angiosarcoma
- Typically lacks pleomorphism that is commonly seen in angiosarcoma
- Found in immunocompromised hosts

REACTIVE VASCULAR PROLIFERATION ASSOCIATED WITH CHRONIC LYMPHEDEMA
- Lacks pleomorphism and mitotic activity seen in angiosarcoma

PEARLS

- *First reported by Stewart-Treves in 1948*
- *Why angiosarcoma develops in a background of chronic lymphedema is unknown*
- *Special stains for vascular endothelium do not distinguish benign from malignant vascular tumors; need to distinguish these entities based on morphology*
- *Amputation and systemic chemotherapy is best treatment*
- *Most patients die from this disease within 2 years; few long-term survivors*

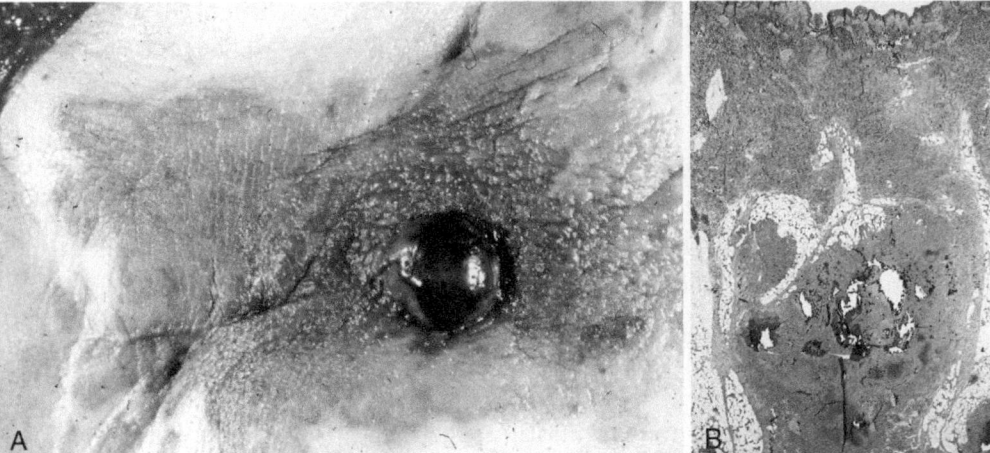

Figure 13-36. Postradiation angiosarcoma. A, Hemorrhagic focus on the skin surface is noted. **B,** Microscopically, there is a proliferation of vascular spaces lined by pleomorphic cells with frequent mitotic figures.

SELECTED REFERENCES

Clements WD, Kirk SJ, Spence RA: A rare late complication of breast cancer treatment. Br J Clin Pract 47:219-220, 1993.

Kindblom LG, Stenman G, Angervall L: Morphological and cytogenetic studies of angiosarcoma in Stewart-Treves syndrome. Virchows Arch 419:439-445, 1991.

Tomita K, Yokogawa A, Oda Y, Terahata S: Lymphangiosarcoma in postmastectomy lymphedema (Stewart-Treves syndrome): ultrastructural and immunohistologic characteristics. J Surg Oncol 38:275-282, 1988.

GYNECOMASTIA

Clinical Features

- Most common physiologic and pathologic change in male breast
- Typically presents as diffuse mammary enlargement, with pain and tenderness
- Both breasts are commonly affected (clinically bilateral in about half of patients)
- Associated with many medical conditions, including cirrhosis, renal failure, chronic pulmonary disease, Klinefelter disease, and various tumors, including Leydig cell, Sertoli cell, and human chorionic gonadotropin–secreting tumors (gonadal and extragonadal germ cell tumors, large cell lung carcinoma, and some gastric and kidney cancers)
- Pathogenesis has been linked to an imbalance between free estrogen and free androgen actions in breast tissues, which can result from multiple mechanisms
- Several drugs can be associated with development of gynecomastia, including herbal products, protease inhibitors, cimetidine, spironolactone, digitalis, alcohol, heroin, anabolic steroids, and alkylating agents

Gross Pathology

- Appears as a firm and rubbery gray-white mass or as ill-defined fibrotic tissue around the nipple-areolar complex

Histopathology (Figure 13-37)

- Ducts show epithelial and myoepithelial cells with varying degrees of hyperplasia that is irregularly distributed
- Lobule formation is usually not seen
- Micropapillary or cribriform pattern is typical
- Increased amount and cellularity of stroma with prominent vessels, edema, and mononuclear infiltrate in initial phase; stromal fibrosis follows
- Epithelial cells may show some atypia with hyperchromatic nuclei
- PASH may develop

Special Stains and Immunohistochemistry

- Noncontributory

Other Techniques for Diagnosis

- Electron microscopy: demonstrates proliferating epithelial and myoepithelial cells

Differential Diagnosis

INTRADUCTAL CARCINOMA

- Epithelial proliferation is more regular and organized
- May show intraductal necrosis

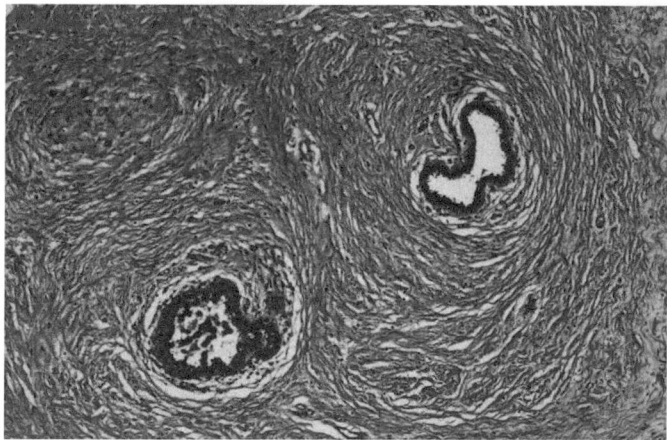

Figure 13-37. Gynecomastia. Proliferation of loose connective tissue around ductal structures.

PEARLS

- *No increased risk for carcinoma is associated with this lesion*
- *Regression occurs with treatment of underlying condition*
- *Tamoxifen use during acute stages has been shown to result in partial or complete regression of gynecomastia*
- *Surgical therapy might be indicated in cases that fail to respond to medical therapy*

SELECTED REFERENCES

Braustein GD: Gynecomastia. N Engl J Med 357:1229-1237, 2007.

Cakan N, Kamat D: Gynecomastia: evaluation and treatment recommendations for primary care providers. Clin Pediatr (Phila) 46:487-490, 2007.

Janes SE, Lengyel JA, Singh S, et al: Needle core biopsy for the assessment of unilateral breast masses in men. Breast 15:273-275, 2006.

Milanezi MF, Saggioro FP, Zanati SG, et al: Pseudoangiomatous hyperplasia of mammary stroma associated with gynecomastia. J Clin Pathol 51:204-206, 1998.

Volpe CM, Raffetto JD, Collure DW, et al: Unilateral male breast masses: cancer risk and their evaluation and management. Am Surg 65:250-253, 1999.

MALE BREAST CARCINOMA

Clinical Features

- About 1000 new cases each year, with about 300 deaths
- Represents less than 1% of all mammary carcinomas
- Risk factors include mutations in high-penetrance genes (more common in *BRCA2* than in *BRCA1* families), Klinefelter syndrome, hyperthyroidism, obesity, liver or testicular damage, and radiation or trauma to chest wall
- Wide age distribution (peak age frequency at 71 years)
- Presents as painless, well-defined, distinct breast mass
- Occasionally patients present with bloody nipple discharge, retraction, or ulceration

Gross Pathology

- Similar features to those seen in female breasts
- Tumors are typically less than 3 cm at time of diagnosis

Histopathology

- Most male breast carcinoma is infiltrating ductal carcinoma
- Typically shows infiltrating tumor with variable degree of gland formation (Figure 13-38)
- Neoplastic cells are pleomorphic and have nuclei showing vesicular, coarse chromatin and distinct nucleoli
- Angiolymphatic or perineural invasion is often present
- Rarely associated DCIS (most are papillary type, of low to intermediate grade)
- Tumor grading is based on same architectural and cytologic features as infiltrating ductal carcinoma in female breasts
- All carcinoma variants identified in female breasts can be seen in male breasts; lobular neoplasia is exceedingly rare in males

Special Stains and Immunohistochemistry

- ER and PR: variable reactivity, usually positive
- AR: variably positive
- HER-2-neu: more frequently positive in high-grade lesions; overall, 2+ or 3+ positivity in 25% to 30% of cases

Other Techniques for Diagnosis

- Noncontributory

Differential Diagnosis

METASTATIC PROSTATE CARCINOMA

- Immunostain for prostate-specific antigen (PSA) is positive
- Presence of bilateral or multifocal disease suggests metastasis

PEARLS

- *No increased risk for carcinoma following diagnosis of gynecomastia*
- *About 50% of cases have axillary node metastases at time of presentation*
- *BRCA2 gene (not BRCA1 gene) is strongly associated with male breast carcinoma*
- *Common sites of metastasis include lung, bone, and central nervous system*

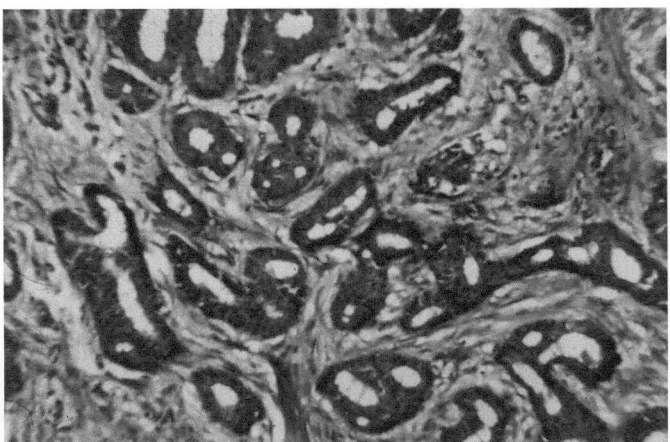

Figure 13-38. Infiltrating ductal carcinoma, grade I (male breast). Tubular structures surrounded by desmoplastic stroma.

- *Initial treatment involves limited surgical excision and chest wall irradiation*
- *Overall 5-year survival rate estimates are about 40% to 65%; prognosis in age-matched, stage-matched breast cancer is the same for men and women*
- *Studies reveal benefits for the use of adjuvant hormonal therapy and chemotherapy for men in intermediate or high-risk categories (as determined by tumor grade, axillary nodal status, and tumor markers)*

SELECTED REFERENCES

Fentiman IS, Fourquet A, Hortobagyi GN: Male breast cancer. Lancet 367:595-604, 2006.
Goss PE, Reid C, Pintilie M, et al: Male breast carcinoma. A review of 229 patients who presented to the Princess Margaret Hospital during 40 years: 1955-1996. Cancer 85:629-639, 1999.
Nahleh Z, Girnius S: Male breast cancer: a gender issue. Natl Clin Pract Oncol 3:428-437, 2006.

METASTATIC TUMORS

Clinical Features

- Metastases to the breast are uncommon in both sexes but are much more common in women
- Most common metastatic carcinoma of the female breast is metastatic tumor from the opposite breast
- Other common metastatic tumors to the breast are malignant melanoma; carcinomas of the lung, ovary, stomach, cervix, kidney, and prostate; and carcinoid tumors
- Most common metastatic tumor of the male breast is metastatic prostate carcinoma
- Secondary lymphomas of the breast are rare; however, they are much more common than primary breast lymphomas, which comprise 0.38% to 0.7% of all non-Hodgkin lymphomas
- Presentation may be similar to primary breast carcinoma with a rapidly growing, painless, firm, palpable mass usually lacking nipple discharge or skin changes
- Bilateral tumors may be the initial clinical manifestation

Gross Pathology

- Well-defined tumors without calcification and spiculation

Histopathology

- Sharply demarcated from adjacent breast tissue
- Infiltrating tumor with the presence of adjacent intraductal carcinoma or LCIS is convincing evidence of a primary breast tumor
- Elastosis is common in primary breast cancer but rare in metastatic tumors
- Calcification is common in primary breast cancer but rare in metastatic tumors, except for metastatic serous papillary carcinoma of the ovary or peritoneum
- Cytoplasmic pigment, intranuclear inclusions, and spindle cells are useful clues to a diagnosis of metastatic melanoma (Figure 13-39A)
- Signet ring, mucin-secreting cells suggest gastric origin
- Clear cell changes and prominent delicate vascularization suggest kidney origin (see Figure 13-39B)

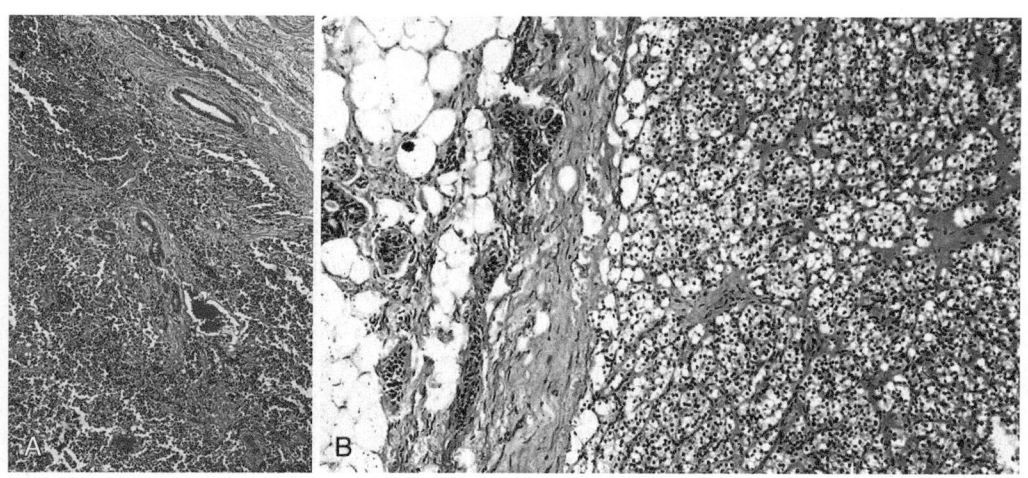

Figure 13-39. Metastasis to the breast. Common metastatic tumors to the breast include melanoma **(A)** and renal cell carcinoma **(B)**.

Special Stains and Immunohistochemistry

- Immunohistochemistry profile should be used in conjunction with clinical history and hematoxylin and eosin stain morphology
- Positivity for S-100 protein, HMB-45, melan-A, microphthalmia transcription factor, and tyrosinase; negativity for EMA and cytokeratin supports a diagnosis of malignant melanoma; melanomas can show aberrant expression of cytokeratins and EMA; breast carcinomas can express S-100
- Expression of WT-1, CA-125, and mesothelin, along with negativity for GCDFP-15, favors a diagnosis of metastatic ovarian carcinoma over primary breast cancer
- Expression of thyroid transcription factor-1, along with negativity for GCDFP-15 and ER, favors a diagnosis of metastatic lung cancer
- PSA and prostatic acid phosphatase are excellent markers of prostatic carcinomas; ER, GCDFP-15, and cytokeratin 7 expression are uncommon in prostate carcinoma
- CDX2 and cytokeratin 20 expressions favor a diagnosis of metastatic gastric cancer over breast cancer primary

Other Techniques for Diagnosis

- Noncontributory

Differential Diagnosis

- Clinical history is important

GASTRIC SIGNET RING CELL CARCINOMA

- May mimic primary signet ring cell carcinoma of breast
- Well-defined mass without infiltrating margins
- No in situ component

OVARIAN CARCINOMA

- Serous papillary carcinoma is the most common type
- Lacks infiltrating margins
- No in situ component
- May grow within ducts and lobules, making distinction from a primary breast carcinoma difficult
- Papillary architecture is not typical for most invasive breast cancers, aside from invasive micropapillary carcinoma
- May be bilateral

PEARLS

- *Identification of metastasis to the breast is usually an indication of widespread disease, and survival is typically less than 2 years*
- *Identification of in situ carcinoma is helpful to diagnose a primary breast lesion*
- *Treatment typically consists of wide excision with radiotherapy; systemic treatment suitable for the primary lesion is most important*

SELECTED REFERENCES

Gaur S, Ayyappan AP, Nahleh Z: Breast metastases from an adrenocorticotropic hormone secreting thymic neuro-endocrine tumor. Breast Dis 34:81-86, 2013.

Jung SP, Lee Y, Han KM, et al: Breast metastasis from rhabdomyosarcoma of the anus in an adolescent female. J Breast Cancer 16:345-348, 2013.

Lee AH: The histological diagnosis of metastases to the breast from extramammary malignancies. J Clin Pathol 60:1333-1341, 2007.

Topalovski M, Domnita C, Mattson JC: Lymphoma of the breast: a clinicopathologic study of primary and secondary cases. Arch Pathol Lab Med 123:1208-1218, 1999.

Yamasaki H, Saw D, Zdanowitz J, et al: Ovarian carcinoma metastasis to the breast: case report and review of the literature. Am J Surg Pathol 17:193-197, 1993.

Chapter 14
Lymph Nodes

ATTILIO ORAZI • JULIA TURBINER GEYER

CHAPTER OUTLINE

NORMAL LYMPH NODE

Histopathology

- A lymph node contains a cortex, a paracortex, a medulla, sinuses, a hilum, and a fibrous capsule
- The cortex is a B-cell area, which contains primary (nonstimulated) lymphoid follicles composed of small mature lymphocytes and secondary (activated) follicles with germinal centers composed of a mixture of small cleaved lymphocytes (centrocytes) and large noncleaved lymphoid cells (centroblasts), as well as numerous tingible-body macrophages
- The paracortex is a T-cell area with a mixture of lymphocytes, antigen-presenting cells, and immunoblasts
- The medulla contains predominantly plasma cells, admixed with small lymphocytes and immunoblasts
- Sinuses contain histiocytes admixed with small lymphocytes

Special Stains and Immunohistochemistry

- B lymphocytes express CD20, Pax-5, and CD79a; whereas T lymphocytes are positive for CD3, CD2, CD5, and CD7
- B lymphocytes of the primary follicles and mantle zones are naïve and memory cells which express Bcl-2 and are negative for CD10 and Bcl-6
- B lymphocytes in the germinal centers express CD10 and Bcl-6 and are negative for Bcl-2
- Follicular dendritic cells form a scaffold of the lymphoid follicle and express CD21 and CD23
- T lymphocytes in the paracortex are predominantly CD4 positive with a smaller number of admixed CD8-positive cells
- The antigen-presenting interdigitating dendritic cells of the paracortex express S-100 protein; Langerhans cells are positive for S-100, CD1a, and Langerin

REACTIVE FOLLICULAR HYPERPLASIA

AUTOIMMUNE DISEASE

Clinical Features

- Autoimmune diseases are chronic systemic illnesses that are frequently characterized by lymphadenopathy
- They usually occur in middle-aged women
- Lymphadenopathy is a common finding, especially during periods of active disease

Histopathology (Figure 14-1)

- Florid reactive follicular hyperplasia with sinus histiocytosis and neutrophilia
- Marked plasmacytic proliferation in the paracortex and medulla
- Rheumatoid arthritis patients who were treated with gold can have scattered nonbirefringent crystal structures associated with foreign body giant cell reaction
- Sjögren syndrome patients may have aggregates of pale-staining monocytoid B cells

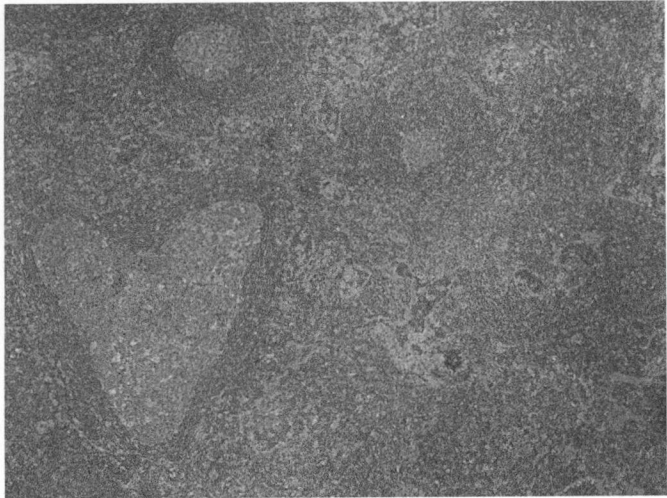

Figure 14-1. Autoimmune disease. Reactive follicular hyperplasia in a patient with Sjögren syndrome.

Special Stains and Immunohistochemistry

- B lymphocytes in the reactive germinal centers express CD10 and Bcl-6 and are negative for Bcl-2
- Proliferation rate with Ki67 immunostain is >90% in the reactive germinal centers and approximately 5% in the interfollicular areas
- Plasma cells are polytypic with staining for kappa and lambda immunoglobulin light chains

Other Techniques for Diagnosis

- Flow cytometry shows evidence of polytypic B cells and T cells that express all the pan-T-cell antigens
- Immunoglobulin heavy chain gene (IgH) rearrangement analysis is typically negative
- A subset of the patients with active autoimmune disease may have evidence of B-cell clonality by polymerase chain reaction (PCR), but this finding by itself does not indicate malignancy
- Cytogenetic analysis shows a normal karyotype

Differential Diagnosis

NONSPECIFIC FOLLICULAR HYPERPLASIA
- A patient without an established clinical diagnosis of autoimmune disease may show identical morphology and immunophenotype

SYPHILIS
- Usually presents with inguinal lymphadenopathy
- Prominent perilymphadenitis with thickening of the capsule, marked plasmacytic infiltration, and vasculitis
- Warthin-Starry stain demonstrates evidence of spirochetes in endothelial cells, within blood vessels, and occasionally in germinal centers

EARLY VIRAL INFECTION
- HIV: frequent follicle lysis
- Mononucleosis: expanded paracortex with numerous immunoblasts
- Cytomegalovirus: monocytoid B-cell hyperplasia and large intranuclear inclusions
- Clinical history and serology confirm the diagnosis

TOXOPLASMA LYMPHADENITIS
- Triad of follicular hyperplasia, monocytoid B-cell hyperplasia and aggregates of epithelioid histiocytes in the lymphoid follicles
- Clinical history and serology confirm the diagnosis

IgG4-RELATED LYMPHADENOPATHY
- Type II is characterized by follicular hyperplasia
- Intrafollicular and paracortical plasmacytosis and scattered eosinophils
- Immunohistochemical stains for IgG and IgG4 quantify the number of plasma cells
  - > 100 IgG4-positive plasma cells per high-power field
  - IgG4/IgG ratio > 40%

FOLLICULAR LYMPHOMA
- Usually in older patients with generalized lymphadenopathy
- Increased number of follicles, which appear monotonous in size and shape

- Neoplastic follicles present throughout the lymph node and may extend outside into the perinodal fat
- Lymph node capsule is thickened and frequently appears split due to the follicular proliferation
- Mantle zone is attenuated or absent
- The cellular composition within the follicles is monomorphic
- Tingible-body macrophages are rare to absent
- Lymphoid cells in the follicles coexpress Bcl-2
- Proliferation rate within the follicles with Ki67 immunostain is < 90% (usually around 10% to 50%)
- Flow cytometry: monotypic B lymphocytes
- PCR for IgH gene rearrangement is monoclonal
- Cytogenetic analysis and fluorescence in situ hybridization (FISH): evidence of t(14;18) translocation and other genetic abnormalities

MARGINAL ZONE LYMPHOMA

- Rare lymphoma that typically presents in middle-aged patients
- Patients may have a history of autoimmune disease, especially Sjögren syndrome and Hashimoto thyroiditis
- Typically, tumor cells are composed of monocytoid B cells, plasma cells, and immunoblasts that surround reactive follicles
- Follicular colonization may be present
- Tumor cells may aberrantly coexpress CD43 and Bcl-2
- Plasma cells frequently show evidence of clonality with immunostains for kappa and lambda light chains
- Flow cytometry: monotypic B lymphocytes
- PCR for IgH gene rearrangement is monoclonal
- Cytogenetic analysis: abnormal karyotype

PLASMA CELL NEOPLASM IN LYMPH NODE

- Very rare
- Suspect in patients with a clinical history of plasma cell myeloma
- Plasma cells always show evidence of clonality with immunostains for kappa and lambda light chains
- Flow cytometry: polyclonal B lymphocytes and monoclonal plasma cells
- PCR for IgH gene rearrangement is monoclonal
- Cytogenetic analysis may show an abnormal karyotype

PEARLS

- *Autoimmune disease is a risk factor for lymphoma, thus lymphoma has to be ruled out in all cases with immunohistochemistry, flow cytometry, and, if indicated, cytogenetics and PCR*
- *Rheumatoid arthritis usually manifests with axillary lymphadenopathy*
- *Correlation with clinical presentation is recommended to rule out infection*

SELECTED REFERENCES

Bagg A: Malleable immunoglobulin genes and hematopathology—the good, the bad, and the ugly: a paper from the 2007 William Beaumont Hospital Symposium on Molecular Pathology. J Mol Diagn 10:396-410, 2008.
Engels K, Oeschger S, Hansmann ML, et al: Bone marrow trephines containing lymphoid aggregates from patients with rheumatoid and other autoimmune disorders frequently show clonal B-cell infiltrates. Hum Pathol 38:1402-1411, 2007.

CYTOMEGALOVIRUS LYMPHADENITIS

Clinical Features

- Can be seen in immunocompetent and immunosuppressed individuals
- Only ~10% of acquired cytomegalovirus (CMV) infections produce symptoms
- The most common presentation in symptomatic patients is with infectious mononucleosis-like illness (fever, fatigue, atypical lymphocytosis)

Histopathology

- Early CMV is characterized by reactive follicular hyperplasia and monocytoid B-cell hyperplasia (Figure 14-2A)
- Subsequently there is predominantly paracortical hyperplasia with many immunoblasts and hypervascularity
- Immunocompromised patients may have necrosis
- Large intranuclear inclusions and cytomegaly are found most often within monocytoid B-cell areas (Figure 14-2B)

Special Stains and Immunohistochemistry

- CMV immunostain confirms the diagnosis
- Cells containing inclusions may express CD15

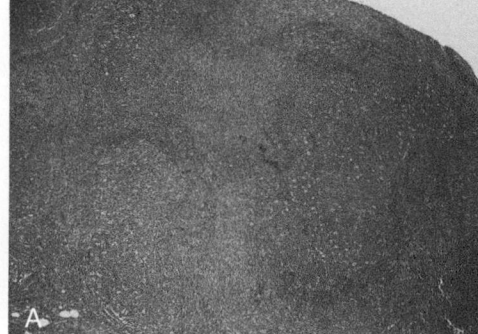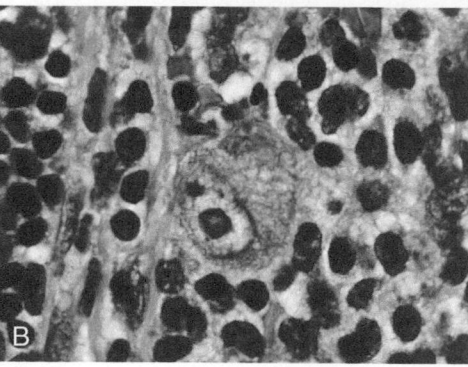

Figure 14-2. Cytomegalovirus lymphadenitis. **A,** Marked reactive follicular hyperplasia and monocytoid B-cell hyperplasia. **B,** Cytomegaly and large intranuclear viral inclusion.

Other Techniques for Diagnosis

- Viral culture
- CMV serology
- Molecular amplification

Differential Diagnosis

NONSPECIFIC FOLLICULAR HYPERPLASIA

- No staining with CMV antibody
- No clinical evidence of CMV infection

TOXOPLASMA LYMPHADENITIS

- Has numerous aggregates of epithelioid histiocytes in the lymphoid follicles in addition to follicular hyperplasia and monocytoid B-cell hyperplasia
- No staining with CMV antibody

CLASSICAL HODGKIN LYMPHOMA

- Cells with viral inclusions may resemble Reed-Sternberg cells and variants
- Reed-Sternberg cells express CD15 and CD30, whereas CMV-infected cells are CD30 negative
- No staining with CMV antibody

SMALL B-CELL LYMPHOMA

- Viral inclusions are not present
- No staining with CMV antibody
- Flow cytometry: monotypic B lymphocytes
- PCR for IgH gene rearrangement is monoclonal
- Cytogenetic analysis: abnormal karyotype

PEARLS

- *Only a few cells with viral inclusions may be found*
- *CMV immunostain is paramount in making the diagnosis*

SELECTED REFERENCES

Navalpotro D, Gimeno C, Navarro D: PCR detection of viral DNA in serum as an ancillary analysis for the diagnosis of acute mononucleosis-like syndrome due to human cytomegalovirus (HCMV) in immunocompetent patients. J Clin Virol 35:193, 2006.

Orasch C, Conen A: Severe primary cytomegalovirus infection in the immunocompetent adult patient: a case series. Scand J Infect Dis 44:987-991, 2012.

TOXOPLASMOSIS

Clinical Features

- Caused by the intracellular protozoan parasite, *Toxoplasma gondii*
- Immunocompetent persons with primary infection are usually asymptomatic
- There is a lifelong risk of reactivation should the individual become immunocompromised
- The most common clinical manifestation is bilateral, symmetrical, nontender cervical adenopathy

Histopathology (Figure 14-3A)

- Triad of reactive follicular hyperplasia, monocytoid B-cell hyperplasia, and aggregates of epithelioid histiocytes
- The histiocytes may be present as single cells or small clusters, typically encroaching on germinal centers
- The organism itself is identified in < 1% of cases
- No evidence of significant necrosis or granuloma formation

Special Stains and Immunohistochemistry

- Toxoplasma immunostain is usually negative due to absence of the parasites but occasionally may be useful (Figure 14-3B)

Other Techniques for Diagnosis

- Serology testing is the most common diagnostic tool
- Toxoplasma DNA identification by PCR in the tissue or blood has been reported

Differential Diagnosis

NONSPECIFIC FOLLICULAR HYPERPLASIA

- Does not have epithelioid histiocytes encroaching on germinal centers

HIV LYMPHADENITIS

- Does not have epithelioid histiocytes encroaching on germinal centers

LEISHMANIASIS

- Can have similar morphology
- Necrotizing or non-necrotizing granulomas with giant cells
- Intracellular organisms can be seen in the histiocytes with hematoxylin and eosin stain (H&E), Giemsa, and other special stains

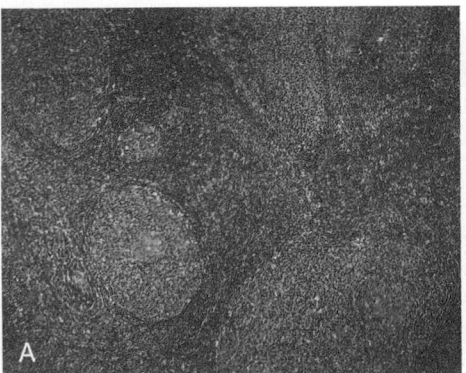 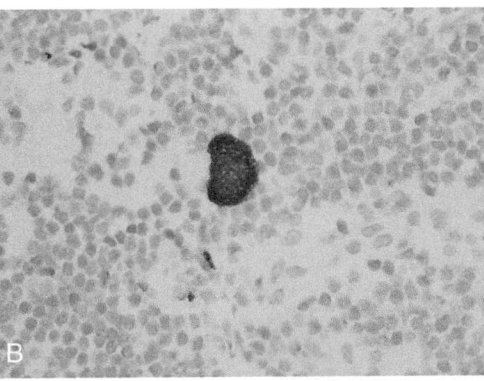

Figure 14-3. Toxoplasmosis. **A,** Reactive follicular hyperplasia, monocytoid B-cell hyperplasia and aggregates of epithelioid histiocytes inside and outside of the germinal centers. **B,** Immunohistochemical stain for Toxoplasma highlights a large tissue cyst and several adjacent small tachyzoites.

CAT SCRATCH DISEASE

- Does not have epithelioid histiocytes encroaching on germinal centers
- Typically has multifocal necrosis with clusters of neutrophils
- Intracellular organisms are detected by Warthin-Starry stain

SARCOIDOSIS

- Granulomas are larger, more numerous, and well-circumscribed
- Frequently the lymph node is partially or wholly replaced by granulomas
- No evidence of follicular hyperplasia or monocytoid B-cell hyperplasia

PEARLS

- *The classic triad is strongly associated with serologic confirmation of infection*
- *In AIDS patients, toxoplasmosis reactivates as toxoplasma encephalitis; lymph node involvement is rare*
- *When toxoplasma infection is acquired for the first time during pregnancy, infection can be transmitted to the fetus, resulting in severe damage*

SELECTED REFERENCES

Eapen M, Mathew CF, Aravindan KP: Evidence based criteria for the histopathological diagnosis of toxoplasma lymphadenopathy. J Clin Pathol 58:1143-1146, 2005.

Lin MH, Kuo TT: Specificity of the histopathological triad for the diagnosis of toxoplasmic lymphadenitis: polymerase chain reaction study. Pathol Int 51:619-623, 2001.

HIV-RELATED LYMPHADENOPATHY

Clinical Features

- Acute symptomatic HIV infection is characterized by fever, lymphadenopathy, sore throat, rash, myalgia/arthralgia, and headache
  - The axillary, cervical, and occipital nodes are primarily enlarged
  - Lymph nodes decrease in size following the acute presentation, but some degree of adenopathy tends to persist
- Persistent generalized lymphadenopathy is defined as lymphadenopathy of > 3-month duration involving at least two noncontiguous lymph node areas in the absence of other illness

Histopathology

- Morphologic features depend on evidence of disease progression
- Early HIV is characterized by florid follicular hyperplasia:
  - Numerous large irregular germinal centers
  - Germinal centers have high mitotic rate, numerous centroblasts, and tingible-body macrophages
  - Follicle lysis is characteristic (fragmented follicles with hemorrhage and invagination by small lymphocytes)
  - Mantle zones are attenuated
  - Monocytoid B cells are frequently prominent

- Paracortex contains plasma cells, immunoblasts, histiocytes, eosinophils, neutrophils, and prominent vasculature
- Sinus histiocytosis with occasional erythrophagocytosis and polykaryocytes
- Well-formed granulomas or scattered epithelioid histiocytes may be seen
- Advanced stages of disease are associated with lymphoid depletion (Figure 14-4):
  - Follicles become small, atrophic, and hyalinized
  - Paracortex is expanded with increased histiocytes and plasma cells and decreased lymphocytes
  - Numerous blood vessels and fibrosis or deposition of amorphous eosinophilic material

Special Stains and Immunohistochemistry

- Reactive germinal centers contain numerous CD8-positive T lymphocytes
- Interfollicular area contains a decreased number of CD4-positive T lymphocytes and an increased number of S-100-positive interdigitating dendritic cells
- Scattered EBV-positive cells are frequently found
- Advanced cases show no evidence of CD21+, CD23+ follicular dendritic cell meshworks

Other Techniques for Diagnosis

- HIV serology
- HIV RNA detection (viral load)
- Flow cytometry for CD4 and CD8 T-cell subsets

Differential Diagnosis

NONSPECIFIC FOLLICULAR HYPERPLASIA

- May be morphologically indistinguishable from early HIV
- Follicles are typically not as large and less irregular
- Well-defined mantle zones

INFECTIOUS MONONUCLEOSIS

- May be morphologically indistinguishable from early HIV
- Epstein-Barr virus (EBV)–positive lymphocytes are much more numerous

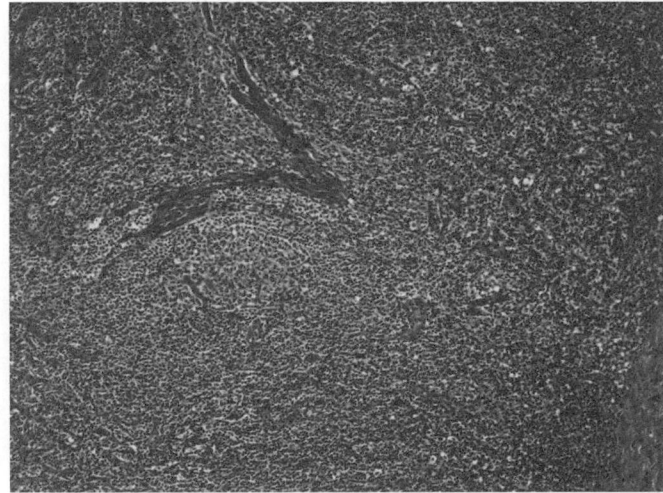

Figure 14-4. HIV-related lymphadenopathy, advanced stage disease. Atrophic germinal center with expanded paracortex and hypervascularity.

FOLLICULAR LYMPHOMA

- Follicles tend to be uniform in size and shape and uniformly distributed throughout the node
- No evidence of tingible-body macrophages in the germinal centers
- Germinal center cells express Bcl-2
- Flow cytometry and PCR: evidence of a monoclonal B-cell population
- Cytogenetics and FISH: t(14;18) translocation and other cytogenetic abnormalities

ANGIOIMMUNOBLASTIC T-CELL LYMPHOMA

- May resemble late-stage HIV due to presence of regressed germinal centers, scattered EBV-positive immunoblasts, lymphoid depletion, and marked proliferation of high endothelial venules
- Morphologic evidence of atypical small to medium-sized lymphocytes with clear cytoplasm
- Tumor cells are CD4-positive T cells that coexpress CD10, Bcl-6, PD-1, and CXCL13 (T-helper cells)
- Follicular dendritic cell meshworks are numerous and expanded

CASTLEMAN DISEASE

- May resemble late-stage HIV due to presence of atrophic follicles and paracortical vascularity and hyalinization
- The follicles are distinctive, with onion-skinning of mantle zones and lollypop appearance
- May express human herpesvirus 8 (HHV-8)

KAPOSI SARCOMA

- Common in HIV patients
- Neoplastic proliferation of lymphatic endothelial cells with evidence of red blood cell extravasation and hyaline globules
- Extensive expression of HHV-8 by the endothelial cells

MYCOBACTERIUM AVIUM INTRACELLULARE INFECTION

- Atypical mycobacterial infection in HIV patients may show a histiocytic proliferation with foamy or spindle histiocytes (mycobacterial pseudotumors)
- HIV-positive patients do not develop well-formed granulomas
- Acid-fast stain reveals numerous intracellular organisms

PEARLS

- *Lymph node excision due to acute HIV is uncommon nowadays due to extensive accumulated clinical experience with HIV*
- *Lymph node excision in patients with known advanced HIV is usually performed to rule out AIDS-associated lymphoma*
- *Histologic features of HIV are highly suggestive but are not pathognomonic*
- *HIV may be detected in follicular dendritic cells even in patients treated with antiretroviral therapy*

SELECTED REFERENCES

Alos L, Naverrete P, Morente V, et al: Immunoarchitecture of lymphoid tissue in HIV-infection during antiretroviral therapy correlates with viral persistence. Mod Pathol 18:127-136, 2005.

Chadburn A, Abdul-Nabi AM, Teruya BS, Lo AA: Lymphoid proliferations associated with human immunodeficiency virus infection. Arch Pathol Lab Med 137:360-370, 2013.

KIMURA DISEASE

Clinical Features

- Kimura disease presents as large painless subcutaneous masses and lymphadenopathy of the head or neck
- East Asian males are classically affected
- Up to 40% of the patients have salivary gland involvement
- Patients have eosinophilia and elevated serum IgE level

Histopathology

- Reactive follicular hyperplasia
- Highly vascular germinal centers and paracortex
- Germinal centers have deposition of eosinophilic proteinaceous material (IgE)
- Germinal centers and paracortex contain numerous eosinophils with eosinophilic microabscesses and polykaryocytes (Figure 14-5)
- Prominent fibrosis may be seen

Special Stains and Immunohistochemistry

- IgE stains the dendritic meshwork of the germinal centers

Other Techniques for Diagnosis

- Laboratory workup reveals eosinophilia

Differential Diagnosis

ANGIOFOLLICULAR HYPERPLASIA WITH EOSINOPHILIA

- Typically presents in middle-aged Caucasian women
- Smaller, more superficial, and better defined lesions
- Has prominent epithelioid endothelial cell proliferation (may represent a benign vascular neoplasm)
- Eosinophilic abscesses are unusual

CLASSICAL HODGKIN LYMPHOMA

- Diagnostic Reed-Sternberg cells are present

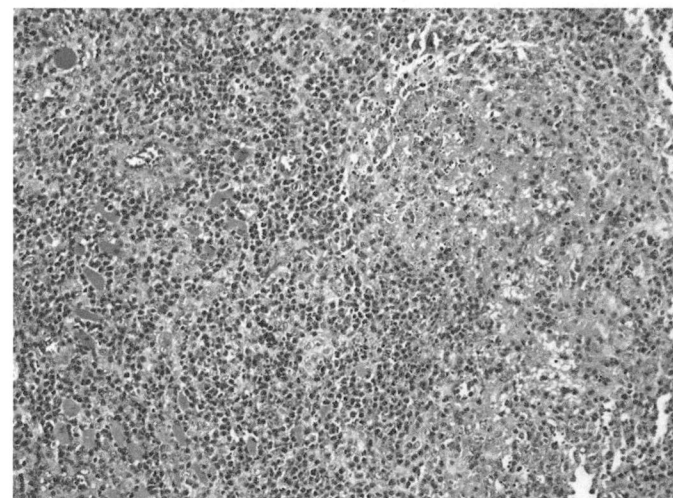

Figure 14-5. Kimura disease. A germinal center with deposition of eosinophilic material and numerous eosinophils. *(Courtesy of Dr. Dennis O'Malley, Clarient, Inc. Aliso Viejo, CA)*

- The inflammatory infiltrate contains eosinophils, but also numerous small lymphocytes, plasma cells, neutrophils, and histiocytes
- Reed-Sternberg cells express CD15 and CD30

LANGERHANS CELL HISTIOCYTOSIS
- Sinusoidal dilation and infiltration
- May have prominent eosinophilia associated with neutrophils, histiocytes, and aggregates of Langerhans cells
- Langerhans cells express CD1a, S-100 protein and Langerin

PARASITIC INFECTION
- Clinical history of active parasitosis

DRUG-RELATED LYMPHADENOPATHY
- Part of a systemic hypersensitivity reaction to medication
- Paracortical proliferation of immunoblasts, with or without follicular hyperplasia
- May have increased number of eosinophils in the paracortex

NONSPECIFIC FOLLICULAR HYPERPLASIA
- Diagnosis of exclusion

PEARLS

- *Kimura disease and angiofollicular hyperplasia with eosinophilia used to be grouped together in the older literature; however, now they are recognized as distinct entities*
- *The triad of florid follicular hyperplasia, eosinophilia, and hypervascularity is considered characteristic of Kimura disease*

SELECTED REFERENCES

Chen H, Thompson LD, Aguilera NS, Abbondanzo SL: Kimura disease: a clinicopathologic study of 21 cases. Am J Surg Pathol 28:505, 2004.
Don DM, Ishiyama A, Johnstone AK, et al: Angiolymphoid hyperplasia with eosinophilia and vascular tumors of the head and neck. Am J Otolaryngol 17:240, 1996.
Mejia R, Nutman TB: Evaluation and differential diagnosis of marked, persistent eosinophilia. Semin Hematol 49:149-159, 2012.

IgG4-RELATED LYMPHADENOPATHY

Clinical Features
- IgG4-related disease is a systemic inflammatory condition characterized by tumefactive sclerosing lesions in multiple organs
- Classic disease presents as autoimmune pancreatitis
- Other frequently involved organs include ocular adnexa, salivary glands, kidney, lung, liver, and gallbladder
- Up to 80% of patients have systemic lymphadenopathy on imaging

Histopathology
- Broad morphologic spectrum
- Type I (multicentric Castleman disease–like) has hyperplastic follicles and atrophic follicles with interfollicular vascular proliferation and eosinophilia
- Type II (follicular hyperplasia) has intrafollicular and paracortical plasmacytosis and scattered eosinophils
- Type III (paracortical expansion) has prominent high endothelial venules, small lymphocytes, immunoblasts, plasmablasts, and eosinophils
- Type IV (progressive transformation of germinal centers) has enlarged follicles with expanded mantle zones and scattered intrafollicular plasma cells
- Type V (inflammatory pseudotumor-like) is extremely rare and has focal node replacement by fibrous tissue with embedded plasma cells and lymphocytes

Special Stains and Immunohistochemistry
- Staining for kappa and lambda light chains demonstrates polytypic plasma cells
- IgG and IgG4 quantify the number of plasma cells (Figure 14-6)
  - > 100 IgG4-positive plasma cells per high power field in at least three high-power fields
  - IgG4/IgG ratio > 40%

Other Techniques for Diagnosis
- Elevated serum level of IgG4
- Imaging to rule out involvement of other organs

Differential Diagnosis
CASTLEMAN DISEASE
- Elevated Il-6 and C-reactive protein (normal levels in IgG4-related disease)
- No significant increase in IgG4-positive plasma cells

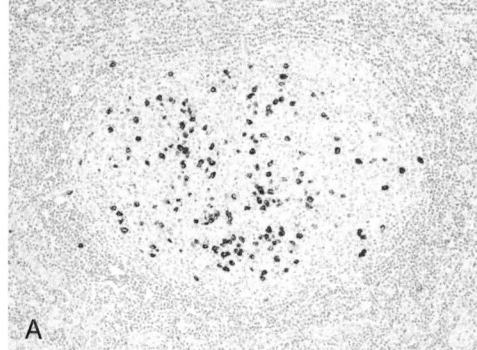
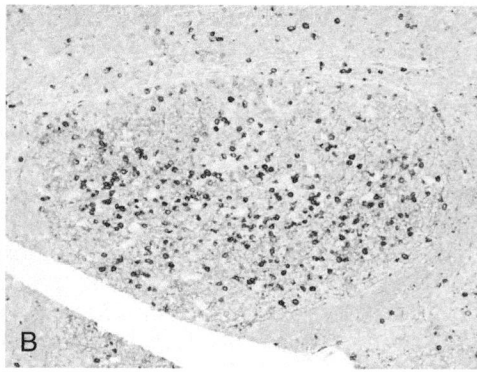

Figure 14-6. IgG4-related lymphadenopathy. A, Immunohistochemical stain for IgG4 highlights numerous positive plasma cells. **B,** Immunohistochemical stain for IgG from the same area.

- May express HHV-8
- May show light-chain restriction in the plasma cells

NONSPECIFIC FOLLICULAR HYPERPLASIA
- No significant increase in IgG4-positive plasma cells
- Diagnosis of exclusion

PROGRESSIVE TRANSFORMATION OF GERMINAL CENTERS
- No significant increase in IgG4-positive plasma cells

INFLAMMATORY PSEUDOTUMOR
- Spindle cell proliferation with a mixed infiltrate of small lymphocytes, immunoblasts, histiocytes, eosinophils, and many plasma cells
- Infectious etiology can be proven in some of these cases (atypical mycobacteria, *Treponema pallidum*, Epstein-Barr virus, and others)
- Immunohistochemical staining to rule out increase in IgG4 plasma cells should be done in all cases of suspected inflammatory pseudotumor

SMALL B-CELL LYMPHOMA WITH PLASMACYTIC DIFFERENTIATION
- Immunohistochemical staining for kappa and lambda light chains shows light chain restriction in the plasma cells
- Flow cytometry and PCR: evidence of a monoclonal B-cell population
- Cytogenetics and FISH: evidence of cytogenetic abnormalities

ANGIOIMMUNOBLASTIC T-CELL LYMPHOMA
- Characteristic morphology with a polymorphous paracortical infiltrate composed of small to medium-sized atypical lymphocytes with moderate pale cytoplasm admixed with numerous reactive small lymphocytes, immunoblasts, eosinophils, plasma cells, and histiocytes
- Paracortical vascular proliferation
- T cells have a follicular T-helper immunophenotype CD10+, BCL6+, PD-1+, and CXCL13+
- CD21 and CD23 highlight expanded follicular dendritic cell meshworks
- No significant increase in IgG4-positive plasma cells

PEARLS

- *IgG4-related disease is a recently described entity that is currently under intense investigation*
- *The pathogenesis of IgG4-related disease is currently unknown, but the likely causes include chronic infection and autoimmune process*
- *Increase in IgG4-positive plasma cells is not entirely specific and may be seen in a variety of otherwise well-characterized conditions (carcinoma, lymphoma, etc.)*
- *If the patient is not known to have systemic IgG4-related disease, the suggested diagnosis is "reactive lymphoid hyperplasia with increased IgG4+ cells"*
- *Clinician should be encouraged to rule out IgG4-related disease clinically*
- *IgG4-related disease is clinically important because the patients have an excellent response to steroids*
- *IgG4-related lymphadenopathy differs from IgG4-related involvement of other sites in that sclerosis is exceptionally rare*

SELECTED REFERENCES

Cheuk W, Chan JK: Lymphadenopathy of IgG4-related disease: an underdiagnosed and overdiagnosed entity. Semin Diagn Pathol 29:226-234, 2012.

Cheuk W, Yuen HK, Chu SY, et al: Lymphadenopathy of IgG4-related sclerosing disease. Am J Surg Pathol 32:671-681, 2008.

Deshpande V, Zen Y, Chan JK et al: Consensus statement on the pathology of IgG4-related disease. Mod Pathol 25:1181-1192, 2012.

Grimm KE, Barry TS, Chizhevsky V, et al: Histopathological findings in 29 lymph node biopsies with increased IgG4 plasma cells. Mod Pathol 25:480-491, 2012.

Rollins-Raval MA, Felgar RE, Krasinskas AM, et al: Increased numbers of IgG4-positive plasma cells may rarely be seen in lymph nodes of patients without IgG4-related sclerosing disease. Int J Surg Pathol 20:47-53, 2012.

Sato Y, Inoue D, Asano N, et al: Association between IgG4-related disease and progressively transformed germinal centers of lymph nodes. Mod Pathol 25:956-967, 2012.

Sato Y, Kojima M, Takata K, et al: Multicentric Castleman's disease with abundant IgG4-positive cells: a clinical and pathological analysis of six cases. J Clin Pathol 63:1084-1089, 2010.

Stone JH, Zen Y, Deshpande V: IgG4-related disease. N Engl J Med 366:539-551, 2012.

PROGRESSIVE TRANSFORMATION OF GERMINAL CENTERS (PTGC)

Clinical Features
- Typically an incidental finding of an isolated enlarged lymph node
- Most common in children and young adults
- Male predominance

Histopathology
- One to several well-defined nodules (transformed germinal centers) with expanded mantle zone (Figure 14-7)
- Residual germinal centers are fragmented or not evident
- No evidence of large atypical lymphoid cells in the nodules
- Background of typical follicular hyperplasia

Special Stains and Immunohistochemistry
- Nodules are composed of CD20+, Pax-5+ B lymphocytes with features of mantle cells (Bcl-2+, IgD+)

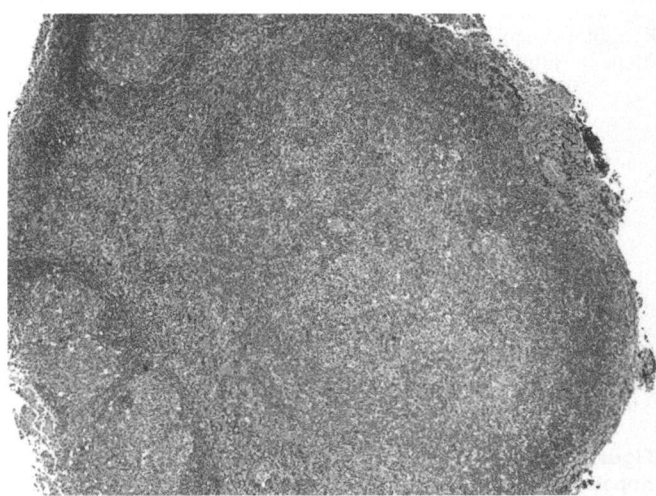

Figure 14-7. PTGC. A large well-defined nodule with expanded mantle zone and a fragmented germinal center.

- No evidence of large atypical B lymphocytes inside or outside the nodules
- Increased number of CD57+ cells in the germinal centers

Other Techniques for Diagnosis

- Flow cytometry may demonstrate a population of CD4+/CD8+ T lymphocytes
- Cytogenetics and PCR: no evidence of B-cell clonality

Differential Diagnosis

NODULAR LYMPHOCYTE-PREDOMINANT HODGKIN LYMPHOMA (NLPHL)

- Generally the entire lymph node is involved by lymphoma
- Characterized by presence of scattered large atypical lymphoid cells with a folded or multilobated nucleus and scant cytoplasm ("popcorn" cell or LP cell)
- LP cells are ringed by CD3+, CD57+, PD-1+ T lymphocytes
- Rarely, may coexist with or have a history of PTGC

FOLLICULAR LYMPHOMA

- Generally the entire lymph node is involved by lymphoma
- The B cells coexpress Bcl-6, CD10, and Bcl-2
- Flow cytometry: B lymphocytes show light chain restriction
- Conventional karyotype and FISH: t(14;18); *BCL2/IGH* gene rearrangement

MANTLE CELL LYMPHOMA

- Generally the entire lymph node is involved by lymphoma
- B lymphocytes coexpress CD5 and Cyclin D1
- Flow cytometry: B lymphocytes show light chain restriction
- Conventional karyotype and FISH: t(11;14); *IGH/ CCND1* gene rearrangement

IgG4-RELATED LYMPHADENOPATHY

- Increased number of plasma cells in the interfollicular area
- >100 IgG4-positive plasma cells per high power field
- IgG4/IgG ratio >40%

PEARLS

- *The differential diagnosis with NLPHL can be challenging and requires careful examination of morphology*
- *Rarely, PTGC can precede, coexist with, or follow the diagnosis of NLPHL*

SELECTED REFERENCES

Chang CC, Osipov V, Wheaton S, et al: Follicular hyperplasia, follicular lysis, and progressive transformation of germinal centers: a sequential spectrum of morphologic evolution in lymphoid hyperplasia. Am J Clin Pathol 120:322-326, 2003.

Hicks J, Flaitz C: Progressive transformation of germinal centers: review of histopathologic and clinical features. Int J Pediatr Otorhinolaryngol 265:195-202, 2002.

Nguyen PL, Ferry JA, Harris NL: Progressive transformation of germinal centers and nodular lymphocyte predominance Hodgkin's disease: a comparative immunohistochemical study. Am J Surg Pathol 23:27-33, 1999.

Rahemtullah A, Harris NL, Dorn ME, et al: Beyond the lymphocyte predominant cell: CD4+CD8+ T cells in nodular lymphocyte predominant Hodgkin lymphoma. Leuk Lymphoma 49:1870-1878, 2008.

Shaikh F, Ngan BY, Alexander S, Grant R: Progressive transformation of germinal centers in children and adolescents: an intriguing cause of lymphadenopathy. Pediatr Blood Cancer 60:26-30, 2013.

REACTIVE PARACORTICAL HYPERPLASIA

INFECTIOUS MONONUCLEOSIS (IM)

Clinical Features

- Most patients are adolescents and young adults
- Patients typically present with fever, pharyngitis, and cervical lymphadenopathy
- Caused by Epstein-Barr virus (EBV)

Histopathology

- Lymph node architecture is distorted
- Expanded paracortex with a polymorphous proliferation of small, medium-sized, and numerous large lymphoid cells (immunoblasts) (Figure 14-8)
- Immunoblasts may be morphologically atypical, sometimes resemble Reed-Sternberg cells, and may form large aggregates
- Increased mitotic activity
- Necrosis may be present

Special Stains and Immunohistochemistry

- Most immunoblasts are CD20+, Mum-1+, CD10- B cells
- Some immunoblasts express CD30, but are always CD15 negative
- The majority of the small and medium-sized lymphocytes are T cells
- In situ hybridization for EBV (EBER) highlights numerous positive small and large lymphocytes

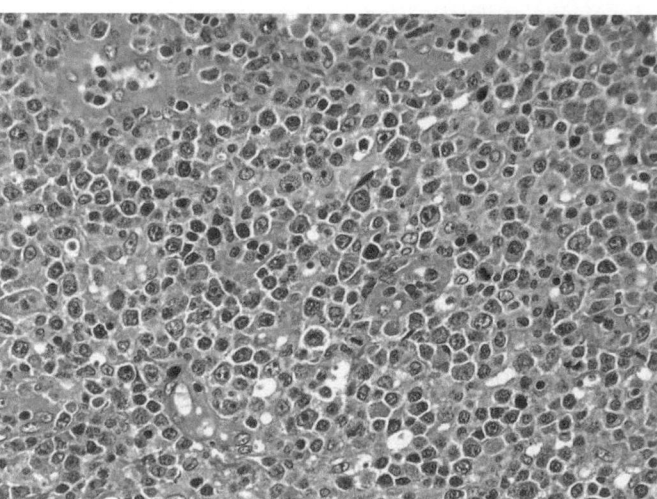

Figure 14-8. Infectious mononucleosis. Expanded paracortex with numerous large immunoblasts.

Other Techniques for Diagnosis

- Monospot (heterophile antibody)
- Serology
- EBV viral load

Differential Diagnosis

DIFFUSE LARGE B-CELL LYMPHOMA

- Occurs in older individuals
- The neoplastic B-cell population is more homogeneous with sheets of large transformed lymphocytes
- EBER may be positive, but only in the large neoplastic cells

PERIPHERAL T-CELL LYMPHOMA

- There is evidence of T-cell antigen loss or aberrant antigen expression
- EBER may be positive, but in a much smaller number of cells and only in the large immunoblasts

CLASSICAL HODGKIN LYMPHOMA

- Even though immunoblasts in IM may appear atypical, most do not resemble Reed-Sternberg cells
- Reed-Sternberg cells express CD30 and CD15
- EBER may be positive, but in a smaller number of cells and only in the large neoplastic cells

CMV LYMPHADENITIS

- Immunohistochemistry for CMV is positive
- EBER is negative

HIV-ASSOCIATED LYMPHADENOPATHY (EARLY PHASE)

- Florid follicular hyperplasia without significant paracortical expansion
- EBER may be positive, but only in rare scattered cells

PEARLS

- *Lymph node biopsy is not indicated in IM, thus the diagnosis is not suspected clinically in the majority of the patients*
- *The combination of immunoblastic proliferation and necrosis frequently raises the possibility of lymphoma*
- *The possibility of IM has to be ruled out in every young patient with suspicion for aggressive high-grade lymphoma or classical Hodgkin lymphoma*
- *IM is a frequent cause of misdiagnosis and second opinion send-out*

SELECTED REFERENCES

Kojima M, Nakamura S, Itoh H, et al: Acute viral lymphadenitis mimicking low-grade peripheral T-cell lymphoma: a clinicopathological study of nine cases. APMIS 109:419-427, 2001.

Louissaint A Jr, Ferry JA, Soupir CP, et al: Infectious mononucleosis mimicking lymphoma: distinguishing morphological and immunophenotypic features. Mod Pathol 2:1149-1159, 2012.

Pittaluga S: Viral-associated lymphoid proliferations. Semin Diagn Pathol 30:130-136, 2013.

HERPES SIMPLEX LYMPHADENITIS

Clinical Features

- Lymphadenopathy can be localized or generalized and is rarely biopsied
- Biopsy is usually performed on the inguinal lymph nodes, when there is a concurrent anogenital infection
- Lymphadenopathy is usually painful
- Many patients are immunosuppressed due to an associated malignancy or immunodeficiency

Histopathology

- Lymph node architecture is distorted but preserved
- Prominent paracortical hyperplasia with many immunoblasts
- Multifocal necrosis with neutrophils, debris, and cells with viral inclusions (Figure 14-9)
- Cells with inclusions contain ground-glass nuclei or intranuclear eosinophilic inclusions with halos, chromatin margination, and multinucleation

Special Stains and Immunohistochemistry

- Herpes simplex virus (HSV) immunostain is positive

Other Techniques for Diagnosis

- Viral culture
- Serology

Differential Diagnosis

HISTIOCYTIC NECROTIZING LYMPHADENITIS (KIKUCHI DISEASE)

- Numerous CD123+ plasmacytoid dendritic cells are present
- There is extensive necrosis with admixed karyorrhectic debris but no neutrophils
- Viral inclusions are absent

CAT SCRATCH DISEASE

- Early lesions contain prominent monocytoid B-cell hyperplasia and neutrophils, but little necrosis
- Late lesions show granulomas
- Viral inclusions are absent
- Warthin-Starry stain shows numerous microorganisms

DIFFUSE LARGE B-CELL LYMPHOMA

- The nodal architecture is effaced with sheets of large transformed lymphoid cells
- Viral inclusions are absent

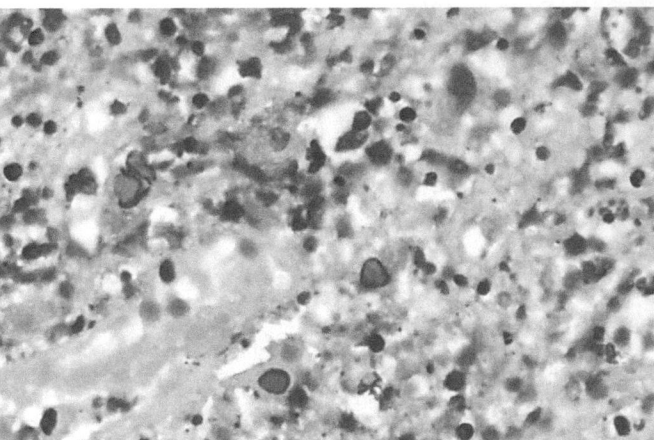

Figure 14-9. HSV lymphadenitis. Necrosis and cells with large viral inclusions. *(Courtesy of Dr. Dennis O'Malley, Clarient, Inc. Aliso Viejo, CA)*

PEARLS

- *Necrosis is not associated with granuloma formation, arguing against most other necrotizing infections*
- *Rare cases of concomitant HSV and EBV infection in the same lymph node have been described in immunosuppressed patients*

SELECTED REFERENCES

Gattenlohner S, Etschmann B, Lippert BM, et al: Concomitant herpes simplex and Epstein-Barr virus lymphadenitis with simultaneous lymph node metastases of an occult squamous cell carcinoma in a patient with chronic lymphocytic leukemia. Leuk Lymphoma 49:2390-2392, 2008.

Higgins J, Warnke R: Herpes lymphadenitis in association with chronic lymphocytic leukemia. Cancer 86:1210-1215, 1999.

Joseph L, Scott MA, Schichman SA, et al: Localized herpes simplex lymphadenitis mimicking large cell (Richter) transformation of chronic lymphocytic leukemia/small lymphocytic lymphoma. Am J Hematol 68:287-291, 2001.

Witt M, Torno M, Sun M, et al: Herpes simplex virus lymphadenitis: case report and review of the literature. Clin Infect Dis 34:1-6, 2002.

DERMATOPATHIC LYMPHADENITIS

Clinical Features

- Found in patients with benign and malignant chronic skin conditions
- Lymphadenitis occurs in the lymph nodes that drain the affected area
- Axillary and inguinal lymph nodes are most commonly affected

Histopathology

- The lymph node architecture is preserved
- Marked diffuse or nodular expansion of the paracortex
- Proliferation of interdigitating dendritic cells, Langerhans cells, and histiocytes that contain melanin pigment (Figure 14-10)

Special Stains and Immunohistochemistry

- The lymphocytes are predominantly CD4+ T cells
- Langerhans cells express S-100 and CD1a

Figure 14-10. Dermatopathic lymphadenitis. Nodular paracortical hyperplasia with numerous admixed dendritic cells and pigment-laden macrophages.

- Interdigitating cells express S-100 and are negative for CD1a
- Histiocytes are highlighted by CD68 and CD163

Other Techniques for Diagnosis

- T-cell receptor gamma gene (TCR) rearrangement shows polyclonal T lymphocytes

Differential Diagnosis

MYCOSIS FUNGOIDES

- Nodal architecture may be preserved or effaced depending on the degree of involvement
- Atypical lymphocytes are present singly, in small clusters, or in large aggregates
- Typical immunophenotype of neoplastic lymphocytes is CD3+, CD2+, CD5+, CD4+, and negative for CD8 and CD7
- PCR: monoclonal TCR gene rearrangement
- Conventional cytogenetics: many cases have a complex karyotype

LANGERHANS CELL HISTIOCYTOSIS

- Numerous Langerhans cells, present singly or in aggregates
- Neoplastic proliferation occurs in the sinuses and is accompanied by eosinophils, neutrophils, plasma cells, and histiocytes

NONSPECIFIC PARACORTICAL HYPERPLASIA

- Dendritic cells and Langerhans cells are less numerous
- No evidence of melanin-containing macrophages

PEARLS

- *Enlarged lymph nodes from patients with mycosis fungoides frequently show dermatopathic changes*
- *Mycosis fungoides can be subtle morphologically, thus PCR for TCR gene rearrangement should be ordered in difficult cases*
- *Melanin pigment particles are darker, smaller and nonrefringent as opposed to hemosiderin*

SELECTED REFERENCES

Winter LK, Spiegel JH, King T: Dermatopathic lymphadenitis of the head and neck. J Cutan Pathol 34:195-197, 2007.

DRUG-RELATED LYMPHADENOPATHY

Clinical Features

- Lymphadenopathy usually occurs 2 to 8 weeks after exposure to the drug
- May be part of drug reaction with eosinophilia and systemic symptoms (DRESS)
- Most often associated with antiepileptic agents (carbamazepine, lamotrigine, phenytoin, phenobarbital) and allopurinol
- Cervical lymph nodes are usually involved, but lymphadenopathy may be systemic

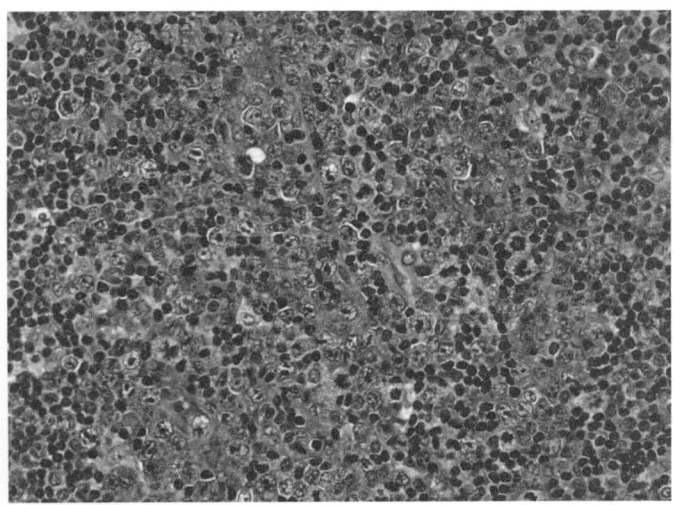

Figure 14-11. Drug-related lymphadenopathy. Paracortical hyperplasia with numerous immunoblasts.

Histopathology

- Paracortical hyperplasia with increased immunoblasts and eosinophilia (Figure 14-11)
- Immunoblasts may form large aggregates

Special Stains and Immunohistochemistry

- Immunoblasts express CD30 and are negative for CD15

Other Techniques for Diagnosis

- Clinical history of exposure to high-risk medication

Differential Diagnosis

DIFFUSE LARGE B-CELL LYMPHOMA
- The lymph node architecture is typically effaced
- Tumor cells rarely express CD30
- Flow cytometry, cytogenetic analysis, and PCR show evidence of B-cell clonality
- Not related to recent exposure to a new medication

NONSPECIFIC PARACORTICAL HYPERPLASIA
- If no history of drug exposure can be documented
- Is a diagnosis of exclusion

PEARLS

- *Complete and accurate clinical history is necessary to make the diagnosis*
- *Cases with a prominent immunoblastic reaction have been called pseudolymphoma in the older literature*

SELECTED REFERENCES

Brown JR, Skarin AT: Clinical mimics of lymphoma. Oncologist 9:406-416, 2004.

Mansur AT, Yaşar SP, Göktay F: Anticonvulsant hypersensitivity syndrome: clinical and laboratory features. Int J Dermatol 47:1184-1189, 2008.

Tas S, Simonart T: Management of drug rash with eosinophilia and systemic symptoms (DRESS syndrome): an update. Dermatology 206:353-356, 2003.

SINUS HISTIOCYTOSIS

ROSAI-DORFMAN DISEASE

Clinical Features

- Also known as sinus histiocytosis with massive lymphadenopathy
- Rare, self-limited histiocytic disorder of unknown etiology
- Most common in children and young adults
- Believed to be a reactive, polyclonal process
- About 90% of patients present with bilateral cervical lymphadenopathy
- Axillary, inguinal, and mediastinal lymph nodes also frequently involved
- Patients also may have fever, weight loss, leukocytosis, anemia, elevated erythrocyte sedimentation rate (ESR)

Histopathology

- Lymph node architecture is preserved
- The capsule is thickened
- There is marked dilation of the sinuses and numerous intrasinusoidal histiocytes (Figure 14-12A)
  - Very large cells with abundant eosinophilic cytoplasm and round nuclei with a single central nucleolus
  - A variable number of the histiocytes contain well-preserved lymphocytes and, occasionally, plasma cells, neutrophils, and erythrocytes in their cytoplasm (emperipolesis) (Figure 14-12B)
- The remaining intrasinusoidal infiltrate consists of small lymphocytes and abundant plasma cells

Special Stains and Immunohistochemistry

- The histiocytes strongly express S-100 protein and other macrophage-associated antigens (CD14, CD68, CD163) (Figure 14-12C)
- The histiocytes are negative for CD1a and langerin
- Some cases have an increased number of IgG4-positive plasma cells

Other Techniques for Diagnosis

- Noncontributory

Differential Diagnosis

NONSPECIFIC SINUS HISTIOCYTOSIS
- Lacks distinctive large histiocytes with round nuclei and prominent nucleoli
- No evidence of emperipolesis
- Histiocytes do not express S-100

LYMPH NODES DRAINING PROSTHETIC IMPLANTS
- Histiocytes contain coarse refractile material
- Lack distinctive large histiocytes with round nuclei and prominent nucleoli
- No evidence of emperipolesis
- Histiocytes do not express S-100

LANGERHANS CELL HISTIOCYTOSIS
- Langerhans cells are smaller and have irregular nuclei with grooves (coffee-bean shape)
- Langerhans cells express CD1a and Langerin in addition to S-100 protein

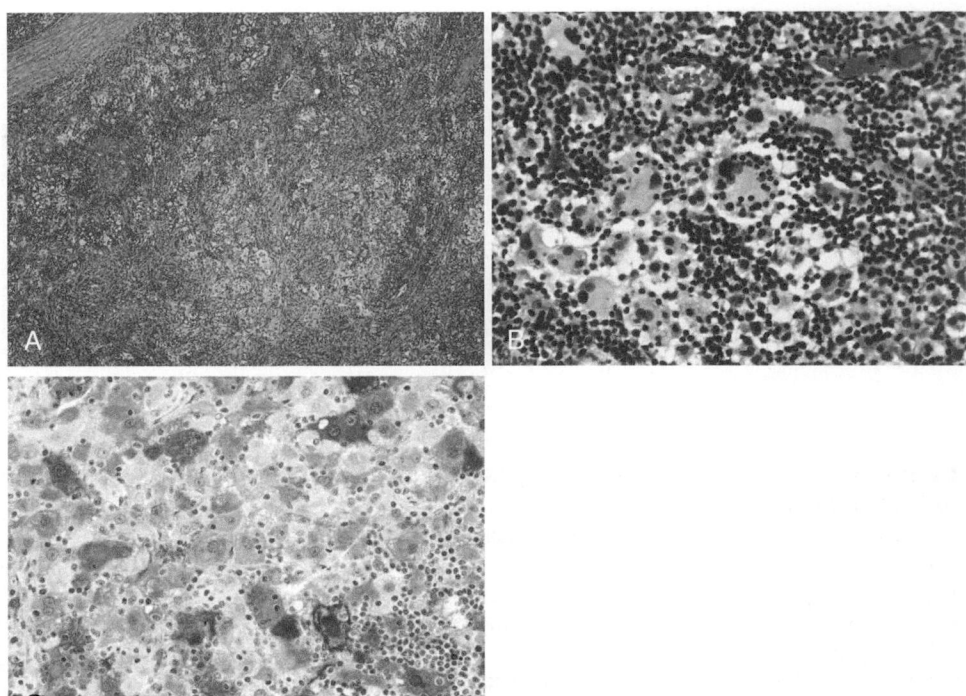

Figure 14-12. Rosai-Dorfman disease. **A,** Dilated sinuses and numerous large histiocytes. **B,** Emperipolesis. **C,** S-100 protein immunostain highlights the abnormal histiocytes.

METASTATIC MELANOMA
- Large atypical cells with prominent macronucleoli and intracytoplasmic melanin pigment
- Express S-100, Melan-A, HMB-45, microphthalmia-associated transcription factor (MITF)

METASTATIC CARCINOMA
- Cohesive clusters of malignant epithelial cells
- Express cytokeratins and epithelial membrane antigen (EMA)
- Adenocarcinoma cells may rarely be positive for S-100

PEARLS
- *The abnormal histiocytic cells are distinctive and are diagnostic of the entity*
- *Up to 40% of the patients have evidence of extranodal disease; the histologic features may be more subtle*

SELECTED REFERENCES

McClain KL, Natkunam Y, Swerdlow SH: Atypical cellular disorders. Hematology. Am Soc Hematol Educ Program 2004: 283-296, 2004.
Zhang X, Hyjek E, Vardiman J: A subset of Rosai-Dorfman disease exhibits features of IgG4-related disease. Am J Clin Pathol 139:622-632, 2013.

WHIPPLE DISEASE

Clinical Features
- Caused by *Tropheryma whipplei,* a gram-positive bacillus related to Actinomycetes
- Predilection for middle-aged white males of European ancestry
- Typically presents with migratory arthralgias, followed by diarrhea, weight loss, and abdominal pain
- Uniform regional and frequent peripheral lymph node involvement

Histopathology
- Dilation of the sinuses (Figure 14-13A)
- Lipogranulomas
- Abundant histiocytes with granular periodic acid-Schiff (PAS)–positive cytoplasm (Figure 14-13B)
  - PAS may be negative in rare lymph nodes with low disease burden
- Non-necrotizing granulomas can be seen, especially in early or extraintestinal disease

Special Stains and Immunohistochemistry
- An immunostain for *T. whipplei* is available

Other Techniques for Diagnosis
- Electron microscopy
- PCR on tissue or fluid (saliva, stool)
- Small intestinal biopsy is the gold standard for diagnosis

Differential Diagnosis
NONSPECIFIC SINUS HISTIOCYTOSIS
- Sinus histiocytes should not stain with PAS

ATYPICAL MYCOBACTERIAL INFECTION
- The organisms are acid-fast bacilli (AFB) positive, whereas *T. whipplei* is AFB negative

SARCOIDOSIS
- PAS staining and electron microscopy are useful in this differential
- In early or atypical cases, the findings may be indistinguishable

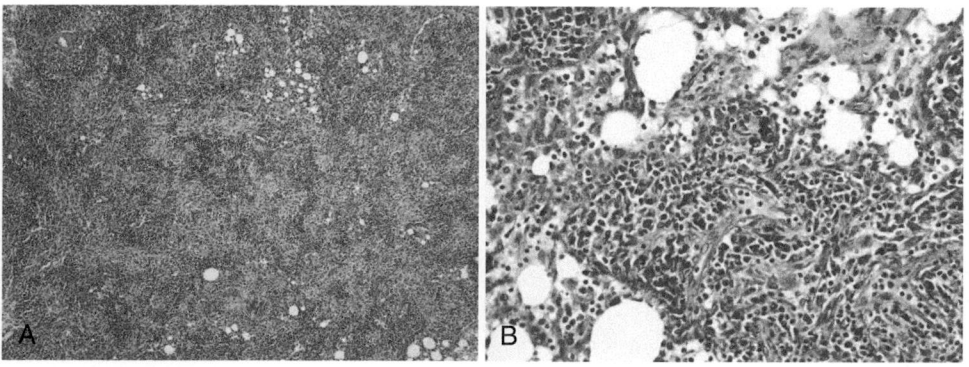

Figure 14-13. Whipple disease. A, The sinuses are distended with numerous histiocytes. **B,** PAS special stain is positive in the histiocytes. *(Courtesy of Dr. Dennis O'Malley, Clarient, Inc. Aliso Viejo, CA)*

LYMPHADENOPATHY DUE TO DEPOSITION OF EXOGENOUS MATERIAL

- Lymphangiography dye, silicone implants, prosthetic material
- Extracellular spaces lined by histiocytes
- Histiocytes contain small vacuoles, may be retractile or birefringent
- Lymph nodes draining prosthesis may contain PAS-positive granular material
- Clinical information is important in this differential diagnosis

LYMPHADENOPATHY DUE TO DEPOSITION OF ENDOGENOUS LIPID MATERIAL

- Typically in porta hepatis and celiac lymph nodes
- Can be due to mineral oil, parenteral nutrition, cholesterol crystals, fat embolism, fat necrosis
- Vacuolated sinus histiocytes, extracellular empty spaces, and giant cells
- Histiocytes are PAS negative

PEARLS

- *T. whipplei is frequently identified in young children with gastroenteritis*
- *T. whipplei DNA has also been detected in stool and saliva specimens from asymptomatic individuals*
- *CNS involvement with varied symptoms is common in Whipple disease*
- *Whipple disease can be fatal if not treated with antibiotics*
- *It is important to consider Whipple disease in patients with characteristic clinical presentation and sarcoidosis-like histopathologic features*
- *Small bowel biopsy should be recommended to make the distinction*

SELECTED REFERENCES

Alkan S, Beals TF, Schnitzer B: Primary diagnosis of Whipple disease manifesting as lymphadenopathy: use of polymerase chain reaction for detection of *Tropheryma whippelii*. Am J Clin Pathol 116:898-904, 2001.

Baisden BL, Lepidi H, Raoult D, et al: Diagnosis of Whipple disease by immunohistochemical analysis: a sensitive and specific method for the detection of *Tropheryma whipplei* (the Whipple bacillus) in paraffin-embedded tissue. Am J Clin Pathol 118:742-748, 2002.

Edouard S, Fenollar F, Raoult D: The rise of *Tropheryma whipplei:* a 12-year retrospective study of PCR diagnoses in our reference center. J Clin Microbiol 50:3917-3920, 2012.

Finzi G, Franzi F, Sessa F, et al: Ultrastructural evidence of *Tropheryma whipplei* in PAS-negative granulomatous lymph nodes. Ultrastruct Pathol 3:169-172, 2007.

Lagier JC, Lepidi H, Raoult D, Fenollar F: Systemic *Tropheryma whipplei:* clinical presentation of 142 patients with infections diagnosed or confirmed in a reference center. Medicine (Baltimore) 89:337-345, 2010.

NECROTIZING LYMPHADENITIS

KIKUCHI DISEASE

Clinical Features

- Rare, benign condition of unknown cause usually characterized by cervical lymphadenopathy and fever
- Typically occurs in young adults with female predominance
- More common in Asians
- Patients may also have fatigue, joint pain, rash, leukopenia, and anemia
- Disease is self-limited in the majority of patients

Histopathology (Figure 14-14 A and B)

- Proliferative phase has patchy nodal involvement
  - Prominent paracortical expansion by immunoblasts, small lymphocytes, plasmacytoid dendritic cells, and histiocytes
  - Single cell necrosis and eosinophilic granular debris
- Necrotizing phase has extensive necrosis with karyorrhectic debris but no intact neutrophils
  - Immunoblasts and histiocytes surround the necrotic areas
  - Histiocytes often have crescentic nuclei and contain phagocytosed debris
- Resolution phase has numerous foamy macrophages
- The inflammatory infiltrate may extend into the perinodal fat

Special Stains and Immunohistochemistry

- CD8+ cytotoxic T lymphocytes are prominent in the necrotic phase
- B lymphocytes are virtually absent outside reactive follicles
- Histiocytes express lysozyme, CD68, and myeloperoxidase
- Plasmacytoid dendritic cells are positive for CD123 (Figure 14-14C)

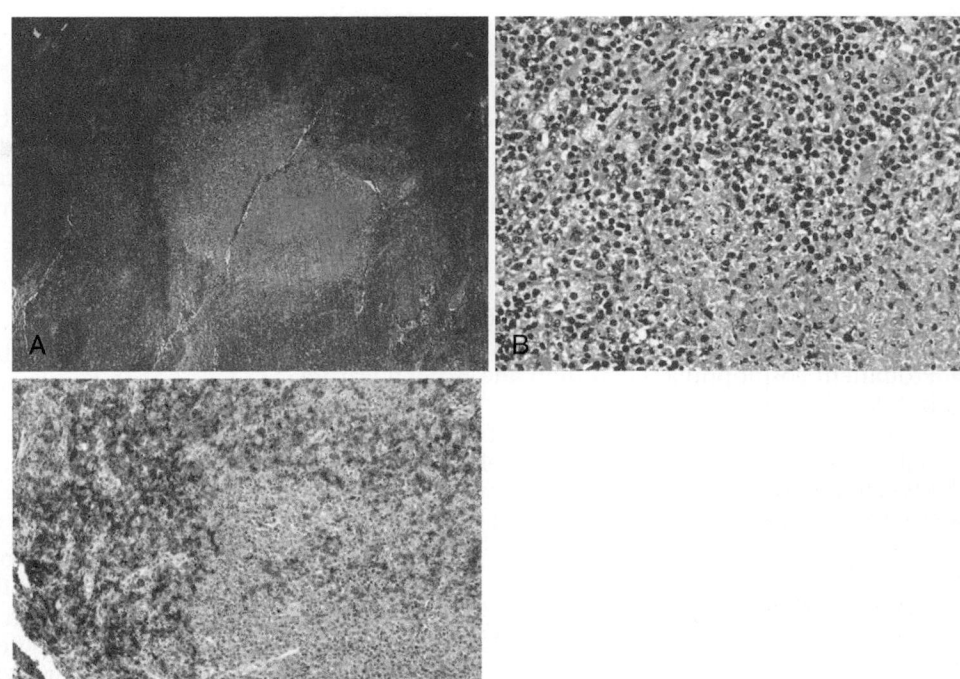

Figure 14-14. Kikuchi disease. **A,** Prominent paracortical hyperplasia with a large area of necrosis. **B,** Immunoblasts, histiocytes and plasmacytoid dendritic cells surround the necrotic foci. No intact neutrophils are present. **C,** CD123 immunostain highlights numerous plasmacytoid dendritic cells around the area of necrosis.

Other Techniques for Diagnosis
- Noncontributory

Differential Diagnosis

SYSTEMIC LUPUS ERYTHEMATOSUS
- Indistinguishable histologic features
- Some cases contain abundant plasma cells
- Hematoxylin bodies (ill-defined purple structures in necrotic foci) are rarely present; these are not seen in Kikuchi disease
- Azzopardi phenomenon (dark blue DNA material deposited on the basement membrane of blood vessels) is rarely present; it is also absent in Kikuchi disease
- Prominent follicular hyperplasia may be seen

HERPES OR CMV LYMPHADENITIS
- Patients are usually immunosuppressed
- Necrotic areas contain neutrophils and are surrounded by granulation tissue with less pronounced histiocytic infiltration
- Viral inclusions are present
- Immunohistochemistry confirms the diagnosis

KAWASAKI DISEASE
- Mainly affects children younger than 5 years
- Characteristic clinical presentation with conjunctivitis, rash, inflammation of the oral mucosa, and lymphadenopathy
- Widespread necrosis with many neutrophils
- Fibrin thrombi in small vessels and arteritis with fibrinoid necrosis are characteristic

FUNGAL LYMPHADENITIS
- Patients are usually immunosuppressed and have disseminated disease
- Well-formed granulomatous reaction is frequently present
- Special stains reveal evidence of fungal forms

TUBERCULOUS LYMPHADENITIS
- Well-formed necrotizing granulomas with many multinucleated giant cells are seen
- AFB stain reveals mycobacteria

CAT SCRATCH DISEASE
- Early disease shows prominent follicular hyperplasia and monocytoid B-cell hyperplasia with focal necrosis
- Late disease has extensive necrosis with many neutrophils and granulomas
- Warthin-Starry and Steiner stains highlight the bacteria

DIFFUSE LARGE B-CELL LYMPHOMA
- May resemble a proliferative phase of Kikuchi disease with numerous immunoblasts
- Extensive necrosis with karyorrhectic debris but no intact neutrophils is rare in diffuse large B-cell lymphoma (DLBCL), but it is typical of Kikuchi disease
- Immunohistochemical stains reveal numerous B lymphocytes, whereas B cells are few in number in Kikuchi disease
- Flow cytometry, cytogenetic analysis, and PCR demonstrate a monoclonal B-cell population

PERIPHERAL T-CELL LYMPHOMA
- Extensive necrosis with karyorrhectic debris but no intact neutrophils is rare in peripheral T-cell lymphoma (PTCL) but is typical of Kikuchi disease

- Nodal T-cell lymphomas are usually CD4-positive, whereas the T lymphocytes in Kikuchi disease are CD8-positive
- Immunohistochemical stains usually show loss of pan-T-cell antigens CD2, CD5, CD7, CD43, or Bcl-2
- Flow cytometry, cytogenetic analysis, and PCR may demonstrate a monoclonal T-cell population

CLASSICAL HODGKIN LYMPHOMA

- Necrosis and a polymorphous inflammatory infiltrate are frequently noted
- Prominent eosinophilia is common and is not a feature in Kikuchi disease
- Presence of classic Reed-Sternberg cells or lacunar cells is required for diagnosis; these cells are absent in Kikuchi disease
- Reed-Sternberg cells express CD30 and CD15

METASTATIC CARCINOMA

- Signet-ring adenocarcinoma cells may be confused with crescentic histiocytes
- Signet ring cells contain mucin, whereas the histiocytes contain phagocytized debris
- Usually presents in elderly patients with widespread metastatic disease
- Immunohistochemical staining for cytokeratins establishes the diagnosis

PEARLS

- *Although it is commonly thought of as a disease of young Asian women, Kikuchi disease can occur in both sexes and in all age and ethnic groups*
- *The relationship of Kikuchi disease and systemic lupus is controversial; some authors believe it is a* forme fruste *of lupus*
- *A subset of patients subsequently develops lupus, thus clinical workup for lupus in all cases is recommended*

SELECTED REFERENCES

Cramer J, Schmiedel S, Alegre NG, et al: Necrotizing lymphadenitis: Kikuchi-Fujimoto disease alias lupus lymphadenitis? Lupus 19:89-92, 2010.

Kim SK, Kang MS, Yoon BY, et al: Histiocytic necrotizing lymphadenitis in the context of systemic lupus erythematosus (SLE): is histiocytic necrotizing lymphadenitis in SLE associated with skin lesions? Lupus 20:809-819, 2011.

O'Malley DP, Grimm KE: Reactive lymphadenopathies that mimic lymphoma: entities of unknown etiology. Semin Diagn Pathol 30:137-145, 2013.

Pileri SA, Facchetti F, Ascani S, et al: Myeloperoxidase expression by histiocytes in Kikuchi's and Kikuchi-like lymphadenopathy. Am J Pathol 159:915-924, 2011.

Rosado FG, Tang YW, Hasserjian RP, et al: Kikuchi-Fujimoto lymphadenitis: role of parvovirus B-19, Epstein-Barr virus, human herpesvirus 6, and human herpesvirus 8. Hum Pathol 44:255-259, 2013.

Seong GM, Kim JH, Lim GC, Kim J: Clinicopathological review of immunohistochemically defined Kikuchi-Fujimoto disease-including some interesting cases. Clin Rheumatol 31:1463-1469, 2012.

SYSTEMIC LUPUS ERYTHEMATOSUS

Clinical Features

- Chronic inflammatory disease of unknown cause that can affect the skin, joints, kidneys, lungs, nervous system, serous membranes, and many other organs
- Enlargement of lymph nodes occurs in approximately 50% of patients
  - Lymph nodes are soft, nontender, and discrete
  - Usually detected in the cervical, axillary, and inguinal areas
  - Lymphadenopathy is more frequently noted at the onset of disease or in association with an exacerbation
- Numerous laboratory abnormalities include neutropenia, anemia, and positive tests for antinuclear antibodies (double-stranded DNA and Smith antigen)

Histopathology

- Edema, hemorrhage, and areas of necrosis surrounded by histiocytes and immunoblasts
- Some cases contain abundant plasma cells
- Hematoxylin bodies (ill-defined purple structures in necrotic foci) are typical of lupus
- Azzopardi phenomenon (dark blue DNA material deposited on the basement membrane of blood vessels) is typical of lupus
- Prominent follicular hyperplasia and capsular inflammation may be present

Special Stains and Immunohistochemistry

- CD8+ cytotoxic T lymphocytes are prominent
- B lymphocytes are virtually absent outside the reactive follicles
- Histiocytes express lysozyme, CD68, and myeloperoxidase
- Plasmacytoid dendritic cells are positive for CD123

Other Techniques for Diagnosis

- Noncontributory

DIFFERENTIAL DIAGNOSIS

- See section on "Differential Diagnosis" for Kikuchi disease

PEARLS

- *Diagnosis requires correlation with the clinical and laboratory findings*
- *Lupus lymphadenitis may precede or follow cases of Kikuchi disease*

SELECTED REFERENCES

Cramer J, Schmiedel S, Alegre NG, et al: Necrotizing lymphadenitis: Kikuchi-Fujimoto disease alias lupus lymphadenitis? Lupus 19:89-92, 2010.

Hu S, Kuo TT, Hong HS: Lupus lymphadenitis simulating Kikuchi's lymphadenitis in patients with systemic lupus erythematosus: a clinicopathological analysis of six cases and review of the literature. Pathol Int 53:221-226, 2003.

Kim SK, Kang MS, Yoon BY, et al: Histiocytic necrotizing lymphadenitis in the context of systemic lupus erythematosus (SLE): is histiocytic necrotizing lymphadenitis in SLE associated with skin lesions? Lupus 20:809-819, 2011.

Zuo Y, Foshat M, Qian YW, et al: A rare case of Kikuchi Fujimoto's disease with subsequent development of systemic lupus erythematosus. Case Rep Rheumatol 2012:325062, 2012.

GRANULOMATOUS LYMPHADENITIS

TUBERCULOSIS

Clinical Features

- Tuberculous lymphadenitis is among the most frequent presentations of extrapulmonary tuberculosis
- Cervical lymphadenitis is the most common site and is known as scrofula
- Tuberculosis is responsible for up to 40% of peripheral lymphadenopathy in the developing world
- In the United States, although the overall number of patients with tuberculosis has decreased, the proportion of tuberculous lymphadenitis has increased
- Isolated peripheral tuberculous lymphadenopathy is usually due to reactivation of disease
- Abdominal tuberculous lymphadenopathy may occur via ingestion of sputum or milk infected with *Mycobacterium tuberculosis* or *M. bovis*

Histopathology (Figure 14-15)

- Gross examination shows areas of white-yellow soft crumbly cheese-like ("caseous") material
- Multiple well-formed granulomas with epithelioid histiocytes and giant cells
- Caseous necrosis with no discernible cell membranes in the center of the granulomas
- AFB stain reveals the mycobacteria

Special Stains and Immunohistochemistry

- Noncontributory

Other Techniques for Diagnosis

- Microbial culture
- PCR

Differential Diagnosis

SARCOIDOSIS

- Granulomas are more uniform, better defined, and compact
- Necrosis is rare, and when present it is focal
- AFB stain is negative

FUNGAL LYMPHADENITIS

- Fungal forms can be identified on the H&E-stained sections
- AFB stain is negative
- Gomori methenamine silver (GMS) and PAS stains highlight the fungal forms

FOREIGN-BODY TYPE GRANULOMA

- Granulomas are non-necrotizing
- Giant cells have a different appearance (foreign-body type)
- Foreign material is usually easily identified in the cytoplasm of the giant cells
- AFB stain is negative

KIKUCHI DISEASE

- No well-formed granulomas or multinucleated giant cells
- Necrosis is coagulative and not caseous
- Numerous immunoblasts, crescentic histiocytes, and plasmacytoid dendritic cells around the areas of necrosis
- AFB stain is negative

AGGRESSIVE B-CELL LYMPHOMA

- May have extensive necrosis
- Lymph node architecture is effaced
- No well-formed granulomas and no multinucleated giant cells
- Sheets of medium-sized or large atypical lymphoid cells surround areas of necrosis

CLASSICAL HODGKIN LYMPHOMA

- Frequently associated with granulomas and necrosis
- Lymph node architecture is effaced
- Mixed inflammatory infiltrate with many small lymphocytes, plasma cells, eosinophils, and neutrophils
- Presence of classic Reed-Sternberg cells or lacunar cells is required for diagnosis

PERIPHERAL T-CELL LYMPHOMA

- Lennert lymphoma (lymphoepithelioid type) is characterized by clusters of epithelioid histiocytes
- No well-formed granulomas or multinucleated giant cells
- Necrosis is very unusual

METASTATIC CARCINOMA

- Can be associated with granulomas
- Nasopharyngeal carcinoma can cause marked necrotizing granulomatous inflammation
- Granulomas can also be seen in lymph nodes that drain carcinoma
- Immunohistochemical staining for cytokeratin highlights the epithelial cells

PEARLS

- *AFB stain needs to be carefully examined under oil (100× magnification) because mycobacteria are usually few in number and are hard to find*
- *Occasionally tuberculous lymphadenitis manifests with non-necrotizing granulomas, thus AFB stain should be performed on all such cases*

Figure 14-15. Tuberculosis. Large necrotizing granulomas are present.

SELECTED REFERENCES

Kato T, Kimura Y, Sawabe M, et al: Cervical tuberculous lymphadenitis in the elderly: comparative diagnostic findings. J Laryngol Otol 123:1343-1347, 2009.

Linasmita P, Srisangkaew S, Wongsuk T, et al: Evaluation of real-time polymerase chain reaction for detection of the 16S ribosomal RNA gene of *Mycobacterium tuberculosis* and the diagnosis of cervical tuberculous lymphadenitis in a country with a high tuberculosis incidence. Clin Infect Dis 55:313-321, 2012.

Marais BJ, Wright CA, Schaaf HS, et al: Tuberculous lymphadenitis as a cause of persistent cervical lymphadenopathy in children from a tuberculosis-endemic area. Pediatr Infect Dis J 25:142-146, 2006.

Peto HM, Pratt RH, Harrington TA, et al: Epidemiology of extrapulmonary tuberculosis in the United States, 1993-2006. Clin Infect Dis 49:1350, 2009.

ATYPICAL MYCOBACTERIAL INFECTION AND LEPROSY

Clinical Features

- Atypical mycobacterial infections are increasing in number and severity in developed countries
- Atypical mycobacteria that cause lymphadenitis include *M. avium* complex (MAC), *M. kansasii, M. scrofulaceum, M. malmoense,* and *M. haemophilum*
  - Found in the environment: water, soil, food products, and domestic and wild animals
- Atypical mycobacterial lymphadenitis typically occurs in immunocompetent children (1 to 5 years old)
  - Isolated cervicofacial nodes, particularly the submandibular nodes, are most frequently involved
  - Presents as a unilateral, nontender node that slowly enlarges over several weeks
- Atypical mycobacterial lymphadenitis may also occur in immunocompromised patients (HIV positive)

- Associated with disseminated infection
- The incidence of leprosy appears to have markedly decreased since the 1990s
  - Countries with high numbers of cases include India, Brazil, Indonesia, Bangladesh, and Nigeria
- Leprosy primarily involves skin and peripheral nerves; if left untreated it may spread to lymph nodes

Histopathology

- Enlarged, matted lymph nodes
- Immunocompetent patients with atypical mycobacterial lymphadenitis or tuberculoid leprosy have necrotizing and non-necrotizing granulomas with Langhans-type giant cells
- Immunosuppressed patients with atypical mycobacterial lymphadenitis may fail to develop well-formed granulomas
  - Small aggregates of histiocytes
  - Rare cases of mycobacterial pseudotumors with a proliferation of foamy or spindle histiocytes, which contain numerous intracellular organisms (Figure 14-16A)
- Immunosuppressed patients with lepromatous leprosy have abundant foamy macrophages that replace the paracortical area (Figure 14-16B and C)
  - These macrophages contain numerous intracellular organisms
- AFB stain or Fite stain highlight the mycobacteria

Special Stains and Immunohistochemistry

- Noncontributory

Other Techniques for Diagnosis

- Microbial culture
- PCR

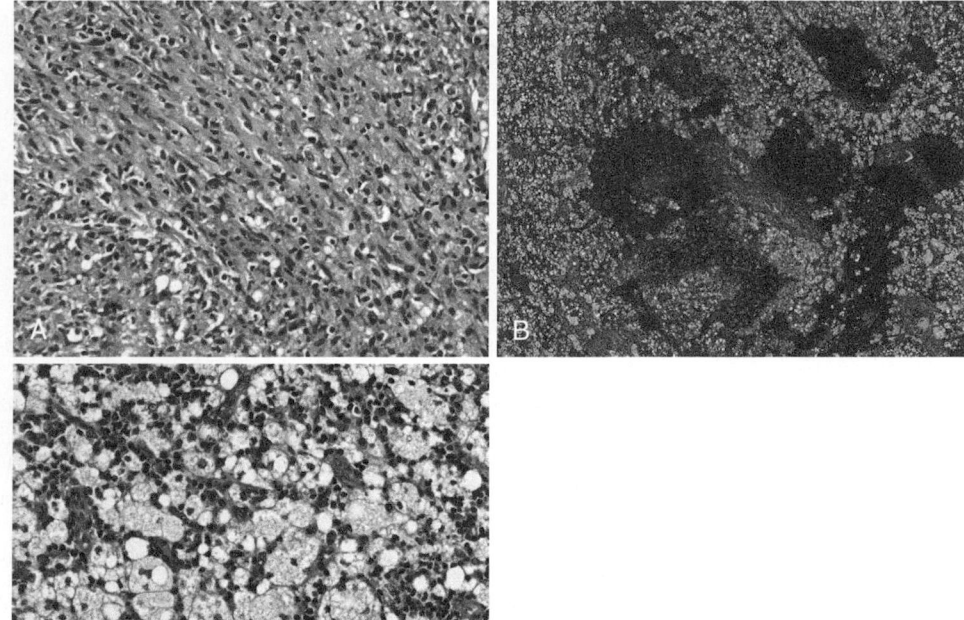

Figure 14-16. Other mycobacterial infections. A, Atypical mycobacterial lymphadenitis with sheets of spindle-shaped histiocytes. **B,** Lepromatous leprosy. Abundant foamy macrophages in the paracortical area, **C,** Lepromatous leprosy and foamy macrophages. *(Courtesy of Dr. Jose Jessurun, Weill Cornell Medical College, New York.)*

Differential Diagnosis

- Inflammatory pseudotumor of lymph node
  - An umbrella term for an ill-defined entity that includes mycobacterial pseudotumor of HIV-positive patients
  - Consists of a spindle cell proliferation with a mixed infiltrate of small lymphocytes, immunoblasts, histiocytes, eosinophils, and many plasma cells (see Figure 14-16A)
  - Infectious etiology can be proven in some of these cases (atypical mycobacteria, *Treponema pallidum*, Epstein-Barr virus and others)
  - Special stains for bacteria, mycobacteria, fungi, and immunohistochemical staining to rule out increase in IgG4 plasma cells should be done in all cases of suspected inflammatory pseudotumor
- Please also see section on "Differential Diagnosis" for "Tuberculosis"

PEARLS

- *Lymph node excision is usually curative in children with atypical mycobacteria*
- *Immunocompetent children have very few scattered mycobacteria, more readily identified at the edge of necrotic areas*
- *On the contrary, immunosuppressed patients have numerous microorganisms that are readily identified by AFB or Fite stains*

SELECTED REFERENCES

Cohen YH, Amir J, Ashkenazi S, et al: Mycobacterium haemophilum and lymphadenitis in immunocompetent children, Israel. Emerg Infect Dis 14:1437, 2008.

Cruz AT, Ong LT, Starke JR: Mycobacterial infections in Texas children: a 5-year case series. Pediatr Infect Dis J 29:772-774, 2010.

Gillis T, Vissa V, Matsuoka M, et al: Characterization of short tandem repeats for genotyping Mycobacterium leprae. Lepr Rev 80:250, 2009.

Jarzembowski JA, Young MB: Nontuberculous mycobacterial infections. Arch Pathol Lab Med 132:1333-1341, 2008.

Penn R, Steehler MK, Sokohl A, Harley EH: Nontuberculous mycobacterial cervicofacial lymphadenitis: a review and proposed classification system. Int J Pediatr Otorhinolaryngol 75:1599-1603, 2011.

Pham-Huy A, Robinson JL, Tapiéro B, et al: Current trends in nontuberculous mycobacteria infections in Canadian children: a pediatric investigators collaborative network on infections in Canada (PICNIC) study. Paediatr Child Health 15:276, 2010.

Scollard DM, Adams LB, Gillis TP, et al: The continuing challenges of leprosy. Clin Microbiol Rev 19:338, 2006.

Zhang FR, Huang W, Chen SM, et al: Genome wide association study of leprosy. N Engl J Med 361:2609, 2009.

CAT SCRATCH DISEASE

Clinical Features

- One of the most common causes of benign lymphadenopathy in the United States
- Occurs in immunocompetent children and young adults
- Caused by *Bartonella henselae* and transmitted by flea bites or cat bites and scratches

- Following inoculation of *B. henselae* into humans, the organism typically causes a local skin infection that manifests as regional lymphadenopathy
- Nodes are tender and often have erythema of the overlying skin

Histopathology

- Early stage: follicular and monocytoid B-cell hyperplasia
  - Small foci of necrosis develop within areas of monocytoid B-cell hyperplasia
  - Microabscesses are also seen within germinal centers
- Late stage: large stellate microabscesses and necrotizing granulomas with palisading histiocytes (Figure 14-17)
  - Areas of necrosis contain neutrophils and debris
  - Necrosis frequently extends outside of the capsule
- Warthin-Starry and Steiner stains identify the bacilli
  - Very small, pleomorphic, slender organisms
  - Present singly, in clusters or chains
  - Most numerous in early cases
  - Found within endothelial cells, macrophages, and areas of necrosis

Special Stains and Immunohistochemistry

- Noncontributory

Other Techniques for Diagnosis

- Serology (low sensitivity and specificity)
- Blood or tissue culture (requires special conditions)
- Tissue PCR (low sensitivity, but high specificity)

Differential Diagnosis

ACUTE SUPPURATIVE LYMPHADENITIS

- Caused by pyogenic cocci
- Follicular hyperplasia may suggest cat scratch disease
- No evidence of palisading histiocytes
- Tissue Gram stain highlights the cocci

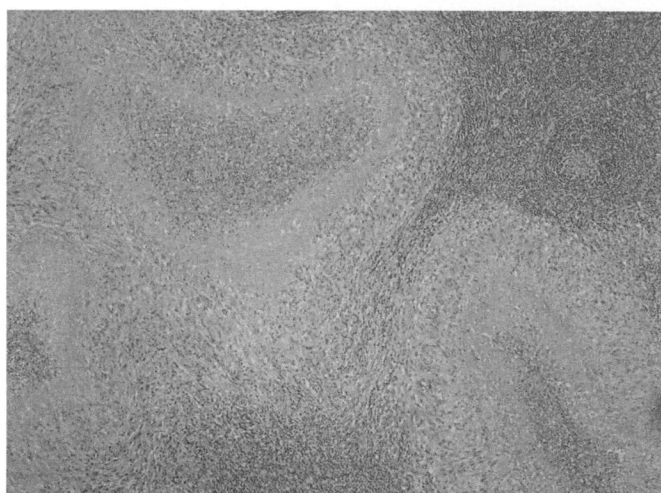

Figure 14-17. Cat-scratch disease, late stage. Large necrotizing granulomas with palisading histiocytes.

OTHER INFECTIOUS NECROTIZING LYMPHADENITIS

- *Chlamydia trachomatis* (lymphogranuloma venereum), *Francisella tularensis* (tularemia), *Hemophilus ducreyi* (chancroid), and *Yersinia enterocolitica* (mesenteric lymphadenitis) may have identical histologic features
- Clinical presentation is distinct
- Patients are systemically ill
- Gram stain, Giemsa stain, and Warthin-Starry stain help identify the respective organisms

MYCOBACTERIAL AND FUNGAL LYMPHADENITIS

- Typically have more extensive necrosis
- Fewer neutrophils
- AFB stain and GMS stain identify the organisms

KIKUCHI DISEASE

- Necrotic areas are surrounded by immunoblasts, crescentic histiocytes, and plasmacytoid dendritic cells
- Neutrophils are absent
- No evidence of organisms on special stains

LYMPHOMA

- Lymph node architecture is effaced
- Sheets of large atypical lymphoid cells or classic Reed-Sternberg cells present

PEARLS

- *Lymphadenitis typically resolves within 2 to 6 months*
- *A positive Warthin-Starry stain does not provide a definitive diagnosis but strongly suggests it in patients with compatible clinical findings*
- *Atypical cases may present with fever, hepatosplenomegaly, abdominal lymphadenopathy, night sweats, and weight loss*
  - *More likely to be biopsied*
- *Immunocompromised patients tend to have widespread granulomatous inflammation, bacillary angiomatosis, or bacillary peliosis*

SELECTED REFERENCES

Lamps LW, Scott MA: Cat-scratch disease: historic, clinical, and pathologic perspectives. Am J Clin Pathol 121(suppl):S71-S80, 2004.

Ridder GJ, Boedeker CC, Technau-Ihling K, et al: Role of cat-scratch disease in lymphadenopathy in the head and neck. Clin Infect Dis 35:643-649, 2002.

Rolain JM, Lepidi H, Zanaret M, et al: Lymph node biopsy specimens and diagnosis of cat-scratch disease. Emerg Infect Dis 12:1338, 2006.

Weinspach S, Tenenbaum T, Schönberger S, et al: Cat scratch disease—heterogeneous in clinical presentation: five unusual cases of an infection caused by Bartonella henselae. Klin Padiatr 222:273-278, 2010.

SARCOIDOSIS

Clinical Features

- Multisystem granulomatous disorder of unknown etiology
- Typically affects young adults
- More common and more severe in blacks
- Classic initial presentation with bilateral hilar adenopathy and pulmonary reticular opacities as well as skin, joint, or eye lesions
- Peripheral lymphadenopathy is present in up to 40% of patients

Histopathology

- Multiple compact well-defined granulomas (Figure 14-18)
- Granulomas are composed of epithelioid histiocytes and multinucleated giant cells
- Necrosis is typically absent
  - Rare cases have small necrotic foci in the granulomas
- Granulomas may become confluent, hyalinized, and replace the lymph node

Special Stains and Immunohistochemistry

- Noncontributory

Other Techniques for Diagnosis

- Noncontributory

Differential Diagnosis

TUBERCULOUS LYMPHADENITIS

- Extensive caseating necrosis
- Granulomas are ill-defined
- Granulomas vary in size and shape
- AFB stain helps highlight the organisms

FUNGAL LYMPHADENITIS

- Granulomatous inflammation with or without caseous necrosis
- The diagnosis is established with GMS stain and cultures

CAT SCRATCH DISEASE

- Granulomas are ill-defined
- Large microabscesses are not a feature of sarcoidosis
- Warthin-Starry stain helps highlight the organisms

BRUCELLOSIS

- Transmitted to humans by contact with fluids from infected animals or derived from food products such as unpasteurized milk
- Systemic infection with a broad clinical spectrum
- Histologically may be indistinguishable from sarcoidosis or tuberculosis
- The organisms are difficult to identify on histology
- Diagnosed based on cultures and serology

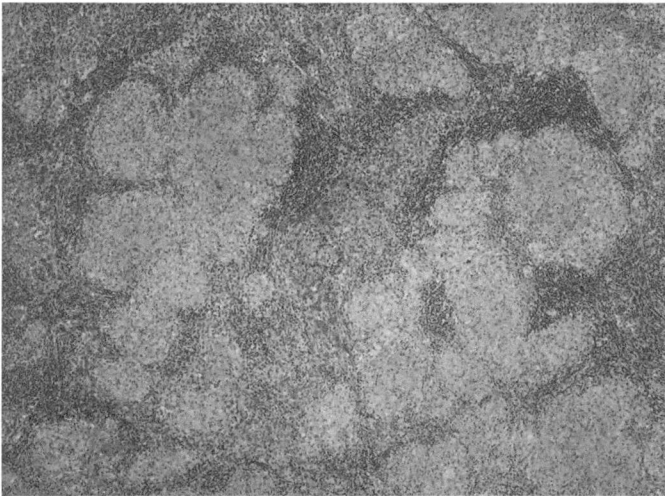

Figure 14-18. Sarcoidosis. Numerous compact epithelioid granulomas with minimal necrosis.

WHIPPLE DISEASE
- PAS staining and electron microscopy are useful in this differential
- In early or atypical cases, the findings may be indistinguishable

SYPHILIS
- Well-formed granulomas frequently present
- Prominent follicular hyperplasia
- Marked interfollicular plasmacytosis
- Capsular thickening and obliterative vasculitis are seen in secondary syphilis
- Warthin-Starry stain demonstrates the spirochetes within the blood vessel walls or inside the granulomas

FOREIGN-BODY TYPE GRANULOMAS
- Foreign material noted within the histiocytes and the giant cells

CLASSICAL HODGKIN LYMPHOMA
- Frequently associated with granulomas
- Lymphoid infiltrate outside of the granulomas should be carefully examined for the presence of Reed-Sternberg cells
- Sarcoid-like granulomas may be present in uninvolved lymph nodes of patients with known Hodgkin lymphoma

PEARLS
- *Sarcoidosis is a diagnosis of exclusion and should be diagnosed histologically with great caution*
- *Presence of fibrinoid necrosis does not exclude the diagnosis*
- *We routinely perform special stains on all cases, in order to rule out an infectious etiology*

SELECTED REFERENCES
Goswami T, Siddique S, Cohen P, Cheson BD: The sarcoid-lymphoma syndrome. Clin Lymphoma Myeloma Leuk 10:241-247, 2010.
Mehrotra R, Dhingra V: Cytological diagnosis of sarcoidosis revisited: a state of the art review. Diagn Cytopathol 39:541-548, 2011.
Rosen Y: Pathology of sarcoidosis. Semin Respir Crit Care Med 28:36-52, 2007.

CASTLEMAN DISEASE

Clinical Features
- Atypical lymphoproliferative disease divided into three subtypes: unicentric hyaline-vascular type, unicentric plasma cell type, and multicentric
- Unicentric hyaline-vascular type is the most common subtype (80% to 90% of cases)
- Isolated benign lymphoproliferative disorder of young adults
  - Usually is an incidental finding
  - Majority occurs in mediastinum
  - Unassociated with HHV-8 infection
  - Curable with surgical resection
- Unicentric plasma cell type (10% to 20% of cases)
  - Similar presentation to unicentric hyaline-vascular type
- Approximately 50% of the patients have systemic findings: anemia, elevated sedimentation rate, hypergammaglobulinemia, and bone marrow plasmacytosis
- Multicentric (very rare)
  - Middle-aged and elderly adults
  - Systemic disease with generalized peripheral lymphadenopathy, hepatosplenomegaly, frequent fevers, and night sweats
  - Strongly associated with immunosuppression (e.g., HIV) and HHV-8 infection
  - May have an associated malignancy (polyneuropathy, organomegaly, endocrinopathy, monoclonal gammopathy, and skin changes [POEMS] syndrome, Kaposi sarcoma, Hodgkin and non-Hodgkin lymphoma)

Histopathology
- Hyaline-vascular type (Figure 14-19A)
  - Abnormal follicles with atrophic or "regressed" hyalinized germinal centers, which contain numerous follicular dendritic cells
  - The follicles are surrounded by broad mantle zones of small lymphocytes, present in an "onion skin" arrangement
  - Two or more adjacent germinal centers may be surrounded by a single mantle zone
  - The regressed germinal centers are often radially penetrated by a hyalinized blood vessel ("lollipop follicle")
  - The interfollicular areas have increased vascularity
  - Sinuses are typically obliterated
- Plasma cell type (Figure 14-19B)
  - A mixture of hyperplastic germinal centers and regressed follicles
  - The interfollicular region is hypervascular and contains sheets of plasma cells
  - Sinuses may be patent
  - The histologic features are similar in the unicentric and multicentric disease
- Occasional cases have mixed features of both hyaline-vascular and plasma cell types
- Plasmablastic type
  - Is part of multicentric disease and occurs in HIV-positive patients
  - Markedly atypical-appearing large cells with plasmablastic morphology (previously called "microlymphoma") (Figure 14-19C)
    - Present inside germinal centers and in interfollicular areas

Special Stains and Immunohistochemistry
- Regressed follicles contain an increased number of CD21-positive, CD23-positive follicular dendritic cell meshworks
- Plasma cell variant may contain monotypic plasma cells, usually of IgGλ or IgAλ isotype (up to half of the cases)
- Plasmablastic type contains IgMλ–restricted atypical large cells
  - Interfollicular plasma cells are polytypic

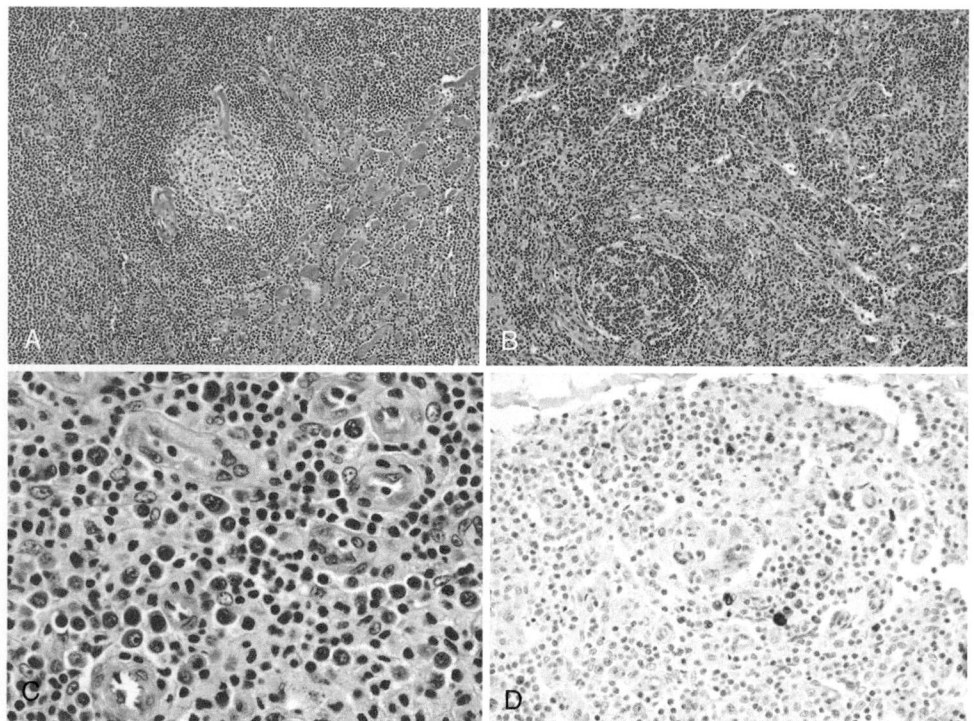

Figure 14-19. Castleman disease. A, Hyaline-vascular type with an atrophic "lollipop" follicle, expanded mantle zone and hyalinized, hypervascular interfollicular area. **B,** Plasma cell type with a regressed follicle and numerous interfollicular plasma cells. **C,** Plasmablastic type with large, atypical-appearing plasmablasts. **D,** HHV-8 immunostain highlights the plasmablasts.

- Up to 40% of patients with multicentric disease (and ~100% of HIV patients) have expression of HHV-8 (Figure 14-19D)
  - Patients with unicentric disease rarely, if ever, have staining with HHV-8 antibody

Other Techniques for Diagnosis

- Elevated serum levels of Il-6
- Tissue PCR for HHV-8
- IgH gene rearrangement shows no evidence of B-cell clonality

DIFFERENTIAL DIAGNOSIS

- Large B-cell lymphoma arising in HHV8-associated multicentric Castleman disease
  - May represent progression of plasmablastic Castleman disease
  - The lymph node architecture is effaced due to large sheets of plasmablast-like cells that express IgMλ
  - IgH gene rearrangement studies reveal a monoclonal population
- Nonspecific follicular hyperplasia
  - Regressed follicles with "onion skin" mantle zones may be part of nonspecific reactive follicular hyperplasia
  - HHV-8 is negative
- HIV-associated lymphadenopathy
  - Late-stage HIV is characterized by follicular regression
  - Follicles have attenuated mantle zones and do not show onion-skin or lollipop appearance
  - The interfollicular areas appear depleted with a decrease of CD4-positive T cells and an increase of plasma cells and histiocytes
  - No evidence of HHV-8 expression

- Low-grade B-cell lymphoma
  - Expanded mantle zones may raise the possibility of mantle cell lymphoma
  - Atrophic hyalinized follicles may be reminiscent of follicular lymphoma
  - Immunophenotyping and presence of typical cytogenetic abnormalities [t(11;14) and t(14;18) respectively] help in this differential diagnosis
- Angioimmunoblastic T-cell lymphoma
  - May resemble hyaline-vascular Castleman disease due to presence of regressed germinal centers, expanded follicular dendritic cell meshworks, lymphoid depletion, and marked proliferation of high endothelial venules
  - Morphologic evidence of atypical small to medium-sized lymphocytes with clear cytoplasm
  - Tumor cells are CD4-positive T cells that coexpress CD10, Bcl-6, PD-1, and CXCL13
- Thymoma
  - Hyaline-vascular follicles resemble Hassall corpuscles
  - The epithelial cells in thymoma are easily highlighted by cytokeratin immunostains
- Autoimmune lymphadenopathy
  - May have sheets of interfollicular plasma cells
  - Clinical correlation is recommended to make this distinction
- IgG4-positive lymphadenopathy
  - Type I (multicentric Castleman disease–like) has hyperplastic and regressed follicles with interfollicular vascular proliferation
  - Characterized by a significant increase in IgG4-positive plasma cells
  - Does not express HHV-8 or have serum elevation of IL-6 or C-reactive protein

- Plasma cell neoplasm
  - Characterized by a marked interfollicular expansion due to a plasma cell proliferation
  - The lymphoid follicles do not have features of Castleman disease
  - Plasma cells are monoclonal, most commonly of IgGκ isotype

PEARLS

- *Hyaline-vascular type is the most common form of disease and is almost invariably localized and HHV-8-negative*
- *Plasma cell type may be localized or multicentric and is frequently associated with HIV and HHV-8 infection*
- *Whereas unicentric disease is indolent, multicentric disease may be rapidly progressive and even fatal*
- *HHV-8-negative Castleman disease is a diagnosis of exclusion*

SELECTED REFERENCES

Bower M, Newsom-Davis T, Naresh K, et al: Clinical features and outcome in HIV-associated multicentric Castleman's disease. J Clin Oncol 29:2481, 2011.

Dargent JL, Lespagnard L, Sirtaine N, et al: Plasmablastic microlymphoma occurring in human herpesvirus 8 (HHV-8)-positive multicentric Castleman's disease and featuring a follicular growth pattern. APMIS 115:869, 2007.

Du MQ, Liu H, Diss TC, et al: Kaposi sarcoma-associated herpesvirus infects monotypic (IgM lambda) but polyclonal naive B cells in Castleman disease and associated lymphoproliferative disorders. Blood 97:2130, 2001.

Powles T, Stebbing J, Bazeos A, et al: The role of immune suppression and HHV-8 in the increasing incidence of HIV-associated multicentric Castleman's disease. Ann Oncol 20:775, 2009.

Talat N, Schulte KM: Castleman's disease: systematic analysis of 416 patients from the literature. Oncologist 16:1316, 2011.

SMALL B-CELL NEOPLASMS

SMALL LYMPHOCYTIC LYMPHOMA/ CHRONIC LYMPHOCYTIC LEUKEMIA (SLL/CLL)

Clinical Features

- Most common adult leukemia in Western countries
- Median age at diagnosis is 70 years

- Most patients present with painless generalized lymphadenopathy with peripheral blood and bone marrow involvement
- Monoclonal B cell lymphocytosis invariably precedes the onset of CLL

Histopathology

- Lymph node architecture is effaced due to a diffuse proliferation of small lymphocytes (Figure 14-20A)
- Lymphocytes have round nuclei with condensed chromatin, inconspicuous nucleoli, and scant cytoplasm
- Proliferation centers are characteristic; these are pale nodular areas composed of a mixture of small, medium-sized (prolymphocytes), and large lymphoid cells (paraimmunoblasts) (Figure 14-20B)
- Rare cases have plasmacytic differentiation

Special Stains and Immunohistochemistry

- Flow cytometry has characteristic features with dim CD20, CD5, CD23, absent FMC-7 and dim monoclonal light chain expression
- Immunohistochemistry: tumor cells aberrantly express CD5 and CD23
- Tumor cells do not express CD10, Bcl-6, or Cyclin D1

Other Techniques for Diagnosis

- PCR: monoclonal IGH gene rearrangement in the majority of cases
- ~80% of cases have cytogenetic abnormalities by FISH
  - Most common chromosomal abnormalities are: deletion 13q14, trisomy 12, deletion 11q22, and deletion 17p13

Differential Diagnosis

FOLLICULAR LYMPHOMA

- Prominent follicular architecture with well-defined abnormal follicles
- The neoplastic cells are a mixture of centrocytes and centroblasts
- Tumor cells express germinal center markers CD10 and Bcl-6 and are negative for CD5
- Flow cytometry: bright CD20 and light chain expression
- Conventional karyotype and FISH: t(14;18); *BCL2/IGH* gene rearrangement

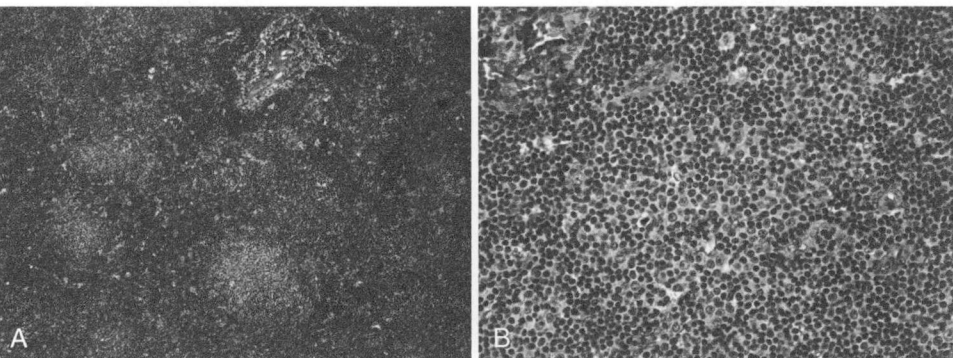

Figure 14-20. CLL. A, Lymph node architecture is effaced with sheets of small lymphocytes and several pale-staining proliferation centers. **B,** Proliferation center is composed of a mixture of small lymphocytes, prolymphocytes, and paraimmunoblasts.

MANTLE CELL LYMPHOMA
- May have a diffuse pattern similar to CLL
- Small cells with irregular nuclei (centrocyte-like)
- No evidence of proliferation centers
- Flow cytometry: tumor cells express bright CD5, CD20, FMC7, and light chain and are negative for CD23
- Immunohistochemistry: Cyclin D1 is positive
- Conventional karyotype and FISH: t(11;14); *IGH/CCND1* gene rearrangement

MARGINAL ZONE LYMPHOMA
- Rare in lymph node
- Tumor cells usually surround reactive lymphoid follicles
- Neoplastic cells are composed of monocytoid B cells (marginal zone B cells) with abundant pale cytoplasm, admixed with plasma cells and scattered immunoblasts
- Prominent plasma cell differentiation may be seen
- Flow cytometry: bright CD20 and monoclonal light chain expression
- Immunohistochemistry: tumor cells are negative for CD5 and CD23
- Conventional karyotype and FISH: trisomy 3, 7, and 18 may be seen in a small subset of cases

DIFFUSE LARGE B-CELL LYMPHOMA (DLBCL)
- Occasional cases of CLL have an increased number of large cells or expanded proliferation centers
- DLBCL contains sheets of large cells, whereas in CLL the large cells are always admixed with intermediate-sized and small lymphocytes
- Five percent to 10% of patients with CLL progress to DLBCL (Richter syndrome)

PEARLS

- *CLL refers to peripheral blood and bone marrow involvement, and SLL represents nodal involvement by the same disease process*
- *Expression of CD38, ZAP70, and p53 has prognostic significance and may influence treatment*
- *CLL cells have slow growth, thus FISH is more informative than conventional karyotype*
- *Rare cases of CLL have dim expression of Cyclin D1 in the proliferation centers; these cases do not have t(11;14) translocation and should not be classified as mantle cell lymphoma*

SELECTED REFERENCES

Gradowski JF, Sargent RL, Craig FE, et al: Chronic lymphocytic leukemia/small lymphocytic lymphoma with cyclin D1 positive proliferation centers do not have CCND1 translocations or gains and lack SOX11 expression. Am J Clin Pathol 138:132-139, 2012.

Landgren O, Albitar M, Ma W, et al: B-cell clones as early markers for chronic lymphocytic leukemia. N Engl J Med 360:659-667, 2009.

O'Malley DP, Vance GH, Orazi A: Chronic lymphocytic leukemia/small lymphocytic lymphoma with trisomy 12 and focal cyclin d1 expression: a potential diagnostic pitfall. Arch Pathol Lab Med 129:92-95, 2005.

Rawstron AC, Bennett FL, O'Connor SJ, et al: Monoclonal B-cell lymphocytosis and chronic lymphocytic leukemia. N Engl J Med 359:575-583, 2008.

Rossi D, Rasi S, Spina V, et al: Integrated mutational and cytogenetic analysis identifies new prognostic subgroups in chronic lymphocytic leukemia. Blood 121:1403-1412, 2013.

FOLLICULAR LYMPHOMA (FL)

Clinical Features
- One of the most common lymphomas in the United States and Europe
- The median age is 60 years
- Most patients present with painless peripheral adenopathy in the cervical, axillary, inguinal, or femoral regions
- Liver, spleen, and bone marrow involvement is present in >50% of the patients
- Pediatric FL is very rare and tends to present with limited stage disease
- Occasional patients have primary extranodal FL (duodenum, breast, skin, and other sites)
- Variable clinical course: some patients have indolent stable disease for many years, whereas others progress rapidly and require treatment

Histopathology
- Closely packed follicles efface the lymph node architecture (Figure 14-21A)
  - Rarely, the infiltrate is follicular and diffuse or predominantly diffuse
- Mantle zones are attenuated or absent
- Follicles appear homogeneous and consist of a mixture of small cleaved lymphocytes (centrocytes) and large lymphoid cells with round nuclei and several small nucleoli (centroblasts)
- Tingible-body macrophages are absent
- The neoplastic infiltrate frequently splits the lymph node capsule and may extend into the perinodal soft tissue
- FL is graded according to the number of centroblasts counted per high-power (40×) field
  - Grade 1 (low-grade): 0 to 5 centroblasts per high-power field (Figure 14-21B)
  - Grade 2 (low-grade): 6 to 15 centroblasts per high-power field (Figure 14-21C)
  - Grade 3 (high-grade): >15 centroblasts per high-power field (Figure 14-21D)
    - Grade 3A contains a mixture of centrocytes and centroblasts
    - Grade 3B contains sheets of centroblasts
- If there is a diffuse area composed predominantly of centroblasts, a separate diagnosis of diffuse large B-cell lymphoma should be made

Special Stains and Immunohistochemistry
- Flow cytometry: bright CD20+ B lymphocytes with CD10 expression and monotypic light chain restriction
- Immunohistochemistry: neoplastic lymphoid cells co-express Bcl-2, Bcl-6, and CD10
  - Bcl-2 may be negative in ~10% of low-grade FL and up to 50% of high-grade FL
  - Some (usually high-grade) cases lack CD10; however, they retain Bcl-6
- Mum-1 is negative in low-grade FL but may be expressed in grade 3 FL
- CD21 and CD23 highlight the follicular dendritic cell meshworks
- Ki67 proliferative fraction typically correlates with grading (<20% in low-grade FL and >20% in high-grade FL)

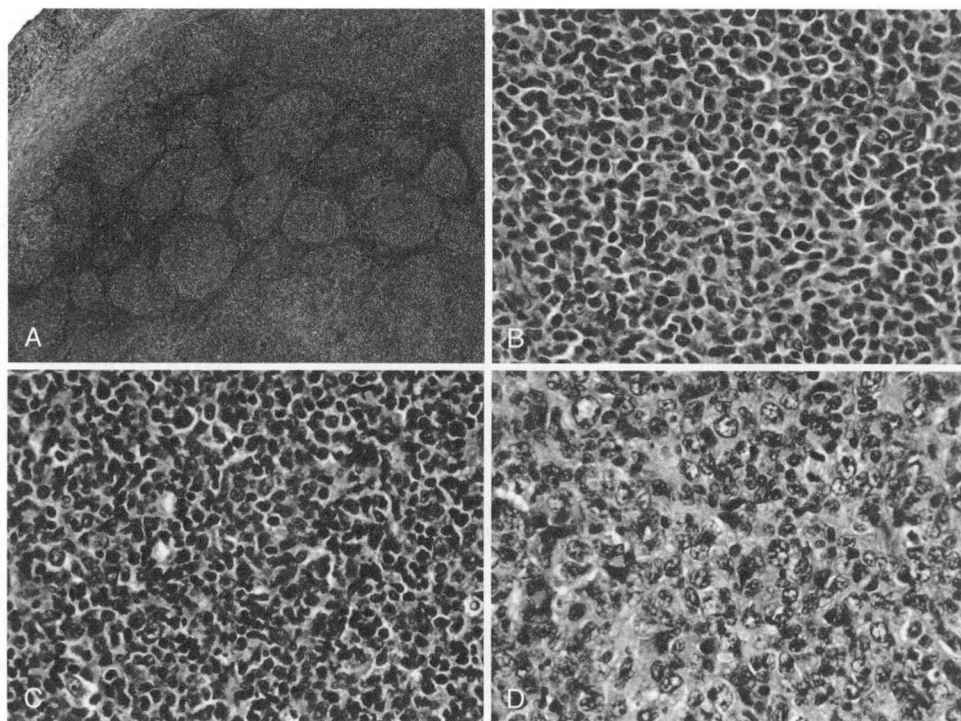

Figure 14-21. Follicular lymphoma.
A, Lymph node architecture is effaced with numerous closely packed follicles. **B,** Follicular lymphoma grade 1. **C,** Follicular lymphoma grade 2. **D,** Follicular lymphoma grade 3.

Other Techniques for Diagnosis

- Conventional karyotype, FISH, and PCR: t(14;18); *BCL2/IGH* gene rearrangement in up to 90% of low-grade FL
- BCL6 gene rearrangement in 5% to 15%, usually present in grade 3B FL
- PCR: monoclonal IGH gene rearrangement in ~80% of cases

Differential Diagnosis

REACTIVE FOLLICULAR HYPERPLASIA

- Lymph node architecture is preserved: capsule is thin, sinuses are patent
- Lymphoid follicles are heterogeneous in size and shape
- Mantle zone is present and well-defined
- Cellular composition within the follicles is heterogeneous with tingible-body macrophages
- Well-defined light and dark zones within germinal centers can be seen
- Lymphoid cells in the follicles express Bcl-6 and CD10, but not Bcl-2
- Proliferation rate within the follicles with Ki67 immunostain is > 90%
- Flow cytometry reveals polytypic B lymphocytes
- PCR for IgH gene rearrangement is polyclonal
- Cytogenetic analysis shows a normal karyotype and no evidence of t(14;18) translocation

MANTLE CELL LYMPHOMA

- May have a nodular pattern similar to FL
- Small cells with irregular nuclei (centrocyte-like); no evidence of centroblasts

- Flow cytometry: tumor cells express CD5, CD20, and light chain and are negative for CD10
- Immunohistochemistry: CD10 and Bcl-6 are negative; CD5 and Cyclin D1 are positive
- Conventional karyotype and FISH: t(11;14); *IGH/CCND1* gene rearrangement

MARGINAL ZONE LYMPHOMA

- Rare in lymph nodes
- Tumor cells usually surround reactive lymphoid follicles
- Neoplastic cells are composed of monocytoid B cells (marginal zone B cells) with abundant pale cytoplasm, admixed with plasma cells and scattered immunoblasts
- Prominent plasma cell differentiation may be seen
- Flow cytometry: bright CD20 and monoclonal light chain expression
- Immunohistochemistry: tumor cells are negative for CD5, CD10, Bcl-6, CD23, Cyclin D1
- Conventional karyotype and FISH: trisomy 3, 7, and 18 may be seen in a small subset

CLL/SLL

- Proliferation centers may resemble neoplastic follicles
- Tumor cells have round nuclei; prolymphocytes and paraimmunoblasts have large central nucleoli
- Flow cytometry: B lymphocytes express CD5, CD23, and have dim CD20 and dim monoclonal light chain expression
- Immunohistochemistry: tumor cells are negative for CD10 and Bcl-6; no abnormal follicles highlighted with CD21 and CD23
- Conventional karyotype and FISH: deletion 13q14, trisomy 12, deletion 11q22, and deletion 17p13 are common abnormalities

DIFFUSE LARGE B-CELL LYMPHOMA (DLBCL)

- May coexist with FL in the same lymph node or represent disease progression in patients with known FL
- DLBCL contains diffuse sheets of large transformed lymphoid cells; there is no evidence of follicular architecture
- CD21 and CD23 are negative in the areas involved by DLBCL

PEARLS

- *When grading, care should be taken to distinguish centroblasts from follicular dendritic cells (large cells with cleared-out chromatin and small or absent nucleoli)*
- *FL grade 1 and FL grade 2 have a similar clinical behavior and are grouped together as low-grade, clinically indolent FL*
- *FL grade 3A and FL grade 3B may represent different entities, with 3B FL being more akin to DLBCL, although this is still controversial*
- *Final diagnosis should mention the different components of lymphoma (i.e., grades 1 and 2 versus grade 3 versus DLBCL) and provide percentage of lymph node involvement by each pattern*
- *Staining with CD21 and CD23 is essential to rule out DLBCL in cases of high-grade FL*
- *Approximately 10% of nodal FL do not harbor the translocation t(14;18) and do not express Bcl-2 protein; these cases are enriched with postgerminal center signature genes by gene expression profiling, but they also show many similarities to conventional germinal center-derived FL*

SELECTED REFERENCES

Díaz-Alderete A, Doval A, Camacho F, et al: Frequency of BCL2 and BCL6 translocations in follicular lymphoma: relation with histological and clinical features. Leuk Lymphoma 49:95, 2008.

Horn H, Schmelter C, Leich E, et al: Follicular lymphoma grade 3B is a distinct neoplasm according to cytogenetic and immunohistochemical profiles. Haematologica 96:1327-1334, 2011.

Karube K, Guo Y, Suzumiya J, et al: CD10-MUM1+ follicular lymphoma lacks BCL2 gene translocation and shows characteristic biologic and clinical features. Blood 109:3076, 2007.

Leich E, Salaverria I, Bea S, et al: Follicular lymphomas with and without translocation t(14;18) differ in gene expression profiles and genetic alterations. Blood 114:826, 2009.

Louissaint A Jr, Ackerman AM, Dias-Santagata D, et al: Pediatric-type nodal follicular lymphoma: an indolent clonal proliferation in children and adults with high proliferation index and no BCL2 rearrangement. Blood 120:2395, 2012.

Misdraji J, Harris NL, Hasserjian RP, et al: Primary follicular lymphoma of the gastrointestinal tract. Am J Surg Pathol 35:1255-1263, 2011.

Schmatz AI, Streubel B, Kretschmer-Chott E, et al: Primary follicular lymphoma of the duodenum is a distinct mucosal/submucosal variant of follicular lymphoma: a retrospective study of 63 cases. J Clin Oncol 29:1445, 2011.

Wahlin BE, Yri OE, Kimby E, et al: Clinical significance of the WHO grades of follicular lymphoma in a population-based cohort of 505 patients with long follow-up times. Br J Haematol 156:225, 2012.

MANTLE CELL LYMPHOMA (MCL)

Clinical Features

- Occurs more commonly in Caucasian men
- Median age at diagnosis is 68 years
- Most patients present with advanced stage disease with lymphadenopathy, hepatosplenomegaly, peripheral blood, and bone marrow involvement
- May involve any region of the gastrointestinal tract (lymphomatous polyposis)
- Generally incurable lymphoma with a median survival of 3 to 4 years
- A subset of the patients have peripheral blood, bone marrow, and spleen involvement without lymphadenopathy; they appear to have an indolent clinical course

Histopathology

- Lymph node architecture is effaced with a vaguely nodular, diffuse, mantle zone or follicular lymphoid proliferation (Figure 14-22A)
- Small to medium-sized lymphoid cells with irregular nuclear shape (centrocytes-like)
- Hyalinized small vessels
- Scattered epithelioid histiocytes devoid of phagocytized nuclear debris (Figure 14-22B)
- Blastoid variant: tumor cells have finely dispersed chromatin with many mitoses (>20 to 30/10 high power fields); is associated with more aggressive behavior
- Pleomorphic variant: larger and pleomorphic cells including cells with prominent nucleoli
- Mitotic rate of >10 to 40/15 high-power fields is an adverse prognostic factor

Special Stains and Immunohistochemistry

- Flow cytometry: B lymphocytes express CD5, CD43, FMC-7, and bright monotypic light chain restriction; tumor cells are negative for CD10 and CD23
- Immunohistochemistry: neoplastic lymphoid cells express Cyclin D1—a diagnostic hallmark of the tumor (Figure 14-22C)
- SOX11, a neuronal transcription factor, has been recently identified as a relatively specific marker of MCL
- Ki67 proliferation rate of >40% to 60% is an adverse prognostic factor

Other Techniques for Diagnosis

- Conventional karyotype and FISH: t(11;14); *IGH/CCND1* gene rearrangement
- PCR: clonal IGH gene rearrangement in the majority of cases

Differential Diagnosis

CLL/SLL

- Proliferation centers may resemble neoplastic nodules of MCL
- Tumor cells have round nuclei; prolymphocytes and paraimmunoblasts have large central nucleoli
- Flow cytometry: B lymphocytes express CD5, CD23, and have dim CD20 and dim monoclonal light chain expression; FMC-7 is negative
- Immunohistochemistry: tumor cells are negative for Cyclin D1
- Conventional karyotype and FISH: deletion 13q14, trisomy 12, deletion 11q22, and deletion 17p13 are common abnormalities

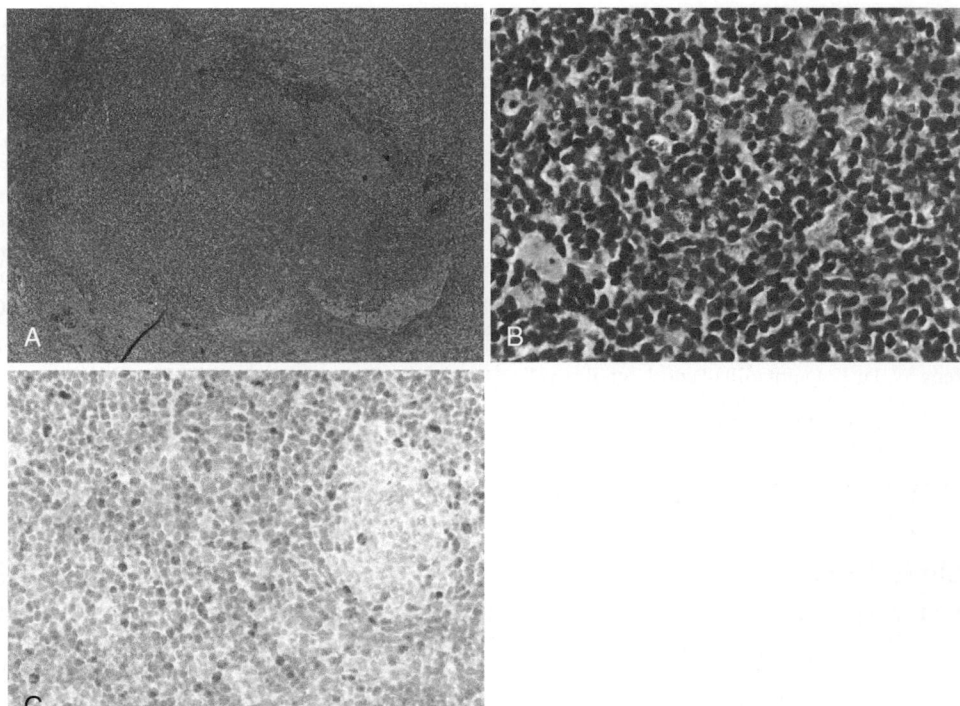

Figure 14-22. Mantle cell lymphoma. A, Vaguely nodular lymphoid proliferation. **B,** Small lymphocytes and scattered epithelioid histiocytes. **C,** Cyclin D1 immunostain is strongly positive in the neoplastic lymphocytes.

FOLLICULAR LYMPHOMA
- Prominent follicular architecture with well-defined abnormal follicles
- The neoplastic cells are a mixture of centrocytes and centroblasts
- Tumor cells express germinal center markers CD10 and Bcl-6 and are negative for CD5 and Cyclin D1
- Flow cytometry: bright CD20, CD10, and bright light chain expression
- Conventional karyotype and FISH: t(14;18); *BCL2/IGH* gene rearrangement

MARGINAL ZONE LYMPHOMA
- Rare in lymph nodes
- Tumor cells usually surround reactive lymphoid follicles
- Neoplastic cells are composed of monocytoid B cells (marginal zone B cells) with abundant pale cytoplasm, admixed with plasma cells and scattered immunoblasts
- Prominent plasma cell differentiation may be seen
- Flow cytometry: bright CD20 and monoclonal light chain expression
- Immunohistochemistry: tumor cells are negative for CD5, CD10, BCL-6, CD23, Cyclin D1
- Conventional karyotype and FISH: trisomy 3, 7, and 18 may be seen in a small subset

LYMPHOBLASTIC LYMPHOMA
- May resemble blastoid variant of MCL
- Neoplastic cells express immature markers (CD34, TdT, CD10), are negative for Cyclin D1 and CD20 and don't express immunoglobulin light chains

DIFFUSE LARGE B-CELL LYMPHOMA (DLBCL)
- May resemble blastoid or pleomorphic variant of MCL

- DLBCL contains sheets of large cells, whereas in MCL the neoplastic cells are intermediate-sized or small; pleomorphic variant of MCL may morphologically overlap with DLBCL
- Do not express Cyclin D1 (with very rare exceptions, see reference)
- Conventional karyotype and FISH: highly complex karyotype with no evidence of t(11;14); *IGH/CCND1* gene rearrangement

PEARLS

- *More aggressive than other small B-cell lymphomas*
- *Rare cases may lack CD5 expression or may express CD23 or CD10, thus Cyclin D1 should be performed on all cases of presumed low-grade B-cell lymphoma*
- *Very rare cases may lack Cyclin D1 expression and t(11;14) translocation; these cases are positive for SOX11 and should be categorized as MCL*
- *Cases of predominantly non-nodal, splenomegalic leukemic MCL may correspond to a different molecular subtype of MCL with a long indolent clinical course*

SELECTED REFERENCES

Dictor M, Ek S, Sundberg M, et al: Strong lymphoid nuclear expression of SOX11 transcription factor defines lymphoblastic neoplasms, mantle cell lymphoma and Burkitt's lymphoma. Haematologica 94:1563-1568, 2009.

Jares P, Colomer D, Campo E: Molecular pathogenesis of mantle cell lymphoma. J Clin Invest 122:3416-3423, 2012.

Mozos A, Royo C, Hartmann E, et al; SOX11 expression is highly specific for mantle cell lymphoma and identifies the cyclin D1-negative subtype. Haematologica 94:1555-1562, 2009.

Ondrejka SL, Lai R, Smith SD, Hsi ED: Indolent mantle cell leukemia: clinicopathologic variant characterized by isolated lymphocytosis, interstitial bone marrow involvement, kappa light chain restriction, and good prognosis. Haematologica 96:1121-1127, 2011.

Royo C, Navarro A, Clot G, et al: Non-nodal type of mantle cell lymphoma is a specific biological and clinical subgroup of the disease. Leukemia 26:1895-1898, 2012.

Tiemann M, Schrader C, Klapper W, et al: Histopathology, cell proliferation indices and clinical outcome in 304 patients with mantle cell lymphoma (MCL): a clinicopathological study from the European MCL Network. Br J Haematol 131:29-38, 2005.

Vela-Chávez T, Adam P, Kremer M, et al: Cyclin D1 positive diffuse large B-cell lymphoma is a post-germinal center-type lymphoma without alterations in the CCND1 gene locus. Leuk Lymphoma 52:458-466, 2011.

Zeng W, Fu K, Quintanilla-Fend L, et al: Cyclin D1-negative blastoid mantle cell lymphoma identified by SOX11 expression. Am J Surg Pathol 36:214-219, 2012.

NODAL MARGINAL ZONE LYMPHOMA (MZL)

Clinical Features

- Primary nodal MZL is a rare lymphoma
  - Most cases represent nodal involvement by extranodal MALT lymphoma
- Similar proportion of men and women
- Median age at diagnosis is 60 years
- Most patients have asymptomatic lymphadenopathy and advanced stage disease at presentation

Histopathology

- Tumor cells usually surround reactive lymphoid follicles (Figure 14-23A)
- Follicular colonization is frequently seen
- Neoplastic cells are composed of monocytoid B cells (also called marginal zone B cells) with abundant pale cytoplasm, admixed with plasma cells and scattered immunoblasts (Figure 14-23B)
- Prominent plasma cell differentiation may be seen (although less common than in extranodal MALT-type lymphomas)

Special Stains and Immunohistochemistry

- Flow cytometry: bright CD20 and monoclonal light chain expression
- Immunohistochemistry: tumor cells are negative for CD5, CD10, Bcl-6, CD23, Cyclin D1
- Tumor cells express CD43 in ~50% and BCL2 in most cases

- CD21 and CD23 show expanded and colonized follicular dendritic cell meshworks
- Plasma cells express monotypic immunoglobulin light chain in cases with plasmacytic differentiation

OTHER TECHNIQUES FOR DIAGNOSIS

- Cytogenetics: trisomy 3, 7, and 18 may be seen in a small subset of cases
- PCR: monoclonal IgH gene rearrangement

Differential Diagnosis

REACTIVE LYMPH NODE WITH MONOCYTOID B-CELL HYPERPLASIA

- Morphologic distinction can be difficult
- Immunohistochemistry: reactive monocytoid B cells are negative for Bcl-2, whereas neoplastic cells are usually positive
- Plasma cells may be increased in number but are always polyclonal
- PCR shows no evidence of IgH gene rearrangement

CLL/SLL

- Proliferation centers are not a feature of MZL
- Prominent plasma cell differentiation is very unusual in CLL
- Tumor cells have round nuclei, prolymphocytes and paraimmunoblasts have large central nucleoli
- Flow cytometry: B lymphocytes express CD5, CD23, and have dim CD20 and dim monoclonal light chain expression; FMC-7 is negative
- Immunohistochemistry: tumor cells express CD5 and CD23; no evidence of follicular dendritic cell meshworks
- Cytogenetics: deletion 13q14, trisomy 12, deletion 11q22, and deletion 17p13 are common abnormalities

FOLLICULAR LYMPHOMA

- Cases of MZL with prominent follicular colonization may appear virtually indistinguishable from FL
- Cases of FL may also have marginal zone differentiation with numerous monocytoid B cells surrounding the neoplastic follicles
- In FL, the neoplastic cells are a mixture of centrocytes and centroblasts
- Tumor cells express germinal center markers CD10 and Bcl-6, whereas neoplastic cells in MZL do not express germinal center antigens

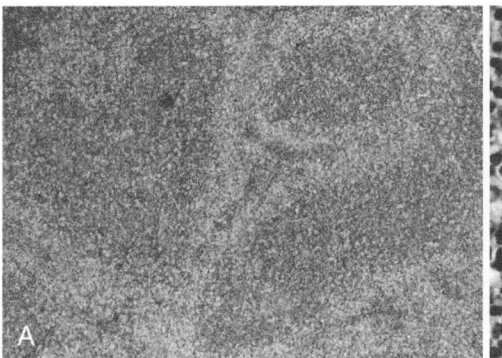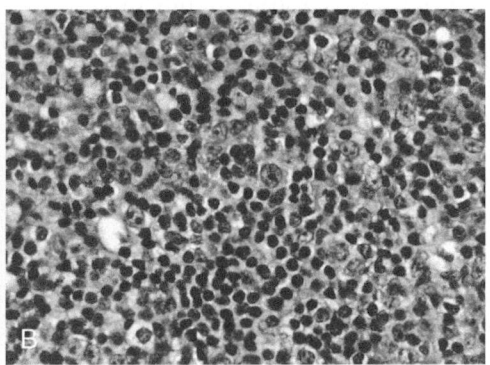

Figure 14-23. Nodal marginal zone lymphoma. A, Neoplastic lymphocytes surround and colonize residual follicles. **B,** Small lymphocytes, plasma cells, and immunoblasts.

- Flow cytometry: neoplastic B cells coexpress CD10 (CD10 is always negative in MZL)
- Conventional karyotype and FISH: t(14;18); *BCL2/IGH* gene rearrangement

MANTLE CELL LYMPHOMA

- May have a mantle zone growth around reactive follicles, similar to MZL
- Does not show plasmacytic differentiation
- Small cells with irregular nuclei (centrocyte-like)
- Flow cytometry: tumor cells express CD5, CD20, and light chain
- Immunohistochemistry: CD5 and Cyclin D1 are positive
- Conventional karyotype and FISH: t(11;14); *IGH/CCND1* gene rearrangement

LYMPHOPLASMACYTIC LYMPHOMA (LPL)

- Distinction between these entities is very problematic
- LPL generally arises in the bone marrow and has high levels of serum IgM with hyperviscosity, whereas MZL generally presents with lymphadenopathy and is rarely associated with hyperviscosity
- LPL classically shows retention of the architecture with dilated sinuses, whereas MZL more typically has monocytoid cellular morphology, a marginal zone growth pattern, and follicular colonization
- Mutations in *MYD88* gene have been found in the large majority of LPLs but are rare in MZLs

DIFFUSE LARGE B-CELL LYMPHOMA

- May arise from a preexisting MZL
- DLBCL contains large sheets of large cells, whereas in MZL the large neoplastic cells are admixed with small lymphocytes

PEARLS

- *MZL does not have a characteristic immunophenotypic abnormality or translocation and thus is a diagnosis of exclusion*
- *Extranodal MZL frequently has specific translocations involving BCL10 and MALT1 genes, which have not been reported in nodal MZL*
- *Primary nodal MZL and nodal involvement by extranodal MALT lymphoma are morphologically similar*
  - *Monocytoid morphology and plasma cell differentiation are more typical of extranodal MALT lymphoma*
- *Patients with Sjögren syndrome and Hashimoto thyroiditis are much more likely to have extranodal mucosa associated lymphoid tissue (MALT) lymphoma presenting in lymph node*
- *Occasionally, exact diagnosis cannot be made after a careful examination and diagnosis of "low-grade B-cell lymphoma with plasmacytic differentiation" is warranted*

SELECTED REFERENCES

Krijgsman O, Gonzalez P, Balague Ponz O, et al: Dissecting the grey zone between follicular lymphoma and marginal zone lymphoma using morphological and genetic features. Haematologica 98:1921-1929, 2013.

Molina TJ, Lin P, Swerdlow SH, Cook JR: Marginal zone lymphomas with plasmacytic differentiation and related disorders. Am J Clin Pathol 136:211-225, 2011.

Naresh KN: Nodal marginal zone B-cell lymphoma with prominent follicular colonization—difficulties in diagnosis: a study of 15 cases. Histopathology 52:331-339, 2008.

Salama ME, Lossos IS, Warnke RA, Natkunam Y: Immunoarchitectural patterns in nodal marginal zone B-cell lymphoma: a study of 51 cases. Am J Clin Pathol 132:39-49, 2009.

Traverse-Glehen A, Bertoni F, Thieblemont C, et al: Nodal marginal zone B-cell lymphoma: a diagnostic and therapeutic dilemma. Oncology (Williston Park) 26:92-99, 2012.

van den Brand M, van Krieken JH: Recognizing nodal marginal zone lymphoma: recent advances and pitfalls: a systematic review. Haematologica 98:1003-1013, 2013.

LYMPHOPLASMACYTIC LYMPHOMA (LPL)

Clinical Features

- Rare lymphoma that occurs in adults with a median age of 60 years
- Majority of patients have a circulating monoclonal IgM that often leads to a hyperviscosity syndrome (Waldenström macroglobulinemia)
- Most patients present with weakness and fatigue, due to anemia
- Some patients have neuropathy, autoimmune manifestations, or cryoglobulinemia
- LPL is a bone marrow-based disease and lymphadenopathy is uncommon

Histopathology

- Lymph node architecture is frequently preserved
- The neoplastic infiltrate is composed of small lymphocytes, plasma cells, and plasmacytoid cells (Figure 14-24)
- Variable number of immunoblasts
- Sinuses are often open and may contain histiocytes containing periodic acid-Schiff (PAS)–positive immunoglobulin
- Other typical characteristics are Dutcher and Russell bodies, mast cells, and hemosiderin-laden macrophages

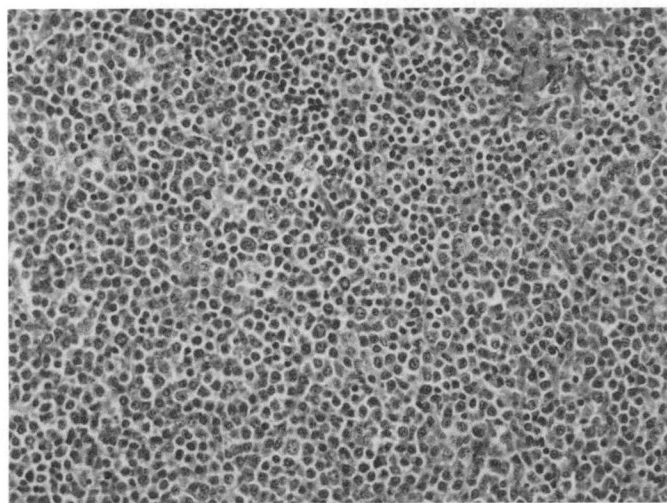

Figure 14-24. LPL. Lymphoplasmacytic lymphoma with a mixture of small lymphocytes, plasmacytoid lymphoid cells, and plasma cells. *(Courtesy of Dr. Dennis O'Malley, Clarient, Inc. Aliso Viejo, CA)*

Special Stains and Immunohistochemistry

- B lymphocytes are negative for CD5, CD10, and CD23
- Plasma cells typically are of IgM isotype and are monotypic

Other Techniques for Diagnosis

- MYD88 L265P somatic mutation is present in > 90% of cases

Differential Diagnosis

MARGINAL ZONE LYMPHOMA

- Distinction may be challenging
- LPL generally presents in the bone marrow with hyperviscosity, whereas MZL generally presents with lymphadenopathy
- LPL classically shows retention of the architecture with dilated sinuses, whereas MZL more typically has monocytoid cellular morphology, a marginal zone growth pattern, and follicular colonization
- Mutations in MYD88 gene are unusual in MZLs

PLASMACYTOMA

- May be seen in patients with known myeloma or be primary in the lymph node
- There are sheets of plasma cells surrounding residual reactive follicles
- B lymphocytes are benign and polyclonal
- Plasma cells are monoclonal

CLL/SLL

- Proliferation centers are not a feature of LPL
- Prominent plasma cell differentiation is very unusual
- Tumor cells have round nuclei, prolymphocytes and paraimmunoblasts have large central nucleoli
- Flow cytometry: B lymphocytes express CD5, CD23, and have dim CD20 and dim monoclonal light chain expression; FMC-7 is negative
- Immunohistochemistry: tumor cells express CD5 and CD23
- Cytogenetics: deletion 13q14, trisomy 12, deletion 11q22, and deletion 17p13 are common abnormalities
- Mutations in the MYD88 gene are very unusual in CLL

MANTLE CELL LYMPHOMA

- Does not show plasmacytic differentiation
- Small cells with irregular nuclei (centrocyte-like)
- Flow cytometry: tumor cells express CD5, CD20, and light chain and are negative for CD10
- Immunohistochemistry: CD10 and BCL6 are negative; CD5 and Cyclin D1 are positive
- Conventional karyotype and FISH: t(11;14); *IGH/CCND1* gene rearrangement
- No evidence of MYD88 L265P somatic mutation

PEARLS

- Waldenström macroglobulinemia *is a clinical term that refers to the presence of IgM paraprotein*
- *LPL is the most common lymphoma associated with Waldenström macroglobulinemia; however, MZL and CLL may also secrete IgM*

- *Alternatively, not all LPLs express IgM and have symptoms related to Waldenström macroglobulinemia (some secrete IgG and rarely IgA)*
- *Precise diagnosis cannot be made in the absence of complete clinical information; in such cases a diagnosis of "low-grade B-cell lymphoma with plasmacytic differentiation" is warranted*

SELECTED REFERENCES

Jiménez C, Sebastián E, Del Carmen Chillón M, et al: MYD88 L265P is a marker highly characteristic of, but not restricted to, Waldenström's macroglobulinemia. Leukemia 27:1722-1728, 2013.

Lin P, Molina TJ, Cook JR, Swerdlow SH: Lymphoplasmacytic lymphoma and other non-marginal zone lymphomas with plasmacytic differentiation. Am J Clin Pathol 136:195-210, 2011.

Treon SP, Xu L, Yang G, Zhou Y, et al: MYD88 L265P somatic mutation in Waldenström's macroglobulinemia. N Engl J Med 367:826-833, 2012.

Varettoni M, Arcaini L, Zibellini S, et al: Prevalence and clinical significance of the MYD88 (L265P) somatic mutation in Waldenstrom's macroglobulinemia and related lymphoid neoplasms. Blood 121:2522-2528, 2013.

Xu L, Hunter ZR, Yang G, et al: MYD88 L265P in Waldenström macroglobulinemia, immunoglobulin M monoclonal gammopathy, and other B-cell lymphoproliferative disorders using conventional and quantitative allele-specific polymerase chain reaction. Blood 121:2051-2058, 2013.

DIFFUSE AGGRESSIVE B-CELL LYMPHOMA

DIFFUSE LARGE B-CELL LYMPHOMA (DLBCL)

Clinical Features

- The most common subtype of lymphoma
  - Heterogeneous disease in terms of morphology, genetics, and biologic behavior
- Median age at presentation is 64 years
- Slightly more common in Caucasian males
- About 60% of patients present with advanced stage disease
- Up to 40% of patients have extranodal disease at presentation
  - Gastrointestinal tract is the most common location
  - May also involve bone, testis, spleen, thyroid, salivary glands, tonsils, skin, uterine cervix, central nervous system, and virtually any other organ
- Frequently represents transformation of a less aggressive lymphoma (i.e., CLL/SLL, MZL, FL)
- Immunosuppression is an important risk factor
  - These lymphomas are typically EBV positive
  - DLBCL is the most common lymphoma in patients with HIV, history of transplant, or primary immunodeficiency
  - EBV + DLBCL of the elderly occurs in patients > 50 years old and is believed to be associated with senescence of the immune system
- DLBCL is aggressive but is also highly curable with intensive chemotherapy

Histopathology

- Lymph node architecture is effaced by sheets of large lymphoid cells

- Cell size is assessed by comparing a tumor cell to admixed histiocytes or endothelial cells
- Tumor cell morphology is variable (Figure 14-25A,B):
  - Cells with round nuclei, several small nucleoli, and scant cytoplasm (centroblasts)
  - Cells with round nuclei, one large central nucleolus, and moderate basophilic cytoplasm (immunoblasts)
  - Cells with bizarre, multilobated nuclei
  - Medium-sized cells
- Numerous mitoses, apoptotic debris, and necrosis are common findings
- T-cell/histiocyte-rich large B-cell lymphoma (THRLBCL) has scattered large tumor cells admixed with numerous reactive small T lymphocytes or histiocytes
- EBV + DLBCL of the elderly commonly contains a polymorphous infiltrate with variably sized tumor cells and many admixed reactive cells, associated with necrosis

Special Stains and Immunohistochemistry

- Tumor cells express B-cell antigens CD20, Pax-5, CD79a, Oct-2, and Bob.1
- CD30 may be positive but is typically weak and only expressed by a subset of tumor cells
- Some cases have aberrant expression of CD5
- The neoplastic B cells have variable expression of CD10, Bcl-2, Bcl-6, and Mum-1
- Hans algorithm (CD10, Bcl-6, Mum-1) or Choi algorithm (CD10, Bcl-6, Mum-1, GCET, FoxP1) are used in some laboratories as a substitute for molecular classification of DLBCL
  - These methods are not standardized and at this point are only used in a research setting
- Proliferative fraction with Ki67 immunostain is high at > 40%
- EBV + DLBCL of the elderly: in situ hybridization for EBV-encoded RNA (EBER) stains the large neoplastic cells; these cells usually coexpress Mum-1 and are negative for CD10 and Bcl-6
- THRLBCL: B-cell antigens highlight a small number of large atypical cells, whereas the small lymphocytes correspond to CD3+ T cells

Other Techniques for Diagnosis

- Flow cytometry: may be insensitive to the presence of large tumor cells
- Cytogenetics: typically shows a highly complex karyotype
  - Presence of c-MYC translocation is an important independent risk factor for poor outcome
  - Cases with c-MYC translocation may have a concurrent IgH-BCL2 translocation or BCL6 break (double-hit lymphoma), these cases have a poor prognosis
- PCR: monoclonal IgH gene rearrangement
- Gene expression profiling is an area of active ongoing research
  - Classifies DLBCL into two groups: germinal center type (superior outcome) and activated B cell type (poor prognosis)
  - Various panels of immunohistochemical markers have been proposed to substitute for DNA microarrays; none has been proven to be entirely concordant

Differential Diagnosis

REACTIVE LYMPH NODE WITH IMMUNOBLASTIC PROLIFERATION

- Benign immunoblasts are scattered and do not form confluent sheets
- Immunoblasts express CD30 and are negative for CD15
- Other features of reactive lymph node are unfailingly present (preserved architecture, follicular hyperplasia, paracortical hyperplasia, etc.)
- No evidence of B-cell clonality with flow cytometry, cytogenetics, or PCR

SMALL B-CELL LYMPHOMA

- CLL may have large expanded proliferation centers, and distinction with DLBCL (Richter transformation) is occasionally difficult
- FL has follicular architecture, highlighted by CD21 and CD23 immunostains
- MZL and LPL frequently contain scattered large transformed lymphoid cells; these do not form confluent sheets

MANTLE CELL LYMPHOMA, BLASTOID, AND PLEOMORPHIC VARIANTS

- Tumor cells are medium sized, not large
- Neoplastic cells express CD5 and Cyclin D1
- Conventional karyotype and FISH: t(11;14); IGH/CCND1 gene rearrangement

BURKITT LYMPHOMA

- Tumor cells are medium sized, not large
- Starry-sky pattern due to very high mitotic rate
- Ki67 proliferation rate is close to 100%
- Characteristic immunophenotype: CD10+, Bcl-6+, Bcl-2-, Mum1-
- Conventional karyotype and FISH: simple karyotype with evidence of c-MYC translocation
- "Gray-zone" lymphomas exist (see section on "B-Cell Lymphoma, Unclassifiable, with Features Intermediate between DLBCL and Burkitt Lymphoma")

LYMPHOBLASTIC LYMPHOMA

- Tumor cells have finely dispersed chromatin and small nucleoli (DLBCL cells have vesicular chromatin)
- Immunophenotype is different from DLBCL with expression of immature markers CD34 and TdT
  - B-lymphoblastic lymphoma cells express CD10, Pax-5, and CD79a; they lack CD20 and light chain expression
  - T-lymphoblastic lymphoma cells express CD1a and CD99; they variably are CD4+/CD8+, CD4–/CD8– or, rarely express only CD4 or CD8

ANAPLASTIC LARGE CELL LYMPHOMA

- May morphologically mimic anaplastic DLBCL
- Immunophenotype is different from DLBCL with lack of B-cell antigen expression
  - DLBCL cells may rarely express CD30 or ALK1
- No evidence of a monoclonal B-cell population by flow cytometry or PCR

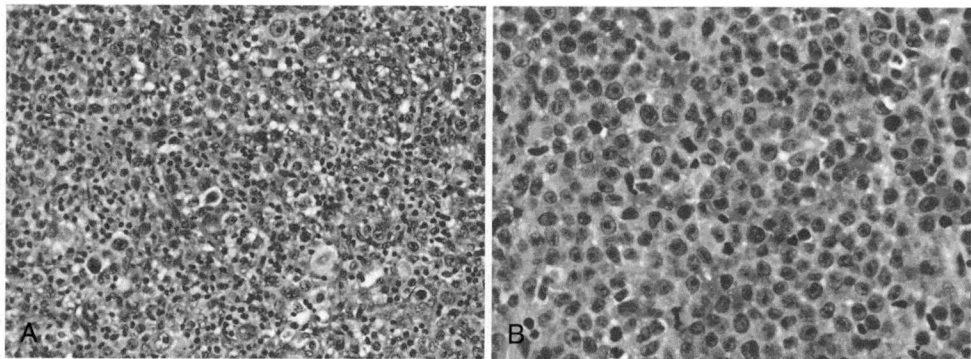

Figure 14-25. DLBCL. **A,** Numerous large cells with vesicular chromatin, irregular nuclei, and one to several nucleoli. **B,** Sheets of immunoblasts.

CLASSICAL HODGKIN LYMPHOMA (CHL)

- May morphologically mimic anaplastic DLBCL
- CHL contains Reed-Sternberg cells admixed with numerous reactive inflammatory cells
- Reed-Sternberg cells are usually scattered and do not form confluent sheets (exception: syncytial variant of nodular sclerosis CHL)
- Immunophenotype is different from DLBCL, with expression of CD30, CD15, weak Pax-5, and lack of CD20
  - Reed-Sternberg cells express either Oct-2 or Bob.1, but not both
- "Gray-zone" lymphomas with intermediate morphology and immunophenotype do, however, exist, especially in the mediastinum
- Nodular lymphocyte-predominant Hodgkin lymphoma (NLPHL)
- Typically present as a localized lymphadenopathy in a young male
- May have a similar appearance to THRLBCL
- THRLBCL may represent disease progression in patients with known NLPHL
- CD21 and CD23 help highlight the expanded nodular architecture in NLPHL
- Large neoplastic cells express CD20, Pax-5, CD79a, and Bcl-6 and are ringed by CD3+, CD57+, PD-1+ T lymphocytes
  - About 50% of cases have EMA expression
- At present, an overlap between the two entities cannot be entirely excluded

METASTATIC NEOPLASM

- The patient usually has a history of a preexisting neoplasm (but not always)
- Morphologic mimics include poorly differentiated carcinoma, melanoma, germ cell tumor, and sarcoma
- An extensive panel of immunohistochemical stains is required for diagnosis
  - CD45, CD20, Pax-5, and CD3 are negative in the large tumor cells
  - Neoplastic cells may express cytokeratins, S-100, HMB-45, MITF1, CD99, Fli1, PLAP, and Oct-4

MYELOID SARCOMA

- The patient usually has a history of preexisting acute myeloid leukemia, myelodysplastic syndrome, or myeloproliferative neoplasm (but not always)
- May appear morphologically identical to DLBCL

- Immunophenotype is very different from DLBCL, with lack of B-cell antigen expression
  - Tumor cells express blast and myeloid cell markers: CD34, CD117, MPO, lysozyme, CD68, CD43
- No evidence of a monoclonal B-cell population by flow cytometry or PCR

PEARLS

- *Numerous immunohistochemical markers have been proposed for use as prognostic indicators; most are being studied in a research setting and are not used in routine clinical practice*
- *Expression of CD30 in DLBCL may become clinically important with increasing use of anti-CD30 antibody-drug conjugate brentuximab vedotin*
- *Rare cases have features intermediate between DLBCL and Burkitt lymphoma and DLBCL and classical Hodgkin lymphoma; these are classified as unique provisional entities in the 2008 World Health Organization (WHO) classification of hematopoietic tumors*

SELECTED REFERENCES

Aukema SM, Siebert R, Schuuring E, et al: Double-hit B-cell lymphomas. Blood 117:2319, 2011.
Choi WW, Weisenburger DD, Greiner TC, et al: A new immunostain algorithm classifies diffuse large B-cell lymphoma into molecular subtypes with high accuracy. Clin Cancer Res 15:5494, 2009.
De Paepe P, Achten R, Verhoef G, et al: Large cleaved and immunoblastic lymphoma may represent two distinct clinicopathologic entities within the group of diffuse large B-cell lymphomas. J Clin Oncol 23:7060, 2005.
Hu S, Xu-Monette ZY, Balasubramanyam A, et al: CD30 expression defines a novel subgroup of diffuse large B-cell lymphoma with favorable prognosis and distinct gene expression signature: a report from the International DLBCL Rituximab-CHOP Consortium Program Study. Blood 121:2715-2724, 2013.
Ott G, Ziepert M, Klapper W, et al: Immunoblastic morphology but not the immunohistochemical GCB/nonGCB classifier predicts outcome in diffuse large B-cell lymphoma in the RICOVER-60 trial of the DSHNHL. Blood 116:4916, 2010.
Salles G, de Jong D, Xie W, et al: Prognostic significance of immunohistochemical biomarkers in diffuse large B-cell lymphoma: a study from the Lunenburg Lymphoma Biomarker Consortium. Blood 117:7070, 2011.
Visco C, Li Y, Xu-Monette ZY, et al: Comprehensive gene expression profiling and immunohistochemical studies support application of immunophenotypic algorithm for molecular subtype classification in diffuse large B-cell lymphoma: a report from the International DLBCL Rituximab-CHOP Consortium Program Study. Leukemia 26:2103-2113, 2012.

LYMPHOBLASTIC LYMPHOMA (LBL)

Clinical Features

- T-lineage lymphoblastic lymphoma (T-LBL) constitutes ~90% of cases; the remainder are B-LBL
- The majority of patients are children and young adults
- Patients with T-LBL present with cervical, supraclavicular, and axillary lymphadenopathy, or with a bulky anterior mediastinal mass associated with pleural effusions
- Patients with B-LBL present with involvement of lymph nodes and extranodal sites (bone, skin, gonads, central nervous system [CNS], other)
- About 50% of patients develop a leukemic phase with bone marrow involvement
- Children with T-LBL have outcomes similar to those for children with B-LBL
- Among adults, T-LBL has a more favorable outcome than B-lineage LBL

Histopathology

- Lymph node architecture is effaced with a diffuse or, rarely, paracortical neoplastic infiltrate (Figure 14-26)
- Tumor cells range from small to large and have finely dispersed chromatin with one to several small nucleoli
- Numerous mitotic figures may be seen

Special Stains and Immunohistochemistry

- B-LBL cells express CD34, TdT, Pax-5, CD79a, and CD10; they usually lack CD20 and light chain expression
- Greater than 90% of T-LBL cases express TdT, CD2, CD3, CD5, and CD7
  - Most cases also express CD1a, CD99, and CD43
  - CD10 is seen in 40% of cases
  - CD34 is seen in ~20% of cases
  - Tumor cells are predominantly double positive for CD4 and CD8, whereas a minority of cases are double negative; rare cases express only CD4 or CD8

Other Techniques for Diagnosis

- Flow cytometry: immature B or T lymphocytes, which may have aberrant expression of myeloid antigens CD13, CD33, or CD117

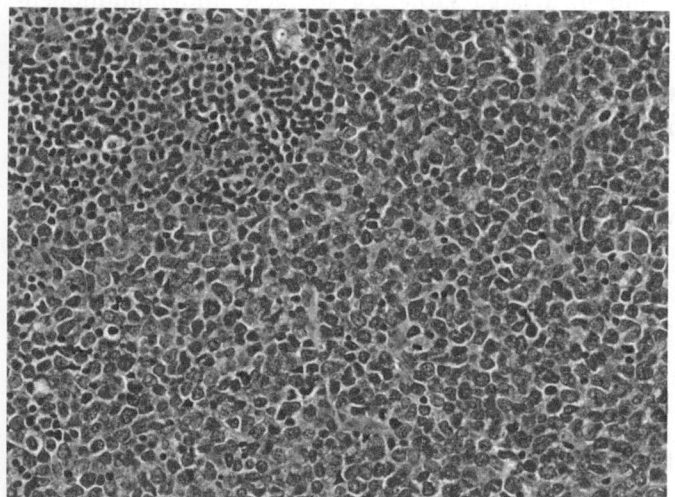

Figure 14-26. Lymphoblastic lymphoma. Sheets of large cells with fine chromatin and scant cytoplasm efface the lymph node architecture.

- Cytogenetics: > 50% of cases have various abnormalities
- PCR: monoclonal IgH gene (B-LBL) or TCR gamma gene rearrangement (T-LBL); many cases have both rearrangements
- Sanger sequencing (fresh frozen tissue): 50% to 60% of T-LBLs have activating mutations of NOTCH1 gene

Differential Diagnosis

DIFFUSE LARGE B-CELL LYMPHOMA

- Tumor cells are large and have vesicular chromatin
- Immunophenotype is very different from LBL, with a lack of immature markers CD34 and TdT and strong expression of CD20
- Flow cytometry: neoplastic B cells show light chain restriction

BURKITT LYMPHOMA

- May be morphologically identical with very high mitotic rate
- Lacks immature markers CD34 and TdT and has strong expression of CD20
- A large subset of cases expresses EBV
- Flow cytometry: neoplastic B cells show light chain restriction
- Conventional karyotype and FISH: t(8;14); c-MYC translocation is characteristic

THYMOMA

- Distinction from a T-cell rich thymoma can be a challenge in a case of a small biopsy from an anterior mediastinal mass
- Thymomas typically occur in middle-aged adults
- Characteristic lobular appearance with separating fibrous bands
- Immunohistochemistry for cytokeratin and EMA highlights the neoplastic thymic epithelial architecture
  - Spindle epithelial cells may express CD20
  - Lymphoid component consists of TdT-positive T lymphoblasts
- Flow cytometry: thymoma has different populations of maturing T cells, whereas LBL cases form tight clusters and may show loss of pan T-cell antigens or aberrant antigen expression

METASTATIC NEOPLASM

- The patient usually has a history of a preexisting neoplasm (but not always)
- Morphologic mimics include small round blue cell tumors (neuroblastoma, alveolar rhabdomyosarcoma, Ewing sarcoma)
- A panel of immunohistochemical stains will reveal that the metastatic malignancy is of nonlymphoid origin and help pinpoint the precise etiology
  - CD45, CD34, TdT, B- and T-cell markers are negative in the tumor cells
  - Neoplastic cells may express CD99, Fli1, chromogranin, synaptophysin, neuron-specific enolase, MyoD1, myogenin, or desmin
  - Conventional karyotype and FISH: characteristic translocations

MYELOID SARCOMA

- The patient usually has a history of preexisting acute myeloid leukemia, myelodysplastic syndrome, or myeloproliferative neoplasm (but not always)
- The blasts usually have more abundant eosinophilic cytoplasm, compared to LBL
- Immunophenotype is very different from LBL, with expression of myeloid blast markers CD34, CD117, MPO, lysozyme, CD68, and lack of B- or T-cell antigens
  - Occasionally myeloid sarcoma cells may express TdT, CD4, CD7, CD43, Pax-5, or CD79a
- Cytogenetic analysis may show monosomy 7, trisomy 8, t(8;21) translocation, and other abnormalities common in myeloid disorders

INDOLENT T-LYMPHOBLASTIC PROLIFERATION

- Rare reports of chronic proliferation of polyclonal precursor T lymphoblasts requiring no therapy
- Associated with other diseases (Castleman disease, follicular dendritic cell sarcoma, angioimmunoblastic T-cell lymphoma, carcinoma)
- Normal lymph node architecture is retained
- TdT-positive lymphoblasts are typically scattered or, rarely, form focal tumor-like sheets
- PCR: no evidence of monoclonal TCR gamma gene rearrangement

PEARLS

- *LBL and acute lymphoblastic leukemia are parts of a disease spectrum, therefore the 2008 WHO classification of hematopoietic tissues advocated the unifying term "B (or T) lymphoblastic leukemia/lymphoma"*
- *The term LBL may be used if the disease is confined to the lymph node with minimal involvement of peripheral blood and bone marrow*
- *Many clinical protocols use the threshold of > 25% bone marrow blasts, with or without a mass lesion for diagnosis of lymphoblastic leukemia*
- *B-LBL and Burkitt lymphoma may have a nearly identical morphology and immunophenotype; presence of immaturity and lack of light chain expression points toward B-LBL*

SELECTED REFERENCES

Cortelazzo S, Ponzoni M, Ferreri AJ, Hoelzer D: Lymphoblastic lymphoma. Crit Rev Oncol Hematol 79:330-343, 2011.

Li S, Juco J, Mann KP, Holden JT: Flow cytometry in the differential diagnosis of lymphocyte-rich thymoma from precursor T-cell acute lymphoblastic leukemia/lymphoblastic lymphoma. Am J Clin Pathol 121:268-274, 2004.

Lin P, Jones D, Dorfman DM, Medeiros LJ: Precursor B-cell lymphoblastic lymphoma: a predominantly extranodal tumor with low propensity for leukemic involvement. Am J Surg Pathol 24:1480-1490, 2000.

Ohgami RS, Zhao S, Ohgami JK, et al: TdT+T-lymphoblastic populations are increased in Castleman disease, in association with follicular dendritic cell tumors, and in angioimmunoblastic T-cell lymphoma. Am J Surg Pathol 36:1619-1628, 2012.

Patel JL, Smith LM, Anderson J, et al: The special stains and immunohistochemistry of T-lymphoblastic lymphoma in children and adolescents: a Children's Oncology Group report. Br J Haematol 159:454-461, 2012.

Weng AP, Ferrando AA, Lee W, et al: Activating mutations of NOTCH1 in human T cell acute lymphoblastic leukemia. Science 306(5694):269-271, 2004.

BURKITT LYMPHOMA (BL)

Clinical Features

- Three distinct clinical forms of BL are recognized: endemic (African), sporadic, and immunodeficiency-associated
- Endemic BL: 30% to 50% of all childhood cancer in equatorial Africa
  - Median age of 6 years
  - Typically presents as an abdominal mass or a jaw tumor
- Sporadic BL: 30% of pediatric lymphomas in the United States and Europe
  - Median age of 11 years in children and 30 years in adults
  - Male predominance
  - Typically extranodal: involves distal ileum, stomach, kidney, testis, ovary, and the like
  - Lymphadenopathy is generally localized
- Immunodeficiency-associated variant is primarily seen in persons with HIV infection
  - Presents in patients with a relatively high CD4 count and no opportunistic infections
  - Rate of BL in the HIV-positive population has not decreased with the advent of highly active antiviral therapy (HAART)
  - More often involves lymph nodes, bone marrow, and CNS
- BL is an extremely aggressive but a highly curable lymphoma; it requires intensive chemotherapy

Histopathology

- Lymph node architecture is effaced by a diffuse infiltrate of monotonous medium-sized cells
- Numerous mitoses and necrosis may be seen
- Abundant apoptotic debris and scattered tingible-body macrophages create a starry-sky appearance (Figure 4-27A)

Special Stains and Immunohistochemistry

- Neoplastic lymphocytes express B-cell antigens and are positive for CD10 and Bcl-6
- Tumor cells do not express Bcl-2 or TdT
- Ki67 proliferation rate is close to 100% (Figure 14-27B)
- In situ hybridization for EBV-encoded RNA (EBER) is strongly diffusely positive in virtually all endemic cases and in a large subset of sporadic and immunodeficiency-associated cases

Other Techniques for Diagnosis

- Flow cytometry: mature B lymphocytes with light chain immunoglobulin restriction, expression of CD10, and no aberrant expression of myeloid antigens
- Conventional karyotype and FISH (break-apart probe): MYC gene rearrangement (chromosome 8q24) in > 90% of cases
  - A simple karyotype with few or no abnormalities besides MYC rearrangement
  - No evidence of BCL2 or BCL6 rearrangement
- PCR: monoclonal IgH gene rearrangement

Differential Diagnosis

DIFFUSE LARGE B-CELL LYMPHOMA

- Tumor cells are large and more pleomorphic with a heterogeneous appearance

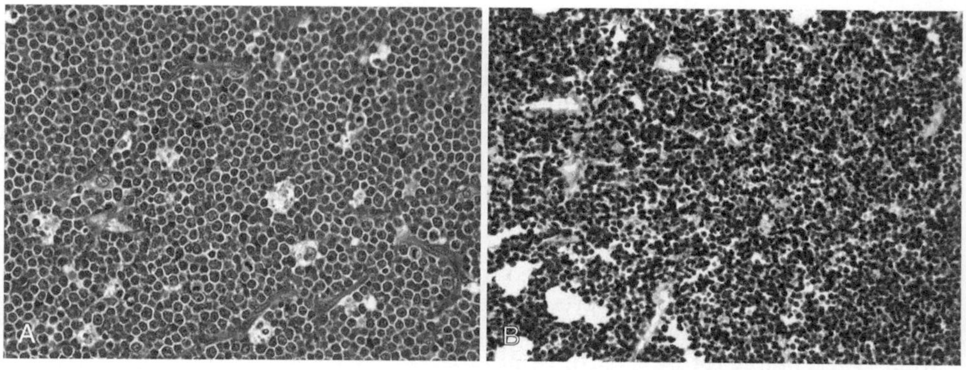

Figure 14-27. Burkitt lymphoma. A, Lymph node architecture is effaced with a starry-sky pattern. **B,** Ki67 immunostain is positive in the majority of the tumor cells.

- Typically lacks the starry-sky pattern
- Immunophenotype may occasionally be similar to BL, but the Ki67 proliferation rate is not as high (< 90%)
- Frequently express strong Bcl-2
- Conventional karyotype and FISH: typically a highly complex karyotype
  - May have MYC, BCL2, or BCL6 rearrangement
- "Gray-zone" lymphomas exist (see section on "B-Cell Lymphoma, Unclassifiable, with features intermediate between DLBCL and Burkitt Lymphoma")

B-Lymphoblastic Lymphoma
- May be morphologically identical with very high mitotic rate
- Immunophenotype is different with immature markers CD34 and TdT and lack of CD20 and EBER
- Flow cytometry: B cells show immature markers, lack light chain restriction, and frequently have aberrant expression of myeloid antigens
- Conventional karyotype and FISH: no evidence of MYC rearrangement

Metastatic Neoplasm
- The patient usually has a history of a preexisting neoplasm (but not always)
- Morphologic mimics include small round blue cell tumors (neuroblastoma, alveolar rhabdomyosarcoma, Ewing sarcoma)
- A panel of immunohistochemical stains will reveal that the metastatic malignancy is of nonlymphoid origin and help pinpoint the precise etiology
  - CD45 and B-cell markers are negative in the tumor cells
  - Neoplastic cells may express CD99, Fli1, chromogranin, synaptophysin, neuron-specific enolase, MyoD1, myogenin, or desmin
- Conventional karyotype and FISH: characteristic translocations

Myeloid Sarcoma
- The patient usually has a history of preexisting acute myeloid leukemia, myelodysplastic syndrome, or myeloproliferative neoplasm (but not always)
- The blasts usually have moderate eosinophilic cytoplasm
- Immunophenotype is very different from BL, with expression of myeloid blast markers CD34, CD117, MPO, lysozyme, and CD68, and a lack of B-cell antigens

- Very rarely myeloid sarcoma cells express Pax-5 or CD79a; these cases typically have a t(8;21) translocation
- Cytogenetic analysis may show monosomy 7, trisomy 8, t(8;21) translocation, and other abnormalities common in myeloid disorders; MYC rearrangement is negative

PEARLS

- *Ki67 immunostain highlights virtually every cell; this finding is extremely unusual in other types of lymphoma*
- *Older age, black race, and advanced stage are associated with worse prognosis and higher mortality*
- *Break sites in the cMYC gene differ between the sporadic and the endemic forms of BL*
- *Although the most common translocation is t(8;14) resulting in fusion of cMYC and IgH genes, the cMYC gene may also become juxtaposed to the kappa light chain gene [t(2;8) translocation] or lambda light chain gene [t(8;22) translocation]*
- *The terms* atypical Burkitt lymphoma *and* Burkitt-like lymphoma *stem from older literature and represent various aggressive lymphomas; their use is no longer recommended*

Selected References

Chuang SS, Ye H, Du MQ, et al: Histopathology and immunohistochemistry in distinguishing Burkitt lymphoma from diffuse large B-cell lymphoma with very high proliferation index and with or without a starry-sky pattern: a comparative study with EBER and FISH. Am J Clin Pathol 128:558-564, 2007.

Costa LJ, Xavier AC, Wahlquist AE, Hill EG: Trends in survival of patients with Burkitt lymphoma/leukemia in the USA: an analysis of 3691 cases. Blood 121:4861-4866, 2013.

Harris NL, Horning SJ: Burkitt's lymphoma: the message from microarrays. N Engl J Med 354:2495-2498, 2006.

Nakamura N, Nakamine H, Tamaru J, et al: The distinction between Burkitt lymphoma and diffuse large B-cell lymphoma with c-myc rearrangement. Mod Pathol 15:771-776, 2002.

Ogwang MD, Bhatia K, Biggar RJ, Mbulaiteye SM: Incidence and geographic distribution of endemic Burkitt lymphoma in northern Uganda revisited. Int J Cancer 123:2658, 2008.

B-CELL LYMPHOMA, UNCLASSIFIABLE, WITH FEATURES INTERMEDIATE BETWEEN DLBCL AND BURKITT LYMPHOMA (BCLU)

Clinical Features

- A heterogeneous category that may be used for cases that have morphologic, immunophenotypic, or genetic

features of both DLBCL and BL but do not fulfill the diagnostic criteria for either entity
- Occurs in older adults, most of whom present at advanced stage with generalized lymphadenopathy or extranodal involvement
- Very aggressive lymphomas with dismal prognosis that are virtually refractory to intensive chemotherapy

Histopathology

- Diffuse proliferation of medium-sized to large cells
- Starry-sky pattern is typically present, resembling BL
- The cells may be larger and more pleomorphic than what is acceptable for BL (Figure 14-28)
- Other cases have typical morphology for BL but an atypical immunophenotype

Special Stains and Immunohistochemistry

- Cases that morphologically resemble BL but have strong expression of Bcl-2 or Ki67 proliferation rate of < 90%
- Cases that morphologically resemble DLBCL but have a typical BL immunophenotype (CD10+, Bcl-6+, Bcl-2-, Mum1-, Ki67 > 90% positive)

Other Techniques for Diagnosis

- Conventional karyotype and FISH:
  - Cases that morphologically resemble BL but have a complex karyotype or MYC associated with BCL2 or BCL6 rearrangements ("double-hit" and "triple-hit" lymphoma)
  - Cases that morphologically resemble DLBCL but have a typical BL immunophenotype and evidence of a simple karyotype with MYC rearrangement

Differential Diagnosis

Diffuse Large B-Cell Lymphoma
- Tumor cells are large and pleomorphic with a heterogeneous appearance
- Typically lacks the starry-sky pattern

- Immunophenotype may occasionally be similar to BL, but the Ki67 proliferation rate is not as high (< 90%)
- Frequently expresses strong Bcl-2
- Conventional karyotype and FISH: typically a highly complex karyotype
  - May have MYC, BCL2, or BCL6 rearrangement

Burkitt Lymphoma
- Tumor cells are medium-sized, not large, and have a monotonous appearance without variation in shape or size
- Starry-sky pattern due to very high mitotic rate
- Ki67 proliferation rate is close to 100%
- Characteristic immunophenotype: CD10+, Bcl-6+, Bcl-2-, Mum1-
- Conventional karyotype and FISH: simple karyotype with a MYC translocation

Follicular Lymphoma (FL)
- A small subset of the "double-hit lymphoma" arises from a preexisting or concurrent FL, presumably by acquisition of MYC rearrangement
- These cases may morphologically resemble low or high-grade FL
- Some cases have unusual morphologic features for FL, such as blastoid morphology, diffuse growth, absence of centrocyte-like cells, very high proliferation, a starry-sky pattern, or focal necrosis

Lymphoblastic Lymphoma (LBL)
- A small subset of the "double-hit lymphoma" expresses TdT and has blastoid morphology
- Although controversial, such cases are currently classified as B-LBL

PEARLS

- *This is a provisional entity in the 2008 WHO classification of hematopoietic tissues; the criteria and characteristics are still evolving*
- *Several large gene expression studies provided additional evidence that some lymphomas are borderline between BL and DLBCL*
- *The term BCLU does not apply to otherwise typical DLBCL cases that have a high proliferation growth fraction, starry-sky macrophages, or MYC translocations*
- *Similarly the term BCLU is not valid in cases of BL that only have an atypical morphology or lack MYC translocation*
  - *About 5% of otherwise typical BL cases lack evidence of MYC rearrangement*
- *Currently the entity of BCLU includes most cases of "double-hit lymphoma" (MYC and BCL2 or MYC and BCL6 rearranged) and "triple-hit lymphoma" (MYC, BCL2 and BCL6 rearranged)*
- *A small subset of the "double-hit lymphomas" does not have morphologic and immunophenotypic features of BCLU and should thus be classified accordingly (follicular lymphoma, lymphoblastic lymphoma, plasma cell myeloma, etc.)*

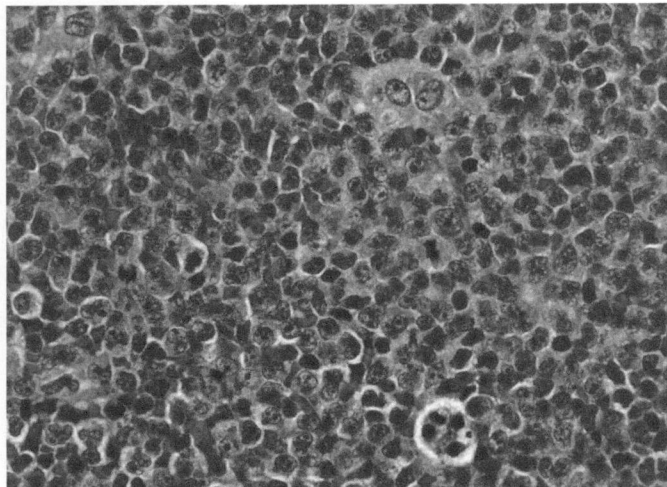

Figure 14-28. BCLU. Tumor cells are larger and more irregular than Burkitt lymphoma. Frequent mitotic figures and apoptotic debris are reminiscent of BL. Immunophenotype and cytogenetic features of this case were compatible with BCLU.

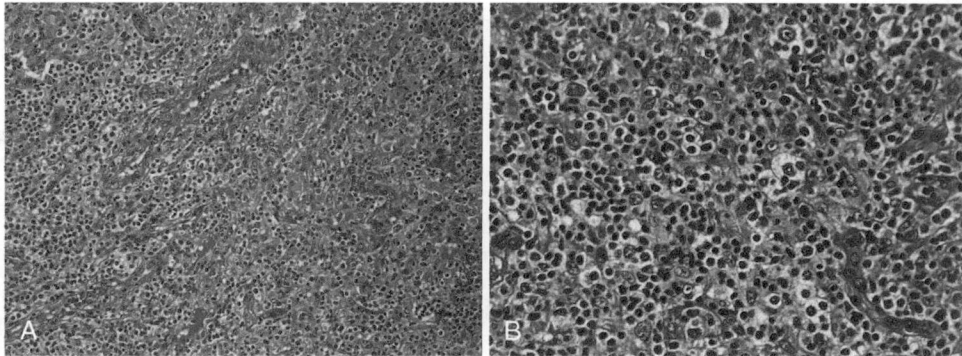

Figure 14-29. Angioimmunoblastic T-cell lymphoma. **A,** Polymorphous infiltrate with small aggregates of atypical lymphoid cells with clear cytoplasm and hypervascularity. **B,** Aggregates of atypical cells (high-magnification).

SELECTED REFERENCES

Johnson NA, Savage KJ, Ludkovski O, et al: Lymphomas with concurrent BCL2 and MYC translocations: the critical factors associated with survival. Blood 114:2273-2279, 2009.

Li S, Lin P, Fayad LE, et al: B-cell lymphomas with MYC/8q24 rearrangements and IGH@BCL2/t(14;18)(q32;q21): an aggressive disease with heterogeneous histology, germinal center B-cell immunophenotype and poor outcome. Mod Pathol 25:145-156, 2012.

Lin P, Dickason TJ, Fayad LE, et al: Prognostic value of MYC rearrangement in cases of B-cell lymphoma, unclassifiable, with features intermediate between diffuse large B-cell lymphoma and Burkitt lymphoma. Cancer 118:1566-1573, 2012.

Perry AM, Crockett D, Dave BJ, et al: B-cell lymphoma, unclassifiable, with features intermediate between diffuse large B-cell lymphoma and Burkitt lymphoma: study of 39 cases. Br J Haematol 162:40-49, 2013.

Pillai RK, Sathanoori M, Van Oss SB, Swerdlow SH: Double-hit B-cell lymphomas with BCL6 and MYC translocations are aggressive, frequently extranodal lymphomas distinct from BCL2 double-hit B-cell lymphomas. Am J Surg Pathol 3:323-332, 2013.

Quintanilla-Martinez L, de Jong D, de Mascarel A, et al: Gray zones around diffuse large B cell lymphoma: conclusions based on the workshop of the XIV meeting of the European Association for Hematopathology and the Society of Hematopathology in Bordeaux, France. J Hematop 2:211-236, 2009.

Said JW: Aggressive B-cell lymphomas: how many categories do we need? Mod Pathol 26(suppl 1):S42-S56, 2013.

Snuderl M, Kolman OK, Chen YB, et al: B-cell lymphomas with concurrent IGH-BCL2 and MYC rearrangements are aggressive neoplasms with clinical and pathologic features distinct from Burkitt lymphoma and diffuse large B-cell lymphoma. Am J Surg Pathol 34:327-340, 2010.

PERIPHERAL T-CELL LYMPHOMA

ANGIOIMMUNOBLASTIC T-CELL LYMPHOMA (AITL)

Clinical Features

- One of the more common subtypes of PTCL
- Occurs in the elderly
- The majority of patients present with advanced disease: generalized lymphadenopathy, hepatosplenomegaly, fever, weight loss, night sweats
- A subset may have rash, polyarthritis, pleural effusion, or ascites
- Most patients have laboratory abnormalities (high LDH, cytopenias, etc.)
- AITL is an aggressive lymphoma and the prognosis is poor

Histopathology

- Partial effacement of lymph node architecture
- Polymorphous paracortical infiltrate composed of small to medium-sized atypical lymphocytes with moderate pale cytoplasm admixed with numerous reactive small lymphocytes, immunoblasts, eosinophils, plasma cells, and histiocytes (Figure 14-29)
- Paracortical vascular proliferation

Special Stains and Immunohistochemistry

- The neoplastic lymphocytes express most pan T-cell antigens (CD, CD2, CD5, CD7) and are CD4+
  - Loss of one or more pan T-cell antigens is common
- Tumor cells have immunophenotype of follicular T-helper cells: CD10+, Bcl-6+, CXCL13+, PD-1+
- CD21 and CD23 highlight expanded follicular dendritic cell meshworks
- The majority of cases have many scattered EBV-positive immunoblasts

Other Techniques for Diagnosis

- PCR: monoclonal TCR gamma gene rearrangement
  - ~10% of cases also have a monoclonal IgH gene rearrangement
- Conventional karyotype: may show trisomy 3, trisomy 5, or additional X chromosome

Differential Diagnosis

PERIPHERAL T-CELL LYMPHOMAS NOT OTHERWISE SPECIFIED (PTCL-NOS)

- PTCL with a follicular growth pattern exhibits immunophenotype of follicular T-helper cells
- The neoplastic cells are located within the germinal center or mantle zone of the follicles
- As opposed to AITL, these cases present in early stage, have no evidence of enlarged follicular dendritic cell meshworks, and lack prominent high endothelial venules
- At present, overlap between the two entities cannot be excluded

CLASSICAL HODGKIN LYMPHOMA

- Occasionally large multinucleated immunoblasts resembling Reed-Sternberg cells are seen in AITL

- Proliferation of atypical small T lymphocytes with clear cytoplasm is not a feature of Hodgkin lymphoma
- No expansion of the follicular dendritic cell meshworks
- No evidence of T-cell clonality by PCR

DLBCL

- T-cell/histiocyte-rich large B-cell lymphoma also has scattered large B cells in the background of T lymphocytes, however, T cells are not atypical and do not show follicular T-helper immunophenotype or antigen loss; the neoplastic B cells do not express EBV
- EBV-positive large B-cell lymphoma of the elderly may have a polymorphous background with scattered neoplastic B cells; however, T cells are not atypical and do not show follicular T-helper immunophenotype or antigen loss
- PCR reveals a monoclonal IgH gene rearrangement and no evidence of T-cell clonality

Reactive Paracortical Hyperplasia

- T cells do not show antigen loss
- Usually the number of CD4+ and CD8+ T lymphocytes is similar
- No evidence of T-cell clonality by PCR

PEARLS

- *Clinical presentation with rash, lymphadenopathy, and fever is nonspecific and frequently suggests an inflammatory process*
- *Lymph node involvement early in disease presentation may be subtle and is easily missed; rebiopsy may be indicated in challenging cases*

Selected References

Abramson JS, Digumarthy S, Ferry JA: Case records of the Massachusetts General Hospital. Case 27-2009: a 56-year-old woman with fever, rash, and lymphadenopathy. N Engl J Med 361:900-911, 2009.

de Leval L, Rickman DS, Thielen C, et al: The gene expression profile of nodal peripheral T-cell lymphoma demonstrates a molecular link between angioimmunoblastic T-cell lymphoma (AITL) and follicular helper T (TFH) cells. Blood 109:4952, 2007.

Federico M, Rudiger T, Bellei M, et al: Clinicopathologic characteristics of angioimmunoblastic T-cell lymphoma: analysis of the international peripheral T-cell lymphoma project. J Clin Oncol 31:240, 2013.

Huang Y, Moreau A, Dupuis J, et al: Peripheral T-cell lymphomas with a follicular growth pattern are derived from follicular helper T cells (TFH) and may show overlapping features with angioimmunoblastic T-cell lymphomas. Am J Surg Pathol 33:682-690, 2009.

ANAPLASTIC LARGE CELL LYMPHOMA (ALCL)

Clinical Features

- One of the most common subtypes of PTCL
- ALCL, anaplastic lymphoma kinase (ALK)-positive presents most frequently in the second and third decades and has a male predominance (6.5:1)
- ALCL, ALK-negative presents in the middle-aged and elderly adults and has a lower male-to-female ratio (0.95:1)
- The majority of the patients present with advanced disease: lymphadenopathy, frequent extranodal involvement, and systemic symptoms
- Patients with ALK+ALCL have a better survival than patients with ALK- ALCL

Histopathology

- ALCL, ALK-positive and ALCL, ALK-negative have identical morphologic features
- Intrasinusoidal infiltration by large tumor cells with eccentric kidney-shaped nuclei (hallmark cells); doughnut- or wreath-like cells can also be seen (Figure 14-30)
- ALCL, common variant (70%): predominant population of pleomorphic large cells with hallmark features
- ALCL, lymphohistiocytic variant (10%): large numbers of admixed histiocytes
- ALCL, small cell variant (5% to 10%): predominant population of small to medium-sized neoplastic cells

Special Stains and Immunohistochemistry

- Tumor cells express CD30
- Most cases express one or more T cell antigens
  - CD45 and EMA are usually positive
  - CD2, CD5, or CD4 are positive in >75% cases
  - Bcl-6 and clusterin are often positive
  - CD3 and Bcl-2 are usually negative
  - Most cases have cytotoxic antigens (TIA1, Granzyme B, perforin)
- Some cases only have evidence of T-cell lineage at the genetic level (so called "null cell")

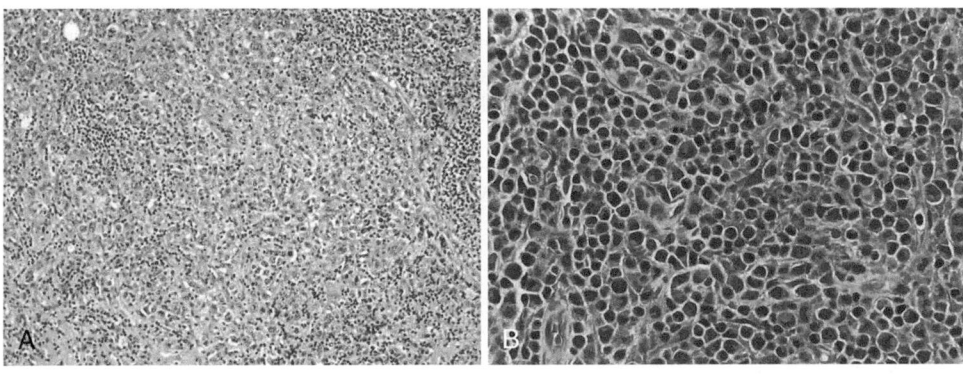

Figure 14-30. Anaplastic large cell lymphoma. A, Sheets of large atypical lymphoid cells fill the sinuses. **B,** Tumor cells have irregular nuclear contours and abundant cytoplasm. Several hallmark cells are present.

- ALK positivity may be nuclear, cytoplasmic, or membranous, depending on the ALK gene rearrangement partner
- Rarely, myeloid cell antigens (e.g., CD13, CD33, CD68) can be expressed
- EBV is negative

Other Techniques for Diagnosis

- Conventional cytogenetics and FISH: t(2;5)(p23;q35) translocation in > 80% of cases
  - Other common ALK abnormalities include t(1;2) and inv(2)
- PCR: monoclonal TCR gamma gene rearrangement

Differential Diagnosis

CLASSICAL HODGKIN LYMPHOMA
- Reed-Sternberg cells express Pax-5 and CD15 (negative in ALCL) in addition to CD30
- Many cases are EBV-positive
- Reed-Sternberg cells do not express T-cell antigens or EMA
- A polymorphous inflammatory background is not a feature of ALCL

DLBCL
- Very rare cases of ALK-positive, EMA-positive DLBCL have been described; they express CD138 and cytoplasmic immunoglobulin and lack CD30 and T-cell antigens
- Some cases of anaplastic DLBCL have similar morphology to ALCL and are CD30-positive; they express B-cell antigens and lack T-cell antigens
  - CD30 is partial and weak

PTCL, NOS
- Some cases have pleomorphic tumor cells with CD30 positivity
- Loss of T-cell antigens is more pronounced in ALCL
- EMA is rarely expressed by PTCL, NOS
- Studies have shown that ALK- ALCL is most likely a separate entity from PTCL, NOS
  - They may be difficult to distinguish in some cases

MYELOID SARCOMA
- Patients with myeloid sarcoma often have a history of preexisting acute myeloid leukemia, myelodysplastic syndrome, or myeloproliferative neoplasm (but not always)
- Lymph node architecture is effaced by sheets of blasts
- Immunophenotypic expression of blast and myeloid markers CD34, CD117, MPO, lysozyme, and lack of EMA and T-cell antigens
  - Myeloid sarcoma cells express CD43 and may frequently have aberrant expression of CD4 or CD7
  - The expression of CD30 is exceptional in myeloid sarcoma and largely restricted to the rare megakaryocytic variant
- Cytogenetic analysis may show monosomy 7, trisomy 8, t(8;21) translocation, and other abnormalities common in myeloid disorders; ALK rearrangement is negative

METASTATIC NEOPLASM
- Metastatic carcinoma and melanoma may have similar morphologic features and a cohesive growth pattern with sinusoidal spread
- Immunohistochemical staining is required to make the diagnosis
  - Carcinomas express cytokeratins
  - Melanomas express S-100 protein, HMB-45, Melan-A
  - Mast cell sarcoma express mast cell tryptase
  - However, it is important to remember that CD30 can be positive in nonhematologic malignancies, including germ cell tumors and aggressive mast cell neoplasms

PEARLS

- *CD30 is a useful marker for workup of a poorly differentiated neoplasm in lymph node, as ALCL may be negative for CD45 and CD3*
- *CD30 is an activation antigen and may be expressed by reactive immunoblasts*
- *Immunohistochemistry for ALK is sensitive and specific, thus genetic confirmation of ALK gene rearrangement is not necessary*
- *Gene expression profiling studies have demonstrated different clustering patterns for ALK+ ALCL, ALK- ALCL and PTCL, NOS*
- *Anti-CD30 antibody-drug conjugate brentuximab vedotin is a promising new agent and has been approved by the Food and Drug Administration (FDA) for treatment of ALCL*

SELECTED REFERENCES

Bovio IM, Allan RW: The expression of myeloid antigens CD13 and/or CD33 is a marker of ALK+anaplastic large cell lymphomas. Am J Clin Pathol 130:628-634, 2008.

Lamant L, de Reyniès A, Duplantier MM, et al: Gene-expression profiling of systemic anaplastic large-cell lymphoma reveals differences based on ALK status and two distinct morphologic ALK+subtypes. Blood 109:2156, 2007.

Piva R, Agnelli L, Pellegrino E, et al: Gene expression profiling uncovers molecular classifiers for the recognition of anaplastic large-cell lymphoma within peripheral T-cell neoplasms. J Clin Oncol 28:1583, 2010.

Pro B, Advani R, Brice P, et al: Brentuximab vedotin (SGN-35) in patients with relapsed or refractory systemic anaplastic large-cell lymphoma: results of a phase II study. J Clin Oncol 30:2190-2196, 2012.

Salaverria I, Beà S, Lopez-Guillermo A, et al: Genomic profiling reveals different genetic aberrations in systemic ALK-positive and ALK-negative anaplastic large cell lymphomas. Br J Haematol 140:516, 2008.

Savage KJ, Harris NL, Vose JM, et al: ALK- anaplastic large-cell lymphoma is clinically and immunophenotypically different from both ALK+ALCL and peripheral T-cell lymphoma, not otherwise specified: report from the International Peripheral T-Cell Lymphoma Project. Blood 111:5496, 2008.

PERIPHERAL T-CELL LYMPHOMA, NOS

Clinical Features

- The most common subtype of T-cell lymphoma
- Occurs in the elderly with median age of 60 years and a male predominance (2:1)

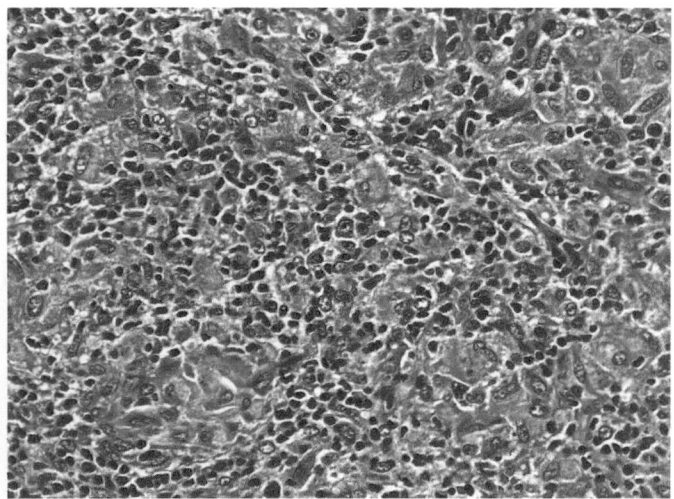

Figure 14-31. PTCL, NOS. Small and large atypical lymphoid cells are admixed with numerous epithelioid histiocytes.

- Most patients present with advanced disease and have B symptoms; generalized lymphadenopathy; and bone marrow, liver, spleen, or extranodal involvement
- Highly aggressive lymphoma with poor response to therapy

Histopathology

- Tumor cell morphology is very heterogeneous
  - Sheets of medium-sized or large, pleomorphic, monotonous-appearing tumor cells
  - Polymorphous infiltrate with small lymphocytes, eosinophils, plasma cells, and histiocytes (Figure 14-31)
  - Clear cells and Reed-Sternberg-like cells may be seen
- Paracortical, follicular, or diffuse involvement of lymph node
- High-endothelial venules may be increased
- Three distinct variants are recognized
  - Lymphoepithelioid (Lennert lymphoma) consists of small neoplastic cells, which may be obscured by numerous epithelioid histiocytes
  - Follicular PTCL occurs when atypical clear cells are located within the germinal centers or mantle zone of the follicles
  - T-zone PTCL is characterized by a perifollicular growth pattern of small lymphocytes with minimal cytologic atypia

Special Stains and Immunohistochemistry

- CD45 positive tumor cells
- Frequent loss of T cell antigens CD5 and CD7
- Usually CD4+, CD8- tumor cells
  - Lymphoepithelioid lymphoma is characterized by CD8+ cells in the majority of cases
- High Ki67 proliferation rate
- Some cases have weak/focal expression of CD30
- A subset of cases (in particular the follicular variant of PTCL) has expression of follicular T-helper markers: CD10, Bcl-6, PD-1, and CXCL13
- Reed-Sternberg-like cells typically express EBV

Other Techniques for Diagnosis

- Conventional cytogenetics: complex karyotype
- PCR: evidence of TCR gamma gene rearrangement

Differential Diagnosis

CLASSICAL HODGKIN LYMPHOMA (CHL)
- Reed-Sternberg cells of CHL express Pax-5 and CD15 in addition to CD30
- Reed-Sternberg cells of CHL do not express CD45 or T-cell antigens
- Very rare cases of PTCL, NOS with true Reed-Sternberg cells of B-cell lineage have also been reported
  - All of these cases had T-cell atypia and abnormal T-cell immunophenotype, allowing for the correct diagnosis

DLBCL
- Immunophenotype is very different from PTCL with expression of B-cell antigens and lack of T-cell antigens
- PCR: evidence of IgH gene rearrangement and lack of TCR gamma gene rearrangement

REACTIVE PARACORTICAL HYPERPLASIA
- Frequent differential diagnosis in T-zone-type PTCL
- No morphologic atypia
- T cells do not show antigen loss
- Similar number of CD4+ and CD8+ T lymphocytes
- No evidence of T-cell clonality by PCR

ANGIOIMMUNOBLASTIC T-CELL LYMPHOMA
- Characteristic morphology with a polymorphous paracortical infiltrate composed of small to medium-sized atypical lymphocytes with moderate pale cytoplasm admixed with numerous reactive small lymphocytes, immunoblasts, eosinophils, plasma cells, and histiocytes
- Paracortical vascular proliferation
- A subset of PTCL, NOS cases may express follicular T-helper immunophenotype (CD10, BCL6, PD1, and CXCL13)
  - These cases include follicular PTCL and, rarely, lymphoepithelioid PTCL
- Presence of expanded follicular dendritic cell meshworks is not a feature of PTCL, NOS
- Some cases are difficult to classify and likely represent a disease spectrum

ANAPLASTIC T-CELL LYMPHOMA
- PTCL, NOS may have pleomorphic tumor cells with CD30 positivity
- Loss of T-cell antigens is more pronounced in ALCL
- EMA is rarely expressed by PTCL, NOS, and ALK1 is always negative
- Studies have shown that ALK- ALCL is most likely a separate entity from PTCL, NOS

PEARLS

- *PTCL, NOS is a diagnosis of exclusion and should only be made if all other, better-defined subtypes of T-cell lymphoma have been excluded*

SELECTED REFERENCES

Nicolae A, Pittaluga S, Venkataraman G, et al: Peripheral T-cell lymphomas of follicular T-helper cell derivation with Hodgkin/Reed-Sternberg cells of B-cell lineage: both EBV-positive and EBV-negative variants exist. Am J Surg Pathol 37:816-826, 2013.

Piccaluga PP, Fuligni F, De Leo A, et al: Molecular profiling improves classification and prognostication of nodal peripheral T-cell lymphomas: results of a phase iii diagnostic accuracy study. J Clin Oncol 31:3019-3025, 2013.

Piva R, Agnelli L, Pellegrino E, et al: Gene expression profiling uncovers molecular classifiers for the recognition of anaplastic large-cell lymphoma within peripheral T-cell neoplasms. J Clin Oncol 28:1583, 2010.

Savage KJ, Harris NL, Vose JM, et al: ALK- anaplastic large-cell lymphoma is clinically and immunophenotypically different from both ALK+ALCL and peripheral T-cell lymphoma, not otherwise specified: report from the International Peripheral T-Cell Lymphoma Project. Blood 111:5496, 2008.

Weisenburger DD, Savage KJ, Harris NL, et al: Peripheral T-cell lymphoma, not otherwise specified: a report of 340 cases from the International Peripheral T-cell Lymphoma Project. Blood 117:3402-3408, 2011.

HODGKIN LYMPHOMA

NODULAR LYMPHOCYTE PREDOMINANT HODGKIN LYMPHOMA (NLPHL)

Clinical Features

- Constitutes ~5% of all Hodgkin lymphoma cases
- Presents in young patients with a strong male predominance
- Most patients have localized cervical, axillary, or inguinal lymphadenopathy

Histopathology

- Nodular proliferation of numerous small lymphocytes admixed with scattered large atypical-appearing cells (Figure 14-32A)
  - Tumor cells have one large folded or multilobated nucleus with multiple nucleoli
- Large cells are called LP (lymphocyte predominant) cells, L&H (lymphocytic and histiocytic) cells or popcorn cells (Figure 14-32B)
- Some nodules may have a rim of epithelioid histiocytes
- Eosinophils, neutrophils, fibrosis, or necrosis are not features of NLPHL
- Many cases have a peripheral rim of uninvolved lymph node tissue

Special Stains and Immunohistochemistry

- The nodules are composed predominantly of small B lymphocytes
- The neoplastic large cells express CD45 and B-cell antigens: CD20, Pax-5, CD79a, Oct-2, and Bob.1
- Bcl-6 and EMA are positive in the majority of cases
- Large cells are negative for CD30, CD15, fascin, and EBV
- Increased number of CD3+, CD4+, CD57+, PD-1+ T lymphocytes in the nodules; these cells may rosette around the LP cells (Figure 14-32C)
- CD21 and CD23 highlight large expanded follicular dendritic cell meshworks in the nodules

Other Techniques for Diagnosis

- Flow cytometry is insensitive to the presence of LP cells but may detect a population of double-positive CD4+/CD8+ T lymphocytes
- Conventional cytogenetics: may show various abnormalities in a subset of cases
- PCR: no evidence of IgH gene rearrangement due to the scarcity of the tumor cells

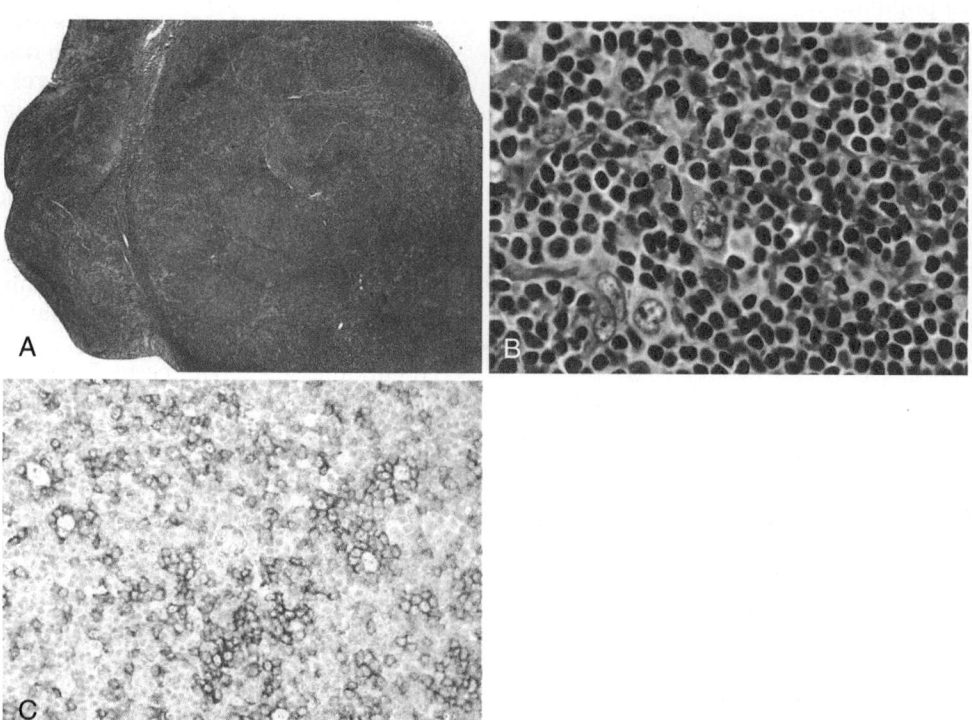

Figure 14-32. Nodular lymphocyte predominant Hodgkin lymphoma. A, Lymph node architecture is effaced by a nodular proliferation of lymphocytes. **B,** LP or popcorn cells. **C,** PD-1 immunostain shows T-cell rosettes around the neoplastic large cells.

Differential Diagnosis

PROGRESSIVE TRANSFORMATION OF GERMINAL CENTERS (PTGC)

- PTGC is a focal finding in a lymph node with reactive follicular hyperplasia
- PTGC does not contain LP cells
- T cells may be increased within the nodules but are scattered, do not form aggregates, and do not rosette
- EMA highlights the LP cells and is negative in PTGC
- The relationship between the two entities is complex and incompletely understood, as they may coexist or precede each other

CLASSICAL HODGKIN LYMPHOMA, LYMPHOCYTE-RICH TYPE

- Both lymphomas have a nodular growth pattern
- Reed-Sternberg cells have a different immunophenotype from LP cells
  - CD45-, CD20-, Pax-5 dim+, CD30+, CD15+
  - EBV is frequently expressed
  - Either Oct-2 or Bob.1 are positive, but not both

T CELL/HISTIOCYTE-RICH LARGE B-CELL (THRLBCL)

- THRLBCL is an aggressive lymphoma with generalized lymphadenopathy, usually present in elderly patients
- The infiltrate is diffuse, not nodular, and completely effaces the lymph node architecture
- CD21 and CD23 are negative
- Small cells are almost exclusively CD3+ T lymphocytes
- Immunophenotype of the large cells may be very similar to NLPHL
- THRLBCL lacks PD-1+ T-cell rosettes around the large tumor cells
- Flow cytometry and PCR are more likely to detect a monoclonal B-cell population
- THRLBCL may represent disease progression in patients with known NLPHL
- At present, an overlap between the two entities cannot be entirely excluded

PEARLS

- *Early stage NLPHL may be curatively treated with excision of the involved lymph node*
- *Frequent relapses and recurrences*
- *Patients are predisposed to develop DLBCL, sometimes 10 to 20 years following the initial presentation*

SELECTED REFERENCES

Al-Mansour M, Connors JM, Gascoyne RD, et al: Tranformation to aggressive lymphoma in nodular lymphocyte-predominant Hodgkin's lymphoma. J Clin Oncol 28:793-799, 2010.

Biasoli I, Stamatoullas A, Meignin V, et al: Nodular lymphocyte-predominant Hodgkin lymphoma: a long-term study and analysis of transformation to diffuse large B-cell lymphoma in a cohort of 164 patients from the Adult Lymphoma Study Group. Cancer 116:631-639, 2010.

Boudova L, Torlakovic E, Delabie J, et al: Nodular lymphocyte predominant Hodgkin lymphoma with nodules resembling T-cell/histiocyte-rich B-cell lymphoma: differential diagnosis between nodular lymphocyte-predominant Hodgkin lymphoma and T-cell/histiocyte-rich B-cell lymphoma. Blood 102:3753-3758, 2003.

Cotta CV, Coleman JF, Li S, Hsi ED: Nodular lymphocyte predominant Hodgkin lymphoma and diffuse large B-cell lymphoma: a study of six cases concurrently involving the same site. Histopathology 59:1194-1203, 2011.

Fan Z, Natkunam Y, Bair E, et al: Characterization of variant patterns of nodular lymphocyte predominant Hodgkin lymphoma with immunohistologic and clinical correlation. Am J Surg Pathol 27:1346-1356, 2003.

Nam-Cha SH, Roncador G, Sanchez-Verde L, et al: PD-1, a follicular T-cell marker useful for recognizing nodular lymphocyte-predominant Hodgkin lymphoma. Am J Surg Pathol 32:1252-1257, 2008.

Rahemtullah A, Reichard KK, Preffer FI, et al: A double-positive CD4+CD8+ T-cell population is commonly found in nodular lymphocyte predominant Hodgkin lymphoma. Am J Clin Pathol 126:805-814, 2006.

CLASSICAL HODGKIN LYMPHOMA, NODULAR SCLEROSIS TYPE (CHL, NS)

Clinical Features

- Most common subtype of CHL in the United States and Europe (~70% of cases)
- Peak incidence is between 15 and 34 years of age
- The majority of patients present with painless localized peripheral lymphadenopathy, typically involving the cervical region
- About 80% of the patients have mediastinal involvement
- Highly curable lymphoma with an excellent prognosis

Histopathology

- Lymph node architecture is effaced
- Nodules composed of Hodgkin and Reed-Sternberg cells (HRS) admixed with numerous reactive small lymphocytes, eosinophils, histiocytes, plasma cells, and, occasionally, neutrophils (Figure 14-33A)
  - Diagnostic Reed-Sternberg cells are large with abundant cytoplasm and at least two nuclear lobes with a prominent nuclear membrane, vesicular chromatin, and eosinophilic macronucleoli (Figure 14-33B)
  - Hodgkin cells: mononuclear variants
  - Wreath cells: multinucleated variants
  - Mummified cells: variants with condensed cytoplasm, and pyknotic hyperchromatic nuclei
  - Lacunar cells: formalin fixation-related artifact that causes retraction of the cytoplasmic membrane, giving the appearance of a lacunar space around the nucleus and the cytoplasm
- The nodules are separated by broad bands of collagen
- Necrosis and granulomas may be seen

Special Stains and Immunohistochemistry

- The HRS cells express Pax-5 (characteristically dim), CD30, CD15 in the majority of cases (~80%) and are negative for CD45 and CD20
  - Weak CD20 in a subset of the tumor cells may be seen in 30% to 40% of cases
  - Mum-1 is consistently positive
  - EMA is negative
- Tumor cells express Oct-2 or Bob.1, but not both
- In situ hybridization for EBV-encoded RNA (EBER) is positive in 10% to 40% of cases

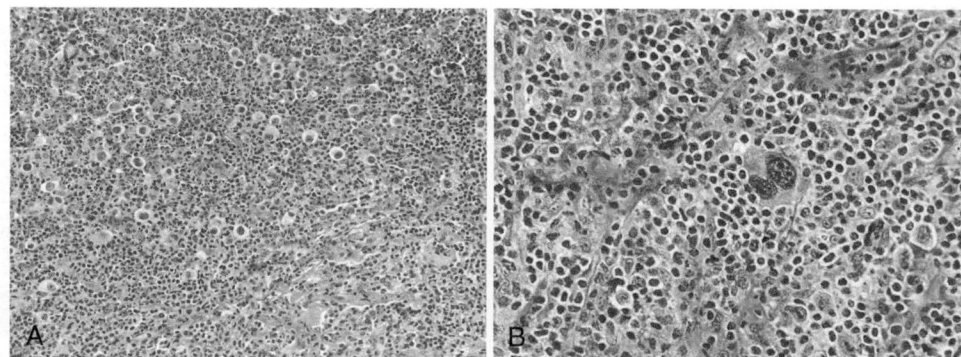

Figure 14-33. Classical Hodgkin lymphoma, nodular sclerosis type. **A,** Polymorphous proliferation of small lymphocytes, eosinophils, neutrophils, and numerous lacunar cells. **B,** Classic Reed-Sternberg cell and lacunar cells.

Other Techniques for Diagnosis

- Flow cytometry: normal B and T lymphocytes (noncontributory)
- Conventional cytogenetics: may show various abnormalities in a subset of cases
- PCR: no evidence of IgH gene rearrangement due to the scarcity of the tumor cells

Differential Diagnosis

CLASSICAL HODGKIN LYMPHOMA, MIXED CELLULARITY TYPE

- The differential diagnosis arises when the bands of sclerosis are not well-developed or are not appreciated
  - CHL is typically not subtyped on small biopsies
- EBV is expressed much more frequently

NODULAR LYMPHOCYTE PREDOMINANT HODGKIN LYMPHOMA

- Both lymphomas have a nodular growth pattern
- LP cells have a different immunophenotype than HRS cells
  - CD45+, CD20+, Pax-5 strong+, CD30+, CD15-
  - EBV is consistently negative
  - Both Oct-2 and Bob.1 are positive

DIFFUSE LARGE B-CELL LYMPHOMA (DLBCL)

- Syncytial variant of CHL has confluent aggregates of lacunar cells, which may morphologically mimic anaplastic DLBCL
- Numerous reactive inflammatory cells are not a features of DLBCL
- Immunophenotype is usually very different from CHL, with expression of CD45, CD20, strong Pax-5, absent or weak/partial CD30, and lack of CD15
  - DLBCL cells express both Oct-2 and Bob.1
- "Gray-zone" lymphomas with intermediate morphology and immunophenotype are well recognized, especially in the mediastinum

ANAPLASTIC LARGE CELL LYMPHOMA (ALCL)

- No evidence of nodules or dense fibrosis
- A polymorphous inflammatory background is not a feature of ALCL
- ALCL tumor cells express CD30 but are negative for Pax5 and CD15

- EBV is consistently negative
- HRS cells do not express T-cell antigens or EMA

PERIPHERAL T-CELL LYMPHOMA (PTCL)

- Some cases of PTCL consist of large Reed-Sternberg like cells; these cells express T-cell antigens and are negative for Pax-5
- PTCL may also contain scattered Reed-Sternberg–like B immunoblasts; these cells express CD45, CD20, strong Pax-5, CD30, and are negative for CD15
- Very rare cases of PTCL with true Reed-Sternberg cells have also been reported
- All PTCL cases have T-cell atypia and abnormal T-cell immunophenotype
- PCR may be useful in difficult cases: monoclonal TCR gamma gene rearrangement

INFECTIOUS MONONUCLEOSIS (IM)

- Even though immunoblasts in IM may appear atypical, most do not resemble HRS cells
- Most IM immunoblasts are CD45+, CD20+, strong Pax-5+ B cells
- Some immunoblasts express CD30; they are always CD15 negative
- EBER highlights numerous positive small and large lymphocytes

REACTIVE LYMPH NODE

- A mistaken diagnosis of benign lymph node may occasionally be rendered on small biopsies, where HRS cells are few in number and may be missed
- Marked fibrosis frequently causes crush artifact precluding optimal evaluation of HRS cells (most commonly seen in small mediastinoscopy biopsy specimens)
  - These cases are usually submitted for frozen section evaluation, where additional tissue should be requested
- If the lymph node appears reactive but the biopsy is small and clinical suspicion for CHL is high, rebiopsy should be recommended (especially relevant for fine-needle aspiration specimens)
- Immunoblasts in reactive lymph node are large but do not have cytologic atypia
  - No diagnostic Reed-Sternberg cells
  - Immunoblasts express CD30 but are negative for CD15

PEARLS

- *Careful morphologic evaluation is paramount to visualize the HRS cells*
- *Avoid ordering CD30 and CD15 in reactive-appearing lymph nodes without morphologic evidence of diagnostic Reed-Sternberg cells*
  - *CD30 stains benign immunoblasts*
  - *CD15 stains neutrophils and histiocytes*
- *The diagnosis of CHL requires a combination of diagnostic Reed-Sternberg cells and the typical polymorphous inflammatory background*
- *HRS cells are particularly numerous at the periphery of necrotic areas*

SELECTED REFERENCES

Browne P, Petrosyan K, Hernandez A, Chan JA: The B-cell transcription factors BSAP, Oct-2, and BOB.1 and the pan-B-cell markers CD20, CD22, and CD79a are useful in the differential diagnosis of classic Hodgkin lymphoma. Am J Clin Pathol 120:767, 2003.

Eberle FC, Mani H, Jaffe ES: Histopathology of Hodgkin's lymphoma. Cancer J 15:129-137, 2009.

Eberle FC, Salaverria I, Steidl C, et al: Gray zone lymphoma: chromosomal aberrations with immunophenotypic and clinical correlations. Mod Pathol 24:1586-1597, 2011.

Harris NL: Shades of gray between large B-cell lymphomas and Hodgkin lymphomas: differential diagnosis and biological implications. Mod Pathol 26(suppl 1):S57-S70, 2013.

Steidl C, Lee T, Shah SP, et al: Tumor-associated macrophages and survival in classic Hodgkin's lymphoma. N Engl J Med 362:875-885, 2010.

Stein H, Marafioti T, Foss HD, et al: Down-regulation of BOB.1/OBF.1 and Oct2 in classical Hodgkin disease but not in lymphocyte predominant Hodgkin disease correlates with immunoglobulin transcription. Blood 97:496, 2001.

CLASSICAL HODGKIN LYMPHOMA, MIXED CELLULARITY TYPE (CHL, MC)

Clinical Features

- Comprises ~25% of cases of CHL
- More frequent in patients with HIV and in developing countries
- Median age is 38 years
- Marked male predominance (~70%)
- Most patients present with painless localized peripheral lymphadenopathy, typically involving the cervical region
  - Mediastinal involvement is uncommon
- Highly curable lymphoma with an excellent prognosis

Histopathology

- Lymph node architecture is effaced
- Diffuse proliferation of HRS cells admixed with numerous reactive small lymphocytes, eosinophils, histiocytes, plasma cells, and neutrophils (Figure 14-34)
- No broad bands of collagen
- Necrosis and granulomas may be seen

Special Stains and Immunohistochemistry

- HRS cells express Pax-5 (characteristically dim), CD30, CD15 in the majority of cases (~80%) and are negative for CD45 and CD20

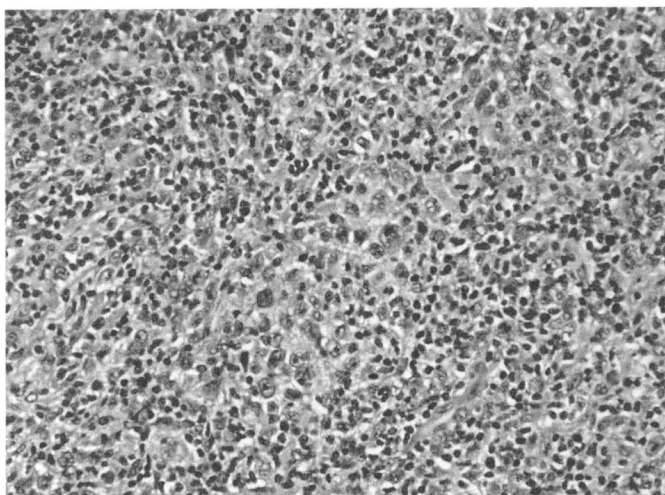

Figure 14-34. Classical Hodgkin lymphoma, mixed cellularity type. Small lymphocytes, eosinophils, histiocytes, and Reed-Sternberg cells and variants.

- Weak CD20 in a subset of the tumor cells may be seen in 30% to 40% of cases
- Mum-1 is consistently positive
- EMA is negative
- Tumor cells express Oct-2 or Bob.1, but not both
- In situ hybridization for EBV-encoded RNA (EBER) is positive in ~75% of cases

Other Techniques for Diagnosis

- Flow cytometry: normal B and T lymphocytes (noncontributory)
- Conventional cytogenetics: may show various abnormalities in a subset of cases
- PCR: no evidence of IgH gene rearrangement due to the scarcity of the tumor cells

Differential Diagnosis

CLASSICAL HODGKIN LYMPHOMA, NODULAR SCLEROSIS TYPE

- The differential diagnosis arises when there is focal interstitial fibrosis
- No evidence of thick bands of sclerosis
- EBV is expressed much less frequently

T CELL/HISTIOCYTE-RICH LARGE B-CELL LYMPHOMA (THRLBCL)

- Contains rare scattered large neoplastic cells surrounded by numerous reactive small T lymphocytes and histiocytes
- Eosinophils, neutrophils, and plasma cells are not features of THRLBCL
- Immunophenotype is very different from CHL, with expression of CD45, CD20, strong Pax-5, absent or weak/partial CD30, and lack of CD15
  - DLBCL cells express both Oct-2 and Bob.1

PEARLS

- *See "Pearls" under "Classical Hodgkin Lymphoma, Nodular Sclerosis Type"*

SELECTED REFERENCES

Browne P, Petrosyan K, Hernandez A, Chan JA: The B-cell transcription factors BSAP, Oct-2, and BOB.1 and the pan-B-cell markers CD20, CD22, and CD79a are useful in the differential diagnosis of classic Hodgkin lymphoma. Am J Clin Pathol 120:767, 2003.

Eberle FC, Mani H, Jaffe ES: Histopathology of Hodgkin's lymphoma. Cancer J 15:129-137, 2009.

Steidl C, Lee T, Shah SP, et al: Tumor-associated macrophages and survival in classic Hodgkin's lymphoma. N Engl J Med 362:875-885, 2010.

Stein H, Marafioti T, Foss HD, et al: Down-regulation of BOB.1/OBF.1 and Oct2 in classical Hodgkin disease but not in lymphocyte predominant Hodgkin disease correlates with immunoglobulin transcription. Blood 97:496, 2001.

CLASSICAL HODGKIN LYMPHOMA, LYMPHOCYTE-RICH TYPE (CHL, LR)

Clinical Features

- Comprises ~5% of cases of CHL
- Median age is higher than in other subtypes of CHL
- Marked male predominance (~70%)
- The majority of patients present with painless localized peripheral lymphadenopathy, typically involving the cervical region
  - Mediastinal involvement is uncommon
- Highly curable lymphoma with an excellent prognosis

Histopathology (Figure 14-35)

- Lymph node architecture is effaced by a nodular proliferation of small lymphocytes
- Small regressed germinal centers usually present in the nodules
- Scattered HRS are present in the nodules
- Eosinophils and neutrophils are rare or absent

Special Stains and Immunohistochemistry

- The HRS cells express Pax-5 (characteristically dim), CD30, CD15 in the majority of cases (~80%) and are negative for CD45 and CD20

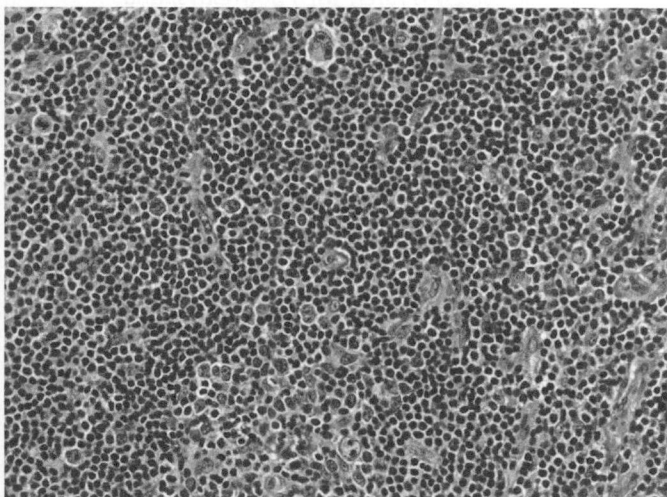

Figure 14-35. Classical Hodgkin lymphoma, lymphocyte-rich type. Nodule with Reed-Sternberg cells and variants amid numerous small lymphocytes.

- Weak CD20 in a subset of the tumor cells may be seen in 30% to 40% of cases
  - Mum-1 is consistently positive
  - EMA is negative
- Tumor cells express Oct-2 or Bob.1, but not both
- Small lymphocytes in the nodules consist of IgD + mantle cell B cells
- CD21 and CD23 highlight small regressed residual germinal centers
- In situ hybridization for EBV-encoded RNA (EBER) is positive in ~50% of cases

Other Techniques for Diagnosis

- Flow cytometry: normal B and T lymphocytes (noncontributory)
- Conventional cytogenetics: may show various abnormalities in a subset of cases
- PCR: no evidence of IgH gene rearrangement due to the scarcity of the tumor cells

Differential Diagnosis

NODULAR LYMPHOCYTE-PREDOMINANT HODGKIN LYMPHOMA (NLPHL)

- Both lymphomas have a nodular growth pattern
- LP cells have a different immunophenotype from HRS cells
  - CD45+, CD20+, strong Pax-5+, EMA+/−, CD30-, CD15-
  - EBV is consistently negative
  - Both Oct-2 and Bob.1 are expressed
- Follicular dendritic cell meshworks are large and expanded, whereas in CHL, LR they are small, round, and tight

FOLLICULAR LYMPHOMA

- Neoplastic cells are a mixture of centrocytes and centroblasts; no HRS cells are seen
- Immunophenotype of small lymphocytes in the nodules represents their germinal center origin: CD10+, Bcl-6+, Bcl-2+, IgD-
- Flow cytometry always identifies a monoclonal B-cell population, whereas flow cytometry in CHL shows polyclonal B lymphocytes

PEARLS

- *CHL, LR is unusual among CHL subtypes in that it does not show the typical polymorphous inflammatory background*
- *Clinical behavior and prognosis appear more similar to NLPHL than to the other subtypes of CHL*

SELECTED REFERENCES

Browne P, Petrosyan K, Hernandez A, Chan JA: The B-cell transcription factors BSAP, Oct-2, and BOB.1 and the pan-B-cell markers CD20, CD22, and CD79a are useful in the differential diagnosis of classic Hodgkin lymphoma. Am J Clin Pathol 120:767, 2003.

de Jong D, Bosq J, MacLennan KA, et al: Lymphocyte-rich classical Hodgkin lymphoma (LRCHL): clinico-pathological characteristics and outcome of a rare entity. Ann Oncol 17:141-145, 2006.

Eberle FC, Mani H, Jaffe ES: Histopathology of Hodgkin's lymphoma. Cancer J 15:129-137, 2009.

Shimabukuro-Vornhagen A, Haverkamp H, Engert A, et al: Lymphocyte-rich classical Hodgkin's lymphoma: clinical presentation and treatment outcome in 100 patients treated within German Hodgkin's Study Group trials. J Clin Oncol 23:5739-5745, 2005.

Steidl C, Lee T, Shah SP, et al: Tumor-associated macrophages and survival in classic Hodgkin's lymphoma. N Engl J Med 362:875-885, 2010.

NONLYMPHOID DISORDERS OF LYMPH NODES

LANGERHANS CELL HISTIOCYTOSIS (LCH)

Clinical Features

- Wide age range with a peak incidence between 1 and 3 years of age
- Localized, multifocal, or disseminated disease with a clonal expansion of Langerhans cells
- Lymph node involvement may be the only site of disease or may be part of multisystem disease (usually with skin and bone involvement)
  - Asymptomatic swelling of cervical, inguinal, mediastinal, or retroperitoneal lymph nodes

Histopathology

- Lymph node architecture is usually preserved with a sinusoidal infiltration
- The infiltrate consists of variable numbers of Langerhans cells, eosinophils, neutrophils, and small lymphocytes (Figure 14-36A)
  - Eosinophils may be numerous enough to form microabscesses
- The Langerhans cells are large and contain abundant, ill-defined acidophilic cytoplasm
  - The nuclei are irregular with an indented, folded, or creased appearance; nucleoli are inconspicuous
  - Many nuclei exhibit a longitudinal groove resulting in a "coffee-bean" appearance (Figure 14-36B)
- Numerous multinucleated giant cells and epithelioid histiocytes containing "coffee bean" nuclei may also be present
- Phagocytosis is not seen

Special Stains and Immunohistochemistry

- The Langerhans cells express S-100 protein, Langerin, CD45, CD1a, perinuclear CD68
- S-100 stains all the cells, whereas only a subset of the tumor cells expresses CD1a and Langerin

Other Techniques for Diagnosis

- BRAF V600E mutation has been identified in 40% to 60% of patients with LCH
- Electron microscopy: characteristic Birbeck granules
- Flow cytometry and cytogenetics are noncontributory

Differential Diagnosis

ROSAI-DORFMAN DISEASE
- Abnormal histiocytic cells are larger and have round nuclei with prominent nucleoli
- Langerhans cells do not exhibit emperipolesis
- Abnormal histiocytic cells express S-100 and are negative for CD1a and Langerin

SINUS HISTIOCYTOSIS
- Histiocytes do not have characteristic indented, folded, or creased "coffee-bean" nuclei
- Eosinophils, neutrophils, and plasma cells are not conspicuous
- Giant cells are absent
- Reactive histiocytes do not express S-100, CD1a, or Langerin

DERMATOPATHIC LYMPHADENITIS
- May contain numerous Langerhans cells
- Paracortical involvement with preserved lymph node architecture; no sinus involvement
- Langerhans cells are admixed with small lymphocytes and histiocytes; there is no evidence of eosinophils, neutrophils, or plasma cells

PEARLS

- *Langerhans cells are weakly phagocytic, antigen-presenting dendritic cells of skin origin*
- *Electron microscopy is rarely used nowadays, and demonstration of Birbeck granules is not required for diagnosis*

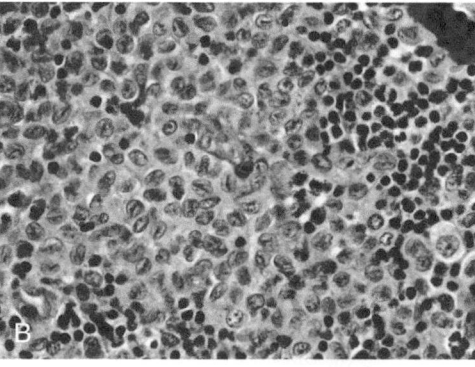

Figure 14-36. Langerhans cell histiocytosis. **A,** Small lymphocytes, numerous eosinophils and sheets of Langerhans cells. **B,** Langerhans cells have irregular folded nuclei with a "coffee bean" appearance.

SELECTED REFERENCES

Badalian-Very G, Vergilio JA, Degar BA, et al: Recurrent BRAF mutations in Langerhans cell histiocytosis. Blood 116:1919-1923, 2010.

Edelweiss M, Medeiros LJ, Suster S, Moran CA: Lymph node involvement by Langerhans cell histiocytosis: a clinicopathologic and immunohistochemical study of 20 cases. Hum Pathol 38:1463-1469, 2007.

Lau SK, Chu PG, Weiss LM: Immunohistochemical expression of Langerin in Langerhans cell histiocytosis and non-Langerhans cell histiocytic disorders. Am J Surg Pathol 32:615-619, 2008.

Sahm F, Capper D, Preusser M, et al: BRAFV600E mutant protein is expressed in cells of variable maturation in Langerhans cell histiocytosis. Blood 120:2700-2703, 2012.

Satoh T, Smith A, Sarde A, et al: B-RAF mutant alleles associated with Langerhans cell histiocytosis, a granulomatous pediatric disease. PLOS One 7:e33891, 2012.

KAPOSI SARCOMA (KS)

Clinical Features

- Benign vascular neoplasm that most frequently involves the skin but also involves the oral cavity, lungs, gastrointestinal tract, and lymph nodes
- AIDS-epidemic KS: most common form in the United States
  - KS is an AIDS-defining condition; it remains the most common neoplasm in this patient population
  - Lymph node involvement is common and may occur in the absence of mucocutaneous disease
- Classic-Mediterranean: rare in the United States and mostly affects elderly men
  - Only involves lymph nodes secondarily and generally late in the course of the disease

Histopathology (Figure 14-37)

- Early lesions are usually observed in or adjacent to the capsule, in the hilum, or, occasionally, in the perinodal adipose tissue
- Vascular channels within the lymph node are prominent, increased in number, and are associated with increased numbers of plasma cells

- Over time, these areas may develop the classic histopathologic features of KS, including interwoven fascicles of spindle cells, vascular slits, and extravasated erythrocytes
- In late stages of disease, the vascular proliferation may replace the entire lymph node

Special Stains and Immunohistochemistry

- Spindle cells and the vascular lining cells express endothelial cell–associated antigens: factor VIII–related antigen, CD34, CD31, and ERG
- HHV-8 latency-associated nuclear antigen (LANA) is expressed in nearly all cases

Other Techniques for Diagnosis

- Noncontributory

Differential Diagnosis

ANGIOSARCOMA

- Metastatic angiosarcoma is much more common than primary angiosarcoma of the lymph node
- Usually replaces the normal lymph node architecture
- Consists primarily of interwoven fascicles of spindle cells displaying prominent cytologic atypia, numerous mitotic figures, and often striking pleomorphism
- Always negative for HHV-8 (LANA)

VASCULAR TRANSFORMATION OF LYMPH NODE

- Congestion of all subcapsular and medullary sinuses
- Anastomosing network of small vascular channels lined by reactive endothelial cells
- Absence of capsular involvement (typical in KS)
- Absence of periodic acid-Schiff (PAS)–positive hyaline globules (typical of KS)
- Always negative for HHV-8 (LANA)

PEARLS

- *AIDS-related KS may frequently coexist with other lymph node abnormalities (high-grade lymphoma, Castleman disease, infection, HIV-associated lymphadenopathy)*
- *Positive immunohistochemical stain for HHV-8 (LANA) is diagnostic of KS and is negative in all its mimickers*

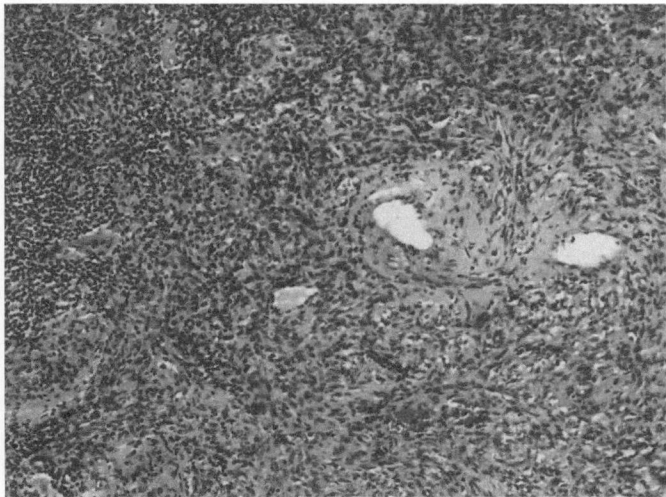

Figure 14-37. Kaposi sarcoma. Lymph node capsule with a proliferation of small vascular channels.

SELECTED REFERENCES

Cheuk W, Wong KO, Wong CS, et al: Immunostaining for human herpesvirus 8 latent nuclear antigen-1 helps distinguish Kaposi sarcoma from its mimickers. Am J Clin Pathol 121:335-342, 2004.

Hong YK, Foreman K, Shin JW, et al: Lymphatic reprogramming of blood vascular endothelium by Kaposi sarcoma-associated herpesvirus. Nat Genet 36:683-685, 2004.

Patel RM, Goldblum JR, Hsi ED: Immunohistochemical detection of human herpes virus-8 latent nuclear antigen-1 is useful in the diagnosis of Kaposi sarcoma. Mod Pathol 17:456-460, 2004.

Robin YM, Guillou L, Michels JJ, Coindre JM: Human herpesvirus 8 immunostaining: a sensitive and specific method for diagnosing Kaposi sarcoma in paraffin-embedded sections. Am J Clin Pathol 121:330-334, 2004.

Schwartz EJ, Dorfman RF, Kohler S: Human herpesvirus-8 latent nuclear antigen-1 expression in endemic Kaposi sarcoma: an immunohistochemical study of 16 cases. Am J Surg Pathol 27:1546-1550, 2003.

Uldrick TS, Whitby D: Update on KSHV epidemiology, Kaposi sarcoma pathogenesis, and treatment of Kaposi sarcoma. Cancer Lett 305:150-162, 2011.

EXTRAMEDULLARY HEMATOPOIESIS (EMH)

Clinical Features

- Typically an incidental finding
- May be normal in small children but is always pathologic in adults
- Most common etiologies include red blood cell disorders (sickle cell anemia, thalassemia, etc.) and myeloproliferative neoplasms
- Cases of EMH in patients treated with neoadjuvant chemotherapy have been reported

Histopathology (Figure 14-38)

- EMH may be seen in the sinuses or in the paracortex
- Erythroid precursors are small cells with round hyperchromatic nuclei and scant cytoplasm; they have a typical intrasinusoidal location
- Myeloid precursors are medium-sized cells with round to irregular nuclear contours and moderate eosinophilic cytoplasm
- Megakaryocytes are large cells with multilobated nuclei and abundant dense eosinophilic cytoplasm
- One, two, or all three lineages may be present

Special Stains and Immunohistochemistry

- Erythroid precursors express Glycophorin C
- Myeloid precursors stain with myeloperoxidase, lysozyme, and CD68
- Occasionally monocytes are part of the EMH; these cells express CD14
- Megakaryocytes are positive for CD42b and CD61

Other Techniques for Diagnosis

- Noncontributory

Differential Diagnosis

MYELOID SARCOMA

- Sheets of myeloid blasts
- No evidence of erythroid precursors or megakaryocytes
- Myeloid blasts express CD34 and CD117 in addition to myeloperoxidase, lysozyme, and CD68

METASTATIC CARCINOMA

- EMH may be seen in axillary lymph nodes of patients with breast cancer
- Immunohistochemical staining with cytokeratin, myeloperoxidase, Glycophorin C, and CD42b helps resolve the diagnostic difficulty

CLASSICAL HODGKIN LYMPHOMA

- Megakaryocytes may occasionally be confused with Reed-Sternberg cells, and maturing myeloid cells may be mistaken for eosinophils
- Megakaryocytes are positive for CD42b and CD61 and do not express Pax-5, CD30, or CD15

PEARLS

- *Presence of an underlying myeloid malignancy or chronic anemia should be carefully investigated in an adult patient*
- *Whereas a unilineage proliferation composed of erythroblasts is typical of a non-neoplastic condition, the presence of trilineage hematopoiesis is more suggestive of myeloproliferative neoplasms*

SELECTED REFERENCES

Millar EK, Inder S, Lynch J: Extramedullary haematopoiesis in axillary lymph nodes following neoadjuvant chemotherapy for locally advanced breast cancer: a potential diagnostic pitfall. Histopathology 54:622-623, 2009.

O'Malley DP: Benign extramedullary myeloid proliferations. Mod Pathol 20:405-415, 2007.

Prieto-Granada C, Setia N, Otis CN: Lymph node extramedullary hematopoiesis in breast cancer patients receiving neoadjuvant therapy: a potential diagnostic pitfall. Int J Surg Pathol 21:264-266, 2013.

MYELOID SARCOMA (MS)

Clinical Features

- Myeloid sarcoma occurs in patients who have acute myeloid leukemia, as a sign of impending blast crisis in chronic myelogenous leukemia or leukemic transformation in patients who have myelodysplastic disorders, as well as a forerunner of acute myeloid leukemia in nonleukemic patients

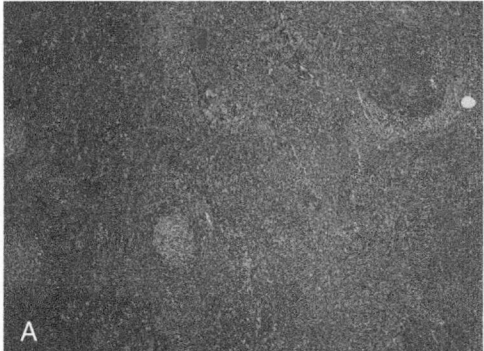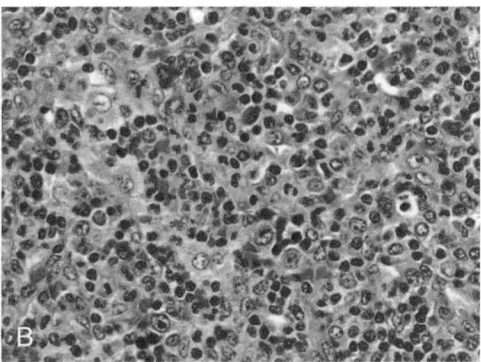

Figure 14-38. Extramedullary hematopoiesis. A, Interfollicular area is markedly expanded. **B,** High magnification of erythroid and myeloid precursors.

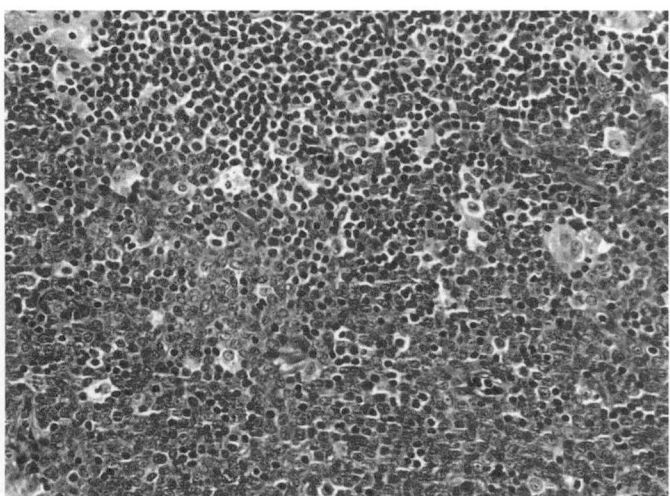

Figure 14-39. Myeloid sarcoma. Sheets of myeloblasts are present in the lower half of the image.

- Myeloid sarcomas most frequently involve soft tissues, lymph nodes, and skin or occur as isolated lytic bone lesions

Histopathology

- Most cases are composed of myeloblasts with or without features of promyelocytic or neutrophilic maturation (Figure 14-39)
- The blasts have round, ovoid, or reniform nuclei with finely stippled chromatin and one or two small nucleoli
- Other cases are characterized by a diffuse monotonous proliferation of myelomonocytic or monoblastic cells

Special Stains and Immunohistochemistry

- CD68/KP1 is the most commonly expressed marker (100%), followed by myeloperoxidase, CD117, CD99, lysozyme, CD34, TdT, and CD56
- About 90% of cases express CD45
- About 50% of myeloid sarcomas express CD43
- Rare cases positive for CD30 have been reported

Other Techniques for Diagnosis

- Cytogenetic analysis: ~50% of cases have chromosomal abnormalities
  - Monosomy 7, trisomy 8, MLL gene rearrangement, inv(16), t(8;21) translocation, and other abnormalities common in myeloid disorders

Differential Diagnosis

Diffuse Large B-Cell Lymphoma
- Tumor cells are large and pleomorphic with vesicular nuclei
- Immunophenotype is different from MS with expression of B-cell antigens and lack of myeloid markers

Burkitt Lymphoma
- Tumor cells are medium sized and have a monotonous appearance
- Starry-sky pattern due to very high mitotic rate
- Immunophenotype is different from MS with expression of B-cell antigens and lack of myeloid markers

Peripheral T-Cell Lymphoma, NOS
- Some tumors may have a monotonous appearance with effacement of lymph node architecture
- Immunophenotype is different from MS with expression of T-cell antigens and lack of myeloid markers

Anaplastic Large Cell Lymphoma (ALCL)
- Many cases of ALCL express myeloid markers CD13 and CD33 by flow cytometry
- Immunophenotypic expression of EMA and T-cell antigens and lack of myeloid blast markers
  - Many cases of ALCL express ALK1
  - Myeloid sarcoma cells may have aberrant expression of T-cell antigens CD43, CD4 or CD7

Lymphoblastic Lymphoma
- Tumor cells also have a blastoid appearance
- Immunophenotype is different from MS with expression of B-cell or T-cell antigens and lack of myeloid markers

Metastatic Neoplasm
- Includes small round blue cell tumors in children and carcinoma and melanoma in adults
- Immunophenotype is different from MS with lack of myeloid markers and blast markers

PEARLS

- *Immunohistochemical stains to rule out MS should be performed in a high-grade lymph node neoplasm that does not express CD20, CD3, and CD138*
- *CD43 is not a reliable marker for MS, as it also stains T cells, plasma cells, and certain B-cell lymphomas*
- *CD34 is much less frequent in MS than in bone marrow-based acute myeloid leukemia*
- *Myeloid sarcoma is considered an extramedullary equivalent of acute myeloid leukemia and is treated in the same fashion*

Selected References

Campidelli C, Agostinelli C, Stitson R, Pileri SA: Myeloid sarcoma: extramedullary manifestation of myeloid disorders. Am J Clin Pathol 132:426-437, 2008.

Pileri SA, Ascani S, Cox MC, et al: Myeloid sarcoma: clinico-pathologic, phenotypic and cytogenetic analysis of 92 adult patients. Leukemia 21:340-350, 2007.

MAST CELL DISEASE

Clinical Features

- May occur at any age
- Mast cell proliferations most commonly involve the dermis, where they form small, localized tumors (mastocytomas) or disseminate (urticaria pigmentosa)
- Other organs that are frequently involved include spleen, liver, and gastrointestinal tract
- Lymph nodes are involved in ~25% of cases of systemic disease

Histopathology

- Complete effacement of the architecture is unusual
- The mast cells preferentially infiltrate the paracortical area but may involve any compartment

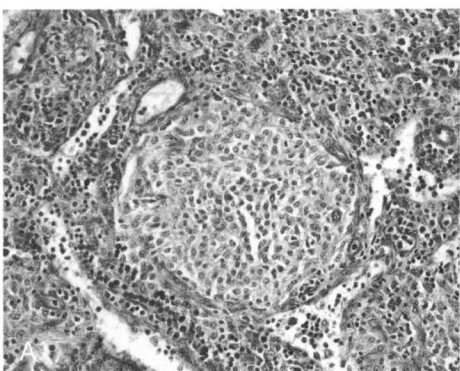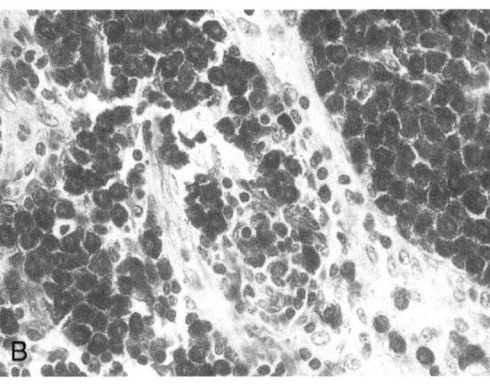

Figure 14-40. Mast cell disease in lymph node. **A,** Aggregate of cells with clear cytoplasm. **B,** Giemsa stain highlights the metachromatic granules of the mast cells. *(Courtesy of Dr. Hans-Peter Horny, Institut für Pathologie, Munich, Germany.)*

- Typically present as small clusters or sheets
- Most mast cells are round and have abundant clear cytoplasm with well-defined cytoplasmic borders (Figure 14-40A)
- Follicular hyperplasia, hypervascularity, increased eosinophils, plasmacytosis, and fibrosis are frequently seen
  - Some cases have eosinophilic abscesses and extreme eosinophilia obscuring other cell types
- Wright-Giemsa–stained touch preparations highlight the metachromatic granules of mast cells (Figure 14-40B)

Special Stains and Immunohistochemistry

- Mast cells express CD117 and mast cell tryptase
- Neoplastic mast cells have aberrant expression of CD2 or CD25
- CD30 may be positive in aggressive subtypes (e.g., mast cell leukemia)

Other Techniques for Diagnosis

- Elevated levels of serum tryptase
- Activating point mutation of codon 816 of KIT gene

Differential Diagnosis

PERIPHERAL T-CELL LYMPHOMA

- May have a component of clear cells, eosinophils, and hypervascularity
- Immunohistochemical staining confirms that the clear cells are T lymphocytes

LANGERHANS CELL HISTIOCYTOSIS

- Polymorphous inflammatory background with eosinophilia is similar
- Immunohistochemical staining highlights the Langerhans cells and shows no evidence of mast cell proliferation

MONOCYTOID B CELLS (IN REACTIVE HYPERPLASIA OR MARGINAL ZONE LYMPHOMA)

- Usually associated with neutrophils, not eosinophils
- Immunohistochemical staining confirms their B-cell origin

PLASMACYTOID DENDRITIC CELLS

- More easily appreciated when present in aggregates

- Plasmacytoid dendritic cells express CD123 and CD68 and are negative for CD117 and mast cell tryptase

FOLLICULAR HYPERPLASIA AND FOLLICULAR LYMPHOMA

- Mast cell aggregates may resemble benign or neoplastic follicles
- Immunohistochemical staining reveals numerous B lymphocytes and shows no evidence of mast cell proliferation

CLASSICAL HODGKIN LYMPHOMA

- Polymorphous inflammatory background with eosinophilia and fibrosis may appear similar
- Diagnostic Reed-Sternberg cells are present

SINUS HISTIOCYTOSIS

- Cases of mast cell leukemia may show striking involvement of the sinuses
- Immunohistochemical staining reveals presence of histiocytes and shows no evidence of mast cell proliferation

PEARLS

- *Mast cells are virtually impossible to recognize on H&E-stained sections, as the granules are not visible*
- *On the H&E-stained sections, aggregates of mast cells may resemble fibrotic foci, histiocytes, or lymphoid aggregates*

SELECTED REFERENCES

Escribano L, Díaz-Agustín B, Bellas C, et al: Utility of flow cytometric analysis of mast cells in the diagnosis and classification of adult mastocytosis. Leuk Res 25:563, 2001.

Garcia-Montero AC, Jara-Acevedo M, Teodosio C, et al: KIT mutation in mast cells and other bone marrow hematopoietic cell lineages in systemic mast cell disorders: a prospective study of the Spanish Network on Mastocytosis (REMA) in a series of 113 patients. Blood 108:2366, 2006.

Valent P, Horny HP, Escribano L, et al: Diagnostic criteria and classification of mastocytosis: a consensus proposal. Leuk Res 25:603-625, 2001.

Valent P, Sperr WR, Schwartz LB, Horny HP: Diagnosis and classification of mast cell proliferative disorders: delineation from immunologic diseases and non-mast cell hematopoietic neoplasms. J Allergy Clin Immunol 114:3, 2004.

Chapter 15
Spleen

ATTILIO ORAZI • SONAM PRAKASH

CHAPTER OUTLINE

NON-NEOPLASTIC DISEASES INVOLVING THE SPLENIC WHITE PULP

REACTIVE FOLLICULAR HYPERPLASIA WITH GERMINAL CENTER FORMATION

CLINICAL FEATURES

- Occurs at any age; more common in children and younger adults
- Caused by a variety of both acute and chronic immunologic stimuli (e.g., bacterial infections, autoimmune diseases including hemolytic processes)
- May represent an incidental finding

Gross Pathology

- May present with splenomegaly, usually mild to moderate in degree (Figure 15-1)
- Prominent white pulp nodularity may be grossly visible

Histopathology

- Tripartite variably prominent germinal centers with well-defined marginal and mantle zones
- Marginal zones may be expanded in chronic cases (Figure 15-2)
- Polarized (dark and light zones) germinal centers with abundant mitoses and tingible body macrophages
- Increased number of plasma cells and small plasma cell aggregates in red pulp

Special Stains and Immunohistochemistry

- Immunohistochemistry may be useful in differential diagnosis from lymphomatous infiltration
- Germinal centers are positive for CD20, CD10, bcl-6, and negative for bcl-2
- Mantle cells are positive for CD20, CD5, and bcl-2 and negative for CD43 and cyclin D1

Other Techniques for Diagnosis

- Evaluation of light-chain expression by flow cytometry may be complicated by high nonspecific binding; nevertheless, polyclonal pattern is always seen supporting the diagnosis of reactive hyperplasia

Differential Diagnosis

FOLLICULAR, MANTLE CELL, AND MARGINAL ZONE LYMPHOMAS

- Neoplastic follicles are less sharply defined, and may coalesce
- Reactive follicles have well-defined marginal and mantle zones with polarized germinal centers, tingible body macrophages, and mitotic figures
- Neoplastic lymphoid infiltrates are often present in red pulp as well as in periarteriolar lymphoid sheaths (PALS) of white pulp
- Immunophenotypic features are dependent on the lymphoma subtype

PEARLS

- *Histologic features of splenic lymphoid hyperplasia are largely similar to those of nodal reactive follicular hyperplasia*
- *Well-developed germinal centers are considered a normal finding in children and young adults. Uncommon in elderly individuals; differential diagnosis includes follicular lymphoma or autoimmune disorders*
- *Localized (nodular) reactive lymphoid hyperplasia is a rare nodular lesion that may grossly simulate lymphoma; histologically, it presents as an aggregation of hyperplastic follicles with typical reactive features*
- *Prominent marginal zone expansion seen in chronic antigenic simulation may resemble marginal zone lymphoma; however, there is no infiltration of the germinal center or red pulp by marginal zone cells and mantle zones are preserved, a feature invariably missing in lymphoma cases*
- *Common findings in patients with splenomegaly associated with systemic lupus erythematosus and rheumatoid arthritis (Felty syndrome) include follicular hyperplasia, plasmacytosis, and red pulp expansion including proliferation of CD3-, CD8-, and CD57-positive cytotoxic T cells, neutropenia, and leg ulcers*

SELECTED REFERENCES

Burke JS, Osborne BM: Localized reactive lymphoid hyperplasia of the spleen simulating malignant lymphoma: a report of seven cases. Am J Surg Pathol 7:373-380, 1983.

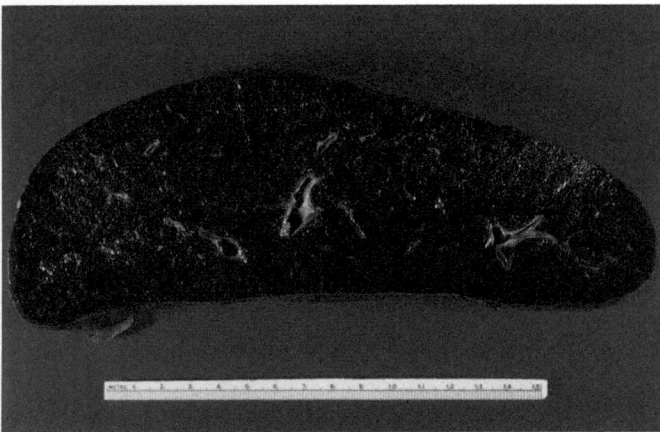

Figure 15-1. Follicular white pulp hyperplasia, gross photograph. The spleen is enlarged. Small indistinct pale foci of hyperplastic white pulp are seen on the cut surface and under the capsule.

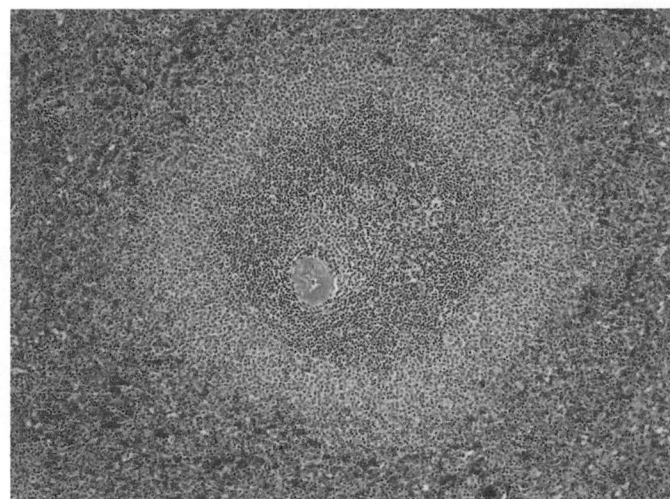

Figure 15-2. Marginal zone hyperplasia.

Burks EJ, Loughran TP Jr: Pathogenesis of neutropenia in large granular lymphocyte leukemia and Felty syndrome. Blood Rev 20:245-266, 2006.

Neiman RS, Orazi A: Reactive lymphoid hyperplasia. In Disorders of the Spleen, 2nd ed. Philadelphia, WB Saunders, 1999, pp 67-84.

REACTIVE LYMPHOID HYPERPLASIA WITHOUT GERMINAL CENTER FORMATION

Clinical Features

- Occurs in any age group
- Most common pattern encountered in viral infections (infectious mononucleosis, herpes simplex virus), transplant recipients, and immunosuppressed individuals (e.g., steroid-treated immune thrombocytopenic purpura, patients with rheumatoid arthritis on methotrexate) and in functional immunodeficiencies encountered in infants and elderly individuals

Gross Pathology

- Modest splenomegaly
- Cut surface may be grossly unremarkable

Histopathology

- White pulp shows a heterogeneous lymphoid population (Figure 15-3)
- Numerous immunoblasts with open chromatin pattern and prominent nucleoli are seen
- Tingible body macrophages may be prominent
- Similar proliferation is seen in white pulp surrounding splenic arterioles (PALS)
- Transformed lymphocytes may infiltrate splenic trabeculae, predisposing to splenic rupture (e.g., in infectious mononucleosis)

Special Stains and Immunohistochemistry

- Immunohistochemistry can be useful in differential diagnosis from lymphomatous infiltration, such as immunoblastic lymphoma

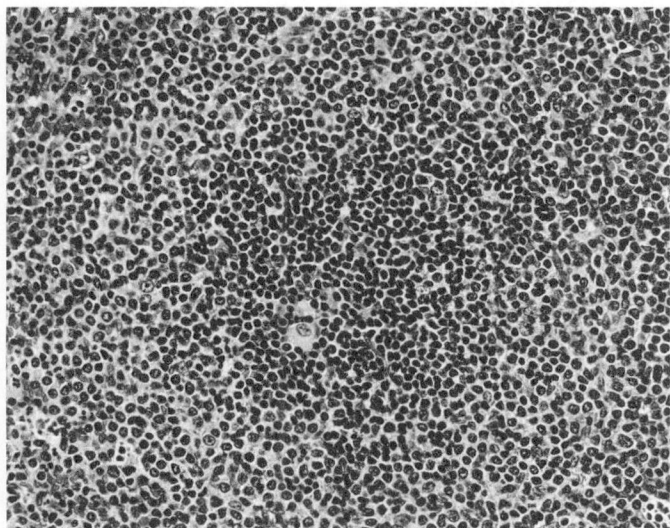

Figure 15-3. Primary (nonfollicular) white pulp hyperplasia. Heterogeneous lymphoid population including immunoblasts with open chromatin pattern.

- Immunohistochemical stains and in situ hybridization studies to exclude viral infection (e.g., Epstein-Barr virus [EBV]) may be helpful

Other Techniques for Diagnosis

- Evaluation of light-chain expression by flow cytometry shows polyclonal B-cell population

Differential Diagnosis

DIFFUSE LARGE B-CELL LYMPHOMA (DLBCL), IMMUNOBLASTIC VARIANT

- Uniform expansive sheets of immunoblasts favor the diagnosis of DLBCL
- Correlation of histologic findings with clinical history and immunohistochemistry, flow cytometry, or molecular analysis is of great value

HODGKIN LYMPHOMA

- Immunoblastic proliferation in infectious mononucleosis may contain Reed-Sternberg–like cells
- Immunoblasts are positive for B- or T-cell markers and CD45, and they may be positive for CD30 antigen; however, in contrast to classical Hodgkin lymphoma, they are negative for CD15 antigen

PEARLS

- *Careful examination of the histologic sections with a high-power objective is mandatory; on low-power examination, nonfollicular lymphoid hyperplasia may superficially resemble an unremarkable unstimulated spleen*

SELECTED REFERENCES

Neiman RS, Orazi A: Reactive lymphoid hyperplasia. In Disorders of the Spleen, 2nd ed. Philadelphia, WB Saunders, 1999, pp 67-84.

Smith EB, Custer RP: Rupture of the spleen in infectious mononucleosis: a clinicopathologic report of seven cases. Blood 61:317-333, 1994.

CASTLEMAN DISEASE (ANGIOFOLLICULAR HYPERPLASIA)

Clinical Features

- Splenic involvement occurs most frequently in multicentric Castleman disease, usually of plasma cell type
- Patients with multicentric Castleman disease present with constitutional symptoms such as fever and frequently show a host of hematologic and immunologic abnormalities (anemia, hypergammaglobulinemia)
- Plasmablastic type of multicentric Castleman disease is a variant associated with human herpesvirus type 8 (HHV-8) seen in human immunodeficiency virus (HIV)-positive patients and in about 40% of HIV-negative cases
- Splenic involvement by Castleman disease of hyaline-vascular type is exceptionally rare and poorly documented

Gross Pathology

- Modest to moderate splenomegaly

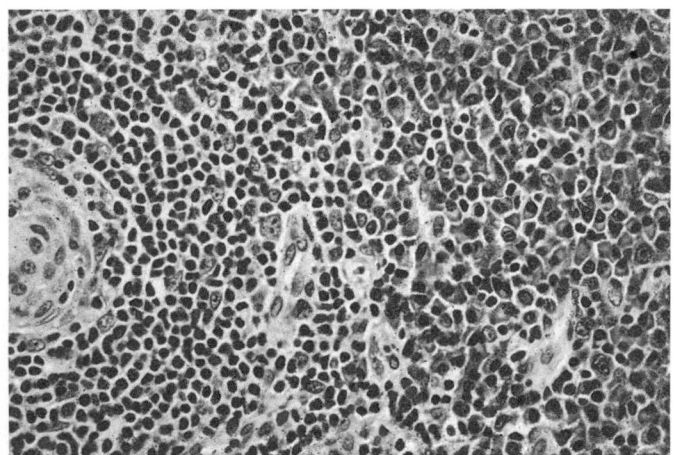

Figure 15-4. Castleman disease (mixed type). Increased plasma cells and hyalinized germinal centers.

Histopathology (Figure 15-4)

- Hyaline-vascular type (see Chapter 14)
- Multicentric Castleman disease
  - Plasma cell type
    - Hyperplastic or regressively transformed follicles
    - Significant red pulp plasmacytosis
  - Plasmablastic type
    - Spectrum of hyperplastic and regressively transformed follicles surrounded by a band of fibrosis with large number of plasma cells
    - Mantle zone with increased number of large lymphoid cells with plasmablastic and immunoblastic features
    - Red pulp is unremarkable
    - Rarely, confluent aggregates of HHV-8–positive plasmablasts are seen, a finding termed *microlymphoma*

Special Stains and Immunohistochemistry

- Plasma cells are usually polyclonal; however, may be monotypic (lambda restricted)
- Usually negative for EBV; only rare cases resembling germinotropic lymphoma are positive for both EBV and HHV-8
- Plasmablasts of plasmablastic type of multicentric Castleman disease are positive for CD20, IgM, lambda light chain, and HHV-8 and are negative for CD30 antigen

Other Techniques for Diagnosis

- Noncontributory

Differential Diagnosis

REACTIVE LYMPHOID HYPERPLASIA
- Hyalinization may be present; however, hyaline-vascular changes associated with follicles characteristic of hyaline-vascular type are not seen

RHEUMATOID ARTHRITIS VERSUS CASTLEMAN DISEASE, PLASMA CELL TYPE
- Germinal centers in the white pulp may be hyperplastic
- Polyclonal plasmacytosis of red pulp may be prominent
- Clinical history and serologic tests are important

SELECTED REFERENCES

Cesarman E, Knowles DM: Kaposi's sarcoma-associated herpesvirus: a lymphotropic human herpesvirus associated with Kaposi's sarcoma, primary effusion lymphoma, and multicentric Castleman's disease. Semin Diagn Pathol 14:54-56, 1997.

Dupin N, Diss TL, Kellam P, et al: HHV-8 is associated with a plasmablastic variant of Castleman disease that is linked to HHV-8-positive plasmablastic lymphoma. Blood 95:1406-1412, 2000.

Frizzera G: Castleman's disease and related disorders. Semin Diagn Pathol 5:346-364, 1998.

Keller AR, Hochholzer L, Castleman B: Hyaline-vascular and plasma-cell types of giant lymph node hyperplasia of mediastinum and other locations. Cancer 29:670-683, 1972.

Menke DM, Tiemann M, Camariano JK, et al: Diagnosis of Castleman's disease by identification of an immunophenotypically aberrant population of mantle zone B lymphocytes in paraffin-embedded lymph node biopsies. Am J Clin Pathol 105:268-276, 1996.

Weisenburger DD: Multicentric angiofollicular lymph node hyperplasia: pathology of the spleen. Am J Surg Pathol 12:176-181, 1988.

COMMON VARIABLE IMMUNODEFICIENCY

Clinical Features

- Presentation in childhood or in an adult patient
- Recurrent infections
- Clinical history necessary for adequate interpretation
- Increased risk for lymphoma

Gross Pathology

- Spleen normal sized to enlarged
- May be grossly unremarkable

Histopathology

- Variable histologic features dependent on the primary pathogenetic deficiency in lymphoid stimulatory molecules (inducible costimulator, transmembrane activator, and calcium modulating cyclophilin ligand [CAML] interactor or CD19 deficiencies)
- Follicular atrophy to hyperplasia
- Atypical follicular hyperplasia may occur
- Granulomas may be prominent
- Immunoblastic proliferation and atypical cells resembling Hodgkin or Reed-Sternberg cells may be present
- There may be lymphoid hyperplasia in the red pulp

Special Stains and Immunohistochemistry

- Most cases are positive for Epstein-Barr virus–encoded latent membrane protein (EBV-LMP) immunostain or Epstein-Barr virus–encoded RNA (EBER) in situ hybridization
- Immunohistochemical stains for T cells and B cells will show a mixed lymphoid population (B and T cells present in variable proportions)
- Polyclonal B-cell population by flow cytometry

Other Techniques for Diagnosis

- Noncontributory

Differential Diagnosis

NONSPECIFIC FOLLICULAR HYPERPLASIA

- Detailed clinical history of immunodeficiency; immunologic and genetic studies

LYMPHOPROLIFERATIVE DISORDERS

- Careful clinical history of immunodeficiency has to be obtained to avoid misinterpretation of significant immunoblastic proliferation associated with common variable immunodeficiency (CVID) as malignant lymphoma
- Often necessary to establish clonality for a firm diagnosis of malignant lymphoma

PEARLS

- *Histologic features are variable and nonspecific*
- *Include special stains for microorganisms in cases with granulomatous presentation*

SELECTED REFERENCES

Cunningham-Rundles C, Bodian C: Common variable immunodeficiency: clinical and immunological features of 248 patients. Clin Immunol 92:34-48, 1999.
Salzer U, Grimbacher B: Common variable immunodeficiency: the power of co-stimulation. Semin Immunol 18:337-346, 2006.
Wang J, Rodriguez-Davalos M, Levi G, et al: Common variable immunodeficiency presenting with a large abdominal mass. J Allergy Clin Immunol 115:1318-1320, 2005.

AUTOIMMUNE LYMPHOPROLIFERATIVE SYNDROME

Clinical Features

- Rare heritable lymphoproliferative syndrome due to mutations in *Fas* (CD95), *Fas ligand, caspase 8,* or *caspase 10* genes
- Presents in early childhood, usually in patients younger than 2 years
- Generalized lymphadenopathy, splenomegaly, and autoimmunity
- Frequent association with immune cytopenias
- Increased risk for development of non-Hodgkin and Hodgkin lymphoma

Gross Pathology

- Massive splenomegaly

Histopathology

- Prominent white pulp with follicular hyperplasia and expansion of marginal zones
- Marked expansion of PALS and red pulp due to the infiltration by a mixed population of small T cells, T-cell immunoblasts, and polyclonal plasma cells (Figure 15-5)

Special Stains and Immunohistochemistry

- Double negative T cells (CD4 and CD8 negative) are the hallmark of the disease and can be predominantly found in the red pulp
- Splenic T cells are also negative for CD25

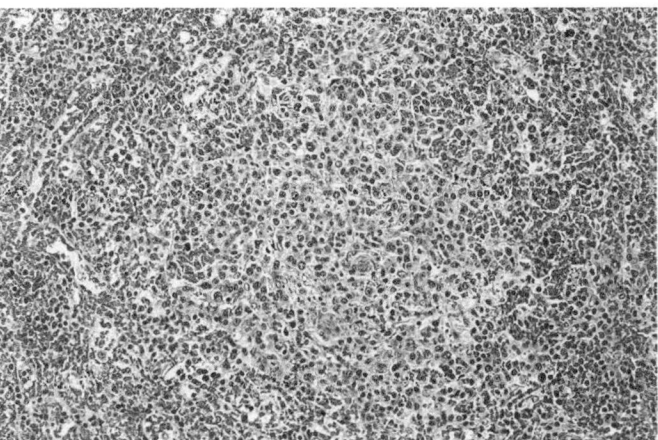

Figure 15-5. Autoimmune lymphoproliferative syndrome. Mixed population of small T cells, T-cell immunoblasts, and polyclonal plasma cells.

Other Techniques for Diagnosis

- Noncontributory

Differential Diagnosis

LYMPHOPROLIFERATIVE DISORDER

- Correlation with clinical history and the presence of splenomegaly in infancy is critical to avoid interpretation of an abnormal T-cell population in the spleen as a T-cell lymphoproliferative disorder

SELECTED REFERENCES

Lim MS, Straus SE, Dale JK, et al: Pathological findings in human autoimmune lymphoproliferative syndrome. Am J Pathol 153:1541-1550, 1998.
Worth A, Thrasher AJ, Gaspar HB: Autoimmune lymphoproliferative syndrome: molecular basis of disease and clinical phenotype. Br J Haematol 133:134-140, 2006.

NEOPLASTIC DISEASES INVOLVING THE SPLENIC WHITE PULP

SPLENIC MARGINAL ZONE LYMPHOMA (SMZL)

Clinical Features

- Most common in middle-aged to elderly patients, without a gender predominance
- Presentation with left upper quadrant pain, anemia, and weight loss
- Most common type of lymphoma to present with massive splenomegaly
- Some cases with autoimmune anemia or thrombocytopenia
- Small monoclonal serum IgM/D paraprotein in one third of cases
- Splenic hilar lymph nodes, peripheral blood, bone marrow, and liver involvement are common at presentation
- Lacks peripheral nodal involvement
- Usually no lymphadenopathy
- Association with hepatitis C, cryoglobulinemia, and autoimmunity
- Splenectomy may produce long-term remission

Gross Pathology

- Prominent lymphoid follicle proliferation producing a miliary pattern of white pulp expansion

Histopathology

- Increase in size and number of white pulp follicles with a variable degree of PALS and red pulp involvement being the rule
- Malignant lymphoid cells may form expanded marginal zones or more often show colonization of germinal centers with attenuated mantle zones; combinations of the two patterns are frequently seen (Figure 15-6A)
- A rare "indolent" variant, which closely simulates marginal zone hyperplasia, has been reported; its diagnosis usually requires demonstration of clonality
- Red pulp involvement either as diffuse pattern or as lymphoid nodules
- Rare cases may display a "red pulp predominant" proliferative pattern

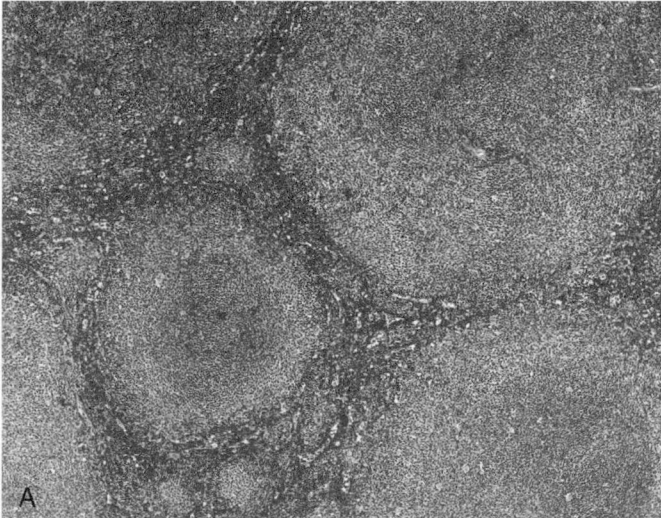

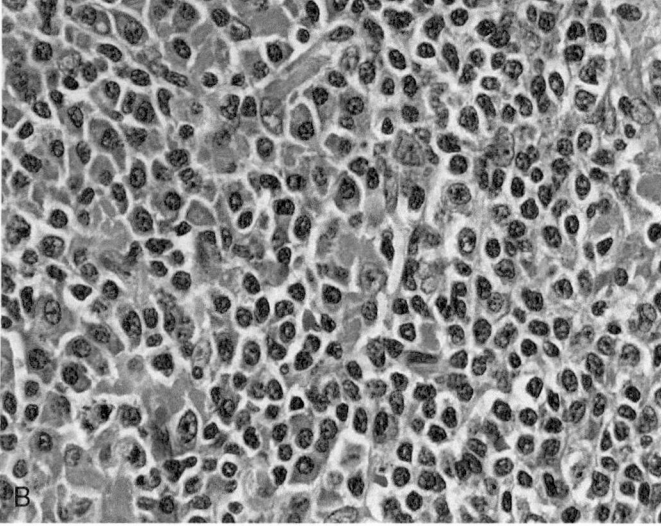

Figure 15-6. Splenic marginal zone lymphoma. A, Histologic section shows expanded marginal zone replaced by tumor cells. **B,** High-power view shows tumor cells with round nuclei and abundant clear cytoplasm and numerous plasma cells.

- Lymphoma cells are medium sized with round to oval nuclei and often abundant clear cytoplasm (Figure 15-6B)
- Larger lymphoid cells are usually seen at the periphery of neoplastic nodules
- Bone marrow infiltration is the rule; may be intrasinusoidal, interstitial, or multinodular
- Peripheral blood may show circulating small lymphocytes with abundant cytoplasm and short polar villi

Special Stains and Immunohistochemistry

- SMZL expresses the B-cell markers CD20, PAX5, and CD79a; CD5, cyclin D1, bcl-6, annexin-A1, and CD10 are absent; CD123 is also usually negative
- Due to the absence of specific markers, the diagnosis of SMZL is based on the absence of immunophenotypic features specific for other lymphoma subtypes

Other Techniques for Diagnosis

- By flow cytometry, the expression of B-cell markers (CD19, CD20, and CD22) and clonal surface light chains is seen
- Molecular studies for immunoglobulin heavy-chain gene show clonal rearrangements
- The *bcl-1* and *bcl-2* genes are not rearranged

Differential Diagnosis (also see Table 15-1)

SPLENIC DIFFUSE RED PULP SMALL B-CELL LYMPHOMA

- Diffuse involvement of red pulp with almost complete obliteration of white pulp
- Cutaneous involvement may be present
- Bone marrow involvement is often subtle with a predominant intrasinusoidal localization of the atypical lymphoid cells
- Strong constant expression of DBA.44 and often of CD11c

HAIRY CELL LEUKEMIA

- Red pulp involvement with prominent blood lakes
- Cells with fine, hairlike cytoplasmic processes may be seen in peripheral blood
- Diffuse pattern of bone marrow involvement (versus nodular in SMZL)
- Distinct immunophenotype: B cells positive for tartrate-resistant acid phosphatase (TRAP), DBA.44, CD25, CD11c, and CD103
- BRAF V600E mutation by polymerase chain reaction (PCR)
- Hairy cell leukemia variant
- Similar to classical hairy cell leukemia but with more pleomorphic cytologic features including a variably prominent nucleolus and lacking CD25, annexin A1, and BRAF V600E mutation

T-CELL LARGE GRANULAR LYMPHOCYTIC LEUKEMIA

- Predominantly a red pulp infiltrate
- Distinct T-cell immunophenotype with varying degrees of loss or decreased density of CD7, CD2, and CD3; CD8 and CD57 positive in most cases; aberrant expression of natural killer receptors for class I major

TABLE 15-1 MORPHOLOGIC AND IMMUNOPHENOTYPIC FEATURES OF B-CELL NON-HODGKIN LYMPHOMAS WITH PROMINENT SPLEEN INVOLVEMENT

| Type of Lymphomas | Morphologic and Immunophenotypic Features | | | |
	Architectural Features	Cytologic Features	Immunophenotype Cytogenetics	Cell of Origin
Chronic lymphocytic leukemia/small lymphocytic lymphoma	White and red pulp involvement; occasional growth centers	Small lymphoid cells with interspersed prolymphocytes and paraimmunoblasts, with or without growth centers	CD20, CD19, CD5, and CD23 positive	Naive or memory B cell
Mantle cell lymphoma	White pulp involvement; nodular or mantle zone pattern	Monotonous population of medium-sized lymphocytes with irregular nuclei; blast like or pleomorphic cells in blastoid variant	CD20, CD19, CD5, FMC7, and cyclin D1 positive; t(11;14)	Mantle zone cell
Follicular lymphoma	White pulp involvement; follicular pattern	Medium-sized lymphocytes with indented nuclei and variable admixture of large lymphoid cells	CD20, CD19, CD10, BCL-6, and BCL-2 positive; t(14;18)	Germinal center cell
Splenic marginal zone lymphoma	Predominantly white pulp involvement; red pulp infiltrates with scattered cells and nodules of lymphoma cells	Medium-sized lymphocytes with clear cytoplasm, indented nuclei, and large lymphoid cells scattered at the periphery of the nodules	CD20 and CD19 positive, CD43 positive or negative	Marginal zone cell
Splenic diffuse red pulp small B-cell lymphoma	Red pulp involvement with usually obliteration of the white pulp	Small to medium-sized lymphoid cells with pale or lightly eosinophilic cytoplasm, round and regular nuclei with only occasional small distinct nucleoli; some cases may show plasmacytoid lymphoid cells	Positive for CD20, DBA.44, BCL2, IgG, often positive for p53, variable positivity for CD11c, CD103 and IgD, and negative for CD25, CD10, CD23, BCL6, and annexin-A1	Not yet ascertained
Hairy cell leukemia	Predominantly red pulp with pseudosinuses	Medium-sized cells with abundant cytoplasm and cytoplasmic projections	CD20, CD19, CD103, CD25, annexin-A1 and CD11c positive,	Suggested origin: post–germinal center memory B cell

histocompatibility complex molecules (of killer cell immunoglobulin-like receptor type, CD158 antigens, and C-type lectin type, CD94 and NKG2 molecules); a minority of cases express CD56, CD16, or both

HEPATOSPLENIC T-CELL LYMPHOMA

- More common in young men
- May occur in the post-transplantation setting and after anti-TNF therapy
- Typically presents with significant hepatomegaly and splenomegaly, abnormal liver function tests, and cytopenias
- Diffuse red pulp infiltration by slightly irregular medium-sized lymphocytes
- T-cell immunophenotype with surface CD3 and associated γδ T-cell receptor (TCR), and absent CD5, CD4, and CD8 antigens; CD56 and CD16 are expressed in some cases

PEARLS

- *Thorough examination of splenectomy specimens with clinical correlation and, if appropriate, with immunohistochemical, flow cytometric, and molecular analysis is mandatory because rare cases of minimal involvement by splenic marginal zone lymphoma have been reported, such as in cases of refractory idiopathic thrombocytopenic purpura (ITP)*
- *Early cases of splenic marginal cell lymphoma may resemble marginal zone hyperplasia; however, in the latter, mantle zones are preserved, a feature invariably missing in lymphoma cases*
- *Subtle lymphomatous infiltrate is also present in the red pulp*
- *Bone marrow involvement is common, often subtle, and intrasinusoidal; sinusoidal infiltrate is best visualized by immunohistochemistry on the marrow core biopsy*

SELECTED REFERENCES

Ngan BY, Warnke RA, Wilson M, et al: Monocytoid B cell lymphoma: a study of 36 cases. Hum Pathol 22:409-421, 1991.

Rosso R, Neiman RS, Paulli M, et al: Splenic marginal zone cell lymphoma: report of an indolent variant without massive splenomegaly presumably representing an early phase of the disease. Hum Pathol 26:39-46, 1995.

Saadoun D, Suarez F, Lefrere F, et al: Splenic lymphoma with villous lymphocytes, associated with type II cryoglobulinemia and HCV infection: a new entity? Blood 105:74-76, 2005.

Traverse-Glehen A, Baseggio L, Callet-Bauchu E, et al: Splenic red pulp lymphoma with numerous basophilic villous lymphocytes: a distinct clinico-pathological and molecular entity? Blood 111:2253-2260, 2008.

Traverse-Glehen A, Verney A, Baseggio L, et al: Analysis of BCL-6, CD95, PIM1, RHO/TTF and PAX5 mutations in splenic and nodal marginal zone B-cell lymphomas suggests a particular B-cell origin. Leukemia 21:1821-1824, 2007.

CHRONIC LYMPHOCYTIC LEUKEMIA/ SMALL LYMPHOCYTIC LYMPHOMA

Clinical Features

- Occur predominantly in elderly individuals
- Patients present with varying degrees of spleen, peripheral blood, and bone marrow involvement

Gross Pathology

- Variable splenomegaly with prominent white pulp (miliary pattern) or more homogeneous diffuse involvement in advanced stages

Histopathology

- Diffuse infiltrate of both red and white pulp; no residual germinal centers are present
- Neoplastic lymphoid cells are small with a coarse chromatin pattern, inconspicuous nucleoli, and scant cytoplasm (Figure 15-7)
- Prolymphocytes and paraimmunoblasts can be intermingled with small lymphoid cells or form ill-defined aggregates; proliferation centers (pseudofollicles) are

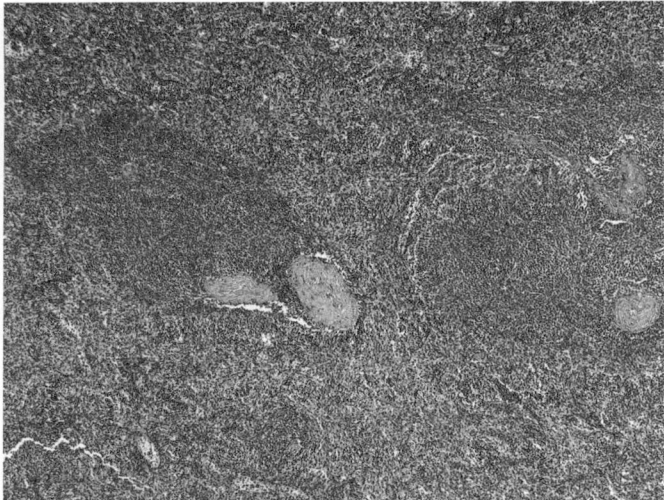

Figure 15-7. Chronic lymphocytic leukemia/small lymphocytic lymphoma. Histologic section shows a neoplasm composed of small uniform lymphoid cells with dense chromatin pattern and scant cytoplasm.

much less common in the spleen than in lymph nodes or bone marrow

Special Stains and Immunohistochemistry

- Neoplastic cells express CD20, CD5, CD23, and CD43

Other Techniques for Diagnosis

- Neoplastic cells express CD19, CD5, CD23, and low-density clonal surface light chain and are weakly positive for CD20 by flow cytometric immunophenotypic analysis
- Clonal immunoglobulin gene rearrangement is present
- Chronic lymphocytic leukemia (CLL) and small lymphocytic lymphoma (SLL) are derived from recirculating CD5 and from immunoglobulin M (IgM) positive and IgD positive or negative B cells normally present in the peripheral blood
- Two groups of CLL/SLL are recognized; this subclassification roughly corresponds to the expression of ZAP-70 and CD38 molecules, which can be quantified by flow cytometry
  - One type corresponding to the pregerminal center phenotype (naive, showing no mutations in the variable region of immunoglobulin heavy-chain $[V_H]$ gene)
  - A second type derived from memory B cells (postgerminal center, mutated V_H gene)

DIFFERENTIAL DIAGNOSIS

SPLENIC MARGINAL ZONE LYMPHOMA

- Predominantly white pulp infiltrate, frequently with marginal zone pattern
- Cells are strongly positive for CD20 and surface light chain (flow cytometry) and negative for CD5 and CD23

FOLLICULAR LYMPHOMA

- Largely a white pulp distribution with only minimal red pulp involvement
- Cytologically composed of a mixture of medium-sized centrocytes and large centroblasts
- Cells are positive for CD19, CD20, CD22, CD10, and bcl-2 [t(14;18)] and negative for CD43, CD5, and CD23

MANTLE CELL LYMPHOMA

- Predominantly white pulp involvement with expansion into the red pulp
- Uniform small to medium-sized cells with irregular nuclear outlines
- Neoplastic cells are positive for CD20, CD19, CD5, CD43, cyclin D1 [t(11;14)], and FMC7 (flow cytometry) and negative for CD23

LYMPHOPLASMACYTIC LYMPHOMA (WALDENSTRÖM MACROGLOBULINEMIA)

- The defining feature is the demonstration of monoclonal IgM protein in the serum, frequently with symptoms related to hyperviscosity
- Prominent plasmacytic component or a mixture of plasma cells and plasmacytoid lymphocytes

- B cell–associated antigens, including CD19, CD20, and CD22, are consistently expressed; the surface IgM expression can be demonstrated in all cases, most cases show dim CD25; coexpression of CD5, CD23, and FMC7 have been reported; a minute monoclonal plasma cell component can be identified by flow cytometry in most cases
- Molecular analysis for MYD88 L265P somatic mutation represents an additional useful diagnostic tool; the mutation that is present in > 90% of LPL cases is only rarely present in other type of small B-cell lymphoma

PROLYMPHOCYTIC LEUKEMIA

- In contrast to small lymphoid cells of CLL/SLL, prolymphocytes are medium-sized atypical lymphoid cells with vesicular nuclei and prominent nucleoli
- Patients typically present with high white blood cell counts
- Splenomegaly may be massive
- CD20 and surface immunoglobulin density are stronger than in typical cases of CLL/SLL; CD5 expression is variable
- Cyclin D1 is positive in 20% cases; these cases are currently considered a splenomegalic form of mantle cell lymphoma

PEARLS

- *White and red pulp infiltrate is composed of uniform small lymphoid cells*
- *Modest splenic enlargement usually occurs; most patients whose disease is dominated by massive splenomegaly have mantle zone lymphoma or SMZL rather than SLL/CLL*
- *Richter transformation may present in the spleen; this appears as fleshy, cream-colored tumor nodules similar to the involvement by DLBCL*

SELECTED REFERENCES

Hollema H, Visser L, Poppema S: Small lymphocytic lymphomas with predominant splenomegaly: a comparison of immunophenotypes with cases of predominant lymphadenopathy. Mod Pathol 4:712-717, 1991.

Pangalis GA, Nathwani BN, Rappaport H: Malignant lymphoma, well-differentiated lymphocytic lymphoma: its relationship with chronic lymphocytic leukemia and macroglobulinemias of Waldenström. Cancer 39:999-1010, 1977.

Treon SP, Xu L, Yang G, et al. MYD88 L265P somatic mutation in Waldenström's macroglobulinemia. N Engl J Med. 367:826-833, 2012.

Van Krieken JH, Feller AC, te Velde J: The distribution of non-Hodgkin's lymphoma in the lymphoid compartments of the human spleen. Am J Surg Pathol 13:757-765, 1989.

PROLYMPHOCYTIC LEUKEMIA

Clinical Features

- Presentation in elderly patients, with male predominance
- Marked lymphocytosis (often greater than $100 \times 10^9/L$) with more than 55% prolymphocytes
- Massive splenomegaly with hypersplenism and resulting cytopenias and the absence of lymphadenopathy are common features

Gross Pathology

- Massive splenomegaly
- Diffuse red pulp infiltration with variable prominence of white pulp

Histopathology

- Diffuse red pulp infiltration associated with involvement of the white pulp in most cases
- Heterogeneous population of lymphoid cells with a predominance of prolymphocytes characterized by medium size, abundant cytoplasm, and prominent nucleoli (Figure 15-8)

Special Stains and Immunohistochemistry

- Eighty percent of prolymphocytic leukemia cases are of B-cell immunophenotype and are positive for CD20, with variable coexpression of CD5 and CD23
- Twenty percent of cases show T-cell immunophenotype (T-cell prolymphocytic leukemia) with a predominant expression of CD3, CD5, and CD4; loss of T-cell antigens may be seen

OTHER TECHNIQUES FOR DIAGNOSIS

- By flow cytometry, a strong expression of CD20, CD19, FMC7, and clonal surface immunoglobulin is seen in most cases

Differential Diagnosis

CLL/SLL

- Massive splenomegaly is relatively uncommon
- Homogeneous population of small lymphoid cells with scant cytoplasm; prolymphocytes are rare
- Weaker expression of surface immunoglobulins and CD20, positivity for CD5 and CD23, negativity for FMC7

SPLENIC MARGINAL ZONE LYMPHOMA

- Significant peripheral lymphocytosis is uncommon
- Neoplastic B-cells usually do not have prominent nucleoli

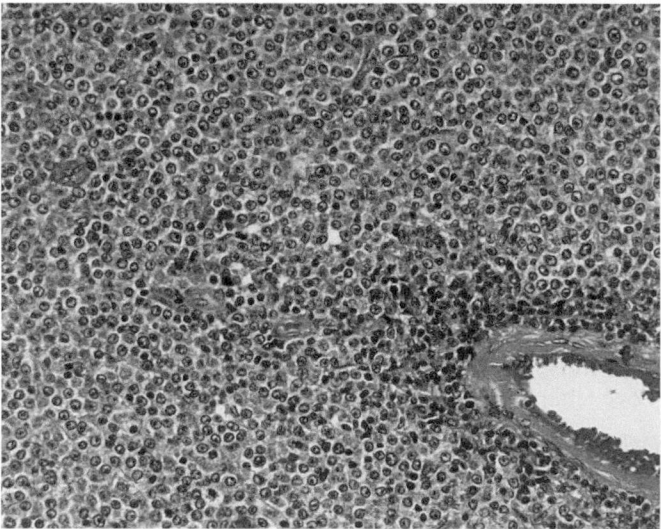

Figure 15-8. Prolymphocytic leukemia. The infiltrate is composed of a heterogeneous population of lymphoid cells, many of which have large nuclei and prominent nucleoli.

- *Prolymphocytic leukemia occurs predominantly in elderly males*
- *Massive splenomegaly with significant lymphocytosis and absence of peripheral lymphadenopathy*
- *Characterized by increased numbers of prolymphocytes (large to medium-sized cells with prominent nucleoli) admixed with the small round lymphocytes*
- *Usually B-cell phenotype*
- *Variable expression of CD5 and CD23 (both positive in CLL/SLL)*

SELECTED REFERENCES

Bearman RM, Pangalis GA, Rappaport H: Prolymphocytic leukemia: clinical, histopathological and cytochemical observations. Cancer 42:2360-2372, 1978.

Lampert I, Catovsky D, Marsh GW, et al: The histopathology of prolymphocytic leukemia with particular reference to the spleen: a comparison with chronic lymphocytic leukemia. Histopathology 4:3-19, 1980.

Ruchlemer R, Parry-Jones N, Brito-Babapulle V, et al: B-prolymphocytic leukaemia with t(11;14) revisited: a splenomegalic form of mantle cell lymphoma evolving with leukaemia. Br J Haematol 125:330-336, 2004.

MANTLE CELL LYMPHOMA

Clinical Features

- Most patients present with widespread peripheral lymphadenopathy and bone marrow involvement
- A splenomegalic variant of mantle cell lymphoma with leukemic peripheral blood involvement and with no appreciable lymphadenopathy has been reported

Gross Pathology

- Prominent white pulp in an enlarged spleen
- Massive splenomegaly may be seen (>1000 g)

Histopathology

- Nodular expansion of white pulp with or without a mantle zone pattern (i.e., lymphoid proliferation surrounding residual germinal centers)
- A pure mantle zone lymphomatous growth pattern is rarely seen
- Homogeneous population of medium-sized lymphoid cells with irregular nuclear outlines
- Blastoid variant of mantle cell lymphoma is composed of blastlike lymphoid cells (lymphoblastoid variant) or of large pleomorphic cells resembling those of DLBCL

Special Stains and Immunohistochemistry

- Neoplastic cells are positive for CD20, CD5, and cyclin D1 [t(11;14)], SOX11, and negative for CD23
- See Chapter 14 for more detailed information

Other Techniques for Diagnosis

- By flow cytometry, the neoplastic cells are positive for CD20 (bright expression), CD19, CD5, and FMC7 and negative for CD23
- The defining feature of mantle cell lymphoma is the presence of t(11;14), the translocation of proto-oncogene

cyclin D1 (*bcl-1*; involved in the regulation of G_1- to S-phase progression) to the immunoglobulin heavy-chain gene locus

Differential Diagnosis

CLL/SLL

- Diffuse red pulp infiltration is prominent
- Small lymphocytes with some large cells (prolymphocytes and paraimmunoblasts)
- Low-density sIg and CD20 positivity; positive for both CD5 and CD23
- Lack of staining for cyclin D1

SPLENIC MARGINAL ZONE LYMPHOMA

- Present with massive splenomegaly without peripheral lymphadenopathy
- Expanded, confluent marginal zones can be difficult to distinguish from expanded mantle zones
- Neoplastic population composed of medium-sized lymphoid cells with rare admixed large cells
- Neoplastic cells do not express CD5 or cyclin D1

LYMPHOBLASTIC LYMPHOMA

- Lymphoblasts are positive for TdT and negative for cyclin-D1

- *Mantle cell lymphoma can present with leukemic peripheral blood involvement and massive splenomegaly*
- *Blastoid mantle cell lymphoma may mimic lymphoblast proliferation or DLBCL*

SELECTED REFERENCES

Angelopoulou MK, Siakantariz MP, Vassilakopoulous TP, et al: The splenic form of mantle cell lymphoma. Eur J Haematol 68:12-21, 2002.

Banks PM, Chan J, Cleary ML, et al: Mantle cell lymphoma: a proposal for unification of morphologic, immunologic and molecular data. Am J Surg Pathol 16:637-640, 1992.

Molina TJ, Delmer A, Cymbalista F, et al: Mantle cell lymphoma, in leukaemic phase with prominent splenomegaly: a report of eight cases with similar clinical presentation and aggressive outcome. Virchows Arch 437:591-598, 2000.

FOLLICULAR LYMPHOMA

Clinical Features

- Patients typically present with multifocal lymphadenopathy and bone marrow involvement (stage IV)
- About half of patients show splenic involvement, often detected only at the microscopic level

Gross Pathology

- Uniform expansion of the white pulp nodules (miliary pattern)

Histopathology (Figure 15-9)

- Uniform multifocal involvement of the white pulp, frequently with small aggregates of lymphoma cells within red pulp
- In grades 1 and 2 follicular lymphoma, neoplastic follicles are composed predominantly of small to

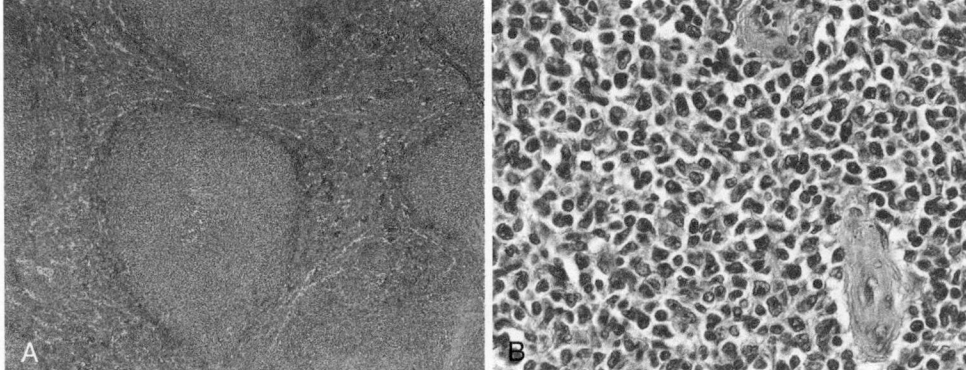

Figure 15-9. Follicular lymphoma. A, Low-power view shows multiple white pulp tumor nodules. **B,** The nodules are composed of predominantly centrocytes.

medium-sized cleaved atypical lymphoid cells (centrocytes) with a variable admixture of large atypical lymphoid cells with vesicular nuclei and multiple nucleoli mostly attached to the nuclear membrane (centroblasts)
- In grade 3 follicular lymphoma, large atypical lymphoid cells predominate

Special Stains and Immunohistochemistry
- The immunophenotype reflects the follicle center cell origin of follicular lymphoma
- B-cell marker CD20 is positive, along with the coexpression of antigens characteristic for germinal center cells, such as CD10 and bcl-6
- Antiapoptotic protein bcl-2 is usually positive
- See Chapter 14 for more detailed information

Other Techniques for Diagnosis
- By flow cytometry, pan B-cell markers (CD19, CD20) and clonal surface immunoglobulin are present along with the coexpression of CD10 antigen in most cases; the coexpression of CD10, similar in intensity to that seen in reactive follicular hyperplasia, in association with a relatively low-intensity CD19, is a characteristic feature of follicular lymphoma
- Expression of bcl-2 is due to the t(14;18)(q32;q21), which places the *bcl-2* gene under a promoter of the immunoglobulin heavy-chain gene; rare cases of bcl-2 protein negative or lacking t(14;18)(q32;q21) follicular lymphoma, however, exist (discussed later).

Differential Diagnosis

REACTIVE FOLLICULAR HYPERPLASIA
- Well-defined follicles with distinct marginal and mantle zones, polarization of germinal center into dark and light zones, tingible body macrophages, and mitotic figures
- Germinal centers negative for bcl-2

CASTLEMAN DISEASE
- Expanded mantle zones
- White pulp follicles are variably expanded or atrophic/hyalinized

- Red pulp is expanded with large numbers of polyclonal plasma cells

MANTLE CELL LYMPHOMA
- Uniform population of small to medium-sized lymphocytes without centroblasts
- Cells express CD5 and are generally CD10 negative
- Overexpression of cyclin D1
- Expression of bcl-2 is not useful in the differential diagnosis

SPLENIC MARGINAL ZONE LYMPHOMA
- More prominent involvement of red pulp
- The expression of markers associated with germinal center origin is not seen

PEARLS
- *Expression of bcl-2 is seen in most types of indolent B-cell lymphomas; however, when seen in nodular proliferation showing germinal center cell immunophenotype, bcl-2 is diagnostic of follicular lymphoma*
- *About 20% of follicular lymphomas are negative for bcl-2 antigen; in a proportion of these cases, molecular studies (polymerase chain reaction [PCR] or fluorescent in situ hybridization [FISH] based) may demonstrate the presence of t(14;18) or bcl-6 rearrangement*
- *Predominantly white pulp involvement, but discrete invasion of red pulp is common*

SELECTED REFERENCES
Gauland P, D'Agay MF, Peuchmar M, et al: Expression of the bcl-2 gene product in follicular lymphoma. Am J Pathol 140:1089-1095, 1992.

Horsman DE, Okamoto I, Ludkovski O, et al: Follicular lymphoma lacking the t(14;18)(q32;q21): identification of two disease subtypes. Br J Haematol 120:424-433, 2003.

Kim H, Dorfman RF: Morphological studies of 84 untreated patients subjected to laparotomy for the staging of non-Hodgkin's lymphoma. Cancer 33:647-674, 1974.

DIFFUSE LARGE B-CELL LYMPHOMA

Clinical Features
- Rare but accounts for about one-third of lymphomas localized to the spleen at presentation
- May arise de novo or represent transformation of low-grade lymphoma

Gross Pathology

- Typically presents as large tumor nodules that may coalesce into larger masses randomly distributed in the splenic parenchyma
- May show large areas of necrosis
- Usually involves hilar and retroperitoneal lymph nodes

Histopathology

- Focal large aggregates or sheets of large atypical lymphoid cells with variable cytologic features (centroblasts, immunoblasts) (Figure 15-10)
- Involves both white and red pulp, effacing the normal splenic architecture

Special Stains and Immunohistochemistry

- DLBCL expresses CD20 and CD79a; as in lymph nodes, it may express other antigens of germinal center derivation (bcl-6 and CD10) or of nongerminal center derivation (MUM-1); some cases may be positive for CD5
- See Chapter 14 for more detailed information

Other Techniques for Diagnosis

- By flow cytometry, DLBCL expresses CD19, CD20, and CD22; most commonly, there is a clonal surface light chain expression, although cases negative for surface light chains are not uncommon
- Immunoglobulin gene rearrangement analysis can be useful (see Chapter 14 for more detailed information)

Differential Diagnosis

HODGKIN LYMPHOMA

- Patients almost always have nodal Hodgkin lymphoma
- Splenic involvement is often associated with liver involvement
- Typical polymorphous cellular background composed of small lymphocytes, plasma cells, eosinophils, neutrophils, and macrophages with large pleomorphic Hodgkin-Reed-Sternberg cells and their variants
- Neoplastic cells are typically negative for CD20, CD45, and CD3 but express PAX-5 (weak) and CD30 with or without CD15

INFLAMMATORY PSEUDOTUMOR (IPT)

- Usually a single, well-demarcated whitish mass
- Histology shows a polymorphous collection of bland spindle cells and inflammatory cells

PEARLS

- *Large tumor nodules often with foci of necrosis*
- *Tumor usually involves hilar and retroperitoneal lymph nodes with or without peripheral lymphadenopathy*

SELECTED REFERENCES

Falk S, Stutte HJ: Primary malignant lymphomas of the spleen: a morphologic and immunohistochemical analysis of 17 cases. Cancer 66:2612-2619, 1990.

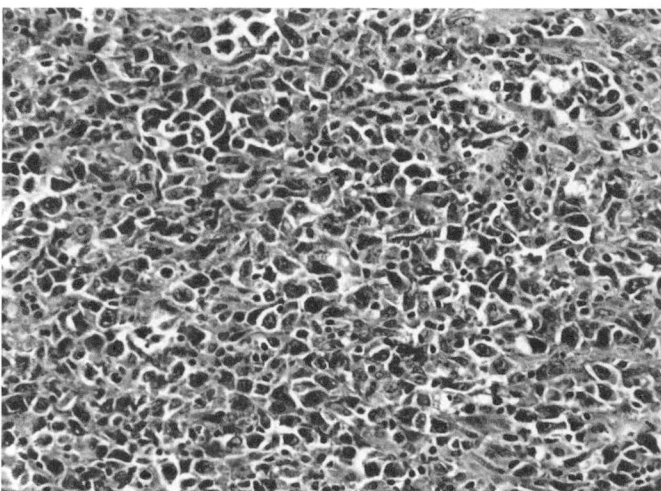

Figure 15-10. Diffuse large B-cell lymphoma. The tumor cells are large with irregular nuclei and high N:C ratio.

Kobrich U, Falk S, Middeke B, et al: Primary large cell lymphoma of the splenic sinuses: a variant of angiotropic B-cell lymphoma (neoplastic angioendotheliomatosis)? Hum Pathol 23:1184-1187, 1992.

Kraemer BB, Osborne BM, Butler JJ: Primary splenic presentation of malignant lymphoma and related disorders: a study of 49 cases. Cancer 54:1606-1619, 1984.

HODGKIN LYMPHOMA

Clinical Features

- Although splenic involvement is not uncommon in cases of nodal-based classical Hodgkin lymphoma, true primary splenic Hodgkin lymphoma is exceedingly rare
- Lymphocyte-predominant Hodgkin lymphoma rarely involves spleen

Gross Pathology

- Focal nodules scattered in spleen parenchyma, often with apparent fibrosis
- Occasionally nodules are small, visible only on thin sectioning of the organ

Histopathology (Figure 15-11)

- Early lesions are found in the T-cell zones of white pulp (PALS) or marginal zones
- Classical Hodgkin lymphoma: typical Hodgkin-Reed-Sternberg cells within a polymorphous background of T cells, histiocytes, and eosinophils
- Lymphocyte-predominant Hodgkin lymphoma: "popcorn" cells characterized by large size and multilobated nucleus with delicate chromatin, within a cellular background of small lymphocytes
- Accompanying fibrosis may be prominent
- Epithelioid granulomas may be present

Special Stains and Immunohistochemistry

- Small lymphocytes are a mixture of CD3-positive T cells (predominantly CD4-positive helper T-cell) and CD20-positive B cells; the former usually predominate

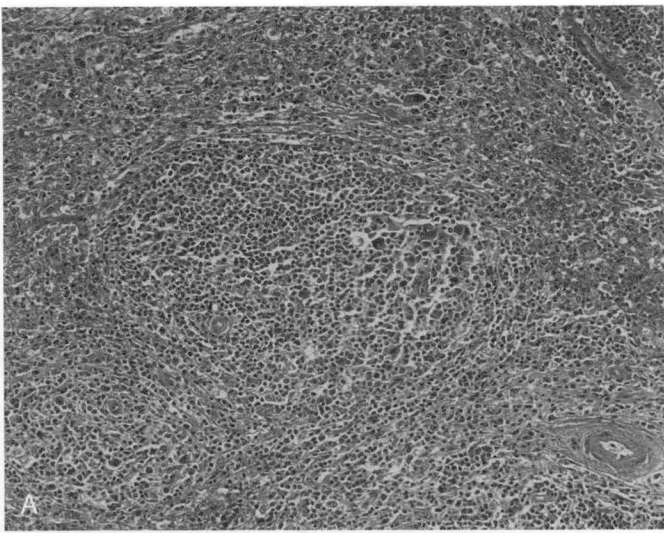

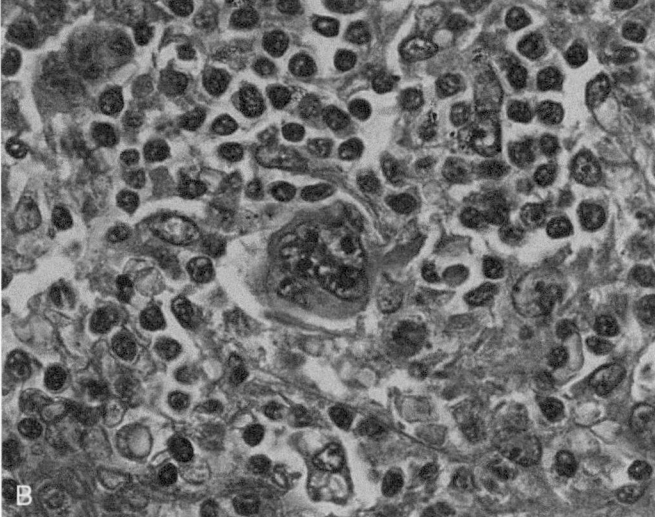

Figure 15-11. Hodgkin lymphoma. A, Low-power view shows multiple distinct white pulp tumor nodules. **B,** The nodules consist of a polymorphous infiltrate, which includes Hodgkin cells, lymphocytes, eosinophils, and epithelioid histiocytes.

- Reed-Sternberg cells and their variants are positive for PAX-5 (weak), CD30 and CD15 and negative for CD45; CD3 and CD20 are usually negative; the latter, however, can be found expressed in a proportion of neoplastic cells with variable staining intensity
- Popcorn cells of lymphocyte-predominant Hodgkin lymphoma are positive for CD20 and CD45 and can be surrounded by CD57- and PD-1-positive T cells (see Chapter 14, lymph nodes for more detailed information)

Other Techniques for Diagnosis

- Noncontributory

Differential Diagnosis

DLBCL

- Similar to CHL, random distribution of tumor nodules
- Composed predominantly of large lymphoid cells
- In most cases, neoplastic cells are positive for CD20 and CD45 and negative for CD15

- Rare cases of Hodgkin lymphoma may be "combined" with DLBCL (composite lymphoma) or rare cases of lymphocyte-predominant Hodgkin lymphoma may show transformation to DLBCL

ANAPLASTIC LARGE CELL LYMPHOMA

- May form tumor masses or diffusely infiltrate the spleen
- Pleomorphic multinucleated large cells with prominent nucleoli may resemble Hodgkin-Reed-Sternberg cells; however, heterogeneous background typical for Hodgkin lymphoma is absent
- Neoplastic cells of anaplastic large cell lymphoma express CD30, at least a few T-cell markers and anaplastic lymphoma kinase (ALK-1) in a subset but are usually negative for CD15 and PAX-5

INFLAMMATORY PSEUDOTUMOR

- Usually a solitary mass with whitish cut surface
- Tumor localized to the spleen; no lymphadenopathy
- Mixture of bland spindle cells, lymphocytes, and plasma cells
- Hodgkin-Reed-Sternberg cells are not identified

SPLENIC HAMARTOMA

- Usually presents as solitary mass with reddish cut surface
- Does not involve tissues other than the spleen
- Typical red pulplike microscopic appearance

METASTATIC CARCINOMA OR MELANOMA

- Almost always a previous history of primary tumor
- Single or multiple randomly distributed tumor nodules
- Microscopy shows sheets of large nonhematopoietic cells (negative for lymphoid antigens)

PEARLS

- *True primary Hodgkin lymphoma of the spleen is rare (<3% of cases)*
- *Modern radiologic imaging techniques have virtually replaced splenectomy for staging of Hodgkin lymphoma; splenectomy, however, remains the single most sensitive method for documenting Hodgkin lymphoma involvement*

SELECTED REFERENCES

Burke JS, Osborne BM: Localized reactive lymphoid hyperplasia of the spleen simulating malignant lymphoma: a report of seven cases. Am J Surg Pathol 7: 373-380, 1983.
Farrer-Brown G, Bennett MH, Harrison CV, et al: The diagnosis of Hodgkin's disease in surgically excised spleens. J Clin Pathol 25: 294-300, 1972.
Lukes RJ: Criteria for involvement of lymph nodes, bone marrow, spleen and liver in Hodgkin's disease. Cancer Res 31:1755-1767, 1971.

NON-NEOPLASTIC DISEASES INVOLVING THE SPLENIC RED PULP

GAUCHER DISEASE AND OTHER STORAGE DISORDERS

Clinical Features

- Gaucher disease has two major forms: infantile and adult

- Infantile form: hepatosplenomegaly and mental deterioration in the first year of life, death in infancy or early childhood
- Adult (later-onset) form
  - Most common form encountered in splenectomy specimens
  - Highest incidence in Ashkenazi Jews
  - Insidious onset in late childhood or adulthood
  - No mental retardation
  - Pancytopenia may be the presenting symptom
  - Hepatomegaly, splenomegaly, and adrenal involvement
  - Bone lesions include pathologic fractures, lytic lesions, and avascular necrosis of the femoral head
- Most other inherited metabolic storage diseases have onset in infancy or childhood; all are extremely rare
- Non-neuronopathic cases of Niemann-Pick disease may also present in adulthood with clinically significant hypersplenism
- Features and differential diagnosis are summarized in Table 15-2

Gross Pathology

- Diffuse enlargement of the spleen with a pale, dry appearance on its cut surface

Histopathology

- Expansion of the red pulp with distention of splenic cords by large pale-stained macrophages (Figure 15-12)
- Gaucher cells have a characteristic "wrinkled-silk" cytoplasm that often appears brownish in H&E-stained sections and is distinguishable from that of Niemann-Pick cells, which is foamy or bubbly owing to the presence of numerous small clear vacuoles (Figure 15-13)

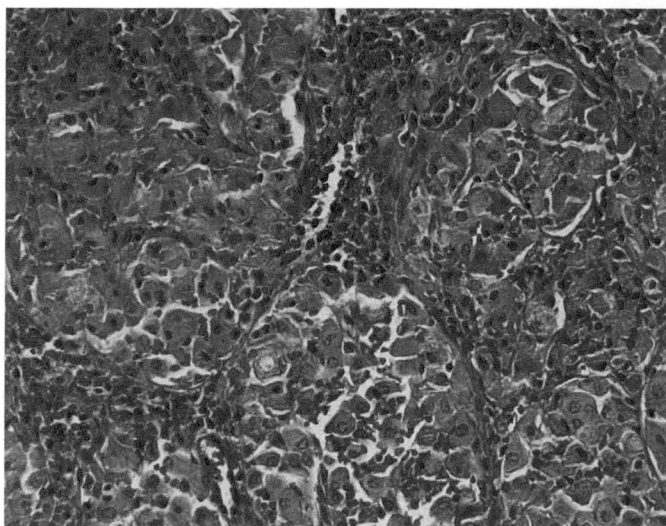

Figure 15-12. Gaucher disease. Gaucher cells occupy the cords of the red pulp. They have abundant cytoplasm and round to oval pale nuclei with uniform nucleoli. This must be distinguished from Langerhans cell histiocytosis, in which the cells are smaller with bean-shaped nuclei. Rarely, macrophages engorged with *Mycobacterium avium* may resemble Gaucher cells.

- Another important distinction is with ceroid histiocytes, which are smaller, faintly yellow-brown (blue-green in Wright-Giemsa stain), and have a distinctive cytoplasmic granularity; typical ceroid containing sea-blue histiocytes are encountered in patients with Hermansky-Pudlak syndrome

Special Stains and Immunohistochemistry

- See Table 15-2

TABLE 15-2	DIFFERENTIAL DIAGNOSIS OF STORAGE DISEASES WITH SPECIAL STAINS AND ADDITIONAL TECHNIQUES			
	Storage Diseases			
Stain or Technique	*Gaucher Disease*	*Niemann-Pick Disease*	*Mucopolysaccharidoses*	*Glycogen Storage Diseases*
Enzyme defect	Glucocerebrosidase (β-glucosidase)	Sphingomyelinase	Varies; multiple types known	Varies; 10 types
Storage product	Glucocerebroside	Sphingomyelin	Varies	Glycogen
Other organs affected	Liver, adrenals, lung, bone; central nervous system in infantile form	Brain, liver, lungs, bone marrow	Central nervous system, tongue, skeleton, liver, cornea, heart valves	Liver, muscle, heart (dependent on type)
Hematoxylin and eosin stain	"Wrinkled silk"	Yellow-green	Clear	Clear
Wright-Giemsa stain	Colorless	Blue-green		
Periodic acid–Schiff stain	Positive	Variable	Weakly positive	Positive
Periodic acid–Schiff with diastase stain	Positive	Variable		Negative
Iron	Positive	Negative		Negative
Acid-fast	Negative	Positive		
Electron microscopy	Lysosomes with twisted helical tubules	Variably sized residual bodies	Membrane-bound vacuoles with lamellar inclusions	Glycogen granules

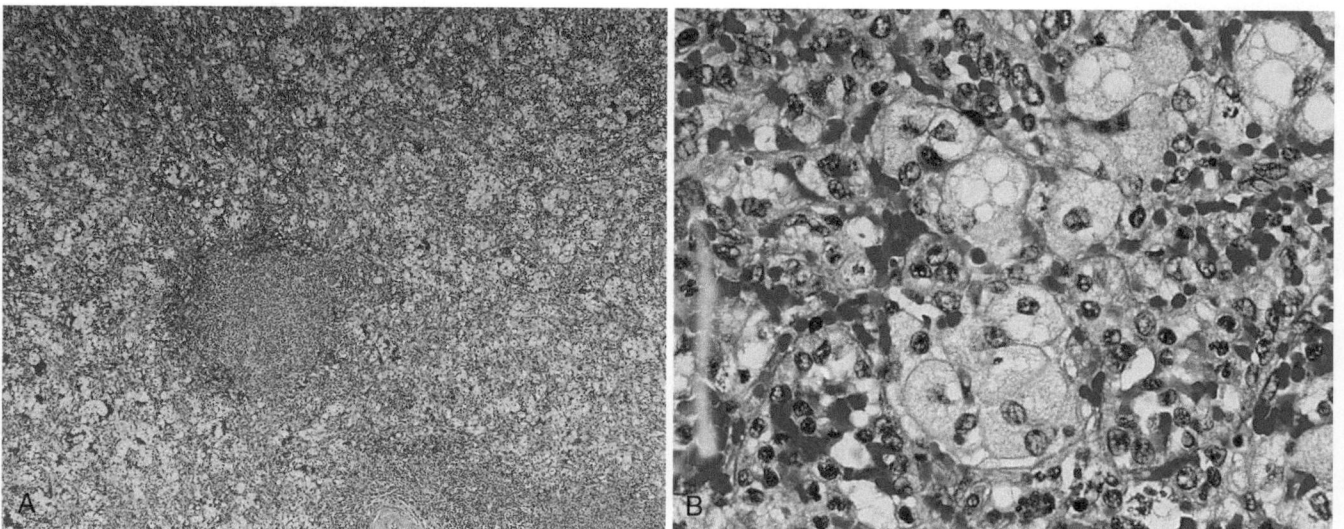

Figure 15-13. **Niemann-Pick disease. A,** Low-power magnification. The histiocytes occupy the cords of the red pulp and surround a splenic follicle. **B,** High-power magnification. The histiocytes have abundant clear multivacuolated cytoplasm and round to oval pale nuclei with uniform nucleoli.

Other Techniques for Diagnosis

- Biochemical analysis of the storage product and determination of the activity of the relevant enzyme in fresh tissue samples are usually necessary for definitive diagnosis
- Detection of the specific gene mutations in patients or in at-risk families is now possible in a large number of metabolic diseases

Differential Diagnosis

- See Table 15-2

PEARLS

- *Pancytopenia may be the presenting clinical feature; it may result from hypersplenism and marrow infiltration by the Gaucher cells*
- *Diagnoses in these diseases are made biochemically from peripheral blood, bone marrow, or other tissues*
- *Patients most often have an established diagnosis by the time the pathologist sees the spleen at autopsy or surgery; thus, the need for clinical correlation cannot be overemphasized*

SELECTED REFERENCES

Barranger JA, Ginns EI: Glucosylceramide lipidoses: Gaucher disease. In Scriver CR, Beaudet AL, Sly WS, et al (eds): The Metabolic Basis of Inherited Diseases, 6th ed. New York, McGraw-Hill, 1989.
Elleder M: Niemann-Pick disease. Pathol Res Pract 185:293-328, 1989.
Lee RE, Peters SP, Glew RH: Gaucher's disease: clinical, morphologic and pathogenetic considerations. Pathol Ann 12:309-339, 1977.

HEMATOLOGIC DISEASES

EXTRAMEDULLARY HEMATOPOIESIS

Clinical Features

- Extramedullary hematopoiesis (EMH) refers to the accumulation of hematopoietic precursor cells in the spleen

- EMH may be divided into two types
  - Non-neoplastic EMH that refers to the accumulation in the splenic red pulp of nonclonal hematopoietic precursor cells
  - A neoplastic form refers to the secondary "spread" to the spleen of a hematologic malignancy capable of manifesting itself as EMH
- Non-neoplastic EMH
  - Normal in the fetus and premature infant
  - Usually an incidental finding in a spleen removed for some other cause
  - Typically seen in patients with severe anemia (e.g., thalassemia major) or in cases where a malignant disease (lymphoma, myeloma, metastatic malignancy) replaces the bone marrow (myelophthisic anemia)
- Neoplastic EMH
  - Often associated with a more marked degree of splenomegaly; in these cases, splenectomy is performed to relieve pain associated with the presence of a large spleen or splenic infarcts or to ameliorate cytopenia due to hypersplenism
  - Typically occurs in patients with classic myeloproliferative neoplasms, particularly primary myelofibrosis, in which EMH is one of the major clinical manifestations
  - It is also seen in other myeloproliferative disorders such as polycythemia vera and, rarely, essential thrombocythemia when they progress to "secondary myelofibrosis"
  - Less frequently, EMH can also be seen in patients with myelodysplastic/myeloproliferative diseases (e.g., chronic myelomonocytic leukemia) and exceptionally, in other types of myeloid neoplasms
- In all patients with myeloid neoplasms, splenic EMH needs to be distinguished from extramedullary (splenic) acute leukemia; when the latter is found superimposed on an EMH background, it may represent disease transformation

Gross Pathology

- Usually an incidental finding without gross features
- May cause diffuse expansion of the red pulp
- Rarely causes multiple soft, bulging, dark-red to brown berry-like nodules; these are most often seen in patients with late stage primary myelofibrosis or postpolycythemia vera (or postessential thrombocythemia) myelofibrosis

Histopathology (Figure 15-14)

- Cellular infiltrates are seen in red pulp cords or within red pulp sinuses, present in a diffuse or nodular growth pattern
- Small clusters of normoblasts are easiest to identify; this is the predominant cell type found in nonclonal EMH. They are most often located intrasinusoidally
- Trilineage EMH is most commonly seen in patients with chronic myeloproliferative neoplasms
- Identification of megakaryocytes and granulocytic precursors may be facilitated by immunohistochemistry (e.g., CD42b and myeloperoxidase)

Special Stains and Immunohistochemistry

- Wright stains (e.g., touch preparations)
- Antihemoglobin (or glycophorin A) immunostaining to highlight the presence of erythroid precursors (erythroblasts)
- Antibodies reactive with myeloperoxidase or lysozyme can be used to highlight myeloid cells
- Antibodies reactive with platelet glycoproteins such as CD42b or CD61 may facilitate the identification of megakaryocytes
- CD34 and CD117 can also be useful in selected cases to identify accumulation of blasts, which may indicate blastic transformation to extramedullary acute myeloid leukemia

Other Techniques for Diagnosis

- Usually not necessary; flow cytometry and cytogenetic techniques may be useful to confirm evolution to acute leukemia

Differential Diagnosis

LYMPHOID INFILTRATE IN RED PULP

- Cells are more pleomorphic; nuclei are not as round as normoblasts and have less dense chromatin (that is, have a more visible chromatin pattern) than normoblasts
- Cell borders are indistinct

ACUTE LEUKEMIA

- Rapid onset usually with severe cytopenias
- Blasts have high nuclear-to-cytoplasmic ratio and display fine chromatin and scant indistinct cytoplasm; however, monoblasts and megakaryoblasts may have more abundant cytoplasm

PEARLS

- *The formerly used term* myeloid metaplasia *to indicate EMH is a misnomer; the phenomenon results from entrapment in the spleen (filtration theory) of circulating immature hematopoietic cells*
- *The identification of early extramedullary (splenic) blastic transformation may be challenging, and immunohistochemistry may be invaluable in these cases*

SELECTED REFERENCES

Neiman RS, Orazi A: Functions of the spleen. In Disorders of the Spleen, 2nd ed. Philadelphia, WB Saunders, 1999, pp 26-38.

O'Malley DP, Kim YS, Perkins SL, et al: Morphologic and immunohistochemical evaluation of splenic hematopoietic proliferations in neoplastic and benign disorders. Mod Pathol 18:1550-1561, 2005.

Prakash S, Hoffman R, Barouk S, et al: Splenic extramedullary hematopoietic proliferation in Philadelphia chromosome-negative myeloproliferative neoplasms: heterogeneous morphology and cytological composition. Mod Pathol 25:815-827, 2012.

HEREDITARY SPHEROCYTOSIS

Clinical Features

PROMINENT SPLENOMEGALY AND ANEMIA

- Patients have familial history of hemolytic anemia (autosomal dominant)

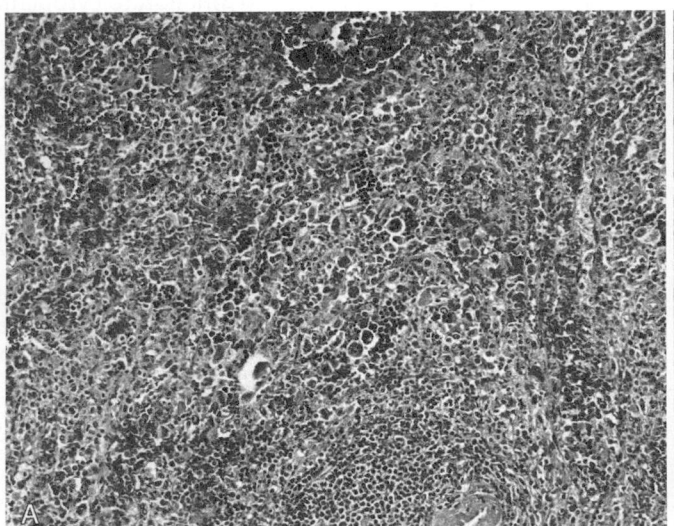
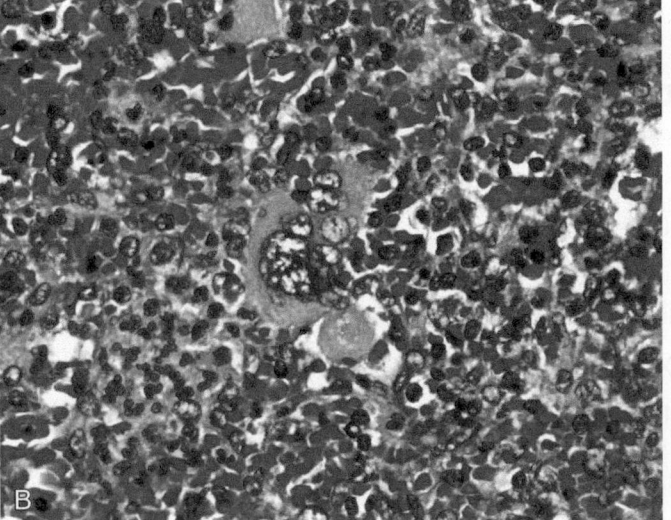

Figure 15-14. Extramedullary hematopoiesis. A, The red pulp and the vascular sinuses contain trilinear hematopoietic cells with a predominance of erythroblasts and megakaryocytes. **B,** Extramedullary hematopoiesis in myelofibrosis. Numerous neutrophils accompany abnormal megakaryocytes.

- Splenectomy in this condition is most often performed in late childhood or early adult years
- At a molecular level this disease is heterogeneous; caused by a variety of mutations involving any of several red cell membrane proteins. More often autosomal dominant inheritance; caused by molecular defects in the genes that code for spectrin, ankyrin, band 3 protein, protein 4.2, and other erythrocyte membrane proteins
- In hereditary spherocytosis, hemolysis and anemia are relieved by splenectomy, but the underlying red cell defect remains

Gross Pathology

- Splenomegaly; usually of moderate degree
- Red pulp shows intense congestion
- Attenuation of the normal white pulp nodularity

Histopathology

- White pulp is normal to atrophic
- Red pulp cords are distended and the sinuses appear empty (Figure 15-15)
- Increased cordal macrophages and hypertrophy of sinus-lining cells
- Erythrophagocytosis is hard to see, and hemosiderin deposition is minimal
- Extramedullary hematopoiesis is not seen
- Spherocytic erythrocytes in peripheral blood

Special Stains and Immunohistochemistry

- Noncontributory

Other Techniques for Diagnosis

- Osmotic fragility test on patient's red cells
- Polyacrylamide gel electrophoresis for molecular subtyping

Differential Diagnosis

AUTOIMMUNE HEMOLYTIC ANEMIA

- No family history
- Acquired disease
- Spleen is of normal size to slightly enlarged

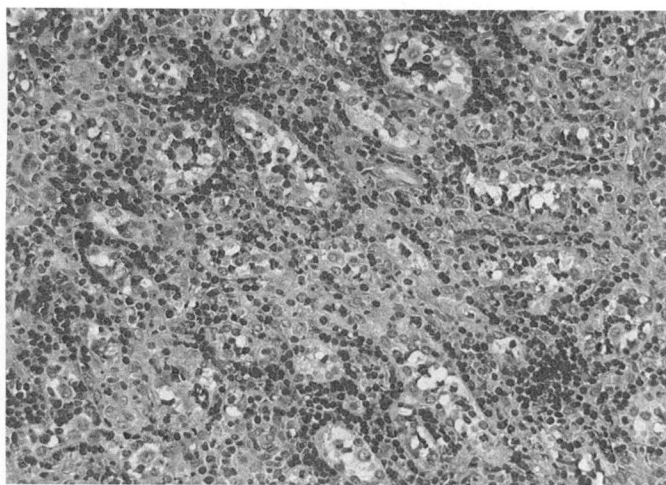

Figure 15-15. Hereditary spherocytosis. The red pulp is expanded and shows accumulation of erythrocytes in the splenic cords, hyperplasia of cordal macrophages and sinus lining cell hypertrophy. The sinuses appear relatively empty.

- If untreated, the spleen shows significant white pulp hyperplasia and red pulp plasmacytosis
- Cords are not as distended, and it is easier to detect erythrophagocytosis both in cordal and in sinus macrophages
- Hemosiderin deposition and extramedullary erythropoiesis may be prominent
- Coombs test positive

SICKLE CELL DISEASE AND VARIANTS

- Usually autosplenectomy due to multiple infarctions by age 7 years (hemoglobin S [HbSS])
- Splenomegaly may be seen in adults with sickle cell variants (e.g., sickle cell and hemoglobin C disease)
- Infarcts much more common; organized infarcts are often iron encrusted (these old infarcts are also termed Gamna-Gandy bodies)
- Stacked, sickled cells in red pulp
- History is important, including ancestry (more common in people of African or Arab ancestry)

FIBROCONGESTIVE SPLENOMEGALY

- Patients usually have liver disease, often with ascites
- Red pulp shows a combination of congestion (due to blood stasis) and fibrosis

PEARLS

- *Rarely, areas of marked red pulp congestion in cases of fibrocongestive splenomegaly may superficially resemble capillary hemangiomas or even a splenic hamartoma; however, the latter two conditions are usually more demarcated focal lesions; additionally, hemangiomas show abnormal vascular channels*

SELECTED REFERENCES

Chang CS, Li CY, Liang YH, Cha SS: Clinical features and splenic pathologic changes in patients with autoimmune hemolytic anemia and congenital hemolytic anemia. Mayo Clin Proc 68:757-762, 1993.

Iolascon A, Miraglia del Giudice E, Perrotta S, et al: Hereditary spherocytosis: from clinical to molecular defects. Haematologica 83:240-257, 1998.

SICKLE CELL DISEASE AND VARIANTS

Clinical Features

- Inherited hemolytic anemia due to mutant HbS molecule produced by the substitution of valine for glutamic acid at the sixth position of the hemoglobin beta chain
- Predominantly in patients of African or Arab ancestry
- Children may have impaired growth
- Disease course is punctuated by various crises
  - Painful (infarcts)
  - Hemolytic crisis
  - Aplastic crisis
  - Splenic sequestration (in young children or in older patients with variant sickling disorders)
  - Hand-foot syndrome
  - Acute chest syndrome
- Patients with homozygous HbSS become functionally asplenic in childhood and are at risk for sepsis from *Haemophilus influenza, Staphylococcus pneumoniae,* and *Neisseria meningitidis*
- Patients may be jaundiced

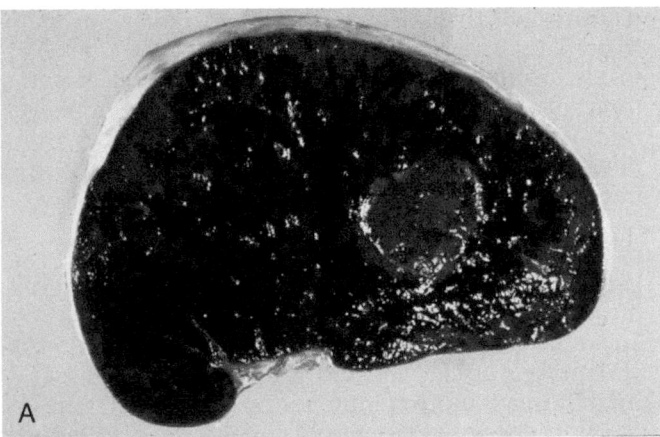

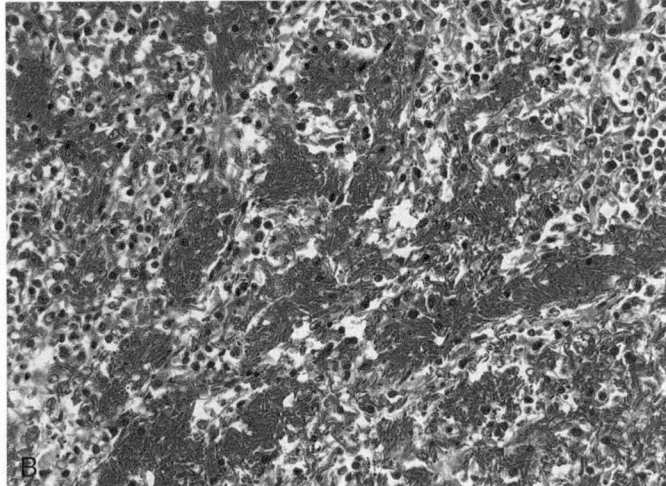

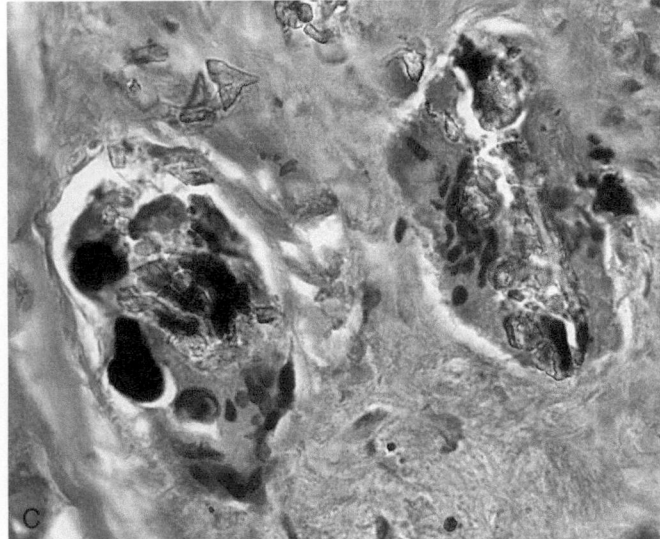

Figure 15-16. A, Hemoglobin SC disease, adult patient with hemolytic crisis, gross photograph. Enlarged spleen with a central round infarct and small peripheral infarcts. **B,** Classic sickle cell disease (hemoglobin SS). Normal red pulp morphology is lost; there are masses of stacked, sickled red cells and pigment-laden macrophages. Evaluation of red cell morphology on tissue sections is not reliable, but the appearance of stacked masses of sickled cells is characteristic of this disease. **C,** Classic sickle cell disease, Gamna-Gandy body. An old organized microinfarct is encrusted by iron and focally calcified.

- Gallstones can develop at an early age
- Increased incidence of *Salmonella* osteomyelitis

Gross Pathology

- HbSS disease: by age 7 years, the spleen has become a small greenish-brown fibrotic nubbin (autosplenectomy)
- With hemoglobin C disease and other variants, the spleen may be enlarged with red pulp congestion; infarcts may occur, but the spleen does not usually totally infarct (Figure 15-16A)

Histopathology (Figure 15-16 B,C)

- Sickling causes stasis and hypoxia, which in turn result in hemorrhagic infarcts; infarcts result in the formation of Gamna-Gandy bodies—that is, fibrotic foci with hemosiderin deposits and calcification; these are not, however, unique to this disease
- HbSS: splenic architecture is progressively destroyed; in the initial stage of the disease, there is a loss of follicular compartment due to preferential sickling of the marginal zone of the white pulp; this is followed by a progressive loss of all splenic tissue; what remains is fibrous tissue with hemosiderin and other pigment deposits and variable numbers of macrophages
- Other sickling diseases
  - Red pulp congestion
  - Sickled red cells in cords and sinuses
  - Increased macrophages with phagocytosed red cells and hemosiderin

Special Stains and Immunohistochemistry

- Noncontributory

Other Techniques for Diagnosis

- Hemoglobin electrophoresis

Differential Diagnosis

SPLENIC INFARCTS
- Extensive loss of splenic parenchyma is rare, especially in children
- Typically subcapsular, wedge-shaped lesions
- Normal hemoglobin electrophoresis
- No sickled red cells

HEREDITARY SPHEROCYTOSIS
- Family history
- Patients usually not of African ancestry
- Splenic enlargement in both children and adults
- Normal hemoglobin electrophoresis
- Red cells spherocytic, not sickled
- Splenic infarcts uncommon

MALARIA
- Acquired disease, usually after residence in or travel to an endemic area
- Periodic fever
- Intermittent hemolysis
- Organisms detectable in peripheral blood
- Sickled cells usually not present
- Hemoglobin electrophoresis usually normal; sickle hemoglobin provides some protection against severe malaria

PEARLS

- *Formalin fixation distorts red cell morphology, but the presence of numerous tactoids and stacked red cells is usually diagnostic*
- *Splenic sequestration crises in children are an indication for splenectomy; this is done for preventing recurrence; these specimens account for most spleens with sickle cell disease seen in pathology*
- *Patients of Arab ancestries with HbSS typically have a higher percentage of hemoglobin F and milder disease*

SELECTED REFERENCES

Bunn HF: Pathogenesis and treatment of sickle cell disease. N Engl J Med 337:762-769, 1997.

Dover GH, Platt OS: Sickle cell disease. In Nathan DG, Orkin SH (eds): Nathan and Oski's Hematology of Infancy and Childhood, 5th ed. Philadelphia, WB Saunders, 1998, pp 762-809.

AUTOIMMUNE HEMOLYTIC ANEMIA

Clinical Features

- Most common in adults
- Female predominance
- May occur as a primary disorder or may coexist with another disease, such as systemic lupus, lymphoid neoplasms (e.g., chronic lymphocytic leukemia), or solid tumors, or may be drug induced
- Increased reticulocytes
- Coombs test positive

Gross Pathology

- Spleen normal to moderately enlarged
- Diffuse process without focal lesions
- White pulp normal to hyperplastic
- Red pulp expanded and congested

Histopathology (Figure 15-17)

- Follicular hyperplasia in white pulp (in untreated patients)
- Variably expanded red pulp

- Increased plasma cells in the red pulp
- Erythrophagocytosis detectable both in cordal and sinus macrophages
- Cords congested; sinuses may appear empty (like in hereditary spherocytosis)

Special Stains and Immunohistochemistry

- Noncontributory

Other Techniques for Diagnosis

- Coombs test on blood

Differential Diagnosis

- History and Coombs test critical for all differential diagnoses

ITP

- Patients have thrombocytopenia but are usually not anemic
- The coexistence of ITP and hemolytic anemia is called *Evans syndrome*
- Antiplatelet antibodies are present in plasma and on patient's platelets
- Histologically, "dirty cords" are due to phagocytosis of platelets (best seen in touch preparations), but there is no evident erythrophagocytosis

CONGESTIVE SPLENOMEGALY

- Patients have portal hypertension and usually have liver disease
- Spleen shows an increased stroma content (fibrocongestive splenomegaly)
- Coombs test negative

HEREDITARY SPHEROCYTOSIS

- Family history
- Lifelong hemolytic anemia
- Abnormal red blood cell morphology
- Coombs test negative

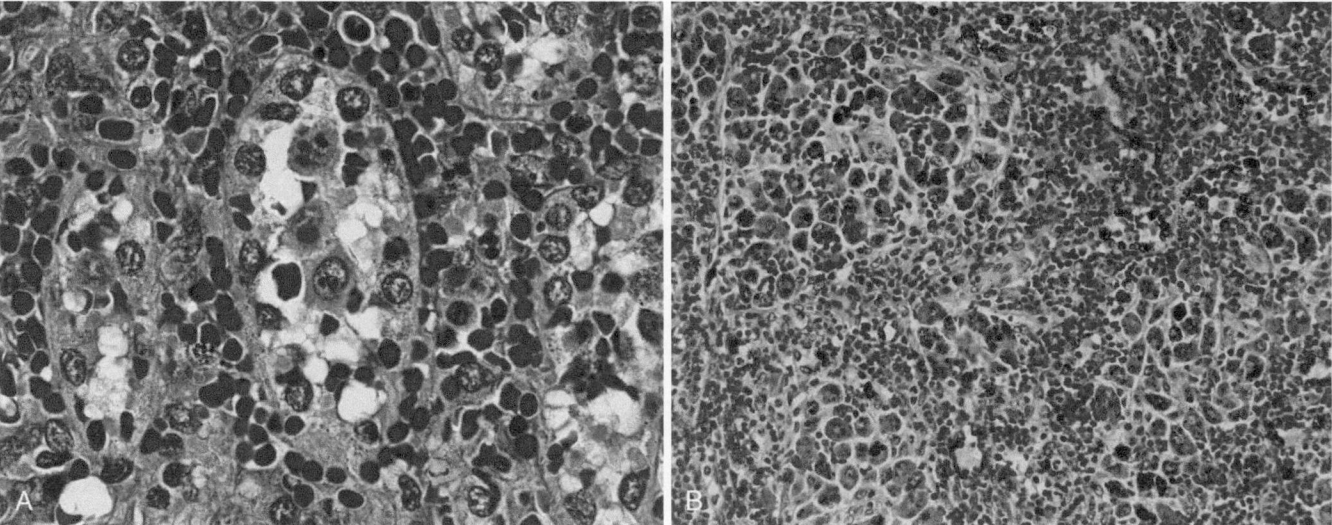

Figure 15-17. Autoimmune hemolytic anemia. **A,** Hemophagocytosis of antibody-covered erythrocytes. **B,** Iron overload. It can be massive and simulate other diseases with severe iron overload (e.g., thalassemia).

- *Most common in women*
- *Check clinical history and Coombs test result*

SELECTED REFERENCES

Chang CS, Li CY, Liang YH, Cha SS: Clinical features and splenic pathologic changes in patients with autoimmune hemolytic anemia and congenital hemolytic anemia. Mayo Clin Proc 68:757-762, 1993.

Sokol RJ, Booker DJ, Stamps R: The pathology of autoimmune haemolytic anaemia. J Clin Pathol 45:1047-1052, 1992.

IDIOPATHIC THROMBOCYTOPENIC PURPURA (AUTOIMMUNE THROMBOCYTOPENIC PURPURA)

Clinical Features

- Seen at any age
- Acute condition, more common in children
- Chronic condition, most common in middle-aged adults
- Female predominance
- Common in HIV infection; the cause of thrombocytopenia is usually multifactorial in these patients

Gross Pathology

- Spleen is usually of normal size
- White pulp may be enlarged

Histopathology (Figure 15-18)

- Follicular hyperplasia in white pulp in untreated patients; absent secondary follicles in patients treated with steroids
- Increased plasma cells
- Granular, dirty appearance of the cordal macrophages (periodic acid–Schiff stain–positive debris in cytoplasm)
- Foamy macrophages in red pulp
- Increased number of neutrophils in red pulp

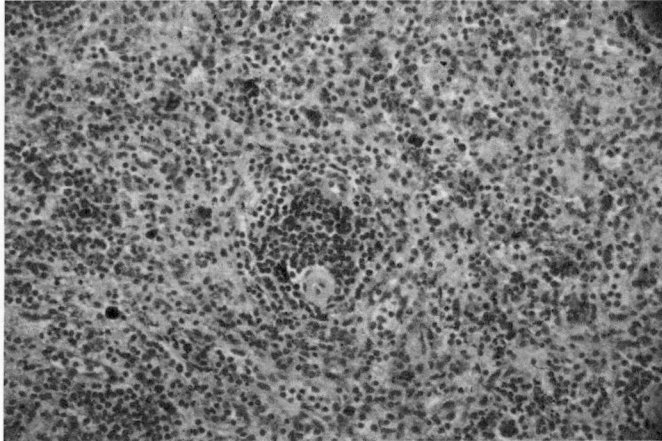

Figure 15-18. Idiopathic (autoimmune) thrombocytopenic purpura (ITP). This photomicrograph shows pale-red pulp with many pale-staining macrophages in the cords. Most patients who undergo splenectomy for ITP have been treated with other modalities first, and thus these features are rarely seen.

- Only minimal extramedullary hematopoiesis
- Bone marrow aspirate and biopsy show normal to increased number of megakaryocytes

Special Stains and Immunohistochemistry

- Noncontributory

Other Techniques for Diagnosis

- Tests for antiplatelet antibodies

Differential Diagnosis

NONSPECIFIC FOLLICULAR HYPERPLASIA

- History and clinical manifestations important
- Complete blood count
- Antiplatelet antibody test negative

- *One of the most common indications for splenectomy*
- *The spleen in these patients is an important site of both platelet destruction and the production of antiplatelet antibodies*
- *Splenectomy is performed only in patients refractory to steroids and other treatment; resected spleens from steroid treated patients rarely show most of the features listed previously*

SELECTED REFERENCES

Hassan NM, Neiman RS: The pathology of the spleen in steroid-treated immune thrombocytopenic purpura. Am J Clin Pathol 84:433-438, 1985.

McMillan R: The pathogenesis of chronic immune (idiopathic) thrombocytopenic purpura. Semin Hematol 37(1 suppl 1):5-9, 2000.

Sandier SG: The spleen and splenectomy in immune (idiopathic) thrombocytopenic purpura. Semin Hematol 37(1 suppl 1):10-12, 2000.

NEOPLASTIC DISEASES INVOLVING THE SPLENIC RED PULP

SPLENIC DIFFUSE RED PULP SMALL B-CELL LYMPHOMA (SDRPBCL)

Clinical Features

- Most patients are over 60 years of age with a slight male predominance
- Massive splenomegaly, low-level lymphocytosis, and infrequent B-symptoms
- Peripheral blood and bone marrow commonly involved, some cases also have cutaneous involvement
- Liver involvement and lymphadenopathy are very rare

Gross Pathology

- Homogeneous red brown cut surface

Histopathology

- Diffuse infiltration of sinusoids and cords in red pulp with atrophic white pulp (Figure 15-19)
- Monomorphous small to medium lymphoid cells with round and regular nuclei with occasional small distinct nucleoli

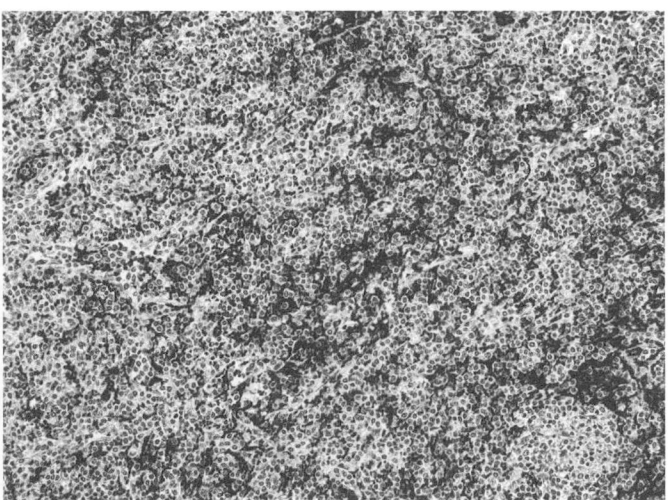

Figure 15-19. Splenic diffuse red pulp small B-cell lymphoma. Diffuse red pulp involvement with infiltration of sinusoids and cords by lymphoma cells.

- Bone marrow with subtle intrasinusoidal infiltrate; peripheral blood with villous lymphocytes
- Skin involvement as dermal infiltrate around cutaneous appendages and blood vessels with epidermotropism

Special Studies and Immunohistochemistry

- Lymphoma cells are positive for CD20, DBA.44, bcl-2, and IgG, show variable positivity for CD103, CD11c, and IgD and are negative for CD25, CD10, CD23, bcl-6, and annexin A1; p53 expression is more common than in SMZL

Differential Diagnosis

SPLENIC MARGINAL ZONE LYMPHOMA (see TABLE 15-1)
- Involves both white pulp and red pulp with a characteristic micronodular growth pattern
- Negative for annexin A-1, usually negative for CD103; rarely positive for DBA.44

HAIRY CELL LEUKEMIA-VARIANT (HCL-v)
- Greater degree of lymphocytosis than SDRPBCL
- At least some lymphoid cells with prominent nucleoli
- White pulp totally atrophic
- Negative for CD25, annexin A-1, and TRAP

HAIRY CELL LEUKEMIA
- White pulp totally atrophic
- Neoplastic cells are positive for CD25, CD11c, CD103, annexin-A1, TRAP, DBA.44, and BRAF V600E mutation

PEARLS

- *SDRPBCL seen predominantly in older males*
- *Red pulp involvement with extensive obliteration of white pulp*
- *Immunohistochemical overlap between SMZL and HCL variant*
- *Distinction from HCL-v relies on morphology of neoplastic cells; this distinction may at times be difficult and such cases should be classified as splenic B-cell leukemia/lymphoma unclassifiable*

SELECTED REFERENCES

Kanellis G, Mollejo M, Montes-Moreno S, et al: Splenic diffuse red pulp small B-cell lymphoma: revision of a series of cases reveals characteristic clinico-pathological features. Haematologica 95:1122-1129, 2010.

Mollejo M, Algara P, Mateo MS, et al: Splenic small B-cell lymphoma with predominant red pulp involvement: a diffuse variant of splenic marginal zone lymphoma? Histopathology 40:22-30, 2002.

Traverse-Glehen A, Baseggio L, Bauchu EC, et al: Splenic red pulp lymphoma with numerous basophilic villous lymphocytes: a distinct clinicopathologic and molecular entity? Blood 111:2253-2260, 2008.

HAIRY CELL LEUKEMIA

Clinical Features

- Occurs in middle age patients with marked male predominance
- Splenomegaly, anemia, and infections
- Lymphadenopathy is absent
- Hairy cells may be rare and hard to see in the blood or marrow aspirate smear
- Monocytopenia is almost always present in the peripheral blood
- Bone marrow is involved in more than 95% of patients; diagnosis is often confirmed by flow cytometry; the most specific marker is CD103
- Bone marrow biopsy shows the characteristic cellular infiltrates associated with fibrosis; in some cases, however, the infiltration might be subtle, and its identification may be greatly facilitated by immunohistology of the bone marrow biopsy (e.g., with CD20, DBA.44, or anti-TRAP antibodies)

Gross Pathology

- Marked splenomegaly
- Diffuse enlargement with uniform firm, dark-red appearance
- Infarcts may be observed

Histopathology

- The atypical lymphoid proliferation homogeneously and diffusely expands the red pulp (Figure 15-20)
- White pulp may be totally obliterated by the expanded red pulp
- Red cell lakes (pseudosinuses) lined by hairy cells
- Hairy cells are found both within the cords and intrasinusoidally
- They have oval nuclei and abundant pale eosinophilic cytoplasm
- Hairlike cytoplasmic projections may be seen on splenic touch preparations or peripheral blood and bone marrow smears
- Virtually lack mitotic activity
- Erythrophagocytosis and extramedullary hematopoiesis are usually absent
- In rare cases, the presence of marked congestion of the red pulp with dispersal of hairy cells can make their recognition difficult (immunohistology beneficial)

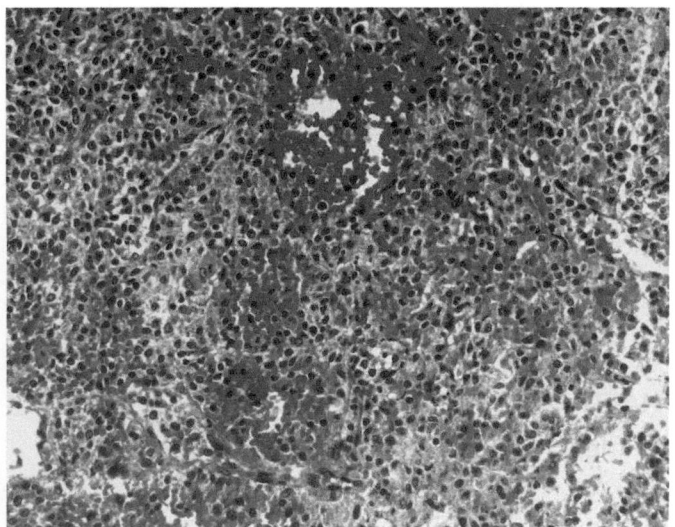

Figure 15-20. Hairy cell leukemia. Monomorphous lymphoid infiltrate is seen in the red pulp. Notice a poorly demarcated red cell lake.

- Rare variants characterized by larger cells or cells with blastic morphology have been reported; in these cases, the diagnosis relies on a hairy cell–like pattern of tissue involvement and an immunophenotypic profile, both consistent with hairy cell leukemia

Special Stains and Immunohistochemistry

- Reticulin: branching network of reticulin that surrounds individual cells
- Hairy cell leukemia is a low-grade B-cell lymphoid neoplasm; the hairy cells are strongly positive with CD20
- TRAP, DBA.44, and annexin A1 positive in hairy cells
- BRAF V600E mutation-specific antibody positive in hairy cells

Other Techniques for Diagnosis

- Flow cytometry: hairy cells express CD103, CD19, CD20, CD11c, CD25, FMC7, and sIg
- Molecular assay for detection of BRAF V600E mutation

Differential Diagnosis

MARGINAL ZONE B-CELL LYMPHOMA
- Predominant infiltration of white pulp (miliary pattern) as opposed to the diffuse red pulp expansion in hairy cell leukemia
- Cells are usually negative for CD103, CD11c, CD25, TRAP, and annexin A1
- Pattern of bone marrow infiltration is different (usually multinodular)

SPLENIC DIFFUSE RED PULP SMALL B-CELL LYMPHOMA
- Lymphoma cells are negative for CD25, annexin A-1

CLL/SLL
- Cells with less cytoplasm
- Weakly positive for CD20 and sIg
- Positive for CD5 and CD23
- Negative for TRAP, CD103, and annexin A1

MASTOCYTOSIS
- Morphologic features are only superficially similar
- Mastocytosis usually has more fibrosis
- Capsular, trabecular, and perifollicular distribution
- Different cytochemistry and immunophenotype results

MYELOID LEUKEMIAS
- Blastic proliferation and high mitotic activity in acute myeloid leukemia and myeloid sarcoma
- Polymorphism and maturation to neutrophils in chronic myeloid leukemias (e.g., chronic myelomonocytic leukemia)
- Different peripheral blood and bone marrow findings
- Different cytochemistry and immunophenotype results

PEARLS
- *HCL seen predominantly in older males*
- *Typical finding: blood lakes*
- *Characteristic flow cytometric and immunohistologic profile*
- *One of the most successfully treatable indolent lymphoproliferative diseases*
- *Splenectomy is now rarely needed for either diagnosis or therapy*

SELECTED REFERENCES

Andrulis M, Penzel R, Weichert W, et al: Application of a BRAF V600E mutation-specific antibody for the diagnosis of hairy cell leukemia. Am J Surg Pathol 36:1796-1800, 2012.

Burke JS, Rappaport H: The diagnosis and differential diagnosis of hairy cell leukemia in bone marrow and spleen. Semin Oncol 11:334-346, 1984.

Tiacci E, Schiavoni G, Forconi F, et al: Simple genetic diagnosis of hairy cell leukemia by sensitive detection of the BRAF-V600E mutation. Blood 119:192-195, 2012.

Tiacci E, Trifonov V, Schiavoni G, et al: BRAF mutations in hairy-cell leukemia. N Engl J Med 364:2305-2315, 2011.

HAIRY CELL LEUKEMIA-VARIANT

Clinical Features

- Usually affects middle-aged to elderly patients with a male predominance
- Splenomegaly with a high white blood count without neutropenia or monocytopenia
- Involves bone marrow less uniformly than classical HCL; marrow is more easily aspirable
- Usually no hepatomegaly or lymphadenopathy

Gross Pathology

- Diffuse enlargement with a homogeneous dark red appearance
- Infarcts may be seen

Histopathology

- Diffuse involvement of red pulp with usually markedly atrophic white pulp
- Blood lakes may be present
- Circulating HCL-v cells are easily identified on peripheral blood smear and show features overlapping prolymphocytic leukemia and hairy cell leukemia: basophilic cytoplasm with abundant villi and central round or bilobed nuclei with prominent nucleoli (Figure 15-21)

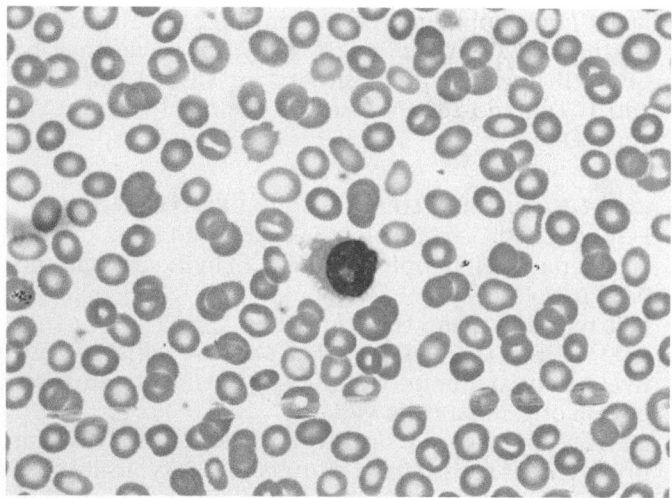

Figure 15-21. Hairy cell leukemia-variant. Peripheral blood showing lymphoid cell with fine cytoplasmic hairy projections and nucleus with prominent nucleolus.

Special Stains and Immunohistochemistry

- Neoplastic cells are positive for CD20, CD22, DBA.44, CD11c; variably positive for CD103; and negative for CD10, CD23, CD25, annexin-A1, TRAP, and CD123

Differential Diagnosis

SPLENIC DIFFUSE RED PULP SMALL B-CELL LYMPHOMA

- Small to medium sized lymphoid cells with round nuclei and occasional small distinct nucleoli
- Immunohistochemical findings largely overlap those seen in HCL-v

CLASSICAL HAIRY CELL LEUKEMIA

- Lymphocytes with circumferential hairy cytoplasmic projections without distinct nucleoli
- Positive for CD25, TRAP, annexin-A1, and BRAF V600E mutation

PEARLS

- *Similar histologic features to those of HCL on spleen sections but distinct lymphoid cell morphology on peripheral blood and touch imprints*
- *Distinct immunophenotype as compared to HCL*
- *Distinct morphology but immunophenotypic overlap with SDRPBCL*

SELECTED REFERENCES

Cawley JC, Burns GF, Hayhoe FG: A chronic lymphoproliferative disorder with distinctive features: a distinct variant of hairy-cell leukaemia. Leuk Res 4:547-559, 1980.

Matutes E, Wotherspoon A, Brito-Babapulle V, et al: The natural history and clinico-pathological features of the variant form of hairy cell leukemia. Leukemia 15:184-186, 2001.

Robak T: Hairy-cell leukemia variant: recent view on diagnosis, biology and treatment. Cancer Treat Rev 37:3-10, 2011.

HEPATOSPLENIC T-CELL LYMPHOMA

Clinical Features

- Occurs in young adults, with male predominance
- May be associated with long-term immunosuppressive therapy (e.g., after transplantation)
- Presents with hepatosplenomegaly, cytopenias, and B symptoms
- May be associated with hemophagocytic syndrome
- Usually no lymphadenopathy is seen at presentation
- Bone marrow involvement is a constant feature

Gross Pathology

- Massive splenomegaly
- Homogeneous cut surface with loss of white pulp

Histopathology (Figure 15-22)

- Diffuse expansion of the red pulp cords and sinuses
- Sinuses filled with sheets of neoplastic cells are commonly seen
- Loss of the white pulp

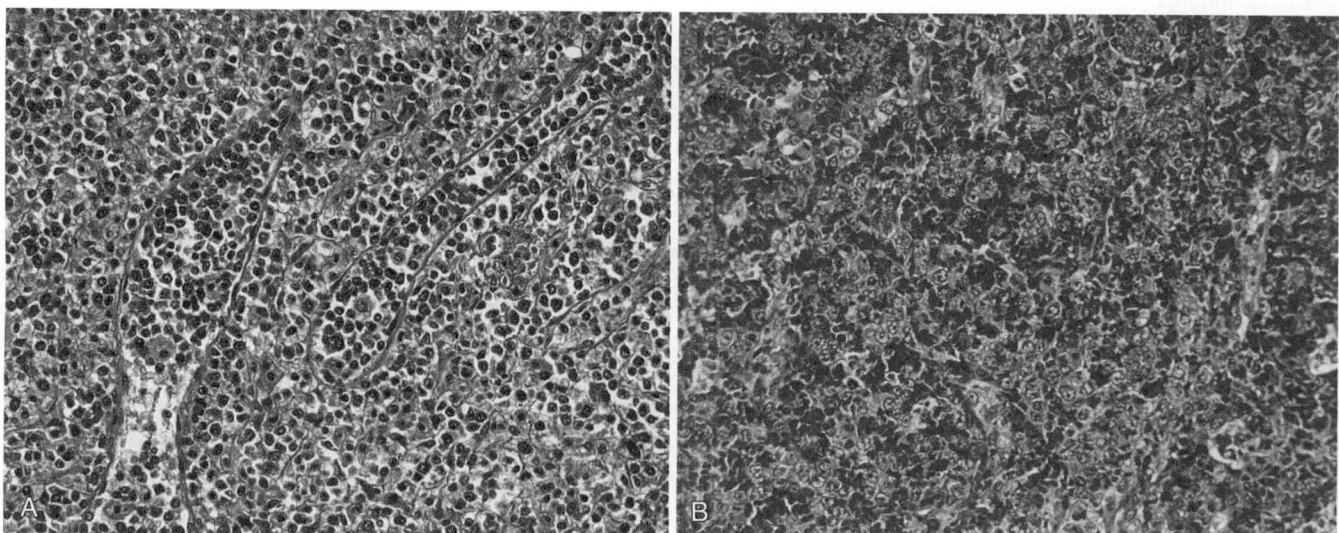

Figure 15-22. Hepatosplenic T-cell lymphoma. A, Numerous neoplastic T cells distending splenic sinuses. **B,** Large neoplastic T cells can be seen in occasional cases of hepatosplenic T-cell lymphoma, particularly at the time of disease progression.

Special Stains and Immunohistochemistry

- Neoplastic cells express CD3 and CD56, TIA-1 and are negative for CD4 and CD8 (double negative), and negative for CD5, CD57, granzyme B, and perforin and frequently for CD7

Other Techniques for Diagnosis

- Expression of γδ TCR can be demonstrated by flow cytometry
- Expression of αβ TCR has been reported in less common cases (demonstrable by flow cytometry or immunohistology with BF1 antibody)
- Isochromosome 7q is a defining cytogenetic abnormality in hepatosplenic T-cell lymphoma

Differential Diagnosis (see also Table 15-3)

CLL/SLL

- Involves both white and red pulp
- Cells weakly positive for CD20 and surface immunoglobulins

HAIRY CELL LEUKEMIA

- Bland cytology and blood lakes
- Cells with fine, hair like cytoplasmic processes may be seen in peripheral blood and bone marrow
- Distinct immunophenotype: B-cells positive for TRAP, DBA.44, CD25, CD11c, annexin-A1, and CD103
- BRAF V600E mutation positive

PROLYMPHOCYTIC LEUKEMIA

- Prolymphocytes are medium-sized cells with vesicular nuclei and prominent nucleoli
- Patients typically present with high white blood cell counts

- B-cell immunophenotype is seen: high-density CD20, CD19, CD22, and sIg; rarely prolymphocytes may be of T-cell lineage with positivity for CD2, CD3, CD7, and TCL-1; and 25% of cases are positive for both CD4 and CD8

LARGE GRANULAR LYMPHOCYTIC LEUKEMIA (LGL)

- LGL cells may occasionally look similar to those of hepatosplenic T-cell lymphoma (HSTCL) in fixed tissue and both neoplasms involve red pulp
- LGL typically spares the white pulp
- CD3, CD8, CD57, CD16, and CD56 are variably positive; potential immunophenotypic overlap in rare cases of LGL of gamma-delta variant
- Marrow appearance is distinct (absence of intravascular involvement with cells in clusters that is typically seen in HSTCL), profoundly different clinical presentation (i.e., indolent versus very aggressive)

PEARLS

- *Massive hepatosplenomegaly in a solid organ transplant recipient on immunosuppression is not an uncommon presentation of hepatosplenic T-cell lymphoma*
- *HSTCL has been reported in children treated with TNF inhibitors (e.g., for rheumatoid arthritis [RA])*
- *Bone marrow involvement is common; the typical intravascular infiltration is best visualized using immunohistochemical stains (e.g., for CD3)*

SELECTED REFERENCES

Macon WR, Levy NB, Kurtin PJ, et al: Hepatosplenic alphabeta T-cell lymphomas: a report of 14 cases and comparison with hepatosplenic gammadelta T-cell lymphomas. Am J Surg Pathol 25:285-296, 2001.

TABLE 15-3 DIFFERENTIAL FEATURES OF HEPATOSPLENIC T-CELL LYMPHOMA, T-CELL PROLYMPHOCYTIC LEUKEMIA, AND LARGE GRANULAR LYMPHOCYTIC LEUKEMIA

Type of Lymphoma/ Leukemia	Age and Sex	Clinical Features	Morphologic Features	Immunophenotype
Hepatosplenic T-cell lymphoma	Adolescents and young adults; male predominance	Hepatosplenomegaly, systemic symptoms, cytopenias, no lymphadenopathy	Red pulp involvement; medium-sized lymphoid cells with oval or folded nuclei and moderate cytoplasm present in red pulp cords and sinuses	Positive for CD2, CD3, CD56, TIA-1, usually gamma/delta TCR, variably positive for CD16 and CD7, usually negative for CD4, CD5, CD8, CD57, CD25, CD30, granzyme-B, perforin
T-cell prolymphocytic leukemia	Adults over the age of 30 years; no sex predominance	Hepatosplenomegaly, generalized lymphadenopathy, lymphocytosis with anemia and thrombocytopenia	Small to medium-sized lymphoid cells with nuclear irregularities, prominent nucleoli, and agranular cytoplasm present in the red pulp and also involving the white pulp	Positive for CD3, CD2, CD7, CD52, TCL-1, 25% cases positive for CD4 and CD8, some cases may show weak surface CD3
Large granular lymphocytic leukemia	45-75 years; no sex predominance	Neutropenia with or without anemia, variable degree of lymphocytosis and moderate splenomegaly	Neoplastic lymphocytes involving cords and sinuses in the red pulp	T-LGL subtype is positive for CD3, CD8, alpha-beta TCR (usually), TIA1, and granzyme-B; NK subtype is positive for CD16, CD56, and cytoplasmic CD3

Neiman RS, Orazi A: Lymphomas of the spleen. In Disorders of the Spleen, 2nd ed. Philadelphia, WB Saunders, 1999, pp 109-136.

Vega F, Medeiros LJ, Gaulard P: Hepatosplenic and other γδ T-cell lymphomas. Am J Clin Pathol 127:869-880, 2007.

Visnyei K, Grossbard ML, Shapira I: Hepatosplenic γδ T-cell lymphoma: an overview. Clin Lymphoma Myeloma Leuk 13:360-369, 2013.

SYSTEMIC MASTOCYTOSIS

Clinical Features

- Spleen is often involved, and most patients have palpable splenomegaly
- Most patients have urticaria pigmentosa or other systemic manifestations of mast cell activity at diagnosis

Gross Pathology

- Splenomegaly
- Thickened splenic capsule
- Multifocal ill-defined nodules with associated fibrosis and sclerosis; calcification may be present

Histopathology

- Mast cells form aggregates and nodules associated with a variable degree of fibrosis, often marked (collagen fibrosis), associated with eosinophils, which are more numerous at the periphery of the aggregates (Figure 15-23A)
- The nodules are often perivascular; they may also display peritrabecular and perifollicular distribution (Figure 15-23B)
- In routine hematoxylin and eosin (H&E)-stained sections, mast cells have mature indented nuclei and abundant cytoplasm
- The mast cells may, however, be spindle shaped or resemble monocytes, monocytoid B cells, or hairy cells, particularly because in routine H&E-stained sections, their granules are difficult to detect
- Occasionally fibrosis of a marked degree (overt collagen sclerosis) may predominate with only rare mast cells being identifiable
- Splenic hilar lymph nodes may also be involved
- Bone marrow is usually involved

Special Stains and Immunohistochemistry

- Mast cells can be detected with Naphthol-AS-D chloroacetate esterase, Giemsa, toluidine blue, or other metachromatic stains, or by immunostains for tryptase, chymase, or CD117

Other Techniques for Diagnosis

- Immunoreactivity with tryptase and CD25 (and often CD2), whose aberrant expression is limited to neoplastic mast cells, is usually sufficient to confirm the diagnosis in the presence of compact mast cell aggregates (> 15 mast cells)
- Serum tryptase persistently elevated (> 20 ng/mL)
- Detection of activating *KITD816V* mutation

Differential Diagnosis

HAIRY CELL LEUKEMIA

- Hairy cells form blood lakes and lack collagen fibrosis
- Lineages are different, myeloid versus lymphoid, demonstrable by immunostains (hairy cells express lymphoid antigens and are negative for tryptase), flow cytometry, or molecular diagnostic techniques

LARGE GRANULAR LYMPHOCYTIC LEUKEMIA

- Cells may occasionally look similar in fixed tissue, and both involve red pulp but only LGL cells are found intrasinusoidally
- No fibrosis in LGL
- CD3, CD8, CD57, CD16, and CD56 are variably positive in LGL
- Mast cell tryptase and CD117 are negative in LGL

PEARLS

- *Splenomegaly is common but splenectomy is only rarely performed*
- *Histologically, the mast cells may superficially resemble monocytes, hairy cells, or monocytoid B cells; however, the low-power appearance with fibrotic nodules and eosinophils is seen only in mastocytosis*
- *Mast cells have a distinctive immunophenotype*

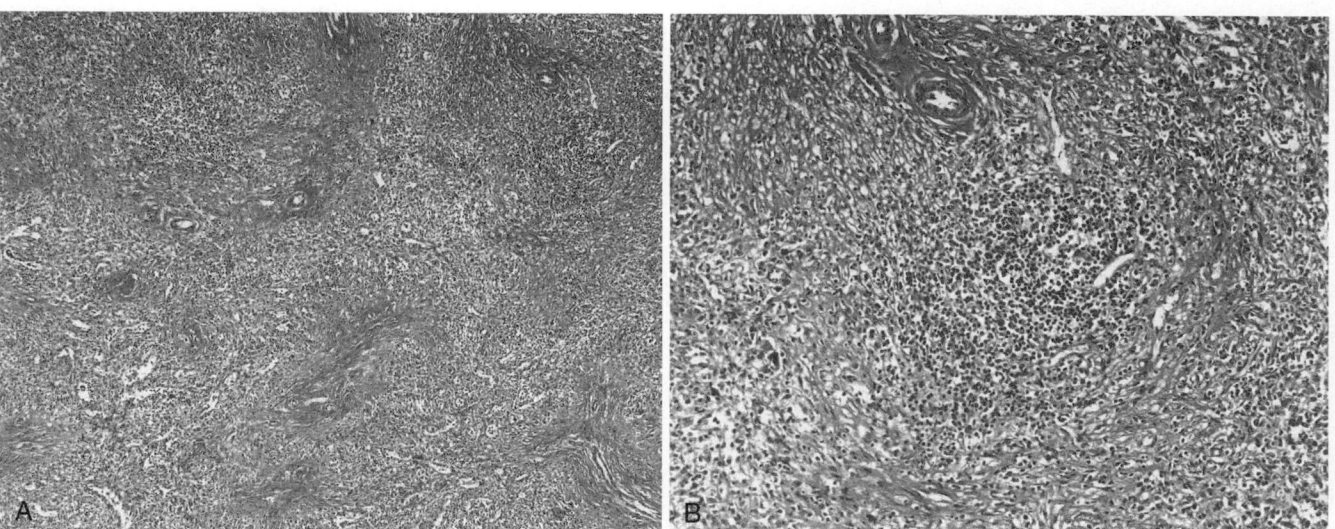

Figure 15-23. Mastocytosis. A, Low power. Aggregates of mast cells within the red pulp. The neoplastic cells have abundant cytoplasm. Note the presence of peritrabecular and perivascular fibrosis. **B,** High power. Perifollicular localization is also characteristically seen.

SELECTED REFERENCES

Brunning RD, McKenna RW, Rosai J, et al: Systemic mastocytosis: extracutaneous manifestations. Am J Surg Pathol 7: 425-438, 1983.
Horny HP, Ruck MT, Kaiserling E: Spleen findings in generalized mastocytosis: a clinicopathologic study. Cancer 70:459-468, 1992.
Horny HP, Sotlar K, Valent P: Mastocytosis: state of the art. Pathobiology 74:121-132, 2007.

CHRONIC MYELOGENOUS LEUKEMIA

Clinical Features

- Patients usually present with leukocytosis with significant neutrophilia, absolute basophilia, and a variable proportion of immature myeloid cells
- Splenomegaly common at presentation

Gross Pathology

- Solid, red, homogeneous appearance
- No lymphoid follicles visible

Histopathology

- White pulp is usually obliterated
- Red pulp cords and sinuses show a polymorphic infiltration by myeloid cells at all stages of maturation with a predominance of mature granulocytes
- Occasionally blastic transformation is first identified in the spleen (Figure 15-24)
- Bone marrow is always involved

Special Stains and Immunohistochemistry

- Naphthol-AS-D chloracetate esterase stain and antibodies such as myeloperoxidase or lysozyme can be used to facilitate the identification of myeloid cells
- Decreased neutrophil alkaline phosphatase (NAP)
- A combination of blastic reactive markers such as CD34, CD117, and TdT can be used to confirm extramedullary (splenic) blastic transformation, and a panel of lineage-specific antibodies (e.g., MPO, lysozyme, CD42b, CD79a, PAX5, CD3) is valuable in characterizing its type (e.g., myeloid transformation versus lymphoid or megakaryocytic)

Other Techniques for Diagnosis

- Identification of Philadelphia chromosome translocation t(9;22) by karyotype analysis, PCR, or FISH for *BCR-ABL1* in blood, marrow, or splenic tissue is necessary to confirm a diagnosis of chronic myelogenous leukemia
- In cases of blastic transformation, flow cytometry is useful to confirm the presence of blast and evaluate their lineage

Differential Diagnosis

- The histologic features are classic, particularly in view of the peripheral blood findings
- In selected cases, cytochemistry for naphthyl butyrate esterase or reactivity with antibody to histiocytic markers may be helpful in separating extramedullary chronic myelogenous leukemia from chronic myelomonocytic leukemia or other types of Ph'-negative myeloid neoplasms

REACTIVE SPLENIC RED PULP HYPERPLASIA

- Usually part of a nonspecific stress response process, which may be associated with a leukemoid reaction in the blood, or related to chronic congestive hypersplenism
- Basophilia is uncommon
- Elevated NAP
- Normal cytogenetics

ACUTE LEUKEMIA

- Differential diagnosis is with blast crisis of chronic myelogenous leukemia
- History of chronic phase disease or cytogenetic demonstration of t(9;22) is needed

PEARLS

- *Associated with the Philadelphia chromosome t(9;22) or BCR-ABL1 gene translocation*
- *Prominent splenomegaly with predominant involvement of red pulp*
- *Patients may undergo a blastic transformation, which is associated with a poor outcome*
- *In pediatric patients, chronic myelogenous leukemia, adult type, needs to be distinguished from juvenile myelomonocytic leukemia (JMML); in spleen sections, however, the two conditions largely overlap morphologically, although JMML displays monocytic differentiation which can be identified by immunohistology with CD68R, CD14, or flow cytometry with histiocytic markers*

SELECTED REFERENCES

Burke JS: Surgical pathology of the spleen: an approach to the differential diagnosis of splenic lymphomas and leukemias. Part II. Diseases of the red pulp. Am J Surg Pathol 5:681-694, 1981.
Pinkus GS, Pinkus JL: Myeloperoxidase: a specific marker for myeloid cells in paraffin sections. Mod Pathol 4:733-741, 1991.
Shepherd PC, Ganesan TS, Galton DA: Haematological classification of the chronic myeloid leukaemias. Baillieres Clin Haematol 1:877-906, 1987.

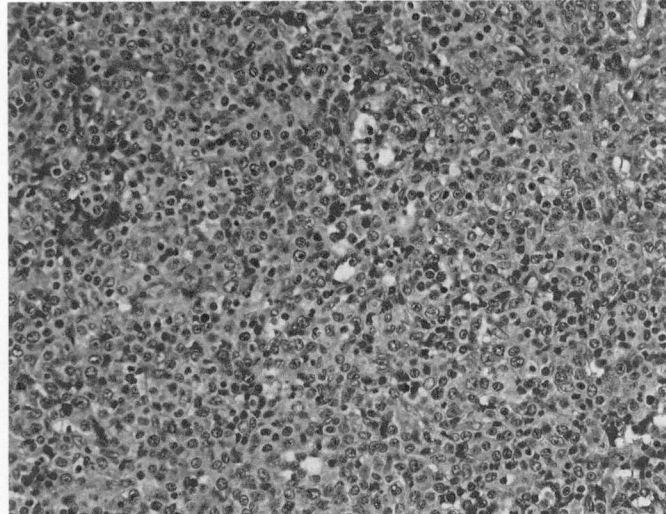

Figure 15-24. Chronic myelogenous leukemia, blastic phase. Diffuse infiltration of the red pulp by leukemic blasts. Acute transformation may manifest itself in the spleen (extramedullary transformation).

LANGERHANS CELL HISTIOCYTOSIS

Clinical Features

- Splenic involvement occurs in infants and young children with the disseminated form of the disease (Letterer-Siwe disease)
- Presenting symptoms include fever and skin lesions

Gross Pathology

- Splenomegaly with diffuse red pulp enlargement

Histopathology

- Langerhans cell infiltration of the red pulp may be diffuse or multinodular (loose aggregates are granuloma-like), only rarely has large discrete tumor masses
- Cells have typical pale, bean-shaped nuclei and pale cytoplasm
- Eosinophils and plasma cells are usually also present, although are much less numerous than in the localized form of the disease (eosinophilic granuloma)

Special Stains and Immunohistochemistry

- CD1a, S-100 protein, and langerin positive
- CD68R (PG-M1) negative

Other Techniques for Diagnosis

- Electron microscopy to demonstrate Birbeck granules

Differential Diagnosis

DISSEMINATED JUVENILE XANTHOGRANULOMA (JXG)

- Nuclei not bean shaped
- Characteristic presence of Touton giant cells; however, these cells may be either absent or present in reduced numbers in the various extracutaneous lesions when compared with JXG in the skin
- Immunohistochemistry: the histiocytic cells are positive for CD68 and factor XIIIa and negative for S-100 protein and CD1a

GAUCHER DISEASE (AND OTHER LYSOSOMAL STORAGE DISEASES)

- Infants present with neurologic deterioration and organomegaly; skin is not involved
- Absence of eosinophils
- Nuclei not bean shaped
- Cells usually larger than Langerhans cells
- Cytoplasm abundant, with wrinkled-silk pattern in Gaucher disease
- Cells periodic acid-Schiff (PAS) positive in most cases; S-100 protein and CD1a negative

HEMOPHAGOCYTIC SYNDROMES

- Patients are systemically ill with cytopenias (similar to Letterer-Siwe disease)
- Macrophages with red cells, leukocytes, and iron
- CD68 positive; S-100 protein and CD1a negative
- Some cases are EBV-related

MYCOBACTERIUM AVIUM-INTRACELLULARE

- Exceptional in children
- Patients usually have evidence of immune deficiency often HIV

- Special stains for acid-fast bacilli, PAS, and Gomori methenamine silver (GMS) reveal organisms in the cells

ACUTE MYELOID LEUKEMIA, PARTICULARLY ACUTE MONOBLASTIC LEUKEMIA

- Presents with cytopenias and peripheral blood or bone marrow involvement
- Blasts have large nuclei with finely dispersed chromatin and scanty to variably abundant cytoplasm depending on the acute myeloid leukemia subtype
- Mitoses more numerous than in Langerhans cell histiocytosis

HISTIOCYTIC SARCOMA (MALIGNANT HISTIOCYTOSIS)

- Patients are seriously ill with profound cytopenias
- Bone marrow usually shows diffuse involvement
- Rarely presents as isolated splenomegaly
- Red pulp infiltration may be associated with prominent necrosis
- Highly atypical cells with pleomorphic nuclei, which can be bean shaped and eccentric with prominent nucleoli and irregularly clumped chromatin; giant cells may resemble Reed-Sternberg cells
- Mitoses much more numerous than in Langerhans cell histiocytosis
- Erythrophagocytosis is seen in reactive macrophages and rarely in the tumor cells
- May express S-100 protein but always CD1a negative; expresses histiocytic markers (e.g., CD68, CD163)

PEARLS

- *Patients usually have skin, liver, and lymph node involvement*
- *Diagnosis is more readily made from bone marrow biopsy*
- *Splenic involvement is more likely to be seen at autopsy than in a surgical specimen*

SELECTED REFERENCES

Herzog KM, Tubbs RR: Langerhans cell histiocytosis. Adv Anat Pathol 5:347-358, 1998.

Pileri SA, Grogan TM, Harris NL, et al: Tumours of histiocytes and accessory dendritic cells: an immunohistochemical approach to classification from the International Lymphoma Study Group based on 61 cases. Histopathology 41:1-29, 2002.

Vardiman JW, Byrne GE Jr, Rappaport H: Malignant histiocytosis with massive splenomegaly in asymptomatic patients: a possible chronic form of the disease. Cancer 36:419-427, 1975.

VASCULAR TUMORS

SPLENIC HEMANGIOMA

Clinical Features

- Most frequent in young to middle-aged adults with no sex predilection
- Usually asymptomatic
- Symptoms and abnormalities reported include the following:
  - Abdominal discomfort
  - Hypersplenism with cytopenias
  - Consumption coagulopathy (disseminated intravascular coagulation)

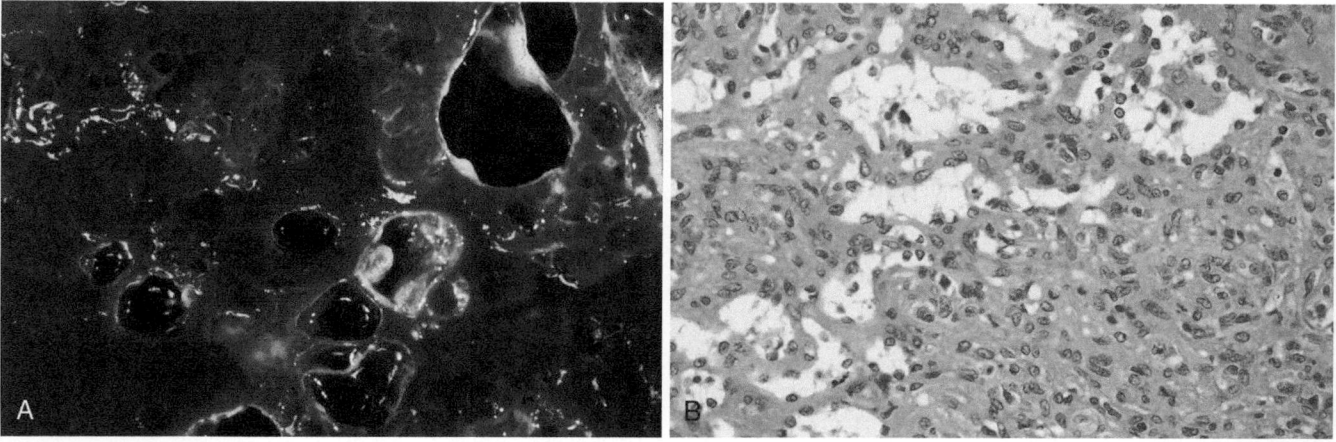

Figure 15-25. Hemangioma. A, Cut surface. In addition to the dilated vessels and cystic spaces, there are pale, spongy tumor nodules around dilated vessels. The intervening parenchyma looks normal. **B,** Photomicrograph. The dilated blood vessels of the tumor are surrounded by red pulp cordal macrophages.

GROSS PATHOLOGY
- Single, sometimes multiple masses
- Spleen normal to moderately enlarged
- Lesions are well circumscribed but not encapsulated
- Reddish-purple and spongy (Figure 15-25A)
- Secondary changes may include infarct or fibrosis
- Angiomatosis is diffuse replacement of the spleen by angiomatous tissue

Histopathology (Figure 15-25B)
- Most are cavernous hemangiomas
- Interconnected vascular channels of varying size
- Channels may be thrombosed with focal infarction
- Endothelium is usually flattened but may be plump; no endothelial tufting
- Mitoses are usually absent (except in children)
- No cellular pleomorphism or hyperchromasia

Special Stains and Immunohistochemistry
- CD34, CD31, and factor VIII positive
- CD8, CD68, CD21, and Ki-67 negative

Other Techniques for Diagnosis
- Noncontributory

Differential Diagnosis
CORD CAPILLARY HEMANGIOMA
- Another benign lesion termed *cordal capillary hemangioma* overlaps morphologically with capillary hemangiomas with sclerosis and may represent the same entity

HEMATOMA
- Few or no blood vessels inside the mass

PELIOSIS
- Often associated with hepatic peliosis
- More often multifocal or diffuse
- May be associated with spontaneous splenic rupture
- Dilated sinuses with attenuated lining cells surrounded by splenic parenchyma; no perilesional fibrosis
- Sinus lining cells: CD8 and CD68 positive

- Concentrated at the periphery of white pulp follicles (not a diffuse red pulp lesion)

LITTORAL CELL ANGIOMA
- More often multifocal or diffuse to almost involving the entire spleen
- Endothelial cells are plump and cuboidal or tall with papillary projections protruding into vascular spaces
- Endothelial cells are CD68 and CD163 positive and CD34 negative, CD21 and S-100 may also be positive; in contrast with normal littoral cells, they are negative for CD8

HEMANGIOENDOTHELIOMA
- Greater cytologic atypia, for example, plump endothelial cells with hyperchromatic nuclei
- Epithelioid and spindle cell variants
- Low to absent mitotic activity and lack of necrosis and invasive growth

ANGIOSARCOMA
- Splenomegaly in elderly patients with fatigue, fever, weight loss, and abdominal pain
- Poorly delineated, large often necrotic tumor masses that may involve the entire organ
- Papillary cell proliferation producing tufts and partially filling vascular spaces
- Anastomosing vascular channels may alternate with solid poorly differentiated areas
- Nuclear pleomorphism, hyperchromasia, and atypia
- Frequent mitoses
- Infiltrative growth pattern
- CD31 is the best marker; expression of other endothelial antigens is variable

SPLENIC HAMARTOMA
- Usually a single bulging and fleshy mass
- Color similar to splenic red pulp
- Contains both cords and sinus structures (the latter CD8 positive)

- Another lesion related to hamartoma is myoid angioendothelioma, a rare benign tumor of the spleen, which is morphologically characterized by a composite of vascular spaces and stromal cells with myoid features

LYMPHANGIOMA
- Mostly occurs in children
- Grossly indistinguishable
- Gross cyst formation is common
- Spaces contain proteinaceous material, lymph, and cholesterol clefts (not blood)
- D2-40, CD31, and factor VIII positive; CD34 usually negative

PEARLS

- *Microangiopathic hemolytic anemia and platelet consumption have been reported with large vascular lesions*

SELECTED REFERENCE

Arber DA, Strickler JG, Chen YY, Weiss LM: Splenic vascular tumors: a histologic, immunophenotypic, and virologic study. Am J Surg Pathol 21:827-835, 1997.

LITTORAL CELL ANGIOMA

Clinical Features
- Rare
- Occurs at any age and in either sex
- May cause splenomegaly and hypersplenism

Gross Pathology
- Single or multiple spongy, purplish-black, well-circumscribed nodules
- Rarely may replace the whole organ; sometimes it s only vaguely multinodular; in other cases, it may appear subdivided into lobules by bands of fibrosis (Figure 15-26A)

Histopathology
- Pleomorphic vascular spaces: from slit-like to dilated and cystic

- Lined by cuboidal to hobnail shaped cells with large vesicular nuclei (Figure 15-26B)
- Papillary projections protruding into the vascular spaces
- Tumor cells can exfoliate into the lumen
- No significant cellular atypia, and mitotic activity is low
- Always lacks solid areas and necrosis

Special Stains and Immunohistochemistry
- Reticulin: annular fibers around vascular spaces
- Occasional PAS-positive cytoplasmic globules
- Distinctive phenotype: CD31, CD68, and CD68R (both KP-1 and PG-M1), CD21, and CD163 positive; negative for CD8 and CD34; may also express S-100 protein

Other Techniques for Diagnosis
- Noncontributory

Differential Diagnosis

HEMANGIOMA
- No irregular anastomosing channels
- More often single
- Vascular spaces lined by flattened cells
- CD68 negative

SPLENIC HAMARTOMA
- Usually a single mass that is bulging and fleshy, color similar to splenic red pulp
- Contains both cords and sinus structures (the latter CD8 positive)
- Endothelia are of littoral cell derivation, positive for CD8 and CD68, and negative for CD34

HEMANGIOENDOTHELIOMA
- Patients may have disease outside the spleen
- Endothelial cells have hyperchromatic nuclei
- Epithelioid or spindle-shaped endothelia
- Endothelial cells are usually negative for CD68

ANGIOSARCOMA
- Elderly patients
- Greater splenic enlargement
- Infiltrative growth pattern and necrosis

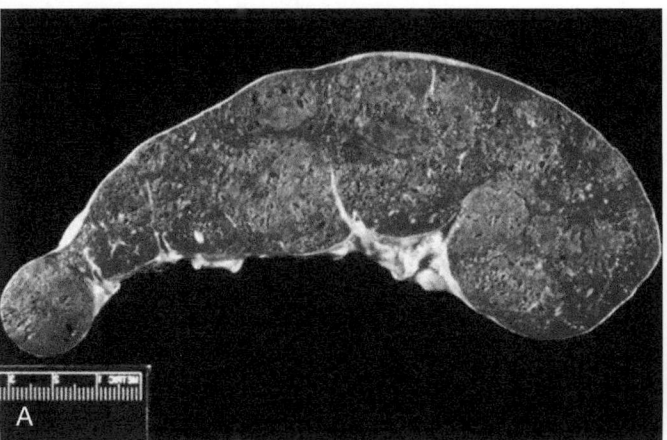
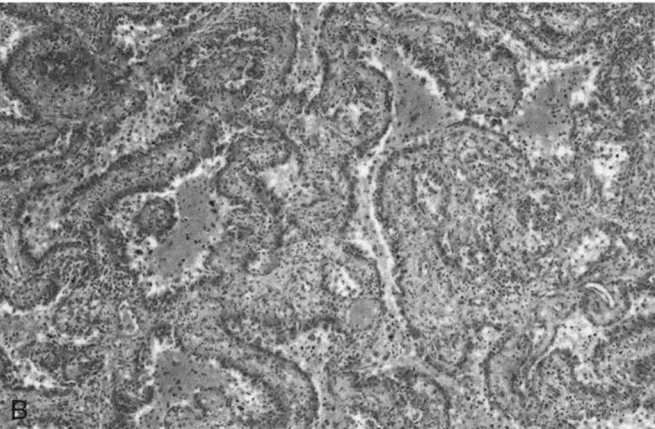

Figure 15-26. Littoral cell angioma. A, Rarely the whole spleen can be replaced by a spongy hemorrhagic, vaguely nodular proliferation. This may raise the possibility of an angiosarcoma. **B,** At this magnification, the larger size and more cuboidal to hobnail pattern of the cells lining the vascular spaces is apparent. These cells do not have the nuclear pleomorphism, atypia, or mitotic activity seen in more aggressive vascular tumors.

- Anastomosing vascular channels lined by a papillary endothelial cell proliferation producing tufts and partially filling vascular spaces
- More mitoses, nuclear pleomorphism, atypia, and hyperchromasia
- Endothelial cells are more often negative for CD68
- Metastases are not uncommon

PEARLS

- *Littoral cell angioma is benign despite its multifocality*
- *No counterpart exists outside the spleen*
- *Extremely rare aggressive counterparts have been described (littoral cell angioendothelioma and littoral cell angiosarcoma)*

SELECTED REFERENCES

Arber DA, Strickler JG, Chen YY, Weiss LM: Splenic vascular tumors: a histologic, immunophenotypic, and virologic study. Am J Surg Pathol 21:827-835, 1997.

Falk S, Stutte HJ, Frizzera G: Littoral cell angioma: a novel splenic vascular lesion demonstrating histiocytic differentiation. Am J Surg Pathol 15:1023-1033, 1991.

Rosso R, Paulli M, Gianelli U, et al: Littoral cell angiosarcoma of the spleen: case report with immunohistochemical and ultrastructural analysis. Am J Surg Pathol 19:1203-1208, 1995.

SPLENIC ANGIOSARCOMA

Clinical Features

- Although it can occur at any age, it is most common in elderly patients; no sex predominance
- Often disseminated at presentation, it may be difficult to ascertain its primary site (splenic versus extrasplenic origin)
- Not associated with vinyl chloride or thorium dioxide (Thorotrast) exposure
- Can cause splenic rupture
- Fatigue, fever, weight loss, and abdominal pain; cytopenias have been reported
- Prognosis is poor: hematogenous metastases to liver and lung

Gross Pathology

- Splenomegaly, often marked (weight > 1000 g common)
- Single or multiple hemorrhagic and necrotic masses or diffuse infiltration, blending with splenic red pulp (Figure 15-27A)

Histopathology

- Cellular appearances, degree of differentiation, and proliferation vary within and among tumors
- Irregular anastomosing vascular channels or solid masses partially or largely occluding vascular spaces
- Cells may be flattened, spindled, polygonal, epithelioid, or small and poorly differentiated; may form papillary projections that protrude into vascular spaces
- Cytologic atypia varies from slightly prominent endothelial cells with slight hyperplasia, pleomorphism, and occasional mitoses to anaplastic cells with numerous mitoses, associated with areas of hemorrhage and necrosis (Figure 15-27B)

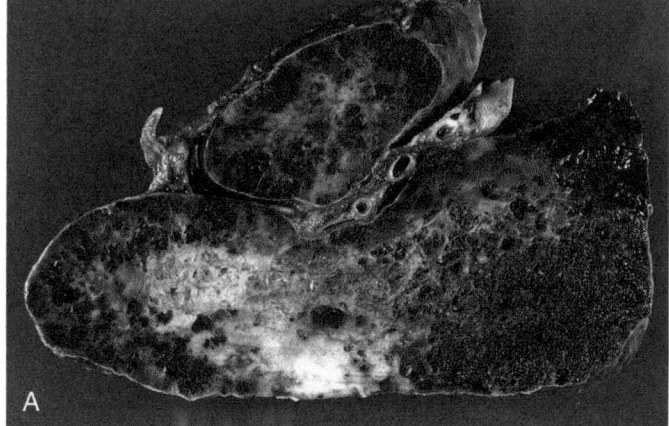

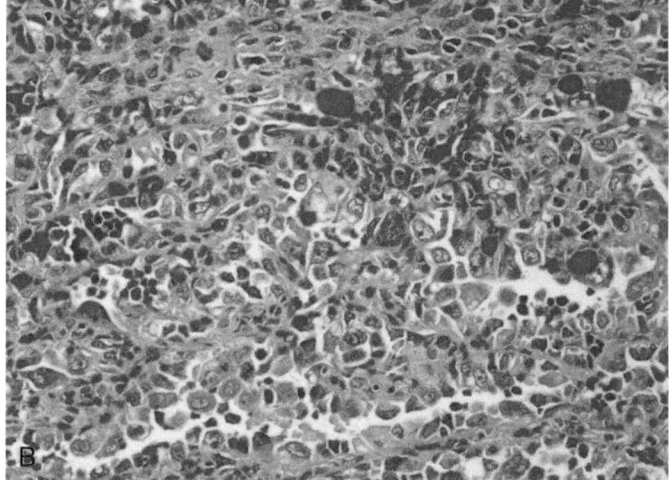

Figure 15-27. Splenic angiosarcoma. A, In this case of splenic angiosarcoma, most of the organ is replaced by a neoplastic proliferation characterized by a mixture of spongy and solid areas with extensive necrosis and hemorrhages. **B,** Pleomorphic neoplastic endothelial cells with a high nuclear-to-cytoplasmic ratio and hyperchromatic nuclei lining the vascular spaces. Some of the cells appear to be floating free in the vascular spaces. Mitotic figures could be found easily. Outside the obvious vascular spaces are solid areas composed of cells similar to those lining the larger vascular spaces. Red cells are present in the vascular lumina.

- Extramedullary hematopoiesis and erythrophagocytosis can both be found in some cases

Special Stains and Immunohistochemistry

- Expression of common endothelial cell antigens is variable but CD31 and *Ulex* lectin are usually positive
- CD34 and factor VIII are usually detected in better differentiated areas only; CD163 is negative
- Positivity for CD68 and CD8 suggests a littoral cell derivation (littoral cell angiosarcoma)
- Expression of D2-40, a marker of differentiation along the lymphatic endothelial lineage, has been reported in some cases; these cases could be classified as lymphangiosarcomas

Other Techniques for Diagnosis

- Electron microscopy: Weibel-Palade bodies

Differential Diagnosis

HEMANGIOMA
- Lacks pleomorphism, mitoses, atypia
- Vascular channels lined by a single layer of uniform cells
- No necrosis or solid areas

HEMANGIOENDOTHELIOMA
- Differentiation from angiosarcoma may be subtle
- No necrosis
- No solid areas
- Less pleomorphism, less atypia, fewer mitoses, and less nuclear hyperchromasia

HEMANGIOPERICYTOMA
- Staghorn vascular channels
- No necrosis
- Usually few mitoses, little or no cellular pleomorphism
- Endothelial cells lining the vascular spaces are a single layer of flattened cells with no atypia
- The proliferating spindle cells surround rather than form the vascular spaces; may be better demonstrated using silver stains
- Positive for vimentin and variable positivity for CD34
- It may correspond to myopericytoma (see "Pearls")

KAPOSI SARCOMA
- Elderly men of Mediterranean ancestry or patients with acquired immunodeficiency syndrome (AIDS)
- Usually forms small nodules
- Composed of spindle cells without papillary formation or vascular channels (except for vessels at the periphery of the nodules)
- No necrosis or hemorrhage
- Slitlike vascular spaces with eosinophilic globules
- Hemosiderin (can also be present in angiosarcoma)
- Immunohistochemistry positivity for D2-40, CD34, and HHV-8

BACILLARY ANGIOMATOSIS
- Typically younger individuals; increased incidence in AIDS patients
- No anastomosing vascular channels
- Few mitoses, little or no pleomorphism
- Grayish interstitial material
- Bacteria identified using Warthin-Starry stain
- HHV-8 negative

METASTATIC MELANOMA
- Patients usually have a history of melanoma elsewhere
- Pigment may be melanin
- No vascular channels
- CD34, CD31, and factor VIII negative
- S-100 protein, HMB-45, and melan-A positive
- Electron microscopy can show melanosomes

MALIGNANT FIBROUS HISTIOCYTOMA
- Rarely primary in spleen
- No anastomosing vascular channels
- Multinucleated giant cells may be present
- Vimentin, α_1-antichymotrypsin, α_1-antitrypsin, and CD68 positive; CD31 and factor VIII negative

PEARLS

- *The existence of hemangiopericytoma as a separate entity has been questioned because a number of neoplasms of different lines of differentiation are characterized by a hemangiopericytoma-like vascular growth pattern*
- *Myopericytoma represents a recently delineated entity showing a hemangiopericytoma-like vascular pattern; it is likely that at least a proportion of cases that have been previously termed* splenic hemangiopericytoma *may represent examples of myopericytoma*
- *Most cases of myopericytoma behave in a benign fashion, but local recurrences and rarely metastases have been reported; more recently, a malignant variant has also been described*

SELECTED REFERENCES

Das A, Arya SV, Soni N, et al: A rare presentation of hepatic and splenic cystic malignant fibrous histiocytoma: a case report and literature review. Int J Surg Case Rep 4:139-141, 2013.

Falk S, Krishnan J, Meis JM: Primary angiosarcoma of the spleen: a clinicopathologic study of 40 cases. Am J Surg Pathol 17:959-970, 1993.

Granter SR, Badizadegan K, Fletcher CD: Myofibromatosis in adults, glomangiopericytoma, and myopericytoma: a spectrum of tumors showing perivascular myoid differentiation. Am J Surg Pathol 22:513-525, 1998.

He L, Zhang H, Li X, et al: Primary malignant fibrous histiocytoma of spleen with spontaneous rupture: a case report and literature review. Med Oncol 28:397-400, 2011.

CYSTS AND PSEUDOTUMORAL LESIONS

EPIDERMOID CYST (TRUE CYSTS)

Clinical Features
- Occurs in children to young adults; no gender predominance
- Most likely of mesothelial derivation

Gross Pathology
- Single or, rarely, multiple lesions
- Cyst has a trabeculated appearance covered by a shiny lining (resembling endocardium) (Figure 15-28)
- Fluid clear to turbid and yellowish; can contain cholesterol crystals

Histopathology
- Thin, fibrous wall with epithelial lining
- Epithelium may be attenuated or denuded
- Epithelium can be squamous (more often), transitional, or columnar

Special Stains and Immunohistochemistry
- Cytokeratin stains highlight the epithelium

Other Techniques for Diagnosis
- Noncontributory

Differential Diagnosis

PSEUDOCYST
- No epithelial lining

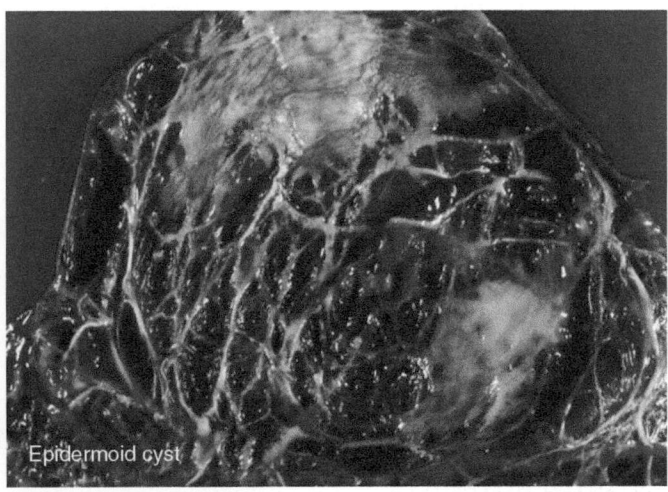

Figure 15-28. Epidermoid splenic cyst. The wall is thicker, and its trabeculation may be reminiscent of the endocardial surface of the ventricular cavities. The cyst contained clear fluid.

PARASITIC (ECHINOCOCCAL) CYST
- Adults are most commonly affected
- Resident in areas of the world where the parasite is endemic (e.g., Greece); in the United States, the disease is rare, but it has been reported in several states (see also "Parasitic [Echinococcal] Cyst")
- Usually requires significant exposure to animal vectors
- Cyst is often multilocular
- Hepatic or peritoneal cysts commonly present
- Granular wall with small granules in cyst contents
- Scolices in wall or secondary cysts

PEARLS

- *True cysts are usually asymptomatic unless infected*
- *Unclear whether these are congenital developmental abnormalities or the result of subtle abdominal trauma with mesothelial entrapment in the spleen*

PSEUDOCYST

Clinical Features
- Four times more common than epithelial cyst
- Clinical presentation identical to that of epithelial cyst
- Believed to result from degradation of a splenic hematoma of posttraumatic origin or to be a consequence of cystic degeneration of a splenic infarct or infarcted hemangioma

Gross Pathology
- Same as for epithelial cyst, but fluid is usually darker reddish brown

Histopathology
- Smooth internal surface (rather than trabeculated)
- Fibrous wall *without* epithelial lining
- Calcification in wall
- Cholesterol clefts can be present

Special Stains and Immunohistochemistry
- Cytokeratin negative

Other Techniques for Diagnosis
- Noncontributory

Differential Diagnosis
Epithelioid Cyst
- Epithelial lining present

Parasitic Cyst
- See "Parasitic (Echinococcal) Cyst"

PEARLS

- *Usually asymptomatic unless infected*
- *Large cysts can rupture; resection is recommended*
- *May be drained under radiologic guidance but are more likely to recur*
- *Thought to be related to splenic trauma and organizing hematoma*

PARASITIC (ECHINOCOCCAL) CYST

Clinical Features
- Occurs in residents of areas of the world where the parasite is endemic (e.g., Greece); in the United States, the disease is rare but has been reported in California, Arizona, New Mexico, and Utah
- Adults are most commonly affected; patients usually have significant exposure to animal vectors; risk factors include exposure to cattle, sheep, pigs, or deer or exposure to the feces of dogs, wolves, or coyotes
- Cysticercosis can produce grossly similar cysts, differing in the nature of the parasite

Gross Pathology
- Often multilocular
- Hepatic or peritoneal cysts commonly present
- Granular wall with small granules in cyst contents

Histopathology
- Fibrous wall
- Daughter cysts or brood capsules containing parasites with scolices
- Inflammatory reaction is usually present

Special Stains and Immunohistochemistry
- Smears of fluid or touch preparations of cyst wall reveal scolices
- Scolices can be highlighted by AFB stain

Other Techniques for Diagnosis
- Noncontributory

Differential Diagnosis
Epithelioid Cyst (see "Epidermoid Cyst [True Cysts]")
- No inflammation
- No scolices
- Epithelial lining

PSEUDOCYST

* No inflammation
* No scolices

PEARLS

* *Intraoperative rupture of the cyst with leakage of cyst contents can cause peritoneal dissemination of the disease and can be fatal*

SELECTED REFERENCES

Garvin DF, King FM: Cysts and nonlymphomatous tumors of the spleen. Pathol Ann 16:61-80, 1981.

Hulzebos CV, Leemans R, Halma C, de Vries TW: Splenic epithelial cysts and splenomegaly: diagnosis and management. Neth J Med 53:80-84, 1998.

SPLENIC HAMARTOMA (SPLENOMA)

Clinical Features

* Occurs at any age
* Usually asymptomatic
* Rarely causes abdominal pain or thrombocytopenia

Gross Pathology

* Usually single nodule (Figure 15-29A)
* Size ranges from less than 1 cm to about 10 cm
* Color usually resembles splenic red pulp
* Bulging from cut surface
* Fleshy consistency
* Well circumscribed but not encapsulated
* Can have foci of infarction and fibrosis

Histopathology (Figure 15-29 B,C)

* A tumor-like lesion composed of structurally disorganized splenic red pulp tissue
* Resembles normal red pulp with no "organized" white pulp within the lesion; may, however, contain scattered lymphocytes
* Consists of both cordal and sinus-like structures
* Compressed red pulp at the periphery, but no true capsule
* Can have foci of infarction and fibrosis, sometimes with hemosiderin deposition

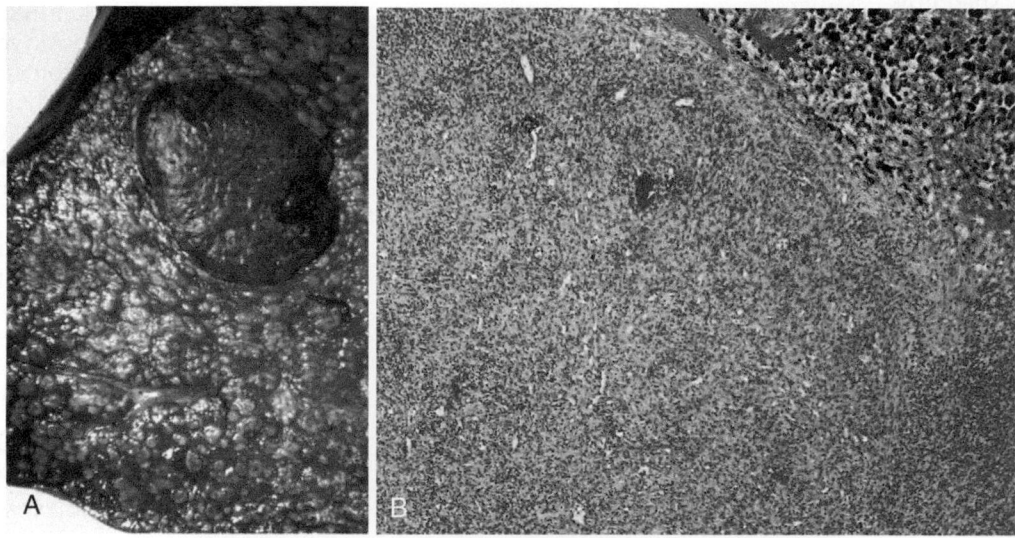

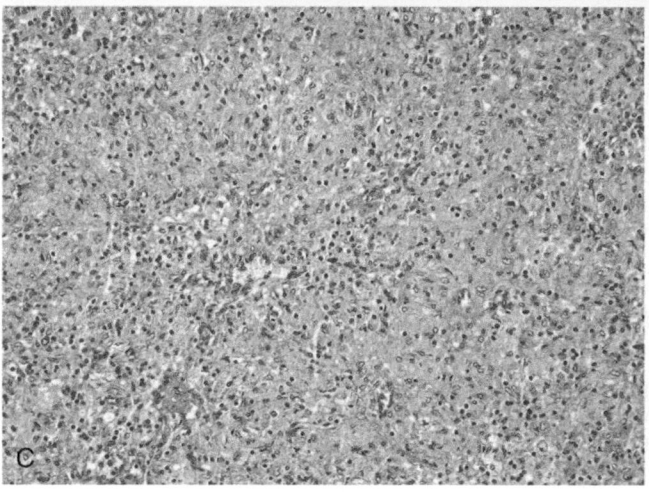

Figure 15-29. A, Splenic hamartoma (splenoma), gross photograph. Hamartoma presents as a well-demarcated, bulging lesion displaying a characteristic "red pulp only" appearance. **B,** Splenic hamartoma. Flattened endothelial cells line irregular vascular spaces, which are surrounded by disorganized red pulp tissue. Unlike a hemangioma, both the blood vessels and other red pulp spaces are disorganized. **C,** Splenic hamartoma (splenoma), cordal variant. A predominance of cordal macrophages is noted. Occasionally, this may resemble an inflammatory pseudotumor.

- May contain immature hematopoietic cells and eosinophils
- May show fibrosis
- A histiocyte-rich variant has also been described

Special Stains and Immunohistochemistry

- Endothelia are positive for CD8 and CD68 and negative for CD34
- Reticulin stain shows a disorganized sinusoidal wall with partial loss of ring fibers

Other Techniques for Diagnosis

- Noncontributory

Differential Diagnosis

HEMANGIOMA

- Hemorrhagic, not fleshy or bulging
- Darker than red pulp
- Vascular endothelial differentiation only, no sinus like structures
- CD34 positive; CD68 and CD8 negative

LITTORAL CELL ANGIOMA

- Usually multifocal dark, purplish black, spongy lesions
- Irregular vascular spaces all of one type
- Mostly polygonal to tall lining cells with luminal shedding
- CD68 and CD21 positive

INFLAMMATORY PSEUDOTUMOR

- Usually paler than surrounding parenchyma
- Lacks sinus structures
- Numerous plasma cells and lymphocytes
- Prominent spindle cell component
- A proportion are EBV positive

PEARLS

- *There is still controversy about whether this is a neoplasm or a "true" hamartoma*
- *Always benign*
- *Occurs only in spleen*

SELECTED REFERENCES

Chiu A, Czader M, Cheng L, et al.: Clonal X-chromosome inactivation suggests that splenic cord capillary hemangioma is a true neoplasm and not a subtype of splenic hamartoma. Mod Pathol 24:108-116, 2011.
Krishnan J, Frizzera G: Two splenic lesions in need of clarification: hamartoma and inflammatory pseudotumor. Semin Diagn Pathol 20:94-104, 2003.

INFLAMMATORY PSEUDOTUMOR OF THE SPLEEN

Clinical Features

- Occurs at any adult age
- Can be asymptomatic or present with fever, weight loss, or abdominal pain
- Rarely present in more than one organ in a given patient

Gross Pathology

- Size ranges from less than 1 cm up to 10 cm
- Usually single but can be multiple; multiple lesions are usually small
- Well circumscribed, pale to white, and bulging often with central necrosis

Histopathology (Figure 15-30)

- Splenic IPT includes the following variants
  - A "truly inflammatory" IPT most commonly seen in older individuals
  - A rare form of IPT containing follicular dendritic cells (FDCs), termed *hepatosplenic IPT-like FDC tumor*, which consistently harbors clonal EBV DNA and shows a marked female predominance
- Irregularly oriented, bland spindle cells intermixed with variable numbers of lymphocytes, plasma cells, macrophages (which can be foamy), and neutrophils with usually, only rare eosinophils
- No proliferative activity or cellular atypia
- Occasional features: sclerosis, hemorrhage, necrosis, calcification, and hemosiderin deposits

Special Stains and Immunohistochemistry

- Spindle cells have smooth muscle differentiation: muscle-specific actin, SMA, sometimes desmin positive
- In the "truly inflammatory IPT," the epithelioid and spindle cells are positive for vimentin and CD68 but lack expression of follicular dendritic cell markers and actin
- A proportion of cases may show an increased IgG4/IgG ratio; in this cases the patient should be evaluated to exclude chronic pancreatitis or other evidence of "IgG4 related disease"
- IPT-like follicular dendritic cell tumor of the spleen shows positivity for dendritic cell markers (CD21, CD23, and CD35) and evidence of EBV infection by EBV-LMP immunostaining or EBV-RNA by in situ hybridization
- Lymphocytes are mostly T cells
- Plasma cells are polyclonal

Other Techniques for Diagnosis

- Gene rearrangement studies
- EBER in situ hybridization

Differential Diagnosis

SPLENIC HAMARTOMA

- Nodules are red and fleshy rather than pale
- Contains sinus-like structures, no solid areas except in foci of fibrosis
- Less inflamed cellular background with fewer lymphocytes and plasma cells

CASTLEMAN DISEASE

- More often multifocal; patients usually have lymph node involvement
- Distinct germinal centers (hyalinized or hyperplastic) in the lesion
- Spindle cells not prominent
- Sheets of plasma cells present in plasma cell and multicentric type

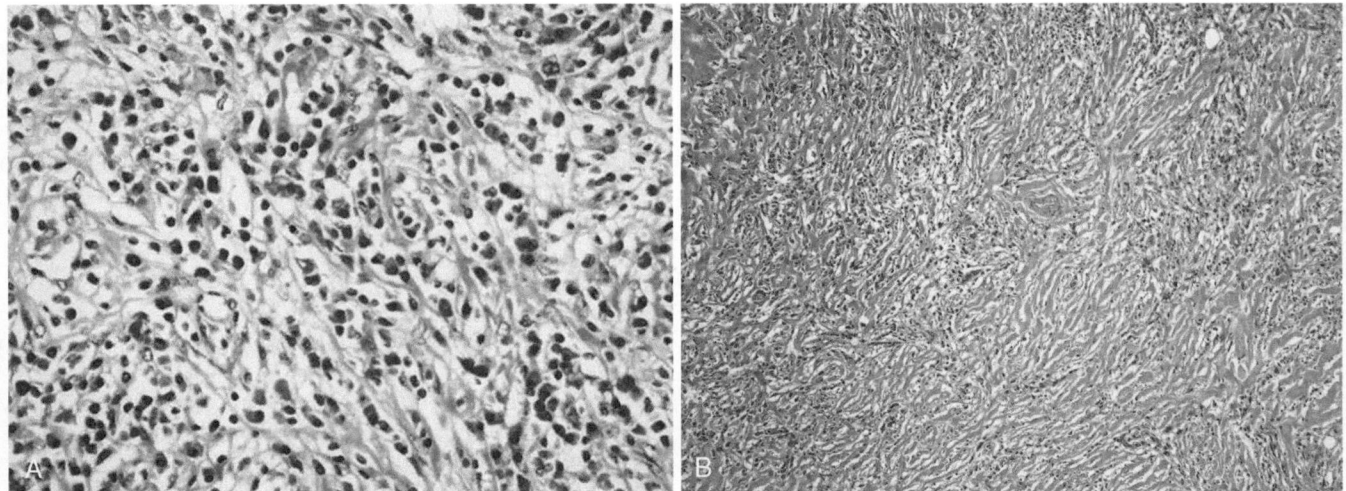

Figure 15-30. Inflammatory pseudotumor. A, Macrophages and relatively rare myofibroblasts are found associated with numerous inflammatory cells, particularly plasma cells. **B,** The lesion has a predominance of spindle cells.

HODGKIN LYMPHOMA
- Patients have Hodgkin lymphoma elsewhere
- Eosinophils often numerous
- Hodgkin-Reed-Sternberg cells present

PLASMACYTOMA
- Occurs in older adults
- Patients usually have known multiple myeloma
- Sclerosis is rare (exception: an osteosclerotic variant associated with hepatosplenomegaly known as POEMS syndrome [polyneuropathy, organomegaly, endocrinopathy, monoclonal paraprotein, and skin hyperpigmentation])
- Plasma cells are monoclonal

FOLLICULAR DENDRITIC CELL SARCOMA (VERSUS IPT-LIKE FOLLICULAR DENDRITIC CELL TUMOR OF THE SPLEEN)
- Sheets of plump spindle cells
- Infiltrative growth pattern
- Cells are CD21 and CD35 positive and SMA negative
- A small proportion of cases have been associated with Castleman disease of the hyaline-vascular type, and others with EBV infection

MYCOBACTERIAL PSEUDOTUMOR
- Patients with AIDS
- Most have mycobacteriosis elsewhere
- Few spindle cells (exception is the rare mycobacterial spindle cell pseudotumor, a lesion seen in immunocompromised patients, composed of proliferative spindle cells admixed with histiocytes and inflammatory cells associated with the presence of *Mycobacterium avium-intracellulare*)
- Sheets of large macrophages with abundant gray cytoplasm, not foamy cells
- Acid-fast stain positive
- Culture for mycobacteria positive

BACILLARY ANGIOMATOSIS
- AIDS patients

- Vascular proliferation
- Gray interstitial material
- Bacteria in interstitial material positive with Warthin-Starry stain
- HHV-8 negative

PEARLS

- *IPT may be truly inflammatory or follicular dendritic cell in origin*
- *Its precise characterization relies on a combination of morphology and immunohistochemistry*
- *It should be distinguished from inflammatory myofibroblastic tumor a clonal myofibroblastic proliferation which is ALK positive; this entity has not yet been reported to occur in the spleen*

SELECTED REFERENCES

Brittig F, Ajtay E, Jakso P, Kelenyi G: Follicular dendritic reticulum cell tumor mimicking inflammatory pseudotumor of the spleen. Pathol Oncol Res 10:57-60, 2004.

Horiguchi H, Matsui-Horiguchi M, Sakata H, et al: Inflammatory pseudotumor-like follicular dendritic cell tumor of the spleen. Pathol Int 54:124-131, 2004.

Lewis JT, Gaffney RL, Casey MB, et al: Inflammatory pseudotumor of the spleen associated with a clonal Epstein-Barr virus genome: case report and review of the literature. Am J Clin Pathol 120:56-61, 2003.

Neiman RS, Orazi A: Splenic cysts, nonhematopoietic tumors, and tumor like lesions. In Disorders of the Spleen, 2nd ed. Philadelphia, WB Saunders, 1999, pp 249-285.

CIRCULATORY ABNORMALITIES

CONGESTIVE SPLENOMEGALY

Clinical Features

- Occurs in patients with liver cirrhosis causing portal hypertension
- Occurs in patients with splenic vein thrombosis (e.g., in paroxysmal nocturnal hemoglobinuria or polycythemia vera)

Gross Pathology

- Moderate, diffuse splenic enlargement; weight usually less than 1 kg
- White pulp inconspicuous
- Red pulp dark, may be firm
- Small infarcts common in larger spleens

Histopathology

- White pulp histology is variable
- Diffuse expansion of the red pulp (Figure 15-31A)
- In early stages, the red pulp is more cellular, becomes fibrotic and hypocellular in later stages
- Increased number of hemosiderin-laden macrophages
- Longstanding cases
  - Fibrosis with excess reticulin deposition in long-standing cases
  - The sinuses may become dilated (pulled open by the fibrosis)
  - It may superficially resemble a capillary hemangioma with sclerosis or a hamartoma but is not circumscribed
  - Gamna-Gandy bodies can occur (for definition of Gamna-Gandy bodies, see "Sickle Cell Disease and Variants")

Special Stains and Immunohistochemistry

- Reticulin stain shows increased fibrosis throughout the red pulp
- A diffuse increased expression of SMA (splenic myoid cells) is typical (Figure 15-31B)

Other Techniques for Diagnosis

- Noncontributory

Differential Diagnosis

LEUKEMIC INFILTRATION

- Red pulp is diffusely infiltrated by blasts, small lymphocytes, or hairy cells depending on the type of leukemia
- Immunohistochemistry to confirm the diagnosis of leukemia

LYMPHOMA

- Subtypes of lymphoid neoplasms involving the red pulp (e.g., hepatosplenic T-cell lymphoma, intravascular large B-cell lymphoma)
- Intrasinusoidal lymphocytosis with cytologic atypia
- Immunohistochemistry to confirm the diagnosis of lymphoma

MYELOFIBROSIS OR OTHER MYELOPROLIFERATIVE DISORDERS

- Lesions are more discrete
- Prominent extramedullary hematopoiesis, usually trilineage
- Atypical megakaryocytes often present in primary myelofibrosis or postpolycythemic myelofibrosis
- Cellularity often increased

PELIOSIS

- Lesions are more discrete
- Dilated sinuses concentrated near white pulp follicles
- Multifocal discrete lesions; sinuses appear dilated but there is no perivascular fibrosis

PEARLS

- *Congestive splenomegaly can cause hypersplenism; splenectomy may be required*
- *Consider additional causes if spleen weight is greater than 1 kg*
- *Coagulation abnormalities in these patients are more commonly the result of liver disease*

SELECTED REFERENCES

Neiman RS, Orazi A: Chronic passive congestion. In Disorders of the Spleen, 2nd ed. Philadelphia, WB Saunders, 1999, pp 238-239.

O'Reilly RA: Splenomegaly in 2,505 patients at a large university medical center from 1913 to 1995. 1963 to 1995:449 patients. West J Med 169:88-97, 1998.

Sheth SG, Amarapurkar DN, Chopra KB, et al: Evaluation of splenomegaly in portal hypertension. J Clin Gastroenterol 22:28-30, 1996.

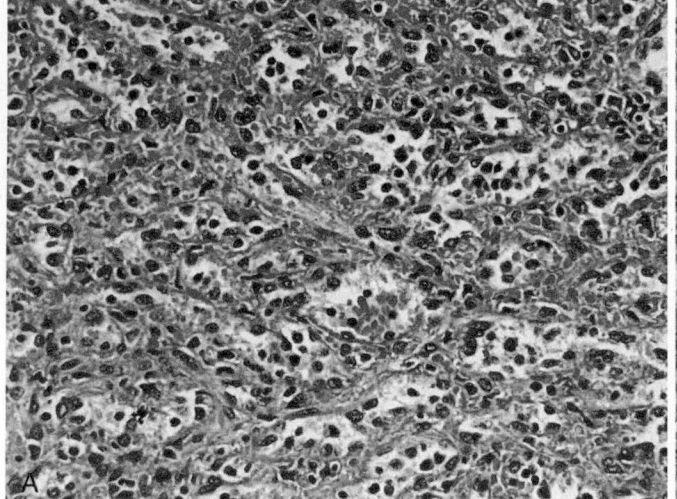
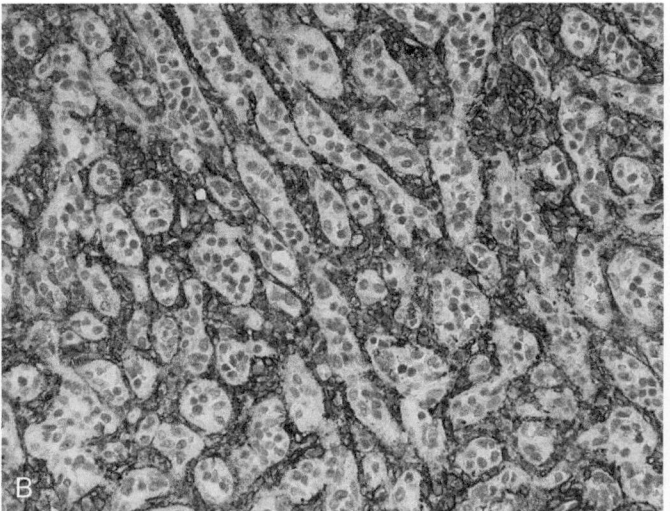

Figure 15-31. **Fibrocongestive splenomegaly (chronic passive congestion). A,** High-power magnification of red pulp. Both cords and sinuses are distended and are surrounded by an increased amount of stroma, which imparts a rigid appearance to the red pulp. **B,** Increased expression of smooth muscle actin due to a reactive hyperplasia of splenic myoid cells is a characteristic finding seen in spleen with chronic passive congestion.

VASCULITIDES

POLYARTERITIS NODOSA, HYPERSENSITIVITY ANGIITIS (CHURG-STRAUSS DISEASE), SYSTEMIC LUPUS ERYTHEMATOSUS, RHEUMATOID ARTHRITIS, AND THROMBOTIC THROMBOCYTOPENIC PURPURA

Clinical Features

- Rarely limited to the spleen; more commonly part of a systemic vasculitis
- Seen in patients with
  - Polyarteritis nodosa
  - Systemic lupus erythematosus
  - Rheumatoid arthritis
  - Thrombotic thrombocytopenic purpura
  - Hypersensitivity angiitis

Gross Pathology

- Multiple infarcts, which can be confluent
- Splenic rupture has been reported

Histopathology

- Vasculitis similar to the manifestation of the basic disease in other organs
- Infarcts can be present

POLYARTERITIS NODOSA

- Small arteries
- Fibrinoid necrosis (Figure 15-32)
- Neutrophils and eosinophils in vessel walls
- Splenic rupture has been reported

HYPERSENSITIVITY ANGIITIS (CHURG-STRAUSS DISEASE)

- Leukocytoclastic vasculitis in arterioles
- Fibrinoid necrosis in small vessels
- Eosinophils in infiltrate

SYSTEMIC LUPUS ERYTHEMATOSUS

- Patchy vascular involvement
- Leukocytoclastic vasculitis in arterioles
- Fibrinoid necrosis in small vessels
- Onion-skin appearance in arterioles owing to concentric perivascular fibrosis (Figure 15-33)
- Plasmacytosis in red pulp

RHEUMATOID ARTHRITIS

- Leukocytoclastic vasculitis in arterioles
- Fibrinoid necrosis in small vessels
- Splenomegaly in Felty syndrome
- Follicular hyperplasia in white pulp
- Lacks concentric perivascular fibrosis

THROMBOTIC THROMBOCYTOPENIC PURPURA

- Platelet-fibrin thrombi in small vessels; no inflammatory infiltrate
- Subendothelial PAS-positive hyaline deposits
- Onion-skin periarteriolar fibrosis may occasionally be observed

Special Stains and Immunohistochemistry

- Elastic stains for vascular damage

Other Techniques for Diagnosis

- Direct immunofluorescence for fibrinogen, immunoglobulin, and complement deposits
- Serologic studies
- Antinuclear antibody test and other anti-DNA tests for lupus
- Rheumatoid factor in rheumatoid arthritis

Differential Diagnosis

- The differential diagnosis in cases of vasculitis includes each of the entities listed previously; additional diseases to consider include the following

THROMBOEMBOLI

- Patients usually have severe atherosclerotic cardiac disease, or left-sided endocarditis
- Thromboembolic or atheroembolic material in arterioles
- True vasculitis only with septic emboli and endocarditis
- Elastic stain may be useful

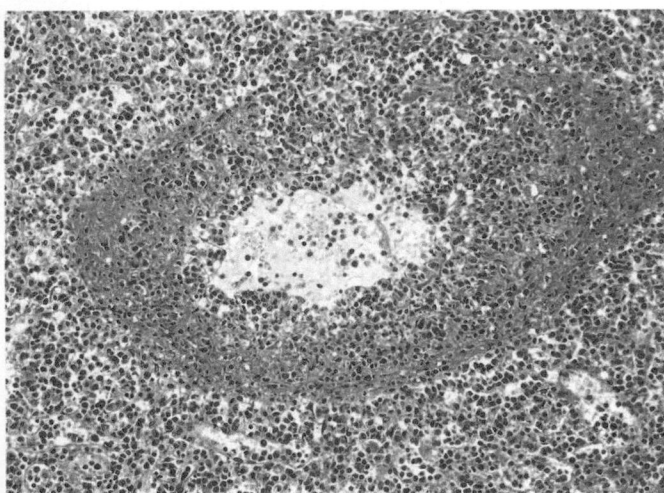

Figure 15-32. Vasculitis in a splenic vessel. The section shows fibrinoid necrosis.

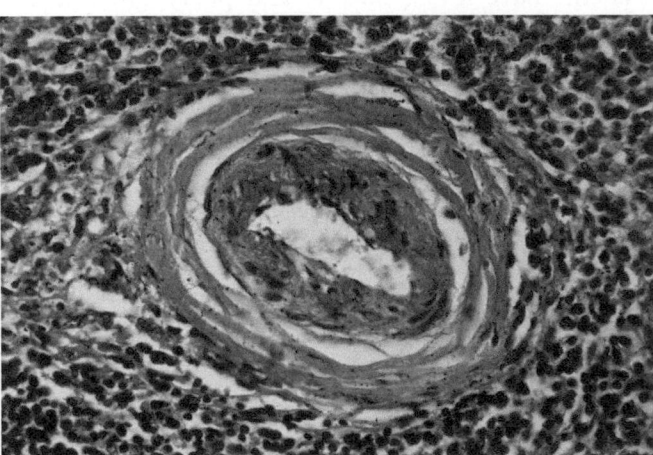

Figure 15-33. Systemic lupus erythematosus. Small artery with concentric collagen formation around a vessel. This is also termed *onion-skinning.*

POSTMORTEM CLOT
- No lines of Zahn
- No true vasculitis
- No changes in splenic parenchyma

AMYLOIDOSIS
- Patients usually have systemic amyloidosis
- Eosinophilic deposits around small blood vessels
- No vasculitis
- Congo red or thioflavin T stains positive

PEARLS

- *Splenic involvement in systemic vasculitis is rarely clinically significant*
- *In lupus and other autoimmune disorders, the changes previously described may have been substantially modified by antecedent therapy (e.g., steroids)*
- *Atypical lymphoid hyperplasia and rarely lymphoma may occur in patients treated with methotrexate for rheumatoid arthritis (methotrexate-associated lymphoproliferative disorders)*
- *Immunohistology for EBV may be helpful to confirm an immunosuppression associated etiology*

SELECTED REFERENCES

Danning CL, Illei GG, Boumpas DT: Vasculitis associated with primary rheumatologic diseases. Curr Opin Rheumatol 10:58-65, 1998.

D'Cruz D: Vasculitis in systemic lupus erythematosus. Lupus 7: 270-274, 1998.

Drenkard C, Villa AR, Reyes E, et al: Vasculitis in systemic lupus erythematosus. Lupus 6:235-242, 1997.

Lhote F, Cohen P, Guillevin L: Polyarteritis nodosa, microscopic polyangiitis and Churg-Strauss syndrome. Lupus 7:238-258, 1998.

VIRAL AND OTHER NONGRANULOMATOUS INFECTIONS

INFECTIOUS MONONUCLEOSIS

Clinical Features

- Most commonly affecting adolescents and young adults
- Patients have fever, malaise, and pharyngitis; rarely, splenic rupture
- May have generalized lymphadenopathy and hepatosplenomegaly
- Caused by primary infection with EBV

Gross Pathology

- Mild to moderate splenomegaly with red pulp congestion and hyperplastic white pulp; rarely, massive spleen enlargement
- Splenectomy may have been performed for spontaneous rupture, which should be documented

Histopathology

- Borders between red and white pulp are blurred
- Variable degree of follicular hyperplasia in white pulp
- Red pulp is expanded by a polymorphic cellular population, which includes pleomorphic lymphocytes, immunoblasts, and plasma cells (Figure 15-34)

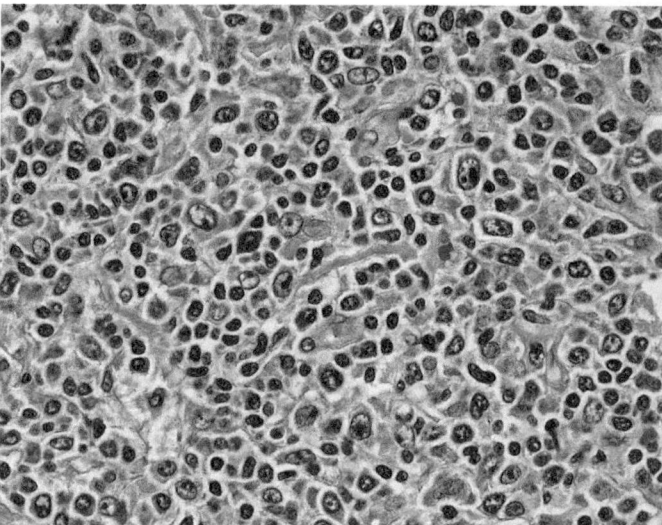

Figure 15-34. Infectious mononucleosis. High-power magnification shows a heterogeneous lymphoid population with numerous immunoblasts.

- PALS may be infiltrated by lymphoid cells, including immunoblasts
- Splenic trabeculae, capsule, and vessels are often infiltrated by lymphoid cells

Special Stains and Immunohistochemistry

- Immunohistochemical stains: large immunoblasts are positive for EBV, CD20, and often CD30
- Activated lymphoid population consists of mixed B cells and T lymphocytes with a predominance of CD8-positive cytotoxic T cells

Other Techniques for Diagnosis

- In situ hybridization for EBER is positive

Differential Diagnosis

LARGE CELL LYMPHOMA OR T-CELL/HISTIOCYTE-RICH LARGE B-CELL LYMPHOMA
- These lymphoid neoplasms generally form discrete masses in splenic parenchyma
- Homogeneous population or B or T cells in large cell lymphomas; in T-cell/histiocyte-rich large B-cell lymphoma, the neoplastic B cells are scattered within a background of small T lymphocytes

HODGKIN LYMPHOMA
- Usually forms discrete, grossly visible nodules rather than causing diffuse splenic enlargement
- Classical Hodgkin-Reed-Sternberg cells are found scattered within lymphohistiocytic nodules; splenic follicles appear normal or reactive
- Eosinophils and plasma cells may be numerous in Hodgkin lymphoma and are rare in infectious mononucleosis

REACTIVE LYMPHOID HYPERPLASIA NOT RELATED TO EBV INFECTION
- May present similar histologic findings
- Immunohistochemical stains to exclude the presence of other viruses (e.g., cytomegalovirus [CMV]) and correlation with viral serology are necessary for definitive diagnosis

- *Patients with acute infectious mononucleosis may have acute splenomegaly and are at risk for spontaneous splenic rupture*
- *Infectious mononucleosis may be misinterpreted as malignant lymphoma or Hodgkin lymphoma owing to the massive immunoblastic proliferation, which may include Hodgkin-Reed-Sternberg-like cells; the immunoblasts usually lack the typical eosinophilic nucleolus of classical Hodgkin-Reed-Sternberg cells*
- *Detailed clinical history, EBV serology, and appropriate immunostains are helpful in the differential diagnosis*

SELECTED REFERENCES

Gowing NFC: Infectious mononucleosis: histopathologic aspects. Pathol Ann 1:1-20, 1975.
Neiman RS, Orazi A: Reactive lymphoid hyperplasia. In Disorders of the Spleen, 2nd ed. Philadelphia, WB Saunders, 1999, pp 67-84.
Reynolds DJ, Banks PM, Gulley ML: New characterization of infectious mononucleosis and a phenotypic comparison with Hodgkin's disease. Am J Pathol 146:379-388, 1995.

CYTOMEGALOVIRUS INFECTION

Clinical Features

- Uncommon
- Occurs most commonly in immunocompromised patients
- Virus-associated hemophagocytic syndrome is a rare complication in early CMV infection; these patients present with general malaise, fever, chills, and leukopenia associated with thrombocytopenia

Gross Pathology

- Congested red pulp
- White pulp usually inconspicuous
- May have small, variably shaped red to pale foci of necrosis

Histopathology

- Necrotic foci in cells with viral inclusions are typically found at the periphery of the lesions
- Scattered neutrophils may be present, but there are usually fewer than in bacterial infections

Special Stains and Immunohistochemistry

- Immunohistochemical stains for CMV

Other Techniques for Diagnosis

- In situ hybridization for CMV
- Viral serology/cultures

Differential Diagnosis

ABSCESS

- Often lacks viral inclusions, but degenerating cells at the periphery can resemble Cowdry (i.e., owl-eye inclusion bodies) type A inclusions
- Neutrophils more numerous
- Bacteria or fungi may be present on appropriate stains or culture

INFARCT

- Peripheral location under capsule and wedge shape
- No viral inclusions

- *Rarely seen in surgical pathology material*
- *Occurs predominantly in immunocompromised patients*

SELECTED REFERENCE

Neiman RS, Orazi A: Reactive lymphoid hyperplasia. In Disorders of the Spleen, 2nd ed. Philadelphia, WB Saunders, 1999, pp 67-84.

MYCOBACTERIUM AVIUM-INTRACELLULARE

Clinical Features

- Occurs in patients with AIDS
- Most patients present with generalized wasting, hepatosplenomegaly, and lymphadenopathy; anemia is the most common laboratory abnormality

Gross Pathology

- Variable degree of splenomegaly
- White pulp variable, atrophic to hyperplastic
- Diffuse, firm expansion of the red pulp

Histopathology (Figure 15-35)

- Diffuse expansion of red pulp by numerous large macrophages with abundant pale-gray–staining cytoplasm
- Erythrophagocytosis may be present

Special Stains and Immunohistochemistry

- AFB, Fite, and PAS stains are used to demonstrate the bacilli in the macrophages
- Wright- or Papanicolaou-stained touch preparations may reveal negative images of the bacilli in macrophage cytoplasm

Other Techniques for Diagnosis

- Cultures

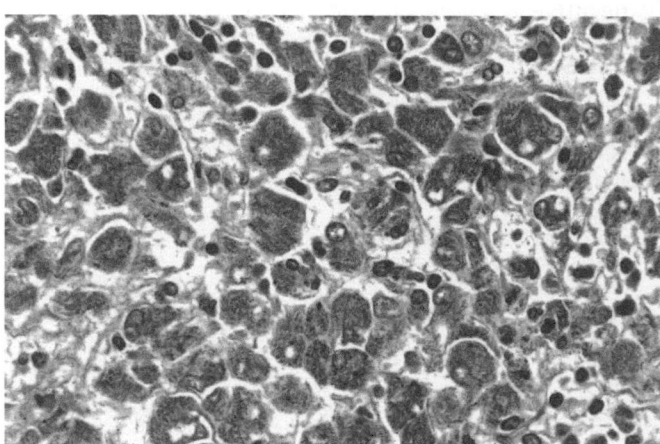

Figure 15-35. *Mycobacterium avium-intracellulare.* Numerous intracellular organisms on periodic acid-Schiff stain.

Differential Diagnosis

LEPROMATOUS LEPROSY
- Involvement is most intense in skin, nerves, and extremities; peripheral disease predominates clinically
- History of residence in area where leprosy is endemic
- Spleen usually contains clusters of macrophages filled with acid-fast organisms (lepra cells)
- Diffuse tumor-like infiltration is exceptional
- Fite stain necessary to demonstrate organisms

HISTOPLASMOSIS
- Most common in the Ohio River Valley and upper Mississippi River areas and adjacent Midwestern states
- GMS and PAS stains demonstrate fungi in macrophages

GAUCHER DISEASE (AND OTHER METABOLIC STORAGE DISEASES)
- Bone, liver, and joints involved (depending on disease type)
- Gaucher cells have wrinkled-silk appearance
- Stains for organisms negative, but storage products may be PAS positive or acid fast

LANGERHANS CELL HISTIOCYTOSIS
- Usually occurs in young children
- Cells have pale pink cytoplasm and bean-shaped nuclei
- Eosinophils are usually prominent
- Acid-fast stain and microbiologic studies negative
- Cells are S-100 protein, langerin, and CD1a positive

PNEUMOCYSTIS CARINII
- Extracellular foamy exudate
- GMS or immunohistochemical stain highlight the organisms

MALARIA
- History of travel or residence in endemic area
- Patients are anemic with intermittent fevers
- Spleen is black with malarial pigment
- Macrophages contain red cells, malarial pigment, or both
- Stains for organisms may be difficult to interpret because of malarial pigment, but acid-fast stain is negative

PEARLS

- *History is important*
- *Look for additional diseases in AIDS patients, including the following:*
  - *Other infections*
  - *Aggressive lymphoma*
  - *Kaposi sarcoma*

SELECTED REFERENCES

Brettle RP: Mycobacterium avium intracellulare infection in patients with HIV or AIDS. J Antimicrob Chemother 40:156-160, 1997.
Horsburgh R Jr: The pathophysiology of disseminated *Mycobacterium avium* complex disease in AIDS. J Infect Dis 179(suppl 3):S461-S465, 1999.

MALARIA

Clinical Features
- Affects children and young adults living in endemic areas
- History of travel or residence in an area where malaria is endemic
- Episodic, recurrent fevers
- Hemolytic anemia
- Hemoglobinuria
- Most common cause of splenic rupture worldwide

Gross Pathology
- Splenomegaly, most prominent in *Plasmodium vivax* infection
- Acute phase: splenomegaly with dark-red parenchyma due to congestion and deposition of malarial pigment (hemozoin); splenic rupture most frequent in acute phase
- Chronic phase: marked splenomegaly, gray discoloration with areas of fibrosis and scarring
- White pulp normal to hyperplastic
- Rarely, development of splenic pseudocyst due to cystic degeneration of hematoma or hemorrhagic infarct

Histopathology

ACUTE PHASE
- Venous sinuses engorged with parasitized red cells
- Proliferation of cordal macrophages and desquamation of sinus lining cells containing phagocytosed erythrocytes
- Increase in small lymphocytes ($\gamma\delta$ T cells) in red pulp
- Macrophages lining the sinuses contain hemosiderin, red cell debris, and malarial pigment
- Erythrocytes containing parasites can be seen in the sinuses in falciparum malaria
- Sinus lining cells may contain malarial organisms

CHRONIC PHASE
- Fibrosis and scarring
- Macrophages with malarial pigment concentrated around periarteriolar lymphoid sheaths
- Syndrome of hyperactive malarial splenomegaly
  - Common presentation of chronic infection in endemic areas
  - Sinusoidal and reticuloendothelial hyperplasia
  - Intense splenic sequestration and phagocytosis of erythrocytes

Special Stains and Immunohistochemistry
- Malarial pigment
  - Refractile
  - Birefringent
  - Not melanin
  - Negative on iron stain (although macrophages will also contain hemosiderin)
- Thick film of peripheral blood stained to look for organisms

Other Techniques for Diagnosis
- Noncontributory

Differential Diagnosis

LEISHMANIASIS
- No malarial pigment in macrophages
- Amastigotes of *Leishmania* species can be detected with Wright-Giemsa staining
- Splenic histology otherwise identical

HEMOCHROMATOSIS
- Prolonged history of dark bronzed skin, arthralgias, and involvement of pancreas, liver, and heart
- Symptoms associated with malaria such as anemia and fevers are not present
- Abundant iron in tissues

FORMALIN PIGMENT
- Artifact of prolonged fixation in unbuffered formalin
- Histologically similar to malarial pigment
- Clinical manifestations of malaria are lacking

PEARLS

- *Diagnosis should be supported by clinical history and peripheral blood smear findings*

SELECTED REFERENCES

Edington GM: Pathology of malaria in West Africa. Br Med J 1:715-718, 1967.

Herwaldt BL: Leishmaniasis. Lancet 354:1191-1199, 1999.

Neiman RS, Orazi A: Non-neoplastic disorders of erythrocytes, granulocytes and platelets. In Disorders of the Spleen, 2nd ed. Philadelphia, WB Saunders, 1999, pp 67-84.

Venizelos I, Tatsiou Z, Papathomas TG, et al: Visceral leishmaniasis in a rheumatoid arthritis patient treated with methotrexate. Int J Infect Dis 13:169-172, 2009.

PYOGENIC BACTERIAL INFECTIONS (ABSCESS)

Clinical Features

- Occurs in patients with acute systemic bacterial infections with hematogenous dissemination (e.g., patients with bacterial endocarditis)
- Most often gram-positive organisms, particularly Staphylococcus species

Gross Pathology

- Follicular hyperplasia with enlarged prominent white pulp follicles; not always present in immunocompromised or clinically septic patients
- Abscesses are localized to white pulp and variably sized, soft to liquid, cream-colored to greenish
- May be surrounded by a thin rim of hyperemic tissue

Histopathology

- Septic emboli produce infarcts as well as abscesses
- Abscesses contain neutrophils and necrotic debris; older abscesses may be surrounded by granulation tissue or fibrous tissue

Special Stains and Immunohistochemistry

- Gram stain or fungal stains for organisms

Other Techniques for Diagnosis

- Microbiologic cultures for organisms

Differential Diagnosis

SPLENIC INFARCT
- Usually larger than abscess
- Peripherally located and wedge shaped rather than round
- Examine arteries carefully for thrombi or emboli
- Infarcts are pale but firm, not liquid
- Inflammation, if present, is most intense at the periphery of the infarct

HODGKIN LYMPHOMA
- Necrotic nodules of Hodgkin lymphoma; these are usually better circumscribed, firm to fibrotic, and elevated above the cut surface of the spleen, but they may also form tumorous lumps under the splenic capsule
- Nodules of Hodgkin lymphoma contain lymphocytes, Reed-Sternberg or Hodgkin cells, eosinophils, and plasma cells

EXTRAMEDULLARY HEMATOPOIESIS
- Rarely forms grossly evident nodules
- Clusters of erythroid precursors are usually evident on microscopic examination and are often the predominant cell type; also look for myeloid cells and megakaryocytes

PEARLS

- *Splenic abscesses are seen more often on autopsy than in surgically resected spleens*
- *When seen in a surgical specimen removed for other indications, consider the possibility of splenic embolization with infarcts*

SELECTED REFERENCE

Neiman RS, Orazi A: Reactive lymphoid hyperplasia. In Disorders of the Spleen, 2nd ed. Philadelphia, WB Saunders, 1999, pp 67-84.

GRANULOMATOUS DISEASES

SARCOIDOSIS, MILIARY TUBERCULOSIS, HISTOPLASMOSIS, COCCIDIOIDOMYCOSIS, AND LIPOGRANULOMAS

Clinical Features

SARCOIDOSIS
- See Chapter 4
- Patients usually have hilar adenopathy, pulmonary symptoms, or other sites of involvement
- Most common in African Americans; female predominance
- Schaumann bodies and asteroid bodies may be present but are not diagnostic
- Small foci of necrosis may be present
- Stains and culture for infectious agents are negative

MILIARY TUBERCULOSIS
- Occurs most often in elderly patients with history of tuberculosis and in immunocompromised patients

HISTOPLASMOSIS

- Occurs at any age
- Clinical spectrum ranging from asymptomatic infection to disseminated disease
- Splenic involvement more common in elderly and immunocompromised patients
- Histoplasmosis is most common in the upper Midwest, upper Mississippi River, and the Ohio River regions
- Organism found in soil
- Pigeons are common vectors; exposure to pigeon droppings can lead to infection

COCCIDIOIDOMYCOSIS

- Occurs at any age
- Splenic involvement is uncommon but can occur in elderly and immunocompromised patients
- Occurs in California in the San Joaquin and Central valleys (valley fever) and in the southwestern United States
- Clinical spectrum ranging from asymptomatic infection to disseminated disease

LIPOGRANULOMAS

- *Lipogranulomatosis* refers to the presence, in lymph nodes and spleen, of lipid material arising from endogenous sources, such as tumors, hematomas, cholesterol deposits, fat embolism, and fat necrosis
- Common in the spleen (seen in 20% of splenectomy specimens and 62% of autopsy specimens; incidence increases with age)
- Usually is an incidental finding without a clear etiology in spleens examined for other indications

Gross Pathology

SARCOIDOSIS

- Often not seen grossly; white pulp inconspicuous
- Occasionally show multiple small, round, well-circumscribed nodules

MILIARY TUBERCULOSIS

- Modest splenomegaly
- Small 1- to 2-mm diameter, whitish nodules resembling white pulp follicles; miliary pattern (Figure 15-36)
- Larger confluent granulomas with dry, caseous to calcified material are uncommon

HISTOPLASMOSIS

- May present with splenomegaly and hypersplenism
- Spherical yellow to white calcified granules, 1 to 2 mm in diameter
- May present as a miliary pattern

COCCIDIOIDOMYCOSIS

- Spherical yellow to white granules, 1 to 2 mm in diameter
- May present as a miliary pattern

LIPOGRANULOMAS

- Not seen on gross examination

Histopathology

SARCOIDOSIS

- More commonly localizes to white pulp
- Small epithelioid granulomas similar to those seen in lung and lymph nodes

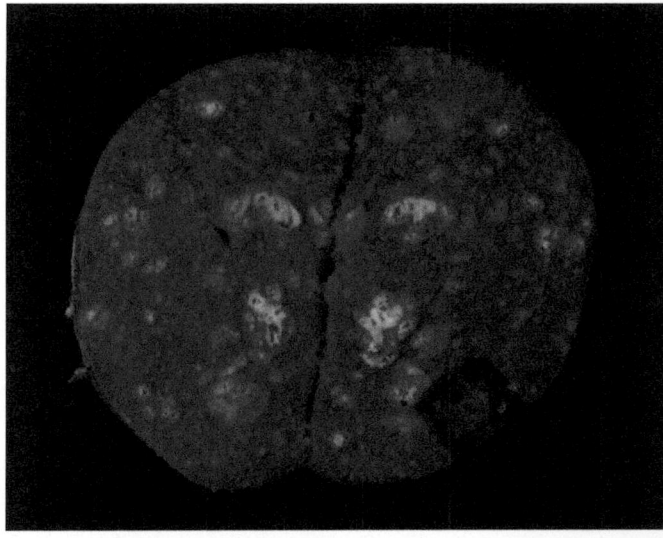

Figure 15-36. Miliary tuberculosis. In this gross photograph, notice the multiple whitish granulomas with necrosis. In patients with miliary tuberculosis, especially immunocompromised patients, the granulomas are often less well formed and lack grossly visible necrosis.

- Schaumann bodies and asteroid bodies may be present but are not diagnostic
- Small foci of necrosis can be seen

MILIARY TUBERCULOSIS

- Scattered randomly in the white and red pulp, may be more frequent in the latter
- Granulomas with central caseous necrosis
- Multinucleated Langhans giant cells are characteristic
- Epithelioid cells and lymphocytes also are present
- Lesions may calcify

HISTOPLASMOSIS

- Scattered randomly in the white and red pulp, may be more frequent in the latter
- In the acute phase, the infection often does not form distinct granulomas but manifests as small collections of histiocytes containing fungal forms, with an infiltrate of plasma cells and lymphocytes
- Neutrophils are usually not seen
- Old inactive lesions are more common; these are partially calcified fibrous nodules with a few lymphocytes at the periphery
- Histiocytes are generally not seen
- Organisms can be detected with GMS stain

COCCIDIOIDOMYCOSIS

- Scattered randomly in the white and red pulp, may be more frequent in the latter
- Granulomas may have central necrosis, and fungal forms may be seen on H&E, GMS, and PAS stains

LIPOGRANULOMAS

- Localized in the white pulp in the vicinity of arterioles, not seen within germinal centers
- Small, ill-defined aggregates of macrophages with single large or numerous small lipid vacuoles

Special Stains and Immunohistochemistry

- GMS, PAS, and acid-fast stains to rule out infectious granulomas required in all cases

- Additional techniques
  - Acid-fast and fungal culture recommended; these organisms can survive snap-freezing

Other Techniques for Diagnosis

- Noncontributory

Differential Diagnosis

- See all "Granulomatous Diseases"

PEARLS

- *Special stains for microorganisms are essential when granulomas are present in the spleen sample*
- *Correlation with results of culture or other microbiology studies from spleen or other source (e.g., blood) is helpful*

SELECTED REFERENCE

Neiman RS, Orazi A: Granulomatous disorders. In Disorders of the Spleen, 2nd ed. Philadelphia, WB Saunders, 1999, pp 85-96.

OTHER CONDITIONS

AMYLOIDOSIS

Clinical Features

- Most occur in older adults
- Occur in patients with systemic amyloidosis
- AL-type amyloid in patients with plasma cell dyscrasia
- AA-type amyloid found in patients with tuberculosis, rheumatoid arthritis, or other chronic inflammatory processes

Gross Pathology

- Three patterns; these do not correlate with amyloid protein type
  - Incidental: seen only on microscopic examination
  - Sago spleen: grayish-white, small, multiple nodules resembling exaggerated white pulp
  - Lardaceous spleen: enlarged spleen with diffuse infiltration; dark, firm, rubbery

Histopathology (Figure 15-37)

- Amyloid is a bright-pink (eosinophilic) amorphous hyaline-like material
- Incidental type: amyloid deposits around small vessels
- Sago spleen: deposits surround cells in the white pulp, eventually with replacement and atrophy of the white pulp
- Lardaceous spleen: deposits in the red pulp adjacent to sinus walls and around small vessels; may become confluent and replace the red pulp

Special Stains and Immunohistochemistry

- Congo red (apple-green birefringence with polarized light) or thioflavin T stain (fluorescent microscope)
- Immunohistochemistry for amyloid chain type and immunoglobulin light chains

Other Techniques for Diagnosis

- Electron microscopy: shows fibrils (generally not needed)

- Mass spectrophotometry to determine type of amyloid-related protein

Differential Diagnosis

CASTLEMAN DISEASE, HYALINE-VASCULAR TYPE

- Rare in spleen
- Hyalinized follicular centers with penetrating arterioles, no perivascular hyaline deposits

INFARCT

- Grossly irregular, wedge-shaped
- Peripheral location, rarely diffuse
- Microscopy shows coagulative necrosis

GRANULOMAS

- Cores contain necrotic material or epithelioid giant cells (no amorphous uniform material); however, old granulomas can be extensively hyalinized

HYALINOSIS

- A common, usually incidental microscopic finding occurring at any age after early childhood
- Eosinophilic hyaline thickening of small arteries and arterioles in the spleen
- Looks like early amyloid
- Deposits are composed of plasma proteins
- Congo red or thioflavin T stains negative

PEARLS

- *Classification of amyloid is based on the protein type; 23 different fibril proteins are described in human amyloidosis and are associated with variable clinical features*
- *AL amyloid is derived from immunoglobulin light chains, more often λ than κ, and is associated with plasma cell dyscrasias or B-cell lymphoproliferative disorders*
- *AA amyloid is derived from SAA protein, an acute-phase reactant; accumulates in chronic inflammatory processes*
- *Amyloid is also present in patients with familial Mediterranean fever (FMF), a febrile disease characterized by acute, spontaneously resolving episodes of fever and pain caused by serosal inflammation and associated with mutations in the FMF gene, MEFV*

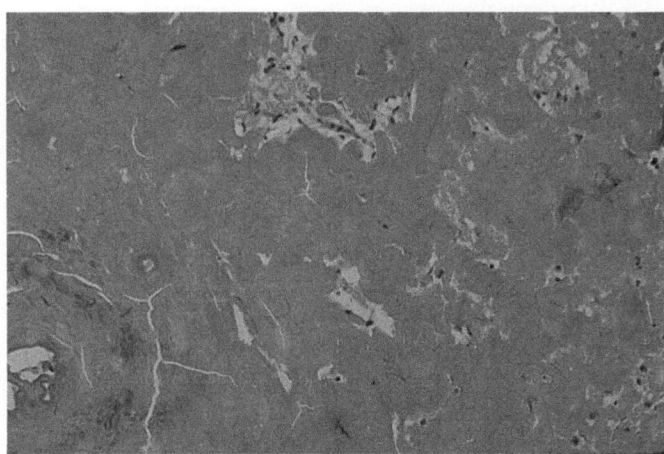

Figure 15-37. Amyloidosis. Masses of amorphous eosinophilic extracellular material (amyloid) replace normal splenic tissue. A few sinuses and blood vessels remain.

SELECTED REFERENCES

Falk RH, Comenzo RL, Skinner M: The systemic amyloidoses. N Engl J Med 337:898-909, 1997.
Westermark P: The pathogenesis of amyloidosis: understanding general principles. Am J Pathol 152:1125-1127, 1998.

HEMATOMA AND TRAUMATIC RUPTURE

Clinical Features

- Hematoma usually follows blunt trauma to the abdomen
- Hematoma results from an internal tear without capsular rupture
- Rupture may follow blunt abdominal trauma or penetrating injury
- Rupture can occur without abdominal trauma in patients with
  - Infections: malaria, infectious mononucleosis
  - Tumors: leukemia, lymphoma, angiosarcoma
  - Congestion
- Rupture can occur "spontaneously" in a patient with a normal spleen (owing to cough, vomiting)

Gross Pathology

HEMATOMA

- Spleen is expanded by an irregularly shaped soft, dark mass of blood
- Capsule is intact
- Parenchyma otherwise grossly normal

RUPTURE

- Capsular tear with adherent blood clot
- Weigh spleen after removal of blood clot and gross examination to exclude spontaneous rupture from underlying splenic pathology

Histopathology

HEMATOMA

- Mass of clotted blood
- Older lesions may have granulation tissue at the periphery and progressive fibrosis
- May be followed by a splenic pseudocyst

RUPTURE

- Similar to hematoma but with capsular tear
- Splenic parenchyma is usually normal

Special Stains and Immunohistochemistry

- Noncontributory

Other Techniques for Diagnosis

- Noncontributory

Differential Diagnosis

SPONTANEOUS RUPTURE

- Spleen normal or enlarged
- No history of abdominal trauma, or minimal abdominal trauma
- Histologic features depend on cause

INFARCT

- Lesion shows coagulative necrosis
- Wedge-shaped, peripheral focal lesions
- Usually does not cause splenomegaly

SPLENIC CYST

- Contents usually clear to turbid liquid (not hemorrhagic)
- Fibrous wall
- Epithelial lining may or may not be present

HEMANGIOMA AND OTHER VASCULAR TUMORS

- No granulation tissue at periphery
- Proliferated blood vessels throughout the lesion

PEARLS

- *Splenic hyalinosis has been reported to be more common in ruptured spleens; however, hyalinosis is present in most spleens, including those of children*

SELECTED REFERENCES

Orloff MJ, Peskin GW: Spontaneous rupture of the normal spleen: a surgical enigma. Int Abstr Surg 106:1-11, 1958.
Pratt DB, Andersen RC, Hitchcock CR: Splenic rupture: a review of 114 cases. Minn Med 54:177-184, 1971.
Rawsthorne GB, Cole TP, Kyle J: Spontaneous rupture of the spleen in infectious mononucleosis. Br J Surg 57:396-398, 1970.

Chapter 16
Bones and Joints

BYRON E. CRAWFORD • JOHN J. SCHMIEG

CHAPTER OUTLINE

OSTEOID TUMORS

OSTEOMA

Clinical Features

- Male predominance (2:1 to 3:1)
- Age ranges from second decade to elderly, with most cases occurring in fourth and fifth decades
- Occurs most commonly in skull bones, including mandible, maxilla, frontal sinuses, ethmoid sinuses, paranasal sinuses, orbital bones, and calvarium; rarely involves the clavicles and long bones
- May be asymptomatic or, if in sinuses, may present with signs of obstruction, including sinusitis and nasal discharges
- Orbital tumors may produce diplopia, exophthalmos, and blindness

Radiographic Findings

- Radiodense, circumscribed surface, or intramedullary mass usually without destructive features

Gross Pathology

- Nodular or dome-shaped, dense cortical bone

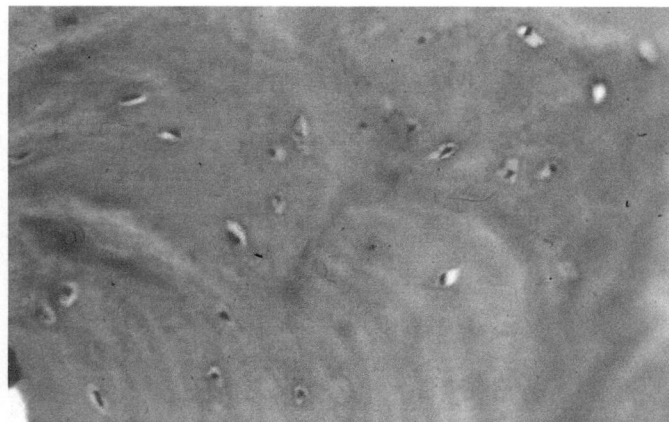

Figure 16-1. Osteoma. Histologic section shows dense lamellar bone.

Histopathology

- Consists of dense lamellar bone with or without haversian canals and usually without a medullary component (Figure 16-1)
- When a medullary component is present, it is represented by hematopoietic tissue or fibroadipose tissue; the process extends up to uninvolved bone and does not blend in with the adjacent normal bone

Special Stains and Immunohistochemistry

- Noncontributory

Other Techniques for Diagnosis

- Noncontributory

Differential Diagnosis

OSTEOBLASTOMA
- Lamellar bone with prominent osteoblastic rimming
- Osteoma may have focal areas of reactive bone with similar features

PAROSTEAL OSTEOSARCOMA
- Tumor osteoid is arranged in parallel arrays and separated by a hypocellular fibroblastic stroma

PEARLS

- *Asymptomatic, nodular, radiodense tumor involving craniofacial bones and composed of mature osteoid is typically an osteoma*
- *Gardner syndrome (colonic polyposis, fibromatoses, osteomas, and epidermal cysts of skin) should be considered in the presence of multiple osteomas or osteomas of long bones*
- *If surgically removed, recurrences rarely develop; no reported cases of malignant transformation*

SELECTED REFERENCES

Larrea-Oyarbide N, Valmaseda-Castellon E, Berini-Aytes L, Gay-Escoda C: Osteomas of the craniofacial region: review of 106 cases. J Oral Pathol Med 37:38-42, 2008.

Unni KK: Dahlin's Bone Tumors: General Aspects and Data on 11,087 Cases. Philadelphia, Lippincott-Raven, 1996, pp 117-120.

OSTEOID OSTEOMA

Clinical Features

- Male-to-female ratio of 3:1
- Usually occurs in second or third decade
- Most commonly occurs in the leg, usually in the proximal femur
- May involve tibia, vertebra (arch more so than body), and small bones of foot and hand
- Typically intracortical tumors
- Classic clinical presentation includes progressive pain that is greater at night and is relieved by aspirin
- Depending on the site, other symptoms may develop
  - Vertebrae: peripheral nerve compression and painful scoliosis owing to muscle spasms (symptoms of intravertebral disk disease)
  - Upper and lower extremities: peritumoral muscular atrophy
  - Epiphyseal tumors: skeletal asymmetry, arthritis, and joint effusions

Radiographic Findings

- Routine radiographs reveal a small, round, central area of radiolucency (nidus) surrounded by sclerosis
- Nidus is usually cortical in location and may exhibit central ossification
- When plain radiographs fail to reveal the tumor (about 25%), tomograms, bone scans, computed tomography (CT), or magnetic resonance imaging (MRI) may be necessary

Gross Pathology

- Dense sclerotic bone surrounds a central nidus that is round, red, soft, and friable; nidus may be granular if ossified
- Typically less than 1 cm

Histopathology

- Central nidus is composed of interlacing thin bone trabeculae or woven bone with variable degrees of mineralization (Figure 16-2)
- Trabeculae may vary in thickness

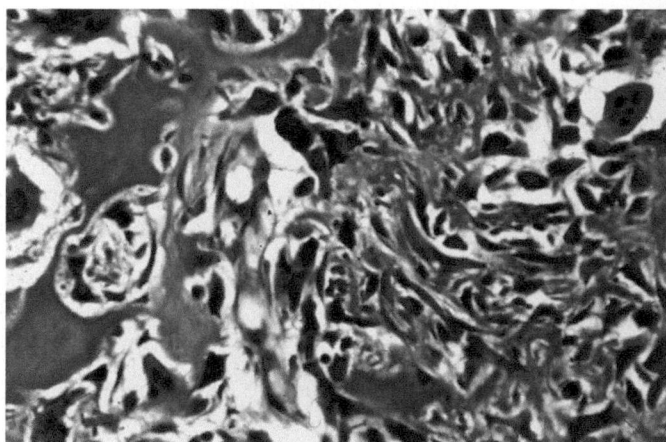

Figure 16-2. Osteoid osteoma. Histologic section shows a central nidus of thin bony trabeculae with prominent benign osteoblastic rimming.

- Prominent benign osteoblastic rimming of the trabeculae and multinucleated osteoclast-like giant cells are present within intervening fibrovascular stroma
- Outside the nidus is an abrupt zone of fibrovascular tissue surrounded by sclerotic compact lamellar bone
- No cartilage in the tumor unless there has been a fracture at the tumor site
- No hematopoietic tissue or adipose tissue within the tumor

Special Stains and Immunohistochemistry

- Noncontributory

Other Techniques for Diagnosis

- Preoperative tetracycline allows osteoblastic incorporation in the nidus, which is fluorescent under ultraviolet light
- Preoperative intravenous technetium-99 m with specimen autoradiography is another technique that may be used to identify a small nidus when curettage is used
- May express *c-fos* and *c-jun* by immunohistochemical analysis; some cases have demonstrated partial deletion of the long arm of chromosome 22 (22q13.1)

Differential Diagnosis

OSTEOMYELITIS AND BONE ABSCESSES
- Lack a central nidus
- Prominent acute inflammatory cell infiltrate

OSTEOBLASTOMA
- Pain is usually not as severe
- Tumor size is usually much greater, and there is evidence of progressive growth
- Lacks a peripheral rim of fibrovascular tissue
- Exhibits variable mineralization and thickness of woven osteoid trabeculae, whereas the nidus of an osteoid osteoma shows a pattern of central maturation toward a more calcified and thicker woven osteoid trabecula

OSTEOSARCOMA
- Lacks the fibrovascular stroma and osteoblastic rimming of osteoid osteoma
- May exhibit chondroid or fibrous differentiation

STRESS FRACTURE
- Zonal pattern with central, more mature, denser bone and peripheral woven bone
- Cartilage with endochondral ossification may be present

PEARLS

- *Pain is related to the presence of unmyelinated nerve fibers in the fibrovascular stroma of the nidus, production of prostaglandin E$_2$, and production of prostacyclin*
- *Clinical pain may precede radiographic evidence of osteoid osteoma*
- *When osteoid osteoma is present in the small bones of the hands and feet, patients are typically treated for an inflammatory process (osteomyelitis, arthritis) first*
- *Intra-articular tumors may produce chronic villous synovitis similar to rheumatoid arthritis*

- *Prostaglandin receptors have been identified within bone, and it has been postulated that prostaglandins may also contribute to the formation of osteoid osteoma*
- *Few reports of spontaneous regression of osteoid osteomas*
- *Treatment is surgical removal*

SELECTED REFERENCES

Baruffi MR, Volpon JB, Neto JB, Casartelli C: Osteoid osteomas with chromosome alterations involving 22q. Cancer Genet Cytogenet 124:127-131, 2001.

Franchi A, Calzolari A, Zampi G: Immunohistochemical detection of c-fos and c-jun expression in osseous and cartilaginous tumors of the skeleton. Virchows Arch [B] 432:515-519, 1998.

Freiberger RH, Loitman BS, Helpern M, Thompson TC: Osteoid osteoma: a report on 80 cases. Am J Roentgenol 82:194-205, 1959.

Sim FH, Dahlin DC, Beabout JW: Osteoid-osteoma: diagnostic problems. J Bone Joint Surg 57A:154-159, 1975.

Unni KK, Inwards CY, Bridge J, et al: Tumors of the Bones and Joints, 4th Series, Fascicle 2. Washington, DC, Armed Forces Institute of Pathology, 2005, pp 119-126.

OSTEOBLASTOMA

Clinical Features

- Male predominance, with a male-to-female ratio of 2:1 to 3:1
- Occurs in first through fourth decades, with most occurring in second and third decades
- Predilection for the vertebral column (arch) and sacrum followed by the mandible and craniofacial bones; the next most common sites are the extremities, where it follows a distribution similar to that of osteoid osteoma
- Typically intramedullary
- Localized pain may be present, but not with the intensity of an osteoid osteoma
- Vertebral tumors may produce scoliosis, muscle atrophy, and neurologic deficits

Radiographic Features

- Round, well-demarcated, expansile, radiolucent zone with a peripheral rim of sclerosis (sclerosis may not be as extensive as in osteoid osteoma)
- Central radiolucent zone (nidus) is greater than 1.5 cm; central stippled calcifications may be present
- Tumor may be surrounded by an area of new bone formation
- About one fourth may exhibit cortical destruction with periosteal new bone formation, suggesting a malignant tumor (osteosarcoma)
- Secondary aneurysmal cyst formation may be present

Gross Pathology

- Features similar to osteoid osteoma; however, these tumors are larger (> 1.5 cm)
- Central nidus is red, soft, and friable; if calcified, the nidus may be yellow and gritty
- Cortical bone may be destroyed or thin, and there may be hemorrhagic cysts within the nidus, representing secondary aneurysmal cyst formation

Histopathology

- Irregular interlacing network of osteoid with prominent osteoblastic rimming and features of woven bone (Figure 16-3)
- Osteoid may be fine and lacelike with variable mineralization
- Osteoblasts have benign cytologic features
- Osteoblasts may exhibit abundant mitotic activity but no atypical forms
- Osteoid is separated by fibrovascular stroma containing multinucleated osteoclast-like giant cells
- Appears well circumscribed, with tumor osteoid merging with adjacent uninvolved bone
- Large blood lakes representing secondary aneurysmal cystic changes may be seen
- Cartilage is usually not present in the tumor, although rare cases have been reported
- Osteoblasts may have epithelioid features represented by large cells with abundant eosinophilic cytoplasm and enlarged nuclei containing large nucleoli
  - When epithelioid cells exceed 75% of the osteoblast population, the diagnosis of aggressive osteoblastoma should be made, which denotes an increased risk for recurrence, although no cases of metastases are reported
- Rare tumors may contain bizarre, cytologically atypical multinucleated giant cells without mitotic activity (these tumors may be designated *bizarre osteoblastoma* or *pseudomalignant osteoblastoma*)

Special Stains and Immunohistochemistry

- Noncontributory

Other Techniques for Diagnosis

- Noncontributory

Differential Diagnosis

OSTEOID OSTEOMA

- Usually smaller than 1 cm; clinically, the pain is of greater intensity
- Periphery of tumor contains a fibrovascular rim
- Nidus exhibits a more zonal pattern with central maturation and less variability in the thickness and degree of mineralization of the osteoid
- No evidence of progressive growth

GIANT CELL TUMOR

- Usually involves the epiphyses of long bones
- Rare in vertebrae, but when they occur in a vertebra, the body and not the arch is usually involved
- Giant cells in giant cell tumors are larger and contain more nuclei
- Often composed of sheets of giant cells
- Giant cell tumors contain mononuclear stromal cells

ANEURYSMAL BONE CYST

- Similar presentation and radiographic findings as osteoblastoma and also tend to involve the vertebra
- Small foci of reactive osteoid may be present in aneurysmal bone cysts, which should not be confused with osteoblastoma

OSTEOBLASTIC OSTEOSARCOMA

- Radiographically, osteosarcoma is poorly circumscribed with cortical destruction and evidence of periosteal reactive bone
- Permeative pattern of growth at the periphery
- Stroma of osteosarcoma is sarcomatoid with cytologic atypia and atypical mitoses
- Sheets or aggregates of atypical osteoblasts are present in osteosarcoma, in contrast to a single rim of osteoblasts around osteoid in osteoid osteoma

PEARLS

- *About one fourth of the cases of osteoblastoma exhibit radiographic evidence suggesting a malignant tumor (osteosarcoma); differentiation from an osteoblastic osteosarcoma can be difficult (see "Differential Diagnosis")*

SELECTED REFERENCES

De Oliveira CR, Mendonca BB, de Camargo OP, et al: Classical osteoblastoma, atypical osteoblastoma, and osteosarcoma: a comparative study based on clinical, histological, and biological parameters. Clinics 62:167-174, 2007.

Jones AC, Prihoda TJ, Kacher JE, et al: Osteoblastoma of the maxilla and mandible: a report of 24 cases, review of the literature, and discussion of its relationship to osteoid osteoma of the jaws. Oral Surg Oral Med Oral Pathol Oral Radiol Endod 102:639-650, 2006.

Unni KK, Inwards CY, Bridge J, et al: Tumors of the Bones and Joints, 4th Series, Fascicle 2. Washington, DC, Armed Forces Institute of Pathology, 2005, pp 126-135.

Vigorita VJ: Orthopaedic Pathology. Philadelphia, Lippincott Williams & Wilkins, 1999, pp 322-325.

CONVENTIONAL INTRAMEDULLARY OSTEOSARCOMA

Clinical Features

- Slight male predominance, with a male-to-female ratio of 1.5:1
- Bimodal age distribution, with most cases occurring in second decade; a second, smaller peak occurs in patients older than 50 years
- Represents the fourth most common cause of malignancy in the pediatric age group
- Patients with hereditary retinoblastoma are at increased risk for developing an osteosarcoma

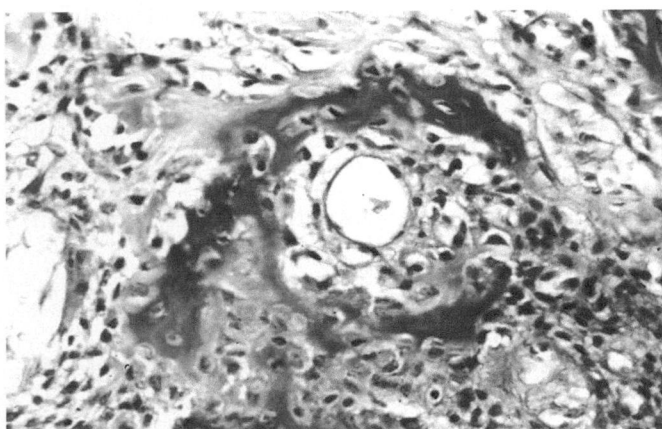

Figure 16-3. Osteoblastoma. Histologic section shows an irregular interlacing network of osteoid with prominent osteoblastic rimming.

- Other conditions that may be associated with the development of osteosarcoma: Li-Fraumeni syndrome, Ollier disease, osteoblastoma, fibrous dysplasia, Paget disease of bone, hereditary multiple exostosis, previous radiation or chemotherapy, hypoplastic or aplasia of thumbs, Werner syndrome, and Rothmund-Thomson syndrome
- Occurs in parts of the skeleton with the highest growth rates
- Predilection for the distal femur, proximal tibia, and proximal humerus
- Approximately 50% of cases occur in the region of the knee
- Typically presents with a history of short-term (several weeks to several months), mild, intermittent pain
- Affected area may be swollen and tender to palpation, and the overlying skin may exhibit telangiectasia and be warm
- Serum alkaline phosphatase may be elevated

Radiographic Features

- Classically shows a large lytic, sclerotic, or mixed lytic-sclerotic mass arising in medullary bone of the metaphysis that extends through the cortex and creates a soft tissue mass
- Variable mineralization within the tumor, which causes cloudy opacities
- Outer cortical surface exhibits prominent periosteal reaction represented by Codman triangle, sunbursts, or onion-skinning
- CT and MRI are used for staging (intramedullary involvement, presence of skip lesions in marrow, and soft tissue involvement)

Gross Pathology

- Resected specimens exhibit an intramedullary metaphyseal mass that has usually penetrated through the cortex and invades into soft tissue (Figure 16-4A)
- Marrow extension of the tumor proximally is usually seen, and there may be skip lesions in which normal marrow separates islands of tumor

- Gross characteristics of the tumor are heterogeneous and variable, depending on the stromal component
  - Highly ossified areas are yellow to white and hard
  - Chondroid areas are lobulated, translucent, and light gray to white
  - Osteoblastic areas are firm, white to yellow, and sometimes gritty
  - Fibroblastic areas are soft and fleshy
  - Tumor may contain areas of necrosis, hemorrhage, and cystic changes

Histopathology

- Microscopic features may vary considerably in different areas of a tumor
  - Tumor is basically composed of sarcomatous, spindle-shaped cells exhibiting evidence of tumor osteoid production (Figure 16-4B)
  - Sarcomatous stroma is hypercellular and may exhibit osteoblastic, chondroblastic, fibroblastic, or malignant fibrous histiocytoma-like differentiation
  - Cells usually have obvious cytologic malignant features, including brisk mitotic activity with atypical forms
  - Some cells may exhibit epithelioid features
- Tumor osteoid is represented by eosinophilic, amorphous, fibrillary deposits between individual tumor cells or small aggregates of tumor cells
- Early tumor osteoid forms a lacelike pattern around tumor cells, whereas the more advanced type is mineralized and has the appearance of woven tumor bone
- As tumor cells become incorporated with tumor osteoid, they tend to become smaller; this feature is regarded as *normalization*
- Some tumors exhibit prominent chondroblastic differentiation requiring careful search for tumor osteoid
- Fibroblastic areas may exhibit a herringbone pattern; diligent search for tumor osteoid is sometimes required
- Some tumors may have large numbers of osteoclast-like giant cells and are designated as *giant cell–rich osteosarcoma*

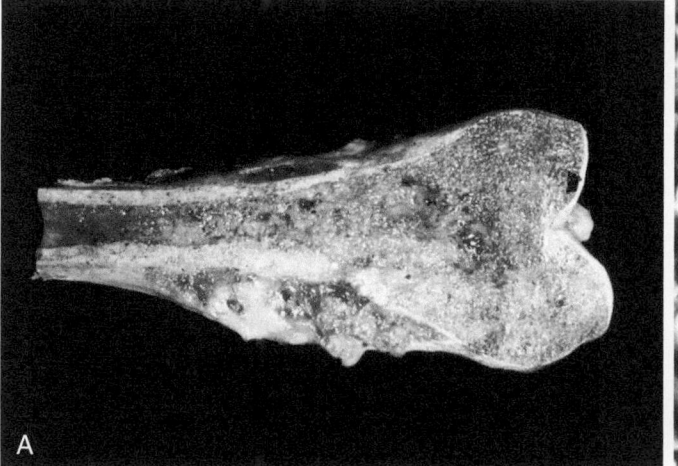 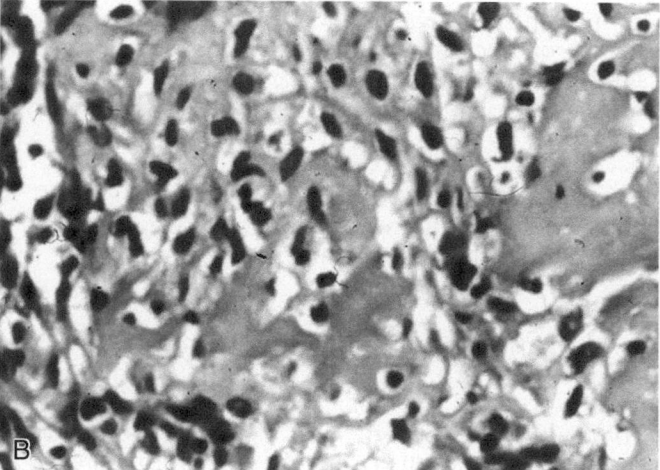

Figure 16-4. Conventional osteosarcoma. A, Gross photograph showing distal femur with destructive tumor mass with medullary and cortical involvement and extension into the surrounding soft tissue. **B,** Histologic section shows a neoplasm composed of sarcomatous stromal cells embedded in a background of osteoid.

- Some tumors may contain foci rich in vascular structures with an hemangiopericytoma-like pattern
- Small cell variant
  - May have features suggestive of Ewing sarcoma/primitive neuroectodermal tumor (PNET), mesenchymal chondrosarcoma, and lymphoma and require immunohistochemistry for differentiation
  - Presence of tumor osteoid
  - Rare cases of small cell variant share genetic features of Ewing sarcoma/PNET
- Preoperative chemotherapy may result in tumor necrosis represented by acellular tumor osteoid, acellular chondroid tissue, fibrosis, or hyalinized vascular stroma; preoperative chemotherapy is considered effective when greater than 90% of the tumor is necrotic

Special Stains and Immunohistochemistry

- SATB2: recently discovered osteoblast transcription factor (nuclear stain) critical for osteoblast lineage commitment
- SATB2 immunohistochemistry can be useful in the diagnosis of osteosarcoma when histologic features of matrix are equivocal (i.e., osteoid vs hyalinized collagen) and when biopsy only samples tumor with undifferentiated appearance

Other Techniques for Diagnosis

- DNA ploidy analysis usually shows prominent aneuploid clones
  - Conversion from pretreatment aneuploidy to predominant diploidy after chemotherapy correlates with subtotal or total necrosis of the tumor
- One case of the small cell variant of osteosarcoma reportedly demonstrated chromosome translocation t(11;22)(q24;q12) typical of Ewing sarcoma/PNET; however, subsequent studies have not replicated this result
- Hereditary form shows a loss of function of the *RB* gene; in nonhereditary form, there may be mutation of the *TP53* gene (about 20% of cases)

Differential Diagnosis

FRACTURE CALLUS

- Callus woven bone or osteoid exhibits a parallel pattern with prominent osteoblastic rimming
- Absence of nuclear atypia and abnormal mitoses in callus
- Cartilage with endochondral ossification is present in callus

OSTEOMYELITIS

- Radiographic findings may mimic osteosarcoma
- Readily differentiated using histologic features

OSTEOBLASTOMA

- Lacks atypical mitoses, infiltrative pattern, and destructive growth pattern

GIANT CELL TUMOR

- Giant cell tumors usually affect skeletally mature patients with closed epiphyses
- Usually involve the epiphyses and extends toward the articular cartilage

- Mononuclear stromal cells without atypia or abnormal mitotic activity
- Radiographic findings can help in differentiating these two entities

CHONDROSARCOMA

- Low-grade chondrosarcoma with areas of ossification may mimic osteosarcoma, whereas chondroblastic osteosarcoma usually contains a high-grade cartilaginous component
- Dedifferentiated chondrosarcoma contains an osteoblastic osteosarcoma component but retains low-grade chondrosarcoma foci
- Clear cell chondrosarcomas may produce bone, thus imitating osteosarcoma
- Presence of clear cells and typical epiphyseal location of clear cell chondrosarcoma help differentiate these two entities

MALIGNANT FIBROUS HISTIOCYTOMA

- Typically occurs in older patients
- Lacks tumor osteoid formation

FIBROSARCOMA

- No production of tumor osteoid

SMALL CELL TUMORS (EWING SARCOMA/PNET, LYMPHOMA, MESENCHYMAL CHONDROSARCOMA)

- Small cell variant of osteosarcoma will have tumor osteoid
- Immunohistochemistry may be helpful in differentiating these tumors (leukocyte common antigen is positive in lymphoma, S-100 protein is positive in mesenchymal chondrosarcoma, CD99 is positive in Ewing sarcoma/PNET, SATB2 is positive in osteosarcomas)

METASTATIC CARCINOMA

- Prostate and mammary carcinomas can elicit a prominent osteoblastic reaction
- Epithelial markers and specific tumor markers by immunohistochemistry can help differentiate metastatic carcinoma

PEARLS

- *Osteosarcoma is the fourth most common malignant tumor found in adolescents; the three most common ones in descending order are leukemia, brain tumors, and lymphoma*
- *If pain has been present for more than 1 year, the diagnosis of osteosarcoma is unlikely*
- *About half of cases of primary osteosarcomas of bone occur in the knee region; osteosarcomas of the hands and feet are rare*
- *Initial clinical presentation of osteosarcoma as a pathologic fracture is rare*
- *Elevated serum alkaline phosphatase levels typically occur in tumors with prominent osteoblastic patterns but may also be elevated in other conditions such as osteoblastoma, osteomyelitis, and callus; a posttherapy increase in serum alkaline phosphatase suggests metastatic disease or recurrence*

- Most osteosarcomas exhibit diagnostic features on routine radiographs, whereas occasionally they may exhibit deceptively benign radiographic features
- Rare cases of epiphyseal osteosarcoma may exhibit radiographic features of clear cell chondrosarcoma or chondroblastoma
- A radiologically malignant metaphyseal tumor in 10- to 30-year-olds is most likely osteosarcoma
- Rare osteosarcomas contain cytologically benign-appearing stromal giant cells that hide the sarcomatous component; careful search is necessary to identify the sarcomatous component and tumor osteoid, which is usually found in a perivascular location
- Osteosarcomas of craniofacial bones, ribs, and vertebrae are usually related to Paget disease or radiation and typically occur in older individuals

SELECTED REFERENCES

Benedict WF, Fung YK, Murphree AL: The gene responsible for retinoblastoma and osteosarcoma. Cancer 62:1691-1694, 1988.

Conner JR, Hornick JL: SATB2 is a novel marker of osteoblastic differentiation in bone and soft tissue tumors. Histopathology 63:36-49, 2013.

Dorfman HD, Czerniak B: Bone Tumors. St. Louis, Mosby, 1998, pp 128-194.

Glasser DB, Lane JM, Huvos AG, et al: Survival, prognosis, and therapeutic response in osteogenic sarcoma: the Memorial Hospital experience. Cancer 69:698-708, 1992.

Martin JW, Squire JA, Zielenska M: The genetics of osteosarcoma. Sarcoma 2012:627254, 2012.

Unni KK, Inwards CY, Bridge J, et al: Tumors of the Bones and Joints, 4th Series, Fascicle 2. Washington, DC, Armed Forces Institute of Pathology, 2005, pp 136-170.

TELANGIECTATIC OSTEOSARCOMA

Clinical Features

- Male-to-female ratio is 2:1
- Most occur in second decade
- Accounts for about 4% of all osteosarcomas
- Similar distribution as conventional intramedullary osteosarcoma
- Predominantly affects distal femur, proximal tibia, and proximal humerus
- Similar symptoms to conventional osteosarcoma, except it is more likely to present as a pathologic fracture (25% of cases)

Radiographic Findings

- Recognizable as a completely lytic lesion involving the metaphysis with infiltrating destructive margins
- May cause cortical expansion of the bone
- Periosteal new bone formation may be represented by onion-skinning or Codman triangle
- Some cases may exhibit benign features and mimic an aneurysmal bone cyst

Gross Pathology

- Hemorrhagic mass that may be multicystic and necrotic
- No areas of fleshy, sarcoma-like tissue or sclerotic areas

Histopathology

- Multiple cystlike spaces resembling an aneurysmal bone cyst, except that the septa of the cysts contain

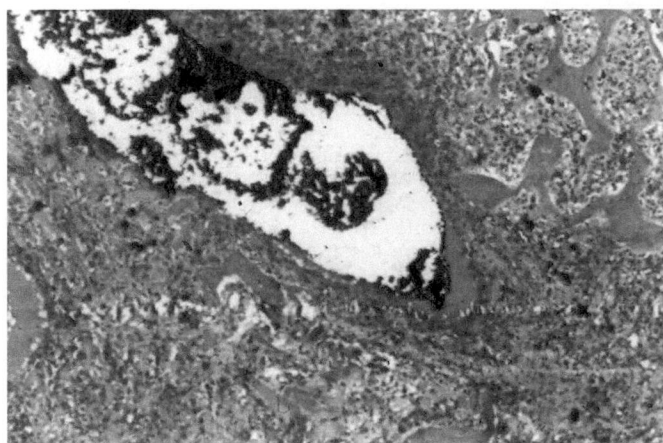

Figure 16-5. Telangiectatic osteosarcoma. Histologic section shows cystlike spaces surrounded by atypical stromal cells and osteoid.

stromal cells (mononuclear and multinucleated) with cytologically malignant features intermixed with benign osteoclast-like giant cells (Figure 16-5)
- Mitotic features are present, including atypical forms
- Sometimes the malignant stromal cells are floating in the center of the hemorrhagic cysts; identification of the stromal cells may be difficult, requiring multiple sections
- Tumor osteoid can be difficult to identify; it is usually focal and found in a delicate lacelike pattern

Special Stains and Immunohistochemistry

- SATB2 immunohistochemistry can be useful in the diagnosis when histologic features of matrix are equivocal (i.e., osteoid vs hyalinized collagen) and when biopsy only samples tumor with undifferentiated appearance

Other Techniques for Diagnosis

- Noncontributory

Differential Diagnosis

ANEURYSMAL BONE CYST

- Stroma may be cellular but typically lacks cytologic atypia and atypical mitoses; may contain reactive bone with atypical osteoblasts
- Definitive cytologic malignant features and atypical mitoses are absent

CONVENTIONAL OSTEOSARCOMA

- Radiographically, these tumors are not purely lytic
- Intramedullary osteosarcoma may contain focal telangiectatic areas, which should not be overinterpreted

PEARLS

- Telangiectatic osteosarcoma is frequently the type of osteosarcoma associated with long-term Paget disease
- Better prognosis than conventional intramedullary osteosarcoma
- When a diagnosis of aneurysmal bone cyst is being considered, all tissue should be evaluated histologically for evidence of malignant stroma to rule out telangiectatic osteosarcoma

SELECTED REFERENCES

Conner JR, Hornick JL: SATB2 is a novel marker of osteoblastic differentiation in bone and soft tissue tumors. Histopathology 63:36-49, 2013.

McCarthy EF: Differential Diagnosis in Pathology: Bone and Joint Disorders. New York, Igaku-Shoin, 1996, pp 44-51, 82-85.

Unni KK, Inwards CY, Bridge J, et al: Tumors of the Bones and Joints, 4th Series, Fascicle 2. Washington, DC, Armed Forces Institute of Pathology, 2005, pp 155-158.

Weiss A, Khoury JD, Hoffer FA, et al: Telangiectatic osteosarcoma: the St. Jude Children's Research Hospital's experience. Cancer 109:1627-1637, 2007.

PAROSTEAL OSTEOSARCOMA

Clinical Features

- Also known as "juxtacortical osteosarcoma"
- Slight female predominance, with a male-to-female ratio of 1:1.5
- Occurs predominantly in third decade
- Involves metaphyses of long bones with approximately three fourths of cases involving the distal posterior femur, with the proximal tibia as the second most common site
- Clinically presents as a painless mass of long duration (slow growing); pain may occur late in the course but is not typical initially
- May also present as an inability to flex the knee

Radiographic Features

- Radiodense, bosselated, or mushroom-shaped mass arising on the surface of a bone (outside of periosteum); in long-term lesions, tumor may encircle the bone
- A separate lucent zone between the tumor and the cortex known as a *string sign* may be seen
- No evidence of periosteal bone reaction
- Peripheral lucent areas may represent a cartilaginous cap
- Central lucent areas may represent high-grade sarcoma or dedifferentiated tumors
- CT or MRI may be necessary to visualize lucent areas

Gross Pathology

- Well-ossified mass that appears attached to the cortical surface of the bone
- Cartilaginous cap may be present and there may be soft foci, which should be sampled; these foci may represent high-grade sarcomatous regions or dedifferentiated tumor

Histopathology

- Tumor osteoid is arranged in parallel arrays and separated by a hypocellular fibroblastic stroma that exhibits minimal cytologic atypia and minimal mitotic activity without atypical forms (Figure 16-6)
- Islands of cartilaginous tissue and a cartilaginous cap may be present
  - Chondrocytes are atypical and do not exhibit orderly arrangement
  - Atypia is mild and reminiscent of chondrocytic atypia seen in enchondromas
- No evidence of periosteal new bone formation
- Areas of dedifferentiated high-grade sarcoma may be seen (about 15% of cases)
- No fatty or hematopoietic marrow is seen in association with the tumor

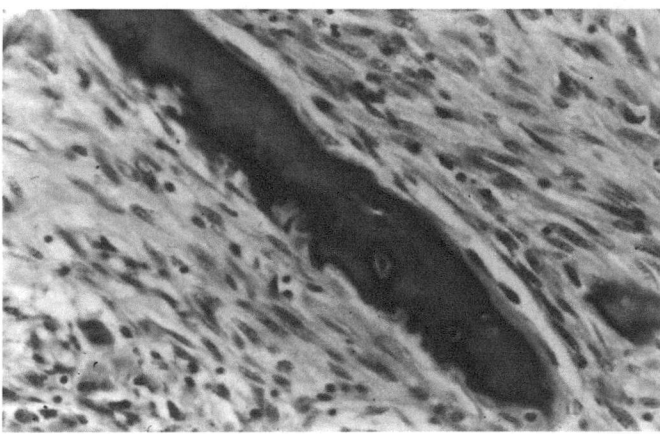

Figure 16-6. Parosteal osteosarcoma. Histologic section shows parallel arrangement of tumor osteoid separated by fibroblastic stroma with only minimal atypia.

Special Stains and Immunohistochemistry

- SATB2 immunohistochemistry can be useful

Other Techniques in Diagnosis

- Cytogenetic studies: a ring chromosome may be seen

Differential Diagnosis

OSTEOCHONDROMA

- Medullary spaces contain adipose tissue or marrow hematopoietic tissue

MYOSITIS OSSIFICANS

- Maturation toward lamellar bone and marrow adipose tissue begins peripherally and extends centrally in this proliferative process, which is the reverse in parosteal osteosarcoma

HIGH-GRADE SURFACE OSTEOSARCOMA

- These are cytologically high-grade tumors that lack residual low-grade areas

PERIOSTEAL OSTEOSARCOMA

- Abundant cartilage is present
- Higher-grade osseous component and evidence of periosteal reaction

PEARLS

- *Symptoms may last up to 10 years*
- *Typically affects an older age group compared with intramedullary osteosarcoma*
- *It is not uncommon for these patients to have a history of recurrence of a previously diagnosed osteochondroma*
- *Radiologic and histologic evidence of periosteal new bone formation is absent*
- *Central lucent areas identified on CT scan or MRI may represent high-grade sarcomatous areas or regions of dedifferentiation*
- *Children may exhibit radiographic lesions that mimic parosteal osteosarcoma of the distal femur; histologically, they have features of fibrous cortical defect*

SELECTED REFERENCES

Conner JR, Hornick JL: SATB2 is a novel marker of osteoblastic differentiation in bone and soft tissue tumors. Histopathology 63:36-49, 2013.

Han I, Oh JH, Na Yg, et al: Clinical outcome of parosteal osteosarcoma. J Surg Oncol 97:146-149, 2008.

Sinovic JK, Bridge JA, Neff JR: Ring chromosome in parosteal osteosarcoma: clinical and diagnostic significance. Cancer Genet Cytogenet 62:50-52, 1992.

Unni KK, Inwards CY, Bridge J, et al: Tumors of the Bones and Joints, 4th Series, Fascicle 2. Washington, DC, Armed Forces Institute of Pathology, 2005, pp 170-177.

PERIOSTEAL OSTEOSARCOMA

Clinical Features

- Slight male predominance, with a male-to-female ratio of 1.7:1
- Typically occurs in second to third decades (later than a conventional osteosarcoma appears and sooner than a parosteal osteosarcoma appears)
- Most occur in the diaphysis and metaphysis of the tibia and femur
- Patients present with pain, swelling, and tenderness; symptoms often present for less than 1 year
- Rare (< 2% of all osteosarcomas)

Radiographic Findings

- Represented by a surface radiolucent tumor containing a spiculated pattern of calcifications that are oriented perpendicular to the long axis of the primary bone
- May see cortical thickening or erosion
- Periosteal reaction may be present
- No medullary involvement

Gross Pathology

- Lobulated surface mass having a cartilaginous appearance
- Cortical erosion may be seen, but the tumor does not extend into the medullary cavity

Histopathology

- Malignant osteoid must be present (may only be focal), but the predominant pattern of tumor is represented by lobulated chondromatous tissue with cytologic features of grade 2 or 3 chondrosarcoma
- Tumor is located on the surface of the bone and may extend into soft tissue
- High-grade anaplastic sarcomatous spindle cell component may separate lobules of the malignant chondroid component
- Periosteal bone formation may be present, and there may be cortical erosion, but the tumor does not involve the medullary cavity

Special Stains and Immunohistochemistry

- SATB2 immunohistochemistry can be useful in the diagnosis of osteosarcoma when histologic features of matrix are equivocal (i.e., osteoid vs hyalinized collagen) and when biopsy only samples tumor with undifferentiated appearance

Other Techniques for Diagnosis

- Cytogenetics: usually diploid

Differential Diagnosis

PERIOSTEAL CHONDROMA

- Usually smaller and better defined
- Composed of benign chondroid tissue; does not contain malignant tumor osteoid

PERIOSTEAL CHONDROSARCOMA

- Radiographically, it contains "popcorn" calcifications
- Histologically, it is a low-grade chondrosarcoma containing no tumor osteoid

PAROSTEAL OSTEOSARCOMA

- Radiographically, these tumors are more radiodense
- Histologically, this is a low-grade malignant fibro-osseous tumor without chondroid differentiation

CONVENTIONAL INTRAMEDULLARY OSTEOSARCOMA

- This is a higher-grade osteosarcoma involving the medullary cavity
- Periosteal osteosarcoma does not involve the medullary cavity

HIGH-GRADE SURFACE OSTEOSARCOMA

- Lacks cartilaginous differentiation
- Osteoid component is pleomorphic and high grade

PEARLS

- *By definition, periosteal osteosarcoma does not involve the medullary cavity*
- *CT scan or MRI may be necessary to rule out medullary involvement*

SELECTED REFERENCES

Conner JR, Hornick JL: SATB2 is a novel marker of osteoblastic differentiation in bone and soft tissue tumors. Histopathology 63:36-49, 2013.

Grimer RJ, Bielack S, Flege S, et al; European Musculo Skeletal Oncology Society. Periosteal osteosarcoma: a European review of outcome. Eur J Cancer 41:2806-2811, 2005.

Rose PS, Dickey ID, Wenger DE, et al: Periosteal osteosarcoma: long-term outcome and risk of late recurrence. Clin Orthop 453:314-317, 2006.

Unni KK, Inwards CY, Bridge J, et al: Tumors of the Bones and Joints, 4th Series, Fascicle 2. Washington, DC, Armed Forces Institute of Pathology, 2005, pp 178-182.

HIGH-GRADE SURFACE OSTEOSARCOMA

Clinical Features

- Very rare tumor, with male-to-female ratio of about 3:1
- Occurs predominantly in third and fourth decades
- Distal and midfemur, proximal humerus, and proximal fibula are most common sites
- Pain and swelling are most common symptoms, with duration from less than a year to many years
- Similar prognosis to conventional intramedullary osteosarcoma, but poorer prognosis than parosteal osteosarcoma

Radiographic Features

- Exhibits a surface mass with features similar to those of periosteal osteosarcoma, except the mineralization

pattern is similar to that of conventional osteosarcoma, revealing a fluffy, cumulus cloud appearance
- May be cortical destruction, periosteal reaction, and focal medullary involvement

Gross Pathology

- Large, lobulated surface mass with variable consistency ranging from soft to firm
- Should not significantly involve the medullary region
- May be hemorrhagic

Histopathology

- Histologically high-grade osteosarcoma with features similar to those of conventional intramedullary osteosarcoma, but lacks significant medullary involvement

Special Stains and Immunohistochemistry

- SATB2 immunohistochemistry can be useful in the diagnosis when histologic features of matrix are equivocal (i.e., osteoid vs hyalinized collagen) and when biopsy only samples tumor with undifferentiated appearance

Other Techniques for Diagnosis

- Noncontributory

Differential Diagnosis

Dedifferentiated Parosteal Osteosarcoma
- Usually has residual low-grade malignant fibroblastic stromal component

Parosteal Osteosarcoma
- Lacks high-grade anaplastic appearance

Conventional Intramedullary Osteosarcoma
- Significant medullary component (minimal medullary component in a high-grade surface osteosarcoma)

PEARLS

- *Radiographically mimics periosteal osteosarcoma, except it has cumulus cloud–like patterns of mineralization*
- *Of all the types of surface osteosarcomas, this has the least favorable prognosis (similar to conventional intramedullary osteosarcoma)*

Selected References

Conner JR, Hornick JL: SATB2 is a novel marker of osteoblastic differentiation in bone and soft tissue tumors. Histopathology 63:36-49, 2013.
Okada K, Unni KK, Swee RG, Sim FH: High grade surface osteosarcoma: a clinicopathologic study of 46 cases. Cancer 85:1044-1054, 1999.
Staals EL, Bacchini P, Bertoni F: High-grade surface osteosarcoma: a review of 25 cases from the Rizzoli Institute. Cancer 112:1592-1599, 2008.

LOW-GRADE CENTRAL OSTEOSARCOMA

Clinical Features

- Male-to-female ratio is about 1:1
- Most cases occur in third and fourth decades; this variant of osteosarcoma can occur in older age groups
- Patients present with a history of pain for many months up to several years; usually no complaint of swelling
- Most common sites include mid- and distal femur and proximal and midtibia

- Some patients may have been previously diagnosed with fibrous dysplasia

Radiographic Features

- Large, poorly marginated intramedullary mass that either is sclerotic or exhibits trabeculations
- Usually no evidence of periosteal reaction
- Medullary tumor may extend along the length of the bone to the subarticular bone
- May have cortical destruction with formation of a soft tissue mass

Gross Pathology

- Tumors are gritty, gray, medullary masses that may have fibrous and fleshy areas
- Cortical destruction may be seen, and the tumor may extend the length of the bone with poor demarcation between tumor and uninvolved medullary bone
- Mean size about 9 cm

Histopathology

- Similar to parosteal osteosarcoma and can also mimic fibrous dysplasia
- Well-differentiated intramedullary fibro-osseous process represented by irregular bony trabeculae separated by fibrous spindly stroma
- Spindle cells are fibroblastic-like and have elongated nuclei with nucleoli
- Nuclei exhibit minimal atypia and infrequent mitoses; atypical mitoses are rare to absent
- Rare chondroid foci may be seen

Special Stains and Immunohistochemistry

- SATB2 immunohistochemistry may be useful

Other Techniques for Diagnosis

- Noncontributory

Differential Diagnosis

Fibrous Dysplasia
- Benign nonaggressive radiographic features with no cortical disruption
- Histologically, the woven bone in fibrous dysplasia is delicate and curved, in contrast to the coarse tumor osteoid in low-grade central osteosarcoma
- Fibrous dysplasia lacks nuclear atypia and mitotic activity

Desmoplastic Fibroma
- No radiographic evidence of matrix formation
- Histologically, the central portion of desmoplastic fibroma will not contain any tumor osteoid

Osteoblastoma
- Typically has benign radiographic features
- Prominent osteoblastic rimming of bony trabeculae

Conventional Intramedullary Osteosarcoma, Fibroblastic Variant
- Nuclear pleomorphism and mitotic activity with atypical forms is greater in this tumor compared with low-grade central osteosarcoma

- Parosteal osteosarcoma
- Surface location with no medullary involvement, but similar histology

PEARLS

- *This variant affects older patients more often than traditional osteosarcomas*
- *Not associated with previous radiation therapy or preexisting Paget disease (typical of osteosarcoma seen in elderly patients)*
- *A small number of these tumors may be interpreted as benign radiographically*
- *Histologically similar to parosteal osteosarcoma*

SELECTED REFERENCES

Andresen KJ, Sundaram M, Unni KK, Sim FH: Imagining features of low-grade central osteosarcoma of the long bones and pelvis. Skeletal Radiol 33:373-379, 2004.

Choong PF, Pritchard DJ, Rock MG, et al: Low grade central osteogenic sarcoma: a long-term follow-up on 20 patients. Clin Orthop 322:198-206, 1996.

Conner JR, Hornick JL: SATB2 is a novel marker of osteoblastic differentiation in bone and soft tissue tumors. Histopathology 63:36-49, 2013.

McCarthy EF: Differential Diagnosis in Pathology: Bone and Joint Disorders. New York, Igaku-Shoin, 1996, pp 44-51, 76-81.

CHONDROID TUMORS

OSTEOCHONDROMA

Clinical Features

- Also known as exostosis
- Most common benign tumor involving bone
- Male-to-female ratio is about 2:1
- Most occur in second and third decades, but can present at any age
- Majority occur in distal femur, proximal tibia, and humerus; pelvis is also a relatively common site
- Extremely rare in craniofacial bones, vertebrae, sacrum, and sternum
- Patients present with a longstanding mass that may be painful or asymptomatic
- Some lesions are asymptomatic and are identified incidentally on radiographs obtained for other reasons

- Pain may be secondary to impingement of a bursa, fracture, or infarction of the lesion
- May develop after radiation treatment (more than 1 year) for other malignant processes
- Hereditary form (autosomal dominant) is called *osteochondromatosis* or *multiple hereditary exostosis* (any bone may be involved except craniofacial bones)
- Other hereditary forms with multiple osteochondromas include Langer-Giedion syndrome and DEFECT-11 syndrome
- Fewer than 2% of osteochondromas undergo malignant transformation; clinical features suggestive of malignant transformation include pain, rapid growth, large tumor size (> 6 cm), and location (axial skeleton)

Radiographic Findings

- Radiographs reveal a pedunculated metaphyseal mass projecting from the surface of a bone (Figure 16-7A)
- Variable smooth or irregular surface and a variable base (narrow to wide); points toward the diaphysis and away from the nearest epiphysis
- Has appearance of mature bone and is continuous with the cortex of the uninvolved adjacent bone
- Surface cap represented by cartilage is not identified with routine radiographs unless calcified; MRI is necessary to evaluate the nonmineralized cartilaginous cap

Gross Pathology

- Pedunculated or broad-based mass containing a smooth, thin (< 1 cm) cartilaginous cap
- In older patients, the cartilaginous cap may be attenuated or absent
- Central part of the mass is represented by normal-appearing medullary bone

Histopathology

- Outer surface is covered by a thin layer of periosteal fibrous tissue
- Cap is represented by hyaline cartilage that contains evenly distributed chondrocytes (Figure 16-7B)
- Nuclei may exhibit atypia and pleomorphism
- Junction of the cap and bone mimics the epiphyseal plate and contains linear rows or columns of chondrocytes

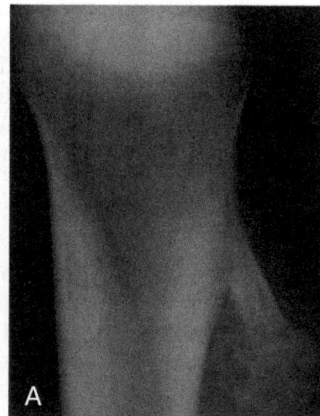
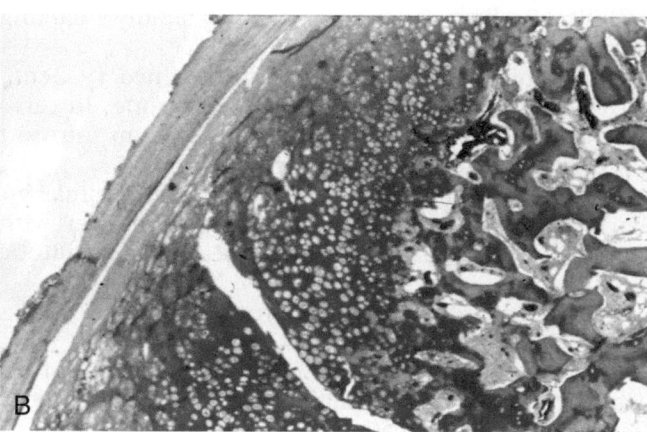

Figure 16-7. Osteochondroma. A, Radiograph of the distal femur shows a pedunculated mass. The cortex and medulla at the base of the stock are continuous with those of the femur. **B,** Low-power view shows a cartilaginous cap overlying bony trabeculae.

- Columns undergo endochondral ossification and form bony trabeculae
- Medullary spaces between the trabeculae of bone contain adipose tissue and sometimes hematopoietic tissue
- Chondrocytic atypia must be evaluated with clinicoradiographic features to determine their significance
  - Nuclear enlargement, variation in nuclear shape, multinucleation, and formation of chondrocytic clusters that are irregularly shaped may cause some concern but can be found in osteochondromas
  - Chondrocytic atypia along with clinical features of malignancy (pain, rapidly enlarging tumor, size > 6 cm) and radiographic features of malignancy (irregular thickened cartilaginous cap > 2 cm, radiolucent areas of the cartilaginous cap, extension through periosteum into soft tissue, and bone destruction) are more ominous and concerning for a secondary chondrosarcoma
  - High mitotic activity is indicative of malignancy

Special Stains and Immunohistochemistry

- Noncontributory

Other Techniques for Diagnosis

- Chromosome rearrangements of 8q24.1 (EXT1) is found in patients with Langer-Giedion syndrome
- Deletions of chromosomal bands 11p11-12 (EXT2) is seen in patients with DEFECT-11 syndrome
- The EXT1 and EXT2 gene products add heparan sulfate to proteoglycans and may have tumor suppressor functions

Differential Diagnosis

PAROSTEAL OSTEOCHONDROMATOUS PROLIFERATION (NORA LESION)

- Usually involves small bones of hands and feet
- Occurs in third and fourth decades of life
- Medullary component of lesion is not in continuity with host bone
- Histologically, the cartilage is hypercellular with atypia and multinucleation
- Chondroid nodules are separated by a spindle cell proliferation that exhibits mitotic activity (no atypical mitoses or nuclear atypia)
- Woven bone with deep basophilia may be present

CHONDROSARCOMA ARISING IN AN OSTEOCHONDROMA

- Clinical findings consist of pain and a rapidly enlarging mass
- Radiographic findings consist of thickened (> 2 cm), irregular cartilaginous cap, radiolucent zones in cartilaginous cap, extension through periosteum into soft tissue, and evidence of bone destruction
- Histologic findings consist of increased cellularity, nuclear atypia represented by enlarged nuclei with open chromatin pattern, multinucleation, and mitotic activity
- Fibroblastic stroma is present in the medullary spaces instead of fat and hematopoietic tissue
- If a cartilaginous cap is present, it is composed of cytologically low-grade malignant chondrocytes without endochondral ossification

PAROSTEAL OSTEOSARCOMA

- Continuity with the medullary component of the parent bone is not present
- Appears to be attached to the surface of the parent bone

PEARLS

- *Clinical and radiographic findings are important in the evaluation of chondrocytic atypia*
- *Radiographically, the long axis of the stalk points away from the nearest epiphysis*
- *Malignant transformation is rare (< 2%)*
- *Cytogenetic abnormalities suggest that osteochondroma represents a true neoplastic process*

SELECTED REFERENCES

Altay M, Bayrakci K, Yildiz Y, et al: Secondary chondrosarcoma in cartilage bone tumors: report of 32 patients. J Orthop Sci 12:415-423, 2007.

Chikhladze R, Nishnianidze T: Clinical-morphological aspects of osteochondroma of long bones. Georgian Med News 152:57-59, 2007.

Nora FE, Dahlin DC, Beabout JW: Bizarre parosteal osteochondromatous proliferations of the hands and feet. Am J Surg Pathol 7:245-250, 1983.

Unni KK, Inwards CY, Bridge J, et al: Tumors of the Bones and Joints, 4th Series, Fascicle 2. Washington, DC, Armed Forces Institute of Pathology, 2005, pp 37-46.

ENCHONDROMA

Clinical Features

- Male-to-female ratio is about equal; affects all age groups (most occur in second to fifth decades)
- Occurs predominantly in the appendicular skeleton, with most occurring in bones of the hands and feet (hands more often affected than feet)
- Proximal humerus and femur and distal femur are also affected; rarely found in the pelvis, ribs, sternum, and vertebrae (no reported cases in craniofacial bones)
- In general, these tumors are asymptomatic and may be identified on routine radiographs or nuclear scans
- Phalangeal tumor may present as a mass
- Pain may be a presenting feature in association with a pathologic fracture or trauma to the tumor

Radiographic Features

- Well-defined, predominantly lucent diaphyseal intramedullary mass (Figure 16-8A)
- Usually lobulated and sharply demarcated with variable mineralization, stippled, ringlike, or flocculent
- Cortical expansion and thinning may be seen, but the cortex should be intact; rare evidence of periosteal reaction

Gross Pathology

- Curettage produces fragments of blue-gray translucent, glistening chondroid tissue intermixed with fragments containing yellow foci representing calcification
- Resected specimens consist of a well-circumscribed medullary, confluent, lobulated, cartilaginous mass; periphery of the tumor may be irregular

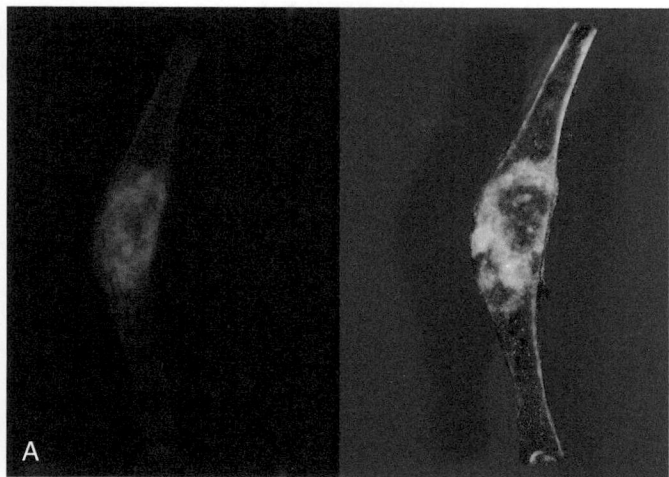

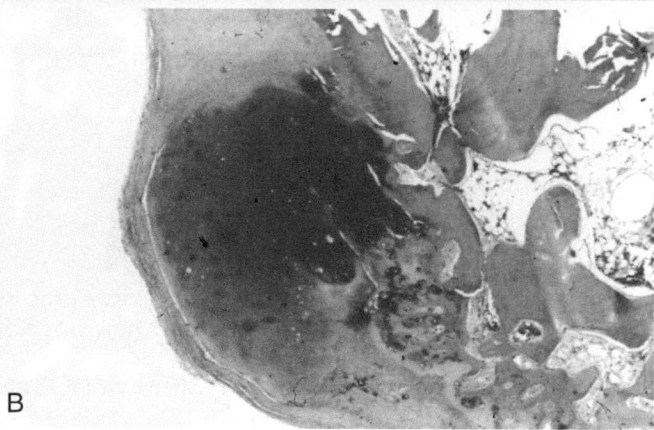

Figure 16-8. Enchondroma. A, Radiograph of the rib shows an expanding radiolucent area with associated calcifications. Gross section of the tumor mass shows a gray-white lesion extending from cortex to cortex. **B,** Low-power view shows a well-circumscribed nodule composed of lobules of mature hyaline cartilage.

Histopathology

- Composed of lobulated, mature, hyaline-like cartilage (Figure 16-8B)
- Lobules may be separated by marrow hematopoietic tissue or endochondral bone
- Chondrocytic cellularity is low and usually evenly distributed
- Bland cytologic features with small, slightly hyperchromatic nuclei without pleomorphism; rare multinucleated forms may be present
- Nuclei with open chromatin patterns and mitoses are generally absent
- Cellularity may be higher in tumors of the hands and feet
- Calcifications and endochondral ossification may be present
- Myxoid areas should arouse suspicion of malignancy except in tumors of the hands and feet

Special Stains and Immunohistochemistry

- Mib-1 (Ki-67): in tumors involving bones other than the hands and feet in which malignancy is suspected clinically or radiologically, Mib-1 may be used to demonstrate proliferative activity
- Proliferative index is low in enchondroma

Other Techniques for Diagnosis

- Enchondromas may exhibit abnormalities of chromosomes 6 and 12
- Molecular studies have shown chromosomal rearrangements involving the *HMGA2* gene localized to 12q15 in some patients with enchondromas

Differential Diagnosis

PROMINENT COSTOCHONDRAL CARTILAGE
- May clinically mimic enchondroma
- Composed of histologically benign chondrocytes with an orderly and regular appearance

FIBROUS DYSPLASIA WITH CHONDROID DIFFERENTIATION
- Radiographs reveal a ground-glass diaphyseal lesion
- Fibro-osseous elements are seen (absent in enchondroma)

LOW-GRADE CHONDROSARCOMA
- Differentiating this tumor from an enchondroma can be extremely difficult and requires clinical, radiographic, and histologic information
- Pain is usually present in low-grade chondrosarcoma; pain is typically absent in enchondroma unless traumatized or pathologically fractured
- Radiographic features of low-grade chondrosarcoma include cortical destruction, cortical thickening due to extension of tumor in haversian canals, and a soft tissue mass
- Increased cellularity and binucleate chondrocytes are more prominent
- Marrow permeation represented by cellular cartilage surrounding mature bone trabeculae and lobules of cartilage separated by fibrous tissue is seen in low-grade chondrosarcoma
- Extension of the tumor into haversian canals (not seen in enchondroma)
- Prominent myxoid features are not typical of enchondromas
- Immunoperoxidase stains for proliferative activity (Mib-1) reveal nuclear positivity in low-grade chondrosarcomas (generally minimal or no staining in enchondromas except for hand and foot tumors)

PEARLS

- *Any cartilaginous neoplasm in the pelvis, ribs, sternum, or vertebrae should be considered a potentially aggressive tumor unless exhibiting completely benign clinical features, benign radiographic features, and benign histologic features*
- *Presence of pain in the absence of trauma or associated pathologic fracture should arouse suspicion of malignancy in a patient with a low-grade chondroid neoplasm*
- *Myxoid features in an enchondroma should raise suspicion of malignancy*
- *Significance of atypical cytologic features, atypical cellularity, and myxoid features in an enchondroma increases as the tumor location gets closer to the axial skeleton*

- Ollier disease (enchondromatosis) *presents with multiple enchondromas and carries a higher risk for malignant transformation*
- Maffucci syndrome: *congenital syndrome consisting of multiple enchondromas and hemangiomas; increased risk for developing chondrosarcomas and malignant vascular tumors (angiosarcoma)*

Selected References

Dorfman HD, Czerniak B: Bone Tumors. St. Louis, Mosby, 1998, pp 253-276.
Gajewski DA, Burnette JB, Murphy MD, Temple HT: Differentiating clinical and radiographic features of enchondroma and secondary chondrosarcoma in the foot. Foot Ankle Int 27:240-244, 2006.
Mirra JM, Gold R, Downs J, Eckardt JJ: A new histologic approach to the differentiation of enchondroma and chondrosarcoma of the bones: a clinicopathologic analysis of 51 cases. Clin Orthop 201:214-237, 1985.
Unni KK, Inwards CY, Bridge J, et al: Tumors of the Bones and Joints, 4th Series, Fascicle 2. Washington, DC, Armed Forces Institute of Pathology, 2005, pp 46-52.

PERIOSTEAL CHONDROMA

Clinical Features

- Male-to-female ratio is 2:1
- Most cases occur in second and third decades
- Proximal humerus, proximal femur, distal femur, and hand bones are most commonly affected
- Usually asymptomatic and often found incidentally on routine radiographs
- Occurs near tendon insertions and thus may cause functional abnormalities and discomfort related to movement
- May occasionally be palpable

Radiographic Features

- Typically a periosteal mass with variable mineralization
- May appear lytic or markedly calcified
- Erodes the outer cortex but does not extend into the medullary cavity
- Periosteal bone formation creating a peripheral buttress causing the tumor to be cup-shaped or crater-like

Gross Pathology

- Cortical, subperiosteal, gray-white lobulated chondroid mass with an outer thin layer of periosteum
- Does not extend into the medullary cavity
- Yellow calcifications may be present

Histopathology (Figure 16-9)

- Similar features to those of an enchondroma composed of hyaline cartilage
- May exhibit higher cellularity, increased nuclear atypia, and more multinucleated chondrocytes than enchondromas
- Myxoid change may be present
- Tumor may appear to extend or push into the medullary cavity, but there is a rim of lamellar bone at the junction of the tumor and medullary cavity

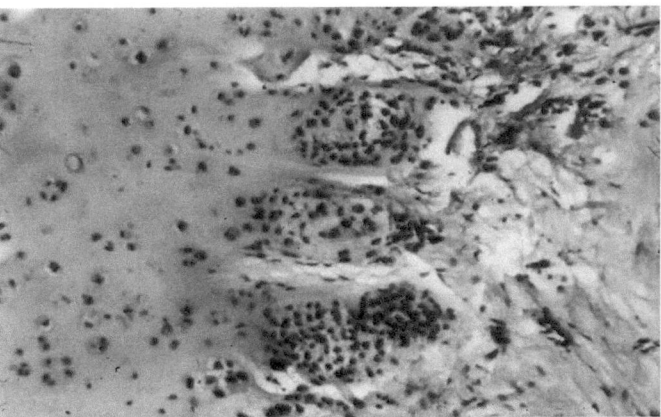

Figure 16-9. Periosteal chondroma. Histologic section shows lobulated cellular hyaline cartilage.

Special Stains and Immunohistochemistry

- Tumor cells express S-100 protein

Other Techniques for Diagnosis

- Noncontributory

Differential Diagnosis

JUXTACORTICAL CHONDROSARCOMA

- Exhibits radiographic features of an aggressive process and does not have buttressing periosteal new bone at the peripheral margins
- May extend into soft tissue and may show variable cytologic atypia

PERIOSTEAL OSTEOSARCOMA

- Radiographically, this tumor exhibits perpendicular feathery calcifications and lacks peripheral buttressing
- Composed of tumor osteoid and has immature mesenchymal stroma between lobules of cartilage

PEARLS

- *Periosteal tumor that creates a cup- or crater-shaped mass extending into the superficial cortex but not into the medullary canal*
- *Composed of hyaline cartilage similar to enchondroma*

Selected References

Bauer TW, Dorfman HD, Latham JT: Periosteal chondroma: a clinicopathologic study of 23 cases. Am J Surg Pathol 6:631-637, 1982.
Nojima T, Unni KK, McLeod RA, Pritchard DJ: Periosteal chondroma and periosteal chondrosarcoma. Am J Surg Pathol 9:666-667, 1985.
Robinson P, White LM, Sundaram M, et al: Periosteal chondroid tumors: radiologic evaluation with pathologic correlation. AJR Am J Roentgenol 177:1183-1188, 2001.
Unni KK, Inwards CY, Bridge J, et al: Tumors of the Bones and Joints, 4th Series, Fascicle 2. Washington, DC, Armed Forces Institute of Pathology, 2005, pp 56-59.

CHONDROBLASTOMA

Clinical Features

- Male-to-female ratio is 1.5:1
- Most cases occur in second decade; 95% occur between ages 5 and 25 years

- Predilection for epiphyses of bones
- Typically involves long bones in skeletally immature patients
- Common sites include distal femur, proximal tibia, and proximal humerus
- Other sites include acetabular area, iliac crest of pelvis, ribs, scapulae, spine, tarsal bones, base of skull, and temporal bone
- Usually presents with pain over months to years; may have muscle wasting, arthralgia of the adjacent joint, and joint effusion
- Rare (< 1% of primary neoplasms involving bone)

Radiographic Findings

- Circumscribed, well-demarcated epiphyseal lytic mass with a rim of sclerotic bone
- Calcifications vary from focal stippling to coarse trabecular patterns
- Periosteal reaction is variable, but never to the degree seen in malignant neoplasms

Gross Pathology

- Curettage reveals friable and gritty red tissue with yellow foci of calcifications
- Resected specimens reveal a well-circumscribed, epiphyseal gray mass containing regional calcification, hemorrhage, and cystic changes
- Usually measure 3 to 6 cm in greatest dimension
- May have bluish-gray areas representing chondroid matrix
- Rim of sclerotic bone surrounds the tumor

Histopathology

- Composed of immature cells with features of fetal chondroblasts (stromal cells), multinucleated giant cells, and chondroid matrix (Figure 16-10)
- Stromal cells are round and have distinct cell membranes
  - Contain predominantly eosinophilic cytoplasm and a centrally placed round nucleus, which gives a fried-egg appearance to the cell
  - Nuclei contain grooves or clefts, and chromatin patterns are finely granular and evenly distributed

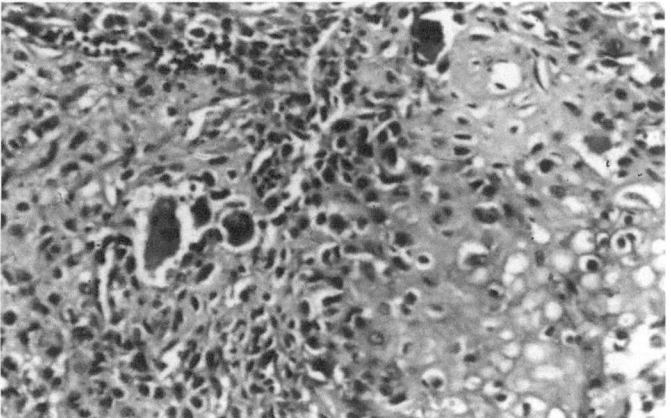

Figure 16-10. Chondroblastoma. Histologic section shows a neoplasm composed of immature chondroblasts, multinucleated giant cells, and chondroid matrix.

- Infrequent mitotic figures without atypical forms are seen
- Regional areas where cells do not have well-demarcated borders and form syncytia may be seen
- Often have areas in which the cells contain larger atypical nuclei
- Multinucleated giant cells containing numerous nuclei (more than 20) are scattered throughout the tumor
- Variable amounts of chondroid matrix, which may contain stromal cells
- Calcification is an important histologic feature and has two patterns
  - Most common pattern is represented by linear calcifications surrounding stromal cells, imparting a chicken-wire appearance
  - Other pattern includes coarse calcifications of the chondroid matrix
- May also have areas of spindle-shaped cells, secondary aneurysmal cystic changes, myxoid changes, and cystic changes containing eosinophilic amorphous material

Special Stains and Immunohistochemistry

- S-100 protein: stromal cells are positive
  - May be helpful to identify the scant numbers of stromal cells in tumors with prominent secondary aneurysmal cystic changes

Other Techniques for Diagnosis

- Noncontributory

Differential Diagnosis

CHONDROMYXOID FIBROMA

- Usually involves the metaphyses
- Lacks calcifications and has more prominent lobulated myxoid stroma

GIANT CELL TUMOR

- Usually occurs in skeletally mature patients
- Stromal cells with nuclear grooves are absent (negative for S-100 protein)
- Lacks chondroid matrix and calcification

LANGERHANS CELL HISTIOCYTOSIS (EOSINOPHILIC GRANULOMA)

- May radiographically and cytologically (nuclear grooves) mimic chondroblastoma
- Contains eosinophils and lacks chondroid matrix and calcifications

ANEURYSMAL BONE CYST

- Chondroblastoma with prominent secondary aneurysmal bone cyst formation may mimic a primary aneurysmal bone cyst
- S-100 protein may be useful in identifying stromal cells in chondroblastoma

CLEAR CELL CHONDROSARCOMA

- Usually seen in older patients
- Composed of cells with clear-staining cytoplasm
- Contains chondrocytic cells with cytologic malignant features
- Tends to be more heavily calcified than chondroblastoma

CHONDROBLASTIC OSTEOSARCOMA

- May rarely involve the epiphyses and mimic chondroblastoma
- Contains tumor osteoid

PEARLS

- *Three common epiphyseal tumors are giant cell tumor, clear cell chondrosarcoma, and chondroblastoma*
- *Rare cases of metastasizing chondroblastoma have been reported without consistent, definitive, and predictable histopathologic features*
- *Aneurysmal lesions of tarsal bones may have minute foci of chondroblastic stroma*

SELECTED REFERENCES

Atalar H, Basarir K, Yildiz Y, et al: Management of chondroblastoma: retrospective review of 28 patients. J Orthop Sci 12:334-340, 2007.

Dahlin DC, Ivins JC: Benign chondroblastoma: a study of 125 cases. Cancer 30:401-413, 1972.

Kurt AM, Unni KK, Sim FH, McLeod RA: Chondroblastoma of bone. Hum Pathol 20:965-976, 1989.

Unni KK, Inwards CY, Bridge J, et al: Tumors of the Bones and Joints, 4th Series, Fascicle 2. Washington, DC, Armed Forces Institute of Pathology, 2005, pp 61-66.

Vigorita VJ: Orthopaedic Pathology. Philadelphia, Lippincott Williams & Wilkins, 1999, pp 363-367.

CHONDROMYXOID FIBROMA

Clinical Features

- Extremely rare benign tumor
- Male-to-female ratio is 1.5:1
- Most cases occur in second and third decades, 80% before the age of 40 years
- Typically occur in the metaphyses of long bones in the lower extremity; most common sites are the distal femur and proximal tibia; may also involve the pelvis or small bones of the feet
- Patients usually present with a long-term history of pain

Radiographic Features

- Eccentric, expansile, lobulated metaphyseal mass that sometimes extends to the epiphysis
- Long axis of the tumor runs parallel to the long axis of the parent bone
- Well-demarcated, completely lytic mass with scalloped margins
- Calcifications on radiographs are rare
- Pelvic tumors have a multiloculated soap-bubble appearance
- Secondary aneurysmal bone cystic changes may be present

Gross Pathology

- Sharply circumscribed, lobulated, soft, gray-white tumor, usually 3 to 8 cm in greatest dimension
- Hemorrhagic and cystic areas may be present
- Myxoid areas may be seen, but are usually not prominent

Histopathology (Figure 16-11)

- At low magnification, the tumor has a lobulated appearance
- Lobulated areas are myxoid and composed of spindled or stellate cells
- The lobules are hypocellular centrally and hypercellular at the periphery
- In the hypercellular peripheral areas, the cells have features of chondroblasts
- In about 30% of cases, bizarre cells with pleomorphic hyperchromatic nuclei are present and may suggest malignancy; however, there is no mitotic activity
- Matrix of the lobules may have chondroid or myxoid characteristics
- Lobules are separated by fibrous tissue containing vessels, multinucleated giant cells, and occasionally osteoid
- Secondary aneurysmal bone cyst changes and foci of necrosis may be seen
- Rare to absent mitotic activity
- Solid cellular areas with features of chondroblastoma may be present
- Although not seen on radiographs, calcifications are extensive histologically and interfere with appreciation of a lobular architecture
- Longstanding tumors may show hyalinization

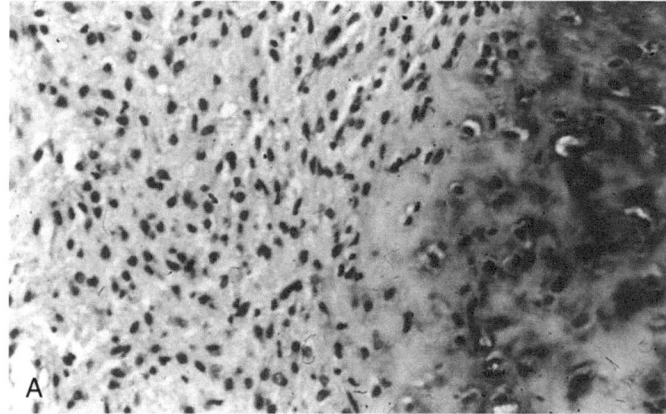
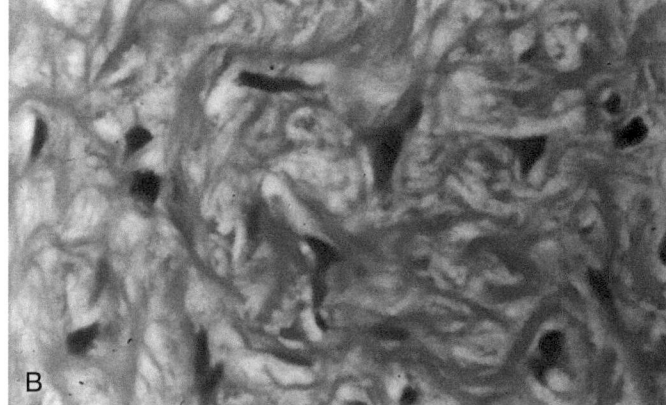

Figure 16-11. Chondromyxoid fibroma. **A,** Histologic section shows a lobulated myxoid neoplasm composed of spindle cells. **B,** Histologic section from another example of chondromyxoid fibroma shows the stellate cells in the stroma.

Special Stains and Immunohistochemistry

- S-100 protein is helpful in demonstrating the presence of chondroid differentiation
- Smooth muscle actin (SMA) and CD34 positivity can be seen in nonchondroid areas

Other Techniques for Diagnosis

- Recurrent anomalies of the long arm of chromosome 6 (6q25), in particular the pericentromeric inversion inv(6)p25q13), have been described

Differential Diagnosis

CHONDROBLASTOMA

- Typically involves the epiphyses
- Calcifications seen both radiographically and histologically (chicken-wire appearance)

MEDULLARY CHONDROSARCOMA

- Most occur in older patients and predominantly in the axial skeleton
- Radiographically, these tumors are poorly circumscribed and contain calcifications; may demonstrate cortical thickening or cortical destruction if high grade
- May cause a soft tissue mass
- Demonstrates marrow extension with chondroid tissue surrounding bony trabeculae
- High-grade tumors may mimic chondromyxoid fibroma but exhibit abundant mitotic activity not seen in the latter
- Multinucleated giant cells and aneurysmal bone cyst changes are usually not present in chondrosarcoma

PEARLS

- *Use low power to appreciate the lobulated or nodular architecture*
- *In curettage, the fibrous septa may be fragmented and go unnoticed histologically*
- *Mitotic activity is not prominent, but if present it supports a diagnosis of chondrosarcoma*

SELECTED REFERENCES

Budny AM, Ismail A, Osher L: Chondromyxoid fibroma. J Foot Ankle Surg 47:153-159, 2008.

Granter SR, Renshaw AA, Kozakewich HP, et al: The pericentromeric inversion, inv(6)(q25q13), is a novel diagnostic marker in chondromyxoid fibroma. Mod Pathol 11:1071-1074, 1998.

Rahima A, Beabout JW, Ivins JC, Dahlin DC: Chondromyxoid fibroma: a clinicopathologic study of 76 cases. Cancer 30:726-736, 1972.

Safar A, Nelson M, Neff JR, et al: Recurrent anomalies of 6q25 in chondromyxoid fibroma. Hum Pathol 31:306-311, 2000.

Unni KK, Inwards CY, Bridge J, et al: Tumors of the Bones and Joints, 4th Series, Fascicle 2. Washington, DC, Armed Forces Institute of Pathology, 2005, pp 68-72.

INTRAMEDULLARY CHONDROSARCOMA (CONVENTIONAL)

Clinical Features

- Male-to-female ratio is 1.5:1
- Usually seen in older adults; most patients are older than 50 years; rare in patients younger than 45 years
- Predilection for the trunk, with pelvis, ribs, proximal femur, and proximal humerus also affected
- Childhood tumors oftentimes involve the extremities
- Dull pain at rest that is often worse at night; symptom duration is typically several months to years

Radiographic Features

- Radiolucent mass with variable calcifications ranging from ring-shaped or punctate calcifications to markedly calcified lesions
- Cortex is thin with endosteal scalloping and erosion through the cortex
- Prominent cortical thickening, representing extension into haversian canals, may be seen
- Periosteal reaction is minimal or absent

Gross Pathology

- Nodular mass with blue-gray, glistening, translucent tissue resembling cartilage (Figure 16-12A)
- Areas of yellow calcifications at the periphery
- May have foci of necrosis, hemorrhage, or myxoid degeneration
- Presence of fleshy tissue indicates a high-grade tumor

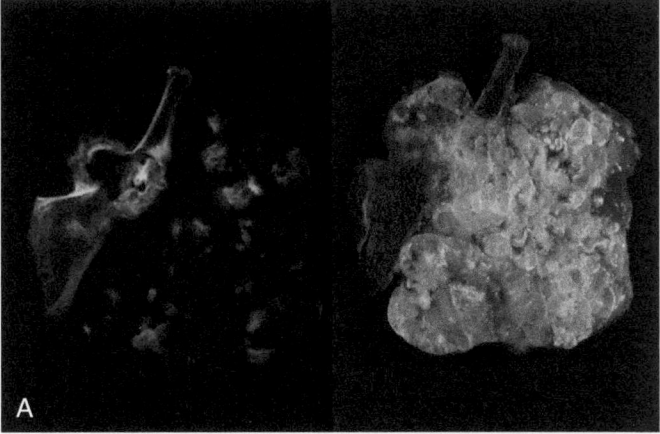

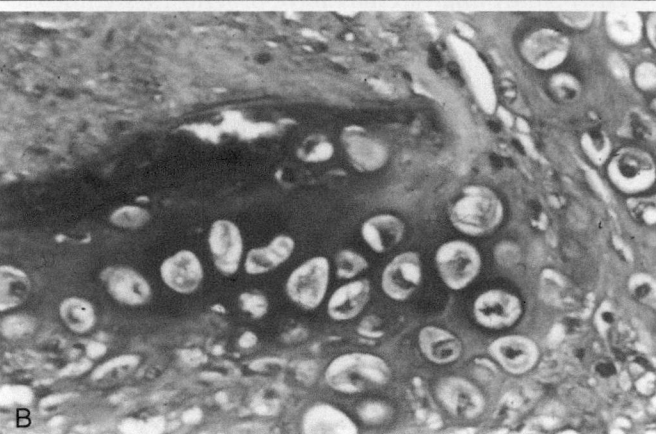

Figure 16-12. Chondrosarcoma. A, Radiograph shows a sacral mass sparsely calcified. Resected specimen shows a smooth, lobulated, gray-white, pearly tumor mass with multiple calcifications. **B,** Histologic section shows a neoplasm composed of chondrocytes with hyperchromatic nuclei and multinucleated forms.

Histopathology

- Significant histologic variation; diagnosis of low-grade tumors requires clinical and radiographic features to correlate with histology
- Large amounts of chondroid matrix with variable cellularity; no tumor osteoid
- Chondrocytes within the matrix form clusters and are swollen as a result of cytoplasmic vacuolization
- Nuclei are mildly pleomorphic, and multinucleated forms are present in variable numbers
- Cells with chondroid differentiation containing nuclei with open chromatin patterns, nucleoli, and mitoses are indicative of malignancy
- The following are criteria for grading based on cellularity and cytology
  - Grade 1: cellularity is low, chondrocytes have small, dark nuclei, and multinucleated forms are rare; no mitotic activity, small foci of necrosis
  - Grade 2: cellularity is increased mainly at the periphery of lobules, myxoid change is present, chondrocytes have more abundant cytoplasm with mildly pleomorphic nuclei, and multinucleated forms are more common; mitoses are rare, foci of necrosis are present
  - Grade 3: cellularity is increased with sparse chondroid matrix; nuclei are large and pleomorphic and contain nucleoli; mitoses are present, and necrosis may be prominent
- Features suggestive of malignancy (hypercellularity, hyperchromasia, binucleated forms, and myxoid changes) may be seen in benign chondroid processes of the hands and feet; must have clinical and radiologic data before rendering diagnosis

Special Stains and Immunohistochemistry

- S-100 protein positive in grades 1 and 2 tumors; grade 3 tumors may be negative in poorly differentiated areas

Other Techniques for Diagnosis

- DNA ploidy analysis may have prognostic significance
  - Grade 1 tumors are diploid
  - Grade 2 tumors may be diploid or aneuploid
  - Grade 3 tumors are aneuploid
  - Gains of the long arms of chromosomes 20 and 8 (20q+ and 8q+) are oftentimes seen

Differential Diagnosis

ENCHONDROMA

- Clinical and radiographic features are needed to differentiate this tumor from grade 1 chondrosarcoma
- Typically not painful
- Radiographically, tumor lacks evidence of an aggressive process (intramedullary lucent lesion without cortical destruction)
- Histologically, tumor may have features similar to those of a grade 1 chondrosarcoma
- Lobules of chondroid tissue are separated by normal hematopoietic tissue, whereas in chondrosarcoma, fibrous tissue separates lobules

FRACTURE CALLUS

- Clinical and radiographic features do not support the diagnosis of chondrosarcoma
- Composed of benign chondrocytes

CHONDROBLASTIC OSTEOSARCOMA (OSTEOSARCOMA WITH PROMINENT CHONDROBLASTIC DIFFERENTIATION)

- Careful sampling of the tumor identifies tumor osteoid
- Radiographically, this tumor exhibits features of an osteoid-producing tumor; prominent periosteal reaction and cumulus cloudlike mineralization
- Occurs in a younger age group than chondrosarcoma

PEARLS

- *Presence of endochondral ossification in a malignant chondroid neoplasm is not indicative of osteosarcoma*
- *About 90% of chondrosarcomas are grade 1 or 2*
- *Cartilaginous tumors of the hands and feet generally behave as benign lesions, whereas cartilaginous tumors of the axial skeleton are usually aggressive*
- *Pain is an important clinical feature that may be used to differentiate benign chondroid processes from malignancy*
- *Chondrosarcomas should be extensively sampled in search of tumor osteoid*
- *Generally, the smaller the amount of calcium seen on radiographs, the higher the grade*
- *Chondrosarcomas are half as common as osteosarcomas*
- *Secondary chondrosarcomas may occur in fibrous dysplasia, enchondromatosis, Maffucci syndrome, and osteochondromas*
- *Juxtacortical chondrosarcoma*
  - *Rare variant*
  - *Periosteal location and lacks tumor osteoid*
  - *May be confused with periosteal chondroma*

SELECTED REFERENCES

Duarte MP, Maldjian C, Katta US, Kenan S: Conventional intramedullary chondrosarcoma with subarticular involvement. Clin Imaging 32:69-72, 2008.

Marco RA, Gitelis S, Brebach GT, Healey JH: Cartilage tumors: evaluation and treatment. J Am Acad Orthop Surg 8:292-304, 2000.

Schiller AL: Diagnosis of borderline cartilage lesions of bone. Semin Diagn Pathol 2:42-62, 1985.

Unni KK, Inwards CY, Bridge J, et al: Tumors of the Bones and Joints, 4th Series, Fascicle 2. Washington, DC, Armed Forces Institute of Pathology, 2005, pp 73-90.

DEDIFFERENTIATED CHONDROSARCOMA

Clinical Features

- Male-to-female ratio is equal
- Most patients older than 50 years
- Femur, pelvis, and humerus are the most common sites
- Recent increase in pain associated with rapid growth is the typical presentation
- Most patients have a pathologic fracture

Radiographic Features

- Exhibits two distinct different components
  - Poorly defined lytic area with a second superimposed area of radiodensity containing calcifications characteristic of chondroid differentiation

- Lytic area is poorly demarcated and exhibits areas of cortical expansion and destruction with formation of a soft tissue mass

Gross Pathology

- As in the radiographs, there are two different components: areas of blue-gray, glistening chondroid tissue admixed with well-demarcated areas of soft, fleshy, tan-yellow tissue with hemorrhagic areas and foci of necrosis

Histopathology

- Cartilaginous component usually has features of a grade 1 chondroid neoplasm (enchondroma or grade 1 chondrosarcoma) and occasionally has features of a grade 2 chondrosarcoma (Figure 16-12B)
- Dedifferentiated component is sharply demarcated from the chondroid component, with no transition or intermediate zone
- Dedifferentiated component usually has features of malignant fibrous histiocytoma, fibrosarcoma, or osteosarcoma; rhabdomyoblastic, angiosarcomatous, and smooth muscle differentiation have also been reported (Figure 16-13)

Special Stains and Immunohistochemistry

- S-100 protein is positive in the chondroid component
- Dedifferentiated areas of the tumor may express SMA, desmin, myoglobin, CD68, or CD34, depending on dedifferentiated tissue type

Other Techniques for Diagnosis

- DNA ploidy analysis typically demonstrates a diploid cartilaginous component and an aneuploid dedifferentiated component

Differential Diagnosis

MALIGNANT FIBROUS HISTIOCYTOMA AND FIBROSARCOMA

- Lack cartilaginous component

MESENCHYMAL CHONDROSARCOMA

- Typically occurs in a younger age group and exhibits a more gradual transition between the cartilaginous

component and the undifferentiated component, and usually demonstrates hemangiopericytoma-like vascular pattern

HIGH-GRADE INTRAMEDULLARY CHONDROSARCOMA

- May contain spindle cell areas suggestive of dedifferentiated chondrosarcoma; however, there is a gradual rather than an abrupt transition between the spindle cell and the chondroid components

METASTATIC SARCOMA TO BONE (LEIOMYOSARCOMA, ANGIOSARCOMA, RHABDOMYOSARCOMA)

- Lacks cartilaginous component

PEARLS

- *Dedifferentiated chondrosarcoma is a rare tumor representing about 10% to 11% of chondrosarcomas*
- *Abrupt and sharply demarcated transition zone between the chondroid and dedifferentiated components is an important histologic feature in the diagnosis of dedifferentiated chondrosarcoma*
- *Prognosis of primary malignant fibrous histiocytoma is significantly better than prognosis for dedifferentiated chondrosarcoma exhibiting malignant fibrous histiocytoma differentiation*
- *When clinical and radiographic features are suggestive of dedifferentiated chondrosarcoma, biopsies of the tumor should include areas of calcification seen on the radiographs, which helps in the identification of the cartilaginous component*

SELECTED REFERENCES

Grimer RJ, Gosheger G, Taminiau A, et al: Dedifferentiated chondrosarcoma: prognostic factors and outcome from a European group. Eur J Cancer 43:2060-2065, 2007.

Sopta J, Dordevic A, Tulic G, Mijucic V: Dedifferentiated chondrosarcoma: our clinico-pathological experience and dilemmas in 25 cases. J Cancer Res Clin Oncol 134:147-152, 2008.

Staals EL, Bacchini P, Bertoni F: Dedifferentiated central chondrosarcoma. Cancer 15:2682-2691, 2006.

Unni KK, Inwards CY, Bridge J, et al: Tumors of the Bones and Joints, 4th Series, Fascicle 2. Washington, DC, Armed Forces Institute of Pathology, 2005, pp 91-95.

MESENCHYMAL CHONDROSARCOMA

Clinical Features

- Male-to-female ratio is equal
- Most cases occur in second and third decades; 80% of cases occur between ages 10 and 40 years (younger patient population than for conventional chondrosarcoma)
- Maxilla, mandible, ribs, vertebrae, and pelvis are the most common sites
- Pain and swelling of variable duration are typical presenting symptoms

Radiographic Features

- Presents as a lucent process with variable mineralization
- Cortical destruction and a soft tissue mass may be seen
- Features similar to those of conventional intramedullary chondrosarcoma may be exhibited

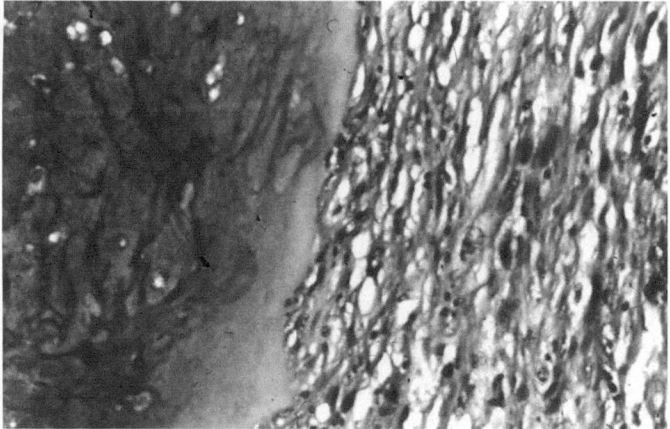

Figure 16-13. Dedifferentiated chondrosarcoma. Histologic section shows a relatively well-differentiated chondrosarcoma surrounded by highly malignant stromal cells.

Gross Pathology

- Gross features are variable
- Tumor is gray to pink and may exhibit lobulated architecture with sharp delineation from adjacent soft tissue and bone
- Foci of hemorrhage and necrosis may be present

Histopathology

- Biphasic pattern consisting of islands of cytologically benign hyaline cartilage with surrounding hypercellular areas containing small, primitive-appearing round and spindled mesenchymal cells (Figure 16-14)
- Mesenchymal cells have scant cytoplasm, mildly pleomorphic nuclei that exhibit irregular chromatin clumping, and small nucleoli; mitotic activity is variable
- Primitive cells surround delicate branching vessels, imparting a hemangiopericytoma-like appearance on low power
- The small cells may have a pattern suggestive of Ewing sarcoma/PNET or embryonal rhabdomyosarcoma, or other small round blue cell tumors
- Chondroid areas may exhibit calcification or endochondral ossification
- Transition zone between the chondroid foci and the mesenchymal component (unlike dedifferentiated chondrosarcoma, which shows an abrupt, sharp demarcation between the two components)

Special Stains and Immunohistochemistry

- S-100 protein: tissue with chondroid differentiation is positive
- Neuron-specific enolase (NSE): primitive mesenchymal cells may be focally positive (negative for S-100 protein)
- Desmin and muscle-specific actin (MSA) positive in tumors with rhabdomyoblastic differentiation
- Small cell component of tumor may express CD99
- Sox9 staining has been shown to distinguish mesenchymal chondrosarcoma from other small round blue cell tumors

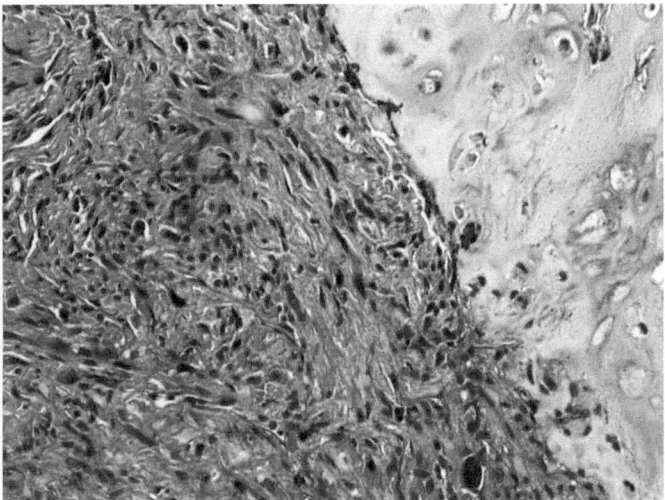

Figure 16-14. Mesenchymal chondrosarcoma. Histologic section shows a biphasic pattern consisting of islands of cartilage surrounded by cellular areas containing small, primitive-appearing mesenchymal cells arranged around blood vessels.

Modern Techniques for Diagnosis

- Cytogenetic studies: some cases show t(11;22)(q24;q12) typical of Ewing sarcoma/PNET, whereas others show t(13;21)(q10;q10)

Differential Diagnosis

DEDIFFERENTIATED CHONDROSARCOMA

- Occurs in older age group and is more likely to affect the appendicular skeleton
- Exhibits abrupt, sharp margins between the chondroid component and the dedifferentiated component; lacks hemangiopericytoma-like pattern

EWING SARCOMA/PNET

- Lacks chondroid component
- Positive for CD99 and t(11;22)(q21;q24), but some mesenchymal chondrosarcomas can also be positive for these

EMBRYONAL RHABDOMYOSARCOMA

- Lacks chondroid component
- Expresses muscle markers (desmin, actin, and myoglobin)

SOLITARY FIBROUS TUMOR (FORMERLY HEMANGIOPERICYTOMA)

- Lacks chondroid component

PEARLS

- *Rare tumor accounting for less than 2% of chondrosarcomas*
- *Biphasic histologic pattern of a chondroid component and a small primitive cell component with hemangiopericytoma-like or Ewing sarcoma/PNET patterns*
- *Should be considered in patients with malignant biomorphic cartilaginous tumors arising in the mandible or maxilla*

SELECTED REFERENCES

Dantonello TM, Int-Veen C, Leuschner I, et al: Mesenchymal chondrosarcoma of soft tissues and bone in children, adolescents, and young adults: experiences of the CWS and COSS study groups. Cancer 112:2424-2431, 2008.
Hameed M: Small round cell tumors of bone. Arch Pathol Lab Med 131:192-204, 2007.
Naumann S, Krallman PA, Unni KK, et al: Translocation der(13;21)(q10;q10) in skeletal and extraskeletal mesenchymal chondrosarcoma. Mod Pathol 15:572-576, 2002.
Pellitteri PK, Ferlito A, Fagan JJ, et al: Mesenchymal chondrosarcoma of the head and neck. Oral Oncol 43:970-975, 2007.
Unni KK, Inwards CY, Bridge J, et al: Tumors of the Bones and Joints, 4th Series, Fascicle 2. Washington, DC, Armed Forces Institute of Pathology, 2005, pp 99-104.
Wehrli BM, Huang W, De Crombrugghe B, et al: Sox9, a master regulator of chondrogenesis, distinguishes mesenchymal chondrosarcoma from other small blue round cell tumors. Hum Pathol 34:263-269, 2003.

CLEAR CELL CHONDROSARCOMA

Clinical Features

- Male-to-female ratio is about 2:1
- Most tumors occur in third and fourth decades
- Predilection for the epiphyses
- More than 50% of these tumors arise in the proximal femur; other common sites include proximal humerus and distal femur

- Pain of variable duration is the usual presentation; range of motion in the adjacent joint may be limited
- May represent malignant counterpart of chondroblastoma
- Relatively low-grade behavior

Radiographic Features

- Typically presents as a lytic lesion in the epiphysis that is sharply demarcated and contains a sclerotic rim
- Cortical expansion may be seen, but the cortex is usually intact
- Secondary aneurysmal bone cyst formation may be present

Gross Pathology

- Soft, gray to red tumor that may contain foci of yellow calcification
- Well circumscribed and may contain foci of hemorrhage and cystic change
- Elements of chondroid tissue may be difficult to identify grossly

Histopathology

- May have a lobular architecture at low power
- Consists of a cellular proliferation of large cells with abundant clear cytoplasm embedded in chondroid matrix (Figure 16-15)
- Cell borders of the clear cells are usually distinct; nuclei are not pleomorphic and contain vesicular chromatin patterns and prominent nucleoli
- Mitotic rate is low
- Multinucleated giant cells may be present
- Scattered bony trabeculae or woven bone is present in the matrix
- May have areas of conventional chondrosarcoma (50% of cases)

Special Stains and Immunohistochemistry

- S-100 protein: clear cells are strongly positive
- Periodic acid-Schiff (PAS) stain: positive in the clear cells (glycogen)

Modern Techniques for Diagnosis

- Noncontributory

Differential Diagnosis

CHONDROBLASTOMA

- Lacks prominent clear cells and bony trabeculae

OSTEOBLASTOMA

- Lacks chondroid differentiation

ANEURYSMAL BONE CYST

- Clear cells and cartilaginous differentiation are absent

INTRAMEDULLARY CHONDROSARCOMA

- Multinucleated giant cells and reactive bony trabeculae are absent within the malignant cartilage

METASTATIC RENAL CELL CARCINOMA

- Clear cells in renal cell carcinoma are positive for vimentin and cytokeratin; typically negative for S-100 protein; however, staining may be variable
- Metastatic renal cell carcinoma has a prominent delicate vascular background surrounding clear cells

PEARLS

- *Three common epiphyseal tumors include giant cell tumor, clear cell chondrosarcoma, and chondroblastoma*
- *May mimic chondroblastoma clinically and radiographically; however, histologically, chondroblastoma lacks prominent clear cells and bony trabeculae*
- *Rare tumor accounting for about 5% of chondrosarcomas*

SELECTED REFERENCES

Bjornsson J, Unni KK, Dahlin DC, et al: Clear cell chondrosarcoma of bone: observations in 47 cases. Am J Surg Pathol 8:223-230, 1984.

Donati D, Yin JQ, Colangeli M, et al: Clear cell chondrosarcoma of bone: long time follow-up of 18 cases. Arch Orthop Trauma Surg 128:137-142, 2008.

Unni KK, Inwards CY, Bridge J, et al: Tumors of the Bones and Joints, 4th Series, Fascicle 2. Washington, DC, Armed Forces Institute of Pathology, 2005, pp 104-108.

VASCULAR TUMORS

HEMANGIOMA

Clinical Features

- Most common vascular tumor of bone
- Male-to-female ratio is about 1:1.5
- Most cases diagnosed between fourth and sixth decades
- Most common sites are craniofacial bones (calvarium) and vertebrae
- Often asymptomatic; if symptomatic, pain and swelling are most common complaints
- May produce neurologic deficits such as facial nerve paralysis (temporal bone) and signs of nerve root and spinal cord compression (vertebral); symptoms of vertebral tumors may be accentuated in women during pregnancy
- Sacral hemangiomas in infants are associated with congenital anomalies elsewhere

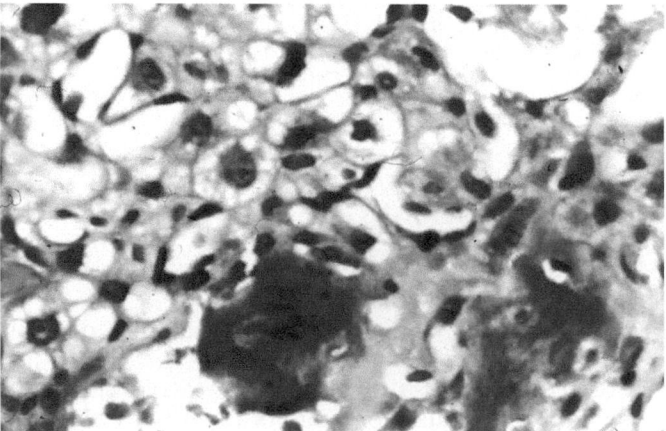

Figure 16-15. Clear cell chondrosarcoma. High-power view shows large cells with abundant clear cytoplasm embedded in a chondroid matrix and scattered foci of osteoid.

Radiographic Features

- Calvarium tumors are lytic and exhibit a sunburst pattern of reactive bone; bulging of the inner and outer tables (outer greater than inner)
- Multiple tumors may be present
- Vertebral tumors present as intramedullary lytic masses with vertical striations ("corduroy cloth"); CT scan of vertebra demonstrates characteristic polka-dot pattern (striations in cross section)

Gross Pathology

- Well-demarcated, intramedullary mass
- Red and spongy with bony trabeculae ("currant jelly" cut surface)

Histopathology

- Composed of a proliferation of delicate, thin-walled vessels lined by flat endothelial cells without atypia (Figure 16-16)
- Most tumors are of cavernous type or mixed cavernous and capillary
- Pure capillary hemangiomas of bone are rare
- Secondary changes may complicate the diagnosis of these tumors
  - Thrombosis of hemangiomas may result in the development of papillary endothelial hyperplasia (so-called Masson tumor), which could cause confusion with angiosarcoma
  - Endothelial cells can undergo epithelioid change, which could lead to a misdiagnosis of epithelioid hemangioendothelioma

Special Stains and Immunohistochemistry

- Vascular endothelial cells express CD31, factor VIII, and CD34
- Also express ERG, a recently characterized endothelial transcription factor (nuclear stain) that is expressed in benign vascular tumors and almost all angiosarcomas and epithelioid hemangioendotheliomas
- ERG is also expressed in other tumors with ERG gene rearrangements such as prostate adenocarcinomas (50%), Ewing sarcoma/PNET (5% to 10%), and some acute myeloid leukemias

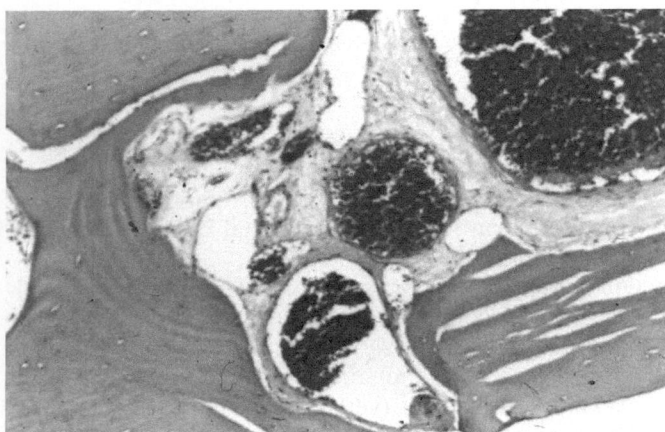

Figure 16-16. Hemangioma. Histologic section shows delicate, thin-walled vessels.

Other Techniques for Diagnosis

- Noncontributory

Differential Diagnosis

EPITHELIOID HEMANGIOENDOTHELIOMA

- Exhibits solid nests of epithelioid endothelial cells that form narrow anastomosing vascular channels

ANGIOSARCOMA

- Composed of vascular spaces lined by atypical endothelial cells that bridge across vascular lumina or form endothelial tufts

PEARLS

- *Only rarely do these tumors become symptomatic*
- *Secondary changes (thrombosis, papillary endothelial hyperplasia, and reactive epithelioid endothelial cells) can be confusing but should still permit the diagnosis of hemangioma*
- *Cystic angiomatosis is a rare condition that includes multiple hemangiomas (predominantly cavernous) of the skeleton, soft tissue, and internal organs (spleen, lung, and liver)*
- *Massive osteolysis (phantom bone disease, Gorham disease) is a rare type of aggressive angiomatosis affecting predominantly trunk bones in children and young adults*
- *Hemangiomas (sometimes lymphangiomas) within bone exhibit osteoclastic reabsorption of trabecular bone at the periphery of the tumor*
- *Extensive involvement of ribs may rarely lead to pulmonary dysfunction and death*

SELECTED REFERENCES

Acosta FL Jr, Sanai N, Chi JH, et al: Comprehensive management of symptomatic and aggressive vertebral hemangiomas. Neurosurg Clin N Am 19:17-29, 2008.

López-Gutiérrez JC, Garcia-Miguel P: Skeletal hemangiomas and vascular malformations. J Pediatr Hematol Oncol 28:634, 2006.

McKay KM, Doyle LA, Lazar AJ, et al: Expression of ERG, an Ets family transcription factor, distinguishes cutaneous angiosarcoma from histiocytic mimics. Histopathology 61:989-991, 2012.

Miettinen M, Wang ZF, Paetau A, et al: ERG transcription factor as an immunohistochemical marker for vascular endothelial tumors and prostatic carcinoma. Am J Surg Pathol 35:432-441, 2011.

Unni KK, Inwards CY, Bridge J, et al: Tumors of the Bones and Joints, 4th Series, Fascicle 2. Washington, DC, Armed Forces Institute of Pathology, 2005, pp 261-264.

Wang WL, Patel NR, Caragea M, et al: Expression of ERG, an Ets family transcription factor, identifies ERG-rearranged Ewing sarcoma. Mod Pathol 25:1378-1383, 2012.

EPITHELIOID HEMANGIOENDOTHELIOMA

Clinical Features

- Male-to-female ratio is about 3.5:1
- Most frequently occurs in second and third decades, but has wide age range
- Most common sites are the lower extremities, axial skeleton, and skull; most tumors are multifocal within the same bone
- Multicentricity has been reported in 50% to 66% of cases

- Synchronous tumors in paired bones (tibia and fibula) is common
- Patients typically present with pain; may have pathologic fractures

Radiographic Features

- Radiographic features are not specific
- Appears as a well-demarcated, lytic lesion with variable peripheral sclerosis
- May see expansion of the bone, cortical erosion, or cortical disruption

Gross Pathology

- Well-demarcated mass with irregular, scalloped peripheral margins
- Soft and bright-red with a hemorrhagic appearance

Histopathology

- Cords and nests of relatively large epithelioid cells that form irregular anastomosing vessels (Figure 16-17)
- Cells are round to polygonal with bland, round nuclei containing small nucleoli and eosinophilic to amphophilic cytoplasm
- Some cells contain intracytoplasmic vacuoles representing primitive vascular lumina; erythrocytes may be present in these vacuoles
- Vacuolization may give the appearance of signet ring cells
- Mitotic activity is rare to absent
- Mixed inflammatory infiltrate is often present, composed of variable numbers of eosinophils, plasma cells, and lymphocytes; sometimes eosinophils predominate
- Foci of myxoid stroma or chondroid-like matrix may be seen

Special Stains and Immunohistochemistry

- Vacuoles are negative for mucin and PAS stains
- Epithelioid cells variably express CD31, CD34, and factor VIII–related antigen
- Some tumors are positive for epithelial membrane antigen (EMA) and cytokeratin (low molecular weight)
- Also express ERG, a recently characterized endothelial transcription factor (nuclear stain) that is expressed in benign vascular tumors and almost all angiosarcomas and epithelioid hemangioendotheliomas
- ERG is also expressed in other tumors with ERG gene rearrangements such as prostate adenocarcinomas (50%), Ewing sarcoma/PNET (5% to 10%), and some acute myeloid leukemias

Other Techniques for Diagnosis

- Noncontributory

Differential Diagnosis

ANGIOSARCOMA

- Exhibits pleomorphic endothelial cells that bridge across lumina or create intraluminal buds
- Prominent mitotic activity

METASTATIC CARCINOMA

- Clinical history is important
- Negative for vascular markers
- Expression of high-molecular-weight cytokeratin
- Immunostains specific to tumor of origin—that is, prostate-specific antigen (prostate) or thyroid transcription factor-1 (lung)

PEARLS

- *In biopsy samples, chondroid-like matrix with myxoid stroma may suggest that the tumor is of cartilaginous differentiation; however, these areas will not express S-100 protein and will be variably positive for endothelial cell markers*
- *Considered an indolent, low-grade malignant vascular tumor*

SELECTED REFERENCES

Bruegel M, Waldt S, Weirich G, et al: Multifocal epithelioid hemangioendothelioma of the phalanges of the hand. Skeletal Radiol 35:787-792, 2006.

Evans HL, Raymond AK, Ayala AG: Vascular tumors of bone: a study of 17 cases other than ordinary hemangioma, with an evaluation of the relationship of hemangioendothelioma of bone to epithelioid hemangioma, epithelioid hemangio-endothelioma and high-grade angiosarcoma. Hum Pathol 34:680-689, 2003.

McKay KM, Doyle LA, Lazar AJ, et al: Expression of ERG, an Ets family transcription factor, distinguishes cutaneous angiosarcoma from histiocytic mimics. Histopathology 61:989-991, 2012.

Unni KK, Inwards CY, Bridge J, et al: Tumors of the Bones and Joints, 4th Series, Fascicle 2. Washington, DC, Armed Forces Institute of Pathology, 2005, pp 273-276.

Yaskiv O, Rubin BP, He H, et al: ERG protein expression in human tumors detected with a rabbit monoclonal antibody. Am J Clin Pathol 138:803-810, 2012.

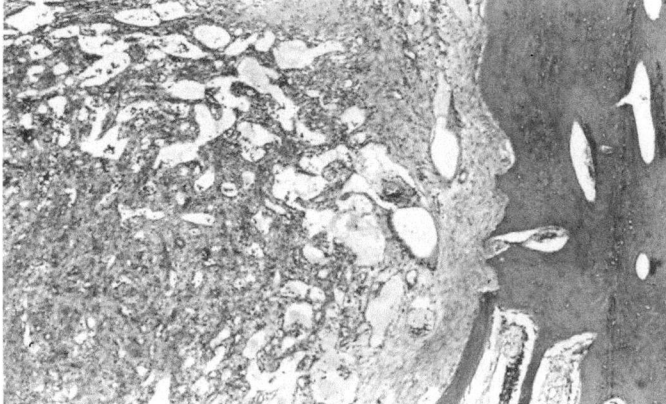

Figure 16-17. Epithelioid hemangioendothelioma. Histologic section shows a neoplasm composed of cords and nests of epithelioid cells forming irregular vascular channels.

SOLITARY FIBROUS TUMOR (FORMERLY HEMANGIOPERICYTOMA)

Clinical Features

- All tumors formerly referred to as hemangiopericytomas are now considered solitary fibrous tumors (hemangiopericytoma=solitary fibrous tumor)
- Male-to-female ratio is 1:1
- Wide variation in age; most occur in fourth and fifth decades

- Pelvis (innominate bone), lower extremities, vertebrae, and mandible are the most common sites
- Usually presents with pain of variable duration
- May be associated with osteomalacia

Radiographic Findings

- Nonspecific radiographic findings
- Consists of an intramedullary lytic mass with variable sharp to ill-defined margins
- Cortical disruption with extension into soft tissue may be seen

Gross Pathology

- Curettage reveals tan to gray, firm tissue

Histopathology

- Solid areas of spindle cells surrounding delicate branching vascular structures lined by benign endothelial cells (Figure 16-18)
- Vascular structures create a deer antler or staghorn pattern ("hemangiopericytoma-like" vascular pattern)
- Variable nuclear atypia, mitotic activity, and necrosis
- Tumors may be graded based on cellularity, presence of nucleoli, nuclear chromatin pattern, mitotic activity, and degree of deer antler pattern
- Most reliable predictor of malignancy: mitotic activity > 4 per 10 high-power fields (HPF)

Special Stains and Immunohistochemistry

- At least variable CD34 is seen in about 95% of cases; however, this is not a specific marker
- Studies have shown that nuclear STAT6 staining is specific for solitary fibrous tumor, which stems from the presence of NAB2-STAT6 fusion gene, a consistent genetic rearrangement discovered in solitary fibrous tumors
- Can also be positive for CD99 and vimentin
- Reticulin stain highlights reticulin fibers surrounding individual pericytes

Other Techniques for Diagnosis

- Cytogenetics/molecular: 12q13 alteration leads to NAB2-STAT6 fusion gene

- The NAB2 and STAT6 genes are both on chromosome 12q13 and are in such close proximity that conventional fluorescence in situ hybridization (FISH) techniques are not useful
- Immunohistochemistry for nuclear STAT6 is currently the best means of detecting the NAB2-STAT6 fusion

Differential Diagnosis

- Diagnosis of solitary fibrous tumor of bone is one of exclusion
  - Metastatic solitary fibrous tumor from a soft tissue primary must be ruled out
  - Other tumors, both primary tumors and metastatic tumors to bone with hemangiopericytoma-like vascular pattern, including mesenchymal chondrosarcoma, small cell osteosarcoma, malignant fibrous histiocytoma, synovial sarcoma, gastrointestinal stromal tumors, and angioblastic meningioma, must be excluded

PEARLS

- *All tumors formerly referred to as hemangiopericytomas are now considered solitary fibrous tumors*
- *Extremely rare bone neoplasm*
- *Diagnosis is one of exclusion*
- *Biologic behavior is difficult to predict but has malignant potential*

SELECTED REFERENCES

Chmielecki J, Crago AM, Rosenberg M, et al: Whole-exome sequencing identified a recurrent NAB2-STAT6 fusion in solitary fibrous tumors. Nat Genet 45:131-132, 2013.

Mohajeri A, Tayebwa J, Collin A, et al: Comprehensive genetic analysis identifies a pathognomonic NAB2/STAT6 fusion gene, nonrandom secondary genomic imbalances, and a characteristic gene expression profile in solitary fibrous tumor. Genes Chromosomes Cancer 52:873-886, 2013.

Robinson DR, Wu YM, Kalyana-Sundaram S, et al: Identification of recurrent NAB2-STAT6 gene fusions in solitary fibrous tumor by integrative sequencing. Nat Genet 45:180-185, 2013.

Schweizer L, Koelsche C, Sahm F, et al: Meningeal hemangiopericytoma and solitary fibrous tumor carry the NAB2-STAT6 fusion protein and can be diagnosed by nuclear expression of STAT6 protein. Acta Neuropathol 125:651-658, 2013.

Unni KK, Inwards CY, Bridge J, et al: Tumors of the Bones and Joints, 4th Series, Fascicle 2. Washington, DC, Armed Forces Institute of Pathology, 2005, pp 276-278.

ANGIOSARCOMA

Clinical Features

- Male-to-female ratio is about 1.5:1
- Occurs in all age groups but rare in patients younger than 30 years
- Most occur in femur, tibia, and humerus; pelvic bones, vertebrae, and ribs are also common sites
- Can present as multicentric tumors, particularly in bones of the lower extremities
- Pain of several months' duration is a typical symptom
- May occur in association with previous bone infarct, chronic osteomyelitis, and radiation exposure
- Distant metastases not uncommon; usually to lung

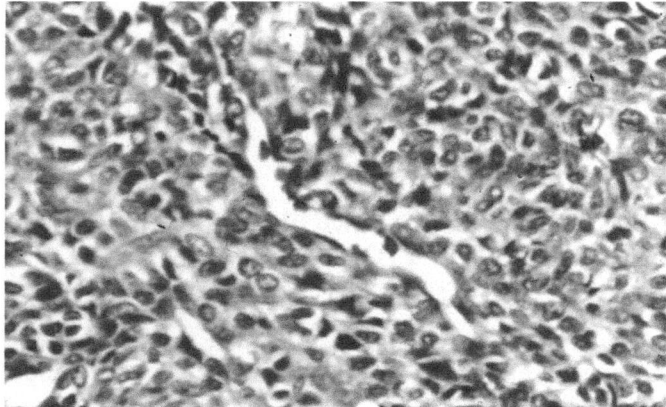

Figure 16-18. Solitary fibrous tumor (formerly hemangiopericytoma). Histologic section shows solid areas of spindle cells surrounded by delicate, branching vascular structures.

Radiographic Features

- Radiographic features are nonspecific
- Presents as a lytic mass with ill-defined borders and little reactive new bone formation
- Cortical erosion and soft tissue extension may be seen
- May be multifocal

Gross Pathology

- Consists of spongy, bloody red tissue containing foci of trabecular bone
- May have solid areas with necrosis

Histopathology

- Only intermediate- and high-grade tumors are considered angiosarcomas
- Tumors contain irregularly shaped vascular structures lined by endothelial cells containing pleomorphic, hyperchromatic nuclei (Figure 16-19)
- Mitotic figures are readily found
- Malignant endothelial cells may be stratified and create intraluminal tufts or papillae; may exhibit epithelioid or histiocytic morphology
- In poorly differentiated tumors, the malignant endothelial cells are closely packed, and the vascular pattern may not be well appreciated
- Necrosis and hemorrhage are not uncommonly seen

Special Stains and Immunohistochemistry

- Reticulin stain highlights endothelial pattern by demonstrating clusters of cells surrounded by a network of reticulin
- CD31, CD34, and factor VIII–related antigen: endothelial cells are positive
- Cytokeratin typically negative; epithelioid angiosarcoma may express cytokeratin
- ERG, a recently characterized endothelial transcription factor (nuclear stain) that is expressed in benign vascular tumors and almost all angiosarcomas and epithelioid hemangioendotheliomas

Other Techniques for Diagnosis

- Noncontributory

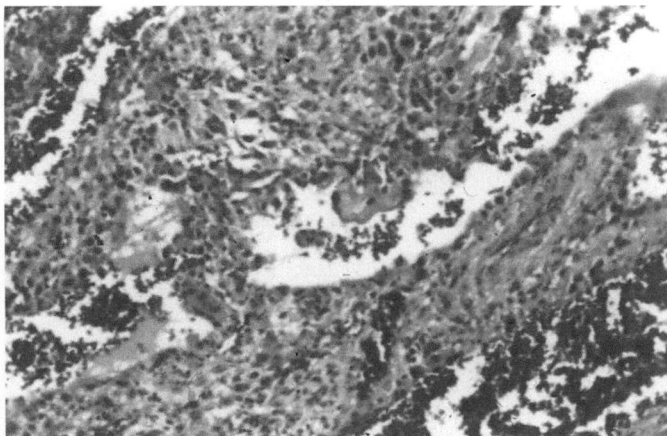

Figure 16-19. Angiosarcoma. Histologic section shows a neoplasm composed of irregular vascular channels.

Differential Diagnosis

EPITHELIOID HEMANGIOENDOTHELIOMA

- Lacks nuclear features of malignancy
- Does not exhibit vascular intraluminal tufting, stratification, or bridging of malignant endothelial cells

METASTATIC CARCINOMA

- Lacks vascular marker expression and shows positivity for epithelial markers

PEARLS

- *Rare tumor that may be seen in association with a previous history of radiation exposure, chronic osteomyelitis, and bone infarcts*

SELECTED REFERENCES

Abraham JA, Hornicek FJ, Kaufman AM, et al: Treatment and outcome of 82 patients with angiosarcoma. Ann Surg Oncol 14:1953-1967, 2007.

McKay KM, Doyle LA, Lazar AJ, et al: Expression of ERG, an Ets family transcription factor, distinguishes cutaneous angiosarcoma from histiocytic mimics. Histopathology 61:989-991, 2012.

Miettinen M, Wang ZF, Paetau A, et al: ERG transcription factor as an immunohistochemical marker for vascular endothelial tumors and prostatic carcinoma. Am J Surg Pathol 35:432-441, 2011.

Unni KK, Inwards CY, Bridge J, et al: Tumors of the Bones and Joints, 4th Series, Fascicle 2. Washington, DC, Armed Forces Institute of Pathology, 2005, pp 266-273.

FIBRO-OSSEOUS, HISTIOCYTIC, AND GIANT CELL LESIONS

FIBROUS DYSPLASIA

Clinical Features

- Believed to be a developmental non-neoplastic disorder of bone forming mesenchyme with maturation arrest at the woven bone stage
- Male-to-female ratio is about equal
- Three fourths of tumors diagnosed before age 30 years
- In monostotic form, the most common sites of involvement are craniofacial bones, femur, tibia, and ribs
- In polyostotic form, the most common sites are femur, tibia, and pelvis
- Symptoms are variable, depending on whether disease is monostotic or polyostotic and on location of lesions; many lesions are asymptomatic
- In polyostotic disease, symptoms usually develop in childhood with pain and recurrent fractures
- Polyostotic form may also present with café-au-lait skin lesions, hyperfunctioning endocrinopathies such as precocious puberty and hyperthyroidism, and soft tissue myxomas
- Other symptoms are as follows
  - Craniofacial bones: facial deformities
  - Long bones: recurrent fractures with shepherd's crook deformity
  - Lesions of the ribs, which are usually asymptomatic

Radiographic Features

- Radiographic features are variable
- Typically an intramedullary metaphyseal or diaphyseal lytic lesion; ground-glass appearance

- Usually symmetrically centered in the medullary canal exhibiting cortical expansion
- If there is cartilaginous differentiation, ringlike and punctate calcifications may be present
- Shepherd's crook deformity may be seen

Gross Pathology

- Intramedullary gritty, gray mass that expands the cortex
- If there is any cartilaginous differentiation, tumor may contain bluish-gray translucent nodules
- May exhibit hemorrhagic foci and cystic regions containing yellow serous fluid

Histopathology

- Spindle cell proliferation with immature woven bone lacking a rim of osteoblasts (maturation arrest)
- Variably cellular tumor composed of fibroblastic, benign spindle cells arranged in a storiform pattern and a variable amount of fibrocollagenous stroma
- Immature woven bone is represented by trabeculae that are thin and irregularly curved, resembling Chinese letters (Figure 16-20)
  - Lacks osteoblastic rimming
  - May undergo mineralization, and in some cases the mineralization forms concentric, laminated bodies reminiscent of cementoid bodies; when prominent, the process has been called *fibrous cementoma* or *cementomatous variant of fibrous dysplasia*
- At the periphery of the tumor adjacent to uninvolved bone is a margin of reactive bone with osteoblastic rimming (this should not inhibit the diagnosis of fibrous dysplasia)
- Foci of cartilaginous differentiation are common in fibrous dysplasia; if prominent, the diagnosis should be fibrocartilaginous dysplasia
- Other features include myxoid stroma, giant cell reaction, prominent foamy histiocytes, and secondary aneurysmal bone cystic changes; more common in rib lesions

Special Stains and Immunohistochemistry

- Noncontributory

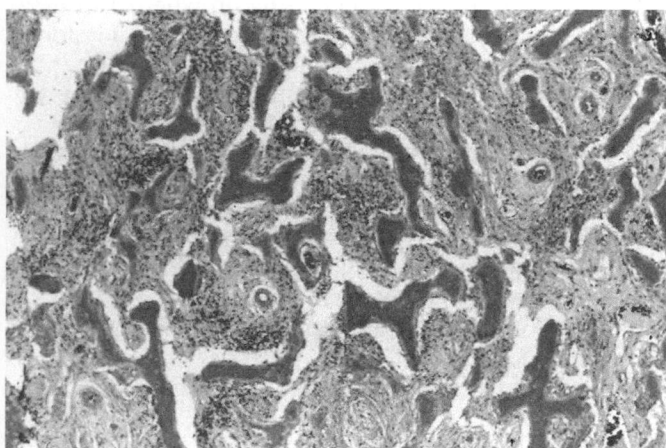

Figure 16-20. Fibrous dysplasia. Histologic section shows immature woven bone composed of thin and irregularly curved trabeculae surrounded by fibroblastic stroma.

Other Techniques for Diagnosis

- *GNAS1* mutations are seen in many cases of fibrous dysplasia and are a specific finding when compared to other fibro-osseus lesions

Differential Diagnosis

OSTEOFIBROUS DYSPLASIA

- Almost universally involves the tibia
- Occurs in younger children
- Cortical location
- Bony trabeculae with osteoblastic rimming
- No *GNAS1* mutations

DESMOPLASTIC FIBROMA

- May be considered in a small biopsy that does not have woven bone (these tumors do not contain woven bone)
- No *GNAS1* mutations

LOW-GRADE INTRAMEDULLARY OSTEOSARCOMA

- Spindle cells in the fibrous stroma are larger and have pleomorphic nuclei with chromatin clumping

PEARLS

- *About 90% of cases of fibrous dysplasia are of the monostotic form*
- *Fibrous dysplasia is a medullary process; rarely it may form an exophytic mass that is attached to or grows on the surface of the bone (fibrous dysplasia protuberans)*
- *In small biopsies, a misdiagnosis of desmoplastic fibroma may be made if no woven bone is present*
- *Presence of woven bone with osteoblastic rimming (reactive bone) at the periphery of the process should not interfere with making the diagnosis of fibrous dysplasia*
- *Regressed lesions of monostotic fibrous dysplasia in females may become reactivated during pregnancy*
- *McCune-Albright syndrome consists of polyostotic fibrous dysplasia and hyperfunctional endocrinopathies such as precocious puberty and hyperthyroidism; patients have café-au-lait skin lesions (irregular borders, said to resemble the coast of Maine)*
- *Cherubism is a variant of fibrous dysplasia that primarily affects the jaws; contains prominent giant cells and causes facial deformities*
- *Mazabraud syndrome consists of polyostotic fibrous dysplasia and soft tissue myxomas*
- *Fibrosarcoma, osteosarcoma, chondrosarcoma, and malignant fibrous histiocytoma can arise as a complication of fibrous dysplasia either de novo or after radiation*

SELECTED REFERENCES

Orcel, P, Chapurlat R: Fibrous dysplasia of bone. Rev Prat 57:1749-1755, 2007.

Riminucci M, Robey PG, Bianco P: The pathology of fibrous dysplasia and the McCune-Albright syndrome. Pediatr Endocrinol Rev 4(suppl 4):401-411, 2007.

Shi RR, Li XF, Zhang R, et al: GNAS mutational analysis in differentiating fibrous dysplasia and ossifying fibroma of the jaw. Mod Pathol 26:1023-1031, 2013.

Tabareau-Delalande F, Collin C, Gomez-Brouchet A, et al: Diagnostic value of investigating GNAS mutations in fibro-osseous lesions: a retrospective study of 91 cases of fibrous dysplasia and 40 other fibro-osseous lesions. Mod Pathol 26:911-921, 2013.

Unni KK, Inwards CY, Bridge J, et al: Tumors of the Bones and Joints, 4th Series, Fascicle 2. Washington, DC, Armed Forces Institute of Pathology, 2005, pp 337-343.

OSTEOFIBROUS DYSPLASIA (OSSIFYING FIBROMA OF LONG BONES)

Clinical Features

- Male-to-female ratio is about 1.5:1
- Most cases diagnosed before age 5 years
- Found exclusively in the tibia and fibula, typically on anterior surfaces
- Usually presents as a painless area of swelling on the anterior surface of the distal lower extremity; may cause anterior or anterolateral bowing of the area or presents as a pathologic fracture

Radiographic Features

- Characteristic features consist of an anterior cortical lucent lesion of the tibial diaphysis that does not involve the medullary canal
- Inner cortical margin may exhibit reactive features
- Anterior bowing may be seen
- May see additional lytic lesions with similar features in the tibia or fibula

Gross Pathology

- Resected lesions consist of an anterior intracortical, soft, sometimes gritty fibrous mass

Histopathology

- Fibroblastic spindle cells with benign cytologic features; may be loosely arranged or may have a storiform architecture (Figure 16-21)
- Bony trabeculae rimmed with osteoblasts exhibit zonal maturation with central immature, thin forms maturing peripherally to thickened mineralized lamellar bone
- Rare cytokeratin positive cells may be seen in the stroma, but nests of epithelial cells are not present
- May have myxomatous stroma, cystic changes, hemorrhage, and aggregates of multinucleated giant cells

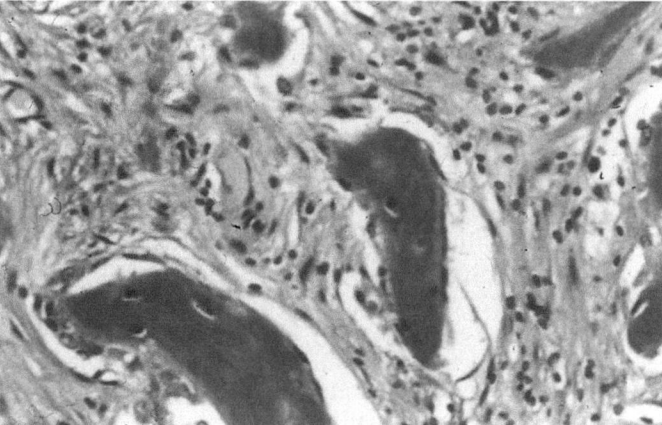

Figure 16-21. Osteofibrous dysplasia. High-power view shows loosely cellular fibroblastic stroma containing bony trabeculae rimmed with osteoblasts.

Special Stains and Immunohistochemistry

- Cytokeratin: rare positive cells may be present within the stroma (not seen in fibrous dysplasia); does not warrant the diagnosis of adamantinoma (believed to be a process closely related to osteofibrous dysplasia)

Other Techniques for Diagnosis

- Noncontributory

Differential Diagnosis

FIBROUS DYSPLASIA

- Occurs in older patients and does not exhibit osteoblastic rimming of osteoid; no bone maturation
- Fibrous dysplasia can have *GNAS1* mutations

ADAMANTINOMA

- Typically occurs in an older age group
- Contains epithelial islands within the stroma that are cytokeratin positive

WELL-DIFFERENTIATED INTRAMEDULLARY OSTEOSARCOMA

- Intramedullary neoplasm
- Spindle cell stroma of this tumor has pleomorphic cells with atypical nuclei with clumped chromatin

PEARLS

- *Osteofibrous dysplasia may be a precursor lesion of adamantinoma*
- *No reported cases of malignant transformation of osteofibrous dysplasia*

SELECTED REFERENCES

Gleason BC, Liegl-Atzwanger B, Kozakewich HP, et al: Osteofibrous dysplasia and adamantinoma in children and adolescents: a clinicopathologic reappraisal. Am J Surg Pathol 32:363-376, 2008.

Grimer RJ, Carter SR, Tillman RM, Abudu A: Osteofibrous dysplasia of the tibia. J Bone Joint Surg Br 89:141, 2007.

Unni KK, Inwards CY, Bridge J, et al: Tumors of the Bones and Joints, 4th Series, Fascicle 2. Washington, DC, Armed Forces Institute of Pathology, 2005, pp 343-345.

Vigorita VJ: Orthopaedic Pathology. Philadelphia, Lippincott Williams & Wilkins, 1999, pp 307-308.

NONOSSIFYING FIBROMA (FIBROUS CORTICAL DEFECT, METAPHYSEAL FIBROUS DEFECT)

Clinical Features

- Male-to-female ratio about 1:1
- Peak incidence in second decade
- Distal femur, proximal tibia, and distal tibia are the most common sites
- Usually asymptomatic and found incidentally on radiographs done for other reasons
- Larger lesions may present with pain or pathologic fractures

Radiographic Features

- Eccentric metaphyseal cortical lytic lesions with well-defined sclerotic margins

- Typically no mineralization except when it is resolving (density of calcification increases)

Gross Pathology

- Curettage produces soft and yellow to tan tissue depending on quantity of foamy histiocytes
- Resected lesions are well-demarcated, eccentric cortical fibrous masses that may be yellow to tan depending on quantity of foamy histiocytes
- Areas of necrosis, hemorrhage, or cystic changes may be present

Histopathology

- Cellular fibroblastic stroma that sometimes exhibits a storiform pattern (Figure 16-22)
- Variable numbers of xanthoma cells, siderophages, and multinucleated giant cells
- Occasional normal mitotic figures
- Hemorrhage with giant cell reaction and cystic changes similar to aneurysmal bone cyst
- Foci of necrosis or reactive bone formation

Special Stains and Immunohistochemistry

- Noncontributory

Other Techniques for Diagnosis

- Noncontributory

Differential Diagnosis

GIANT CELL TUMOR

- Occurs in skeletally mature patients
- Located in the epiphysis

DESMOPLASTIC FIBROMA

- Exhibits dense collagenous stroma

FIBROUS DYSPLASIA

- Usually does not exhibit reactive bone with osteoblastic rimming of osteoid and lacks multinucleated giant cells
- Fibrous dysplasia can have *GNAS1* mutations

BENIGN FIBROUS HISTIOCYTOMA

- Histologically, this tumor is identical to nonossifying fibroma

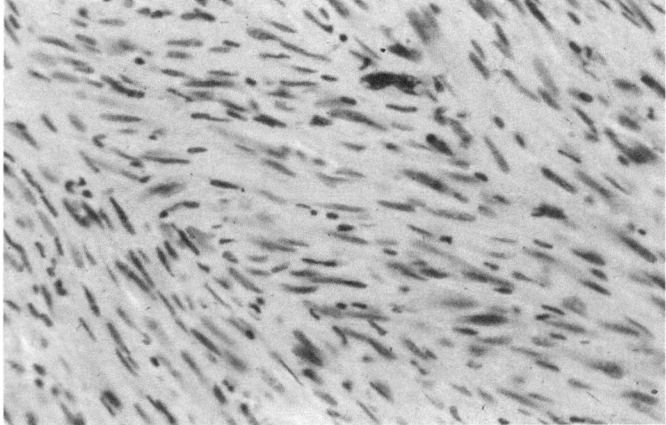

Figure 16-22. Nonossifying fibroma. Histologic section shows a cellular fibroblastic proliferation with a vague storiform pattern.

- *Benign fibrous histiocytoma* is the term used when the features of nonossifying fibroma are found in ribs, vertebrae, or flat bones

PEARLS

- *Most cases of nonossifying fibroma are asymptomatic and are treated only if large enough to become symptomatic*
- *Multifocal nonossifying fibromas may occur in neurofibromatosis and Jaffe-Campanacci syndrome (multifocal nonossifying fibroma, café-au-lait pigmentation, mental retardation, and nonskeletal anomalies)*
- *Presence of necrosis and mitotic activity with typical forms is not indicative of an aggressive process*

SELECTED REFERENCES

Betsy M, Kupersmith LM, Springfield DS: Metaphyseal fibrous defects. J Am Acad Orthop Surg 12:89-95, 2004.
Biermann JS: Common benign lesions of bone in children and adolescents. J Pediatr Orthop 22:268-273, 2002.
Unni KK, Inwards CY, Bridge J, et al: Tumors of the Bones and Joints, 4th Series, Fascicle 2. Washington, DC, Armed Forces Institute of Pathology, 2005, pp 334-336.

DESMOPLASTIC FIBROMA

Clinical Features

- Male-to-female ratio is about equal
- Most cases occur in second decade
- Most common sites are the mandible (mental region), pelvis, and metaphyses of the humerus, femur, and tibia
- Patients present with pain and swelling
- About one fifth of patients present with a pathologic fracture, and some patients present with a deformity of the affected bone

Radiographic Features

- Well-delineated, expansile, lucent mass
- May be multicystic with trabeculations, giving it a soap-bubble appearance
- Cortical destruction with extension into the surrounding soft tissue may be seen

Gross Pathology

- Typically has features similar to a soft tissue desmoid and appears as a solid, firm, gray mass sometimes exhibiting a whorled pattern

Histopathology

- Histologic features are similar to those of fibromatosis (desmoid tumor)
- Variably cellular mass composed of spindle-shaped fibroblasts intermixed with collagenous stroma (Figure 16-23)
- Fibroblasts are haphazardly arranged and with slightly enlarged oval to fusiform, mildly hyperchromatic nuclei with inconspicuous nucleoli
- Mitotic figures are usually absent
- May exhibit infiltrative borders, including extension into haversian canals, permeation of bone marrow, and extension into soft tissue

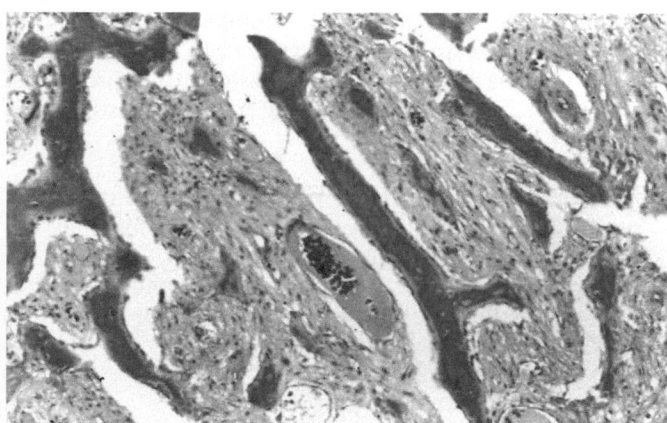

Figure 16-23. Desmoplastic fibroma. Histologic section shows bony trabeculae separated by a proliferation of fibroblastic cells embedded in a collagenous stroma.

Special Stains and Immunohistochemistry

- Vimentin and MSA positive

Other Techniques for Diagnosis

- Trisomy 8 and trisomy 20 may be found in desmoplastic fibroma of bone

Differential Diagnosis

LOW-GRADE FIBROSARCOMA

- Lacks multicystic appearance radiographically
- Histologically, the fibroblasts are arranged in herringbone pattern rather than haphazardly
- Cells with variable nuclear pleomorphism, hyperchromasia, nucleoli, and mitotic activity

FIBROUS DYSPLASIA

- In a small biopsy that does not demonstrate osteoid, desmoplastic fibroma may be diagnosed
- Fibrous dysplasia can have *GNAS1* mutations

PEARLS

- *Extremely rare tumor*
- *Should be suspected clinically in a young patient with a lytic lesion of the mandible*
- *Mitotic activity of any significant degree (greater than rare) should raise concern for well-differentiated fibrosarcoma*
- *Desmoplastic fibromas are rarely associated with Paget disease and fibrous dysplasia*

SELECTED REFERENCES

Bridge JA, Swarts SJ, Buresh C, et al: Trisomies 8 and 20 characterize a subgroup of benign fibrous lesions arising in both soft tissue and bone. Am J Pathol 154:729-733, 1999.

Dahlin DC, Hoover NW: Desmoplastic fibroma of bone. JAMA 188:685-687, 1964.

Hauben EI, Jundt G, Cleton-Jansen AM, et al: Desmoplastic fibroma of bone: an immunohistochemical study including beta-catenin expression and mutational analysis for beta-catenin. Hum Pathol 36:1025-1030, 2005.

Unni KK, Inwards CY, Bridge J, et al: Tumors of the Bones and Joints, 4th Series, Fascicle 2. Washington, DC, Armed Forces Institute of Pathology, 2005, pp 193-196.

West R, Huvos AG, Levine AM, et al: Desmoplastic fibroma of bone arising in fibrous dysplasia. Am J Clin Pathol 79:630-633, 1983.

FIBROSARCOMA

Clinical Features

- Male-to-female ratio is equal
- Cases occur in all age groups; rare in first decade
- Most common sites are distal femur, proximal tibia, pelvis, mandible, and proximal femur and humerus; multicentric forms have been described
- Patients usually present with pain and swelling of several months' duration

Radiographic Features

- Large, eccentric, metaphyseal or diaphyseal lesion that is purely lytic and poorly demarcated
- May see cortical destruction and soft tissue extension
- Tumor may extend to the articular cartilage in skeletally mature patients

Gross Pathology

- Dependent on degree of differentiation
  - Well-differentiated tumors are usually better-delineated, firm, white masses
  - Poorly differentiated tumors are fleshy, gray to brown with ill-defined, infiltrative margins
  - Higher-grade tumors contain areas of necrosis, hemorrhage, and myxoid features

Histopathology

- Well-differentiated tumors are composed of spindle cell fibroblasts arranged in interlacing fascicles within collagenous stroma (Figure 16-24)
  - Tumor cells typically arranged in a herringbone pattern
  - Mild nuclear atypia and occasional mitotic figures
- Higher-grade tumors exhibit less collagenous stroma
  - More significant nuclear atypia
  - Greater mitotic activity
  - Necrosis, hemorrhage, and myxoid areas
- Tumors are graded as follows
  - Grade 1
    - Fibroblasts are of normal size with little nuclear atypia
    - Mitotic activity ranging from one to four mitotic figures/high-power field
    - Abundant collagenous tissue

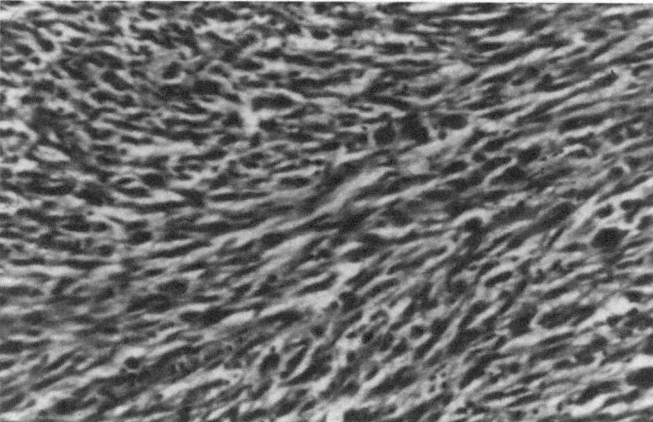

Figure 16-24. Fibrosarcoma. Histologic section shows a proliferation of spindle-shaped cells arranged in interlacing fascicles within a collagenous stroma.

- Grade 2
  - Numerous mitotic figures
  - Increased nuclear atypia
  - Less collagen with greater cellularity
- Grade 3
  - High cellularity with marked nuclear pleomorphism and prominent nucleoli
  - Abundant mitotic activity with atypical forms
  - Necrosis, hemorrhage, and myxoid change

Special Stains and Immunohistochemistry

- Vimentin strongly positive

Other Techniques for Diagnosis

- Gain of the platelet-derived growth factor-β (*PDGF*-β) gene located at 22q12.3-q13.1

Differential Diagnosis

DESMOPLASTIC FIBROMA

- Radiographically has a multicystic appearance not seen in fibrosarcoma
- Less cellular tumor composed of benign, bland spindle cells arranged haphazardly; lacks herringbone pattern
- Contains tumor osteoid
- Lacks mitotic activity and nuclear pleomorphism

DEDIFFERENTIATED CHONDROSARCOMA

- Contains areas of low-grade chondrosarcoma

MALIGNANT FIBROUS HISTIOCYTOMA

- Tumor cells are typically arranged in a storiform pattern and contains neoplastic multinucleated giant cells; lacks herringbone pattern

PEARLS

- *Fibrosarcoma may be a secondary tumor arising most commonly after irradiation of a previous giant cell tumor and also in Paget disease, enchondroma, osteochondroma, fibrous dysplasia, chronic osteomyelitis, bone infarct, and ameloblastic fibroma*

SELECTED REFERENCES

Hattinger CM, Tarkkanen M, Benini S, et al: Genetic analysis of fibrosarcoma of bone, a rare tumor entity closely related to osteosarcoma and malignant fibrous histiocytoma of bone. Eur J Cell Biol 83:483-491, 2004.

Huvos AG, Higinbotham NL: Primary fibrosarcoma of bone: a clinicopathologic study of 130 patients. Cancer 37:939-945, 1976.

Papageloupoulos PJ, Galanis EC, Trantafyllidis P, et al: Clinicopathologic features, diagnosis, and treatment of fibrosarcoma of bone. Am J Orthop 31:253-257, 2002.

Unni KK, Inwards CY, Bridge J, et al: Tumors of the Bones and Joints, 4th Series, Fascicle 2. Washington, DC, Armed Forces Institute of Pathology, 2005, pp 196-199.

MALIGNANT FIBROUS HISTIOCYTOMA

Clinical Features

- Male-to-female ratio is equal
- Found in all age groups; rare in patients younger than 20 years
- Most common sites are distal femur, proximal femur, proximal tibia, pelvis, and skull

- Patients present with pain of variable duration
- May rarely arise as a secondary tumor in enchondromas, fibrous dysplasia, Paget disease, bones with infarcts, radiated bones, and bones containing metallic prostheses

Radiographic Features

- Radiographic findings are not diagnostic but show a poorly defined, metaphyseal, lytic mass that may exhibit mottled-appearing calcifications
- Cortical expansion causes destruction and extension into soft tissue, resulting in an extraskeletal mass
- Periosteal reaction is minimal or absent
- Tumor may extend into epiphysis
- Pathologic fracture may be present

Gross Pathology

- Poorly demarcated tumor that may be firm and fibrous or soft and fleshy
- Varies in color from gray to tan to yellow
- Regional necrosis and hemorrhage are common

Histopathology

- Composed of a malignant proliferation of giant cells, histiocytes, fibroblasts, and myofibroblasts arranged in a storiform, swirling, cartwheel, or irregular pattern (Figure 16-25)
- Intermixed are variable numbers of foamy macrophages, siderophages, inflammatory cells, and collagenous matrix
- Spindle fibroblastic cells are usually arranged in storiform pattern and exhibit prominent nuclear pleomorphism, hyperchromasia, and abundant mitotic activity, often with atypical forms
- Mononuclear histiocytic cells also have pleomorphic nuclei and brisk mitotic activity
- Admixed lymphocytic infiltrate; occasional plasma cells and eosinophils may be seen
- May have areas with hemangiopericytoma-like pattern
- Foci of thick eosinophilic fibrillary deposits surrounding individual tumor cells and mimicking tumor osteoid may be seen
- Any of the variants of malignant fibrous histiocytoma in soft tissue may be found in bone tumors

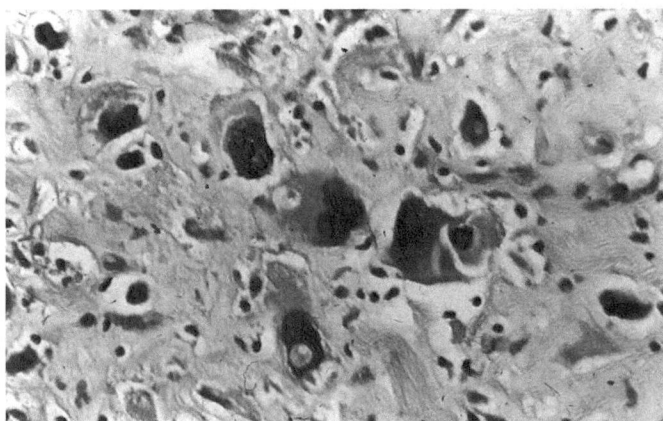

Figure 16-25. Malignant fibrous histiocytoma. High-power view shows atypical multinucleated cells with focally vacuolated eosinophilic cytoplasm.

- Most common types are the storiform-pleomorphic variant and the giant cell–rich variant
- By definition, no areas of osteosarcoma or chondrosarcoma

Special Stains and Immunohistochemistry

- Vimentin positive
- CD68 typically positive

Other Techniques for Diagnosis

- Increased levels of C-myc protein

Differential Diagnosis

GIANT CELL TUMOR

- Giant cell–rich variant of malignant fibrous histiocytoma may be misdiagnosed as a giant cell tumor
- Giant cell tumor does not exhibit significant nuclear pleomorphism and atypical mitoses

OSTEOSARCOMA

- Contains tumor osteoid

DEDIFFERENTIATED CHONDROSARCOMA

- Contains areas of low-grade chondrosarcoma

FIBROSARCOMA

- Composed of spindle cells arranged in a herringbone pattern
- Does not contain neoplastic multinucleated giant cells

PEARLS

- *Presence of definitive tumor osteoid within a bone tumor with features of malignant fibrous histiocytoma should be categorized as osteosarcoma*
- *Diagnosis of malignant fibrous histiocytoma should only be made after exclusion of tumors with myoid, lipomatous, chondroid, and osteoid differentiation; also rule out metastatic spindle cell carcinomas and melanoma*

SELECTED REFERENCES

Capanna R, Bertoni F, Bacchini P, et al: Malignant fibrous histiocytoma of bone: the experience at the Rizzoli Institute: report of 90 cases. Cancer 54:177-187, 1984.
Dahlin DC, Unni KK, Matsuno T: Malignant (fibrous) histiocytoma of bone—fact or fancy? Cancer 39:1508-1516, 1977.
Huvos AG, Heilweil M, Bretsky, SS: The pathology of malignant fibrous histiocytoma of bone: a study of 130 patients. Am J Surg Pathol 9:853-871, 1985.
Tarkkanen M, Larramendy ML, Böhling T, et al: Malignant fibrous histiocytoma of bone: analysis of genomic imbalances by comparative genomic hybridisation and C-MYC expression by immunohistochemistry. Eur J Cancer 42:1172-1180, 2006.
Unni KK, Inwards CY, Bridge J, et al: Tumors of the Bones and Joints, 4th Series, Fascicle 2. Washington, DC, Armed Forces Institute of Pathology, 2005, pp 202-207.

GIANT CELL TUMOR

Clinical Features

- Sometimes referred to as "osteoclastoma"
- Typically occurs in skeletally mature patients
- Slight female predominance

- Most occur in second, third, and fourth decades
- Most common sites are distal femur, proximal tibia, distal radius, and sacrum
- Patients typically present with localized pain
- Muscular atrophy with decreased range of motion of the adjacent joint may be present
- Some patients may present with a pathologic fracture

Radiographic Features

- Lytic epiphyseal mass without sclerosis or periosteal reaction (Figure 16-26A)
- May appear to extend into soft tissue but contains an outer rim of thin periosteal bone

Gross Pathology

- Curettage reveals friable, soft tissue of variable color
- Resected specimens reveal an epiphyseal mass that is red, brown, gray, and focally yellow (Figure 16-26B)

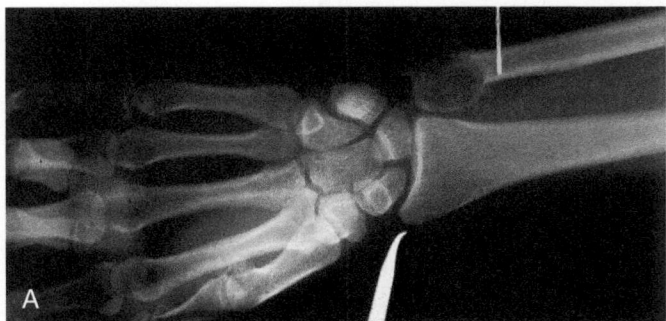

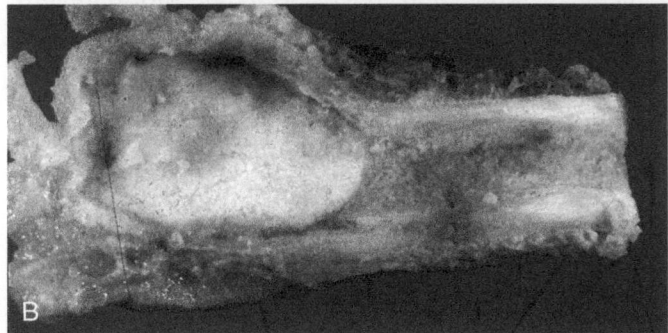

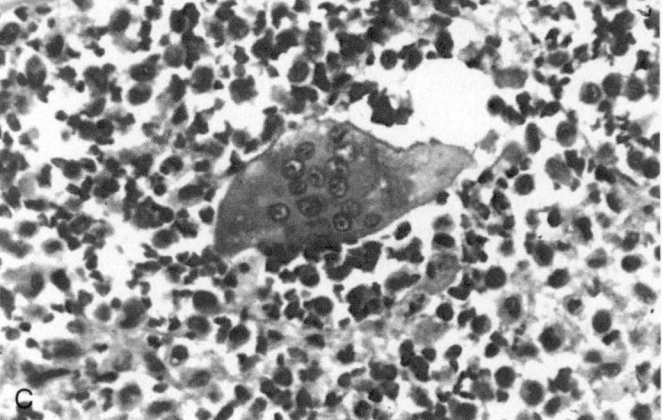

Figure 16-26. Giant cell tumor of the ulna. A, Typical circumscribed lytic lesion. **B,** Resected specimen shows a well-defined, fleshy tumor mass. **C,** Histologic section shows a single multinucleated giant cell with multiple nuclei in a background of sheets of mononuclear histiocytic cells and red blood cells.

- Can extend to the articular cartilage
- May contain fleshy areas, foci of necrosis, and cystic changes suggestive of aneurysmal bone cyst

Histopathology

- Typically consists of large numbers of evenly distributed multinucleated osteoclast-like giant cells in a background of sheets of mononuclear histiocytic cells (Figure 16-26C)
- Mononuclear histiocytic cells (believed to be the neoplastic cell population) are polygonal or round to oval with cytologically benign nuclei; variable mitotic rate with no atypical forms
- Multinucleated giant cells have features of osteoclasts
  - May contain numerous nuclei, sometimes greater than 100
  - Nuclei have benign cytologic features similar to the mononuclear cells
  - Giant cells are not mitotically active
- Foamy histiocytes, siderophages, reactive bone, and delicate vascular structures containing intravascular tumor may be seen
- Cartilaginous tissue is not found in giant cell tumors unless associated with a fracture

Special Stains and Immunohistochemistry

- Noncontributory

Other Techniques for Diagnosis

- Cytogenetically, giant cell tumors may demonstrate telomeric associations (tas), end-to-end fusion of cytogenetically appearing intact chromosomes; telomeres most commonly involved include 19q, 1p, 15p, 21p, 20q, and 18p
- Overexpression of *c-myc*, hepatocyte growth factor receptor, and vascular endothelial growth factor gene has been associated with more aggressive behavior

Differential Diagnosis

Giant Cell Reparative Granuloma

- Lacks uniform distribution of giant cells
- Giant cells contain much fewer nuclei and tend to aggregate around foci of hemorrhage
- Stroma is more fibrotic and contains more abundant hemosiderin and hemorrhage
- Stromal cells are spindle shaped rather than round to oval

Nonossifying Fibroma

- Radiographically shows peripheral sclerosis
- Typically affects younger patients
- Usually metaphyseal lesions

Aneurysmal Bone Cyst

- Does not typically involve epiphyses
- Giant cells are arranged around cystic spaces

Giant Cell–Rich Osteosarcoma

- Though present only focally, delicate strands of osteoid can be found surrounding aggregates of pleomorphic mononuclear cells exhibiting atypical mitotic activity

Metastatic Carcinoma Containing Giant Cells

- Positive for epithelial markers: cytokeratin and EMA

PEARLS

- *Three common epiphyseal tumors, which include giant cell tumor, clear cell chondrosarcoma, and chondroblastoma*
- *Complete evaluation of clinicopathologic and radiographic features is essential in the diagnosis of giant cell tumor*
- *Account for about one fifth of all benign bone tumors*
- *Diagnosis of giant cell tumor in a skeletally immature patient should be questioned*
- *Paramyxovirus-like nuclear inclusions have been reported in some giant cell tumors*
- *May be associated with Paget disease of bone (craniofacial bones and pelvis)*
- *Serum chemistry may be helpful in the differential diagnosis of giant cell tumors*
  - *Elevated serum calcium and parathyroid hormone suggest hyperparathyroidism (brown tumor)*
  - *Elevated alkaline phosphatase and normal calcium may indicate a giant cell tumor arising in Paget disease of bone*
- *Benign pulmonary metastases (e.g., tumor embolization) may occur in patients with giant cell tumors that show intratumoral vascular invasion; however, this is an uncommon event*
- *Malignant giant cell tumors arise from benign giant cell tumors or in sites of prior benign giant cell tumors*
- *Tumors with radiographic evidence of aggressive growth should be evaluated carefully histologically*

SELECTED REFERENCES

Balke M, Schremper L, Gebert C, et al: Giant cell tumor of bone: treatment and outcome of 214 cases. J Cancer Res Clin Oncol 134:969-973, 2008.

Bridge JA, Neff JR, Mouron BJ: Giant cell tumor of bone: chromosomal analysis of 48 specimens and review of the literature. Cancer Genet Cytogenet 58:2-13, 1992.

Brimo F, Aziz M, Rosen G, et al: Malignancy in giant cell tumour of bone: is there a reproducible histological threshold? A study of three giant cell tumours with worrisome features. Histopathology 51:864-866, 2007.

Dahlin DC, Cupps RE, Johnson EW: Giant cell tumor: a study of 195 cases. Cancer 25:1061-1070, 1970.

Junming M, Cheng Y, Dong C, et al: Giant cell tumor of the cervical spine: a series of 22 cases and outcomes. Spine 33:380-388, 2008.

Unni KK, Inwards CY, Bridge J, et al: Tumors of the Bones and Joints, 4th Series, Fascicle 2. Washington, DC, Armed Forces Institute of Pathology, 2005, pp 281-298.

GIANT CELL GRANULOMA (GIANT CELL REPARATIVE GRANULOMA)

Clinical Features

- Male-to-female ratio is equal
- About 75% of patients are younger than 30 years
- Most common sites are phalanges, metatarsals, metacarpals, mandible, and maxilla
- Patients usually present with pain and swelling of variable duration

Radiographic Features

- Expansile, purely lytic lesion with cortical thinning
- May exhibit trabeculation and periosteal bone formation

Gross Pathology

- Curettage produces fragments of reddish brown friable tissue

Histopathology

- Consists of spindle cells within collagenous stroma and multinucleated giant cells exhibiting clustering around areas of hemorrhage (Figure 16-27)
- Multinucleated giant cells are fewer in number and contain fewer nuclei than seen in giant cell tumors; mitoses are not seen in this cell population
- Mitotic figures (no atypical forms) may be found but typically are fewer than in giant cell tumors
- Scattered chronic inflammatory cells may be found in the stroma
- Reactive osteoid and bone may be present with and without osteoblastic rimming
- Siderophages, giant cells with phagocytized erythrocytes, and intravascular giant cells may be seen
- Secondary aneurysmal bone cyst formation may be found
- Cartilage is not present unless associated with a fracture

Special Stains and Immunohistochemistry

- Mononuclear stromal cells and multinucleated giant cells express α_1-antitrypsin, α_1-antichymotrypsin, and CD68

Other Techniques for Diagnosis

- Noncontributory

Differential Diagnosis

ANEURYSMAL BONE CYST

- May share histologic features with giant cell reparative granuloma; typically giant cells surround cystic spaces
- In tumors of the hands and feet, the presence of solid foci stromal cells and giant cells is more consistent with a diagnosis of giant cell reparative granuloma over primary aneurysmal bone cyst

BROWN TUMOR IN HYPERPARATHYROIDISM

- Histologically indistinguishable from giant cell reparative granuloma
- Patients have elevated serum calcium and parathyroid hormone levels

GIANT CELL TUMOR

- Greater numbers of giant cells, which are generally evenly distributed without clustering
- Giant cells contain greater numbers of nuclei

NONOSSIFYING FIBROMA

- Aggregate of giant cells is not typical in these tumors
- Rare in bones of hands, feet, mandible, and maxilla

GIANT CELL–RICH OSTEOSARCOMA

- Contains delicate strands of osteoid, which can be found focally surrounding aggregates of pleomorphic mononuclear cells exhibiting atypical mitotic activity

MALIGNANT FIBROUS HISTIOCYTOMA

- Cytologic features of malignancy can be found even if low grade
- Radiographic features include cortical destruction with soft tissue extension

PEARLS

- *May enlarge rapidly during pregnancy*
- *Giant cell granulomas have been found in association with polyostotic fibrous dysplasia and Paget disease of bone*
- *Any patient with the clinical diagnosis of giant cell reparative granuloma of bone should have serum calcium, phosphorous, alkaline phosphatase, and parathyroid hormone levels evaluated to rule out hyperparathyroidism*

SELECTED REFERENCES

De Lange J, van den Akker HP, van den Berg H: Central giant cell granuloma of the jaw: a review of the literature with emphasis on therapy options. Oral Surg Oral Med Oral Pathol Oral Radiol Endod 104:603-615, 2007.

Motamedi MH, Eshghyar N, Jafari SM, et al: Peripheral and central giant cell granulomas of the jaws: a demographic study. Oral Surg Oral Med Oral Pathol Oral Radiol Endod 103:e39-e43, 2007.

Unni KK, Inwards CY, Bridge J, et al: Tumors of the Bones and Joints, 4th Series, Fascicle 2. Washington, DC, Armed Forces Institute of Pathology, 2005, pp 357-358.

Vigorita VJ: Orthopaedic Pathology. Philadelphia, Lippincott Williams & Wilkins, 1999, pp 272-273.

ADAMANTINOMA

Clinical Features

- Male-to-female ratio is equal
- Most cases occur in second and third decades
- Most common site is the diaphysis of the tibia (> 80%)
- Patients present with pain of variable duration from several weeks to several years

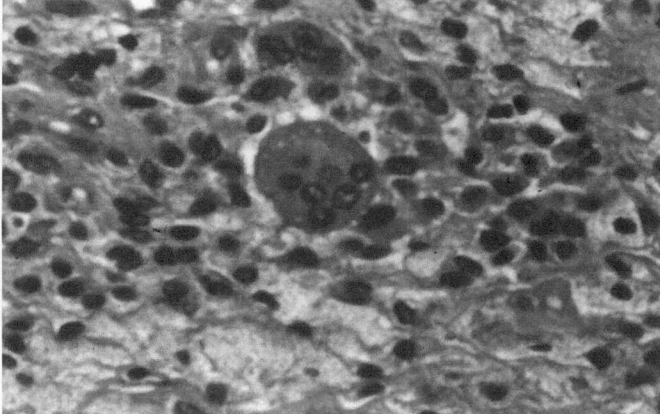

Figure 16-27. Giant cell granuloma. Histologic section shows a single multinucleated giant cell containing few nuclei and surrounded by mononuclear stromal cells and foam cells.

- May be swelling and pathologic fracture at presentation
- Significant number of patients report a history of trauma, which is most likely coincidental

Radiographic Features

- Eccentric, multicystic (soap-bubble appearance), lobulated, lytic diaphyseal tibial defect
- Usually involves both the cortical and medullary portions of the bone and may be multifocal in the same bone
- Peripheral sclerosis may connect multiple lesions
- Cortical expansion with thinning
- Occasionally cortical penetration with development of a soft tissue mass is seen

Gross Pathology

- Well-circumscribed, lobulated gray mass
- Variable consistency from soft to granular to fibrous
- May contain regional hemorrhage and cystic changes

Histopathology (Figure 16-28)

- Characterized by a hypocellular fibrous stroma containing epithelioid cellular islands
- Epithelioid cellular islands may be composed of various cell types, including basaloid, squamoid, tubular, or spindle cells
  - Nests with basaloid patterns exhibit central loose spindle cells (stellate reticulum-like) with peripheral palisading of cuboidal cells
  - Squamoid cell nests may show keratinization
  - Tubular pattern consists of branching and anastomosing tubular structures lined by a single layer of epithelioid cells, imparting a vascular appearance
  - Spindle cell pattern consists of plump, fibroblast-like spindle cells within a fibrous stroma reminiscent of the sclerosing variant of basal cell carcinoma
- These cells are generally bland without atypia and mitotic activity; rare cases may exhibit mild atypia and occasional mitotic figures

Special Stains and Immunohistochemistry

- Cytokeratin: epithelioid islands are positive

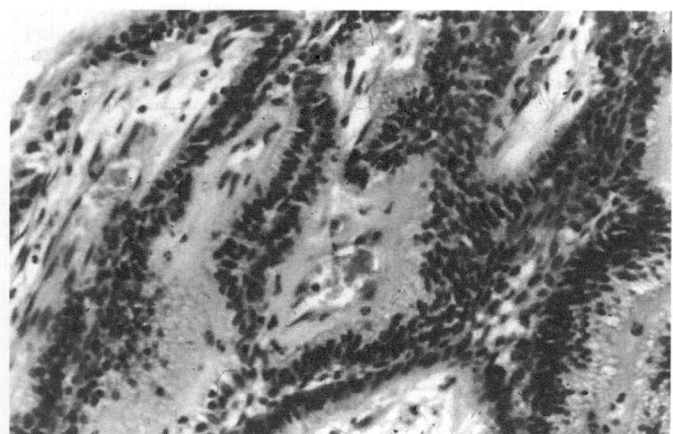

Figure 16-28. Adamantinoma. Histologic section slows strands of epithelial cells with peripheral palisading and stellate reticulum-like stroma.

Other Techniques for Diagnosis

- Extra copies of chromosomes 7, 8, 12, 19, and 21 are reported in adamantinoma; inversions, translocations, deletions, and marker chromosomes may also be detected

Differential Diagnosis

OSTEOFIBROUS DYSPLASIA

- Lacks epithelioid cell islands
- Stroma may contain individual cytokeratin positive cells
- Cytogenetics may be similar to adamantinoma; osteofibrous dysplasia lacks structural abnormalities such as translocations, inversions, and deletions
- May be precursor lesion to adamantinoma of long bones

FIBROUS DYSPLASIA

- Lacks cytokeratin-positive epithelial cells

METASTATIC CARCINOMA

- Usually older population
- Tumor cells typically show significantly more cytologic atypia with nuclear pleomorphism
- High mitotic rate often with atypical forms

PEARLS

- *Slow-growing, locally destructive tumors with low metastatic potential*
- *Typically cured by local resection*

SELECTED REFERENCES

Jain D, Jain VK, Vasishta RK, et al: Adamantinoma: a clinicopathological review and update. Diagn Pathol 3:8, 2008.
Papagelopoulos PJ, Mavrogenis AF, Galanis EC, et al: Clinicopathological features, diagnosis, and treatment of adamantinoma of the long bones. Orthopedics 30:211-217, 2007.
Unni KK, Inwards CY, Bridge J, et al: Tumors of the Bones and Joints, 4th Series, Fascicle 2. Washington, DC, Armed Forces Institute of Pathology, 2005, pp 299-307.
Vigorita VJ: Orthopaedic Pathology. Philadelphia, Lippincott Williams & Wilkins, 1999, pp 401-403.

SMALL CELL NEOPLASMS

EWING SARCOMA/PRIMITIVE NEUROECTODERMAL TUMOR (PNET)

Clinical Features

- Ewing sarcoma and PNET are considered the same tumor
- Male-to-female ratio is about 1.3:1
- Most patients present between ages 5 and 20 years; rare in patients younger than 5 or older than 30 years
- Second most common bone sarcoma in the pediatric age group (most common is osteosarcoma)
- Bones in the lower extremities and pelvis are the most common sites; rare in the upper extremities
- Patients present with progressively increasing pain and swelling

- Presence of fever, increased sedimentation rate, leukocytosis, anemia, and malaise may indicate disseminated disease

Radiographic Features

- Poorly marginated lytic or sclerotic diaphyseal mass with periosteal reaction (sunburst or onion-skin pattern) (Figure 16-29A)
- Soft tissue mass may be present
- Extensive permeation of bone marrow may be seen on MRI

Gross Pathology

- Intact tumor is a gray-white intramedullary mass that is soft, glistening, and moist
- May be watery and have the appearance of pus
- Regional areas of cystic changes and hemorrhage may be present

Histopathology

- Broad sheets of small, uniform cells with hyperchromatic nuclei with inconspicuous nucleoli, scant cytoplasm, and indistinct cell borders; minimal surrounding stroma (Figure 16-29B)
- Occasional mitotic activity

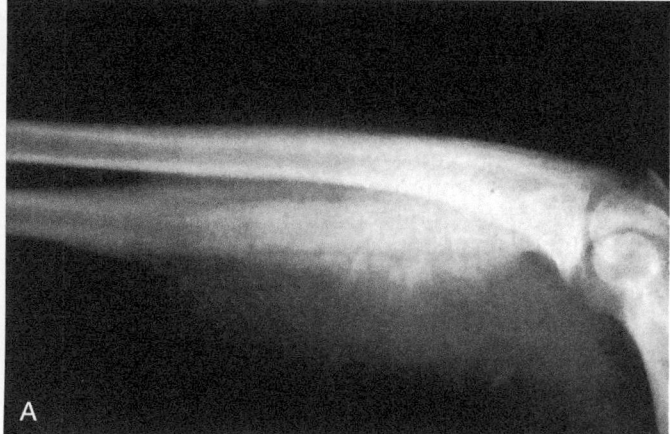

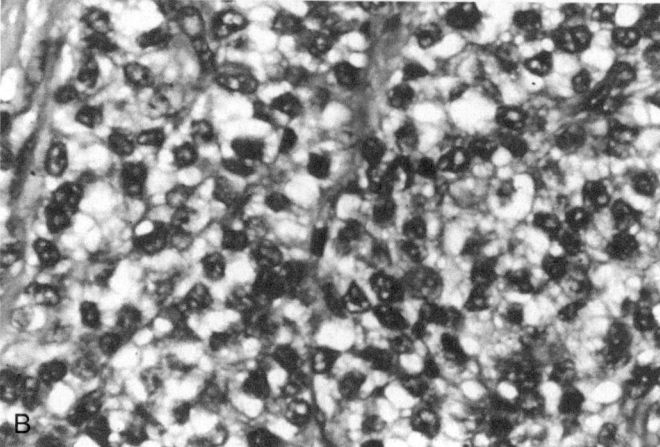

Figure 16-29. Ewing sarcoma/PNET. A, Radiograph of the radius shows a medullary lesion with expansion and permeation of the cortex, giving a sunburst appearance. **B,** Histologic section shows small, uniform cells with hyperchromatic nuclei and scant, vacuolated cytoplasm.

- A subgroup of degenerate or apoptotic cells that have hyperchromatic pyknotic nuclei usually present
- Rosettes, lobular architecture, focal spindle cells, and metaplastic bone (not osteoid) or cartilage may be present
- Areas of geographic necrosis or small foci of necrosis are usually seen
- Chemotherapy and radiation may cause tumor cells to be more pleomorphic and have larger nuclei with folded forms, multinucleated forms, and prominent nucleoli
- Large cell variant may morphologically resemble lymphoma

Special Stains and Immunohistochemistry

- CD99 (MIC2) positive
- PAS: most tumors exhibit intracytoplasmic glycogen (diastase sensitive)
- Vimentin and cytokeratin: variable expression
- Neuron specific enolase (NSE), synaptophysin, and chromogranin: variable expression
- Leukocyte common antigen (LCA), SMA, MSA, and vascular markers negative

Other Techniques for Diagnosis

- Cytogenetic studies demonstrate characteristic chromosomal translocation t(11;22)(q24;q12) in 95% of cases; t(21;22)(q22;q12) usually found in the remaining 5% of cases
- Presence of type 1 *EWS/FLI1* fusion gene as opposed to type 2 has prognostic significance, with type 1 exhibiting significantly longer survival time
- MIC2 overexpression may be demonstrated by in situ hybridization

Differential Diagnosis

METASTATIC NEUROBLASTOMA

- Typically occurs in children younger than 5 years
- Urinary catecholamine metabolites may be elevated
- Tends to metastasize to the skull
- Contains Homer-Wright rosettes with fibrillary background
- Expresses neuroendocrine markers but is negative for CD99

LYMPHOMA, LEUKEMIA

- Expresses lymphoid markers; negative for CD99

OSTEOSARCOMA, SMALL CELL VARIANT

- Foci of tumor osteoid should be present
- Positive for SATB2
- Negative for CD99

MESENCHYMAL CHONDROSARCOMA

- Foci of chondroid differentiation should be present
- Tumor expresses S-100 protein
- Negative for CD99

PEARLS

- *Rare in blacks, patients younger than 5 years, and patients older than 30 years*
- *In patients younger than 5 years, metastatic neuroblastoma and leukemia-lymphoma are more common and should be ruled out*

- *In patients older than 30 years, metastatic small cell carcinoma and large cell lymphoma are more common and should be ruled out*
- *Multiple bone involvement at time of diagnosis is not uncommon*

SELECTED REFERENCES

Fletcher C, Bridge JA, Hogendoorn P, et al (eds): WHO Classification of Tumours of Soft Tissue and Bone, 4th ed. Lyon, France, International Agency for Research on Cancer, 2013, pp 298-300.

Kissane JM, Askin FB, Foulkes M, et al: Ewing's sarcoma of bone: clinicopathologic aspects of 303 cases from the Intergroup Ewing's Sarcoma Study. Hum Pathol 14:773-779, 1983.

Riggi N, Suvá ML, Suvá D, et al: EWS-FLI-1 expression triggers a Ewing's sarcoma initiation program in primary human mesenchymal stem cells. Cancer Res 68:2176-2185, 2008.

Unni KK, Inwards CY, Bridge J, et al: Tumors of the Bones and Joints, 4th Series, Fascicle 2. Washington, DC, Armed Forces Institute of Pathology, 2005, pp 209-222.

LYMPHOMA

Clinical Features

- Male-to-female ratio is 1.5:1
- Most bone lymphomas occur in second through eighth decades
- Pelvis and bones of the lower extremities are the most common sites
- Patients present with pain, typically of long duration (> 1 year)
- Primary bone lymphomas have a good prognosis even when they are the large cell type
- Stage is the most important prognostic factor regardless of subtype

Radiographic Features

- Lytic lesion with a moth-eaten appearance
- May be sclerotic, suggesting Paget disease of bone
- Usually no periosteal reaction
- Soft tissue mass may be present; MRI, CT, and isotope scans may be helpful in delineating the extent of disease

Gross Pathology

- Typically a soft, white, fleshy mass
- Permeates the medullary cavity
- Cyst formation, necrosis, and hemorrhagic foci may be present

Histopathology

- Diffuse large cell lymphomas are the most common type
- Composed of sheets of large cells that may or may not have cleaved nuclei; most are noncleaved (Figure 16-30)
- Some tumors may contain multilobate nuclei or cells with immunoblastic features
- May exhibit a prominent inflammatory infiltrate consisting of neutrophils and mature lymphocytes, which may suggest a diagnosis of osteomyelitis
- Small cell lymphomas and mixed small cell–large cell lymphomas may also occur

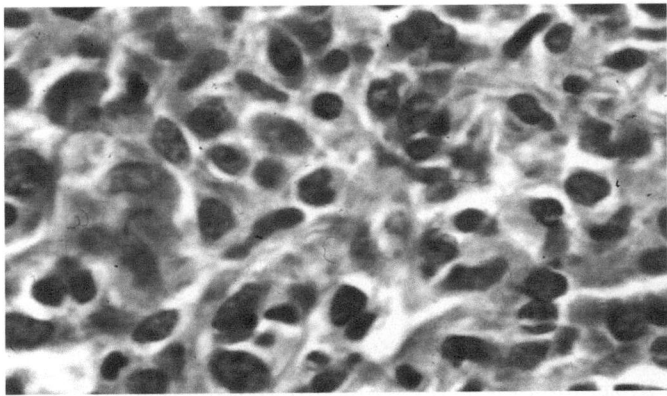

Figure 16-30. Lymphoma, large cell type. High-power view shows sheets of large, atypical lymphoid cells.

- Spindle cell patterns suggestive of sarcoma or clear cell patterns, signet ring cell variants, and clustering of epithelioid cells suggestive of metastatic carcinoma may occur
- Starry-sky pattern (Burkitt lymphoma) occurs in the maxilla and mandible

Special Stains and Immunohistochemistry

- Tumor cells express lymphoid markers and are usually of B-cell type
  - CD19, CD20, CD79a, CD45, and PAX-5 positive
  - Large cell lymphomas may express bcl-2
- Classical Hodgkin lymphoma expresses CD30 and usually CD15
- Anaplastic large cell lymphoma (a T-cell lymphoma) expresses CD30 and may express ALK1
- Reticulin stain highlights fine network of reticulin around individual tumor cells

Other Techniques for Diagnosis

- Phenotyping by flow cytometry and gene rearrangement studies may be helpful in ruling out benign processes that may mimic lymphoma
- About 80% of non-Hodgkin lymphomas have clonal chromosome abnormalities, some of which are disease specific

Differential Diagnosis

NEUROECTODERMAL TUMOR OF BONE
- Typically have prominent rosettes
- Positive for NSE, chromogranin, synaptophysin, CD99
- Negative for LCA

METASTATIC NEUROBLASTOMA
- Usually occurs in children younger than 5 years
- May have elevated urinary catecholamine metabolites
- Tends to metastasize to the skull
- Characterized by Homer-Wright rosettes with fibrillary background
- Positive for NSE, chromogranin, and synaptophysin

OSTEOSARCOMA, SMALL CELL VARIANT
- Foci of tumor osteoid should be seen

MESENCHYMAL CHONDROSARCOMA
- Foci of chondroid differentiation
- Tumor cells express S-100 protein; negative for LCA

METASTATIC SMALL CELL CARCINOMA
- Positive for cytokeratin and neuroendocrine markers

LANGERHANS CELL HISTIOCYTOSIS
- Composed of histiocytes with a prominent eosinophilic cellular infiltrate
- Histiocytes express S-100 protein and CD1a and are negative for B- and T-cell markers and CD30

SARCOMA
- Occasionally lymphomas will have a spindle cell component, mimicking sarcoma
- Sarcomas do not express lymphoid markers

CHRONIC OSTEOMYELITIS
- Typically composed of a polymorphous inflammatory cell infiltrate with lymphocytes, eosinophils, and neutrophils; lacks large neoplastic lymphocytes
- Immunophenotypically consists of a mixed population of B and T cells
- Absence of clonal population by flow cytometry or gene rearrangement

PEARLS

- *T-cell lymphomas of bone are extremely rare and are most common in Japan*
- *Primary Hodgkin disease of bone is rare, with the most common types being nodular sclerosing and mixed cellularity; axial skeletal involvement is much more common than appendicular involvement*
- *Primary lymphoma of bone is diagnosed only if there is no evidence of extraskeletal lymphoma 6 months after original diagnosis of the bone lesion and there is no prior history of extraskeletal lymphoma*
- *Primary lymphoma of bone is more common in the appendicular skeleton, whereas secondary osseous lymphoma is more common in the axial skeleton*
- *Low-grade secondary osseous lymphomas do not necessarily have a worse prognosis, whereas secondary high-grade osseous lymphomas do have a worse prognosis*

SELECTED REFERENCES

Lima FP, Bousquet M, Gomez-Brouchet A, et al: Primary diffuse large B-cell lymphoma of bone displays preferential rearrangements of the c-MYC or BCL2 gene. Am J Clin Pathol 129:723-726, 2008.

Swerdlow SH, Campo E, Harris NL, et al (eds): WHO Classification of Tumours of Haematopoietic and Lymphoid Tissues, 4th ed. Lyon, France, International Agency for Research on Cancer, 2008, pp 179-195, 214-366.

Unni KK, Inwards CY, Bridge J, et al: Tumors of the Bones and Joints, 4th Series, Fascicle 2. Washington, DC, Armed Forces Institute of Pathology, 2005, pp 231-240.

MULTIPLE MYELOMA AND SOLITARY PLASMACYTOMA OF BONE

Clinical Features

- Male-to-female ratio is about 2:1
- Most cases occur between ages 50 and 80 years
- Solitary plasmacytoma tends to occur at a slightly younger age
- Vertebrae, ribs, skull, pelvis, and long bones are the most common sites
- Patients with multiple myeloma present with pain, usually of less than 6 months' duration
  - May cause weight loss, peripheral neuropathy, pathologic fracture, fever, anemia, bleeding, hypercalcemia, hypergammaglobulinemia, and renal dysfunction
- Patients with solitary plasmacytoma of bone usually present with pain; about 10% of patients with solitary plasmacytoma are asymptomatic
- Some cases may be associated with POEMS syndrome (*p*olyneuropathy, organomegaly [hepatosplenomegaly and lymphadenopathy], *e*ndocrinopathy [amenorrhea, diabetes, gynecomastia, hirsutism, or impotence], *M*-protein, and *s*kin changes [hyperpigmentation, hypertrichosis, or clubbing of digits])

Radiographic Features

- In multiple myeloma, there are multiple punched-out lytic lesions, typically without sclerosis or periosteal reaction (Figure 16-31A and B)
- Solitary plasmacytoma may exhibit a lytic lesion in vertebrae with cortical ridging (corduroy cloth) or a bubbly appearance in long bones; cortical expansion may be seen

Gross Pathology

- Soft, gray-red tissue involving the marrow space

Histopathology

- Tumor is composed of sheets of small cells with plasmacytic features (Figure 16-31C)
  - Eccentric nuclei with stippled chromatin patterns (cartwheel or clock face)
  - Cytoplasm is eosinophilic with perinuclear clearing (perinuclear Golgi zone)
- Intracytoplasmic immunoglobulins may produce grapelike structures (Mott cells or morula)
- Extracytoplasmic immunoglobulins may be found and are represented as Russell bodies (extracellular eosinophilic spherical bodies)
- Plasma cells may be atypical, multinucleated, or immature (plasmablasts have large nuclei and prominent nucleoli)
- Generally, mitotic activity is not prominent unless atypical forms or plasmablasts are present
- Amyloid may be present accompanied by giant cell reaction

Special Stains and Immunohistochemistry

- Predominance of either κ or λ light chains (clonal process)
- CD38, CD138 positive
- Positive for immunoglobulin (Ig) G or IgA, less commonly for either IgM or IgE
- Tumor cells may express EMA but are cytokeratin negative
- Congo red stain with apple-green birefringence is seen if amyloid is present

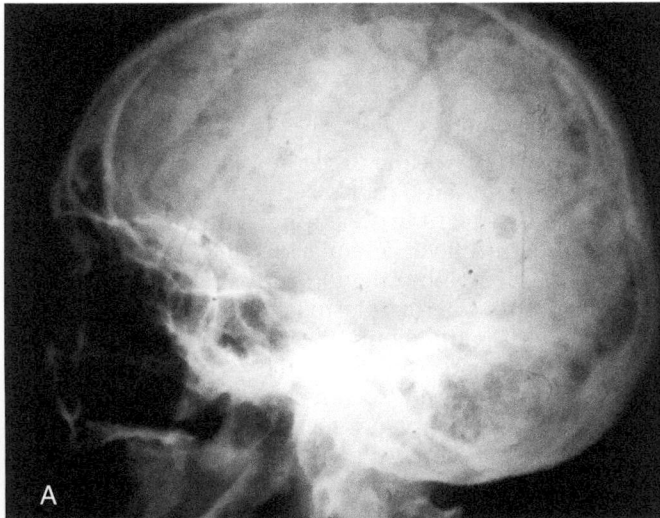

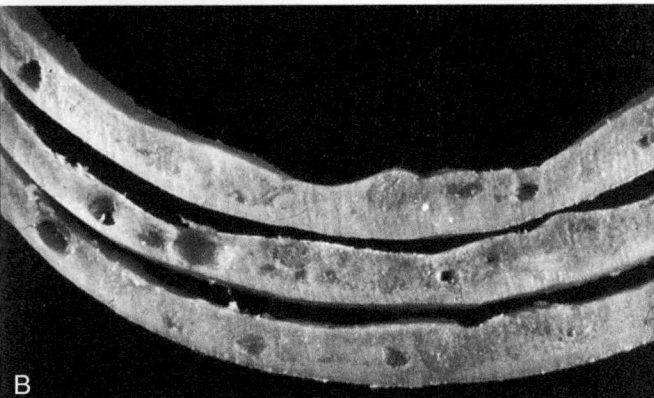

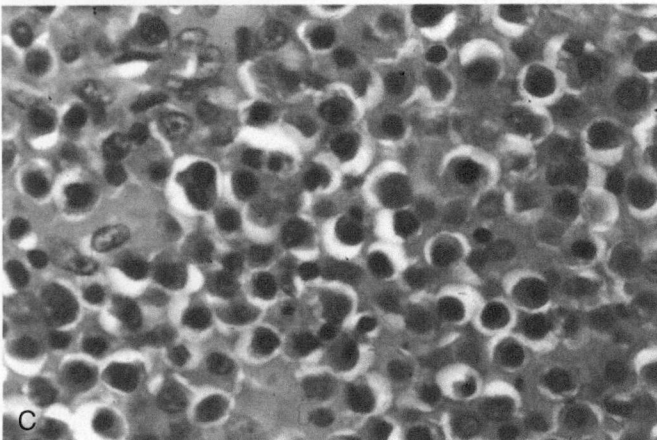

Figure 16-31. Multiple myeloma involving the skull. A, Multiple osteolytic, defined round lesions. **B,** Cross section of the scalp shows punched-out lesions. **C,** Histologic section shows sheets of plasma cells.

- Aberrant loss of CD19 and CD45 is common
- Aberrant gain of CD56, CD117, and CD20 can also be seen

Other Techniques for Diagnosis

- Serum and urine protein electrophoresis is used to demonstrate the presence and quantity of a paraprotein (M spike)
  - M spike usually seen in the gamma region on serum protein electrophoresis (SPEP) but can be seen in the beta region in some IgA myelomas

- Serum and urine immunofixation electrophoresis (IFE) is used to demonstrate specific monoclonal light chains and heavy chains
- Flow cytometry can be used to demonstrate light chain restriction and the aberrant loss or gain of markers
- Gene rearrangements usually found in IgG heavy chain
- Clonal cytogenetic abnormalities are common and have prognostic significance

Differential Diagnosis

CHRONIC OSTEOMYELITIS

- Typically composed of a polymorphous inflammatory cell infiltrate with lymphocytes, eosinophils, and neutrophils
- Prominent fibrosis
- κ-to-λ light chain ratio is normal or slightly elevated (about 3:1)

METASTATIC CARCINOMA

- Occasionally the plasma cell infiltrate will mimic an epithelial neoplasm
- Epithelial cells are cytokeratin positive
- EMA is not helpful because myeloma cells can be EMA positive

B-CELL IMMUNOBLASTIC LYMPHOMA

- Positive for B-cell markers

PEARLS

- *In most patients, cases of solitary plasmacytoma of the bone progress to multiple myeloma*
- *About 4% of cases of multiple myeloma are nonsecretory; paraprotein is made, but it is not secreted outside the cell (these patients tend to have a better prognosis than do those with the secretory form of myeloma)*
- *Most common sites of solitary plasmacytoma of bone are thoracic and lumbar vertebrae*
- *κ Light chains are the most common type of light chain produced in multiple myeloma*
- *IgG and IgA are the most common monoclonal gammopathies seen in multiple myeloma (IgG more common than IgA)*
- *About 75% of patients with solitary plasmacytoma do not have a serum paraprotein*
- *A preponderance of immature plasmablastic cells is pathognomonic for myeloma in a subset of the literature*
- *Multinucleated forms of plasma cells are not diagnostic of myeloma or solitary plasmacytoma; may be found in reactive and inflammatory processes*
- *Multiple myeloma is the most common primary malignant bone tumor*
- *Osteosclerotic myeloma is a rare form that presents in younger patients with sclerotic bone lesions*

SELECTED REFERENCES

Bilsky MH, Azeem S: Multiple myeloma: primary bone tumor with systemic manifestations. Neurosurg Clin N Am 19:31-40, 2008.

Edwards CM, Zhuang J, Mundy GR: The pathogenesis of the bone disease of multiple myeloma. Bone 42:1007-1013, 2008.

Sawyer JR: The prognostic significance of cytogenetics and molecular profiling in multiple myeloma. Cancer Genet 204:3-12, 2011.

Swerdlow SH, Campo E, Harris NL, et al (eds): WHO Classification of Tumours of Haematopoietic and Lymphoid Tissues, 4th ed. Lyon, France, International Agency for Research on Cancer, 2008, pp 196-213.

Unni KK, Inwards CY, Bridge J, et al: Tumors of the Bones and Joints, 4th Series, Fascicle 2. Washington, DC, Armed Forces Institute of Pathology, 2005, pp 222-231.

MISCELLANEOUS BONE LESIONS

CHORDOMA

Clinical Features

- Malignant midline bone tumor arising from fetal notochord remnants
- Male-to-female ratio is 2:1
- Most occur in fourth to seventh decades; occurrence in patients younger than 30 years is rare
- Spheno-occipital tumors tend to occur at a slightly younger age (10 years younger) than sacral tumors
- Half of cases involve the sacrum, and one third occur in the spheno-occipital region; remainder occur in cervical and lumbar regions of the spinal cord
- Symptoms are dependent on site of tumor
  - Sacral tumors present with pain, bladder dysfunction, and constipation
  - Spheno-occipital tumors present with cranial nerve deficits, hypopituitarism, and diplopia
  - Slow growing with frequent recurrences and late distant metastases to skin, bone, and ovary

Radiographic Features

- Midline lytic destructive tumor that may contain intralesional calcifications
- In spheno-occipital tumors, there may be erosion of the sella turcica, clivus, and sphenoid bones

Gross Pathology

- Lobulated gelatinous gray tissue that may appear encapsulated

Histopathology

- Lobulated mass containing vacuolated cells forming nests and cords or strands within a myxoid mucoid matrix (Figure 16-32)

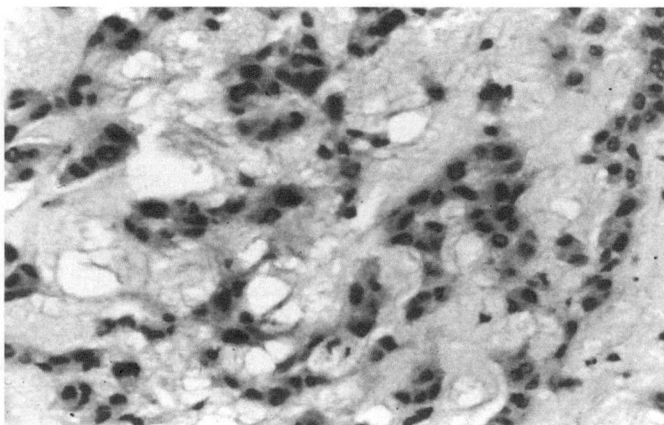

Figure 16-32. Chordoma. Histologic section shows nests and cords of large vacuolated cells within a myxoid mucoid matrix.

- Cellularity is variable, and some tumors may contain solid areas
- Rare mitoses may be present
- Classic *physaliphorous* cells are round to oval and have a central nucleus with a prominent nucleolus; cytoplasm is abundant and eosinophilic with circumferential perinuclear vacuoles imparting a bubbly appearance to the cell cytoplasm; typically found in a myxoid matrix and may form syncytia
- May exhibit foci of chondroid differentiation, especially in spheno-occipital tumors; designated *chondroid chordoma*
- Rare cases exhibit a malignant spindle cell component with features of malignant fibrous histiocytoma; designated *dedifferentiated chordoma*

Special Stains and Immunohistochemistry

- Brachyury: recently identified marker that is highly sensitive and specific for chordoma
- Brachyury shows nuclear positivity in chordomas but is negative in potential mimics including chondrosarcoma and metastatic carcinoma
- Also positive for cytokeratin (CAM-5.2), EMA, vimentin, and S-100 protein

Other Techniques for Diagnosis

- Cytogenetics: tumors commonly aneuploid

Differential Diagnosis

CHONDROSARCOMA

- Tumor cells are negative for cytokeratin, EMA, and brachyury

METASTATIC ADENOCARCINOMA

- Does not have a physaliphorous pattern
- Often exhibits glandular differentiation
- Metastatic adenocarcinoma will not be positive for brachyury

LIPOSARCOMA

- Tumor cells are negative for cytokeratin, EMA, and brachyury

PEARLS

- *Chordoma is not an uncommon neoplasm; follows osteosarcoma, chondrosarcoma, and Ewing sarcoma/PNET in frequency of primary malignant bone tumors*
- *Classic physaliphorous cells may be rare in some cases*
- *In some studies, chondroid chordoma has a higher survival rate than traditional chordoma*
- *Dedifferentiated chordomas typically occur after several recurrences of a classic chordoma; some of these patients have been irradiated, suggesting that these tumors are radiation induced*

SELECTED REFERENCES

Jambhekar NA, Rekhi B, Thorat K, et al: Revisiting chordoma with brachyury, a "new age" marker: analysis of a validation study on 51 cases. Arch Pathol Lab Med 134:1181-1187, 2010.

Oakley GJ, Fuhrer K, Seethala RR: Brachyury, SOX-9, and podoplanin, new markers in the skull based chordoma vs chondrosarcoma differential: a tissue microarray-based comparative analysis. Mod Pathol 21:1461-1469, 2008.

Sangoi AR, Karamchandani J, Lane B, et al: Specificity of brachyury in the distinction of chordoma from clear cell renal cell carcinoma and germ cell tumors: a study of 305 cases. Mod Patgol 24:425-429, 2011.

Sell M, Sampaolo S, Di Lorio G, Theallier A: Chordomas: a histological and immunohistochemical study of cases with and without recurrent tumors. Clin Neuropathol 23:277-285, 2004.

Tirabosco R, Mangham DC, Rosenberg AE, et al: Brachyury expression in extra-axial skeletal and soft tissue chordomas: a marker that distinguishes chordoma from mixed tumor/myoepithelioma/parachondroma in soft tissue. Am J Surg Pathol 32:572-580, 2008.

ANEURYSMAL BONE CYST

Clinical Features

- Male-to-female ratio is about 1.3:1
- More than 75% of cases occur in first two decades
- Three fourths occur in vertebrae (posterior aspect and spinous process), distal femur, and proximal tibia
- Small bones of the hands and feet and craniofacial bones are also relatively common sites
- Pain of variable duration and swelling are presenting symptoms

Radiographic Features

- Eccentric metaphyseal or posterior vertebral cystic lytic lesion that initially exhibits a permeative growth pattern with cortical destruction
- Periosteal bone formation may be seen
- In older lesions, a thin outer bony shell (eggshell) develops, and the cyst becomes trabeculated

Gross Pathology

- Hemorrhagic, cystic, honeycomb mass (Figure 16-33A)
- Fibrous septa separating the cavernous cystic spaces are gritty
- Spaces are filled with blood or serosanguineous fluid
- Solid, soft-gray to white mass may be present, representing a precursor lesion in secondary aneurysmal bone cysts

Histopathology

- Composed of numerous cavernous or cystic spaces filled with blood and lacking an endothelial lining
- Spaces are separated by fibrous septa lacking smooth muscle and containing fibroblasts, capillaries, inflammatory cells, giant cells, benign osteoid (may resemble osteoblastoma), and benign chondroid tissue (Figure 16-33B)
- Chondroid areas may have myxoid features, which is characteristic of aneurysmal bone cysts
- Mitotic activity may be brisk, but no atypical mitosis or stromal cell nuclear anaplasia is present
- Secondary aneurysmal bone cysts have solid areas exhibiting histologic features of the precursor lesion
- Secondary aneurysmal bone cyst may occur in many tumors, including the following: osteosarcoma, malignant fibrous histiocytoma, metastatic carcinoma, osteoblastoma, chondroblastoma, chondromyxoid fibroma, giant cell tumor, nonossifying fibroma, fibrous histiocytoma, fibrous dysplasia, eosinophilic

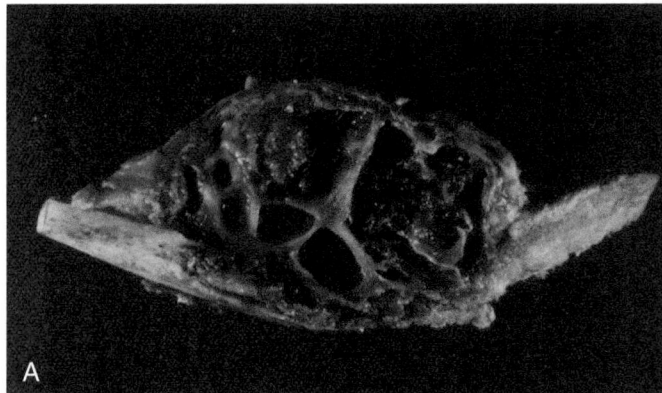

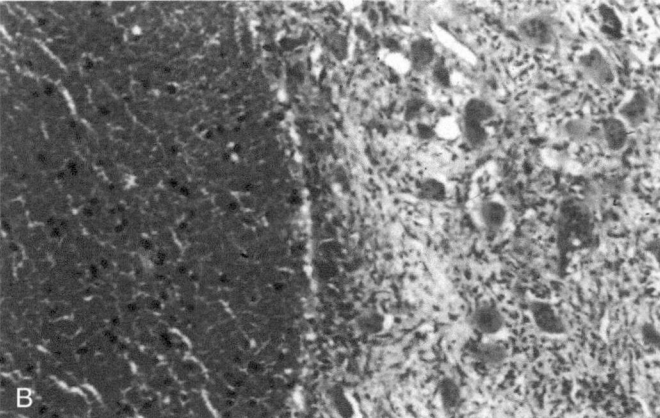

Figure 16-33. Aneurysmal bone cyst. A, Cross section shows complex, multiloculated cystic spaces filled with blood. **B,** Histologic section shows cystic spaces filled with red blood cells surrounded by giant cells, fibroblasts, and inflammatory cells.

granuloma, hemangioma, giant cell reparative granuloma, and unicameral bone cyst

Special Stains and Immunohistochemistry

- Noncontributory

Other Techniques for Diagnosis

- In one study, FISH detected abnormalities of chromosome 17p13.2 in 63% of primary aneurysmal bone cysts

Differential Diagnosis

UNICAMERAL BONE CYST

- Fibrous septa are usually hypocellular, with foci containing occasional giant cells
- Fibrous septa lack inflammatory cells, osteoid, and chondroid tissue

GIANT CELL TUMOR

- Located in the epiphyses in skeletally mature patients
- Stromal mononuclear cells and numerous evenly spaced multinucleated giant cells are present

TELANGIECTATIC OSTEOSARCOMA

- Uncommon in vertebrae, craniofacial bones, and bones of hands and feet
- Anaplastic tumor with production of tumor osteoid
- May show complex karyotypic abnormalities not found in aneurysmal bone cyst

SECONDARY ANEURYSMAL BONE CYST
- Histologic evidence of a precursor lesion (see "Histopathology") should be identified

PEARLS

- *Curettings and any solid areas of an excised tumor should be processed completely to evaluate for the presence of a precursor lesion*
- *Clinicoradiographic correlation is necessary to determine whether the histology represents a secondary aneurysmal bone cyst*
- *Precursor lesion is found in about half of aneurysmal bone cysts; most common preexisting lesions are giant cell tumor, chondroblastoma, fibrous dysplasia, and chondromyxoid fibroma*
- *Radiographic features of an aneurysmal bone cyst may mimic a malignant process*

SELECTED REFERENCES

Althof PA, Ohmori K, Zhou M, et al: Cytogenetic and molecular cytogenetic findings in 43 aneurysmal bone cysts: aberrations of 17p mapped to 17p13.2 by fluorescence in situ hybridization. Mod Pathol 17:518-525, 2004.

Basrir K, Piskin A, Guclü B, et al: Aneurysmal bone cyst recurrence in children: a review of 56 patients. J Pediatr Orthop 27:938-943, 2007.

Martinez V, Sissons HA: Aneurysmal bone cyst: a review of 123 cases including primary lesions and those secondary to other bone pathology. Cancer 61:2291-2304, 1988.

Mendenhall WM, Zlotecki RA, Gibbs CP, et al: Aneurysmal bone cyst. Am J Clin Oncol 29:311-315, 2006.

Saccomanni B: Aneurysmal bone cyst of spine: a review of literature. Arch Orthop Trauma Surg 128:1145-1147, 2007.

Unni KK, Inwards CY, Bridge J, et al: Tumors of the Bones and Joints, 4th Series, Fascicle 2. Washington, DC, Armed Forces Institute of Pathology, 2005, pp 324-330.

UNICAMERAL BONE CYST (SIMPLE CYST)

Clinical Features

- Male-to-female ratio is about 2:1
- Most cases occur in first two decades
- Most common sites are proximal humerus, midhumerus, and proximal femur
- Most are asymptomatic, but some patients present with sudden onset of pain due to pathologic fracture

Radiographic Features

- Elongated medullary expanding cystic lesion without cortical disruption
- Bone fragment may be present in the dependent area of the cyst (fallen-fragment sign)
- Cyst may contain fluid that has the density of water

Gross Pathology

- Intramedullary cyst containing clear or straw-colored, nonviscous, serous-like fluid
- May be multiloculated
- Cyst is composed of thin, delicate fibrous tissue

Histopathology

- Cyst wall is composed of thin, hypocellular fibrous tissue

- Occasional giant cells may be seen in the fibrous septa
- Inflammatory changes are absent or minimal
- No osteoid or chondroid tissue

Special Stains and Immunohistochemistry

- Noncontributory

Other Techniques for Diagnosis

- Noncontributory

Differential Diagnosis

ANEURYSMAL BONE CYST
- Hemorrhagic cyst contents contain osteoid and chondroid tissue with fibromyxoid features, and giant cells

GIANT CELL TUMOR
- Occurs in the epiphyses of bones in skeletally mature patients
- Composed of mononuclear stromal cells and many more giant cells than are normally seen in unicameral bone cyst

PEARLS

- *Fracture of unicameral bone cyst may complicate the histology because of the presence of reactive bone; may result in misinterpretation as aneurysmal bone cyst*

SELECTED REFERENCES

Dorfman HD, Czerniak B: Bone Tumors. St. Louis, Mosby, 1998, pp 879-891.

McCarthy EF: Differential Diagnosis in Pathology: Bone and Joint Disorders. New York, Igaku-Shoin, 1996, pp 105-107.

Unni KK, Inwards CY, Bridge J, et al: Tumors of the Bones and Joints, 4th Series, Fascicle 2. Washington, DC, Armed Forces Institute of Pathology, 2005, p 330.

Vigorita VJ: Orthopaedic Pathology. Philadelphia, Lippincott Williams & Wilkins, 1999, pp 256-261.

PAGET DISEASE OF BONE

Clinical Features

- Also known as osteitis deformans
- Male-to-female ratio is 2:1
- Most cases occur in fifth and sixth decades; rarely found in patients younger than 40 years
- Most common sites are pelvis, skull, femur, vertebrae, and tibia; rare in hands and feet
- About 85% are polyostotic, 15% monostotic
- Patients may be asymptomatic or present with pain
- Other symptoms that may occur at presentation or develop later are largely due to hypercalcemia and include deafness and other cranial nerve deficits, high-output heart failure, nephrolithiasis, hyperuricemia, arthritis, fractures, leonine facies, and femoral, tibial, or vertebral bowing
- Increased risk of developing a sarcoma (usually osteosarcoma)

Radiographic Features

- Bones show increased density with cotton-wool appearance intermixed with lucent areas

- Flame-shaped or V-shaped lytic areas may be seen in long bones; known as a *flame sign* or *blade of grass sign*
- Increased bone density or cortical thickening (window-frame appearance); round occipital and frontal bone radiolucencies (osteitis circumscripta) may be present

Gross Pathology

- Pinkish discoloration of bone due to increased vascularity
- Coarse, irregular, thickened cortex (Figure 16-34A)
- Irregular, thickened medullary cancellous bone
- Mosaic pattern of cement lines with rock-hard, dense bone in late stages

Histopathology

- Initially prominent osteoclastic activity with clustering of osteoclasts (large multinucleate forms)
  - Bony trabeculae with Howship lacunae formation
  - Intratrabecular fibrosis with increased vascularization
- Later, prominent osteoblastic activity and production of osteoid with abnormal collagen deposition are seen
- In the final inactive stage, the bony trabeculae are irregularly thickened, and cement lines form a mosaic pattern (Figure 16-34B)

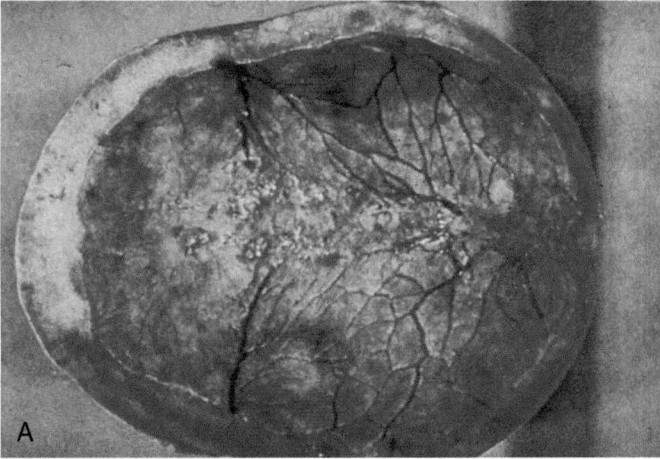

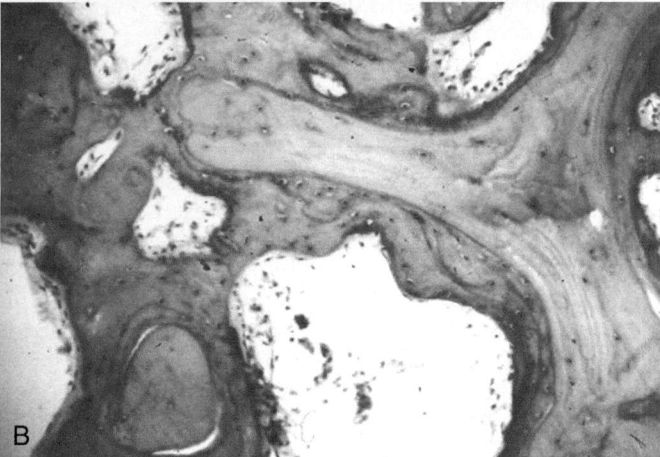

Figure 16-34. Paget disease of bone. A, Gross section of the calvarium shows marked overgrowth of the cortex. **B,** Histologic section shows irregularly thickened bony trabeculae with prominent cement lines.

Special Stains and Immunohistochemistry

- Noncontributory

Other Techniques for Diagnosis

- Genetic factors may play an important role, with mutations affecting different components of RANK-NF-κB signaling pathway
- Increased serum alkaline phosphatase and urinary hydroxyproline; normal or elevated serum calcium and serum phosphate

Differential Diagnosis

OSTEOBLASTIC METASTATIC CARCINOMA

- Tumor cells positive for cytokeratin

CHRONIC OSTEOMYELITIS

- Mixed inflammatory infiltrate consisting of intratrabecular plasma cells, lymphocytes, and occasional neutrophils

FIBROUS DYSPLASIA

- Osteoid islands do not exhibit osteoclastic or osteoblastic activity and do not contain abnormal cement lines

OSTEOBLASTOMA

- Usually occurs in a younger age group
- May involve the jaw bones but usually does not involve the calvarium
- Radiographic evidence of calcification may be present within the tumor
- Histologically, osteoblastoma is sharply demarcated from uninvolved bone

PEARLS

- *Paget disease of bone is a manifestation of an imbalance in bone metabolism; dysregulated osteoclastic activity followed by osteoblastic activity*
- *Symptoms may result from hypercalcemia when present*
- *Measles virus has been found in osteoclast precursors in Paget disease of bone*
- *Sarcoma occurs in about 1% of patients with Paget disease of bone; increases to about 20% in patients with polyostotic disease for more than 20 years*
- *Most common sarcoma arising in Paget disease of bone is osteosarcoma; other tumors that may arise are malignant fibrous histiocytoma, fibrosarcoma, chondrosarcoma, and malignant giant cell tumor*
- *Survival rate of patients with osteosarcoma arising in Paget disease of bone is much lower than that of classic osteosarcoma*
- *An increase in the baseline serum alkaline phosphatase level in a patient with Paget disease of bone is suggestive of sarcomatous transformation*

SELECTED REFERENCES

Deyrup AT, Montag AG, Inwards CY, et al: Sarcomas arising in Paget disease of bone: a clinicopathologic analysis of 70 cases. Arch Pathol Lab Med 131:942-946, 2007.

Josse RG, Hanley DA, Kendler D, et al: Diagnosis and treatment of Paget's disease of bone. Clin Invest Med 30:E210-223, 2007.

Layfield R: The molecular pathogenesis of Paget disease of bone. Expert Rev Mol Med 9:1-13, 2007.

Sharma H, Mehdi SA, MacDuff E, et al: Paget sarcoma of the spine: Scottish Bone Tumor Registry experience. Spine 31:1344-1350, 2006.

Unni KK, Inwards CY, Bridge J, et al: Tumors of the Bones and Joints, 4th Series, Fascicle 2. Washington, DC, Armed Forces Institute of Pathology, 2005, pp 368-370.

METASTATIC TUMORS

Clinical Features

- Most common sites are axial and proximal appendicular skeleton in adults and include pelvis, ribs, vertebrae, skull, and proximal femur and humerus
- Pain, swelling, and tenderness are the most common symptoms; some patients present with a pathologic fracture
- Most patients (about 80%) present with a history of a primary malignancy

Radiographic Features

- Consist of multiple, irregular, moth-eaten destructive lesions that are usually lytic but can be blastic or mixed lytic-blastic
- Periosteal reaction may be present

Gross Pathology

- Usually poorly delineated with infiltrative margins
- Variable in appearance, color, and consistency, depending on their primary tumor type
- Prostatic metastases are osteoblastic and may be dense

Histopathology (Figure 16-35)

- Most metastatic lesions exhibit histologic features suggestive of some line of differentiation (squamous, glandular, mesenchymal, or melanocytic)
- Clear cell patterns, glandular patterns with follicular features, and pigmented spindle cell tumors are indicative of renal cell carcinoma, follicular carcinoma of thyroid, and melanoma, respectively, and generally pose no problems in identifying the primary
- Some tumors are undifferentiated and require immunohistochemistry for determination of the site of origin

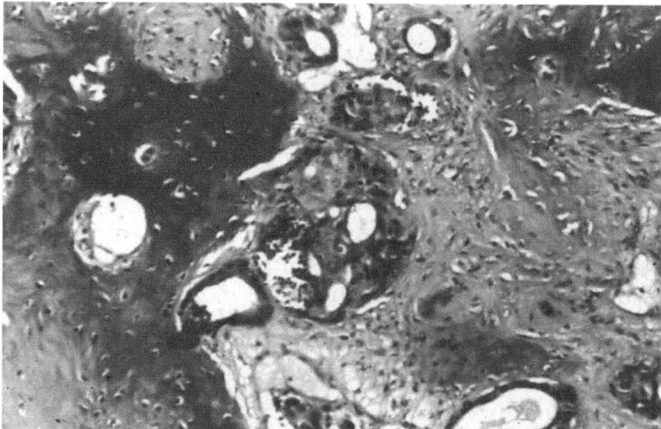

Figure 16-35. Metastatic adenocarcinoma. Histologic section shows bone with metastatic adenocarcinoma in a patient with a lung primary.

- Spindle cell tumors require immunohistochemistry to differentiate true sarcomas from the spindle cell variant of renal cell carcinoma and other spindle cell carcinomas

Special Stains and Immunohistochemistry

- Battery of immunohistochemical stains may be necessary to delineate primary tumor origin, depending on clinical history and morphology

Other Techniques for Diagnosis

- Noncontributory

Differential Diagnosis

OSTEOSARCOMA

- Metastatic carcinoma may produce prominent osteoid, suggesting osteosarcoma
- Negative for cytokeratin

PRIMARY BONE SARCOMAS

- Differentiation of primary bone sarcomas (malignant fibrous histiocytoma and fibrosarcoma) can be difficult and requires clinical correlation

PAGET DISEASE

- May mimic osteoblastic metastases
- Osteoblasts lining trabecular bone may appear atypical but do not express cytokeratin

PEARLS

- *Metastatic tumor cells reach bone through arterial embolization or retrograde flow through venous plexuses (e.g., Batson plexus, which lacks valves) or through veins with defective valves*
- *Metastases to bones distal to the elbows and knees are rare in adults*
  - *Metastatic acral bone tumors are usually due to metastatic lung carcinoma*
  - *Metastatic tumors to bone are more common in the appendiceal skeleton in children*
- *The most common primary malignancies in adults to metastasize to bone are prostate, kidney, thyroid, lung, pancreas, and breast*
- *In children, the most common are rhabdomyosarcoma, clear cell carcinoma of kidney, and neuroblastoma*
- *Osteolytic lesions on radiographs are usually thyroid, kidney, lung, or gastrointestinal tract in origin*
- *Osteoblastic lesions on radiographs are usually metastatic prostate, medulloblastoma, or carcinoid*
- *Tumor cells of prostatic adenocarcinoma metastases to bone in patients previously treated may appear histiocytic and require immunohistochemistry (prostate-specific antigen, prostatic acid phosphatase) to identify prostatic origin*

SELECTED REFERENCES

Ricco AI, Wodajo FM, Malawer M: Metastatic carcinoma of the long bones. Am Fam Physician 76:1489-1494, 2007.

Unni KK, Inwards CY, Bridge J, et al: Tumors of the Bones and Joints, 4th Series, Fascicle 2. Washington, DC, Armed Forces Institute of Pathology, 2005, pp 321-324.

Vigorita VJ: Orthopaedic Pathology. Philadelphia, Lippincott Williams & Wilkins, 1999, pp 472-489.

JOINT AND SYNOVIAL DISEASES

OSTEOARTHRITIS

Clinical Features

- Also known as degenerative joint disease (DJD)
- Male-to-female ratio is equal
- Greater than 80% occur in patients older than 55 years
- Interphalangeal joints of the hands; metacarpophalangeal joint of the thumb, hips, and knees; cervical and lumbar vertebrae; and metatarsophalangeal joint of great toe may be affected
- Other joints may be affected in secondary osteoarthritis
- Patients complain of arthralgia, limitation of motion, joint enlargement, and swelling
- Vertebral involvement may produce paresthesias, muscle weakness, and hyperreflexia
- Secondary osteoarthritis may result from Legg-Calvé-Perthes disease, previous history of gouty arthritis, rheumatoid arthritis, infectious arthritis, pseudogout, Paget disease of bone, osteonecrosis, hemarthrosis, trauma, hemochromatosis, and Wilson disease

Radiographic Features

- Diagnostic features include osteophyte formation, asymmetric joint space narrowing, subchondral osteosclerosis, and subchondral cyst formation

Gross Pathology

- Cartilaginous articular surface is thinned, irregular, or denuded, giving a polished ivory appearance to the outer subchondral bone (bony eburnation)
- Subchondral bone is thickened and sclerotic
- Peripheral osteophyte formation is common

Histopathology

- Articular cartilaginous surface is fibrillated, frayed, and thinned or denuded
- Chondrocytic hyperplasia is represented by aggregates of chondrocytes surrounded by basophilic staining matrix
- Subchondral bone is represented by thickened trabeculae
- Intratrabecular granulation tissue is present and may contain few lymphocytes and plasma cells
- Intratrabecular granulation tissue may undergo myxoid changes, with coalescence producing subchondral cysts
- May be superficial foci of osteonecrosis, subcortical fibrocartilaginous production, and marginal cartilage proliferation, with endochondral ossification producing osteophytes
- Mild synovial cell hyperplasia with subsynovial lymphocytosis
- Fragments of bone and cartilage may become embedded in synovium
- Cartilage may ultimately form loose bodies or "joint mice" by proliferation of chondrocytes, with subsequent fragmentation into the joint space

Special Stains and Immunohistochemistry

- Noncontributory

Other Techniques for Diagnosis

- Noncontributory

Differential Diagnosis

RHEUMATOID ARTHRITIS

- Contains a subchondral intratrabecular infiltrate of plasma cells
- Pannus formation

OSTEOARTHRITIS SECONDARY TO AVASCULAR NECROSIS

- Segmental osteonecrosis with bony trabeculae containing empty lacunae

OSTEOARTHRITIS SECONDARY TO CHONDROCALCINOSIS

- Contains clusters of calcium pyrophosphate crystals within chondroid matrix
- Crystals are rhomboid and are weakly birefringent

PEARLS

- *Denervation of joints, most commonly associated with diabetes, may produce osteoarthritic changes and is called neuropathic joint*
- *Spondylosis deformans is a form of osteoarthritis that involves the disks and vertebral bodies of the spine; disk cartilage herniates into the vertebral body (Schmorl node)*

SELECTED REFERENCES

Benjamin M, McGonagle D: Histopathologic changes at "synovio-entheseal complexes" suggesting a novel mechanism for synovitis in osteoarthritis and spondylarthritis. Arthritis Rheum 56:3601-3609, 2007.

Cushner FD, La Rosa DF, Vigorita VJ, et al: A quantitative histologic comparison: ACL degeneration in the osteoarthritic knee. J Arthroplasty 18:687-692, 2003.

McCarthy EF, Frassica FJ: Pathology of Bone and Joint Disorders with Clinical and Radiographic Correlation. Philadelphia, WB Saunders, 1998, pp 324-337.

RHEUMATOID ARTHRITIS

Clinical Features

- Male-to-female ratio is 1:3
- Can occur in all age groups, with most cases occurring in fourth and fifth decades
- Most commonly affects joints of hands, feet, and knees but eventually may involve other joints, including hips, shoulders, ankles, and sternoclavicular joint
- Patients present with arthralgia, stiffness, swelling, erythema, limitation of motion, and joint tenderness
- Extra-articular manifestations involving the heart, lung, pleura, skin/subcutaneous tissue, and hematolymphoid system can also be seen

Radiographic Features

- Concentric joint space narrowing, osteopenia, and marginal bony erosions

Gross Pathology

- Synovium is edematous with prominent villous architecture

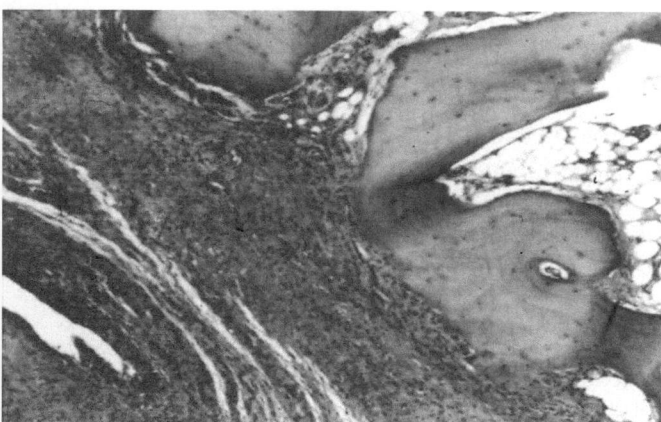

Figure 16-36. Rheumatoid arthritis. Histologic section shows a pannus covering the degenerated articular surface.

- Surfaces may have fibrinous deposits
- Articular cartilaginous surface is irregular and fibrillated and may be denuded, resulting in exposure of subchondral bone
- Pannus is present in subchondral bone and extends to the surface of the articular cartilage
- Rice bodies (detached inflamed fibrinous exudate) may be present

Histopathology (Figure 16-36)

- Subsynovial connective tissue contains plasma cell and lymphocytic infiltrate with lymphoid follicle formation
- Perifollicular cuffing of plasma cells and multinucleated giant cells (Grimley-Sokoloff synovial giant cells) may be present
- Pannus is represented by inflamed granulation tissue that undermines and covers the articular cartilaginous surface
- Chondrolysis is represented by cartilage exhibiting decreased staining of chondroid matrix and loss of chondrocytic nuclei
- Subchondral intratrabecular spaces may contain plasma cell infiltrates

Special Stains and Immunohistochemistry

- Noncontributory

Other Techniques for Diagnosis

- Serologic tests for serum autoantibodies: rheumatoid factor (RF) (low specificity); anti-citrullinated protein antibodies (high specificity)
- Class II major histocompatibility complex alleles DR4, DR1, or both

Differential Diagnosis

Osteoarthritis

- Osteophytes are more prominent, and articular surface pannus is absent
- Subchondral granulation tissue may exhibit myxoid changes, and subchondral cysts may be present
- Chondrolysis is not present
- Serology studies are typically negative

Chronic Osteomyelitis

- Presence of intratrabecular plasma cell infiltrates may mimic chronic osteomyelitis
- Clinical and radiographic features are different
- Serology studies are typically negative

PEARLS

- *There are no pathognomonic histologic changes of rheumatoid arthritis*
- *About 20% of patients with rheumatoid arthritis develop subcutaneous rheumatoid nodules*
- *Clinical history and laboratory findings provide helpful clinicopathologic correlations*

Selected References

Gynther GW, Holmlund AB, Reinholt FP, Lindblad S: Temporomandibular joint involvement in generalized osteoarthritis and rheumatoid arthritis: a clinical, arthroscopic, histologic, and immunohistochemical study. Int J Oral Maxillofac Surg 26:10-16, 1997.

McCarthy EF, Frassica FJ: Pathology of Bone and Joint Disorders with Clinical and Radiographic Correlation. Philadelphia, WB Saunders, 1998, pp 337-345.

McPherson RA, Pincus MR (eds): Henry's Clinical Diagnosis and Management by Laboratory Methods, 22nd ed. Philadelphia, Elsevier/Saunders, 2011, pp 980-983.

Vigorita VJ: Orthopaedic Pathology. Philadelphia, Lippincott Williams & Wilkins, 1999, pp 588-609.

GOUT

Clinical Features

- Male-to-female ratio is 2:1
- Peak incidence in fifth decade
- Usually monoarticular and involves large peripheral joints of the lower extremities
- Great toe is the most common site
- Acute gout presents with joint redness, swelling, and tenderness
- Chronic gout consists of painless tophi that may involve the ear helix, feet, hands, fingers, tibia, olecranon bursa, and Achilles tendon

Radiographic Features

- In acute phase, only subcutaneous swelling is seen
- In chronic phase, subcutaneous and periarticular masses adjacent to eroded bone are present
- Bone erosions are most common in the hands and feet

Gross Pathology

- Synovial pasty and chalk-white deposits in the soft tissue

Histopathology

- Specimens should be fixed in alcohol rather than formalin so as not to dissolve the crystals
- Polarizable needle-shaped uric acid crystals may be found within neutrophils and macrophages of synovial fluid
- In acute gout, the synovium contains neutrophilic and lymphocytic infiltrates

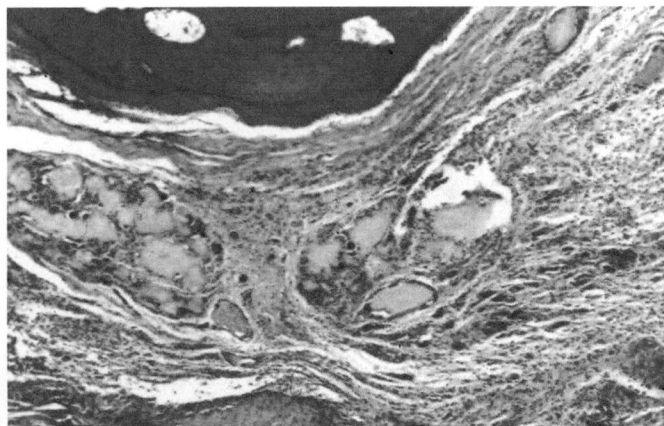

Figure 16-37. Gout. Histologic section shows amorphous material surrounded by histiocytic and multinucleated giant cells.

- In chronic gout, tophi are represented by pale-staining amorphous material surrounded by histiocytes and multinucleated foreign body–like giant cells (Figure 16-37)

Special Stains and Immunohistochemistry

- Noncontributory

Other Techniques for Diagnosis

- Polarized light and compensated polarized light have been used to identify crystals and categorize as uric acid (needle-shaped crystals that are blue when perpendicular and yellow when parallel to compensated polarized light)

Differential Diagnosis

PSEUDOGOUT (CALCIUM PYROPHOSPHATE DEPOSITION DISEASE)

- Crystals are rhomboid and birefringent
- Crystals appear blue when parallel and yellow when perpendicular to compensated polarized light
- Granulomatous inflammation is absent

INFECTIOUS GRANULOMATOUS SYNOVITIS

- Special stains (acid-fast bacilli, Gomori methenamine silver, PAS) may be positive, but negative stains do not rule out infectious granulomatous synovitis
- Cultures and clinicoradiographic correlation are necessary to rule out an infectious etiology

PEARLS

- *If a surgeon is suspicious of gout, recommend submitting surgical tissue specimen in 100% ethanol to prevent uric acid crystals from dissolving (uric acid crystals are soluble in formalin and will dissolve)*

SELECTED REFERENCES

Lam HY, Cheung KY, Law SW, Fung KY: Crystal arthropathy of the lumbar spine: a report of 4 cases. J Orthop Surg (Hong Kong) 15:94-101, 2007.

McCarthy EF, Frassica FJ: Pathology of Bone and Joint Disorders with Clinical and Radiographic Correlation. Philadelphia, WB Saunders, 1998, pp 346-348.

Vigorita VJ: Orthopaedic Pathology. Philadelphia, Lippincott Williams & Wilkins, 1999, pp 533-537.

PSEUDOGOUT (CHONDROCALCINOSIS–CALCIUM PYROPHOSPHATE DEPOSITION DISEASE)

Clinical Features

- Male-to-female ratio is 1.4:1
- Mean age of 72 years
- Rare before the age of 30 years
- Typically affects the distal radioulnar joint, symphysis pubis, knee, and intervertebral disks
- Many patients are asymptomatic
- Patients may present with symptoms of acute arthritis, including pain, swelling, and redness of the affected joint
- Associated conditions include hyperparathyroidism, hemochromatosis, hypophosphatasia, hypomagnesemia, hypothyroidism, gout, neuropathic joints, amyloidosis, trauma, osteochondritis desiccans, and familial hypocalciuric hypercalcemia

Radiographic Features

- Exhibits linear, punctate intra-articular calcifications within tendons, articular cartilage, and menisci

Gross Pathology

- Articular cartilage contains linear white deposits
- Synovium exhibits white deposits of crystalline material

Histopathology

- Aggregates of crystals are present within cartilage and synovium
- Crystals are rhomboid and birefringent; the crystals appear blue when parallel and yellow when perpendicular to compensated polarized light
- Inflammation is absent
- If crystals are absent, the chondroid matrix may exhibit reduced basophilia and mucoid changes, which are considered diagnostic of pseudogout

Special Stains and Immunohistochemistry

- Noncontributory

Other Techniques for Diagnosis

- Polarized light and compensated polarized light have been used to identify crystals and categorize as calcium pyrophosphate, which appears yellow when parallel and blue when perpendicular to compensated polarized light

Differential Diagnosis

GOUT

- Crystals are needle shaped and not birefringent; they are yellow when parallel and blue when perpendicular to compensated polarized light
- Granulomatous inflammation is present

TUMORAL CALCINOSIS (CALCIUM HYDROXYAPATITE DEPOSITION; METASTATIC CALCIFICATION)

- Radiographically, this process is represented by fused, round to oval soft tissue radiodensities
- Composed of nodular calcifications surrounded by macrophages and giant cells

- Intracytoplasmic giant cell calcifications, metaplastic bone, and psammoma bodies may be present
- No polarizable crystals are present
- May be associated with a history of chronic renal dialysis

PEARLS

- *By the age of 80 years, 20% of patients have joint deposits of calcium pyrophosphate*
- *About 25% of patients who undergo knee replacement surgery have deposits of calcium pyrophosphate in the native joints*

SELECTED REFERENCES

Fenoy AJ, Menezes AH, Donovan KA, Kralik SF: Calcium pyrophosphate dihydrate crystal deposition in the craniovertebral junction. J Neurosurg Spine 8:22-29, 2008.

McCarthy EF, Frassica FJ: Pathology of Bone and Joint Disorders with Clinical and Radiographic Correlation. Philadelphia, WB Saunders, 1998, pp 348-350.

Ryan LM, McCarty DJ: Arthritis associated with calcium containing crystals. In Stein JH (ed): Internal Medicine. St. Louis, Mosby, 1998, pp 1276-1279.

Saffer P: Chondrocalcinosis of the wrist. J Hand Surg [Br] 29:486-493, 2004.

SYNOVIAL CHONDROMATOSIS

Clinical Features

- Male-to-female ratio is 2:1
- Most cases occur in fourth and fifth decades
- Most commonly affected joints are knees (70%), hips, and elbows
- Most cases are monarticular
- Patients present with pain, swelling, and limitation of motion of variable duration (averaging 5 years)

Radiographic Features

- Well-marginated ring-shaped and stippled radiodensities in the joint or bursa
- May be fusion of these densities, forming a mass
- Bone erosion may be seen

Gross Pathology

- Synovium contains single or multiple well-circumscribed nodules of cartilaginous tissue
- Detached free cartilaginous nodules may be in the joint space
- Bosselated, larger nodules with outer granular surfaces representing fused smaller nodules may be identified
- Tendons and bursa may be involved

Histopathology

- Synovium contains multiple discrete nodules of hyaline cartilage, which may exhibit myxoid changes, calcification, or peripheral ossification (Figure 16-38)
- Clusters of atypical chondrocytes showing nuclei with open chromatin; small multinucleated forms, and mitotic figures can also be seen
- Cartilaginous nodules may exhibit endochondral ossification
- Chondrocytes with clear cell features and prominent eosinophilic cytoplasm may be seen

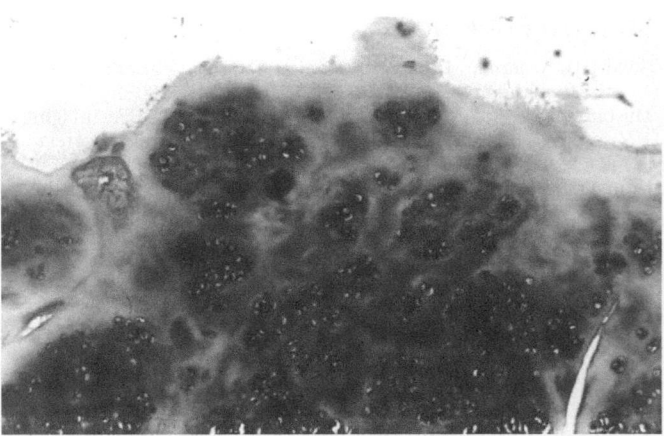

Figure 16-38. Synovial chondromatosis. Histologic section shows discrete nodules of mature hyaline cartilage.

Special Stains and Immunohistochemistry

- Noncontributory

Other Techniques for Diagnosis

- Noncontributory

Differential Diagnosis

SECONDARY SYNOVIAL CHONDROMETAPLASIA

- Evidence of preexisting joint disease (history or radiographic features of chondral fracture, osteonecrosis, or osteoarthritis)
- Histologically, the cartilaginous nodule has a central nidus of detached hypocellular articular cartilage or detached, necrotic subchondral bone that is surrounded by concentric rings of metaplastic cartilage composed of benign-appearing chondrocytes

SYNOVIAL CHONDROSARCOMA

- May mimic synovial chondrometaplasia radiographically, but the radiodensities are poorly circumscribed or demarcated
- Histologically, the cellularity is increased without clusters or cloning
- Solid sheets of crowded chondrocytes exhibit more significant atypia and mitotic activity
- Spindle-shaped forms are located around the periphery of nodules, and necrosis may be present
- Myxoid features may be more prominent

SECONDARY JOINT INVOLVED CHONDROSARCOMA

- Clinical and radiographic features suggest that the tumor is not arising in synovium but rather in bone with extension into the joint space

PEARLS

- *Chondrocytic atypia can be present in synovial chondrometaplasia to the degree that, in a different location (proximal or axial skeleton, not synovium), the diagnosis of chondrosarcoma might be made*
- *Clinicoradiographic correlation is important for evaluating these lesions so that they are not overdiagnosed as chondrosarcomas*
- *Malignant transformation has been reported*

SELECTED REFERENCES

Galat DD, Ackerman DB, Spoon D, et al: Synovial chondromatosis of the foot and ankle. Foot Ankle Int 29:312-317, 2008.

Murphey MD, Vidal JA, Fanburg-Smith JC, Gajewski DA: Imaging of synovial chondromatosis with radiologic pathologic correlation. Radiographics 27:1465-1488, 2007.

Unni KK, Inwards CY, Bridge J, et al: Tumors of the Bones and Joints, 4th Series, Fascicle 2. Washington, DC, Armed Forces Institute of Pathology, 2005, pp 386-389.

PIGMENTED VILLONODULAR SYNOVITIS (PVNS)

Clinical Features

- Male-to-female ratio is 1:2
- Majority occur in third and fourth decades
- Knee is the most common joint involved (80%)
- Hip, shoulder, and ankle are also commonly involved
- Usually presents with a long history of pain, swelling, limitation of motion, and joint stiffness
- Some patients present with hemarthroses

Radiographic Features

- Routine radiographs usually reveal soft tissue swelling
- May exhibit evidence of degenerative joint disease, represented by subchondral cysts and erosions on both sides of the joint
- Lucent bone lesions may be present
- CT or MRI reveals pedunculated lesions in the joint

Gross Pathology

- Synovium is brown and thickened; contains papillary villous projections and nodular structures
- Cut surface shows variable coloring, including yellow and red areas, depending on lipid and hemosiderin content
- Pedunculated or polypoid masses may be seen

Histopathology

- Cellular infiltrates of mononuclear cells within the subsynovial connective tissue
  - Mononuclear cells have oval nuclei with vesicular or clumped chromatin and prominent cytoplasm
  - Mitotic activity may be brisk
- Hemosiderin-laden mononuclear cells, multinucleated giant cells, and foam cells are present (Figure 16-39)
- In older lesions, areas of fibrosis are common

Special Stains and Immunohistochemistry

- Mononuclear cells and multinucleated giant cells express CD68 and HAM-56

Other Techniques for Diagnosis

- Cytogenetic studies: trisomy 7, trisomy 5, and aneuploid mononuclear cell lines may be seen
- Structural rearrangements of 1p11-13 may be seen

Differential Diagnosis

HEMOSIDEROTIC SYNOVITIS

- Usually occurs in patients with hemophilia, on anticoagulant therapy, or having a past history of post-traumatic hemarthroses, or in the presence of synovial vascular tumors (hemangioma)

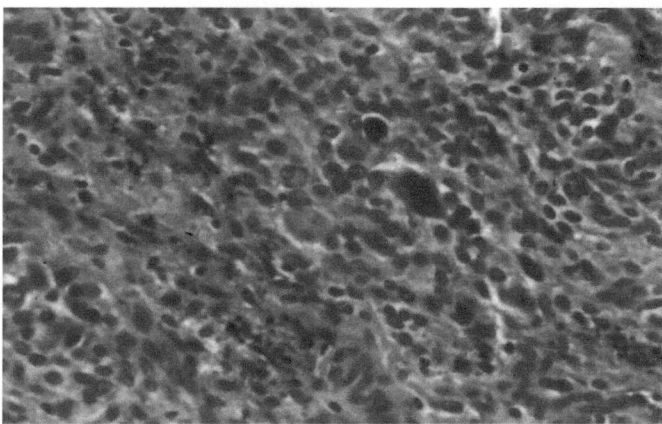

Figure 16-39. Pigmented villonodular synovitis. Histologic section shows subsynovial cellular infiltrate of mononuclear cells, multinucleated giant cells, foam cells, and scattered hemosiderin-laden macrophages.

- Villous synovial projections are delicate and do not form nodules
- Mononuclear cells in pigmented villonodular synovitis are not present, and foam cells and multinucleated giant cells are not typical

GIANT CELL TUMOR

- Does not exhibit radiolucent lesions on both sides of the joint
- Giant cells are larger, have many more nuclei, and do not stain with histiocytic markers

RHEUMATOID SYNOVITIS

- Synovial plasma cell and lymphocytic infiltrates with follicle formation
- Hemosiderin is not prominent

TRAUMATIC SYNOVITIS

- Foam cells and multinucleated giant cells are not present

DETRITIC SYNOVITIS

- Foreign material is found associated with an inflammatory response

PEARLS

- *Extra-articular nodular form of pigmented villonodular synovitis is called* giant cell tumor of tendon sheath; *occurs most often in older males and more commonly involves the fingers*
- *Secondary bone invasion occurs in about one fourth to half of patients*
- *Most cases are monoarticular*
- *Polyarticular involvement may occur, but it is seen in younger patients, tends to be familial, and may be associated with multiple lentigines syndrome, pectus excavatum, or fibrous dysplasia*
- *Malignant pigmented villonodular synovitis has been reported*
  - *Histologic features suggesting malignancy include cells with large, atypical nuclei containing large nucleoli and prominent eosinophilic cytoplasm; areas of necrosis and infiltrative borders are seen*

Selected References

Carpintero P, Gascon E, Mesa M, et al: Clinical and radiologic features of pigmented villonodular synovitis of the foot: report of eight cases. J Am Podiatr Med Assoc 97:415-419, 2007.

McCarthy EF, Frassica FJ: Pathology of Bone and Joint Disorders with Clinical and Radiographic Correlation. Philadelphia, WB Saunders, 1998, pp 310-312.

Somerhausen NS, Flecher CD: Diffuse-type giant cell tumor: clinico-pathologic and immunohistochemical analysis of 50 cases with extraarticular disease. Am J Surg Pathol 24:479-492, 2000.

Unni KK, Inwards CY, Bridge J, et al: Tumors of the Bones and Joints, 4th Series, Fascicle 2. Washington, DC, Armed Forces Institute of Pathology, 2005, pp 383-384.

Chapter 17
Soft Tissue

ROBIN D. LEGALLO • MARK R. WICK

CHAPTER OUTLINE

NODULAR FASCIITIS

Clinical Features

- Primarily affects young adults aged 20 to 40 years; occasionally seen in children

- Presents as a rapidly growing solitary mass; may be painful
- Inconsistently associated with recognized previous trauma (10% to 15%)
- Can involve any site; flexor aspect of forearm, chest, and back are common sites

Gross Pathology

- Located in the deep dermis or subcutis; occasionally occurs intramuscularly
- Round to oval, nodular, well-circumscribed mass; usually smaller than 3 cm
- Cut surface may be fibrous, myxoid, or cystic

Histopathology

- Usually well circumscribed but occasionally infiltrative
- "Tissue culture" appearance with long fascicles of spindled cells with a whorled growth pattern; extravasated red blood cells are a helpful feature (Figure 17-1)
- Newer lesions have a loose, feathery collagenous stroma with myxoid or microcystic appearance, whereas older lesions are less cellular and more densely collagenized
- Zonal pattern with cellular periphery and loose, feathery center that may be cystic
- Scattered inflammatory cells, typically lymphocytes and macrophages
- Frequent mitotic figures; no abnormal mitotic figures
- Variants
  - Intravascular fasciitis
    - Primarily affects children and adolescents
    - Involves arteries and veins
  - Cranial fasciitis
    - Affects infants younger than 1 year
    - Involves the scalp and skull
    - Often shows osseous metaplasia
  - Ossifying fasciitis
    - Periosteal location
    - Similar to myositis ossificans but lacks triphasic zonal pattern

Special Stains and Immunohistochemistry

- Vimentin and smooth muscle actin (SMA) positive
- Immunohistochemistry does not help to exclude other myofibroblastic or smooth muscle proliferations

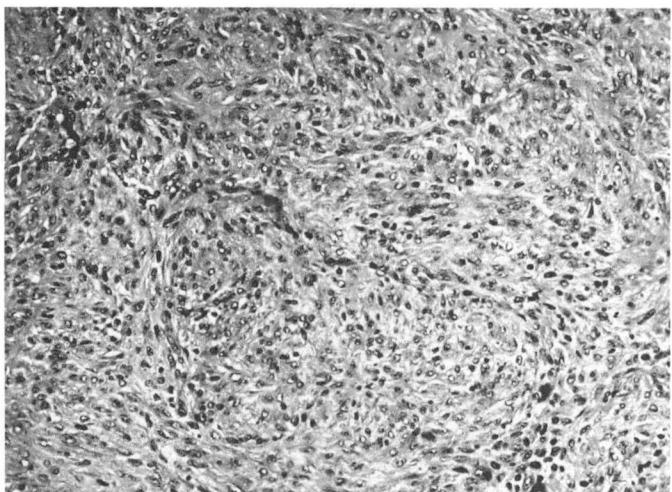

Figure 17-1. Nodular fasciitis. Bland, plump spindle cells show a "cell culture" growth pattern. Rare extravasated red cells are present.

Other Techniques for Diagnosis

- Translocation t(17;22)(p13;q13.1), producing a *MYH9-UPS6* fusion demonstrable by molecular or in situ hybridization studies, typically cryptic by karyotype
- Only seen in nodular fasciitis, not its variants

Differential Diagnosis

Kaposi Sarcoma

- Ill-defined margins
- Prominent vasculature, extravasated red blood cells
- Found in immunocompromised individuals; typically patients with acquired immunodeficiency syndrome (AIDS)
- Immunoreactive for human herpesvirus type 8 (HHV-8) and latent nuclear antigen 1 (LNA-1)

Myxoma

- Characterized by a paucity of cells, myxoid matrix, and sparse vascularity

Fibrous Histiocytoma (Dermatofibroma)

- Spindle cell proliferation admixed with epithelioid and foamy histiocytes
- Typically arranged in a storiform pattern
- Lacks prominent vasculature and extravasated red blood cells

Fibromatosis (Desmoid Tumor)

- Typically involves the abdomen or trunk
- Usually shows infiltrative margins
- Dense collagenous stroma usually lacking inflammatory component or myxoid areas
- Lacks thin-walled vessels and extravasated red blood cells
- Nuclear immunoreactivity for β-catenin

PEARLS

- *Nodular fasciitis is commonly misdiagnosed as a sarcoma*
- *Confirmed as a neoplastic condition*
- *Benign lesion with an excellent prognosis*
- *May progress through myxoid, cellular, and fibrous phases*
- *Conservative surgical resection is the treatment of choice*

Selected References

Amary MF, Ye H, Berisha F, Tirabosco R, et al: Detection of USP6 gene rearrangement in nodular fasciitis: an important diagnostic tool. Virchows Arch 463:97-98, 2013.

Erickson-Johnson MR, Chou MM, Evers BR, et al: Nodular fasciitis: a novel model of transient neoplasia induced by MYH9-USP6 gene fusion. Lab Invest 91:1427-1433, 2011.

Montgomery EA, Meis JM: Nodular fasciitis: its morphologic spectrum and immunohistochemical profile. Am J Surg Pathol 15:942-948, 1991.

Price EB Jr, Sillaphant WM, Shuman R: Nodular fasciitis: a clinicopathologic analysis of 65 cases. Am J Clin Pathol 35:122-136, 1961.

Sarangarajan R, Dehner LP: Cranial and extracranial fasciitis of childhood: a clinicopathologic and immunohistochemical study. Hum Pathol 30:87-92, 1999.

PROLIFERATIVE FASCIITIS AND MYOSITIS

Clinical Features

- Typically occurs in adults (usually about 50 years of age)
- Firm, palpable, rapidly growing subcutaneous or intramuscular nodule; may be painful
  - Proliferative fasciitis

- Most common site is forearm, followed by leg and trunk
  - Often associated with a history of trauma
- Proliferative myositis
  - Commonly located in the flat muscles of the trunk and shoulder girdle

Gross Pathology

- Poorly circumscribed, gray-white soft tissue mass
- Typically measures 1 to 3 cm in diameter
- Proliferative myositis is commonly a pale, gray, scarlike induration involving muscle and overlying fascia

Histopathology

- Ill-defined lesions characterized by large myofibroblasts that have large vesicular nuclei, prominent nucleoli, and abundant eosinophilic cytoplasm (ganglion-like cells) admixed with immature spindle cells in a matrix composed of varying proportions of mucoid material and collagen
- Often numerous mitotic figures in spindled and ganglion-like cells; they are not atypical (Figure 17-2)
  - Proliferative fasciitis
    - Histologic features similar to those of proliferative myositis except for a lack of intramuscular location
    - Typically grows along fibrous septa with an interlobular distribution
  - Proliferative myositis
    - Endomysial and epimysial growth separates bundles of atrophic skeletal muscle, creating a checkerboard pattern

Special Stains and Immunohistochemistry

- Ganglion-like cells are often nonreactive toward muscle markers and react with vimentin only

Other Techniques for Diagnosis

- Noncontributory

Differential Diagnosis

RHABDOMYOSARCOMA

- Tumor of children, rarely seen in adults
- Presence of rhabdomyoblasts rarely with cytoplasmic cross-striations

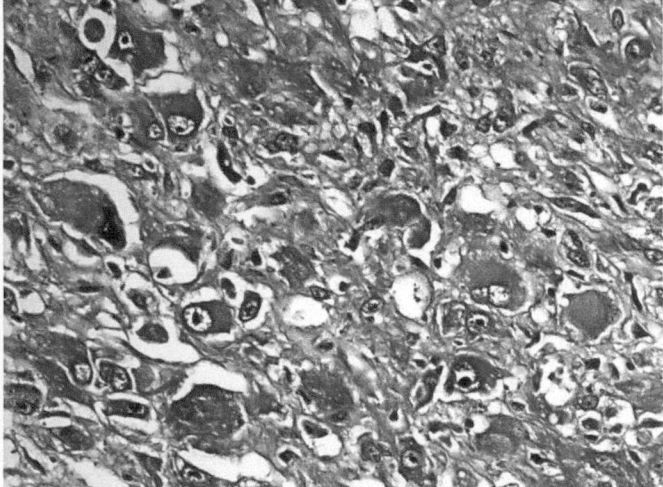

Figure 17-2. Proliferative fasciitis. Numerous ganglion-like cells are seen in a collagenous stroma.

- Immunoreactivity for desmin, muscle-specific actin (MSA), myogenin, and MyoD1

GANGLIONEUROBLASTOMA

- Intermixed neuroblasts and ganglion cells in a background of schwannian spindle cell stroma
- S-100 protein is present in the schwannian stroma
- Tumor of young children; extremities an unusual location

NODULAR FASCIITIS

- Typically has well-defined margins
- Spindle cell proliferation with scattered inflammatory cells and extravasated red blood cells
- Lacks prominent ganglion-like cells
- *MYH9-USP6* translocation

PEARLS

- *Pathogenesis of proliferative fasciitis and myositis remains unexplained; fascial or muscular injury is thought to be a likely contributor*
- *Benign, self-limited, reactive process treated with conservative surgical excision*
- *Proliferative fasciitis and proliferative myositis are similar reactive proliferations that are best distinguished by their locations*

SELECTED REFERENCES

Chung EB, Enzinger FM: Proliferative fasciitis. Cancer 36:1450-1458, 1975.

El-Jabbour JN, Bennett MH, Burke MM, et al: Proliferative myositis: an immunohistochemical and ultrastructural study. Am J Surg Pathol 15:654-659, 1991.

Enzinger FM, Dulcey F: Proliferative myositis: report of thirty-three cases. Cancer 20:2213-2223, 1967.

Meis JM, Enzinger FM: Proliferative fasciitis and myositis of childhood. Am J Surg Pathol 16:364-372, 1992.

Wong NL: Fine needle aspiration cytology of pseudosarcomatous reactive proliferative lesions of soft tissue. Acta Cytol 46:1049-1055, 2002.

MYOSITIS OSSIFICANS

Clinical Features

- Commonly affects young, athletic adults; usually involves the extremities
- Uncommon in children
- Presents as a solitary, tender mass; often associated with a history of trauma (> 50% of cases)
- Radiographic findings show characteristic zonal ossification

Gross Pathology

- Well-circumscribed, gray-yellow lesions with gritty areas

Histopathology

- Typically shows a triphasic pattern with distinct zonation
  - Central cellular region
    - Resembles nodular fasciitis
    - Cells have bland nuclear features and a variable mitotic rate
    - Occasional multinucleated giant cells
  - Intermediate region is composed of immature osteoid
  - Peripheral zone is composed of mature, "purposeful" lamellar bone

Special Stains and Immunohistochemistry

- Noncontributory

Other Techniques for Diagnosis

- Noncontributory

Differential Diagnosis

EXTRASKELETAL OSTEOSARCOMA

- Characterized by disorderly growth of hyperchromatic, pleomorphic cells with delicate lacelike osteoid formation, often with faint bluish calcification
- Absence of zonation

PEARLS

- *Myositis ossificans is a benign, self-limited process with an excellent prognosis*
- *Spontaneous regression can occur*

SELECTED REFERENCES

Ackerman LV: Extra-osseous localized non-neoplastic bone and cartilage formation (so-called myositis ossificans): clinical and pathological confusion with malignant neoplasms. J Bone Joint Surg Am 40:279-298, 1958.

Clapton WK, James CL, Morris LL, et al: Myositis ossificans in childhood. Pathology 24:311-314, 1992.

Nuovo MA, Norman A, Chumas J, Ackerman LV: Myositis ossificans with atypical clinical, radiographic, or pathologic findings: a review of 23 cases. Skeletal Radiol 21:87-101, 1992.

Wilson JD, Montague CJ, Salcuni P, et al: Heterotopic mesenteric ossification ("intraabdominal myositis ossificans"): report of five cases. Am J Surg Pathol 23:1464-1470, 1999.

ISCHEMIC FASCIITIS

Clinical Features

- Also referred to as *atypical decubital fibroplasia*
- Occurs over bony prominences or other pressure points in debilitated patients
- Almost exclusively seen in late adulthood and rarely in younger patients
- More commonly found in females

Gross Pathology

- Poorly circumscribed, multinodular mass up to 10 cm in diameter
- May have overlying ulceration

Histopathology

- Typical zonation pattern
  - Central necrotic region
    - Liquefactive or coagulative necrosis with fibrin deposition (Figure 17-3)
  - Peripheral fibroblastic and vascular proliferation
    - Granulation tissue–like with plump endothelial cells
    - Atypical fibroblasts with abundant eosinophilic cytoplasm and ganglion-like features
    - Vascular thrombosis and fibrinoid necrosis

Special Stains and Immunohistochemistry

- Noncontributory

Other Techniques for Diagnosis

- Noncontributory

Differential Diagnosis

EPITHELIOID SARCOMA

- Typically seen on the extremities of younger patients
- Atypical cells are immunoreactive for keratin and epithelial membrane antigen (EMA), loss of INI1

MYXOID LIPOSARCOMA

- Lacks the zonation of ischemic fasciitis
- Delicate plexiform vasculature and presence of lipoblasts
- *FUS-DDIT3* translocation

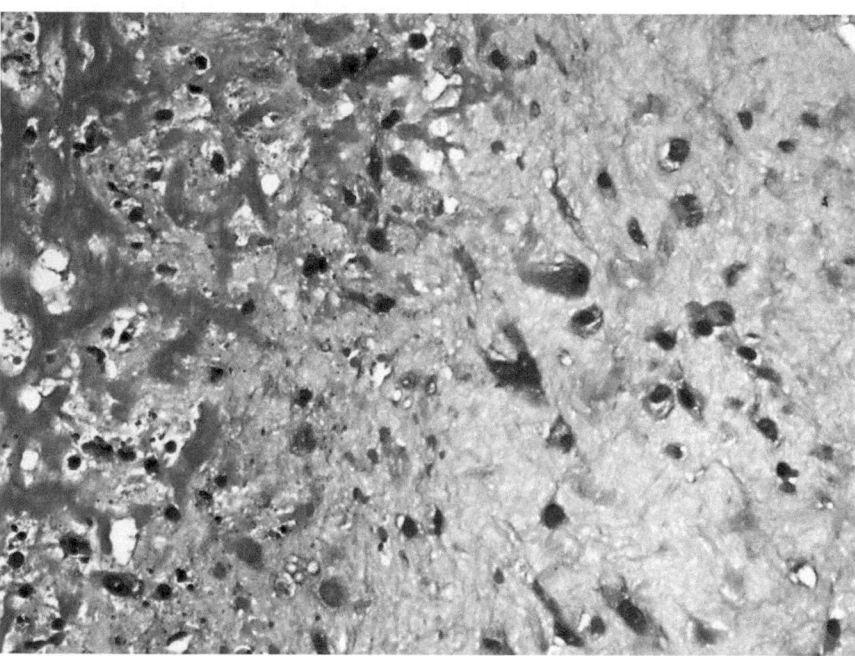

Figure 17-3. Ischemic fasciitis. A transition is seen between fibrin-rich necrosis and stellate myofibroblastic cells.

SELECTED REFERENCES

Ilaslan H, Joyce M, Bauer T, Sundaram M: Decubital ischemic fasciitis: clinical, pathologic, and MRI features of pseudosarcoma. Am J Roentgenol 187:1338-1341, 2006.

Liegl B, Fletcher CD: Ischemic fasciitis: analysis of 44 cases indicating an inconsistent association with immobility or debilitation. Am J Surg Pathol 32:1546-1552, 2008.

Perosio PM, Weiss SW: Ischemic fasciitis: a juxta-skeletal fibroblastic proliferation with a predilection for elderly patients. Mod Pathol 6:69-72, 1993.

ELASTOFIBROMA

Clinical Features

- Usually presents as a deeply seated mass located in the lower subscapular area
- Almost exclusively seen in late adulthood and rarely in younger patients
- More commonly found in females

Gross Pathology

- Firm, rubbery soft tissue mass with ill-defined margins
- Cut surface is gray-white and glistening with entrapped foci of fat
- Focal cystic degeneration often seen

Histopathology

- Poorly defined lesion composed of thickened, coarse slightly basophilic elastic fibers and scant fibroblastic cells embedded in a heavily collagenized stroma (Figure 17-4A)
- Entrapped mature adipose tissue is typically seen

Special Stains and Immunohistochemistry

- Verhoeff-Van Gieson elastic stain: Highlights elastic fibers (Figure 17-4B)

Other Techniques for Diagnosis

- Noncontributory

Differential Diagnosis

FIBROLIPOMA

- Characterized by predominance of mature adipocytes with intervening fibrous connective tissue
- Lacks elastic fibers

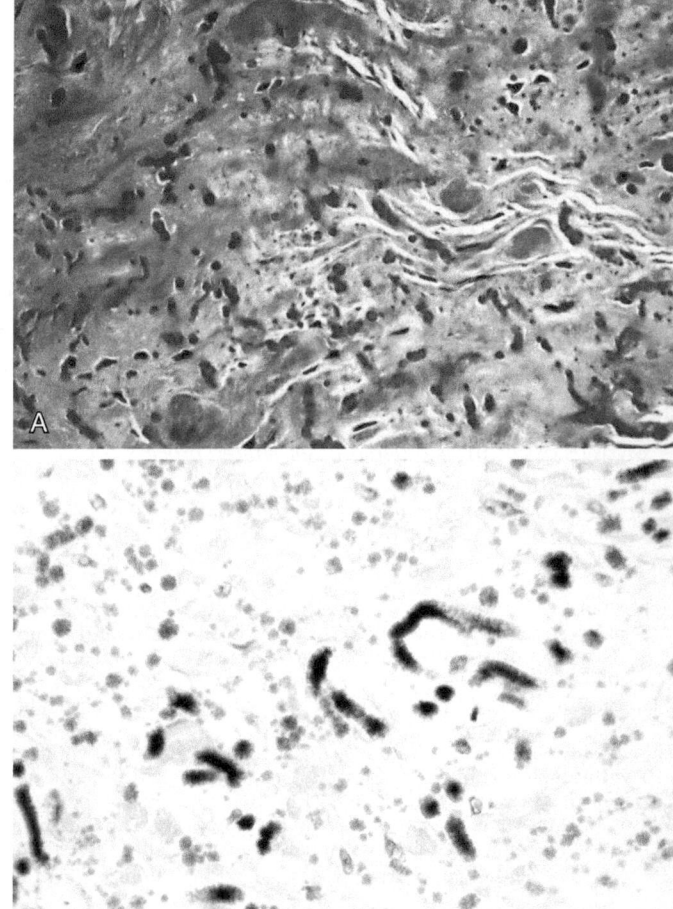

Figure 17-4. Elastofibroma. A, Thick and fragmented elastic fibers are seen in a collagenous background. **B,** Verhoeff-van Gieson elastic stain highlights the abnormal elastic fibers.

SELECTED REFERENCES

Lococo F, Cesario A, Mattei F, et al: Elastofibroma dorsi: clinicopathological analysis of 71 cases. Thorac Cardiovasc Surg 61:215-222, 2013.

Vincent J, Maleki Z: Elastofibroma: cytomorphologic, histologic, and radiologic findings in five cases. Diagn Cytopathol 40(Suppl 2):E99-E103, 2012.

Yamazaki K: An ultrastructural and immunohistochemical study of elastofibroma: CD 34, MEF-2, prominin 2 (CD133), and factor XIIIa-positive proliferating fibroblastic stromal cells connected by Cx43-type gap junctions. Ultrastruct Pathol 31:209-219, 2007.

SUPERFICIAL FIBROMATOSES

Clinical Features

- Presents as a small, slow-growing, subcutaneous nodule or thickening
  - Palmar fibromatosis (Dupuytren contracture)
    - Palmar surface of the hand; may result in contractures
    - Almost exclusively in adults, males affected more than females
    - Often bilateral, especially in alcoholics
  - Plantar fibromatosis (Ledderhose disease)
    - Plantar, non-weight-bearing area of the foot
    - Occurs in both children and adults
    - Often multinodular

- Penile fibromatosis (Peyronie disease)
  - Dorsal aspect of the shaft of the penis
  - Exclusively seen in adults

Gross Pathology

- Single or multiple, gray-white, firm nodules or scarlike tissue in the subcutis

Histopathology

- Proliferative and involutional phases
- Proliferative phase shows variably cellular fascicles of bland, spindled cells often arranged in a nodular pattern
- Occasionally prominent giant cells in plantar lesions
- Mitotic figures may be seen
- Involutional or residual phase shows paucicellular, densely collagenized tissue

Special Stains and Immunohistochemistry

- SMA positive
- Immunohistochemistry does not help to exclude other myofibroblastic or smooth muscle proliferations

Other Techniques for Diagnosis

- Noncontributory

Differential Diagnosis

CALCIFYING APONEUROTIC FIBROMA

- Primarily affects children and adolescents
- Characterized by an infiltrative growth pattern
- Hyalinized nodules with stippled calcification, often with chondroid features

FIBROMA OF TENDON SHEATH

- Well-circumscribed, sometimes multinodular mass firmly attached to tendon sheath
- Hypocellular with bland spindle cells widely separated by hyalinized collagenous stroma (Figure 17-5)

FIBROSARCOMA (INFANTILE AND ADULT TYPES)

- Infantile fibrosarcoma usually affects children younger than 1 year

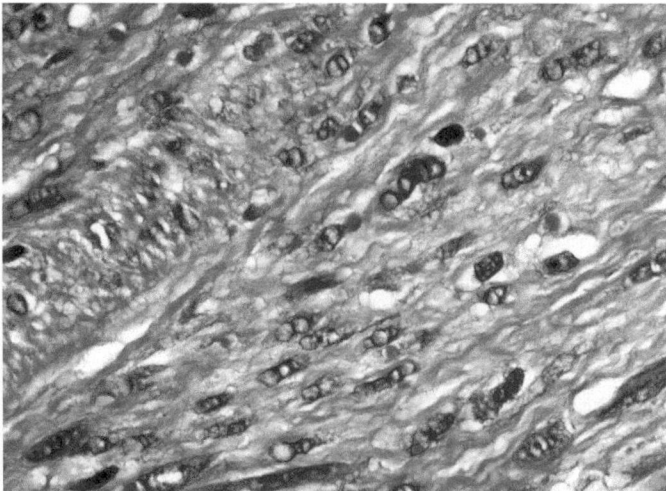

Figure 17-5. Inclusion body fibromatosis. Plump spindle cells contain cytoplasmic round, eosinophilic inclusions.

- Adult fibrosarcoma is only rarely found in distal extremities
- Highly cellular, infiltrative tumor composed of uniform fibroblasts with hyperchromatic nuclei and scant cytoplasm, arranged in a distinctive herringbone pattern
- High mitotic rate is common; atypical mitotic figures may be seen
- Areas of necrosis or hemorrhage may be seen

PEARLS

- *Superficial fibromatosis may be multifocal*
- *Plantar or palmar fibromatosis may be highly cellular and mistaken for sarcoma*
- *Associated conditions may include diabetes, cirrhosis, and epilepsy; some fibromatoses may have a hereditary component*
- *Surgical excision is the treatment of choice*

SELECTED REFERENCES

Allen PW: The fibromatoses: a clinicopathologic classification based on 140 cases. Am J Surg Pathol 1:255-270, 1977.
Evans HL: Multinucleated giant cells in plantar fibromatosis. Am J Surg Pathol 26:244-248, 2002.
Montgomery E, Lee JH, Abraham SC, Wu TT: Superficial fibromatoses are genetically distinct from deep fibromatoses. Mod Pathol 14:695-701, 2001.

FIBROUS HAMARTOMA OF INFANCY

Clinical Features

- Rapidly growing, painless subcutaneous mass in young children, sometimes congenital
- Common sites include trunk, shoulder, axilla, and groin
- Most cases occur within the first 2 years of life

Gross Pathology

- Poorly defined deep dermal or subcutaneous mass
- Gray, firm cut surface with yellow flecks
- Usually 2 to 5 cm but may be larger

Histopathology

- Triphasic appearance comprising an admixture of fibrous tissue, adipose tissue, and bundles of immature mesenchymal cells (Figure 17-6)
- Often has a stellate configuration and infiltrates surrounding fat

Special Stains and Immunohistochemistry

- SMA positive
- Immunohistochemistry does not help to exclude other myofibroblastic or smooth muscle proliferations

Other Techniques for Diagnosis

- Noncontributory

Differential Diagnosis

LIPOFIBROMATOSIS

- Lacks a primitive mesenchymal component

LIPOBLASTOMA

- Lobulated mass with fat lobules separated by fibrous bands
- Lacks a primitive mesenchymal component
- Myxoid stroma and lipoblasts are present

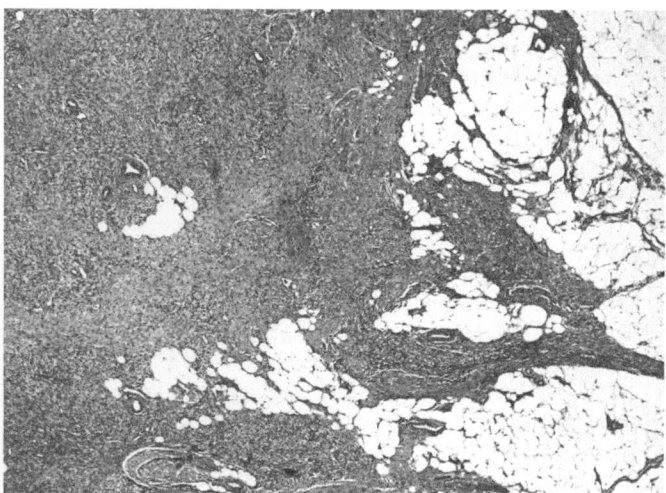

Figure 17-6. Fibrous hamartoma of infancy. The triphasic population of collagen fascicles, primitive myoid bundles, and fat forms a stellate lesion.

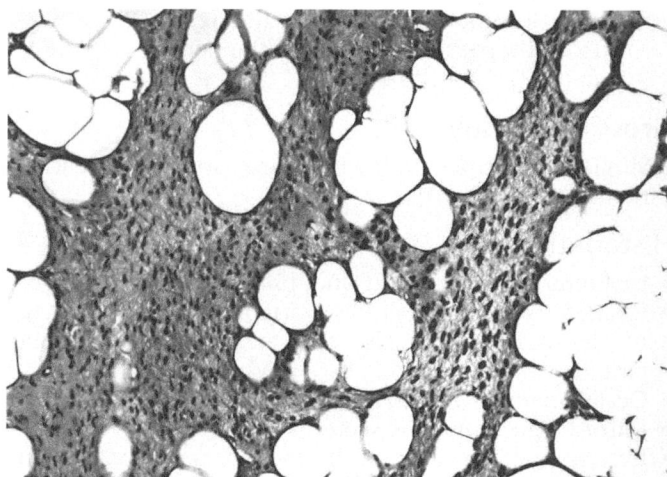

Figure 17-7. Lipofibromatosis. Fascicles of bland spindle cells and collagen are admixed with mature adipose tissue.

EMBRYONAL RHABDOMYOSARCOMA
- Lacks fibrous and adipose tissue
- Positive for desmin, myogenin, and MyoD1

PEARLS

- *Fibrous hamartoma of infancy is a benign lesion usually cured with local excision*

SELECTED REFERENCES

Coffin CM, Dehner LP: Fibroblastic-myofibroblastic tumors in children and adolescents: a clinicopathologic study of 108 examples in 103 patients. Pediatr Pathol 11:569-588, 1991.
Dickey GE, Sotelo-Avila C: Fibrous hamartoma of infancy: current review. Pediatr Dev Pathol 2:236-243, 1999.
Groisman G, Lichtig C: Fibrous hamartoma of infancy: an immunohistochemical and ultrastructural study. Human Pathol 22:914-918, 1991.

LIPOFIBROMATOSIS

Clinical Features

- Previously referred to as *infantile fibromatosis, nondesmoid type*
- Occurs in childhood, between birth and second decade; males affected more than females
- Slowly growing, painless mass most commonly presenting in an extremity or on the trunk; rare cases in the head and neck
- May cause isolated macrodactyly

Gross Pathology

- Poorly defined subcutaneous mass with admixed adipose tissue
- Usually 1 to 3 cm

Histopathology

- Bands of bland spindled cells and collagen traversing through mature adipose tissue (Figure 17-7)
- Infiltrative borders

Special Stains and Immunohistochemistry

- SMA positive
- Immunohistochemistry does not help to exclude other myofibroblastic or smooth muscle proliferations

Other Techniques for Diagnosis
- Noncontributory

Differential Diagnosis

FIBROUS HAMARTOMA OF INFANCY
- Contains a primitive mesenchymal component

LIPOBLASTOMA
- Lobulated mass with fat lobules separated by fibrous bands
- Myxoid stroma and presence of lipoblasts

DESMOID-TYPE FIBROMATOSIS
- Contains moderately cellular areas of fibrous growth, which infiltrates into fat; adipose tissue is not a primary component

PEARLS

- *Lipofibromatosis has a high rate of local recurrence but no metastatic potential*
- *Wide local excision is the standard treatment*

SELECTED REFERENCES

Deepti AN, Madhuri V, Walter NM, Cherian RA: Lipofibromatosis: report of a rare paediatric soft tissue tumour. Skeletal Radiol 37:555-558, 2008.
Fetsch JF, Miettinen M, Laskin WB, et al: A clinicopathologic study of 45 pediatric soft tissue tumors with an admixture of adipose tissue and fibroblastic elements, and a proposal for classification as lipofibromatosis. Am J Surg Pathol 24:1491-1500, 2000.
Kenney B, Richkind KE, Friedlaender G, Zambrano E: Chromosomal rearrangements in lipofibromatosis. Cancer Genet Cytogenet 179:136-139, 2007.

CALCIFYING APONEUROTIC FIBROMA

Clinical Features

- Also known as *juvenile aponeurotic fibroma* or *Keasby tumor*
- Most commonly affects children but may also occur in adults
- Presents as a slow-growing, painless mass, usually on the palmar or plantar surfaces of the hands or feet, rarely in other locations

Gross Pathology

- Poorly circumscribed, firm, gray-white, rubbery nodule usually smaller than 3 cm
- Gritty cut surface

Histopathology

- Bland oval plump fibroblasts in a heavily collagenized stroma
- Foci of stippled to confluent amorphous calcifications surrounded by rounded chondrocyte-like cells (Figure 17-8)
- Infiltrative margins with extension into adipose tissue
- Osteoclast-like giant cells may be associated with calcification

Special Stains and Immunohistochemistry

- Noncontributory

Other Techniques for Diagnosis

- Noncontributory

Differential Diagnosis

FIBROMATOSIS (PALMAR, PLANTAR)

- Characterized by fascicles of spindled uniform-appearing fibroblasts with varying amount of collagen
- Growth along fascial planes and tendons
- Absence of calcification or chondroid differentiation
- Usually found in adults, but plantar fibromatosis occasionally seen in children

CHONDROMA

- Typically occurs in adults
- Characteristically a lobulated lesion composed of mature hyaline cartilage
- Undergoes calcification in a diffuse rather than in a focal manner

GIANT CELL TUMOR OF TENDON SHEATH

- Numerous giant cells, plump mononuclear cells, and variable amounts of xanthoma cells
- Not calcified and no chondroid differentiation

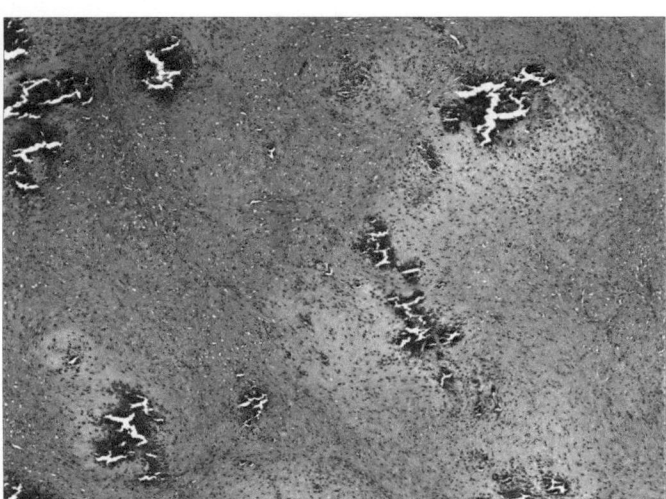

Figure 17-8. Calcifying aponeurotic fibroma. Nodular calcifications are surrounded by chondrocyte-like cells with intervening spindle cells in a hyalinized stroma.

SELECTED REFERENCES

Allen PW, Enzinger FM: Juvenile aponeurotic fibroma. Cancer 26:857-867, 1970.
Coffin CM, Dehner LP: Fibroblastic-myofibroblastic tumors in children and adolescents: a clinicopathologic study of 108 examples in 103 patients. Pediatr Pathol 11:569-588, 1991.
Fetsch JF, Miettinen M: Calcifying aponeurotic fibroma: a clinicopathologic study of 22 cases arising in uncommon sites. Hum Pathol 29:1504-1510, 1998.

FIBROMA OF TENDON SHEATH

Clinical Features

- Most commonly affects the hands of young to middle-aged adults; slight male predominance
- Presents as a slow-growing, painless mass, usually on the preaxial digits or wrist but may affect foot or knee joint

Gross Pathology

- Circumscribed, firm, gray-white, lobulated nodule attached to the tendon, usually smaller than 3 cm
- Fibrous, often multinondular cut surface separated by clefts

Histopathology

- Spindled to stellate cells embedded in a collagenous stroma, sometimes myxoid
- Clefted, pseudovascular spaces separate the nodules
- Degenerative cytologic atypia may be present; giant cells are rare

Special Stains and Immunohistochemistry

- Positive for smooth muscle actin (SMA)
- Negative for CD34, EMA, S100

Other Techniques for Diagnosis

- t (2;11)(q31;q12) has been reported but is not typically used for diagnosis; suggests a genetic link to collagenous fibroma

Differential Diagnosis

FIBROMATOSIS (PALMAR, PLANTAR)

- Growth along fascial planes and tendons with infiltrative borders

NODULAR FASCIITIS

- Rarely occurs in the hands
- Loose, feathery stroma with "tissue culture" appearance, extravasated red cells and scattered inflammatory cells
- Presence of t(17;22)(p13;q13.1), producing an *MYH9-UPS6*

- Giant cell tumor of tendon sheath
- Numerous giant cells, plump mononuclear cells, and variable amounts of xanthoma cells

PEARLS

- *Fibroma of tendon sheath is benign and typically cured by surgical excision; recurrence is rare*

SELECTED REFERENCES

Maluf HM, DeYoung BR, Swanson PE, Wick MR: Fibroma and giant cell tumor of tendon sheath: a comparative histological and immuno-histological study. Mod Pathol 8:155-159, 1995.

Pulitzer DR, Martin PC, Reed RJ: Fibroma of tendon sheath: a clinico-pathologic study of 32 cases. Am J Surg Pathol 13:472-479, 1989.

Sciot R, Samson I, van den Berghe H, et al: Collagenous fibroma (desmoplastic fibroblastoma): genetic link with fibroma of tendon sheath? Mod Pathol 12:565-568, 1999.

COLLAGENOUS FIBROMA

Clinical Features

- Also known as *desmoplastic fibroblastoma*
- Most commonly presents as slow growing painless mass in subcutaneous or deep tissues of upper extremities
- The majority occur in late adulthood but can occur in childhood

Gross Pathology

- Well circumscribed mass, usually less than 5 cm
- Cut surface gray-white with a lobulated or whorled appearance

Histopathology

- Hypocellular spindle to stellate cell mass embedded in a loose collagenous stroma
- Mitotic figures are typically not seen

Special Stains and Immunohistochemistry

- Spindle cell typically stain for vimentin only

Other Techniques for Diagnosis

- 11q21 rearrangements involving the *FOSL1* gene are frequently found
- Most common translocation t(2;11)(q31;q12)
- Differential diagnosis

DESMOID FIBROMATOSIS

- Typically seen in younger patients
- Infiltrative borders that entrap connective tissues
- Nuclear immunoreactivity for beta-catenin

PEARLS

- *Surgical resection is the standard treatment, typically does not recur*
- *May have a genetic link to fibroma of tendon sheath*

SELECTED REFERENCES

Evans HL: Desmoplastic fibroblastoma: a report of seven cases. Am J Surg Pathol 19:1077-1081, 1995.

Macchia G, Trombetta D, Moller E, et al: FOSL1 as a candidate target gene for 11q12 rearrangements in desmoplastic fibroblastoma. Lab Invest 92:735-743, 2012.

Miettinen M, Fetsch JF: Collagenous fibroma (desmoplastic fibroblastoma): a clinicopathologic analysis of 63 cases of a distinctive soft tissue lesion with stellate-shaped fibroblasts. Human Pathol 29:676-682, 1998.

Nishio J, Akiho S, Iwasaki H, Naito M: Translocation t(2;11) is characteristic of collagenous fibroma (desmoplastic fibroblastoma). Cancer Genet 204:569-571, 2011.

MYOFIBROMA AND MYOFIBROMATOSIS

Clinical Features

- Also known as *infantile congenital myofibromatosis* or *congenital myofibromatosis* in children
- Most common fibrous tumor of infancy
- About 90% occur within the first 2 years of life; however, adults may be affected
- *Myofibroma* refers to a solitary lesion (common), whereas *myofibromatosis* denotes multiple skin and soft tissue lesions with variable visceral involvement
  - Solitary subcutaneous nodules typically involve the head and neck but can occur anywhere
  - Multicentric form may involve the lungs, heart, bones, and gastrointestinal tract

Gross Pathology

- Cut surface is rubbery gray-white with a lobulated or whorled appearance
- May have central necrosis or cyst formation
- Margins may be well defined or focally infiltrative
- Size from 0.5 cm up to 8 cm

Histopathology

- Typically shows a biphasic pattern or zonal phenomenon
  - *Peripheral areas* show fascicular or whorled growth of plump, spindled cells with eosinophilic cytoplasm (myofibroblasts)
  - *Central areas* of the lesion are more cellular with oval cells and a staghorn-appearing, hemangiopericytoma-like vasculature (Figure 17-9)
- Variable mitotic activity but no atypical division figures
- Scattered lymphoplasmacytic infiltrate typically present

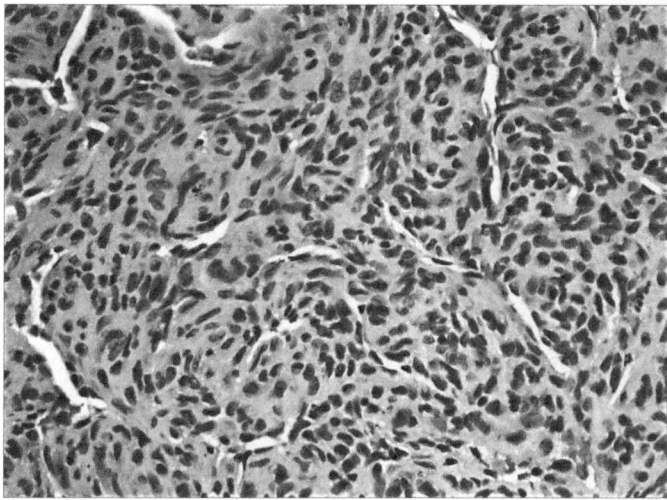

Figure 17-9. Myofibroma. Plump, bland ovoid cells are arranged in a hemangiopericytomatous growth pattern.

- Polypoid protrusion into vascular spaces is typical at the edge of the lesion
- Focal areas of hemorrhage, calcification, and necrosis may be seen centrally
- May be well circumscribed or infiltrative

Special Stains and Immunohistochemistry

- SMA and MSA positive
- Desmin variable
- Immunohistochemistry does not help to exclude other myofibroblastic or smooth muscle proliferations

Other Techniques for Diagnosis

- Noncontributory aside from ruling out other selected lesions such as infantile fibrosarcoma

Differential Diagnosis

NODULAR FASCIITIS

- Usually seen in older children
- Solitary, well-circumscribed nodule
- Zonation tends to be reversed, with a more cellular periphery and collagenized center
- Tends to be more myxoid, with more inflammatory cells and extravasated red blood cells

INFANTILE FIBROSARCOMA

- Most commonly involves the extremities or trunk
- Highly cellular, infiltrative tumor with herringbone pattern of growth
- Numerous mitotic figures
- Translocation t(12;15)(p13;q26), producing an *ETV6-NTRK* fusion demonstrable by molecular or cytogenetic studies

PEARLS

- *Patients with solitary and multiple lesions of myofibroma or myofibromatosis confined to soft tissues have an excellent prognosis; visceral involvement imparts a worse prognosis depending on the particular locations and extent of growth*
- *Lesions may spontaneously regress*
- *Surgical resection is the standard treatment*

SELECTED REFERENCES

Chung EB, Enzinger FM: Infantile myofibromatosis. Cancer 48:1807-1818, 1981.
Coffin CM, Dehner LP: Fibroblastic-myofibroblastic tumors in children and adolescents: a clinicopathologic study of 108 examples in 103 patients. Pediatr Pathol 11:569-588, 1991.
Daimaru Y, Hashimoto H, Enjoji M: Myofibromatosis in adults (adult counterpart of infantile myofibromatosis). Am J Surg Pathol 13:859-865, 1989.
Zand DJ, Huff D, Everman D, et al: Autosomal dominant inheritance of infantile myofibromatosis. Am J Med Genet 126:261-266, 2004.

GARDNER FIBROMA

Clinical Features

- Benign lesion of childhood and early adulthood that has a strong association with desmoid-type fibromatosis and familial adenomatous polyposis (Gardner syndrome)

- Poorly defined, plaquelike soft tissue mass in superficial and deep tissues of back and paraspinal region, head and neck, extremities, and chest

Gross Pathology

- Ill-defined firm mass with a white-gray, rubbery cut surface
- Ranges in size from 1 to 12 cm

Histopathology

- Sheets of densely hyalinized bundles of collagen containing scant, small spindle cells
- Collagen fibers are separated by cracks or clefts
- Infiltrative borders are seen with entrapped connective tissue

Special Stains and Immunohistochemistry

- CD34 positive
- β-Catenin: most are positive with nuclear labeling

Other Techniques for Diagnosis

- Noncontributory

Differential Diagnosis

DESMOID-TYPE FIBROMATOSIS

- More cellular spindle cell proliferation with fascicular growth pattern

NUCHAL FIBROMA

- Bundles of hyalinized collagen with entrapped adnexal structures and connective tissues
- Frequently has proliferation of small nerves similar to traumatic neuroma
- Distinct clinical presentation, occurs in the posterior neck of middle-aged adult (males affected more than females); associated with diabetes mellitus in about half of cases
- CD34 and β-catenin stains typically negative

ELASTOFIBROMA

- Densely eosinophilic elastic fibers intermixed with collagen as highlighted with the Verhoeff-van Gieson elastic stain
- Occurs in older patients, frequently in subscapular location
- Not associated with familial adenomatous polyposis

PEARLS

- *Gardner fibroma may be the first presentation of familial adenomatous polyposis (Gardner syndrome)*
- *About half of patients will develop desmoid-type fibromatosis*
- *Surgical resection is the standard treatment*

SELECTED REFERENCES

Allen PW: Nuchal-type fibroma appearance in a desmoid fibromatosis. Am J Surg Pathol 25:828-829, 2001.
Coffin CM, Hornick JL, Zhou H, Fletcher CD: Gardner fibroma: a clinicopathologic and immunohistochemical analysis of 45 patients with 57 fibromas. Am J Surg Pathol 31:410-416, 2007.
Wehrli BM, Weiss SW, Yandow S, Coffin CM: Gardner-associated fibromas (GAF) in young patients: a distinct fibrous lesion that identifies unsuspected Gardner syndrome and risk for fibromatosis. Am J Surg Pathol 25:645-651, 2001.

DESMOID-TYPE FIBROMATOSIS

Clinical Features

- Also referred to as aggressive or deep fibromatosis
- Typically occurs in adolescents and young adults, but age range is wide
- Comprises a group of proliferative tumors that present as deep-seated masses
- Shoulder region, chest wall, thigh, and mesentery are favored sites
  - Musculoaponeurotic fibromatosis
    - Lesions are associated intimately with muscular aponeuroses
  - Abdominal fibromatosis
    - Rectus muscle is the favored location
    - Occurs almost exclusively in women who are pregnant or postpartum
  - Mesenteric fibromatosis
    - Found in mesentery of the bowel or retroperitoneum
    - Often associated with previous history of abdominal surgery
    - May be associated with Gardner syndrome (familial adenomatous polyposis, mesenteric fibromatosis, osteomas, and multiple epidermal inclusion cysts)

Gross Pathology

- May appear well defined but actually has infiltrative margins
- Often grows along fascial planes
- Firm tumor that often has a gritty cut surface
- Sectioning reveals a glistening, white, trabeculated surface

Histopathology

- Composed of uniform-appearing, spindle-shaped fibroblasts and abundant collagen (Figure 17-10)
- Infiltrative margins
- Extremely rare mitotic figures
- Delicate, thin-walled vessels with open lumens
- Myxoid matrix may be seen, primarily in abdominal fibromatosis

Special Stains and Immunohistochemistry

- β-Catenin: positive nuclear immunoreactivity
- SMA positive

Other Techniques for Diagnosis

- Recurrent chromosomal abnormalities include trisomies 8 and 20 and loss of 5q, not usually needed for diagnosis

Differential Diagnosis

NODULAR FASCIITIS

- Usually smaller than 3 cm
- Loose, feathery collagenous stroma with myxoid or microcystic appearance
- Scattered chronic inflammatory cells
- Frequent mitotic figures may be seen
- Extravasated red blood cells

LOW-GRADE FIBROMYXOID SARCOMA

- Alternating collagenized and myxoid zones with prominent curvilinear vessels
- May contain hyaline collagen rosettes
- Negative for nuclear β-catenin
- Presence of t(7;16)(q33;p11), producing an *FUS-CREB3L2* fusion in molecular or cytogenetic analysis

FIBROSARCOMA (INFANTILE AND ADULT TYPES)

- Most commonly affects children younger than 1 year; occasionally seen in adults
- Highly cellular, infiltrative tumor composed of fibroblasts with hyperchromatic nuclei and scant cytoplasm arranged in a herringbone pattern
- Mitoses are obvious, and atypical mitotic figures may be seen
- Areas of necrosis or hemorrhage may be present
- Infantile fibrosarcoma harbors t(12;15)(p13;q26), producing an *ETV6-NTRK* fusion demonstrable by molecular or cytogenetic studies

PEARLS

- *Desmoid-type fibromatosis has a high recurrence rate and may be locally aggressive but typically has no metastatic potential*
- *Surgical removal with a wide margin of resection is the preferred treatment*
- *Recurrence rate ranges between 25% and 80%*
- *There are no pathologic features that can predict recurrence*

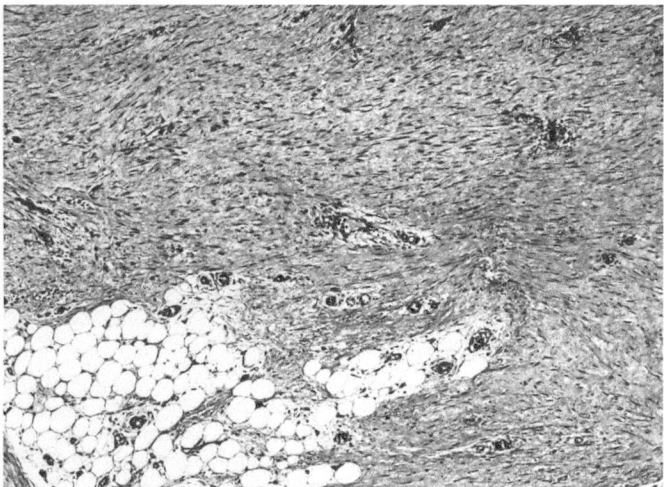

Figure 17-10. Desmoid-type fibromatosis. Moderately cellular fascicles of bland spindle cells in a collagenized stroma diffusely infiltrate surrounding fat.

SELECTED REFERENCES

Bhattacharya B, Dilworth HP, Iacobuzio-Donahue C, et al: Nuclear beta-catenin expression distinguishes deep fibromatosis from other benign and malignant fibroblastic and myofibroblastic lesions. Am J Surg Pathol 29:653-659, 2005.

Carlson JW, Fletcher CD: Immunohistochemistry for beta-catenin in the differential diagnosis of spindle cell lesions: analysis of a series and review of the literature. Histopathology 51:509-514, 2007.

De Wever I, Dal Cin P, Fletcher CD, et al: Cytogenetic, clinical, and morphologic correlations in 78 cases of fibromatosis: a report from the CHAMP Study Group. Chromosomes and Morphology. Mod Pathol 13:1080-1085, 2000.

CALCIFYING FIBROUS (PSEUDO) TUMOR

Clinical Features

- Benign fibrous tumor that occurs predominantly in adolescents and young adults
- Most common in subcutaneous and deep soft tissues of extremities, trunk, groin, and neck but has been described in many locations, including viscera
- Originally thought to be pseudoneoplastic, but not currently

Gross Pathology

- Typically a circumscribed solid mass, 3 to 5 cm, but may be larger
- Cut surface is solid, firm, and gray-white

Histopathology

- Hypocellular, sclerotic tissue with a sparse lympho-plasmacytic infiltrate and discrete calcifications (Figure 17-11)
- Calcification may be psammomatous or dystrophic
- Germinal center formation may be seen at lesion periphery

Special Stains and Immunohistochemistry

- Noncontributory

Other Techniques for Diagnosis

- Noncontributory

Differential Diagnosis

INFLAMMATORY MYOFIBROBLASTIC TUMOR

- Typically more cellular and less densely collagenized
- Calcifications are extremely uncommon
- Frequently positive for anaplastic lymphoma kinase-1 (ALK-1) in 40% of cases by immunohistochemistry

NODULAR FASCIITIS

- Typically more cellular with a myxedematous stroma
- Lacks calcifications
- Loosely apposed lesional cells

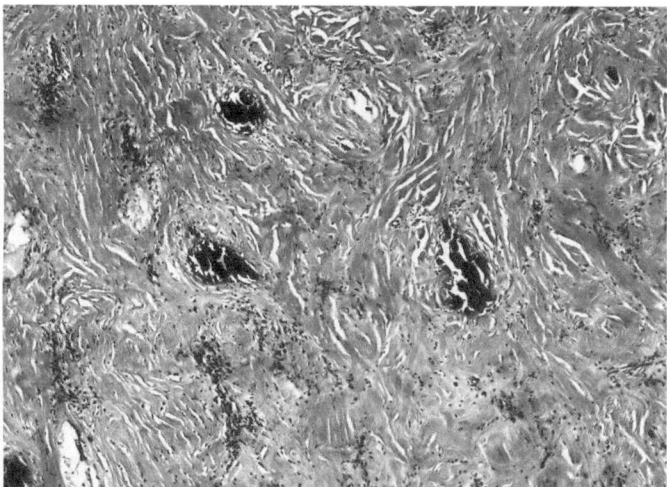

Figure 17-11. Calcifying fibrous tumor. Paucicellular, sclerotic lesion contains lymphoplasmacytic infiltrate and psammomatous calcifications.

DESMOID-TYPE FIBROMATOSIS

- Characterized by fascicles of spindle-shaped fibroblasts with varying amounts of collagen and infiltrative borders
- Calcifications are uncommon
- Positive for β-catenin nuclear reactivity

CALCIFYING APONEUROTIC FIBROMA

- Stippled calcification with surrounding chondroid differentiation
- Infiltrative margins
- Inflammation not typical
- Typically seen on hands and feet of young children

PEARLS

- *Calcifying (pseudo) tumor is a benign lesion with rare reports of recurrence*
- *Treatment is complete surgical resection*

SELECTED REFERENCES

Hill KA, Gonzalez-Crussi F, Chou PM: Calcifying fibrous pseudotumor versus inflammatory myofibroblastic tumor: a histological and immunohistochemical comparison. Mod Pathol 14:784-790, 2001.

Kirby PA, Sato Y, Tannous R, Dehner LP: Calcifying fibrous pseudotumor of the myocardium. Pediatr Dev Pathol 9:384-387, 2006.

Lau SK, Weiss LM: Calcifying fibrous tumor of the adrenal gland. Human Pathol 38:656-659, 2007.

Nascimento AF, Ruiz R, Hornick JL, Fletcher CD: Calcifying fibrous "pseudotumor": clinicopathologic study of 15 cases and analysis of its relationship to inflammatory myofibroblastic tumor. Int J Surg Pathol 10:189-196, 2002.

INFLAMMATORY MYOFIBROBLASTIC TUMOR

Clinical Features

- Previously known as *inflammatory pseudotumor* and *plasma cell granuloma*
- Most often occurs in children and young adults but has a wide age range
- Commonly seen in the lung; the most frequent extra-pulmonary sites are mesentery and omentum, but it can involve any location
- Systemic symptoms and signs may be present, including fever, weight loss, anemia, increased erythrocyte sedimentation rate, and elevated C-reactive protein levels

Gross Pathology

- Typically circumscribed, but nonencapsulated; often multinodular
- Cut surface is solid, firm, and gray-white

Histopathology

- Variably cellular tumor comprising spindle cells and mixed inflammatory cells in a myxoid or collagenized background (Figure 17-12)
- Some lesions contain large histiocytoid ganglion-like cells
- May be hypocellular and resemble scars
- Mitotic figures may be numerous but are not atypical

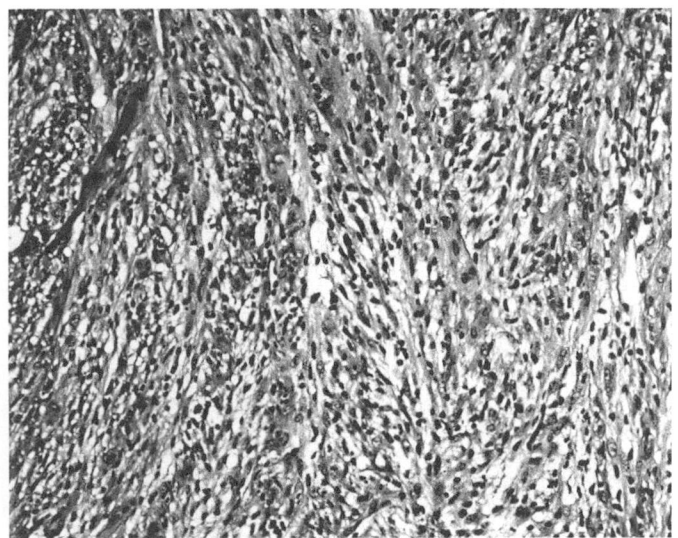

Figure 17-12. Inflammatory myofibroblastic tumor. Loose fascicles of spindled cells with large vesicular nuclei are admixed with an inflammatory infiltrate.

Special Stains and Immunohistochemistry

- SMA positive
- ALK-1 protein present in about 40% of cases, more frequently in childhood tumors

Other Techniques for Diagnosis

- Rearrangement of *ALK* locus at 2p23 by molecular or cytogenetic analysis

Differential Diagnosis

LEIOMYOMA

- Characterized by fascicles of uniform, spindle-shaped smooth muscle cells in short interlacing fascicles with negligible mitotic activity
- Well circumscribed
- Extremely rare in the deep soft tissues
- Lacks a mixed inflammatory infiltrate
- Immunohistochemistry not useful for differential diagnosis unless ALK-1 is positive (favoring a diagnosis of inflammatory myofibroblastic tumor)

LEIOMYOSARCOMA

- Characterized by fascicles of cytologically atypical spindle cells with hyperchromatic nuclei and variable but present mitotic activity
- Lacks a mixed inflammatory infiltrate
- Typically, middle-aged and elderly adults are affected

DESMOID-TYPE FIBROMATOSIS

- Fascicles of spindle-shaped fibroblasts with variable amounts of collagen and infiltrative borders
- Positive for β-catenin with nuclear labeling

EMBRYONAL RHABDOMYOSARCOMA

- Primitive spindle cells, usually in a myxoid background; focal strap cells may be present
- Usually lacks inflammation
- Positive for myogenin and MyoD1

INFLAMMATORY MALIGNANT FIBROUS HISTIOCYTOMA

- Usually occurs in older adults; retroperitoneum is the most common location
- Atypical hyperchromatic cells with prominent mixed inflammation rich in xanthomatous cells
- Negative for SMA and ALK-1

METASTATIC SARCOMATOID CARCINOMA

- May have areas of squamous differentiation
- At least focally positive for keratin, EMA, MOC31, or p63

SPINDLE CELL MELANOMA

- Variably cellular spindle cell lesion with variable cellular pleomorphism, prominent nucleoli, and nuclear pseudoinclusions
- May show perineural invasion extending beyond the tumoral component
- Positive for S-100 protein; rarely for tyrosinase, melan-A, or HMB-45

PEARLS

- *Inflammatory myofibroblastic tumor is currently considered a neoplastic process*
- *Treatment is based on surgical resection*
- *May recur after excision*

SELECTED REFERENCES

Coffin CM, Dehner LP, Meis-Kindblom JM: Inflammatory myofibroblastic tumor, inflammatory fibrosarcoma, and related lesions: an historical review with differential diagnostic considerations. Semin Diagn Pathol 15:102-110, 1998.

Coffin CM, Hornick JL, Fletcher CD: Inflammatory myofibroblastic tumor: comparison of clinicopathologic, histologic, and immunohistochemical features including ALK expression in atypical and aggressive cases. Am J Surg Pathol 31:509-520, 2007.

Cook JR, Dehner LP, Collins MH, et al: Anaplastic lymphoma kinase (ALK) expression in the inflammatory myofibroblastic tumor: a comparative immunohistochemical study. Am J Surg Pathol 25:1364-1371, 2001.

SOLITARY FIBROUS TUMOR

Clinical Features

- Typically occurs in middle-aged adults but has a wide age range
- Presents as a localized, slow-growing, painless mass
- Most commonly involves the pleura; extrapleural sites include subcutaneous and deep soft tissues, orbit, retroperitoneum, mediastinum, pericardium, and other locations

Gross Pathology

- Ranges in size from 1 to 27 cm
- Typically well circumscribed with a firm, tan-white cut surface; sometimes multinodular
- Focal necrosis, hemorrhage, and cystic degeneration may be seen

Histopathology

- Characterized by uniform spindle cells with attenuated nuclei, haphazardly arranged in a collagenized background; collagen focally surrounds individual cells (Figure 17-13)

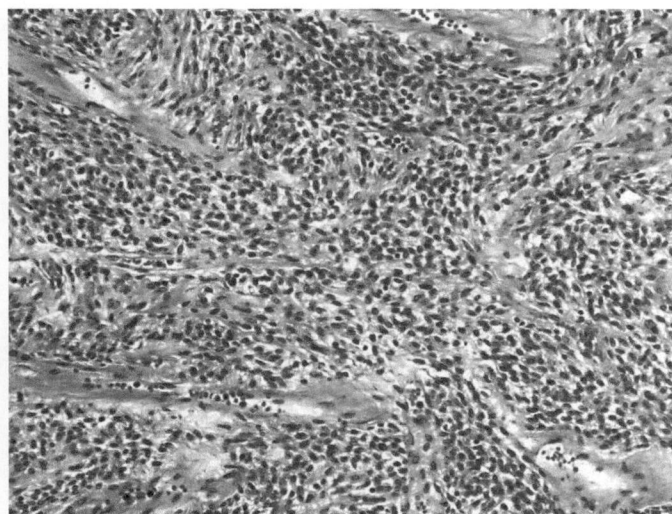

Figure 17-13. Solitary fibrous tumor. Monotonous ovoid and spindle tumor cells arranged in a "patternless pattern" around a hyalinized vasculature.

- Alternating hypercellular and hypocellular areas
- Hemangiopericytoma-like vasculature
- Epithelioid areas may be present
- Low mitotic activity (< 3 mitotic figures/10 high-power fields [hpf])
- Criteria for malignancy include dense cellularity, numerous mitotic figures, obvious cytologic atypia, necrosis, and infiltrative growth; dedifferentiation has been reported

Special Stains and Immunohistochemistry

- CD34 positive in about 85% of cases, CD99 and bcl-2 positive in about 75% of cases
- Nuclear immunoreactivity for STAT6 in 98% of cases

Other Techniques for Diagnosis

- Genomic inversion at 12q13 leading to fusion *NAB2-STAT6* in majority of cases

Differential Diagnosis

HEMANGIOPERICYTOMA

- Characterized by staghorn vascular spaces of varying sizes lined by flattened endothelium
- Perivascular and intervascular proliferation of uniform spindle-shaped tumor cells
- May show faint positivity for CD34; CD57 also positive in 50% to 60% cases
- Negative for keratin, EMA, and CD99

SYNOVIAL SARCOMA

- Monophasic spindle cell or biphasic spindle cell and epithelioid tumors with high nuclear-to-cytoplasmic ratios
- Herringbone growth pattern is common
- May show myxoid, squamoid, or collagenized images focally
- Mitotic activity is usually easily seen
- Intratumoral calcifications are sometimes present
- Immunoreactive for keratin or EMA, CD99, and bcl-2; CD34 negative

FIBROSARCOMA (INFANTILE AND ADULT TYPES)

- Usually found in children younger than 1 year; occasionally seen in adults
- Infantile form most commonly involves the extremities
- Highly cellular, infiltrative tumor composed of spindle cells with hyperchromatic nuclei and scant cytoplasm
- Mitotic figures are usually seen
- Tumor cells are arranged in a herringbone pattern, at least focally
- May show areas of hemorrhage and necrosis
- Negative for CD34, CD99, and bcl-2

PEARLS

- *Solitary fibrous tumor can occur at any location*
- *Has "patternless pattern" of spindle cells with hemangiopericytoma-like vasculature*
- *Usually behaves in an indolent manner but may recur or metastasize even if histologically banal; borderline tumor*
- *Surgical resection is the preferred treatment*

SELECTED REFERENCES

Doyle LA, Vivero M, Fletcher CD, et al: Nuclear expression of STAT6 distinguishes solitary fibrous tumor from histologic mimics. Modern Pathol 27:390-395, 2014.
Mohajeri A, Tayebwa J, Collin A, et al: Comprehensive genetic analysis identifies a pathognomonic NAB2/STAT6 fusion gene, nonrandom secondary genomic imbalances, and a characteristic gene expression profile in solitary fibrous tumor. Genes Chromosomes Cancer 52:873-886, 2013.
Mosquera JM, Fletcher CD: Expanding the spectrum of malignant progression in solitary fibrous tumors: a study of 8 cases with a discrete anaplastic component: is this dedifferentiated SFT? Am J Surg Pathol 33:1314-1321, 2009.

HEMOSIDEROTIC FIBROLIPOMATOUS TUMOR (HFLT)/MYXOINFLAMMATORY FIBROBLASTIC SARCOMA (MIFS)

Clinical Features

- HFLT (also known as *hemosiderotic fibrohistiocytic lipomatous lesion*) and MIFS are discussed together due to their clinicopathologic and molecular similarities; hybrid tumors have been reported
- Presents as a localized, slow-growing mass of the distal extremities; HFLT is more common on the ankles
- Adults are affected more often than children, and HFLT is more common in women

Gross Pathology

- Ranges in size from 1 to 20 cm and has infiltrative borders
- Tan to yellow cut section but may be gelatinous or fatty; hemorrhage may be present

Histopathology

- HFLT is characterized by spindle cells admixed with mature adipose tissue
- Abundant hemosiderin laden macrophages and scattered inflammatory cells are present in the spindle cell component
- MIFS is heterogenous with a myxoid component containing pseudolipoblasts, neutrophilia and lymphocytes, and a bland spindle cell proliferation

- Large ganglion or Reed-Sternberg like cells may be present throughout the tumor in MIFS
- Low mitotic activity (< 3 mitotic figures/10 high-power fields [hpf])
- Mitotic figures are sparse and atypical mitoses are not present

Special Stains and Immunohistochemistry

- CD34 immunoreactivity in the spindle cell component in both HFLT and MIFS
- Smooth muscle actin (SMA), desmin, and S100 are negative

Other Techniques for Diagnosis

- Presence of t(1;10) (p22;q24) producing a *TGFBR3-MGEA5* fusion has been reported in both HFLT and MIFS
- Both have also shown amplification of 3p, typically as a ring chromosome

Differential Diagnosis

WELL-DIFFERENTIATED LIPOSARCOMA
- Presents in the retroperitoneum and deep soft tissues of proximal extremities
- Typically lacks prominent spindle cell component; variation in size of adipocytes and lipoblasts may be present
- *MDM2* amplification

SPINDLE CELL LIPOMA
- Most common on upper back of elderly men; fairly well circumscribed
- Lacks inflammatory component; spindle cells are often in background of myxoid stroma
- Coarse collagen bundles are a helpful feature

PLEXIFORM FIBROHISTIOCYTIC TUMOR
- Subcutaneous mass in the extremities of young adults
- Distinct nodules composed of mononuclear cells and osteoclast-like giant cell connected by a spindle cell proliferation

HIGH-GRADE MYXOFIBROSARCOMA (HIGH-GRADE PLEOMORPHIC SARCOMA, MYXOID MALIGNANT FIBROUS HISTIOCYTOMA [MFH])
- Deep seated large tumors in adults
- Hemorrhage and necrosis often present, brisk mitotic activity with atypical mitotic figures

PEARLS

- *HFLT and MIFS are genetically linked tumors*
- *Considered benign but locally aggressive, with up to a 50% recurrence rate*
- *Metastasis is rare and more common in those with MIFS histology, and dedifferentiation of HFLT has been reported*

SELECTED REFERENCES

Antonescu CR, Zhang L, Nielsen GP, et al: Consistent t(1;10) with rearrangements of TGFBR3 and MGEA5 in both myxoinflammatory fibroblastic sarcoma and hemosiderotic fibrolipomatous tumor. Genes Chromosomes Cancer 50:757-764, 2011.

Elco CP, Marino-Enriquez A, Abraham JA, et al: Hybrid myxoinflammatory fibroblastic sarcoma/hemosiderotic fibrolipomatous tumor: report of a case providing further evidence for a pathogenetic link. Am J Surg Pathol 34:1723-1727, 2010.

Laskin WB, Fetsch JF, Miettinen M: Myxoinflammatory fibroblastic sarcoma: a clinicopathologic analysis of 104 cases, with emphasis on predictors of outcome. Am J Surg Pathol 38:1-12, 2014.

Solomon DA, Antonescu CR, Link TM, et al: Hemosiderotic fibrolipomatous tumor, not an entirely benign entity. Am J Surg Pathol 37:1627-1630, 2013.

Weiss VL, Antonescu CR, Alaggio R, et al: Myxoinflammatory fibroblastic sarcoma in children and adolescents: clinicopathologic aspects of a rare neoplasm. Pediatr Dev Pathol 16:425-431, 2013.

Wettach GR, Boyd LJ, Lawce HJ, et al: Cytogenetic analysis of a hemosiderotic fibrolipomatous tumor. Cancer Genet Cytogenet 182:140-143, 2008.

LOW-GRADE FIBROMYXOID SARCOMA

Clinical Features

- Also known as *Evans tumor*, related to "hyalinizing spindle cell tumor with giant rosettes"
- Typically seen in young adults but can occur in children and elderly
- Deep soft tissue mass most often in proximal extremities or trunk
- May be present for several years before diagnosis

Gross Pathology

- Usually a large and nonencapsulated but well-circumscribed mass
- Cut surface is firm, white, or tan, sometimes with a myxoid appearance

Histopathology

- Biphasic low-grade spindle cell proliferation
- Myxoid nodules of bland fusiform cells with a prominent arcade of hyalinized vessels, around which tumor cells aggregate (Figure 17-14)
- Collagenized areas are arranged in short haphazard fascicles with a whorling growth pattern
- Rosettes may be present, characterized by hyalinized nodules cuffed by tumor cells

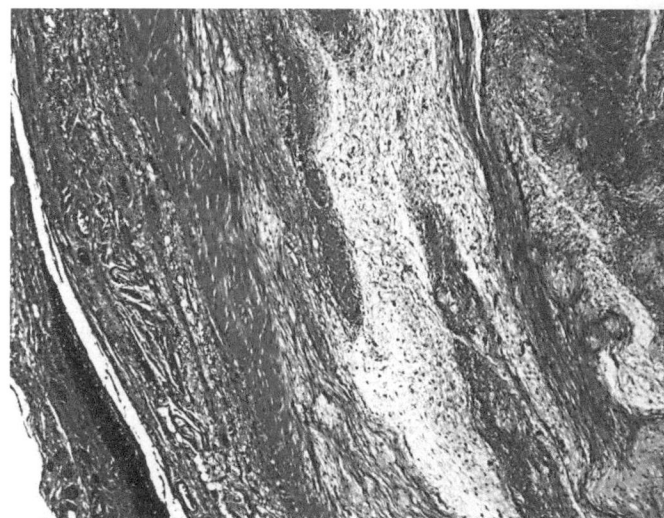

Figure 17-14. Low-grade fibromyxoid sarcoma. Well-circumscribed tumor with alternating hyalinized and myxoid tumor fascicles.

- Mitotic figures are absent or sparse
- Higher-grade foci may be present; this does not appear to affect prognosis adversely

Special Stains and Immunohistochemistry

- Immunoreactive toward MUC4
- Variably positive for EMA, SMA, desmin, and CD34
- Areas of higher cellularity may be positive or bcl-2

Other Techniques for Diagnosis

- Presence of t(7;16)(q34;p11), producing an *FUS-CREBL2* fusion, can be demonstrated by cytogenetic or molecular analysis in most cases

Differential Diagnosis

LOW-GRADE MYXOFIBROSARCOMA

- Almost exclusively myxoid with long, curvilinear vessels
- Mild cytologic atypia and pseudolipoblasts
- Older patients; more superficial location

SYNOVIAL SARCOMA

- Monophasic spindle cell or biphasic spindle cell and epithelioid tumors with high nuclear-to-cytoplasmic ratios
- Herringbone growth pattern is common
- May show myxoid, squamoid, or collagenized images focally
- Mitotic activity usually easily seen
- Intratumoral calcifications sometimes present
- Immunoreactive for keratin or EMA

DESMOID-TYPE FIBROMATOSIS

- Lacks alternating myxoid and collagenized zonation
- Highly infiltrative borders
- Positive for β-catenin by nuclear labeling

MYXOID NEUROFIBROMA

- Lacks zonation
- Slender, wavy nuclei with tapered ends
- Positive for S-100 protein, CD56, and CD57

PEARLS

- *Histologic link to sclerosing epithelioid fibrosarcoma; however, they appear to be separate entities*
- *Cellular, mitotically active areas are relatively common but do not seem to predict prognosis*
- *Low-grade fibromyxoid sarcoma can be deceptively poorly circumscribed; margins are usually positive if shelled out*
- *Recurrence is common with and an average duration of 3 years after excision (up to 15), and metastases can occur averaging 5 years after resection (up to 45)*
- *Wide surgical excision is the standard therapy*

SELECTED REFERENCES

Billings SD, Giblen G, Fanburg-Smith JC: Superficial low-grade fibromyxoid sarcoma (Evans tumor): a clinicopathologic analysis of 19 cases with a unique observation in the pediatric population. Am J Surg Pathol 29:204-210, 2005.

Doyle LA, Moller E, Dal Cin P, et al: MUC4 is a highly sensitive and specific marker for low-grade fibromyxoid sarcoma. Am J Surg Pathol 35:733-741, 2011.

Evans HL: Low-grade fibromyxoid sarcoma: a clinicopathologic study of 33 cases with long-term follow-up. Am J Surg Pathol 35:1450-1462, 2011.

Evans HL: Low-grade fibromyxoid sarcoma: a report of 12 cases. Am J Surg Pathol 17:595-600, 1993.

Guillou L, Benhattar J, Gengler C, et al: Translocation-positive low-grade fibromyxoid sarcoma: clinicopathologic and molecular analysis of a series expanding the morphologic spectrum and suggesting potential relationship to sclerosing epithelioid fibrosarcoma: a study from the French Sarcoma Group. Am J Surg Pathol 31:1387-1402, 2007.

Rekhi B, Deshmukh M, Jambhekar NA: Low-grade fibromyxoid sarcoma: a clinicopathologic study of 18 cases, including histopathologic relationship with sclerosing epithelioid fibrosarcoma in a subset of cases. Ann Diagn Pathol 15:303-311, 2011.

LOW-GRADE MYOFIBROBLASTIC SARCOMA

Clinical Features

- Also known as *myofibrosarcoma*
- Distinctive low-grade tumor with myofibroblastic differentiation
- Tumor of middle-aged adults, rarely reported in children
- Most commonly involves head and neck

Gross Pathology

- Firm mass with white cut surface and poorly defined margins

Histopathology

- Moderately cellular spindle cell lesion arranged in fascicles and whorls
- Modest nuclear hyperchromasia and mild cellular pleomorphism
- Infiltrates adjacent tissues
- Mitotic figures are variable in number

Special Stains and Immunohistochemistry

- Desmin, MSA, SMA: at least one is positive

Other Techniques for Diagnosis

- Electron microscopy shows intercellular fibronexuses, cytoplasmic thin filaments, dense bodies, and intermediate-type gap junctions

Differential Diagnosis

DEEP FIBROMATOSIS

- Lacks cellular pleomorphism
- Positive for β-catenin with nuclear labeling

LOW-GRADE FIBROMYXOID SARCOMA

- Alternating hypocellular myxoid areas and collagenized foci
- Possible presence of hyalinizing rosettes
- Margins usually less infiltrative
- Presence of t(7;16)(q34;p11), producing an *FUS-CREBL2* fusion, is characteristic

INFANTILE FIBROSARCOMA

- Almost exclusively seen in young children
- Lacks myogenic differentiation by immunohistochemistry and electron microscopy
- Presence of t(12;15)(p13;q26), producing an *ETV6-NTRK3* fusion, is typical

MYOFIBROMA AND MYOFIBROMATOSIS

- Almost exclusively seen in young children
- Less cellular and lacks significant pleomorphism
- Hemangiopericytoma-like growth pattern
- Biphasic growth, in terms of cellularity

PEARLS

- *Wide surgical resection is necessary for low-grade myofibroblastic sarcoma*
- *Local recurrence is common; metastases are rare but may be seen after many years*
- *High-grade myofibroblastic sarcomas are likely a different clinicopathologic entity, synonymous with* malignant fibrous histiocytoma *or high-grade pleomorphic sarcoma*

SELECTED REFERENCES

Cai C, Dehner LP, El-Mofty SK. In myofibroblastic sarcomas of the head and neck, mitotic activity and necrosis define grade: a case study and literature review. Virchows Arch 463:827-836, 2013.

Fisher C: Myofibrosarcoma. Virchows Arch 445:215-223, 2004.

Gonzalez-Campora R, Escudero AG, Rios Martin JJ, et al: Myofibrosarcoma (low-grade myofibroblastic sarcoma) with intracytoplasmic hyaline (fibroma-like) inclusion bodies. Ultrastruct Pathol 27:7-11, 2003.

Mentzel T, Dry S, Katenkamp D, Fletcher CD: Low-grade myofibroblastic sarcoma: analysis of 18 cases in the spectrum of myofibroblastic tumors. Am J Surg Pathol 22:1228-1238, 1998.

INFANTILE FIBROSARCOMA

Clinical Features

- Occurs primarily in children younger than 2 years; about 25% are congenital
- Most common on extremities, followed by trunk and head and neck
- May mimic a vascular lesion both clinically and radiographically; large "hemangiomas" in young children should undergo biopsy if they enlarge

Gross Pathology

- Infiltrative borders
- Firm, fleshy, lobulated mass, often large
- Cut surface is gray-white to tan-yellow

Histopathology

- Cellular tumor is characterized by apposed, spindle-shaped fibroblasts arranged in interlacing fascicles or a herringbone pattern (Figure 17-15)
- Frequent mitotic activity is seen, sometimes with atypical forms
- Necrosis and hemorrhage are common
- Myxoid or collagenous stroma may be seen
- May have focal hemangiopericytoma-like vasculature
- Scattered chronic inflammatory cells and focal extramedullary hematopoiesis are seen

Special Stains and Immunohistochemistry

- Negative for epithelial, myogenous, and neural markers, CD34, bcl-2, and CD99

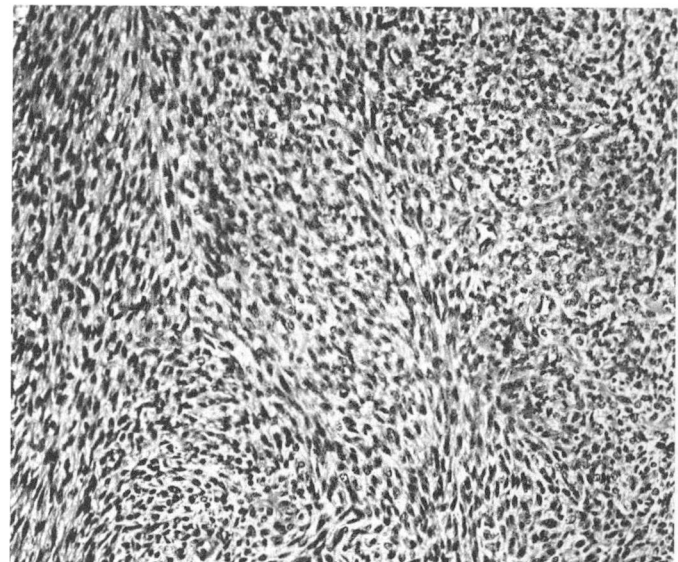

Figure 17-15. Infantile fibrosarcoma. Cellular fascicles of spindle cells are arranged in herringbone growth pattern.

Other Techniques for Diagnosis

- Up to 90% of cases have t(12;15)(p13;q26) that creates a fusion gene, *ETV6-NTRK3* (*TEL-TRCKC*): this may be cryptic on conventional karyotyping and requires reverse transcription polymerase chain reaction or fluorescent in situ hybridization studies
- Trisomy 11 is the most common additional chromosomal abnormality, followed by trisomies 8, 17, and 20

Differential Diagnosis

FIBROMATOSIS

- Lacks dense cellularity, mitotic figures, and herringbone pattern of growth
- No hemorrhage or necrosis

MYOFIBROMA AND MYOFIBROMATOSIS

- Infantile fibrosarcoma may contain foci indistinguishable from those of myofibroma; shows more cellular and atypical areas as well
- Biphasic areas of cellular density
- Possible intravascular polypoid projections

SPINDLE CELL RHABDOMYOSARCOMA

- Intersecting short cellular fascicles with variable stromal collagen
- Possible presence of strap cells
- Positive for desmin, myogenin, and MyoD1

SYNOVIAL SARCOMA (MONOPHASIC)

- May have herringbone or hemangiopericytoma-like growth patterns
- Immunoreactivity for cytokeratin, EMA, CD99, and bcl-2
- Presence of t(X;18) is characteristic
- Extremely rare in infancy

MALIGNANT PERIPHERAL NERVE SHEATH TUMOR

- Composed of elongated cells with variably pleomorphic, serpentine nuclei

- Cellular growth in fascicles and whorls, with possible neural "tactoid" formation
- Nuclear palisading potentially present
- May be positive for S-100 protein, CD56, CD57, or collagen type IV
- Extremely rare in infancy

PEARLS

- *Wide surgical excision is the preferred treatment for infantile fibrosarcoma*
- *Chemotherapy is reserved for unresectable tumors*
- *About 15% to 30% of cases recur, but metastases are rare*
- *Presence of t(12;15) is also seen in cellular mesoblastic nephroma of the kidney*

SELECTED REFERENCES

Bourgeois JM, Knezevich SR, Mathers JA, Sorensen PH: Molecular detection of the ETV6-NTRK3 gene fusion differentiates congenital fibrosarcoma from other childhood spindle cell tumors. Am J Surg Pathol 24:937-946, 2000.
Coffin CM, Jaszcz W, O'Shea PA, Dehner LP: So-called congenital-infantile fibrosarcoma: does it exist and what is it? Pediatr Pathol 14:133-150, 1994.
Sandberg AA, Bridge JA: Updates on the cytogenetics and molecular genetics of bone and soft tissue tumors: congenital (infantile) fibrosarcoma and mesoblastic nephroma. Cancer Genet Cytogenet 132:1-13, 2002.

ADULT FIBROSARCOMA

Clinical Features

- Rare malignant spindle cell tumor with possible herringbone growth pattern
- Tumor of middle-aged to elderly adults
- Located in deep tissue of extremities, trunk, or head and neck; rarely other locations
- In rare cases seen as a second pattern in dermatofibrosarcoma protuberans or other low-grade sarcomas
- May be seen as a postirradiation neoplasm

Gross Pathology

- Firm, lobulated mass usually 3 to 10 cm in diameter
- Small tumors may be well circumscribed
- Cut surface is gray-white to tan-yellow with hemorrhage or necrosis

Histopathology

- Variably hyperchromatic spindle cells with eosinophilic or amphophilic cytoplasm, may show a herringbone growth pattern; some lesions resemble desmoid fibromatosis but have mitotic figures
- Variable mitotic activity
- Lacks significant pleomorphism
  - Well-differentiated fibrosarcoma: shows an orderly arrangement of spindle cells with minimal pleomorphism and variable amounts of collagen; mitotic figures are infrequent
  - Poorly differentiated fibrosarcoma: a cellular lesion with nuclear hyperchromasia, mild pleomorphism, and numerous mitotic figures; hemorrhage and necrosis are common

Special Stains and Immunohistochemistry

- Negative for epithelial, myogenous, and neural markers as well as CD34, CD99, bcl-2, and nuclear β-catenin

Other Techniques for Diagnosis

- Noncontributory except to rule out other tumors, especially monophasic synovial sarcoma (t X;18)

Differential Diagnosis

DESMOID-TYPE FIBROMATOSIS
- Lacks dense cellularity, nuclear hyperchromasia, and herringbone growth
- No hemorrhage or necrosis
- Positive for nuclear β-catenin

SYNOVIAL SARCOMA (MONOPHASIC)
- May have herringbone or hemangiopericytoid growth patterns
- Commonly shows areas of hypercellularity and hypocellularity
- Immunoreactivity for cytokeratin, EMA, TLE1, CD99, bcl-2, and CD57
- Presence of t(X;18)

MALIGNANT PERIPHERAL NERVE SHEATH TUMOR
- Composed of elongated cells with variably pleomorphic, serpentine nuclei
- Cells arranged in fascicles or whorls; possible formation of neural tactoids
- Nuclear palisading sometimes seen
- May be positive for S-100 protein, CD56, CD57, and collagen type IV

DEDIFFERENTIATED AND SPINDLE CELL LIPOSARCOMA
- May be seen de novo through the clonal evolution of well-differentiated liposarcoma
- Dedifferentiated areas may mimic fibrosarcoma, but extensive sampling reveals low-grade adipocytic component
- Most commonly occurs in the retroperitoneum

LOW-GRADE FIBROMYXOID SARCOMA
- Alternating hypocellular myxoid areas and collagenized spindle cell foci
- Lacks herringbone and desmoid-like patterns of growth
- Presence of t(7;16) or FUS rearrangement by fluorescence in situ hybridization (FISH)

PEARLS

- *Wide resection, with or without adjuvant radiotherapy, for adult fibrosarcoma is standard therapy; chemotherapy may be indicated for high-grade tumors*
- *Local recurrence in 10% to 50% of cases, and high-grade tumors may produce hematogenous metastases*
- *Fibrosarcoma is a pathologic diagnosis of exclusion and likely makes up less than 1% of sarcomas*

SELECTED REFERENCES

Bahrami A, Folpe AL: Adult-type fibrosarcoma: a reevaluation of 163 putative cases diagnosed at a single institution over a 48-year period. Am J Surg Pathol 34:1504-1513, 2010.

Hansen T, Katenkamp K, Brodhun M, Katenkamp D: Low-grade fibrosarcoma: report on 39 not otherwise specified cases and comparison with defined low-grade fibrosarcoma types. Histopathology 49:152-160, 2006.

Pritchard DJ, Soule EH, Taylor WF, Ivins JC: Fibrosarcoma: a clinicopathologic and statistical study of 199 tumors of the soft tissues of the extremities and trunk. Cancer 33:888-897, 1974.

SCLEROSING EPITHELIOID FIBROSARCOMA

Clinical Features

- Distinctive variant of fibrosarcoma
- Tumor of middle-aged adults, but has been reported in children
- Common locations include deep soft tissue of extremities, trunk, chest wall, or head and neck; may be painful

Gross Pathology

- Firm, oval, or lobulated soft tissue mass ranging in size from 2 to 20 cm
- Cut surface is gray-white; may have myxoid or cystic areas

Histopathology

- Nests or cords of uniform, round to oval tumor cells with eosinophilic to clear cytoplasm embedded in a densely hyalinized stroma (Figure 17-16)
- May have fascicular, myxoid, or cystic areas and hemangiopericytoma-like vasculature
- Mitotic figures are infrequent

Special Stains and Immunohistochemistry

- Positive for MUC4, variably for EMA

Other Techniques for Diagnosis

- Electron microscopy confirms fibroblastic/myofibroblastic differentiation with abundant rough endoplasmic reticulum and skeins of thin filaments that are helpful in distinguishing this tumor from mimics of other cell lineages
- Few chromosomal and molecular abnormalities have been reported, two of which showed rearrangements of 10p11

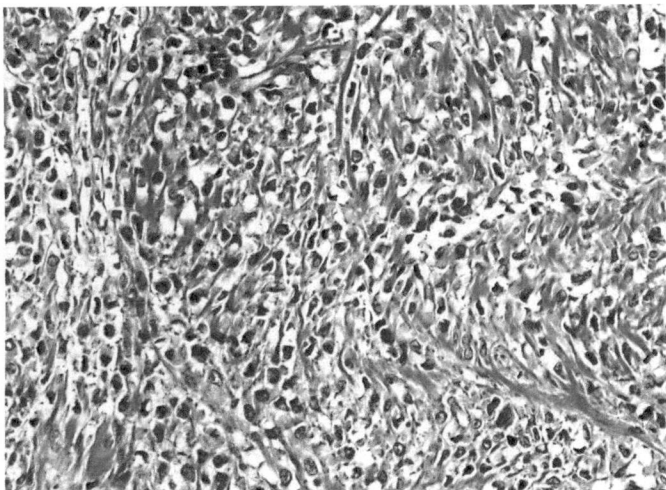

Figure 17-16. Sclerosing epithelioid fibrosarcoma. Small epithelioid cells with nuclear atypia are set in a sclerotic matrix.

- Rearrangements in FUS have been reported, similar to that of low-grade fibromyxoid sarcoma

Differential Diagnosis

METASTATIC CARCINOMA

- Histology may suggest lobular breast carcinoma or signet ring cell adenocarcinoma
- Positive for keratin, p63, MOC31, or CA72.4

SCLEROSING LYMPHOMA

- Positive for leukocyte common antigen (CD45) and B-cell markers (CD20, CD79a, and PAX5)

DEEP FIBROMATOSIS

- Cells tend to be more fusiform, and margins are infiltrative
- Positive for β-catenin (nuclear)

SCLEROSING RHABDOMYOSARCOMA

- Eosinophilic, hyperchromatic, and pleomorphic cells
- Positive for desmin, myogenin, and MyoD1

SCLEROSING, WELL-DIFFERENTIATED LIPOSARCOMA

- Usually contains lipomatous areas if well sampled
- Nuclear pleomorphism and lipoblasts are present

LOW-GRADE FIBROMYXOID SARCOMA

- Shows clinical and histologic overlap with sclerosing epithelioid fibrosarcoma, and distinction may be difficult
- Alternating bundles of hypocellular myxoid areas with collagenized spindle cells
- Presence of (7;16)

PEARLS

- *Wide surgical resection is mainstay of therapy for sclerosing epithelioid fibrosarcoma*
- *Local recurrence in about 50% of cases; distant metastases are common*
- *Overlap with low-grade fibromyxoid sarcoma, although likely distinct entities*

SELECTED REFERENCES

Antonescu CR, Rosenblum MK, Pereira P, et al: Sclerosing epithelioid fibrosarcoma: a study of 16 cases and confirmation of a clinicopathologically distinct tumor. Am J Surg Pathol 25:699-709, 2001.

Doyle LA, Wang WL, Dal Cin P, et al: MUC4 is a sensitive and extremely useful marker for sclerosing epithelioid fibrosarcoma: association with FUS gene rearrangement. Am J Surg Pathol 36:1444-1451, 2012.

Guillou L, Benhattar J, Gengler C, et al: Translocation-positive low-grade fibromyxoid sarcoma: clinicopathologic and molecular analysis of a series expanding the morphologic spectrum and suggesting potential relationship to sclerosing epithelioid fibrosarcoma: a study from the French Sarcoma Group. Am J Surg Pathol 31:1387-1402, 2007.

Ogose A, Kawashima H, Umezu H, et al: Sclerosing epithelioid fibrosarcoma with der(10)t(10;17)(p11;q11). Cancer Genet Cytogenet 152:136-140, 2004.

MYXOFIBROSARCOMA

Clinical Features

- Also known as *myxoid malignant fibrous histiocytoma*
- Almost exclusively occurs in older adults and elderly people

- Usually presents as a slow-growing, painless mass in subcutaneous or deep tissues of the proximal extremities, rarely on trunk or head and neck

Gross Pathology

- Multilobulated or single ill-defined mass with gelatinous, myxoid cut surface

Histopathology

- Multilobulated lesion demarcated with incomplete fibrous septa containing a myxoid stroma and pleomorphic cells
  - Low-grade myxofibrosarcoma
    - Abundant myxoid matrix with scattered spindled or stellate hyperchromatic tumor cells with irregular borders and eosinophilic cytoplasm (Figure 17-17)
    - Pseudolipoblasts show eccentric, pleomorphic nuclei and abundant vacuolated cytoplasm
    - Presence of long curvilinear blood vessels with perivascular condensation of tumor cells is characteristic
  - High-grade myxofibrosarcoma
    - Cellular tumor composed of fascicles or sheets of highly pleomorphic fusiform or stellate cells, many of which are multinucleated
    - Myxoid stroma that is less apparent but variable throughout the lesion
    - Numerous mitotic figures and atypical mitoses
    - Hemorrhage and necrosis common
    - Rarely, has an epithelioid phenotype

Special Stains and Immunohistochemistry

- Vimentin positive

Other Techniques for Diagnosis

- Karyotypes tend to be complex but with no specific recurrent abnormalities

Differential Diagnosis

LOW-GRADE FIBROMYXOID SARCOMA

- Alternating bundles of hypocellular myxoid areas with collagenized spindle cells
- Delicate, plexiform vasculature
- Presence of hyalinizing rosettes
- Tends to be in younger patients
- Presence of t(7;16)(q33;p11), producing an *FUS-CREB3L2* fusion

MYXOID LIPOSARCOMA

- Bland spindled or fusiform cells with presence of true lipoblasts
- Tumor cells are less pleomorphic
- Vasculature is delicate and arborizing and lacks condensed perivascular tumor cells
- Deeply seated tumor that most commonly occurs in the thighs of adults
- Presence of t(12;16)(q13;p11), producing an *FUS-DDIT3* fusion

MYXOMA

- Paucicellular lesion with small, bland nuclei that lack pleomorphism
- Usually intramuscular

PEARLS

- *Wide surgical resection with radiation, chemotherapy, or both for high-grade lesions is the standard therapy for myxofibrosarcoma*
- *Low-grade tumors show local recurrence in up to 50% of cases but rarely metastasize*
- *High-grade tumors have a high rate of local recurrence and metastasize in about one third of cases*

SELECTED REFERENCES

Mentzel T, Calonje E, Wadden C, et al: Myxofibrosarcoma: clinicopathologic analysis of 75 cases with emphasis on the low-grade variant. Am J Surg Pathol 20:391-405, 1996.

Nascimento AF, Bertoni F, Fletcher CD: Epithelioid variant of myxofibrosarcoma: expanding the clinicomorphologic spectrum of myxofibrosarcoma in a series of 17 cases. Am J Surg Pathol 31:99-105, 2007.

Willems SM, Debiec-Rychter M, Szuhai K, et al: Local recurrence of myxofibrosarcoma is associated with increase in tumour grade and cytogenetic aberrations, suggesting a multistep tumour progression model. Mod Pathol 19:407-416, 2006.

GIANT CELL TUMOR OF TENDON SHEATH

Clinical Features

- Also referred to as *nodular tenosynovitis*; diffuse form is termed *pigmented villonodular synovitis*
- Typically found in adults but may affect persons of any age; more commonly occurs in women
- Presents as a slow-growing, small mass usually in the hands, but may affect feet, wrists, knees, and rarely other joints

Gross Pathology

- Well-circumscribed, lobulated, gray-white mass

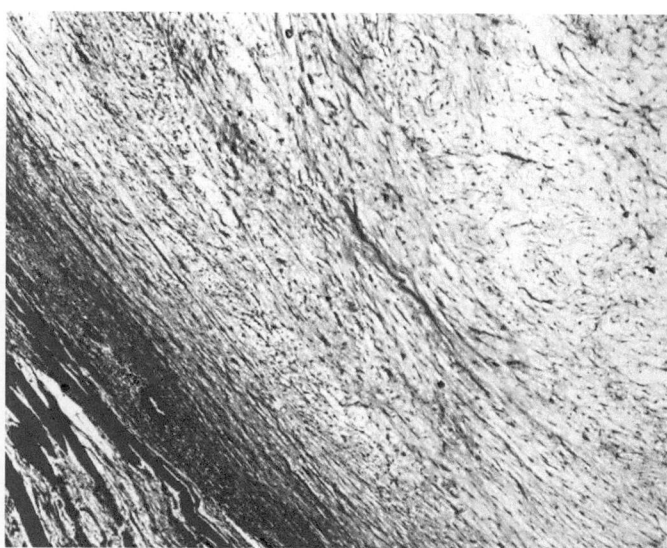

Figure 17-17. Low-grade myxofibrosarcoma. Demarcated, paucicellular tumor with small spindle cells in abundant myxoid matrix.

Histopathology

- Cellular tumors with a nodular architecture composed of varying amounts of mononuclear stromal cells admixed with osteoclast-like giant cells, xanthoma cells, and inflammation (Figure 17-18)
- Stroma may be hyalinized, and hemosiderin is invariably present
- Mitotic figures are usually present
- Malignant giant cell tumor of tendon sheath
  - Rare tumors
  - Typical giant cell tumor of tendon sheath containing or recurring as frank sarcomatous elements
  - Destructive localized growth, increased mitotic activity (more than 10 mitotic figures/20 hpf), and extensive necrosis are typically seen in clinically malignant cases

Special Stains and Immunohistochemistry

- CD68 positive
- MSA and desmin variably positive

Other Techniques for Diagnosis

- Structural abnormalities of chromosome 1p are common
- Most common translocation is t(1;2)(p13;q37) resulting in *COL6A3-CSF1* fusion gene

Differential Diagnosis

GIANT CELL MALIGNANT FIBROUS HISTIOCYTOMA

- Characterized by bizarre, pleomorphic tumor cells arranged in a storiform pattern
- High mitotic rate and necrosis

FIBROMA OF TENDON SHEATH

- Typically hypocellular lesion composed of spindled fibroblasts in a collagenized stroma
- Lacks osteoclast-like giant cells and inflammatory cells

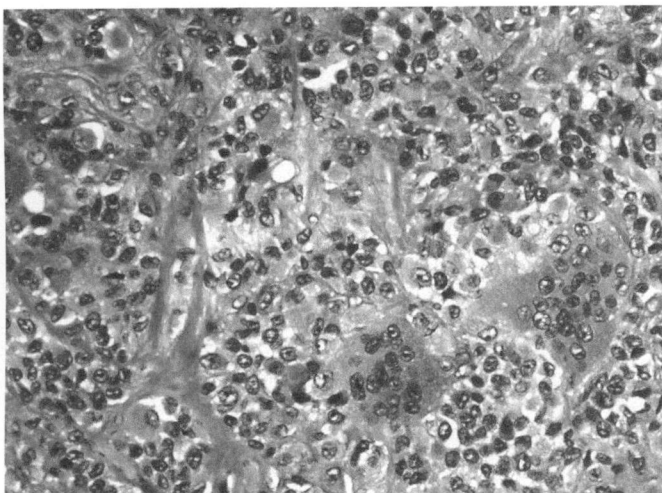

Figure 17-18. Giant cell tumor of tendon sheath. High-power view shows osteoclast-like giant cells and mononuclear cells with eccentric nuclei and eosinophilic cytoplasm.

PEARLS

- *Giant cell tumor of tendon sheath is a benign lesion but may recur in 5% to 30% of cases, usually in a nondestructive fashion amenable to repeat excision*
- *Rare malignant forms that tend to have multiple local recurrences have been reported and may metastasize to the same extremity, lymph nodes, and lung*
- *Complete surgical resection is the preferred treatment*
- *The use of imatinib mesylate has been explored in metastatic disease with some effect*

SELECTED REFERENCES

Cassier PA, Gelderblom H, Stacchiotti S, et al: Efficacy of imatinib mesylate for the treatment of locally advanced and/or metastatic tenosynovial giant cell tumor/pigmented villonodular synovitis. Cancer 118:1649-1655, 2012.

Moller E, Mandahl N, Mertens F, Panagopoulos I: Molecular identification of COL6A3-CSF1 fusion transcripts in tenosynovial giant cell tumors. Genes Chromosomes Cancer 47:21-25, 2008.

Sciot R, Rosai J, Dal Cin P, et al: Analysis of 35 cases of localized and diffuse tenosynovial giant cell tumor: a report from the Chromosomes and Morphology (CHAMP) study group. Mod Pathol 12:576-579, 1999.

Somerhausen NS, Fletcher CD: Diffuse-type giant cell tumor: clinicopathologic and immunohistochemical analysis of 50 cases with extraarticular disease. Am J Surg Pathol 24:479-492, 2000.

Ushijima M, Hashimoto H, Tsuneyoshi M, Enjoji M: Giant cell tumor of the tendon sheath (nodular tenosynovitis): a study of 207 cases to compare the large joint group with the common digit group. Cancer 57:875-884, 1986.

DEEP BENIGN FIBROUS HISTIOCYTOMA

Clinical Features

- Rare benign fibrohistiocytic tumor usually presenting in early adulthood
- Slow-growing, painless nodule, predominantly on head and neck and lower extremities
- Most often involves subcutaneous tissue; deep lesions rare

Gross Pathology

- Well-defined lesion with a tan-white cut surface
- Focal areas of hemorrhage may be seen

Histopathology

- Well-defined or focally infiltrative margins
- Bland spindle cells arranged in short fascicles or storiform pattern; hemangiopericytoma growth pattern may be seen
- Scattered chronic inflammatory cells are common; foam cells and giant cells may be seen
- Typically has few mitotic figures; no atypical mitoses

Special Stains and Immunohistochemistry

- Noncontributory

Other Techniques for Diagnosis

- Noncontributory

Differential Diagnosis

NODULAR FASCIITIS

- Loose, feathery collagenous stroma with myxoid or microcystic appearance

Differential Diagnosis

INVOLUTING JUVENILE HEMANGIOMA

- Regressive change in preexisting juvenile hemangioma; usually seen in children
- Lobular lesion with ectatic vessels infiltrated by mature adipose tissue; microthrombi are not a component

INTRAMUSCULAR HEMANGIOMA AND HEMANGIOMATOSIS

- Also called *infiltrating angiolipoma* in older literature
- Deep vascular lesion infiltrating muscle, which has largely been replaced by fat
- Poorly circumscribed lesion lacking microthrombi

Kaposi Sarcoma

- Ill-defined tumors with infiltrative margins
- Slitlike vascular spaces with lymphoplasmacytic inflammation and extravasated red blood cells; adipose tissue is not a major component
- Intralesional hyaline globules may be seen
- Seen in HIV patients or on the legs of elderly patients
- HHV-8 and LNA-1 immunoreactivity in 85% of cases

PEARLS

- *Angiolipoma is one of the painful lesions associated with the ANGEL mnemonic (angiolipoma, neuroma, glomus tumor, eccrine spiradenoma, leiomyoma)*
- *Angiolipomas are benign and cured by surgical excision*

SELECTED REFERENCES

Hunt SJ, Santa Cruz DJ, Barr RJ: Cellular angiolipoma. Am J Surg Pathol 14:75-81, 1990.
Sciot R, Akerman M, Dal Cin P, et al: Cytogenetic analysis of subcutaneous angiolipoma: further evidence supporting its difference from ordinary pure lipomas. A report of the CHAMP Study Group. Am J Surg Pathol 21:441-444, 1997.

SPINDLE CELL LIPOMA AND PLEOMORPHIC LIPOMA

Clinical Features

- Tumor of older individuals; seen on the posterior neck or shoulders
- Mobile, subcutaneous mass

Gross Pathology

- Well-circumscribed mass with yellow to tan cut surface

Histopathology

- Spindle cell lipoma
  - Mature fat admixed with haphazardly arranged fascicles of bland spindle cells; ropy collagen is characteristic; myxoid change is common
  - No mitotic figures
- Pleomorphic lipoma
  - Variably numerous multinucleated hyperchromatic floret-like cells admixed with mature fat (Figure 17-22)
  - Ropy collagen characteristic
  - No mitotic figures

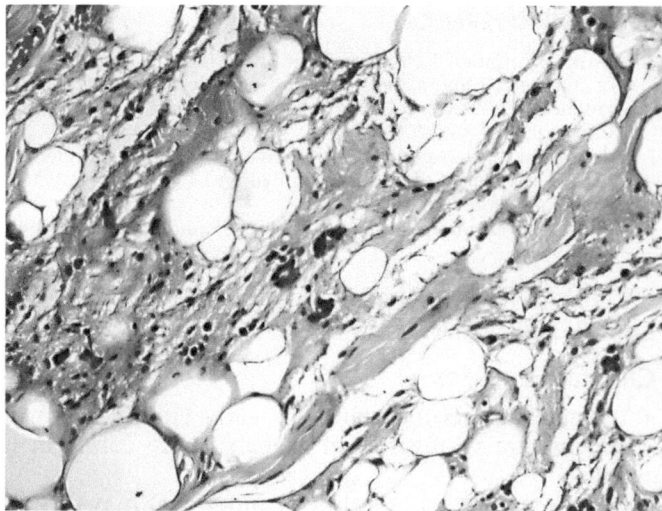

Figure 17-22. Pleomorphic lipoma. Mature fat, floret-like giant cells, and ropy collagen are characteristic.

Special Stains and Immunohistochemistry

- S-100 protein positive in adipocytes
- CD34 positive in spindle and pleomorphic cells

Other Techniques for Diagnosis

- Karyotype is often diploid, but partial loss of chromosomes 13 and 16 is common

Differential Diagnosis

WELL-DIFFERENTIATED LIPOSARCOMA OR ATYPICAL LIPOMATOUS TUMOR

- Deeply seated lesion in the extremities or retroperitoneum
- Atypical stromal cells are variably prominent
- Rare mitotic figures and no ropy collagen as seen in spindle cell or pleomorphic lipoma
- Amplification of 12q14-15 as a supernumerary ring chromosome

PLEOMORPHIC LIPOSARCOMA

- Extremities are the most common location
- Pleomorphic lipoblasts in an otherwise high-grade sarcoma
- Mitotically active
- Negative for CD34

LIPOFIBROMATOSIS

- Poorly circumscribed lesion, usually on extremities of children
- Organized fascicles of bland spindle cells with abundant collagen admixed with mature adipose tissue
- Infiltrative borders

PEARLS

- *Spindle cell or pleomorphic lipoma represents a morphologic spectrum of clinically and genetically similar tumors, and features of both can be seen in the same lesion*
- *Benign lesion cured by surgical excision*

SELECTED REFERENCES

Domanski HA, Carlen B, Jonsson K, et al: Distinct cytologic features of spindle cell lipoma: a cytologic-histologic study with clinical, radiologic, electron microscopic, and cytogenetic correlations. Cancer 93:381-389, 2001.

Fanburg-Smith JC, Devaney KO, Miettinen M, Weiss SW: Multiple spindle cell lipomas: a report of 7 familial and 11 nonfamilial cases. Am J Surg Pathol 22:40-48, 1998.

Yue XH, Liu YQ: Pleomorphic lipoma. Am J Surg Pathol 20:898-899, 1996.

LIPOBLASTOMA AND LIPOBLASTOMATOSIS

Clinical Features

- Typically occurs in infancy or early childhood; most patients are younger than 5 years; more common in boys
- Usually presents as a painless, superficial mass on the extremities but may occur in any location
- Lipoblastomatosis
  - Diffuse form of lipoblastoma
  - Tends to infiltrate muscle

Gross Pathology

- Well-circumscribed, lobular tumors averaging 5 cm (1 to 20 cm); lipoblastomatosis has infiltrative borders
- Cut surface often shows myxoid to gelatinous tissue with fibrous strands

Histopathology

- Typically has a lobular architecture separated by fibrous septa of variable cellularity
- Adipose tissue in various stages of maturation; usually with identifiable lipoblasts (Figure 17-23)
- Variably myxoid stroma

Special Stains and Immunohistochemistry

- Noncontributory

Other Techniques for Diagnosis

- Cytogenetic and molecular studies: associated with re-arrangements of chromosome 8q11-13 involving the *PLAG1* gene

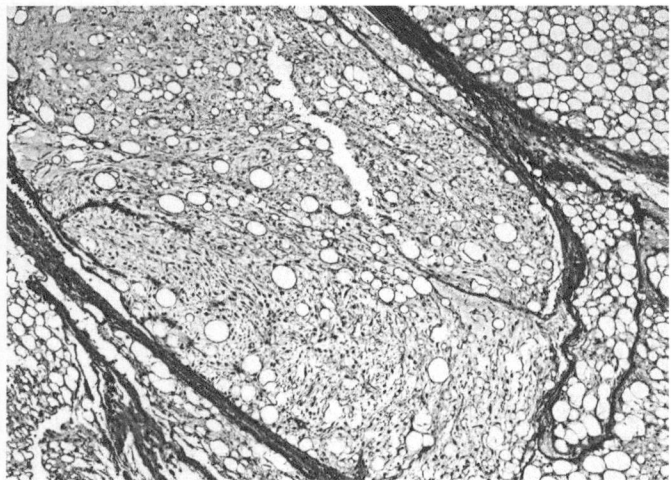

Figure 17-23. Lipoblastoma. Nodular growth of mature adipose tissue admixed with lipoblasts in a highly myxoid stroma.

Differential Diagnosis

MYXOID LIPOSARCOMA
- Found primarily in adults
- Prominent myxoid matrix with a characteristic delicate plexiform capillary network
- Presence of lipoblasts and mild nuclear atypia
- Lacks the lobular configuration of lipoblastoma
- Presence of t(12;16)(q13;p11), producing an *FUS-CHOP* fusion

LIPOFIBROMATOSIS
- Ill-defined tumors with infiltrative margins
- Composed of mature adipocytes with cellular fascicles of spindled cells
- Lacks lobular architecture, myxoid stroma, and lipoblasts

PEARLS

- *Lipoblastoma and lipoblastomatosis are benign lesions that may recur if not completely excised*
- *Recurrences are often less myxoid and more lipoma-like*

SELECTED REFERENCES

Bartuma H, Domanski HA, Von Steyern FV, et al: Cytogenetic and molecular cytogenetic findings in lipoblastoma. Cancer Genetics Cytogenetics 183:60-63, 2008.

Chen Z, Coffin CM, Scott S, et al: Evidence by spectral karyotyping that 8q11.2 is nonrandomly involved in lipoblastoma. J Mol Diagn 2:73-77, 2000.

Collins MH, Chatten J: Lipoblastoma/lipoblastomatosis: a clinicopathologic study of 25 tumors. Am J Surg Pathol 21:1131-1137, 1997.

Morerio C, Nozza P, Tassano E, et al: Differential diagnosis of lipoma-like lipoblastoma. Pediatric Blood Cancer 52:132-134, 2009.

WELL-DIFFERENTIATED LIPOSARCOMA AND ATYPICAL LIPOMATOUS TUMOR

Clinical Features

- Most common form of liposarcoma
- Primarily occurs in adult life; peak incidence between 50 and 70 years
- Common sites include thigh, retroperitoneum, spermatic cord, and posterior mediastinum
- Usual presentation is that of an insidiously growing, ill-defined mass that has attained a large size by the time it is identified

Gross Pathology

- Well-circumscribed to irregular mass that may exceed 30 cm
- Cut surface is usually fatty with fibrous bands but may be predominantly fibrous or myxoid
- Areas of fat necrosis are common

Histopathology

- Composed of variably sized adipocytes with variable nuclear atypia and hyperchromasia
- Varying numbers of vacuolated or signet ring cell lipoblasts
- Fibrous septa containing occasional hyperchromatic stromal cells with nuclear atypia; floret-like cells may be seen

- Lipoma-like liposarcoma
  - Predominantly mature fat, atypical cells are hard to find; most common in retroperitoneum
- Sclerosing liposarcoma
  - Collagenous stroma admixed with variable amounts of adipose-tissue containing pleomorphic, hyperchromatic stromal cells and rare lipoblasts
- Inflammatory liposarcoma
  - Dense chronic inflammatory infiltrate superimposed on lipoma-like or sclerosing forms of liposarcoma
  - Hyperchromatic, atypical stromal cells are scattered throughout

Special Stains and Immunohistochemistry

- S-100 protein positive
- *MDM2* variably positive

Other Techniques for Diagnosis

- Giant supernumerary marker ring chromosome composed of the 12q14-15 region represents *MDM2* amplification; commonly identified by FISH

Differential Diagnosis

PANNICULITIS

- Mature adipose tissue showing fat necrosis, acute inflammation, and lipid-laden macrophages

SPINDLE CELL OR PLEOMORPHIC LIPOMA

- Typically seen on upper trunk superficially
- Uniform spindle cells admixed with mature adipose tissue
- Pleomorphic lipoma pattern is characterized by hyperchromatic, multinucleated, floret-like giant cells
- Both often contain ropy collagen fibers
- CD34 positive in spindled and pleomorphic cells
- Lacks *MDM2* amplification

ANGIOMYOLIPOMA

- Typically seen in the kidney but may occur in the soft tissues
- Composed of mature fat, smooth muscle, and thick-walled vessels
- Positive for HMB-45, MART-1, or PNL2

PEARLS

- *The nomenclature for well-differentiated liposarcoma (WDL) and atypical lipomatous tumor (ALT) is not always consistent, but WDL is often used for deep masses, whereas ALT is reserved for more superficial lesions that are amenable to complete surgical resection*
- *The identification of lipoblasts is neither necessary nor sufficient to warrant a diagnosis of WDL or ALT*
- *Lipoma-like, sclerosing, and inflammatory patterns often coexist in liposarcomas of the retroperitoneum*
- *WDL and ALT rarely metastasize but show frequent recurrences and have the potential to dedifferentiate*
- *Surgical excision with wide margins of resection is the treatment of choice*

SELECTED REFERENCES

Binh MB, Sastre-Garau X, Guillou L, et al: MDM2 and CDK4 immunostainings are useful adjuncts in diagnosing well-differentiated and dedifferentiated liposarcoma subtypes: a comparative analysis of 559 soft tissue neoplasms with genetic data. Am J Surg Pathol 29:1340-1347, 2005.

Evans HL: Atypical lipomatous tumor, its variants, and its combined forms: a study of 61 cases, with a minimum follow-up of 10 years. Am J Surg Pathol 31:1-14, 2007.

Rosai J, Akerman M, Dal Cin P, et al: Combined morphologic and karyotypic study of 59 atypical lipomatous tumors: evaluation of their relationship and differential diagnosis with other adipose tissue tumors (a report of the CHAMP Study Group). Am J Surg Pathol 20:1182-1189, 1996.

Sirvent N, Coindre JM, Maire G, et al: Detection of MDM2-CDK4 amplification by fluorescence in situ hybridization in 200 paraffin-embedded tumor samples: utility in diagnosing adipocytic lesions and comparison with immunohistochemistry and real-time PCR. Am J Surg Pathol 31:1476-1489, 2007.

Thway K, Flora R, Shah C, et al: Diagnostic utility of p16, CDK4, and MDM2 as an immunohistochemical panel in distinguishing well-differentiated and dedifferentiated liposarcomas from other adipocytic tumors. Am J Surg 36:462-469, 2012.

MYXOID AND ROUND CELL LIPOSARCOMA

Clinical Features

- Represents 30% to 50% of liposarcomas
- Primarily occurs in young to middle-aged adults; rare in children
- Most common site is deep tissue of thigh; rare in retroperitoneum or superficial locations

Gross Pathology

- Poorly circumscribed mass with fatty to myxoid cut surface
- Areas of hemorrhage or necrosis are common and may represent more poorly differentiated areas (round cell component)

Histopathology (Figures 17-24 and 25)

- Composed of lipoblasts in various stages of maturation, ranging from primitive mesenchymal cells to well-differentiated lipoblasts
- Prominent myxoid matrix; large pools of myxoid material may be seen

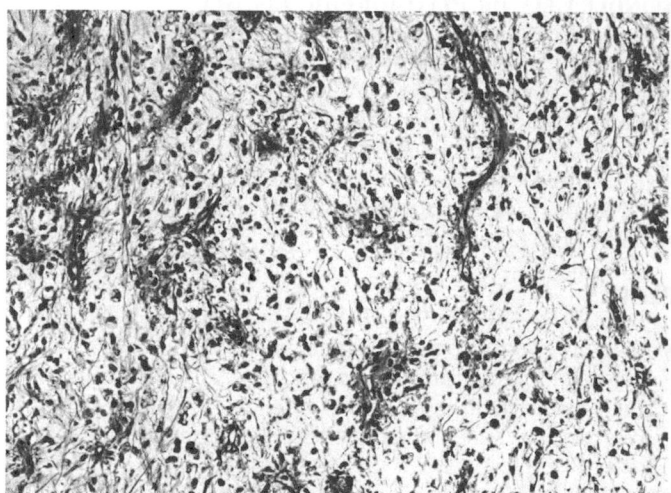

Figure 17-24. Myxoid liposarcoma. Numerous vacuolated lipoblasts are seen in a loose myxoid stroma with a characteristic chicken-wire vasculature.

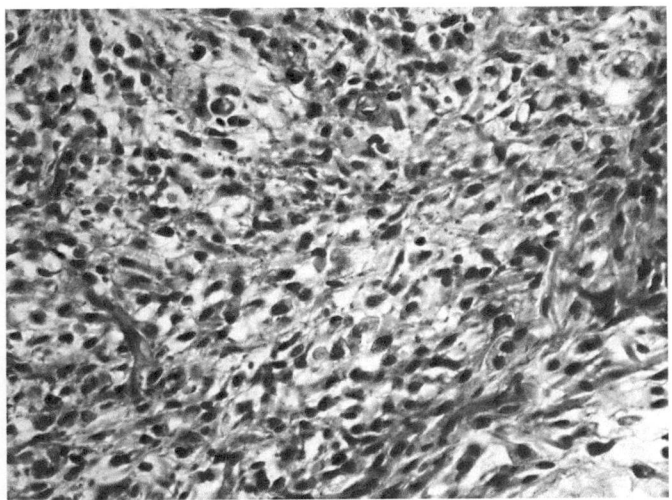

Figure 17-25. Round cell myxoid liposarcoma. The tumor cells have hyperchromatic round nuclei, and there is little myxoid stroma.

- Arborizing, plexiform capillary network
- Rare mitotic activity
- Mast cells are common

Special Stains and Immunohistochemistry

- S-100 protein positive
- *MDM2* variably positive

Other Techniques for Diagnosis

- Presence of t(12;16)(q13;p11), producing an *FUS-DDIT3* fusion (also called *TLS-CHOP*) in 90% of cases, identified by cytogenetic or molecular genetic techniques
- Less commonly, t(12;22)(q13;p11), producing an *EWS-DDIT3* fusion

Differential Diagnosis

LIPOBLASTOMA
- Lobulated mass with fibrous septa
- Lacks delicate vascular network
- Lesion of young children; extremely rare in adults
- Alterations at 8q11-13 involving *PLAG1*

SPINDLE CELL OR PLEOMORPHIC LIPOMA
- Typically presents on superficial upper trunk in adults
- Uniform spindle-shaped cells admixed with mature adipose tissue
- Pleomorphic lipoma pattern is characterized by hyperchromatic, multinucleated floret-like giant cells
- Both often contain ropy collagen fibers
- CD34 positive in spindled and pleomorphic cells
- Lacks *MDM2* amplification

PEARLS

- *Round cell liposarcoma is considered a higher-grade variant of myxoid liposarcoma, and a transition between the histologic features of both is often present; more than 5% round cell sarcoma represents an adverse prognostic factor*
- *Surgical excision with wide margins of resection is the treatment of choice*
- *Myxoid liposarcoma is essentially nonexistent in retroperitoneum, almost universally well differentiated liposarcoma with myxoid features*

SELECTED REFERENCES

Antonescu CR, Elahi A, Humphrey M, et al: Specificity of TLS-CHOP rearrangement for classic myxoid/round cell liposarcoma: absence in predominantly myxoid well-differentiated liposarcomas. J Mol Diagn 2:132-138, 2000.

de Vreeze RS, de Jong D, Tielen IH, et al: Primary retroperitoneal myxoid/round cell liposarcoma is a nonexisting disease: an immunohistochemical and molecular biological analysis. Mod Pathol 22:223-231, 2009.

Downs-Kelly E, Goldblum JR, Patel RM, et al: The utility of fluorescence in situ hybridization (FISH) in the diagnosis of myxoid soft tissue neoplasms. Am J Surg Pathol 32:8-13, 2008.

Fiore M, Grosso F, Lo Vullo S, et al: Myxoid/round cell and pleomorphic liposarcomas: prognostic factors and survival in a series of patients treated at a single institution. Cancer 109:2522-2531, 2007.

Hoffman A, Ghadimi MP, Demicco EG, et al: Localized and metastatic myxoid/round cell liposarcoma: clinical and molecular observations. Cancer 119:1868-1877, 2013.

PLEOMORPHIC LIPOSARCOMA

Clinical Features

- High-grade sarcoma representing about 10% of liposarcomas
- Most common site is extremities; occasionally occurs in the abdomen or retroperitoneum
- Tumor occurs in elderly people

Gross Pathology

- Large, multinodular mass with yellow to tan cut surface
- Areas of hemorrhage or necrosis common

Histopathology

- Pleomorphic, multivacuolated lipoblasts with scalloped hyperchromatic nuclei
- Background lesion is a high-grade spindle cell and pleomorphic sarcoma (Figure 17-26)
- Mitotic figures are easily identified, and necrosis is common
- Eosinophilic hyaline globules may be present
- Epithelioid variant shows pleomorphic lipoblasts in a background of cohesive hyperchromatic polygonal cells with variable amounts of eosinophilic cytoplasm

Special Stains and Immunohistochemistry

- S-100 protein and MDM2 variably positive

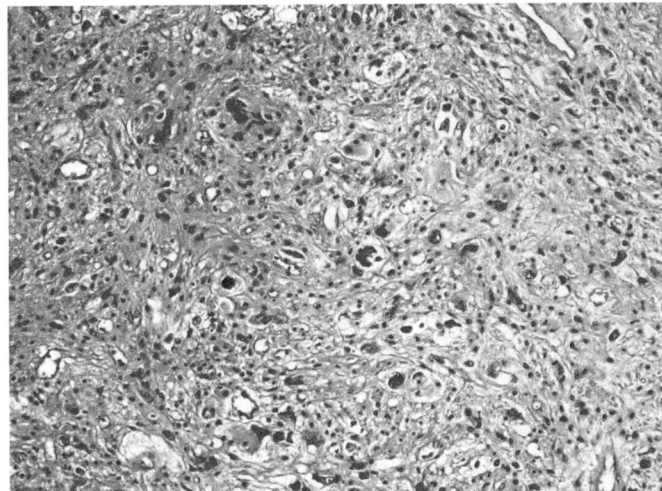

Figure 17-26. Pleomorphic liposarcoma. Haphazard growth of markedly pleomorphic cells without discernible lipoblasts.

Other Techniques for Diagnosis

- Complex karyotype, often with large ring-marker chromosomes or double minutes
- MDM2 nonamplified but often polysomic

Differential Diagnosis

PLEOMORPHIC LIPOMA

- Posterior neck and shoulder most common location; superficial
- Basic histologic image is that of lipoma
- Presence of ropy collagen
- Mitotic figures extremely rare or absent

DEDIFFERENTIATED LIPOSARCOMA

- Pleomorphic lipoblasts
- Has a coexisting or preexisting lower-grade liposarcoma component

HIGH-GRADE PLEOMORPHIC SARCOMA OR MALIGNANT FIBROUS HISTIOCYTOMA

- No lipoblasts
- Lacks S-100 protein immunoreactivity

PLEOMORPHIC RHABDOMYOSARCOMA

- Pleomorphic rhabdomyoblasts may mimic lipoblasts
- Immunoreactivity for desmin, myogenin, MyoD1, or myoglobin

PEARLS

- *Pleomorphic liposarcoma is a high-grade sarcoma with a high propensity for local recurrence and metastasis, usually to the lungs*
- *Surgical excision with wide margins of resection is the treatment of choice, often with adjuvant radiotherapy*

SELECTED REFERENCES

Downes KA, Goldblum JR, Montgomery EA, Fisher C: Pleomorphic liposarcoma: a clinicopathologic analysis of 19 cases. Mod Pathol 14:179-184, 2001.

Fiore M, Grosso F, Lo Vullo S, et al: Myxoid/round cell and pleomorphic liposarcomas: prognostic factors and survival in a series of patients treated at a single institution. Cancer 109:2522-2531, 2007.

Gardner JM, Dandekar M, Thomas D, et al. Cutaneous and subcutaneous pleomorphic liposarcoma: a clinicopathologic study of 29 cases with evaluation of MDM2 gene amplification in 26. Am J Surg Pathol 36:1047-1051, 2012.

Gebhard S, Coindre JM, Michels JJ, et al: Pleomorphic liposarcoma: clinicopathologic, immunohistochemical, and follow-up analysis of 63 cases: a study from the French Federation of Cancer Centers Sarcoma Group. Am J Surg Pathol 26:601-616, 2002.

DEDIFFERENTIATED LIPOSARCOMA

Clinical Features

- Nonlipomatous component arising from low-grade liposarcoma
- Occurs in about 10% of well-differentiated liposarcomas, most commonly in retroperitoneum
- Majority arise de novo in a primary liposarcoma; less frequently, they are seen in recurrences

- Most dedifferentiated liposarcomas show high-grade dedifferentiation, but low-grade dedifferentiation (actually divergent differentiation) can occur

Gross Pathology

- Large, multinodular mass, often with a distinct solid component in an overtly fatty background

Histopathology

- The dedifferentiated component has conventionally been defined by a nonlipogenic tumor that often has the appearance of a high-grade pleomorphic sarcoma but may show pleomorphic liposarcomatous differentiation
- An abrupt transition with the well-differentiated liposarcoma is common, but the transition may be gradual (Figure 17-27)
- Heterologous differentiation along myogenic, osseous, or neurogenic lines can be seen
- Low-grade dedifferentiation is represented by a low-grade myogenous or fibroblastic or myofibroblastic component

Special Stains and Immunohistochemistry

- Dedifferentiated component is often only positive for vimentin but may show immunoreactivity for heterologous lineage markers

Other Techniques for Diagnosis

- Usually shows the same ring-marker chromosomes composed of 12q14-15, as seen in well-differentiated liposarcoma

Differential Diagnosis

HIGH-GRADE PLEOMORPHIC SARCOMA OR MALIGNANT FIBROUS HISTIOCYTOMA

- May be indistinguishable from high-grade dedifferentiated liposarcoma if low-grade areas have not been sampled
- Lacks adjacent low-grade liposarcoma

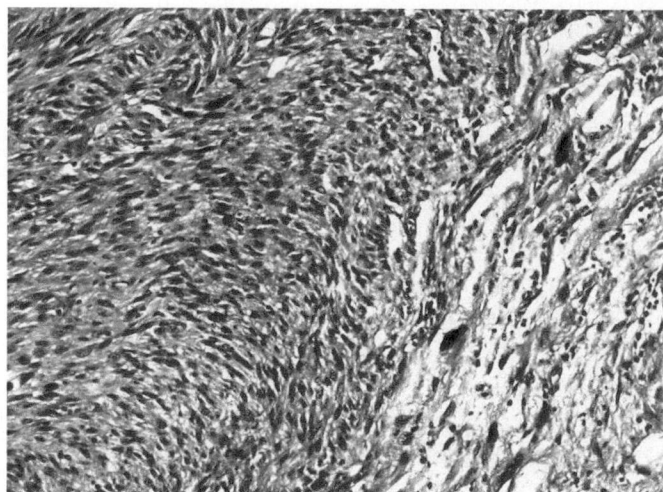

Figure 17-27. Dedifferentiated liposarcoma. An abrupt transition is seen between the well-differentiated sclerosing liposarcoma and a high-grade nonlipogenic component.

PEARLS

- *Dedifferentiated liposarcoma is usually a high-grade sarcoma but has a less aggressive course than other pleomorphic sarcomas*
- *Sampling should be thorough to recognize the low-grade liposarcoma component*
- *Presence of heterologous elements does not affect prognosis*
- *Surgical excision with wide margin is preferred treatment, with or without adjuvant therapy*

SELECTED REFERENCES

Binh MB, Guillou L, Hostein I, et al: Dedifferentiated liposarcomas with divergent myosarcomatous differentiation developed in the internal trunk: a study of 27 cases and comparison to conventional dedifferentiated liposarcomas and leiomyosarcomas. Am J Surg Pathol 31:1557-1566, 2007.

Boland JM, Weiss SW, Oliveira AM, et al: Liposarcomas with mixed well-differentiated and pleomorphic features: a clinicopathologic study of 12 cases. Am J Surg Pathol 34:837-843, 2010.

Henricks WH, Chu YC, Goldblum JR, Weiss SW: Dedifferentiated liposarcoma: a clinicopathological analysis of 155 cases with a proposal for an expanded definition of dedifferentiation. Am J Surg Pathol 21:271-281, 1997.

Marino-Enriquez A, Fletcher CD, Dal Cin P, Hornick JL: Dedifferentiated liposarcoma with "homologous" lipoblastic (pleomorphic liposarcoma-like) differentiation: clinicopathologic and molecular analysis of a series suggesting revised diagnostic criteria. Am J Surg Pathol 34:1122-1131, 2010.

RHABDOMYOMA

Clinical Features

- Rare benign extracardiac tumor with skeletal muscle differentiation; less than 2% of all skeletal muscle tumors
- Three distinct clinical and morphologic subtypes exist
  - Fetal rhabdomyoma
    - Typically occurs in children younger than 3 years; may be congenital
    - Mass in the subcutaneous or mucosal tissue of the head and neck
  - Adult rhabdomyoma
    - Average age is 60 years; more common in males
    - Polypoid mass in the head and neck region; may present with upper airway obstruction
    - May be multinodular and rarely multifocal
  - Genital rhabdomyoma
    - Presents as a polypoid mass in the vagina or vulva of young to middle-aged women
    - May cause vaginal bleeding

Gross Pathology

- Circumscribed, lobulated tumor with a finely granular, red-brown cut surface
- Typically ranges in size from 2 to 10 cm

Histopathology

FETAL RHABDOMYOMA

- Classic or myxoid form shows primitive spindle cells in a loose myxoid stroma
- Intermediate or cellular form has a fascicular growth pattern with strap cells or plump rhabdomyoblasts

- Both forms contain cells with cross-striations, negligible mitotic figures, and a lack of necrosis

ADULT RHABDOMYOMA

- Large, round to polygonal rhabdomyocytes with eosinophilic, granular, or vacuolated cytoplasm and small peripheral nuclei
- Tumor cells show variable cross-striation and focal vacuolization owing to glycogen content; "spider" cells are common

GENITAL RHABDOMYOMA

- Plump polygonal or fusiform cells in various stages of myogenic differentiation in a fibrous stroma with dilated vessels

Special Stains and Immunohistochemistry

- MSA, desmin, and myoglobin positive
- Myogenin and MyoD1 may be positive in scattered cells

Other Techniques for Diagnosis

- Electron microscopy: cells with large nuclei and prominent nucleoli; thick and thin myofilaments with Z lines and A and I bands

Differential Diagnosis

ADULT RHABDOMYOMA

GRANULAR CELL TUMOR

- Sheet of polygonal cells with coarsely granular eosinophilic cytoplasm and small central nuclei; no strap cells
- Positive for S-100 protein in 85% of cases; no myogenic markers

HIBERNOMA

- Characterized by round to oval cells with central nuclei and granular or vacuolated cytoplasm containing lipofuscin pigment (brown fat)

PARAGANGLIOMA

- Organoid arrangement of round to oval cells with central nuclei, eosinophilic granular cytoplasm, and a delicate capillary network
- Positive for chromogranin, synaptophysin, and CD56; lacks myogenic markers

RHABDOMYOSARCOMA

- In adults, usually pleomorphic; poorly circumscribed lesion with marked nuclear pleomorphism, mitotic activity, and necrosis
- A higher percentage of cells are positive for myogenin and MyoD1; infrequent staining for myoglobin

FETAL AND GENITAL RHABDOMYOMA

EMBRYONAL RHABDOMYOSARCOMA (ERMS)

- A distinction between fetal rhabdomyoma and ERMS may be difficult
- ERMS lacks circumscription, shows less differentiation, and manifests mitotic figures or necrosis
- Myogenin and MyoD1 stain less than 50% of the tumor cells; rare cell positivity for myoglobin

BOTRYOID RHABDOMYOSARCOMA

- Spindled to rounded rhabdomyoblasts in an abundant myxoid matrix with a condensed cambium layer under an epithelial surface

SELECTED REFERENCES

Braaten K, Young RH: Ovarian serous cystadenoma with associated genital rhabdomyoma. Hum Pathol 36:1240-1241, 2005.

Cronin CT, Keel SB, Grabbe J, Schuler JG: Adult rhabdomyoma of the extremity: a case report and review of the literature. Hum Pathol 31:1074-1080, 2000.

Walsh SN, Hurt MA: Cutaneous fetal rhabdomyoma: a case report and historical review of the literature. Am J Surg Pathol 32:485-491, 2008.

RHABDOMYOSARCOMA

Clinical Features

- Tumors with almost exclusive skeletal muscle differentiation
- Most common sarcomas of childhood
  - Embryonal rhabdomyosarcoma
    - Common sites include the head and neck, genitourinary tract, abdomen, retroperitoneum, and paratesticular region
    - Primarily affects young children
    - Botryoid rhabdomyosarcoma is a favorable variant that occurs beneath the mucosal surfaces of the genitourinary tract or head and neck in young children
    - Spindle cell rhabdomyosarcoma is a favorable subtype when seen in the paratesticular soft tissue of adolescents
  - Alveolar rhabdomyosarcoma
    - Most commonly presents as a deep mass in the extremities or buttocks
    - Typically affects adolescents
  - Pleomorphic rhabdomyosarcoma
    - Presents as a deep mass in the extremities
    - Typically affects adults

Gross Pathology

- Soft, poorly circumscribed lobulated mass with a gray-tan cut surface
- Focal areas of necrosis are common
- Botryoid rhabdomyosarcomas are polypoid, grapelike masses with a gray-white cut surface

Histopathology

EMBRYONAL RHABDOMYOSARCOMA

- Hyperchromatic, primitive spindled cells, often with a myxoid stroma (Figure 17-28)
- Alternating hypocellular and hypercellular areas with cells condensed around blood vessels
- Rare strap cells with eosinophilic cytoplasm, tapered ends, and cross-striations
- Anaplasia is defined by large hyperchromatic tumor cells at least 3 times the size of neighboring nuclei, with atypical mitotic figures
  - Botryoid rhabdomyosarcoma

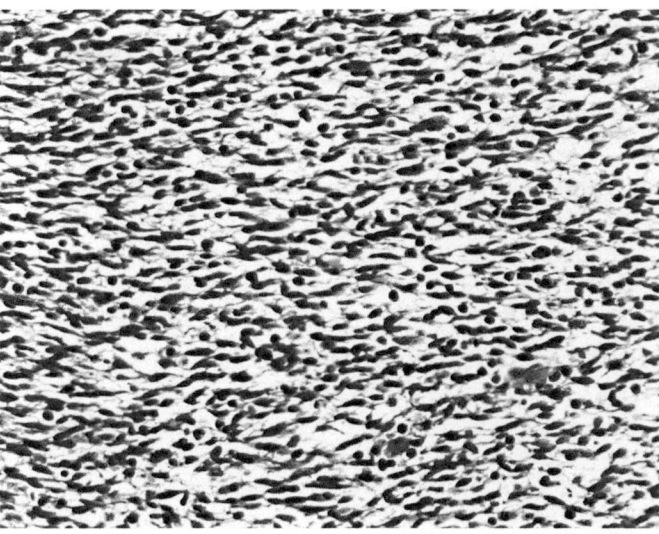

Figure 17-28. Embryonal rhabdomyosarcoma. Pleomorphic, primitive spindle cells with tapered eosinophilic cytoplasm are seen in myxoid stroma.

    - Polypoid architecture
    - Cambium layer (condensation of tumor cells) under intact epithelium in at least one microscopic field
  - Spindle cell rhabdomyosarcoma
    - Fascicular growth pattern within a variably collagenized background

ALVEOLAR RHABDOMYOSARCOMA

- Classic alveolar pattern shows round hyperchromatic tumor cells clinging to fibrovascular cores with central dyshesion (Figure 17-29)
- Solid alveolar pattern represented by sheets or nests of monomorphic tumor cells with round nuclei and a fine chromatin pattern
- Scattered tumor giant cells
- Differentiating rhabdomyoblasts are oval cells with eccentric eosinophilic cytoplasm

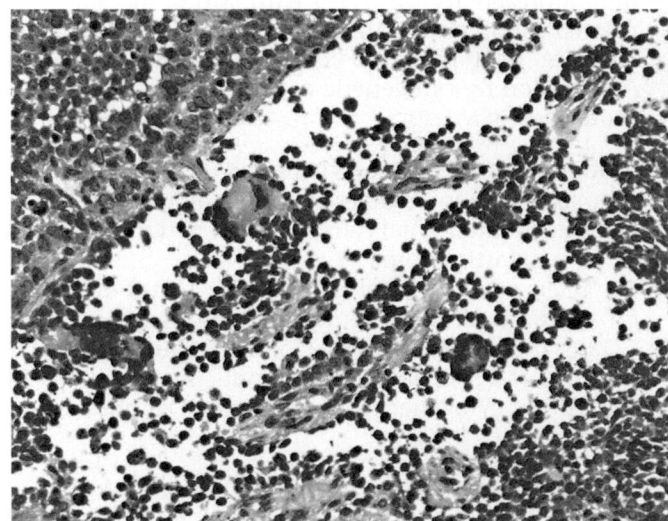

Figure 17-29. Alveolar rhabdomyosarcoma. Monomorphic, hyperchromatic round cells cling to fibrovascular septa. Tumor giant cells are abundant.

PLEOMORPHIC RHABDOMYOSARCOMA

- Large, pleomorphic cells with abundant eosinophilic cytoplasm
- Admixture of small, primitive, undifferentiated cells and spindle cells

Special Stains and Immunohistochemistry

- Desmin and MSA positive
- Myogenin and MyoD1: nuclear reactivity
- Myoglobin positive only in cells with overt skeletal muscle differentiation

Other Techniques for Diagnosis

- Electron microscopy: rhabdomyoblasts show cytoplasmic thick and thin filaments and dilated endoplasmic reticulum
- Cytogenetic and molecular studies
  - Alveolar rhabdomyosarcoma: 75% have either t(2;13)(q35;q14) or t(1;13)(p36;q14), producing a *PAX3* or *PAX7-FKHR* fusion
  - Embryonal rhabdomyosarcoma: commonly show loss of heterozygosity at 11q15 or hyperdiploidy with gains of chromosome 2, 7, 8, 12, and 13

Differential Diagnosis

NEUROBLASTOMA

- Usually in patients younger than 5 years, occurring in the adrenal or along the sympathetic chain
- Small round cells with variable neuropil and ganglion cell differentiation; rosettes may be seen
- Nests of tumor cells separated by delicate curvilinear vascular network
- Immunoreactivity for neuron-specific enolase (NSE), synaptophysin, and NB84; lacks myogenic markers

EWING SARCOMA (EWS) AND PRIMITIVE NEUROECTODERMAL TUMOR (PNET)

- Sheets of monomorphic round cells with a rim of eosinophilic to clear cytoplasm
- Rosettes may be seen
- Lacks tumor giant cells and rhabdomyoblasts
- Immunoreactivity for CD99 with strong membranous pattern and nuclear Fli-1; lacks myogenic markers
- Presence of t(11;22)(q24;q12), producing an *EWS-FLI-1* fusion by cytogenetic or molecular techniques is characteristic

DESMOPLASTIC SMALL ROUND CELL TUMOR (DSRCT)

- Characteristically involves abdomen of adolescents
- Undifferentiated small cells in nested pattern separated by desmoplastic stroma
- Polyphenotypic immunophenotype with reactivity for keratin and EMA, neural markers (synaptophysin, CD56), and desmin; negative for myogenin and MyoD1
- Presence of t(11;22)(p13;q12), producing an *EWS-WT1* fusion by cytogenetic or molecular techniques, is characteristic

INFLAMMATORY MYOFIBROBLASTIC TUMOR

- Can mimic the spindle cell or embryonal rhabdomyosarcoma
- Ganglion cell–like myofibroblasts and mixed inflammatory background

- Immunoreactivity for SMA and ALK-1 (40%); negative for myogenin and MyoD1

MONOPHASIC SYNOVIAL SARCOMA

- In the differential diagnosis of spindle cell rhabdomyosarcoma
- Cellular lesion with herringbone or hemangiopericytoma-like pattern of growth
- Immunoreactive for cytokeratin, EMA, bcl-2, or CD99; negative for myogenin and MyoD1
- The presence of t(X,18)(p11.2;q11.2), producing an *SYT-SSX1/2* fusion by cytogenetic or molecular techniques, is characteristic

MALIGNANT LYMPHOMA

- Diffuse population of atypical lymphoid cells
- Tumor cells are immunoreactive for CD45

PEARLS

- *Surgical excision with adjuvant chemotherapy and radiotherapy is the standard therapy for rhabdomyosarcoma*
- *Risk stratification for rhabdomyosarcoma is based on histology, patient age, tumor stage, and site of origin*
- *Alveolar rhabdomyosarcoma has a worse prognosis than other subtypes; may involve bone marrow*
- *Anaplasia is considered a poor prognosis in intermediate-risk embryonal rhabdomyosarcomas*
- *Metastases usually involve the lungs and regional lymph nodes*

SELECTED REFERENCES

Ferrari A, Dileo P, Casanova M, et al: Rhabdomyosarcoma in adults: a retrospective analysis of 171 patients treated at a single institution. Cancer 98:571-580, 2003.

Folpe AL, McKenney JK, Bridge JA, Weiss SW: Sclerosing rhabdomyosarcoma in adults: report of four cases of a hyalinizing, matrix-rich variant of rhabdomyosarcoma that may be confused with osteosarcoma, chondrosarcoma, or angiosarcoma. Am J Surg Pathol 26:1175-1183, 2002.

Furlong MA, Mentzel T, Fanburg-Smith JC: Pleomorphic rhabdomyosarcoma in adults: a clinicopathologic study of 38 cases with emphasis on morphologic variants and recent skeletal muscle-specific markers. Mod Pathol 14:595-603, 2001.

Morotti RA, Nicol KK, Parham DM, et al: An immunohistochemical algorithm to facilitate diagnosis and subtyping of rhabdomyosarcoma: the Children's Oncology Group experience. Am J Surg Pathol 30:962-968, 2006.

Nishio J, Althof PA, Bailey JM, et al: Use of a novel FISH assay on paraffin-embedded tissues as an adjunct to diagnosis of alveolar rhabdomyosarcoma. Lab Invest 86:547-556, 2006.

Parham DM, Qualman SJ, Teot L, et al: Correlation between histology and PAX/FKHR fusion status in alveolar rhabdomyosarcoma: a report from the Children's Oncology Group. Am J Surg Pathol 31:895-901, 2007.

LEIOMYOMA (CUTANEOUS AND DEEP SOFT TISSUE)

Clinical Features

- Clinical presentation depends on location and can range from painful cutaneous swellings to deep masses in the extremities, abdomen, or retroperitoneum

- Based on their location, leiomyomas are categorized as follows
  - Cutaneous leiomyoma
    - Most commonly involves extensor surfaces of extremities or genital skin
    - Extremity lesions differentiate toward the pilar arrector muscle; they are often multiple and usually painful
    - Typically seen in adolescents and young adults but may occur in childhood
  - Angioleiomyoma
    - Differentiates toward vascular smooth muscle
    - Typically found in women
    - Solitary, often painful mass, usually on the extremities
  - Deep leiomyoma
    - Arises in the deep tissues of the extremities, abdomen, or retroperitoneum
    - Rare tumor found almost exclusively in adults
    - Radiograph often shows intralesional calcification
    - A diagnosis to be made with caution; most deep smooth muscle tumors of soft tissue are malignant

Gross Pathology

- Typically measures less than 2 cm; deep tumors may be larger
- Sectioning shows a firm, trabeculated, gray-white, bulging surface
- Focal areas of calcification or hyalinization may be present

Histopathology

CUTANEOUS LEIOMYOMA

- Typically has ill-defined margins
- Well-differentiated smooth muscle cells arranged in interlacing fascicles (Figure 17-30)
- Eosinophilic cytoplasm and oval, blunt-ended nuclei with perinuclear vacuoles
- Focal calcification, hyalinization, ossification, and myxoid degeneration may be seen
- No mitotic activity
- Atrophic epidermis

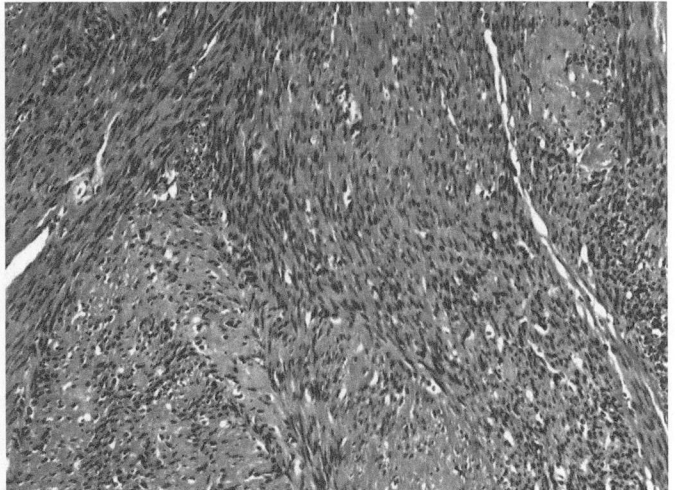

Figure 17-30. Leiomyoma. Interlacing fascicles of well-differentiated smooth muscle without nuclear atypia or mitotic figures.

ANGIOLEIOMYOMA

- Well-defined margins
- Prominent, irregular, interconnecting vascular spaces surrounded by well-differentiated smooth muscle; may be solid or contain large vascular spaces

DEEP LEIOMYOMA

- Interlacing fascicles of well-differentiated smooth muscle spindle cells with blunt ends and perinuclear vacuoles
- Variable degenerative atypia, calcification, and ossification apparent, but true pleomorphism should be absent
- Mitotic figures should be absent

Special Stains and Immunohistochemistry

- SMA and desmin positive

Other Techniques for Diagnosis

- Noncontributory

Differential Diagnosis

CUTANEOUS FIBROUS HISTIOCYTOMA (DERMATOFIBROMA)

- Characterized by spindle cells arranged in a storiform pattern with entrapment of collagen
- Immunoreactive for factor XIIIa

LEIOMYOSARCOMA

- Characterized by spindle-shaped cells with cigar-shaped nuclei, atypical nuclear features, and mitotic activity
- Cells are arranged in interlacing fascicles
- Focal necrosis, hyalinization, and myxoid change may be seen

PEARLS

- *Cutaneous leiomyomas are benign tumors that are treated by surgical excision*
- *Cutaneous leiomyomas may show an autosomal dominant pattern of inheritance*
- *Retroperitoneal smooth muscle tumors in women are often estrogen dependent*
- *Diagnosis of retroperitoneal leiomyoma is controversial, and some observers regard all smooth muscle tumors in that location as sarcomas de facto*

SELECTED REFERENCES

Billings SD, Folpe AL, Weiss SW: Do leiomyomas of deep soft tissue exist? An analysis of highly differentiated smooth muscle tumors of deep soft tissue supporting two distinct subtypes. Am J Surg Pathol 25:1134-1142, 2001.

Fletcher CD, Kilpatrick SE, Mentzel T: The difficulty in predicting behavior of smooth-muscle tumors in deep soft tissue. Am J Surg Pathol 19:116-117, 1995.

Sandberg AA: Updates on the cytogenetics and molecular genetics of bone and soft tissue tumors: leiomyoma. Cancer Genet Cytogenet 158:1-26, 2005.

LEIOMYOSARCOMA (CUTANEOUS AND DEEP SOFT TISSUE)

Clinical Features

- Usually seen in patients between 40 and 70 years of age, but can occur at any age

- Retroperitoneum or pelvis is the most common location, but leiomyosarcoma may also arise from large veins and in deep tissues of extremities
- Retroperitoneal and intra-abdominal tumors are more common in women
- Usual presentation is that of an enlarging mass with symptoms related to displacement of adjacent organs

Gross Pathology

- Relatively well-circumscribed, fleshy mass with a gray-white, whorled, cut surface
- Focal hemorrhage, necrosis, or cystic change may be seen

Histopathology

- Variably cellular tumor composed of fascicles of spindle cells with eosinophilic cytoplasm and cigar-shaped nuclei with perinuclear vacuoles (Figure 17-31)
- Cellular pleomorphism may be minimal to marked; tumor giant cells and osteoclast-like giant cells possible
- Mitotic rate usually 5 mitotic figures/10 hpf, but any mitotic activity should raise suspicion of malignancy
- Areas of hyalinization and coagulative tumor necrosis often seen
- Epithelioid differentiation, myxoid change, nuclear palisading, or prominent lymphoid inflammation may occasionally be present

Special Stains and Immunohistochemistry

- SMA, h-caldesmon positive
- Desmin typically positive

Other Techniques for Diagnosis

- Electron microscopy: thin filaments (actin and myosin) with dense bodies, pinocytosis, and external basal lamina
- Cytogenetic studies: most leiomyosarcomas have complex karyotypes but no diagnostic abnormality
- Alterations in the Rb1–cyclin D pathway are common

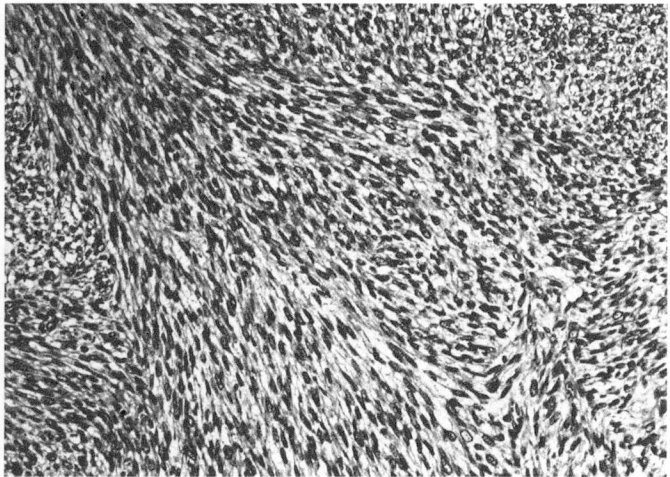

Figure 17-31. Leiomyosarcoma. Cellular tumor with short intersecting fascicles composed of hyperchromatic spindle cells with bluntly tapered ends.

Differential Diagnosis

LEIOMYOMA
- Low-power appearance similar to that of well-differentiated leiomyosarcoma
- Absent mitotic activity and minimal cytologic atypia
- No coagulative necrosis

CELLULAR SCHWANNOMA OR MALIGNANT PERIPHERAL NERVE SHEATH TUMOR
- Elongated cells with wavy, serpentine nuclei
- Nuclear palisading is common, but this can also be seen in leiomyosarcoma
- At least focal positivity for S-100 protein or CD56 with a lack of smooth muscle markers

MALIGNANT FIBROUS HISTIOCYTOMA (PLEOMORPHIC SARCOMA)
- Pleomorphic and spindle cells arranged in a storiform pattern, often in a collagenized or myxoid stroma
- High-grade leiomyosarcomas may have a similar appearance
- Negative for SMA, MSA, desmin, and h-caldesmon

MONOPHASIC SYNOVIAL SARCOMA
- Fascicles of spindle cells with variable nuclear pleomorphism and a herringbone or hemangiopericytoma-like growth pattern
- Variable mitotic rate
- Immunoreactivity for cytokeratin, EMA, bcl-2, or CD99; lacks smooth muscle markers
- The presence of t(X;18)(p11.2;q11.2), producing an *SYT-SSX1/2* fusion by cytogenetic or molecular techniques, is characteristic

SPINDLE CELL RHABDOMYOSARCOMA
- Often occurs in the paratesticular region in adolescent males
- Focal strap cell differentiation may be seen
- Nuclear immunoreactivity for myogenin and MyoD1

EXTRAGASTROINTESTINAL STROMAL TUMOR
- May have an epithelioid, spindle cell, or mixed phenotype; myxoid change may be present
- Fascicular growth is not prominent
- Immunoreactive for C-kit (CD117) and CD34

INFLAMMATORY MYOFIBROBLASTIC TUMOR
- Spindle cell lesion with ganglion cell–like myofibroblasts and prominent inflammation
- Usually lacks the fascicular growth pattern of leiomyosarcoma
- Immunoreactive for SMA, but lacks desmin and h-caldesmon; positive for ALK-1 (40%)

FIBROSARCOMA (INFANT AND ADULT TYPE)
- Most often affects children younger than 1 year; occasionally seen in adults
- Usually found in the extremities
- Highly cellular, infiltrative tumor with hyperchromatic nuclei and scant cytoplasm; herringbone growth pattern

- High mitotic rate; atypical mitotic figures may be seen
- Negative for SMA, desmin, and h-caldesmon

PEARLS

- *Leiomyosarcoma is often a large tumor; local recurrence and metastases to lungs and liver are common*
- *Tumor location, depth, and size are more important prognostic factors than histologic features*
- *Surgical excision with wide resection margins is the treatment of choice*
- *Deep smooth muscle tumors with discernible mitotic activity should be considered malignant*

SELECTED REFERENCES

Kraft S, Fletcher CD: Atypical intradermal smooth muscle neoplasms: clinicopathologic analysis of 84 cases and a reappraisal of cutaneous "leiomyosarcoma." Am J Surg Pathol 35:599-607, 2011.

Oda Y, Miyajima K, Kawaguchi K, et al: Pleomorphic leiomyosarcoma: clinicopathologic and immunohistochemical study with special emphasis on its distinction from ordinary leiomyosarcoma and malignant fibrous histiocytoma. Am J Surg Pathol 25:1030-1038, 2001.

Rubin BP, Fletcher CD: Myxoid leiomyosarcoma of soft tissue, an underrecognized variant. Am J Surg Pathol 24:927-936, 2000.

Sandberg AA: Updates on the cytogenetics and molecular genetics of bone and soft tissue tumors: leiomyosarcoma. Cancer Genet Cytogenet 161:1-19, 2005.

GRANULAR CELL TUMOR

Clinical Features

- Typically occurs in adults (fourth through sixth decades); females are affected more than males
- Presents as a dermal, subcutaneous, or submucosal mass, infrequently multiple
- Tongue is a common site of involvement

Gross Pathology

- Poorly circumscribed nodule
- Typically small (< 3 cm) and firm with a yellow-white cut surface

Histopathology

- Composed of sheets of large, polygonal cells with abundant coarse, eosinophilic, granular cytoplasm (Figure 17-32)
- May grow in sheets, nests, or trabeculae; occasionally exhibit pronounced desmoplasia
- May have small nuclei or larger vesicular nuclei with nucleoli
- Minimal nuclear pleomorphism and rare mitotic activity
- Pseudoepitheliomatous hyperplasia often seen in overlying squamous epithelium
- Histologic features worrisome for malignancy include necrosis, more than 2 mitotic figures/10 hpf, tumor cell spindling, vesicular chromatin with large nucleoli, and cellular pleomorphism

Special Stains and Immunohistochemistry

- S-100 protein, CD68 positive
- Periodic acid–Schiff (PAS): cells typically show cytoplasmic positivity

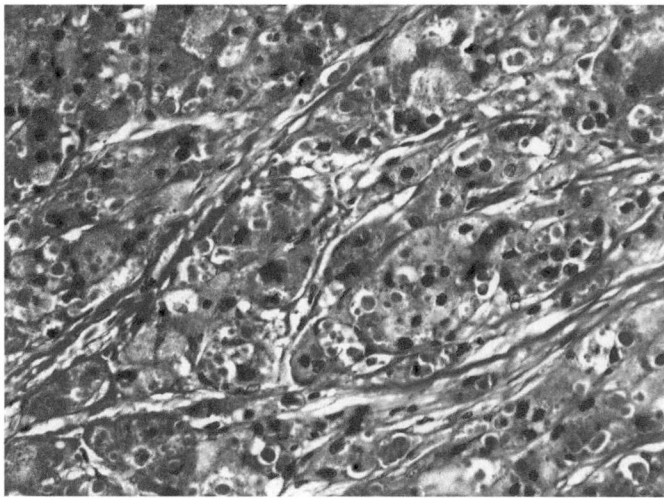

Figure 17-32. Granular cell tumor. Large polygonal cells with small vesicular nuclei have abundant eosinophilic, granular cytoplasm.

Other Techniques for Diagnosis

- Electron microscopy shows cytoplasmic membrane-bound granules consistent with phagolysosomes

Differential Diagnosis

ADULT RHABDOMYOMA

- Characterized by round to polygonal cells with cytoplasmic cross-striations
- Immunoreactivity for desmin, myogenin, and myoglobin

HIBERNOMA

- Cells have vacuolated to granular cytoplasm with distinct cell borders
- Lipid droplets can be detected by oil red O stain

PEARLS

- *Granular cell tumor is a benign neural tumor typically treated by local excision*
- *Most granular cell tumors behave in a benign manner; however, malignant granular cell tumors do exist (about 1%); histologic criteria to differentiate between benign and malignant tumors are not well established*
- *Metastasis is the only definitive feature of malignant tumors*
- *Pseudoepitheliomatosis may be mistaken for squamous cell carcinoma*

SELECTED REFERENCES

Fanburg-Smith JC, Meis-Kindblom JM, Fante R, Kindblom LG: Malignant granular cell tumor of soft tissue: diagnostic criteria and clinicopathologic correlation. Am J Surg Pathol 22:779-794, 1998.

Filie AC, Lage JM, Azumi N: Immunoreactivity of S100 protein, alpha-1-antitrypsin, and CD68 in adult and congenital granular cell tumors. Mod Pathol 9:888-892, 1996.

SCHWANNOMA

Clinical Features

- Also called *neurilemmoma*
- Can occur at any age; typically in adulthood

- Common sites of involvement are intracranial sites (cerebellopontine angle), posterior mediastinum, retroperitoneum, flexor surface of extremities, and head and neck
- Slow-growing, usually painless tumors
- Most often sporadic; less than 5% occur in patients with neurofibromatosis type 2 (NF2)

Gross Pathology

- Ovoid or fusiform mass, usually smaller than 5 cm
- Well-defined and typically encapsulated with pink to tan, firm cut surface
- Focal areas of cystic degeneration may be seen

Histopathology

- Well-defined capsule consisting of epineurium
- Presence of compact hypercellular areas (Antoni A areas) and hypocellular, myxoid areas (Antoni B areas) (Figure 17-33)
- Nuclear palisading around fibrillary processes (Verocay bodies)
- Cells are spindled and contain elongated, wavy nuclei with tapered ends
- Hyalinized vessels are characteristic
- Focal areas of hemorrhage, hemosiderin deposition, and xanthomatous change
- Rarely have glandular structures or pure epithelioid morphology
- Ancient schwannoma
  - Prominent degenerative changes, including cyst formation, calcification, hyalinized vessels, hemorrhage, and cytologic atypia
- Cellular schwannoma
  - Composed almost entirely of Antoni A areas (must be distinguished from malignant peripheral nerve sheath tumor)
  - Mitotically active but cellularity exceeds mitotic figures
- Melantoic schwannoma
  - Associated with Carney complex, usually arises from spinal nerve roots but may occur in other locations
- Cytoplasmic melanin deposits, often has psammoma bodies

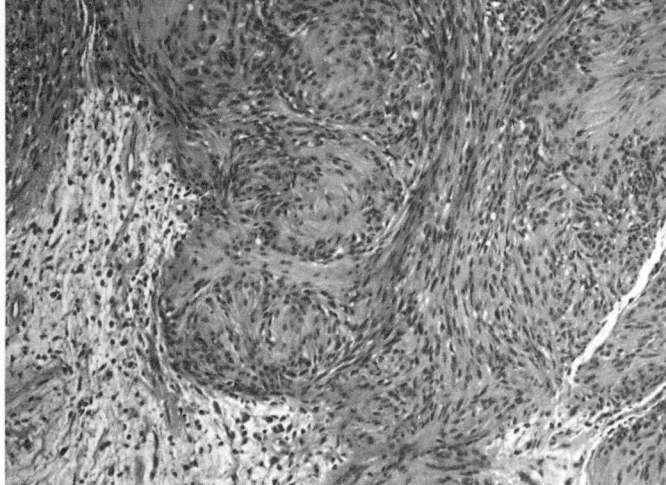

Figure 17-33. Schwannoma. Loose Antoni B areas alternate with cellular Antoni A foci with nuclear palisading and Verocay bodies.

- May have local recurrence, and metastasis is rare but recognized

Special Stains and Immunohistochemistry

- S-100 protein strongly positive
- Leu-7 (CD57), CD56, and glial fibrillary acidic protein (GFAP) positive
- Collagen IV: surround individual tumor cells
- Loss of INI1 in syndromic schwannomatosis

Other Techniques for Diagnosis

- Electron microscopy: tumor cells contain electron-dense basement membrane material and characteristic Luse bodies (long-spaced collagen)
- Schwannomatosis often associated with biallelic loss of NF2 and SMARCB1; subset of patients have germline SMARCB1 mutations

Differential Diagnosis

NEUROFIBROMA

- Characterized by fascicles and whorls of elongated cells with wavy, serpentine nuclei with wavy collagen fibers; often has a myxoid stroma
- Lacks Antoni A and Antoni B areas

LEIOMYOMA

- Characterized by interlacing bundles of spindle cells with oval, blunt-ended nuclei
- Lacks Antoni A and Antoni B areas
- Positive for SMA

MALIGNANT PERIPHERAL NERVE SHEATH TUMOR

- Infiltrative, highly cellular tumors characterized by elongated cells with pleomorphic nuclei
- Prominent mitotic activity
- Necrosis is common
- Less intense positivity for S-100 protein

PEARLS

- *Schwannoma is a benign tumor showing almost exclusively Schwann cell differentiation; malignant transformation is exceedingly rare*
- *Surgical removal with nerve preservation is the recommended treatment*
- *Cellular schwannoma may be misclassified as a malignant peripheral nerve sheath tumor; strong S-100 protein reactivity favors cellular schwannoma*

SELECTED REFERENCES

Begnami MD, Palau M, Rushing EJ, et al: Evaluation of NF2 gene deletion in sporadic schwannomas, meningiomas, and ependymomas by chromogenic in situ hybridization. Hum Pathol 38:1345-1350, 2007.

Harder A, Wesemann M, Hagel C, et al: Hybrid neurofibroma/schwannoma is overrepresented among schwannomatosis and neurofibromatosis patients. Am J Surg Pathol 36:702-709, 2012.

Rizzo D, Freneaux P, Brisse H, et al: SMARCB1 deficiency in tumors from the peripheral nervous system: a link between schwannomas and rhabdoid tumors? Am J Surg Pathol 36:964-972, 2012.

Torres-Mora J, Dry S, Li X, et al: Malignant melanotic schwannian tumor: a clinicopathologic, immunohistochemical, and gene expression profiling study of 40 cases, with a proposal for the reclassification of "melanotic schwannoma." Am J Surg Pathol 38:94-105, 2014.

NEUROFIBROMA

Clinical Features

- Usually occur in the dermal or subcutaneous tissues throughout the body
- People of any age can be affected, but seen most commonly in young adults
- Lesions may be localized, diffuse, or plexiform, the latter two having a strong association with NF1
  - NF1, von Recklinghausen disease
    - Autosomal dominant, chromosome 17
    - Positive family history in most cases
    - Multiple neurofibromas at different areas of the body
    - Café-au-lait spots (hyperpigmented skin lesions)
    - Lisch nodules (pigmented iris hamartomas)

Gross Pathology

- Well-defined fusiform lesion often in association with a nerve trunk
- Firm, gray-white cut surface
- Diffuse lesions show ill-defined, plaquelike thickening of the subcutaneous tissues
- Plexiform lesions are a multinodular conglomerate of lesions likened to a "bag of worms"

Histopathology

- Low to moderately cellular lesion composed of cells with wavy nuclei and eosinophilic cytoplasm interspersed with wisps of collagen (Figure 17-34)
- Stroma may show small amounts of mucoid material or be myxoid and is occasionally hyalinized
- Tumor is well circumscribed but usually not encapsulated
- Mild nuclear atypia is common and does not mean malignant transformation
- May contain melanin pigment (pigmented neurofibroma) or show epithelioid morphology (epithelioid neurofibroma)
- Plexiform neurofibroma
  - Almost exclusively associated with NF1
  - Irregularly expanded nerve bundles giving a multinodular appearance
  - Tend to be hypocellular with a prominent myxoid matrix
  - Variable degrees of nuclear pleomorphism may be seen
  - Infrequent mitotic activity
- Diffuse neurofibroma
  - Neoplastic cells expand the dermal and subcutaneous tissues and envelop subcutaneous and adnexal structures

Special Stains and Immunohistochemistry

- S-100 protein positive

Other Techniques for Diagnosis

- Biallelic loss of *NF1* tumor suppressor gene on chromosome 17q11.2 may be demonstrated by molecular techniques

Differential Diagnosis

SCHWANNOMA

- Encapsulated by epineurium and composed almost exclusively of fascicles of Schwann cells
- Lacks the myxoid background, and hyalinized vessels are common
- Presence of both Antoni A and Antoni B areas

MYXOMA

- May be intramuscular, cutaneous, or juxta-articular
- Composed of spindled to stellate cells in a prominent myxoid background
- Negative for S-100 protein

MALIGNANT PERIPHERAL NERVE SHEATH TUMOR

- Cellular tumor characterized by pleomorphic cells with wavy nuclei
- Prominent mitotic activity
- Areas of tumor necrosis
- Less strongly positive for S-100 protein

PEARLS

- *Localized, sporadic neurofibroma is a benign lesion treated by conservative excision; malignant transformation is exceedingly rare*
- *Malignant transformation occurs in about 3% of neurofibromas associated with NF1, most commonly in deep-seated and plexiform lesions, and is characterized by increased cellularity, mitotic activity, and diffuse nuclear atypia*
- *May have hybrid areas of schwannoma, frequently associated with neurofibromatosis or schwannomatosis*

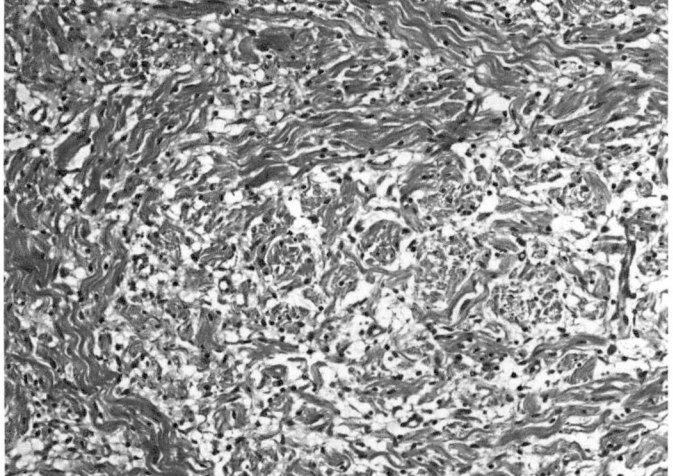

Figure 17-34. Neurofibroma. Small wavy spindle cells are admixed with dense collagen bundles.

SELECTED REFERENCES

De Luca A, Bernardini L, Ceccarini C, et al: Fluorescence in situ hybridization analysis of allelic losses involving the long arm of chromosome 17 in NF1-associated neurofibromas. Cancer Genet Cytogenet 150:168-172, 2004.

Fetsch JF, Michal M, Miettinen M: Pigmented (melanotic) neurofibroma: a clinicopathologic and immunohistochemical analysis of 19 lesions from 17 patients. Am J Surg Pathol 24:331-343, 2000.

Harder A, Wesemann M, Hagel C, et al: Hybrid neurofibroma/schwannoma is overrepresented among schwannomatosis and neurofibromatosis patients. Am J Surg Pathol 36:702-709, 2012.

SOFT TISSUE PERINEURIOMA

Clinical Features

- Most common in adults, but children and elderly can be affected
- Extremities are most common, site followed by trunk, retroperitoneum, and head and neck
- Most frequently subcutaneous or deep seated but may be dermal

Gross Pathology

- Grossly well circumscribed, ranging in size from 1 to 20 cm
- Firm, gray-white cut surface

Histopathology

- Low to moderately cellular lesion, although hypercellular tumors are not uncommon; mitoses typically not seen but may reach up to 4 per 10 hpf
- Storiform or fascicular growth pattern; sclerosing variant is well recognized
- Stroma typically collagenous but may be myxoid or mixed
- Nuclear atypia may be seen and does not mean malignant transformation

Special Stains and Immunohistochemistry

- EMA, Claudin1, Glut 1, and CD34 positive
- Negative for S100, GFAP, neurofilament protein, and desmin

Other Techniques for Diagnosis

- 22q abnormalities are common
- Deletions or rearrangements of 10q seem to be unique to sclerosing perineuriomas

Differential Diagnosis

BENIGN NERVE SHEATH TUMOR (SCHWANNOMA OR NEUROFIBROMA)

- Nerve sheath tumors are positive for S100 and negative for EMA

LOW-GRADE FIBROMYXOID SARCOMA (LGFMS)

- LGFMS shows an abrupt transition between myxoid and collagenous areas
- May be EMA positive but typically negative for Claudin1 and Glut1
- MUC4 positive and FUS translocation

MYXOMA

- Typically intramuscular, cutaneous, or juxta-articular
- Composed of spindled to stellate cells in a prominent myxoid background
- Negative for EMA, Glut1, and Claudin1

MENINGIOMA

- Extracranial meningioma typically arises in skin or soft tissue of scalp or near the vertebral column
- EMA positive but typically negative for Glut1 and Claudin1
- Often progesterone receptor or somatostatin receptor 2 positive

PEARLS

- *Benign lesion with low recurrence risk and little to no metastatic potential; histologic features do not predict recurrence*
- *May have hybrid areas of schwannoma; no clear association with neurofibromatosis*

SELECTED REFERENCES

Brock JE, Perez-Atayde AR, Kozakewich HP, et al: Cytogenetic aberrations in perineurioma: variation with subtype. Am J Surg Pathol 29:1164-1169, 2005.

Folpe AL, Billings SD, McKenney JK, et al: Expression of claudin-1, a recently described tight junction-associated protein, distinguishes soft tissue perineurioma from potential mimics. Am J Surg Pathol 26:1620-1626, 2002.

Hornick JL, Bundock EA, Fletcher CD: Hybrid schwannoma/perineurioma: clinicopathologic analysis of 42 distinctive benign nerve sheath tumors. Am J Surg Pathol 33:1554-1561, 2009.

Hornick JL, Fletcher CD: Soft tissue perineurioma: clinicopathologic analysis of 81 cases including those with atypical histologic features. Am J Surg Pathol 29:845-858, 2005.

PARAGANGLIOMA

Clinical Features

- Occurs in patients between 40 and 60 years of age
- Presents with different symptoms depending on location
  - Carotid body tumor
    - Painless, slowly enlarging mass in the neck
  - Jugulotympanic paraganglioma
    - Dizziness, tinnitus, cranial nerve palsy, and conductive hearing loss
  - Vagal paraganglioma
    - Horner syndrome and vocal cord paralysis
  - Retroperitoneal paraganglioma
    - Back pain and a palpable mass

Gross Pathology

- Lobular, red-brown, well-circumscribed masses
- May measure from a few centimeters up to 20 cm in diameter

Histopathology

- Trabecular or organoid arrangement of round to polygonal cells (Zellballen) with central nuclei and eosinophilic, faintly granular cytoplasm (Figure 17-35)
- Variable nuclear hyperchromasia and pleomorphism
- Extensive delicate vascular network
- Infrequent mitotic activity
- Malignant paraganglioma
  - No reliable histologic criteria can predict malignancy
  - Aggressive behavior has been associated with tumor necrosis, vascular invasion, and increased mitotic activity
  - Metastatic spread is the only reliable criterion for malignancy

Special Stains and Immunohistochemistry

- NSE, chromogranin positive
- S-100 protein highlights sustentacular network surrounding tumor nests
- Cytokeratin typically negative

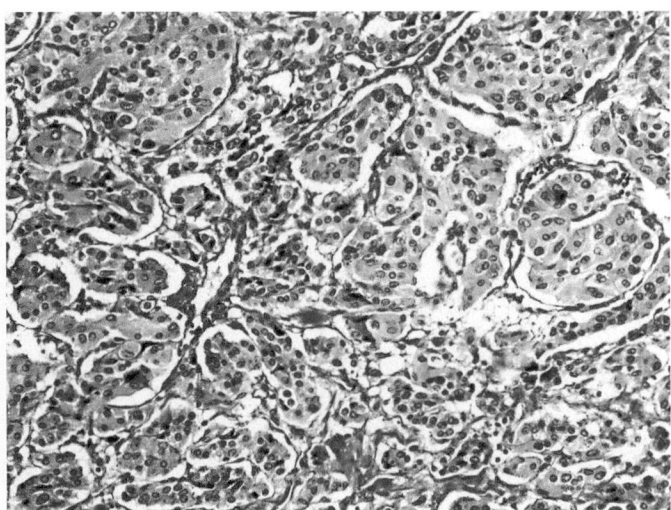

Figure 17-35. Paraganglioma. Nests of polygonal tumor cells with nuclear atypia and eosinophilic cytoplasm create a Zellballen pattern.

Other Techniques for Diagnosis

- Electron microscopy: cytoplasmic dense-core neurosecretory granules

Differential Diagnosis

CARCINOID TUMOR

- Sheets of small, uniform cells with central nuclei, stippled chromatin, and abundant finely granular cytoplasm
- Immunoreactivity for cytokeratin

ALVEOLAR SOFT PART SARCOMA

- Occurs in the deep soft tissue; usually thigh
- Characterized by uniform, polygonal cells with eosinophilic, granular, cytoplasm, and central nuclei
- Organoid growth pattern
- Vascular invasion commonly seen

PEARLS

- *Paraganglioma usually follows a benign clinical course*
- *Overall incidence of malignant transformation is about 10%; no reliable histologic criteria can predict malignancy*
- *About 10% to 20% of patients have germline mutations, associated with von Hippel-Lindau disease, multiple endocrine neoplasia syndromes, NF1, and germline succinate dehydrogenase mutations*
- *May be associated with Carney triad: paraganglioma, pulmonary chondroma, and gastric leiomyosarcoma*

SELECTED REFERENCES

Carney JA: Gastric stromal sarcoma, pulmonary chondroma, and extraadrenal paraganglioma (Carney Triad): natural history, adrenocortical component, and possible familial occurrence. Mayo Clin Proc 74:543-552, 1999.

Cascon A, Landa I, Lopez-Jimenez E, et al: Molecular characterization of a common SDHB deletion in paraganglioma patients. J Med Genet 45:233-238, 2008.

Fishbein L, Nathanson KL: Pheochromocytoma and paraganglioma: understanding the complexities of the genetic background. Cancer Genet 205:1-11, 2012.

Papathomas TG, de Krijger RR, Tischler AS: Paragangliomas: update on differential diagnostic considerations, composite tumors, and recent genetic developments. Semin Diagn Pathol 30:207-223, 2013.

Plaza JA, Wakely PE Jr, Moran C, et al: Sclerosing paraganglioma: report of 19 cases of an unusual variant of neuroendocrine tumor that may be mistaken for an aggressive malignant neoplasm. Am J Surg Pathol 30:7-12, 2006.

MALIGNANT PERIPHERAL NERVE SHEATH TUMOR

Clinical Features

- Typically presents as an enlarging mass arising in association with a major nerve trunk, frequently on the proximal extremities
- About 3% to 10% of patients with NF1 develop a malignant peripheral nerve sheath tumor (MPNST)
- About 50% of cases are found in patients with NF1; often develops after 10 to 20 years
- Sporadic cases typically develop in adults, with a male-to-female ratio of 1:1
- Cases associated with neurofibromatosis occur at a younger age and show a 4:1 male-to-female ratio

Gross Pathology

- Arises as a fusiform, deep-seated mass, often within a major nerve
- Tumors are typically poorly defined and frequently infiltrate along adjacent nerve or into adjacent soft tissue
- Tan-white, fleshy cut surface with focal areas of hemorrhage and necrosis

Histopathology

- Cellular spindle cell tumor with fascicular growth pattern (Figure 17-36)
- Alternating hypercellular and hypocellular zones often with areas of myxoid stroma
- Nuclear palisading and whorled nodules of spindle cells may be seen
- Perivascular tumor cell condensation and growth along nerve twigs is common

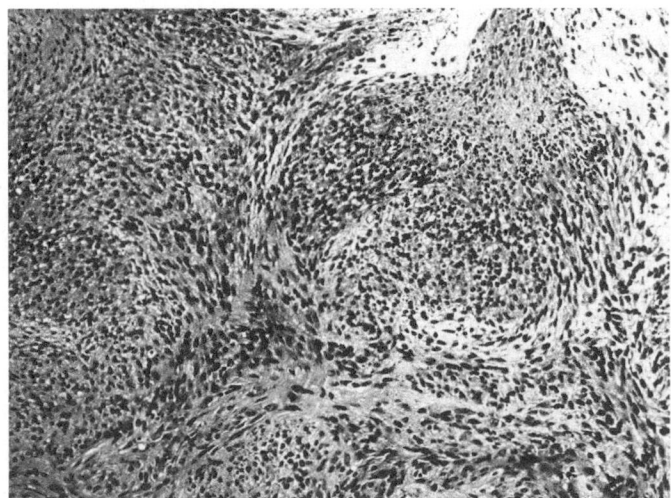

Figure 17-36. Malignant peripheral nerve sheath tumor. Fascicles of pleomorphic spindle cells with dense cellularity alternate with less cellular areas. Focal necrosis is present.

- Spindle cells show hyperchromatic wavy or buckled nuclei and show minimal to marked pleomorphism
- High mitotic activity and necrosis are common
- Benign or malignant heterologous elements such as bone, cartilage, and skeletal muscle may be seen

MALIGNANT TRITON TUMOR
- Presence of rhabdomyoblastic differentiation

MPNST
- Tumor showing areas of conventional MPNST admixed with nests of round to polygonal epithelioid cells with round nuclei, prominent nucleoli, and clear to eosinophilic cytoplasm

Special Stains and Immunohistochemistry
- S-100 protein focally and weakly positive in most cases
- CD56 and CD57 variably positive
- Collagen IV positive around individual tumor cells

Other Techniques for Diagnosis
- Electron microscopy reveals interdigitating cell processes, complete or partial external lamina, cell junctions, and pinocytotic vesicles
- Cytogenetic studies show numerous structural and numeral abnormalities, none of which are diagnostic

Differential Diagnosis

CELLULAR SCHWANNOMA
- Hypercellular tumor composed almost entirely of Antoni A areas
- Typically well circumscribed rather than infiltrative
- Tumor cells are more uniform with less nuclear pleomorphism
- Mitotic activity and necrosis are infrequent
- Strong positivity for S-100 protein

LEIOMYOSARCOMA
- Characterized by spindle cells with eosinophilic cytoplasm and atypical cigar-shaped nuclei arranged in short interlacing fascicles
- Cellular pleomorphism is often pronounced, and mitotic figures are numerous
- Immunoreactivity for SMA and desmin

FIBROSARCOMA
- Highly cellular, infiltrative tumor composed of fibroblasts with hyperchromatic nuclei and scant cytoplasm arranged in an almost exclusive herringbone pattern
- High mitotic rate; atypical mitotic figures may be seen
- Negative for markers of neural differentiation

SYNOVIAL SARCOMA (MONOPHASIC)
- Characterized by fascicles and whorls of spindle-shaped cells with a high nuclear-to-cytoplasmic ratio
- Immunoreactivity for cytokeratin, EMA, CD99, and bcl-2
- Presence of t(X;18)(p11;q11)

CLEAR CELL SARCOMA (MELANOMA OF SOFT PARTS)
- Characterized by uniform cells with central round to oval nuclei, prominent basophilic nucleoli, and clear to eosinophilic cytoplasm with glycogen

- Intracellular melanin (frequently inconspicuous)
- Groups of cells separated by delicate fibrous septa; collagen IV stain surrounds groups rather than individual tumor cells
- Immunoreactivity for S-100 protein, HMB-45, and melan-A
- Presence of t(12;22)(q13:q12), producing an *EWS-ATF1* fusion

PEARLS

- *MPNSTs have a high likelihood of local recurrence and distant metastasis*
- *Metastases usually involve the lungs, liver, and bone; lymph node involvement is rare*
- *These tumors have a propensity to spread for considerable distances along the nerve sheath*

SELECTED REFERENCES

Allison KH, Patel RM, Goldblum JR, Rubin BP: Superficial malignant peripheral nerve sheath tumor: a rare and challenging diagnosis. Am J Clin Pathol 124:685-692, 2005.

Anghileri M, Miceli R, Fiore M, et al: Malignant peripheral nerve sheath tumors: prognostic factors and survival in a series of patients treated at a single institution. Cancer 107:1065-1074, 2006.

Rodriguez FJ, Folpe AL, Giannini C, Perry A: Pathology of peripheral nerve sheath tumors: diagnostic overview and update on selected diagnostic problems. Acta Neuropathologica 123:295-319, 2012.

Stasik CJ, Tawfik O: Malignant peripheral nerve sheath tumor with rhabdomyosarcomatous differentiation (malignant triton tumor). Arch Pathol Lab Med 130:1878-1881, 2006.

Zhou H, Coffin CM, Perkins SL, et al: Malignant peripheral nerve sheath tumor: a comparison of grade, immunophenotype, and cell cycle/growth activation marker expression in sporadic and neurofibromatosis 1-related lesions. Am J Surg Pathol 27:1337-1345, 2003.

HEMANGIOMA

Clinical Features

CAPILLARY HEMANGIOMA (INFANTILE AND JUVENILE HEMANGIOMA)
- Most common vascular tumor of infancy, usually presenting in the first few weeks of life
- Commonly occurs in the head and neck; may involve the subcutaneous tissue or occasionally the viscera; diffuse soft tissue growth is termed *hemangiomatosis*
- Typically presents as a crimson skin lesion that becomes raised over time (strawberry hemangioma)
- Usually grows through first year of life and regresses over time

CAVERNOUS HEMANGIOMA
- Commonly seen in children, with a predilection for skin of the head and neck (port-wine nevus)
- Typically involves deeper tissue than capillary hemangiomas do
- May occur in abdominal viscera, notably liver and spleen
- Less likely to regress over time
- Occasionally associated with Maffucci syndrome (multiple enchondromas and vascular proliferations)

EPITHELIOID HEMANGIOMA
- Also termed *angiolymphoid hyperplasia with eosinophilia*
- Presents in head and neck as a pruritic red lesion; may be multifocal

- Most common in third to fifth decades; slightly more common in men
- May recur after excision

PYOGENIC GRANULOMA (LOBULAR CAPILLARY HEMANGIOMA [LCH])

- Essentially the same as a capillary hemangioma, although LCH does not usually present in infancy
- Typically a polypoid growth in the skin or oral mucosa
- Commonly associated with pregnancy or use of oral contraceptives

SPINDLE CELL HEMANGIOMA

- Typically presents as a subcutaneous nodule on a distal extremity; may be multifocal
- Most common in the second to third decades but can occur at any age

INTRAMUSCULAR HEMANGIOMA

- Presents as a slowly growing deep mass that may be painful
- Lower extremities are most commonly affected, followed by head and neck, upper extremities, and trunk
- Most common in adolescents and young adults
- Has a tendency to recur if incompletely excised

Gross Pathology

- Hemangiomas may be dermal or deeply seated and well circumscribed or infiltrative
- Most have a spongy, dark-red cut surface

Histopathology

CAPILLARY HEMANGIOMA

- Lobular architecture with arborizing, small vascular channels lined by plump to flattened endothelial cells, separated by scant connective tissue stroma (Figure 17-37)
- Cellular lesions show inconspicuous capillary lumina; solid growth pattern and variable mitotic activity (*cellular hemangioma*)
- Involutional changes include vascular ectasia and replacement by fat or fibrous tissue

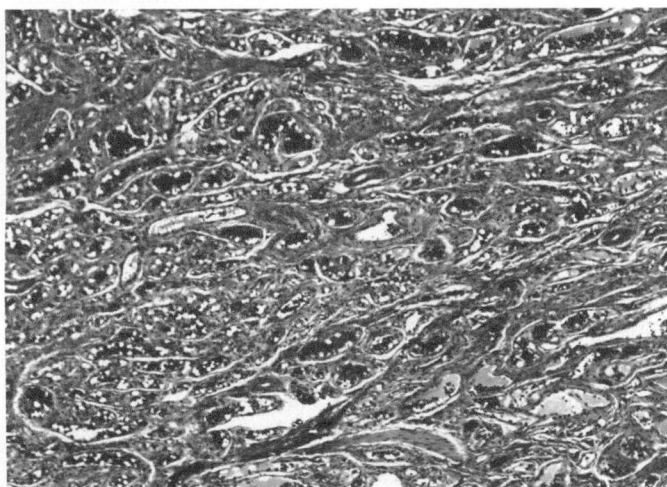

Figure 17-37. Hemangioma. Tightly packed small vascular channels are lined by a flattened endothelium.

CAVERNOUS HEMANGIOMA

- Typically found in subcutaneous tissue
- Characterized by dilated, blood-filled, medium- to large-caliber vascular spaces, lined by flat endothelial cells

EPITHELIOID HEMANGIOMA

- Well-circumscribed dermal lesion comprising small to medium-sized blood vessels
- Vascular channels lined by plump endothelial cells with abundant eosinophilic cytoplasm and vesicular oval nuclei
- Background typically shows a lymphocytic infiltrate, sometimes with germinal centers; variable numbers of interspersed mast cells, eosinophils, and plasma cells

PYOGENIC GRANULOMA

- Well circumscribed with a lobular architecture
- Characterized by small, arborizing vascular channels and bland endothelium

SPINDLE CELL HEMANGIOMA

- Poorly circumscribed lesion
- Biphasic population of solid masses of spindle cells combined with cavernous vascular channels; may contain thrombi
- Cells lining ectatic channels are attenuated, whereas spindle cells tend to be plump, often with cytoplasmic vacuoles

INTRAMUSCULAR ANGIOMA

- Capillary or cavernous channels admixed with mature skeletal muscle and a variable amount of fat

Special Stains and Immunohistochemistry

- Thrombomodulin, CD34, CD31, and Fli-1 highlight endothelial cells
- GLUT1 positive in capillary hemangioma of juvenile type only

Other Techniques for Diagnosis

- Noncontributory

Differential Diagnosis

HEMANGIOPERICYTOMA

- Almost always seen in adult population
- Typically occurs in deep soft tissue of legs, pelvis, or retroperitoneum
- Cellular blunt spindle cell tumor characterized by staghorn blood vessels
- Perivascular and intervascular proliferation of uniform pericytic cells

ANGIOSARCOMA

- Angiosarcomas are extraordinarily rare in children
- Typically found in skin or viscera; rare in deep soft tissue
- Characterized by irregular anastomosing vascular channels lined by atypical endothelial cells
- Mitotic activity usually present
- Hemorrhage and necrosis are common

KAPOSI SARCOMA

- Fascicles of uniform spindle cells forming slitlike vascular spaces
- Extravasated red blood cells common
- PAS-positive hyaline globules (intracellular and extracellular)
- Most common in AIDS patients and elderly patients of Mediterranean descent
- Immunoreactive for HHV-8 and LNA-1 in 80% to 85% of cases

PEARLS

- *Von Hippel-Lindau disease is characterized by cerebellar hemangioblastomas, widespread visceral angiomatous lesions, and renal cell carcinoma*
- *Sturge-Weber syndrome is characterized by venous angiomatous lesions in the leptomeninges and ipsilateral port-wine nevi of the face*
- *Strawberry hemangiomas tend to resolve spontaneously without treatment*
- *Epithelioid hemangiomas and intramuscular angiomas are more likely to recur following excision*

SELECTED REFERENCES

Brenn T, Fletcher CD: Cutaneous epithelioid angiomatous nodule: a distinct lesion in the morphologic spectrum of epithelioid vascular tumors. Am J Dermatopathol 26:14-21, 2004.

Calonje E, Fletcher CD: Sinusoidal hemangioma: a distinctive benign vascular neoplasm within the group of cavernous hemangiomas. Am J Surg Pathol 15:1130-1135, 1991.

Goh SG, Calonje E: Cutaneous vascular tumours: an update. Histopathology 52:661-673, 2008.

North PE, Waner M, Mizeracki A, Mihm MC Jr: GLUT1: a newly discovered immunohistochemical marker for juvenile hemangiomas. Hum Pathol 31:11-22, 2000.

GLOMUS TUMOR

Clinical Features

- Tumor differentiates toward modified smooth muscle of the glomus body
- Typically seen in young adults
- Usually involves distal extremities, especially fingers and toes; deep or visceral tumors are rare
- Red and blue subcutaneous nodule that is painful; may be multifocal

Gross Pathology

- Typically smaller than 1 cm; well-circumscribed dermal or subcutaneous nodule

Histopathology

- Sheets or nests of uniform, round cells with oval nuclei and pale eosinophilic cytoplasm (Figure 17-38)
- Groups of glomus cells may surround dilated vessels (*glomangioma*)
- Minimal mitotic activity
- May show focal degenerative nuclear atypia

Special Stains and Immunohistochemistry

- SMA and h-caldesmon positive
- CD34 variably positive
- CD31 and thrombomodulin negative in tumor cells

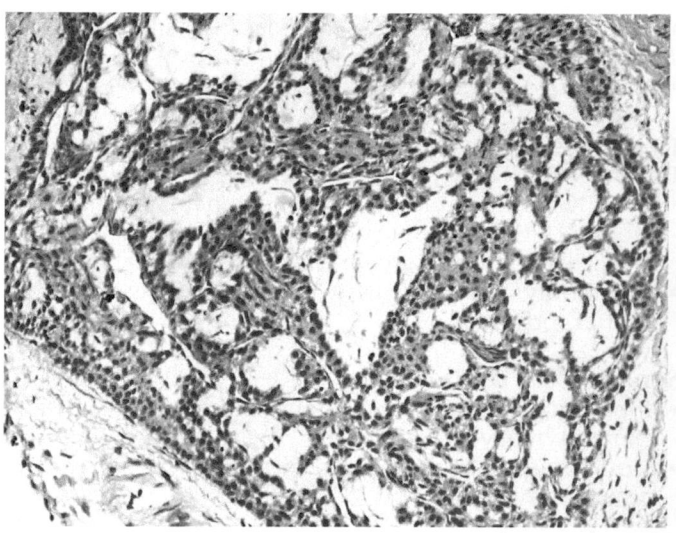

Figure 17-38. Glomus tumor. Nodular proliferation of uniform round cells with central nuclei and pale cytoplasm.

Other Techniques for Diagnosis

- Noncontributory

Differential Diagnosis

CELLULAR OR CAVERNOUS HEMANGIOMA

- Cellular hemangioma is characterized by small, arborizing vascular channels lined by flat endothelial cells
- No glomus cells
- Focal cavernous hemangioma-like areas may be present in glomangioma
- Positive for thrombomodulin, CD31, and CD34; negative for SMA

PARAGANGLIOMA

- Trabecular or organoid arrangement of round to polygonal cells with oval nuclei and eosinophilic, granular cytoplasm
- Extensive and delicate capillary network, dividing tumor into compartments (Zellballen)
- Positive for neuroendocrine markers (synaptophysin, chromogranin, and NSE); negative for keratin and SMA

PEARLS

- *Glomus tumor is benign and typically treated by excision; about 5% to 10% recur*
- *Malignant glomus tumors (glomangiosarcoma) are exceedingly rare; they are typically large, in deep or visceral locations, with infiltrative growth, nuclear atypia, and brisk mitotic activity*

SELECTED REFERENCES

Folpe AL, Fanburg-Smith JC, Miettinen M, Weiss SW: Atypical and malignant glomus tumors: analysis of 52 cases, with a proposal for the reclassification of glomus tumors. Am J Surg Pathol 25:1-12, 2001.

Mentzel T, Dei Tos AP, Sapi Z, Kutzner H: Myopericytoma of skin and soft tissues: clinicopathologic and immunohistochemical study of 54 cases. Am J Surg Pathol 30:104-113, 2006.

Miettinen M, Paal E, Lasota J, Sobin LH: Gastrointestinal glomus tumors: a clinicopathologic, immunohistochemical, and molecular genetic study of 32 cases. Am J Surg Pathol 26:301-311, 2002.

HEMANGIOPERICYTOMA AND MYOPERICYTOMA

Clinical Features

HEMANGIOPERICYTOMA

- Has at least borderline malignant potential; shows differentiation toward modified pericytes
- Occurs in adults; usually deep, most frequently in legs, pelvis, or retroperitoneum
- Often large on clinical detection
- Hypoglycemia may be associated with tumors of the pelvis or retroperitoneum (Doege-Potter syndrome)

MYOPERICYTOMA

- Same as hemangiopericytoma, except that lesion is subcutaneous, usually on distal extremities

Gross Pathology

- Solitary, well-circumscribed, often lobulated mass with gray-white to red-brown cut surface
- Focal hemorrhage or cystic degeneration may be seen

Histopathology

HEMANGIOPERICYTOMA

- Thin-walled staghorn vascular channels lined by a single layer of flat endothelium, surrounded by perivascular and intervascular proliferation of uniform-appearing oval to spindle-shaped pericytes showing ill-defined cytoplasmic borders (Figure 17-39)
- Reticulin-rich network surrounding individual pericytes
- Focal hyalinization and myxoid change may be present
- Mitotic rate typically fewer than four mitotic figures/10 hpf
- May have variable admixed adipose tissue "lipomatous hemangiopericytoma"
- Criteria characterizing "malignant" hemangiopericytomas are not clearly defined, but aggressive behavior associated with brisk mitotic activity, nuclear atypia, necrosis, and hemorrhage; *all* hemangiopericytomas have at least borderline malignant potential

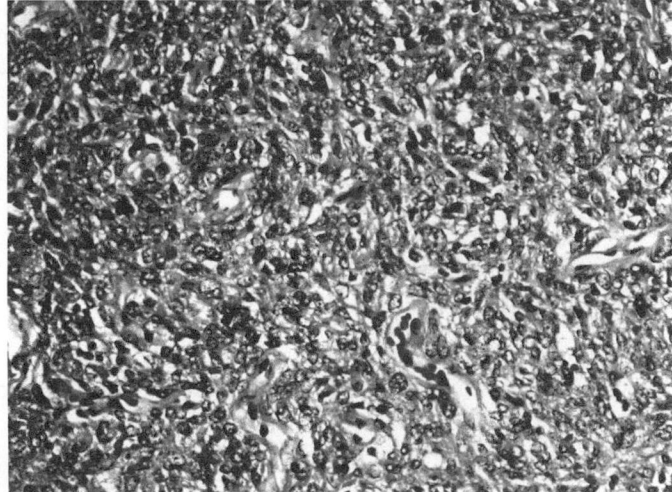

Figure 17-39. Hemangiopericytoma. Bland ovoid tumor cells with indistinct cytoplasmic borders are arranged around a ramifying vascular network.

MYOPERICYTOMA

- Same as hemangiopericytoma, except with plump, spindled to round myoid cells that surround vessels with a hemangiopericytoid pattern

Special Stains and Immunohistochemistry

- CD34: equivocal positivity
- SMA positive in myopericytoma but negative in conventional hemangiopericytoma

Other Techniques for Diagnosis

- Electron microscopy: pericytes contain rough endoplasmic reticulum, mitochondria, free polyribosomes, and thin filaments
- Cytogenetic studies: hemangiopericytoma may be associated with structural aberrations involving the long arm of chromosome 12

Differential Diagnosis

SOLITARY FIBROUS TUMOR

- Semantic difference; the World Health Organization has combined hemangiopericytoma and solitary fibrous tumor into one entity
- Patternless architecture of spindle cells in a variably hyalinized stroma; hemangiopericytoid vasculature is common
- Often pleural but can occur in any location
- Positive for CD34, CD99, and bcl-2

FIBROUS HISTIOCYTOMA WITH HEMANGIOPERICYTOMA-LIKE AREAS

- Spindle cells and histiocytoid cells arranged in a storiform pattern
- Often shows admixed inflammatory cells
- "Dissection" of collagen by tumor cells at lesion periphery

GLOMANGIOMA

- Dilated vessels surrounded by sheets of round cells with central nuclei and pale eosinophilic cytoplasm
- Positive for SMA

SYNOVIAL SARCOMA (MONOPHASIC)

- Composed of hyperchromatic blunt spindle cells with a hemangiopericytoma-like growth pattern
- Immunoreactivity for cytokeratin or EMA; positivity for CD99 and bcl-2, but not CD34
- Presence of t(X;18)(p11;q11)

PEARLS

- *Hemangiopericytoma is a diagnosis of exclusion because the hemangiopericytoma-like pattern may be seen in a variety of other tumors*
- *Long-term survival following surgical resection is typical; metastases may appear 10 to 20 years later and usually involve lung or bone*
- *Natural history is difficult to predict; occasional tumors with aggressive morphologic characteristics may have more rapid evolution*
- *Tumor recurrence often precedes the appearance of distant metastases*

SELECTED REFERENCES

Ferrari A, Casanova M, Bisogno G, et al: Hemangiopericytoma in pediatric ages: a report from the Italian and German Soft Tissue Sarcoma Cooperative Group. Cancer 92:2692-2698, 2001.

Gengler C, Guillou L: Solitary fibrous tumour and haemangio-pericytoma: evolution of a concept. Histopathology 48:63-74, 2006.

Guillou L, Gebhard S, Coindre JM: Lipomatous hemangiopericytoma: a fat-containing variant of solitary fibrous tumor? Clinicopathologic, immunohistochemical, and ultrastructural analysis of a series in favor of a unifying concept. Hum Pathol 31:1108-1115, 2000.

Thompson LD, Miettinen M, Wenig BM: Sinonasal-type hemangiopericytoma: a clinicopathologic and immuno-phenotypic analysis of 104 cases showing perivascular myoid differentiation. Am J Surg Pathol 27:737-749, 2003.

HEMANGIOENDOTHELIOMA

Clinical Features

- Considered to be a low-grade variant of endothelial malignancy; may be seen in several anatomic locations

EPITHELIOID HEMANGIOENDOTHELIOMA

- Occurs in any age group but is rare in children
- Usually involves dermal or subcutaneous tissues of extremities; rarely multicentric; bone or visceral involvement is possible
- Often surrounds a preexisting blood vessel, most commonly a vein, and may be associated with edema or thrombophlebitis

KAPOSIFORM HEMANGIOENDOTHELIOMA

- Occurs principally in children, often in first year of life
- Most common locations are superficial and deep soft tissues of extremities or retroperitoneum
- Often associated with consumptive coagulopathy and thrombocytopenia (Kasabach-Merritt syndrome), especially with deep lesions

RETIFORM HEMANGIOENDOTHELIOMA AND PAPILLARY INTRALYMPHATIC ANGIOENDOTHELIOMA (DABSKA TUMOR)

- Seen at all ages; retiform hemangioendothelioma is more common in adults, and Dabska tumor is more common in children
- The limbs are the most commonly affected

Gross Pathology

- Violaceous plaques or subcutaneous nodules; often multinodular
- Infiltrative borders and gray to white variegated cut surfaces
- Epithelioid hemangioendotheliomas associated with large vessels may resemble organizing thrombi

Histopathology

EPITHELIOID HEMANGIOENDOTHELIOMA

- Cords and nests of polygonal endothelial cells with eosinophilic cytoplasm and oval nuclei (Figure 17-40)
- Intracellular cytoplasmic lumens with intraluminal red blood cells
- Intramural growth into preexisting vessels with perivascular extension of tumor

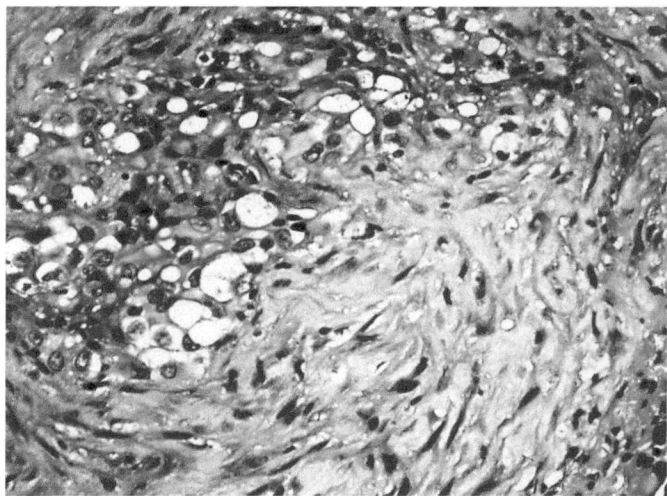

Figure 17-40. Epithelioid hemangioendothelioma. Nests of epithelioid cells with cytoplasmic vacuoles are embedded in a fibro-myxoid stroma.

- Tumor cells typically have bland, round to oval nuclei but may show some pleomorphism
- Background stroma is myxoid or hyalinized
- Typically low mitotic rate

KAPOSIFORM HEMANGIOENDOTHELIOMA

- Tumor nodules separated by fibrous septa; nodules may resemble capillary hemangioma or have the spindle cell morphology of Kaposi sarcoma
- Glomeruloid structures, consisting of small nodules of tumor cells, are characteristic
- Extravasated red blood cells, intratumoral hemorrhage, and hemosiderin are common

RETIFORM HEMANGIOENDOTHELIOMA AND PAPILLARY INTRALYMPHATIC ANGIOENDOTHELIOMA (DABSKA TUMOR)

- Both tumors are characterized by plump cells lining lymphatic-like vascular channels, with or without intraluminal papillary projections
- Retiform hemangioendothelioma shows narrow, arborizing vascular spaces lined by the plump endothelium and separated by sclerotic stroma, often containing a lymphocytic infiltrate
- Dabska tumor contains intraluminal tufts of plump endothelium and resembles deep lymphangioma; characteristic deposits of basement membrane are seen in cellular tufts

Special Stains and Immunohistochemistry

- Factor VIIIa, CD31, CD34, thrombomodulin, podoplanin, and Fli-1 positive
- GLUT1 negative
- Keratin may be focally positive in epithelioid hemangioendothelioma
- Reticulin highlights constituent vessels

Other Techniques for Diagnosis

- Recurrent t(1;3)(p36;q25) has been reported in epithelioid hemangioendothelioma

Differential Diagnosis

EPITHELIOID SARCOMA

- Usually occurs in the distal extremities of adolescents and young adults
- Coalescing nodules of polygonal cells with central areas of necrosis
- Positive for cytokeratin and EMA; negative for endothelial markers except for CD34

EPITHELIOID ANGIOSARCOMA

- Solid growth with sievelike vascular channels rather than the architectural patterns of hemangioendothelioma
- Greater nuclear atypia, mitotic activity, and necrosis than are seen in epithelioid hemangioendothelioma

KAPOSIFORM HEMANGIOENDOTHELIOMA AND KAPOSI SARCOMA

- Kaposi sarcoma
  - Extraordinarily rare in children; typically associated with immunosuppression
  - Lacks areas reminiscent of cellular hemangioma
  - Positive for HHV-8 and LNA-1, unlike hemangioendotheliomas

PEARLS

- *Hemangioendotheliomas have borderline biologic behavior with the ability to recur but rare metastasis; epithelioid hemangioendotheliomas are the most aggressive of the group, metastasizing in up to 33% of cases*
- *Surgical excision is standard treatment; medical therapy may be indicated for unresectable lesions or to treat consumptive coagulopathy*

SELECTED REFERENCES

Dabska M: Malignant endovascular papillary angioendothelioma of the skin in childhood: clinicopathologic study of 6 cases. Cancer 24:503-510, 1969.

Debelenko LV, Perez-Atayde AR, Mulliken JB, et al: D2-40 immunohistochemical analysis of pediatric vascular tumors reveals positivity in kaposiform hemangioendothelioma. Mod Pathol 18:1454-1460, 2005.

Fukunaga M, Suzuki K, Saegusa N, Folpe AL: Composite hemangioendothelioma: report of 5 cases including one with associated Maffucci syndrome. Am J Surg Pathol 31:1567-1572, 2007.

Lyons LL, North PE, Mac-Moune Lai F, et al: Kaposiform hemangioendothelioma: a study of 33 cases emphasizing its pathologic, immunophenotypic, and biologic uniqueness from juvenile hemangioma. Am J Surg Pathol 28:559-568, 2004.

Zukerberg LR, Nickoloff BJ, Weiss SW: Kaposiform hemangioendothelioma of infancy and childhood: an aggressive neoplasm associated with Kasabach-Merritt syndrome and lymphangiomatosis. Am J Surg Pathol 17:321-328, 1993.

ANGIOSARCOMA

Clinical Features

- Rare tumor comprising less than 1% of sarcomas; usually seen in adults
- Predilection for skin and superficial soft tissue, breast, bone, liver, and spleen; rare in deep soft tissue
- May be associated with chronic lymphedema (typically postmastectomy), previous therapeutic radiation, or arteriovenous fistulas in renal transplant recipients
- Angiosarcomas of the liver are associated with prior exposure to polyvinyl chloride and thorium dioxide (Thorotrast)

Gross Pathology

- Cutaneous angiosarcomas present as an ill-defined, bruiselike lesion or ulcerated hemorrhagic nodules, or plaques simulating erysipelas
- Commonly large hemorrhagic, ill-defined masses with spongy quality and blood-filled spaces

Histopathology

- Primarily constituted by epithelioid or fusiform cells with rudimentary vascular differentiation; pleomorphism, mitoses, and widespread tissue infiltration are common
- Tumor cells in vascular spaces may be attenuated or plump with hyperchromatic nuclei (Figure 17-41)
- Spindle cell areas may resemble fibrosarcoma or other spindle cell tumors

Special Stains and Immunohistochemistry

- Thrombomodulin, CD31, CD34, Fli-1, factor VIII and Claudin-5 positive
- Cytokeratin may be positive in epithelioid variant of angiosarcoma

Other Techniques for Diagnosis

- Electron microscopy may demonstrate cytoplasmic Weibel-Palade bodies in roughly 25% of cases
- *CMYC* amplification in radiation-induced angiosarcoma and some cases of cutaneous angiosarcoma

Differential Diagnosis

HEMANGIOMA

- Complete tubular vascular channels lined by uniform, flattened endothelial cells
- Lacks pleomorphism, mitotic activity, necrosis, and irregular tissue infiltration

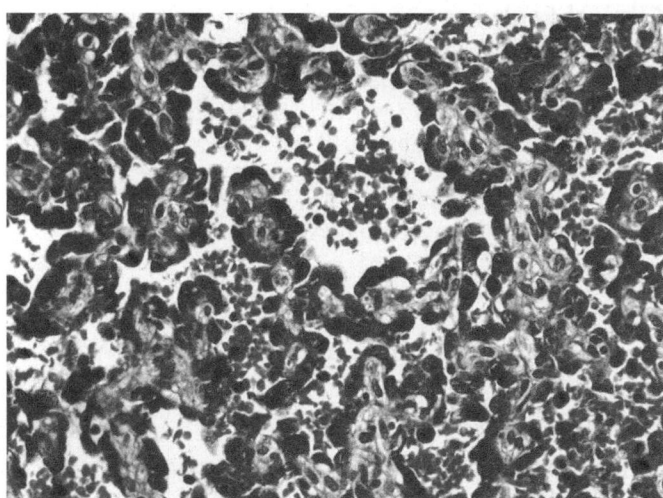

Figure 17-41. Angiosarcoma. Hyperchromatic, pleomorphic tumor cells form primitive vascular channels containing red blood cells.

Papillary Endothelial Hyperplasia (Intravascular Hemangioendothelioma of Masson)

- An unusual variant of organizing thrombus characterized by numerous intravascular anastomosing pseudopapillae lined by endothelial cells
- Lacks nuclear pleomorphism and mitotic activity; no extravascular component

Epithelioid Hemangioendothelioma

- Polygonal epithelioid endothelial cells in cords and clusters, eosinophilic cytoplasm, and oval, bland nuclei
- Little if any nuclear pleomorphism and limited mitotic activity; cytoplasmic vacuoles

PEARLS

- *Angiosarcomas are treated with radical surgery and radiation therapy*
- *Clinical course is characterized by frequent recurrence and distant metastasis, most commonly to lungs, lymph nodes, and bone*
- *Prognosis is related to size, multifocality, and ability to achieve a complete excision*

SELECTED REFERENCES

Deyrup AT, McKenney JK, Tighiouart M, et al: Sporadic cutaneous angiosarcomas: a proposal for risk stratification based on 69 cases. Am J Surg Pathol 32:72-77, 2008.

Guo T, Zhang L, Chang NE, et al: Consistent MYC and FLT4 gene amplification in radiation-induced angiosarcoma but not in other radiation-associated atypical vascular lesions. Genes Chromosomes Cancer 50:25-33, 2011.

Meis-Kindblom JM, Kindblom LG: Angiosarcoma of soft tissue: a study of 80 cases. Am J Surg Pathol 22:683-697, 1998.

Miettinen M, Sarlomo-Rikala M, Wang ZF: Claudin-5 as an immunohistochemical marker for angiosarcoma and hemangioendotheliomas. Am J Surg 35:1848-1856, 2011.

Shon W, Sukov WR, Jenkins SM, Folpe AL: MYC amplification and overexpression in primary cutaneous angiosarcoma: a fluorescence in-situ hybridization and immunohistochemical study. Mod Pathol 27:509-515, 2014.

LYMPHANGIOMA

Clinical Features

- Rare tumors typically occurring as congenital tumors; most present before the age of 2 years
- Typically present as a poorly defined soft tissue or cutaneous mass in the head and neck or axillary region
- Abdominal or visceral involvement may be found
- Subcategorized into the following types
  - Cystic lymphangioma (cystic hygromas)
    - Superficially located
    - Commonly involves the neck region
  - Cavernous lymphangioma
    - Commonly involves skeletal muscle or deeper soft tissue

Gross Pathology

- Commonly appears as a soft, cystic, gray-white tumor
- Cystic lymphangiomas are typically well circumscribed, whereas cavernous lymphangiomas have infiltrative margins

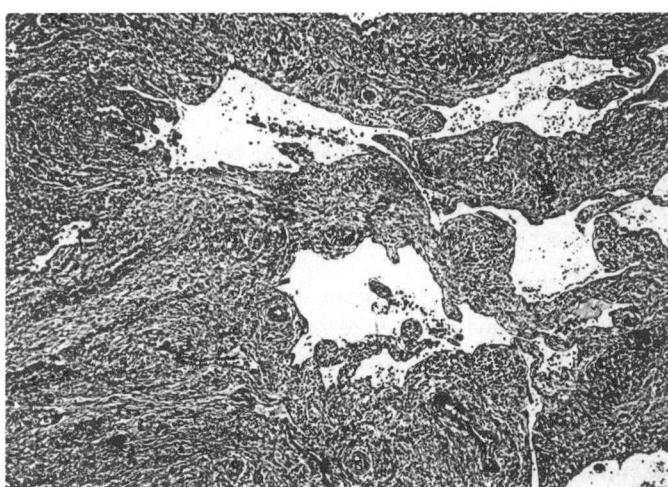

Figure 17-42. Lymphangioma. Dilated lymphatic channels are separated by inflamed fibrous stroma.

Histopathology

- Characterized by anastomosing, thin-walled, irregular lymphatic channels lined by flat endothelial cells (Figure 17-42)
- Proteinaceous intraluminal fluid containing lymphocytes and red blood cells
- Stromal fibrosis and chronic inflammatory infiltrate are common; lymphoid aggregates are often seen
- Cavernous lymphangiomas have infiltrative margins and often extend into adjacent adipose tissue

Special Stains and Immunohistochemistry

- Noncontributory

Other Techniques for Diagnosis

- Noncontributory

Differential Diagnosis

HEMANGIOMA

- Arborizing, small vascular channels lined by flattened endothelial cells

PEARLS

- *Lymphangiomas are treated by surgical excision*
- *Overall excellent prognosis; may rarely recur*

SELECTED REFERENCES

Fukunaga M: Expression of D2-40 in lymphatic endothelium of normal tissues and in vascular tumours. Histopathology 46:396-402, 2005.

Galambos C, Nodit L: Identification of lymphatic endothelium in pediatric vascular tumors and malformations. Pediatr Dev Pathol 8:181-189, 2005.

Gomez CS, Calonje E, Ferrar DW, et al: Lymphangiomatosis of the limbs: clinicopathologic analysis of a series with a good prognosis. Am J Surg Pathol 19:125-133, 1995.

Guillou L, Fletcher CD: Benign lymphangioendothelioma (acquired progressive lymphangioma): a lesion not to be confused with well-differentiated angiosarcoma and patch stage Kaposi's sarcoma. Clinicopathologic analysis of a series. Am J Surg Pathol 24:1047-1057, 2000.

MYXOMA

Clinical Features

- Usually well-defined, deep mass; may be intramuscular, cutaneous, or juxta-articular
- Intramuscular tumors are common in older patients and are found within the large muscles of the body
- Juxta-articular tumors typically occur around the knee or other large joints
- May be associated with Carney complex
  - Autosomal dominant
  - Characterized by myxomas, skin pigmentation, and endocrine hyperactivity

Gross Pathology

- Round to ovoid tumors with a gray-white, gelatinous cut surface

Histopathology

- Hypocellular tumor with well-circumscribed margins; often with a pseudocapsule at the interface of tumor and surrounding soft tissue
- Few stellate or bipolar cells with oval nuclei (spider cells)
- Abundant loose, paucicellular, myxoid stroma (Figure 17-43)

Special Stains and Immunohistochemistry

- Vimentin positive

Other Techniques for Diagnosis

- Noncontributory

Differential Diagnosis

NERVE SHEATH MYXOMA

- Characterized by parallel layers of spindle cells with wavy nuclei at the periphery

MYXOID NEUROFIBROMA

- Wavy, spindle nuclei; often areas show a collagenized stroma
- Positive for S-100 protein

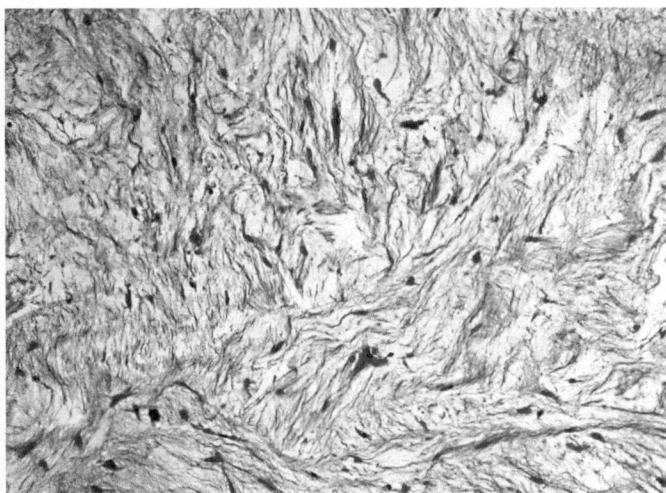

Figure 17-43. Myxoma. Paucicellular lesion shows bland spindle cells in abundant myxoid stroma.

AGGRESSIVE ANGIOMYXOMA

- Most common in the vulvar region in women of reproductive age but may be seen in the perineum of males; intramuscular location is unusual
- Prominent thick- and thin-walled vessels
- Matrix is often collagenized
- Usually positive for SMA and desmin

PEARLS

- *Myxomas are benign tumors with rare local recurrence; surgical excision is the preferred treatment and is usually curative*

SELECTED REFERENCES

Nielsen GP, O'Connell JX, Rosenberg AE: Intramuscular myxoma: a clinicopathologic study of 51 cases with emphasis on hypercellular and hypervascular variants. Am J Surg Pathol 22:1222-1227, 1998.

Okamoto S, Hisaoka M, Meis-Kindblom JM, et al: Juxta-articular myxoma and intramuscular myxoma are two distinct entities: activating Gs alpha mutation at Arg 201 codon does not occur in juxta-articular myxoma. Virchows Arch 440:12-15, 2002.

van Roggen JF, McMenamin ME, Fletcher CD: Cellular myxoma of soft tissue: a clinicopathological study of 38 cases confirming indolent clinical behaviour. Histopathology 39:287-297, 2001.

OSSIFYING FIBROMYXOID TUMOR (OFMT)

Clinical Features

- Occurs primarily in adults; slight male predominance
- Painless, well-defined mass in the upper and lower extremities; may also occur in the head and neck
- Typically affects the deep subcutis

Gross Pathology

- Well-circumscribed, lobulated, subcutaneous mass
- May be partially surrounded by a shell of bony tissue

Histopathology

- Variably cellular tumor with uniform, round to polygonal cells arranged in nests or cords
- Cells have uniform, bland, round to oval nuclei with eosinophilic to clear cytoplasm and ill-defined cytoplasmic borders (Figure 17-44)
- Abundant myxoid to hyaline matrix
- Metaplastic bone formation is common and is typically seen at the periphery
- Malignant features include high cellularity, high N:C ratio, brisk mitotic activity, increased intralesional bone, and absence of bony shell

Special Stains and Immunohistochemistry

- Vimentin and S-100 protein positive
- Variably positive for desmin, CD10, Leu-7, NSE, and GFAP

Other Techniques for Diagnosis

- 6p21 rearrangements are frequently found in OFMT; present in about half of both benign and malignant cases by *PHF1* interphase break apart FISH
- Most common translocation t(6;12) (p21;q24) resulting in *PHF1-EP400* fusion gene

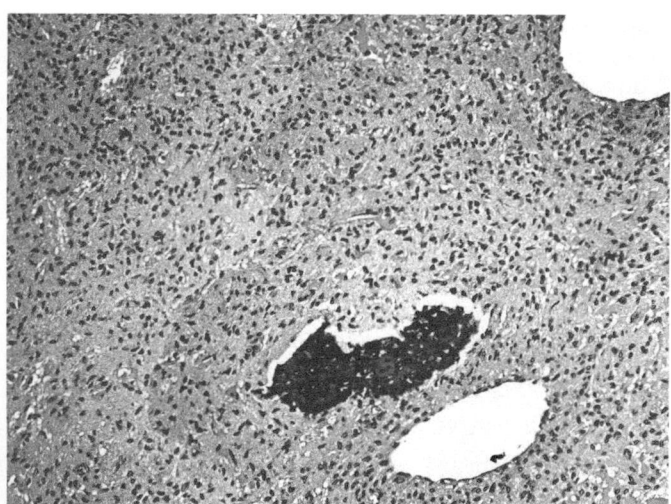

Figure 17-44. Ossifying fibromyxoid tumor. Bland ovoid cells are randomly arranged in a fibromyxoid stroma. Focal calcification is present.

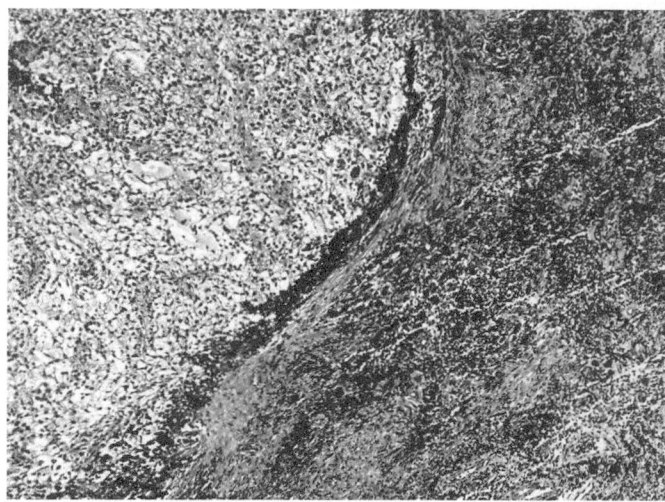

Figure 17-45. Angiomatoid fibrous histiocytoma. Nodule of bland spindle cells with myxoid change surrounded by a fibrous pseudocapsule with a dense lymphocytic infiltrate.

Differential Diagnosis

MYXOID CHONDROSARCOMA (EXTRASKELETAL)

- Anastomosing cords of round to oval, atypical chondrocytes
- Abundant myxoid matrix and intervening fibrous septa
- *EWSR1* translocation

PEARLS

- *Surgical excision is the preferred treatment for ossifying fibromyxoid tumor*
- *Local recurrence is seen in about 25% of patients; metastases are exceedingly rare*

SELECTED REFERENCES

Endo M, Kohashi K, Yamamoto H, et al: Ossifying fibromyxoid tumor presenting EP400-PHF1 fusion gene. Hum Pathol 44:2603-2608, 2013.

Enzinger FM, Weiss SW, Liang CY: Ossifying fibromyxoid tumor of soft parts: a clinicopathological analysis of 59 cases. Am J Surg Pathol 13:817-827, 1989.

Folpe AL, Weiss SW: Ossifying fibromyxoid tumor of soft parts: a clinicopathologic study of 70 cases with emphasis on atypical and malignant variants. Am J Surg Pathol 27:421-431, 2003.

Graham RP, Weiss SW, Sukov WR, et al: PHF1 Rearrangements in ossifying fibromyxoid tumors of soft parts: a fluorescence in situ hybridization study of 41 cases with emphasis on the malignant variant. Am J Surg Pathol 37:1751-1755, 2013.

ANGIOMATOID FIBROUS HISTIOCYTOMA

Clinical Features

- Typically seen in children and young adults but can occur at any age
- The extremities, head and neck, and trunk are common locations; often occur in locations of normal lymph nodes

Gross Pathology

- Well-circumscribed, lobulated, multicystic mass; usually about 5 cm in size
- Cystic spaces are often filled with hemorrhagic fluid

Histopathology

- Low-power appearance shows multinodular proliferation, often with central cystic spaces with a prominent lymphoid cuff
- Cells are spindle or ovoid and often surround pseudoangiomatoid spaces (Figure 17-45)
- Cells are usually cytologically bland, but nuclear atypia and mitotic activity may be seen
- A prominent fibrous pseudocapsule contains a prominent lymphoplasmacytic infiltrate

Special Stains and Immunohistochemistry

- Desmin and CD68 are usually positive
- EMA and CD99 may be positive

Other Techniques for Diagnosis

- Presence of t(2;22)(q34;q12), producing an *EWSR1-CREB1* fusion; t(12;22)(q13;q12), producing an *EWSR1-ATF1* fusion, or t(12;16)(q13;p11), producing an *FUS-ATF1* fusion, can be demonstrated in most cases by cytogenetic or molecular techniques

Differential Diagnosis

BENIGN FIBROUS HISTIOCYTOMA

- Lacks the inflammatory fibrous pseudocapsule and pseudoangiomatoid spaces
- Well-circumscribed nodular lesion with storiform architecture

PEARLS

- *Angiomatoid fibrous histiocytoma is a low-grade lesion that occasionally recurs; metastases are exceedingly rare*
- *Surgical excision is the standard therapy*

SELECTED REFERENCES

Fanburg-Smith JC, Miettinen M: Angiomatoid "malignant" fibrous histiocytoma: a clinicopathologic study of 158 cases and further exploration of the myoid phenotype. Hum Pathol 30:1336-1343, 1999.

Hasegawa T, Seki K, Ono K, Hirohashi S: Angiomatoid (malignant) fibrous histiocytoma: a peculiar low-grade tumor showing immunophenotypic heterogeneity and ultrastructural variations. Pathol Int 50:731-738, 2000.

Rossi S, Szuhai K, Ijszenga M, et al: EWSR1-CREB1 and EWSR1-ATF1 fusion genes in angiomatoid fibrous histiocytoma. Clin Cancer Res 13:7322-7328, 2007.

Thway K: Angiomatoid fibrous histiocytoma: a review with recent genetic findings. Arch Pathol Lab Med 132:273-277, 2008.

SYNOVIAL SARCOMA

Clinical Features

- Typically found in adolescents or young adults but can occur at any age
- Presents as a deep-seated, often painful mass; has often been present for years
- Usually arises near the joint in close relation to tendons and bursa but not in the joint space itself; lower extremities are commonly affected
- Synovial sarcoma has been described in virtually every location, including viscera

Gross Pathology

- Typically a well-circumscribed mass with a gray-white or variegated cut surface; rapidly growing tumors tend to be more infiltrative
- Variably sized cyst formation may be seen
- Attachment to surrounding tendons or walls of joint capsules may be present

Histopathology

BIPHASIC SYNOVIAL SARCOMA

- Characterized by fascicles of spindle cells admixed with groups of epithelial cells that form clefts, cysts, cords, nests, tubules, or papillae (Figure 17-46)
- Epithelial cells are cuboidal to columnar with ovoid nuclei and a moderate amount of cytoplasm
- Eosinophilic or mucinous secretions are common in overtly epithelial cell groups; squamous metaplasia can occur
- Spindle cell component shows herringbone-like or hemangiopericytoma-like growth

- Calcification is seen in about 25% of cases; myxoid, chondroid, or osseous foci are less common
- Mast cells are common

MONOPHASIC SYNOVIAL SARCOMA

- Spindle cell form predominates over purely epithelial synovial sarcoma
- Fascicles of spindle cells, often with herringbone or hemangiopericytoid growth pattern; epithelial component is inconspicuous (Figure 17-47)
- At low power, a biphasic pattern of alternating loose and dense areas is seen
- Calcification, myxoid change, hyalinization, and mast cell infiltration may be present
- Mitotic figures can be identified but usually are not numerous

POORLY DIFFERENTIATED SYNOVIAL SARCOMA

- Small cell tumor composed of hyperchromatic round to spindled cells with high nuclear-to-cytoplasmic ratios; hemangiopericytoma-like growth is common
- Mitotic figures are readily identified and necrosis is common
- Rhabdoid differentiation may be present

Special Stains and Immunohistochemistry

- Cytokeratin, EMA, E-cadherin: epithelial component is positive, and mesenchymal-like component often shows focal positivity for at least one of these markers
- CD99: membranous staining in either or both components
- CD56, CD57, and bcl-2: cytoplasmic staining in either or both components
- SYT: nuclear staining
- S-100 protein: focal nuclear staining in 33% of cases
- CD34, Fli-1, and CD117 negative

Other Techniques for Diagnosis

- Presence of t(X;18)(p11;q11) can be demonstrated in greater than 90% of synovial sarcomas by cytogenetic or molecular techniques; fusion genes are *SYT-SSX1/SSX2* or *SSX4*

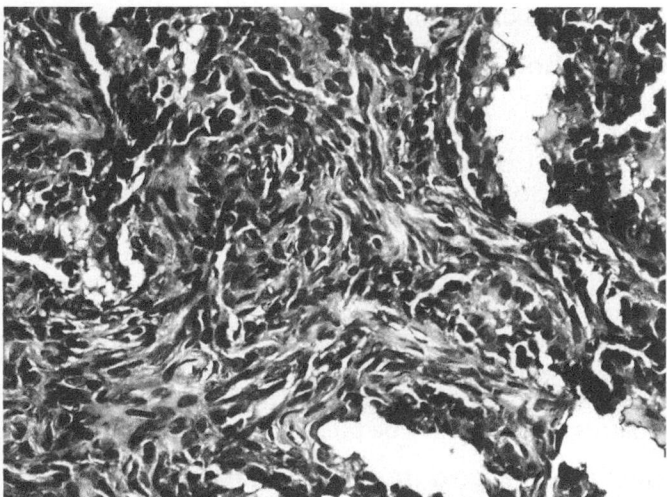

Figure 17-46. Biphasic synovial sarcoma. Glandular structures are seen interspersed with spindle cells.

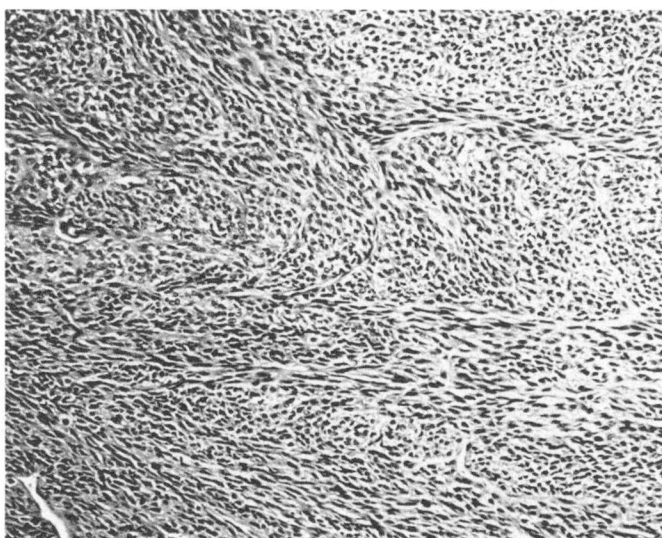

Figure 17-47. Monophasic synovial sarcoma. Fascicles of uniform spindle cells exhibit a herringbone growth pattern.

Differential Diagnosis

HEMANGIOPERICYTOMA

- Characterized by numerous thin-walled and branching staghorn vessels of variable caliber lined by a single layer of flattened endothelium; this vascular pattern is present throughout the tumor
- Reticulin network surrounding individual tumor cells
- Lacks epithelial differentiation by immunohistochemistry and is positive for CD34 in 70% to 80% of cases
- Absence of t(X:18)
- Rare lesion; diagnosis is one of ultimate exclusion

EWS AND PNET

- May be difficult to distinguish from poorly differentiated synovial sarcoma, especially in a small biopsy
- Monomorphic round cell tumor with high nuclear-to-cytoplasmic ratios and fine chromatin; cellular rosettes may be present
- Spindle cell change may occur but is usually focal
- Like synovial sarcoma, PNET is positive for CD99 and may express epithelial antigens, especially low-molecular-weight keratins
- Usually negative for CD56 and bcl-2; positive for Fli-1
- Presence of t(11;22)(q24;q12) can be demonstrated by cytogenetic or molecular techniques and is diagnostic

FIBROSARCOMA

- Most often affects children younger than 1 year; occasionally seen in adults
- Typically found in the extremities
- Variably cellular, infiltrative tumor composed of fusiform cells with hyperchromatic nuclei and eosinophilic or amphophilic cytoplasm, arranged in a herringbone pattern
- Variable mitotic rate; atypical mitotic figures may be seen
- Lacks a biphasic growth pattern
- Negative for epithelial antigens, CD99, and t(X;18)

MPNST

- Characterized by fascicles of elongated cells with serpiginous nuclei; nuclear palisading or cellular tactoids may be present
- Typically shows at least some nuclear pleomorphism and high mitotic activity
- Often associated with a major nerve or neurofibromatosis
- Immunophenotype may overlap with that of synovial sarcoma; both may show focal S-100 protein positivity; MPNST may show focal epithelial differentiation but lacks CD99 and SYT

SOLITARY FIBROUS TUMOR

- Frequently pleural but has been reported in soft tissue sites as well
- Well-circumscribed, often exophytic mass with gray-white firm cut surface
- Short fascicles or "patternless pattern" of spindle cells in variably collagenized stroma, often with hemangiopericytoma-like vasculature
- Positive for CD34, bcl-2, and CD99 in 85% to 90% of cases; lacks epithelial immunoreactivity

SELECTED REFERENCES

Ferrari A, Gronchi A, Casanova M, et al: Synovial sarcoma: a retrospective analysis of 271 patients of all ages treated at a single institution. Cancer 101:627-634, 2004.

Hartel PH, Fanburg-Smith JC, Frazier AA, et al: Primary pulmonary and mediastinal synovial sarcoma: a clinicopathologic study of 60 cases and comparison with five prior series. Mod Pathol 20:760-769, 2007.

He R, Patel RM, Alkan S, et al: Immunostaining for SYT protein discriminates synovial sarcoma from other soft tissue tumors: analysis of 146 cases. Mod Pathol 20:522-528, 2007.

Kanemitsu S, Hisaoka M, Shimajiri S, et al: Molecular detection of SS18-SSX fusion gene transcripts by cRNA in situ hybridization in synovial sarcoma using formalin-fixed, paraffin-embedded tumor tissue specimens. Diagn Mol Pathol 16:9-17, 2007.

EPITHELIOID SARCOMA

Clinical Features

- Typically seen in adolescents and young adults (usually in second and third decades); males affected more than females
- Presents as a slowly growing, painless nodule or plaque, usually occurring on the flexor surfaces of the extremities; epithelioid sarcoma is the most common sarcoma of distal extremities
- Central, deeply seated lesions in pelvis and genital tract have been termed *proximal epithelioid sarcomas*

Gross Pathology

- Poorly defined multinodular mass with infiltrating margins, ranging in size from 0.5 to 5 cm
- Gray-white cut surface; focal areas of necrosis and hemorrhage are common
- Overlying skin may be ulcerated

Histopathology

- Multinodular proliferation of epithelioid and spindle cells commonly with central necrosis
- Epithelioid cells have round vesicular nuclei, prominent nucleoli, and ample eosinophilic cytoplasm; proximal epithelioid sarcoma may exhibit a rhabdoid phenotype (Figure 17-48)
- Spindle cells have similar cytologic features in a collagenized stroma
- Central zones of degeneration and necrosis resemble infectious or palisading granuloma
- Extensive hyalinization and scattered chronic inflammatory infiltrate may be present

Special Stains and Immunohistochemistry

- Cytokeratin or EMA positive in more than 90% of cases
- Vimentin positive

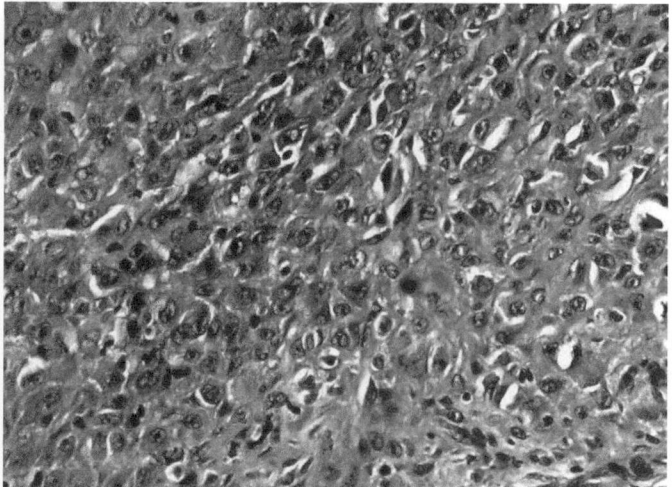

Figure 17-48. Epithelioid sarcoma. Cytologic features of epithelioid sarcoma include round, eccentric vesicular nuclei with prominent nucleoli and eosinophilic cytoplasm.

- CD34 positive in about 50% of cases
- S-100 protein may be focally positive
- INI1/SMARCB1: loss of immunoreactivity in proximal type of epithelioid sarcoma

Other Techniques for Diagnosis

- Electron microscopy: tumor cells show prominent masses of filaments, cell processes, and intercellular junctions
- Although loss of INI1 protein expression is common, molecular alterations of the *SMARCB1* gene appear rare

Differential Diagnosis

GRANULOMA ANNULARE
- Palisading histiocytes around central zones of necrobiotic collagen and stromal mucin
- May be dermal or subcutaneous
- Cells are negative for epithelial markers (cytokeratin and EMA) and positive for CD68 or factor XIIIa

SYNOVIAL SARCOMA
- Deeper and usually more proximal than epithelioid sarcoma
- Characterized by fascicles of spindle cells admixed with obvious nests of epithelial cells (biphasic pattern), but purely epithelioid synovial sarcoma may resemble epithelioid sarcoma
- Lacks nodular growth with central necrosis; cells usually have less abundant cytoplasm than those of epithelioid sarcoma
- Shows vimentin and epithelial marker immunoreactivity; negative for CD34
- Presence of t(X;18)(p11;q11) is diagnostic of synovial sarcoma as demonstrated by cytogenetic or molecular techniques

EPITHELIOID ANGIOSARCOMA
- Most often affects the scalp of elderly patients but can occur at other sites, especially in the setting of lymphedema

- Hemorrhagic, multinodular, and infiltrative tumor with solid growth or with rudimentary vascular channels
- Tumor cells are plump and hyperchromatic with distinct nucleoli and eosinophilic cytoplasm
- Immunoreactive for CD34, CD31, thrombomodulin, and Fli-1; may "aberrantly" express keratin but not EMA

EPITHELIOID MALIGNANT PERIPHERAL NERVE SHEATH TUMOR
- Usually a deep tumor associated with a major nerve but may be cutaneous; superficial lesions are usually well circumscribed and not multinodular
- Tumor cells are round to polygonal with large vesicular nuclei and prominent central or eccentric nucleoli
- Positive for S-100 protein, CD56, CD57, and nestin and may show focal positivity for epithelial markers; negative for CD34

RHABDOID TUMOR
- Typically seen in the deep soft tissues or kidney in children younger than 1 year; skin is a rare site
- CD34 tends to be negative in rhabdoid tumor
- Both may show loss of INI1 protein expression, but rhabdoid tumor also shows biallelic molecular alterations of the *SMARCB1* gene

MALIGNANT MELANOMA
- Frequently has an in situ component at the dermoepidermal junction
- Positive for S-100 protein, HMB-45, melan-A, tyrosinase, and PNL2; negative for epithelial markers and CD34

PEARLS

- *Epithelioid sarcoma is an aggressive neoplasm with a propensity for multiple recurrences before metastasizing*
- *Most common metastatic site is the lung, but it may involve regional lymph nodes as well*
- *Overall prognosis is poor; survival is related to tumor size, depth, mitotic rate, and necrosis and presence of vascular invasion*

SELECTED REFERENCES

Casanova M, Ferrari A, Collini P, et al: Epithelioid sarcoma in children and adolescents: a report from the Italian Soft Tissue Sarcoma Committee. Cancer 106:708-717, 2006.

Chase DR, Enzinger FM: Epithelioid sarcoma: diagnosis, prognostic indicators, and treatment. Am J Surg Pathol 9:241-263, 1985.

Chbani L, Guillou L, Terrier P, et al: Epithelioid sarcoma: a clinicopathologic and immunohistochemical analysis of 106 cases from the French sarcoma group. Am J Surg Pathol 131:222-227, 2009.

Guillou L, Wadden C, Coindre JM, et al: "Proximal-type" epithelioid sarcoma, a distinctive aggressive neoplasm showing rhabdoid features: clinicopathologic, immunohistochemical, and ultrastructural study of a series. Am J Surg Pathol 21:130-146, 1997.

Hornick JL, Dal Cin P, Fletcher CD: Loss of INI1 expression is characteristic of both conventional and proximal-type epithelioid sarcoma. Am J Surg Pathol 33:542-550, 2009.

Kohashi K, Izumi T, Oda Y, et al: Infrequent SMARCB1/INI1 gene alteration in epithelioid sarcoma: a useful tool in distinguishing epithelioid sarcoma from malignant rhabdoid tumor. Hum Pathol 40:349-355, 2009.

Miettinen M, Fanburg-Smith JC, Virolainen M, et al: Epithelioid sarcoma: an immunohistochemical analysis of 112 classical and variant cases and a discussion of the differential diagnosis. Hum Pathol 30:934-942, 1999.

EXTRASKELETAL EWING SARCOMA AND PERIPHERAL NEUROECTODERMAL TUMOR

Clinical Features

- Primarily affects adolescents and young adults but has a wide age range; makes up 15% of pediatric sarcomas
- Often presents as a rapidly growing deep mass; occasionally painful
- Common sites include chest, paravertebral region, abdomen and pelvis, and extremities

Gross Pathology

- Typically a lobulated, soft, tan-gray tumor with focal hemorrhage and necrosis
- Usually measures 5 to 10 cm in maximum diameter

Histopathology

- Cellular tumor comprising monomorphic round cells with finely dispersed chromatin, small nucleoli, and scant clear or amphophilic cytoplasm (Figure 17-49)
- Growth is in sheets, nests, or islands, but EWS and PNET may have an alveolar pattern or show focal spindle cell change; cellular discohesion is common
- Tumor cells often contain intracytoplasmic glycogen with PAS staining
- Variable mitotic rate and apoptosis are often present
- Cellular rosettes may be seen

Special Stains and Immunohistochemistry

- CD99 strongly positive with a membrane pattern
- FLi-1 and ERG: nuclear positivity (ERG cross reacts with Fli-1)
- Neural markers, including NSE, synaptophysin, CD57, and PGP 9.5 variably positive
- Keratin: 20% of cases positive for low-molecular-weight keratins
- PAS: intracytoplasmic positivity with abrogation of staining after pretreatment with diastase

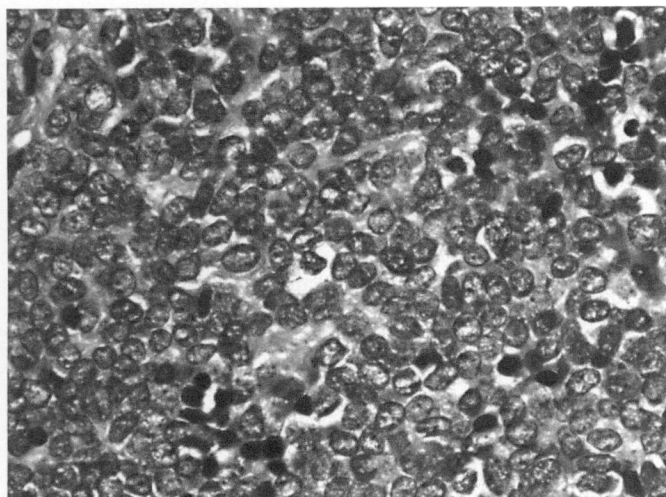

Figure 17-49. Ewing sarcoma. Sheets of overlapping uniform undifferentiated round cells represent only one pattern of this tumor.

Other Techniques for Diagnosis

- Electron microscopy: tumor cells have intracytoplasmic glycogen pools, primitive organelles, and macular junctions
- Presence of t(11;22)(q24;q12), producing an *EWS-FLI1* fusion (80% to 85%) or t(21;22)(q12;q12), producing an *EWS-ERG* fusion (5% to 10%) can be demonstrated by cytogenetic or molecular techniques; other variant translocations involving EWS or FUS have been reported

Differential Diagnosis

NEUROBLASTOMA

- Typically seen in young children arising from adrenal gland or sympathetic nerve trunk
- Characterized by the presence of cellular neuropil or ganglion cell differentiation
- Absence of intracellular glycogen
- Positive for CD56 and NB84; negative for keratin, CD99, and Fli-1
- Frequent chromosomal aberrations involve 17q, 1p, and 11q; *MYCN* amplification is present in 15% of cases but is not seen in EWS or PNET

ALVEOLAR RHABDOMYOSARCOMA

- May have solid or alveolar architecture; monomorphic round tumor cells adhere to fibrovascular septa
- Focal overt rhabdomyoblastic differentiation may be seen with abundant eccentric pink cytoplasm; tumor giant cells are common
- Immunoreactivity for desmin, myogenin, and MyoD1; may be positive for CD99 but with a cytoplasmic pattern
- Presence of t(2;13)(q35;q14) or t(1;13)(p36;q14) can be demonstrated by cytogenetic or molecular techniques in 75% of cases

LYMPHOMA

- Characterized by diffuse growth of atypical round cell with irregular nuclear membranes
- Most lymphomas show immunoreactivity for leukocyte common antigen (LCA; CD45), and lymphoblastic lymphoma expresses CD34, CD99, CD117, and TdT; either B-cell or T-cell antigens are also present
- Lymphoblastic lymphoma is frequently positive for CD99 and Fli-1, and additional markers must be used (e.g., TdT) to distinguish it from EWS and PNET

DESMOPLASTIC SMALL ROUND CELL TUMOR

- Most common in the abdomen of adolescent and young adult males
- Diffuse peritoneal spread
- Nests of small round cells with uniform, hyperchromatic nuclei, indistinct nucleoli, and scant cytoplasm, separated by a desmoplastic stroma
- Polyphenotypic immunoprofile with coexpression of vimentin, keratin, neural markers, and desmin, the latter with a dotlike pattern
- Presence of t(11;22)(p13;q12), producing an *EWS-WT1* fusion, can be demonstrated by cytogenetic or molecular techniques

Poorly Differentiated Synovial Sarcoma
- Difficult to distinguish from EWS and PNET, especially in a small biopsy
- Hyperchromatic tumor cells, often with a hemangiopericytoma-like growth pattern
- Positive for CD99, bcl-2, CD57, and EMA and keratin; negative for Fli-1
- Presence of t(X;18)(p11;q11) demonstrable by cytogenetic or molecular techniques

PEARLS

- *EWS and PNET are high-grade sarcomas, but current therapy has significantly improved the prognosis*
- *Common sites of distant metastasis include lung and bone*
- *Large tumor size and necrosis are factors that adversely affect the prognosis*

Selected References

Dehner LP: Primitive neuroectodermal tumor and Ewing's sarcoma. Am J Surg Pathol 17:1-13, 1993.

Folpe AL, Hill CE, Parham DM, et al: Immunohistochemical detection of FLI-1 protein expression: a study of 132 round cell tumors with emphasis on CD99-positive mimics of Ewing's sarcoma/primitive neuroectodermal tumor. Am J Surg Pathol 24:1657-1662, 2000.

Gamberi G, Cocchi S, Benini S, et al: Molecular diagnosis in Ewing family tumors: the Rizzoli experience—222 consecutive cases in four years. JMD 13:313-324, 2011.

Lewis TB, Coffin CM, Bernard PS: Differentiating Ewing's sarcoma from other round blue cell tumors using a RT-PCR translocation panel on formalin-fixed paraffin-embedded tissues. Mod Pathol 20:397-404, 2007.

Tomlins SA, Palanisamy N, Brenner JC, et al: Usefulness of a monoclonal ERG/FLI1 antibody for immunohistochemical discrimination of Ewing family tumors. Am J Surg Pathol 139:771-779, 2013.

DESMOPLASTIC SMALL ROUND CELL TUMOR

Clinical Features

- Primarily affects young adults
- More commonly occurs in males (4:1 ratio)
- Usually found in the abdomen with extensive peritoneal spread, but also has been reported in other locations
- Presents with abdominal pain, distention, and ascites

Gross Pathology

- Large lobulated tumors with a gray-white cut surface
- Myxoid and necrotic areas are typically seen

Histopathology

- Well-demarcated nests of small round cells with uniform, hyperchromatic nuclei, indistinct nucleoli, and scant cytoplasm, separated by desmoplastic stroma
- Nests vary in size, and cords or individual tumor cells also may infiltrate fibrous stroma (Figure 17-50)
- High mitotic rate and necrosis
- Occasional rhabdoid features or overt epithelial differentiation may be seen

Special Stains and Immunohistochemistry

- Cytokeratin and EMA positive in most cases
- NSE typically positive

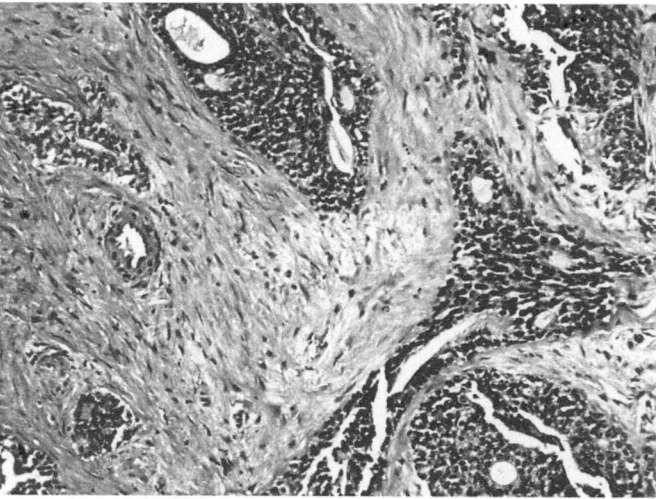

Figure 17-50. Desmoplastic small round cell tumor. Variably sized islands of hyperchromatic tumor cells separated by abundant desmoplastic stroma. This case shows overt epithelial differentiation.

- Vimentin positive
- Desmin positive (perinuclear dotlike pattern)
- WT-1 (C-terminus) positive

Other Techniques for Diagnosis

- Electron microscopy: tumor cells show minimal differentiation with scant organelles; perinuclear whorls of microfilaments are common, and dense core neurosecretory granules may be seen
- Presence of t(11;22)(p13;q12), producing an *EWS-WT1* fusion, can be demonstrated by cytogenetic or molecular techniques

Differential Diagnosis

Extraskeletal EWS and PNET
- Usually seen in chest wall, extremities, paravertebral region, or retroperitoneum
- Cellular tumor characterized by sheets or nests of uniform round cells with finely dispersed chromatin, small nucleoli, and scant cytoplasm
- Tumor cells may contain intracytoplasmic glycogen
- Rich, delicate vasculature surrounding groups of tumor cells
- Lacks desmoplastic stroma
- Positive for CD99 and Fli-1
- Presence of t(11;22)(q24;q12), producing an *EWS-FLI1* fusion or variants, can be demonstrated by cytogenetic or molecular techniques

Alveolar Rhabdomyosarcoma
- May have solid or alveolar architecture; monomorphic round tumor cells adhere to fibrovascular septa
- Focal overt rhabdomyoblastic differentiation with abundant plump eosinophilic cytoplasm; tumor giant cells are common
- Diffuse cytoplasmic staining for desmin and nuclear labeling for myogenin and MyoD1
- Presence of t(2;13)(q35;q14) or t(1;13)(p36;q14) can be demonstrated by cytogenetic or molecular techniques in 75% of cases

SMALL CELL CARCINOMA

- Large intra-abdominal tumor is an atypical presentation of carcinoma
- Positive for cytokeratin, EMA, NSE, chromogranin, CD56, or synaptophysin; negative for vimentin and desmin

PEARLS

- *The line of differentiation of DSRCT is uncertain*
- *DSRCT is an aggressive tumor and often unresectable at the time of presentation; most patients die within 5 years*
- *Variant chromosomal translocations have been described and are often associated with an atypical histology*

SELECTED REFERENCES

Chang F: Desmoplastic small round cell tumors: cytologic, histologic, and immunohistochemical features. Arch Pathol Lab Med 130:728-732, 2006.

Lae ME, Roche PC, Jin L, et al: Desmoplastic small round cell tumor: a clinicopathologic, immunohistochemical, and molecular study of 32 tumors. Am J Surg Pathol 26:823-835, 2002.

Sandberg AA, Bridge JA: Updates on the cytogenetics and molecular genetics of bone and soft tissue tumors: desmoplastic small round-cell tumors. Cancer Genet Cytogenet 138:1-10, 2002.

Zhang PJ, Goldblum JR, Pawel BR, et al: Immunophenotype of desmoplastic small round cell tumors as detected in cases with EWS-WT1 gene fusion product. Mod Pathol 16:229-235, 2003.

ALVEOLAR SOFT PART SARCOMA

Clinical Features

- Rare malignant soft tissue tumor presenting in late adolescence and young adulthood; rarely affects young children and elderly people
- Arises predominantly in the upper extremity and less often in the retroperitoneum, mesentery, and omentum; tumors in younger patients often involve the head and neck region
- Typically presents as a slow-growing, painless mass but may present with symptoms related to distant metastases usually involving lung and brain

Gross Pathology

- Poorly defined soft tissue mass
- Yellow-gray cut surface, often with focal areas of hemorrhage and necrosis

Histopathology

- Organoid or nested growth pattern with islands of cells separated by delicate sinusoidal spaces (Figure 17-51)
- Central cellular discohesion may impart an alveolar appearance
- Epithelioid cells with abundant eosinophilic, granular, or clear cytoplasm and regular, uniform nuclei, often with central nucleoli
- Intracytoplasmic crystals and intracytoplasmic glycogen often present; best seen with PAS stain
- Typically low mitotic rate
- Vascular invasion is typically present

Special Stains and Immunohistochemistry

- Desmin variably positive
- MyoD1 often positive in cytoplasm only

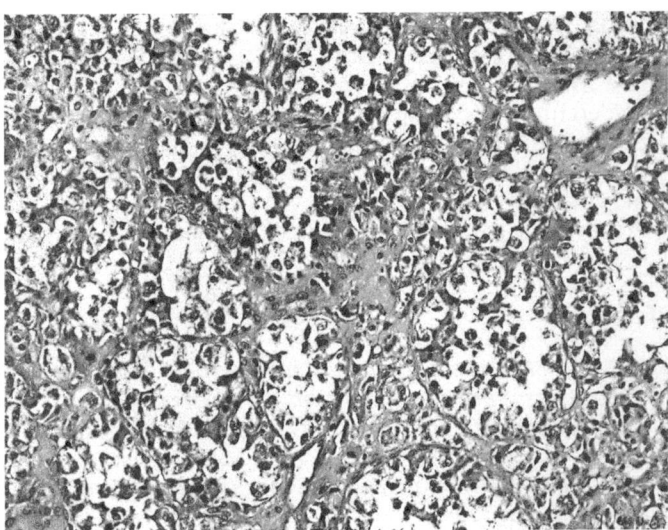

Figure 17-51. Alveolar soft part sarcoma. Organoid growth pattern of polygonal cells with cellular dyshesion.

- TFE3: positive nuclear staining
- PAS highlights intracytoplasmic glycogen and crystals

Other Techniques for Diagnosis

- Electron microscopy: may show characteristic membrane-bound or free rhomboid crystals
- Presence of t(X;17)(p11;q25), producing an *ASPL-TFE3* fusion, can be demonstrated by cytogenetic or molecular techniques

Differential Diagnosis

ALVEOLAR RHABDOMYOSARCOMA

- Organoid architecture is not as prominent
- Cells have higher nuclear-to-cytoplasmic C ratios and nuclear hyperchromasia; rhabdomyoblasts and giant cells may be seen
- Nuclear immunoreactivity toward myogenin and MyoD1
- Alveolar rhabdomyosarcoma shows t(2:13) or t(1:13) in 75% of cases

PARAGANGLIOMA

- Characterized by trabecular or organoid arrangement of round to polygonal cells with central nuclei and eosinophilic granular cytoplasm
- Uncommon in extremity, usually seen along sympathetic chain
- Positive for neuroendocrine markers (synaptophysin, chromogranin, and NSE)

GRANULAR CELL TUMOR

- Composed of sheets of large, polygonal cells with abundant coarse, eosinophilic, granular cytoplasm; lacks organoid pattern seen in alveolar soft part sarcoma
- Cells have small vesicular nuclei with prominent nucleoli
- Positive for S-100 protein

METASTATIC RENAL CELL CARCINOMA (CLEAR CELL)

- Tumor cells typically show more prominent cytoplasmic clearing
- Lacks PAS positive crystals
- Positive for epithelial membrane antigen (EMA), renal cell carcinoma (RCC), and CD10

- *Alveolar soft part sarcoma is a high-grade sarcoma with a poor prognosis, although it may have a prolonged course*
- *Distant metastases to lung and brain are present at diagnosis in up to one third of cases but may occur late in the course*
- *Large tumor size, older age, and metastases at diagnosis portend a worse prognosis*

Selected References

Cullinane C, Thorner PS, Greenberg ML, et al: Molecular genetic, cytogenetic, and immunohistochemical characterization of alveolar soft-part sarcoma: implications for cell of origin. Cancer 70:2444-2450, 1992.

Hodge JC, Pearce KE, Wang X, et al: Molecular cytogenetic analysis for TFE3 rearrangement in Xp11.2 renal cell carcinoma and alveolar soft part sarcoma: validation and clinical experience with 75 cases. Mod Pathol 27:113-127, 2014.

Lieberman PH, Brennan MF, Kimmel M, et al: Alveolar soft-part sarcoma: a clinico-pathologic study of half a century. Cancer 63:1-13, 1989.

Tsuji K, Ishikawa Y, Imamura T: Technique for differentiating alveolar soft part sarcoma from other tumors in paraffin-embedded tissue: comparison of immunohistochemistry for TFE3 and CD147 and of reverse transcription polymerase chain reaction for ASPSCR1-TFE3 fusion transcript. Hum Pathol 43:356-363, 2012.

Weiss SW: Alveolar soft part sarcoma: are we at the end or just the beginning of our quest? Am J Pathol 160:1197-1199, 2002.

CLEAR CELL SARCOMA (CCS)

Clinical Features

- Also referred to as *malignant melanoma of soft parts*
- Typically occurs in adults aged 20 to 40 years
- Extremities are most common location (lower affected more than upper), often distal; frequently associated with tendons or aponeuroses
- Usually presents as a slowly enlarging mass; may be painful

Gross Pathology

- Lobulated mass with a gray-white cut surface
- Focal areas of hemorrhage, necrosis, and dark-brown pigmentation may be seen

Histopathology

- Nests and fascicles of round or fusiform cells with vesicular nuclei showing a single, prominent, basophilic nucleolus and clear to eosinophilic cytoplasm (Figure 17-52)
- Thin fibrous septa typically surround nests, but background may be hyalinized
- Multinucleated giant cells are common; rhabdoid cells may be present
- Variable mitotic rate, typically fewer than two mitotic figures/10 hpf
- Intracellular melanin pigment occasionally seen

Special Stains and Immunohistochemistry

- S-100 protein, HMB-45 positive
- HMB-45, melan-A, tyrosinase, and Mart-1 variably positive

Other Techniques for Diagnosis

- Electron microscopy: schwannian cell features including interdigitating cell processes and melanosomes

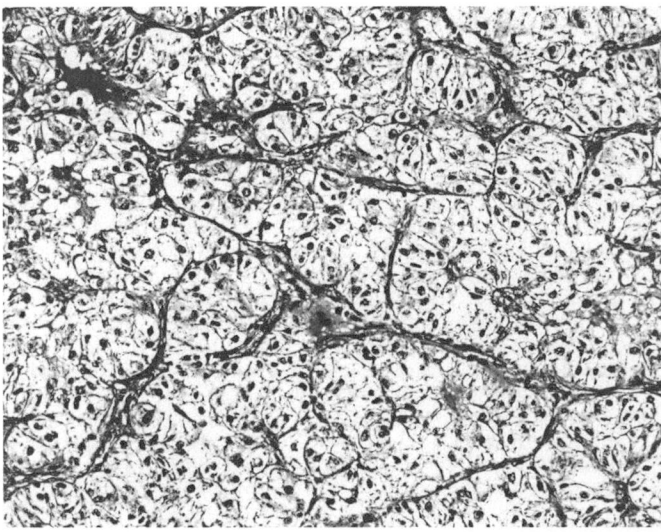

Figure 17-52. Clear cell sarcoma. Nests of polygonal cells with abundant clear cytoplasm are separated by a delicate fibrovascular network.

- Presence of t(12;22)(q13;q12), producing an *EWS-ATF1* fusion, can be demonstrated by cytogenetic or molecular techniques

Differential Diagnosis

Malignant Melanoma

- Typically located within the dermis; often associated with junctional activity and pagetoid spread, the latter being rare in CCS
- More heterogenous in appearance than CCS, although multinucleated giant cells are rare
- *BRAF* mutations common; *EWS* translocation absent

Fibrosarcoma

- Most often affects children younger than 1 year; occasionally seen in adults
- Typically found in the extremities
- Highly cellular, infiltrative tumor composed of fibroblasts with hyperchromatic nuclei and scant cytoplasm arranged in a distinctive herringbone pattern
- High mitotic rate; atypical mitotic figures may be seen

Epithelioid Malignant Peripheral Nerve Sheath Tumor

- Characterized by cords and nests of polygonal cells with round nuclei, prominent nucleoli, and clear to eosinophilic cytoplasm
- Positive for S100 protein but not other melanocytic markers
- Absent *EWS* translocation

- *Clear cell sarcoma is a highly aggressive tumor with a poor prognosis*
- *Local recurrence and metastases are common; metastases often occur within 3 years*
- *Common sites of metastasis include lungs, lymph nodes, and bone*
- *Adverse prognostic factors include large tumor size, vascular invasion, and tumor necrosis*

SELECTED REFERENCES

Enzinger FM: Clear-cell sarcoma of tendons and aponeuroses: an analysis of 21 cases. Cancer 18:1163-1174, 1965.

Ferrari A, Casanova M, Bisogno G, et al: Clear cell sarcoma of tendons and aponeuroses in pediatric patients: a report from the Italian and German Soft Tissue Sarcoma Cooperative Group. Cancer 94:3269-3276, 2002.

Hantschke M, Mentzel T, Rutten A, et al: Cutaneous clear cell sarcoma: a clinicopathologic, immunohistochemical, and molecular analysis of 12 cases emphasizing its distinction from dermal melanoma. Am J Surg Pathol 34:216-222, 2010.

Hisaoka M, Ishida T, Kuo TT, et al: Clear cell sarcoma of soft tissue: a clinicopathologic, immunohistochemical, and molecular analysis of 33 cases. Am J Surg Pathol 32:452-460, 2008.

Kawai A, Hosono A, Nakayama R, et al: Clear cell sarcoma of tendons and aponeuroses: a study of 75 patients. Cancer 109:109-116, 2007.

Wang WL, Mayordomo E, Zhang W, et al: Detection and characterization of EWSR1/ATF1 and EWSR1/CREB1 chimeric transcripts in clear cell sarcoma (melanoma of soft parts). Mod Pathol 22:1201-1209, 2009.

PERIVASCULAR EPITHELIOID CELL TUMOR

Clinical Features

- Tumor with putative perivascular cell differentiation composed of clear epithelioid cells with coexpression of smooth muscle and melanocytic markers ("myomelanocytes")
- Most common locations are uterus and falciform ligament; other soft tissue and visceral sites are rare; marked female predominance
- The perivascular epithelioid cell tumor (PEComa) family includes angiomyolipoma, lymphangioleiomyoma and lymphangioleiomyomatosis, and clear cell "sugar" tumor of lung, all of which may be associated with tuberous sclerosis
  - PEComa of internal female genitalia
    - Tumor of middle-aged women
    - May present with pelvic pain or vaginal bleeding
  - Clear cell myomelanocytic tumor of the falciform ligament or ligamentum teres
    - Occurs in young women during first or second decade
    - Presents as painful abdominal mass

Gross Pathology

- Firm, gray-white mass; may show cystic change, hemorrhage, or necrosis
- Maximum size ranges from 1 to 20 cm; intra-abdominal and retroperitoneal tumors tend to be largest

Histopathology

- Highly vascular tumor with thin-walled vessels, the walls of which blend with ovoid or fusiform neoplastic cells
- Epithelioid tumor cells often contain clear cytoplasm; spindle cells have more granular eosinophilic cytoplasm (Figure 17-53)
- Falciform ligament tumors tend to have an exclusively spindle cell morphology
- Small centrally placed nuclei and small nucleoli are typical, although pleomorphism and high nuclear grade may be seen
- Mitotic activity tends to be low; numerous mitotic figures or atypical forms may indicate more aggressive behavior

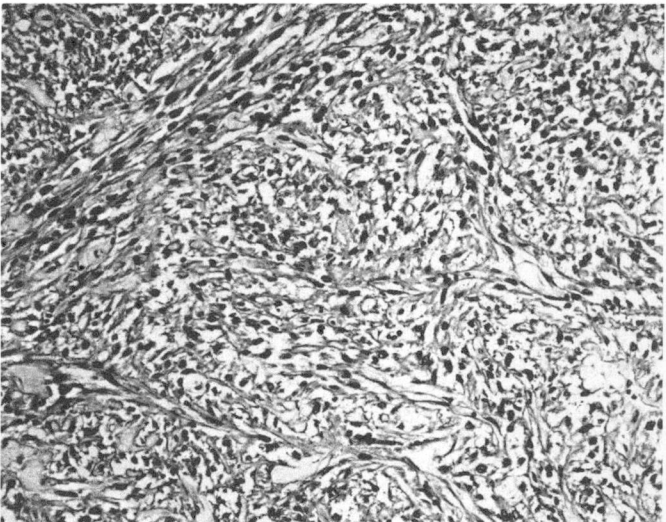

Figure 17-53. Perivascular epithelioid cell tumor (PEComa). Haphazard arrangement of spindle and epithelioid cells has cleared out cytoplasm.

Special Stains and Immunohistochemistry

- HMB-45 positive in more than 95% of cases
- Melan-A, MiTF, S-100 protein, tyrosinase, and PNL2 variably positive
- SMA positive
- Desmin variably positive
- Cytokeratin, CD117, and CD34 typically negative

Other Techniques for Diagnosis

- Electron microscopy: smooth muscle and melanocytic differentiation with premelanosomes
- Cytogenetics: numeric and structural abnormalities including loss of 1p, 16p, 17p, 18p, and 19p and gains of 2q, 3q, 5, 12q, and X
- *TFE3* translocations associated with the clear cell variant; may represent a distinct entity

Differential Diagnosis

CLEAR CELL SARCOMA (MALIGNANT MELANOMA OF SOFT PARTS)

- Most commonly seen in the extremities; rare in abdomen or visceral organs
- Tends to be strongly positive for S-100 protein but lacks evidence of smooth muscle differentiation
- Presence of t(12;22)(q13:q12), producing an *EWS-ATF1* fusion, can be demonstrated in most cases

GASTROINTESTINAL STROMAL TUMOR

- Positive for CD117 and CD34 and lacks melanocytic differentiation

LEIOMYOMA AND LEIOMYOSARCOMA

- Epithelioid and clear cells usually make up only part of the tumor
- Lacks melanocytic differentiation

CLEAR CELL CARCINOMAS

- Positive for keratin; lack melanocytic and smooth muscle differentiation

PEARLS

- *PEComas are rare tumors, and criteria for malignancy are not well established; about 10% to 20% behave in a malignant fashion*
- *Large size, infiltrative borders, high nuclear grade, greater than 1 mitotic figure/50 hpf, necrosis, and vascular invasion may be indicative of aggressive behavior*
- *Falciform ligament tumors are usually indolent*
- *Common sites of metastases include liver, lung, and bone*

SELECTED REFERENCES

Folpe AL, Kwiatkowski DJ: Perivascular epithelioid cell neoplasms: pathology and pathogenesis. Hum Pathol 41:1-15, 2010.

Folpe AL, Mentzel T, Lehr HA, et al: Perivascular epithelioid cell neoplasms of soft tissue and gynecologic origin: a clinicopathologic study of 26 cases and review of the literature. Am J Surg Pathol 29:1558-1575, 2005.

Malinowska I, Kwiatkowski DJ, Weiss S, et al: Perivascular epithelioid cell tumors (PEComas) harboring TFE3 gene rearrangements lack the TSC2 alterations characteristic of conventional PEComas: further evidence for a biological distinction. Am J Surg Pathol 36:783-784, 2012.

Pan CC, Jong YJ, Chai CY, et al: Comparative genomic hybridization study of perivascular epithelioid cell tumor: molecular genetic evidence of perivascular epithelioid cell tumor as a distinctive neoplasm. Hum Pathol 37:606-612, 2006.

MALIGNANT FIBROUS HISTIOCYTOMA/ HIGH-GRADE PLEOMORPHIC SARCOMA

Clinical Features

- *Malignant fibrous histiocytoma* (MFH) often used synonymously with *high-grade pleomorphic sarcoma*
- Most common malignant soft tissue tumor in adults, usually occurring in the sixth and seventh decades
- Common sites include proximal extremities and retroperitoneum; inflammatory MFH usually found in the retroperitoneum
- Presents as an enlarging, painless mass

Gross Pathology

- Solitary, multilobulated, fleshy, tan-white to gray mass; often large
- Most are located in the deep soft tissue, usually within skeletal muscle
- Areas of hemorrhage and necrosis are common

Histopathology

- Cellular tumor characterized by large pleomorphic cells with large, hyperchromatic nuclei and prominent nucleoli
- May show a storiform architecture
- Abundant mitotic activity; often, atypical mitoses are present
- Areas of hyalinization and necrosis may be seen; xanthoma cells are also common
- Various subtypes are described
  - Myxoid MFH
    - Greater than 50% of tumor composed of myxoid areas
    - Combination of myxoid areas and conventional MFH
    - Prominent vascularity
    - Numerous xanthoma cells may be present
  - Inflammatory MFH
    - Presence of an intense, acute, and chronic inflammatory infiltrate
  - Pleomorphic MFH
    - Displays bizarre giant cells
    - Numerous mitotic figures, including atypical mitoses
  - Giant cell MFH
    - Presence of osteoclast-like giant cells admixed with conventional MFH areas
    - Must differentiate from giant cell tumor of bone with extraosseous extension; giant cell component is similar; however, background cells appear malignant in giant cell MFH

Special Stains and Immunohistochemistry

- Vimentin positive
- CD68 often positive

Other Techniques for Diagnosis

- Electron microscopy reveals histiocyte-like cells with prominent lysosomes, Golgi, and surface ruffles
- Cytogenetic studies: MFH may be associated with deletion of chromosome 1

Differential Diagnosis

MYXOID LIPOSARCOMA

- Composed of vacuolated lipoblasts in a myxoid matrix
- Delicate plexiform capillary pattern is common
- Typically immunoreactivity for S-100 protein

PLEOMORPHIC LIPOSARCOMA

- Characterized by bizarre giant lipoblasts
- May be immunoreactive for S-100 protein

PLEOMORPHIC RHABDOMYOSARCOMA

- Large, pleomorphic rhabdomyoblasts, which may show cytoplasmic cross-striations
- Rhabdomyoblasts are immunoreactive for desmin, myogenin, and MyoD1

LEIOMYOSARCOMA

- Prominent fascicular growth pattern
- Immunoreactive for SMA and desmin

PEARLS

- *MFH is an aggressive tumor with a tendency to recur (myxoid and inflammatory types have lower rates of metastatic spread)*
- *Distant metastases occur most commonly in the lung, followed by the bone and liver*
- *Depth and location are important prognostic factors*
- *Surgical resection with wide margins is the treatment of choice*
- *MFH may be associated with previous radiation exposure*

SELECTED REFERENCES

Coindre JM, Mariani O, Chibon F, et al: Most malignant fibrous histiocytomas developed in the retroperitoneum are dedifferentiated liposarcomas: a review of 25 cases initially diagnosed as malignant fibrous histiocytoma. Mod Pathol 16:256-262, 2003.

Daw NC, Billups CA, Pappo AS, et al: Malignant fibrous histiocytoma and other fibrohistiocytic tumors in pediatric patients: the St. Jude Children's Research Hospital experience. Cancer 97:2839-2847, 2003.

Nakayama R, Nemoto T, Takahashi H, et al: Gene expression analysis of soft tissue sarcomas: characterization and reclassification of malignant fibrous histiocytoma. Mod Pathol 20:749-759, 2007.

Fletcher CD: The evolving classification of soft tissue tumours: an update based on the new WHO classification. Histopathology 48:3-12, 2006.

Chapter 18
Heart, Pericardium, and Blood Vessels

CARMELA D. TAN • E RENE RODRIGUEZ

CHAPTER OUTLINE

HEART

CARDIOMYOPATHY

Clinical Features

HYPERTROPHIC CARDIOMYOPATHY

- Myocardial disease characterized by left ventricular hypertrophy in the absence of systemic hypertension, aortic valve stenosis, or overt infiltrative diseases
- Associated with normal systolic function and diastolic dysfunction; systolic dynamic obstruction of the left ventricular outflow tract occurs in 25%
- Estimated prevalence of unexplained left ventricular hypertrophy on echocardiography compatible with a diagnosis of hypertrophic cardiomyopathy is 1 in 500
- Clinical presentation varies from asymptomatic to congestive heart failure, syncope, dyspnea, chest pain, and sudden death
- Associated with sudden death in athletes during exercise

DILATED CARDIOMYOPATHY

- Most common cause of congestive heart failure in young patients and one of the leading indications for heart transplantation
- Patient presentation related to systolic dysfunction and progressive cardiac chamber enlargement with secondary mitral or tricuspid regurgitation

- Usually idiopathic, but can be caused by toxins, drugs, and metabolic derangements; can be associated with myocarditis, alcohol abuse, pregnancy, familial incidence, nutritional deficiencies, neuromuscular disorders, and endocrine abnormalities
- Idiopathic dilated cardiomyopathy is a diagnosis of exclusion; heart failure is out of proportion to the presence of any concomitant coronary artery disease, systemic hypertension, or valvular heart disease

RESTRICTIVE CARDIOMYOPATHY

- Patients present with symptoms associated with diastolic dysfunction, reduced diastolic volume, and normal systolic function
- Caused by endomyocardial scarring (idiopathic restrictive cardiomyopathy, endomyocardial fibrosis, Löffler syndrome, and endocardial fibroelastosis), storage disease (hemochromatosis, glycogen storage disease, Fabry disease), or myocardial infiltrate (amyloidosis, sarcoidosis, and radiation fibrosis)
- Idiopathic restrictive cardiomyopathy
  - Rare entity with autosomal dominant transmission and associated with skeletal myopathy
- Endomyocardial fibrosis
  - Recognized as a tropical disease, occurring most often in sub-Saharan Africa, affecting children and young adults

- Löffler syndrome (Löffler endomyocarditis and endocarditis parietalis fibroplastica)
  - Occurs in older patients and in men (more often than women) who live in the temperate zone
  - Often associated with reactive or neoplastic eosinophilia
- Endocardial fibroelastosis
  - Classified as primary or secondary; secondary form is much more common
  - Primary form may be related to intrauterine myocardial injury with left ventricular dilation
  - Secondary form is most often associated with congenital heart disease involving the left ventricle such as aortic stenosis, hypoplastic left heart syndrome, and coarctation of the aorta
- Hemochromatosis
  - Primary hemochromatosis is an autosomal recessive disorder in which excessive iron absorption leads to iron overload
  - Secondary hemochromatosis is associated with ineffective erythropoiesis, chronic liver disease, or multiple blood transfusions

ARRHYTHMOGENIC RIGHT VENTRICULAR DYSPLASIA/ CARDIOMYOPATHY

- Inherited heart muscle disease that may present with arrhythmias, heart failure, or sudden death
- Arrhythmias are usually of right ventricular origin associated with global or regional dysfunction of the right ventricle
- Increasingly recognized as an important cause of sudden cardiac death
- Clinical diagnosis is based on diagnostic criteria originally proposed in 1994 by the European Society of Cardiology and Scientific Council on Cardiomyopathies of the International Society and Federation of Cardiology and revised in 2010

Gross Pathology

HYPERTROPHIC CARDIOMYOPATHY

- Left ventricular hypertrophy, which may be symmetrical or asymmetrical
- Asymmetrical forms include thickening of subaortic ventricular septum (which is at least 1.5 times that of the left ventricular free wall), midventricular segment, or apical region
- Systolic anterior motion of the anterior mitral leaflet leads to a contact lesion in the septum seen as an area of endocardial fibroelastosis
- Mechanical trauma to the anterior mitral leaflet and chordae result in thickening and fibrosis
- Foci of small scars often observed in the septum do not correspond to areas supplied by the major epicardial coronary arteries

DILATED CARDIOMYOPATHY

- Increased cardiac weight with four-chamber dilation
- Normal or decreased left ventricular wall thickness due to chamber dilation
- Mural thrombi may be present
- Endocardial thickening is focal and may be related to organized thrombus or jet lesions from valvular regurgitation

- Valves are normal or may exhibit secondary changes associated with insufficiency such as dilated annulus or thickening of free edges
- Coronary arteries are normal or may exhibit mild atherosclerotic change within limits expected for the patient's age

RESTRICTIVE CARDIOMYOPATHY

- Idiopathic restrictive cardiomyopathy
  - Firm myocardium with normal left ventricular wall thickness
  - Normal left ventricular cavity size
  - Often biatrial dilation
  - Endocardium is not grossly thickened
- Endomyocardial fibrosis
  - Thick, white scarring of the left ventricular endocardium at the inflow tract and apex with encasement of papillary muscles and subvalvular apparatus resulting in valvular regurgitation
  - Fibrosis of right ventricular apex seen in half of the cases
- Löffler syndrome
  - Fibrosis of endocardium characteristically with large mural thrombi at the inflow tract and apex of both ventricles
- Endocardial fibroelastosis
  - Left ventricle is usually contracted but may be dilated
  - Diffusely thickened pearly white endocardium that may obscure trabeculae carneae
- Hemochromatosis
  - Left ventricular hypertrophy with rusty-brown discoloration of myocardium

ARRHYTHMOGENIC RIGHT VENTRICULAR DYSPLASIA/ CARDIOMYOPATHY

- Replacement of right ventricular myocardium by adipose and fibrous tissue
- In early disease, these changes are segmental and present in the apex, right ventricular inlet, and right ventricular outflow tract
- Progressive loss of myocardium leads to diffuse involvement with right ventricular dilation and localized ventricular aneurysms
- Left ventricular involvement is seen in advanced stages with preferential involvement of the posterolateral wall

Histopathology

HYPERTROPHIC CARDIOMYOPATHY

- Hypertrophy and disarray of myocytes with interstitial fibrosis (Figures 18-1A and B)
- Disarray is maximal in the middle or deeper region of the interventricular septum
- Intramural small coronary arteries are dysplastic with narrowed lumens due to medial hyperplasia with or without intimal thickening (Figure 18-1C)
- Replacement fibrosis and myocardial scars
- Should not be diagnosed on the basis of a right ventricular endomyocardial biopsy as disarray is common in the trabeculae of the right ventricle

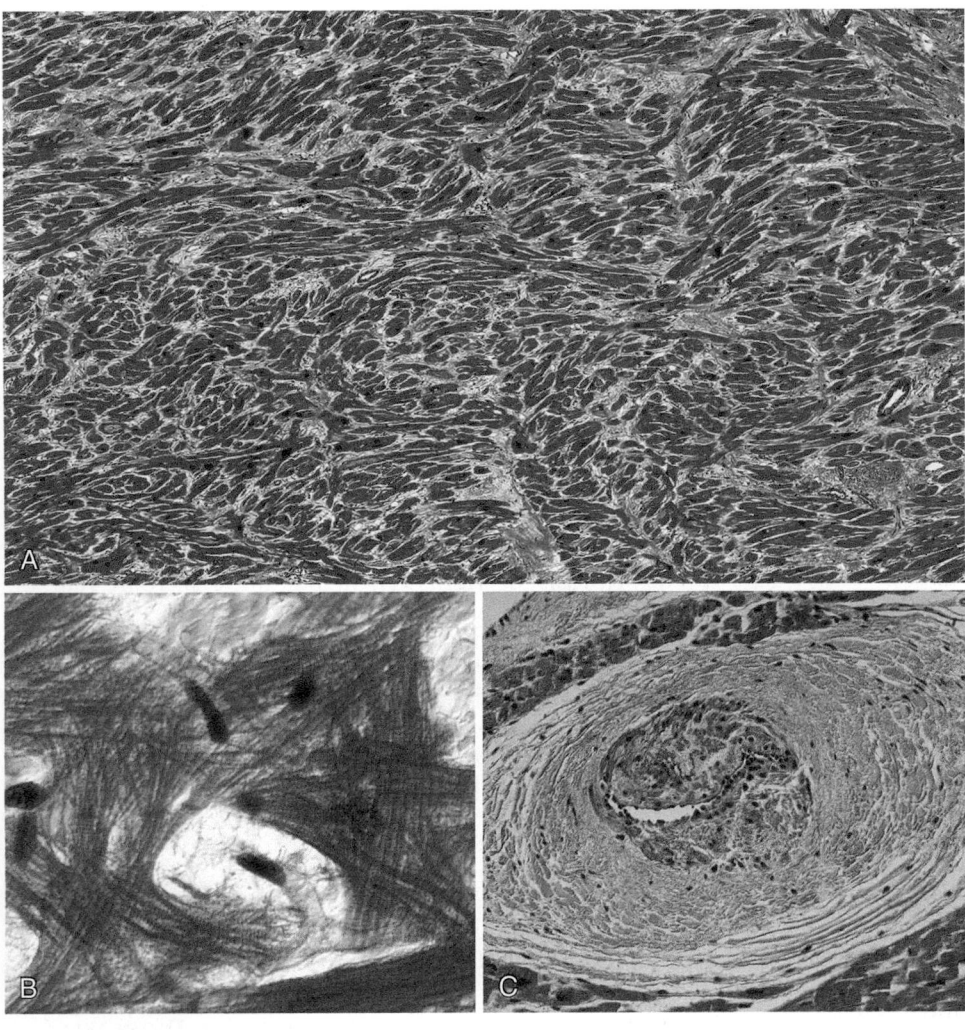

Figure 18-1. Hypertrophic cardio-myopathy. **A,** Movat-stained histologic section shows disorganization in the arrangement of myocyte bundles with interstitial fibrosis. **B,** Disarray can also be observed in the myofibrils of individual myocytes. **C,** Dysplastic small intramural coronary arteries are often observed with a narrowed lumen, irregularly thickened wall, and adventitial fibrosis.

DILATED CARDIOMYOPATHY
- Histopathologic findings are nonspecific
- Myocyte hypertrophy with enlarged hyperchromatic nuclei, mixed with myocyte atrophy and degeneration
- Interstitial fibrosis sometimes associated with sparse inflammatory cell infiltrates

RESTRICTIVE CARDIOMYOPATHY
- Idiopathic restrictive cardiomyopathy
  - Diffuse interstitial fibrosis that surrounds individual myocytes
- Endomyocardial fibrosis
  - Hyalinized collagen scarring of the endocardium with few mesenchymal cells
  - Fibrosis extends into the inner myocardium
- Löffler syndrome
  - Three stages have been described
    - Acute necrotic stage: shows intense eosinophilic infiltrate in myocardium with arteritis
    - Thrombotic stage: characterized by superimposed thrombosis on thickened endocardium and thrombi in intramyocardial vessels
    - Fibrotic stage: shows thick endocardium with loosely arranged vascularized fibrous tissue in the

deepest layer; vessels show intimal thickening and perivascular fibrosis
  - Once the fibrotic stage is reached, the distinction between endomyocardial fibrosis and Löffler syndrome based on pathologic features may not be possible
- Endocardial fibroelastosis
  - Diffuse fibrosis of endocardium with prominent elastic fibers
- Hemochromatosis
  - Hemosiderin deposition within myocytes (Figure 18-2A)

ARRHYTHMOGENIC RIGHT VENTRICULAR DYSPLASIA/ CARDIOMYOPATHY
- Transmural extensive fatty replacement of the myocardium with fibrosis and myocyte atrophy (Figure 18-3A)
- Lymphocytic infiltrates associated with myocyte damage may be present

Special Stains and Immunohistochemistry
- Masson trichrome highlights interstitial fibrosis and myofibrillar loss
- Movat pentachrome highlights fibrosis and elastosis (Figure 18-3B)
- Prussian blue highlights iron deposition in myocytes and macrophages (Figure 18-2B)

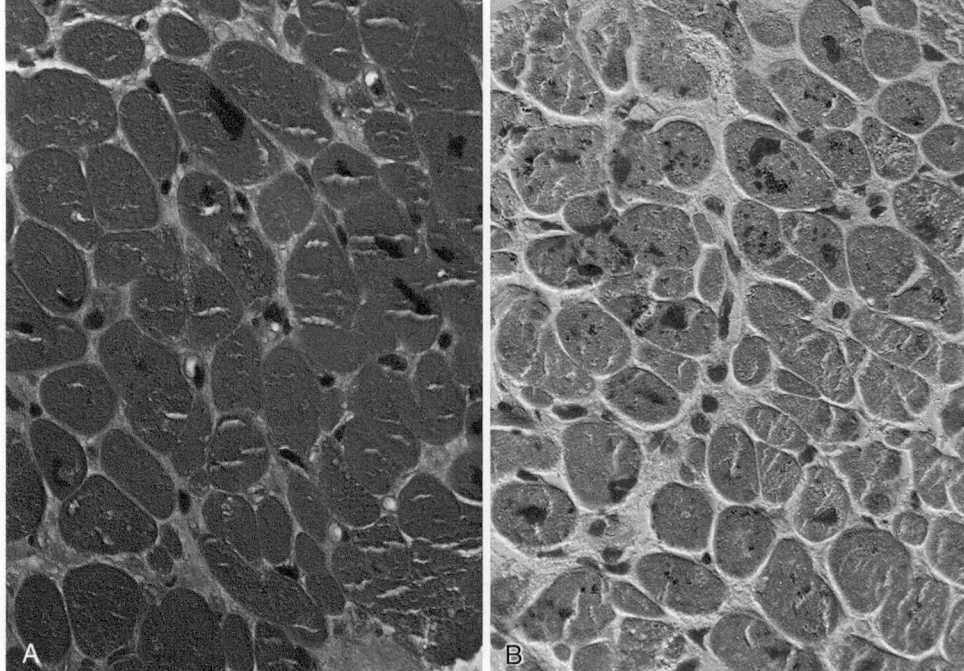

Figure 18-2. Hemochromatosis. A, Iron deposits in the form of hemosiderin accumulate in the sarcoplasm of the myocytes as brown pigment, usually in the perinuclear region of the sarcoplasm where secondary lysosomes accumulate. In contrast to lipofuscin pigment, which is yellow, the hemosiderin pigment is brown and may be birefringent upon polarization. **B,** Perls Prussian blue stain highlights ferric iron in these secondary lysosomes, which are seen in the perinuclear and peripheral areas of the myocyte sarcoplasm.

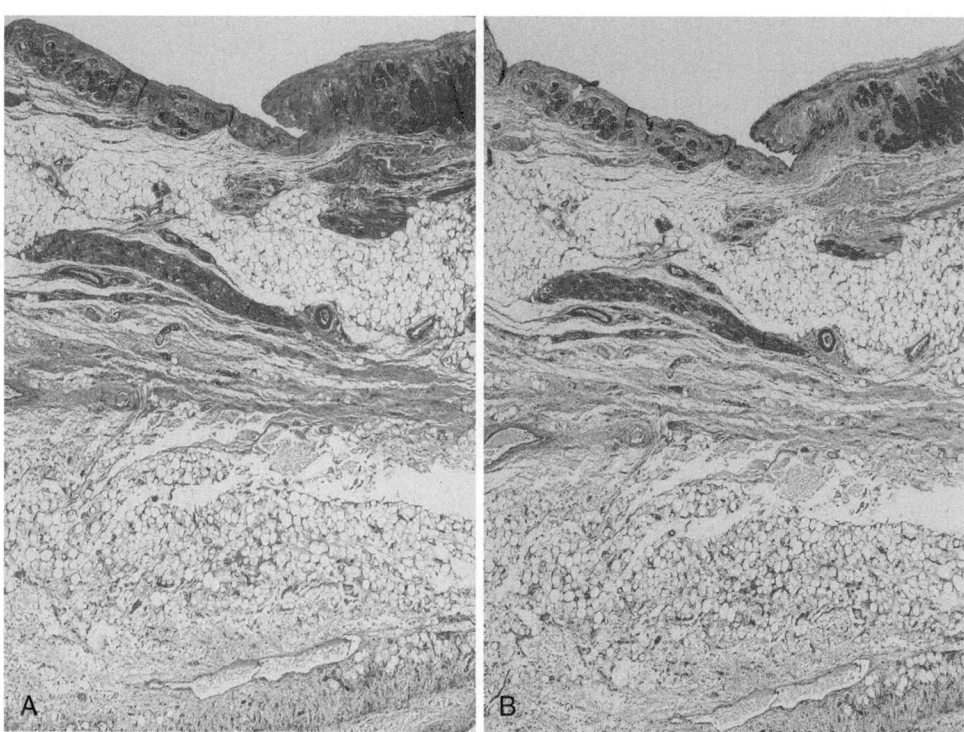

Figure 18-3. Arrhythmogenic right ventricular cardiomyopathy. A, Histologic section of right ventricular wall shows a markedly thinned myocardium with fatty infiltration of the wall. **B,** Movat stain shows fibrous replacement of the myocytes.

- Periodic acid–Schiff (PAS) with and without diastase highlights glycogen accumulation in myocytes, including basophilic degeneration

Other Techniques for Diagnosis

DILATED CARDIOMYOPATHY
- Electron microscopy: myocyte degeneration with myofibrillar loss in some myocytes and myocyte hypertrophy in others; dilation of T tubules, increased

number of mitochondria, and increased glycogen, lipid vacuoles, myelin figures, and phagolysosomes

TOXIC CARDIOMYOPATHY (SPECIFICALLY DOXORUBICIN)
- Grading of doxorubicin endomyocardial biopsies requires at least three pieces of myocardium and examination of 10 plastic-embedded semithin sections stained with toluidine blue

- Grade 0: normal myocardium by light and electron microscopy
- Grade 1: occasional isolated myocytes with myofibrillar loss or vacuolar degeneration (distended sarcoplasmic reticulum and T-tubular system) involving less than 5% of cells
- Grade 1.5: scattered, single myocytes with myofibrillar loss or vacuolar degeneration affecting 5% to 15% of myocytes
- Grade 2: clusters of affected myocytes affecting 16% to 25% of cells
- Grade 2.5: 26% to 35% of myocytes affected
- Grade 3: diffuse myocyte damage affecting more than 35% of cells; myocyte cell necrosis (total loss of contractile elements, loss of organelles, and mitochondrial and nuclear degeneration)

METABOLIC CARDIOMYOPATHY

- Fabry disease
  - Electron microscopy: electron-dense intracellular lamellar bodies or myelin figures corresponding to the accumulation of glycolipids
- Mitochondrial cardiomyopathy
  - Electron microscopy: proliferation of mitochondria, which are pleomorphic in size and shape and have abnormal cristae and paracrystalline inclusions
- Glycogen storage disease
  - Electron microscopy: markedly increased sarcoplasmic free glycogen; glycogen in lysosomes; vacuoles containing autophagic material

Differential Diagnosis

HYPERTROPHIC CARDIOMYOPATHY VERSUS METABOLIC CARDIOMYOPATHY

- Myocyte sarcoplasmic vacuolization or granularity should raise suspicion for storage disease and mitochondrial abnormalities; electron microscopy is necessary for complete evaluation
- Fabry disease due to mutations in lysosomal α-galactosidase A
- Adult-onset glycogen storage disease with left ventricular hypertrophy and Wolff-Parkinson-White syndrome due to mutations in the γ2 regulatory subunit of the adenosine monophosphate-activated protein kinase (PRKAG2)
- X-linked hypertrophic cardiomyopathy (Danon disease) with skeletal myopathy and mental retardation due to mutations in lysosome-associated membrane protein (LAMP2)
- Mitochondrial cardiomyopathy due to mutations in mitochondrial DNA

SYMMETRICAL HYPERTROPHIC CARDIOMYOPATHY VERSUS PHYSIOLOGIC HYPERTROPHY IN RESPONSE TO EXERCISE ("ATHLETE'S HEART")

- Differentiation of physiologic cardiac hypertrophy induced by athletic training from those with structural disease may require extensive non-invasive and invasive clinical screening tests

HYPERTROPHIC CARDIOMYOPATHY VERSUS AGE-RELATED SUBAORTIC BULGING OF THE INTERVENTRICULAR SEPTUM (SIGMOID OR CATENOID SEPTUM)

- Anatomic variant commonly seen in elderly patients, which may be accentuated by concomitant systemic hypertension, simulating asymmetrical hypertrophic cardiomyopathy

HYPERTROPHIC CARDIOMYOPATHY VERSUS DISEASES ASSOCIATED WITH LEFT VENTRICULAR HYPERTROPHY IN INFANTS AND YOUNG CHILDREN

- Infiltrative cardiomyopathies including type II Pompe disease, Hunter disease, and Hurler disease
- Noonan syndrome resulting from *PTPN11* (protein-tyrosine phosphatase, nonreceptor type 11) gene mutation presenting with cardiofacial abnormalities, including pulmonic valve stenosis and atrial septal defect
- Infants of insulin-dependent diabetic mothers

RESTRICTIVE CARDIOMYOPATHY VERSUS CONSTRICTIVE PERICARDITIS

- Diastolic filling is restricted in constrictive pericarditis by rigid, thickened pericardium with fibrous pericardial adhesions
- Endomyocardial biopsy has proved useful in establishing diagnosis of infiltrative cardiomyopathies
- A normal endomyocardial biopsy would direct the clinical workup to reevaluate the pericardium

PEARLS

- *Traditional functional classification of cardiomyopathies has been challenged as the genetic basis of a number of cardiomyopathies has become evident; moreover, hypertrophic cardiomyopathy and some infiltrative diseases may progress to a dilated form late in the course of the disease.*
- *Hypertrophic cardiomyopathy*
  - *Familial in at least 50% of cases with autosomal dominant mode of inheritance but variable clinical expression as to age of onset and severity*
  - *Sometimes referred to as disease of the sarcomere because mutations are most common in genes that encode sarcomeric proteins*
  - *Most common gene mutations involve the β-myosin heavy chain (MYH7, chromosome locus 14q12) and myosin-binding protein C (MYBPC3, chromosome locus 11p11.2)*
  - *Endomyocardial biopsy is almost never diagnostic but can be helpful to rule out other diagnoses*
  - *Disarray may be absent in small myectomy specimens, but presence of coronary artery dysplasia, replacement, and interstitial fibrosis is suggestive of hypertrophic cardiomyopathy*
- *Dilated cardiomyopathy*
  - *Studies indicate that at least 30% of dilated cardiomyopathy cases may be familial*
  - *Pattern of inheritance is variable and includes autosomal dominant, autosomal recessive, and X-linked*
  - *Mutations are more varied and are found in genes encoding sarcomeric proteins, intermediate filaments, dystrophin-associated protein complex components, nuclear membrane proteins, and phospholamban*

- *Arrhythmogenic right ventricular dysplasia/cardiomyopathy*
  - *Familial occurrence in about 30% to 50% of cases with predominantly autosomal dominant pattern of inheritance and incomplete penetrance*
  - *Most common mutations are in genes encoding desmosomal proteins (desmoplakin, plakophilin-2, desmoglein-2, desmocollin-2, and plakoglobin)*
- *There are considerable overlap and variation in the phenotypic expression of genetic mutations associated with cardiomyopathies*
- *Endomyocardial biopsy is able to establish the diagnosis in patients with unexplained cardiomyopathy with a high degree of sensitivity and specificity*

SELECTED REFERENCES

Arad M, Maron BJ, Gorham JM, et al: Glycogen storage diseases presenting as hypertrophic cardiomyopathy. N Engl J Med 352:362-372, 2005.

Chimenti C, Pieroni M, Maseri A, Frustaci A: Histologic findings in patients with clinical and instrumental diagnosis of sporadic arrhythmogenic right ventricular dysplasia. J Am Coll Cardiol 43:2305-2313, 2004.

Felker GM, Hu W, Hare JM, et al: The spectrum of dilated cardiomyopathy: the Johns Hopkins experience with 1,278 patients. Medicine (Baltimore) 78:270-283, 1999.

Hershberger RE, Hedges DJ, Morales A: Dilated cardiomyopathy: the complexity of a diverse genetic architecture. Nat Rev Cardiol 10:531-547, 2013.

Leone O, Veinot JP, Angelini A, et al: 2011 consensus statement on endomyocardial biopsy from the Association for European Cardiovascular Pathology and the Society for Cardiovascular Pathology. Cardiovasc Pathol 21:245-274, 2012.

Maron BJ, Towbin JA, Thiene G, et al: Contemporary definitions and classification of the cardiomyopathies: an American Heart Association scientific statement from the Council on Clinical Cardiology, Heart Failure and Transplantation Committee; Quality of Care and Outcomes Research and Functional Genomics and Translational Biology Interdisciplinary Working Groups; and Council on Epidemiology and Prevention. Circulation 113:1807-1816, 2006.

Olsen EG, Spry CJ: Relation between eosinophilia and endomyocardial disease. Prog Cardiovasc Dis 27:241-254, 1995.

Seki A, Patel S, Ashraf S, et al: Primary endocardial fibroelastosis: an underappreciated cause of cardiomyopathy in children. Cardiovasc Pathol 22:345-350, 2013.

MYOCARDITIS

Clinical Features

LYMPHOCYTIC MYOCARDITIS

- Frequently asymptomatic or has a subclinical course that later progresses to dilated cardiomyopathy
- May present as chest pain, unexplained acute onset of congestive heart failure, ventricular arrhythmias, or sudden death
- Viruses are the most common cause of myocarditis, particularly in children

GIANT CELL MYOCARDITIS

- Typically affects young and middle-aged adults
- Most patients present with rapidly progressive heart failure, often with refractory ventricular arrhythmia, rarely with heart block or chest pain mimicking myocardial infarction
- Poor prognosis and often fatal if untreated

EOSINOPHILIC MYOCARDITIS

- Hypersensitivity myocarditis
  - Believed to be an allergic delayed hypersensitivity reaction to diverse pharmacologic drugs and nutritional supplements
  - Reported complication of smallpox vaccination in young individuals
  - Associated with prolonged continuous administration of vasopressors, particularly dobutamine
  - Signs and symptoms are nonspecific and include typical allergic reaction (fever, rash, and blood eosinophilia), arrhythmias, sudden death, and congestive heart failure
- Acute necrotizing eosinophilic myocarditis
  - Thought to represent the most severe form of hypersensitivity myocarditis but can also be associated with viral infections, cancer, connective tissue diseases, and Churg-Strauss syndrome
  - Presents with fulminant heart failure and can be rapidly fatal
- Hypereosinophilic syndrome
  - Characterized by eosinophilia in the blood and bone marrow and tissue infiltration with eosinophils in multiple organs
  - Predominantly affects males between 20 and 50 years old
  - Cardiac involvement is most common and can present with restrictive physiology
  - Mural thrombi are frequently formed and can lead to systemic embolization

Gross Pathology

- Variable degrees of cardiac hypertrophy and possible chamber dilation may be seen
- Affected myocardium appears as pale foci, sometimes with minute hemorrhages
- Irregular and geographic fibrous scars without predilection to particular sites and affecting both ventricles and interventricular septum develop in giant cell myocarditis if patient survives
- In hypereosinophilic syndrome, endocardial damage leads to mural thrombosis
- Associated fibrinous pericarditis and pericardial effusion

Histopathology

LYMPHOCYTIC MYOCARDITIS

- Focal to diffuse interstitial mononuclear cell infiltrate, predominantly lymphocytes, with associated myocyte necrosis (Figure 18-4)
- In endomyocardial biopsies, sparse lymphocytic infiltrate not associated with myocyte damage is diagnosed as borderline myocarditis based on the Dallas criteria
- Repeat biopsies showing persistent lymphocytic infiltrate is called *persistent myocarditis*, a less intense infiltrate is *resolving myocarditis*, and absence of inflammatory infiltrate is *resolved myocarditis*

GIANT CELL MYOCARDITIS

- Multifocal to diffuse infiltrate consisting of lymphocytes and macrophages with multinucleated giant cells (Figure 18-5A and B)

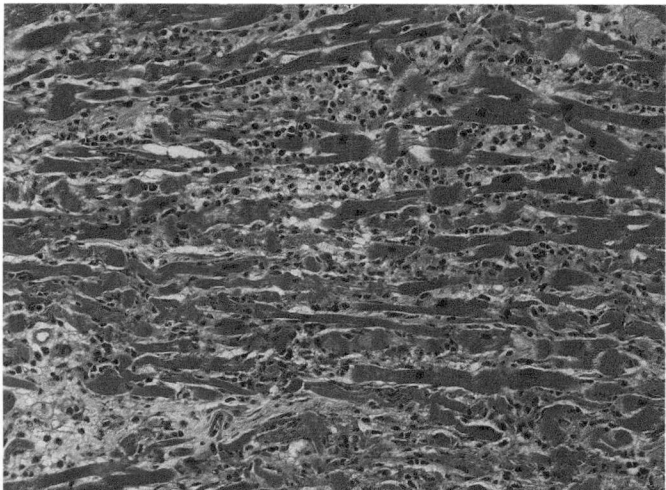

Figure 18-4. Lymphocytic myocarditis. Histologic section shows interstitial infiltrate of lymphocytes with rare eosinophils. Note the thinning of the myocytes in areas of myocyte necrosis.

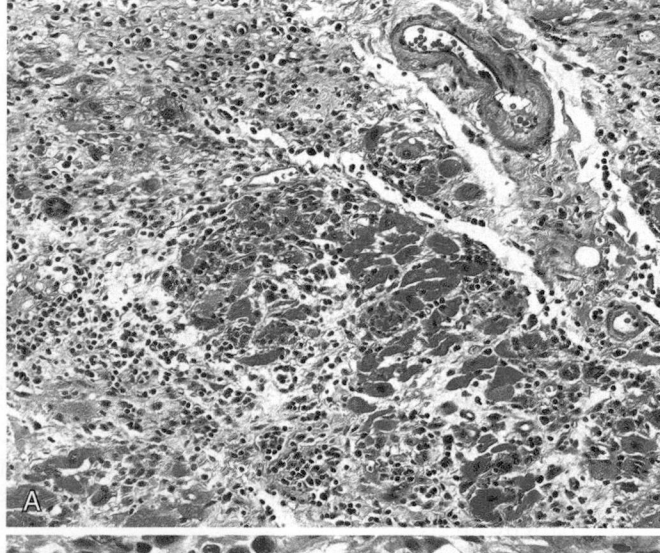

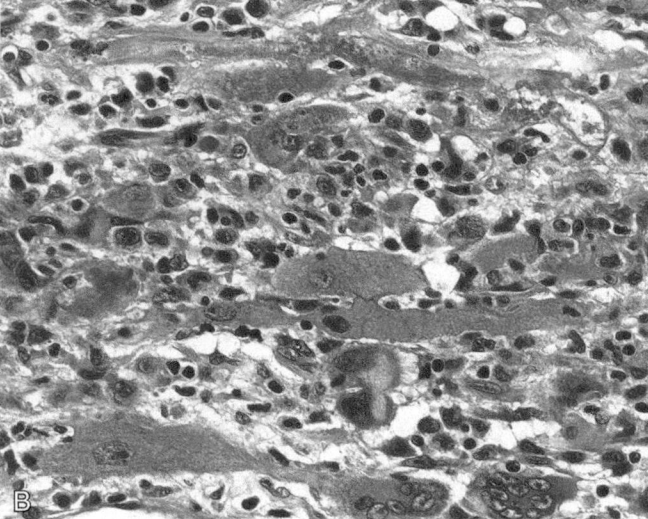

Figure 18-5. Giant cell myocarditis. A, Histologic section shows extensive areas of myocyte dropout with a mixed inflammatory infiltrate. **B,** Conspicuous giant cells admixed with macrophages, lymphocytes, and eosinophils do not form discrete granulomas.

- Eosinophils are often present
- Occasional poorly formed granuloma-like structures may be seen
- Geographic areas of myocyte damage or necrosis with varying degrees of fibrosis are evident on low magnification

EOSINOPHILIC MYOCARDITIS
- Patchy interstitial and perivascular infiltrates consisting of many eosinophils mixed with histiocytes, lymphocytes, and plasma cells
- May involve the endocardium and epicardium
- Lesions are all of the same age
- Usually only minimal myocyte necrosis and interstitial fibrosis
- Acute necrotizing eosinophilic myocarditis shows intense and diffuse infiltrates with extensive myocyte necrosis
- Hypereosinophilic syndrome also shows eosinophilic infiltrates with myocyte necrosis
- Charcot-Leyden crystals can be seen

Special Stains and Immunohistochemistry
- Gram, Gomori methenamine silver (GMS), PAS, and Ziehl-Neelsen stains to demonstrate causative organisms in infectious myocarditis
- The utility of immunohistochemical staining and quantitation of inflammatory cells using T and B cell markers, CD68, and HLA-DR is not yet firmly established

Other Techniques for Diagnosis
- In situ hybridization and polymerase chain reaction for viral detection; most commonly detected viruses are enteroviruses (Coxsackie B), parvovirus B19, adenovirus, human herpesvirus type 6, cytomegalovirus, influenza virus A and B, Epstein-Barr virus, and hepatitis C virus (HCV)

Differential Diagnosis

LYMPHOCYTIC MYOCARDITIS
- Myocarditis associated with infectious agents including Lyme disease, leptospirosis, typhoid fever, syphilis, chlamydia and rickettsial infections, and AIDS
- Myocarditis associated with collagen vascular disease and autoimmune disorders
- Toxic myocarditis
  - Includes toxin-induced myocardial injury (e.g., diphtheria exotoxin) and dose-related, direct toxic effects of drugs to myocardium
  - Can be seen in patients who are on vasopressor agents, have elevated endogenous catecholamines, or are cocaine abusers
  - Small foci of myocardial necrosis with contraction bands
  - Inflammatory infiltrates are predominantly macrophages
  - Lesions are of varying ages
- Microbiologic, serologic, and clinical correlation help make the diagnosis

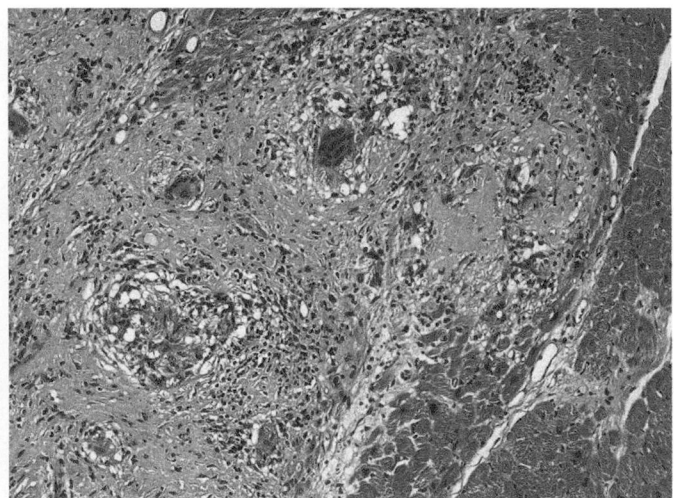

Figure 18-6. Cardiac sarcoidosis. Epithelioid granulomas with multinucleated giant cells are seen in areas of replacement fibrosis. Unlike giant cell myocarditis, the granulomas are discrete in a background of dense fibrous tissue.

GIANT CELL MYOCARDITIS

- Sarcoidosis
  - Dense fibrous scars toward the base of the heart involving the septum more heavily than the free wall of the left or right ventricle can be seen in sarcoidosis
  - Characterized by well-formed granulomas and fibrosis with few or no eosinophils (Figure 18-6)
  - Generally lacks myocyte necrosis
  - Rarely present as isolated cardiac involvement; lymph node or lung involvement almost always present
- Rheumatic myocarditis
  - Endocardial and interstitial Aschoff granulomas with giant cells
- Infectious granulomatous diseases
  - Giant cells may be seen in tuberculosis, cryptococcosis, syphilitic myocarditis, or measles myocarditis
  - Myocardial involvement is rarely isolated
  - Special stains for microorganisms should be performed
- Foreign-body reaction
  - Birefringent material under polarized light
  - Myocardial reaction to pacemaker leads, assist devices

EOSINOPHILIC MYOCARDITIS

- Parasitic infestation with peripheral eosinophilia (e.g., *Trichinella* species)

NEUTROPHILIC INFILTRATES

- Usually seen in systemic bacterial and fungal infections in the immunocompromised host or spread by direct extension
  - Focal neutrophilic infiltrates with myocyte necrosis and microabscesses
- Myocardial infarction
  - A zone of necrosis with neutrophilic infiltration at the periphery corresponding to a territory supplied by an epicardial coronary artery

PEARLS

- *Lymphocytic myocarditis*
  - *Detection of viral genome, specifically enteroviruses, is an independent predictor of poor clinical outcome in patients with dilated cardiomyopathy*
  - *Detection of autoantibodies directed against myocardial structural, sarcoplasmic, or sarcolemmal proteins suggests immune-mediated myocarditis*
- *Giant cell myocarditis*
  - *Up to 20% of patients have other inflammatory diseases, especially inflammatory bowel disease or autoimmune disorders*
  - *Most commonly associated tumor is thymoma*
  - *Giant cell myocarditis is known to recur in transplanted hearts*
- *Hypersensitivity myocarditis*
  - *Diagnosis requires high clinical index of suspicion*
  - *Endomyocardial biopsy necessary to establish the diagnosis*
  - *No correlation between the duration and dose of the drug and the severity of myocarditis*
  - *Treatment requires removal of the offending substance; immunosuppressive therapy may be indicated in severe cases*

SELECTED REFERENCES

Caforio AL, Pankuweit S, Arbustini E, et al: Current state of knowledge on aetiology, diagnosis, management, and therapy of myocarditis: a position statement of the European Society of Cardiology Working Group on Myocardial and Pericardial Diseases. Eur Heart J 34:2636-2648, 2648a-2648d, 2013.

Calabrese F, Thiene G: Myocarditis and inflammatory cardiomyopathy: microbiological and molecular biological aspects. Cardiovasc Res 60:11-25, 2003.

Ginsberg F, Parrillo JE: Eosinophilic myocarditis. Heart Fail Clin 1: 419-429, 2005.

Kuhl U, Pauschinger M, Seeberg B, et al: Viral persistence in the myocardium is associated with progressive cardiac dysfunction. Circulation 112:1965-1970, 2005.

AMYLOIDOSIS

Clinical Features

- Amyloid deposition in the cardiovascular system may be local (isolated atrial, valvular or aortic amyloidosis) or be part of a systemic involvement
- When symptomatic, patients can present with restrictive cardiomyopathy, congestive heart failure, atypical chest pain, and arrhythmias
- Preponderance of male patients

Gross Pathology

- Cardiac amyloidosis usually leads to cardiomegaly with biventricular hypertrophy
- Cut surface may show a variable appearance ranging from normal to firm and rubbery myocardium depending on extent of amyloid deposition
- Tiny, semitranslucent, waxy yellow-ochre nodules may be seen on the endocardium, more prominent in the left atrium; in severe cases, they are visible in all chambers and on the valvular endocardium

Histopathology

- Characteristic interstitial deposition of extracellular eosinophilic material surrounding individual myocytes results in atrophy and loss of myocytes (Figure 18-7A)
- Other patterns of infiltration are nodular, subendocardial, vascular, and mixed
- Mononuclear inflammatory cell infiltrates can be found and correlate with poor prognosis

Special Stains and Immunohistochemistry

- Congo red: apple-green birefringence under polarized light
- Thioflavin T or thioflavin S: ultraviolet fluorescence of the amyloid deposits (Figure 18-7B)
- Sulfated alcian blue: highlights green-staining amyloid surrounding individual myocytes and red-staining interstitial fibrosis
- Immunohistochemical staining by immunoperoxidase or immunofluorescence method with the following antibodies is useful in cardiac amyloidosis: transthyretin, κ and λ light chains, heavy chains, amyloid A, and atrial natriuretic peptide (Figure 18-7C)

Other Techniques for Diagnosis

- Electron microscopy: interstitial expansion by extracellular, nonbranching, randomly oriented fibrils measuring 8 to 10 nanometers in diameter
- Laser microdissection and tandem mass spectrometry-based proteomic analysis can be useful in establishing the type of amyloid

Differential Diagnosis

HYALINIZED COLLAGEN

- May appear similar to amyloid on hematoxylin and eosin-stained sections but exhibits periodic banding pattern on polarization

- Congo red may have false-positive birefringence in collagen if staining method is not optimal
- Blue collagen fibers can be differentiated from the blue-gray hue of amyloid on Masson trichrome stain

PEARLS

- *Amyloidosis involving the heart can be divided into primary (light and heavy chains), secondary (amyloid A), hereditary (mutant transthyretin), senile systemic (wild-type transthyretin), isolated atrial (atrial natriuretic peptide), and hemodialysis-related (β_2-microglobulin)*
- *Deposits in the heart are most common in primary (immunoglobulin light chain) and transthyretin amyloidosis*
- *Localized forms of amyloidosis in the atria, valves, and aorta are generally incidental findings not associated with significant clinical disease*
- *Endomyocardial biopsy is a safe method to establish the diagnosis*
- *In early disease, amyloid deposits may be visible only with electron microscopy*
- *The type of protein needs to be identified by immunophenotyping or by mass spectroscopy, as it has prognostic and therapeutic implications*
- *Thioflavin T or S is more sensitive than Congo red and easy to perform but requires fluorescence microscopy*

SELECTED REFERENCES

Tan CD, Rodríguez ER: Cardiac amyloidosis. In Picken MM, Dogan A, Herrera G (eds): Amyloid and Related Disorders: Surgical Pathology and Clinical Correlations. New York, Humana Press, 2012, pp 319-338.

Vrana JA, Gamez JD, Madden BJ, et al: Classification of amyloidosis by laser microdissection and mass spectrometry-based proteomic analysis in clinical biopsy specimens. Blood 114:4957-4959, 2009.

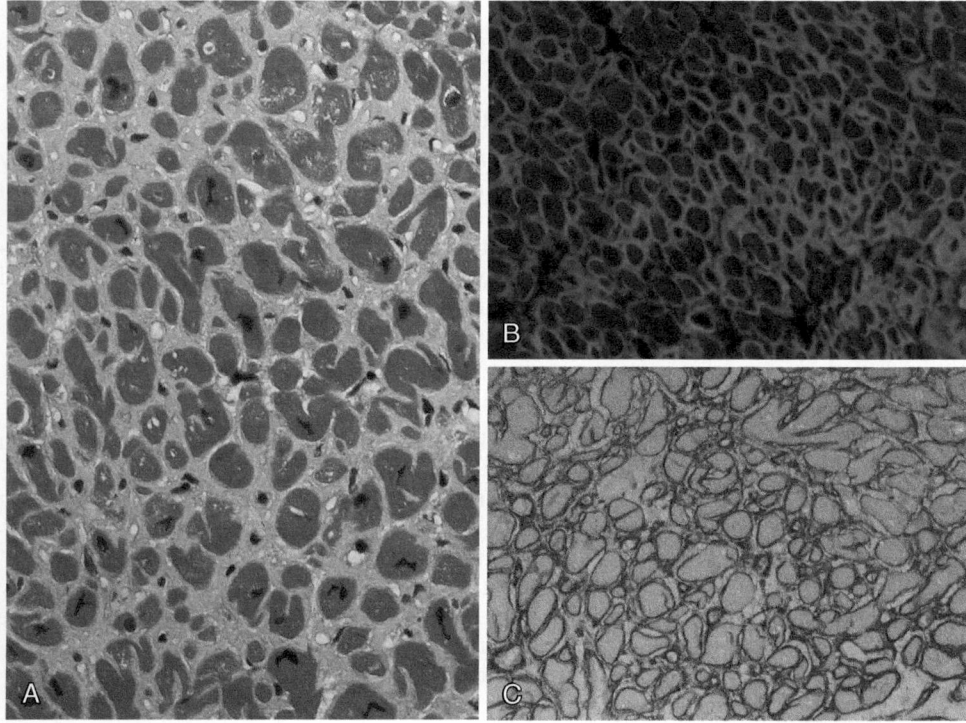

Figure 18-7. Amyloidosis. A, Abundant eosinophilic material is deposited around myocytes, which show marked variation in size on cross section, indicating hypertrophy and degeneration. **B,** Individual myocytes are outlined by amyloid deposits that fluoresce with thioflavin stain. **C,** Immunohistochemical staining with λ light chains is positive in this case.

SARCOIDOSIS

Clinical Features

- Affects young or middle-aged adults of either sex
- Lung, lymph nodes, skin, and eyes commonly involved; rarely, isolated cardiac involvement has been reported
- Cardiac involvement present in about 25% of sarcoidosis patients in autopsy series, with less than 5% having associated symptoms
- Patients present with arrhythmias, heart block, and heart failure, or sudden death

Gross Pathology

- Granulomatous infiltration may be visible as patchy, irregular white firm areas
- Transmural myocardial scars not associated with coronary atherosclerosis represent healed granulomas
- Preferential sites of involvement, in decreasing order of frequency, are left ventricular free wall at the base of and including papillary muscles, basal and cephalic portion of interventricular septum, and right ventricular free wall

Histopathology

- Noncaseating, well-formed granulomas composed of epithelioid histiocytes and multinucleated giant cells with or without lymphocytic infiltrates and no stainable microorganisms (Figure 18-6)
- Granulomas may involve the endocardium, myocardium, epicardium, and pericardium
- Typically minimal associated myocyte necrosis
- Collagenous stroma around granulomas
- Myocardial scars with few or no residual granulomas in burned-out or treated cases

Special Stains and Immunohistochemistry

- Noncontributory

Other Techniques for Diagnosis

- Noncontributory

Differential Diagnosis

GIANT CELL MYOCARDITIS

- Poorly formed granulomas with greater extent of myocyte necrosis and increased eosinophils compared with sarcoidosis
- Appears clinically distinct with a more fulminant course and shorter time from symptom onset to death or transplantation

INFECTIOUS MYOCARDITIS

- Infectious etiology should be excluded by performing stains for fungi and mycobacteria

MYOCARDIAL INFARCTION

- Scarring and thinning of the ventricle may be mistaken for healed myocardial infarcts, but normal coronary arteries should rule out ischemic heart disease

PEARLS

- *Endomyocardial biopsy has poor sensitivity in detecting cardiac sarcoidosis; therefore, a negative endomyocardial biopsy does not exclude the diagnosis of sarcoidosis*
- *Extensive myocardial scarring and ventricular aneurysm may be related to the natural history of the disease or previous corticosteroid therapy*

SELECTED REFERENCES

Ardehali H, Howard DL, Hariri A, et al: A positive endomyocardial biopsy result for sarcoid is associated with poor prognosis in patients with initially unexplained cardiomyopathy. Am Heart J 150:459-463, 2005.

Okura Y, Dec GW, Hare JM, et al: A clinical and histopathologic comparison of cardiac sarcoidosis and idiopathic giant cell myocarditis. J Am Coll Cardiol 41:322-329, 2003.

Roberts WC, McAllister HA Jr, Ferrans VJ: Sarcoidosis of the heart: a clinicopathologic study of 35 necropsy patients (group 1) and review of 78 previously described necropsy patients (group 11). Am J Med 63:86-108, 1977.

VALVULAR DISEASES

Morphologic and Functional Correlations

STENOTIC VALVES WITH OR WITHOUT REGURGITATION

- Diffuse fibrous thickening with a variable amount of calcification
- No valvular tissue loss, perforations, or vegetations
- No valvular tissue excess
- Fusion of valve commissures
- Chordae tendineae are fibrotic, fused, and shortened
- Attached papillary muscle is normal

PURELY REGURGITANT VALVES

- Usually mild and focal fibrous thickening and absent calcification
- Perforations or vegetations may be present
- Excess valvular tissue may be present
- No commissural fusion
- Chordae tendineae are elongated or ruptured
- Attached papillary muscle may be ruptured

Etiology of Valvular Dysfunction

MITRAL VALVE

- Mitral stenosis
  - Congenital
  - Acquired
    - Postinflammatory and rheumatic
    - Mitral annular calcification
- Mitral regurgitation
  - Congenital
  - Acquired
    - Mitral valve prolapse
    - Postinflammatory and rheumatic
    - Mitral annular calcification
    - Infective endocarditis
    - Ruptured papillary muscle
    - Papillary muscle dysfunction secondary to ischemia and infarct
    - Distortion of left ventricular geometry

AORTIC VALVE

- Aortic stenosis
  - Congenital
    - Unicuspid aortic valve
    - Calcification of bicuspid aortic valve
  - Acquired
    - Senile calcific aortic stenosis
    - Postinflammatory and rheumatic

- Aortic regurgitation
  - Congenital
    - Bicuspid aortic valve
  - Acquired
    - Postinflammatory and rheumatic
    - Infective endocarditis
    - Aortic dilation and aneurysm
    - Aortic dissection

Clinical Features

RHEUMATIC HEART DISEASE

- Findings of acute rheumatic fever include pericardial friction rubs, weak heart sounds, tachycardia, and arrhythmias; usually occur 10 days to 6 weeks after the pharyngitis episode
- Findings in chronic rheumatic heart disease include evidence of valvular stenosis or regurgitation, congestive heart failure, arrhythmias, thromboembolic complications, and infective endocarditis; usually occur 20 to 25 years after the acute disease

MITRAL VALVE PROLAPSE

- Prevalence is estimated at 2% to 3% of the population, with equal distribution among men and women
- Most patients do not develop symptoms
- Prolapse occurs most commonly in the middle scallop of the posterior mitral valve leaflet as identified on echocardiography
- Commonly idiopathic
- Known association with connective tissue disorders including Marfan syndrome, Ehlers-Danlos syndrome, osteogenesis imperfecta, and pseudoxanthoma elasticum
- Men appear to have a higher incidence of complications, which include severe mitral regurgitation, infective endocarditis, thromboembolic events, and sudden death

CALCIFIC AORTIC VALVE DISEASE

- Senile calcific aortic stenosis is more common in males, with a peak incidence in the seventh and eighth decades of life
- Calcification of a congenital bicuspid aortic valve peaks in the fifth and sixth decades of life
- Calcific disease of the aortic valve results in left ventricular hypertrophy, with symptoms including angina, syncope, and congestive heart failure

MITRAL ANNULAR CALCIFICATION

- More common and more severe in women, primarily those older than 60 years
- Associated with aging, hypertension, aortic stenosis, chronic renal disease, and atherosclerosis
- Often asymptomatic, but potential complications include acquired mitral stenosis or regurgitation, conduction system disturbances, endocarditis, and systemic embolism

PURE AORTIC REGURGITATION

- Pure aortic insufficiency can be due to lesions of the valve or the aorta
- Aortic root dilation is currently the most common cause of aortic insufficiency, followed by congenital bicuspid valve associated with ascending aortic aneurysm

CARCINOID HEART DISEASE

- Carcinoid syndrome is characterized by episodic bronchospasm, flushing of the skin, telangiectasia, and diarrhea, usually associated with gastrointestinal carcinoid tumors that have metastasized to the liver
- Cardiac involvement manifests as right-sided valvular disease that progresses to right-sided heart failure
- Valvular dysfunction results in pure regurgitation of the tricuspid valve and predominantly regurgitation of the pulmonic valve
- Left-sided involvement is rare and associated with the presence of right-to-left shunt, pulmonary metastases, or bronchial carcinoids

Gross Pathology

RHEUMATIC HEART DISEASE

- Involves, in descending order of frequency, mitral, aortic, tricuspid, and pulmonic valves
- Acute rheumatic fever may show small verrucous vegetations along the lines of closure
- Chronic rheumatic heart disease shows diffuse thickening and fibrous retraction of valve leaflets with or without calcification, fusion of the commissures, and shortened, fused, and thickened chordae (Figure 18-8)
- Narrowed valvular orifice due to commissural fusion
- Calcific deposits are found at the commissures, which may become ulcerated

MITRAL VALVE PROLAPSE

- Myxomatous degeneration may involve any valve but most frequently involves the mitral valve
- Diffuse leaflet thickening and redundancy with increased surface area (Figure 18-8)
- Interchordal hooding or billowing (parachute) deformity may be seen
- Cut surface reveals abundant gray translucent myxoid material in the spongiosa layer affecting the base, midportion, and free edge of the leaflet
- Elongated chordae with irregular thickening are commonly seen, and sometimes rupture occurs
- Often with annular dilation

CALCIFIC AORTIC VALVE DISEASE

- Senile calcific aortic stenosis shows fibrosis and calcification of the base and body of the cusps often protruding into the sinuses of Valsalva and rarely involving the free edge (Figure 18-9)
- Calcification of a congenital bicuspid aortic valve typically begins in the median raphe or false commissure and extends to the body of the cusps
- Absent or minimal commissural fusion is seen in degenerative aortic valve stenosis

MITRAL ANNULAR CALCIFICATION

- Calcification develops in the ring of the mitral valve, usually at the base of the posterior leaflet, forming a solid bar causing distortion and elevation of the posterior leaflet
- Lesion may also extend into the myocardium and medially into the septum, where it may cause disruption of the bundle of His
- Calcium mass may erode through the valve leaflet, ulcerate, and predispose to thrombosis and infection

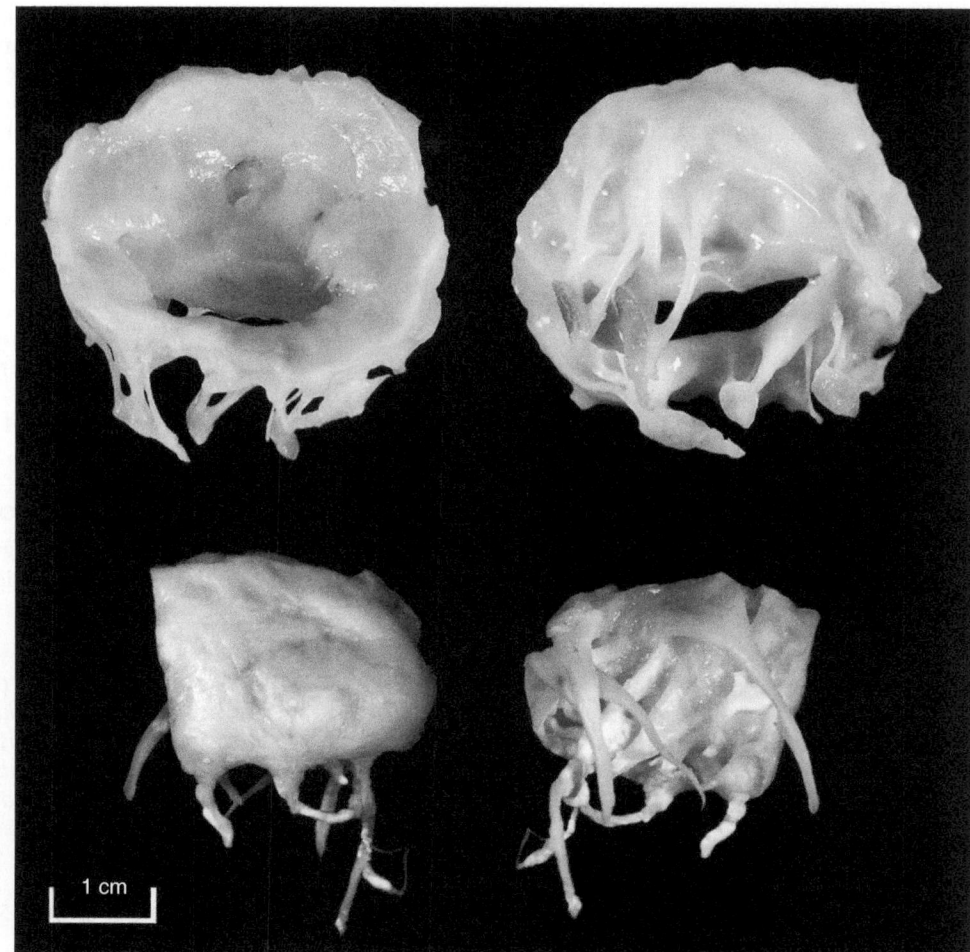

Figure 18-8. Mitral valve. In the upper specimen, postinflammatory scarring in rheumatic mitral valve disease results in commissural fusion and stenosis of the orifice. The chordae are fused, thickened, and shortened. Shown at the same magnification, the lower specimen, a segmental resection of a mitral valve, shows a diffusely thickened, expanded leaflet with mild billowing typical of mitral valve prolapse. The chordae are elongated and irregularly thickened, as seen on the ventricular aspect of the right lower specimen.

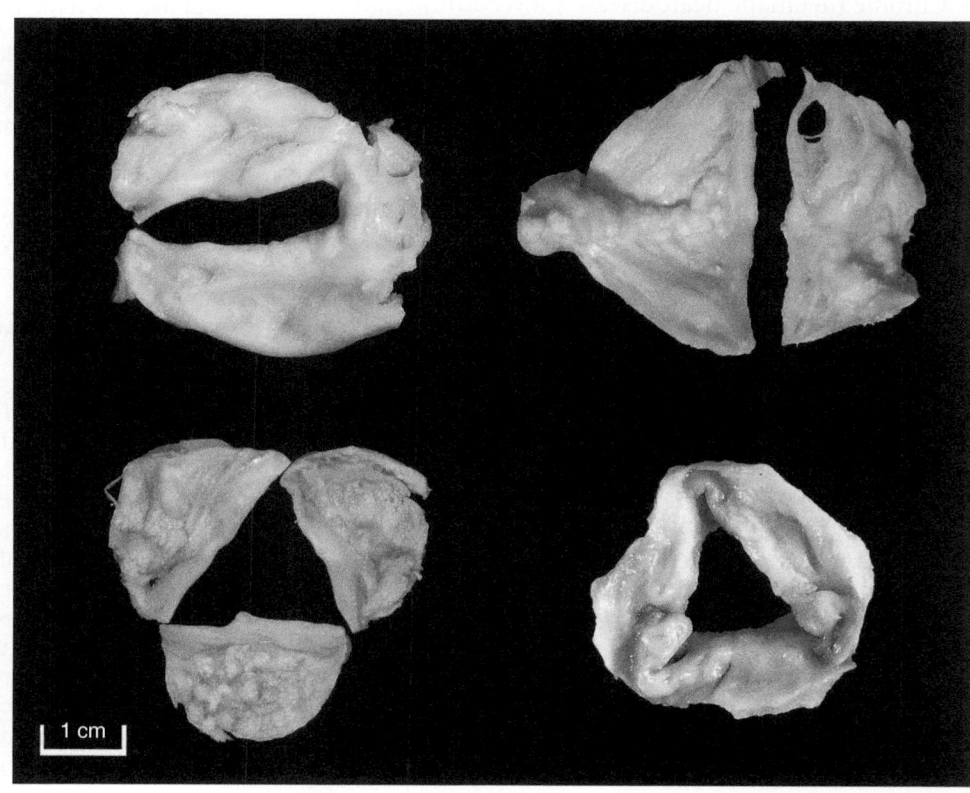

Figure 18-9. Aortic valve. Only one commissure is identified in this surgically excised congenitally malformed unicommissural aortic valve with eccentrically located orifice (*upper left*). A bicuspid aortic valve has two cusps with a slitlike opening of the valve. The larger of the cusps termed the conjoined cusp shows a calcified median raphe, which represents the site of failed cusp division. A fenestration is present in the smaller cusp (*upper right*). Calcific aortic stenosis due to severe nodular calcification of all three cusps is shown (*lower left*). Rheumatic aortic stenosis shows fusion of all the commissures with thick retracted cusps resulting in a fixed triangular orifice (*lower right*).

- Central softening and liquefaction of the calcification may occur and should not be mistaken for an abscess

PURE AORTIC REGURGITATION

- Floppy valves are large, redundant, mildly thickened, and gelatinous in consistency
- In aortic regurgitation secondary to dilation of the aortic root, the aortic cusps can be normal, with only focal and minimal fibrosis in the body; free edges are thickened; commissures are not fused

CARCINOID HEART DISEASE

- White fibrotic plaques on the tricuspid and pulmonic valve, mural endocardium, and occasionally intima of great vessels
- Fibrous plaques located predominantly on the ventricular aspect of tricuspid valve and almost exclusively on the arterial aspect of pulmonic valve
- Plaques cause thickening and retraction of the leaflets
- Plaques may also cause adherence of the valve to the mural endocardium of the right ventricle or intima of the pulmonary artery

Histopathology

RHEUMATIC HEART DISEASE

- Acute rheumatic fever may show inflammation and Aschoff bodies in all layers of the heart, including valves and papillary muscles
- Aschoff bodies consist of foci of fibrinoid degeneration surrounded by lymphocytes, occasional plasma cells, and Anitschkow or Aschoff cells
- Anitschkow cells are macrophages with abundant cytoplasm and central round to oval vesicular nuclei with a central bar of condensed chromatin (caterpillar-like); may become multinucleated to form Aschoff giant cells
- Chronic rheumatic heart disease shows diffuse fibrosis, neovascularization, or calcification of the valve
- Focal chronic inflammatory cell infiltrate (mainly lymphocytic) may be seen

MITRAL VALVE PROLAPSE

- Accumulation of mucopolysaccharides in the spongiosa layer with disruption of the collagenous bundles in the fibrosa and fragmentation of elastic fibers
- Absence of neovascularization or inflammation
- Mucopolysaccharide infiltration of the chordae tendineae

CALCIFIC AORTIC VALVE DISEASE

- Calcification begins in the fibrosa layer
- Lipid deposits, neovascularization, and chronic inflammatory cell infiltrates are commonly found
- Osseous metaplasia may develop in the calcium deposits

MITRAL ANNULAR CALCIFICATION

- Calcification may be associated with mild inflammation and foreign-body giant cells

PURE AORTIC REGURGITATION

- Fibrous thickening of the free edges
- Myxomatous degeneration with accumulation of mucopolysaccharides in the spongiosa

CARCINOID HEART DISEASE

- Plaque is cellular and contains fibroblasts, myofibroblasts, smooth muscle cells, and collagen embedded in a myxoid matrix
- Plaques have a stuck-on appearance on the underlying valve and endocardium, which are intact
- Usually there are no elastic lamellae (i.e., no fibroelastosis) within the carcinoid plaque

Special Stains and Immunohistochemistry

- Movat delineates the different layers of the valve and highlights mucopolysaccharide accumulation, fibrosis, and disruption and fragmentation of elastic fibers

Other Techniques for Diagnosis

- Noncontributory

Differential Diagnosis

- Stenosis versus regurgitant: see "Morphologic and Functional Correlations" under "Valvular Diseases"

PEARLS

- *An etiologic diagnosis can be formulated in most instances with careful gross evaluation of operatively excised valves*
- *Histologic evaluation is necessary to establish diagnosis in infective endocarditis and metabolic diseases involving cardiac valves (e.g., Fabry disease, mucopolysaccharidoses, carcinoid syndrome)*

SELECTED REFERENCES

Feldman T: Rheumatic heart disease. Curr Opin Cardiol 11:126-130, 1996.
Hayek E, Gring CN, Griffin BP: Mitral valve prolapse. Lancet 365:507-518, 2005.
Roberts WC, Ko JM: Frequency by decades of unicuspid, bicuspid, and tricuspid aortic valves in adults having isolated aortic valve replacement for aortic stenosis, with or without associated aortic regurgitation. Circulation 111:920-925, 2005.
Simula DV, Edwards WD, Tazelaar HD, et al: Surgical pathology of carcinoid heart disease: a study of 139 valves from 75 patients spanning 20 years. Mayo Clin Proc 77:139-147, 2002.
Waller B, Howard J, Fess S: General concepts in the morphologic assessment of operatively excised cardiac valves. Part I. Clin Cardiol 17:41-46, 1994.
Waller B, Howard J, Fess S: General concepts in the morphologic assessment of operatively excised cardiac valves. Part II. Clin Cardiol 17:208-214, 1994.

INFECTIVE ENDOCARDITIS

Clinical Features

- Risk factors for infective endocarditis are structural valvular abnormalities, congenital heart diseases, prosthetic heart valves, and injection drug use
- *Staphylococcus aureus* has become the most common cause of infective endocarditis owing to nosocomial infections and medical and surgical interventions including indwelling catheters and devices
- Most subacute cases of native valve endocarditis are due to *Streptococcus viridans*
- Prosthetic valve endocarditis is usually caused by *Staphylococcus epidermidis* and *S. aureus*
- Endocarditis caused by fastidious gram-negative bacilli of the HACEK group (*Haemophilus parainfluenzae*,

Aggregatibacter (formerly Haemophilus) aphrophilus, H. paraphrophilus, H. influenzae, Aggregatibacter (formerly Actinobacillus) actinomycetemcomitans, Cardiobacterium hominis, Eikenella corrodens, Kingella kingae, and *K. denitrificans*) accounts for about 5% to 10% of native valve community-acquired endocarditis in patients who are not injection drug users
- Symptoms are nonspecific and include fever, chills, fatigue, and weight loss
- Special attention to potential sources of bacteremia, new regurgitant murmurs, and embolic phenomena including septic lung emboli is emphasized
- Infection of a mechanical prosthetic valve may lead to valve dehiscence or paravalvular leak

Gross Pathology

- Aortic and mitral valves are most commonly affected
- Valvular insufficiency is caused by destruction or perforation of the valve and bulky vegetations that prevent proper coaptation of the leaflets (Figure 18-10A)
- Cusp or leaflet may have an irregular, ulcerated free border or perforation of the body and ruptured chordae
- Healed endocarditis may result in aneurysms or perforation with smooth borders
- Tissue prosthetic valve usually shows vegetations on both inflow and outflow surfaces

- Mechanical prosthetic valve infection starts at the sewing ring and results in a periprosthetic or ring abscess

Histopathology

- Acute vegetations consist of fibrin, platelets, neutrophils, and bacteria (Figure 18-10B)
- Subacute vegetations have granulation tissue at the base with both acute and chronic inflammatory cells as well as histiocytes and occasionally multinucleated giant cells (Figure 18-10C)

Special Stains and Immunohistochemistry

- Gram, PAS, GMS, Warthin-Starry, Fite, and Ziehl-Neelsen stains are useful in detecting microorganisms in tissues
- Antibodies to *Tropheryma, Chlamydia, Bartonella,* and *Coxiella* species are available only in specialized laboratories

Other Techniques for Diagnosis

- Serologic tests are useful for the diagnosis of *Bartonella, Coxiella,* and *Legionella* endocarditis
- Polymerase chain reaction followed by direct sequencing of 16S recombinant RNA genes from valve tissue are also used to detect *Tropheryma, Bartonella,* and *Coxiella* species and other etiologic agents of culture-negative endocarditis

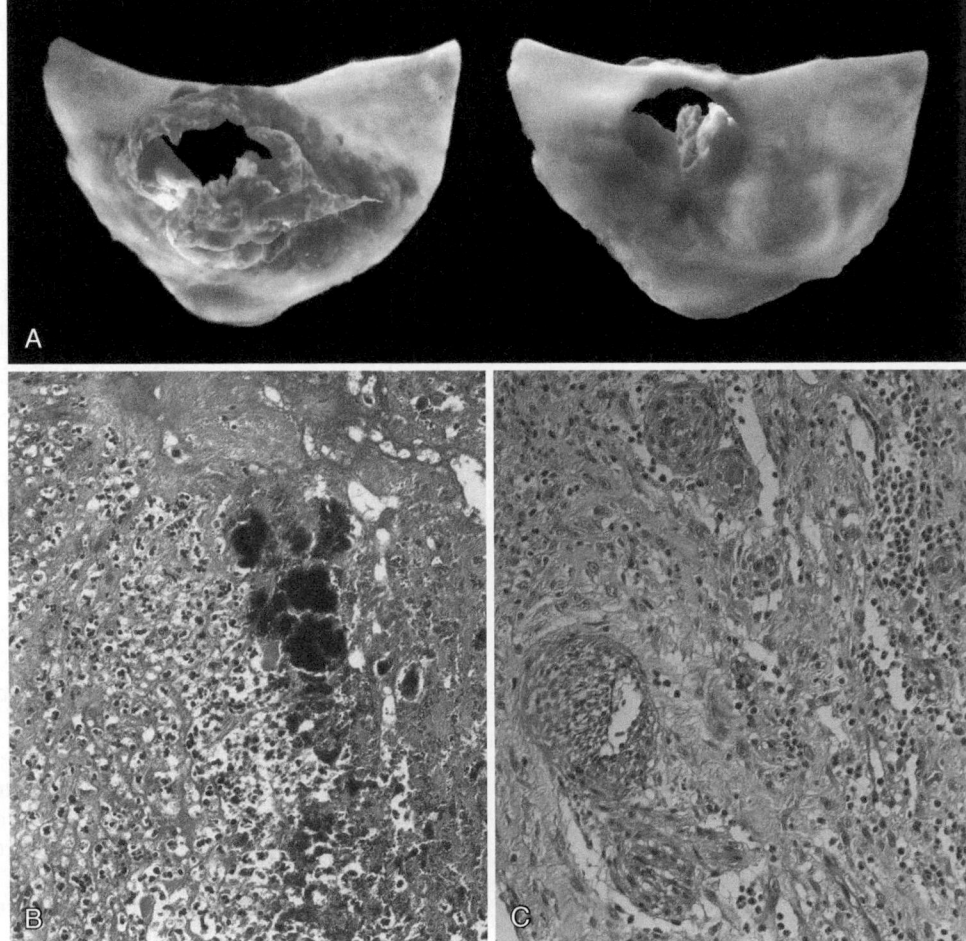

Figure 18-10. Infective endocarditis. A, An aortic cusp shows perforation with large yellow-red vegetations on the ventricular aspect. **B,** Vegetation shows fibrin with acute inflammatory exudate with bacterial colonies in a case of Staphylococcal endocarditis. **C,** Granulation tissue with neovascularization and neutrophilic infiltrates is commonly seen in Streptococcal endocarditis.

Differential Diagnosis

NONBACTERIAL THROMBOTIC ENDOCARDITIS

- Usually occurs in association with chronic inflammatory disease, hypercoagulable state, and underlying malignancy, especially adenocarcinomas
- Aseptic vegetation may embolize or serve as a substrate for infection
- Aortic and mitral valves are most commonly affected
- Right-sided lesions are usually associated with intravenous catheters
- Vegetations are present on the atrial surfaces of atrioventricular valves and ventricular surfaces of semilunar valves
- Small (1- to 5-mm), multiple, nondestructive vegetations are loosely attached to the underlying valve leaflets, usually on previously normal valves
- Composed of platelets mixed with fibrin and a few red blood cells
- Inflammatory reaction is absent
- Organization may be seen at the base of the lesion with fibroblastic proliferation

LIBMAN-SACKS ENDOCARDITIS

- Occurs in patients with systemic lupus erythematosus (SLE)
- Only 6% to 20% of cases are symptomatic
- Rare source of emboli
- Most often develops on mitral and tricuspid valves
- Relatively adherent, sessile, small (3- to 4-mm), pink to yellow-tan vegetations occurring singly or in clusters on the atrial and ventricular surfaces of the valve, anywhere from the free edge to the base, with extension onto the endocardium, chordae tendineae, and papillary muscles
- Sterile vegetations consist of fibrin and mononuclear cells with fibroblastic proliferation and neovascularization
- Necrosis with hematoxylin bodies rarely seen
- Healed endocarditis results in fibrous plaque

PEARLS

- *Up to 20% of patients with infective endocarditis have negative blood cultures, which may result from previous antibiotic administration or infection with highly fastidious bacteria and unusual organisms such as* Bartonella *species,* Coxiella burnetii, Brucella *species,* Tropheryma whippelii, Chlamydia, *and* Legionella *species*

SELECTED REFERENCES

Baddour LM, Wilson WR, Bayer AS, et al: Infective endocarditis: diagnosis, antimicrobial therapy, and management of complications: a statement for healthcare professionals from the Committee on Rheumatic Fever, Endocarditis, and Kawasaki Disease, Council on Cardiovascular Disease in the Young, and the Councils on Clinical Cardiology, Stroke, and Cardiovascular Surgery and Anesthesia, American Heart Association, endorsed by the Infectious Diseases Society of America. Circulation 111:e394-e434, 2005.

Fowler VG Jr, Miro JM, Hoen B, et al: Staphylococcus aureus endocarditis: a consequence of medical progress. JAMA 293:3012-3021, 2005.

Houpikian P, Raoult D: Blood culture-negative endocarditis in a reference center: etiologic diagnosis of 348 cases. Medicine (Baltimore) 84:162-173, 2005.

PROSTHETIC VALVES

Most Commonly Implanted Prosthetic Heart Valves

BIOPROSTHETIC VALVES

- Stented bioprosthetic valves
  - Leaflets made from bovine pericardium or porcine aortic valve treated with a chemical preservative
  - Mounted on flexible plastic or titanium metal frame (stent) covered with synthetic fabric (sewing cuff); three stent posts (struts) further support the cusps
- Stentless bioprosthetic valve
  - Chemically treated porcine aortic valve and a portion of the aortic root reinforced with a pliable exterior cuff

MECHANICAL VALVES

- Hinged bileaflet D-shaped tilting disks made of pyrolytic carbon
- Housing made of a short hollow tube with a sewing cuff
- Previous designs included caged ball, caged disk, and tilting disk

HOMOGRAFTS

- Cryopreserved human aortic roots

TRANSCATHETER AORTIC VALVE IMPLANTATION

- Expandable stent housing a trileaflet pericardial tissue valve that is delivered percutaneously via a catheter for patients with severe aortic stenosis who are not open surgery candidates

Common Complications and Modes of Failure of Prosthetic Heart Valves

THROMBUS FORMATION

- May become a source of thromboemboli or become infected
- May hinder or entrap leaflets at hinge points in mechanical valves
- Thrombi usually form in the outflow side of bioprosthetic valves, filling up the concave aspect of the cusps

INFECTION

- Infection at the sewing ring may progress to ring abscess, leading to valve dehiscence or paravalvular leak
- Infection of bioprosthetic valve cusps may be bacterial or fungal

PANNUS OVERGROWTH

- Fibrous tissue overgrowth from the sewing ring extends to valvular cusps, resulting in stiff thickened cusps, commissural fusion, and stenosis
- Retraction of cusps results in insufficiency

PARAVALVULAR LEAK

- Early leaks are complications arising from suturing technique or separation from an annulus with calcification or infection
- Late paravalvular leak results from tissue retraction during healing

STRUCTURAL DETERIORATION

- Most frequent cause of failure in bioprosthetic valves
  - Mineralization of tissue valves causes stiffening and often tearing of cusps
  - Connective tissue matrix degradation leads to cuspal tears and perforations or cuspal stretching
  - Tears also occur at flexure sites and at attachment sites to the stent and stent posts
- Fracture of metallic components of mechanical valves rarely occurs

PEARLS

- *Most patients with bioprosthetic valves do not require lifetime anticoagulation, but valves wear out or become stenotic with mineralization and pannus overgrowth*
- *Mechanical valves are more durable but require anticoagulation*
- *Homografts are efficient in terms of hemodynamics and usually do not require prolonged anticoagulation but are of limited availability and require more demanding surgical technique; no homograft valves are available for mitral position*
- *Ross procedure is advantageous in children with congenital heart disease; this technique uses the patient's pulmonic valve and pulmonary trunk (autograft) to replace the aortic valve and aortic root with a homograft implanted in the pulmonary position*

SELECTED REFERENCES

Schoen FJ: Pathology of bioprostheses and other tissue heart valve replacements. In Silver MD (ed): Cardiovascular Pathology, 2nd ed. New York, Churchill Livingstone, 1991, pp 1547-1606.

Silver MD, Wilson GJ: Pathology of mechanical heart valve prostheses and vascular grafts made of artificial materials. In Silver MD (ed): Cardiovascular Pathology, 2nd ed. New York, Churchill Livingstone, 1991, pp 1487-1546.

MYXOMA

Clinical Features

- Most common primary cardiac tumor in adults
- Clinical manifestations include constitutional symptoms, an embolic phenomenon, and valvular stenosis
- Sporadic tumors more prevalent in women; peak incidence in fifth decade
- Familial tumors often present earlier, with equal sex distribution and more frequent right atrial or multiple site involvement

Gross Pathology

- Most frequently found in the left atrium attached to the fossa ovalis but may be found in any cardiac chamber and sometimes attached to valves
- Usually pedunculated with short stalk; rarely sessile
- Varies from a soft, gelatinous, papillary mass to a firm, smooth mass (Figure 18-11A)
- Cut surface shows a variegated appearance, frequently with areas of hemorrhage and cyst formation
- Calcification may be focal or extensive

Histopathology

- Tumor is composed of polygonal, bipolar, or stellate myxoma or lepidic cells that have round to oval nuclei with inconspicuous nucleoli, eosinophilic cytoplasm, and indistinct borders (Figure 18-11B)
- Cells may be scattered singly, aggregate in small nests or cords, or form rings surrounding vascular channels
- Minimal pleomorphism and mitoses
- Background typically consists of myxoid and loose fibrous tissue with scattered lymphocytic and histiocytic infiltrate, especially hemosiderin-laden macrophages
- Surface thrombus may be identified
- Rarely, ossification and mucinous glands may be seen

Special Stains and Immunohistochemistry

- Reactive with calretinin, vimentin, CD34, and α_1-antichymotrypsin

Other Techniques for Diagnosis

- Noncontributory

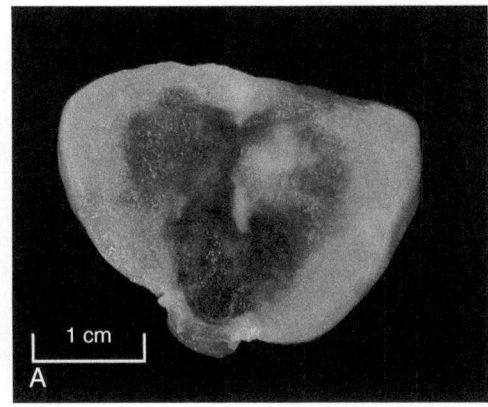
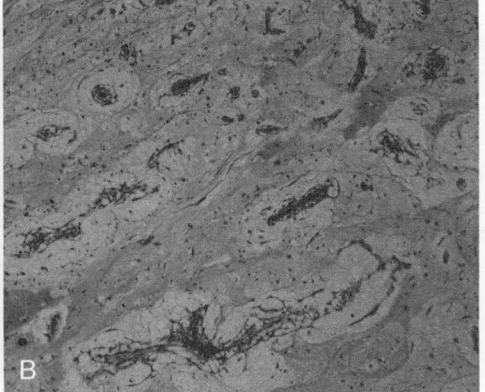

Figure 18-11. Cardiac myxoma. A, Gross photograph of a myxoma with a smooth outer surface and a short pedicle. Cut surface is myxoid with areas of hemorrhage. **B,** The histologic section shows concentrically arranged layers of elongated neoplastic (lepidic) cells around blood vessels and cords of tumor cells in abundant eosinophilic stroma.

Differential Diagnosis

ORGANIZED THROMBUS

- Hypocellular fibrous endocardial tumors or organized intravascular thrombi
- Spindle mesenchymal cells are not arranged in cords, nests, or ring structures
- Base of endocardial lesions does not contain the lymphocytic infiltrates or prominent thick-walled vessels that are often present in myxoma
- Differentiation between thromboembolus and myxoma embolus may not be possible at times

MYXOID SARCOMAS

- Most cardiac sarcomas are also found in the left atrium and often have myxoid stroma
- Foci of atypical spindle cells with nuclear pleomorphism, hypercellularity, and increased mitotic activity
- Tumor cells do not form cords or ring structures around blood vessels
- Tumor cells often exhibit a storiform growth pattern with arborizing vessels

PAPILLARY FIBROELASTOMA

- Typically located on valves
- Soft and papillary tumors can be grossly misdiagnosed as myxoma but are readily distinguished from myxoma on histology

PEARLS

- *Neoplastic nature is supported by demonstration of chromosomal abnormalities and aneuploidy*
- *Villous or papillary surface is associated with embolic events*
- *Tumor production of interleukin-6 is correlated with constitutional symptoms, including fever, weight loss, and fatigue*
- *Surgical excision is curative; recurrence is more frequent in familial tumors*
- *Some familial myxomas are manifestations of Carney complex (myxomas at various sites, endocrine tumors, and spotty pigmentation of the skin)*

SELECTED REFERENCES

Acebo E, Val-Bernal JF, Gomez-Roman JJ, Revuelta JM: Clinicopathologic study and DNA analysis of 37 cardiac myxomas: a 28-year experience. Chest 123:1379-1385, 2003.

Burke AP, Virmani R: Cardiac myxoma: a clinicopathologic study. Am J Clin Pathol 100:671-680, 1993.

Dewald GW, Dahl RJ, Spurbeck JL, et al: Chromosomally abnormal clones and non-random telomeric translocations in cardiac myxomas. Mayo Clin Proc 62:558-567, 1987.

RHABDOMYOMA

Clinical Features

- Benign congenital cardiac tumor believed to be a hamartoma
- Most common cardiac tumor in infancy and childhood; most are found in infants aged 1 year or younger
- Usually occurs in patients with tuberous sclerosis but may be sporadic or arise in patients with structural congenital heart disease
- Symptoms related to tuberous sclerosis, fetal hydrops, congestive heart failure, arrhythmias, and intracardiac obstruction in the perinatal period

Gross Pathology

- White, solid, well-circumscribed nodules
- Multiple tumors can measure less than 0.1 cm
- Most often found in the interventricular septum or the left ventricle

Histopathology

- Well-circumscribed tumors composed of large, vacuolated, atypical myocytes with central nuclei and a thin peripheral rim of cytoplasm
- Radial cytoplasmic strands extending from the nucleus to the cell wall are responsible for the term *spider cells*
- Intervening clear cytoplasm contains abundant glycogen

Special Stains and Immunohistochemistry

- PAS highlights abundant glycogen content in cells
- Reactive with muscle markers desmin, smooth muscle actin, and myoglobin; also reactive with hamartin, tuberin, and ubiquitin

Other Techniques for Diagnosis

- Electron microscopy: intercalated disklike structures around the cell periphery with abundant glycogen and a decreased number of small mitochondria

Differential Diagnosis

GLYCOGEN STORAGE DISEASE (E.G., Pompe Disease)

- Myocytes show vacuolization owing to abundant cytoplasmic glycogen
- Involves the myocardium in a more diffuse manner; distinct tumor nodules are not seen

HISTIOCYTOID CARDIOMYOPATHY

- Cardiac hamartoma often manifesting as ventricular tachyarrhythmias or sudden death in infants and children
- Clusters of large round to oval cells with pale granular cytoplasm resembling histiocytes
- Ultrastructural studies show myocytes with proliferation of mitochondria, absence of T tubules, and few myofibrils

PEARLS

- *Tumors increase in size until 32 weeks of gestation and then regress progressively*
- *Multiple rhabdomyomas are associated with tuberous sclerosis in 50% to 80% of cases*
- *Cardiac rhabdomyomas may be the earliest marker of disease in tuberous sclerosis caused by mutations in TSC1, encoding the protein hamartin, and TSC2, encoding the protein tuberin*
- *Surgical excision is recommended only in patients with severe hemodynamic compromise or persistent arrhythmias*

SELECTED REFERENCES

Bader RS, Chitayat D, Kelly E, et al: Fetal rhabdomyoma: prenatal diagnosis, clinical outcome, and incidence of associated tuberous sclerosis complex. J Pediatr 143:620-624, 2003.

Becker AE: Primary heart tumors in the pediatric age group: a review of salient pathologic features relevant for clinicians. Pediatr Cardiol 21:317-323, 2000.

Burke AP, Virmani R: Cardiac rhabdomyoma: a clinicopathologic study. Mod Pathol 4: 70-74, 1991.

FIBROMA

Clinical Features

- Rare, benign, congenital cardiac tumor, probably a fibrous hamartoma
- Usually seen in infancy and childhood
- Clinical presentation is related to left ventricular outflow obstruction, ventricular dysfunction, and conduction disturbances, depending on the location and extent of tumor involvement
- Cardiomegaly is the most common radiologic finding

Gross Pathology

- Usually a single large mural lesion in the interventricular septum or left ventricular free wall
- Round, homogeneous mass of whorled, rubbery, white fibrous tissue
- May show circumscribed or infiltrative borders

Histopathology

- Cellular tumor consisting of spindle-shaped fibroblasts and mild to extensive stromal collagen deposition, commonly with elastic fibers
- Minimal pleomorphism and rare mitotic figures
- Often shows irregular, infiltrating margin
- Calcification is common
- Lymphocytic infiltrate around small vessels may be seen
- Tumor cellularity decreases with age, and collagen content increases with age

Special Stains and Immunohistochemistry

- Reactive with vimentin; may be focally reactive with smooth muscle actin

Other Techniques for Diagnosis

- Noncontributory

Differential Diagnosis

FIBROSARCOMA

- Frequent site of involvement is the left atrium
- May resemble a cellular fibroma in newborns and infants but contains more frequent mitoses

INFLAMMATORY PSEUDOTUMOR

- Rare cardiac tumor
- Less cellular mass showing a prominent mixed inflammatory cell infiltrate

PEARLS

- *Residual tumor after incomplete resection usually remains stable for years*
- *Spontaneous regression has been reported*

- *Occasional association with nevoid basal cell carcinoma syndrome (Gorlin-Goltz syndrome) manifesting with enlarged occipital circumference, odontogenic keratocysts of the jaws, epidermal cysts, rib anomalies, ovarian fibromas, and multiple basal cell carcinomas of the skin*

SELECTED REFERENCES

Burke AP, Rosado-de-Christenson M, Templeton PA, Virmani R: Cardiac fibroma: clinicopathologic correlates and surgical treatment. J Thorac Cardiovasc Surg 108:862-870, 1994.

Cho JM, Danielson GK, Puga FJ, et al: Surgical resection of ventricular cardiac fibromas: early and late results. Ann Thorac Surg 76:1929-1934, 2003.

Thomas-de-Montpreville V, Nottin R, Dulmet E, Serraf A: Heart tumors in children and adults: clinicopathological study of 59 patients from a surgical center. Cardiovasc Pathol 16:22-28, 2007.

PAPILLARY FIBROELASTOMA

Clinical Features

- Benign endocardial tumor that seldom causes symptoms and usually is an incidental finding on echocardiography or at autopsy
- Most commonly located on the aortic valve but can be found anywhere on any valve, endocardial surfaces, or chordae tendineae
- Right-sided papillary fibroelastomas are usually asymptomatic; left-sided tumors may present with symptoms of embolization or prolapse into coronary ostia
- Most commonly diagnosed in the fifth and sixth decades of life

Gross Pathology

- Typically small, frondlike, soft to fibrotic outgrowths that may be sessile or attached by a short stalk
- Soft polypoid lesions are best examined underwater to appreciate the papillary villous configuration of the tumor, which has been likened to a sea anemone
- May occasionally be multiple

Histopathology

- Branching papillary fronds composed of an avascular dense central core surrounded by a myxoid loose connective tissue stroma (Figure 18-12A)
- Papillae are covered by an endothelial cell lining
- Central core contains collagen and concentric aggregates of elastin

Special Stains and Immunohistochemistry

- Movat highlights elastic fibers and collagenous core (Figure 18-12B and C)

Other Techniques for Diagnosis

- Noncontributory

Differential Diagnosis

PAPILLARY MYXOMA

- Contains typical polygonal or stellate myxoma cells arranged in ringlike structures around vascular channels
- Usually attached to the atrial septum; rarely seen on valve surfaces
- Most do not contain elastic tissue

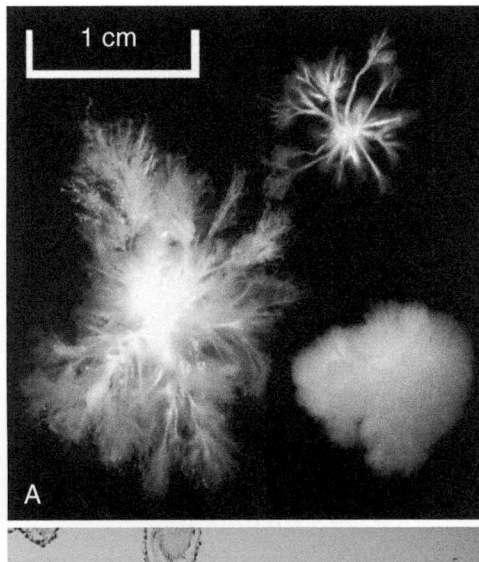

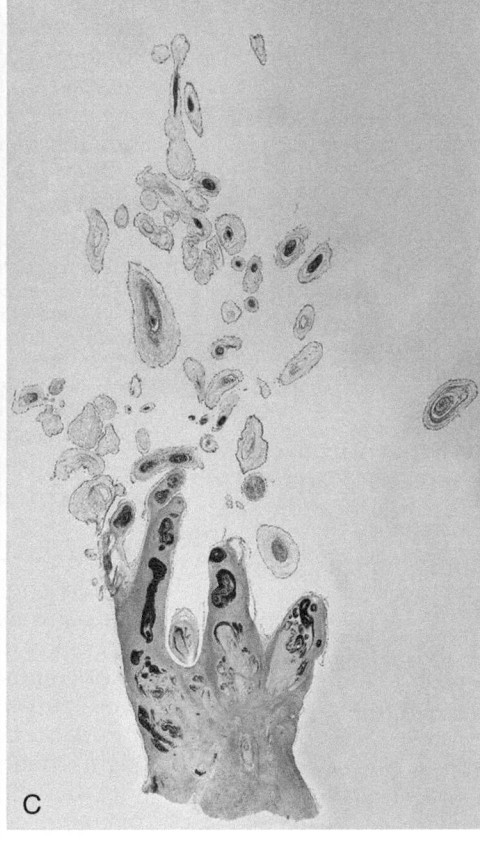

Figure 18-12. Papillary fibroelastoma. A, Gross photograph of papillary fibroelastomas shows delicate branching papillary structures best appreciated when examined under water. **B** and **C,** Movat-stained section shows a dense central core of collagen at the base. The papillary fronds consist of fibrous cores surrounded by concentric layers of elastic fibers. A thin myxoid layer rich in acid mucopolysaccharides and an overlying layer of endothelial cells surround the fibroelastic core.

LAMBL EXCRESCENCES

- Probably related to age, typically found in elderly patients
- Often multiple, usually smaller than 0.5 cm, and found on cardiac valves along the line of closure and nodule of Arantius
- Not seen on the arterial side of semilunar valves or on mural endocardium
- Characterized by broad-based filiform processes without a central stalk

PEARLS

- *Tumor resembles large Lambl excrescences, both grossly and microscopically*
- *Pathogenesis is unknown; suggested mechanisms are a reaction to prior endocardial damage, hamartomatous origin, and organizing thrombi*
- *Mobile tumors as detected on echocardiography are independent predictors of risk for embolic events and sudden cardiac death*
- *Surgical excision is curative*

SELECTED REFERENCES

Gowda RM, Khan IA, Nair CK, et al: Cardiac papillary fibroelastoma: a comprehensive analysis of 725 cases. Am Heart J 146:404-410, 2003.

Rubin MA, Snell JA, Tazelaar HD, et al: Cardiac papillary fibroelastoma: an immunohistochemical investigation and unusual clinical manifestations. Mod Pathol 8:402-407, 1995.

Sun JP, Asher CR, Yang XS, et al: Clinical and echocardiographic characteristics of papillary fibroelastomas: a retrospective and prospective study in 162 patients. Circulation 103:2687-2693, 2001.

CARDIAC SARCOMAS

Clinical Features

- Most common primary malignant tumors of the heart are sarcomas, representing about 95% of cases; the other 5% are hematologic malignancies (primarily non-Hodgkin lymphomas)
- Cardiac sarcomas include angiosarcoma, myxosarcoma, liposarcoma, fibrosarcoma, leiomyosarcoma, rhabdomyosarcoma, osteosarcoma, synovial sarcoma, neurofibrosarcoma, malignant mesenchymoma, and undifferentiated pleomorphic sarcoma
- Tumors are often asymptomatic until advanced stage
- Symptoms are related to intracavitary obstruction, embolic phenomena, local invasion causing arrhythmia, congestive heart failure, or pericardial effusion; constitutional symptoms are frequent
- Left atrium is commonly involved in most sarcomas
- Angiosarcoma
  - Most common primary malignant tumor of the heart
  - Characteristically located in the right-sided chambers, commonly originating from the right atrium
  - More common in males, with a peak incidence in the fourth decade
  - Patients often present with signs and symptoms of cardiac tamponade, pericardial constriction, right ventricular outflow obstruction, or pulmonary metastases
- Rhabdomyosarcoma
  - Occurs in infants, children, and young adults, with mean age at presentation in the second to third decade

- Slightly more common in males
- Can involve any chamber, with no predilection for left atrium

Gross Pathology

- Bulky, invasive masses that can have both intramural and intracavitary extension and epicardial infiltration
- Some tumors can have polypoid growth
- Tend to be multicentric
- Involvement of valvular structures by direct extension
- Firm cut surface with hemorrhages, cysts, or calcifications
- Angiosarcoma
  - Large, dark, multilobular hemorrhagic mass
  - May diffusely infiltrate local structures and pericardium
- Rhabdomyosarcoma
  - Can be found either in atrium or in ventricle
  - Soft, gray, bulky, invasive tumor that may appear myxoid or gelatinous

Histopathology

- Classified similar to soft tissue sarcomas (see Chapter 17)
- About 24% of primary cardiac sarcomas are unclassifiable and designated as undifferentiated pleomorphic sarcomas (malignant fibrous histiocytoma)
- Undifferentiated pleomorphic sarcomas are composed of epithelioid or small cells with marked cellular atypia (Figure 18-13)
- If the tumor is predominantly composed of pleomorphic spindle cells arranged in storiform pattern, the term undifferentiated pleomorphic spindle cell sarcoma may be used
- Myxofibrosarcomas are intermediate-grade tumors composed of spindle cells without marked atypia and with a fibrous or myxoid matrix
- Sarcomas with more than 10 mitoses per high-power field and tumors with necrosis are considered high grade

Special Stains and Immunohistochemistry

- Vimentin positive in undifferentiated pleomorphic sarcomas

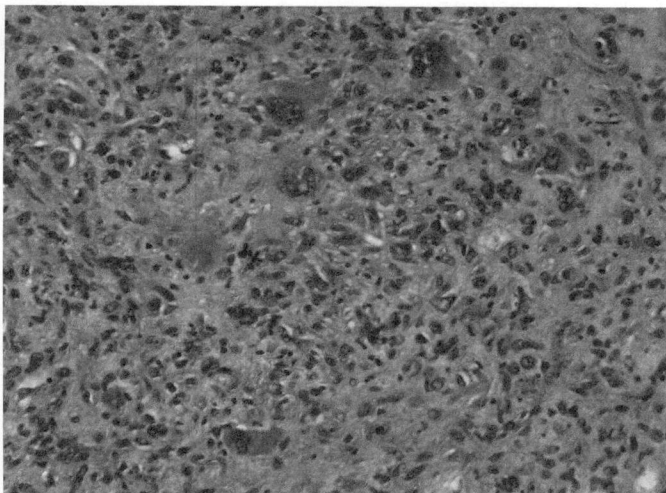

Figure 18-13. Undifferentiated pleomorphic sarcoma. A polypoid left atrial mass shows discohesive pleomorphic cells in a fibrous stroma with scattered giant cells.

- Smooth muscle actin and muscle-specific actin focally positive in undifferentiated pleomorphic sarcomas and myxofibrosarcomas, not specific for leiomyosarcoma
- CD34 and CD31 highlight endothelial cells
- Desmin highlights rhabdomyoblasts; also positive in some leiomyosarcomas
- Cytokeratin positive in epithelial cell component of synovial sarcoma
- S-100 focally positive in malignant peripheral nerve sheath tumors (neurofibrosarcoma)

Other Techniques for Diagnosis

- Synovial sarcoma: cytogenetic analysis for t(X;18) (p11.2;q11.2) chromosomal translocation

Differential Diagnosis

MYXOMA

- Lacks cellular pleomorphism and hypercellularity
- Absence of mitoses
- Absence of necrosis (groups of cells with neutrophilic infiltrate)
- Presence of capillary vessels surrounded by myxoma cells
- Chondroid differentiation not seen

PEARLS

- *Extensive sampling of tumor is important because some sarcomas can have hypocellular myxoid areas*
- *Prognosis for cardiac sarcomas is poor owing to advanced stage at presentation*
- *Reported survival rates at 1 and 3 years are 47% and 24%, respectively*
- *Histologic type and presence of differentiation do not correlate well with prognosis*
- *Surgical approach ranges from open biopsy to complete resection to tumor debulking*

SELECTED REFERENCES

Bakaeen FG, Reardon MJ, Coselli JS, et al: Surgical outcome in 85 patients with primary cardiac tumors. Am J Surg 186:641-647, 2003.
Burke AP, Cowan D, Virmani R: Primary sarcomas of the heart. Cancer 69:387-395, 1992.
Burke AP, Virmani R: Tumors of the Heart and Great Vessels. Atlas of Tumor Pathology, 3rd Series, Fascicle 16. Washington, DC, Armed Forces Institute of Pathology, 1996, pp 127-170.
Tazelaar HD, Locke TJ, McGregor CG: Pathology of surgically excised primary cardiac tumors. Mayo Clin Proc 67:957-965, 1992.

PERICARDIUM

ACUTE PERICARDITIS

Clinical Features

- Patients present with chest pain, pericardial friction rub, electrocardiographic changes, and constitutional symptoms

Gross Pathology

- Fibrinous and serofibrinous pericarditis are most common and cause a dry, dull, roughened pericardial surface with fibrinous adhesions

- Variable type and amount of effusion in pericardial sac, including serous, fibrinous, purulent, bloody, and caseous accumulations, depending on cause

Histopathology

- Histology generally not helpful in determining underlying cause
- Inflammatory cell infiltrates with neutrophils and lymphocytes, proliferation of capillaries, edema, and fibrin deposition

Special Stains and Immunohistochemistry

- Special stains for microorganisms (GMS, PAS, Ziehl-Neelsen) may identify causative organisms in infectious cases

Other Techniques for Diagnosis

- Noncontributory

Differential Diagnosis

- Etiology of pericarditis: Idiopathic, viral infection, acute myocardial infarction, Dressler syndrome, uremia, bacterial infection (tuberculous and nontuberculous), chest irradiation, rheumatic fever, connective tissue diseases (rheumatoid arthritis, SLE, scleroderma), trauma, drugs, and neoplasms

PEARLS

- *Normal pericardium is a fibroelastic tissue lined by mesothelium*
- *Normal pericardial sac contains 15 to 50 mL of clear, straw-colored fluid*
- *Acute pericarditis that subsides in a few days is most often idiopathic*
- *Hemorrhagic effusions are often caused by malignancy and infection*

SELECTED REFERENCES

Klein AL, Abbara S, Agler DA, et al: American Society of Echocardiography clinical recommendations for multimodality cardiovascular imaging of patients with pericardial disease: endorsed by the society for cardiovascular magnetic resonance and society of cardiovascular computed tomography. J Am Soc Echocardiogr 26:965-1012, 2013.

Waller BF, Taliercio CP, Howard J, et al: Morphologic aspects of pericardial heart disease: part I. Clin Cardiol 15:203-209, 1992.

Waller BF, Taliercio CP, Howard J, et al: Morphologic aspects of pericardial heart disease: part II. Clin Cardiol 15:291-298, 1992.

Zayas R, Anguita M, Torres F, et al: Incidence of specific etiology and role of methods for specific etiologic diagnosis of primary acute pericarditis. Am J Cardiol 75:378-382, 1995.

CONSTRICTIVE PERICARDITIS

Clinical Features

- Idiopathic in about half of cases
- A restrictive or constrictive clinical picture, with biventricular equalization of pressures, elevated jugular venous pressure, and significantly decreased cardiac output
- Effect on ventricular contraction may be mild to marked, depending on degree of constriction
- Enlarged congested liver or hypoperfused lungs may be seen

Gross Pathology

- Significant fibrous thickening of pericardium, with or without calcification
- Dense pericardial adhesions with obliteration of pericardial space

Histopathology

- Marked fibrosis, associated calcifications, neovascularization, and mild chronic lymphoplasmacytic cell infiltrate
- Hemosiderin-laden macrophages may be seen
- Occasional granulomas in constrictive tuberculous pericarditis

Special Stains and Immunohistochemistry

- Noncontributory

Other Techniques for Diagnosis

- Noncontributory

Differential Diagnosis

- Most common identifiable causes include Chest irradiation and previous cardiac surgery; classically caused by tuberculosis

PEARLS

- *Histology is generally not helpful in differentiating among underlying causes*
- *Occasional patients with clinically constrictive physiology will have pericardial biopsy showing no fibrosis or calcification*

SELECTED REFERENCES

Myers RB, Spodick DH: Constrictive pericarditis: clinical and pathophysiologic characteristics. Am Heart J 138:219-232, 1999.

Oh KY, Shimizu M, Edwards WD, et al: Surgical pathology of the parietal pericardium: a study of 344 cases (1993-1999). Cardiovasc Pathol 10:157-168, 2001.

PERICARDIAL CYSTS

Clinical Features

- Asymptomatic except when large; chest pain is the most common symptom
- Often found incidentally on chest radiographs
- Most commonly located in the cardiophrenic angle but may also be seen in the any of the mediastinal compartments

Gross Pathology

- Thin-walled, uniloculated cysts with smooth lining and filled with clear fluid
- Typically small but may vary in size and weigh up to 300 g
- May occasionally communicate with the pericardial sac

Histopathology

- Cyst wall composed of fibrous connective tissue and lined by a layer of flattened mesothelial cells

Special Stains and Immunohistochemistry

- Noncontributory

Other Techniques for Diagnosis

- Noncontributory

Differential Diagnosis

LOCULATED EFFUSION

- Does not have a cyst wall with lining

BRONCHOGENIC CYST

- Most commonly found in the anterior or middle mediastinum, may be intracardiac or intrapericardial
- Contains mucoid material
- Lined by pseudostratified ciliated columnar cells with smooth muscle and cartilage in the wall

PEARLS

- *Pericardial cysts are considered congenital lesions but are diagnosed in adulthood*

SELECTED REFERENCES

Patel J, Park C, Michaels J, et al: Pericardial cyst: case reports and a literature review. Echocardiography 21:269-272, 2004.

Wick MR: Cystic lesions of the mediastinum. Semin Diagn Pathol 22:241-253, 2005.

LOCALIZED FIBROUS TUMOR OF THE PERICARDIUM

Clinical Features

- Extremely rare benign pericardial tumor
- Often are incidental findings; some patients present with dyspnea and pericardial effusion

Gross Pathology

- May be broad based or attached to the pericardium by a stalk; rarely, arise from the epicardium and encase the heart
- Round to ovoid, white, well-circumscribed mass with a firm, whorled cut surface
- Cystic change may be seen
- No invasion into the myocardium

Histopathology

- Consists of patternless proliferation or short fascicles of spindled fibroblasts with thick collagen bundles
- Alternating hypocellular and hypercellular areas
- Hemangiopericytoma-like vascular pattern
- Minimal pleomorphism, mitotic activity, and necrosis
- May have focal calcification

Special Stains and Immunohistochemistry

- Vimentin and CD34 positive
- Cytokeratin, actin, and S-100 negative

Other Techniques for Diagnosis

- Noncontributory

Differential Diagnosis

SARCOMATOID MESOTHELIOMA

- Invasion of underlying tissue
- Presence of marked nuclear pleomorphism and hyperchromasia
- Negative for CD34

PEARLS

- *Surgical excision is usually curative*

SELECTED REFERENCES

Andreani SM, Tavecchio L, Giardini R, Bedini AV: Extrapericardial solitary fibrous tumour of the pericardium. Eur J Cardiothorac Surg 14:98-100, 1998.

el-Naggar AK, Ro JY, Ayala AG, et al: Localized fibrous tumor of the serosal cavities: immunohistochemical, electron-microscopic, and flow-cytometric DNA study. Am J Clin Pathol 92:561-565, 1989.

PRIMARY MALIGNANT TUMORS OF THE PERICARDIUM

Clinical Features

- Clinical findings of dyspnea, constrictive pericarditis, pericardial effusion, and cardiac tamponade are frequent
- Male predominance
- Pericardial mesothelioma
  - Represents less than 2% of malignant mesotheliomas of serosal membranes
  - May be localized or diffuse
  - Male predominance
- Pericardial angiosarcoma
  - Less common than primary angiosarcoma of the heart

Gross Pathology

- Tumors are found in the parietal and visceral pericardium (epicardium) as coalescent nodules that obliterate the pericardial space and may diffusely encase the heart and great vessels
- Pericardial mesothelioma
  - Solitary or localized mesothelioma is rare
  - Usually invades the heart only superficially
- Pericardial angiosarcoma
  - Invades the myocardium, and in one fourth of cases, intracavitary extension is seen

Histopathology

PERICARDIAL MESOTHELIOMA

- Epithelioid, sarcomatoid, and mixed types have all been reported
- Histology similar to mesothelioma of pleura and peritoneum

PERICARDIAL ANGIOSARCOMA

- Anastomosing vascular channels lined by atypical endothelial cells with abundant mitotic activity and areas of necrosis
- Solid areas of epithelioid anaplastic cells or spindle cells are often present

Special Stains and Immunohistochemistry

- Reticulin stain highlights a vascular pattern in angiosarcoma
- CK5/6, calretinin, WT-1, HBME-1, thrombomodulin, mesothelin, podoplanin, D2-40, and h-caldesmon are considered positive markers in mesothelioma
- CD31, CD34, and von Willebrand factor are positive in angiosarcoma

Other Techniques for Diagnosis

- Pericardial mesothelioma
  - Electron microscopy: numerous long, slender, smooth microvilli on cellular surface and intracellular and intercellular lumens with a length-to-diameter ratio greater than 10 in epithelioid mesothelioma; epithelial differentiation of sarcomatoid mesotheliomas includes presence of intercellular junctions, surface microvilli, tonofilaments, and basal lamina formation
- Pericardial angiosarcoma
  - Electron microscopy: vasoformative structures and Weibel-Palade bodies

Differential Diagnosis

METASTATIC ADENOCARCINOMA

- A panel of positive markers for adenocarcinomas arising from different sites (thyroid transcription factor-1, carcinoembryonic antigen, Leu-M1, MOC-31, BG-8, B72.3, Ber-EP4, and CA19-9) can be used in the evaluation of malignant pericardial tumors

EPITHELIOID ANGIOSARCOMA VERSUS MESOTHELIOMA

- Epithelioid angiosarcoma shows strong and diffuse reactivity for vimentin and absent to weak staining with cytokeratin
- Mesotheliomas will have more intense staining with cytokeratin and less intense vimentin staining
- Additional immunohistochemical stains (see "Special Stains and Immunohistochemistry") can establish the diagnosis in most instances

PEARLS

- *No definite association has been found between asbestos exposure and pericardial mesothelioma*
- *Pericardial mesothelioma may spread to adjacent pleura, mediastinum, diaphragm, and lymph nodes but rarely presents with distant metastases*
- *In advanced disease, differentiation between primary cardiac and pericardial angiosarcoma may not be possible*

SELECTED REFERENCES

Lin BT, Colby T, Gown AM, et al: Malignant vascular tumors of the serous membranes mimicking mesothelioma: a report of 14 cases. Am J Surg Pathol 20:1431-1439, 1996.

Suster S, Moran CA: Applications and limitations of immunohistochemistry in the diagnosis of malignant mesothelioma. Adv Anat Pathol 13:316-329, 2006.

Thomason R, Schlegel W, Lucca M, et al: Primary malignant mesothelioma of the pericardium: case report and literature review. Tex Heart Inst J 21:170-174, 1994.

Val-Bernal JF, Figols J, Gomez-Roman JJ: Incidental localized (solitary) epithelial mesothelioma of the pericardium: case report and literature review. Cardiovasc Pathol 11:181-185, 2002.

METASTATIC TUMORS OF THE HEART AND PERICARDIUM

Clinical Features

- Twenty to 40 times more common than primary tumors of the heart
- Signs and symptoms vary but include dyspnea on exertion, cough, chest pain, pericardial effusion, and conduction abnormalities
- Most commonly develop through lymphatic spread from primary epithelial tumors (lung and breast) in the thoracic cavity and usually metastasize to the pericardium
- Hematogenous spread occurs from melanoma, leukemia, sarcoma, and renal cell carcinoma and shows small myocardial metastases
- Intracavitary extension from the inferior vena cava into the right atrium most commonly occurs with renal cell carcinoma and hepatocellular carcinoma

Gross Pathology

- Metastatic tumors most commonly involve the pericardium
- In the heart, lesions are commonly found as epicardial and myocardial nodules or bulky intracavitary masses
- Valves and endocardium are relatively spared

Histopathology

- Carcinomas, lymphomas, and leukemias, in descending order of frequency, are the most common histologic types of malignancy seen
- Melanoma also often metastasizes to the heart

Special Stains and Immunohistochemistry

- Identical to primary tumor

Other Techniques for Diagnosis

- Identical to primary tumor

Differential Diagnosis

- See "Primary Malignant Tumors of the Pericardium"

PEARLS

- *In children, common metastatic tumors include non-Hodgkin lymphoma, neuroblastoma, sarcomas, Wilms tumor, and hepatoma*
- *Clinical evidence of cardiac involvement by metastatic neoplasms is found in only about 10% of patients; most of the cardiac symptoms result from pericardial effusions and pericardial constriction*

SELECTED REFERENCES

Abraham KP, Reddy V, Gattuso P: Neoplasms metastatic to the heart: review of 3314 consecutive autopsies. Am J Cardiovasc Pathol 3: 195-198, 1990.

Butany J, Leong SW, Carmichael K, Komeda M: A 30-year analysis of cardiac neoplasms at autopsy. Can J Cardiol 21:675-680, 2005.

Chan HS, Sonley MJ, Moes CA, et al: Primary and secondary tumors of childhood involving the heart, pericardium, and great vessels: a report of 75 cases and review of the literature. Cancer 56:825-836, 1985.

Roberts WC: Primary and secondary neoplasms of the heart. Am J Cardiol 80:671-682, 1997.

BLOOD VESSELS

THE VASCULITIDES

- Widely used criteria for classification of vasculitis are those of the American College of Rheumatology and the Chapel Hill Consensus Conference on the Nomenclature of Systemic Vasculitis

- Classification criteria were developed for use in clinical trials and epidemiologic studies; they were not intended for use as diagnostic criteria
- Useful information for the classification of vasculitis includes
  - Size of predominant vessels involved
    - Large vessels include the aorta and its major branches
    - Medium vessels include muscular arteries and small arteries that can be observed with the naked eye or visualized by arteriography
    - Small vessels include small arteries, arterioles, capillaries, and postcapillary venules, vessels that are typically 500 μm or less
    - Overlap in the size of involved vessels is often observed, but predominant vessels involved usually produce the typical clinical manifestations
  - Demographic profile, particularly age group and ethnicity
  - Organ tropism
  - Immune complex deposition
  - Presence of antineutrophil cytoplasmic and antiglomerular basement membrane antibodies in serum
- Pathologic evaluation alone is usually insufficient and may not always be required to make a clinical diagnosis

LARGE-VESSEL VASCULITIS

Clinical Features

GIANT CELL ARTERITIS
- Frequently involves the aorta and its major branches
- More commonly found in older females; rare in blacks and Asians
- Patients present with a variety of symptoms, including fatigue, headaches, jaw claudication, diplopia, and vision loss; common cause of fever of unknown origin in elderly patients
- Often associated with polymyalgia rheumatica
- Aortic involvement results in aneurysms, less often leads to stenosis, and is clinically manifest in only a minority of patients
- End-organ ischemia may result from luminal stenosis or occlusion of extracranial branches of the external and internal carotid arteries and vertebral arteries; most commonly involves the temporal artery

TAKAYASU ARTERITIS
- Typically occurs in patients younger than 40 years with female predominance; worldwide distribution, but higher frequency in Japan, Southeast Asia, and India
- Involvement of the aorta and its major branches, with frequent involvement of the subclavian and carotid arteries; may also involve coronary, pulmonary, mesenteric, and renal arteries
- Patients often present with fever, malaise, arthralgia, myalgia, and weight loss
- Causes ischemic symptoms (pulselessness, claudication, and blindness), loss or asymmetry of pulses and blood pressure, bruits, renovascular hypertension, and sometimes aortic aneurysms

Gross Pathology

- Aortic aneurysms will show wrinkled intima with a tree-bark appearance, indistinct medial layer, and variably thickened adventitia
- Stenotic lesions show fibrous thickening of the vessel wall with reduction in the lumen caliber of the aorta and major arteries; thrombosis may occur

Histopathology

GIANT CELL ARTERITIS
- Characterized by focal granulomatous inflammation of large and medium-sized arteries (Figure 18-14A)

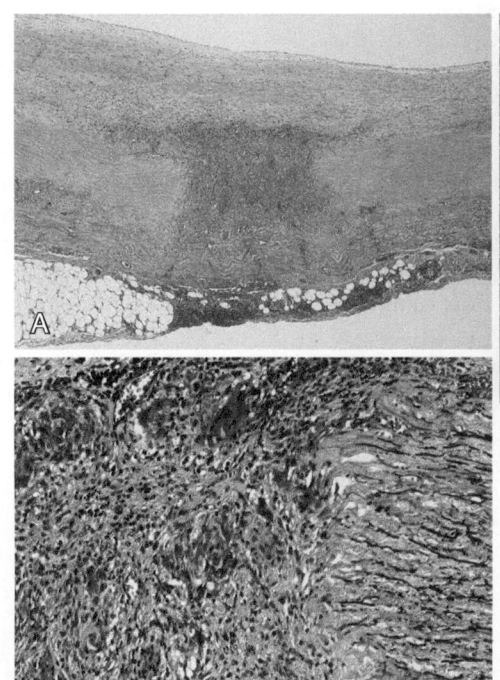
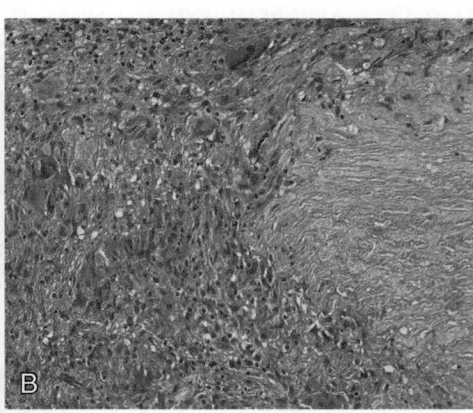

Figure 18-14. Giant cell aortitis. A, Aorta shows a central area of inflammation disrupting the media, which in turn is acellular. The areas of absent smooth muscle cells correspond to laminar necrosis. In addition, there is fibrointimal hyperplasia, adventitial fibrosis, and mononuclear inflammation. **B,** Numerous multinucleated giant cells are admixed with the lymphohistiocytic infiltrates. **C,** Movat stain shows elastic lamellae within the eosinophilic areas of laminar medial necrosis.

- In the aorta, areas of laminar medial necrosis surrounded by granulomatous inflammation are common; adventitial involvement by the inflammatory process is not common (Figure 18-14B and C)
- In temporal arteries, infiltrates are centered along the internal elastic lamina (Figure 18-15)
- Mixed inflammatory cell infiltrate consisting mainly of lymphocytes, plasma cells, and histiocytes with occasional neutrophils and eosinophils
- Giant cells are variably present, ranging from 44% to 100% of cases
- Healing or healed lesions show irregular fibrointimal proliferation, focal fibrosis, and scarring of the media and diminished inflammatory cell infiltrate

TAKAYASU ARTERITIS
- Variable inflammatory response, including a necrotizing acute inflammatory cell infiltrate, granulomatous inflammation with giant cells, or a chronic lymphocytic infiltrate
- Acute phase shows inflammation and neovascularization in the outer two thirds of media, adventitia, and adventitial fat
- Healing lesions may show minimal inflammatory component; often shows only medial scarring with focal loss of elastic lamellae and marked intimal and adventitial thickening and fibrosis

Special Stains and Immunohistochemistry
- Movat highlights the disrupted internal elastic lamina, aortic elastic lamellae, and fibrosis
- Trichrome demonstrates scarring in the vessel wall

Other Techniques for Diagnosis
- Noncontributory

Differential Diagnosis
GIANT CELL ARTERITIS AND TAKAYASU DISEASE
- Major discriminating clinical feature is the age of the patient; giant cell arteritis is common after 50 years, and Takayasu disease rarely occurs after 50 years

CHRONIC SCLEROTIC PHASE OF AORTITIS
- Healed phase of Takayasu or giant cell arteritis may not be diagnosed with certainty
- Other causes of inflammatory aortitis, including infectious (syphilitic) disease and rheumatologic diseases (rheumatoid arthritis, ankylosing spondylitis, relapsing polychondritis, SLE, Behçet disease, and sarcoidosis), need to be considered in the differential diagnosis with correlative clinical information necessary to arrive at a diagnosis

IgG4-RELATED AORTITIS/PERIAORTITIS
- Transmural dense lymphoplasmacytic infiltrate with occasional eosinophils
- Granulomas, giant cells, and prominent neutrophilic infiltrates are absent
- Moderate to severe adventitial fibrosis; obliterative phlebitis usually not observed
- IgG4+/IgG+ plasma cell ratio of >50% and >50 IgG4+ plasma cells/high power field are highly suggestive of IgG4-related aortitis

BEHÇET DISEASE
- Relapsing autoimmune disorder with recurrent oral and genital ulcers, eye and skin lesions commonly in young adult males
- Involves both large (aorta and pulmonary arteries) to small caliber arteries and veins
- Aortic aneurysm with arterial occlusion and aortitis similar to Takayasu arteritis may be seen
- Intense mixed inflammatory infiltrates with giant cells are described in the active stage associated with medial destruction
- Venous occlusion due to thrombophlebitis

AGE-RELATED CHANGES (ARTERIOSCLEROSIS)
- Concentric intimal thickening, fragmentation, and reduplication of the internal elastic lamina and foci of calcification may be seen in temporal arteries
- Lacks inflammatory cell component

PEARLS

- *Giant cell arteritis and Takayasu arteritis cannot always be confidently differentiated based on histopathologic features only*
- *Because of the frequent involvement of temporal arteries in giant cell arteritis,* temporal arteritis *has often been used interchangeably with* giant cell arteritis *in the literature; however,* giant cell arteritis *is the preferred term because not all patients with giant cell arteritis have temporal arteritis, and not all cases of temporal arteritis are caused by giant cell arteritis*

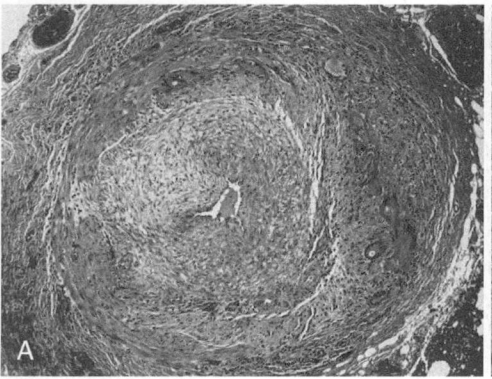
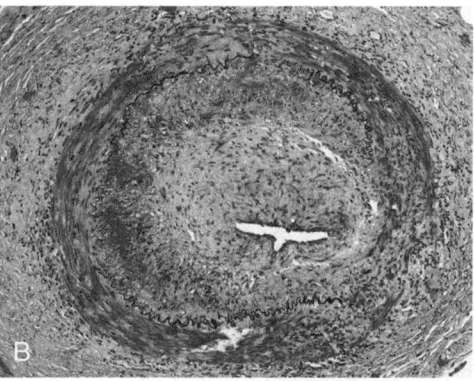

Figure 18-15. Giant cell arteritis. A, A temporal artery biopsy shows transmural granulomatous inflammation with giant cells in the media and adventitia of this muscular artery. **B,** Movat stain shows disruption of the internal elastic lamina in the areas with inflammation and marked intimal hyperplasia. Fibrinoid necrosis is occasionally observed.

- *Rate of positive temporal artery biopsies ranges between 10% and 20% of specimens; negative predictive value of temporal artery biopsy is about 90%*
- *Lesions of giant cell arteritis are typically segmental*
  - *At least three hematoxylin and eosin stained levels and one elastic stain of the temporal artery must be evaluated*
  - *Multiple sections of the aorta should be submitted*
- *Takayasu arteritis*
  - *Frequently diagnosed by clinical criteria and vascular imaging*
  - *Stenotic lesions are found in up to 98% of patients and aneurysms in 27%*
  - *Abdominal aorta is affected in about 40% of patients*
  - *Most common sites requiring surgical intervention are aortic arch and branch vessels*
- *Isolated aortitis*
  - *Most often discovered after surgical resection of ascending aortic aneurysms*
  - *Histopathologic features similar to those of giant cell aortitis, but patients lack evidence of systemic disease*
  - *Favorable outcome even without medical therapy*

SELECTED REFERENCES

Deshpande V, Zen Y, Chan JK, et al: Consensus statement on the pathology of IgG4-related disease. Mod Pathol 25:1181-1192, 2012.

Genereau T, Lortholary O, Pottier MA, et al: Temporal artery biopsy: a diagnostic tool for systemic necrotizing vasculitis. French Vasculitis Study Group. Arthritis Rheum 42:2674-2681, 1999.

Jennette JC, Falk RJ, Bacon PA, et al: 2012 revised International Chapel Hill Consensus Conference Nomenclature of Vasculitides. Arthritis Rheum 65:1-11, 2013.

Miller DV, Isotalo PA, Weyand CM, et al: Surgical pathology of noninfectious ascending aortitis: a study of 45 cases with emphasis on an isolated variant. Am J Surg Pathol 30:1150-1158, 2006.

MEDIUM-VESSEL VASCULITIS

Clinical Features

POLYARTERITIS NODOSA (PAN)

- Idiopathic systemic disease characterized by vasculitis involving medium-sized and small muscular arteries
- Most patients are in the fourth to sixth decades; male-to-female ratio is 2:1
- Patients usually have nonspecific systemic symptoms of weight loss and fever with focal symptoms in the specific organ involved (peripheral neuropathy, testicular pain, livedo reticularis, myalgias, and gastrointestinal infarction)
- Associated with deposition of circulating immune complexes in hepatitis B infection
- May become manifest in the course of hairy cell leukemia, rheumatoid arthritis, and Sjögren syndrome
- Arteriography detects aneurysms or occlusions of visceral arteries; commonly involved vessels are renal, coronary, hepatic, and mesenteric arteries; lung involvement (bronchial arteries) in up to 30% of patients

KAWASAKI DISEASE (MUCOCUTANEOUS LYMPH NODE SYNDROME, INFANTILE PAN)

- Acute self-limited disease typically affects infants and children (range, 6 months to 15 years; peaks at 13 to 24 months)

- Increased incidence in Japan and Korea
- In the United States, children of American Asian and Pacific Island origin have higher incidence compared with African American and white children
- Clinical criteria include fever for at least 5 days and at least four of the following clinical features: conjunctival injection, cervical lymphadenopathy, oral mucosal changes, polymorphous rash, and swelling or redness of the extremities
- Typically affects coronary arteries, but any muscular artery may be involved; subclavian, axillary, iliac, femoral, renal, and superior mesenteric artery involvement has been observed

Gross Pathology

PAN

- Tendency to occur at arterial branching sites
- Aneurysms or stenosis of the arteries may be seen
- Thrombosis is common

KAWASAKI DISEASE

- Coronary ectasia or aneurysm can be seen in the acute stage
- Regression of aneurysms is seen in half of the cases within 1 to 2 years
- Progression of aneurysms to stenotic lesions occurs in about 10%

Histopathology

PAN

- Lesions are usually in various stages of development
- Acute injury is characterized by transmural inflammation with focal segmental destruction of the wall and deposition of amorphous eosinophilic material (fibrinoid necrosis) (Figure 18-16)
- Inflammation is initially neutrophilic but later is composed predominantly of lymphocytes and macrophages
- Healing lesions consist of granulation tissue within the vessel wall and may show luminal narrowing owing to thrombosis or fibrointimal proliferation

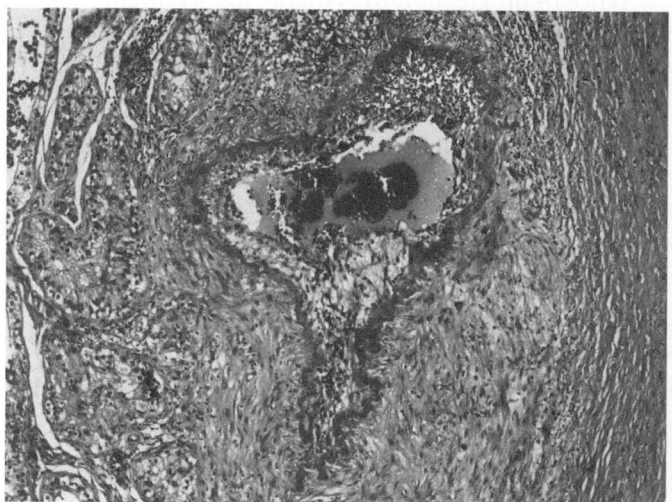

Figure 18-16. Necrotizing arteritis. A testicular muscular-type artery shows fibrinoid necrosis with focal transmural acute inflammation.

- Aneurysms and pseudoaneurysms may develop owing to weakening of the vessel wall

KAWASAKI DISEASE

- Inflammation consisting of lymphocytes and macrophages is first seen in the intima and adventitia, then progresses into the media
- Panarteritis is associated with neutrophilic infiltration, disruption of the internal elastic lamina, smooth muscle degeneration, and edema in the media
- Healed lesions show fibrointimal proliferation, recanalization, thinning of the media, destruction of the internal elastic lamina, and fibrosis in the adventitia

Special Stains and Immunohistochemistry

- Elastic highlights destruction of the elastic lamina
- Trichrome stains fibrin red
- Movat highlights both elastin and collagen

Other Techniques for Diagnosis

- Noncontributory

Differential Diagnosis

PAN

- Isolated or single-organ vasculitis
  - Often an unexpected finding in surgical specimens resected for inflammatory processes or mass lesions
  - Isolated vasculitis has been reported from the gastrointestinal tract, gallbladder, appendix, breast, uterus, ovary, and testis
  - Although the histologic features are similar to those of PAN, use of PAN in the diagnosis is discouraged because it can be misleading
  - Necrotizing or granulomatous inflammation of the vessels can be present
  - Cured with resection and does not require systemic therapy
  - May be the first manifestation of a systemic vasculitis; clues to systemic disease include the presence of systemic symptoms, acute-phase reactants, and serologic autoimmune markers
  - Long-term follow-up is necessary to confirm the absence of progression to systemic involvement
- Kawasaki disease
  - Fibrinoid necrosis is absent, and inflamed media is edematous
  - Predominance of mononuclear cells (T lymphocytes and macrophages) rather than neutrophils in the acute phase
- Small-vessel vasculitis
  - If involvement of only small arteries is seen in a biopsy, differentiation between medium-vessel and small-vessel vasculitis cannot be made accurately because small arteries can be affected in both conditions
- Vasculitis associated with connective tissue disorders
  - Most commonly arises in the setting of rheumatoid arthritis, SLE, or Sjögren syndrome and is correlated with disease activity
  - May involve vessels of any size; small-vessel involvement predominates
  - Clinically manifest with cutaneous or visceral organ involvement (usually renal or gastrointestinal)

- Cholesterol atheroembolism
  - Can present with multiorgan involvement including renal failure, tissue necrosis, or visceral organ infarction
  - Cholesterol emboli derived from ulcerated plaques in the aorta often affect the kidneys, intestines, and extremities
  - Embolization can occur spontaneously but is often triggered by invasive procedures, cardiovascular surgery, anticoagulation, and thrombolytic therapy
  - Occlusion of small arteries and arterioles by cholesterol emboli; cholesterol crystals induce foreign-body giant cell reaction and variable infiltrates of neutrophils, eosinophils, and mononuclear cells
- Segmental mediolytic arteriopathy
  - Presence of visceral ischemia, intra-abdominal hemorrhage, and multiple arterial aneurysms is usually mistaken for PAN
  - Abrupt gaps in the arterial wall due to loss of medial smooth muscle; gaps are bridged by fibrin deposits and hemorrhage
  - Vacuolar degeneration of smooth muscle cells results in intramural hemorrhage and dissection
  - Inflammation if present is minimal and limited to the adventitial fibrinous deposits

PEARLS

- *PAN*
  - *Involvement of arterioles, venules, or capillaries (including pulmonary capillaritis and glomerulonephritis) is not consistent with a diagnosis of PAN as proposed in the Chapel Hill Consensus Conference*
  - *Classic PAN is not associated with antineutrophil cytoplasmic antibodies (ANCA)*
  - *Fibrinoid necrosis should not be equated with PAN*
  - *Most patients have a chronic relapsing course; high-dose corticosteroids and often cyclophosphamide are typically beneficial*
  - *Factors associated with a poor prognosis include age greater than 50 years and gastrointestinal, renal, or cardiac involvement*
  - *Five-year survival rate approaches 80% in treated patients; often fatal if untreated*
- *Kawasaki disease*
  - *Diagnosis is usually based on clinical criteria rather than tissue biopsy or angiography*
  - *Coronary artery aneurysm develops in 15% to 25% of untreated cases; male patients, infants younger than 6 months of age, children older than 8 years, patients who did not receive intravenous immunoglobulin treatment or who have persistent fever despite treatment are at highest risk for this complication*
  - *Giant aneurysms (diameter of coronary lumen > 8 mm) are at risk for rupture in the acute phase and become stenotic with progressive intimal hyperplasia and thrombosis in the chronic phase*

SELECTED REFERENCES

Colmegna I, Maldonado-Cocco JA: Polyarteritis nodosa revisited. Curr Rheumatol Rep 7: 288-296, 2005.

Kato H, Sugimura T, Akagi T, et al: Long-term consequences of Kawasaki disease: a 10- to 21-year follow-up study of 594 patients. Circulation 94:1379-1385, 1996.

Lightfoot RW Jr, Michel BA, Bloch DA, et al: The American College of Rheumatology 1990 criteria for the classification of polyarteritis nodosa. Arthritis Rheum 33:1088-1093, 1990.

Newburger JW, Takahashi M, Gerber MA, et al: Diagnosis, treatment, and long-term management of Kawasaki disease: a statement for health professionals from the Committee on Rheumatic Fever, Endocarditis and Kawasaki Disease, Council on Cardiovascular Disease in the Young, American Heart Association. Circulation 110:2747-2771, 2004.

Takahashi K, Oharaseki T, Naoe S, et al: Neutrophilic involvement in the damage to coronary arteries in acute stage of Kawasaki disease. Pediatr Int 47:305-310, 2005.

PAUCI-IMMUNE SMALL-VESSEL VASCULITIS

Clinical Features

GRANULOMATOSIS WITH POLYANGIITIS, FORMERLY WEGENER GRANULOMATOSIS (GPA)

- Syndrome characterized by a necrotizing granulomatous vasculitis involving the upper and lower respiratory tract and glomerulonephritis
  - Head and neck involvement includes the nose, middle ear, eyes, sinuses, and subglottis, with symptoms of sinusitis, rhinitis, proptosis, septal perforation, or airway stenosis
  - Pulmonary manifestations include cough, hemoptysis, cavitary nodular densities, and lung infiltrates
  - Renal disease characterized by hematuria and proteinuria; occasionally renal failure
- Typically affects individuals in their fifth and sixth decades, with equal male-to-female distribution
- Strong association with ANCA
  - Autoantibodies directed against components of neutrophil granules and monocytes lysosomes
  - c-ANCA (cytoplasmic): antiproteinase-3 antibodies; present in up to 90% of cases
  - p-ANCA (perinuclear): antimyeloperoxidase antibodies; nonspecific; found in 5% to 10% of cases
  - Up to 20% of patients are negative for ANCA, especially those with the limited form of the disease confined to the respiratory tract or the eye

EOSINOPHILIC GRANULOMATOSIS WITH POLYANGIITIS, FORMERLY CHURG-STRAUSS SYNDROME (EGPA)

- Systemic necrotizing vasculitis associated with severe asthma, peripheral blood and tissue eosinophilia, extravascular granulomas, and multiple organ involvement
- Typically diagnosed in middle age, with slight male predominance
- Symptoms of allergic disease, eosinophilia, and systemic vasculitis usually do not occur simultaneously, and time interval between asthma and vasculitis is variable
- Affects multiple organ systems
  - Pulmonary infiltrates often noted on radiography; granulomatous pulmonary mass lesions and capillaritis causing alveolar hemorrhage more unusual in EGPA than in GPA or microscopic polyangiitis
  - Mononeuritis multiplex, polyneuropathy, and central nervous system vasculitis

- Nodules on extensor surfaces of joints; rash and palpable purpura on the lower extremities
- Cardiac involvement is a significant cause of mortality; may be complicated by small coronary artery vasculitis and myocardial ischemia, mural thrombosis, endomyocardial fibrosis, cardiomyopathy, and acute or constrictive pericarditis
- Gastrointestinal symptoms are related to eosinophilic gastroenteritis and mesenteric artery vasculitis
- Kidneys are affected in one fourth of patients
- Associated with p-ANCA in 40% to 60% of cases and less commonly with c-ANCA (10%)
- ANCA-positive patients tend to have glomerulonephritis, pulmonary hemorrhage, and peripheral neuropathy; ANCA-negative patients manifest with cardiac involvement

MICROSCOPIC POLYANGIITIS (MPA)

- Syndrome characterized by necrotizing small-vessel vasculitis with few or no immune deposits affecting arterioles, venules, and capillaries in the skin, kidneys, and lungs (glomeruli and pulmonary capillaries)
- Mean age of onset is 50 years, with slight male predominance
- Symptoms are nonspecific and include hemoptysis, hematuria, proteinuria, palpable purpura, neuropathy, myalgias, and arthralgias
- Serum-positive p-ANCA is characteristic (70% of cases)

Gross Pathology

- Noncontributory

Histopathology

GRANULOMATOSIS WITH POLYANGIITIS

- Geographic areas of parenchymal necrosis (coagulative or suppurative), often surrounded by epithelioid histiocytes, are frequently seen in nasal and oral cavities, paranasal sinuses, trachea, or lung parenchyma
- Neutrophilic microabscesses with necrotic centers and nuclear debris
- Granulomas are small and poorly formed with palisading histiocytes around microabscesses or necrotic foci
- Hyperchromatic multinucleated giant cells are randomly dispersed
- Lymphocytes and plasma cells are typically present; eosinophils may be seen but are not abundant
- Necrotizing vasculitis affects small to medium-sized arteries and veins and may be minimal or absent in biopsy tissue
- Necrotizing vasculitis with partial or complete destruction of the vessel wall by granulomatous or nongranulomatous inflammation
- Other variants of pulmonary involvement include bronchocentric injury, intense stromal eosinophilia, bronchiolitis obliterans-organizing pneumonia-like, and pulmonary hemorrhage with capillaritis
- Head and neck lesions show similar changes of tissue necrosis, granulomatous inflammation, and vasculitis, but these changes often are not found concurrently in biopsies, probably because of sampling limitations

- Kidney lesions include focal segmental necrotizing glomerulonephritis, crescentic glomerulonephritis, glomerular thrombosis, interstitial granulomatous inflammation, and papillary necrosis

EOSINOPHILIC GRANULOMATOSIS WITH POLYANGIITIS

- Typically affects small and medium-sized arteries and veins
- Vasculitis is characterized by fibrinoid necrosis with eosinophil-rich infiltrate; can be granulomatous or nongranulomatous
- Inflammatory cells are an admixture of eosinophils, neutrophils, lymphocytes, plasma cells, histiocytes, and multinucleated giant cells
- Pulmonary lesions consist of eosinophilic pneumonia, extravascular eosinophilic granuloma, and necrotizing vasculitis
- Skin biopsies reveal eosinophil-rich leukocytoclastic vasculitis, dermal eosinophilia, and extravascular necrotizing granuloma
- Cardiac involvement is that of eosinophilic myocarditis
- Glomerulonephritis can be focal, segmental, or crescentic glomerulonephritis

MICROSCOPIC POLYANGIITIS

- Destruction of the vessel wall by polymorphonuclear and mononuclear infiltrates, often with leukocytoclasia and segmental fibrinoid necrosis
- Associated hemorrhage is common
- Cutaneous lesions often involve upper and middle dermal venules with a histologic pattern of leukocytoclastic vasculitis
- Pulmonary lesions show inflammation and necrosis of interalveolar septa and capillaries with neutrophils, nuclear dusts, and intra-alveolar hemorrhage
- Renal lesions are those of necrotizing and crescentic glomerulonephritis
- Lesions are typically of the same age
- May affect small and medium-sized arteries, but arterial involvement is not necessary for diagnosis
- Occasional thrombosis present in arteritis results in tissue infarction and ulceration
- Granulomatous inflammation is not seen

Special Stains and Immunohistochemistry

- Trichrome stains fibrin red
- Movat highlights both elastin and collagen

Other Techniques for Diagnosis

- Immunofluorescence microscopy: little or no staining with immunoglobulins (immunoglobulin G [IgG]) in the affected vessels (including glomeruli) for GPA, EGPA, and MPA; hence, these vasculitides are often referred to as *pauci-immune (ANCA-associated) small-vessel vasculitis*
- Electron microscopy: no immune complex–type deposits are detected

Differential Diagnosis

- There are no histologic features that are specific for the different types of small-vessel vasculitis; further classification is based on clinical criteria and serology in conjunction with biopsy of the relevant organ

POLYARTERITIS NODOSA

- Proposed distinguishing feature of PAN is the absence of involvement of small vessels (i.e., arterioles, venules, or capillaries)
- Vasculitis is characterized by lesions of varying ages, including focal and segmental fibrinoid necrosis and occasional multinucleated giant cells, but granulomatous inflammation is not seen
- Does not cause pulmonary capillaritis or glomerulonephritis
- When small and medium-sized arteries are involved, necrotizing arteritis as a component of MPA is histologically indistinguishable from that of PAN
- Not associated with positive ANCA

ANTIGLOMERULAR BASEMENT MEMBRANE DISEASE (GOODPASTURE SYNDROME)

- Clinical presentation of pulmonary-renal syndrome of alveolar hemorrhage and rapidly progressive glomerulonephritis similar to MPA
- Associated with glomerular and alveolar capillary basement membrane antibodies; antigen target is an α_3 chain of type IV collagen
- Linear immunoglobulin deposition of IgG, often with C3, in glomerular and alveolar capillary basement membrane on immunofluorescence microscopy

DRUG-INDUCED VASCULITIS

- Associated with recent medication use, most commonly antibiotics and diuretics
- Manifestations range from isolated skin involvement to multiorgan involvement; time interval from drug exposure to onset of clinical manifestations is highly variable
- Neutrophilic or lymphocytic vasculitis in superficial small vessels; if present, tissue eosinophilia is a clue to possible drug etiology
- Usually no ANCA association
- Drug-related vasculitis with positive ANCA: hydralazine, pantoprazole, propylthiouracil, carbimazole, minocycline, and cimetidine

INFECTION-INDUCED VASCULITIS

- Commonly implicated infectious agents are hepatitis B, mycoplasma, meningococci, streptococci, *Staphylococcus aureus, Pseudomonas* species, *Yersinia* species, *Legionella* species, *Helicobacter pylori*, herpesvirus, adenovirus, cytomegalovirus, parvovirus B19, *Mycobacterium tuberculosis, Rickettsia* species, and fungi
- Histology shows superficial neutrophilic small-vessel vasculitis
- Septic vasculitis will show luminal thrombosis with neutrophils, hemorrhage, microabscesses, and necrosis
- Eccentric or segmental vessel wall necrosis is more characteristic of systemic vasculitides

VASCULITIS ASSOCIATED WITH CIRCULATING IMMUNE COMPLEXES

- Immune complex deposition can occur in solid organ and hematologic malignancies, connective tissue disorders, chronic active hepatitis, and inflammatory bowel diseases

SARCOIDOSIS

- Characterized by tight, compact granulomas usually without necrosis
- Granulomas typically distributed along interlobular septa and bronchovascular pathways
- Non-necrotizing granulomas within the media of vessels are frequently seen
- Necrosis is not a prominent feature
- Commonly lung involvement; rarely kidney involvement
- No association with c-ANCA or p-ANCA

EOSINOPHILIC PULMONARY INFILTRATES

- EGPA needs to be differentiated from eosinophilic pneumonia, idiopathic hypereosinophilic syndrome, allergic bronchopulmonary aspergillosis, parasitic infections, and Hodgkin disease

EPSTEIN-BARR VIRUS–ASSOCIATED LYMPHOPROLIFERATIVE DISORDERS WITH PROPENSITY FOR ANGIOINVASION

- Extranodal natural killer and T-cell lymphoma, nasal type (angiocentric lymphoma)
  - Most commonly involves the nasal and nasopharyngeal areas
  - Atypical lymphoid cells are small to medium in size
  - Tumor necrosis often present; neutrophilic infiltration rare
- Lymphomatoid granulomatosis
  - T cell–rich, B cell–proliferative disorder
  - Predilection for lung, but skin and central nervous system can also be affected
  - Destructive nodular infiltrates with central necrosis and prominent vascular and perivascular infiltration
  - Infiltrates consist of small lymphocytes, histiocytes, plasma cells, and atypical intermediate to large B cells
  - Absence of granulomatous inflammation

PEARLS

- *Vasculitis involving arterioles, capillaries, and venules allows for the diagnosis of small-vessel vasculitis*
- *ANCA testing by indirect immunofluorescence microscopy confirmed by enzyme-linked immunosorbent assay has about 99% sensitivity and 70% specificity; negative ANCA test does not rule out a diagnosis of pauci-immune small-vessel vasculitis*
- *Induction and remission therapy in pauci-immune ANCA-positive small-vessel vasculitis is similar for all subtypes and consists of systemic glucocorticoids and cyclophosphamide*

Granulomatosis with Polyangiitis

- Etiology is unknown; evidence suggests an immune-mediated mechanism with a synergistic effect of ANCA and proinflammatory stimuli most likely of infectious origin
- Chronic carriage of *S. aureus* in the upper airways is associated with increased risk for relapses
- Evolution of inflammatory vascular lesions and symptoms over time may cause a change in the diagnosis of patients from MPA to GPA if patients subsequently develop granulomatous lesions

- Limited forms of GPA spare the kidney
- c-ANCA levels are often used to monitor disease activity

Eosinophilic Granulomatosis with Polyangiitis

- Clinical manifestations may evolve over time or be suppressed by oral glucocorticoid therapy for asthma; sometimes, vasculitis precedes development of asthma
- More frequent involvement of peripheral nerves, skin, and heart; less frequent involvement of kidneys; less frequently positive for ANCA than are GPA and MPA
- Eosinophils may not be found or become less abundant in biopsies from patients treated with corticosteroids
- Increased mortality rate is seen when two or more of the following are present at the time of diagnosis: elevated serum creatinine, proteinuria, and gastrointestinal, cardiac, and central nervous system involvement

Microscopic Polyangiitis

- Previously referred to as *microscopic polyarteritis* and *microscopic periarteritis*; however, arterial involvement is not a constant feature
- Known clinical and histologic overlap with GPA

SELECTED REFERENCES

Guillevin L, Pagnoux C, Mouthon L: Churg-Strauss syndrome. Semin Respir Crit Care Med 25:535-545, 2004.

Jennette JC, Thomas DB, Falk RJ: Microscopic polyangiitis (microscopic polyarteritis). Semin Diagn Pathol 18:3-13, 2001.

Leavitt RY, Fauci AS, Bloch DA, et al: The American College of Rheumatology 1990 criteria for the classification of Wegener's granulomatosis. Arthritis Rheum 33:1101-1107, 1990.

Masi AT, Hunder GG, Lie JT, et al: The American College of Rheumatology 1990 criteria for the classification of Churg-Strauss syndrome (allergic granulomatosis and angiitis). Arthritis Rheum 33:1094-1100, 1990.

Sable-Fourtassou R, Cohen P, Mahr A, et al: Antineutrophil cytoplasmic antibodies and the Churg-Strauss syndrome. Ann Intern Med 143:632-638, 2005.

Travis WD: Pathology of pulmonary vasculitis. Semin Respir Crit Care Med 25:475-482, 2004.

IMMUNE COMPLEX SMALL-VESSEL VASCULITIS

Clinical Features

IgA VASCULITIS, FORMERLY HENOCH-SCHÖNLEIN PURPURA (IgAV)

- Most common form of small-vessel vasculitis in children (typically ages 3 to 15 years); males affected twice as commonly as females; rarely affects adults
- Commonly preceded by an upper respiratory tract infection
- Manifestations include nonthrombocytopenic palpable purpura, arthralgias, arthritis, colicky abdominal pain, and bloody diarrhea
- Renal involvement with hematuria or mild proteinuria in up to 50% of cases; rarely a progressive renal disease
- Serum IgA levels are increased in more than 50% of patients

CRYOGLOBULINEMIC VASCULITIS

- Mixed cryoglobulins are composed of monoclonal IgM and polyclonal IgG in type II and polyclonal IgM and IgG in type III
- Can be essential or secondary to connective tissue diseases, hematologic malignancies, and infections

- Mixed cryoglobulins are found in 55% to 90% of patients with chronic HCV infection, but cryoglobulinemic vasculitis is present in fewer than 5% of these patients
- Syndrome is characterized by purpura, arthralgias, and weakness, usually with peripheral nervous system and renal involvement
- Serologic tests show HCV viremia, anti-HCV antibodies, mixed cryoglobulins, high titers of rheumatoid factor, and low complement levels
- Clonal B-lymphocyte expansion is responsible for autoantibody production with increased incidence of developing non-Hodgkin lymphoma

Gross Pathology

- Noncontributory

Histopathology

IgA VASCULITIS

- Small-vessel vasculitis involving postcapillary venules, arterioles, and capillaries
- Characterized by neutrophilic infiltrate with fibrin deposits and nuclear debris in small, predominantly superficial dermal vessels
- Renal lesions vary from focal to diffuse mesangial proliferation to crescentic glomerulonephritis

CRYOGLOBULINEMIC VASCULITIS

- Skin biopsy shows leukocytoclastic vasculitis in superficial and deep dermal plexus
- Some patients have lymphocytic vasculitis and involvement of medium-sized arteries
- Membranoproliferative glomerulonephritis type I is the most common renal lesion; fibrinoid necrosis and crescents are absent to rare

Special Stains and Immunohistochemistry

- Noncontributory

Other Techniques for Diagnosis

IMMUNOFLUORESCENCE MICROSCOPY

- IgA vasculitis: glomerular (mesangial, capillary wall, arteriolar) and dermal vascular staining with IgA and C3
- Cryoglobulinemic vasculitis: vascular staining with IgM, IgG, or C3

ELECTRON MICROSCOPY

- IgA vasculitis: with renal involvement, prominent electron-dense mesangial deposits are seen
- Cryoglobulinemic vasculitis: mesangial and subendothelial deposits and intraluminal monocytes

Differential Diagnosis

CUTANEOUS LEUKOCYTOCLASTIC VASCULITIS (HYPERSENSITIVITY VASCULITIS)

- Localized, self-limited cutaneous vasculitis often triggered by drugs or preceding infection
- Similar histologic features of leukocytoclastic vasculitis in superficial vessels
- Ulcers or subcutaneous nodules uncommon and suggest involvement of arteries in the dermal-subcutis interface in other systemic vasculitis
- Diagnosis of exclusion; no systemic vasculitis or glomerulonephritis

HYPOCOMPLEMENTEMIC URTICARIAL VASCULITIS

- Chronic or recurrent urticaria with leukocytoclastic vasculitis and deposition of immunoglobulins and complement around vessels
- Hypocomplementemia observed in patients with systemic manifestations including arthralgia or arthritis, uveitis or episcleritis, glomerulonephritis, recurrent abdominal pain, chronic obstructive pulmonary disease, and positive lupus band test on skin biopsy
- Low serum C1q levels with anti-C1q autoantibodies
- Associated with SLE and Sjögren syndrome

DRUG-INDUCED VASCULITIS

- See "Differential Diagnosis" under "Pauci-immune Small-Vessel Vasculitis"

INFECTION-INDUCED VASCULITIS

- See "Differential Diagnosis" under "Pauci-immune Small-Vessel Vasculitis"

MALIGNANCY-ASSOCIATED (PARANEOPLASTIC) VASCULITIS

- Most common underlying malignancies are lymphomas and leukemias
- Histopathology shows leukocytoclastic vasculitis, rarely lymphocytic vasculitis

CONNECTIVE TISSUE DISEASE–ASSOCIATED VASCULITIS

- Frequently associated with SLE, rheumatoid arthritis, and Sjögren syndrome, and less commonly with dermatomyositis, scleroderma, and relapsing polychondritis
- Affects small and medium-sized vessels
- Can have neutrophilic, lymphocytic, or granulomatous infiltrates
- Can be complicated by the presence of antiphospholipid antibodies that lead to vascular thrombosis
- Can be positive for p-ANCA and, less commonly, c-ANCA

PAUCI-IMMUNE SMALL-VESSEL VASCULITIS

- Skin lesions can be part of the initial presentation in GPA, EGPA, and MPA
- Absence or paucity of immunoglobulin or complement deposits in vascular lesions

IgA NEPHROPATHY (BERGER DISEASE)

- Renal lesions are histologically indistinguishable from IgA vasculitis
- Disease localized to the kidney; no systemic manifestations

PEARLS

- *IgA vasculitis*
  - *Etiologic agent is currently unknown*
  - *Typically self-limited; most cases spontaneously regress in 2 to 3 weeks without sequelae*
  - *Renal failure is the most common cause of morbidity and mortality; poor prognostic features include development of nephrotic syndrome and renal biopsy showing more than 50% of glomeruli with crescents*
  - *Treatment involves supportive therapy; corticosteroids only for severe systemic symptoms*

- *Cryoglobulinemic vasculitis*
  - *There is no established classification or diagnostic criteria for cryoglobulinemic vasculitis*
  - *Diagnosis is established with serologic and histopathologic examination*
  - *Overlap of symptoms with Sjögren syndrome, autoimmune hepatitis, and B-cell lymphoproliferative disorders is recognized*

SELECTED REFERENCES

Carlson JA, Chen KR: Cutaneous vasculitis update: small vessel neutrophilic vasculitis syndromes. Am J Dermatopathol 28:486-506, 2006.

Ferri C, Sebastiani M, Giuggioli D, et al: Mixed cryoglobulinemia: demographic, clinical, and serologic features and survival in 231 patients. Semin Arthritis Rheum 33:355-374, 2004.

Mills JA, Michel BA, Bloch DA, et al: The American College of Rheumatology 1990 criteria for the classification of Henoch-Schonlein purpura. Arthritis Rheum 33:1114-1121, 1990.

BUERGER DISEASE (THROMBOANGIITIS OBLITERANS)

Clinical Features

- Inflammatory and occlusive vascular disorder affecting small and medium-sized arteries and veins
- Typically involves the vessels of the distal upper and lower extremities; rare involvement of mesenteric arteries and veins
- Found almost exclusively in young men who are heavy smokers; occasionally reported in women smokers
- Onset before age of 40 years
- Patients with advanced disease may present with claudication, ischemic ulcers, or gangrene

Gross Pathology

- Segmental involvement of arteries or veins with acute or organized thrombosis and luminal narrowing

Histopathology

- Involves both small and medium-sized arteries and veins
- Acute lesions are diagnostic and consist of cellular inflammatory thrombus and mild acute transmural inflammation without fibrinoid necrosis
- Microabscesses are noted within the thrombus, often with multinucleated giant cells
- Older lesions show organizing thrombosis with chronic inflammation resulting in luminal occlusion; recanalization is often seen
- Internal elastic lamina remains intact in acute and chronic lesions
- Superficial migratory thrombophlebitis with or without inflammatory thrombus is seen in fewer than half of the patients

Special Stains and Immunohistochemistry

- Elastic highlights the intact elastic lamina

Other Techniques for Diagnosis

- Noncontributory

Differential Diagnosis

ORGANIZING THROMBOEMBOLI

- Giant cells and prominent inflammatory infiltrate within the organizing thrombus are not seen
- Acute inflammation within the vessel wall is not seen

NECROTIZING ARTERITIS

- Characterized by granulomatous or nongranulomatous inflammation with fibrinoid necrosis and destruction of the internal elastic lamina

PEARLS

- *Tobacco use appears to be a universal factor associated with this condition*
- *No laboratory or serologic tests are useful in establishing diagnosis*
- *Cessation of smoking with or without steroid therapy usually renders a good prognosis*

SELECTED REFERENCES

Ohta T, Ishioashi H, Hosaka M, Sugimoto I: Clinical and social consequences of Buerger disease. J Vasc Surg 39:176-180, 2004.

Olin JW, Shih A: Thromboangiitis obliterans (Buerger's disease). Curr Opin Rheumatol 18:18-24, 2006.

FIBROMUSCULAR DYSPLASIA

Clinical Features

- Noninflammatory, nonatherosclerotic vascular diseases that affect medium and small muscular arteries
- Can affect any artery, but the most commonly involved are the renal arteries (60% to 75%, bilateral in 35%) and carotid or vertebral arteries (25% to 30%)
- About 28% of cases have multiple arteries involved
- Most patients are asymptomatic; most common presentations are renovascular hypertension, cervical or epigastric systolic and diastolic bruit
- Multisystem involvement mimics systemic necrotizing vasculitis with mesenteric ischemia, renal failure, syncope, stroke, end-organ ischemia, or extremity ischemia
- Typically affects young adults, more commonly women in the third and fourth decades
- Angiography shows the classic string-of-beads appearance

Gross Pathology

- Artery may show stenosis or segmental narrowing with or without dilations

Histopathology

MEDIAL FIBROMUSCULAR DYSPLASIA

- Is divided into three subtypes
- Medial fibroplasia is the most common histologic type and characterized by thick fibromuscular ridges alternating with areas of medial thinning
  - Smooth muscle cells are disorganized and separated by moderate accumulation of collagen and ground substance
  - External elastic lamina is frequently fragmented
  - Intima is normal
  - Internal elastic lamina is disrupted in advanced lesions with microaneurysm formation

- Medial hyperplasia causes concentric luminal stenosis by proliferation of smooth muscle exhibiting minimal disorganization
- Perimedial fibroplasia shows excessive accumulation of elastic tissue between the outer media and adventitia with effacement of the external elastic lamina

INTIMAL FIBROPLASIA
- Segmental concentric or eccentric accumulation of loose fibrous tissue without lipids or inflammatory cells
- Internal elastic lamina is frequently fragmented or reduplicated
- Media and adventitia are normal

ADVENTITIAL (PERIARTERIAL) FIBROPLASIA
- Dense collagen replaces the adventitia and extends into the periadventitial soft tissue
- Intima and media including external elastic lamina are intact

Special Stains and Immunohistochemistry
- Elastic stain highlights destruction of the elastic lamina

Other Techniques for Diagnosis
- Noncontributory

Differential Diagnosis

ATHEROSCLEROSIS
- Occurs in older population with high atherosclerotic risk factors
- Atherosclerotic disease tends to affect the renal artery ostia and proximal portion; in contrast, fibromuscular dysplasia affects the distal two thirds and branches of the artery
- Fibroatheromatous plaques with focal disruption of the elastic lamina and medial atrophy

HEALED ARTERITIS
- Medial destruction and focal loss of the elastic lamina may lead to aneurysm
- Often granulation tissue or fibrosis is seen in the media
- Residual inflammatory cell infiltrate may be seen

NEUROFIBROMATOSIS
- Aneurysms and stenotic arterial lesions often involve the renal arteries, aorta, carotid, vertebral, and mesenteric vessels
- Nodular intimal proliferation of spindle cells in a mucoid matrix, with disruption of the internal elastic lamina and attenuation of the media
- Characteristic skin and skeletal abnormalities and tumorous growths in neurofibromatosis allows for clinical differentiation

PEARLS

- *Dissections, aneurysms, and arteriovenous fistulas are complications of fibromuscular dysplasia*
- *Classic angiographic findings are suggestive of this condition*
- *Percutaneous balloon angioplasty is performed for arterial stenosis; surgery is used to treat microaneurysms*

SELECTED REFERENCES
Luscher TF, Lie JT, Stanson AW, et al: Arterial fibromuscular dysplasia. Mayo Clin Proc 62:931-952, 1987.
Slovut DP, Olin JW: Fibromuscular dysplasia. N Engl J Med 350:1862-1871, 2004.

HERITABLE DISORDERS OF BLOOD VESSELS
Clinical Features
MARFAN SYNDROME
- Autosomal dominant trait with variable clinical manifestations, including bilateral ectopia lentis, tall stature, long slender limbs, arachnodactyly, pectus excavatum or carinatum, and scoliosis
- Aortic dissection follows a period of progressive aortic dilation
- Patients with a second type of Marfan syndrome exhibit some of the cardiovascular and skeletal manifestations of Marfan syndrome but lack ocular abnormalities

LOEYS-DIETZ SYNDROME
- Autosomal dominant disorder characterized by a triad of arterial tortuosity and aneurysm, hypertelorism, and bifid uvula or cleft palate
- Aneurysms in thoracic arterial branches are common, in addition to thoracic aortic aneurysm
- High incidence of pregnancy-related complications and aortic dissection or rupture in young patients

EHLERS-DANLOS SYNDROME TYPE IV (VASCULAR EHLERS-DANLOS SYNDROME)
- Autosomal-dominant group of heritable connective tissue disorders characterized by skin hyperextensibility, joint hypermobility, and tissue fragility
- Only form of Ehlers-Danlos syndrome associated with increased risk for premature death owing to arterial, intestinal, or uterine ruptures
- A major event is the presenting feature in about 70% of patients

FAMILIAL THORACIC AORTIC ANEURYSMS AND AORTIC DISSECTIONS
- Aortic dilatation and aneurysm with positive family history and absence of clinical features of Marfan, Loeys-Dietz, or Ehlers-Danlos syndrome

Gross Pathology
- Aneurysmal aortic wall may be thin with a bluish tinge of the intima
- Dissection may be evident with a hematoma between the split media
- Chronic dissection shows a false lumen lined by white opalescent neointima
- Occasional intimal lacerations are not associated with intramural dissection and heal with neointima lining an ellipsoid intimal depression

Histopathology
- Cystic medial degeneration shows fragmentation and loss of elastic lamellae with or without significant proteoglycan deposition (Figure 18-17A)

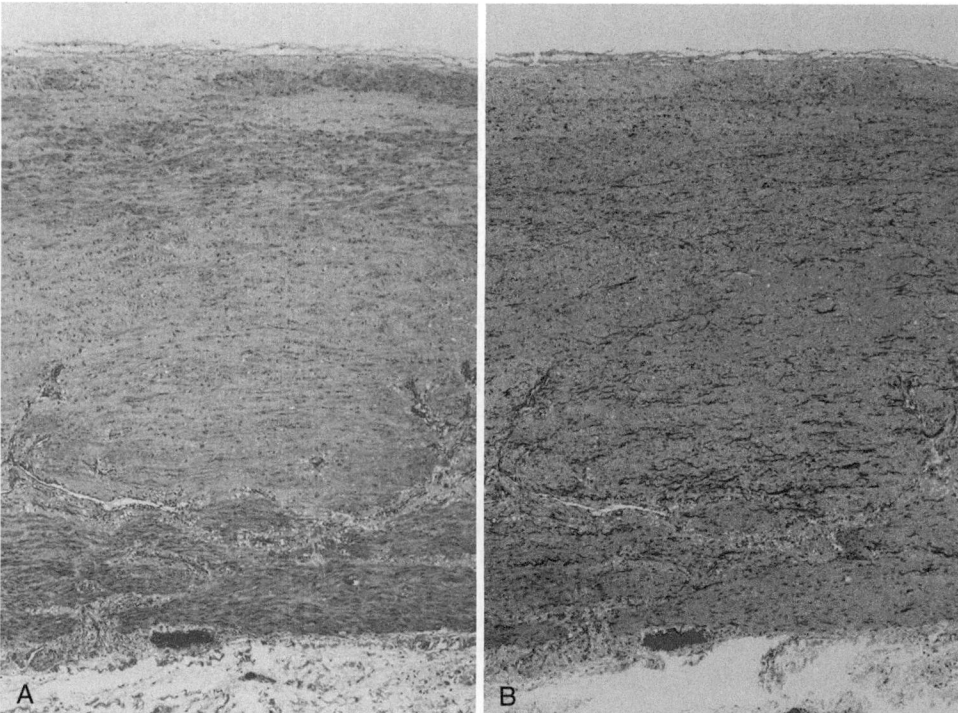

Figure 18-17. Cystic medial degeneration. A, The hematoxylin and eosin stain shows areas of blue discoloration in the media. **B,** Movat stain shows corresponding mucopolysaccharide deposits with fragmentation and loss of elastic lamellae.

- Laminar medial necrosis is characterized by loss of smooth muscle cells in the media with collapse of the elastic lamellae and fibrosis
- Aortic dissection
  - Dissection typically occurs between the inner two thirds and outer one third of the media
  - False lumen may be lined by blood, fibrin and thrombus, granulation tissue, or neointima, depending on the age of the lesion (Figure 18-18A and B)
  - Inner media usually shows medial necrosis
  - Acute inflammation is usually limited to fibrinous deposits and adventitia, extending minimally into the media
  - Healed dissection is recognized by a linear vascularized collagenous scar tissue in the media

Special Stains and Immunohistochemistry

- Movat demonstrates loss of the elastic lamellae, loss of smooth muscle cells with fibrosis, and proteoglycan deposition (Figure 18-17B)

Other Techniques for Diagnosis

MARFAN SYNDROME
- Classic Marfan syndrome patients have mutations in the *fibrillin 1* gene, *FBN1*
- Marfan syndrome type 2 is linked to mutations in the gene encoding transforming growth factor-β receptor 2 (*TGFBR2*)

LOEYS-DIETZ SYNDROME
- Associated with mutations in *TGFBR1* and *TGFBR2*

EHLERS-DANLOS SYNDROME
- Caused by mutations in type III procollagen gene, *COL3A1*

FAMILIAL THORACIC AORTIC ANEURYSMS AND AORTIC DISSECTIONS
- Associated mutations reported in *TGFBR1*, *TGFBR2*, *MYH11* (myosin heavy chain), *ACTA2* (alpha-actin), *MYLK* (myosin light chain kinase), *SMAD3* (mothers against decapentaplegic homolog 3), *FBN1*

Figure 18-18. Aortic dissection. A, An acute dissection shows a false lumen filled with recent thrombus in the media. **B,** The intimomedial flap of a chronic dissection is shown with a thick neointima lining the plane of dissection.

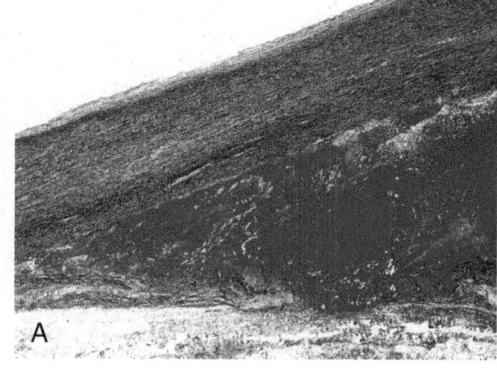
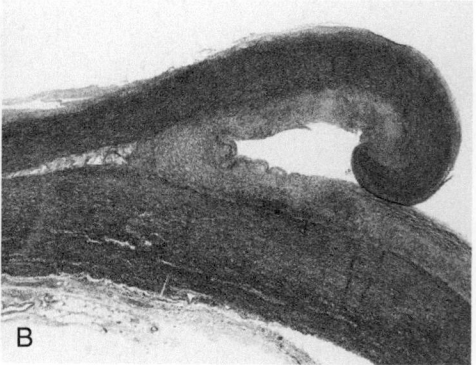

Differential Diagnosis

- Medial changes are nonspecific, but quantitative differences are found between normal, aging aorta, and diseased or dilated aorta
- Conditions associated with cystic medial degeneration include the normal aging process, systemic hypertension, bicuspid aortic valve, and Marfan syndrome

INFECTIOUS AORTITIS

- Etiologic agents include *Staphylococcus aureus,* streptococci, *Salmonella* species, *Escherichia coli,* and Mycobacteria and *Clostridium* species
- Results from hematogenous seeding, septic embolization from infective endocarditis, or direct extension of infection from a contiguous site
- Abdominal aorta and femoral arteries are more commonly affected than thoracic aorta
- Causes aortic rupture or produces mycotic aneurysms
- Medial necrosis with marked acute inflammatory infiltrates in the media
- Inflammatory reaction in the adventitia common and includes neutrophilic infiltrates, microabscesses, edema, and granulation tissue

PEARLS

- *Ascending aortic aneurysms are clinically distinct from descending thoracic and abdominal aortic aneurysms*
- *Pathologic changes in the media vary considerably from one area to the next, necessitating multiple and extensive histologic sampling of the specimen*

SELECTED REFERENCES

Hahn RT, Roman MJ, Mogtader AH, Devereux RB: Association of aortic dilation with regurgitant, stenotic and functionally normal bicuspid aortic valves. J Am Coll Cardiol 19:283-288, 1992.

Homme JL, Aubry MC, Edwards WD, et al: Surgical pathology of the ascending aorta: a clinicopathologic study of 513 cases. Am J Surg Pathol 30:1159-1168, 2006.

Loeys BL, Schwarze U, Holm T, et al: Aneurysm syndromes caused by mutations in the TGF-beta receptor. N Engl J Med 355:788-798, 2006.

Pepin M, Schwarze U, Superti-Furga A, Byers PH: Clinical and genetic features of Ehlers-Danlos syndrome type IV, the vascular type. N Engl J Med 342:673-680, 2000.

Robinson PN, Arteaga-Solis E, Baldock C, et al: The molecular genetics of Marfan syndrome and related disorders. J Med Genet 43:769-787, 2006.

Chapter 19
Central Nervous System

ELIZABETH J. COCHRAN

CHAPTER OUTLINE

ASTROCYTIC TUMORS

DIFFUSE ASTROCYTOMA, ANAPLASTIC ASTROCYTOMA, GLIOBLASTOMA, GIANT CELL GLIOBLASTOMA, GLIOSARCOMA, AND GLIOMATOSIS CEREBRI (WORLD HEALTH ORGANIZATION [WHO] GRADES II, III, AND IV)

Clinical Features

- Astrocytic tumors account for 23% of all primary brain tumors and 76% of all gliomas
- Commonly produce headaches, seizures, or focal neurologic deficits; symptoms related to the location of the tumor
- Magnetic resonance imaging (MRI) shows an ill-defined area of low signal on T1
  - Low-grade astrocytomas do not show contrast enhancement; higher-grade tumors, including anaplastic astrocytomas, gliosarcoma, and glioblastoma, typically enhance and frequently show ring enhancement
  - Gliomatosis cerebri shows diffuse enlargement of involved areas without a focal mass identifiable (T1 hypointensity, T2 hyperintensity); no enhancement
- Diffuse astrocytomas occur commonly in cerebral hemispheres in adults (mean age, 30 to 40 years) and in the brain stem in children; occasionally in the cerebellum or spinal cord
- Anaplastic astrocytoma is typically found in adults (mean age, 45 years); pontine lesions are more common in children
- Glioblastoma
  - Most frequently occurring glioma (54%)
  - Overall, usually occurs in individuals between ages 45 and 75 years (80% occur in those older than 50 years); most commonly involves the cerebral hemispheres
  - Usually affects the brain stem in children
  - Primary glioblastomas occur de novo as a grade IV neoplasm
    - Most glioblastomas are primary and have a short (< 3 months) clinical history
    - Usually occur at older ages (mean age, 62 years)
  - Secondary glioblastomas occur in the setting of a previously diagnosed grade II or III astrocytoma
    - Mean age of occurrence is 45 years

- Gliomatosis cerebri
  - Glioma, usually astrocytic, which involves at least three cerebral lobes of the brain; usually bilateral involvement and without defined focal mass identifiable
  - Peak occurrence between ages 40 and 50 years
  - Wide-ranging signs and symptoms; generalized cognitive impairment, often without focal neurologic deficits

Gross Pathology

- Low-grade tumors have a variable appearance ranging from subtle, barely visible lesions to large, soft, gelatinous, gray-white ill-defined masses that blur the gray-white border and expand the cortex or white matter
- Glioblastomas are typically large and often involve more than one lobe
  - Extension across the corpus callosum results in involvement of both hemispheres (*butterfly glioma*)
  - Hemorrhage and large areas of necrosis are characteristic
- Gliomatosis cerebri: diffuse enlargement of affected brain regions; usually, no distinct mass is seen
- Giant cell glioblastomas and gliosarcoma may each be sharply circumscribed and firm owing to presence of connective tissue components

Histopathology (Figure 19-1)

ASTROCYTOMA (WHO GRADE II)

- Hypercellular (relative to normal brain), infiltrative, ill-defined lesions typically centered in the white matter or less commonly the cerebral cortex
- Presence of a single mitosis should not prompt designation as an anaplastic astrocytoma
- Sample size is important in this determination; a small sample with mitosis suggests an anaplastic designation, but a single mitosis in a large resection should not prompt a higher-grade diagnosis

FIBRILLARY ASTROCYTOMAS: MOST COMMON TYPE

- Neoplastic astrocytes are slightly pleomorphic and enlarged, with hyperchromatic angular cigar-shaped nuclei
- Cytoplasm is often not visible, or scant asymmetrical cell processes are evident
- Loose fibrillary glial matrix is present in more cellular areas

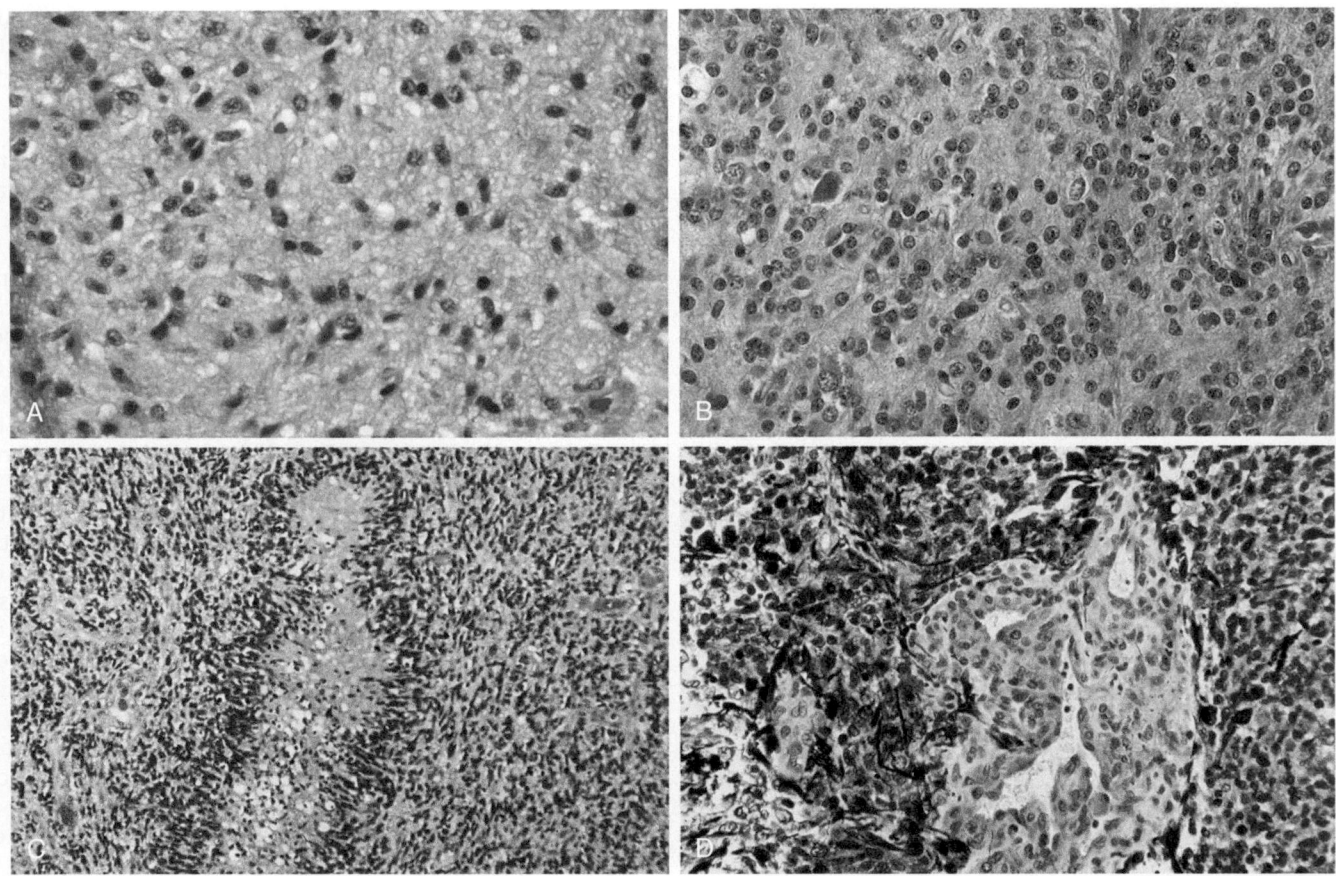

Figure 19-1. A, Low-grade astrocytoma. Cellular infiltrate of neoplastic astrocytes showing nuclear enlargement, nuclear membrane irregularity, and slight hyperchromasia. **B,** Anaplastic astrocytoma. Highly cellular tumor composed of neoplastic astrocytes with moderate nuclear pleomorphism, hyperchromatism, nuclear membrane irregularity, and mitoses. **C,** Glioblastoma multiforme (GBM). Notice the prominent area of necrosis with pseudopalisading. **D,** GBM. Neoplastic astrocytes surrounding endothelial proliferation (glial fibrillary acidic protein stain).

PROTOPLASMIC ASTROCYTOMAS: RARE VARIANT OF LOW-GRADE ASTROCYTOMA

- Nuclei are round to oval, and fibrillary processes are not evident
- Cells reside in loose mucoid matrix with prominent microcysts

GEMISTOCYTIC ASTROCYTOMA

- Neoplastic astrocytes have large cell bodies with abundant eosinophilic cytoplasm and short fibrillary processes and eccentric nuclei
- Presence of at least 20% of gemistocytes is necessary for this designation
- This subtype has a high tendency to progress to anaplastic astrocytoma
- Mitotic figures are typically scant or absent

ANAPLASTIC ASTROCYTOMA (WHO GRADE III)

- Tumor shows higher cellularity, increased nuclear pleomorphism, and hyperchromasia
- Mitotic figures are present (see the previous discussion of mitoses in astrocytoma)

GLIOMATOSIS CEREBRI (WHO GRADE III)

- Growth pattern of diffuse glioma, most often astrocytoma, but may be mixed or oligodendroglioma

- Astrocytic cells often contain elongated nuclei (may be confused with microglia)
- Mitoses are usually sparse; endothelial proliferation and necrosis are absent
- With longer survival, autopsy may show focal areas of higher grade (glioblastoma)

GLIOBLASTOMA (WHO GRADE IV)

- Infiltrative, highly cellular tumor with a wide range of abnormal cytology
- Cells with hyperchromatic, pleomorphic nuclei and ill-defined fibrillary cytoplasm are usually present
- The following may also be seen: multinucleated cells, lipidized cells, granular cells, and epithelioid change
- Numerous mitotic figures are always present
- Rarely, metaplastic elements are present, including squamous or adenoid differentiation, bone, or cartilage (more common in gliosarcoma)
- Required for diagnosis
  - Endothelial cell proliferation or areas of necrosis with or without pseudopalisading

Variants of Glioblastoma

- Giant cell glioblastoma (WHO grade IV)
  - Large, bizarre cells with markedly pleomorphic nuclei and multinucleation

- May have increased reticulin network and appear more circumscribed
- Gliosarcoma (WHO grade IV)
  - Defined by the presence of a sarcomatous component in addition to a malignant astrocytic component in the neoplasm; molecular studies support a common origin of both cell types
  - Astrocytic component is high grade and may occasionally display adenoid or squamous metaplasia
  - Sarcomatous component most often shows histology suggesting fibrosarcoma
- Small cell astrocytoma (WHO grade III or IV)
  - Monomorphous oval nuclei, mild nuclear hyperchromasia, occasional small nucleoli, scant cytoplasm, many mitoses
  - Endothelial proliferation or pseudopalisading necrosis may be present (if present, grade IV; if absent, grade III)
  - May exhibit architectural features causing confusion with oligodendroglioma, such as chicken-wire vasculature, clear halos, perineuronal satellitosis, and calcifications
- Glioblastoma with primitive neuroectodermal component (WHO grade IV)
  - Presence of hypercellular nodules of cells with hyperchromatic carrot-shaped nuclei, high nuclear-to-cytoplasmic ratios, presence of abundant mitoses and karyorrhexis, and Homer Wright rosettes, within a glioblastoma; desmoplasia or large cell/anaplastic cytology may also be present

Special Stains and Immunohistochemistry

- Glial fibrillary acidic protein (GFAP) positive in grade II; higher-grade tumors are highly variable in expression
- MIB-1 (Ki-67): labeling index is low in low-grade astrocytomas (< 5%) and high in anaplastic astrocytomas (5% to 10%) and glioblastomas (15% to 20%)
- Isocitrate dehydrogenase-1 (*IDH1*) (R132H): antibody identifies mutated IDH1 protein present in low-grade diffuse gliomas and secondary glioblastomas but not in primary glioblastomas (see section on cytogenetics, presented later)
  - Extremely helpful in confirming presence of low-grade glioma in biopsy tissue in cases where distinction from reactive astrocytosis is difficult
  - Also helpful in distinguishing a diffuse astrocytoma from a pilocytic astrocytoma (pilocytic astrocytomas do not have *IDH1* [R132H] mutation)
- Cytokeratin: high-grade astrocytomas may show cross-reactivity to AE1/AE3 cytokeratin
- Epithelial membrane antigen (EMA) typically negative
- Synaptophysin: often positive in glioblastoma with primitive neuroectodermal tumor (PNET) component in primitive cells; these foci are usually also GFAP and neuron-specific enolase (NSE) positive and have high MIB-1 labeling
- Positive for p53; may help distinguish a low-grade astrocytoma from reactive astrocytosis and from a pilocytic astrocytoma
- Reticulin highlights mesenchymal and sarcomatous components in gliosarcoma and desmoplastic component in giant cell glioblastoma

- Periodic acid–Schiff (PAS) and CD68 positive in granular cell change

Other Techniques for Diagnosis

- Electron microscopy
  - Astrocytes show cytoplasmic intermediate filaments and cell processes; poorly formed cell junctions may be seen
- Cytogenetics
  - *TP53* mutation: in 59% of astrocytomas, 53% of anaplastic astrocytomas, 65% of secondary glioblastomas, 84% of giant cell glioblastoma multiforme types (GBMs), 26% of primary gliosarcomas, and 28% of primary glioblastomas
  - *IDH1* gene mutation occurs with high frequency in low-grade gliomas and secondary glioblastomas and confers a prognostic benefit
  - Of the *IDH1* gene mutation, R132H has been identified in 73% of diffuse astrocytomas, 64% anaplastic astrocytomas, 82% of oligodendrogliomas, 70% of anaplastic oligodendrogliomas, 40% of gliomatosis cerebri, 85% of secondary glioblastomas, 0.05% of primary glioblastomas, 15% of GBM with PNET foci, and 7% of gliosarcomas, but not in small cell or giant cell GBMs
  - *IDH2* gene mutations are much less common in astrocytomas than *IDH1* gene mutations: < 1% in grade 2 and 3 astrocytomas
  - Gain of chromosome 7: identified in two thirds of astrocytomas
  - Loss of heterozygosity of chromosome 10q: 35% to 60% of anaplastic astrocytomas, and about equal frequencies in primary and secondary glioblastomas (60% to 70%)
  - *PTEN* mutation: 4% of secondary GBMs, 32% of primary GBMs, 37% of primary gliosarcomas, and 33% of giant cell GBMs
  - *EGFR* gene amplification, 8% of secondary glioblastomas, 5% of giant cell GBMs, < 8% of gliosarcomas, 36% of primary glioblastomas, and a high frequency of occurrence in small-cell type astrocytomas
  - O⁶-methylguanine methyltransferase (*MGMT*) promoter gene methylation: methylation decreases levels of *MGMT* protein resulting in increased response with temozolomide treatment; *MGMT* methylation also confers an improved response to other therapies that may be due to the molecular phenotype

Differential Diagnosis

METASTASIS (METASTATIC CARCINOMA OR METASTATIC MELANOMA)

- Metastatic carcinoma: cytokeratin and EMA positive
- Metastatic melanoma: S-100, MelanA, and HMB-45 typically positive
- GFAP negative

LYMPHOMA

- May show radiologic findings similar to those in GBM
- Typically located in periventricular regions and multifocal
- Angiocentric distribution
- Leukocyte common antigen (LCA) positive; most are of B-cell lineage (CD20 positive)

REACTIVE ASTROCYTOSIS

- Small cyst like spaces are not typically seen in reactive processes
- Cellularity is not as high as in astrocytomas
- Reactive astrocytes lack hyperchromatic and pleomorphic nuclei
- More regular arrangement of cells
- Absence of *IDH1 (R132H)* mutated protein on immunohistochemistry

OLIGODENDROGLIOMA

- Cells show cytologic features of oligodendrocytes, including perinuclear halos
- Composed of uniform round cells with minimal cytologic atypia
- Negative for GFAP
- Characteristic genetic profile: deletions of chromosomes 1p and 19q

DEMYELINATING DISEASES

- Characteristically have numerous foamy macrophages and inflammatory cells
- Areas of demyelination may be identified with myelin stains

PEARLS

- *Patients with well-differentiated diffuse astrocytomas may be treated with surgery, alkylating agents (most often temozolomide), and radiation; most patients die of the disease within 10 years; progression to a high-grade tumor commonly occurs (secondary glioblastoma)*
- *Both anaplastic astrocytoma and glioblastoma are usually treated with surgery, temozolomide, radiation, and possibly bevacizumab; patients with anaplastic astrocytoma typically die in 2 to 3 years, and those with glioblastoma usually die on average within 2 years of diagnosis*
- *Astrocytomas of the brain stem occur most commonly in the first decade in the ventral pons, encasing the basilar artery and associated with a poor prognosis*

SELECTED REFERENCES

Hartmann C, Meyer J, Balss J, et al: Type and frequency of IDH1 and IDH2 mutations are related to astrocytic and oligodendroglial differentiation and age: a study of 1,010 diffuse gliomas. Acta Neuropathol 118:469-474, 2009.

Jansen M, Yip S, Louis DN: Molecular pathology in adult neuro-oncology: an update on diagnostic, prognostic and predictive markers. Lancet Neurol 9:717-726, 2010.

Joseph NM, Phillips J, Dahiya S, et al: Diagnostic implications of IDH1-R132H and OLIG2 expression patterns in rare and challenging glioblastoma variants. Mod Pathol 26:315-326, 2013.

Perry A, Aldape KD, George DH, Burger PC: Small cell astrocytoma: an aggressive variant that is clinicopathologically and genetically distinct from anaplastic oligodendroglioma. Cancer 101:2318-2326, 2004.

Perry A, Miller CR, Gujrati M, et al: Malignant gliomas with primitive neuroectodermal tumor-like components: a clinicopathologic and genetic study of 53 cases. Brain Pathol 19:81-90, 2009.

PILOCYTIC ASTROCYTOMA (WHO GRADE I)

Clinical Features

- Occurs predominantly in children and young adults; usually presents in the first two decades
- Most common glioma in children
- Most frequently occurs in the cerebellum; may be seen in the optic nerve, third ventricle, hypothalamus, brain stem, cerebral hemispheres, or thalamus
- When arising in the brain stem, it is usually exophytic dorsally or extends into the cerebellopontine angle
- Patients can present with either focal or nonlocalized neurologic deficits or symptoms of increased intracranial pressure; may present with seizures
- MRI scans show a well-circumscribed contrast enhancing mass commonly associated with a cyst (multiple or solitary)

Gross Pathology

- Typically well-circumscribed, soft, gray, discrete tumors
- Cyst formation in about 50% of cases

Histopathology

- Most commonly demonstrates a biphasic pattern consisting of pilocytic areas and microcystic components (Figure 19-2A)
  - Loose, microcystic areas typically contain eosinophilic granular bodies or protein droplets
  - Pilocytic component shows elongated cells with densely packed fibrillary cytoplasm and Rosenthal fibers (tapered, eosinophilic, corkscrew-shaped hyaline structures); Rosenthal fibers are not always seen or necessary for diagnosis (Figure 19-2B)
- A diffuse variant of pilocytic astrocytomas with a dense fibrillary component and lacking microcystic areas has been described and has a good prognosis
- Neoplastic astrocytes are usually piloid and have uniform nuclei with minimal pleomorphism
- Multinucleated giant cells are commonly seen
- Mitotic activity is rare; more frequently seen in tumors of infants
- Endothelial proliferation and areas of hyalinization are common features
- Focal areas of calcification may be seen, but necrosis is uncommon
- Although grossly circumscribed, the tumor may have microscopic infiltration into adjacent brain tissue
- Occasionally hypercellular tumors with increased pleomorphism and multinucleation (features associated with long-standing lesions) are seen
- Pilomyxoid areas (see complete histologic description in the section on pilomyxoid astrocytomas) may be found in varying amounts in a pilocytic astrocytoma; no prediction of tumor behavior is possible at present based on the quantity of these intermixed elements; given the possibility of aggressive behavior, a pilomyxoid component should be communicated to the clinician

Special Stains and Immunohistochemistry

- GFAP positive
- Synaptophysin positivity may be found
- Negative for p53
- MIB-1 labeling index ranges from 0% to 4% (mean 1%)

Other Techniques for Diagnosis

- Electron microscopy: pilocytic astrocytes show abundant intermediate filaments; eosinophilic granular

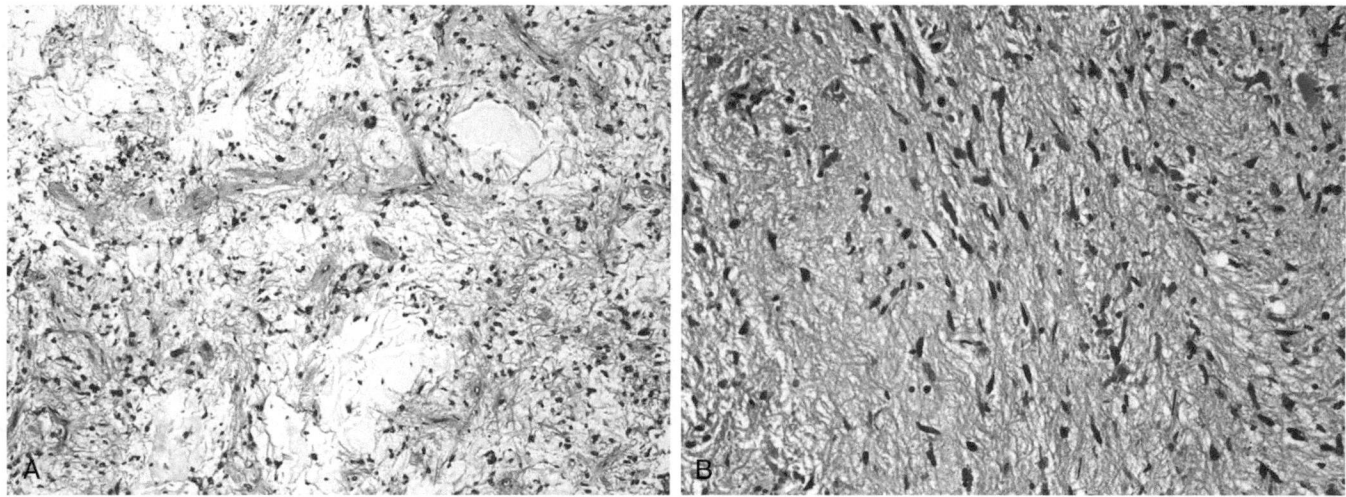

Figure 19-2. Pilocytic astrocytoma. A, Classic architecture of densely fibrillated areas alternating with microcystic areas. **B,** Diffuse pilocytic astrocytoma consisting only of densely packed elongated cells. Rosenthal fibers are also present.

bodies contain intermediate filaments, osmiophilic granules, and myelin figures
- Cytogenetics
  - Most pilocytic astrocytomas have *BRAF-KIAA1549* gene fusion, which is not present in low-grade diffuse astrocytomas and may be useful in distinguishing pilocytic astrocytomas from diffuse astrocytomas; gains are also seen in chromosomes 5 and 7
  - High frequency of underexpression of *ALDH1L1* gene in aggressive pilocytic astrocytomas
  - Presence of mutation in *BRAF V600E* has been identified in 33% of diencephalic pilocytic astrocytomas

Differential Diagnosis

DIFFUSE ASTROCYTOMA
- Typically lack circumscription and contrast enhancement
- Tissue infiltration and malignant behavior are much more common
- Usually lacks biphasic pattern, Rosenthal fibers, and eosinophilic granular bodies

PILOMYXOID ASTROCYTOMA
- May be difficult to exclude as focal areas of pilomyxoid morphology may be present in a pilocytic astrocytoma
- Pilomyxoid astrocytomas typically do not have fibrillar areas, eosinophilic granular bodies, Rosenthal fibers, or calcifications; they do have a myxoid background, pseudorosette pattern, and monomorphic cells

PLEOMORPHIC XANTHOASTROCYTOMA
- Lacks biphasic pattern
- Typically more cellular and has increased nuclear pleomorphism
- Xanthomatous cells are present that are not seen in pilocytic astrocytoma

GANGLION CELL TUMORS
- Show clustered atypical neurons, which are immunohistochemically positive for neuronal markers

HEMANGIOBLASTOMA
- Also associated with cyst formation

- Highly vascular with abundant reticulin formation
- Contains foamy cells filled with lipid

PEARLS

- *Important to distinguish pilocytic astrocytomas from fibrillary or diffuse astrocytomas because treatment and prognosis are different*
- *Typically cured by complete resection; overall prognosis is excellent*
- *Rare tumors have an aggressive clinical course, and transformation to glioblastoma has been reported*

SELECTED REFERENCES

Korshunov A, Meyer J, Capper D, et al: Combined molecular analysis of BRAF and IDH1 distinguishes pilocytic astrocytoma from diffuse astrocytoma. Acta Neuropathol 118:401-405, 2009.

Rodriguez FJ, Giannini C, Asmann YW, et al: Gene expression profiling of NF-1-associated and sporadic pilocytic astrocytoma identifies aldehyde dehydrogenase 1 family member L1 (ALDH1L1) as an underexpressed candidate biomarker in aggressive subtypes. J Neuropathol Exp Neurol 67:1194-1204, 2008.

Schindler G, Capper D, Meyer J, et al: Analysis of BRAF V600E mutation in 1,320 nervous system tumors reveals high mutation frequencies in pleomorphic xanthoastrocytoma, ganglioglioma, and extra-cerebellar pilocytic astrocytoma. Acta Neuropathol 121:397-405, 2011.

Tihan T, Davis R, Elowitz E, et al: Practical value of Ki-67 and p53 labeling indexes in stereotactic biopsies of diffuse and pilocytic astrocytomas. Arch Pathol Lab Med 124:108-113, 2000.

Tomlinson FH, Scheithauer BW, Hayostek CJ, et al: The significance of atypia and histologic malignancy in pilocytic astrocytomas of the cerebellum: a clinicopathologic and flow cytometric study. J Child Neurol 9:301-310, 1994.

PILOMYXOID ASTROCYTOMA (WHO GRADE II)

Clinical Features

- Closely related to pilocytic astrocytoma but may have a more aggressive clinical course
- Occurs predominantly in infants and young children (mean age, 18 months) and involves the chiasm and

hypothalamus most often; it occasionally occurs in adults and the elderly

- Reported in temporal lobe, thalamus, posterior fossa, and spinal cord
- Symptoms may be nonlocalizing: failure to thrive, developmental delay, vomiting and feeding difficulties, generalized weakness, and altered levels of consciousness
- Focal neurologic symptoms also occur: visual disturbances and endocrine dysfunction
- Tendency to disseminate through cerebrospinal fluid and to recur
- MRI scans show hypointensity on T1-weighted and hyperintensity on T2-weighted images with homogeneous contrast enhancement

Gross Pathology

- Myxoid ill-defined mass

Histopathology

- Monomorphous, hypercellular, compact small bipolar cells set in a myxoid and fibrillary background
- Angiocentric pattern of arrangement of cells suggestive of perivascular pseudorosettes is often evident
- Limited peripheral parenchymal involvement
- Rare nuclear pleomorphism
- Usually lacks Rosenthal fibers and eosinophilic granular bodies
- Mitotic figures may be present
- Endothelial proliferation and necrosis reported in some cases
- Tumors exhibiting features of both pilomyxoid astrocytoma (PMA) and pilocytic astrocytoma (PA) are reported and identified as intermediate lesions (see the section on pilocytic astrocytomas)

Special Stains and Immunohistochemistry

- GFAP: diffuse positivity
- Synaptophysin: positivity has been reported
- Neuronal markers: negative
- MIB-1 labeling index ranges from 2% to 20%

Other Techniques for Diagnosis

- Cytogenetics: regional chromosome loss on 2p, 2q, and 3q and high frequency of underexpression of *ALD1L1* gene

Differential Diagnosis

PILOCYTIC ASTROCYTOMA

- Occurs also in the chiasm and hypothalamus
- Rosenthal fibers and eosinophilic granular bodies present
- Biphasic architecture

PEARLS

- *Reports of transition of a pilomyxoid astrocytoma to a pilocytic astrocytoma and tumors with features of both entities suggest that a pilomyxoid astrocytoma may transition in time to a pilocytic astrocytoma*
- *Pilomyxoid astrocytoma is locally aggressive with a tendency to recur (76%) and disseminate through the cerebrospinal fluid (14%); overall survival is 63 months*

SELECTED REFERENCES

Brat DJ, Scheithauer BW, Fuller GN, Tihan T: Newly codified glial neoplasms of the 2007 WHO classification of tumours of the central nervous system: angiocentric glioma, pilomyxoid astrocytoma and pituicytoma. Brain Pathol 17:319-324, 2007.

Johnson MW, Eberhart CG, Perry A, et al: Spectrum of pilomyxoid astrocytomas, intermediate pilomyxoid tumors. Am J Surg Pathol 34:1783-1791, 2010.

Komotar RJ, Mocco J, Jones JE, et al: Pilomyxoid astrocytoma: diagnosis, prognosis, and management. Neurosurg Focus 18:E7, 2005.

Marko NF, Weil RJ: The molecular biology of WHO grade II gliomas. Neurosurg Focus 34:E1, 2013.

Tihan T, Fisher PG, Kepner JL, et al: Pediatric astrocytomas with monomorphous pilomyxoid features and a less favorable outcome. J Neuropath Exp Neurol 58:1061-1068, 1999.

PLEOMORPHIC XANTHOASTROCYTOMA (WHO GRADE II)

Clinical Features

- Rare astrocytic neoplasm usually found in children and young adults (66% are younger than 18 years)
- Superficial location in the cerebral hemisphere (most frequently temporal lobe) often involving the meninges; rare involvement of the deep gray matter, cerebellum, spinal cord, sella, suprasellar region, and retina
- Patients present typically with a long history of seizures and occasional headaches; seldom with focal neurologic signs
- Computed tomography (CT) and magnetic resonance imaging (MRI) show a well-defined enhancing mass, adjacent to the meninges, that is solid or cystic with a mural nodule

Gross Pathology

- Well-defined, cystic mass with a mural nodule or a solid mass
- Often attached to the meninges; may spread along brain surface

Histopathology

- Varied histologic pattern ranging from single or multinucleated giant cells to irregular spindle cells showing intracellular lipid accumulation (xanthomatous change) (Figure 19-3)
- Reticulin network surrounding individual tumor cells; desmoplasia often present
- Patchy lymphocytic infiltrates often seen
- Variable degrees of vascular sclerosis
- Eosinophilic granular bodies or protein droplets prominent
- Usually absent or inconspicuous mitotic activity and necrosis
- When numerous mitoses (> 5 mitoses/10 high-power fields [hpf]) and necrosis are present, high rates of recurrence are seen (pleomorphic xanthoastrocytoma with anaplastic features)
- Neuronal differentiation may be present

Special Stains and Immunohistochemistry

- GFAP, S-100 protein, and CD34 positive

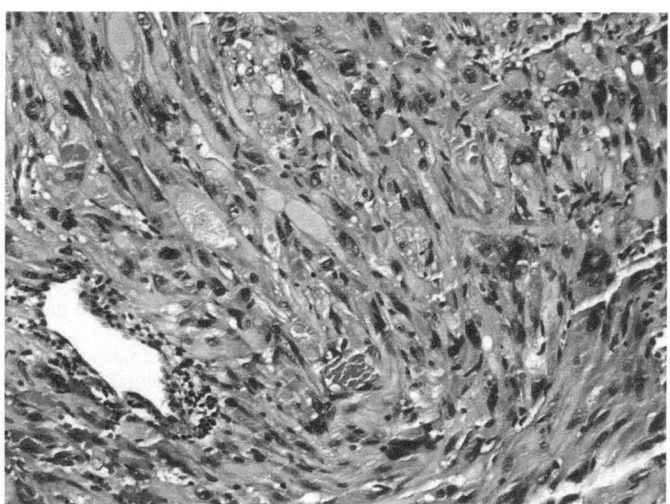

Figure 19-3. Pleomorphic xanthoastrocytoma. Infiltrate of neoplastic astrocytic cells with marked nuclear pleomorphism and xanthomatous changes. Eosinophilic granular bodies are present.

- Reticulin highlights fibrous network surrounding tumor cells
- Synaptophysin and neurofilament variably positive
- MIB-1 labeling index: less than 1% (unless anaplastic)

Other Techniques for Diagnosis

- Electron microscopy: cells typically show abundant intermediate filaments, lysosomes, lipid droplets, basal lamina, and secondary lysosomes
- Approximately 20% show ultrastructural features indicating neuronal differentiation: microtubules, dense core granules, and clear vesicles
- Cytogenetic analyses: *BRAF(V600E)* mutations have been found in 66% of grade 2 pleomorphic xanthoastrocytomas and 65% of grade 3 anaplastic pleomorphic xanthoastrocytomas

Differential Diagnosis

GLIOBLASTOMA

- Important distinction from pleomorphic xanthoastrocytoma because of poor prognosis associated with glioblastoma
- Most lack reticulin investment and eosinophilic granular bodies
- Usually not cystic with mural nodules; always a high mitotic index and endothelial proliferation or necrosis

PILOCYTIC ASTROCYTOMA

- Biphasic pattern is characteristic
- Rosenthal fibers are commonly found
- Usually less cellular and without xanthomatous changes

GANGLION CELL TUMORS

- Atypical neurons that are positive for neuronal markers (synaptophysin and neurofilament) are a defining feature
- Usually lack xanthomatous changes

- *Surgical resection is primary treatment with overall good prognosis, especially when gross total resection is possible*
- *Elderly patients and those with anaplastic (grade III), subtotally resected, or recurrent tumors have worse prognosis*
- *Hypothesized to arise from subpial astrocytes and often display neuronal differentiation*

SELECTED REFERENCES

Giannini C, Scheithauer BW, Lopes MBS, et al: Immunophenotype of pleomorphic xanthoastrocytoma. Am J Surg Pathol 26:479-485, 2002.

Kepes JJ: Pleomorphic xanthoastrocytoma: the birth of a diagnosis and a concept. Brain Pathol 3:269-274, 1993.

Marko NF, Weil RJ: The molecular biology of WHO Grade II gliomas. Neurosurg Focus 34:E1, 2013.

Perkins SM, Mitra N, Fei W, et al: Patterns of care and outcomes of patients with pleomorphic xanthoastrocytoma: a SEER analysis. J Neurooncol 110:99-104, 2012.

Schindler G, Capper D, Meyer J, et al: Analysis of *BRAF V600E* mutation in 1,320 nervous system tumors reveals high mutation frequencies in pleomorphic xanthoastrocytoma, ganglioglioma, and extra-cerebellar pilocytic astrocytoma. Acta Neuropathol 121:397-405, 2011.

SUBEPENDYMAL GIANT CELL ASTROCYTOMA (WHO GRADE I)

Clinical Features

- Most common neoplastic process involving the brain in patients with tuberous sclerosis (TS)
  - TS is an autosomal dominant disorder with markedly variable penetrance and an incidence between 1 per 9000 and 1 per 10,000 births
  - Central nervous system (CNS) abnormalities include cortical hamartomas (tubers), subcortical glioneuronal hamartomas, subependymal glial nodules, subependymal giant cell astrocytoma (SEGA); other organs affected are skin, lung, retina, kidney, and heart
  - Neurologic symptoms in TS usually occur shortly after birth and include seizures and infantile spasms; cognitive disability and autism may become evident at older ages
  - Mutations in either of two genes, *TSC1* (encoding hamartin) on chromosome 9 and *TSC2* (encoding tuberin) on chromosome 16, are found in > 85% of patients with the TS complex
- SEGA rarely occurs without association with TS
  - Occurs in 5% to 20% of persons with TS
  - Usually develops during childhood or adolescence
  - Clinical symptoms are usually secondary to obstructive hydrocephalus and occur when large SEGAs block cerebrospinal fluid (CSF) flow

Gross Pathology

- Typically an exophytic, solid, fleshy, well-defined, tan mass arising in the wall of the lateral ventricle

Histopathology

- Variable cellular morphology, including the following:
  - Polygonal cells with abundant eosinophilic cytoplasm suggestive of gemistocytic astrocytes (Figure 19-4)

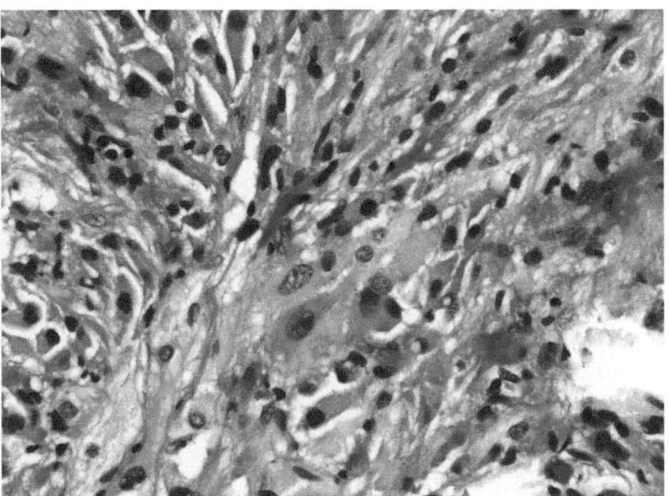

Figure 19-4. Subependymal giant cell astrocytoma. Infiltrate of astrocytic-appearing cells with abundant, frequently spindled eosinophilic cytoplasm. Prominent nucleoli are frequent.

- Spindle-shaped cells with fibrillary cytoplasm forming streams and bundles
- Large pleomorphic cells with nuclei exhibiting prominent nucleoli, suggestive of neuronal differentiation (sometimes multinucleated)
- Focal microcalcifications and scattered mast cells are common features
- Ill-defined pseudorosette formation may be seen
- Variable mitotic activity
- Vascular proliferation and necrosis are uncommon
- High-grade cytologic features do not appear to impose an adverse clinical course

Special Stains and Immunohistochemistry

- GFAP, S-100 protein, synaptophysin, and neurofilament positive
- Class III β-tubulin and neuropeptides (somatostatin and met-enkephalin) positive
- MIB-1 (Ki-67): few positive cells (low proliferative index)

Other Techniques for Diagnosis

- Cytogenetics: deletion mutations in *TSC1* or *TSC2* cause a constitutive up-regulation of mTOR complex 1 tumor suppressor complex, resulting in abnormal cellular proliferation

Differential Diagnosis

GEMISTOCYTIC ASTROCYTOMA

- May be confused because both lesions contain astrocytic cells with abundant pink glassy cytoplasm
- Intraparenchymal tumor rather than an exophytic intraventricular mass
- Typically shows an infiltrative architecture
- No mast cell infiltrate and microcalcifications

SUBEPENDYMAL GLIAL NODULE

- Considered to be a precursor to SEGA
- More frequently calcified than SEGA
- Usually asymptomatic; shows no growth on serial brain scans
- Histologically identical to SEGA

PEARLS

- *Debate still exists as to whether SEGAs can occur outside the setting of TS*
- *Believed to be an astrocytic neoplasm; however, studies have shown that many tumors show a more glioneuronal phenotype*
- *Tumors occasionally recur, but unlike gemistocytic astrocytoma, no malignant transformation has been shown, although local invasion has been reported*
- *Approximately 50% of TS patients have a positive family history, suggesting a high rate of spontaneous mutation*
- *Current standard treatment is surgical resection; studies have shown reduction in tumor size with administration of everolimus, an inhibitor of the mTOR complex 1*

SELECTED REFERENCES

Chan JA, Zhang H, Roberts PS, et al: Pathogenesis of tuberous sclerosis subependymal giant cell astrocytomas: biallelic inactivation of TSC1 or TSC2 leads to mTOR activation. J Neuropathol Exp Neurol 63:1236-1242, 2004.

Goh S, Butler W, Thiele EA: Subependymal giant cell tumors in tuberous sclerosis complex. Neurology 63:1457-1461, 2004.

Krueger DA, Care MM, Holland K, et al: Everolimus for subependymal giant-cell astrocytomas in tuberous sclerosis. N Engl J Med 363:1801-1811, 2010.

GLIONEURONAL TUMOR WITH NEUROPIL-LIKE ISLANDS (WHO GRADES II AND III)

Clinical Features

- Occur typically in cerebrum in adults, males more often than females, ranging from 23 to 65 years old (mean, 42 years)
- Present with new-onset seizures or focal neurologic deficit
- MRI scan typically shows solid, infiltrative, nonenhancing masses (contrast enhancement has been identified in recurrent tumors)
- Occurs usually in cerebrum but also reported in spinal cord
- Gross pathology: not reported

Histopathology

- Diffusely infiltrative fibrillary or gemistocytic astrocytic components alternate with islands of neuropil-like tissue surrounded by cells (in a subset, forming rosettes) that may appear oligodendroglial or neurocytic; mature-appearing neurons may also be present in the glial or neuropil-like areas
- Mitoses seen in glial component
- Anaplasia has been reported with increased mitoses, endothelial proliferation, and necrosis

Special Stains and Immunohistochemistry

- GFAP: positive in the glial appearing component; neuropil islands and neurocytic/neuronal cells are negative
- Synaptophysin and Neu-N: positive in neuropil-like islands and neurocytic/neuronal cells
- P53: may be positive in both glial and neuronal components
- MIB-1 is < 4% to 5% in lower-grade tumors; up to 18% has been reported in anaplastic neoplasms

Other Techniques for Diagnosis

- Cytogenetics: positive for *IDH1 (R132H)* mutation; no co-deletions of chromosomes 1p and 19q

Differential Diagnosis

GANGLIOGLIOMA

- Lacks rosetting pattern and small round cell component found in glioneuronal tumors with neuropil-like islands (GTNI)
- Presence of eosinophilic granular bodies and Rosenthal fibers not seen in GTNI

GRADE 2 OR 3 DIFFUSE ASTROCYTOMA

- Absence of neuropil islands, neurons, small round cell component, and positive staining with neuronal markers

EPENDYMOMA

- Location is most often intraventricular rather than intraparenchymal
- Presence of perivascular pseudorosettes and ependymal rosettes rather than neuropil islands

OLIGODENDROGLIOMA

- Morphologically more monomorphic than GTNI
- Most have deletions of 1p and 191 (not seen in GTNI)

PEARLS

- *Behavior is comparable to diffuse astrocytomas of the same grade*
- *Leptomeningeal dissemination reported*

SELECTED REFERENCES

Allende DS, Prayson RA: The expanding family of glioneuronal tumors. Adv Anat Pathol 16:33-39, 2009.

Barbashina V, Salazar P, Ladanyi M, et al: Glioneuronal tumor with neuropil-like islands (GTNI): A report of 8 cases With chromosome 1p/19q deletion analysis. Am J Surg Pathol 31:1196-1202, 2007.

Huse JT, Nafa K, Shukla N, et al: High frequency of IDH-1 mutation links glioneuronal tumor with neuropil-like islands to diffuse astrocytomas. Acta Neuropathol 122:367-369, 2011.

Teo JG, Gultekin SH, Bilsky M, et al: A distinctive glioneuronal tumor of the adult cerebrum with neuropil-like (including "rosette") islands: report of 4 cases. Am J Surg Pathol 23:502-510, 1999.

OLIGODENDROGLIAL TUMORS

OLIGODENDROGLIOMA (WHO GRADE II) AND ANAPLASTIC OLIGODENDROGLIOMA (WHO GRADE III)

Clinical Features

- Reported to represent between 12% and 20% of all infiltrating gliomas
- Typically occurs in middle-aged adults between 35 to 50 years in age; there is a slight predominance in males
- Patients present with a long history of progressively worsening neurologic symptoms
- Commonly cause severe headache and seizures
- CT and MRI show a well-defined mass, often with calcifications; presence of contrast-enhancement suggests anaplastic morphology

Gross Pathology

- Frontal lobe is the lobe most commonly involved; typically white-matter tumors; infiltration into the cortex is common, and infiltration into leptomeninges may be seen
- Soft, ill-defined, gray-pink tumors, which often expand gray matter and blur gray-white matter junction
- Mucoid degeneration with a gelatinous appearance may be seen
- Cyst formation and focal intratumoral hemorrhage are common

Histopathology

OLIGODENDROGLIOMA

- Low to moderately cellular tumor composed of cells with round nuclei that are larger than normal oligodendrocytes and show atypia; nuclei are hyperchromatic and may appear lobate (cytologic features are well demonstrated with smear preparations) (Figure 19-5A)

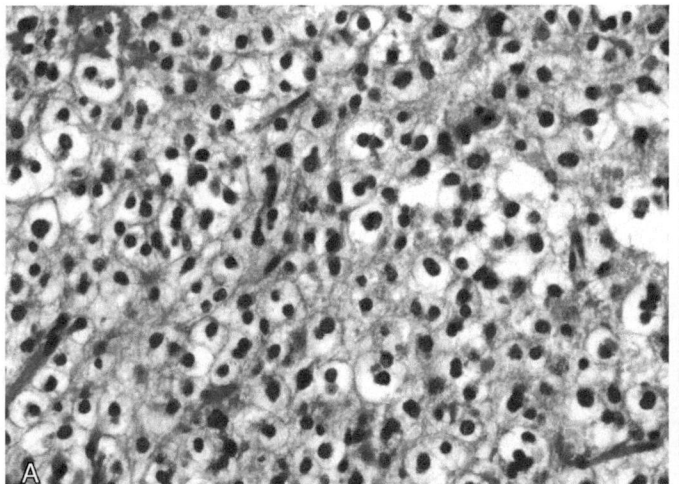
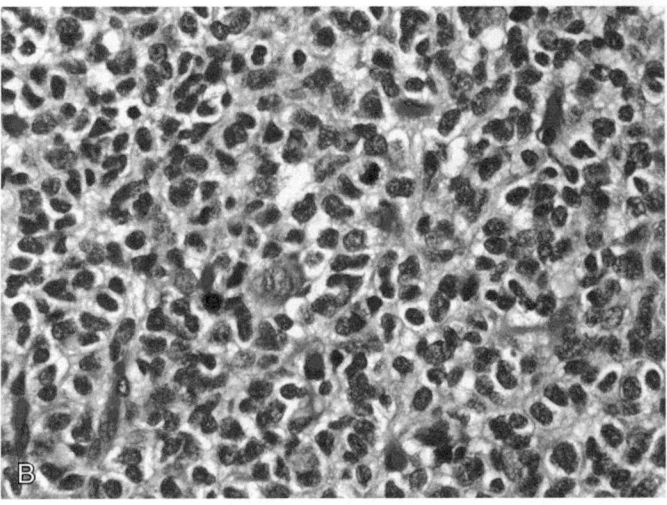

Figure 19-5. A, Low-grade oligodendroglioma. Moderately cellular tumor composed of cells with round hyperchromatic nuclei and clear cytoplasm, giving the characteristic fried-egg appearance. **B,** Anaplastic oligodendroglioma. Notice the mitoses, high cellularity, nuclear enlargement, and hyperchromatism.

- Formalin-fixed, paraffin-embedded tissue often causes the tumor cells to swell, resulting in an enlarged cell with well-defined cell membranes and clear cytoplasm; fried-egg appearance (not seen on smear preparations, frozen sections, or quickly fixed tissue)
- Few glial fibrillary processes are seen
- Two morphologic variants of oligodendroglial cells may also be present (especially in anaplastic tumors)
  - Minigemistocytes or microgemistocytes, exhibiting small pools of eosinophilic cytoplasm
  - Gliofibrillary oligodendrocytes, exhibiting paranuclear eosinophilic fibrils
- A dense network of branching capillaries (chicken-wire appearance) is seen throughout the tumor
- Mitotic activity is usually low
- Microcalcifications and mucoid and microcystic degeneration are helpful diagnostic features
- Focal hemorrhage is commonly seen
- Cortex is often involved; perineuronal satellitosis, perivascular satellitosis, or subpial aggregation (secondary structures of Scherer) are often present

ANAPLASTIC OLIGODENDROGLIOMA
- Same cytologic features described previously but with increased nuclear atypia and cellular pleomorphism while retaining round nuclear outlines
- Increased cellularity is evident, but this finding is not sufficient for anaplastic designation (Figure 19-5B)
- Mitotic activity is marked (minimum of 6 mitoses/10 hpf)
- Several studies have shown endothelial vascular proliferation to correlate with aggressive behavior and poor prognosis
- Presence of geographic necrosis (with or without pseudopalisading) has also been found to correlate with aggressive behavior and poor prognosis but is not an independent prognostic factor in all studies

OLIGODENDROGLIOMA WITH NEUROCYTIC DIFFERENTIATION
- Foci of Homer Wright rosettes and perivascular pseudorosettes associated with small round dark nuclei (reminiscent of internal granular cell layer neurons) have been reported in otherwise typical oligodendrogliomas

Special Stains and Immunohistochemistry
- GFAP positive in reactive astrocytes, gliofibrillary oligodendrocytes, and minigemistocytes
- Synaptophysin, Neu-N, and neurofilament negative except in rare specimens with foci of neurocytic differentiation
- p53: weak to absent in low-grade tumors; may be present in high-grade tumors, especially after treatment
- Cytokeratin negative
- MIB-1: disease-free survival is significantly shorter in patients with a labeling index of more than 5% compared with patients with a labeling index of less than 5%

Other Techniques for Diagnosis
- Electron microscopy: presence of microtubules

- Cytogenetics
  - Losses of 1p and 19q are almost always found together in oligodendrogliomas (50% to 80%); co-deletions are much less common in pediatric cases
  - Oligodendrogliomas with neurocytic differentiation have co-deletions of 1p and 19q in 75% of cases
  - Mutations in the *IDH1* gene is usually present (82% of grade 2 oligodendrogliomas and 69.5% of grade 3 anaplastic oligodendrogliomas)
  - Mutations in the *IDH2* gene are much less common than in *IDH1* gene but more common in oligodendrogliomas (4.7% in grade 2 oligodendrogliomas and 5.2% in grade 3 anaplastic oligodendrogliomas) than astrocytomas
  - *TP53* mutations are rare

Differential Diagnosis
DIFFUSE ASTROCYTOMA
- Tumor cells have greater nuclear irregularity and pleomorphism, no perinuclear halos, and fibrillary cytoplasm
- GFAP positive
- *TP53* mutations; no losses of chromosomes 1p and 19q

SMALL CELL VARIANT OF ANAPLASTIC ASTROCYTOMA AND GLIOBLASTOMA
- Cytologically monotonous, but oval, not round, nuclei
- Numerous mitoses, pseudopalisading necrosis, vascular proliferation
- GFAP positive cytoplasmic processes
- No loss of chromosomes 1p and 19q or presence of *IDH1* gene mutation
- Amplification of *EGFR* and *EGFRvIII*, loss of chromosome 10q

CENTRAL NEUROCYTOMA OR EXTRAVENTRICULAR NEUROCYTOMA
- Central neurocytoma is usually within the ventricle attached to the septum pellucidum
  - Well-circumscribed without infiltrative borders, neurocytic rosettes
  - Positive for synaptophysin
  - Lack of co-deletions of chromosomes 1p and 19q
- Extraventricular neurocytoma
  - Positive for synaptophysin
  - From 17% to 24% of extraventricular neurocytomas have deletions of 1p and 19q

DYSEMBRYOPLASTIC NEUROEPITHELIAL TUMOR (DNT)
- Usually found in younger individuals with a long history of seizures
- Most are located in the temporal lobe
- Histologically consists of a glioneuronal element, glial nodules, and cortical dysplasia
- Distinction from an oligodendroglioma may be impossible on a fragmented specimen

CLEAR CELL EPENDYMOMA
- Usually affects younger individuals
- Forms perivascular pseudorosettes consisting of cells with elongated, tapering processes and ependymal rosettes and canals

- GFAP positive
- Often anaplastic and exhibits noninfiltrative growth pattern

PILOCYTIC ASTROCYTOMA
- Affects children usually
- Cerebellar location, but also in hypothalamus, optic nerve, and brain stem
- Elongated cells with prominent fibrillary cytoplasm, Rosenthal fibers, and eosinophilic granular bodies
- GFAP positive

CHRONIC SEIZURE DISORDERS WITH OLIGODENDROCYTE HYPERPLASIA
- Numerous oligodendrocytes are frequently evident in resections in patients with chronic epilepsy
- Lack of cytologic atypia and subpial extension; perineuronal satellitosis may be seen

PEARLS

- *Loss of 1p and 19q is a strong predictor of response to chemotherapy (procarbazine, lomustine, vincristine [PCV], and temozolomide), possibly radiation therapy, and long survival in low- and high-grade oligodendrogliomas*
- *Testing for deletions of 1p and 19q and IDH gene mutations may be indicated to help in diagnostic classification when a glioma does not clearly show morphologic features allowing definitive designation as oligodendroglioma*
- *Overall, patients have a survival time of 3 to 5 years for all oligodendrogliomas*
- *Other factors associated with increased survival: younger age, frontal location, tumor size, complete surgical removal, and lack of enhancement*
- *Most patients with anaplastic oligodendroglioma die of local recurrence; CSF dissemination or systemic metastases occur rarely*

SELECTED REFERENCES

Aldape K, Burger PC, Perry A: Clinicopathologic aspects of 1p/19q loss and the diagnosis of oligodendroglioma. Arch Pathol Lab Med 131:242-251, 2007.

Cairncross JG, Ueki K, Zlatescu MC, et al: Specific genetic predictors of chemotherapeutic response and survival in patients with anaplastic oligodendrogliomas. J Natl Cancer Inst 90:1473-1479, 1998.

Hartmann C, Meyer J, Balss J, et al: Type and frequency of IDH1 and IDH2 mutations are related to astrocytic and oligodendroglial differentiation and age: a study of 1,010 diffuse gliomas. Acta Neuropathol 118:469-474, 2009.

Rodriguez FJ, Giannini C: Oligodendroglial tumors: diagnostic and molecular pathology. Semin Diagn Pathol 27:136-145, 2010.

OLIGOASTROCYTOMA (WHO GRADE II), ANAPLASTIC OLIGOASTROCYTOMA (WHO GRADE III), AND GLIOBLASTOMA MULTIFORME WITH OLIGODENDROGLIAL FEATURES (WHO GRADE IV)

Clinical Features

- Account for 5% to 10% of gliomas
- Clinical signs and symptoms at presentation are similar to those seen in pure gliomas

Gross Pathology

- Gross features similar to those seen with pure gliomas

Histopathology

- May exhibit distinct areas of astrocytic and oligodendroglial differentiation or have intermingled astrocytic and oligodendroglial cells
- Percentages of each glial component necessary to qualify the glioma as mixed are not universally agreed on

OLIGOASTROCYTOMA (WHO GRADE II)
- Low to moderate cellularity and cytologic atypia
- Rare mitotic figures

ANAPLASTIC OLIGOASTROCYTOMA (WHO GRADE III)
- Higher cellularity and increased cytologic atypia
- Abundant mitotic activity
- Endothelial proliferation
- Anaplastic features may be present in either glial component

GLIOBLASTOMA MULTIFORME WITH OLIGODENDROGLIAL FEATURES (WHO GRADE IV)
- Study has found that the presence of necrosis with or without pseudopalisading is associated with a worse prognosis than an anaplastic oligoastrocytoma without necrosis, and suggested use of designation *GBM with oligodendroglial features*

Special Stains and Immunohistochemistry

- See "Special Stains and Immunohistochemistry" for astrocytomas and oligodendrogliomas

Other Techniques for Diagnosis

- Cytogenetics
  - Mixed tumors usually exhibit homogeneous genetic profiles
  - Analysis of oligoastrocytomas suggests two distinct genetic subsets
    - Mutation in *TP53* gene or loss of heterozygosity of 17p indicates relationship to astrocytomas
    - Loss of heterozygosity of 1p and 19q indicates genetic resemblance to oligodendrogliomas (reported in 20% to 30% of oligoastrocytomas)
  - Mutations in *IDH1* gene at codon 132 (R132H) have been identified in 82% of oligoastrocytomas, 66% of anaplastic oligoastrocytomas, and 55% of GBM with oligodendroglial features
  - Mutations in *IDH2* gene have been identified in 1.3% and 6%, respectively, of oligoastrocytoma and anaplastic oligoastrocytoma

Differential Diagnosis

PURE ASTROCYTOMA
- Only a neoplastic astrocytic component is present
- Lacks unequivocal neoplasia in other glial cell line

PURE OLIGODENDROGLIOMA
- Only a neoplastic oligodendroglial component is present
- Lacks unequivocal neoplasia in other glial cell line

PEARLS

- *Prognosis in this neoplasm is still better than that of a glioma without an oligodendroglioma component, independent of 1p and 19q deletion status*
- *Some studies show that oligoastrocytomas and pure oligodendrogliomas respond similarly to chemotherapy and show no significant differences in survival; in addition, it has been reported that patients with pure oligodendrogliomas or oligoastrocytomas do better than those with pure astrocytomas*
- *Combined loss of 1p and 19q is associated with improved survival in oligoastrocytomas compared with oligoastrocytomas without deletions of 1p and 19q*
- *Pathologic diagnosis of oligoastrocytomas is subject to marked interobserver variability*

SELECTED REFERENCES

Hartmann C, Meyer J, Balss J, et al: Type and frequency of IDH1 and IDH2 mutations are related to astrocytic and oligodendroglial differentiation and age: a study of 1,010 diffuse gliomas. Acta Neuropathol 118:469-474, 2009.

Joseph NM, Phillips J, Dahiya S, et al: Diagnostic implications of IDH1-R132H and OLIG2 expression patterns in rare and challenging glioblastoma variants. Mod Pathol 26:315-326, 2013.

Miller CR, Dunham CP, Scheithauer BW, Perry A: Significance of necrosis in grading of oligodendroglial neoplasms: a clinicopathologic and genetic study of newly diagnosed highgrade gliomas. J Clin Oncol 24:5419-5426, 2006.

Perl A, Fuller CE, Banerjee R, et al: Ancillary FISH analysis for 1p and 19q status: preliminary observations in 287 gliomas and oligodendroglioma mimics. Front Biosci 8:a1-a9, 2003.

EPENDYMAL TUMORS

EPENDYMOMA (WHO GRADE II) AND ANAPLASTIC EPENDYMOMA (WHO GRADE III)

Clinical Features

- Occur most commonly in children and young adults
- Account for about 3% to 9% of all neuroepithelial tumors; most frequent neuroepithelial tumors of the spinal cord (50% to 60% of spinal gliomas)
- Occur at any site along the ventricular system; most commonly in the fourth ventricle and spinal cord, followed by the lateral ventricles
- Tumors in children are more commonly in the infratentorial region at a mean age of 6.4 years
- Spinal and supratentorial tumors occur in adults
- Patients often present with symptoms of hydrocephalus, including nausea, vomiting, and headache; patients occasionally develop seizures
- Posterior fossa tumors may cause visual disturbances or cerebellar ataxia

Gross Pathology

- Soft gray-pink tumors that may be solid or cystic
- Areas of hemorrhage or necrosis may be present
- Typically protrude from the ventricular lining and fill the ventricular lumen; well demarcated, but may invade the adjacent brain parenchyma

Histopathology (Figure 19-6)

EPENDYMOMA

- Cellular tumors composed of monomorphic cells with round to oval hyperchromatic nuclei and long fibrillary cell processes
- Perivascular pseudorosettes consisting of tumor cells radially arranged around blood vessels are prominent
- True ependymal rosettes consisting of columnar cells radially arranged around a central lumen are less common than perivascular pseudorosettes
- Calcification, as well as metaplastic cartilage or bone, may be seen
- Histologic features of grade II: less than five mitotic figures per 10 hpf, absence of endothelial vascular proliferation and pseudopalisading necrosis, focal areas of 5 to 10 mitoses per 10 hpf and necrosis without pseudopalisading may be present

EPENDYMOMA VARIANTS

- Cellular ependymoma (WHO grade II)
  - Increased cellularity without appreciable increase in mitotic rate or other features associated with anaplasia
  - Increased occurrence in extraventricular sites
- Papillary ependymoma (WHO grade II)
  - Extensive papillary formations
- Clear cell ependymoma
  - Cells exhibit round nuclei and perinuclear halos
  - Anaplastic histologic features are often present
  - Occurs more frequently in supratentorial compartment than in infratentorial compartment
- Tanycytic ependymoma (WHO grade II)
  - Occurs more commonly in spinal cord
  - Composed of elongated spindled glial cells forming fascicles
  - Ependymal rosettes often not present; perivascular pseudorosettes may be ill-defined

ANAPLASTIC EPENDYMOMA

- Morphologic criteria that consistently correlate with prognosis are still debated
- Features associated with poor outcome: (1) hypercellularity with nuclear hyperchromasia and pleomorphism, (2) "brisk" mitotic activity (greater than 10 per 10 hpf), (3) endothelial proliferation, or (4) necrosis with pseudopalisading
- Perivascular pseudorosettes persist

Special Stains and Immunohistochemistry

- GFAP: marked cytoplasmic immunoreactivity, especially prominent in the perivascular pseudorosettes
- Cytokeratin: AE1/AE3 immunoreactivity present in most ependymomas; focal and variably strong positivity with other keratin antibodies
- EMA: dotlike cytoplasmic immunoreactivity present in most neoplastic cells
- CD99: diffuse and dotlike cytoplasmic immunoreactivity with accentuation at membrane surface
- MIB-1 labeling index: more than 5% associated with decreased survival
- Nestin immunoreactivity is associated with a poor prognosis

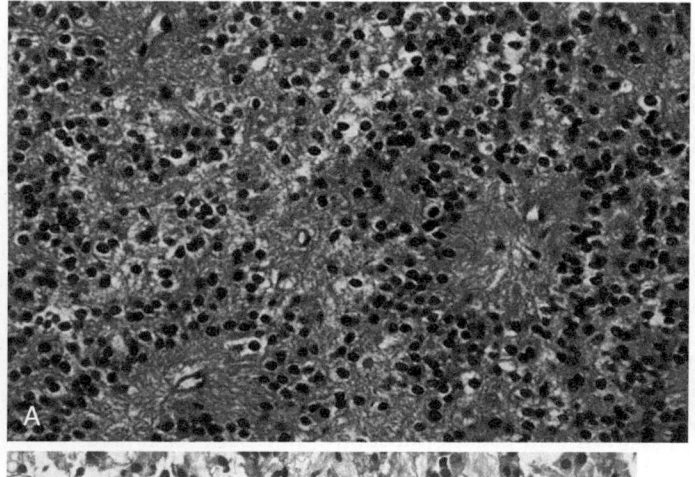

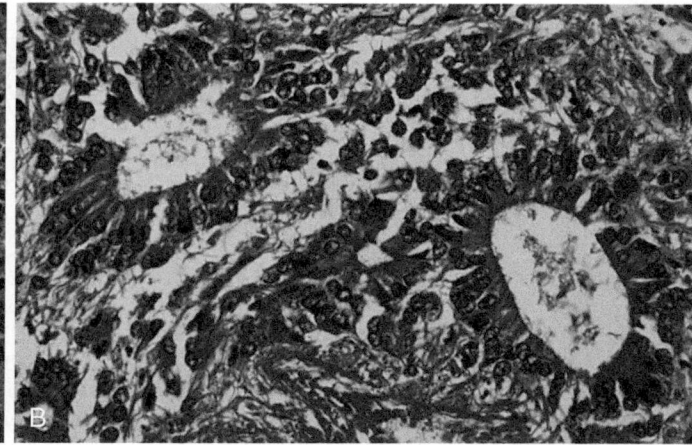

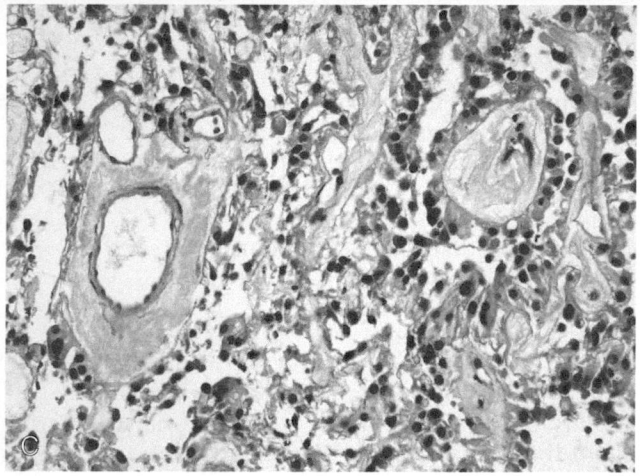

Figure 19-6. Ependymoma. A, Low-power view shows a moderately cellular glial tumor with classic perivascular pseudorosettes. **B,** High-power view shows classic ependymal rosettes. Notice glial cells radially arranged to form a canal (phosphotungstic acid–hematoxylin stain). **C,** Myxopapillary ependymoma. Glial cells exhibiting perivascular arrangement with abundant interposed mucin deposition.

Other Techniques for Diagnosis

- Electron microscopy: cells show polarity with well-formed terminal bars; typically have surface microvilli, cilia, intercellular junctions (zonula adherens), and blepharoplasts
- Cytogenetics: studies have identified two subgroups of ependymoma: group A shows up-regulation of *LAMA2* and chromosome 1q gain, associated with younger age, lateral location, recurrence, and poor survival relative to group B; group B shows up-regulation of *NELL2*, loss of chromosome 22, and lower likelihood of recurrence or metastasis

Differential Diagnosis

METASTATIC ADENOCARCINOMA

- Morphology more consistently epithelial
- Cytokeratin positivity specific for site of origin; less likely positive in ependymoma

FIBRILLARY OR DIFFUSE ASTROCYTOMA

- Poorly defined infiltrative tumor
- Lacks rosette formation
- EMA typically negative

ASTROBLASTOMA

- Rare tumor
- Located away from the ventricle
- Shows marked and diffuse vascular sclerosis

- Tumor cells have short, broad processes
- Lacks true rosette formation

CHOROID PLEXUS PAPILLOMA OR CARCINOMA

- Papillary architecture and no rosette formation (Figure 19-7)
- Negative or only focally positive for GFAP
- Carcinomas have a loose papillary architecture and consist of sheets of pleomorphic cells with a high mitotic rate; extensive necrosis is common

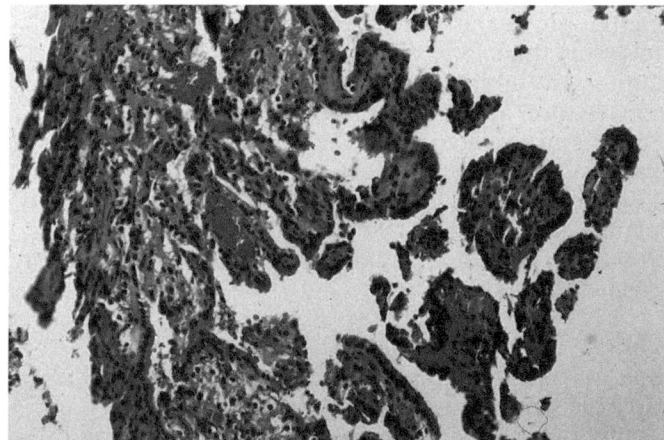

Figure 19-7. Choroid plexus papilloma. Columnar epithelium overlying classic papillary architecture with central fibrovascular core.

PEARLS

- *Extent of surgical resection, age, and histologic grade are significantly associated with progression-free survival, but only extent of surgical resection and age are associated with overall survival*
- *Children < 3 years of age have a survival disadvantage compared to those > 3 years*
- *Patients with spinal ependymomas do much better because complete surgical resection is more feasible*
- *May occasionally occur in the deep white matter away from the ventricle*

SELECTED REFERENCES

Foulade M, Helton K, Dalton J, et al: Clear cell ependymoma: a clinicopathologic and radiographic analysis of 10 patients. Cancer 98:2232-2244, 2003.

Kurt E, Zheng POP, Hop WCJ, et al: Identification of relevant prognostic histopathologic features in 69 intracranial ependymomas, excluding myxopapillary ependymomas and subependymomas. Cancer 106:388-395, 2006.

Tihan T, Zhou T, Holmes E, et al: The prognostic value of histological grading of posterior fossa ependymomas in children: a Children's Oncology Group study and a review of prognostic factors. Mod Pathol 21:165-177, 2008.

Witt H, Korshunov A, Pfister SM, et al: Molecular approaches to ependymoma: the next step(s). Curr Opin Neurol 25:745-750, 2012.

MYXOPAPILLARY EPENDYMOMA (WHO GRADE I)

Clinical Features

- Represents about 10% to 13% of all ependymomas
- Typically presents in young adults at an average age of 36 years
- Occurs more frequently in males (2.5:1)
- Occurs almost exclusively in the conus-cauda-filum terminale region and rarely in the fourth or lateral ventricles or brain parenchyma
- Also reported in subcutaneous tissue overlying the sacrococcyx and in the presacral and postsacral regions
- Signs and symptoms include low back pain, sciatica, and focal neurologic deficits referable to the tumor location

Gross Pathology

- Lobulated, circumscribed, soft gray tumors in the filum terminale or attached to nerve roots

Histopathology

- Composed of papillae lined by monotonous elongated or columnar cells surrounding a central vascular core
- Occasionally fascicular architecture is present
- Abundant perivascular mucin pools and a fibrillary background

Special Stains and Immunohistochemistry

- GFAP, vimentin, and S-100 protein positive
- PAS and Alcian blue highlight perivascular mucin
- Cytokeratin and EMA: each variably reported as positive and negative in literature
- MIB-1: low (< 2%)

Other Techniques for Diagnosis

- Ultrastructural examination shows collagen-rich stroma, cells with basal lamina, and cellular interdigitation
- Cytogenetics: *HOXB13, NEFL,* and *PDGFRα* genes are overexpressed in pediatric cases

Differential Diagnosis

METASTATIC ADENOCARCINOMA (MUCIN SECRETING)

- Rarely involves the filum terminale
- Consists of pleomorphic tumor cells with high mitotic rate
- Hemorrhage and necrosis are typical
- Strong cytokeratin positivity

CHORDOMA

- Characterized by a lobular architecture with cords of epithelial and physaliphorous cells
- Lacks papillary architecture and fibrillary background
- GFAP negative

SCHWANNOMA

- Abundant reticulin
- GFAP negative

PARAGANGLIOMA

- Morphologic features of neuroendocrine differentiation
- Immunoreactive for neuroendocrine markers
- GFAP usually negative tumor cells

PEARLS

- *Typically slow-growing tumors with a favorable prognosis, but dissemination within neural axis is described*
- *Recurrence or dissemination occurs more frequently in children and with incomplete resections; radiation treatment usually given in these settings*
- *Tumors occurring in soft tissues have been associated with aggressive behavior and metastases*

SELECTED REFERENCES

Barton VN, Donson AM, Kleinschmidt-DeMasters BK, et al: Unique molecular characteristics of pediatric myxopapillary ependymoma. Brain Pathol 20:560-570, 2010.

Schittenhelm J, Becker R, Capper D, et al: The clinic-surgico-pathological spectrum of myxopapillary ependymomas: report of four unusual cases and review of the literature. Clin Neuropathol 27;:21-28, 2008.

Sonneland PRL, Scheithauer BW, Onofrio BM: Myxopapillary ependymoma: a clinicopathologic and immunocytochemical study of 77 cases. Cancer 56:883-893, 1985.

SUBEPENDYMOMA (WHO GRADE I)

Clinical Features

- Most frequently found in adult males (male-to-female ratio, 4:1)
- Most occur in the fourth (50% to 60%) or lateral (40% to 50%) ventricles; less commonly in the spinal cord

- Many found incidentally at autopsy, but some cause symptoms, usually related to increased intracranial pressure due to obstruction of the ventricular system
- Mean age at presentation of symptomatic tumors is 47 years
- Symptoms related to mass effect may also be seen (focal neurologic signs, seizures)
- MRI scans of symptomatic lesions show hypointense or isointense signals on T1 images, hyperintensity on T2 images, and heterogeneous contrast enhancement

Gross Pathology

- Firm, tan-white, polypoid nodules of varying size
- Arise from the lining of the ventricle or from the septum pellucidum and protrude in the ventricular lumen; usually well circumscribed
- Focal hemorrhage, calcifications, and cystic changes may be present

Histopathology

- Characterized by clusters of monomorphic tumor cells (resembling normal ependymal cells) in a dense fibrillary matrix of glial cell processes
- Microcystic architecture is a common feature
- Small blood vessel proliferation or focal hemorrhage may be seen within the tumor
- Mitotic activity is rare to absent
- Ependymal pseudorosettes may be seen but are not a typical finding; true rosettes are rare
- Microcalcifications are common
- Microcysts filled with basophilic amorphous material are common

Special Stains and Immunohistochemistry

- GFAP positive, but may be variable in extent
- S-100 protein diffusely positive
- MIB-1: usually less than 1%

Other Techniques for Diagnosis

- Ultrastructural examination shows surface microvilli, intercellular junctions, and cilia
- Initial studies with comparative genomic hybridization have shown varied chromosomal copy number abnormalities

Differential Diagnosis

EPENDYMOMA

- Generally found in younger individuals
- Usually symptomatic, producing hydrocephalus, visual disturbances, or cerebellar ataxia
- More cellular and characterized by rosette and prominent pseudorosette formation

PEARLS

- *For symptomatic lesions, surgical resection is the treatment of choice and is often curative*
- *Tumors showing both ependymal and subependymal features are generally classified as ependymomas*
- *Hypothesized to arise from subependymal glial cells (tanycytes) or astrocytes of the subependymal plate; may be a hamartomatous proliferation*

SELECTED REFERENCES

Brown DF, Rushing EJ: Subependymomas: clinicopathological study of 14 tumors. Arch Pathol Lab Med 123:873, 1999.

Jain A, Amin AG, Jain P, et al: Subependymoma: clinical features and surgical outcomes. Neurol Res 34:677- 684, 2012.

Kurian KM, Jones DTW, Marsden F: Genome-wide Analysis of subependymomas shows underlying chromosomal copy number changes involving chromosomes 6, 7, 8, and 14 in a proportion of cases. Brain Pathol 18:469-473, 2008.

OTHER NEUROEPITHELIAL TUMORS

ASTROBLASTOMA (NO ASSIGNED WHO GRADE)

Clinical Features

- Rare neoplasm occurring most frequently in children and young adults; uncommon in older adults; one study has noted a female predominance
- Patients typically present with symptoms of mass effect; may have focal neurologic deficits, headache, or seizures
- Usually located near or at the surface of the cerebral hemispheres; may arise in the corpus callosum, cerebellum, optic nerves, brain stem, or cauda equina
- MRI shows a well-defined, contrast-enhancing mass with solid or cystic components; the solid component has a characteristic bubbly appearance and little associated T2 hyperintensity

Gross Pathology

- Small cyst formation and focal necrosis may be seen, especially in larger tumors

Histopathology

- Key feature is the astroblastic pseudorosette composed of broad, nontapering, nonfibrillar processes that radiate toward a central blood vessel
- Depending on the tumor grade, cells may be monomorphic with inconspicuous nucleoli or show pleomorphic, hyperchromatic nuclei with obvious nucleoli
- Marked perivascular hyalinization is characteristic and may coalesce to occupy extensive areas
- Typically noninfiltrative interface with surrounding brain tissue
- Low grade
  - Uniform distribution of perivascular pseudorosettes
  - Low mitotic activity (mean 1 mitosis/10 hpf)
  - Minimal cellular pleomorphism
  - No vascular proliferation or necrosis with pseudopalisading
- High grade
  - Increased cellularity (focal or multifocal)
  - High mitotic rate (> 5 mitoses/10 hpf)
  - Nuclear anaplasia
  - Endothelial proliferation and necrosis with pseudopalisading

Special Stains and Immunohistochemistry

- GFAP, S-100, and vimentin: strong immunoreactivity
- EMA: focal membranous immunoreactivity
- Cytokeratin (low molecular weight): variable
- MIB-1 index: low grade, 3%; high grade, 15%

Other Techniques for Diagnosis

- Electron microscopy: tumor cells contain abundant intermediate filaments and exhibit microvilli, poorly developed intercellular junctions, and rare cilia
- In comparative genomic hybridization studies, most frequently found was gain of chromosome 20q, and slightly less frequent was gain of chromosome 19

Differential Diagnosis

EPENDYMOMA

- Most are infratentorial and within or close to a ventricle
- Lacks vascular hyalinization
- Shows formation of true rosettes
- Cells have elongated fibrillary processes and fibrillary background

ANGIOCENTRIC GLIOMA

- In contrast to astroblastoma, angiocentric gliomas are infiltrating lesions composed of piloid cells that exhibit circumferential arrangements of neoplastic cells around vessels in addition to radial arrangements (as seen in astroblastomas)

PAPILLARY MENINGIOMA

- Contain distinct areas of meningothelial differentiation
- Characteristically EMA positive
- GFAP negative

PEARLS

- *Cell of origin is debated because astroblastomas exhibit features of both astrocytes and ependymal cells; they are suggested to be of tanycytic derivation*
- *Complete resection typically results in long-term survival; in high-grade lesions, adjuvant radiotherapy or chemotherapy is indicated*
- *Focal astroblastic features may be seen in low-grade and high-grade astrocytomas*

SELECTED REFERENCES

Brat DJ, Hirose Y, Cohen KJ, et al: Astroblastoma: clinicopathologic features and chromosomal abnormalities defined by comparative genomic hybridization. Brain Pathol 10:342-352, 2000.

Port JD, Brat DJ, Burger PC, Pomper MG: Astroblastoma: radiologic-pathologic correlation and distinction from ependymoma. Am J Neuroradiol 23:243-247, 2002.

Salvati M, D'Elia A, Brogna C, Frati A, et al: Cerebral astroblastoma: analysis of six cases and critical review of treatment options. J Neurooncol 93:369-378, 2009.

CHORDOID GLIOMA (WHO GRADE II)

Clinical Features

- Uncommon glioma arising in region of third ventricle
- Mean age, 46 years; range, 12 to 70 years
- Females affected more than males
- Signs and symptoms usually secondary to obstructive hydrocephalus; reported symptoms include headache, weight loss, endocrine disturbances, autonomic disturbances, psychosis, and focal neurologic deficits

Gross Pathology

- Well-circumscribed, fusiform, ovoid shape containing cysts; may be attached to the hypothalamus

Histopathology

- Clusters of epithelioid cells and cords of spindle cells in a myxoid and mucinous background
- Sparse to abundant lymphoplasmacytic infiltrates with Russell bodies
- Rare mitotic figures, no necrosis, and endothelial proliferation
- Does not infiltrate into surrounding brain, but Rosenthal fibers are present in adjacent brain

Special Stains and Immunohistochemistry

- PAS and Alcian blue positive background; mucin negative
- Reticulin surrounds clusters of epithelioid cells
- GFAP and vimentin: strong diffuse immunoreactivity
- CD34, EMA, and S100 focal positivity
- Cytokeratin, E-cadherin, neuron-specific enolase (NSE), neurofilament, CD31, and synaptophysin: variable positivity
- MIB-1 labeling index: generally less than 2%

Other Techniques for Diagnosis

- Electron microscopy: abundant intermediate filaments in cytoplasm, apical microvilli, abnormal cilia, focal basal lamina, and hemidesmosomes
- Cytogenetics: preliminary investigations have shown alterations on 9q and 11q and absence of typical molecular abnormalities presence in diffuse gliomas

Differential Diagnosis

CHORDOMA

- Limited cytokeratin immunoreactivity in chordoid glioma, compared with diffuse and strong reactivity in chordoma
- Physaliferous cells characteristic

CHORDOID MENINGIOMA

- Presence of whorls and psammoma bodies, nuclear pseudoinclusions
- No immunoreactivity for GFAP; usually positive for EMA
- Both may have inflammatory infiltrates

PEARLS

- *Gross total resection is the optimal treatment, but adherence to hypothalamus may prevent complete resection and lead to significant morbidity and poor outcome*
- *Cell of origin is hypothesized to be the tanycyte (glial progenitor cell with astrocytic and ependymal features) found in circumventricular organs (lamina terminalis in anterior third ventricular wall)*
- *Metaplastic elements have been reported (chondroid)*

SELECTED REFERENCES

Buccoliero AM, Caldarella A, Gallina P, et al: Chordoid glioma: clinicopathologic profile and differential diagnosis of an uncommon tumor. Arch Pathol Lab Med 128:e141-e145, 2004.

Cenacchi G, Roncaroli F, Cerasoli S, et al: Chordoid glioma of the third ventricle: an ultrastructural study of three cases with a histogenetic hypothesis. Am J Surg Pathol 25:401-405, 2001.

Horbinski C Dacic S, McLendon RE, et al: Chordoid glioma: a case report and molecular characterization of five cases. Brain Pathol 19:439-448, 2009.

ANGIOCENTRIC GLIOMA (WHO GRADE I)

Clinical Features

- Slow-growing glioma
- Reported in patients ranging in age from 2 to 70 years, but occurs most commonly in childhood and adolescence
- Most present with seizures; longstanding history of seizures is common
- Occurs most commonly in cerebral cortex
- MRI of tumor shows a homogeneous not well-demarcated lesion of the cortex and white matter with focal extension to the ventricular surface; a peripheral rim of hyperintensity on T1-weighted images and hyperintensity on T2-weighted and fluid-attenuated inversion recovery images without enhancement are evident

Gross Pathology

- Not yet described

Histopathology

- Superficial cortical location with subpial accumulation
- Infiltration of surrounding parenchyma
- Monomorphous slender bipolar cells with angiocentricity
- Circumferential (more common) or radial arrangements around vessels of all sizes
- Occasional fascicular architecture
- Rare mitoses; no necrosis or endothelial proliferation
- Palmini and colleagues' type 1 cortical dysplasia has been described adjacent to the tumors

Special Stains and Immunohistochemistry

- GFAP: variable degrees of positivity, often around vessels
- S-100 and vimentin positive
- EMA surface and paranuclear dotlike positivity
- Neu-N, chromogranin, and synaptophysin negative
- MIB-1 index: 1%to 5%

Other Techniques for Diagnosis

- Electron microscopy: perivascular cells contain cytoplasmic intermediate filaments and exhibit basement membrane; cell junctions, cilia, and microvilli are described, suggesting ependymal differentiation
- Cytogenetics: *IDH1* (R132H) mutation not present

Differential Diagnosis

ASTROCYTOMA

- Lacks monomorphic nuclear appearance of angiocentric glioma
- No angiocentricity

PILOCYTIC ASTROCYTOMA

- Not infiltrative
- EMA negative

PILOMYXOID ASTROCYTOMA

- Mucinous and myxoid background
- Usual location in hypothalamus
- Contrast enhancing
- Occurs in very young patients

EPENDYMOMA

- Usually in or adjacent to a ventricle
- Exhibits only radially arranged perivascular pseudorosettes and ependymal rosettes

ASTROBLASTOMA

- Radially arranged perivascular pseudorosettes with marked vessel sclerosis

PEARLS

- *Excellent prognosis; gross total resection is usually curative with termination of seizures*
- *Hypothesized to be of ependymal or radial glial cell origin*

SELECTED REFERENCES

Brat DJ, Scheithauer BW, Fuller GN, Tihan T: Newly codified glial neoplasms of the 2007 WHO classification of tumors of the central nervous system: angiocentric glioma, pilomyxoid astrocytoma, and pituicytoma. Brain Pathol 17:319-324, 2007.

Lellouch-Tubiana A, Boddaert N, Bourgeois M, et al: Angiocentric neuroepithelial tumor (ANET): a new epilepsy-related clinicopathological entity with distinctive MRI. Brain Pathol 15:281-286, 2005.

Marburger T, Prayson R: Angiocentric glioma: a clinicopathologic review of 5 tumors with identification of associated cortical dysplasia. Arch Pathol Lab Med 135:1037-1041, 2011.

Raghunathan A, Olar A, Vogel H, et al: Isocitrate dehydrogenase 1 R132H mutation is not detected in angiocentric glioma. Ann Diagn Pathol 16:255-259, 2012.

Wang M, Tihan T, Fojiani AM, et al: Monomorphous angiocentric glioma: a distinctive epileptogenic neoplasm with features of infiltrating astrocytoma and ependymoma. J Neuropath Exp Neurol 64:875-881, 2005.

NEURONAL AND GLIONEURONAL NEOPLASMS

GANGLIOCYTOMA (WHO GRADE I) AND GANGLIOGLIOMA (WHO GRADES I AND III)

Clinical Features

- Gangliocytomas are WHO grade I; most gangliogliomas are WHO grade I; criteria for grade II gangliogliomas are not yet established and anaplastic gangliogliomas are uncommon (WHO grade III)
- Low incidence (1.3% of all brain tumors), but the most common neoplasm in patients with chronic intractable focal epilepsy
- Typically supratentorial and usually involves the temporal lobe (70%)
- Most present in the first three decades; may be found in all ages
- CT and MRI usually show a complex solid or cystic mass; often with calcification

Gross Pathology

- Well-circumscribed gray granular mass that is variably solid and cystic; mural nodule within the cystic component is often seen
- May extend into the leptomeninges and subarachnoid space
- Extensive calcification, hemorrhage, or necrosis may be seen

Histopathology

GANGLIOCYTOMA

- Composed entirely of neurons forming ill-defined groups
- Often exhibits cytologic atypia

GANGLIOGLIOMA

- Tumor composed of atypical ganglion cells as well as a neoplastic glial component (Figure 19-8)
- Neoplastic neurons are characterized by haphazard clustering, lack of orderly distribution, and, often, an abnormal location (in white matter)
- Abnormal neurons may be small or large; often they are binucleated and have large nuclei and prominent nucleoli
- Glial component is variably cellular and most commonly consists of a neoplastic astrocytic population; pilocytic morphology may be seen and oligodendroglial foci are rarely seen
- Rosenthal fibers and eosinophilic granular bodies are often present
- Atypical glial cells with large, bizarre, hyperchromatic nuclei with intranuclear cytoplasmic inclusions may be seen
- Tumor cells may be located in a reticulin-rich stroma
- Foci of perivascular chronic inflammation is a common histologic feature
- Microcalcifications are often present
- Microcystic cavities may be present
- Mitotic figures are rare
- Atypical ganglioglioma (WHO grade II): increased cellularity and mitoses in the astrocytic component
- Anaplastic ganglioglioma (WHO grade III): further increased mitotic activity in the astrocytic component

Special Stains and Immunohistochemistry

- Synaptophysin, S-100 protein, NSE, and Neu-N: neurons are positive
- Neurofilament: neurons may be positive
- Silver stain (Bielschowsky) highlights cell processes of ganglion cells
- CD 34: neuronal component is positive
- GFAP: astrocytic component is positive
- MIB-1: low index (< 3%) in typical ganglioglioma (grade I); elevated in atypical (grade II) and anaplastic (grade III) gangliogliomas

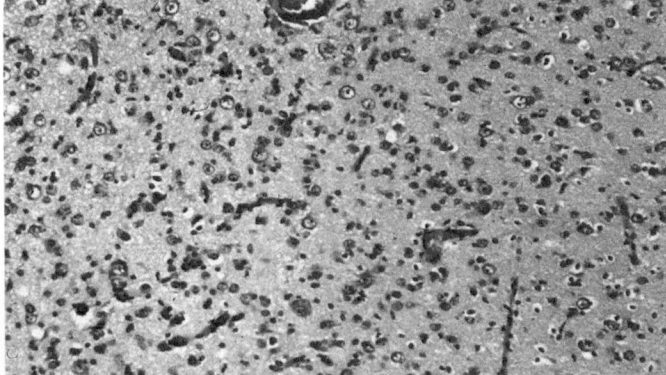

Figure 19-8. Ganglioglioma. Mixed glial-neuronal neoplasm composed of neoplastic astrocytes intermixed with atypical clustered ganglion cells.

Other Techniques for Diagnosis

- Electron microscopy: neurons contain dense-core neurosecretory granules and occasionally exhibit synapses
- Cytogenetic analyses: gangliogliomas
  - Gains of chromosome 7 are most often found, and *TSC2* gene mutation is reported in glial component
  - *IDH1 R132H* gene mutations occur in a minority of gangliogliomas (< 10%) and have been associated with older age of presentation, higher rate of recurrence, malignant transformation, or death
  - Mutation of *BRAF (V600E)* has been identified in 18% of gangliogliomas and 50% of anaplastic gangliogliomas

Differential Diagnosis

VARIANTS OF GANGLIOGLIOMA

- Desmoplastic infantile ganglioglioma and astrocytoma, WHO grade I
  - Most occur before 2 years of age
  - Large cystic masses, superficially located, most often occurring in frontal and parietal lobes, may involve more than one lobe
  - Dense fibrotic masses
  - Fibrous stroma with intermixed clusters or scattered astrocytes
  - Eosinophilic granular bodies and Rosenthal fibers
  - Ganglion cells and small neurocytic cells present in desmoplastic infantile ganglioglioma but may be sparse
- Dysplastic gangliocytoma of the cerebellum (Lhermitte-Duclos)
  - Benign cellular proliferation of dysplastic ganglion cells
  - Diffusely enlarged cerebellar folia secondary to ganglion cells that enlarge and distort the molecular and internal granular cell layers
  - Pathognomonic of Cowden disease

PILOCYTIC ASTROCYTOMA

- Similar radiographic findings
- Biphasic tumor consisting of pilocytic areas and a microcystic background
- Lacks clusters of atypical neurons

DNT

- Both tumors show similar clinical picture
- Composed of a multinodular architecture with a mucoid collagenous background
- Neurons in DNT are typically normal; lacks clustering of pleomorphic neurons

FIBRILLARY OR DIFFUSE ASTROCYTOMA

- Entrapped non-neoplastic neurons may suggest ganglioglioma
- Tumor cells are negative for neuronal markers; positive for GFAP
- MIB-1 index: higher in astrocytomas than gangliogliomas

PLEOMORPHIC XANTHOASTROCYTOMA

- Pleomorphic, xanthomatous cells characterize the neoplasm
- Exhibits both CD34 and GFAP positivity
- Usually lacks a neuronal component

PEARLS

- *Surgical resection for gangliocytoma and ganglioglioma is usually curative; no radiation or chemotherapy is needed; over 90% have a recurrence-free survival > 7 years*
- *Eosinophilic granular bodies are evidence of chronicity and slow growth; they are not diagnostic of gangliogliomas and may be seen in pilocytic astrocytoma, pleomorphic xanthoastrocytoma, and other low-grade astrocytomas*
- *Malignant transformation of the glial cells is extremely rare (anaplastic ganglioglioma)*
- *Ganglion cells may be difficult to appreciate on frozen section; patient age, radiographic findings, and clinical history are helpful*

SELECTED REFERENCES

Blumcke I, Wiestler OD: Gangliogliomas: an intriguing tumor entity associated with focal epilepsies. J Neuropathol Exper Neurol 61:575-584, 2002.

Horbinski C, Kofler J, Yeaney G, et al: Isocitrate dehydrogenase 1 analysis differentiates gangliogliomas from infiltrative gliomas. Brain Pathol 21:564-574, 2011.

McLendon RE, Provenzale J: Glioneuronal tumors of the central nervous system. Brain Tumor Pathol 19:51-58, 2002.

Prayson RA, Khajavi K, Comair YG: Cortical architecture abnormalities and MIB-1 immunoreactivity in gangliogliomas: a study of 60 patients with intracranial tumors. J Neuropathol Exper Neurol 54:513-520, 1995.

Schindler G, Capper D, Meyer J, et al: Analysis of BRAF V600E mutation in 1,320 nervous system tumors reveals high mutation frequencies in pleomorphic xanthoastrocytoma, ganglioglioma, and extra-cerebellar pilocytic astrocytoma. Acta Neuropathol 121:397-405, 2011.

DYSEMBRYOPLASTIC NEUROEPITHELIAL TUMOR (DNT) (WHO GRADE I)

Clinical Features

- Typically found in the first decade in the setting of drug-resistant epilepsy
- Occurs most often in the temporal lobe cortex; also reported in frontal, parietal, and occipital cortexes and selected infratentorial areas

Gross Pathology

- May be well defined or poorly demarcated
- Variable size; most measure a few centimeters
- Gyral expansion with vague multinodular formation and mucoid viscous appearance
- Small cyst formation often seen
- Distortion of the overlying skull may be present

Histopathology

- Cortical, multinodular, microcystic, mucoid tumor
- Three classic histologic features
  - Glioneuronal element ("specific component")
    - Oligodendroglial-like cells (OLC) form clusters and satellites around normal-appearing neurons floating in mucin-rich spaces (Figure 19-9)
    - If only this element is present, it is called a "simple" DNT
  - Glial nodules
    - Aggregates of oligodendroglial-like cells mixed with astrocytes resembling an oligoastrocytoma

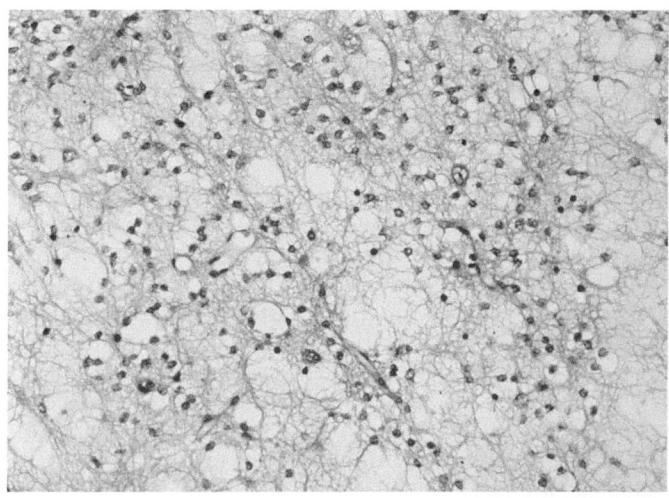

Figure 19-9. Dysembryoplastic neuroepithelial tumor. Neurons floating in a mucoid matrix with oligodendroglial-like cells.

- Presence of the glioneuronal element and glial nodules is called a "complex" DNT
- Cortical dysplasia (variably present)
  - Architectural disarray with loss of normal laminations
- Presence of only a diffuse pattern of growth without glial nodules or glioneuronal elements is referred to as a "nonspecific" or "diffuse" DNT; controversy exists over this distinction
- Eosinophilic granular bodies may be present
- Endothelial proliferation may be present

Special Stains and Immunohistochemistry

- Synaptophysin, NSE, and Neu-N highlight neuronal component
- GFAP stains astrocytic component
- S-100, nestin, and CD34 protein stains oligodendroglial-like cells
- Alcian blue highlights mucoid background (acid mucopolysaccharide)
- MIB-1: usually low index, but up to 8% reported

Other Techniques for Diagnosis

- Electron microscopy
  - Oligodendroglial-like cells in the glial nodules or specific glial neuronal component have round or oval nuclei and scant cytoplasm with short processes
  - Cytoplasm contains mitochondria, free ribosomes, rough endoplasmic reticulum, and lysosomes
  - Occasional astrocytic (intermediate filaments) and neuronal differentiation (dense core granules) are seen
- Cytogenetics: co-deletions of 1p and 19q have been reported in 10% of DNT and mutations in *IDH1/2* genes have been reported in < 5%

Differential Diagnosis

GANGLIOGLIOMA

- Dominant feature is bizarre, pleomorphic, or binucleate neurons
- Shows a neoplastic glial component in addition to the abnormal neurons

- Lacks multinodular architecture
- Typically shows perivascular lymphoid infiltrate and may have abundant collagenous stroma

OLIGODENDROGLIOMA

- Lacks distinct multinodular architecture
- No glioneuronal element
- Difficult to distinguish from DNT in small biopsies

OLIGOASTROCYTOMA

- Lacks distinct multinodular architecture
- No glioneuronal element

PILOCYTIC ASTROCYTOMA

- Composed of biphasic dense and loose piloid astrocytes without floating neurons or associated cortical dysplasia

PEARLS

- *Histogenesis remains unknown; may be hamartomatous or a benign neoplasm*
- *Surgical resection is reserved for patients with intractable seizures*
- *Most patients remain seizure free and without tumor recurrence after resection*
- *Recurrence and transformation to a higher-grade diffuse glioma are each uncommon but have been reported*

SELECTED REFERENCES

Daumas-Duport C, Scheithauer BW, Chodkiewicz JP, et al: Dysembryoplastic neuroepithelial tumor: a surgically curable tumor of young patients with intractable partial seizures. Report of 39 cases. Exp Clin Studies 23:545-556, 1988.

Ray WZ, Blackburn SL, Casavilca-Zambrano S, et al: Clinicopathologic features of recurrent dysembryoplastic neuroepithelial tumor and rare malignant transformation: a report of 5 cases and review of the literature. J Neurooncol 94:283-292, 2009.

Thom M, Toma A, An S, et al: One hundred and one dysembryoplastic neuroepithelial tumors: an adult epilepsy series with immunohistochemical, molecular genetic, and clinical correlations and a review of the literature. J Neuropathol Exp Neurol 70:859-878, 2011.

CENTRAL AND EXTRAVENTRICULAR NEUROCYTOMA (WHO GRADE II)

Clinical Features

- Incidence is 0.25% to 0.50% of all brain tumors
- Typically occurs in young adults (ages 20 to 40 years)
- Central neurocytoma: intraventricular tumors are usually found in the lateral or third ventricles, adjacent to the foramen of Monro
  - Central neurocytomas present with signs of increased intracranial pressure: headache, nausea, vomiting, seizures, visual disturbance, and papilledema
  - Extraventricular neurocytomas occur in parenchyma, away from the ventricular system; reported in cerebrum, cerebellum, deep gray matter, brain stem, spinal cord, pineal gland, and retina
  - Presentation of extraventricular neurocytomas is dependent on location of the tumor

- Cerebellar liponeurocytoma
  - Rare low-grade (WHO grade II) neoplasm, usually occurring in cerebellar hemispheres composed of neurocytes with focal lipomatous differentiation
  - Mean age of occurrence, 50 years
  - CT and MRI characteristically show a heterogeneously contrast-enhancing, partially calcified intraventricular (or in extraventricular lesions, parenchymal) mass; cysts and calcification are common
  - MRI scans show an isointense or slightly hypointense mass on T1-weighted images and hyperintensity on T2-weighted images

Gross Pathology

- Well-circumscribed, lobulated, soft, gray tumor
- Typically, infiltration into the surrounding brain parenchyma is not seen
- Often hemorrhagic, focally calcified, and cystic

Histopathology

CENTRAL NEUROCYTOMAS

- Hypercellular tumor composed of diffuse sheets of monotonous uniform cells punctuated by anuclear areas composed of a fibrillar matrix, reminiscent of neuropil (Figure 19-10)
- Perivascular arrangement of cell processes resembling ependymal pseudorosettes may be seen
- Delicate vascular stroma and microcalcifications are often present
- Nuclei have regular outlines with salt and pepper chromatin and small inconspicuous nucleoli
- Mitotic activity, endothelial proliferation, and necrosis are rare
- Rare cases exhibit ganglion cells

ATYPICAL NEUROCYTOMAS

- Defined by elevation of MIB-1 index (> 2%) with or without the presence of endothelial proliferation, necrosis, and increased cytologic atypia

EXTRAVENTRICULAR NEUROCYTOMAS

- Cytologically similar to central neurocytomas
  - Architectural pattern is more varied, such as clusters, ribbons, or rosettes, in addition to sheets

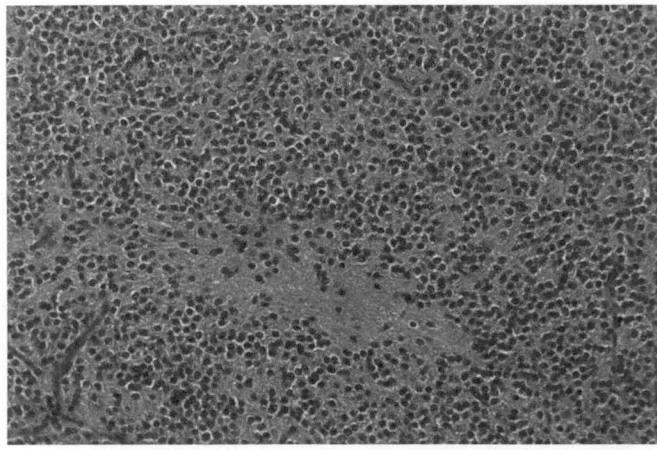

Figure 19-10. Central neurocytoma. The neoplasm is composed of a monotonous population of small round cells with a fine chromatin pattern and occasional nuclei-free islands suggesting neuropil.

- Higher degree of ganglionic differentiation and possibly glial differentiation

CEREBELLAR LIPONEUROCYTOMA
- Composed of neurocytes, some showing lipidization

Special Stains and Immunohistochemistry
- Synaptophysin: diffusely positive
- NSE and Neu-N positive
- Chromogranin and neurofilament usually negative
- GFAP negative in central neurocytomas; variable in extraventricular neurocytomas
- MIB-1 index: less than 2% in typical neurocytomas; more than 2% shortens recurrence-free survival
- Cerebellar liponeurocytoma: in addition to neuronal markers, focal GFAP positivity is often present

Other Techniques for Diagnosis
- Electron microscopy: membrane bound dense core neurosecretory granules, cytoplasmic microtubular arrays
- Cytogenetic analyses: most central neurocytomas do not have deletions of chromosomes 1p and 19q, but extraventricular neurocytomas do frequently have this co-deletion (identified in approximately 25% and studies suggest association with aggressive behavior)
- Mutations in p53 gene have not been identified

Differential Diagnosis

OLIGODENDROGLIOMA
- Poorly circumscribed with an infiltrative border
- Typically not located in the ventricle
- Lacks salt-and-pepper nuclei, neuropil islands, and ganglion cell differentiation
- Synaptophysin negative

EPENDYMOMA (ESPECIALLY CLEAR CELL VARIANT)
- Cells have long fibrillary processes
- Characteristically shows true rosettes
- Typically protrudes from ventricular lining
- GFAP positive and synaptophysin negative

NEUROBLASTOMA (PRIMITIVE NEUROECTODERMAL TUMOR)
- Hyperchromatic atypical cells with frequent mitoses
- Lack of fine chromatin and neuropil islands
- Intraparenchymal with tendency to seed neuraxis
- Immunohistochemical profiles are the same

PEARLS

- *Most are slow-growing tumors that are essentially cured by surgical resection; associated with an excellent prognosis*
- *Recurrence and adverse outcomes are associated with subtotal resection and elevated MIB-1 proliferation index*

SELECTED REFERENCES

Choudhari K, Kaliaperumal C, Jain A, et al: Central neurocytoma: a multi-disciplinary review. Br J Neurosurg 23:585-595, 2009.
Giangaspero F, Cenacchi G, Losi L, et al: Extraventricular neoplasms with neurocytoma features. Am J Surg Pathol 21:206-212, 1997.
Kane AJ, Sughrue ME, Rutkowski MJ, et al: The molecular pathology of central neurocytomas. J Clin Neurosci 18:1-6, 2011.
Rodriguez FJ, Mota RA, Scheithauer BW, et al: Interphase cytogenetics for 1p19q and t(1;19)(q10;p10) may distinguish prognostically relevant subgroups in extraventricular neurocytoma. Brain Pathol 19:623-629, 2009.

PAPILLARY GLIONEURONAL TUMOR (WHO GRADE I)

Clinical Features
- Usually low grade
- Rare neoplasm; wide age range, from 4 to 75 years (mean age, 23 years)
- Seizures, headaches, visual disturbances, language or gait disturbances, and mood changes have been reported as presenting symptoms
- Occurs in cerebral parenchyma, most commonly in frontal and temporal lobes
- MRI shows a well-circumscribed solid and cystic mass with contrast enhancement; may have a cyst with a mural nodule

Gross Pathology
- Well-circumscribed solid and cystic mass, may have a mural nodule in a cyst

Histopathology
- Architecturally composed of pseudopapillae and solid areas
- Pseudopapillae exhibit pseudostratified, small cuboidal cells without atypia around hyalinized vessels
- Solid areas contain mixtures of neurocytes and ganglion cells and cells intermediate between the two within a fibrillar or basophilic mucoid matrix
- Rosenthal fibers, calcification, and old hemorrhage are seen
- Mitoses are rare or absent
- No endothelial proliferation or necrosis

Special Stains and Immunohistochemistry
- GFAP: cells of pseudopapillae positive
- Synaptophysin, Neu-N, and neurofilament: cells from solid areas (neurocytes and ganglion cells) positive
- S100, nestin, and galectin-3: positive
- Chromogranin and CD34: negative
- MIB-1 index: range, 1% to 3%; reports of up to 26%
- EGFR and *IDH1 (R132H)* immunohistochemistry: negative
- p53: most often negative

Other Techniques for Diagnosis
- Ultrastructural examination: pseudopapillae lining cells show astrocytic features with intermediate filaments; solid area cells show neuronal features such as microtubules, dense core, and clear vesicles and occasionally synaptic junctions
- Cytogenetic analyses: no co-deletions of 1p or 19q or reports of *IDH1* gene mutations

Differential Diagnosis
PAPILLARY EPENDYMOMA
- Lacks solid component exhibiting neuronal elements

PAPILLARY MENINGIOMA

- EMA positive
- GFAP negative
- Synaptophysin and Neu-N negative

CHOROID PLEXUS PAPILLOMA

- Papillary formation not consistently GFAP positive
- Lacks solid areas composed of neuronal elements

METASTATIC PAPILLARY ADENOCARCINOMA

- Cytokeratin positive
- GFAP, synaptophysin, and Neu-N negative

ASTROBLASTOMA

- Lacks neuronal elements

PEARLS

- *Good prognosis*
- *No reports of recurrence after gross total resection*

SELECTED REFERENCES

Agarwal S, Sharma MC, Singh G, et al: Papillary glioneuronal tumor—a rare entity: report of four cases and brief review of literature. Childs Nerv Syst 28:1897-1904, 2012.

Edgar M, Rosenblum MK: Mixed glioneuronal tumors, recently described entities. Arch Pathol Lab Med 131:228-233, 2007.

Komori T, Scheithauer BW, Anthony DC, et al: Papillary glioneuronal tumor: a new variant of mixed neuronal-glial neoplasm. Am J Surg Pathol 22:1171-1183, 1998.

ROSETTE-FORMING GLIONEURONAL TUMOR OF THE FOURTH VENTRICLE (WHO GRADE I)

Clinical Features

- Rare neoplasm occurring at mean age of 32 years (range, 12 to 70 years)
- Women affected more than men
- Signs and symptoms secondary to obstructive hydrocephalus, headaches, ataxia, visual disturbances, and vertigo
- MRI scan T1-weighted images show a heterogeneous (cystic or solid) isointense or hypointense lesion; it is hyperintense on T2-weighted images and usually shows focal contrast enhancement; calcifications may be seen on CT scan
- Most often occur in the fourth ventricle, but they have been described in the spinal canal, pons, cerebellar vermis, and thalamus

Gross Pathology

- Soft, gelatinous, well demarcated

Histopathology

- Composed of neurocytic and glial cells
- Neurocytic component exhibits small round nuclei and scant cytoplasm and forms perivascular pseudorosettes and Homer Wright rosettes, often accompanied by a microcystic, myxoid background; rarely, ganglion cells may be seen
- Glial component exhibits piloid and spindle-shaped cells, may be more extensive than the neuronal component

- Rosenthal fibers and eosinophilic granular bodies may be seen
- Degenerative changes are often seen consisting of sclerotic vessels, collagen, calcifications, and hemosiderin-laden macrophages
- Endothelial proliferation may be seen
- Mitoses are rare
- Well-defined tumor-parenchyma interface

Special Stains and Immunohistochemistry

- Synaptophysin: positive granular staining of neurocytic component
- NSE positive in neurocytic component
- GFAP and S-100 positive in glial component
- MIB-1 index: less than 3%

Other Techniques for Diagnosis

- Electron microscopy: glial component has bundles of intermediate filaments; neurocytic component exhibits cells with small round nuclei, ribosomes, and rough endoplasmic reticulum; Golgi apparatus, sparse dense core granules, and microtubules in the rosette formations; occasional presynaptic specializations are seen
- Cytogenetics: presence of *PIK3CA* mutation and absence of *KIAA1549-BRAF* fusions, *BRAF (V600E)* mutation, co-deletions of 1p/19q, or pathogenic mutations of *IDH1/2*

Differential Diagnosis

PILOCYTIC ASTROCYTOMA

- Usually occurs in younger individuals
- Lacks neurocytic component and Homer Wright rosettes
- Presence of *KIAA1549-BRAF* fusion

CENTRAL NEUROCYTOMA

- Does not have a biphasic appearance with the piloid astrocytic component alternating with the neurocytic component

PAPILLARY GLIONEURONAL NEOPLASM

- More often occurs in cerebrum rather than fourth ventricle
- Does not display Homer Wright rosettes
- Exhibits pseudopapillary architecture formed by astrocytic cells
- Ependymoma
- Not biphasic (does not have the neurocytic component)
- Homogeneously enhancing
- Medulloblastoma
- Not biphasic (typically does not have the glial component) and is composed of primitive appearing cells
- Homogeneously enhancing

PEARLS

- *Indolent growth; excellent prognosis with surgical resection*
- *Multifocal tumor nodules have been reported*

SELECTED REFERENCES

Gessi M, Lambert SR, Lauriola L, et al: Absence of *KIAA1549-BRAF* fusion in rosette-forming glioneuronal tumors of the fourth ventricle (RGNT). J Neurooncol 110:21-25, 2012.

Komori T, Scheithauer BW, Hirose T: A rosette-forming glioneuronal tumor of the fourth ventricle: infratentorial form of dysembryoplastic neuroepithelial tumor? Am J Surg Pathol 26:582-591, 2002.

Thommen F, Hewer E, Schafer SC, et al: Rosette-forming glioneuronal tumor of the cerebellum in statu nascendi: an incidentally detected diminutive example indicates derivation from the internal granule cell layer. Clin Neuropathol 32:370-376, 2013.

Zhang J, Babu R, McLendon RE, et al: A comprehensive analysis of 41 patients with rosette-forming glioneuronal tumors of the fourth ventricle. J Clin Neurosci 20:335-341, 2013.

PARAGANGLIOMA OF THE SPINAL CORD (WHO GRADE I)

Clinical Features

- Benign, encapsulated neoplasm arising from neural crest cells, occurring in cauda equina and filum terminale
- Constitutes 3.5% of all neoplasms in this location
- Mean age of occurrence is 48 years
- Patients most commonly present with back pain or sciatica and urinary or fecal incontinence; sensory or motor deficits are less common; symptoms secondary to hormonal manifestations are uncommon

Gross Pathology

- Most are intradural and encapsulated (80%)
- Red-brown soft tissue; may contain cysts
- Usually attached to filum terminale

Histopathology

- Nests (Zellballen) of small uniform cells surrounded by sustentacular cells
- Delicate vascular network (organoid pattern)
- Cells are polygonal or columnar with round nuclei and fine chromatin and granular eosinophilic cytoplasm
- Perivascular pseudorosette formation may occur
- Mitoses and necrosis are infrequent
- Ganglion cell differentiation present in up to 45%
- Divergent differentiation is reported (homologous or heterologous components)
- Melanotic and oncocytic variants have been described

Special Stains and Immunohistochemistry

- Chromogranin, synaptophysin, and NSE positive
- Neurofilament: variable staining
- GFAP: sustentacular cells positive
- Cytokeratin: positive and negative staining reported
- S-100: variably positive sustentacular cells; tumor cells often positive
- MIB-1 index: low

Other Techniques for Diagnosis

- Electron microscopy: cytoplasmic dense core secretory granules and intermediate filaments
- Cytogenetics
  - Mutations in succinic dehydrogenase genes (part of mitochondrial complex II)
  - Comparative genomic hybridization on one specimen has shown a normal DNA profile
  - Associated with the following autosomal dominant syndromes: von Hippel-Lindau disease (VHL), multiple endocrine neoplasia type 2 (MEN2), and neurofibromatosis type 1 (NF1)

Differential Diagnosis

EPENDYMOMA
- GFAP positive
- Fibrillary pattern with perivascular pseudorosettes and ependymal rosettes

METASTATIC CARCINOMA
- Cytologically anaplastic, lacking organoid pattern of uniform cells
- Not encapsulated

PEARLS
- *Most are slow growing and curable with complete resection*
- *Recurrence may occur with subtotal resection*
- *Subarachnoid space dissemination reported*
- *Morphologic criteria to distinguish between benign and aggressive tumors not described*

SELECTED REFERENCES

Gutenberg A, Wegner C, Pilgram-Pastor SM, et al: Paraganglioma of the filum terminale: review and report of the first case analyzed by CGH. Clin Neuropathol 29:227-223, 2010.

Miliaras GC, Kyritsis AP, Polyzoidis KS: Cauda equina paraganglioma: a review. J Neurooncol 65:177-190, 2003.

Pytel P, Krausz T, Wollmann R, Utset MF: Ganglioneuromatous paraganglioma of the cauda equina: a pathological case study. Hum Pathol 36:444-446, 2005.

EMBRYONAL TUMORS

MEDULLOBLASTOMA (WHO GRADE IV)

Clinical Features

- Malignant neoplasm of cerebellum composed of primitive cells usually with neuronal differentiation
- Most occur before 16 years of age (peak, 7 years)
- May occur in adulthood; most often between 21 and 40 years
- Symptoms include signs of cerebellar dysfunction (gait abnormalities, ataxia) or increased intracranial pressure

Gross Pathology

- Most occur in vermis and may bulge into or fill the fourth ventricle
- Involvement of the hemispheres is more common in older individuals
- Hemispheric lesions are more likely desmoplastic
- Solid, variably demarcated (from well to poorly defined), homogeneous mass

Histopathology

- Highly cellular tumor composed of undifferentiated cells with variable growth patterns (Figure 19-11)
- Classical type consists of small, round to carrot-shaped uniform cells with hyperchromatic nuclei and wispy cytoplasm, often with distinct fibrillary background composed of cell processes
- Homer Wright rosettes may be seen (40%) but are often absent
- High mitotic rate is common

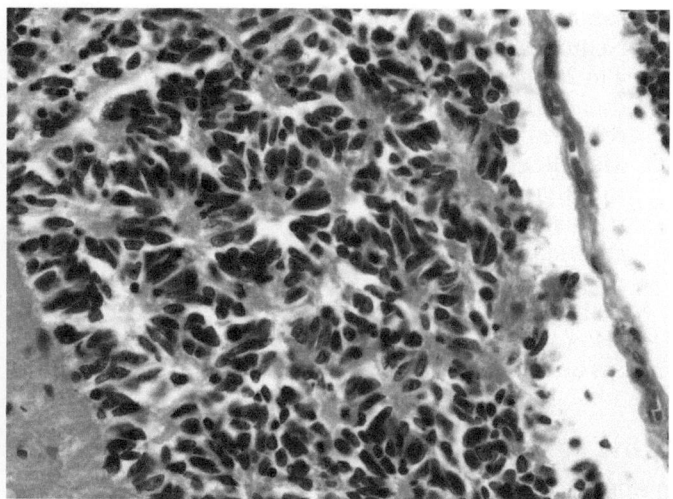

Figure 19-11. Medulloblastoma. Highly cellular tumor, spreading in the subarachnoid space, composed of small cells with carrot-shaped nuclei and indistinct cytoplasm forming Homer Wright rosettes.

- Individual cell and small areas of necrosis are frequently present
- Distinct streaming (single-filing) or palisading of tumor cells is often seen
- Morphologic subtypes
  - Desmoplastic/nodular medulloblastoma (previously called *cerebellar neuroblastoma*)
    - Pale nodular areas lacking reticulin are surrounded by hypercellular sheets containing abundant reticulin
    - Nodules contain cells with neuronal maturation, and often a neuropil formation is present
    - Surrounding cells are more primitive and have high mitotic rates
  - Medulloblastoma with extensive nodularity
    - Large pale areas composed of neurocytic cells and neuropil with scant internodular component
  - Large cell and anaplastic medulloblastoma
    - Anaplastic changes are the presence of marked nuclear pleomorphism, cell wrapping and molding, high mitotic and MIB-1 indexes, and abundant apoptosis
    - Large cell changes are defined by cells with large round nuclei with prominent nucleoli, abundant mitoses, and apoptosis
    - Often, both large cells and anaplastic changes are found in the same neoplasm
  - Medullomyoblastoma
    - Rhabdomyoblastic differentiation is present
    - Spindle cells or globular cells, which are positive for desmin, actin, or myoglobin
  - Melanotic medulloblastoma
    - Contains cells with melanin pigment
    - May also see ill-defined tubules or papillary formations

Special Stains and Immunohistochemistry

- Synaptophysin, microtubule-associated protein 2, neurofilament (low- and intermediate-molecular-weight), vimentin, NSE positive
- Cytokeratin negative

- GFAP may show focal positivity in tumors with astrocytic differentiation or may represent entrapped astrocytes
- MIB-1 index: more than 20%
- Subtype (see molecular subtypes described as follows) specific immunohistochemistry:
  - WNT tumors: filamin A: cytoplasmic positivity; YAP1 and β-catenin: nuclear and cytoplasmic positivity; GAB1: negative
  - SHH tumors: filamin A, β-catenin and GAB1: cytoplasmic positivity, YAP1: nuclear and cytoplasmic positivity
  - Non–WNT/SHH tumors: filamin A, YAP1 and GAB1: negative; β-catenin: cytoplasmic positivity

Other Techniques for Diagnosis

- Electron microscopy: undifferentiated neuroepithelial cells with scant cytoplasm and few organelles; may show prominent cytoplasmic processes; more differentiated neoplasms have microtubules, dense core vesicles, and synapses
- Four distinct molecular subtypes of medulloblastoma have been described with distinct clinical, prognostic, and immunohistochemical characteristics but overlap morphologically:
  - Activation of Wingless pathway (WNT) and monosomy 6: associated with classic histology, progression-free survival and overall survival rates of > 90%, occurrence in older children (girls more than boys)
  - Activation of sonic hedgehog pathway (SHH) and *PTCH1* loss: associated with classic or desmoplastic histology, occurrence in infants (good prognosis) and adults (intermediate prognosis)
  - Group C (classic or large cell histology): *MYCC* or *MYCN* amplification and chromosome 17 imbalance; occurs in young children and has poor prognosis
  - Group D (classic or large cell histology): *MYC* or *MYCN* amplification and chromosome 17 imbalance; occurs in children and has an intermediate prognosis

Differential Diagnosis

ATYPICAL TERATOID/RHABDOID TUMOR
- Usually in children younger than 2 years
- Presence of rhabdoid cells
- Unique immunohistochemical profile positive for EMA, vimentin, smooth muscle actin (SMA), cytokeratin, and synaptophysin; negative INI1 protein antibody
- *hSNF5/INI1* deletion or mutation (found in 85%)

PERIPHERAL PRIMITIVE NEUROECTODERMAL TUMOR (pPNET) AND EXTRAOSSEOUS EWING SARCOMA OF THE CRANIOSPINAL VAULT
- Morphologically indistinguishable from medulloblastoma and supratentorial PNET
- CD99: membranous staining
- *EWS-FLI1* fusion gene detectable by fluorescent in situ hybridization (FISH)

EPENDYMOMA
- Generally less cellular, and cells have more cytoplasm; infrequent mitotic activity
- Form perivascular pseudorosettes and ependymal rosettes

- GFAP positive
- Synaptophysin and chromogranin negative

PILOCYTIC ASTROCYTOMA

- Similar location and age range
- Less cellular tumor consisting of biphasic pattern with elongated astrocytic areas (piloid) and a microcystic architecture
- GFAP diffusely positive
- Synaptophysin and chromogranin negative

LYMPHOMA AND LEUKEMIA

- History of lymphoma and leukemia is often known
- Lack nodular architecture and rosette formation
- Lymphomatous infiltrate is positive for LCA (CD45) and, if B-cell type, CD20

METASTATIC NEUROENDOCRINE CARCINOMA

- Typically found in older individuals
- Lacks rosette formation
- Positive for cytokeratin

PEARLS

- *Propensity for leptomeningeal dissemination*
- *Surgical resection followed by craniospinal radiation and chemotherapy is the typical treatment*

SELECTED REFERENCES

Ellison DW, Dalton J, Kocak M, et al: Medulloblastoma: clinicopathological correlates of SHH, WNT, and non-SHH/WNT molecular subgroups. Acta Neuropathol 121:381-396, 2011.

Giangaspero F, Wellek S, Masuoka J, et al: Stratification of medulloblastoma on the basis of histopathological grading. Acta Neuropathol 112:5-12, 2006.

Kazmi SA, Perry A, Pressey JG, et al: Primary Ewing sarcoma of the brain: a case report and literature review. Diagn Mol Pathol 16:108-111, 2007.

McLendon R, Adekunle A, Rajaram V, et al: Embryonal central nervous system neoplasms arising in infants and young children: a pediatric brain tumor consortium study. Arch Pathol Lab Med 135:984-993, 2011.

Northcott PA, Korshunov A, Witt H, et al: Medulloblastoma comprises four distinct molecular variants. J Clin Oncol 29:1408-1414, 2011.

Pfister SM, Korshunov A, Kool M, et al: Molecular diagnostics of CNS embryonal tumors. Acta Neuropathol 120:553-566, 2010.

CNS PRIMITIVE NEUROECTODERMAL NEOPLASMS (NEUROBLASTOMA, GANGLIONEUROBLASTOMA, EPENDYMOBLASTOMA, MEDULLOEPITHELIOMA, EMBRYONAL TUMOR WITH ABUNDANT NEUROPIL AND TRUE ROSETTES) (WHO GRADE IV)

Clinical Features

- All are composed of primitive neuroepithelial cells occurring in hemispheres, brain stem, or spinal cord
- May display differentiation along neuronal (neuroblastoma, ganglioneuroblastoma), neural, glial, and mesenchymal lines (medulloepithelioma) or may lack clear lines of differentiation (embryonal tumor with abundant neuropil and true rosettes [ETANTR])

- Mean age at presentation and usual locations:
  - Neuroblastoma/ganglioneuroblastoma: 5.5 years (range, 4 to 20 years); adult cases have been reported; location is usually the cerebrum; they have been reported in spinal cord and suprasellar region
  - Medulloepithelioma: 45 months (range, < 1 month to 23 years). They are usually in cerebrum (periventricular), but also occur in ventricles, sella, cauda equina, presacral region, orbit, and optic nerve
  - ETANTR: 24 months (range 9 to 48 months), females > males; most often supratentorial location, but also found in brain stem, cerebellum and spinal cord
- Signs and symptoms are referable to the site of the mass lesion

Gross Pathology

- Appear as a well-circumscribed, tan-gray, homogeneous mass
- Small cyst formation and calcification are common
- Hemorrhage and necrosis may be present
- Medulloepitheliomas are often massive lesions with abundant necrosis and hemorrhage and arise close to the ventricular system
- ETANTR: also large (2 to 8 cm) with solid and cystic components; may disseminate through subarachnoid space

Histopathology

NEUROBLASTOMA

- Hypercellular tumors that appear well circumscribed but are infiltrative
- Homer Wright rosettes are often present, but poorly formed pseudorosettes consisting of perivascular anuclear zones showing loose fibrillary processes are more common
- Presence of fibrous connective tissue stroma will produce a lobular pattern; this is most prominent when leptomeninges are invaded (desmoplastic form)
- Tumor cells are usually small (round to carrot shaped) and have monomorphic but hyperchromatic nuclei and inconspicuous nucleoli; a moderate degree of nuclear pleomorphism is occasionally seen; anaplastic or large cell features may be present, as also described in medulloblastoma
- Neuronal differentiation is seen in 25% to 50% of cases involving the brain

GANGLIONEUROBLASTOMA

- Cells will have larger nuclei, vesicular chromatin, nucleoli, and more abundant cytoplasm
- Mitotic activity is variable (usually numerous)

MEDULLOEPITHELIOMA

- Neural tubelike structures composed of primitive cells and pseudostratified epithelium arranged in tubular, papillary, or trabecular architecture

ETANTR

- Hypercellular areas (containing small cells with hyperchromatic round/oval nuclei and indistinct cell borders) alternating with hypocellular areas composed of a fibrillary matrix similar to neuropil; these areas may contain neurocytic cells, ganglion cells, or calcifications; ependymoblastic rosettes (pseudostratified elongate cells arranged around a lumen) are seen in both hypercellular and neuropil-like areas; Homer Wright rosettes and perivascular pseudorosettes may be present in the hypercellular areas; mitoses are usually seen and necrosis may be present

Special Stains and Immunohistochemistry

GANGLIONEUROBLASTOMA AND NEUROBLASTOMA
- Synaptophysin and S-100 positive
- NSE and neurofilament positive
- GFAP and cytokeratin negative
- MIB-1 index: markedly variable, 0% to 85%

MEDULLOEPITHELIOMA
- Nestin and vimentin positive
- GFAP, EMA, cytokeratin, and NF variably positive

ETANTR
- MIB-1 proliferative index: 10% to 80%
- Neuropil-like areas: synaptophysin and neurofilament positive
- Neurocytic and ganglion cells in neuropil areas: Neu-N positive
- GFAP: usually negative
- INI1: positive

Other Techniques for Diagnosis
- Electron microscopy: tumor cells have microtubules within bipolar processes; typically few neurosecretory granules and sparse cytoplasmic organelles
- Cytogenetics
  - Neuroblastomas: genetic abnormalities of *CDK/CYCLIND* loci, in neuroblastomas are reported
  - TP53 and IDH1 (R132H) mutations have been identified in a subset of adult supratentorial PNETs
  - *MYCN* amplification has also been identified in approximately 40% of noncerebellar PNETs
  - ETANTR: amplification at 19q13.42 has been identified

Differential Diagnosis

CENTRAL NEUROCYTOMA
- Located within the lateral or third ventricle
- Lacks distinct rosette formation
- Cells are uniform and have low mitotic activity

PERIPHERAL PNET AND EXTRAOSSEOUS EWING SARCOMA OF THE CRANIOSPINAL VAULT
- Morphologically indistinguishable from medulloblastoma and supratentorial PNET
- CD99: membranous staining
- *EWS-FLI1* fusion gene detectable by FISH

METASTATIC NEUROENDOCRINE CARCINOMA
- Typically found in older individuals
- Lacks rosette formation
- Positive for cytokeratin

DESMOPLASTIC INFANTILE GANGLIOGLIOMA
- Large cystic mass in infancy (usually younger than 18 months)
- Typically involves frontal and parietal lobes
- Usually involves leptomeninges, prominent collagenous stroma

- Divergent differentiation along astrocytic and neuronal lines
- Composed of GFAP-positive spindle cells and often inconspicuous ganglion cells

GLIOBLASTOMA WITH PNET FOCI
- Exhibits areas of malignant GFAP positive astrocytoma (variably sized nuclei with pleomorphism and hyperchromatism, often abundant eosinophilic cytoplasm), necrosis with or without pseudopalisading, and endothelial proliferation

ESTHESIONEUROBLASTOMA (OLFACTORY NEUROBLASTOMA)
- Occurs most often in the region of the cribriform plate in adults
- Composed of primitive neuroectodermal cells with scant ill-defined cytoplasm, forming nests or lobules or sheetlike growth; well-formed rosettes are rare
- Synaptophysin positive; S100 positive sustentacular cells are edges of nests

PEARLS

- *Neuroblastoma: children younger than 2 years have a poorer prognosis than those older than 2 years*
- *Cerebrospinal pathway seeding does occur (neuroblastoma, medulloepithelioma, and ETANTR), and metastases outside the CNS have been reported*
- *Ependymoblastoma: no longer considered a distinct entity; ependymoblastic rosettes are found in other embryonal tumors, most often embryonal tumors with abundant neuropil and true rosettes*
- *Medulloepithelioma has a poor prognosis (unlike intraorbital medulloepithelioma, which has a benign course)*
- *ETANTR: mean survival 9 months*

SELECTED REFERENCES

Behdad A, Perry A: Central nervous system primitive neuroectodermal tumors: a clinicopathologic and genetic study of 33 cases. Brain Patholo 20:441-450, 2010.

Eberhart CG, Brat DJ, Cohen KJ, et al: Pediatric neuroblastic brain tumors containing abundant neuropil and true rosettes. Pediatr Dev Pathol 3:346-352, 2000.

Gessi M, Giangaspero F, Lauriola L, et al: Embryonal tumors with abundant neuropil and true rosettes: a distinctive CNS primitive neuroectodermal tumor. Am J Surg Pathol 33:211-217, 2009.

Judkins AR, Ellison DW: Ependymoblastoma: dear, damned, distracting diagnosis, farewell! Brain Pathol 20:133-139, 2010.

Li M, Lockwood W, Zielenska M et al: Multiple CDK/CYCLING genes are amplified in medulloblastoma and supratentorial primitive neuroectodermal brain tumor. Cancer Genet 205:220-231, 2012.

Molloy PT, Yachnis AT, Rorke LB, et al: Central nervous system medulloepithelioma: a series of eight cases including two arising in the pons. J Neurosurg 84:430-436, 1996.

ATYPICAL TERATOID/RHABDOID TUMOR (WHO GRADE IV)

Clinical Features
- Rare malignant neoplasm occurring most commonly in children younger than 3 years

- About 50% of cases occur in the posterior fossa, with a predilection for the cerebellopontine angle; other reported sites include suprasellar region, pineal region, cerebrum, and spinal cord
- May be intra-axial or extra-axial, with predilection for leptomeningeal dissemination
- Symptoms may be nonlocalizing, consisting of lethargy, vomiting, and failure to thrive; in posterior fossa tumors, focal signs are usually cranial nerve palsies

Gross Pathology

- Gray-white tissue with necrosis and hemorrhage

Histopathology

- Sheets or nests of large cells, each with a round nucleus, prominent nucleolus, plump cell body with homogeneous cytoplasm, or a dense round distinct cytoplasmic inclusion (rhabdoid cells)
- Frequently co-occurrence of foci or sheets of primitive neuroectodermal neoplastic cells, most often a minority component
- Epithelial (adenomatous or papillary pattern) or mesenchymal (loosely packed spindle cells) neoplastic components may also be present (about 33%); epithelial component is least common
- Abundant mitoses and necrosis
- Leptomeningeal spread is common and may be evident on the surface of the cerebellum

Special Stains and Immunohistochemistry

- EMA, vimentin, and smooth muscle actin positive
- GFAP, synaptophysin, and cytokeratin (high and low-molecular-weight cocktail) frequently positive
- Neurofilament, chromogranin, S-100, desmin, and HMB-45 may be positive
- INI1 negative
- MIB-1 index: more than 50%

Other Techniques for Diagnosis

- Electron microscopy: rhabdoid cell cytoplasm contains bundles of intermediate filaments
- Cytogenetics: *hSNF5/INI1* deletion or mutation (found in 85%)

Differential Diagnosis

Medulloblastoma

- Rhabdoid cells not seen, EMA negative, INI1 positive

Choroid Plexus Carcinoma

- Not usually in posterior fossa; cytokeratin positive, EMA negative

PEARLS

- *Resistant to standard therapy for primitive neuroectodermal neoplasms; mean survival time is 10 to 15 months*
- *Presence of rhabdoid cells is not diagnostic of atypical teratoid/rhabdoid tumor*
- *Immunohistochemistry and evaluation for the presence of a mutation of the hSNF5/INI1 gene should be performed*

SELECTED REFERENCES

Bambakidis NC, Robinson S, Cohen M, Cohen AR: Atypical teratoid/rhabdoid tumors of the central nervous system: clinical, radiographic and pathologic features. Pediatr Neurosurg 37:64-70, 2002.

Judkins AR: Immunohistochemistry of INI1 expression: a new tool for old challenges in CNS and soft tissue pathology. Adv Anat Pathol 14:335-339, 2007.

Packer RJ, Biegel JA, Blaney S, et al: Atypical teratoid/rhabdoid tumor of the central nervous system: report on workshop. J Pediatr Hematol Oncol 24:337-342, 2002.

Rorke LB, Packer RJ, Biegel JA: Central nervous system atypical teratoid/rhabdoid tumors of infancy and childhood: definition of an entity. J Neurosurg 85:56-65, 1996.

CHOROID PLEXUS TUMORS

CHOROID PLEXUS PAPILLOMA (WHO GRADE I), ATYPICAL CHOROID PLEXUS PAPILLOMA (WHO GRADE II), AND CHOROID PLEXUS CARCINOMA (WHO GRADE III)

Clinical Features

- Choroid plexus papillomas (WHO grades I and II)
  - Slow-growing benign tumors account for less than 1% of brain tumors overall but constitute 13% of brain tumors occurring in the first year of life
  - Characteristically found in the fourth ventricle (40%), lateral ventricle (50%), or third ventricle (5%) or at the cerebellopontine angle
  - Commonly found in the first and second decades (50% found before age 20); more often occur in the lateral ventricles when in young individuals and in the fourth ventricle and cerebellopontine angle in adults
  - Choroid plexus papilloma grade II (atypical choroid plexus papilloma) is defined histologically (discussed later)
- Choroid plexus carcinomas (WHO grade III)
  - Typically occur in patients younger than 10 years; rare in adults
  - Most carcinomas affecting the choroid plexus in adults are metastatic carcinomas
- Patients often present with signs and symptoms secondary to hydrocephalus owing to the overproduction of cerebrospinal fluid or obstruction

Gross Pathology

- Well-demarcated, pedunculated, or cauliflower-like masses
- Papillomas do not invade into the adjacent tissue
- Carcinomas characteristically invade the surrounding tissue and are often necrotic and hemorrhagic

Histopathology

Choroid Plexus Papilloma (WHO Grade I)

- Papillary architecture is composed of a single orderly layer of columnar cells surrounding a distinct fibrovascular core
- A mild degree of nuclear stratification, crowding of the nuclei, focal necrosis, and nuclear atypia may be seen
- Stromal calcifications; may see metaplastic bone or cartilage
- Mitotic activity is typically minimal
- Small foci of ependymal differentiation may be seen

ATYPICAL CHOROID PLEXUS PAPILLOMA (WHO GRADE II)

- Defined by increase in mitoses ($\geq$ 2 mitoses/10 randomly selected hpf)
- Hypercellularity, nuclear pleomorphism, solid growth pattern, and necrosis may also be present

CHOROID PLEXUS CARCINOMA

- Typically show a loose papillary architecture consisting of sheets of pleomorphic cells
- Extensive necrosis and high mitotic activity (> 5 mitoses/hpf)
- Brain invasion

Special Stains and Immunohistochemistry

- S-100 protein positive (more uniform in papillomas than in carcinomas)
- Cytokeratin 8 and 18, vimentin positive
- Transthyretin (prealbumin): approximately 70% are positive
- GFAP: papillomas may be focally positive; carcinomas typically negative
- EMA variable to negative
- Carcinoembryonic antigen (CEA) usually negative
- INI1 protein positive
- Synaptophysin variable positivity
- MIB-1 index: range in papillomas is 2% to 5%; range in carcinomas is 14% to 18%

Other Techniques for Diagnosis

- Electron microscopy: cells of both papillomas and carcinomas typically show cilia, microvilli, basement membrane, and desmosomes
- Cytogenetics
  - Inactivating mutation of the *hSNF5/INI1* gene has been reported in several series of choroid plexus carcinomas and in one series of papillomas
  - Somatic *TP53* mutations have been identified in 50% of choroid plexus carcinomas and 5% of choroid plexus papillomas in a recent series

Differential Diagnosis

NORMAL CHOROID PLEXUS

- Apical hobnail cuboidal cells instead of crowded, more columnar cells with some atypia are present in normal choroid plexus

METASTATIC CARCINOMA

- Usually found in older adults
- Not usually associated with the ventricle
- Typically positive for EMA and often also for CEA
- Usually negative for S-100 protein and GFAP

EPENDYMOMA (ESPECIALLY PAPILLARY SUBTYPE)

- Intraventricular location is common for both tumors
- Solid nonpapillary areas may be evident with both perivascular pseudorosette and true rosette formation
- GFAP positive; usually more diffuse than in choroid plexus neoplasms

ATYPICAL TERATOID AND RHABDOID TUMORS

- Important part of differential diagnosis in children with posterior fossa tumors

- Epithelial areas form part, not all, of the neoplasm
- Rhabdoid cells and primitive neuroectodermal cell components are also present
- INI1 protein negative

PAPILLARY ENDOLYMPHATIC SAC TUMOR

- Occurs in inner ear and extends to cerebellopontine angle most often in middle age with symptoms of hearing loss and tinnitus
- Histologically and immunohistochemically similar to choroid plexus papillomas occurring at cerebellopontine angle
- Positive for pan-cytokeratin, CK7, EMA, S-100 and variably to GFAP; it is negative with transthyretin antibody which may help in distinction from choroid plexus papilloma

PEARLS

- *GFAP positivity demonstrates that choroid plexus tumors may show ependymal differentiation*
- *Overall prognosis in surgically resected choroid plexus papilloma is good, but incompletely resected tumors occasionally recur*
- *Leptomeningeal spread may occur in both papillomas and carcinomas but is rare in papillomas*
- *Choroid plexus carcinoma has an overall poor prognosis*
  - *Brain invasion and cerebrospinal fluid spread is typically seen*
  - *Systemic metastases are rarely seen*

SELECTED REFERENCES

Jeibmann A, Hasselblatt M, Gerss J, et al: Prognostic implications of atypical histologic features in choroid plexus papilloma. J Neuropathol Exp Neurol 65:1069-1073, 2006.

Krishnan S, Brown PD, Scheithauer BW, et al: Choroid plexus papillomas: a single institutional experience. J Neurooncol 68:49-55, 2004.

Safaee M, Oh MC, Bloch O: Choroid plexus papillomas: advances in molecular biology and understanding of tumorigenesis. Neuro-Oncology 15:255-267, 2013.

Sun YH, Wen W, Wu JH, et al: Endolymphatic sac tumor: case report and review of the literature. Diagn Pathol 7:36, 2012.

PINEAL PARENCHYMAL TUMORS

PINEOCYTOMA (WHO GRADE I) AND PINEAL PARENCHYMAL TUMOR OF INTERMEDIATE DIFFERENTIATION (WHO GRADES II AND III)

Clinical Features

- Rare tumors accounting for less than 1% of all intracranial neoplasms
- Typically occur in adults with slight female predominance
- Localized to the region of the pineal gland and surrounding structures, may extend into the third ventricle and compress the colliculi and cerebral aqueduct
- Variable clinical presentations: eye movement abnormalities, mental status changes, and symptoms related to increased intracranial pressure or endocrine abnormalities
- CT and MRI scans show a round, homogeneous, contrast-enhancing mass

Gross Pathology

- Well-circumscribed tumor typically less than 3 cm in diameter
- Gray-tan homogeneous tumor often with small cyst formation
- Small areas of hemorrhage may be present
- Necrosis is not a typical finding

Histopathology

PINEOCYTOMA

- Sheets of tumor cells without a distinct pattern or an irregular lobular arrangement with large aggregates of tumor cells separated by fibrous septa
- Small and uniform cells with hyperchromatic nuclei, finely granular chromatin, inconspicuous nucleoli, and eosinophilic cytoplasmic processes
- Forms large (pineocytomatous) rosettes with abundant fibrillary cell processes in the center, sometimes with cytoplasmic club-shaped terminal expansion; may or may not be centered around blood vessels
- Calcification may be present
- Ganglion cells and multinucleated giant cells are occasionally seen
- Mitotic activity is minimal, and necrosis is not seen

PINEAL PARENCHYMAL TUMOR OF INTERMEDIATE DIFFERENTIATION

- Diffuse or lobulated tumors of moderate cellularity
- Mild to moderate nuclear atypia, with less cytoplasm than typically seen in pineocytomas, sparse to moderately frequent mitoses, endothelial proliferation is often present, and necrosis may be seen

Special Stains and Immunohistochemistry

- Synaptophysin, chromogranin, neurofilament, NSE, and S-100 protein positive
- Retinal S antigen and rhodopsin positive
- GFAP highlights background residual reactive astrocytes
- MIB-1 labeling index
  - Pineocytoma: average is < 2%
  - Pineal parenchymal tumor of intermediate differentiation: 8% to 11%

Other Techniques for Diagnosis

- Electron microscopy: cells have oval nuclei and cytoplasm containing numerous organelles, including smooth and rough endoplasmic reticulum, Golgi complexes, mitochondria, lysosomes, intermediate filaments, microtubules, synapse-like junctions, and membrane-bound electron-dense granules; cell processes are typically prominent
- Cytogenetic analyses
  - Pineocytomas: no consistent chromosomal abnormalities have been identified
  - Pineal parenchymal tumor of intermediate differentiation: cytogenetically more similar to pineoblastoma than pineocytoma; gains of 12q and losses of chromosome 22 reported

Differential Diagnosis

NORMAL PINEAL GLAND

- Normal lobular architecture is a helpful distinguishing feature
- May show irregular calcifications

PINEAL CYST

- Radiographically shows a distinct cystic structure
- Rarely symptomatic; mean age of symptomatic occurrence is 30 years
- Women are affected more than men
- Lacks large rosettes typically seen in pineocytoma
- Consists of a glial-lined cavity surrounded by reactive glial tissue

PINEOBLASTOMA

- Occurs typically in young individuals
- Shows well-formed, small perivascular rosettes
- Consists of undifferentiated, monomorphic, small round blue cells

ASTROCYTOMA

- Lacks lobular architecture and rosettes
- GFAP positive
- Synaptophysin negative

PAPILLARY TUMORS OF THE PINEAL REGION

- Presence of papillary formation help to distinguish it from pineal parenchymal tumors
- Cytokeratin positive; focal (rather than diffuse) synaptophysin positivity

PEARLS

- *Pineocytoma*
  - *Slow-growing neoplasm with excellent prognosis; metastases are not reported with these tumors*
  - *Treatment consists of conservative surgery after the development of symptoms*
- *Five-year survival rate for pineal parenchymal tumor of intermediate differentiation ranges from 39% to 74%*
- *Factors associated with improved survival are presence of neurofilament immunoreactivity, low mitoses, and absence of necrosis*

SELECTED REFERENCES

Dahiya S, Perry A: Pineal tumors. Adv Anat Pathol 17:419-427, 2010.
Hirato J, Nakazato Y: Pathology of pineal region tumors. J Neurooncol 54:239-249, 2001.
Jouvet A, Sainte-Pierre G, Fauchon F, et al: Pineal parenchymal tumors: a correlation of histological features with prognosis in 66 cases. Brain Pathol 10:49-60, 2000.
Taylor MD, Mainprize TG, Squire JA, Rutka JT: Molecular genetics of pineal region neoplasms. J Neurooncol 54:219-238, 2001.

PINEOBLASTOMA (WHO GRADE IV)

Clinical Features

- Constitute 45% of all pineal tumors
- Typically found in children within the first two decades
- Variable clinical presentations: ophthalmologic dysfunction; mental status changes, symptoms related to increased intracranial pressure, or endocrine abnormalities
- CT and MRI show a large, lobulated, poorly defined, heterogeneously contrast-enhancing mass

Gross Pathology

- Poorly defined soft, friable mass with hemorrhage and necrosis

- Infiltration into adjacent brain parenchyma and meninges (45% of cases) is common

Histopathology

- Highly cellular neoplasm composed of primitive, poorly differentiated tumor cells
- Diffuse sheets of neoplastic cells with focal rosette formation
- Round or oval hyperchromatic nuclei, typically with single nucleoli, scant cytoplasm, and indistinct cell borders
- Homer Wright rosettes or, less commonly, Flexner-Wintersteiner true rosettes
- Mitotic activity is often prominent; hemorrhage and necrosis are common

Special Stains and Immunohistochemistry

- Synaptophysin: positive, diffuse, or dotlike
- Chromogranin, neurofilament, and NSE positive, but may be focal
- Retinal S antigen positive
- GFAP variable and focal
- MIB-1 labeling index: average is 27% (range 17% to 40%)

Other Techniques for Diagnosis

- Electron microscopy: cells are typically poorly differentiated with round to oval nuclei, scant cytoplasm containing occasionally microtubules and intermediate filaments; dense core granules are sparse; junctional complexes and cilia may be present whereas synapses are not
- Cytogenetic analyses: patients with germline mutations in *Rb* gene (chromosome 13q14) are predisposed to tumor occurrence as part of trilateral retinoblastoma disease; this mutation has not been reported in sporadic pineoblastomas; many other genes are highly expressed in pineoblastomas, and chromosome 1p rearrangements are frequently found

Differential Diagnosis

PINEOCYTOMA AND PINEAL PARENCHYMAL TUMOR OF INTERMEDIATE DIFFERENTIATION

- Pineocytomas have better-differentiated cells with more abundant cytoplasm and pineocytomatous rosettes
- Pineal parenchymal tumors of intermediate differentiation have moderate cellularity, less atypia, and fewer mitoses

PEARLS

- *Aggressive tumor typically with craniospinal seeding; rare extracranial metastases*

SELECTED REFERENCES

Dahiya S, Perry A: Pineal Tumors. Adv Anat Pathol 17:419-427, 2010.
Hirato J, Nakazato Y: Pathology of pineal region tumors. J Neurooncol 54:239-249, 2001.
Taylor MD, Mainprize TG, Squire JA, Rutka JT: Molecular genetics of pineal region neoplasms. J Neurooncol 54:219-238, 2001.

PAPILLARY TUMOR OF THE PINEAL REGION (WHO GRADES II AND III)

Clinical Features

- Wide age range (5 to 66 years); mean, 32 years

- Presentation is usually with headache due to obstructive hydrocephalus, without focal neurologic signs
- MRI shows a well-circumscribed T1-hyper- or isointense, T2-hyperintense enhancing mass in the pineal region, ranging in size from 1.7 to 5 cm

Gross Pathology

- Well-circumscribed, usually solid

Histopathology

- Papillary architecture with perivascular pseudorosettes; ependymal rosettes have been reported; solid areas also usually present
- Cells are cuboidal to columnar and have well-defined cytoplasm
- Necrosis is usually present; mitoses are sparse, and vascular proliferation is not usually present

Special Stains and Immunohistochemistry

- Cytokeratin (AE1/AE3, CAM5.2, CK18) and S-100 positive
- GFAP: focal positivity
- Synaptophysin, chromogranin, and NSE weakly and focally positive
- EMA variably positive
- MIB-1 labeling index: 4% to 5%

Other Techniques for Diagnosis

- Electron microscopy: microvilli, zipper-like junctions, abundant rough endoplasmic reticulum, dilated cisternae, annulatae lamellae, dense core vesicles, and microtubules
- Cytogenetics: most commonly found are losses of chromosomes 10 and 22q and gain of chromosome 4

Differential Diagnosis

CHOROID PLEXUS PAPILLOMA

- Distinctly epithelial morphology and well-defined papillary formations
- No ependymal rosettes
- Usually no necrosis

EPENDYMOMA

- Fibrillary cytoplasm
- GFAP: prominent perivascular pseudorosette positivity
- EMA: consistent dotlike positivity
- Cytokeratin: focally positive

PEARLS

- *Tumor recurrence and progression is frequent (72%) and is associated with incomplete resection and increased mitoses*

SELECTED REFERENCES

Dahiya S, Perry A: Pineal tumors. Adv Anat Pathol 17:419-427, 2010.
Fèvre-Montange M, Hasselblatt M, Figarella-Branger D, et al: Prognosis and histopathologic features in papillary tumors of the pineal region: a retrospective multicenter study of 31 cases. J Neuropathol Exp Neurol 65:1004-1011, 2006.
Jouvet A, Fauchon F, Liberski P, et al: Papillary tumor of the pineal region. Am J Surg Pathol 27:505-512, 2003.

OTHER NEOPLASMS AND RELATED ENTITIES

PERIPHERAL NERVE SHEATH TUMORS

Clinical Features

SCHWANNOMA (WHO GRADE I)
- Benign tumor composed of Schwann cells; also called *neurilemmoma*
- Found in all ages, most commonly in the fourth through sixth decades
- Most commonly involves peripheral nerves in skin and subcutaneous tissues of the head and neck region and flexor surfaces of extremities
- Accounts for about 10% of intracranial tumors (usually arises from sensory cranial nerves, most often the eighth cranial nerve) and about 30% of spinal tumors
- Associated with neurofibromatosis type 2 (NF2) (bilateral vestibular schwannomas)
- Peripheral tumors typically present as asymptomatic masses; spinal tumors often present with radicular pain or signs of spinal cord compression; tumors of cranial nerve VIII cause hearing difficulties, tinnitus, or facial paresthesias

NEUROFIBROMA (WHO GRADE I)
- Common benign tumor composed of Schwann cells, fibroblasts, and perineural cells
- Most frequently occur sporadically but associated with NF1 in 10%
- Occur anywhere in the central or peripheral nervous systems, most often on flexor surfaces of extremities, retroperitoneum, neck, thorax, and cranium
- Multiple subtypes
  - Localized cutaneous neurofibroma: most common subtype, usually solitary and not associated with NF; cases associated with NF1 are often multiple
  - Diffuse cutaneous neurofibroma: uncommon, occurs primarily in children and young adults, forms large, ill-defined plaques
  - Localized intracranial neurofibroma: causes segmental, fusiform enlargement of the nerve; multiple lesions occur primarily in a background of NF1
  - Plexiform neurofibroma: transformation of multiple fascicles of nerve into neurofibroma with preservation of normal anatomic configuration, affecting larger nerves or a nerve plexus and occurring almost exclusively in patients with NF1
  - Massive soft tissue neurofibroma: the least common variant, found in patients with NF1, typically massive tumors resulting in marked enlargement of the affected extremity or regional soft tissue

MALIGNANT PERIPHERAL NERVE SHEATH TUMOR (MPNST) (WHO GRADE II, III, OR IV)
- May arise from Schwann cells, fibroblasts, or perineural cells
- Most present as mass lesions in association with medium to large peripheral nerves of the extremities
- Intracranial lesions usually involve the vagus or vestibular nerves
- About 50% are associated with NF1
- Tumors occur most commonly in third to sixth decades, but earlier in association with NF1

PERINEURIOMA (WHO GRADE I, II, OR III)
- Present in teens or young adulthood with muscle weakness in distribution of a peripheral nerve or as mass lesion in deep soft tissue
- Several types described with varying presentations
  - Extraneural soft tissue perineurioma: subcutaneous tissues of trunk and limbs; painless mass, in children or adults
  - Sclerosing perineurioma: hands of young adult men
  - Reticular perineurioma: in upper limbs of women (31 to 61 years)
  - Intraneural perineurioma: in children and young adults, in extremities

Gross Pathology

SCHWANNOMA
- Typically solitary, encapsulated, round to oval mass measuring up to 10 cm (multiple lesions are seen in NF)
- Cut surface shows firm, tan-white to bright yellow, glistening tissue
- Small cyst formation and focal hemorrhage may be seen (cysts are typically absent in cellular schwannomas)
- Nerve may be identified at periphery of mass

NEUROFIBROMA
- Solid, tan-white, soft to mucoid tumors surrounded by a thin capsule when intraneural or diffusely infiltrative when extraneural
- Tumor incorporates the nerve, so no nerve is typically identified

PLEXIFORM NEUROFIBROMA
- Typically forms a complex tangle of enlarged nerves resembling a bag of worms

MALIGNANT PERIPHERAL NERVE SHEATH TUMOR
- Large infiltrative, nonencapsulated mass with a fleshy, tan cut surface
- Hemorrhage and necrosis are common

PERINEURIOMA
- Circumscribed and firm; intraneural subtype is associated with peripheral nerve

Histopathology

SCHWANNOMA
- Shows biphasic pattern alternating between highly cellular, compact areas and loose, spongy areas of low cellularity
- Compact, cellular areas are termed *Antoni A* and consist of interlacing fascicles of elongated, regular spindle cells with long, pencil-shaped nuclei (Figure 19-12A)
- Sparsely cellular areas consisting of loose, spongy tissue with small, uniform cells termed *Antoni B*
- Tumors showing marked nuclear pleomorphism, hyperchromasia (degenerative atypia), and thick, hyalinized blood vessels are called *ancient schwannomas*
- Areas of nuclear palisading with nuclei arranged in linear stacks are called *Verocay bodies*; more commonly seen in spinal schwannomas
- Axons may be seen at the periphery of the tumor
- Mitotic activity is minimal

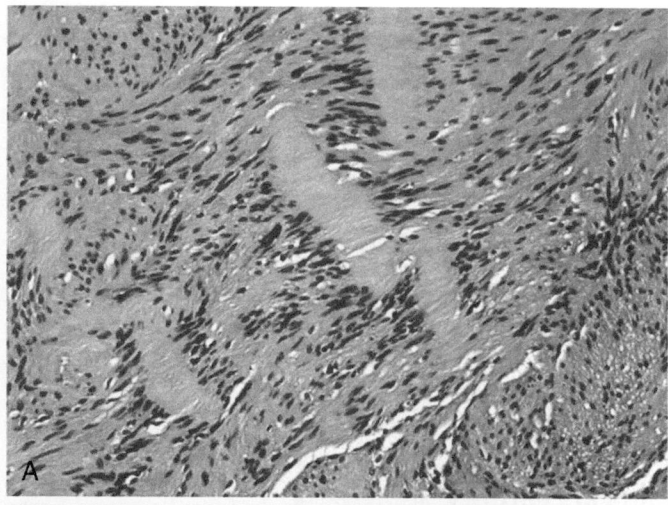

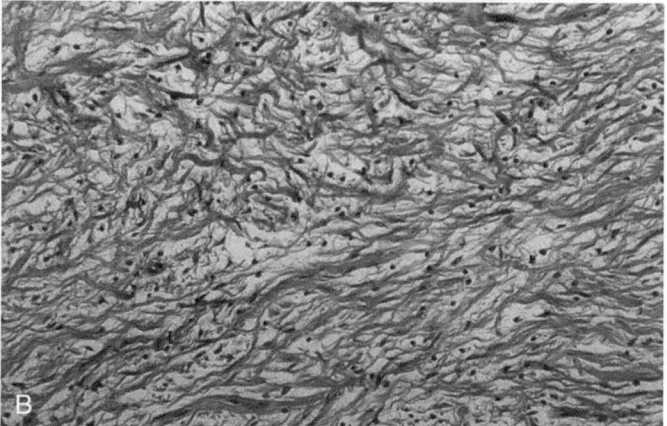

Figure 19-12. A, Schwannoma. Compact spindle cells (Antoni A tissue) and Verocay bodies. **B,** Neurofibroma. Sparsely cellular proliferation of spindle cells with wavy nuclei and cytoplasmic processes.

- Perivascular whorls resembling meningioma may occasionally be seen
- Vessels are often hyalinized, and foci of lipid-laden macrophages may be present
- Two subtypes
  - Cellular schwannoma
    - Increased likelihood of recurrence, but lacks ability to metastasize
    - Highly cellular, consisting predominantly of Antoni A areas (< 10% Antoni B areas)
    - Variable mitotic activity; typically show 1 to 4 mitoses/10 hpf
    - Frequent capsular, subcapsular, and perivascular lymphocytic infiltrates
    - Small foci of necrosis may be seen
    - Often contains aggregates of foamy histiocytes
  - Melanotic schwannoma
    - Usually grossly pigmented and contains Schwann cells with melanosomes
    - About 10% behave more aggressively than the nonmelanotic schwannomas

NEUROFIBROMA
- Typically hypocellular tumor consisting of interlacing fascicles of elongated spindle cells with wavy nuclei; minimal nuclear pleomorphism is typical (Figure 19-12B)

- Background shows variable degrees of mucopolysaccharide matrix, collagen ("shredded carrot type"), and reticulin
- May show degenerative cytologic atypia (ancient change) or increased cellularity (cellular neurofibroma)
- Minimal mitotic activity
- Plexiform neurofibroma: consists of multiple hypocellular, pale fascicles of spindle cells
- Mucinous or myxoid background

MALIGNANT PERIPHERAL NERVE SHEATH TUMOR
- Highly cellular tumor with moderate to marked nuclear pleomorphism (sarcomatous appearance)
- High mitotic rate (more than 5/10 hpf)
- Areas of geographic necrosis may be seen
- Greatly variable morphology, but often spindle cells forming a herringbone or fascicular pattern are seen
- Up to 20% of cases show unusual histologic features, including epithelioid cells and divergent mesenchymal (cartilage, bone, or skeletal muscle) or glandular differentiation

PERINEURIOMA
- Extraneural and sclerosing subtypes: vary from spindle-shaped elongated cells to epithelioid; variable architectural patterns, including whorling, lamellar, and storiform
- Reticular subtype: prominent myxoid stroma, netlike growth pattern
- Intraneural subtype: spindle cells arranged in pseudo onion-bulb arrangement around axons and Schwann cells

Special Stains and Immunohistochemistry
SCHWANNOMA
- S-100, CD34, calretinin, Sox10, and podoplanin positive
- GFAP: variable focal positivity
- Neurofilament may be positive at periphery of tumor
- EMA negative
- Cellular schwannomas retain strong diffuse S100 positivity
- SMA, desmin, and CD117 negative

NEUROFIBROMA
- S-100, CD34, and Sox10 positive
- Collagen IV, laminin, podoplanin, and calretinin variably positive
- Neurofilament may show sparse positivity within the tumor
- EMA: few positive cells

PERINEURIOMA
- EMA, collagen IV, laminin, claudin-1, and GLUT1 positive
- S-100 negative
- MIB-1 index: ranges from 5% to 15%

MPNST
- S-100 positive in up to 70%, but higher-grade lesions show less positivity
- MIB-1 index: ranges from 5% to 65%

Other Techniques for Diagnosis

CONVENTIONAL AND CELLULAR SCHWANNOMA

- Electron microscopy: well-differentiated, elongated cells with long cytoplasmic processes surrounded by a complete basal lamina; characteristically shows intercellular long-spacing collagen (Luse bodies)
- Cytogenetics: loss of the *NF2* gene product on chromosome 22 (also called *Merlin*) in 60%

NEUROFIBROMA

- Electron microscopy: mixture of cells including Schwann cells and perineurial cells
- Cytogenetics: plexiform subtype associated with NF1; sporadic neurofibromas commonly also have mutations in the *NF1* gene; structural rearrangements of chromosome 9 have been reported

MPNST

- Electron microscopy: poorly differentiated cells showing nuclear pleomorphism and an incomplete basement membrane; usually no Luse bodies
- Cytogenetics: 50% associated with NF1; other abnormalities identified include mutations in *TP53*, *CDKN2A*, and amplification of *EGFR* gene

PERINEURIOMA

- Electron microscopy: elongated cells and nuclei, delicate chromatin, pinocytotic vesicles, basal lamina, and tight junctions
- Cytogenetics: loss of chromosome 22 or 22q

Differential Diagnosis

SCHWANNOMA VERSUS MENINGIOMA

- Meningioma usually show prominent whorled pattern and psammoma bodies
- Rare in lumbosacral region (common site for schwannomas)
- Negative or faint staining for S-100 protein
- Positive staining for EMA (70%)

NEUROFIBROMA VERSUS TRAUMATIC NEUROMA

- Disorganized and haphazardly arranged variably sized clusters of axons and Schwann cells in fibrous tissue characterize a traumatic neuroma and distinguish it from a neurofibroma with its loose matrix and elongated wavy nuclei in a "shredded carrots" background

MPNST VERSUS SYNOVIAL SARCOMA

- Presence of *SS18-SSX1* or *SS18-SSX2* gene fusions in synovial sarcomas but not MPNST

PEARLS

- *Large neurofibromas associated with NF and plexiform neurofibromas have an increased potential for malignant transformation (MPNST)*
- *Multiple schwannomas may be seen in various syndromes (schwannomatosis, NF2, Carney complex); isolated bilateral schwannomas of cranial nerve VIII are pathognomonic of NF2*
- *MPNSTs are high-grade, aggressive tumors with tendency to recur and metastasize (often metastasize to lung)*
- *EMA positivity in perineuriomas may be faint and difficult to see because of thin processes*
- *Perineuriomas are usually cured with complete resection, but rare malignant cases are reported*

SELECTED REFERENCES

Macarenco RS, Ellinger F, Oliveira AM: Perineurioma: A distinctive and underrecognized peripheral nerve sheath neoplasm. Arch Pathol Lab Med 31:625-636, 2007.

Rodriguez FJ, Folpe AL, Giannini C, Perry A: Pathology of peripheral nerve sheath tumors: diagnostic overview and update on selected diagnostic problems. Acta Neuropathol 123:295-319, 2012.

Scheithauer BW, Erdogan S, Rodriguez FJ, et al: Malignant peripheral nerve sheath tumors of cranial nerves and intracranial contents: a clinicopathologic study of 17 cases. Am J Surg Pathol 33:325-338, 2009.

MENINGIOMA (WHO GRADE I), ATYPICAL MENINGIOMA (WHO GRADE II), AND ANAPLASTIC MENINGIOMA (WHO GRADE III)

Clinical Features

- Common tumor accounting for 24% to 30% of all primary intracranial neoplasms
- Typically found in middle-aged adults; occasionally seen in children
- More commonly occurs in females (3:2); intraspinal tumors show a 10:1 female-to-male ratio
- About 90% of tumors are intracranial
- Patients usually present with symptoms related to an enlarging intracranial mass or increased intracranial pressure; may have focal neurologic deficits or rarely seizures
- CT and MRI show dura-based, richly vascular, contrast-enhancing, well-defined masses; clusters of calcifications may be seen
- Rarely arise from the optic nerve, causing visual symptoms, or within the spinal cord, causing radicular pain; may also rarely involve the ventricular system
- Most (80%) meningiomas are benign (WHO grade 1)

Gross Pathology

- Firm, well-defined, tan-white tumor often showing attachment to a segment of dura; may show a yellow or gelatinous cut surface owing to lipid or mucin accumulation
- Frequent infiltration of bone and scalp
- Frequently causes hyperostosis of skull adjacent to the tumor
- Calcification is commonly seen
- Atypical or anaplastic meningioma
  - Typically causes considerable cerebral edema
  - Brain invasion is frequently present

Histopathology

- Extremely diverse tumor with numerous histologic variants

CLASSIC MENINGIOMA (WHO GRADE I)

- Syncytial, fibrous, and transitional variants (transitional variant is most common): *syncytial pattern* is created by sheets of tumor cells that have indistinct cell borders; *fibrous meningiomas* show elongated cells in a collagenous background; *transitional meningiomas* show a pattern that is intermediate between the syncytial and fibrous types or composed of a mixture of syncytial and fibrous patterns (Figure 19-13)

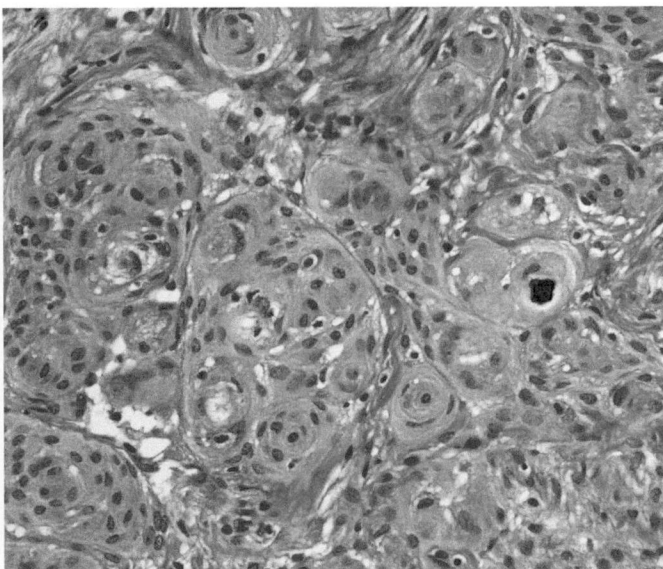

Figure 19-13. Meningioma. Syncytial pattern of neoplastic cells displaying a classic meningothelial appearance with round to oval nuclei. Several whorls are present.

- Neoplastic cells are arranged in a whorled or lobulated architecture
- Tumor cells have a meningothelial appearance with round to oval nuclei, dispersed chromatin, inconspicuous nucleoli, and eosinophilic cytoplasm
- Prominent round intranuclear inclusions are typical
- Psammoma bodies (round accumulation of calcium) are often noted throughout the tumor; less commonly seen in pure fibrous types
- Focal nuclear pleomorphism is often present
- Scattered mitotic figures may be seen
- Other variants
  - Psammomatous meningioma (WHO grade I)
    - Shows abundant psammoma bodies throughout the tumor
  - Secretory meningioma (WHO grade I)
    - Cytoplasm contains round, eosinophilic, hyaline structures resembling psammoma bodies (pseudopsammoma bodies)
    - Structures are PAS positive and diastase resistant
  - Microcystic meningioma (WHO grade I)
    - Consists of a delicate, microcystic architecture with cystic spaces filled with clear fluid
    - Often shows greater degree of cytologic atypia or areas of xanthomatous cells with vacuolated cytoplasm
  - Lymphoplasmacytic meningioma (WHO grade I)
    - Shows a pronounced lymphoplasmacytic response
  - Metaplastic meningioma (WHO grade I)
    - Metaplastic areas may consist of myxoid, chordoid, osteoblastic, lipoblastic, or xanthomatous differentiation
  - Angiomatous meningioma (WHO grade I)
    - Abundant vessels with sparse meningothelial cells
    - Vessels are usually hyalinized, and degenerative nuclear atypia is common
- Prognostically important variants
  - Chordoid meningioma (WHO grade II)
    - Rare variant
    - Consists of small groups or cords of epithelioid cells in a mucin-rich background (resembles a chordoma)
  - Clear cell meningioma (WHO grade II)
    - Composed of cells with clear cytoplasm
    - Cytoplasm contains glycogen (PAS positive)
    - Occurs more frequently in the spinal canal or cerebellopontine angle than in cerebrum
    - More aggressive growth and recurrence compared to grade 1 meningiomas
  - Papillary meningioma (WHO grade III)
    - Typically occurs in younger individuals
    - Tumor cells arranged around blood vessels resembling ependymoma-like pseudorosettes
    - Aggressive clinical course (55% recurrence rate; 20% metastasis rate)
  - Rhabdoid meningioma (WHO grade III)
    - Tumors that exhibit > 50% or exclusively rhabdoid cellular morphology qualify for designation as rhabdoid meningioma, WHO grade III; presence of small rhabdoid foci intermixed with typical meningioma cells is of uncertain significance
    - Rhabdoid cells have eccentric nuclei and hyaline paranuclear inclusions
    - Reported cases have high MIB-1 index and many mitoses, which have been associated with a high rate of recurrence and aggressive growth

ATYPICAL MENINGIOMA (WHO GRADE II)

- Exhibits increased mitoses (≥ 4 mitoses/10 hpf), brain invasion, or the presence of at least three of following five microscopic features: tumor showing sheetlike growth pattern, nuclei with macronucleoli, hypercellularity, and small cell formation or spontaneous necrosis

ANAPLASTIC MENINGIOMA (WHO GRADE III)

- Exhibits focal or diffuse loss of meningothelial differentiation at the light microscopic level (areas showing sarcomatous, carcinomatous, or melanoma-like appearance) *or* marked elevation in mitotic rate (≥ 20 mitoses/10 hpf)

Special Stains and Immunohistochemistry

- EMA, claudin-1: most are positive
- S-100 protein: occasionally positive; fibrous meningiomas: 80% are positive
- Cytokeratin: usually negative; secretory meningiomas usually positive
- CEA: positive in secretory meningiomas
- GFAP negative
- MIB-1: labeling index correlates with grade and recurrence rate; in general, an index greater than 4% is associated with increased recurrence; mean values of MIB-1 index: benign, 3.8%; atypical, 7.2%; anaplastic, 14.7%
- CD34: 60% of fibrous meningiomas are positive
- Progesterone receptor: variably positive; less likely to be positive in atypical or anaplastic meningiomas

Other Techniques for Diagnosis

- Electron microscopy: cells have nuclei with interdigitating, irregular membranes, desmosomes, and intranuclear cytoplasmic inclusions

- Cytogenetics
  - Meningiomas are found in NF2 (NF2 locus on chromosome 22q), and mutations in the *NF2* gene on chromosome 22 are found in 80% of sporadic meningiomas
  - Additional chromosome abnormalities associated with increased grade are loss of heterozygosity for chromosome 1p, loss of 14q, deletion of 9q21, and abnormalities of chromosomes 6q, 10, 14q, and 17q

Differential Diagnosis

SCHWANNOMA

- Biphasic tumor consisting of highly cellular areas (Antoni A) admixed with loose spongy areas of lower cellularity (Antoni B)
- Usually lacks distinct whorled architecture and psammoma bodies
- Typically found in posterior fossa or spinal cord
- S-100 protein and EMA usually positive

EPENDYMOMA

- Located within the ventricle; not usually associated with the meninges
- Typically occurs in children or young adults
- Cells have long fibrillary processes
- Perivascular pseudorosettes are commonly seen
- GFAP positive

MENINGEAL HYPERPLASIA

- Single or multiple foci of meningothelial cells (more than 10 cell layers thick)
- Usually associated with a predisposing factor (hemorrhage, chronic renal failure, trauma)
- Discontinuous growth pattern and no invasion or adjacent tissue

SOLITARY FIBROUS TUMOR AND HEMANGIOPERICYTOMA/CELLULAR SOLITARY FIBROUS TUMOR

- Contains numerous variably sized, slitlike and staghorn vessels
- No psammoma bodies
- Negative for EMA and varying CD34 positivity (diffuse and strong in solitary fibrous tumor; patchy, weak positivity in hemangiopericytoma/cellular solitary fibrous tumor)

PEARLS

- *Treatment is complete surgical resection; typically offers an excellent prognosis with classic meningiomas*
- *Radiation therapy has been shown to be beneficial in recurrent or unresectable tumors*
- *Preoperative embolization is often performed to reduce operative blood loss; it may cause alteration of tumor morphology (small cell change, clear cell-like, rhabdoid cell-like or pseudopapillary pattern) or increased MIB-1 positive cells adjacent to areas of embolism-induced necrosis*
- *Benign meningiomas have a recurrence rate of up to 25%; atypical meningiomas are associated with a 29% to 52% recurrence rate; anaplastic meningiomas have a recurrence rate of 50% to 94%*

SELECTED REFERENCES

Alahmadi H, Croul SE: Pathology and genetics of meningiomas. Semin Diagn Pathol 28:314-324, 2011.

Matsuda K, Takeuchi H, Arai Y, et al: Atypical and ischemic features of embolized meningioma. Brain Tumor Pathol 29:17-24, 2012.

Mawrin C, Perry A: Pathological classification and molecular genetics of meningiomas. J Neurooncol 99:379-391, 2012.

Nakasu S, Li DH, Okabe H, et al: Significance of MIB-1 staining indices in meningiomas. Am J Surg Pathol 25:472-478, 2001.

Perry A, Scheithauer BW, Nascimento AG: The immunophenotypic spectrum of meningeal hemangiopericytoma: a comparison with fibrous meningioma and solitary fibrous tumor of meninges. Am J Surg Pathol 21:1354-1360, 1997.

Vranic A, Peyre M, Kalamarides M: New insights into meningioma: from genetics to trails. Curr Opin Oncol 24:660-665, 2012.

SOLITARY FIBROUS TUMOR AND HEMANGIOPERICYTOMA/CELLULAR SOLITARY FIBROUS TUMOR

Clinical Features

- Dura/meninges-based neoplasms occurring more often intracranially rather than spinal, account for less than 1% of all CNS tumors
- No clinical features distinguish between solitary fibrous tumor and hemangiopericytoma
- Most originate in the meninges and often mimic meningiomas
- Usually found in adults; no sex predilection
- Most patients present with headache and focal neurologic deficits
- CT and MRI scans show a diffusely enhancing, sharply defined lesion with dural attachment suggestive of meningioma; bone destruction may be seen

Gross Pathology

- Typically forms a discrete, lobulated, tan-gray, fleshy mass
- May show invasive architecture with destruction of adjacent bone; usually no calcifications
- Markedly vascular tumor that bleeds profusely at surgery
- Cut surface is solid, focally hemorrhagic, and often with large vascular spaces

Histopathology

- Variably cellular tumors with numerous small slitlike and large staghorn vascular channels (Figure 19-14)
- Some tumors show predominantly spindle cells with a patternless architecture containing thick bands of collagen (fibrous or conventional solitary fibrous tumor)
- Others are hypercellular, monotonous, and less fibrous (hemangiopericytoma/cellular solitary fibrous tumor) with plump oval or elongated nuclei with inconspicuous nucleoli and scant cytoplasm
- Lacks tight whorls, psammoma bodies, or nuclear pseudoinclusions as seen in meningiomas
- May be further divided based on the presence/absence of necrosis or mitoses (none, greater than 5 mitoses/10 hpf, or fewer than 5 mitoses/10 hpf)

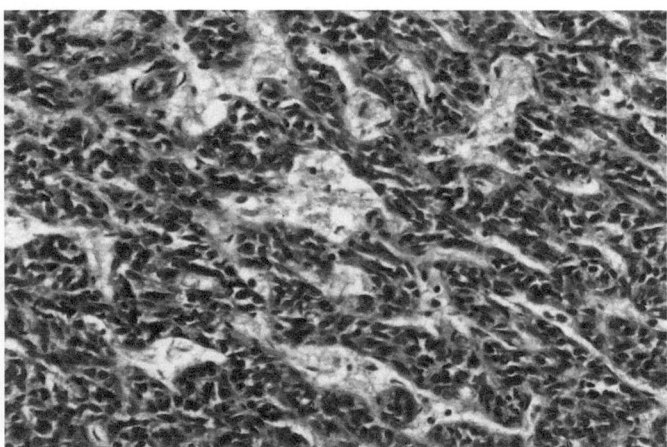

Figure 19-14. Hemangiopericytoma. Classic staghorn vascular pattern is evident in this neoplasm composed of polygonal to spindle-shaped cells.

Special Stains and Immunohistochemistry

- Reticulin: surrounds individual cells
- CD34: patchy positivity in hemangiopericytoma/cellular solitary fibrous tumor and diffuse positivity in conventional or fibrous solitary fibrous tumor
- Bcl-2, and vimentin: strong diffuse positivity
- CD99: positive in most cases
- Progesterone receptor: reports vary from 33% to 82%; estrogen receptor: reports vary from negative to 40% positive
- Factor XIIIa, variably positive
- S100 and EMA: usually negative
- Factor VIII and CD31: endothelial cells are positive; tumor cells are negative
- MIB-1 labeling index: conventional solitary fibrous tumor: usually < 5%; hemangiopericytoma/cellular solitary fibrous tumor: > 5%

Other Techniques for Diagnosis

- Electron microscopy: cells with basal lamina, primitive intercellular junctions, and whorled masses of intermediate filaments
- Molecular analysis: both conventional solitary fibrous tumors and hemangiopericytoma/cellular solitary fibrous tumors occurring in the meninges show fusion of the *NAB1-STAT6* gene supporting their likely common origin

Differential Diagnosis

MENINGIOMA

- Presence of psammoma bodies, whorls, calcification, and pseudoinclusions
- Typically lacks large staghorn blood vessels and abundant reticulin
- EMA positive, CD34 negative, CD99 negative, bcl-2 negative

MESENCHYMAL CHONDROSARCOMA

- Cartilage is present (not found in hemangiopericytoma/solitary fibrous tumor)

- *Progress in morphologic and molecular analyses of hemangiopericytoma and solitary fibrous tumors of meninges has supported that they are a single entity, each with a fibroblastic cell of origin*
- *Hemangiopericytoma/cellular solitary fibrous tumors, in general, have a higher rate of local recurrence with frequent late distant metastases typically involving the bone, liver, or lung than a conventional solitary fibrous tumor; this behavior has been associated with necrosis and increased mitoses, but a new grading system to apply to the previously separate, but now merged, entities of hemangiopericytoma and solitary fibrous tumor has not been created*
- *Surgical resection followed by radiotherapy is the usual treatment*
- *Postoperative radiation, chemotherapy, or both decrease tumor recurrence and may increase survival*

SELECTED REFERENCES

Couvier C, Metellus P, Maues de Paul A, et al: Solitary fibrous tumors and hemangiopericytomas of the meninges: overlapping pathological features and common prognostic factors suggest the same spectrum of tumors. Brain Pathol 22:511-521, 2012.

Fargen KM, Opalach KJ, Wakefield D, et al: The central nervous system solitary fibrous tumor: a review of clinical, imaging, and pathologic findings among all reported cases from 1996 to 2010. Clin Neurol Neurosurg 113:703-710, 2011.

Park MS, Araujo DM: New insights into the hemangiopericytoma/solitary fibrous tumor spectrum of tumors. Curr Opin Oncol 21:327-331, 2009.

Schweizer L, Koelsche C, Sahm F, et al: Meningeal hemangiopericytoma and solitary fibrous tumors carry the *NAB2-STAT6* fusion and can be diagnosed by nuclear expression of STAT6 protein. Acta Neuropathol 135:651-658, 2013.

Tihan T, Viglione M, Rosenblum MK, et al: Solitary fibrous tumors in the central nervous system: a clinicopathologic review of 18 cases and comparison to meningeal hemangiopericytomas. Arch Pathol Lab Med 127:432-439, 2003.

HEMANGIOBLASTOMA (WHO GRADE I)

Clinical Features

- Low-grade neoplasm, associated with VHL, autosomal dominant disorder characterized by hemangioblastomas of the CNS and retina, renal cell carcinoma, pheochromocytoma, pancreatic islet cell tumor, endolymphatic sac tumor, and visceral cysts
- Approximately 25% of cerebellar hemangioblastomas occur in patients with VHL
- In patients with VHL, 70% develop hemangioblastomas
- Sporadic cases are typically found in adults (fourth and fifth decades) and are usually single; multiple tumors are commonly seen in patients with VHL and occur at younger ages (third and fourth decades)
- Typically occur in the cerebellum (80%); less commonly found in the spinal cord, brain stem, or cerebrum
- Symptoms are usually related to increased intracranial pressure when the tumor is in the posterior fossa; back pain and weakness or pain in extremities are seen in spinal cord tumors
- Tumor production of erythropoietin may cause secondary polycythemia

Gross Pathology

- Well-circumscribed, highly vascular mass, usually largely cystic with a solid mural nodule
- Cyst fluid is clear, often yellow, and may be hemorrhagic
- Neoplasm may be yellow owing to a high lipid content and commonly has areas of hemorrhage

Histopathology

- Characteristically shows a prominent dense network of capillaries lined by hyperplastic endothelial cells and pericytes; interspersed large thin-walled vessels are also present
- Interstitial stromal cells are large and have abundant vacuolated lipid-rich pale cytoplasm; nuclei are large, usually without nucleoli, and occasionally show slight to moderate pleomorphism (Figure 19-15)
- Cellular and reticular variants of hemangioblastoma have been identified; the cellular variant is more uncommon and composed of epithelioid cells in large clusters with more limited capillaries, whereas the reticular variant contains more abundant capillary network
- Cyst wall is composed of reactive astrocytes and Rosenthal fibers that may resemble a pilocytic astrocytoma
- Mitotic activity is rare to absent

Special Stains and Immunohistochemistry

- GFAP: entrapped astrocytes positive; stromal cells negative
- Inhibin A, brachyury, vimentin, and oil red O (on fresh tissue): stromal cells positive
- S-100 and NSE: stromal cells variably positive
- EMA, cytokeratin, CD34, and factor VIII: stromal cells negative
- Reticulin highlights vessels and is present around tumor cells
- MIB-1 index: sparse positive nuclei (< 2%)

Other Techniques for Diagnosis

- Electron microscopy: three cell types are identified: endothelial cells, pericytes, and stromal cells; the stromal cells contain lipid droplets, microfilaments, and electron-dense granules (associated with erythropoietin-like substance)

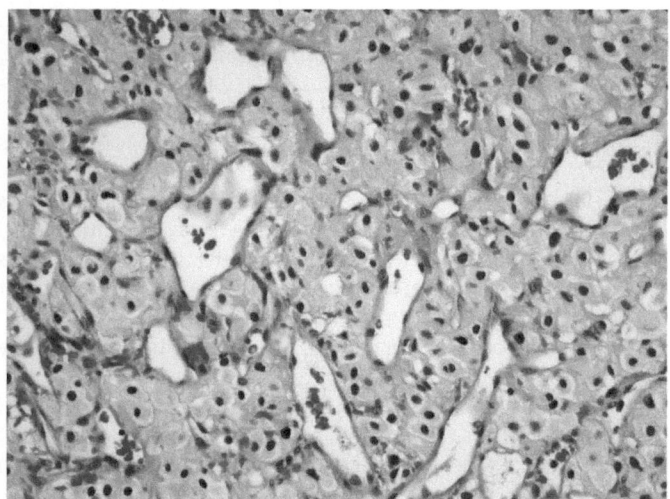

Figure 19-15. Hemangioblastoma. Abundant vascular channels and numerous lipid-laden stromal cells.

- Cytogenetics: VHL is caused by deletions or mutations in the VHL tumor suppressor gene (chromosome 3p25-26); germline mutations in this gene are found in some individuals presenting with hemangioblastoma and loss or inactivation of the gene is found in up to 50% of patients with sporadic neoplasms

Differential Diagnosis

PILOCYTIC ASTROCYTOMA
- Classically cells have elongated nuclei and fibrillary cytoplasm
- GFAP diffusely positive

METASTATIC CLEAR CELL RENAL CELL CARCINOMA
- May occur in association with hemangioblastoma in VHL
- Usually not cystic
- Mitotic figures usually abundant
- Typically positive for EMA, cytokeratin (CAM5.2), CD10, PAX2, and PAX8; negative for inhibin A and NSE

PARAGANGLIOMA
- Typically synaptophysin and chromogranin positive

MENINGIOMA (ANGIOMATOUS)
- EMA positive and inhibin A negative

PEARLS

- *Stromal cells are considered neoplastic components of the tumor, but its histogenesis has not been clarified*
- *Complete surgical resection offers excellent results; rare reports of tumor recurrence after incomplete resection exist*
- *Study suggests that symptom progression is secondary to the increasing size of the cyst rather than growth of the neoplasm*
- *Preliminary studies have suggested that the cellular type of hemangioblastoma has a higher risk of recurrence than the reticular type*

SELECTED REFERENCES

Carney EM, Banerjee P, Ellis CL, et al: PAX2(-)/PAX8(-)/InhibinA(+) immunoprofile of hemangioblastoma: a helpful combination in the differential diagnosis with metastatic clear cell renal carcinoma to the central nervous system. Am J Surg Pathol 35:262-267, 2011.

Hasselblatt M, Jeibmann A, Gerb J, et al: Cellular and reticular variants of haemangioblastoma revisited: a clinicopathologic study of 88 cases. Neuropathol Appl Neurobiol 31:618-622, 2005.

Hoang MP, Amirkhan MH: Inhibin alpha distinguishes hemangioblastoma from clear cell renal cell carcinoma. Am J Surg Pathol 27:1152-1156, 2003.

Takei H, Bhattacharjee MB, Rivera A, et al: New immunohistochemical markers in the evaluation of central nervous system tumors: a review of seven selected adult and pediatric brain tumors. Arch Pathol Lab Med 131:234-241, 2007.

MALIGNANT LYMPHOMA (NON-HODGKIN AND HODGKIN)

Clinical Features

- Primary CNS lymphomas (PCNSLs) make up 6.6% of all primary brain tumors and occur in both immunocompetent and immunocompromised hosts
- PCNSL is predominantly non-Hodgkin type, and about 5% of primary cases are associated with acquired immunodeficiency syndrome (AIDS)

- Incidence of PCNSL has increased since the late 1980s, only partially attributable to occurrence in those with the human immunodeficiency virus (HIV) infection
- Peak ages of occurrence in the immunocompetent individual are in the sixth and seventh decades, with a slightly higher occurrence in men than women
- Immunocompromised host mean age is 37 years in transplant recipients and 39 years in AIDS patients
- Most common location is in the parenchyma of the cerebral hemispheres, forming discrete or diffuse lesions
  - Occurs, with decreasing frequency, in the thalamus and basal ganglia, corpus callosum, ventricles, and cerebellum
  - Less common sites of occurrence are the leptomeninges, eye, and spinal cord
- Overall, up to 50% are multiple, but multifocality is more common in the immunocompromised patient (85%)
- Meningeal involvement is more common in secondary lesions
- The typical clinical presentation of PCNSL is with focal neurologic signs or symptoms (70%), followed by neuropsychiatric symptoms (43%) and increased intracranial pressure (33%)
- Primary Hodgkin disease in the CNS is extremely rare; more common is to have CNS involvement with known systemic disease

Gross Pathology

- An ill-defined mass involving the deep periventricular tissue or occurring superficially in the brain, causing thickening of the cortex, is most common
- Tumor may be yellow or gray-white, show areas of hemorrhage or necrosis, and be solid or cystic
- Hodgkin disease typically involves the dura, meninges, and skull-base structures

Histopathology

NON-HODGKIN LYMPHOMA

- In both the immunocompetent and immunocompromised hosts, most are diffuse large B-cell type (> 95%)

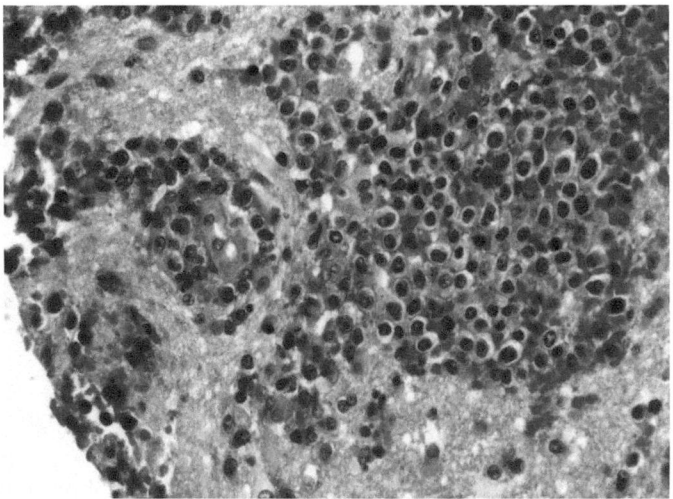

Figure 19-16. Malignant lymphoma. Classic angiocentric pattern for a malignant lymphoma involving the brain.

- Less commonly, low-grade B-cell type, marginal zone B-cell lymphoma, Burkitt lymphoma, or T-cell types
- Patchy clusters of cells with a predilection for perivascular spaces (evokes a deposition of reticulin fibers); diffuse sheets may also be seen (Figure 19-16)
- Individual cells are usually large and round with scant circumscribed cytoplasm and pleomorphic nuclei with nucleoli
- Mitoses, apoptosis, and geographic necrosis are common

HODGKIN DISEASE

- Most common subtypes involving the brain are nodular sclerosing and mixed cellularity
- Characterized by neoplastic Reed-Sternberg cells (large, binucleated cells with each nucleus containing a single prominent nucleolus; abundant eosinophilic cytoplasm) in a background of mixed inflammatory cells, including lymphocytes, plasma cells, neutrophils, eosinophils, and macrophages

Special Stains and Immunohistochemistry

- LCA (CD45) positive
- B- and T-cell markers: CD20/CD3 positive depending on lineage
- In situ hybridization for EBV RNA (EBER) is positive in lymphomas in AIDS patients and other immunocompromised hosts

Other Techniques for Diagnosis

- Cytogenetics: gains of chromosomes 12, 1, 18, and 7 have been identified; in addition, homozygous deletion and promoter hypermethylation of *CDKN2A* have been identified

Differential Diagnosis

METASTATIC NEUROENDOCRINE CARCINOMA

- Well-defined tumors typically lacking an infiltrative margin
- Cell cohesion and nuclear molding typically present
- Cytokeratin, synaptophysin, and chromogranin positive
- LCA and CD20 negative

OLIGODENDROGLIOMA

- Monomorphic oligodendroglial cells with perinuclear halos and less well-defined cytoplasm compared with lymphoma cells
- Cells typically do not infiltrate through the vessel walls as in lymphoma
- Microcalcifications are characteristic
- LCA and CD20 negative
- Deletions of chromosomes 1p and 19q are usually frequent

REACTIVE LYMPHOCYTOSIS (AS IN VIRAL ENCEPHALITIS, VASCULITIS, AND DEMYELINATING DISEASES)

- Lymphocytes do not show significant cytologic atypia
- Lacks monoclonality (usually predominantly T lymphocytes, less often B lymphocytes)
- Cluster in perivascular regions, but do not form solid sheets of cells in the parenchyma
- Consider progressive multifocal leukoencephalopathy (PML) and toxoplasmosis in the immunocompromised host

MEDULLOBLASTOMA AND PNET
- Rosette formation may be seen
- Positive for synaptophysin, NSE, and neurofilament
- Negative for LCA

PEARLS

- *Treatment with steroids before biopsy is to be avoided if possible because it may disrupt cellular morphology so completely that pathologic diagnosis is not possible*
- *Prognostic markers: the following have been associated with a poor prognosis:*
  - *Age greater than 60 years*
  - *Poor performance status*
  - *Increased lactate dehydrogenase level*
  - *Increased CSF protein*
  - *Deep location of tumor mass in the brain*
- *PCNSL occasionally presents without focal signs/symptoms due to wide infiltration of neoplastic cells and lack of a distinct mass lesion evident on MRI scans; this has been termed lymphomatosis cerebri*

SELECTED REFERENCES

Batchelor T, Loeffler JS: Primary CNS lymphoma. J Clin Oncol 24:1281-1288, 2006.
Bhagavathi S, Wilson JD: Primary central nervous lymphoma. Arch Pathol Lab Med 132:1830-1834, 2008.
Commins DL: Pathology of primary central nervous system lymphoma. Neurosurg Focus 21:E2, 2006.
Ferreri AJM, Reni M: Prognostic factors in primary central nervous lymphomas. Hematol Oncol Clin N Am 19:629-649, 2005.
Rollins KE, Kleinschmidt-DeMasters BK, Corboy JR, et al: Lymphomatosis cerebri as a cause of white matter dementia. Hum Pathol 36:282-290, 2005.
Scott BJ, Douglas VC, Tihan T, et al: A systematic approach to the diagnosis of suspected central nervous system lymphoma. JAMA Neurol 70:311-319, 2013.

GERM CELL TUMORS

Clinical Features

- Central nervous system counterpart of germ cell tumors found in gonads and other extracranial sites
- About 90% of patients present before age 20; more common in males
- Symptoms include signs of increased intracranial pressure, hydrocephalus, visual abnormalities (gaze palsies or visual field cuts), or various endocrinopathies, including diabetes insipidus, hypopituitarism, or precocious puberty
- Typically located in the midline; most often involving the pineal or pituitary region (two thirds in pineal region, one third in pituitary region)
- In germinomas, MRI scans show a well defined mass with hypointensity on T1-weighted images and hyperintensity on T2-weighted images

Gross Pathology

- See Chapters 11 and 12 for descriptions of germinoma, choriocarcinoma, yolk sac tumor, embryonal carcinoma, teratoma (benign, immature, mature, and malignant)

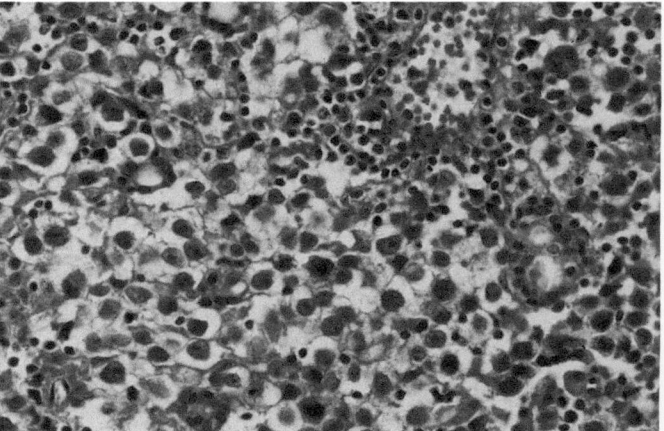

Figure 19-17. Germinoma. Large polygonal and well-defined cells with abundant clear cytoplasm and nuclei with prominent nucleoli, intermixed with lymphocytes.

Histopathology (Figure 19-17)

- See Chapters 11 and 12

Special Stains and Immunohistochemistry

- See Chapters 11 and 12

Other Techniques for Diagnosis

- Cytogenetic analysis: most frequent chromosomal abnormalities in germinomas of the pineal region are loss of 13q and 18q

Differential Diagnosis

PINEOCYTOMA AND PINEOBLASTOMA
- Presence of pineocytomatous rosettes or small blue cells
- Human chorionic gonadotropin, human placental lactogen, placental alkaline phosphatase, and cytokeratin negative

PEARLS

- *Overall, intracranial germ cell tumors are rare; represent 3% to 11% of all brain tumors in children and 1% in adults*
- *Sacrococcygeal teratomas are often identified in the neonatal period; more common in females and usually benign*

SELECTED REFERENCES

Balmaceda C, Modak S, Finlay J: Central nervous system germ cell tumors. Semin Oncol 25:243-250, 1998.
Hirato J, Nakazato Y: Pathology of pineal region tumors. J Neurooncol 54:239-249, 2001.
Rickert CH, Simon R, Bergmann M, et al: Comparative genomic hybridization in pineal region germ cell tumors. J Neuropathol Exp Neurol 59:815-821, 2000.

NEURAXIAL CYSTS: RATHKE CLEFT CYST, COLLOID CYST, AND ENTEROGENOUS CYST

Clinical Features

RATHKE CLEFT CYST (RCC)
- Usually located in the sella or suprasellar region
- Often asymptomatic and found at autopsy, but may produce compressive symptoms (headache, hypopituitarism, hyperprolactinemia, and visual disturbance) owing to accumulated colloid secretions

COLLOID CYST (CC)

- Usually within third ventricle near the foramen of Monro
- May cause obstructive hydrocephalus
- Rarely associated with sudden death
- Mean age of occurrence is 40 years

ENTEROGENOUS CYST (ENTC)

- Also known as neurenteric cyst, endodermal cyst, foregut, respiratory, or bronchogenic cyst
- Usually located within the spinal canal, usually in the cervical and upper thoracic levels
- Rarely located intracranially
- Usually intradural, extramedullary, and anterior to the cord
- May be associated with vertebral abnormalities
- Usually occurs in children and young adults

Gross Pathology

- Each cyst is thin walled with a smooth lining and filled with gray-white mucoid material
- CC often contains particularly dense cyst contents

Histopathology (Figures 19-18 and 19-19)

- Cysts are lined by epithelium ranging from simple columnar or cuboidal cells to a pseudostratified layer of cells; cilia and mucin production are typically seen

- In RCC, cyst often overlies anterior pituitary gland cells, and squamous metaplasia may be seen
- Enterogenous cyst epithelium resembles gastrointestinal or respiratory epithelium

Special Stains and Immunohistochemistry

- Cytokeratin and EMA: RCC, CC, and EntC lining cells positive
- Vimentin: RCC is positive; CC and EntC variably positive
- GFAP: RCC, CC, and EntC negative

Other Techniques for Diagnosis

- Electron microscopy: ciliated and nonciliated epithelial cells with junctional complexes and microvilli, resting on a continuous basal lamina

Differential Diagnosis

CRANIOPHARYNGIOMA VERSUS RCC

- Presence of squamous metaplasia in RCC may make distinction difficult, but RCC lacks wet keratin formation typical of craniopharyngioma
- Craniopharyngiomas contain solid epithelial islands, distinctive stellate reticulum, and basally palisaded epithelium

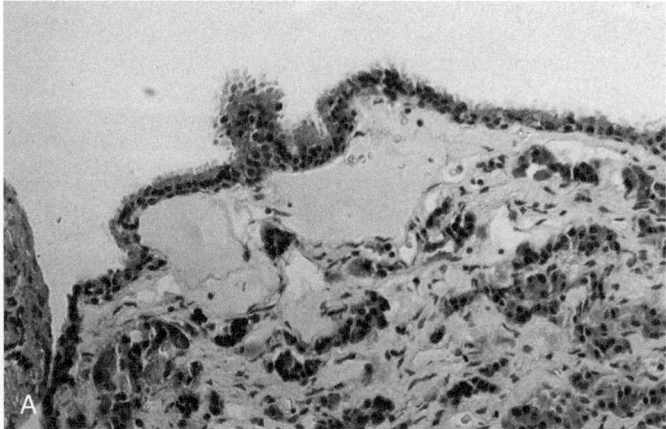
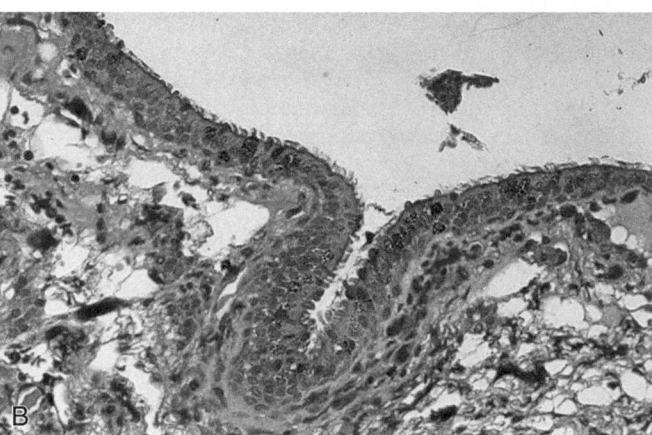

Figure 19-18. Rathke cleft cyst. A, The cyst wall is lined by ciliated columnar epithelium overlying anterior pituitary tissue. **B,** Mucin stain showing positive goblet cells.

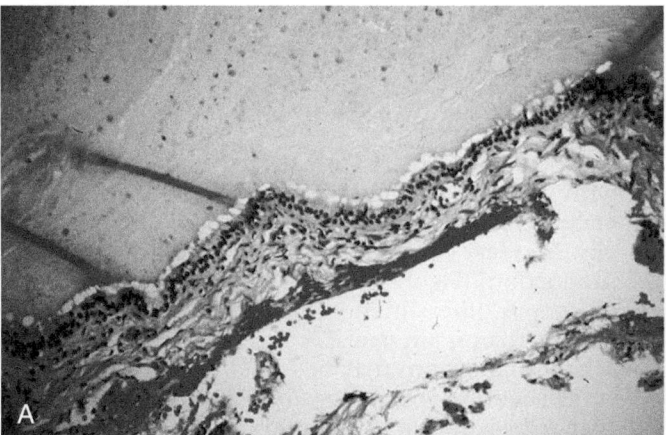
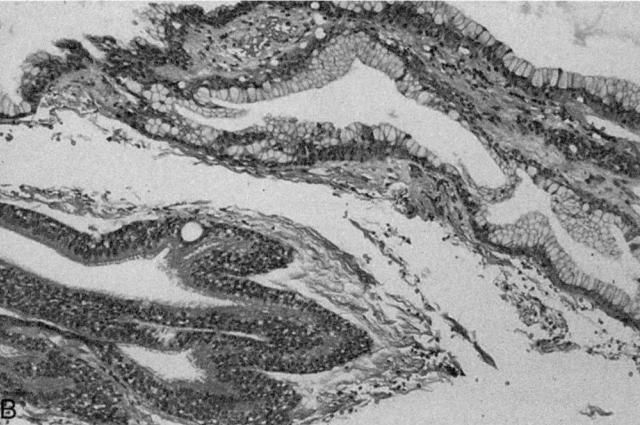

Figure 19-19. A, Colloid cyst. The cyst wall is lined by cuboidal to columnar epithelium, overlying a fibrous stroma. **B,** Enterogenous cyst. The cyst wall is lined by ciliated or mucin-secreting columnar epithelium reminiscent of respiratory or intestinal linings, respectively.

EPIDERMOID OR DERMOID CYSTS

- Both cysts are lined by keratinized squamous epithelium; dermoid cysts also contain skin appendages (hair follicles, sebaceous glands, sweat glands)
- Dermoid cysts are more likely to occur in the midline and epidermoid cysts in a lateral position (often in cerebellopontine angle or parasellar region)

DISTINCTION BETWEEN RCC, CC, AND EntC

- Difficult to distinguish histologically
- Location is likely to be helpful

EPENDYMAL CYST

- Most are in the deep white matter
- Epithelial lining of low cuboidal to columnar cells that are frequently ciliated
- Cyst lining is positive for GFAP and S-100 protein

ARACHNOID CYST

- No epithelial lining; lined by meningothelial cells
- Lining cells positive for EMA; negative for GFAP and S-100 protein

CYSTICERCOSIS OF VENTRICULAR SYSTEM OR SUBARACHNOID SPACE

- Presence of fragments of parasite on biopsy indicates correct diagnosis

PEARLS

- *Each cyst is benign and usually cured by complete excision*
- *Co-occurrence of pituitary adenoma and Rathke cleft cyst has been reported*

SELECTED REFERENCES

Caldarelli M, Massimi L, Kondageski C, et al: Intracranial midline dermoid and epidermoid cysts in children. J Neurosurg 100:473-480, 2004.

Gauden AJ, Khurana VG, Tsui AE, et al: Intracranial neuroenteric cysts: a concise review including an illustrative patient. J Clin Neurosc 19:352-359, 2012.

Kleinschmidt-DeMasters BK, Lillehei KO, Stears JC: The pathologic, surgical, and MR spectrum of Rathke cleft cysts. Surg Neurol 44:19-27, 1995.

Osborn AG, Preece MT: Intracranial cysts: radiologic-pathologic correlation and imaging approach. Radiology 239:650-664, 2006.

Trifanescu R, Ansorge O, Wass JAH, et al: Rathke's cleft cysts. Clin Endocrinol 76:151-160, 2012.

PITUITARY ADENOMA (INCLUDING TYPICAL AND ATYPICAL ADENOMAS), PITUITARY CARCINOMA, AND PITUITARY HYPERPLASIA

Clinical Features

PITUITARY ADENOMAS

- Most frequently found in women in their third through sixth decades; rarely seen in children
- Represent about 15% of all intracranial neoplasms
- May occasionally be found incidentally at autopsy
- Patients present with endocrinopathy in two thirds of the cases (hormone secretion by tumor or pressure on stalk or hypothalamus) or with visual complaints (a nonsecretory tumor is more likely to grow large enough to compress optic tracts)
- Functional tumors have variable presentation depending on what hormone they secrete
  - Growth hormone (GH)–secreting adenomas produce acromegaly
  - Prolactin (PRL)–secreting adenomas produce galactorrhea
  - Adrenocorticotropic hormone (ACTH)–secreting adenomas produce Cushing disease or Nelson syndrome
  - Gonadotrophic adenomas (follicle-stimulating hormone [FSH] or luteinizing hormone [LH] producing) are not usually biochemically active and present as nonfunctioning tumors
  - Thyroid-stimulating hormone (TSH)-producing adenomas produce hyperthyroidism
- May be associated with MEN1
- Atypical pituitary adenoma
  - Accounts for about 5% of adenomas
  - Defined histopathologically (see "Histopathology")

PITUITARY CARCINOMA

- Defined only by the presence of metastasis

PITUITARY HYPERPLASIA

- Clinical presentation is the same as for adenomas
- Radiologic studies may show diffuse enlargement of pituitary gland without a discernible rim of normal tissue

Gross Pathology

- Range in size from microadenomas to several centimeters, with enlargement of the sella and occasionally extrasellar extension
- Soft masses with occasional cystic degeneration or necrosis in larger lesions
- Invasive pituitary adenoma
  - Shows extensive dural, vascular, osseous, neural, or sinus invasion; this designation is best made radiographically or intraoperatively
  - Invasion is present in about 50% of all adenomas

Histopathology

- Tumor has a nested, sheetlike, or trabecular architecture with large groups of cells surrounded by incomplete reticulin network; may show focal papillary architecture
- Compression of adjacent normal pituitary gland may be seen
- Tumor is generally composed of monomorphic cells with round nuclei and inconspicuous nucleoli; a moderate degree of nuclear pleomorphism may occasionally be seen (see characteristics specific to hormone production) (Figure 19-20)
- Oncocytic differentiation may occasionally be present
- Mitotic figures are rare
- Microcalcifications may be present
- Large adenomas may show focal necrosis, infarction, or hemorrhage (pituitary apoplexy)
- Complete tumor infarction may rarely occur

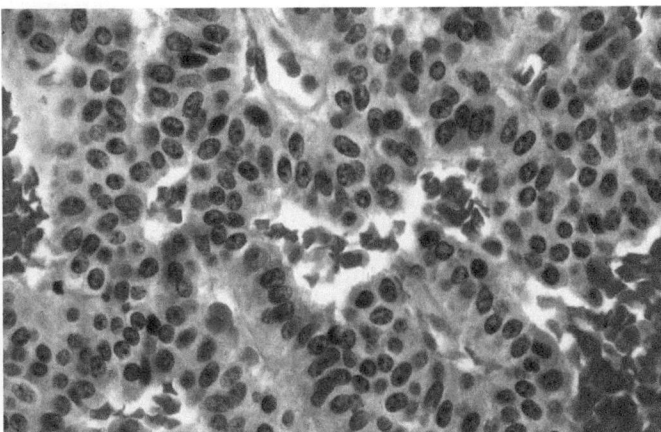

Figure 19-20. Pituitary adenoma. Sinusoidal pattern of uniform cells with distinct cytoplasm and round nuclei containing salt-and-pepper chromatin.

- Characteristics specific to hormone production
  - PRL-containing adenomas (30% of all adenomas)
    - Sparsely granulated adenomas
      - Usually are responsive to dopamine agonists and show changes secondary to treatment (small cells in fibrous stroma and focal staining for PRL)
      - Untreated tumors are chromophobic with abundant cytoplasm and strong juxtanuclear PRL positivity
      - Prolactinomas are associated with dystrophic calcification and eosinophilic bodies (amyloid deposits)
    - Densely granulated adenomas: acidophilic to chromophobic cells with strong diffuse positivity to PRL; much less common than the sparsely granulated PRL-containing adenomas
    - Acidophil stem cell adenoma: aggressive behavior, chromophobic with oncocytic change, clear cytoplasmic vacuoles, variably positivity to PRL and GH with CAM5.2 fibrous bodies and characteristic electron microscopy
  - GH-containing adenomas (10% to 15% of all adenomas)
    - Sparsely granulated adenomas: chromophobic to lightly eosinophilic cells with weak positivity for GH, and CAM5.2 identifies characteristic fibrous bodies; distinction from densely granulated GH-containing adenomas is important as these exhibit more aggressive behavior
    - Densely granulated adenomas: eosinophilic cytoplasm and strong diffuse cytoplasmic immunoreactivity with CAM5.2
    - Mammosomatotroph adenoma: may also produce and secrete prolactin in addition to GH or PRL and TSH (plurihormonal adenoma)
      - Cells have eosinophilic cytoplasm and GH and prolactin immunostaining in the same tumor cells
  - ACTH-containing adenomas (10% to 15% of all adenomas)
    - May be sparsely or densely granulated
      - Sparsely granulated ACTH adenomas are composed of chromophobic cells, usually macroadenomas, and are aggressive tumors

- Most microadenomas are densely granulated and composed of basophilic cells with strong PAS positivity, CAM5.2 positivity, and strong diffuse positivity for ACTH
  - Adjacent nonadenomatous gland shows Crooke hyaline change (concentric whorls of hyaline material in cytoplasm)
  - Silent corticotroph adenomas may be densely or sparsely granulated and have a high recurrence rate with increased occurrence of hemorrhage and infarction
  - Crooke cell adenoma is rare and aggressive and is composed of cells with an accumulation of cytoplasmic keratin filaments, which pushes the secretory granules to the cell periphery
- TSH-secreting adenomas (< 1% of all adenomas)
  - Usually large infiltrative masses with fibrosis, atypia, and aggressive behavior
  - Composed of chromophobic polygonal, angulated, or spindle-shaped cells with nuclear pleomorphism and a solid growth pattern
- Nonfunctioning adenomas and null cell adenomas
  - Most nonfunctioning adenomas are of gonadotrophic origin (30% of all adenomas) without clinical evidence of hormonal secretion
    - Solid sheets, nests, or sinusoidal pattern of acidophilic cells; pseudopapillae and rosettes may also be seen
    - FSH and LH: multifocal and variable positivity
  - Null cell adenomas do not show any evidence of specific cell-type differentiation
    - Oncocytic change may be present
- Plurihormonal adenomas
  - Most frequent combinations include GH, PRL, and one or more of the following: TSH, FSH, or LH
- Silent subtype 3 adenoma
  - Often positive for PRL, GH, and TSH (all may be focal)
  - Intense stromal fibrosis and high vascularity
  - Characteristic electron microscopy
  - Aggressive behavior and poor prognosis
- Atypical adenomas
  - Usually show invasive growth
  - Increased mitoses, and MIB-1 labeling index greater than 3%
  - Extensive nuclear positivity for p53
- Invasive pituitary adenoma
  - Defined by invasion into bone, sphenoid or cavernous sinus, and diaphragm sellae; same histologic features as typical pituitary adenomas; no reliable light or electron microscopic findings help distinguish this subtype
  - May show elevation of MIB-1 and p53 positivity
- Pituitary hyperplasia
  - Pituitary acini expanded by cells of one hormonal type with intermixed cells staining for all hormones
  - Reticulum network remains intact but expanded
  - Often difficult to distinguish from normal gland
- Pituitary carcinoma
  - Rare pituitary tumor
  - Morphologically cannot be separated from typical pituitary adenoma

- Two thirds are functional and produce PRL or ACTH
- Definitive diagnosis is based on the presence of cerebrospinal or systemic metastases

Special Stains and Immunohistochemistry

- PAS stain identifies granules of corticotrophs, thyrotrophs and gonadotrophs
- Variably positive or negative staining for anterior pituitary gland hormones (see detailed description under "Histopathology")
- "Densely" versus "sparsely" granulated adenomas usually correlate with the extent of immunoreactivity for the specific antibody
- MIB-1: a positive correlation between invasiveness and high MIB-1 index is inconsistently reported; labeling index of greater than 3% defines atypical adenomas
- Extensive positivity for p53 in atypical adenomas

Other Techniques for Diagnosis

- Electron microscopy: distribution and morphology of secretory granules help to classify adenomas
  - Silent subtype III adenomas have characteristic nuclear inclusions called spheridia (nuclear inclusions)
  - Acidophil stem cell adenomas have abundant enlarged mitochondria
- Loss of chromosome 11p is reported to be associated with recurrence and metastasis in prolactinomas and GH-producing neoplasms
- An activating mutation of the *gsp* oncogene is found in approximately 40% of sporadic GH-secreting adenomas

Differential Diagnosis

NORMAL PITUITARY GLAND

- Small clusters of monomorphic cells with uniform nuclei completely surrounded by reticulin network

CRANIOPHARYNGIOMA

- Distinctive morphology: cords and solid areas of squamous epithelium with palisaded basal cells, keratin formation, and calcification

HYPOPHYSITIS

- May occur as a primary process confined to the gland or secondary to systemic disease
  - Lymphocytic hypophysitis (primary)
    - More common in women, especially peripartum
    - Partial or total pituitary hypofunction
    - Lymphoplasmacytic infiltrate of gland; lymphoid follicles may be seen
  - Granulomatous hypophysitis (primary)
    - Well-formed granulomas composed of epithelioid histiocytes, giant cells, and lymphocytes
    - Infectious etiology should be considered
    - May be the primary manifestation of sarcoidosis
    - Idiopathic form exists; hypothesized to be of autoimmune origin

RCC

- Single layer of ciliated cuboidal to columnar cells forming a cyst wall, often overlying pituitary gland
- Squamous metaplasia may occur

SPINDLE CELL ONCOCYTOMA OF THE ADENOHYPOPHYSIS (WHO GRADE I)

- Suspected to derive from folliculostellate cells of anterior pituitary gland
- Interlacing spindle and epithelioid cells with eosinophilic oncocytic cytoplasm
- May see nuclear atypia
- TTF-1, EMA galectin-3, and S-100 positive
- Pituitary hormones, GFAP, cytokeratin, chromogranin, and synaptophysin negative

GRANULAR CELL TUMOR OF THE NEUROHYPOPHYSIS

- Polygonal cells with granular cytoplasm
- TTF-1 and galectin-3 positive and GFAP, EMA, and cytokeratin negative

PEARLS

- *Hemorrhagic necrosis of a pituitary adenoma (pituitary apoplexy) constitutes a surgical emergency (occurs in less than 1% of cases)*

SELECTED REFERENCES

Al-Brahim NYY, Asa SL: My approach to pathology of the pituitary gland. J Clin Pathol 59:1245-1253, 2006.
Asa SL, Ezzat S: The pathogenesis of pituitary tumors. Annu Rev Path Mech Dis 4:97-126, 2009.
Lopes MBS: Growth hormone-secreting adenomas: pathology and cell biology. Neurosurg Focus 29:E2, 2010.
Mete O, Asa SL: Clinicopathological correlations in pituitary adenomas. Brain Pathol 22:443-453, 2012.
Mete O, Ezzat S, Asa SL: Biomarkers of aggressive pituitary adenomas. J Mol Endocrinol 49:R69-R78, 2012.
Ogiwara H, Dubner S, Shafizadeh S, et al: Spindle cell oncocytoma of the pituitary and pituicytoma: two tumors mimicking pituitary adenoma. Surg Neurol Int 2:116, 2011.

PITUICYTOMA (WHO GRADE I)

Clinical Features

- Low-grade glial neoplasm arising in the neurohypophysis or infundibulum
- Extremely rare; occurs in adults (mean age at presentation is 50 years with a range from 17 to 83 years); men are affected more than women
- Signs and symptoms are secondary to mass effect: visual disturbance, headache, and hypopituitarism; may also see compression of infundibulum and secondary hyperprolactinemia
- MRI scans of pituicytomas show isointensity on T1-weighted images and hyperintensity on T2 and proton-density images and the majority enhance with contrast

Gross Pathology

- Circumscribed solid mass

Histopathology

- Spindle cells forming fascicles or storiform pattern
- Cells range from elongated to rounded and contain nuclei with little atypia
- No mitoses
- No intermixed axons or axonal swellings

Special Stains and Immunohistochemistry

- GFAP positive, but may vary in intensity and extent
- TTF-1, galectin-3, vimentin and S-100 positive
- EMA, neurofilament, synaptophysin, and chromogranin negative
- Cytokeratin and pituitary hormones negative
- MIB-1 labeling: 0.5% to 2.0%

Other Techniques for Diagnosis

- Electron microscopic examination shows cytoplasmic intermediate filaments, but no desmosomes or basal lamina
- Cytogenetic analysis of one patient showed a loss of 1p, 14q, and 22q with overrepresentation of chromosome 5p

Differential Diagnosis

PITUITARY ADENOMA

- Morphologically composed of epithelial cells forming sheets, trabeculae, or ribbons
- Cytokeratin positive
- GFAP negative

GRANULAR CELL TUMOR OF THE NEUROHYPOPHYSIS (WHO GRADE I)

- Polygonal cells with abundant granular cytoplasm forming nodules or sheets
- S-100, CD68, α_1-antitrypsin, and α_1-antichymotrypsin positive
- Pituitary hormones, GFAP, cytokeratin, synaptophysin chromogranin negative

SPINDLE CELL ONCOCYTOMA OF THE ADENOHYPOPHYSIS (WHO GRADE I)

- Spindle and epithelioid cells
- TTF-1, EMA galectin-3, and S-100 positive
- Pituitary hormones, GFAP, cytokeratin, chromogranin, and synaptophysin negative

PILOCYTIC ASTROCYTOMA

- Characteristically has dense and loose architecture
- Presence of Rosenthal fibers and eosinophilic granular bodies

PEARLS

- *Pituicytomas are hypothesized to arise from neurohypophysial cells*
- *Indolent growth and no reports of malignant transformation, but recurrences are documented*
- *Gross total surgical removal is indicated; role of adjuvant therapy remains to be defined*

SELECTED REFERENCES

Brat DJ, Scheithauer BW, Staugaitis SM, et al: Pituicytoma: a distinctive low-grade glioma of the neurohypophysis. Am J Surg Pathol 24:362-368, 2000.

Figarella-Branger D, Dufour H, Fernandez C, et al: Pituicytomas, a misdiagnosed benign tumor of the neurohypophysis: report of three cases. Acta Neuropathol (Berlin) 104:313-319, 2002.

Ogiwara H, Dubner S, Shafizadeh S, et al: Spindle cell oncocytoma of the pituitary and pituicytoma: two tumors mimicking pituitary adenoma. Surg Neurol Int 2:116, 2011.

Secci F, Merciadri P, Criminelli Rossi D, et al: Pituicytomas: radiological findings, clinical behavior and surgical management. Acta Neurochir 154:649-657, 2012.

Ulm AJ, Yachnis AT, Brat DJ, et al: Pituicytoma: report of two cases and clues regarding histogenesis. Neurosurgery 54:753-758, 2004.

CRANIOPHARYNGIOMA (WHO GRADE I)

Clinical Features

- Represents approximately 3% of all intracranial tumors
- Usually suprasellar; may be found within the sella, both suprasellar and infrasellar (dumbbell shape) or in the third ventricle, or rarely in the pineal region
- Two peaks of incidence: children and older adults (fifth and sixth decades)
- Two histologic subtypes
  - Adamantinomatous variant usually presents in the first or second decade
  - Papillary variant typically occurs in adults (mean age, 45 years)
- Presenting symptoms are of three types
  - Visual abnormalities
  - Symptoms secondary to pituitary or hypothalamic dysfunction (typically short stature, diabetes insipidus, delayed sexual development, obesity, psychomotor retardation)
  - Symptoms secondary to increased intracranial pressure
- On MRI, adamantinomatous subtypes show cystic lesions frequently with calcifications; the solid areas are isointense and enhancing; papillary subtypes do not calcify

Gross Pathology

- Classically forms a variably sized, lobulated suprasellar mass that may distort the roof of the third ventricle and infiltrate adjacent brain; usually interdigitates with surrounding brain tissue
- Adamantinomatous type shows cysts filled with thick, dark-brown fluid (resembling motor oil) and small glistening cholesterol crystals, and calcification; poorly circumscribed and frequently infiltrates surrounding brain tissue
- Papillary type is entirely solid or has a small cystic component; more circumscribed than the adamantinomatous variant

Histopathology

- Two subtypes; mixture of both subtypes may be seen
  - Adamantinomatous variant
    - Lobules of basally palisading squamous epithelium underlying a stellate reticulum of loose cells topped by keratin formation (Figure 19-21)
    - Keratin pearls or wet keratin (nodules of plump eosinophilic, keratinized cells with ghost nuclei) are characteristic histologic features; often associated with calcification
    - Degeneration results in cystic cavities filled with fluid or acellular debris
    - These tumors typically show local invasion of the surrounding brain tissue
    - Adjacent brain tissue usually shows marked chronic inflammation, cholesterol clefts, foreign-body giant cells, and Rosenthal fiber–rich astrocytosis

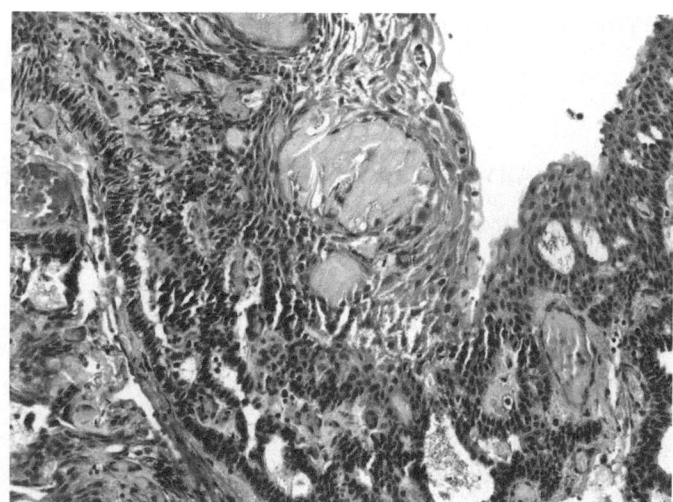

Figure 19-21. Craniopharyngioma. Section shows adamantinomatous squamous epithelium exhibiting keratinization and typical peripherally palisading nuclei.

- Papillary variant
  - Papillary architecture composed of well-differentiated epithelial cells with distinct fibrovascular cores
  - No microcyst formation, nuclear palisading, keratin pearls, wet keratin, calcification, or significant inflammatory component

Special Stains and Immunohistochemistry

- Cytokeratin highlights epithelial component
- β-catenin: nuclear and cytoplasmic positivity in adamantinomatous craniopharyngiomas (may be focal); membranous positivity in papillary craniopharyngiomas
- MIB-1 labeling index: no association between index and recurrence

Other Techniques for Diagnosis

- Electron microscopy: epithelial component shows well-formed desmosomes and bundles of tonofilaments
- Cytogenetics: mutations in *CTNNB1* gene (for β-catenin) are present in more than 70% (adamantinomatous type)

Differential Diagnosis

RCC

- Well-defined, thin-walled, fluid-filled cyst lined by a single layer of columnar and mucus-secreting cells
- Lacks papillary or solid architecture, keratin formation, and calcification
- β-catenin membranous positivity when squamous metaplasia is present

EPIDERMOID OR DERMOID CYSTS

- Both are cysts lined by keratinized squamous epithelium; dermoid cysts also contain skin appendages (hair follicles, sebaceous glands, sweat glands)
- Dermoid cysts are more likely to occur in the midline and epidermoid cysts in a lateral position (often in cerebellopontine angle or parasellar region)
- Neither contain wet keratin or exhibit basal palisading or stellate reticulum

PILOCYTIC ASTROCYTOMA

- Confusion with pilocytic astrocytoma may arise because of reactive astrocytosis and Rosenthal fibers surrounding the neoplasm
- Consists of pilocytic areas (elongated astrocytic cells with Rosenthal fibers) and a microcystic background
- Lacks cholesterol crystals and chronic inflammatory infiltrate
- Negative for cytokeratin, positive for GFAP

XANTHOGRANULOMA

- Composed of chronic inflammation, macrophages, and cholesterol clefts
- No significant component of epithelium

PEARLS

- *Histogenesis is debated; one hypothesis is that craniopharyngiomas occur from a developmental remnant of the Rathke cleft pouch; the other is that they arise from metaplastic squamous cells of the anterior pituitary gland*
- *Incomplete resection leads to recurrence even though most lesions are slow growing; postoperative radiotherapy may be given to tumors that are incompletely resected or recurrent, with improved patient survival*
- *One report stated that papillary craniopharyngiomas are smaller and behave more indolently than adamantinomatous types, which are more frequently recurrent*
- *Malignant change of an existing craniopharyngioma or de novo occurrence of a malignant craniopharyngioma is extremely rare, with only a few cases reported in the literature, two occurring in the setting of prior radiation therapy*

SELECTED REFERENCES

Crotty TB, Scheithauer BW, Young WF Jr, et al: Papillary craniopharyngioma: a clinicopathological study of 48 cases. J Neurosurg 83:206-214, 1995.

Edgar MA, Rosenblum MK: The differential diagnosis of central nervous system tumors. Arch Path Lab Med 132:500-509, 2008.

Larkin SJ, Ansorge O: Pathology and pathogenesis of craniopharyngiomas. Pituitary 16:9-17, 2013.

Rodriguez FJ, Scheithauer BW, Tsunoda S, et al: The spectrum of malignancy in craniopharyngioma. Am J Surg Pathol 31:1020-1028, 2007.

Tavangar SM, Larijani B, Mahta A, et al: Craniopharyngioma: a clinicopathological study of 141 cases. Endocr Pathol 15:339-344, 2004.

CHORDOMA

Clinical Features

- Rare tumors (1% of all intracranial tumors; 4% of primary bone tumors)
- Arise from notochord remnants, usually in or near the midline, anywhere from the sella turcica to the sacrum
- Approximately one third occur in the sacrum, one third in the spheno-occipital region or clivus, and one third in the vertebrae

- Occur in adults (peak in fourth decade) typically; rare in children
- Patients with sacral chordomas present with pain, anal sphincter dysfunction, or neurologic symptoms secondary to pressure on the adjacent nerve roots
- Intracranial tumors generally produce headache and cranial nerve palsies
- Radiographically, tumors are expansile, are destructive of bone, and extend into soft tissue; MRI scans show hypointense signal on T1-weighted images and high signal intensity on T2-weighted images and enhancement after contrast administration

Gross Pathology

- Locally invasive and destructive lesions that commonly destroy adjacent bone and entrap regional nerves
- Typically lobulated gelatinous or mucoid gray masses

Histopathology

- Divided into conventional, chondroid, or dedifferentiated subtypes
  - Conventional chordoma
    - Well-defined, lobular architecture separated by bands of fibrous tissue that may exhibit chronic inflammation
    - Lobules are composed of cords of epithelial-appearing cells and a mucoid background (Figure 19-22)
    - Cells have variably sized central nuclei and abundant, pale-pink to clear, vacuolated cytoplasm (physaliphorous cells)
    - Necrosis and recent or old hemorrhage may be present
    - Mitoses are infrequent
  - Chondroid chordoma
    - Variant of chordoma that contains cartilaginous areas resembling chondrosarcoma
    - Distinction is important because it usually has a better prognosis than either typical chordoma or high-grade chondrosarcoma

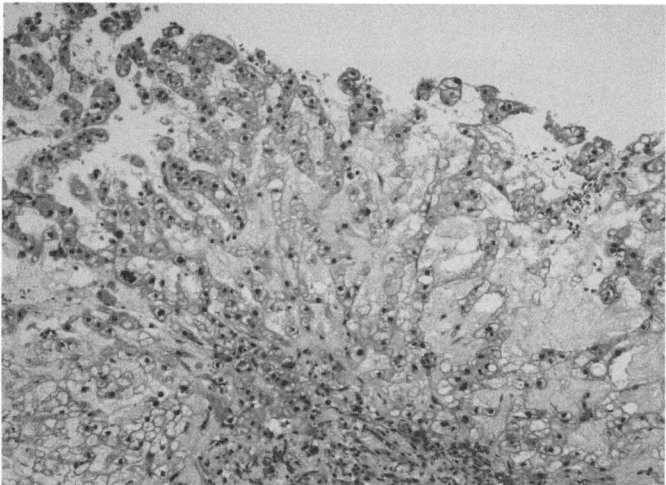

Figure 19-22. Chordoma. Classic trabecular pattern of the physaliferous cells in a mucoid background.

- Dedifferentiated chordoma
  - Rarely, chordomas show transformation into a malignant tumor with features of malignant fibrous histiocytoma, chondrosarcoma, or malignant undifferentiated spindle cell tumor or dedifferentiated chordoma

Special Stains and Immunohistochemistry

- PAS and PAS with diastase stains identify glycogen in cytoplasm (PAS positive; diastase sensitive)
- Mucin stain: stroma stains lightly
- Alcian blue: stroma strongly positive
- Mixed mesenchymal and epithelial immunophenotype of neoplastic cells
  - Vimentin positive
  - Cytokeratin (CK8, CK15, CK18, and CK19) positive
  - S-100 protein: most are positive
  - Brachyury (newly described protein found in notochord and notochord-derived tumors) positive

Other Techniques for Diagnosis

- Electron microscopy: distinct features of epithelial cells, including well-formed desmosomes and intracytoplasmic lumens; extracellular mucin is typically abundant
- Cytogenetic analyses have shown losses in chromosomes 1 and 3 and gains in chromosome 7; in familial chordoma, duplications in the 6q27 region (containing the brachyury gene) have been identified in tumor samples
- Discoveries of the expression of various receptors and signaling molecules (receptor tyrosine kinases PDGFR, EGFR, c-Met, and downstream effectors PI3K/ATK and mTOR) have prompted the use of therapy targeting several of these molecules

Differential Diagnosis

CHONDROSARCOMA

- Vacuolated (physaliphorous) cells are not found
- Negative for cytokeratin and EMA, positive for S-100

MYXOPAPILLARY EPENDYMOMA

- Almost exclusively found in the filum terminale
- Pseudopapillary architecture with elongated monomorphic cells
- Positive for GFAP

METASTATIC MUCINOUS ADENOCARCINOMA

- Cytologically more anaplastic appearing with pleomorphism, hyperchromatism
- Necrosis and mitoses
- Likely S-100 negative

CHORDOID MENINGIOMA

- Foci of whorls, intranuclear pseudoinclusions, and psammoma bodies
- Cytokeratin negative

CHORDOID GLIOMA

- Typically arise in third ventricular and suprasellar regions
- GFAP positive; most cells are negative for EMA and cytokeratin

PEARLS

- *Treatment typically involves an attempt at complete resection and postoperative radiotherapy*
- *Chordomas often recur and occasionally show distant metastases to lymph nodes, lung, or skin*
- *Chondroid chordomas occur more frequently in the skull base than the sacrum*
- *Dedifferentiated chordomas occur more frequently in the sacrum*
- *Factors associated with a worse prognosis include the following:*
  - *Female sex*
  - *Age more than 40 years at time of diagnosis*
  - *Presence of mitotic activity or necrosis*
  - *Large tumor volume*
  - *Incomplete resection*

SELECTED REFERENCES

Barry JJ, Jian BJ, Sughrue ME, et al: The next step: innovative molecular targeted therapies for treatment of intracranial chordoma patients. Neurosurgery 68:231-241, 2011.

Radner H, Katenkamp D, Reifenberger G, et al: New developments in the pathology of skull base tumors. Virchows Arch 438:321-335, 2001.

Walcott BP, Nahed BV, Mohyeldin A, et al: Chordoma: current concepts, management, and future directions. Lancet Oncol 13: e69-e76, 2012.

Vujovic S, Handerson S, Presneau N, et al: Brachyury, a crucial regulator of notochordal development, is a novel biomarker for chordomas. J Pathol 209:157-165, 2006.

SECONDARY TUMORS

Clinical Features

- Metastases typically occur through hematogenous route or by direct extension from skull or spinal column lesions
- Direct extension
  - Carcinomas metastatic to bone (commonly breast, prostate, or lung) may expand and compress brain or spinal cord
  - May also metastasize directly to dura
  - Head and neck neoplasms may extend discontinuously along nerves, appearing metastatic
- Hematogenous route
  - Up to 10% of carcinomas metastatic to CNS are not recognized before presentation of CNS metastasis
  - Metastatic tumors are the most common neoplasms of the CNS
  - About 30% of intracranial brain tumors in adults are due to metastatic carcinoma
  - Common primary sites of malignancy that may metastasize to the brain in adults include, in decreasing order of frequency, lung carcinoma (especially small cell and adenocarcinoma), breast carcinoma, melanoma, renal cell carcinoma, and colon carcinoma
  - Metastases are usually multiple and radiographically show distinct, contrast-enhancing masses with a surrounding zone of cerebral edema
  - Patients often present with headaches, focal neurologic deficits, or altered mental status

- Carcinomatous meningitis
  - Metastases involving the meninges, predominantly the subarachnoid space, without an intraparenchymal mass lesion
  - More commonly occurs with adenocarcinoma of the lung, breast, or stomach
  - Headache, stroke, encephalopathy, and cranial nerve deficit are typical presenting symptoms
  - Cytologic examination of the CSF is positive in about 60% of cases

Gross Pathology

- Typically gray-white to tan and well-circumscribed masses with a pushing rather than an infiltrative margin
- Hemorrhage and necrosis are common, especially in melanoma, choriocarcinoma, and renal cell carcinoma
- Brown-black pigmentation is common in metastatic melanoma

Histopathology (Figure 19-23)

- Histologic features similar to those of the primary tumors
- Discrete lesions usually displacing rather than infiltrating the adjacent brain tissue; small cell carcinoma often shows limited infiltrative borders
- Neoplastic cells often have prominent perivascular distribution with more viable tumor located around blood vessels
- Necrosis is typically extensive
- Vascular proliferation is not a characteristic feature
- Meningeal carcinomatosis shows tumor cells freely floating within the subarachnoid space with extension along Virchow-Robin spaces and into superficial brain parenchyma

Special Stains and Immunohistochemistry

- Cytokeratins, EMA: carcinomas
- S-100 protein, HMB-45, Melan-A: malignant melanoma
- LCA (CD45), T and B cell and lymphocyte subset markers: lymphoma
- Vimentin, actin, desmin, myoD1, myogenin, CD34: sarcoma

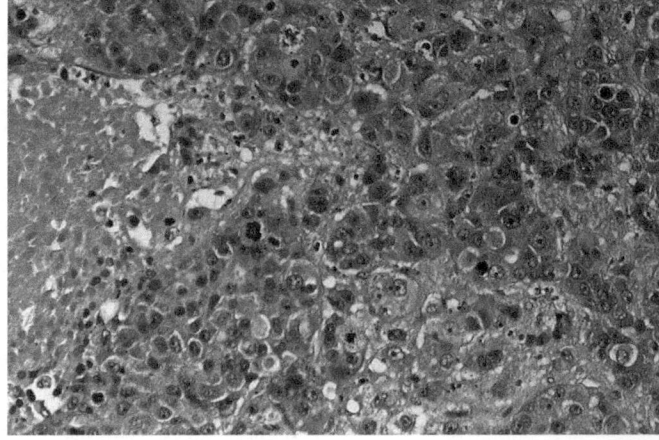

Figure 19-23. Metastatic ductal carcinoma from the breast. Solid proliferation of malignant epithelial cells with focal necrosis.

- Antibodies with high site specificity: PSA and PAP (prostate), TTF-1/napsin (lung adenocarcinoma), thyroglobulin (follicular and papillary thyroid carcinomas), calcitonin (medullary thyroid carcinomas), HepPar1 (hepatocellular carcinoma), CDX-2 (gastrointestinal tract adenocarcinomas), GCDFP-15 and mammaglobin (breast carcinoma), renal cell carcinoma (RCC)
- GFAP negative in most metastatic neoplasms

Other Techniques for Diagnosis

- Electron microscopy: features similar to those of the primary neoplasm
- Cytogenetics: same genetic abnormalities as found in primary neoplasm

Differential Diagnosis

GLIAL NEOPLASMS WITH EPITHELIOID, SARCOMATOUS, OR SMALL-CELL DIFFERENTIATION
- Infiltrative tumors with areas morphologically typical for glioma
- Positive for GFAP
- May be positive for cytokeratin AE1/AE3, but usually not other cytokeratins
- EMA positivity reported in some gliomas
- TTF-1 is negative in most primary brain tumors, but has been described in a few third ventricular neoplasms

PRIMITIVE NEUROECTODERMAL NEOPLASMS INCLUDING MEDULLOBLASTOMAS
- Cytokeratin negative
- CD99 and EWS/FLI-1 negative
- Uncommon in adults

ANAPLASTIC MENINGIOMA
- Cytokeratin usually negative
- EMA positive
- Usually focal areas morphologically suggestive of meningioma

CHOROID PLEXUS CARCINOMA (VERSUS METASTATIC PAPILLARY ADENOCARCINOMA)
- Choroid plexus carcinomas are rare in adults
- S-100 variably positive
- GFAP positive in 20%

PEARLS

- *Features reliably used to distinguish metastatic carcinomas from primary CNS tumors on frozen section include cell cohesion, tumor circumscription, and prominent fibrous septa around groups of tumor cells; smear preparations are usually better for evaluating cytologic characteristics*
- *Use of a panel of immunohistochemical markers including antibodies expected to be positive and negative is recommended for accurate determination of neoplasm origin*

SELECTED REFERENCES

Giordana MT, Cordera S, Boghi A: Cerebral metastases as first symptom of cancer: a clinico-pathologic study. J Neurooncol 50:265-273, 2000.

Krishna M: Diagnosis of metastatic neoplasms: an immunohistochemical approach. Arch Pathol Lab Med 134:207-215, 2010.
Marchevsky AM, Gupta R, Balzer B: Diagnosis of metastatic neoplasms: a clinicopathologic and morphologic approach. Arch Pathol Lab Med 134:194-206, 2010.
Oien K: Pathologic evaluation of unknown primary cancer. Semin Oncol 36:8-37, 2009.

NON-NEOPLASTIC CONDITIONS

VASCULAR MALFORMATIONS

Clinical Features

ARTERIOVENOUS MALFORMATION (AVM)
- Commonly found in adults; occasionally seen in children
- Presentation is usually before 40 years of age
- Two thirds are discovered when the patient presents with signs or symptoms of intracerebral hemorrhage; most of the remaining are discovered during evaluation for headache, seizures, or focal neurologic deficits; few are discovered incidentally

CAVERNOUS HEMANGIOMA
- Patients may present with seizures or focal neurologic deficits
- Average age of onset is 30 years
- Hemorrhages are common but are usually small and do not cause significant mass effect
- About 20% are incidental findings at autopsy
- Most are found in the cerebrum; other common locations include the brain stem, cerebellum, spinal cord, and leptomeninges

CAPILLARY TELANGIECTASIA
- Usually found in the brain stem (basis pontis) or spinal cord
- Typically an incidental postmortem finding and of little clinical significance

VENOUS HEMANGIOMA
- Typically found in the subarachnoid space of the spinal cord (usually lower thoracic); may be seen within the brain
- Rarely symptomatic; typically an incidental postmortem finding
- Angiography shows veins with a caput medusa appearance

Gross Pathology

AVM
- Variable size with large lesions causing displacement of the adjacent brain tissue
- Typically arises in the vicinity of the middle cerebral artery
- Consists of a mass of tangled and tortuous vessels with intervening and surrounding brain parenchyma
- Often has thrombosed or dilated vessels
- Necrosis of the brain parenchyma and of old and recent hemorrhage is common

CAVERNOUS HEMANGIOMA
- Most commonly found in the subcortical white matter or brain stem

- Well-defined mass composed of compact tangles of vessels
- Typically measures less than 3 cm in diameter
- Thrombosis is commonly found
- Evidence of prior bleeding in the form of a peripheral rim of hemosiderin is present in virtually all lesions

CAPILLARY TELANGIECTASIA
- Usually small with a diameter of less than 2 cm
- Poorly defined lesions typically causing an ill-defined stippling or discoloration of the brain parenchyma

VENOUS HEMANGIOMA
- Composed of a network of thin-walled, dilated, blood-filled veins

Histopathology

AVM
- Composed of variably sized arteries and veins without intervening capillaries (Figure 19-24A)
- Vessel walls show varying degrees of fibrosis, thinning, and dilation
- Necrosis and hemosiderin-laden macrophages are often seen in brain tissue if thrombosed vessels are present

CAVERNOUS HEMANGIOMA
- Compact network of vessels without smooth muscle or elastic lamella
- Vessels are tightly packed with no brain parenchyma between the vascular network (Figure 19-24B)
- Hemosiderin and reactive gliosis seen in the surrounding brain parenchyma
- Calcification is common

CAPILLARY TELANGIECTASIA
- Composed of thin-walled, delicate, dilated vessels without smooth muscle (Figure 19-24C)
- Hemorrhage is rare
- Intervening and adjacent brain parenchyma is unremarkable without gliosis or hemosiderin

VENOUS HEMANGIOMA
- Consists of a small collection of delicate veins formed of endothelium and collagen without smooth muscle
- Veins lie within brain parenchyma that only rarely shows gliosis or hemorrhage

Special Stains and Immunohistochemistry
- Elastic highlights elastic lamella of the arteries seen in AVMs
- Trichrome highlights collagen and smooth muscle of vessel walls

Other Techniques for Diagnosis
- Cytogenetic analysis:
  - Hereditary hemorrhagic telangiectasia is associated with brain, lung, and liver AVMs and skin telangiectasias; mutations in three genes have been described (endoglin, *ACVRL1*, and *SMAD4*)
  - Familial forms of cavernous angiomas have been associated with mutations in three genes (*KRIT1*, *CCM2*, and *PDCD10*)

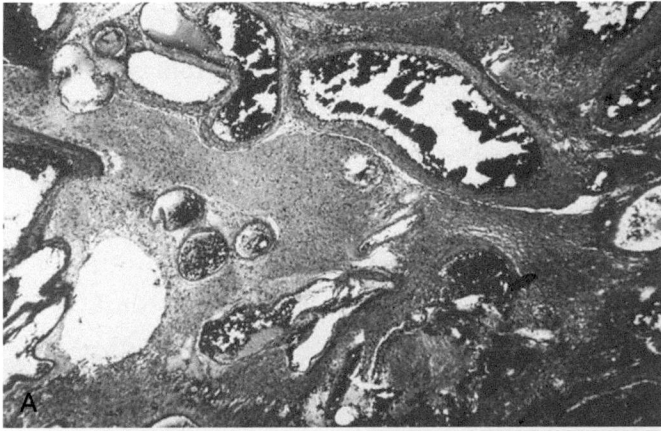
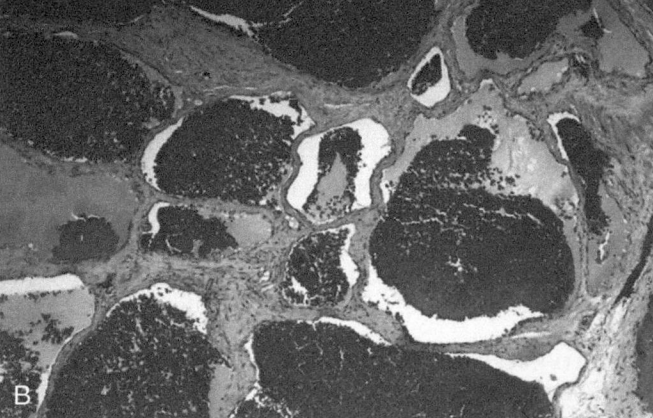
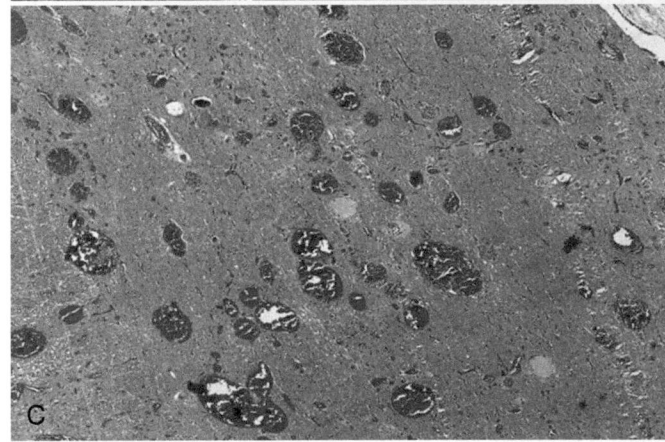

Figure 19-24. A, Arteriovenous malformation. Numerous intraparenchymal arteries and veins. **B,** Cavernous hemangioma. Numerous dilated thin-walled blood vessels without intervening brain parenchyma. **C,** Capillary telangiectasia. Numerous capillaries are scattered in the basis pontis.

Differential Diagnosis
- Discussed earlier under "Histopathology"
- Difficult to distinguish venous angioma from capillary telangiectasia

PEARLS

- *AVMs are the most dangerous because of their size and likelihood to rupture*
- *First hemorrhage from AVMs carries 10% to 15% mortality rate*

- *Surgical removal, stereotactic radiotherapy, and embolization are common methods of treatment for AVMs*
- *Increased occurrence of aneurysms in patients with AVMs*
- *AVMs with prior hemorrhage, deep location, deep venous drainage, and associated aneurysms have a greater risk of hemorrhage than AVMs without these characteristics*

SELECTED REFERENCES

Arteriovenous Malformation Study Group: Arteriovenous malformations of the brain in adults. N Engl J Med 340:1812-1818, 1999.

Challa VR, Moody DM, Brown WR: Vascular malformations of the central nervous system. J Neuropathol Exper Neurol 54:609-621, 1995.

Gross BA, Du R: Natural history of cerebral arteriovenous malformations: a meta-analysis. J Neurosurg 118:437-443, 2013.

Labauge P, Denier C, Bergametti F, Tournier-Lasserve E: Genetics of cavernous angiomas. Lancet Neurol 6:237-244, 2007.

Whitehead KJ, Smith MCP, Li DY: Arteriovenous malformations and other vascular malformation syndromes. Cold Spring Harb Perspect Med 3:a006635, 2012.

CEREBRAL INFARCTION AND INTRACEREBRAL HEMATOMAS

Clinical Features

ISCHEMIC CEREBRAL INFARCTIONS

- Patients typically present with sudden onset of neurologic impairment
- Neurologic deficits vary depending on location and size of infarction
- Atherosclerosis, cardiac emboli (mural thrombi or valvular heart disease and hypertension-associated hyaline arteriolar sclerosis) are the most common causes; multiple infarcts are often related to emboli and lacunar infarcts (≤1.5 cm) most often occur in deep gray, deep white matter, cerebellum, and pons.
- May radiographically mimic malignant glioma
- Multiple ischemic infarcts may cause dementia (multi-infarct dementia; see "Dementia" for further discussion)

VENOUS CEREBRAL INFARCTS

- Result from thrombosis of the dural sinuses and cerebral veins; classified as primary or secondary; most often hemorrhagic
- Primary (aseptic) infarcts are associated with hypercoagulable states, including dehydration, pregnancy, oral contraceptive use, and hemolytic anemias
- Secondary (septic) infarcts are associated with bacterial infections of the face or sinuses, subdural abscesses, and meningitis

INTRACEREBRAL HEMATOMAS

- Associated with hypertension, aneurysms (hematomas occur secondary to blood under high pressure from ruptured or leaking aneurysm), vascular malformations (see the previous section), amyloid angiopathy, and neoplasms (most commonly metastatic, occasionally primary)
- Bleeding typically causes significant mass effect with compression of adjacent structures
- Hypertension-associated hemorrhages most commonly develop in deep gray matter, cerebellum, or pons

- Amyloid-associated hemorrhages are typically lobar (frontal, temporal, parietal, or occipital), occur in elderly individuals, and occur secondary to weakening of the arterial walls owing to deposition of Aβ amyloid

Gross Pathology

ISCHEMIC INFARCTS

- Grossly recognizable 2 to 4 days after stroke
- Acute lesions are discolored, soft, and swollen; confined to the distribution of a single blood vessel
- Subacute infarcts contain soft, friable necrotic brain tissue
- Old infarcts show cavitation

VENOUS INFARCTS

- More commonly involve white matter and are often hemorrhagic
- Bilateral parasagittal hemorrhagic infarcts are associated with superior sagittal sinus occlusion

INTRACEREBRAL HEMATOMAS

- Well-defined lesion consisting of fresh or organizing blood
- With organization, a fibrous capsule is formed around the hematoma
- In older lesions, adjacent brain tissue is yellow-brown (accumulation of hemosiderin-laden macrophages)

Histopathology

ISCHEMIC INFARCTS DUE TO ARTERIAL COMPROMISE

- Show varying features, depending on the age of the infarct (Figure 19-25)
  - *In 6 to 24 hours:* eosinophilic neurons become visible
  - *In 12 to 24 hours:* polymorphonuclear leukocyte infiltrate (peaks at about 24 hours and gone by 7 days) and cerebral edema (peaks at 3 to 4 days)
  - *Days 2 to 3:* infiltration of lipid-laden macrophages and vascular proliferation
  - *Day 7:* beginning of cavitation is evident; proliferation of surrounding astrocytes
  - *Days 14 to 30:* sheets of lipid-laden macrophages; clustering of macrophages around blood vessels is common
  - *More than 3 months:* cystic space surrounded by numerous fibrillary astrocytes
- General rule is that a 1-cm infarct takes 3 months to become cystic
- Exact timing of microscopic changes varies from brain to brain and is dependent on infarct size

VENOUS INFARCTS

- Similar histologic features as described previously, but typically more hemorrhagic

INTRACEREBRAL HEMATOMAS

- Consist of organizing hemorrhage with numerous hemosiderin-laden macrophages
- Proliferation of fibroblasts at periphery forms capsule
- Reactive astrocytosis is evident in surrounding brain
- Underlying cause of hematoma should be looked for: vascular malformation, neoplasm, hyaline arteriolosclerosis in hypertension, and acellular thickening of the small and medium-sized arteries in amyloid angiopathy (Figure 19-26A)

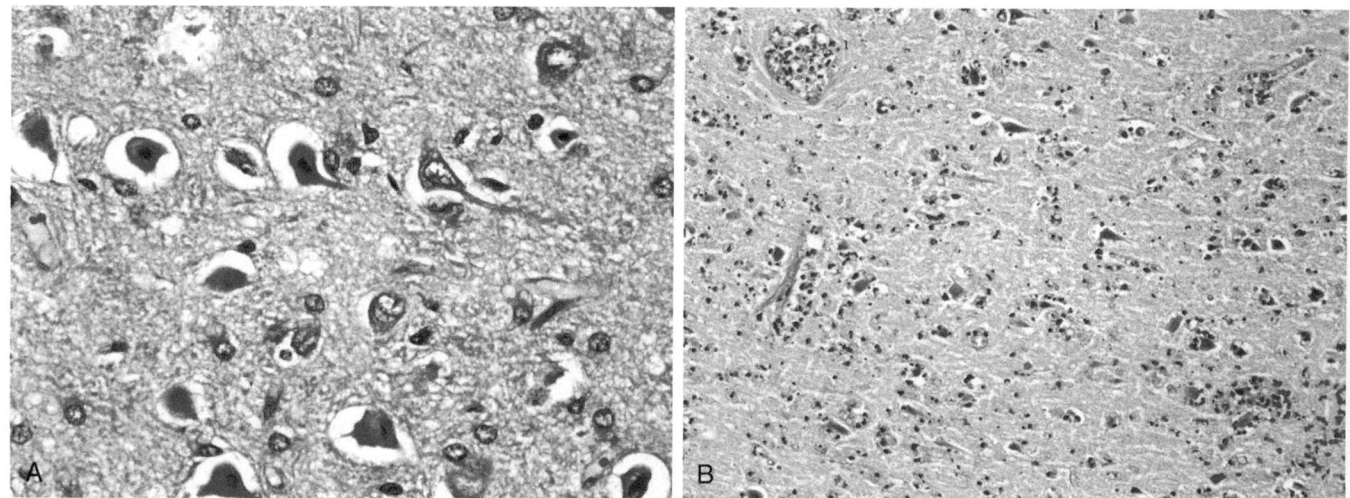

Figure 19-25. Acute cerebral infarct. A, Several acutely hypoxic neurons are present. Note the brightly eosinophilic cytoplasm and the pyknotic nucleus. **B,** Acutely infarcted brain tissue showing red neurons, necrosis, and acute inflammation.

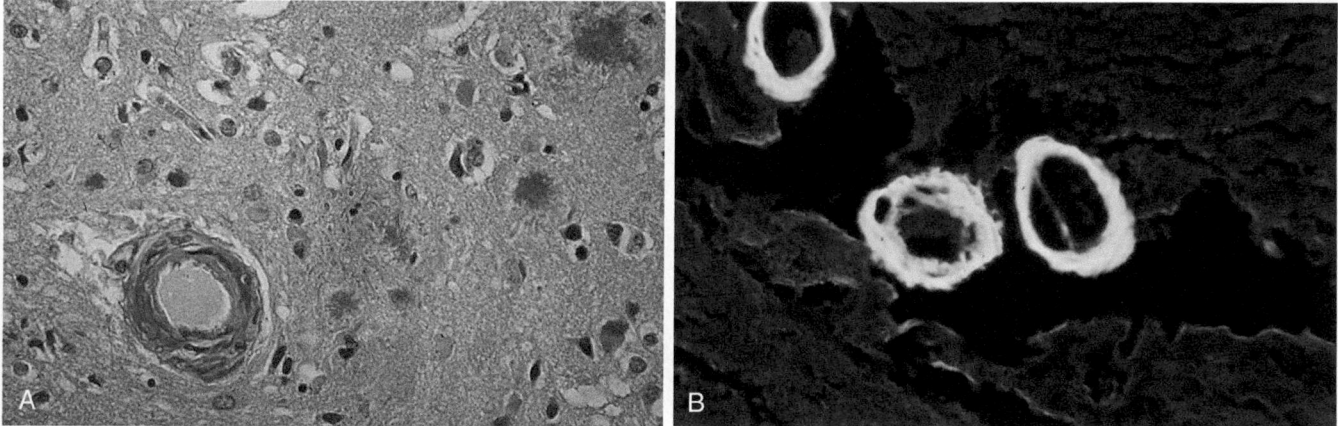

Figure 19-26. Amyloid angiopathy. A, Intraparenchymal arteriole containing amorphous eosinophilic material in the media. **B,** Thioflavin S-stained arterioles viewed under ultraviolet light are positive for amyloid deposition.

Special Stains and Immunohistochemistry

- CD68, (PGM1-more specific or KP-1) highlight macrophages
- PAS: myelin debris within macrophages is positive
- GFAP: reactive astrocytes are positive
- Congo red identifies vascular amyloid deposition; shows apple-green birefringence in polarized light
- Thioflavin-S identifies vascular amyloid and is fluorescent under ultraviolet light (Figure 19-26B)
- Aβ amyloid immunohistochemistry: positive in vessels in amyloid angiopathy

Other Techniques for Diagnosis

- Electron microscopy: vessels containing Aβ amyloid show bundles of 10-nm filaments in the adventitia at the media-adventitia interface

Differential Diagnosis

GLIOMA (OLIGODENDROGLIOMA OR ASTROCYTOMA)
- Distinction from reactive process is difficult in small biopsies
- Typically lacks macrophages (macrophage markers are negative)

GBM
- Foamy macrophages and necrosis may be seen
- Shows marked cytologic atypia, which is absent in areas of infarction
- Mitoses present; elevated MIB-1 staining

DEMYELINATING DISEASES
- Usually occur in younger individuals
- Multiple sclerosis (MS) has lesions disseminated in time and space with numerous small plaques without respect for vascular territory
- Axons are relatively preserved (neurofilament positive) in areas of demyelination and are destroyed in areas of infarction
- Presence of T lymphocytes in perivascular distribution

ENCEPHALITIS
- Areas of necrosis typically seen
- Abundant acute and chronic inflammatory cells
- Organisms (bacteria, viral inclusions, parasites) may be seen

PEARLS

- *Uncommonly, cerebral infarctions may radiographically mimic a neoplasm, prompting biopsy to rule out a neoplasm*
- *Lymphocytes are typically scant or absent in infarcts; if present within lesion or around blood vessels, consider vasculitis (primary or secondary)*

SELECTED REFERENCES

Garcia JH, Menan H: Vascular diseases. In Garcia JH, Budka H, McKeever PE, Sarnat HB (eds): Neuropathology: The Diagnostic Approach. St. Louis, Mosby, 1997, pp 263-320.

Vinters HV: Cerebrovascular disease—practical issues in surgical and autopsy pathology. Curr Top Pathol 95:51-99, 2001.

VASCULITIS

Clinical Features

- Involvement of the CNS by vasculitis may be divided into primary or secondary; secondary vasculitis may occur in systemic vasculitis, often in association with collagen vascular diseases or in infectious processes

INFECTIOUS VASCULITIS

- Associated with tuberculous meningitis and syphilitic meningoencephalitis
- Associated with cerebritis due to aspergillosis and mucormycosis infections
- Viral infections of the brain causing vasculitis include varicella-zoster virus (VZV), cytomegalovirus (CMV), herpes simplex virus (HSV), and HIV

VASCULITIS IN ASSOCIATION WITH COLLAGEN VASCULAR DISEASES AND OTHER NONINFECTIOUS CAUSES

- Brain involvement is uncommon in patients with systemic vasculitides
- Occurs in polyarteritis nodosa and Wegener granulomatosis and less commonly in Takayasu arteritis, Behçet disease, Kawasaki disease, and Sjögren syndrome
- Systemic lupus erythematosus (SLE) is more likely to cause vasculopathy and is rarely associated with cerebral vasculitis; similar morphologic findings to malignant hypertension
- CNS vasculitis may be associated with radiation damage and illicit drugs (e.g., amphetamines, cocaine)
- Vasculitis also uncommonly occurs in association with deposition of Aβ protein (amyloid angiopathy) in the cerebral cortical and leptomeningeal vessels

PRIMARY (OR ISOLATED) VASCULITIS OF THE CNS, ALSO KNOWN AS *GRANULOMATOUS VASCULITIS*, OCCURS WITHOUT SYSTEMIC INVOLVEMENT

- Occurs in fourth to sixth decades (mean age of onset is 50 years)
- Affects leptomeningeal, cortical, and subcortical small and medium-sized arteries and less frequently veins and venules
- Radiologic evaluation includes cerebral angiogram; it has been found to have low sensitivity and specificity

- MRI is usually abnormal but nonspecific; it may show lesions indicative of ischemia and inflammation involving the meninges, cortex, and white matter, bilaterally
- Headaches and encephalopathy are the most common presenting symptoms, focal or multifocal neurologic deficits and stroke are less common
- Cerebrospinal fluid is usually abnormal due to elevation of protein and slight elevation in white blood cell count; signs of systemic inflammation are often absent
- Definitive diagnosis is made by positive brain biopsy

Gross Pathology

- Uncomplicated vasculitis may not be recognized grossly
- Complications include brain infarction and hemorrhage

Histopathology

PRIMARY VASCULITIS

- Segmental acute or chronic inflammation of small arteries and arterioles with intimal proliferation and fibrosis in association with fibrinoid necrosis of the vessel wall (Figure 19-27)
- Granulomatosis response (multinucleated giant cells) may be present (< 50%)
- Thrombosis of the affected vessels may be evident
- Brain adjacent to affected vessels may show ischemia, infarction, or hemorrhage

SECONDARY VASCULITIS

- In infection-associated processes, viral inclusions or fungal organisms occasionally seen in the parenchyma or vessel walls, respectively
- Special stains (discussed later) may help identify microorganisms
- Occasionally, affected vessels show aneurysmal dilation due to septic emboli (mycotic aneurysms); usually due to fungal and bacterial infections

Special Stains and Immunohistochemistry

- Special stains for organisms: PAS, Gomori methenamine silver (GMS), and acid-fact bacilli (AFB)
- Elastic and Movat stains highlight elastic lamina

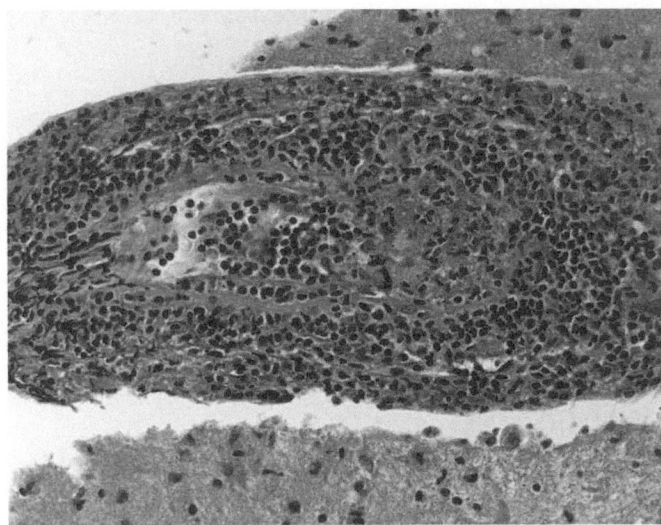

Figure 19-27. Vasculitis. Section of a medium-sized blood vessel showing fibrinoid necrosis of the wall and chronic inflammation.

Other Techniques for Diagnosis

- In situ hybridization: DNA or RNA radioactive probes may be useful in identifying viral agents

Differential Diagnosis

PRIMARY CNS LYMPHOMA

- Perivascular lymphoid cells have atypical morphology and are mostly of B-cell origin

MS AND ACUTE DEMYELINATING ENCEPHALOMYELITIS (ADEM)

- Inflammatory infiltrate is typically perivascular and is not associated with wall destruction
- Both MS and ADEM are characterized by areas of demyelinated (not usually necrotic) brain parenchyma

VIRAL ENCEPHALITIS

- Perivascular and parenchymal lymphocytic inflammation without vessel wall destruction
- Microglial nodules are characteristic

SARCOIDOSIS

- Characterized by perivascular and parenchymal granulomas without necrosis; no destruction of the vessel walls
- Predilection for hypothalamic and suprasellar regions

NONVASCULITIC AUTOIMMUNE INFLAMMATORY MENINGOENCEPHALITIS (NAIM)

- Clinical presentation with acute or subacute encephalopathy that may or may not be associated with systemic autoimmune illness
- Clinical manifestations are variable but usually include cognitive impairment and behavioral changes
- Typically steroid responsive
- Pathologic studies are few; perivascular lymphocytic infiltrates and microglial cell proliferation without vasculitis and variable parenchymal involvement has been described

PEARLS

- *Primary CNS vasculitis is typically focal and segmental; a negative biopsy does not exclude the diagnosis*

SELECTED REFERENCES

Birnbaum J, Hellmann DB: Primary angiitis of the central nervous system. Arch Neurol 66:704-709, 2009.

Josephs KA, Rubino FA, Dickson DW: Nonvasculitic autoimmune inflammatory meningoencephalitis. Neuropathology 24:149-152, 2004.

Lyons MK, Castelli RJ, Parisi JE: Nonvasculitic autoimmunory meningoencephalitis as a cause of potentially reversible dementia: report of 4 cases. J Neurosurg 108:1024-1027, 2008.

Miller DV, Salvarani C, Hunder GG, et al: Biopsy findings in primary angiitis of the central nervous system. Am J Surg Pathol 33:35-43, 2009.

Parisi JE, Moore PM: The role of biopsy in vasculitis of the central nervous system. Semin Neurol 14:341-349, 1994.

BRAIN ABSCESS

Clinical Features

- Most occur during the third and fourth decades; males are affected more than females
- May be due to local extension from an extracerebral infection, including ear, sinus, or dental infections; hematogenous spread from a systemic infection is less common; penetrating head trauma may also cause brain abscess
- Immunosuppressed individuals (AIDS patients, transplant recipients, cancer patients) are at greater risk
- Occasionally brain abscess may be a complication of neurosurgery
- Features of local or systemic infections are often absent
- Presenting signs and symptoms are often nonspecific but may include headache, fever, and altered level of consciousness
- Various organisms, including bacteria, fungi, mycobacteria, and parasites (cysticercosis and toxoplasmosis), are the causative agents; bacteria are the most frequently isolated organisms (*Streptococci, Staphylococci, Fusobacterium,* and *Bacteroides* species are most common) in patients with intact immune systems
- Gram-negative rods, *Aspergillus, Candida,* and *Mucor* species occur in the neutropenic patient; T-cell dysfunction is associated with *Toxoplasma, Listeria, Nocardia, Cryptococcus,* and *Mycobacteria* species
- Typically found in the white matter or at the gray-white junction; usually seen in the frontal, temporal, or parietal lobes
- CT shows a cystic mass with ring enhancement and surrounding edema; MRI gives better resolution

Gross Pathology

- Well-defined area of central necrosis surrounded by hyperemic and edematous brain tissue
- Older lesions show a distinct organized fibrous capsule surrounding the necrotic tissue
- *Aspergillus* infection especially associated with hemorrhagic necrosis

Histopathology

- Characteristically shows three distinct zones
  - Central area of necrosis with abundant acute inflammatory cells
  - Zone of acute or chronically inflamed granulation tissue, consisting of fibroblastic and vascular proliferation (Figure 19-28)
  - Peripheral area of edematous brain tissue with a reactive gliosis and a fibrous capsule in later stages
- Organisms may be identified within or adjacent to the necrotic tissue
- Caseating granulomas are characteristic of tuberculosis
- Multinucleated giant cells are usually seen in fungal or tuberculous infection
- May identify parasite (most commonly cysticercosis and toxoplasmosis)
- Gummas in syphilis are rare tumor-like, nonsuppurative lesions

Special Stains and Immunohistochemistry

- Special stains: Gram, PAS, GMS, AFB, Fite, and Warthin-Starry may identify microorganisms

Other Techniques for Diagnosis

- Culture of the necrotic tissue may yield positive results
- Polymerase chain reaction (PCR) may identify mycobacteria (tuberculosis) and selected other bacteria

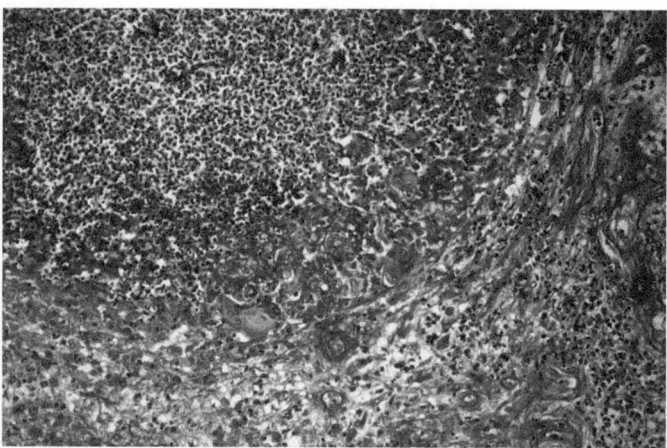

Figure 19-28. Brain abscess. Section shows a central area of purulent material, surrounded by vascular and fibroblast proliferation and numerous chronic inflammatory cells (periodic acid-Schiff stain).

- Immunohistochemistry: available for identification of toxoplasmosis

Differential Diagnosis

GBM AND METASTASIS

- On imaging studies, high-grade astrocytoma, brain metastasis, and brain abscess may have similar characteristics
- Histologic examination shows high cellularity, neoplastic cells and associated mitoses, necrosis, and endothelial proliferation (in GBM)

PEARLS

- *Mortality rates are variable depending on the etiologic agent; overall mortality rates have dropped dramatically owing to better diagnostic and treatment modalities*
- *Tissue for culture should be taken in operating room rather than in pathology laboratory*
- *Aspergillus species brain infection has been reported in patients with asthma and chronic steroid use as their only risk factor*

SELECTED REFERENCES

Calfee DP, Wispelwey B: Brain abscess. Semin Neurol 20:353-360, 2000.
Kleinschmidt-DeMasters BK: Central nervous system aspergillosis: a 20-year retrospective series. Hum Pathol 33:116-124, 2002.
Muzumdar D, Jhawar S, Goel A: Brain abscess: an overview. Int J Surg 9:136-144, 2011.
Pendlebury WW, Perl DP, Munoz DG: Multiple microabscesses in the central nervous system: a clinicopathologic study. J Neuropathol Exper Neurol 48:290-300, 1989.

ENCEPHALITIS AND MENINGOENCEPHALITIS

Clinical Features

- Infection of the cerebral parenchyma characterized by altered level of consciousness, seizures, and focal neurologic deficits
- Infection of both the meninges and parenchyma often occurs (meningoencephalitis)

COMMON CAUSATIVE AGENTS: VIRAL

- Viral encephalitis: togaviruses (Eastern equine encephalitis), flaviviruses (St. Louis encephalitis), enteroviruses, and herpesvirus are the most common causative agents

- Herpesvirus infections of the nervous system include herpes simplex virus types 1 and 2 (HSV-1, HSV-2), EBV, CMV, VZV, and human herpesvirus type 6 (HHV-6)
  - HSV-1
    - Causes frontotemporal lobe encephalitis (usually asymmetrical) occurring in immunocompetent older children and adults
    - Most common sporadic encephalitis without seasonal occurrence
  - HSV-2
    - Usually causes aseptic meningitis in adults (women are affected more than men) and neonates; less commonly a cause of encephalomyelitis in adult immunocompetent or immunocompromised hosts
  - CMV
    - Encephalitis occurs most often in AIDS patients; congenital CMV infection also occurs (meningitis and encephalitis)
  - EBV
    - Variable CNS involvement: meningitis, encephalitis, cranial nerve involvement, cerebellitis, and neuromuscular involvement; usually severe neurologic impairment does not occur
  - HHV-6
    - Meningoencephalitis occurs in immunosuppressed patients
- West Nile virus encephalitis
  - Currently the most common cause of epidemic viral encephalitis in the United States
- HIV infection
  - Brain impairment secondary to HIV virus usually occurs in late-stage AIDS patients

COMMON CAUSATIVE AGENTS: BACTERIAL

- Tuberculous meningitis
- Spirochete infections include both syphilis (*Treponema pallidum*) and Lyme disease (*Borrelia burgdorferi*)
- Whipple disease caused by *Tropheryma whippelii*
  - Systemic disease; often intestinal dysfunction with weight loss, lymphadenopathy, and arthralgias

COMMON CAUSATIVE AGENTS: PARASITIC

- Parasite infections are numerous and include trichinosis, strongyloidiasis, cysticercosis, echinococcosis, toxoplasmosis, schistosomiasis, and amebiasis (*Entamoeba histolytica* and *Naegleria, Acanthamoeba* species)
  - Cysticercosis is the most common parasite worldwide
    - Patients present with seizures
    - Parasite may localize in the subarachnoid space, parenchyma, or ventricles
  - Toxoplasmosis and most fungal infections are seen in immunocompromised hosts (e.g., patients with AIDS)

COMMON CAUSATIVE AGENTS: FUNGAL

- Common fungal infections include candidiasis, histoplasmosis, blastomycosis, cryptococcosis, aspergillosis, mucormycosis, and coccidioidomycosis

Gross Pathology

ENCEPHALITIS

- Brain may appear normal or be edematous
- Herpes simplex type 1 infection most commonly affects the temporal lobes, orbital and insular cortexes, and cingulate gyri causing hemorrhagic necrosis

- AIDS dementia complex: generalized cortical atrophy; gray discoloration of white matter

MENINGOENCEPHALITIS
- If meninges are involved, exudate may be present in subarachnoid space

Histopathology (Figure 19-29)

VIRAL ENCEPHALITIS
- Predominantly lymphocytic infiltrate involving the leptomeninges with extension into the underlying brain parenchyma
- Infiltrate is primarily located in a perivascular distribution
- Microglial nodules are characteristic histologic findings

HERPESVIRUS ENCEPHALITIS
- Extensive hemorrhage and tissue destruction
- Cowdry type A inclusions (nuclear inclusions consisting of an eosinophilic body surrounded by a clear halo)
- Inclusions may be found in neurons, astrocytes, or oligodendrocytes

CYTOMEGALOVIRUS
- Cowdry type A inclusions (may be nuclear or cytoplasmic) most commonly involving ependymal cells, neurons, or glial cells

RABIES ENCEPHALITIS
- Negri bodies (large intracytoplasmic eosinophilic inclusions typically involving neurons of the Purkinje cells, and pyramidal cells of the hippocampus)

HIV ENCEPHALITIS AND LEUKOENCEPHALOPATHY
- Diffuse microglial activation and microglial nodules containing multinucleated giant cells
- Diffuse astrocytosis and perivascular chronic inflammation
- Diffuse pallor of white matter

TUBERCULOUS MENINGITIS AND TUBERCULOMA
- Caseating granulomas with a lymphoplasmacytic inflammation
- Parenchymal involvement consists of granulomatous inflammation with central necrosis
- Endarteritis obliterans may cause ischemic infarction
- Meningeal involvement is particularly severe on base of brain

NEUROSYPHILIS: MENINGOVASCULAR AND PARENCHYMAL FORMS
- Meningovascular
  - Meninges show a lymphoplasmacytic infiltrate predominantly around blood vessels; may progress to a vasculitis with intimal proliferation and luminal narrowing, resulting in ischemic changes

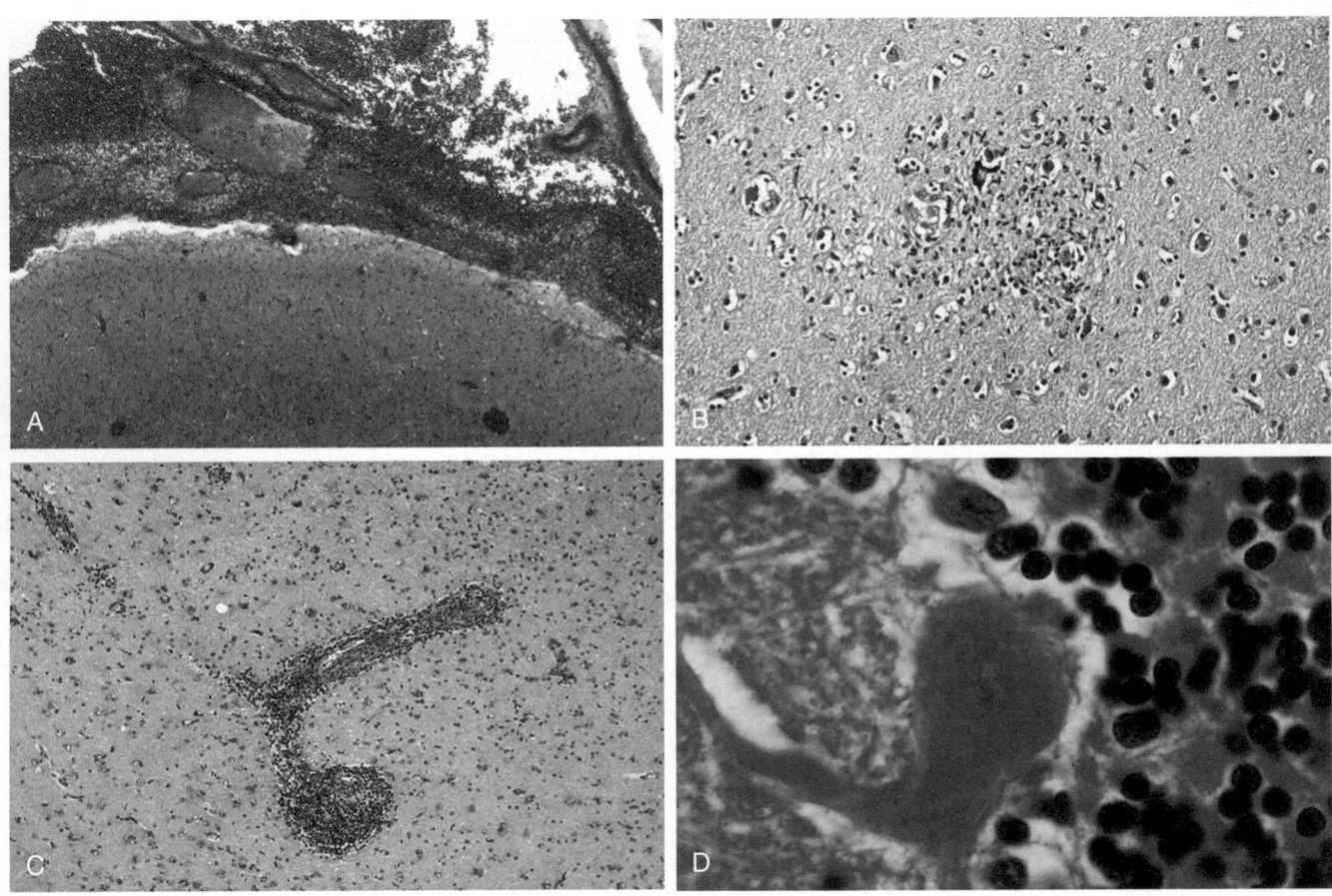

Figure 19-29. A, Acute meningitis. Low-power view shows dense acute inflammatory infiltrate of the leptomeninges. **B,** HIV encephalitis. A microglial nodule containing a multinucleated giant cell. **C,** Viral encephalitis. Low-power view shows classic perivascular lymphocytic infiltrate of the brain parenchyma. **D,** Rabies encephalitis. Classic intracytoplasmic inclusions in cytoplasm of the Purkinje cell of the cerebellum.

Continued

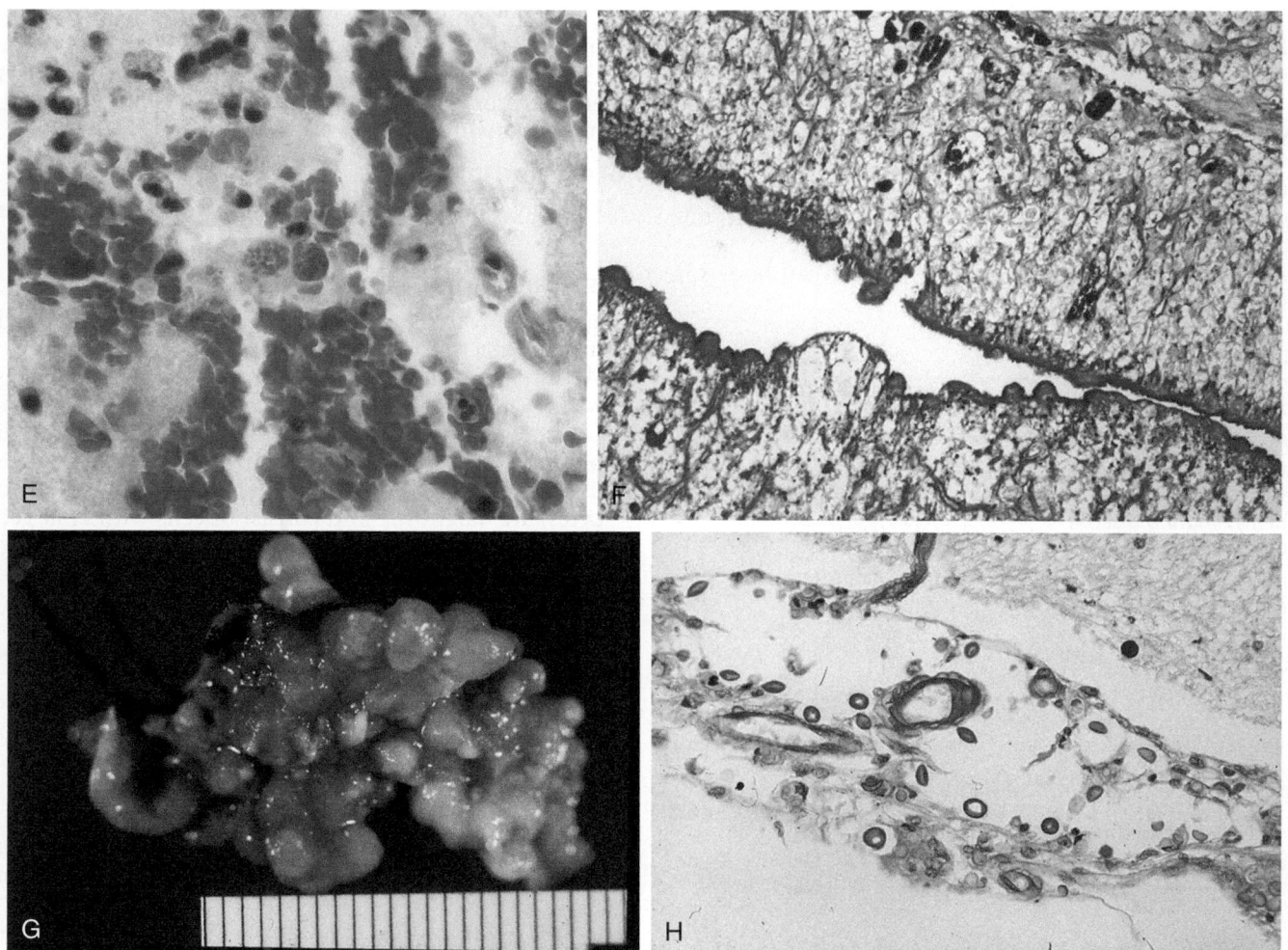

Figure 19-29—Cont'd. E, Toxoplasmosis. An area of encephalitis showing acute inflammation and a cyst containing *Toxoplasma bradyzoites.* **F,** Cysticercosis. Shown is the wall of a cyst of cysticercus. **G,** Cysticercosis, gross photograph. A cluster of cysts (racemose form) of cysticercosis occurs in the ventricles and cisterns of the brain. **H,** *Cryptococcus* meningitis. Mucin stain shows numerous round microorganisms. Notice the lack of staining of the capsule and the absent inflammatory response (periodic acid–Schiff stain).

- Spirochetes may be present in the meninges
- Parenchymal form (general paresis)
  - Invasion of the brain leads to neuronal loss and a reactive gliosis
  - Many rod-shaped microglia in brain parenchyma; perivascular lymphocytes and plasma cells
  - Spirochetes may be present

OTHER CAUSES OF MENINGITIS AND ENCEPHALITIS
- In fungal and parasitic infections, a predominantly chronic inflammatory infiltrate is in subarachnoid space or parenchyma
- Parenchymal infection with fungi or parasites consists of cerebritis, which may progress to abscess (dependent on host immune response)
- *Aspergillus* species cause hemorrhagic necrosis owing to vessel infiltration by hyphae
- In Whipple disease, aggregates of PAS-positive macrophages
- In West Nile encephalitis, involvement of the temporal lobes, basal ganglia, thalamus, brainstem and anterior horns is often prominent

Special Stains and Immunohistochemistry
- Special stains for microorganisms such as Gram, PAS, GMS, AFB, and Fite
- Immunohistochemistry for selected agents such as herpesvirus, *Toxoplasma* species

Other Techniques for Diagnosis
- Culture of the CSF or the necrotic brain tissue
- In situ hybridization using DNA or RNA probes or PCR on CSF or tissue for organisms (e.g., mycobacteria, treponemes [Lyme disease], *Tropheryma whippelii,* etc.)

Differential Diagnosis
SARCOIDOSIS
- Only rarely involves the CNS and is usually limited to the meninges
- Characterized by noncaseating granulomas
- Special stains for organisms are negative

NONINFECTIOUS VASCULITIS
- No organisms identified
- Inflammation likely to be primarily in vessel wall

NONSPECIFIC AUTOIMMUNE ENCEPHALOMYELITIS
- May be associated with autoimmune disorders
- Characteristically steroid responsive

PARANEOPLASTIC ENCEPHALITIS
- Clinical signs and symptoms may precede diagnosis of underlying neoplasm
- Characterized by perivascular lymphocytes and microglial modules
- Analysis of cerebrospinal fluid for related antibodies is indicated (e.g., anti-Hu, anti-Jo)

PEARLS

- *Patients with viral or bacterial meningitis typically do not undergo brain biopsy; with clinical features of encephalitis, biopsy may be performed to isolate the causative organism and to rule out a vasculitis or demyelinating disease*
- *Cowdry type A inclusions are usually only found during the first few days of herpes infection; later, only nonspecific features of encephalitis are found*

SELECTED REFERENCES

Davis LE, DeBiasi R, Goade DE, et al: West Nile virus neuroinvasive disease. Ann Neurol 60:286-300, 2006.
Gyure KA: West Nile virus infections. J Neuropathol Exp Neurol 68:1053-1060, 2009.
Kleinschmidt-DeMasters BK, Gilden DH: The expanding spectrum of herpesvirus infections of the nervous system. Brain Pathol 11:440-451, 2001.
Scaravilli F, Bazille C, Gray F: Neuropathologic contributions to understanding AIDS and the central nervous system. Brain Pathol 17:197-208, 2007.

PROGRESSIVE MULTIFOCAL LEUKOENCEPHALOPATHY (PML)

Clinical Features

- Demyelinating disease typically seen in immunocompromised patients, such as those with AIDS, hematologic cancer, or organ transplantation
- Caused by infection of oligodendrocytes with a papovavirus that produces focal areas of demyelination
- Patients present with visual deficits, personality changes (dementia), and motor deficits
- Typically multifocal; when single, may mimic a neoplasm on CT or MRI
- CT and MRI show white matter lesions without mass effect; most often involve occipital lobe; typically nonenhancing

Gross Pathology

- Variably sized, patchy areas of softening or discoloration of the white matter

Histopathology

- Sparse perivascular lymphocytes and moderate to numerous macrophages are seen
- Within the areas of demyelination, reactive gliosis, with both oligodendrocytes and astrocytes showing considerable nuclear atypia (may mimic glial neoplasm) (Figure 19-30A)
- Infected glial cells (mostly oligodendrocytes and astrocytes) are diagnostic and consist of cells with enlarged, glassy, dark, round nuclei; best appreciated at the edge of the lesion (Figure 19-30B)

Special Stains and Immunohistochemistry

- JC virus immunohistochemistry positive in infected cells
- Klüver stain shows areas of demyelination
- Neurofilament shows relative preservation of axons; there may be axonal loss in the center of a lesion

Other Techniques for Diagnosis

- Electron microscopy: characteristic intranuclear inclusions consisting of stick-and-ball shaped virion particles
- In situ hybridization for JC virus DNA on CSF or tissue sample confirms the diagnosis

Differential Diagnosis

MALIGNANT GLIOMA (ASTROCYTOMA OR OLIGODENDROGLIOMA)
- Lacks macrophage component, areas of demyelination, inflammation, and inclusions

MS
- May create a difficult diagnostic problem
- Oligodendrocytes with characteristic inclusions are not visible

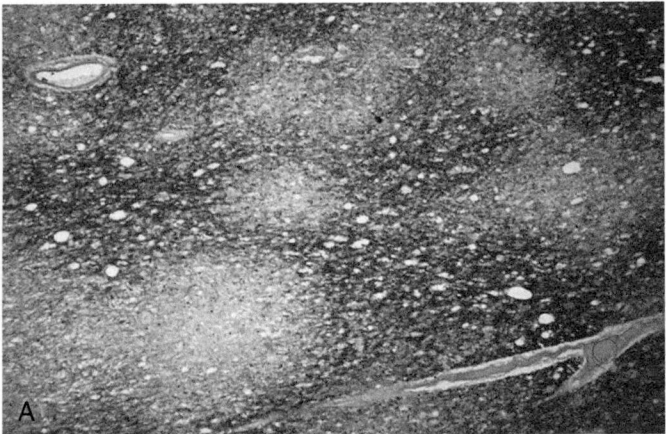 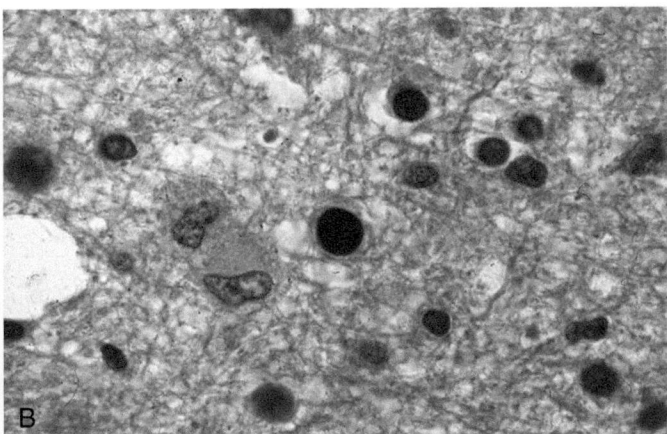

Figure 19-30. Progressive multifocal leukoencephalopathy. A, Low-power view shows multiple irregular areas of demyelination (myelin stain). **B,** Classic intranuclear viral inclusion in oligodendroglial cell is evident in the center of the photomicrograph.

- Immunohistochemistry and in situ hybridization for JC virus are negative

PEARLS

- *PML is associated with reactivation of JC virus in an immunocompromised patient*
- *JC virus is a polyomavirus believed to be acquired in most individuals at a young age, persisting in a latent form in the kidney*
- *PML has an aggressive clinical course, with death usually resulting in a few months*
- *PML has been reported to develop after treatment with natalizumab (a monoclonal antibody to α_4-integrins) in patients with MS and Crohn disease*

SELECTED REFERENCES

Aksamit AJ Jr: Progressive multifocal leukoencephalopathy: a review of the pathology and pathogenesis. Microsc Res Tech 32:302-311, 1995.

Kleinschmidt-DeMasters BK, Tyler KL: Progressive multifocal leukoencephalopathy complicating treatment with natalizumab and interferon beta-1a for multiple sclerosis. N Engl J Med 353:369-374, 2005.

Koralnik IJ, Schellingerhout D, Frosch MP: Case 14-2004: a 66-year-old man with progressive neurologic deficits. N Engl J Med 350:1882-1893, 2004.

Steiner I, Berger JR: Update on progressive multifocal leukoencephalopathy. Curr Neurol Neurosci Rep 12 :680-686, 2012.

Weber T, Major EO: Progressive multifocal leukoencephalopathy: molecular biology, pathogenesis and clinical impact. Intervirology 40:98-111, 1997.

DEMYELINATING DISEASES

Clinical Features

MULTIPLE SCLEROSIS

- Signs and symptoms are markedly variable: visual symptoms, paralysis, ataxia, motor and sensory disturbances, optic neuritis, bladder and bowel dysfunction
- Classically disseminated in space and time
- Wide range of onset: 15 to 55 years
- Women are more commonly affected
- Plaques are commonly located adjacent to the lateral ventricles: optic pathway, cerebellum, and spinal cord are also often affected
- Large plaques causing significant mass effect may radiographically mimic brain tumors

MARBURG TYPE OF MS (ACUTE MS)

- Rare variant set apart because of its aggressive course
- Death occurs usually 1 to 6 months after onset
- Usually involves cerebral hemispheres; large confluent lesions

CONCENTRIC SCLEROSIS OF BALÓ

- Distinguished by separate concentric rings of demyelinated and myelinated white matter visible, in some instances, on MRI and seen microscopically
- Clinically similar to Marburg variant

DEVIC DISEASE (NEUROMYELITIS OPTICA [NMO]): INVOLVEMENT OF OPTIC NERVE AND SPINAL CORD PREDOMINATES

- Pathogenetically distinct from MS
- Associated with serum autoantibody NMO-IgG

ADEM

- Found in both children and adults
- Acute demyelinating disease, usually monophasic, may be associated with or follow infection or vaccination; may also occur without identified predisposing factors
- Acute presentation with neurologic symptoms: ataxia, headache, and weakness

ACUTE HEMORRHAGIC LEUKOENCEPHALITIS (HURST DISEASE)

- Believed to be a hyperacute form of ADEM
- Clinical presentation: fever, nausea, vomiting, focal neurologic deficits, and seizures
- Progression to coma and death or recovery with severe disability

Gross Pathology

MS

- Plaques appear as well-defined, pink to gray gelatinous lesions
- Plaques are often periventricular

ACUTE DEMYELINATING ENCEPHALOMYELITIS

- Lesions are usually in cerebral white matter bilaterally and brain stem

ACUTE HEMORRHAGIC LEUKOENCEPHALITIS

- Brain swelling
- White matter exhibits scattered petechial hemorrhages and necrotic foci

Histopathology

MS

- Active plaques are discrete, hypercellular lesions composed primarily of macrophages and reactive astrocytes (Figure 19-31A)
- Macrophages have round uniform nuclei, vacuolated or granular cytoplasm (containing myelin debris), and distinct cell borders
- Occasional mitotic figures may be seen (in astrocytes called *Creutzfeldt cells*)
- Perivascular cuffs of lymphocytes (predominantly T cells) are prominent in active lesions
- Inactive plaques are hypocellular and exhibit fibrillary astrocytosis and few macrophages
- Marburg variant shows abundant Luxol fast blue (LFB)-containing macrophages in the demyelinated plaques
- Baló concentric sclerosis variant shows alternating bands of myelinated and unmyelinated white matter with myelin stain
- Devic disease: lesions are particularly destructive and may cavitate, contain abundant macrophages and inflammatory cells, and axonal loss in addition to myelin loss

ADEM

- Characterized by foci of demyelination, which are usually perivenous or perivenular
- Numerous lipid-laden macrophages and a perivascular, mononuclear cell infiltrate
- All lesions show similar levels of activity or age

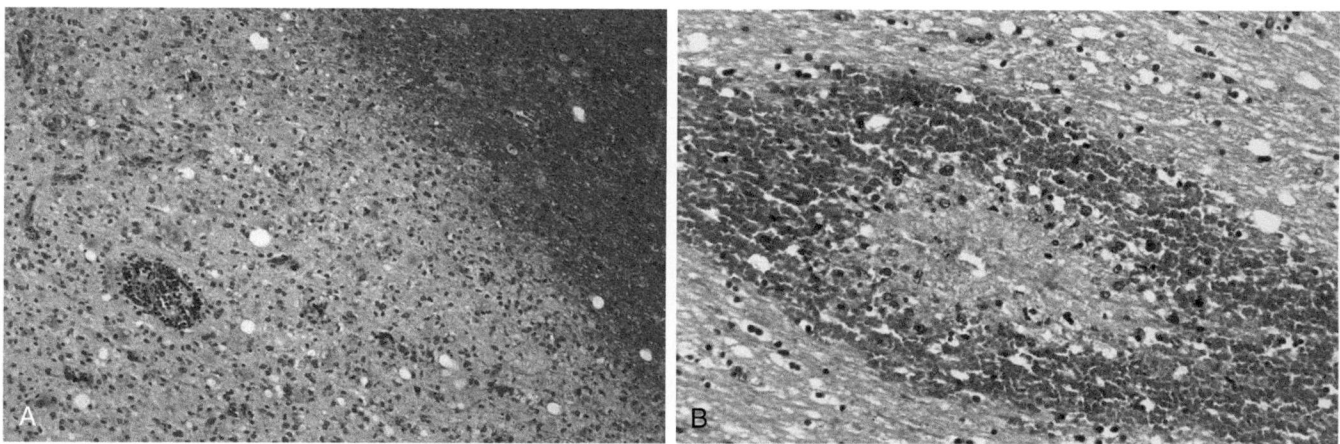

Figure 19-31. A, Multiple sclerosis. Edge of an active plaque of multiple sclerosis showing abrupt loss of myelin, macrophages, reactive astrocytes, and perivascular lymphocytes (myelin stain). **B,** Acute hemorrhagic leukoencephalitis. An area of acute parenchymal hemorrhage is evident surrounding a necrotic vessel.

ACUTE HEMORRHAGIC LEUKOENCEPHALITIS
- Fibrinoid necrosis of white matter blood vessels with surrounding hemorrhage and demyelination or necrosis (Figure 19-31B)
- Neutrophils and lymphocytes surround vessels

Special Stains and Immunohistochemistry
- LFB with PAS shows discrete areas of demyelination and highlights macrophages containing myelin debris (LFB-positive debris implies acute process, PAS-positive debris implies subacute process)
- Neurofilament: shows relative preservation of axons in demyelinated areas

Other Techniques for Diagnosis
- Electron microscopy: breakdown of myelin and ingestion by macrophages, demyelinated axons, sparse oligodendrocytes, and inflammatory cells

Differential Diagnosis
CEREBRAL INFARCTION
- Symptoms are typically acute
- Variable histologic features depending on the age of the infarct
- Neurofilament immunostain shows axonal loss equal to myelin loss

PROGRESSIVE MULTIFOCAL LEUKOENCEPHALOPATHY
- Typically found in an immunocompromised host
- Glial cells have characteristic nuclear inclusions
- Immunohistochemistry and in situ hybridization for JC virus confirms diagnosis

ASTROCYTOMA
- Do not see macrophage component that characterizes demyelinating diseases
- Lacks areas of demyelination
- No perivascular lymphocytes

LEUKODYSTROPHIES
- Adrenoleukodystrophy or adrenomyeloneuropathy
  - Presence of inflammatory cells may lead to confusion with MS
  - Clinical features are distinct from MS
  - Diffuse nature of lesion rather than focal plaques
  - Elevated levels of long-chain fatty acids in plasma
- Other leukodystrophies
  - Often inherited and with distinctive clinical presentations
  - Diffuse nature of lesion rather than focal plaques
  - Morphologic findings may also be distinctive (metachromatic deposits or globoid cells)

PEARLS

- *In MS, solitary plaques may radiographically resemble a neoplasm (tumefactive MS), prompting biopsy of the lesion*
- *In ADEM, most patients eventually recover with resolution of symptoms and eventual remyelination*
- *In acute hemorrhagic leukoencephalitis, there is a much higher fatality rate*

SELECTED REFERENCES

Love S: Demyelinating diseases. J Clin Pathol 59:1151-1159, 2006.
Lucchinetti CF, Brueck W, Rodriguez M, Lassmann H: Multiple sclerosis: lessons from neuropathology. Semin Neurol 18:337-349, 1998.
Morales Y, Parisi JE, Lucchinetti CF: The pathology of multiple sclerosis: evidence for heterogeneity. Adv Neurol 98:27-45, 2006.
Zagzag D, Miller DC, Kleinman GM, et al: Demyelinating disease versus tumor in surgical neuropathology: clues to a correct pathologic diagnosis. Am J Surg Pathol 17:537-545, 1993.

DEMENTIA

Clinical Features

ALZHEIMER DISEASE
- Most common cause of dementia
- Affects adults of all ages; older age is an important risk factor
- Patients present with memory loss and cognitive impairment; progresses over several years

LEWY BODY DEMENTIA

- Presents with cognitive impairment with prominent behavioral abnormalities, hallucinations, and fluctuating clinical course followed by parkinsonian signs and symptoms

VASCULAR DEMENTIA

- Pathologic substrate of vascular dementia is variable
- Presence of infarcts in brain regions strategically critical for cognition; multiple lacunar infarcts in deep gray matter (less frequently cortex) or white matter, and multiple large infarcts have each been shown to cause dementia
- Presence of multiple white matter infarcts often in association with hypertension has been called *subcortical arteriosclerotic leukoencephalopathy* (*Binswanger disease*)
- Clinical course is more variable than in Alzheimer disease: usually relatively sudden onset of impairment and tendency for stepwise progression and fluctuation
- Cerebral autosomal dominant arteriopathy with subcortical infarcts and leukoencephalopathy (CADASIL)
  - Most common form of hereditary (autosomal dominant) stroke leading to dementia
  - Characteristic white matter hyperintensities on MRI
  - Wide range of onset of first stroke: 28 to 60 years of age

CREUTZFELDT-JAKOB DISEASE

- Believed to be caused by a proteinaceous, infectious particle called a *prion*
- Classic nonfamilial patients develop a rapidly progressive dementia with myoclonus and ataxia
- Characteristic electroencephalogram findings of periodic sharp wave complexes

FRONTOTEMPORAL LOBAR DEGENERATION (FTLD)

- *FTLD* is a general term that encompasses several neurodegenerative diseases in which the most severe pathology involves the frontal and temporal lobes
- Included in this category are the following entities:
  - FTLD-tau (subtypes follow)
    - Frontotemporal dementia with parkinsonism linked to chromosome 17
    - Pick disease (PiD)
    - Corticobasal degeneration (CBD)
    - Progressive supranuclear palsy (PSP)
    - Argyrophilic grain disease (AGD)
    - Sporadic multiple system tauopathy with dementia
    - Tangle predominant dementia
    - Unclassifiable tauopathies
  - FTLD-ubiquitin (FTLD-U) (subtypes follow)
    - FTLD-TAR DNA-binding protein of 43 kDa (FTLD-TDP-43)
    - FTLD-fused in sarcoma protein (FTLD-FUS)
    - FTLD-FUS-neuronal intermediate filament inclusion dementia (NIFID)
    - FTLD-FUS-basophilic inclusion body disease (BIBD)
    - FTLD-ubiquitin protease system (FTLD-UPS): includes familial and sporadic types
    - FTLD-no inclusions (FTLD-ni)
- Clinical presentation is usually frontotemporal dementia (FTD), which presents in two general ways: behavioral abnormalities or primary progressive aphasia; positive family history is present in 25% to 50% of patients; amyotrophic lateral sclerosis is associated with a subset of FTLD-TDP-43 cases

Gross Pathology

ALZHEIMER DISEASE

- Brain weight is decreased
- Gyral atrophy is usually generalized affecting all cerebral lobes; atrophy of the inferior temporal lobe, amygdala, and hippocampus is usually prominent
- Increased size of lateral ventricles is typical, especially temporal horns

LEWY BODY DEMENTIA

- Marked depigmentation of the substantia nigra and locus ceruleus
- Usually diffuse cortical atrophy and ventricular enlargement

VASCULAR DEMENTIA

- Caused by multiple cerebral infarcts in various combinations of size and location (cortical, subcortical)
- Multiple white matter infarcts suggest subcortical arteriosclerotic leukoencephalopathy or CADASIL

CREUTZFELDT-JAKOB DISEASE

- Mild cerebral cortical or cerebellar atrophy

FTLD

- Generally frontal and temporal lobes usually show more gyral atrophy than other lobes and anterior basal ganglia are atrophic; may be asymmetric
- PiD: particularly severe atrophy of frontal lobes, anterior middle and inferior temporal gyri, and hippocampus
- CBD: Perirolandic cortical atrophy and substantia nigra pallor
- PSP: Substantia nigra pallor and atrophy of midbrain, subthalamic nucleus, and cerebellar peduncles

Histopathology

ALZHEIMER DISEASE

- Characteristically, two major histologic lesions are seen; semiquantitative estimates of density and locations of neuritic plaques and neurofibrillary tangles form the basis of the pathologic diagnosis of Alzheimer disease (Figure 19-32A)
  - Neurofibrillary tangles: intraneuronal cytoplasmic fibrillary accumulations especially prominent within the association cortexes and mesial temporal lobe (entorhinal cortex and hippocampus)
    - Flame-shaped or globose, depending on whether location is cortical or subcortical
  - Senile plaques: found throughout the cerebral cortex; less dense in subcortical gray matter and cerebellum
    - Multiple subtypes
    - Diffuse plaque contains Aβ protein
    - Neuritic plaque composed of Aβ protein and tau protein

LEWY BODY DEMENTIA

- Cortical Lewy bodies
  - Eosinophilic, cytoplasmic round inclusions with no halo

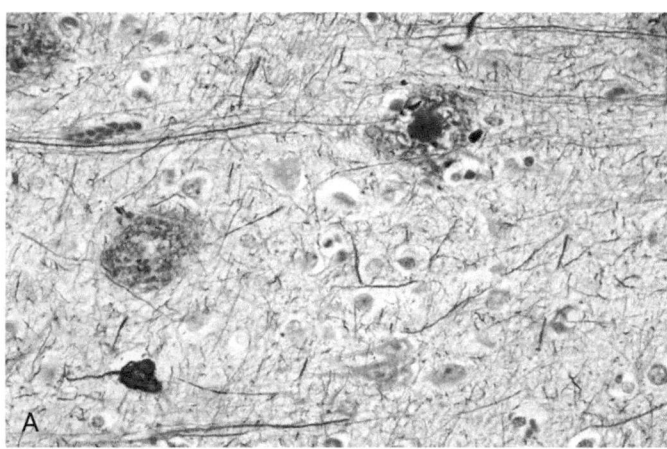 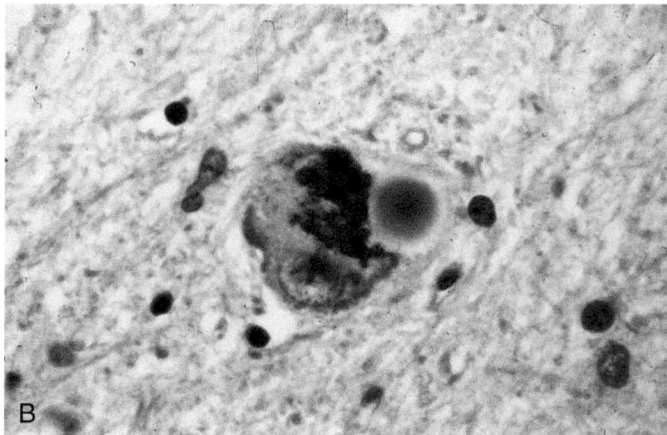

Figure 19-32. A, Alzheimer disease. A neuritic plaque, diffuse plaque, and neurofibrillary tangle in the cerebral cortex (modified Bielschowsky stain). **B,** Parkinson disease. A pigmented substantia nigra neuron containing a classic Lewy body in the cytoplasm. Note the brightly eosinophilic body surrounded by a halo.

- Found in lower layers of cortex, especially prominent in the anterior cingulate gyrus and parahippocampal gyrus
- Lewy bodies are also in pigmented nuclei (most commonly in the substantia nigra) and consist of intracytoplasmic eosinophilic inclusions surrounded by a clear halo that are found within the affected neurons (Figure 19-32B)

VASCULAR DEMENTIA
- Ischemic necrosis of varying ages; acute (eosinophilic neurons and edema) to old (cystic cavity with glial scar)
- Arteriolosclerosis is typically severe when multiple lacunes are present
- CADASIL: thickening of the walls of arteries due to the deposition of granular eosinophilic material (PAS positive) associated with infarcts in the white matter

CREUTZFELDT-JAKOB DISEASE
- Spongiform degeneration with neuronal loss and astrocytosis seen in the affected gray matter; white matter is typically not involved; no inflammatory cells
- Approximately 10% of cases have prion amyloid plaques in cerebellum
- Familial form of prion disease (Gerstmann-Sträussler-Scheinker disease) exhibits plaques and neurofibrillary tangles in the neocortex

FRONTOTEMPORAL LOBAR DEGENERATION
- In most types of FTLD: neuronal loss and astrocytosis in frontal and temporal lobes, anterior basal ganglia and substantia nigra; the hippocampus is less affected than typically evident in Alzheimer disease
- PiD: severe neuronal loss and astrocytosis in frontotemporal lobes with Pick bodies and Pick cells and severe neuronal loss of hippocampus
- PSP: neuronal loss in substantia nigra, subthalamic nucleus, dentate nucleus, and additional deep gray matter and brain stem nuclei
- CBD: neuronal loss in substantia nigra, basal ganglia, and motor and sensory cortexes
- FTLD-TDP-43: often show hippocampal sclerosis (severe neuronal loss and astrocytosis of hippocampus);

may be associated with pathologic findings of amyotrophic lateral sclerosis
- NIFID: neuronal loss, astrocytosis, and neuronal cytoplasmic inclusions (eosinophilic) in neocortex, hippocampus, and basal ganglia
- BIBD: well defined basophilic neuronal cytoplasmic inclusions in neocortex, hippocampus, dentate granule cells, globus pallidus, and thalamus

Special Stains and Immunohistochemistry
ALZHEIMER DISEASE
- Bielschowsky silver stain identifies neurofibrillary tangles and neuritic plaques (see Figure 19-32A)
- Aβ antibodies identify amyloid component of plaque; tau antibodies identify neuritic plaques and neurofibrillary tangles

LEWY BODY DEMENTIA
- α-Synuclein antibodies identify cortical and subcortical Lewy bodies

VASCULAR DEMENTIA
- Klüver and neurofilament immunostain in white matter
- CADASIL: granular eosinophilic deposits may be visualized immunohistochemically with NOTCH3 antibody

CREUTZFELDT-JAKOB DISEASE
- Prion protein immunohistochemistry positive

FRONTOTEMPORAL LOBAR DEGENERATION
- FTDP-17 and sporadic multisystem tauopathy with dementia: tau positive deposits in neurons or neurons and glia of the cerebral cortex, white matter, subcortical nuclei, brain stem, and cerebellum; these may be in various forms including neurofibrillary tangles, Pick-like bodies, tufted astrocytes, astrocytic plaques, globular glial inclusions, or oligodendroglial coiled bodies
- PiD: Pick bodies (cytoplasmic neuronal inclusions): silver (Bielschowsky, Bodian, Gallyas, and King stains) and tau positive; Pick cells (ballooned neurons) are neurofilament positive

- PSP: a variety of tau-positive structures are present; most prominent are the neurofibrillary tangles and tufted astrocytes
- CBD: a variety of tau-positive structures are present; most prominent are the astrocytic plaques and thread-like processes
- AGD: tau and silver positive small elongated grains, coiled bodies, and short filaments are found in mesial temporal lobe structures and basal ganglia
- Tangle predominant dementia: tau and silver positive neurofibrillary tangles in the hippocampus, entorhinal cortex, amygdala, and substantia nigra
- FTLD-TDP-43: tau negative, TDP-43 and ubiquitin positive neuronal nuclear and cytoplasmic inclusions and dystrophic neurites
- FTLD-FUS: tau negative, TDP-43 negative, ubiquitin positive and FUS positive
- NIFID: tau negative, TDP-43 negative, ubiquitin positive, FUS positive, and neurofilament positive neuronal cytoplasmic inclusions
- BIBD: tau negative, TDP-43 negative, ubiquitin positive, FUS positive neuronal cytoplasmic inclusions
- FTLD-UPS: tau, TDP-43, and FUS negative; ubiquitin positive
- FTLD-ni: negative for silver stains, tau, TDP-43, FUS, and ubiquitin

Other Techniques for Diagnosis

ALZHEIMER DISEASE
- Several gene mutations identified in early onset familial (autosomal dominant) Alzheimer disease
  - Amyloid precursor protein (chromosome 21)
  - Presenilin 1 (chromosome 14)
  - Presenilin 2 (chromosome 1)
  - Apolipoprotein E gene allele ε4: dose-dependent risk factor for development of Alzheimer disease

VASCULAR DEMENTIA
- CADASIL
  - Ultrastructural examination of the brain or vessels from skin biopsy shows deposition of specific granular osmiophilic material (GOM) evident in basal lamina adjacent to degenerating smooth muscle cells of arteries
  - Cytogenetics: mutation in *Notch3* gene on chromosome 19

CREUTZFELDT-JAKOB DISEASE
- Western blot for protease-resistant prion protein
- Genetic analysis for mutation in prion protein gene

FRONTOTEMPORAL LOBAR DEGENERATION
- FTDP-17: familial cases associated with mutation in *MAPT* gene (for tau protein)
- FTLD-TDP-43: many associated genes with mutations: *GRN, VCP, TARDBP, UBQLN2, C9ORF72,)*

- FTLD-FUS: familial cases associated with mutations in *FUS* or *CHMP2B* genes

Differential Diagnosis

KUFS DISEASE (ADULT FORM OF NEURONAL CEROID LIPOFUSCINOSIS)
- Rare storage disease involving the central nervous system of adults
- Age of onset is about 30 years
- Slowly progressive disease with dementia; some patients have myoclonic epilepsy and ataxia, whereas others have behavioral and motor disturbances
- Excessive deposition of lipofuscin-like substance in neurons and gastrointestinal tract

STATUS SPONGIOSUS
- May be mistaken for spongiform degeneration of Creutzfeldt-Jakob disease
- Found in acute infarcts and end-stage neurodegenerative diseases
- Vacuoles are predominantly pericellular rather than in the neuropil or intraneuronal

PEARLS

- *Premortem diagnosis of probable Alzheimer disease is usually based primarily on clinical symptoms; definitive diagnosis can only be made on tissue examination*
- *Dementia with atypical clinical presentation is more likely to warrant biopsy*
- *In prion disease, infectious agent is resistant to formalin fixation; treatment of fixed tissue with formic acid before processing, embedding, and cutting is suggested to decrease infectivity of tissue*
- *Important to snap-freeze portion of brain biopsy for possible genetic or biochemical studies when clinical history is dementia*

SELECTED REFERENCES

Bigio EH: Making the diagnosis of frontotemporal lobar degeneration. Arch Pathol Lab Med 137:314-325, 2013.

Kalimo H, Ruchous M-M, Viitanen M, Kalaria RN: CADASIL: a common form of hereditary arteriopathy causing brain infarcts and dementia. Brain Pathol 12:371-384, 2002.

McKeith IG, Galaski D, Kosaka K, et al: Consensus guidelines for the clinical and pathologic diagnosis of dementia with Lewy bodies (DBL): report of the consortium on DBL international workshop. Neurology 47:1113-1124, 1996.

Montine TJ, Phelps CH, Beach TG, et al: National Institute on Aging-Alzheimer's Association guidelines for the neuropathologic assessment of Alzheimer's disease: a practical approach. Acta Neuropathol 123:1-11, 2012.

Rademakers R, Neumann M, Mackenzie IRA: Recent advances in the molecular basis of frontotemporal dementia. Nat Rev Neurol 8:423-434, 2012.

Schott JM, Reiniger L, Thom M, et al: Brain biopsy in dementia: clinical indications and diagnostic approach. Acta Neuropathol 120:327-341, 2010.

Chapter 20
Eye and Orbit

HREEM N. PATEL • RICHARD J. GROSTERN

CHAPTER OUTLINE

ADULT OCULAR LESIONS

EXTERNAL LESIONS

MALIGNANT MELANOMA OF THE CONJUNCTIVA

Clinical Features

- Usually pigmented (may be amelanotic), nodular, elevated lesion, anywhere on conjunctiva
- Usually movable, but may be fixed to sclera
- Indistinct edges
- Rare in dark-skinned people
- Spreads through lymphatics
- Incidence increasing in the United States

Gross Pathology

- Noncontributory

Histopathology

- Mixtures of cell types, including small polyhedral cells, spindle cells, epithelioid cells, and balloon cells (Figure 20-1)
- Normal polarity is lost
- Invasion of overlying epithelium by tumor cells
- May have epithelial cysts if arising from nevus
- Often inflammation is found at the base of the lesion

Special Stains and Immunohistochemistry

- S-100 protein (low specificity, high sensitivity)
- HMB-45 antigen is less sensitive but more specific for melanomas; can be used to distinguish between benign and malignant lesions
- Melan-A (MART-1) staining can be used to determine the extent of the lesion
- Bcl-2 (antiapoptotic cell death protein) is a more robust and consistent marker
- MIB-1 (Ki-67) used to assess proliferative index and is a marker for aggressive behavior

Other Techniques for Diagnosis

- Noncontributory

Differential Diagnosis

PRIMARY ACQUIRED MELANOSIS (PAM)

- Unique to conjunctiva; equivalent to melanoma in situ of skin
- PAM usually lacks mitotic activity but has varying degrees of atypia

NEVUS

- Congenital lesion, without growth
- May become pigmented only in adulthood
- Cysts present on histopathology about 50% of time

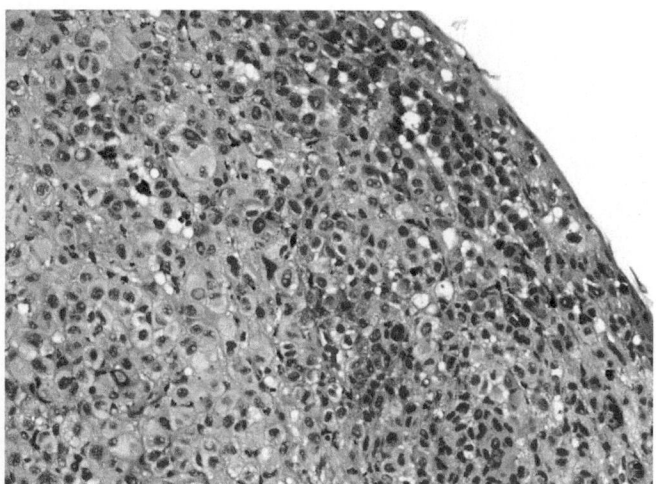

Figure 20-1. Conjunctival melanoma. Numerous polyhedral and spindle cells are present in this conjunctival melanoma.

SECONDARY MELANOMA
- Metastatic from skin or uvea
- Direct extension of intraocular uveal melanoma

RACIAL (CONGENITAL) OCULAR MELANOSIS
- Seen in heavily pigmented individuals
- Histopathologically completely benign

PEARLS

- *Two thirds arise from preexisting PAM; one third arise de novo or from preexisting nevi*
- *Thickness can predict prognosis: less than 1.5 mm, excellent prognosis; more than 1.5 mm, high mortality from metastases*
- *Sentinel node biopsy (preauricular and deep cervical nodes) should be considered in melanomas more than 2-mm thick as well as > 10 mm in diameter*
- *Local recurrence can occur in 36% to 62% of patients; frequency of lymph node metastasis is 36% to 40%*
- *Adjuvant radiotherapy can decrease the incidence of local recurrences*
- *Anecdotal data of successful treatment using recombinant interferon α-2b as adjuvant therapy*
- *Breslow and Clark staging is difficult to apply*

SELECTED REFERENCES

Kurli M, Finger PT: Melanocytic conjunctival tumors. Ophthalmol Clin N Am 18:15-24, 2005.
Liesegang TJ: Pigmented conjunctival and scleral lesions. Mayo Clin Proc 69:151-161, 1994.
Lim LA, Madigan MC, Conway RM: Conjunctival melanoma: a review of conceptual and treatment advances. Clin Ophthalmol 6:521-531, 2013.
Seregard S: Conjunctival melanoma. Surv Ophthalmol 42:321-350, 1998.

PRIMARY ACQUIRED MELANOSIS OF THE CONJUNCTIVA

Clinical Features

- Acquired unilateral diffuse or patchy pigmentation, flat and noncystic
- More common in fair-skinned individuals
- Can arise anywhere on conjunctiva
- Freely mobile
- Indistinct edges with dusty pigmentation
- Average age of onset, 40 to 50 years
- Potential for malignant degeneration into melanoma

Gross Pathology

- Noncontributory

Histopathology

- Atypical melanocytes near basal layer of epithelium (Figure 20-2)
- Usually divided into PAM without atypia and PAM with atypia
- Ranges from mild hyperpigmentation of the epithelium (epithelial cells) with no atypical melanocytes to clusters of deep atypical melanocytes (crossover with malignant melanoma), usually arranged in pagetoid configuration
- Atypical melanocytes will replace basal epithelium in the most aggressive lesions
- Prominent nucleoli (in atypical lesions)
- Lacks epithelial cysts of nevi and some melanomas
- May be arranged in nests, which may indicate poorer prognosis
- Similar to melanoma in situ of skin

Special Stains and Immunohistochemistry

- HMB-45 immunostaining may help distinguish benign from malignant lesions
- See "Malignant Melanoma of the Conjunctiva" for staining patterns

Other Techniques for Diagnosis

- Noncontributory

Differential Diagnosis

CONJUNCTIVAL MELANOMA
- More atypia than PAM
- Loss of normal polarity with mitotic figures
- Melanocytes invade overlying epithelium or underlying stroma

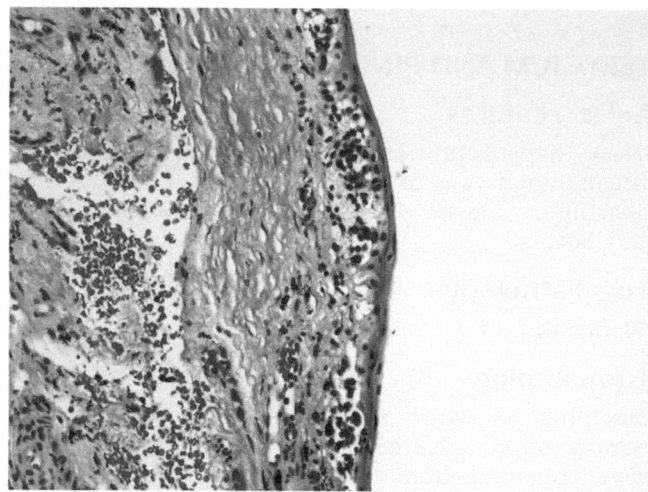

Figure 20-2. Primary acquired melanosis of the conjunctiva. Atypical melanocytes replace many of the deeper layers of the conjunctival epithelium.

CONJUNCTIVAL NEVUS

- Cells always arranged in nests
- Benign appearance
- Congenital
- Adjacent epithelial cells lack pigmentation

RACIAL MELANOSIS

- Bilateral
- Occurs in dark-skinned people

PIGMENTED PAPILLOMA

- Benign papillomatous lesion with pigmented mono-layer of basal cells
- Lacks malignant features
- Drug deposits (adrenochrome granules from epinephrine use)
- Mascara deposits (inadvertent and intentional tattooing)

PEARLS

- *About 46% chance of malignant transformation (into melanoma) if atypical melanocytes are in the basal epithelial layer; much greater chance if melanocytes invade the epithelium in a pagetoid manner or are arranged in deep nests (75% to 90%)*
- *Can consider using topical mitomycin C as an alternative treatment for PAM with atypia*
- *Some sources advocate biopsy of all PAM lesions; others advocate biopsy only with proven growth or if obviously thick*

SELECTED REFERENCES

Jakobiec FA, Folberg R, Iwamoto T: Clinicopathologic characteristics of premalignant and malignant melanocytic lesions of the conjunctiva. Ophthalmology 96:147-166, 1989.

Kurli M, Finger PT: Melanocytic conjunctival tumors. Ophthalmol Clin N Am 18:15-24, 2005.

Liesegang TJ: Pigmented conjunctival and scleral lesions. Mayo Clin Proc 69:151-161, 1994.

Shields JA, Shields CL, Mashayekhi A, et al: Primary acquired melanosis of the conjunctiva: risks for progression to melanoma in 311 eyes. The 2006 Lorenz E. Zimmerman Lecture. Ophthalmology 115:511-519, 2008.

PTERYGIUM AND PINGUECULA

Clinical Features

- Fleshy hypertrophic lesions of ocular surface overlying sclera (pinguecula) or sclera and cornea (pterygium)
- Usually over nasal globe, occasionally temporal, usually bilateral

Gross Pathology

- Noncontributory

Histopathology

- Basophilic (elastotic or actinic) degeneration of substantia propria (Figure 20-3)
- Overlying epithelium may have acanthosis, dyskeratosis, or orthokeratosis
- Histopathologically similar to each other; however, pterygium invades superficial cornea, pinguecula does not

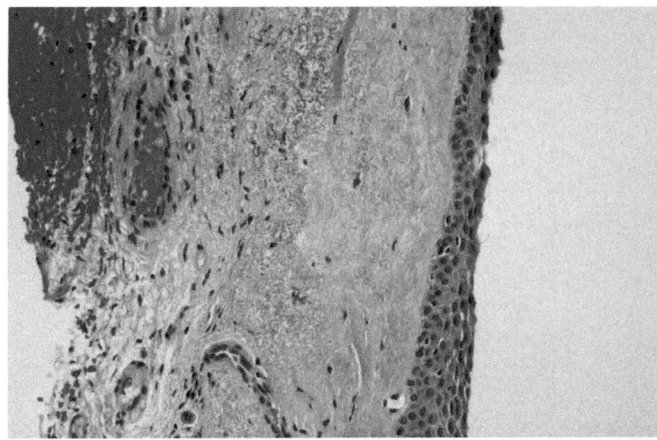

Figure 20-3. Pterygium and pinguecula. Conjunctival epithelium with underlying actinic (elastotic) degeneration.

Special Stains and Immunohistochemistry

- Noncontributory

Modern Techniques for Diagnosis

- Noncontributory

Differential Diagnosis

SQUAMOUS CELL CARCINOMA OF CONJUNCTIVA AND CORNEA (INVASIVE OR IN SITU)

- Easily differentiated by lack of dysplasia in pterygium and pinguecula
- Pseudopterygium as a result of previous penetrating injury with superficial scar formation

PEARLS

- *Commonly removed, commonly recur*
- *Less chance of recurrence if excision is combined with conjunctival autograft or with amniotic graft*

SELECTED REFERENCE

Robin JB, Schanzlin DJ, Verity SM, et al: Peripheral corneal disorders (review). Surv Ophthalmol 31:1-36, 1986.

SQUAMOUS CELL CARCINOMA OF THE CONJUNCTIVA AND CORNEA

Clinical Features

- Gelatinous, with superficial vessels
- Papilliform or leukoplakic lesion
- Usually in the interpalpebral fissure at the corneal limbus, extending into the corneal center
- Uncommonly, incompletely excised lesions can invade through corneoscleral lamellae into the anterior chamber
- Thickened, well-demarcated area

Gross Pathology

- Noncontributory

Histopathology

- Replacement of epithelium by atypical pleomorphic epithelial cells

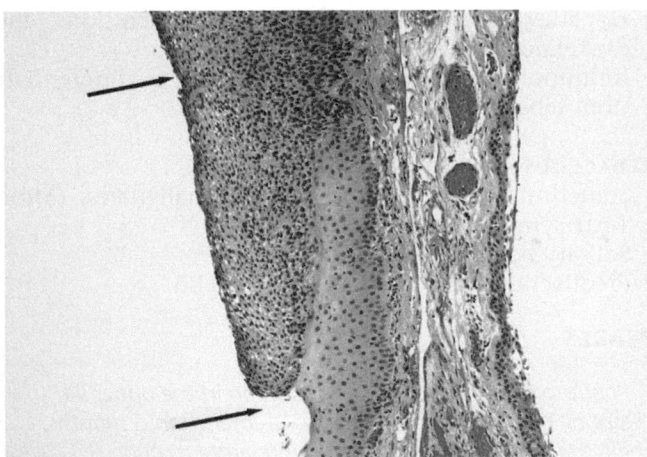

Figure 20-4. Squamous cell carcinoma. Nonkeratinized epithelium of conjunctiva with conjunctival intraepithelial neoplasia. *Upper arrow* indicates a dysplastic region with a sharp line of demarcation to normal-appearing conjunctiva (*lower arrow*).

- Mitoses are common
- Usually will stay within the epithelium (in situ, also known as conjunctival or corneal intraepithelial neoplasia [CIN]), occasionally invades deeper structures, including globe (Figure 20-4)
- Three types of invasive conjunctival squamous cell carcinoma have been reported
  - Spindle cell: spindle-shaped cells are difficult to distinguish from fibroblasts
  - Mucoepidermoid carcinoma: yellow globular cystic component secondary to mucous secreting cells within cysts; in older patients, more aggressive
  - Adenoid squamous carcinoma: extracellular hyaluronic acid but no intracellular mucin; aggressive form and may invade globe or orbit
- Cells can gain access to blood vessels and lymphatics but rarely metastasizes

Special Stains and Immunohistochemistry

- Pancytokeratin staining to confirm surface ectodermal lineage

Other Techniques for Diagnosis

- Noncontributory

Differential Diagnosis

SEBACEOUS CARCINOMA
- More common in conjunctiva and eyelid than is squamous cell carcinoma
- Similar dysplasia, but tends to have a more malignant appearance with a high proportion of cells that display intracytoplasmic vacuolization (sebaceous differentiation)
- May be a more malignant variant of squamous cell carcinoma

PTERYGIUM AND PINGUECULA
- No dysplasia in pterygium and pinguecula

SQUAMOUS PAPILLOMA
- Typical finger-like projections with fibrovascular cores

- Goblet cells common
- Often associated with human papillomavirus (HPV)

ONCOCYTOMA
- Rare tumor of the caruncle
- Cystic cavities lined by proliferating epithelium

Lipodermoid

- Congenital lesion with typical clinical appearance
- Histopathologically similar to dermoid cyst

PEARLS

- *Exposure to solar ultraviolet radiation is a major etiologic factor*
- *HPV and human immunodeficiency virus (HIV) are also etiologic factors*
- *Diagnosis is usually known before excision*
- *May recur, but usually stays in situ if the primary tumor was in situ*

SELECTED REFERENCES
Pe'er J: Ocular surface squamous neoplasia. Ophthalmol Clin N Am 18:1-13, 2005.
Robin JB, Schanzlin DJ, Verity SM, et al: Peripheral corneal disorders (review). Surv Ophthalmol 31:1-36, 1986.
Shields CL, Shields JS: Tumors of the conjunctiva and cornea. Surv Ophthalmology 49:3-24, 2004.
Waring GO III, Roth AM, Ekins MB: Clinical and pathological descriptions of 17 cases of corneal intraepithelial neoplasia. Am J Ophthalmol 97:547-549, 1984.

SEBACEOUS CARCINOMA

Clinical Features

- More common in women
- Most common in patients 60 to 80 years of age
- Genetic factors: Muir Torre syndrome, p53, LEF1 mutations
- Represents 5% of all malignant eyelid tumors
- Second most common eyelid tumor after basal cell carcinoma (more common than squamous cell carcinoma of the eyelid)
- Wide range of presentations, from a small, firm nodule resembling chalazion to diffuse plaque like thickening of the tarsus, to unilateral chronic diffuse blepharitis or conjunctivitis, have loss of cilia
- Overall mortality of about 20%
- May spread through direct extension into adjacent structures (orbit, nasal cavity, sinuses, intracranial cavity) or by the intraepithelial route (pagetoid invasion), lending an impression of multiple primary tumors
- Originates from sebaceous glands of the eyelid and conjunctiva, usually meibomian glands of the tarsus, and from the glands of Zeis (accessory lacrimal glands in conjunctival fornix)
- More common in upper eyelid
- Regional metastasis through lymphatics with the upper eyelid lesions spreading to the preauricular and parotid lymph nodes and the lower eyelid lesions spreading to the submandibular and cervical lymph nodes

Gross Pathology

- Noncontributory

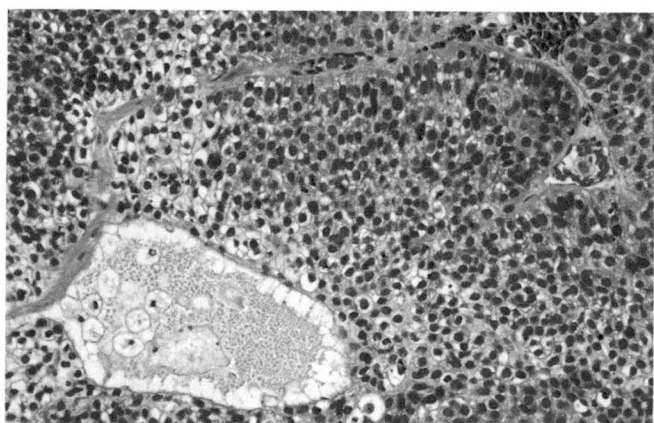

Figure 20-5. Sebaceous carcinoma with typical comedo pattern. Notice numerous cells with vacuolated cytoplasms and many mitotic figures.

Histopathology

- Irregular lobular masses of cells with sebaceous differentiation indicated by prominent cytoplasmic vacuolizations (Figure 20-5)
- Frequent mitoses, nuclear atypia, pleomorphism
- Varies from highly differentiated to poorly differentiated (which may resemble anaplastic carcinoma)
- Four histologic patterns have been identified
  - Lobular: neoplastic cells form well-demarcated lobules
  - Comedocarcinoma: large lobules with central necrotic foci
  - Papillary: fronds of neoplastic cells, sometimes mistaken for squamous carcinoma or squamous papilloma, although careful examination reveals sebaceous differentiation
  - Mixed: mixture of previous three
- Small biopsies may identify strictly intraepithelial tumors, which may be manifestations of pagetoid spread; more extensive biopsy is usually advised

Special Stains and Immunohistochemistry

- Fat stains of frozen tissue show that many cells contain lipid but typically not necessary
- BRST1 marker is positive in sebaceous carcinoma, negative in basal cell carcinoma and squamous carcinoma
- EMA, CK7, Cam 5.2 are typically expressed

Other Techniques for Diagnosis

- Noncontributory

Differential Diagnosis

CHALAZION (STYE)
- Lipogranulomatous inflammation on biopsy

BASAL CELL CARCINOMA
- Spreads only through direct extension (unifocal)
- Lacks sebaceous differentiation

SQUAMOUS CELL CARCINOMA
- Can be difficult to differentiate histopathologically
- Lacks sebaceous differentiation

- Hyperkeratosis, parakeratosis, keratin inclusions, and dyskeratosis
- Immunohistochemistry can be useful to differentiate from sebaceous carcinoma

SEBACEOUS ADENOMA
- Sometimes associated with visceral malignancy (Muir-Torre syndrome)
- Solitary benign nodule
- Predilection for the eyebrow and eyelid

PEARLS

- *Poor prognosis is indicated by location in the upper lid, size of 10 mm or more, duration greater than 6 months, infiltrative growth pattern, and moderate to poor sebaceous differentiation*
- *Early diagnosis and treatment with wide local excision may improve prognosis*
- *Sometimes referred to as "the great masquerader" because it can mimic many other conditions*
- *Can be found in younger patients who have undergone orbital irradiation (e.g., for retinoblastoma) as well as patients who are immunosuppressed*

SELECTED REFERENCES

Burnier MN Jr, Burnier SV, Correia CP, et al: The immunohistochemical profile of sebaceous cell carcinomas of the eyelid. Presented at the Association for Research in Vision and Ophthalmology (ARVO), May 2000.

Kass LG, Hornblass A: Sebaceous carcinoma of the ocular adnexa. Surv Ophthalmol 33:477-490, 1989.

Rao NA, Hidayat AA, McLean IW, Zimmerman LE: Sebaceous gland carcinoma of the ocular adnexa: a clinicopathologic study of 104 cases with five-year follow-up data. Hum Pathol 13:113-122, 1982.

Shields JA, Shields CL: Sebaceous adenocarcinoma of the eyelid. Int Ophthalmol Clin fall; 49:45-61, 2009.

INTERNAL LESIONS

MALIGNANT MELANOMA

Clinical Features
- Most common primary malignant intraocular tumor
- Incidence of 5 to 7 per 1 million general population per year
- Incidence of 20 per million per year in Caucasians older than 50 years
- Unlike cutaneous melanomas, incidence rates do not vary by latitude
- Lifetime risk of 1 in 2500 for whites
- Median age at presentation is in the sixth decade
- About 1% occur in patients younger than 20 years
- Slightly more prevalent in men and in blue-eyed patients
- No known hereditary component, although a few familial occurrences have been reported
- Pregnancy is suggested to enhance growth of melanoma and metastases
- With oculodermal melanocytosis (Nevus of Ota) in a white person, there is an increase in the rate of uveal melanoma by 30-fold
- About 50% harbor mutations in GNAQ gene, which is also seen in precursor lesions

- Patient may be asymptomatic or may complain of blurred vision because of direct tumor involvement of macula, detachment of retina from subretinal fluid produced by tumor, vitreous hemorrhage, or massive size of tumor obscuring vision
- Elevated lesion noted in fundus, sometimes with orange pigment on its surface
- Slow growing
- Anterior (ciliary body) position may be associated with segmental cataract
- Anterior (ciliary body) tumors
  - More difficult to visualize
  - Can attain a large size before clinically recognized
  - Associated with ≥ 1 dilated episcleral blood vessels, epibulbar pigmented lesion, cataractous lens, secondary glaucoma
  - Can be dome shaped or have a diffuse circumferential growth pattern (ring melanoma)
- Choroidal melanomas can be flat and diffuse, making clinical diagnosis more difficult
- Ultrasonography demonstrates solid tumor with low to medium internal reflectivity

Gross Pathology

- Mushroom-shaped or dome-shaped pigmented mass in choroid or ciliary body
- When these tumors arise in the choroid (as opposed to the ciliary body), they may rupture through the overlying Bruch membrane and extend into the subretinal space (giving a mushroom or collar-button shape)
- Size and location are important prognostic factors (size greater than $1 cm^3$ and location at the ciliary body or over the optic nerve are poor prognosticators)
- Extrascleral extension can be seen, usually through scleral canals with vortex veins; this too is an important poor prognosticator
- Occasionally may extend into the subconjunctival space and be mistaken for a primary conjunctival lesion

Histopathology (Figure 20-6)

- Most tumors probably arise from preexisting nevi in the choroid (not retinal pigment epithelium); others arise de novo
- Cell types (Callender histologic classification is most commonly used)
  - Spindle A
    - About 5% of melanomas (second least common)
    - Highly cohesive cells with spindle-shaped nuclei having a central stripe of chromatin (caused by nuclear fold)
    - Cell boundaries not easily identified
    - Rare mitoses
    - High survival rate (> 90%)
    - Pure spindle A tumors behave more like nevi than malignant melanomas
  - Spindle B
    - Common type (about 35% to 40% of all melanomas)
    - Plump spindle cells with prominent nucleoli but without chromatin bar
    - Indistinct cell boundaries

- Mitotic figures are rare, although more common than in spindle A
- Often arranged in fascicular (herringbone) pattern
- Moderate survival rate (about 75%)
- Epithelioid
  - Rarest type (about 3%)
  - Noncohesive, large cells with large nuclei and abundant cytoplasm
  - High degree of pleomorphism
  - Mitoses are common
  - Poor prognosis; survival of about 28%
- Mixed
  - Most common type (about 45%)
  - By definition contains a mixture of epithelioid and spindle cell types
  - Usually spindles predominate, but the occasional epithelioid cell classifies the tumor as mixed and negatively affects prognosis
  - Survival rate about 40%
- Necrotic
  - Rare
  - Tumor is so necrotic as to be unidentifiable in cell type
  - Survival approximates that of mixed cell type
  - Most tumors have some necrosis
  - Balloon cells commonly found and may represent aging apoptotic cells
  - Inflammatory infiltrates commonly seen within tumor, composed mostly of T-cell lymphocytes
  - Macrophages (melanophages) are commonly seen scattered throughout melanomas
  - Degree of pigmentation varies between tumors and even within an individual tumor (varies from amelanotic to deeply pigmented)

Special Stains and Immunohistochemistry

- Frequently HMB-45 positive (about 50%)
- Commonly S-100 positive (> 90%)

Other Techniques for Diagnosis

- Gene expression profile (GEP) identified two classes of tumors:
  - Class 1 melanoma resembles melanocytes, and < 5% of these metastasize
  - Class 2 melanoma resembles primitive neural or ectodermal stem cells, and 90% of these metastasize

Differential Diagnosis

CHOROIDAL NEVUS

- Smaller than melanoma
- Exclusively spindle cell type (usually spindle A)
- Uncommonly has serous subretinal fluid associated
- Never extends out of globe
- Mitoses not present

CAVERNOUS HEMANGIOMA OF THE CHOROID

- Hamartoma that may occur in isolation or in association with Sturge-Weber syndrome (encephalotrigeminal angiomatosis)
- Round or oval, slightly elevated orange-red lesion, usually 3 to 15 mm in diameter
- Occasional leakage of fluid, similar to melanoma

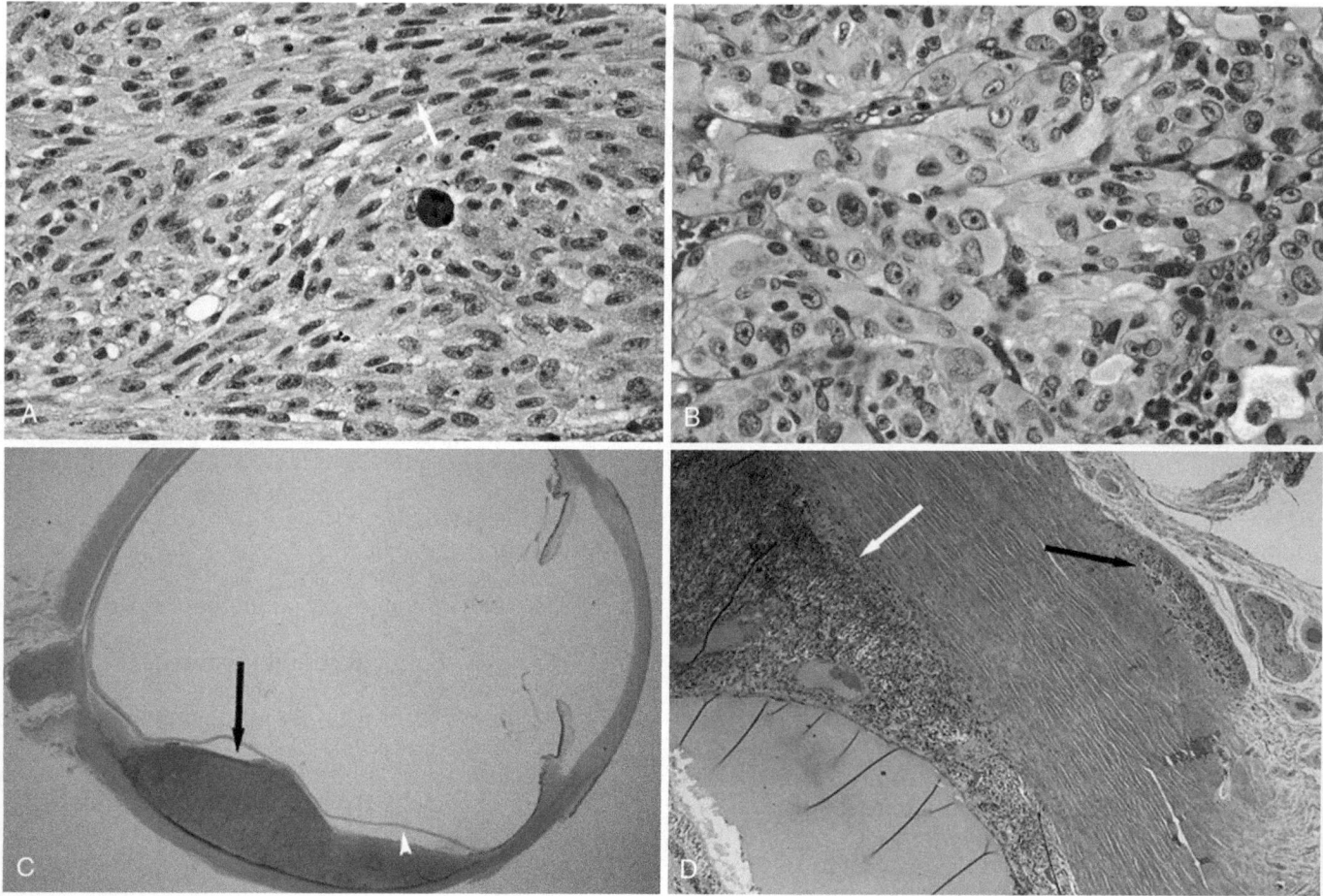

Figure 20-6. A, Typical spindle B choroidal melanoma. *White arrow* indicates a spindle A cell, whereas most of the cells are of the spindle B variety. **B,** Epithelioid melanoma. Large flat cells with prominent nucleoli and marked pleomorphism. This histopathologic appearance is an ominous prognosticator. **C,** Cross section of whole globe with choroidal melanoma. *Arrow* indicates a dome-shaped mass under the retina (*arrowhead*). **D,** Choroidal melanoma with extraocular extension. Choroidal tumor is indicated by *white arrow*, extraocular tumor by *black arrow*.

- Ultrasound helpful in differentiating from melanoma (high versus medium internal reflectivity)
- Histopathologically shows many large cavernous blood-filled spaces

METASTATIC CARCINOMA
- Most common intraocular tumor
- Usually in posterior pole, near vascular arcades
- Fast growing
- May be multifocal
- Ultrasonography may help to differentiate from melanoma
- Breast and lung are the two most common metastatic tumors to the eye
- Up to 12% of all carcinomas may metastasize to choroid (based on autopsy studies)
- In 20% to 45% of cases, ocular findings precede the diagnosis of the primary tumor
- Histopathology varies depending on site of primary tumor

CHOROIDAL MELANOCYTOMA (MAGNOCELLULAR NEVUS)
- Deeply pigmented (jet-black) benign tumor of choroidal melanocytes
- Usually occurs adjacent to optic nerve
- Tends to be flat or minimally elevated

- More common in heavily pigmented people
- Probably has the same low malignant potential as nevus
- Histologically composed of deeply pigmented plump polyhedral nevus cells containing large melanosomes

SUBRETINAL HEMORRHAGE
- Deep red, may appear brown or black
- Ultrasonography useful in differentiating from melanoma

SCHWANNOMA
- Rare tumor of Schwann cells surrounding ciliary nerves
- Clinically and ultrasonographically similar to choroidal melanoma
- Histologically difficult to differentiate from spindle cell melanoma, although characteristically lacks the prominent nucleoli of melanoma
- Electron microscopy may be helpful in making diagnosis (Antoni patterns)

CHOROIDAL OSTEOMA
- An unusual benign osseous, creamy-white lesion of posterior pole
- Usually relatively flat
- Ultrasonography shows calcification

PEARLS

- *About 4% of eyes enucleated from white patients with blind, painful eyes and opaque media harbor unsuspected choroidal melanoma (which may provoke pain, leading to enucleation more commonly than in nonpainful blind eyes)*
- *Monosomy 3 or amplification of long arm of chromosome 8 are also associated with poorer prognosis*
- *Metastases are usually a late occurrence and may happen years after enucleation*
- *Liver is by far the most common site of metastasis (90%)*
- *Mistaken clinical diagnosis rate by experienced ophthalmologists of approximately 1%*
- *Overall 15-year mortality rate is about 40% to 50%, significantly worse for large tumors and better for small tumors*
- *Treatment options include external-beam irradiation, plaque brachytherapy with iodine-125, transpupillary thermal therapy, local excision, and enucleation*
- *Choroidal melanomas are not known to be chemoresponsive, nor are the metastases*

SELECTED REFERENCES

Albert DM: The ocular melanoma story. LIII Edward Jackson memorial lecture: Part II. Am J Ophthalmol 123:729-741, 1997.

Albert DM, Rubenstein RA, Scheie HG: Tumor metastasis to the eye. I. Incidence in 213 adult patients with generalized malignancy. Am J Ophthalmol 63:723-726, 1967.

The Collaborative Ocular Melanoma Study Group: Histopathologic characteristics of uveal melanomas in eyes enucleated from the Collaborative Ocular Melanoma Study: COMS report no. 6. Am J Ophthalmol 125:745-766, 1998.

The Collaborative Ocular Melanoma Study Group: The COMS randomized trial of iodine 125 brachytherapy for choroidal melanoma. V. Twelve-year mortality rates and prognostic factors: COMS report no 28. Arch Ophthalmol 124:1683-1693, 2006.

Eagle RC: The pathology of ocular cancer. Eye 27:128-136, 2013.

Laver NV, McLaughlin ME, Duker JS: Ocular melanoma. Arch Pathol Lab Med 134:1778-1784, 2010.

CILIARY BODY ADENOMA

Clinical Features

- Also known as Fuchs adenoma, Fuchs reactive hyperplasia, coronal adenoma, Fuchs epithelioma, and benign ciliary epithelioma
- Present in more than 25% of older people
- Can cause local symptoms including secondary cataracts, secondary glaucoma, inflammation, vitreous hemorrhage, neovascularization of the optic disk, and cystoid macular edema

Gross Pathology

- Small mass in ciliary body sometimes noted on dissection of an eye in the pathology laboratory

Histopathology

- Benign proliferation of cords of nonpigmented ciliary epithelium separated by septae of extracellular material (Figure 20-7)
- Abundant eosinophilic basement membrane material is present among the cords

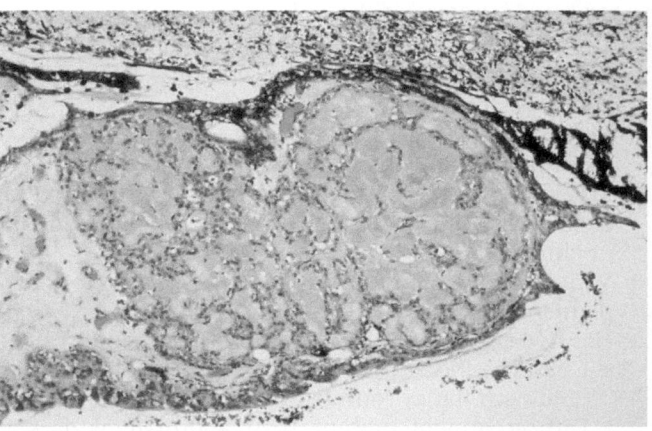

Figure 20-7. Ciliary body (Fuchs) adenoma. Chords of ciliary epithelium interspersed with abundant eosinophilic material.

Special Stains and Immunohistochemistry

- S-100, vimentin, cytokeratin positive
- HMB-45 negative

Other Techniques for Diagnosis

- Noncontributory

Differential Diagnosis

AMELANOTIC MELANOMA

- Spindle or epithelioid cell types
- Usually has some pigment

MEDULLOEPITHELIOMA

- Congenital lesion
- Slowly enlarging
- Made up of poorly differentiated neuroectodermal tissue

METASTATIC CARCINOMA

- Usually rapidly growing
- Most commonly breast and lung carcinomas

PEARLS

- *Proliferative rather than neoplastic*
- *May rarely cause occlusion of the anterior chamber angle*
- *Rarely misdiagnosed as a ciliary body melanoma*

SELECTED REFERENCES

Bateman JB, Foos RY: Coronal adenomas. Arch Ophthalmol 97:2379-2384, 1979.

Chen Z. Fang X: Adenoma of nonpigmented epithelium in ciliary body: literature review and case report. J Zhejiang Univ Sci B 8:612-615, 2007.

Shields JA, Eagle RC, Shields CL, DePotter PD: Acquired neoplasms of the nonpigmented ciliary epithelium (adenoma and adenocarcinoma). Ophthalmology 103:2007-2016, 1996.

IRIS NEVUS AND MELANOMA

Clinical Features

- Included as a separate entity because of distinct behavior compared with ciliary body and choroidal melanoma
- Nevi and melanoma are the most common tumors of the iris but only account for 3% to 10% of all uveal melanoma
- No sex predilection

- Average age of involvement is between 40 and 50 years, 10 years younger than uveal melanoma
- Nonaggressive tumor (overall chance of metastasis about 2% to 4%)
- May have prominent vascularity
- Predisposition for inferior iris (80%)
- May present as a discrete mass, a diffuse mass (cottage cheese-like), iris heterochromia, hyphema, glaucoma, or chronic uveitis
- Varies in pigmentation from amelanotic to deeply pigmented
- Has two types of growth: circumscribed and diffuse
  - Circumscribed tumors are yellow, tan, or brown colored with flat or rounded-out contour
  - Diffuse tumors present with a unilateral dark iris without focal thickening
- Difficult to distinguish nevus from melanoma
  - The presence of vascularity, increased intraocular pressure, or tumor seeding within the anterior chamber will increase the likelihood of malignancy

Gross Pathology

- Noncontributory

Histopathology

- Varies from more benign to purely malignant
  - More benign tumors usually have an abundance of slender spindle cells with few prominent nucleoli (may be considered a nevus)
  - More malignant tumors have plump spindle cells with prominent nucleoli or epithelioid cells (worst prognosis) (Figure 20-8)
- Arises from iris stroma, not from posterior pigment epithelium

Special Stains and Immunohistochemistry

- Most tumors show positive staining for HMB-45, but this does not predict prognosis and does not help distinguish melanoma from nevus

Other Techniques for Diagnosis

- Noncontributory

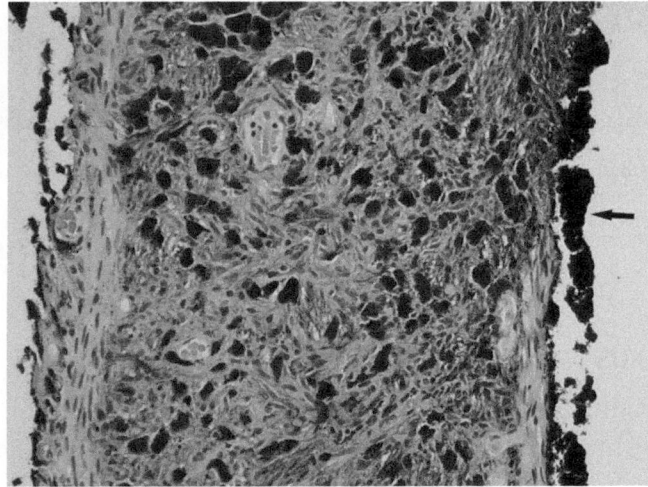

Figure 20-8. Iris melanoma. *Black arrow* indicates posterior pigment epithelium of iris. Note the overall hypercellularity of the stroma with a population of spindle-shaped melanocytes displaying moderate pleomorphism.

Differential Diagnosis

IRIS NEVUS
- Benign-appearing spindle cells
- May slowly enlarge, but usually does not lead to glaucoma or hyphema
- Increased incidence in people who have neurofibromatosis type 1 (called a *Lisch nodule*, histopathologically identical to nevus)

CILIARY BODY MELANOMA WITH ANTERIOR EXTENSION
- Much more malignant in histopathologic appearance with poor prognosis

IRIDOCORNEAL ENDOTHELIAL SYNDROME (ICE) VARIANT
- Iris nevus syndrome—diffuse hyperpigmentation with inflammation
- Usually associated with glaucoma or corneal decompensation

CYST OF POSTERIOR IRIS EPITHELIUM
- May follow surgery or trauma
- Ultrasound will detect fluid-filled cavity

METASTATIC TUMORS TO THE IRIS
- Most commonly lung and breast carcinoma

IRIS FRECKLE (EPHELIS)
- Small, without discrete mass
- Increase in pigmentation without an increase in the number of melanocytes

INFLAMMATORY MASS
- Collection of lymphocytes and plasma cells

PENETRATING OCULAR TRAUMA
- Foreign body with inflammatory reaction
- Iris prolapse simulating iris mass

IRIS LEIOMYOMA
- Rare
- May be difficult to differentiate from nevus and melanoma (all spindle cell tumors)

PEARLS

- *Most arise from preexisting nevi*
- *Constitute 5% to 10% of all uveal melanomas*
- *Rate of metastasis up to 10%*
- *Can often be successfully excised; some may require enucleation if large and diffuse involving more than 6 clock hours of the iris and invading the trabecular meshwork*

SELECTED REFERENCES

Arentsen JJ, Green WR: Melanoma of the iris: report of 72 cases treated surgically. Ophthalmic Surg 6:23-27, 1975.

Henderson E, Margo CE: Iris melanoma. Arch Pathol Lab Med 132:268-272, 2008.

Kersten RC, Tse DT, Anderson R: Iris melanoma: nevus or malignancy? Surv Ophthalmol 29:423, 1985.

Yap-Veloso MI, Simmons RB, Simmons RJ: Iris melanomas: diagnosis and management. Int Ophthalmol Clin 37:87-100, 1997.

CHILDHOOD OCULAR LESIONS

RETINOBLASTOMA

Clinical Features

- A common childhood malignancy, occurring in 1 in 16,000 to 23,000 live births
- Third most common intraocular malignancy after metastasis and uveal melanoma
- No racial or sex predilection
- Bilateral in 20% to 30% of cases
- Average age of diagnosis is between 12 and 18 months, with 89% diagnosed before age 3 years
- Average age at diagnosis is lower in bilateral cases
- Rare after age 10 years; has rarely been reported in adults
- Usually presents as leukocoria (literally, "white pupil") but may present as strabismus, intraocular inflammation, hemorrhage, or trauma
- Highly malignant with great metastatic potential
- Most common method of spread is by direct invasion of optic nerve with extension into central nervous system
- May spread by invasion of leptomeninges and dissemination into cerebrospinal fluid
- Hematogenous spread can lead to distant metastases throughout the entire body
- May spread through lymphatics
- Retinoblastoma has one of the highest rates of spontaneous regression of any malignant tumor (regressed retinoblastoma, also called *retinocytoma* or *retinoma*)
- Heredity
  - The retinoblastoma (*RB*) gene is a tumor suppressor gene on the long arm of chromosome 13 (13q14), and retinoblastoma arises as a result of mutations in both copies of the gene
  - May arise in a sporadic or inherited fashion
  - Sporadic cases with germline mutation in RB1 will present at an earlier age, ~12 months old, whereas sporadic cases with a somatic mutation in RB1 gene will present around 24 months old
  - Somatic mutation results in unilateral tumor
  - Germline mutation is likely to result in bilateral or multifocal tumors
  - Can be inherited as a genotypically recessive gene, but phenotypically behaves like a dominant gene; if one faulty copy of the gene is transmitted, there is greater than a 90% chance of acquiring the second mutation
  - *Trilateral retinoblastoma* refers to retinoblastoma tumor arising in the pineal gland in addition to bilateral retinoblastoma; this occurs with germline mutations
  - About one third of tumors are germline, and two thirds are somatic
  - About 10% of all retinoblastoma cases are familial
  - The risk for a bilateral (germline) retinoblastoma survivor's having an affected offspring is about 45%
  - The risk for a unilateral (somatic) retinoblastoma survivor's having an affected offspring is about 7% to 15%

Gross Pathology

- Chalky-white tumor arising from the retina
- May grow in an endophytic pattern (into vitreous) or an exophytic pattern (into subretinal space), or more commonly in some combination of both

Histopathology

- Basic cell type has a large basophilic nucleus of variable size and shape and scanty cytoplasm (Figure 20-9A)
- Mitoses are frequent
- Tumor cells are clustered around blood vessels with intervening areas of necrosis and scattered calcification ("Islands of blue tumor in a sea of pink necrosis with purple flecks of calcium"— M.E. Smith) (Figure 20-9B)
- The Flexner-Wintersteiner rosette is pathognomonic of retinoblastoma and consists of a single row of tumor cells surrounding a central lumen; these are found exclusively in retinoblastoma (Figure 20-9C)
- The Homer-Wright rosette is also commonly found and consists of a single row of tumor cells surrounding a jumbled eosinophilic center; these are found in retinoblastoma, neuroblastoma, and medulloblastoma
- Groups of partially differentiated retinoblasts elongate and resemble photoreceptors; they then form a flower-like configuration known as a *fleurette*
- Blood vessels commonly have a cuff of basophilia, which most likely represents the accumulation of DNA from necrotic and apoptotic retinoblastoma cells
- Calcification is usually present
- Histopathologic factors that help determine the chance of metastases include extension of the tumor into the optic nerve beyond the lamina cribrosa, extension of tumor to the surgical margin of optic nerve, massive invasion of the choroid by the tumor, and extraocular tumor (Figure 20-9D)
- Fully differentiated forms of retinoblastoma are referred to as *retinocytomas* and lack malignant characteristics

Special Stains and Immunohistochemistry

- The typical histopathologic appearance of these tumors makes special stains clinically unimportant

Other Techniques for Diagnosis

- Noncontributory

Differential Diagnosis

- The differential diagnosis of leukocoria (white pupil) in a young child is broad and includes cataract, developmental ocular abnormalities, ocular inflammation and infection, other tumors, vascular abnormalities, trauma, and retinal detachment
- Retinoblastoma is usually an easy histopathologic diagnosis

PEARLS

- *Treatment of unilateral cases is usually by enucleation, with adjuvant chemotherapy and radiation therapy reserved for cases with evidence of extraocular spread or cases with histopathologic risk factors for metastasis*
  - *With small tumors (<3 mm) and little subretinal fluid, treat with plaque radiotherapy*
  - *With larger tumors (>3 mm) and extensive seeding or subretinal fluid, treat with chemoreduction and consolidation*
- *Treatment of bilateral cases usually involves enucleation of the more severely affected eye (if there is no potential*

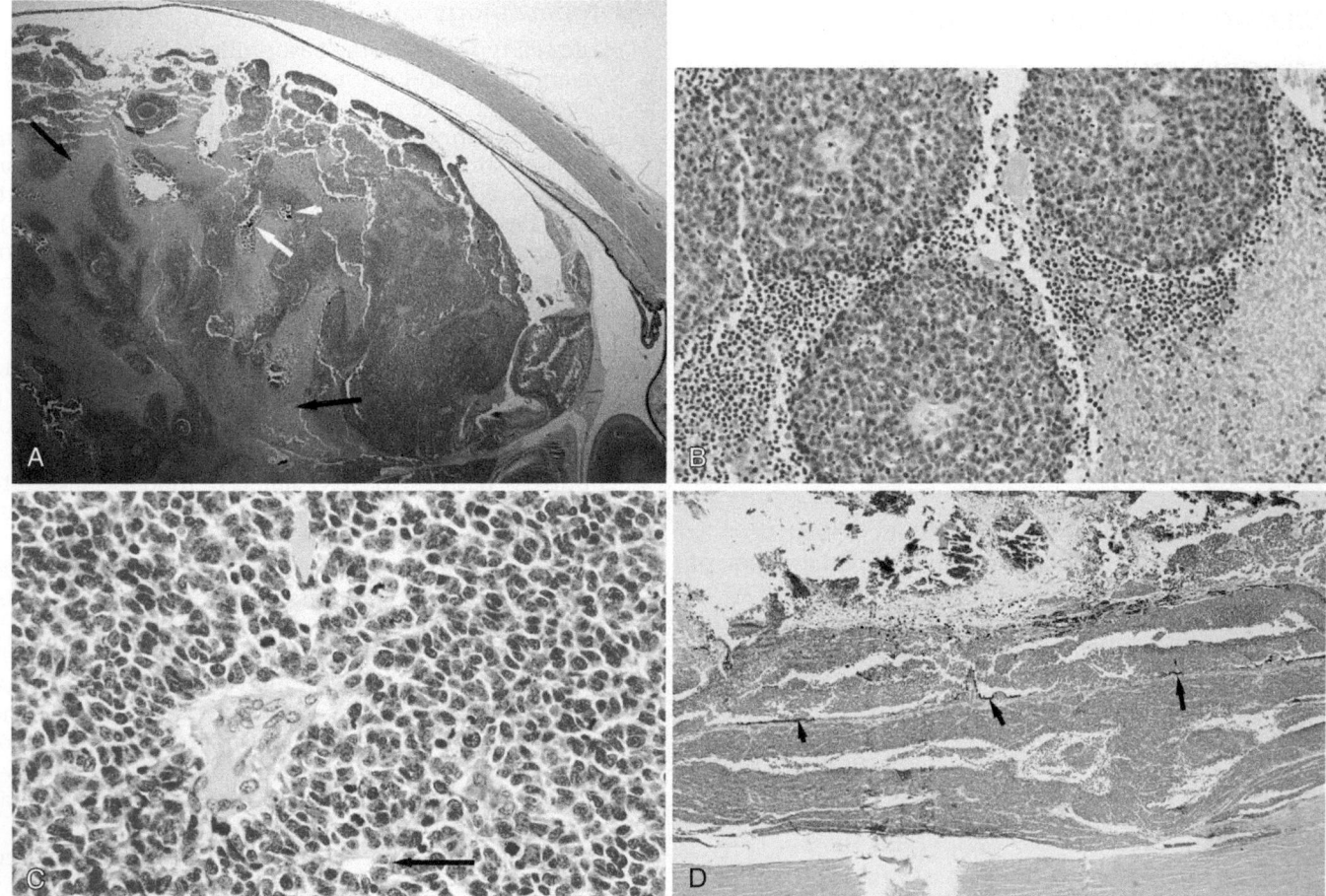

Figure 20-9. Large retinoblastoma. A, Low-power view. Notice the overall architecture of the tumor with basophilic tumor cells clustered around blood vessels within a background of necrosis (*black arrows*). *White arrows* indicate areas of calcification within the tumor. **B,** Tumor cells clustered around blood vessel in a pseudorosette pattern with adjacent necrosis. **C,** High-power view demonstrating many mitotic figures, a fleurette (*yellow arrow*) and a Flexner-Wintersteiner rosette (*black arrow*). **D,** Invasion of the tumor into the choroid. Retinal pigment epithelium (*black arrows*) separates the retina from the choroid, and there is a tumor on both sides.

for useful vision) with subsequent chemotherapy (chemoreduction) combined with radiation, cryotherapy, or laser photocoagulation; bilateral enucleation is also a consideration

- *New treatment with intra-arterial chemotherapy reports of favorable outcomes; however, long-term complications remain unknown and no clinical trial has established its role*
- *Disseminated leptomeningeal disease is the most difficult type of extraocular retinoblastoma to cure secondary to craniospinal radiation doses and the volume needed for treatment*
- *The risk for subsequent neoplasms in germline retinoblastoma survivors is high, and the overall mortality rate from second tumors is as high as 30%*
- *The most common second neoplasm is osteosarcoma, especially in irradiated fields (orbit); however, soft tissue sarcomas, malignant melanoma, carcinomas, malignancies of the hematopoietic system, and brain tumors occur at a higher rate in individuals with germline mutations*
- *Overall long-term survival rate is about 85%, although a mortality rate as high as 60% after 35 years has been reported in patients with bilateral retinoblastoma*

SELECTED REFERENCES

Abramson DH: Second nonocular cancers in retinoblastoma: unified hypothesis. The Franceschetti Lecture. Ophthalmic Genet 20:193-204, 1999.

Albert DM: Historic review of retinoblastoma. Ophthalmology 94:654-662, 1987.

Dimaras H, Kimani K, Dimba EA, et al: Retinoblastoma. Lancet 379:1436-1446, 2012.

Eagle RC: The pathology of ocular cancer. Eye 27:128-136, 2013.

Shields CL, Shields JA: Retinoblastoma management: advances in enucleation, intravenous chemoreduction, and intra-arterial chemotherapy. Curr Opin Ophthalmol 21:203-212.

Usalito M, Wheeler S, O'Briend J: New approaches in the clinical management of retinoblastoma. Ophthalmol Clin North Am 12:255-264, 1999.

ADULT ORBITAL LESIONS

ORBITAL LYMPHOMA, INCLUDING LYMPHOID HYPERPLASIA AND MALIGNANT LYMPHOMA OF THE ORBIT

Clinical Features

- Average age of onset is 50 to 70 years; rare before age 20 years

- Females slightly more affected than males
- Insidious presentation
- No inflammatory signs; little (if any) pain
- May present with gradually progressive proptosis or as a visible "salmon patch" of the conjunctiva (Figure 20-10A)
- Lacrimal sac involvement can present with epiphora, swelling over the lacrimal gland or dacryocystitis
- Lacrimal gland involved in 30% of cases
- Imaging reveals an infiltrative lesion, which molds to surrounding structures (globe, orbital bones)
- Most common in superior anterior orbit

Gross Pathology

- Noncontributory

Histopathology

- Range of features depends on degree of malignancy of lesion
- More benign lesions (lymphoid hyperplasia)
  - Dense lymphoid infiltrate consisting of mature-appearing lymphocytes
  - Cell population has benign features (no pleomorphism, low mitotic activity, moderate amount of polyclonality and polymorphism)
  - Well-defined germinal centers
- True lymphomas
  - Usually non-Hodgkin B-cell lymphomas
  - Cells can be small or large, cleaved or noncleaved
  - Mucosa-associated lymphoid tissue (MALT) lymphomas account for up to 50% of all orbital lymphomas (Figure 20-10B)
  - May be classified according to the Modified Rappaport Classification or the Revised European-American Lymphoma Classification
- Differentiation between lymphoid hyperplasia and true lymphoma is often difficult; occasionally pathologists evoke the term *atypical lymphoid hyperplasia*

Special Stains and Immunohistochemistry

- Because most are B-cell tumors, they express CD20
- κ and λ light chains may indicate monoclonality

- Polymorphism among the populations of more benign lesions may show positive T-cell, plasma cell, or macrophage markers

OTHER TECHNIQUES FOR DIAGNOSIS

- Noncontributory

Differential Diagnosis

INFLAMMATORY ORBITAL PSEUDOTUMOR (IDIOPATHIC ORBITAL INFLAMMATION)

- More inflammatory onset
- Varies according to stage and type, but usually a polymorphic infiltrate of benign-appearing lymphocytes with or without fibrosis
- May include germinal centers
- Occasionally, granulomatous inflammation

ORBITAL CELLULITIS

- Imaging usually reveals a periosteal abscess or adjacent sinusitis
- More likely to occur in younger individuals
- In most cases does not come to biopsy, although true abscesses of orbit are often drained
- Acute inflammatory signs

SOLID TUMORS OF ORBIT

- Including lacrimal gland tumors, primary and metastatic orbital tumors

GRAVES ORBITOPATHY

- Extraocular muscles are always the site of primary involvement
- Interstitial edema and lymphocytic inflammatory infiltrate within the endomysial connective tissue are early findings
- May lead to edema and inflammatory infiltration around muscles and eventually fibrosis
- Lacks germinal centers

VASCULAR LESIONS

- Includes hemangioma, lymphangioma, varix, and arteriovenous fistula

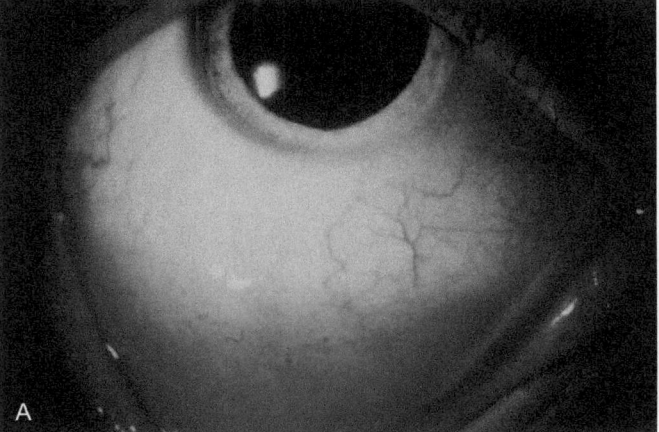 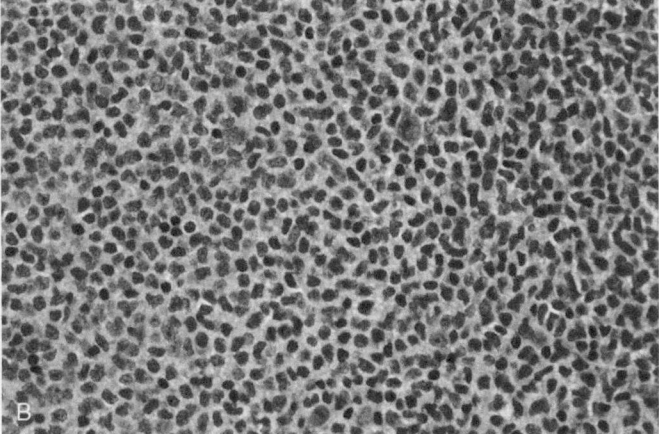

Figure 20-10. A, Lymphoma of the anterior orbit. Clinical photograph of a patient showing a typical "salmon patch" in the inferior conjunctival fornix. **B,** Lymphoid infiltrate with marked pleomorphism. Orbital biopsy from the patient in Figure 20-2.

PEARLS

- *Strictly conjunctival and epibulbar tumors are less likely to be associated with systemic disease*
- *About 13% to 19% of patients have known systemic lymphoma at the time of diagnosis*
- *Up to 25% of all patients with orbital lymphoma can be expected to have evidence of systemic lymphoma within 5 years*
- *Bilaterality is not uncommon and does not necessarily predict a higher likelihood of systemic disease*
- *Treatment is usually with orbital external-beam irradiation; alternative treatments include local cryotherapy, chemotherapy, interferon treatment, and surgical excision*
- *Systemic evaluation should be performed and may include hematologic evaluation with bone marrow biopsy, bone scan, and head, chest, and abdomen radioimaging*

SELECTED REFERENCES

Bardenstain DS: Ocular adnexal lymphoma: classification, clinical disease, and molecular biology. Ophthalmol Clin N Am 18:187-197, 2005.

Bernardini FP, Bazzan M: Lymphoproliferative disease of the orbit. Curr Opin Ophthalmol 18:398-401, 2007.

Knowles DM, Jakobiec FA, McNally L, et al: Lymphoid hyperplasia and malignant lymphoma occurring in the ocular adnexa (orbit, conjunctiva, and eyelids): A prospective multiparametric analysis of 108 cases during 1977 to 1987. Hum Pathol 21:959-973, 1990.

Mederios LJ, Harris NL: Lymphoid infiltrates of the orbit and conjunctiva: a morphologic and immunophenotypic study of 99 cases. Am J Surg Pathol 13:459-471, 1989.

INFLAMMATORY ORBITAL PSEUDOTUMOR (IDIOPATHIC ORBITAL INFLAMMATION)

Clinical Features

- Lymphoid tumors are not included as part of this topic
- Non-neoplastic, nonspecific inflammatory space-occupying orbital lesion
- Presents as proptosis, chemosis, lid swelling, and erythema, usually accompanied by pain
- Usually unilateral, but may be bilateral (especially in children)
- Equal sex incidence
- Most common in fourth to sixth decades
- May present acutely, subacutely, or chronically
- May be recurrent
- May present as myositis, dacryoadenitis, nonspecific connective tissue inflammation, or deep orbital inflammation with accompanying cranial nerve dysfunction
- Can also involve the eye and produce optic nerve edema, scleritis, and intraocular inflammation
- First-line treatment is usually oral prednisone in high doses (60 to 80 mg)

Gross Pathology

- Noncontributory

Histopathology

- Histopathologic findings vary depending on which tissue is primarily involved

- Early disease
  - Edema
  - Paucicellular polymorphic inflammatory infiltrate consisting of mature lymphocytes, plasma cells, eosinophils (especially in children), and neutrophils
  - Frequent perivascular lymphocytic cuffing
- Late disease
  - Increasing fibrosis (Figure 20-11)
  - Less inflammatory infiltrate
  - Germinal centers occasionally found
- Lymphoid elements are usually widely separated by fibrosis (in contrast to sheets of lymphoid elements found in lymphoid tumors)
- Granulomatous foci are occasionally found

Special Stains and Immunohistochemistry

- Markers for monoclonality will usually not be positive

Other Techniques for Diagnosis

- Noncontributory

Differential Diagnosis

ORBITAL CELLULITIS

- Imaging will usually reveal a periosteal abscess or adjacent sinusitis
- More likely to occur in younger individuals
- In most cases does not come to biopsy, although true abscesses of orbit are often drained

THYROID ORBITOPATHY

- Extraocular muscles are almost always the site of primary involvement
- Usually lacks eosinophils and germinal centers

ORBITAL LYMPHOMA

- More insidious onset
- Monoclonal tumor

POSTERIOR SCLERITIS

- May present with acute pain, proptosis, and ocular and periocular inflammation
- Imaging reveals no orbital mass or infiltration

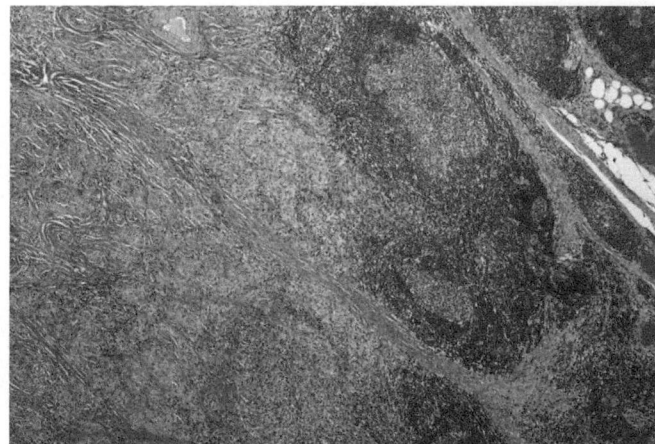

Figure 20-11. Sclerosing orbital pseudotumor. Dense fibrosis and inflammatory infiltrate with germinal centers are present.

Solid Tumor of Orbit
- Includes lacrimal gland tumors and primary and metastatic orbital tumors

Granulomatous Disease
- Sinus involvement expected

Ruptured Dermoid Cyst
- May present in an adult with no prior knowledge of the dermoid
- See "Dermoid and Epidermoid Cysts"

Vascular Lesion
- Includes hemangioma, lymphangioma, varix, and arteriovenous fistula

PEARLS

- *About 6% to 15% of orbital pseudotumors occur during the first two decades of life*
- *More likely to be bilateral in children*
- *First line of therapy is with systemic steroids, second line is with radiation as acute pseudotumor is extremely radiosensitive, and third line is with immunomodulators*

Selected References

Chavis RM, Garner A, Wright JE: Inflammatory orbital pseudotumor: a clinicopathologic study. Arch Ophthalmol 96:1817-1822, 1978.
Espinoza GM: Orbital inflammatory pseudotumors: etiology, differential diagnosis, and management. Curr Rheumatol Rep 12:443-447, 2010.
Kennerdell JS, Dresner SC: The nonspecific orbital inflammatory syndromes. Surv Ophthalmol 29:93-103, 1984.

THYROID ORBITOPATHY (THYROID OPHTHALMOPATHY, DYSTHYROID ORBITOPATHY, AND GRAVES ORBITOPATHY)

Clinical Features

- Graves disease: autoimmune process that includes any combination of hyperthyroidism, ophthalmopathy, and infiltrative dermatopathy
- Usually associated with hyperthyroidism, although patient may be hypothyroid or euthyroid
- Ophthalmopathy is clinically apparent in 50% of patients with Graves disease but requires intervention in only 3% to 5% of cases
- Women are affected three to four times more often than men
- Usually begins as mild irritation of the eyes, followed by upper eyelid retraction, proptosis, and diplopia
- Acute anterior orbital inflammatory signs and symptoms may develop
- Advanced disease can lead to glaucoma, compressive optic neuropathy, and corneal blindness from exposure
- A detailed classification of ocular changes in thyroid orbitopathy is included in the NOSPECS classification
- Imaging will reveal enlargement of extraocular muscle bellies without involvement of the tendons
- Diagnosis is usually clinical, although biopsy of extraocular muscles or orbital fat is occasionally performed

Gross Pathology

- Thin strips of extraocular muscle or small pieces of orbital fat and connective tissue

Histopathology

- Inflammation and enlargement of extraocular tissues, most commonly the extraocular muscles (Figure 20-12)
- Histologic findings vary with the stage and extent of disease
- Interstitial edema and lymphocytic inflammatory infiltrate within the endomysial connective tissue are early findings
- Inflammatory infiltrate consists mostly of lymphocytes and plasma cells with scattered mast cells
- Eosinophils and germinal centers are not a prominent feature
- Later the inflammation spreads to perimysium and epimysium
- Eventual fibrosis and fatty infiltration of the muscle occurs

Special Stains and Immunohistochemistry

- Noncontributory

Other Techniques for Diagnosis

- Noncontributory

Differential Diagnosis

Orbital Pseudotumor
- Involvement usually not restricted to muscles
- When muscles are involved, the tendon is not spared as it is in thyroid orbitopathy
- Eosinophils and germinal centers are more common than in thyroid orbitopathy

Orbital Cellulitis
- Imaging usually reveals a periosteal abscess or adjacent sinusitis
- More likely to occur in younger individuals
- In most cases does not come to biopsy, although true abscesses of the orbit are often drained

Metastatic Tumors to Extraocular Muscles
- Most commonly carcinoma of breast and lung

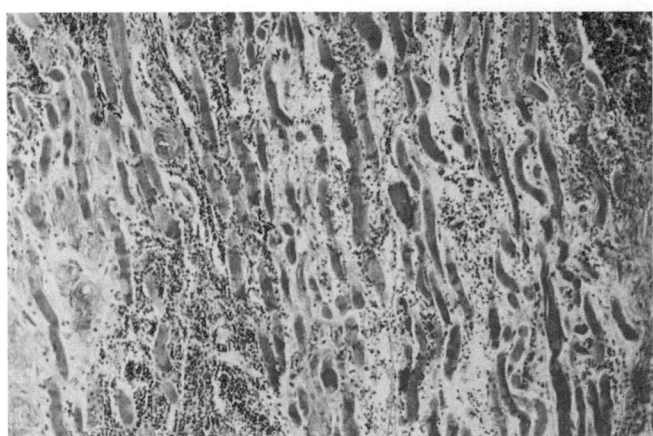

Figure 20-12. Thyroid orbitopathy. Interstitial inflammatory infiltrate within striated extraocular muscle.

OTHER ORBITAL INFLAMMATORY, INFILTRATIVE, AND NEOPLASTIC CONDITIONS

- Usually do not present with muscular involvement, and the diagnosis is made clinically

PEARLS

- *Most common cause of unilateral and bilateral proptosis in adults*
- *Smoking is a known risk factor for the development and progression of thyroid orbitopathy*
- *Investigation with TNFα's role in TED may help decrease inflammation and help improve vision*
- *Treatment is aimed at the predominant sign or symptom*
  - *Eyelid procedures for corneal exposure*
  - *Radiotherapy and a systemic steroid for acute cases of massive swelling of the extraocular muscles can improve diplopia and resolve optic nerve compression*
  - *Strabismus surgery for stable symptomatic diplopia unresponsive to other treatment*
  - *Orbital decompression surgery for acute optic nerve compression unresponsive to radiotherapy and steroids*

SELECTED REFERENCES

Jakobiec FA, Bilyk JR, Font RL: Orbit: noninfectious orbital inflammations—thyroid-related orbitopathy. In Spencer W (ed): Ophthalmic Pathology: An Atlas and Textbook, 4th ed, vol 4. Philadelphia, WB Saunders, 1996, pp 2811-2828.

Naik VM, Naik MN, Goldberg RA, et al: Immunopathogenesis of thyroid eye disease: emerging paradigms. Surv Ophthalmol 55:215-226, 2010.

Trokel SL, Jakobiec FA: Correlation of CT scanning and pathologic features of ophthalmic Graves' disease. Ophthalmology 88:553-564, 1981.

Werner SC: Modification of the classification of the eye changes of Graves' disease. Am J Ophthalmol 83:725-727, 1977.

CHILDHOOD ORBITAL LESIONS

CYSTIC

DERMOID AND EPIDERMOID CYSTS

Clinical Features

- Most common cystic orbital tumors
- Most common orbital tumors in pediatric age group
- Choristomatous tumors
- Result from primitive epithelial or dermal elements that are sequestered in fetal suture lines
- Propensity for superotemporal location at the zygomaticofrontal suture and superonasal anterior quadrants of the orbit
- Firm on palpation, deep and fixed to underlying bone
- Always present from birth, but may become apparent only during first decade of life

Gross Pathology

- Large single or multiloculated cystic cavity
- Keratin center has cheesy yellow appearance

Histopathology

- Single or multilobulated cyst lined by stratified squamous epithelium

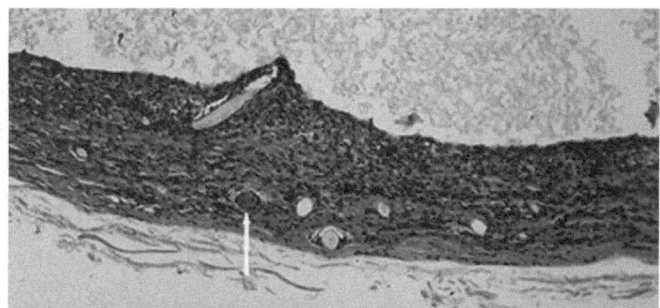

Figure 20-13. Dermoid cyst. The wall of the cyst with a lumen appears toward the top of the photograph. A pilosebaceous apparatus is seen in the wall of this cyst, which had previously ruptured and provoked an intense granulomatous giant cell reaction (*arrow*).

- Dermoid has accompanying pilosebaceous apparatus (hair shafts, sebaceous glands); epidermoid contains only epidermal elements, which is thought to occur when the epidermis becomes entrapped in deeper tissues during embryonic development (Figure 20-13)
- May have extensive foreign-body giant cell reaction within wall of cyst if the cyst has previously ruptured
- Center is filled with keratin, hair shafts, and lipid material

Special Stains and Immunohistochemistry

- Noncontributory

Other Techniques for Diagnosis

- Noncontributory

Differential Diagnosis

RHABDOMYOSARCOMA
- Solid mass
- Rapidly progressive
- Rhabdomyoblasts with malignant features

HEMANGIOMA
- Densely packed capillaries with plump endothelial lining
- May have a lobular pattern

MICROPHTHALMOS WITH CYST
- See "Microphthalmos with Cyst"

ORBITAL CELLULITIS
- Inflamed dermoid may mimic cellulitis
- Imaging will usually help with diagnosis

PEARLS

- *Ultrasound and radiography useful in detecting cystic nature of lesion; computed tomography (CT) will demonstrate a well-defined lesion with an enhancing wall and a non-enhancing lumen*
- *Dumbbell-shaped dermoid may project anteriorly from lateral orbit, erode lateral wall of orbit, and straddle the temporal fossa and orbit, which can cause a pulsating proptosis with mastication*

SELECTED REFERENCES

Sherman RP, Rootman J, LaPoint JS: Dermoids: clinical presentation and management. Br J Ophthalmol 68:642-652, 1984.

Shields JA, Shields CL: Orbital cysts of childhood: classification, clinical features, and management. Surv Ophthalmol 49:281-299, 2004.

Yanoff M, Fine BS: Ocular Pathology, 4th ed. Chicago, Mosby-Wolfe, 1996, pp 505-507.

CAPILLARY HEMANGIOMA OF THE ORBIT

Clinical Features

- Also known as hemangioma of infancy, strawberry hemangioma, and benign hemangioendothelioma
- Most common periocular vascular tumor in infancy and childhood
- More common in females (2:1)
- About 30% of these tumors are evident at birth and 95% by 6 months of age, often with explosive growth for 3 to 6 months
- Most spontaneously involute by 4 to 8 years of age
- Usually presents with proptosis
- Mass may increase in size with crying, owing to increased venous congestion
- Half may develop amblyopia, either from deprivation caused by occlusion or from astigmatism
- When located near the surface, diagnosis is easy, and the tumor is commonly referred to as strawberry nevus
- Generally occurs in otherwise healthy children; at 1% to 2% overall incidence

Gross Pathology

- Circumscribed soft, red lobular mass
- Feeding vessels may be apparent

Histopathology

- Densely packed capillaries lined by plump endothelial cells (Figure 20-14)
- May have lobular pattern
- Lumens often difficult to identify
- Mitotic figures may be seen during active phase
- With time, fibrosis develops within each lobule, effacing the endothelial cells

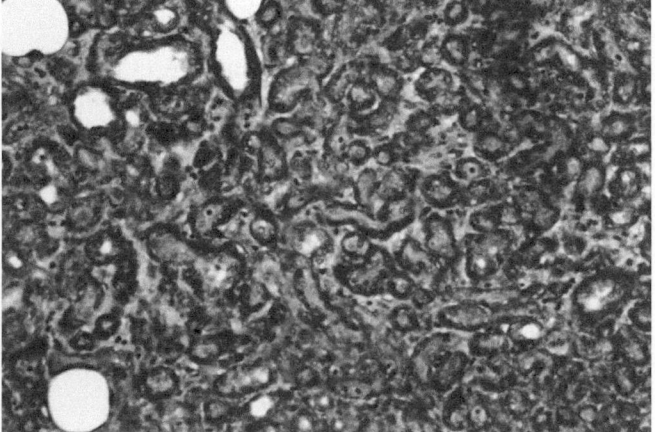

Figure 20-14. Capillary hemangioma of the orbit. Numerous densely packed capillaries lined by plump endothelial cells. Periodic acid-Schiff staining helps delineate individual vessels.

Special Stains and Immunohistochemistry

- Reticulin stain sometimes necessary to help delineate the lumens

Other Techniques for Diagnosis

- Noncontributory

Differential Diagnosis

RHABDOMYOSARCOMA

- See "Orbital Rhabdomyosarcoma"

LYMPHANGIOMA

- See "Lymphangioma"

CONGENITAL HYDROPS

EPIDERMOID AND DERMOID CYSTS

- See "Epidermoid and Dermoid Cysts"

PEARLS

- *Deep tumors can be difficult to differentiate from rhabdomyosarcoma, necessitating biopsy*
- *Superficial tumors were treated in the past with intralesional steroid injections or systemic steroid; now the preferred treatment is with beta-blockers: oral propranolol or topical timolol*
- *Small superficial tumors may also be surgically excised*
- *Deep orbital injection of steroid has been associated with central retinal artery occlusion and is thus contraindicated*
- *Because of a high rate of spontaneous involution, treatment is instituted only under vision-threatening circumstances*
- Kasabach-Merritt syndrome *refers to a large sequestration of platelets (usually) in gastrointestinal hemangiomas leading to thrombocytopenia and hemorrhage*

SELECTED REFERENCES

Haik BG, Jakobiec FA, Ellsworth RM, Jones IS: Capillary hemangioma of the lids and orbit: an analysis of the clinical features and therapeutic results in 101 cases. Ophthalmology 86:760-792, 1979.

Kushner BJ: Hemangiomas. Arch Ophthalmol 118:835-836, 2000.

Kushner BJ: Intralesional corticosteroid injection for infantile adnexal hemangioma. Am J Ophthalmol 93:496-506, 1982.

Mulliken JB, Young AE: Vascular birthmarks: hemangiomas and malformations. Philadelphia, JB Lippincott, 1988.

Ni N, Guo S, Langer P: Current concepts in the management of periocular infantile (capillary) hemangioma. Curr Opin Ophthalmol 22:419-425, 2011.

LYMPHANGIOMA

Clinical Features

- Defined as a choristoma of the orbit because lymphatics are not normally found there
- Frequently presents in a child younger than 10 to 15 years (although may present in adulthood) with acute onset of fulminant proptosis, presumably secondary to spontaneous hemorrhage
- Fluctuating clinical course with multiple recurrences is typical

- During severe exacerbations, may lead to compressive optic neuropathy, glaucoma, or large refractive shift
- Mass may enlarge during or after an upper respiratory infection

Gross Pathology

- Diffusely infiltrating mass, usually not removed in total because of inaccessible location

Histopathology

- Unencapsulated lesion affecting any orbital structure
- Blood- and lymph-filled, thin-walled vascular channels of varying caliber (Figure 20-15)
- Channels lined by an attenuated endothelial layer with interrupted basement membrane, anchoring fibrils, and general absence of pericytes

Special Stains and Immunohistochemistry

- Noncontributory

Other Techniques for Diagnosis

- Noncontributory

Differential Diagnosis

HEMANGIOMA

- Capillary hemangiomas found in children usually present in the first year of life
- Histopathologically distinct—see "Capillary Hemangioma of the Orbit"

PRIMARY AND METASTATIC MALIGNANCIES OF THE ORBIT

- Include primary rhabdomyosarcoma, metastatic neuroblastoma, other metastatic tumors of childhood, and solid tumor of leukemia (chloroma)

CEPHALOCELE

- Continuous with central nervous system
- Contains cerebrospinal fluid
- Imaging helps to differentiate
- Microphthalmos usually not present
- Neural tissue with overlying meninges present on histopathology

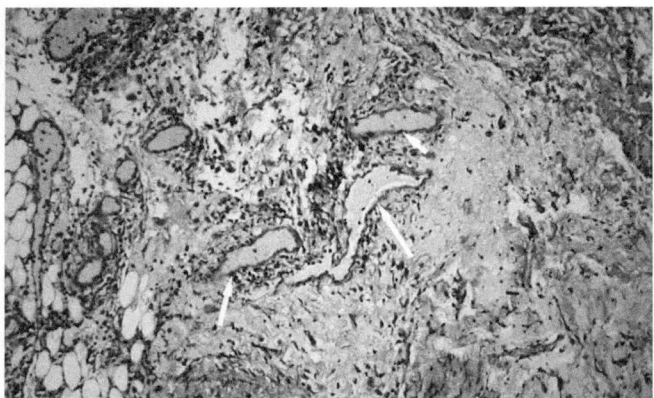

Figure 20-15. Lymphangioma. Within a background of connective tissue, many thin-walled structures are identified *(arrows),* some of which are filled with faint eosinophilic material.

ORBITAL PSEUDOTUMOR

- See "Inflammatory Orbital Pseudotumor (Idiopathic Orbital Inflammation)"

PEARLS

- *Clinical management is difficult*
- *Systemic steroids have little effect*
- *Surgery is usually reserved for cases of acute optic nerve compression*
- *Diagnosis can usually be made with close clinical observation and orbital imaging*

SELECTED REFERENCES

Iliff WJ, Green WR: Orbital lymphangiomas. Ophthalmology 86:914-929, 1979.

Jakobiec FA, Jones IS: Vascular tumors, malformations, and degenerations. In Jones IS, Jakobiec FA (eds): Diseases of the Orbit. Hagerstown, MD, Harper & Row, 1979, pp 269-308.

Jones IS: Lymphangioma of the ocular adnexa: an analysis of 62 cases. Trans Am Ophthalmol Soc 57:602-665, 1959.

MICROPHTHALMOS WITH CYST

Clinical Features

- Congenital malformation resulting from incomplete closure of the embryonic fissure at the 7 to 20 mm stage of development during 6 to 7 weeks of gestation
- Usually unilateral but may be bilateral
- Bilateral cases can be associated with systemic abnormalities

Gross Pathology

- Thin-walled cystic structure adjacent to (and adherent to) globe
- Histologically, the eye may range from relatively normal to small and disorganized

Histopathology

- Cyst wall usually composed of fibrous tissue (Figure 20-16A)
- Cyst usually lined with neural elements, including gliotic retina, nonspecific glial cells, or poorly differentiated retina (Figure 20-16B)

Special Stains and Immunohistochemistry

- Primitive retinal elements within the cyst will stain with typical neural stains like synaptophysin or glial fibrillary acidic protein (glial elements)

Other Techniques for Diagnosis

- Noncontributory

Differential Diagnosis

DERMOID AND EPIDERMOID CYSTS

- Associated with adjacent normal eye
- See "Dermoid and Epidermoid Cysts"

CEPHALOCELE

- Continuous with central nervous system
- Contains cerebrospinal fluid
- Imaging helps to differentiate

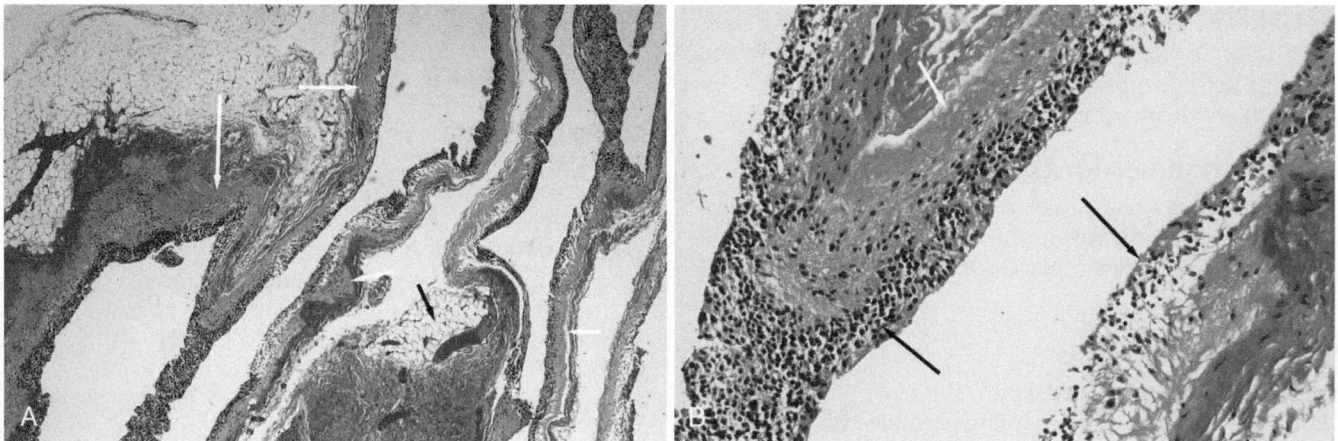

Figure 20-16. Microphthalmos with cyst. A, Low-magnification view. *Black arrow* indicates orbital fat. *White arrows* show the fibrous wall of this cystic lesion. **B,** High-magnification view. *White arrow* indicates the fibrous coat of this lesion (analogous to sclera). *Black arrows* indicate neural retina.

- Microphthalmos usually not present
- Neural tissue with overlying meninges present on histopathology

PEARLS

- *Usually a sporadic occurrence but may be associated with 13q deletion, chromosome 18 deletion, and trisomy*

SELECTED REFERENCES

Mann I: Developmental Abnormalities of the Eye, 2nd ed. Philadelphia, JB Lippincott, 1957.

Shields JA. Shields CL: Orbital cysts of childhood: classification, clinical features, and management. Surv Ophthalmol 49:281-299, 2004.

Waring GO, Roth AM, Rodriques MM: Clinicopathologic correlation of microphthalmos with cyst. Am J Ophthalmol 82:714-721, 1976.

SOLID ORBITAL RHABDOMYOSARCOMA

Clinical Features

- Most common primary malignant orbital tumor in children
- Annual incidence of 4.3 cases per million
- Found elsewhere in the body but has a predilection for the orbit (about 10% of all rhabdomyosarcomas present in the orbit)
- Average age of onset is 8 years; most occur before 10 years of age; extremely rare after age 25 years
- Males are affected more than females
- Usually presents as rapidly progressive proptosis or a rapidly enlarging orbital mass (progressing daily); predilection for the superior nasal quadrant
- Important to determine bone invasion and extension into intracranial cavity and paranasal sinuses, therefore necessary to obtain CT/magnetic resonance imaging (MRI)

Gross Pathology

- Firm, rubbery, solid mass
- Arises not from extraocular muscles but from undifferentiated mesenchymal cells that can mature into striated muscle

Histopathology

- Divided into three main types
  - Embryonal
    - Most common type
    - Malignant rhabdomyoblasts in a loose, haphazard arrangement
    - Frequent mitoses
    - Round, oval, spindled, or stellate cells, some with prominent eosinophilic cytoplasm (may see cross-striations typical of striated muscle)
    - Hyperchromatic, atypical nuclei with many mitotic figures (Figure 20-17)
  - Alveolar
    - Poorest prognosis
    - Pattern resembles alveolar architecture of the lung with loosely arranged cells forming trabecular pattern
    - Difficult-to-find cross-striations
  - Differentiated
    - Rarest, but best prognosis
    - Easily found cross-striations, fewer mitoses

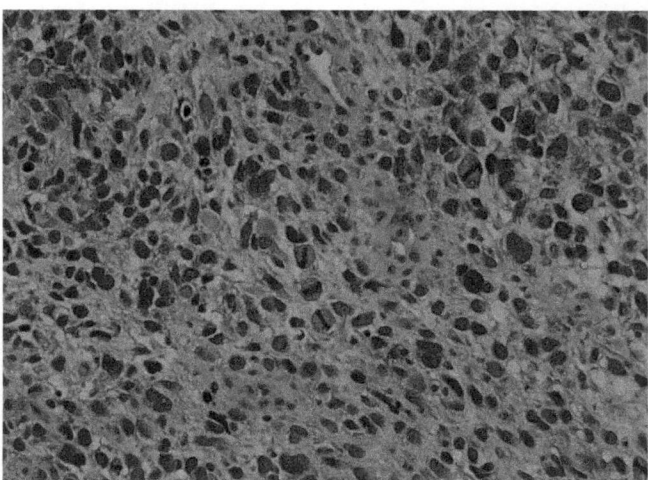

Figure 20-17. Embryonal rhabdomyosarcoma. Highly pleomorphic specimen with numerous mitotic figures.

Special Stains and Immunohistochemistry

- Positivity for vimentin, myosin, myoglobin, muscle-specific actin, and desmin
- Masson trichrome positive

Other Techniques for Diagnosis

- Electron microscopy may reveal typical myofibrillary differentiation; however, the classic light-microscopic appearance makes electron microscopy largely unnecessary

Differential Diagnosis

METASTATIC NEUROBLASTOMA

- Usually occurs late in the disease, once the primary is known
- Histopathologic findings are typical with small, undifferentiated cells, Homer-Wright rosettes, pseudorosettes, and neuropil
- Can occur in up to 20% of children with adrenal neuroblastoma

LEIOMYOMA AND LEIOMYOSARCOMA

- Rare tumors in the orbit
- Electron microscopy can aid in differentiation

ORBITAL CAPILLARY HEMANGIOMA

- Congenital lesion, but may become apparent later in life

ORBITAL DERMOID CYST

CEPHALOCELE

LYMPHANGIOMA

ORBITAL PSEUDOTUMOR (IDIOPATHIC ORBITAL INFLAMMATION)

- Uncommon in children

ORBITAL CELLULITIS

- Imaging usually reveals a periosteal abscess or adjacent sinusitis
- In most cases, does not come to biopsy, although true abscesses of the orbit are often drained

PEARLS

- *Survival rate of up to 90% if the tumor is confined to the orbit*
- *Most deaths occur within 3 years*
- *Treatment options include chemotherapy, external beam radiation, and surgery*

SELECTED REFERENCES

Jakobiec FA, Bilyk JR, Font RL: Orbit: mesenchymal tumors: striated muscle neoplasms. In Spencer W (ed): Ophthalmic Pathology: An Atlas and Textbook, 4th ed, vol 4. Philadelphia, WB Saunders, 1996, pp 2573-2587.

Karcioglu ZA, Hadjistilianou D, Rozans M, DeFrancesco S: Orbital rhabdomyosarcoma. Cancer Control 11:328-333, 2004.

Knowles DM, Jakobiec FA, Potter G, Jones IS: Ophthalmic striated muscle neoplasms: a clinico-pathologic review. Surv Ophthalmol 21:219-261, 1976.

Index

Note: Page numbers followed by *f* indicate figures and *t* indicate tables.

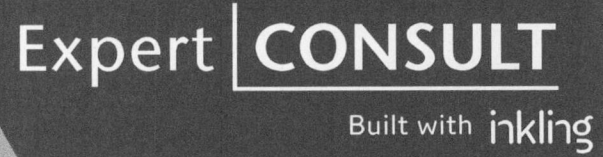

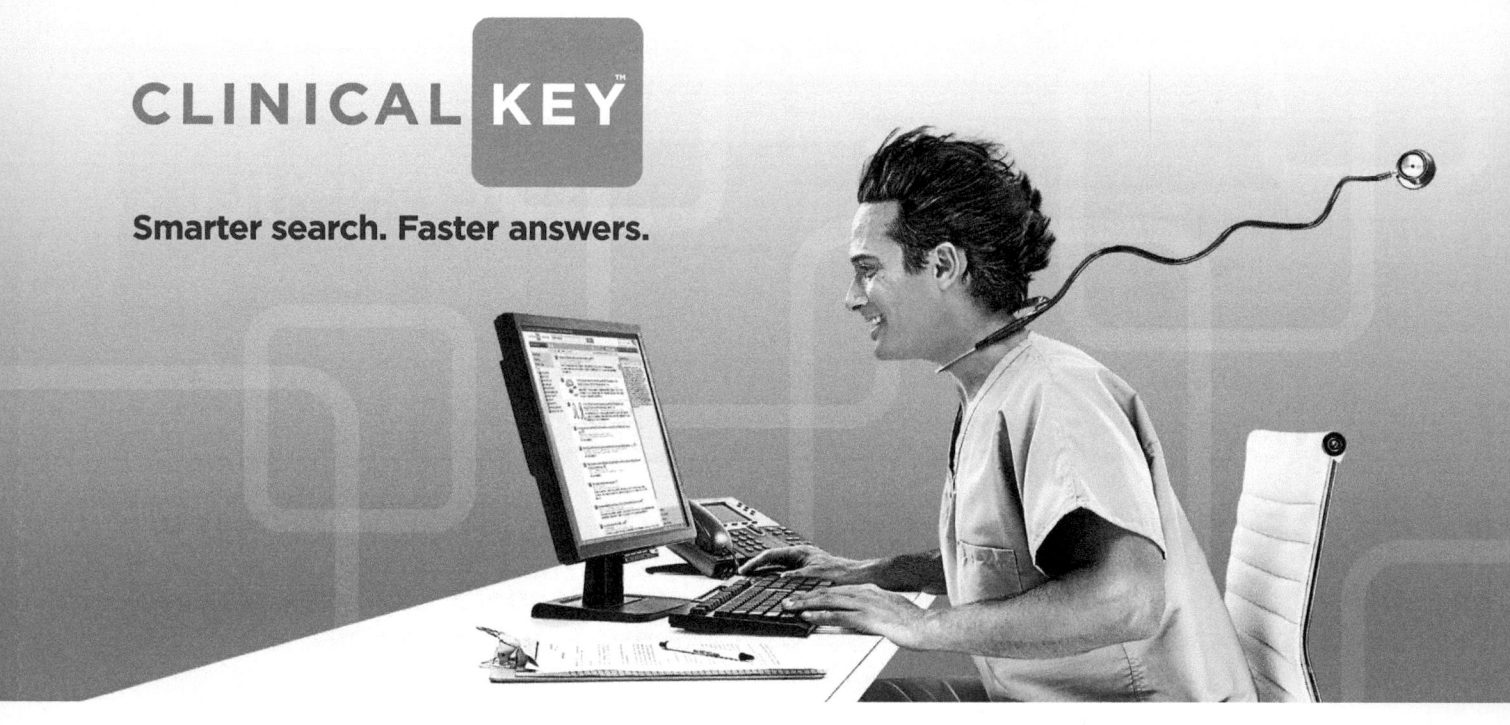

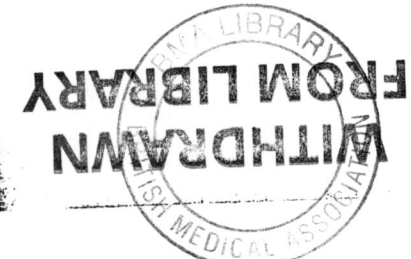